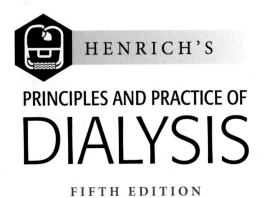

HENRICH'S

PRINCIPLES AND PRACTICE OF
DIALYSIS

FIFTH EDITION

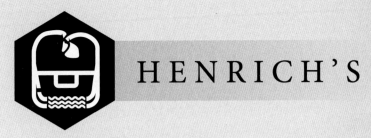

HENRICH'S
PRINCIPLES AND PRACTICE OF
DIALYSIS

FIFTH EDITION

EDITED BY

Edgar V. Lerma, MD, FACP, FASN, FNKF
Clinical Professor of Medicine
Section of Nephrology
University of Illinois at Chicago/Advocate Christ Medical Center
Oak Lawn, Illinois
Associates in Nephrology
Chicago, Illinois

Matthew R. Weir, MD
Professor and Director
Division of Nephrology
Department of Medicine
University of Maryland School of Medicine
Baltimore, Maryland

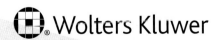

. Wolters Kluwer

Philadelphia • Baltimore • New York • London
Buenos Aires • Hong Kong • Sydney • Tokyo

Acquisitions Editor: Kel McGowan
Product Development Editor: Leanne Vandetty
Editorial Assistant: Diane Solomon
Production Project Manager: David Saltzberg
Design Coordinator: Holly McLaughlin
Manufacturing Coordinator: Beth Welsh
Marketing Manager: Rachel Mante Leung
Prepress Vendor: Absolute Service, Inc.

Fifth edition

9 8 7 6 5 4 3 2 1

Printed in China

Library of Congress Cataloging-in-Publication Data

Names: Lerma, Edgar V., editor. | Weir, Matthew R., 1952- editor.
Title: Henrich's principles and practice of dialysis / edited by Edgar V.
  Lerma, Matthew R. Weir.
Other titles: Principles and practice of dialysis.
Description: Fifth edition. | Philadelphia : Wolters Kluwer, [2017] |
  Preceded by Prinicples and practice of dialysis / edited by William L.
  Henrich. 4th ed. c2009. | Includes bibliographical references and index.
Identifiers: LCCN 2016027838 | ISBN 9781496318206
Subjects: | MESH: Renal Dialysis | Kidney Failure, Chronic—complications |
  Kidney Failure, Chronic—therapy
Classification: LCC RC901.7.H45 | NLM WJ 378 | DDC 617.4/61059—dc23 LC record available at
  https://lccn.loc.gov/2016027838

To all my mentors, and friends, at the University of Santo Tomas Faculty of Medicine and Surgery in Manila, Philippines; Mercy Hospital & Medical Center in Chicago, Illinois; and Northwestern University Feinberg School of Medicine in Chicago, Illinois; who have in one way or another influenced and guided me to become the physician that I am.

To all the medical students, interns, and residents at University of Illinois at Chicago/Advocate Christ Medical Center whom I have taught or learned from, especially those who eventually decided to pursue nephrology as a career. . . .

To my parents and my brothers, without whose unwavering love and support through the good and bad times, I would not have persevered and reached my goals in life. . . . Most especially to my two lovely and precious daughters, Anastasia Zofia and Isabella Ann, whose smiles and laughter constantly provide me unparalleled joy and happiness, and my very loving and understanding wife Michelle, who has always been supportive of my endeavors, both personally and professionally, and who sacrificed a lot of time and exhibited unwavering patience as I devoted a significant amount of time and effort to this project. Truly, they provide me with motivation and inspiration.

- EVL

For my wonderful wife, Duffy, and my three amazing children, Ryan, Courtney, and Kerry, who have generously shared me with my career as a caregiver for patients with kidney disease, I am eternally grateful.

- MRW

CONTENTS

CONTRIBUTING AUTHORS

Rajiv Agarwal, MD, FASN, FAHA, FASH
Professor of Medicine, Indiana University School of Medicine, Indianapolis, Indiana

Imran I. Ali, MD, FAAN Professor of Neurology, Senior Associate Dean for Academic Affairs; Director, Comprehensive Epilepsy Program, University of Toledo College of Medicine and Life Sciences, Toledo, Ohio

Stephen J. Bander, MD Medical Director, Vascular Access Centers, St. Luke's Hospital; Adjunct Professor of Medicine, St. Louis University School of Medicine, St. Louis, Missouri

Shweta Bansal, MBBS, MD, FASN Assistant Professor of Medicine, Division of Nephrology, Department of Medicine, University of Texas Health Science Center at San Antonio, San Antonio, Texas

William M. Bennett, MD, MACP, FASN Medical Director, Legacy Transplant Services, Legacy Good Samaritan Medical Center, Portland, Oregon

Ruth Berggren, MD Marvin Forland, M.D., Distinguished Professor in Medical Ethics, Director, The Center for Medical Humanities & Ethics, The University of Texas Health Science Center at San Antonio, San Antonio, Texas

Jeffrey S. Berns, MD Professor of Medicine and Pediatrics, Renal, Electrolyte, and Hypertension Division, Perelman School of Medicine at the University of Pennsylvania, Philadelphia, Pennsylvania

Paola Boccardo, BiolSciD Head, Laboratory Regulatory Affairs for Clinical Studies, IRCCS - Istituto di Ricerche Farmacologiche Mario Negri, Clinical Research Centre for Rare Diseases "Aldo e Cele Daccò", Ranica BG, Italy

Wendy Weinstock Brown, MD, MPH, FACP, FAHA, FNKF Professor of Medicine, Northwestern University Feinberg School of Medicine and University of Illinois Chicago College of Medicine, Chicago, Illinois

John M. Burkart, MD Professor of Medicine/Nephrology, Wake Forest University Medical Center, Winston Salem, North Carolina; Chief Medical Officer, Health Systems Management, Tifton, Georgia

Charles B. Cangro, MD, PhD Assistant Professor, Department of Medicine, University of Maryland School of Medicine, Baltimore, Maryland

Juan Jesus Carrero, Pharm, PhD Pharm, PhD Med, MBA Associate Professors of Renal Medicine, Karolinska Institutet, Stockholm, Sweden; Clinical Fellow, Division of Nephrology and Hypertension, Vanderbilt University School of Medicine, Nashville, Tennessee

Celina Cepeda, MD Pediatric Nephrology Fellow, Department of Pediatric Nephrology, Rady Children's Hospital/University of California San Diego, San Diego, California

Rafia Chaudhry, MD Assistant Professor, Division of Nephrology and Hypertension, Albany Medical College, Albany, New York

Yusra Cheema, MD Instructor of Medicine, Division of Nephrology and Hypertension, Northwestern University Feinberg School of Medicine, Chicago, Illinois

Andrew I. Chin, MD Clinical Professor of Medicine, Division of Nephrology, University of California Davis School of Medicine, Sacramento, California

Tushar Chopra, MBBS Assistant Professor of Medicine, Division of Nephrology, University of Virginia Medical Center, Charlottesville, Virginia

Gabriela Cobo, MD Specialist in Nephrology, Clinical Researcher, Divisions of Renal Medicine and Baxter Novum, Department of Clinical Science, Intervention and Technology, Karolinska Institutet, Stockholm, Sweden

William J. Dahms, Jr., DO, FASN Nephrology Associates, P.A., Newark, Delaware

Thomas A. Depner, MD Professor of Medicine, Division of Nephrology, University of California Davis School of Medicine, Sacramento, California

George T. Fantry, MD Associate Professor of Medicine, Assistant Dean for Student Research and Education, Division of Gastroenterology and Hepatology, University of Maryland School of Medicine, Baltimore, Maryland

William H. Fissell, MD Associate Professor, Division of Nephrology and Hypertension, Vanderbilt University Medical Center, Nashville, Tennessee

Miriam Galbusera, BiolScid Head, Unit of Platelet Endothelial Cell Interaction, IRCCS - Istituto di Ricerche Farmacologiche Mario Negri, Bergamo, Italy

F. John Gennari, MD Professor Emeritus, University of Vermont College of Medicine, Burlington, Vermont

Thomas A. Golper, MD, FACP, FASN Professor of Medicine, Division of Nephrology and Hypertension, Vanderbilt University Medical Center, Nashville, Tennessee

Edward R. Gould, MD Clinical Instructor of Medicine, Division of Nephrology, Vanderbilt University Medical Center, Nashville, Tennessee

Donna S. Hanes, MD, FACP Clinical Associate Professor of Medicine, Division of Nephrology, University of Maryland School of Medicine, Baltimore, Maryland

William L. Henrich, MD, MACP President and Professor of Medicine, University of Texas Health Science Center at San Antonio, San Antonio, Texas

Dirk M. Hentschel, MD Director, Interventional Nephrology, Assistant Professor, Department of Medicine, Division of Renal Medicine, Brigham and Women's Hospital, Harvard Medical School, Boston, Massachusetts

Kathy L. Jabs, MD Associate Professor of Pediatrics, Vanderbilt University School of Medicine; Director, Pediatric Nephrology and Hypertension, Vanderbilt University Medical Center, Nashville, Tennessee

Kamyar Kalantar-Zadeh, MD, MPH, PHD Chief, Division of Nephrology and Hypertension, Professor of Medicine, Pediatrics and Public Health, University of California Irvine School of Medicine, Orange and Irvine, California; Adjunct Professor of Epidemiology, Department of Epidemiology, UCLA Fielding School of Public Health, Los Angeles, California; Staff Physician and Principal Investigator, Veterans Affairs Long Beach Healthcare System, Long Beach, California

Lakshmi Kannan, MD Clinical Fellow, Division of Endocrinology, Hospital of University of Pennsylvania, Philadelphia, Pennsylvania

Feras F. Karadsheh, MBBS Assistant Professor, Department of Internal Medicine, University of Maryland Medical Center, Baltimore, Maryland

Fathima Konari, MBBS Fellow, Department of Medicine, Division of Nephrology, University of Maryland Medical Center, Baltimore, Maryland

Joel D. Kopple, MD Professor of Medicine and Public Health, David Geffen School of Medicine at UCLA, UCLA Fielding School of Public Health, Division of Nephrology and Hypertension, Los Angeles Biomedical Research Institute at Harbor-UCLA Medical Center, Torrance, California

Andrew Kowalski, MD, MPH Resident Physician, Department of Internal Medicine, University of Illinois at Chicago/Advocate Christ Medical Center, Chicago, Illinois

Armand Krikorian, MD, FACE Program Director, Internal Medicine, University of Illinois at Chicago/Advocate Christ Medical Center; Associate Professor of Clinical Medicine, University of Illinois at Chicago, Oak Lawn, Illinois

Jay I. Lakkis, MD, FACP, FASN Assistant Clinical Professor of Medicine, University of Hawaii John A. Burns School of Medicine; Consulting Nephrologist at Maui Memorial Medical Center-Pacific Nephrology, LLC, Wailuku, Hawaii

L. Richard A. Lange, MD, MBA President, Dean, Paul L. Foster School of Medicine, Texas Tech University Health Sciences Center El Paso, El Paso, Texas

Edgar V. Lerma, MD, FACP, FASN, FNKF Clinical Professor of Medicine, Section of Nephrology, University of Illinois at Chicago/Advocate Christ Medical Center, Oak Lawn, Illinois; Associates in Nephrology, Chicago, Illinois

Bengt Lindholm, MD, PhD Adjunct Professor, Division of Baxter Novum and Renal Medicine, Department of Clinical Science, Intervention and Technology, Karolinska Institutet, Stockholm, Sweden

Yaakov Liss, MD Nephrology Fellow, Department of Nephrology, Hospital of the University of Pennsylvania, Philadelphia, Pennsylvania

Naim Maalouf, MD Associate Professor of Medicine, University of Texas Southwestern Medical Center, VA North Texas Health Care System, Dallas, Texas

Michael Achilles Markos, MD Attending Physician, Mercy Hospital & Medical Center; Clinical Instructor of Medicine, University of Illinois Medical Center, Chicago, Illinois

Sean P. Martin, MD FRCPC Medical Renal Transplant Fellow, Dalhousie University, Halifax, Nova Scotia, Canada

Piyush Mathur, MBBS, DNB (Internal Medicine), DNB (Nephrology) Consultant Nephrologist, Department of Nephrology, Santokba Durlabhji Memorial Hospital, Jaipur, India

Ravindra L. Mehta, MD, FACP, FASN, FRCP Professor of Clinical Medicine, Associate Chair for Clinical Research Department of Medicine, University of California, San Diego Medical Center, San Diego, California

Susan R. Mendley, MD Division Chief, Pediatric Nephrology, Associate Professor of Pediatrics and Medicine, University of Maryland School of Medicine, Baltimore, Maryland

Federica Mescia, MD Nephrology fellow, Unit of Nephrology and Dialysis, Azienda Socio Sanitaria Territoriale (ASST) Papa Giovanni XXIII, Bergamo, Italy

Brent W. Miller, MD Professor of Medicine, Director of Dialysis Home Modalities, Division of Nephrology, Washington University School of Medicine, Saint Louis, Missouri

R. Tyler Miller, MD Professor of Medicine, University of Texas Southwestern Medical School; Chief Medical Service, Dallas VA Medical Center, Dallas, Texas

Sean W. Murphy, MD, FRCP(C) Associate Professor of Medicine, Division of Nephrology, Memorial University of Newfoundland, St. John's, Newfoundland, Canada

Dana Negoi, MD Associate Professor of Medicine, Division of Nephrology, University of Vermont Medical Center, Burlington, Vermont

Iheanyichukwu Ogu, MD Clinical Fellow, Division of Nephrology and Hypertension, Vanderbilt University Medical Center, Nashville, Tennessee

Ali J. Olyaei, PharmD Professor of Medicine and Pharmacotherapy, Nephrology & Hypertension, Oregon State University/Oregon Health & Sciences University, Portland, Oregon

Yin Oo, MD Associate Professor of Medicine in Endocrinology, University of Texas Southwestern Medical Center, Dallas VA Medical Center, Dallas, Texas

Biff F. Palmer, MD Professor of Internal Medicine, University of Texas Southwestern Medical Center, Dallas, Texas

Patrick S. Parfrey, MD, FRCPC, FASN, OC, FRSC John Lewis Paton Distinguished University Professor, Division of Nephrology, Health Sciences Centre, St. John's, Newfoundland, Canada

Ami M. Patel, MD Assistant Professor of Medicine, Division of Nephrology, University of Maryland School of Medicine, Baltimore, Maryland

Ruchita Patel, DO Resident Physician, Internal Medicine, University of Illinois at Chicago, Advocate Christ Medical Center, Chicago, Illinois

Seema Patil, MD Assistant Professor of Medicine, Division of Gastroenterology and Hepatology, University of Maryland School of Medicine, Baltimore, Maryland

Andreas Pierratos, MD, FRCPC Nephrologist, Humber River Hospital; Professor of Medicine, University of Toronto, Toronto, Ontario, Canada

Noor A. Pirzada, MD Professor, Residency Program Director of EMG Services, Department of Neurology, University of Toledo Medical Center, Toledo, Ohio

Robert Provenzano, MD, FACP, FASN Clinical Professor of Medicine, Wayne State University School of Medicine; Chief of Nephrology, Hypertension & Transplantation, St. John Hospital & Medical Center, Detroit, Michigan

Wajeh Y. Qunibi, MD, FACP Professor of Medicine, Division of Nephrology, Department of Medicine, University of Texas Health Science Center at San Antonio, San Antonio, Texas

Janani Rangaswami, MD, FACP Associate Program Director, Department of Medicine, Einstein Medical Center; Clinical Assistant Professor of Medicine, Sidney Kimmel Medical College of Thomas Jefferson University, Philadelphia, Pennsylvania

Giuseppe Remuzzi, MD, FRCP Head, Unit of Nephrology and Dialysis, Azienda Socio Sanitaria Territoriale (ASST) Papa Giovanni XXIII, Bergamo, Italy; Director, IRCCS - Istituto di Ricerche Farmacologiche Mario Negri, Bergamo, Italy; "Chiara fama" Professor of Nephrology, Department of Biomedical and Clinical Sciences, University of Milan, Milan, Italy

Sharmeela Saha, MD Assistant Professor of Medicine, University Hospitals Case Medical Center, Cleveland, Ohio

Daniel Jay Salzberg, MD, FACP Assistant Professor of Medicine, Division of Nephrology, University of Maryland Medical Center, Baltimore, Maryland

William Salzer, MD Professor of Clinical Medicine, Division of Infectious Disease, University of Missouri School of Medicine, Columbia, Missouri

Gerald Schulman, MD, FASN Professor of Medicine, Co-Director of Clinical Trials in Nephrology, Vanderbilt University School of Medicine, Nashville, Tennessee

Steve Schwab, MD Chancellor, Professor, Department of Medicine, Nephrology Division, The University of Tennessee Health Science Center, Memphis, Tennessee

Anuja Shah, MD Assistant Professor, David Geffen School of Medicine at UCLA, Division of Nephrology and Hypertension, Harbor-UCLA Medical Center, Torrance, California

Jonathan Silverman, MD Resident Physician, Department of Internal Medicine, University of Illinois at Chicago College of Medicine/Advocate Christ Medical Center, Chicago, Illinois

Vibhu Sharma, MD, MS Attending Physician, John H. Stroger Hospital of Cook County, Assistant Professor of Medicine, Rush University Medical College, Chicago, Illinois

Arjun D. Sinha, MD, MS Assistant Professor of Clinical Medicine, Indiana University School of Medicine, Division of Nephrology, Richard L. Roudebush VA Medical Center, Indianapolis, Indiana

Amy L. Skversky, MD, MSc Assistant Professor, Pediatric Nephrology, The Children's Hospital at Montefiore, Bronx, New York

Peter Stenvinkel, MD, PhD, FERA Clinical Professor of Nephrology, Department of Renal Medicine, Karolinska University Hospital, Stockholm, Sweden

Judy K. Tan, MD Fellow, Division of Nephrology, Mount Sinai Hospital, New York, New York

Isaac Teitelbaum, MD, FACP Professor of Medicine, University of Colorado School of Medicine; Director, Home Dialysis Program, University of Colorado Hospital, Aurora, Colorado

Beje Thomas, MD Assistant Professor of Medicine, Division of Nephrology, University of Maryland Medical Center, Baltimore, Maryland

Peter Noel Van Buren, MD, MSCS Dedman Family Scholar in Clinical Care, Assistant Professor of Internal Medicine, Division of Nephrology, University of Texas Southwestern Medical Center, Dallas, Texas

Ravinder K. Wali, MD, MRCP Medical Director, Abdominal Transplant Center, Inova Health System; Clinical Professor of Medicine, Virginia Commonwealth University School of Medicine, Richmond, Virginia; Clinical Professor of Medicine, The George Washington University Medical Center, Washington, DC; Associate Professor of Medicine, University of Maryland School of Medicine, Baltimore, Maryland

Bradley A. Warady, MD Professor of Pediatrics, University of Missouri-Kansas City School of Medicine; Senior Associate Chairman, Department of Pediatrics; Director, Division of Pediatric Nephrology; Director, Dialysis and Transplantation, Children's Mercy Hospital, Kansas City, Missouri

Matthew R. Weir, MD Professor and Director, Division of Nephrology, Department of Medicine, University of Maryland School of Medicine, Baltimore, Maryland

Jay B. Wish, MD Professor of Clinical Medicine, Indiana University School of Medicine; Medical Director, Outpatient Dialysis Unit, Indiana University Health University Hospital, Indianapolis, Indiana

PREFACE

The first edition of *Principles and Practice of Dialysis* was published in 1994. The practice of dialysis has evolved substantially since that first edition.

As in previous editions, the fifth edition carries on the tradition of prior editions to achieve a balance between scholarship, clarity, and practicality. The text is written by several acknowledged experts with a view to providing clinical direction built on a platform of the best scientific and clinical evidence. In this edition, we welcome contributions from new authors as well as new topics (home hemodialysis, wearable artificial kidney, respiratory disorders in dialysis patients, dialysis and reproduction, cystic kidney diseases in dialysis patients) and have reworked each chapter to reflect the changing nature of modern dialysis practice.

From personal experience, we are cognizant that for a variety of reasons, the majority of readers would read only one or a few chapters at any given time. In this vein, we considered that each chapter would complement each other yet be complete in itself. Therefore, in this multiauthored text, it is unavoidable to have some overlap in the information presented in a few chapters. However, we feel that this was necessary to provide sufficiently complete information on a particular topic.

This book would not have been possible were it not for many people. First, we would like to thank all of our wonderful contributing authors who have spent countless hours in producing high-quality, up-to-date information. We express our sincere gratitude for their openness to this collegial collaboration, which has been a truly rewarding learning experience for us. We also thank the staff of Wolters Kluwer who helped us in this production, most especially Leanne Vandetty, our Product Development Editor; and Kel McGowan and Julie Goolsby, our Acquisitions Editors.

We are indebted to our teachers and mentors who devoted their own time to educate and train us. We thank all the medical students, residents, and fellows who in one way or another have given us the inspiration to persevere in this profession. Mostly, of course, we are grateful to our patients who are and have been instrumental in our education. On behalf of all the contributors to this book, we sincerely hope that our efforts will contribute to relieving suffering.

It is the wish of all the authors and staff associated with this book that it will continue to serve as a valuable reference and guide for busy practitioners and for trainees at all levels. It is through the accomplishment of these missions that we trust dialysis therapy will improve so that the quality of life for all of our patients with kidney disease may improve.

WILLIAM L. HENRICH, MD, MACP
EDGAR V. LERMA, MD, FACP, FASN, FNKF
MATTHEW R. WEIR, MD

CHAPTER 1

Choice of the Hemodialysis Membrane

Jay I. Lakkis and Matthew R. Weir

Although renal replacement therapy (RRT) has been successful at simulating the kidneys' capacity for solute regulation and volume management, significant limitations persist, which continue to challenge the successes of this therapy when compared to normal kidney physiology. In hemodialysis (HD) therapy, the most prevalent form of RRT (>90%) in the United States (1), both ultrafiltration and solute clearance are driven at the level of the dialysis membrane. In addition to dialysis time and frequency, solute clearance remains an integral part of the ongoing quest to establish the optimal dialysis dose and to set clearly defined adequacy measures that correlate with survival, less chronic inflammation, better nutritional status, and improved well-being. Some of the byproducts of this pursuit are a plethora of techniques and mathematical models that simulate target solute kinetics (e.g., urea, index Kt/V) and the continuing development of newer high-performance membranes (HPM) and dialysate solutions to improve clinical outcomes.

The dialysis membrane is manufactured from semipermeable compounds, which may be geometrically designed in coil (1946) (2), parallel-plate (1948), or most commonly hollow-fiber (1956) structure (TABLE 1.1), then stabilized mechanically into a potting compound (e.g., polyurethane), and finally encased in a housing material (e.g., polypropylene or polycarbonate). This design creates a barrier between the blood and the dialysate during HD while allowing a bidirectional exchange of solute (e.g., potassium from blood to dialysate and bicarbonate in the opposite direction); the major mechanisms that govern solute clearance in HD are diffusive transport, convective transport, and adsorption. The ideal dialysis membrane is perfectly biocompatible with no proinflammatory effects, achieves the desired ultrafiltration and the highest clearance of all uremic toxins, is associated with the most optimal nutritional status, and does not result in any short-term or long-term complications.

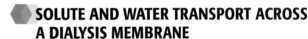

SOLUTE AND WATER TRANSPORT ACROSS A DIALYSIS MEMBRANE

The net clearance of any specific solute, or of water, from a patient's blood at the end of a dialysis treatment is the sum total of a complex interplay between diffusive transport, convective transport, and adsorption, all of which are in turn determined by solute properties, membrane characteristics, solute concentration gradients, transmembrane pressure (TMP) gradients, blood and dialysate flow rates, ultrafiltration rate, patient's hematocrit (Hct) and protein concentrations, and temperature. These processes are described in this section.

Solute Classification by Molecular Weight

A small molecular weight (SMW) solute is one whose molecular weight is less than 500 Da. Examples include most nitrogen-based solutes such as creatinine and urea, lactic acid, cholesterol, most vitamins (A, B_1, B_2, B_3, B_5, B_6, B_7, B_9, C, D_2, D_3, E, K_1, K_2, K_3), and all electrolytes (TABLE 1.2).

A middle molecular weight (MMW) solute is a solute with a molecular weight between 500 Da and 15 kDa. Examples include β_2-microglobulin (β_2-MG), cystatin C, vitamin B_{12}, inulin, hemoglobin (Hb) and myoglobin, and bilirubin (TABLE 1.2).

A large molecular weight (LMW) solute has a molecular weight greater than 15 kDa. Examples include albumin, immunoglobulins, kappa and lambda free light chains, and ferritin (TABLE 1.2).

Diffusion

Diffusion is a mass transfer process that describes the transport of matter from one part of a system to another as a result of random molecular motion triggered by thermally induced agitation; in HD, such transport occurs between the blood and the dialysate across the semipermeable dialysis membrane from a region of high

TABLE 1.1	**Choice of Dialysis Membrane**

Geometric design
  Hollow fiber
  Parallel plate
  Coil
	Hollow fiber is the most widely used.

Chemical composition
  Cellulosic, unmodified, regenerated
  Cellulosic, modified, substituted
  Synthetic, noncellulosic
	Free hydroxyl groups on surface of unmodified cellulosic membranes contribute to blood–membrane interactions and degree of bioincompatibility.
	Hydrophobicity of a membrane enhances adsorptive capacity.

Solute clearance: efficiency
  Low efficiency
  High efficiency
	Efficiency is measured by K_oA urea and can be increased by increasing membrane surface area.
	 • Low efficiency K_oA urea <500 mL/min
	 • High efficiency K_oA urea >600 mL/min

Solute clearance: flux
  Low flux
  High flux
  Super high flux
	Flux is measured by β_2-MG or water clearance and can be increased by increasing membrane pore size/permeability.
	 • Low flux: $K_{\beta_2\text{-MG}}$ <10 mL/min or K_{UF} ≤12 mL/h/mm Hg
	 • Medium flux: $K_{\beta_2\text{-MG}}$ 10–20 mL/min
	 • High flux: $K_{\beta_2\text{-MG}}$ >20 mL/min or K_{UF} >12 mL/h/mm Hg
	 • Super high flux: $K_{\beta_2\text{-MG}}$ >50 mL/min, clearance high MW cutoff up to 65 kDA

Biocompatibility
  Biocompatible
  Bioincompatible
	Inflammation: anaphylatoxins, granulocyte activation, cytokines
	Thrombogenicity
	Worse nutritional status
	Accelerated atherosclerosis and cardiovascular disease
	Erythropoietin resistance
	Deposition of β_2-MG fibrils and dialysis-related amyloidosis
	Sterilization technique

Performance
  Low performance
  High performance
	High-performance membranes are very highly biocompatible, have enhanced adsorptive capacity, and clear solutes with a high MW cutoff very close to the native kidney, for example, low MW proteins.

K_oA, membrane permeability-area coefficient; K, clearance; β_2-MG, β_2-microglobulin; K_{UF}, ultrafiltration coefficient; MW, molecular weight.

concentration to a region of low concentration. This is best represented by Fick's first law of diffusion:

$$J_{Diffusion} = dn/dt = -D \cdot A \cdot \Delta C / \Delta X$$

where $J_{Diffusion}$ (dn/dt) is flux in mol/s, D is diffusion constant in cm^2/s, A is membrane surface area in cm^2, ΔC is the concentration gradient in moles/cm^3, and ΔX is thickness of the barrier to diffusion in cm. Since flux remains positive while the concentration gradient is dissipating, a minus sign is added to D.

For a specific dialysis membrane, D and ΔX are constant at any preset temperature, and thus, the above equation can simplified as follows:

$$J_{Diffusion} = -K_o \cdot A \cdot \Delta C$$

where K_o is the overall mass transfer coefficient in cm/min. If rearranged, $K_o = (J_{Diffusion} / A) / -\Delta C$ = flux per unit area / driving force of the concentration gradient; furthermore, this can be rewritten as $(J_{Diffusion} / A) = -\Delta C/(1 / K_o) = -\Delta C / R_o$, which can be read as mass transfer per unit area = driving force / resistance to transport. For any specific solute to diffuse from the blood to the dialysate, the total resistance R_o would be the sum of the resistance to move from the bloodstream to the blood surface of the membrane R_B, the resistance to move across the dialysis membrane R_M, and the resistance to move from the dialysis side of the membrane to the dialysate R_D: $R_o = R_B + R_M + R_D$ (3). R_B can be minimized by the maximization of the blood-flow rate Q_B and shear rate, R_D can be attenuated by increasing the dialysate flow rate Q_D, and R_M can be optimized by an even packing density of the membrane fibers and spacer compounds during production.

In intermittent HD, diffusion is the major process for small solute clearance; is governed by concentration gradients; and depends mainly on membrane surface area and thickness, blood-flow rate, dialysate flow rate, and temperature (4). Q_B is usually slower than Q_D and as such has the greatest impact on diffusive solute clearance; at a Q_B of 400 mL/min, any increase in the Q_D above 600 mL/min will only offer a mediocre increase in diffusive solute clearance (5).

Convection

Convection is a mass transfer process that describes the bulk transport of molecules within fluids where transport is dependent upon factors such as changes in hydrostatic or osmotic pressure and membrane porosity; in HD, this is represented by a solute following the bulk transport of water (solvent drag phenomenon) during ultrafiltration triggered by a positive TMP. Said bulk transport follows Poiseuille's law for hydrodynamic flow, which describes laminar flow of a Newtonian fluid through a pipe (e.g., hollow fiber); Newtonian fluids, such as water, have a constant viscosity in time and at different rates of shear stress.

$$Q = dV/dt = \pi \cdot \Delta P \cdot r^4 / 8 \cdot \eta \cdot L$$

where Q is the volume flow rate under laminar flow conditions, ΔP is the pressure drop across a pipe, r is the radius of the pipe, η is the viscosity coefficient (a constant that is dependent on temperature but independent of the speed of flow), and L is the length of the pipe.

However, blood does not obey Poiseuille's law, owing to its being a non-Newtonian viscoelastic fluid with cells, which can deform, and proteins, both of which make its viscosity variable at different Hct and protein concentrations. Viscosity would be at its highest when the blood-flow rate and the shear rate applied are at their lowest (4). For blood flowing in a laminar fashion

| TABLE 1.2 | Clinically Relevant Solutes and Their Molecular Weights | | | | |

Molecule	Formula	MW Da	Molecule	Formula	MW Da
Albumin	—	66,500	Lambda free light chain (dimer)	—	45,000
β_2-Microglobulin	—	11,815	Magnesium	Mg(2+)	24.305
Bilirubin	$C_{33}H_{36}N4O_6$	584.66214 (CID: 5280352)	Myoglobin	—	17,200
Calcium	Ca(2+)	40.078	Phosphate	—	134
Carbon dioxide	CO_2	44.0095 (CID: 280)	Phosphorus	P(3−)	30.973761
Chloride	Cl(−)	35.453	Potassium	K(+)	39.0983
Cholesterol	$C_{27}H_{46}O$	386.65354 (CID: 5997)	Sodium	Na(+)	22.9898
Creatinine	$C_4H_7N_3O$	113.11788 (CID: 588)	Urea[a](1)	CH_4N_2O	60.05526 (CID: 1176)
Cystatin C	$C_{22}H_{40}N_8O_5$	13,359 (PMID: 9574456)	Vitamin A (retinol)	$C_{20}H_{30}O$	286.4516 (CID: 445354)
Ferritin (24 subunits)	—	474,000	Vitamin B_1 (thiamine)	$C_{12}H_{17}N_4OS+$	265.35458 (CID: 1130)
Glucose	$C_6H_{12}O_6$	180.15588 (CID: 53782692)	Vitamin B_{12} (cyanocobalamin)[a](3)	$C_{63}H_{88}CoN_{14}O_{14}P$	1,355.365177 (CID: 5311498)
Hemoglobin tetramer	—	64,458	Vitamin B_2 (riboflavin)	$C_{17}H_{20}N_4O_6$	376.3639 (CID: 493570)
Immunoglobulin A (monomer)	—	162,000	Vitamin B_3 (niacin, nicotinic acid)	$C_6H_5NO_2$	123.1094 (CID: 938)
Immunoglobulin A secretory (dimer)	—	380,000	Vitamin B_5 (pantothenic acid)	$C_9H_{17}NO_5$	219.23498 (CID: 6613)
Immunoglobulin D	—	184,000	Vitamin B_6 (pyridoxine)	$C_8H_{11}NO_3$	169.17784 (CID: 1054)
Immunoglobulin E	—	188,000	Vitamin B_7 (biotin)	$C_{10}H_{16}N_2O_3S$	244.31064 (CID: 171548)
Immunoglobulin G	—	153,000	Vitamin B_9 or folic acid	$C_{19}H_{19}N_7O_6$	441.39746 (CID: 6037)
Immunoglobulin G1	—	146,000	Vitamin C (ascorbic acid)	$C_6H_8O_6$	176.12412 (CID: 54670067)
Immunoglobulin G2	—	146,000	Vitamin D_2 (ergocalciferol)	$C_{28}H_{44}O$	396.64836 (CID: 5280793)
Immunoglobulin G3	—	170,000	Vitamin D_3 (cholecalciferol)	$C_{27}H_{44}O$	384.63766 (CID: 5280795)
Immunoglobulin G4	—	146,000	Vitamin E (α-tocopherol)	$C_{29}H_{50}O_2$	430.7061 (CID: 14985)
Immunoglobulin M	—	970,000	Vitamin K_1 (phylloquinone)	$C_{31}H_{46}O_2$	450.69574 (CID: 5284607)
Inulin	$C_{228}H_{382}O_{191}$	6,179.35808 (CID: 18772499)	Vitamin K_2 (sub20) (menaquinone)	$C_{31}H_{40}O_2$	444.6481 (CID: 5282367)
Kappa free light chain (monomer)	—	22,500	Vitamin K_3 (menadione)	$C_{11}H_8O_2$	172.18002 (CID: 4055)
Lactic acid	$C_3H_6O_3$	90.07794 (CID: 612)			

MW, molecular weight.
[a]National Center for Biotechnology Information. PubChem Compound Database; CID.

across a hollow-fiber dialysis membrane under preset condition that makes its viscosity constant, convection is reflected by the Hagen-Poiseuille equation:

$$\Delta P = (8 \cdot \eta \cdot L \cdot Q_B) / (N \cdot \pi \cdot r^4)$$

where ΔP is the pressure gradient across the dialysis membrane, η is the blood viscosity, L is the length of the dialyzer membrane, Q_B is the blood-flow rate, N is the number of hollow fibers in a dialyzer, and r is the radius of the hollow fiber.

Thus, convective clearance across a dialysis membrane is better achieved with a higher pressure gradient ΔP along the length of the dialysis membrane, a higher blood viscosity η which is dependent on Hct, a higher blood-flow rate Q_B exceeding 300 mL/min, a smaller diameter of individual hollow fibers.

Convective clearance can be represented by the following equation:

$$J_{Convection} = SC \cdot Q_F$$

where SC is the apparent solute sieving coefficient and Q_F is the ultrafiltration rate (6).

In HD, convective solute transport is driven by TMP and ultrafiltration (Q_F) and accentuates diffusive transport; convective transport gains greater clinical significance as the solute's molecular weight increases (7) and is the cornerstone of therapies such as hemodiafiltration (HDF) (8).

Adsorption

Adsorption refers to solute removal via solute deposition, predominantly low molecular weight proteins (LMWPs), and adhesion to the dialysis membrane. An initial phase of competitive adsorption of high molecular weight proteins (HMWPs) to the inner layer of the dialysis membrane occurs until saturation is reached; this process results in a surface biofilm consistent of HMWP such as albumin, globulins, and fibrinogen. A second dynamic and slower phase of adsorption involves LMWP, such as β_2-MG, cytokines, and anaphylatoxins, and involves the inner layers of the dialysis membrane and is completely dependent on membrane porosity and charge-dependent selective permeability (9). Synthetic membranes have a higher adsorption clearance than cellulosic membranes owing in part to their higher hydrophobicity and porosity; examples include polysulfone, polyacrylonitrile (PAN), and polymethylmethacrylate (PMMA) (10).

Clearance

The clearance of any specific solute is the sum total of its diffusive clearance, convective clearance, and adsorptive clearance. Clearance K = solute mass removal rate per unit time / plasma solute concentration. Based on prior discussion, solute clearance can be increased in the majority of instances by maximizing Q_B and Q_F.

Membrane Efficiency

Membrane efficiency refers to SMW solute permeability, most commonly, urea. It is the capacity of any one specific membrane to clear any one specific solute from the blood when other HD variables are preset, namely, blood-flow rate (Q_B) and dialysate flow rate (Q_D); urea has been traditionally the solute of choice to report efficiency in the dialysis membrane industry.

Efficiency is determined by a membrane's surface area and its solute permeability and is quantitatively measured by the membrane permeability-area coefficient K_oA, where K_o is the mass transfer coefficient and A is the membrane's surface area (11). As mentioned earlier, most dialysis membrane manufacturers report the values for K_oA measurements for urea when all other dialysis conditions are preset *in vitro*, namely, the Q_B, the Q_D, the ultrafiltration rate Q_F, dialysate temperature, and blood percent Hct. The K_oA of a membrane indicates its urea clearance when Q_B and Q_D are infinite.

In vivo membrane efficiency may fall short of the *in vitro* performance due to blood-to-dialysate flow mismatch; for example, this may be caused by a higher blood viscosity on the luminal side of the membrane and thus affecting the blood-flow distribution, or to an uneven fiber density in a heterogeneously packed hollow-fiber membrane, thus affecting the dialysate flow distribution and resulting in a decreased dialysate flow velocity in the more densely packed areas, usually in the center, and a higher flow velocity in the less densely packed areas (4). Synthetic membrane fibers are usually distributed in an undulated or rippled pattern and thus result in a lesser blood-to-dialysate flow mismatch than the straight and unevenly packed fibers seen in cellulose membranes (12). It is also worth noting that the performance of many membranes is reported by the manufacturer based on an Hct of 32%, and higher *in vivo* values may also affect dialyzer efficiency (13,14). When *in vitro* experiments use a fluid other than blood, the manufacturer's reported efficiency or K_oA tends to overestimate the *in vivo* values; for instance, the Hemodialysis (HEMO) Study Group reported an *in vivo* K_oA at $80 \pm 7\%$ (SD) of the *in vitro* values ($p <0.001$) in the 1,208 patients with arteriovenous accesses at first use and at a Q_D of 500 mL/min, and this further declined to $74.8 \pm 6.6\%$ when other variables were accounted for, namely, effects of Q_D and reuse number (11).

Synthetic and asymmetric membranes also tend to be more efficient due to a lesser resistance to water and solute transport conferred by their lower membrane thickness when compared to homogeneous and symmetric membranes (15).

Membrane Flux

Membrane flux refers to MMW solute permeability. This measure of permeability by molecular size cutoff is routinely reported in reference to a specific MMW or high molecular weight (HMW) solute, most commonly β_2-MG and less commonly vitamin B_{12} or inulin.

Current dialysis membranes in order of permeability are high-cutoff membranes or super high-flux membranes > high-flux membranes > low-flux membranes.

Membrane flux has also been reported as a membrane's capacity at ultrafiltration, or water flux, the major determinant of convective solute clearance across the membrane. The measure of the ultrafiltration capacity of a membrane, and thus its designation as low or high flux, is based on the ultrafiltration coefficient (K_{UF}):

$$K_{UF} \text{ (mL/min/mm Hg)} = \text{water flux / transmembrane pressure} = Q_F / (P_B - P_D)$$

where Q_F is the ultrafiltration rate in mL/min, and $P_B - P_D$ refers to the TMP gradient between the blood and the dialysis compartments. K_{UF} is measured *in vitro* by the ultrafiltration of bovine blood at different TMPs (16). K_{UF} is naturally dependent on membrane permeability to water, and thus, pore size is the major determinant of membrane flux; a membrane with larger pore sizes has the advantage of higher rates of water flux and a higher ultrafiltration capacity as well as a better removal of HMW solutes than membranes with smaller pore size.

Both parameters used to report membrane flux, MMW solute clearance and ultrafiltration capacity (K_{UF}), correlate well as membrane performance measures (17).

Internal Filtration and Backfiltration

Internal filtration/backfiltration (IF/BF) is the phenomenon that describes the automatic and uncontrolled convective transport of solute with water from the dialysate compartment to the blood compartment when the driving force of filtration is dissipated under countercurrent flow conditions; this occurs when the oncotic pressure balances the hydrostatic pressure due to the high ultrafiltration rate characteristic of high-flux dialyzers (18). During a typical HD treatment with a high-flux membrane, the ongoing balance between hydrostatic and oncotic pressures along the membrane results in an ongoing process of IF/BF even when the ultrafiltration rate is nil; it is estimated that 6 to 8 L are internally filtered and backfiltered during a 4-hour treatment when no ultrafiltration is prescribed.

Theoretically, this IF/BF may result in the transport of bacterial byproducts or inflammatory mediators from a contaminated dialysate to the patient's blood and result in bioincompatibility of the membrane; thus, it is recommended that ultrapure dialysate be used with high-flux HD to avoid potential proinflammatory effects (19).

This IF/BF phenomenon contributes to an automatic, uncontrolled form of convective solute transport, a convection-enhanced or IF-enhanced HD with its own internal hemodiafiltration (iHDF) component and without a replacement solution. IF/BF promotes MMW and LMW solute clearance, such as β_2-MG, and LMWP clearance, in a process that is dependent on the IF flow rate Q_{IF}, which can be augmented by increasing Q_B (20–22). Several membrane developers have used this same phenomenon in the development of a newer generation of iHDF membranes that enhances the clearance of aforementioned solutes. A quantifying mathematical model has also been developed (23).

Dialysis Membrane Biocompatibility

Biocompatibility refers to the magnitude of the reaction of the human body upon exposure of blood to the dialysis membrane, triggering a cascade of events and generating a proinflammatory status, via activation of cellular and humoral immunity, and/or a thrombogenic effect. Thus, a hypothetically perfect biocompatible membrane would not trigger any human response (immune or thrombogenic or otherwise) and a bioincompatible membrane would mobilize all components of the immune and coagulation systems among others. For example, membranes made of the naturally abundant, unmodified cellulose polysaccharide (a D-glucose linear homopolymer $(C_6H_{10}O_5)_n$) (24) are among the least biocompatible membranes and, while at one point of time were the most widely used dialyzer membrane worldwide, have since been discontinued in 2006 and largely replaced by more biocompatible synthetic membranes, largely made of polysulfone (25).

 CLASSIFICATION OF DIALYSIS MEMBRANES

There is no one classification of dialysis membranes by geometric design, chemical composition, efficiency, flux, or biocompatibility. With the continued development of newer membranes, there is a considerable overlap when considering all these criteria (**TABLE 1.1**).

Classification of Dialysis Membranes by Geometry, Design, and Structure

Coil Dialyzers have the highest resistance for solute mass transport from the blood to the dialysate (16) and are mostly of historical interest at this time.

Parallel-Plate Dialyzers have a lesser resistance for solute mass transport from the blood to the dialysate (16).

Hollow-Fiber Dialyzers have the lowest resistance for solute mass transport from the blood to the dialysate (16) and are the most widely used all over the world. Cross-sectionally, hollow-fiber dialyzers may be symmetric or asymmetric. Symmetric fibers are homogenous in cross-section with similar pore sizes across all layers. Asymmetric fibers are designed with a thin inner layer on the blood side of the membrane, which is the major determinant for solute permeability, and a thick outer supporting layer (the stroma) with larger pores toward the dialysate side of the membrane. The internal distribution of the hollow fibers plays an important role in its performance, and as mentioned earlier, asymmetric design is associated with less blood-to-dialysate flow mismatch (12).

Classification of Dialysis Membranes by Chemical Composition/Material

Dialysis membranes may be made of unmodified or regenerated cellulose, synthetically modified cellulose (SMC), or synthetic polymers (**TABLES 1.1** and **1.3**). Polymer-based synthetic membranes became commercially available in the 1970s and have since dominated the dialysis membrane industry; they tend to have higher performance, are more biocompatible, and their availability in high flux made it possible for patients to have a shorter HD time without jeopardizing dialysis adequacy (26). It must be noted though, that a dissociation between solute and water flux for membranes of any specific composition makes any simplified model of flux/composition classification almost impossible.

Unmodified or Standard Cellulose

The first described dialysis membrane was made of collodion, a polymer of cellobiose, an unmodified cellulose-trinitrate derivative (27); cellulose comprises 90% of cotton and 50% of wood and is as such the most abundant of all naturally occurring organic compounds. It is this low-flux membrane that Adolf Fick and Thomas Graham, among other scientists, used to lay out the principles of HD in the 19th century and early 20th century to selectively separate SMW solutes from blood through the process of diffusion (28). In 1914, a team of scientists led by Abel (29) developed and tested the first efficient *in vivo* dialysis system in a living animal at Johns Hopkins University School of Medicine, and in 1924, the first human HD was performed in a uremic patient by George Haas in 1924 at the University of Giessen in Germany (30,31).

Unmodified cellulose membranes are mechanically stable, have symmetric fibers, and are homogenous in cross-section with similar pore sizes across all layers; they are also hydrophilic enabling lower membrane thickness (6 to 15 μm dry thickness) (15,25), have small pores, and as such a good efficiency/performance on LMW or small solute diffusive clearance. However, they have a low flux with a K_{UF} of <10 mL/h/mm Hg and perform poorly on middle-molecule clearance (molecular cutoff clearance of 5,000 Da; e.g., β_2-MG); this, along with their bioincompatibility, driven by a high degree of alternative complement pathway activation as a result of complement protein interaction with the free cellulose hydroxyl moiety (25), eventually led to their replacement and the development of more biocompatible membranes with better clinical performance measures and clinical outcomes.

Regenerated Cellulose

Regenerated cellulose is obtained from cellulose that has been liquefied, purified, and extruded and changed by physical, rather than chemical, treatment such as cellophane, rayon, and viscose; their chemical structure remains identical to cellulose. One prototype dialysis membrane manufactured from regenerated cellulose is Cuprophan (CU, manufactured by Membrana); other examples include cellophane and cuprammonium rayon. In 1947, Cuprophan flat sheets were established as wrapping foil, and by 1965, the first flat sheet HD membranes were developed, but it was only in 1966 that Cuprophan was used in the world's first industrially manufactured artificial kidney. Regenerated cellulose membranes replaced collodion because they offered better performance at the time and were more stable mechanically; they also had the same advantage of a low membrane thickness owing to their strong hydrophilic characteristics (15).

Modified Cellulose
Substituted Cellulose

This membrane is made by the chemical treatment of cellulose, for example, with acetic acid, where acetate replaces the free hydroxyl groups on the surface of the cellulose molecule. The replacement of the hydroxyl group decreases the availability of free nucleophilic moieties and is thought to reduce complement protein binding and activation and hence enhance biocompatibility (25).

TABLE 1.3 Examples of Dialysis Membranes Used in the United States

Membrane Information			Specifications			Performance		
Series	Membrane Example	Composition Membrane/ Potting Compound/ Housing	ESA (m²) – PV (mL)	HFID (μm) – HFWT (μm)	Max. TMP (mm Hg) – Sterilization	K_oA (Urea) (mL/min)	K_{UF} (mL/h/ mm Hg)	Other
Manufacturer: Asahi Kasei Medical America Inc								
REXEED-S / R	REXEED-18S / R[a]	REXBRANE	1.8 – 95	185 – 45	500 – GR	1,483[b]	71[c]	—
REXEED-L	REXEED-18L		1.8 – 103	185 – 45	500 – GR	1,145[d]	13[e]	—
REXEED-A	REXEED-18A		1.8 – 103	185 – 45	500 – GR	1,415[d]	80[f]	0.85 – 0.002[g]
ViE	ViE-18	VitabranE	1.8 – 105	200 – 45	500 – GR	836[d]	70[h]	0.70 – ≤0.002[g]
ViE-L	ViE-18L		1.8 – 103	185 – 45	500 – GR	1,145[d]	13[e]	
Manufacturer: Fresenius Medical Care								
Fresenius Optiflux	Optiflux F180NR	Advanced Fresenius Polysulfone, PU, PC	1.8 – 98	200 – 40	? – EB	1,239[i]	60[j]	74[k]
Manufacturer: Baxter								
CA single-use	CA 70	Cellulose acetate	0.7 – 45	200 – 15	? – ETO	330[l]	3.6	—
EXELTRA single-use	EXELTRA 170	Cellulose triacetate	1.7 – 105	200 – 15	? – GR	1,103[l]	33.80	—
DICEA single-use	DICEA 170	Cellulose diacetate	1.7 – 105	200 – 15	? – GR	961[l]	12.5	—
CT reuse	CT 190G	Cellulose triacetate	1.9 – 115	200 – 15	? – GR	1,214[l]	36.42	—
CA-HP Reuse	CA-HP 170	Cellulose diacetate	1.7 – 105	200 – 15	? – ETO	945[l]	10.0	—
Xenium XPH single-use	Xenium XPH 170	Polynephron	—	—	—	—	—	—
Manufacturer: Gambro								
Polyflux L	Polyflux 17L	Polyamix PU, PC	1.7 – 104	215 – 50	600 – Steam	1,026[d]	12.5[m]	—
Polyflux H	Polyflux 170H		1.7 – 115	215 – 50	600 – Steam	1,153[d]	70[n]	1.0 – 1.0 – 0.70 – <0.01[o]
Polyflux 2H Gambro	Polyflux 2H		0.2 – 17	—	600 – Steam		15[m]	1.0 – 1.0 – 0.70 – <0.01[o]
Polyflux 6H Gambro	Polyflux 6H	Polyflux PU, PC	0.6 – 52	215 – 50	600 – Steam	465[p]	33 ± 20%[m]	1.0 – 0.99 – 0.63 – <0.01[o]
Polyflux Revaclear	Polyflux Revaclear MAX	Poracton PU, PC	1.8 – 100	190 – 35	600 – Steam	1,487[d]	60 ± 20%[m]	1.0 – 1.0 – 0.7 – <0.01[o]
Polyflux R (reuse)	Polyflux 17R	Polyflux PU, PC	1.7 – 121	215 – 50	600 – Steam	880[d]	71 ± 20%[m]	—
Evodial	Evodial 1.6	HeprAN, PU, PC	1.65 – 100	210 – 45	450 – GR	—	50 ± 20%[m]	? – 0.96 – ? – <0.01[o]

(Continued)

TABLE 1.3 (*Continued*)								
Membrane Information			**Specifications**			**Performance**		
Series	**Membrane Example**	**Composition Membrane/ Potting Compound/ Housing**	**ESA (m^2) – PV (mL)**	**HFID (μm) – HFWT (μm)**	**Max. TMP (mm Hg) – Sterilization**	**K$_o$A (Urea) (mL/min)**	**K$_{UF}$ (mL/h/ mm Hg)**	**Other**
Nephral ST	Nephral ST 400	AN69 ST, PU, PC	1.65 – 98	210 – 42	450 – GR	–	50 ± 20%^{m}	1.00 – 0.96 – ? – <0.01^o
Crystal (Plate)	Crystal ST	AN69 ST, PU, PC						

ESA, effective surface area; PV, priming volume; HFID, inside diameter of hollow fiber; HFWT, wall thickness of hollow fiber; TMP, transmembrane pressure; K$_o$A, membrane permeability-area coefficient; K$_{UF}$, ultrafiltration coefficient; REXBRANE, Asahi polysulfone; GR, gamma ray; EB, electron beam; ETO, ethylene oxide; Polynephron, polyethersulfone; Polyflux, blend of Polyarylethersulfone, Polyvinylpyrrolidone, Polyamide; Polyamix membrane, three-layered blended polymer of polyarylethersulfone, polyvinylpyrrolidone, and polyamide; PU, polyurethane; PC, polycarbonate; Poracton, polyarylethersulfone, polyvinylpyrrolidone; HeprAN, AN69 ST heparin grafted; AN69 ST, acrylonitrile and sodium methallyl sulfonate copolymer–polyethylenimine.

^{a}S, single use; R, multiple use.
^{b}K$_o$A: Q$_B$ = 400 mL/min, Q$_D$ = 800 mL/min.
^{c}K$_{UF}$: with bovine plasma, TP = 6.5 ± 0.5 g/dL, TMP = 50mm Hg.
^{d}K$_o$A: Q$_B$ = 300 mL/min, Q$_{BD}$ = 500 mL/min, Q$_F$ = 0 mL/min.
^{e}K$_{UF}$: with bovine blood, TP = 60 ± 5 g/L, Hct = 32 ± 2%, Q$_B$ = 300 mL/min, TMP = 100 mm Hg.
^{f}K$_{UF}$: with bovine blood, TP = 60 ± 5 g/L, Hct = 32 ± 2%, Q$_B$ = 300 mL/min, TMP = 50 mm Hg.
^{g}Sieving coefficient for β$_2$-microglobulin (β$_2$-MG) – albumin bovine plasma, TP = 60 ± 5g/L.
^{h}K$_{UF}$: with bovine blood, TP = 60 ± 5 g/L, Hct = 32 ± 2%, Q$_B$ = 300 mL/min.
^{i}Q$_B$, Q$_D$, Q$_F$ settings not specified in manufacturer's brochure.
^{j}K$_{UF}$: with bovine blood, hematocrit = 32 ± 2%.
^{k}Middle molecule clearance mL/min: molecular weight 14,800 Da, surrogate for middle molecule clearance measured with lysozyme.
^{l}K$_o$A: Q$_B$ = 300 mL/min, Q$_D$ = 500 mL/min.
^{m}K$_{UF}$: Measured with bovine blood, hematocrit = 32%, protein 60 g/L, at 37°C.
^{n}K$_{UF}$: Measured with bovine blood, hematocrit of (32 ± 3) % and a protein content of (60 ± 5) g/L.
^{o}Sieving coefficient for vitamin B$_{12}$ – inulin – β$_2$-MG – albumin. Typical values measured with Polyflux 170H dialyzer, with hematocrit of (32 ± 3) % and a protein content of (60 ± 5) g/L.
^{p}K$_o$A: Q$_B$ = 200 mL/min, Q$_D$ = 500 mL/min, Q$_F$ = 0 mL/min.

A prototype of substituted cellulose membrane is cellulose triacetate (molecular formula $C_{40}H_{54}O_{27}$; molecular weight: 966.84056 g/mol) (32) (e.g., CT190G, Baxter Healthcare Corp, Deerfield, IL) where there is a total replacement of all hydroxyl groups with acetate; other examples include cellulose acetate, cellulose diacetate, and cellulose hydrate. When replaced with acetate, there is an increase in membrane porosity and hence water and solute permeability; furthermore, the substituted cellulose triacetate membrane is highly hydrophobic and the absence of swelling decreases the membrane thickness (15,16). The cellulose triacetate dialysis membrane is the most biocompatible of all cellulosic membranes has a similar biocompatibility to that of the polysulfone membrane (16).

Semisynthetic Cellulose

This modification aims at replacing the free surface hydroxyl group with a bulky moiety that sterically hinders blood–membrane interactions. One prototype of modified semisynthetic membranes is Hemophan (manufactured by Membrana), in which a synthetic material, diethylaminoethyl (DEAE), is mixed with liquefied cellulose during its regeneration for membrane formation. This membrane retains the high-efficiency characteristics of the unmodified cellulose membrane and is available in low flux and high flux and has an affinity to bind anions, such as heparin and phosphate, and hence a decrease in thrombogenicity and phosphate clearance when compared to nonmodified cellulose membranes (33) but no change in phosphorus kinetics when compared to synthetic membranes (34).

Other examples of semisynthetic cellulose membranes include benzyl-modified cellulose (SMC, Membrana GmbH, Wuppertal, Germany), polyethylene glycol-grafted cellulose (AM-BIO, Asahi Medical Co, Ltd, Tokyo, Japan), and vitamin E (Excebrane, Asahi Medical Co, Ltd, Tokyo Japan).

Noncellulose Synthetic

Synthetic membranes are manufactured with a noncellulosic polymers but are more often than not alloys or copolymers of more than one polymer; this latter point is extremely important for the accurate interpretation of the physical and chemical properties of any synthetic membrane, especially that membrane nomenclature may be often misleading as it refers to only to one of the polymers used.

The first synthetic dialysis membrane was developed in the early 1970s and was a PAN membrane, namely, AN69 (Gambro, Lakewood, CO; Hospal, Meyzieu, France), an alloy of the acrylonitrile and sodium methallyl sulfonate polymers; at the time, the rationale was to develop a membrane with a high ultrafiltration coefficient for high-flux HD and hemofiltration (35).

Currently, the majority of dialysis membranes in use are synthetic. Of the synthetic membranes used, 93% are polymers from the polyarysulfone family with 71% being polysulfone and 22% being polyethersulfone (36).

Prototypes of noncellulose synthetic dialysis membrane include polysulfone (molecular formula: $C_{27}H_{26}O_6S$; molecular weight: 478.55674 g/mol) (32) (e.g., F80A, Fresenius, Lexington, MA) which is the most widely used membrane, polyarylethersulfone

(PAES) or polyethersulfone [molecular formula: $(C_{12}H_8O_3S)_n$; molecular weight: $(232.258)_n$ g/mol], polyacrylonitrile (PAN) [molecular formula: $(C_3H_3N)_n$; molecular weight: $(53.06262)_n$ g/mol] (32) (e.g., AN69), polycarbonate [molecular formula: $(CO_3^{i2})_n$; molecular weight: $(60.0089)_n$ g/mol] (32), polyamide (molecular formula: $C_{18}H_{35}N_3O_3$; molecular weight: 341.4888 g/mol) (32), PMMA membranes [molecular formula: $(C_5H_8O_2)_n$; molecular weight: $(100.11582)_n$ g/mol] (32), and poly(vinyl alcohol-co-ethylene) (EVOH) (linear molecular formula: $(CH_2CH_2)_x[CH_2CH(OH)]_y$). Synthetic membranes are thicker than cellulose membranes (35 µm or more dry thickness) (25), their fibers may be symmetric (AN69, PMMA) or asymmetric (polysulfone, polyamide) with various structures (sponge- or fingerlike) of the supportive stromal layer (16). During the polymerization process of predominantly hydrophobic synthetic membranes, such as polysulfone, polyamide, and polyethersulfone, a wetting hydrophilic agent polyvinylpyrrolidone (PVP, a widely used pharmaceutical excipient) is added to enhance the overall membrane's hydrophilic properties making its clinical use feasible; PVP also promotes the alloyed membrane's porosity and also determines membrane integrity upon reuse.

Bioactive Membranes

Bioactive membranes are synthetic or cellulosic membranes, which are coated with a bioactive compound such as heparin or vitamin E, with a hypothetical intent to decrease thrombogenicity or oxidant stress in these two instances.

Classification of Dialysis Membranes by Flux and Water Ultrafiltration Coefficient

Membrane flux is measured by the permeability of the membrane to water and other molecules typically β_2-MG.

Low-Flux Membranes

The HEMO study defines such a membrane as one with low permeability to β_2-MG and a mean clearance <10 mL/min (17). The U.S. Food and Drug Administration (FDA) describes a low-flux "conventional" membrane as one with an *in vitro* permeability to water molecules K_{UF} equal or less to 12 mL/h/mm Hg (37).

High-Flux Membranes

The HEMO study defines such a membrane as one with high permeability to β_2-MG and mean clearance >20 mL/min and a K_{UF} of more than 14 mL/h/mm Hg (17). The FDA describes a high-flux "high-permeability" membrane as one with an *in vitro* permeability to water molecules K_{UF} of more than 12 mL/h/mm Hg (37).

Super High-Flux or High-Cutoff Membranes

These membranes have the ability to clear LMW solutes, naturally larger than β_2-MG, such as LMWP including protein-bound uremic toxins. These membranes can clear solutes with a molecular weight cutoff very close to the native kidney and as high as 65,000 Da; they have the ability to clear cytokines in sepsis syndromes, myoglobin in rhabdomyolysis, and kappa and lambda free light chains in multiple myeloma and other plasma cell dyscrasias and dysproteinemias (38,39).

In Japan and for health insurance reimbursement purposes, dialysis membranes are stratified into five different classes based on their β_2-MG clearance (mL/min), when Q_B is set at 200 mL/min, Q_D is set at 500 mL/min, and Q_F is set at 10 mL/min, as follows: type I <10, 10 ≤ type II <30, 30 ≤ type III <50, 50≤

type IV <70, and type V ≥70. As such, types IV and V are super high-flux dialyzers (40,41).

Classification of Dialysis Membranes by Efficiency

A dialysis membrane whose K_oA urea <500 mL/min is considered a low-efficiency membrane and one whose urea KoA >600 mL/min is considered a high-efficiency membrane. Membrane efficiency increases with increasing membrane surface area, optimizing Q_B and Q_D, and a dialysis access capable of providing the prescribed blood-flow rate. Since the potential for augmentation of Q_B, Q_D, or access is quite limited, high-efficiency membranes have traditionally been higher surface area membranes, usually more than 1.5 m².

Classification of Dialysis Membranes by Performance

The performance of a dialysis membrane is based on its solute clearance effectiveness and its biocompatibility. An HPM would have the following features: (a) ability to clear target solutes including MMW and LMW uremic toxins, such as β_2-MG and LMWPs; (b) larger pore size and high molecular weight cutoff, thus enhancing its convective clearance capacity, the pore sizes ought to be highly uniform and with minimal variability resulting in a shaper sieving coefficient cutoff and augmented clearance of LMWP-bound uremic toxins (while minimizing albumin losses) as well as MMW and LMW uremic toxins with clearances approaching those of the native kidney; (c) enhanced adsorptive capacity; and (d) superb biocompatibility profile.

The Japanese Society of Dialysis Therapy (JSDT) favors an HPM pore size that is permissive of albumin losses of less than 3 g during one treatment (Q_B 200 mL/min; Q_D 500 mL/min) to enhance albumin turnover (12,40,42,43).

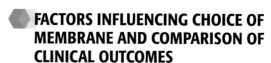

FACTORS INFLUENCING CHOICE OF MEMBRANE AND COMPARISON OF CLINICAL OUTCOMES

Geometric Design

Coil dialysis membranes have been associated with a higher incidence of intradialytic hypotension than parallel-plate and hollow-fiber dialysis membranes (44). Hollow-fiber dialysis membranes were associated with less thrombocytopenia and a higher mean postdialysis platelet count (93% of predialysis platelet count) when compared to parallel-plate dialysis membranes (postdialysis platelet count 69% of predialysis platelet count) (45). There was no statistically significant difference in the blood levels of anaphylotoxins C3a, C4a, and C5a or their des-Arg forms as measured by radioimmunoassay between patients who were dialyzed with parallel-plate or hollow-fiber membranes (46). In contrast, Lins et al. (47) studied the effects of dialysis membrane geometry on platelet count, whole blood activated coagulation time, heparin dose requirement, and complement C3a activation; they found no statistically significant differences between hollow-fiber and parallel-plate Cuprophan dialyzers for any measure at any time.

Currently, the overwhelming majority of dialysis membranes are manufactured in hollow fiber; as such, geometric design hardly plays any significant role in choosing the desired membrane.

Membrane Biocompatibility

The continuing advances in the design of dialysis membranes, aiming to manufacture the perfectly biocompatible dialysis membrane for patients on maintenance HD, can be viewed as yet another application of "Primum non nocere" or "first, do no harm." Membrane and dialysis biocompatibility may have various clinical implications, some known and others not, that include patient's well-being, inflammatory status, nutritional status, and degree of thrombogenicity among others.

Well-described aspects of bioincompatibility include (a) an enhanced chronic inflammatory status resulting from the activation of the alternative complement system with subsequent activation of granulocytes and release of cytokines, (b) enhanced thrombogenicity resulting in blood loss and worsening anemia or blood-to-dialysate flow mismatch and reduced uremic toxin clearance, (c) erythropoietin resistance, (d) declining nutritional status and loss of muscle and body mass, (e) accelerated atherosclerosis and cardiovascular disease, and (f) deposition of β_2-MG fibrils resulting in dialysis-related amyloidosis (DRA) (10,48,49). These aspects will be discussed below.

Inflammation

Activation of the alternative complement pathway during HD with a bioincompatible membrane is triggered by the spontaneous production of C3b, covalent bonding of C3b to the free nucleophilic groups on the dialysis membrane, limiting the C3b-binding of inhibitory regulatory factor H and favoring its binding to activating regulatory factors (e.g., factor B), and an amplification positive feedback loop perpetuated by the generation of C3-convertase which in turn results in more C3b production. The end result is the extracorporeal production of anaphylatoxins C3a, C4a, and C5a in the dialysis membrane, which induce granulocytes to release cytokines such as interleukin 1 (IL1), interleukin 6 (IL6), and tumor necrosis factor (TNF). C5a upregulates platelet adhesion molecules, binds and activates granulocytes (neutrophils and monocytes) and lymphocytes, and induces neutrophil degranulation with release of lysosomes and reactive oxygen species creating a state of oxidative stress which in turn results in lipid and protein peroxidation and toxic-radical induced endothelial cell activation leading to vascular injury and atherosclerosis. The activated granulocytes in the dialysis circuit are removed immediately upon their return to the circulation, resulting in a transient granulocytopenia in the first half hour after starting HD. In addition to C5a-induced granulocytopenia, C5a-induced pulmonary hypertension/pulmonary dysfunction has been described in patients dialyzed with older less biocompatible membranes, mostly unmodified cellulose (9,50–52). First-use syndrome, an anaphylactoid reaction, is mediated by activation of the complement pathway (53).

Activation of the classical and the lectin complement pathway has also been reported but is thought to play a minor role.

The water affinity of the dialysis membrane has been associated with different degrees of biocompatibility with hydrophilic membranes showing greater degrees of complement activation than hydrophobic membranes (16); similarly, chemical composition plays an important role in the degree of biocompatibility with some surface moieties readily accessible for covalent bonding with C3b (e.g., hydroxyl OH, ammonia NH_3) triggering a stronger immune response.

Other important factors that influence biocompatibility and trigger a proinflammatory response include the purity level of the dialysate water, especially with high-flux dialysis membranes where BF is known to occur, and the use of chemicals. In the absence of ultrapure dialysate, bioincompatibility has been described with various scenarios such as dialysate bacterial products and endotoxins

backfiltering into the bloodstream where they trigger a potent inflammatory response.

Similar reactions may be observed with leaching of chemicals into the bloodstream, such as residues of ethylene oxide (ETO) used to sterilize the membrane leaching from the polyurethane potting compound and triggering an anaphylactoid reaction (54–57). Chemicals applied for reuse such as formaldehyde have also been described to result in hypersensitivity reactions (58).

Spallation due to insoluble solutes entering the bloodstream, as has been described with silicone released from the tubing of the blood pump under mechanical stress and triggering inflammation with clinical manifestations such as hepatitis, granuloma formation, and hypercalcemia (25,59,60).

An atypical presentation of a polysulfone membrane hypersensitivity was recently described in a patient with recurrent fevers during and posthemodialysis, with a negative infectious workup (61).

Thrombogenecity

Upon the extracorporeal flow of blood through the dialysis membrane, some plasma proteins immediately adsorb to the inner layer of the membrane creating a secondary membrane, a biofilm. This biofilm is thought to play a key role in the degree of activation of the immune and coagulation systems. Since membranes with hydrophobic surfaces enhance this adsorption process, they are generally associated with a higher degree of thrombogenicity (16). The binding of fibrinogen (factor I) to the inner surface of the dialysis membrane activates the coagulation cascade and results in its conversion of insoluble fibrin which in turn upregulated platelet activation and aggregation, the end result being blood clotting and increased thrombogenicity; to offset this rise in thrombogenicity, most dialysis patients receive some form of anticoagulation during dialysis. This protein biofilm may also adversely affect the diffusive and convective clearance of various solutes across the membrane. On the other hand, it has been suggested that this biofilm may limit complement activation in some cases and, as mentioned earlier, plays an essential role in the clearance of some LMWP. No cellulose of synthetic membrane has been proven to our knowledge to avoid this aspect of bioincompatibility triggered by blood–dialyzer interaction (10,25).

Since a dominantly hydrophilic inner surface of a dialysis membrane promotes complement activation, whereas a hydrophobic surface favors thrombogenicity, there seems to be a theoretical benefit to biocompatibility offered by a balanced combination of hydrophilic and hydrophobic microdomains. Clinical examples include the benzyl SMC membrane, polycarbonate/polyether membrane, and other synthetic membranes (16).

A hypersensitivity reaction has been well described in HD patients who were taking angiotensin-converting enzyme inhibitors (ACEIs) and dialyzed with negatively charged membranes, such as AN69. In the first few minutes after blood flows through the dialysis membrane, the anionic surface binds and activates coagulation factor XII (Hageman factor) triggering a chain reaction that culminates in the production of bradykinin. Since ACEI also inhibit kininase II, the enzyme responsible for the degradation of kinins, bradykinin levels may increase more than 100-fold and the anaphylactoid reaction ensues (62). Thus, it is advised to avoid anionic dialysis membranes, especially AN69, in patients who are taking ACEI. This has led to the development of a modified AN69 membrane, the AN69-ST, the surface of which is treated and coated with polyethylenimine to prevent such hypersensitivity reactions (63).

Composition/Material

Membrane composition and biocompatibility are closely interconnected. There is an abundance of publications that evaluate the impact of dialysis membrane composition on biocompatibility and performance measures. For example, Chiappini et al. (64) reported that cellulose membranes were associated with higher mortality and morbidity when compared to middle- and high-flux biocompatible membranes; morbidity was reflected by a worse nutritional status, higher levels of inflammatory marker C-reactive protein, and higher pre- and postdialysis levels of β_2-MG. Maintenance HD with a Cuprophan membrane was associated with a higher rate of cystic bone lesions and bone amyloidosis than with an AN69 synthetic membrane (65).

However, unfortunately, there are not many large randomized controlled trials that have evaluated the impact of the material and composition of the dialysis membranes on clinical measures. In a Cochrane Database meta-analysis, MacLeod et al. (26) analyzed data from 32 randomized and quasi-randomized controlled trials, which evaluated impact of the dialysis membrane composition (synthetic vs. cellulose/modified cellulose) on various clinical measures in patients with end-stage kidney disease (ESKD) on HD. They found no difference in mortality rates or dialysis-related complications; synthetic membranes were associated with the most favorable albumin (regardless of flux) and lipid profile (high-flux only), while cellulose membranes were associated with a significantly higher urea reduction ratio (URR) than synthetic and modified cellulose membranes. β_2-MG levels seemed to be lower with high-flux synthetic membranes but the heterogeneity between trials (number of patients, membrane flux) rendered the data insufficient to make any reliable conclusions. The authors noted that the clinical trials included were heterogeneous and that the numbers of patients included in many of the trials with outcome measures were low.

Flux

β_2-MG is the only MMW solute, LMWP that has been associated with adverse complications due to the deposition of β_2-MG fibrils in the joints and juxta-articular structures, bones, and gastrointestinal viscera of patients with ESKD. Higher flux membranes have resulted in lower pre- and posthemodialysis β_2-MG blood levels and the amelioration of these clinical manifestations (66–70); however, whether enhanced β_2-MG clearance translates into improved survival in this population remains to be proven.

Hyperphosphatemia has been associated with higher mortality rates in patients on RRT (71,72). High-flux dialysis has been shown to provide better control of phosphorus control than low-flux dialysis but less than HDF (73–77).

Similarly, anemia is associated with increased mortality and morbidity in this patient population. The use of high-flux dialysis in 48 erythropoietin-hyporesponsive patients (dose $\geq$200 IU/kg/wk) resulted in lower erythropoietin requirements ($p < 0.001$) and improved anemia markers ($p < 0.001$) as well as greater reductions in β_2-MG and phosphorus levels when compared to low-flux dialysis (73). However, Badve et al. (78) conducted a systematic review of two clinical trials to evaluate the efficacy of intervention in the management of erythropoietin-resistant anemia, including high-flux dialysis, highlighted the absence of any randomized controlled trials powered enough to make evidence-based recommendations in favor of any specific intervention.

Koda et al. (67) reported improved survival, lower predialysis β_2-MG levels and risk for carpal tunnel syndrome in a retrospective

analysis of among 819 patients who were switched from conventional low-flux to high-flux dialysis.

In the HEMO study, a randomized controlled trial, Eknoyan et al. (17) noted that high-flux membranes did not improve survival or reduce morbidity when compared to low-flux membranes in their primary data analysis, despite the fact that the high-flux membranes resulted in a clear improvement in both urea and β_2-MG clearances. Of interest, secondary analysis showed a possible trend toward a decrease in cardiovascular mortality and hospitalizations in the high-flux membrane group and a possible benefit in women and patients with higher dialysis vintage (>3.7 years) (79).

Similarly, the Membrane Permeability Outcome (MPO) Study Group found no statistically significant survival benefit among 738 incident HD patients randomized to use high-flux and low-flux membranes over a follow-up period of 3 to 7.5 years (80). High-flux membranes were associated with a statistically significant higher survival rates among patients whose serum albumin levels were less than or equal to 4 g/dL; subgroup analysis revealed that there was a possible survival benefit in diabetics as well.

Finally, Palmer et al. (81) conducted a Cochrane Database meta-analysis which included 33 randomized and quasi-randomized controlled trials which evaluated the impact of membrane flux in 3,820 HD patients on all-cause mortality, cause-specific mortality (cardiovascular mortality, infection-related mortality), and hospitalization. Membrane flux did not have any effect on all-cause mortality, infection-related mortality, or hospitalizations; however, high-flux membrane resulted in a 17% reduction in cardiovascular mortality, thus preventing three cardiovascular deaths for each 100 patients treated with high-flux HD for 2 years.

There was no difference between online hemodiafiltration (OL-HDF) and high-flux HD in regard to blood pressure, serum albumin, erythropoietin resistance index, bone, and mineral parameters in a retrospective cohort of 858 patients followed over 18 years, but there was a reduction in mortality rates in patients treated predominantly with HDF (82). Similarly, in a cohort of 906 maintenance HD patients, those who received postdilution OL-HDF had a reduction in all-cause mortality risk by 30% (NNT 8), of cardiovascular mortality by 33%, and of infection-related mortality by 55%, and in intradialytic hypotension when compared to high-flux HD (83). In contrast, Ok et al. (84) did not find any survival benefit between OL-HDF and high-flux HD except when replacement volumes exceeded 17.4 L. OL-HDF is also hypothesized to improve vascular endothelial function and decrease vascular stiffening and inflammation (85); it has also been associated with a more favorable left ventricular ejection fraction and phosphorus control (74). There are no randomized controlled prospective studies that we know of yet to confirm the superiority of HDF.

The European best practice guidelines on HD strategies recommend the use of high-flux synthetic membranes to avoid long-term complications such as dialysis-related amyloidosis and accelerated cardiovascular disease and to improve phosphate and anemia control (86).

Effect on Residual Kidney Function

The raison d'être of high-performance dialysis membranes, with their high flux and excellent biocompatibility, may generate a hypothesis that they are associated with a better preservation of residual kidney function, owing to their attenuated proinflammatory profile.

Biocompatible high-flux polysulfone membranes are associated with better preservation of residual kidney function than cellulose membranes (87).

However, Hakim et al. (88) reported no statistically significant difference in residual renal function among 159 incident hemodialysis patients who were randomized for HD with a low-efficiency biocompatible dialysis membrane or a low-efficiency bioincompatible dialysis. Similarly, Richardson et al. (89) failed to show any difference in residual kidney function at 7 months in 177 HD patients randomized to a medium-flux modified cellulose triacetate membrane (SF170E, Nipro, Osaka, Japan) or a high-flux polysulfone membrane, Fresenius (HF80LS, Bad Homburg, Germany).

Nutritional Status and Protein Loss

Protein malnutrition (serum albumin <3.5 g/dL) is a known clinical manifestation in patients with ESKD on maintenance HD. Over a period of 18 months, the effect of membrane biocompatibility on various surrogates of nutritional status was evaluated in 158 incident HD patients; dialysis with a biocompatible membrane as opposed to a bioincompatible membrane was associated with an improved dry weight ($p < 0.05$) and an earlier and more significant increase in serum albumin levels (90).

Tayeb et al. (91) reported improved serum albumin levels in patients with protein malnutrition, who were switched from a cuprammonium to a more biocompatible polysulfone dialysis membrane ($p < 0.002$).

In a prospective cohort of 138 maintenance HD patients, middle- and high-flux dialysis were associated with improved nutritional indices, C-reactive protein, pre- and postdialysis β_2-MG, and survival when compared to low-flux dialysis (62).

A decline in body mass index has been associated with increased mortality in maintenance dialysis patients (92–94). Thus, it has been hypothesized that a dialysis membrane that decreases protein loss and associated loss of muscle mass may be associated with enhanced survival. Masakane (70) reports preservation of body and muscle mass, and lower protein loss, in patients who were dialyzed with an ethylene vinyl alcohol copolymer (EVAL) membrane when compared with a PMMA membrane; similar results were observed when predilution OL-HDF was sued with a polysulfone membrane.

Membrane Bioactivity

No study has shown improved survival with any of the available bioactive membranes such as vitamin E– or heparin-coated membranes.

Vitamin E

Several small studies, however, have pointed the favorable outcome of vitamin E–coated membranes on oxidative stress and biocompatibility, thought to be mediated by the binding of vitamin E to oxygen free radicals in the fiber lumen (95). Examples of such antioxidant activity included prevention of erythrocyte oxidative stress (96,97) and reduction of asymmetric dimethylarginine (ADMA, an endogenous inhibitor of nitric oxide synthase) (98) upon treatment with vitamin E–coated polysulfone membrane. In a prospective randomized Japanese trial, which followed 305 patients from 48 different centers, there was no difference in the erythropoiesis resistance index (ERI = total weekly ESA dose / Hb) at 1 year of follow-up between patients who were dialyzed with a vitamin E–bonded polysulfone and an uncoated polysulfone membrane (99).

In a systematic review, Huang et al. (100) reported that vitamin E–coated membranes may decrease ERI but failed to find any definitive benefit with respect to anemia, nutritional status, lipid profile, or atherosclerosis.

Heparin

The HepZero study is a multinational prospective open-label randomized controlled trial of 251 HD patients, who were randomized to dialyze with a heparin-grafted membrane (HGM), a polyacrylonitrile sodium methallyl sulfonate copolymer (Evodial, Gambro-Hospal, Meyzieu, France), or no-heparin HD with saline flushes or predilution HDF (control group); HGM membrane was noninferior but not superior to saline flushes (101). This provides a reasonable therapeutic alternative to HD patients who are at high risk for bleeding (102).

Sterilization Methods

Dialyzer membranes may be sterilized by the manufacturer in various ways such as gas chemical sterilization with ETO, autoclave or steam heat sterilization, and gamma ray or electron beam irradiation.

Different sterilization techniques did not affect small solute clearances but altered vitamin B_{12} clearance due to membrane shrinkage during the process (103).

Steam sterilization had more favorable biocompatibility surrogate measures when compared to ETO, such as white blood cell and platelet counts, anaphylatoxin levels (C3a and C5a), and polymorphonuclear neutrophil elastase plasma concentration (104).

Yamashita et al. (105) reported improved solute clearance in super high-flux dialyzers which underwent sterilization as compared to no sterilization at all. Kiaii et al. (106) reported that patients who received dialysis with an electron beam sterilized dialyzer had an odds ratio of 3.57 of developing thrombocytopenia on HD, defined by a decline in platelet count exceeding 15%.

Golli-Bennour et al. (107) reported improved viability of endothelial cell and less lipid peroxidation in 10 patients when steam sterilization was used as compared to gamma ray or ETO sterilization.

Dialysis Membrane Reuse

The effect of reprocessing and reuse of the dialysis membrane has been a topic of continued controversy. During reuse, the dialysis membrane is reprocessed with germicides and disinfectants; examples include formaldehyde, hypochlorite, glutaraldehyde, peracetic acid, heated citric acid, Renalin, and bleach.

Reuse is more common in the United States and reached a peak in 1997 when 82% of dialysis facilities implemented a reuse policy and has been declining since (39% in 2005) (108); most European countries and Japan implement no-reuse policies. The rationales for membrane reuse has varied and examples include improved biocompatibility, reduced cost, reduced nonbiodegradable waste production and a more favorable environmental impact (part of a green dialysis or eco-dialysis). On the other hand, concerns over effect of mortality, a possible promotion of the proinflammatory status, infections, and leaching resulting from improper reprocessing procedure with chemicals and germicides, and loss of functional membrane surface area have been described (109,110).

The use of formaldehyde to reprocess less biocompatible membranes, such as unmodified cellulosic membranes, has been associated with less complement activation and neutropenia, owing to the continued saturation of membrane receptors with C3b during the first use (111). In contrast, bleach is capable of effective removal of the C3b from its binding sites resulting in effects similar to first use all over again after each reuse (112).

A systematic review of 14 studies found no difference in mortality between single-use dialysis membrane and reuse (average number of reuses 2.54 to 15) among 956,807 patients with ESKD on HD (113).

There remains an increased risk with reuse inherent to the reprocessing technique with chemical disinfectants and outbreaks of bloodstream infections or sensitivity reactions continue to be reported continually (114).

Environmental Considerations

Biomedical waste from single-use dialyzer membrane poses a huge environmental burden and takes several forms; it has been estimated that in 1997 when reuse was its peak, single-use dialysis membranes alone generated 17 to 18 million pounds of waste (110,115).

 CONCLUSIONS

There has been great progress in HD membrane technology. This has eliminated many of the concerns about biocompatibility. Moreover, advances in flux, minimizing protein losses, and enhancing clearance, while reducing the need for anticoagulation requirements has helped improve the clinical care.

 REFERENCES

1. Saran R, Li Y, Robinson B, et al. US Renal Data System 2014 Annual Data Report: epidemiology of kidney disease in the United States. *Am J Kidney Dis* 2015;66(1 Suppl 1):S1–S305.
2. McKellar S. Gordon Murray and the artificial kidney in Canada. *Nephrol Dial Transplant* 1999;14:2766–2770.
3. Maher JF. *Replacement of Renal Function by Dialysis: A Textbook of Dialysis.* 3rd ed. Dordrecht, The Netherlands: Kluwer Academic Publishers, 1989.
4. Ronco C, Brendolan A, Crepaldi C, et al. Blood and dialysate flow distributions in hollow-fiber hemodialyzers analyzed by computerized helical scanning technique. *J Am Soc Nephrol* 2002;13(Suppl 1):S53–S61.
5. Bhimani JP, Ouseph R, Ward RA. Effect of increasing dialysate flow rate on diffusive mass transfer of urea, phosphate and beta2-microglobulin during clinical haemodialysis. *Nephrol Dial Transplant* 2010;25:3990–3995.
6. Jaffrin MY. Convective mass transfer in hemodialysis. *Artif Organs* 1995;19:1162–1171.
7. Hootkins R, Bourgeois B. The effect of ultrafiltration on dialysance. Mathematical theory and experimental verification. *ASAIO Trans* 1991;37:M375–M377.
8. Ledebo I, Blankestijn PJ. Haemodiafiltration-optimal efficiency and safety. *NDT Plus* 2010;3:8–16.
9. Chanard J, Lavaud S, Randoux C, et al. New insights in dialysis membrane biocompatibility: relevance of adsorption properties and heparin binding. *Nephrol Dial Transplant* 2003;18:252–257.
10. Huang Z, Gao D, Letteri JJ, et al. Blood-membrane interactions during dialysis. *Semin Dial* 2009;22:623–628.
11. Depner TA, Greene T, Daugirdas JT, et al. Dialyzer performance in the HEMO study: in vivo K0A and true blood flow determined from a model of cross-dialyzer urea extraction. *ASAIO J* 2004;50:85–93.
12. National Kidney Foundation. *A Clinical Update on Dialyzer Membranes: State-of-the-Art Considerations for Optimal Care in Hemodialysis.* Basel, Switzerland: Karger, 2013.
13. Buur T, Lundberg M. Secondary effects of erythropoietin treatment on metabolism and dialysis efficiency in stable hemodialysis patients. *Clin Nephrol* 1990;34:230–235.
14. Paganini EP, Latham D, Abdulhadi M. Practical considerations of recombinant human erythropoietin therapy. *Am J Kidney Dis* 1989;14:19–25.
15. Mineshima M. The past, present and future of the dialyzer. *Contrib Nephrol* 2015;185:8–14.
16. Clark WR, Hamburger RJ, Lysaght MJ. Effect of membrane composition and structure on solute removal and biocompatibility in hemodialysis. *Kidney Int* 1999;56:2005–2015.
17. Eknoyan G, Beck GJ, Cheung AK, et al. Effect of dialysis dose and membrane flux in maintenance hemodialysis. *N Engl J Med* 2002;347:2010–2019.
18. Ronco C, Feriani M, Chiaramonte S, et al. Backfiltration in clinical dialysis. Nature of the phenomenon and possible solutions. *Contrib Nephrol* 1990;77:96–105.
19. Schiffl H. High-flux dialyzers, backfiltration, and dialysis fluid quality. *Semin Dial* 2011;24:1–4.
20. Fiore GB, Ronco C. Principles and practice of internal hemodiafiltration. *Contrib Nephrol* 2007;158:177–184.
21. Lucchi L, Fiore GB, Guadagni G, et al. Clinical evaluation of internal hemodiafiltration (iHDF): a diffusive-convective technique performed with internal filtration enhanced high-flux dialyzers. *Int J Artif Organs* 2004;27:414–419.
22. Sakiyama R, Ishimori I, Akiba T, et al. Effect of blood flow rate on internal filtration in a high-flux dialyzer with polysulfone membrane. *J Artif Organs* 2012;15:266–271.
23. Schneditz D, Zierler E, Jantscher A, et al. Internal filtration in a high-flux dialyzer quantified by mean transit time of an albumin-bound indicator. *ASAIO J* 1992;59:505–511.
24. Klemm D, Heublein B, Fink HP, et al. Cellulose: fascinating biopolymer and sustainable raw material. *Angew Chem Int Ed Engl* 2005;44:3358–3393.
25. Ward RA. Do clinical outcomes in chronic hemodialysis depend on the choice of a dialyzer? *Semin Dial* 2011;24:65–71.
26. Macleod AM, Campbell M, Cody JD, et al. Cellulose, modified cellulose and synthetic membranes in the haemodialysis of patients with end-stage renal disease. *Cochrane Database Syst Rev* 2005;(3):CD003234.
27. Vienken J, Diamantoglou M, Henne W, et al. Artificial dialysis membranes: from concept to large scale production. *Am J Nephrol* 1999;19:355–362.
28. Eggerth AH. The preparation and standardization of collodion membranes. *J Biol Chem* 1921;48:203–221.
29. Abel JJ, Rowntree LG, Turner BB. On the removal of diffusable substances from the circulating blood by means of dialysis. Transactions of the Association of American Physicians, 1913. *Transfus Sci* 1990;11:164–165.
30. Benedum J. Pioneer of dialysis, George Haas (1886-1971). *Med Hist* 1979;14:196–217.
31. Haas G. Versuche der Blutauswaschung am Lebenden mit Hilfe der Dialyse [in German]. *Klin Wochenschr* 1925;4:13–14.
32. National Center for Biotechnology Information, U.S. National Library of Medicine. *Cellulose Triacetate.* Bethesda, MD: National Center for Biotechnology Information, U.S. National Library of Medicine, 2009.
33. Falkenhagen D, Bosch T, Brown GS, et al. A clinical study on different cellulosic dialysis membranes. *Nephrol Dial Transplant* 1987;2:537–545.
34. Katopodis KP, Chala A, Koliousi E, et al. Role of the dialyzer membrane on the overall phosphate kinetics during hemodialysis. *Blood Purif* 2005;23:359–364.
35. Thomas M, Moriyama K, Ledebo I. AN69: evolution of the world's first high permeability membrane. *Contrib Nephrol* 2011;173:119–129.
36. Bowry SK, Gatti E, Vienken J. Contribution of polysulfone membranes to the success of convective dialysis therapies. *Contrib Nephrol* 2011;173:110–118.
37. U.S. Food and Drug Administration. *Guidance for Industry and CDRH Reviewers. Guidance for the Content of Premarket Notifications for Conventional and High Permeability Hemodialyzers.* Silver Spring, MD: U.S. Food and Drug Administration, 1998.
38. Gondouin B, Hutchison CA. High cut-off dialysis membranes: current uses and future potential. *Adv Chronic Kidney Dis* 2011;18:180–187.
39. Hutchison CA, Cockwell P, Reid S, et al. Efficient removal of immunoglobulin free light chains by hemodialysis for multiple myeloma: in vitro and in vivo studies. *J Am Soc Nephrol* 2007;18:886–895.
40. Saito A. Definition of high-performance membranes—from the clinical point of view. *Contrib Nephrol* 2011;173:1–10.
41. Saito A, Kawanishi H, Yamashita AC, et al. *High-Performance Membrane Dialyzers.* Basel, Switzerland: Karger, 2011.
42. Niwa T. Update of uremic toxin research by mass spectrometry. *Mass Spectrom Rev* 2011;30:510–521.
43. Tsuchida K, Minakuchi J. Albumin loss under the use of the high-performance membrane. *Contrib Nephrol* 2011;173:76–83.

44. Degoulet P, Reach I, Rozenbaum W, et al. Society of Nephrology, Computer Technology Commission. Dialysis computer program. VI.—survival and risk factors. *J Urol Nephrol* 1979;85:909–962.
45. Lynch RE, Bosl RH, Streifel AJ, et al. Dialysis thrombocytopenia: parallel plate vs hollow fiber dialyzers. *Trans Am Soc Artif Intern Organs* 1978;24:704–708.
46. Miranda VM, Miranda RM, Guerra L, et al. The influence of the geometry of the dialyzer and the composition of the dialysate in activating the complement system. *Nephron* 1990;54:26–31.
47. Lins LE, Boberg U, Jacobson SH, et al. The influence of dialyzer geometry on blood coagulation and biocompatibility. *Clin Nephrol* 1993;40:281–285.
48. Nilsson B, Ekdahl KN, Mollnes TE, et al. The role of complement in biomaterial-induced inflammation. *Mol Immunol* 2007;44:82–94.
49. Uda S, Mizobuchi M, Akizawa T. Biocompatible characteristics of high-performance membranes. *Contrib Nephrol* 2011;173:23–29.
50. Amadori A, Candi P, Sasdelli M, et al. Hemodialysis leukopenia and complement function with different dialyzers. *Kidney Int* 1983;24:775–781.
51. Chenoweth DE. Complement activation in extracorporeal circuits. *Ann N Y Acad Sci* 1987;516:306–313.
52. Ivanovich P, Chenoweth DE, Schmidt R, et al. Symptoms and activation of granulocytes and complement with two dialysis membranes. *Kidney Int* 1983;24:758–763.
53. Cheung AK. Biocompatibility of hemodialysis membranes. *J Am Soc Nephrol* 1990;1:150–161.
54. Bellucci A. Shortness of breath and abdominal pain within minutes of starting hemodialysis. *Semin Dial* 2004;17:417–421.
55. Bommer J, Ritz E. Ethylene oxide (ETO) as a major cause of anaphylactoid reactions in dialysis (a review). *Artif Organs* 1987;11:111–117.
56. Masin G, Polenaković M, Ivanovski N, et al. Hypersensitivity reactions to ethylene oxide: clinical experience. *Nephrol Dial Transplant* 1991;6(Suppl 3):50–52.
57. Pearson F, Bruszer G, Lee W, et al. Ethylene oxide sensitivity in hemodialysis patients. *Artif Organs* 1987;11:100–103.
58. Maurice F, Rivory JP, Larsson PH, et al. Anaphylactic shock caused by formaldehyde in a patient undergoing long-term hemodialysis. *J Allergy Clin Immunol* 1986;77:594–597.
59. Altmann P, Dodd S, Williams A, et al. Silicone-induced hypercalcaemia in haemodialysis patients. *Nephrol Dial Transplant* 1987;2:26–29.
60. Bommer J, Ritz E. Spallation of dialysis materials—problems and perspectives. *Nephron* 1985;39:285–289.
61. Mukaya JE, Jacobson MS, Esprit D, et al. Allergic reaction to polysulphone membrane dialyser masquerading as infection. *BMJ Case Rep* 2015:2015.
62. Schaefer RM, Schaefer L, Hörl WH. Anaphylactoid reactions during hemodialysis. *Clin Nephrol* 1994;42(Suppl 1):S44–S47.
63. Cerqueira A, Martins PA, Carvalho BA, et al. AN69-ST membrane, a useful option in two cases of severe dialysis reactions. *Clin Nephrol* 2015;53:100–103.
64. Chiappini MG, Ammann T, Selvaggi G, et al. Effects of different dialysis membranes and techniques on the nutritional status, morbidity and mortality of hemodialysis patients. *G Ital Nefrol* 2004;21(Suppl 30):S190–S196.
65. van Ypersele de Strihou C, Jadoul M, Malghem J, et al. Effect of dialysis membrane and patient's age on signs of dialysis-related amyloidosis. The Working Party on Dialysis Amyloidosis. *Kidney Int* 1991;39:1012–1019.
66. Ayli M, Ayli D, Azak A, et al. The effect of high-flux hemodialysis on dialysis-associated amyloidosis. *Ren Fail* 2005;27:31–34.
67. Koda Y, Nishi S, Miyazaki S, et al. Switch from conventional to high-flux membrane reduces the risk of carpal tunnel syndrome and mortality of hemodialysis patients. *Kidney Int* 1997;52:1096–1101.
68. Küchle C, Fricke H, Held E, et al. High-flux hemodialysis postpones clinical manifestation of dialysis-related amyloidosis. *Am J Nephrol* 1996;16:484–488.
69. Locatelli F, Marcelli D, Conte F, et al. Comparison of mortality in ESRD patients on convective and diffusive extracorporeal treatments. The Registro Lombardo Dialisi E Trapianto. *Kidney Int* 1999;55:286–293.
70. Masakane I. High-quality dialysis: a lesson from the Japanese experience: effects of membrane material on nutritional status and dialysis-related symptoms. *NDT Plus* 2010;3:i28–i35.
71. Block GA, Hulbert-Shearon TE, Levin NW, et al. Association of serum phosphorus and calcium x phosphate product with mortality risk in chronic hemodialysis patients: a national study. *Am J Kidney Dis* 1998;31:607–617.
72. Cozzolino M, Messa P, Brancaccio D, et al. Achievement of NKF/K-DOQI recommended target values for bone and mineral metabolism in incident hemodialysis patients: results of the FARO-2 cohort. *Blood Purif* 2014;38:37–45.
73. Ayli D, Ayli M, Azak A, et al. The effect of high-flux hemodialysis on renal anemia. *J Nephrol* 2004;17:701–706.
74. Francisco RC, Aloha M, Ramón PS. Effects of high-efficiency postdilution online hemodiafiltration and high-flux hemodialysis on serum phosphorus and cardiac structure and function in patients with end-stage renal disease. *Int Urol Nephrol* 2013;45:1373–1378.
75. Lornoy W, De Meester J, Becaus I, et al. Impact of convective flow on phosphorus removal in maintenance hemodialysis patients. *J Ren Nutr* 2006;16:47–53.
76. Minutolo R, Bellizzi V, Cioffi M, et al. Postdialytic rebound of serum phosphorus: pathogenetic and clinical insights. *J Am Soc Nephrol* 2002;13:1046–1054.
77. Tuccillo S, Bellizzi V, Catapano F, et al. Acute and chronic effects of standard hemodialysis and soft hemodiafiltration on interdialytic serum phosphate levels. *G Ital Nefrol* 2002;19:439–445.
78. Badve SV, Beller EM, Cass A, et al. Interventions for erythropoietin-resistant anaemia in dialysis patients. *Cochrane Database Syst Rev* 2013;(8):CD006861.
79. Cheung AK, Levin NW, Greene T, et al. Effects of high-flux hemodialysis on clinical outcomes: results of the HEMO study. *J Am Soc Nephrol* 2003;14:3251–3263.
80. Locatelli F, Martin-Malo A, Hannedouche T, et al. Effect of membrane permeability on survival of hemodialysis patients. *J Am Soc Nephrol* 2009;20:645–654.
81. Palmer SC, Rabindranath KS, Craig JC, et al. High-flux versus low-flux membranes for end-stage kidney disease. *Cochrane Database Syst Rev* 2012;(9):CD005016.
82. Vilar E, Fry AC, Wellsted D, et al. Long-term outcomes in online hemodiafiltration and high-flux hemodialysis: a comparative analysis. *Clin J Am Soc Nephrol* 2009;4:1944–1953.
83. Maduell F, Moreso F, Pons M, et al. High-efficiency postdilution online hemodiafiltration reduces all-cause mortality in hemodialysis patients. *J Am Soc Nephrol* 2013;24:487–497.
84. Ok E, Asci G, Toz H, et al. Mortality and cardiovascular events in online haemodiafiltration (OL-HDF) compared with high-flux dialysis: results from the Turkish OL-HDF Study. *Nephrol Dial Transplant* 2013;28:192–202.
85. Bellien J, Fréguin-Bouilland C, Joannidès R, et al. High-efficiency online haemodiafiltration improves conduit artery endothelial function compared with high-flux haemodialysis in end-stage renal disease patients. *Nephrol Dial Transplant* 2014;29:414–422.
86. Tattersall J, Martin-Malo A, Pedrini L, et al. EBPG guideline on dialysis strategies. *Nephrol Dial Transplant* 2007;22:ii5–ii21.
87. Hartmann J, Fricke H, Schiffl H. Biocompatible membranes preserve residual renal function in patients undergoing regular hemodialysis. *Am J Kidney Dis* 1997;30:366–373.
88. Hakim RM, Wingard RL, Husni L, et al. The effect of membrane biocompatibility on plasma beta 2-microglobulin levels in chronic hemodialysis patients. *J Am Soc Nephrol* 1996;7:472–478.
89. Richardson D, Lindley EJ, Bartlett C, et al. A randomized, controlled study of the consequences of hemodialysis membrane composition on erythropoietic response. *Am J Kidney Dis* 2003;42:551–560.
90. Parker TF III, Wingard RL, Husni L, et al. Effect of the membrane biocompatibility on nutritional parameters in chronic hemodialysis patients. *Kidney Int* 1996;49:551–556.
91. Tayeb JS, Provenzano R, El-Ghoroury M, et al. Effect of biocompatibility of hemodialysis membranes on serum albumin levels. *Am J Kidney Dis* 2000;35:606–610.

92. Kalantar-Zadeh K, Kopple JD, Block G, et al. A malnutrition-inflammation score is correlated with morbidity and mortality in maintenance hemodialysis patients. *Am J Kidney Dis* 2001;38:1251–1263.

93. Kopple JD, Zhu X, Lew NL, et al. Body weight-for-height relationships predict mortality in maintenance hemodialysis patients. *Kidney Int* 1999;56:1136–1148.

94. Port FK, Ashby VB, Dhingra RK, et al. Dialysis dose and body mass index are strongly associated with survival in hemodialysis patients. *J Am Soc Nephrol* 2002;13:1061–1066.

95. Panagiotou A, Nalesso F, Zanella M, et al. Antioxidant dialytic approach with vitamin E-coated membranes. *Contrib Nephrol* 2011;171:101–106.

96. Bargnoux AS, Cristol JP, Jaussent I, et al. Vitamin E-coated polysulfone membrane improved red blood cell antioxidant status in hemodialysis patients. *J Nephrol* 2013;26:556–563.

97. Yang CC, Hsu SP, Wu MS, et al. Effects of vitamin C infusion and vitamin E-coated membrane on hemodialysis-induced oxidative stress. *Kidney Int* 2006;69:706–714.

98. Morimoto H, Nakao K, Fukuoka K, et al. Long-term use of vitamin E-coated polysulfone membrane reduces oxidative stress markers in haemodialysis patients. *Nephrol Dial Transplant* 2005;20:2775–2782.

99. Sanaka T, Mochizuki T, Kinugasa E, et al. Randomized controlled open-label trial of vitamin E-bonded polysulfone dialyzer and erythropoiesis-stimulating agent response. *Clin J Am Soc Nephrol* 2013;8:969–978.

100. Huang J, Yi B, Li AM, et al. Effects of vitamin E-coated dialysis membranes on anemia, nutrition and dyslipidemia status in hemodialysis patients: a meta-analysis. *Ren Fail* 2015;37:398–407.

101. Laville M, Dorval M, Fort Ros J, et al. Results of the HepZero study comparing heparin-grafted membrane and standard care show that heparin-grafted dialyzer is safe and easy to use for heparin-free dialysis. *Kidney Int* 2014;86:1260–1267.

102. Meijers BK, Poesen R, Evenepoel P. Heparin-coated dialyzer membranes: is non-inferiority good enough? *Kidney Int* 2014;86:1084–1086.

103. Takesawa S, Ohmi S, Konno Y, et al. Varying methods of sterilisation, and their effects on the structure and permeability of dialysis membranes. *Nephrol Dial Transplant* 1987;1:254–257.

104. Müller TF, Seitz M, Eckle I, et al. Biocompatibility differences with respect to the dialyzer sterilization method. *Nephron* 1998;78:139–142.

105. Yamashita AC, Fujita R, Hosoi N. Effect of sterilization on solute transport performances of super high-flux dialyzers. *Hemodial Int* 2012;16(Suppl 14):S10–S14.

106. Kiaii M, Djurdjev O, Farah M, et al. Use of electron-beam sterilized hemodialysis membranes and risk of thrombocytopenia. *JAMA* 2011;306:1679–1687.

107. Golli-Bennour EE, Kouidhi B, Dey M, et al. Cytotoxic effects exerted by polyarylsulfone dialyser membranes depend on different sterilization processes. *Int Urol Nephrol* 2011;43:483–490.

108. Denny GB, Golper TA. Does hemodialyzer reuse have a place in current ESRD care: "to be or not to be?" *Semin Dial* 2014;27:256–258.

109. Robinson BM, Feldman HI. Dialyzer reuse and patient outcomes: what do we know now? *Semin Dial* 2005;18:175–179.

110. Upadhyay A, Sosa MA, Jaber BL. Single-use versus reusable dialyzers: the known unknowns. *Clin J Am Soc Nephrol* 2007;2:1079–1086.

111. Chenoweth DE, Cheung AK, Ward DM, et al. Anaphylatoxin formation during hemodialysis: comparison of new and re-used dialyzers. *Kidney Int* 1983;24:770–774.

112. Cheung AK, Parker CJ, Janatova J. Analysis of the complement C3 fragments associated with hemodialysis membranes. *Kidney Int* 1989;35:576–588.

113. Galvao TF, Silva MT, Araujo ME, et al. Dialyzer reuse and mortality risk in patients with end-stage renal disease: a systematic review. *Am J Nephrol* 2012;35:249–258.

114. Oyong K, Marquez P, Terashita D, et al. Outbreak of bloodstream infections associated with multiuse dialyzers containing O-rings. *Infect Control Hosp Epidemiol* 2014;35:89–91.

115. Hoenich NA, Levin R, Pearce C. Clinical waste generation from renal units: implications and solutions. *Semin Dial* 2005;18:396–400.

CHAPTER 2

Dialysate Composition in Hemodialysis and Peritoneal Dialysis

Peter Noel Van Buren and Biff F. Palmer

Patients with end-stage kidney disease (ESKD) depend on dialysis to maintain fluid and electrolyte balance. In both hemodialysis and peritoneal dialysis, solutes diffuse between blood and dialysate such that, over the course of the procedure, plasma composition is restored toward normal values. The makeup of the dialysate is of paramount importance in accomplishing this goal. This chapter reviews recent developments on how the dialysate can be manipulated to improve patient tolerance and outcome. Individualizing the dialysate composition is likely to gain increasing importance given the advancing age and increasing number of comorbid conditions found in ESKD patients.

DIALYSATE COMPOSITION IN HEMODIALYSIS

In most outpatient settings, patients receive hemodialysis using dialysate prepared in bulk and delivered via a central delivery system so that the composition of the dialysate is the same for all patients. Although most patients tolerate the procedure when administered in this fashion, many patients suffer from hemodynamic instability or symptoms of dialysis disequilibrium. One strategy to improve the clinical tolerance to dialysis is to adjust the dialysate composition according to the individual characteristics of the patient.

Dialysate Sodium

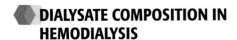

As dialysis has evolved, there has been continued interest in adjusting the dialysate sodium (Na) concentration in an attempt to improve the tolerability of the procedure. In the early days of dialysis, fluid removal was accomplished by a process of osmotic ultrafiltration. High concentrations of glucose were placed in the dialysate in order to create an osmotic driving force for fluid removal, as the coil

dialyzers utilized at the time were unable to withstand high transmembrane hydrostatic pressures. In order to prevent the development of hypernatremia as water moved from plasma to dialysate, the Na concentration in dialysate was purposely set low, usually in the range of 125 to 130 mEq/L. With the development of more resilient membranes capable of withstanding high transmembrane pressures, osmotic ultrafiltration was replaced by hydrostatic ultrafiltration. Initially, a low dialysate Na concentration continued to be used in order to avoid the problems of chronic volume overload such as hypertension and heart failure. With the institution of shorter treatment times, volume removal became more rapid and symptomatic hypotension emerged as a common and often disabling problem during dialysis. It soon became apparent that changes in the serum Na concentration, and more specifically changes in serum osmolality, were playing a role in the development of this hemodynamic instability. Subsequent studies demonstrated that raising dialysate Na to between 139 and 144 mEq/L was associated with improved hemodynamic stability and general tolerance to the procedure (1,2).

The importance of a stable plasma osmolality in maintaining hemodynamic stability was first suggested when the hemodynamic profiles of ultrafiltration were compared to diffusional solute clearance. Ultrafiltration alone (the removal of iso-osmolar fluid by exerting a transmembrane pressure across the dialyzer) decreases cardiac output primarily due to a reduction in the stroke volume but is accompanied by an increase in peripheral vascular resistance such that arterial pressure is maintained. By contrast, diffusional dialysis results in a fall in arterial pressure while peripheral vascular resistance remains the same. With conventional dialysis (ultrafiltration and dialysis), less volume removal can be achieved before hypotension occurs as compared to ultrafiltration alone. The primary and characteristic difference between these two processes with respect to plasma osmolality is that plasma osmolality remains relatively constant during ultrafiltration but declines during dialysis due to the rapid intradialytic fall in plasma urea.

The decline in plasma osmolality during regular hemodialysis favors a fluid shift from the extracellular space to the intracellular space, thereby exacerbating the volume-depleting effects of dialysis. In animal studies, both conventional dialysis and sequential ultrafiltration dialysis result in an ultrafiltrate volume which is less than the decrease in extracellular fluid volume consistent with a shift of fluid into the intracellular compartment (3). In addition, during sequential ultrafiltration hemodialysis, this shift only occurs during the diffusive phase. With the advent of high clearance dialyzers and more efficient dialysis techniques, this decline in plasma osmolality becomes more apparent as solute is more rapidly removed.

Use of a low dialysate sodium concentration would tend to further augment the intracellular shift of fluid, as plasma tends to become even more hyposmolar consequent to the movement of sodium from plasma to dialysate. Older studies that employed maneuvers designed to minimize the decline in plasma osmolality such as infusing hypertonic mannitol, placement of high concentrations of dextrose in the dialysate, or placement of glycerol in the dialysate found that hemodynamic stability became comparable to that seen with ultrafiltration. While maneuvers to minimize the decline in plasma osmolarity using mannitol or glycerol can optimize hemodynamic stability during hemodialysis (4,5), the main and, perhaps the most physiologic, approach adopted to reduce the extent of change in the osmolality of body fluids during dialysis has been to increase the sodium concentration of the dialysate. Indeed, numerous investigators have now demonstrated that hemodynamic tolerance to dialysis is improved when the dialysate sodium concentration is increased to at least 135 mEq/L.

The mechanism by which raising the dialysate Na concentration improves hemodynamic stability is depicted in **Figure 2.1**. As discussed previously, a high dialysate Na concentration has been shown effective in maintaining a relatively constant plasma osmolality, thereby minimizing intracellular water movement during dialysis. In this regard, Van Stone et al. (6) measured changes in body water compartments as a function of low or high dialysate sodium concentrations in a group of dialysis patients in which 2-kg volumes were removed. With a low dialysate sodium (7% lower than serum sodium concentration), there was a dramatic decrease in extracellular water and a 21% decline in plasma volume while intracellular water increased. Use of a high dialysate sodium (7% greater than the serum sodium concentration) resulted in proportional decreases in intra- and extracellular water, and plasma volume only fell by 13%. By preventing a decrease in plasma osmolality, the higher sodium dialysate leads to mobilization of fluid from the intracellular space, resulting in better preservation of plasma volume. These findings have been confirmed by more recent studies utilizing bioimpedance measurements to study changes in body fluid compartments (7). As the dialysate-to-plasma Na gradient increases, there is a greater contraction of the intracellular fluid compartment. The shift of fluid into the extracellular fluid space increases the hydrostatic pressure of the interstitium, thus increasing the capacity for vascular refilling during volume removal resulting in a reduced frequency of hypotension and cramps.

A high Na dialysate may also more favorably influence compensatory mechanisms involved in maintaining peripheral vascular resistance during volume reduction. Decreased plasma osmolality has been associated with impaired peripheral vasoconstriction during volume removal possibly due to an inhibitory effect of hyposmolality on afferent sensing mechanisms. This effect would compound the tendency toward hemodynamic instability, as many

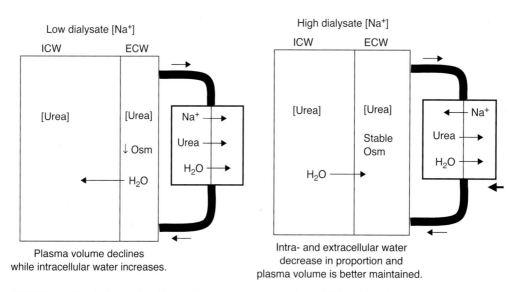

FIGURE 2.1 Use of a low sodium dialysate is more commonly associated with intradialytic hypotension. In the initial period of dialysis, the extracellular urea concentration falls, creating an osmotic driving force for water movement into the cell due to the higher intracellular urea concentration. This drop in extracellular osmolality and movement of water into the intracellular space is exacerbated in the setting of a low dialysate Na concentration. As a result, plasma volume falls and the risk of hypotension increases. A high sodium dialysate helps to minimize the development of extracellular hyposmolality allowing for better refilling of the intravascular compartment. Plasma volume remains better preserved and the risk of hypotension is reduced. ICW, intracellular weight; ECW, extracellular weight.

chronic dialysis patients have baseline abnormalities in autonomic function. In addition, central nervous system abnormalities due to cellular swelling are more likely to result during low osmolality dialysis, potentially further impairing autonomic function. A low Na dialysis solution has also been shown to increase prostaglandin E_2 levels. This prostaglandin has venodilatory properties that could lead to venous pooling, thus contributing to hemodynamic instability (8).

The primary concern with use of a higher dialysate Na concentration is the potential to stimulate thirst and cause increased weight gain and poor blood pressure control in the interdialytic period. Studies addressing this issue confirmed that a higher dialysate Na modestly increased interdialytic weight gain. However, this excess weight was found to be readily removed with improved tolerance to ultrafiltration (1).

More recently, there has been interest in varying the concentration of Na in the dialysate during the procedure to minimize the potential complications of a high Na solution while retaining the beneficial hemodynamic effects. A high dialysate Na concentration is used initially with a progressive reduction toward isotonic or hypotonic levels by the end of the procedure. This method allows for a diffusive Na influx early in the session to prevent the rapid decline in plasma osmolality resulting from the efflux of urea and other small molecular weight solutes. During the remainder of the procedure, when the reduction in osmolality accompanying urea removal is less abrupt, the lower dialysate Na level minimizes the development of hypertonicity and any resultant excessive thirst, fluid gain, and hypertension in the interdialytic period.

Several studies have compared the hemodynamic and symptomatic effects of a dialysate in which the Na concentration is varied during the procedure to that in which the Na concentration is fixed. Dumler et al. (9) used a dialysate Na of 150 mEq/L during the initial 3 hours of dialysis at the time of ultrafiltration; the dialysate Na was decreased to 130 mEq/L for the last hour. The control group was dialyzed against Na concentration fixed at 140 mEq/L. Use of the high/low Na hemodialysis was associated with a smaller decline in systolic pressure as well as fewer symptomatic hypotensive episodes.

Other investigators have varied dialysate Na according to a Na gradient protocol in which the Na is set to decrease from a high to a low level over the course of a dialysis session. Raja et al. (10) and Daugirdas et al. (11) found no measurable benefit. Acchiardo and Hayden (12) found a reduction in hypotensive episodes, and Sadowski et al. (13) had similar results in young patients. The linear and step Na modeling programs have been found to be better in lowering the risk of intradialytic headache as compared with the exponential program. The linear program was the only individual program that alleviated interdialytic cramps; the most striking reduction in the risk for posttreatment hypotension occurred with the step program.

Differences in the incidence of symptomatic hypotension during dialysis or in the degree of interdialytic weight gain between the fixed or variable Na protocols have been difficult to demonstrate. Levin and Goldstein (14) studied a group of patients who were specifically selected because of the frequent occurrence of symptoms on dialysis such as headaches, cramps, and light-headedness. In a crossover trial, these patients were assigned either to a fixed Na dialysate and a constant rate of ultrafiltration or to a gradient protocol in which the initial Na concentration and ramping pattern were individually adjusted to minimize thirst. Use of the patient-specific Na gradient profiles was associated with improvement in all patients with headache and in 70% of patients with light-headedness.

Most patients reported an increase in thirst, but there were no differences in interdialytic weight gain or in predialysis and postdialysis mean arterial pressure. Using a more general dialysis population, Sang et al. (15) compared a linear or step Na gradient (155 to 140 mEq/L) protocol with a fixed Na dialysate (140 mEq/L). In this study, Na modeling was associated with a significant reduction in cramps and symptomatic hypotension. However, these benefits were followed by increasing thirst, fatigue, and weight gain between dialysis sessions as well as a higher predialysis blood pressure. The authors concluded that only 22% of patients had a significant benefit from the modeling programs. Finally, a study by Movilli et al. (16) found improved blood volume preservation by using a pattern of high to low Na change (160 to 133 mEq/L); the changes in blood pressure were similar between this high to low variation and conventional dialysis.

In summary, the available data suggest that in most chronic dialysis patients, changing the dialysate Na during the course of the treatment offers little advantage over a constant dialysate Na of between 140 and 145 mEq/L. The inability to clearly demonstrate a superiority of Na modeling may be due to the fact that the time-averaged concentration of Na was similar in many of the comparative studies. For example, a linear decline in dialysate Na from 150 to 140 mEq/L will produce approximately the same postdialysis serum Na as occurs when a dialysate Na of 145 mEq/L is used throughout the procedure. In addition, the optimal time-averaged Na concentration whether administered in a modeling protocol or with a fixed dialysate concentration is likely to vary from patient to patient as well as in the same patient during different treatment times (17). This variability is supported by studies demonstrating wide differences in the month-to-month predialysis Na concentration in otherwise stable dialysis patients (18).

Nevertheless, in selected patients, Na modeling may be of benefit (**TABLE 2.1**). Patients initiating dialysis with marked azotemia are often deliberately dialyzed to decrease the urea concentration slowly over the course of several days to avoid the development of the dialysis disequilibrium syndrome. The use of a high/low Na dialysate in these patients may minimize fluid shifts into the intracellular compartment and decrease the tendency for neurologic complications. Na modeling may also be beneficial in patients suffering frequent intradialytic hypotension, cramping, nausea, vomiting, fatigue, or headache. In such patients, the modeling protocol can be individually tailored to minimize increased thirst, weight gain, and hypertension. Combining dialysate Na profiling with a varying rate of ultrafiltration may provide additional benefit in particularly

TABLE 2.1	**Indications and Contraindications for Use of Na Modeling (High/Low Programs)**

A. Indications
- Intradialytic hypotension
- Cramping
- Initiation of hemodialysis in setting of severe azotemia
- Hemodynamically unstable patient (as in intensive care unit setting)

B. Contraindications
- Intradialytic development of hypertension
- Large interdialytic weight gain induced by high Na dialysate
- Hypernatremia

symptomatic patients (19). Use of this combined approach may be of particular benefit in ensuring hemodynamic stability in patients with acute kidney injury in the intensive care unit (20).

When prescribing a Na gradient protocol, it is important to monitor the patient for evidence of a progressive increase in total body Na. In some patients, a high/low Na protocol can lead to large interdialytic weight gain or cause intradialytic hypertension (**TABLE 2.1**). Such adverse effects are more likely to occur when the time-averaged Na concentration is greater than the patient's predialysis serum Na concentration (21). In this setting, use of a low dialysate Na during the terminal phase of the procedure does not guarantee negative Na balance. In hypertensive patients, adjusting the protocol to achieve negative Na balance may be of therapeutic benefit in the long-term control of blood pressure. In this regard, Flanigan et al. (22) recently compared a fixed dialysate Na of 140 mEq/L to a gradient protocol in which the dialysate Na was lowered in an exponential fashion from 155 to 135 mEq/L and then held constant at 135 mEq/L for the final half hour of the procedure. Ultrafiltration was discontinued during the final half hour of the session. Use of the variable Na dialysate permitted a 50% reduction in the dose of antihypertensive medications without significant changes in predialysis blood pressure or interdialytic weight gain. Although not specifically measured, use of the terminal low Na period may have caused a decrease in the total body exchangeable Na, thus accounting for improved blood pressure control in Na-sensitive patients. A recent report from a single dialysis facility also described a beneficial effect on blood pressure when the dialysate Na was simply lowered from a set value of 141 to 138 mmol/L (23). As in the study by Flanigan et al. (22), this effect occurred in the absence of a change in interdialytic weight again consistent with a volume independent effect.

Profiled hemodialysis is a recent attempt to make the dialysate Na even more patient specific. This technique is based on a mathematical model in which baseline patient characteristics are used to construct a patient-specific Na profile dialysate before each treatment. Initial experience with this procedure has shown improved cardiovascular hemodynamics when compared with a fixed dialysate Na concentration despite the same total mass of Na being removed (24).

In dialysis patients, interdialytic Na and water loads vary from one patient to another and from treatment to treatment. Water balance can be achieved by making total ultrafiltrate volume equal to interdialytic weight gain. Current research is focusing on ways in which the dialysate Na concentration can be adjusted to more accurately match intradialytic Na removal with interdialytic Na intake. The ability to achieve zero Na balance would enhance the ability to control hypertension in the interdialytic intervals and minimize the risk of hypotension during the dialysis procedure.

The ability of dialysis to accurately regulate fluid balance has become highly refined over the years (although choosing the target dry weight and reaching it are more problematic). A similar accuracy in the maintenance of Na balance requires that the dialysate Na concentration be individualized such that with each treatment, a constant end-session plasma Na concentration is reached. If over time end-dialysis weight and plasma Na concentration are kept constant (assuming no change in Na distribution volume), one can assume that the patient will be in Na balance. As currently practiced, the dialysate Na concentrations whether fixed or varied are not chosen with the primary aim of achieving Na balance. This approach risks a pathologic excess in the total Na mass, which over time can lead to clinical manifestations of volume overload such as hypertension or congestive heart failure.

To properly calculate the dialysate Na concentration required to maintain Na balance, measurement of the patient's plasma water Na concentration at the beginning of the treatment is required. Given the linear correlation between the conductivity of dialysate and its Na content, conductivity measurements can be used as a surrogate of Na concentration. Locatelli et al. (25,26) have recently described the use of a biofeedback system that allows for the automatic determination of plasma water and dialysate conductivity such that blood sampling can be avoided. With these measurements, along with session time, desired weight loss, and expected end-treatment plasma water conductivity, the dialysate conductivity is automatically adjusted to achieve the prescribed final plasma water conductivity. Application of this conductivity kinetic model to patients treated with a variant of hemodiafiltration has allowed for near zero hydro-sodium balance to be achieved. At the same time, cardiovascular stability was improved (25). Newer technologies capable of repetitive measurements of plasma water and dialysate conductivity will allow for the dialysate Na to be adjusted throughout the procedure (27).

With increased ability to individualize the dialysate Na concentration, one can envision a scenario in which a patient initiated on hemodialysis is initially treated with a dialysate Na concentration designed to achieve negative Na balance. Once the patient becomes normotensive or requires minimal amounts of antihypertensive medications, the dialysate Na can be adjusted on a continual basis to ensure that Na balance is maintained. However, a universal approach to prescribing the dialysate sodium relative to the serum remains controversial. Recent epidemiologic data show that, similar to the nondialysis population, lower serum sodium levels (measured predialysis) are associated with increased mortality (28). Despite the known effects on weight gain from high dialysate sodium, large dialysis cohort data show that use of a lower dialysate sodium is actually associated with further increase in mortality compared to higher dialysate sodium (29) among those patients with the lower tertile of serum sodium (<137 mEq/L). Identifying the appropriate dialysate sodium requires consideration of numerous factors including intradialytic symptoms and interdialytic habits. Achieving the optimal total body Na content will likely become just as important as determining an accurate dry weight.

Dialysate Potassium

In most chronic outpatient dialysis centers, there is little individualization of the dialysate potassium concentration. Rather, most patients are dialyzed with a potassium bath that is prepared centrally and delivered with a concentration fixed at 1 or 2 mEq/L. When using a fixed dialysate potassium, it is difficult to predict the exact amount of potassium that will be removed in a given dialysis session. Typically, one should not expect more than about 80 to 100 mEq of potassium removal even with the use of a potassium-free dialysate. In addition, there will be marked variability in the amount of potassium removed from patient to patient despite similar predialysis potassium levels and dialysis regimens. This variability can be explained by the fact that potassium movement from the intracellular to the extracellular space and ultimately into the dialysate is influenced by several patient-specific factors.

The removal of excess potassium by dialysis is achieved by the use of a dialysate with a potassium concentration lower than that of plasma creating a gradient favoring potassium removal; its rate is largely a function of this gradient. Plasma potassium concentration falls rapidly in the early stages of dialysis, but as the plasma concentration falls, potassium removal becomes less efficient. Because potassium is

TABLE 2.2	Factors Affecting Potassium Removal during Hemodialysis

A. Shifts K into cell thereby ↓ dialytic K removal
- Exogenous insulin
- Glucose containing dialysate versus glucose-free dialysate
- β-Agonists
- Correction of metabolic acidosis during dialysis

B. Shifts K to extracellular space or impairs cell K uptake thereby ↑ dialytic K removal
- β-Blockers
- α-Adrenergic receptor stimulation
- Hypertonicity

↓, decrease; ↑, increase.

freely permeable across the dialysis membrane, movement of potassium from the intracellular space to the extracellular space appears to be the limiting factor in potassium removal. Factors that importantly dictate the distribution of potassium between these two spaces include changes in acid–base status, tonicity, glucose and insulin concentration, and catecholamine activity (TABLE 2.2).

The movement of potassium between the intracellular and extracellular space is influenced by changes in acid–base balance that occur during the dialysis procedure (30). Extracellular alkalosis causes a shift of potassium into cells, whereas acidosis results in potassium efflux from cells. During a typical dialysis, there is net addition of base to the extracellular space, which promotes cellular uptake of potassium and therefore attenuates the removal of potassium during dialysis. The degree to which potassium shifts into the cell is directly correlated with the bicarbonate concentration of the dialysate (31). However, with routine dialysis, the change in blood pH is of small magnitude and the effect on potassium removal is not profound. By contrast, dialysis in patients who are acidotic will result in less potassium removal because potassium is shifted into cells as the serum bicarbonate rises. Wiegand et al. (32) described five patients in whom the serum potassium concentration decreased during dialysis even though the dialysate potassium concentration was higher than the original serum potassium concentration. The decline in potassium concentration occurred in association with a marked rise in the pH. In one patient, the decline in potassium concentration was of such a magnitude that she became quadriplegic and developed respiratory failure. There appears to be no difference in potassium removal whether acetate or bicarbonate is chosen as the dialysate buffer.

Insulin is known to stimulate the cellular uptake of potassium and can therefore influence the amount of potassium removal during dialysis. This effect of insulin was demonstrated in studies comparing potassium removal using glucose-containing and glucose-free dialysates (33). The use of a glucose-free dialysate was found to result in greater amounts of potassium removal when compared with the use of a glucose-containing bath. The use of a glucose-free dialysate would be expected to result in lower levels of insulin. However, another study showed little difference in intradialytic or postdialysis serum potassium levels between high and low glucose baths in diabetic and nondiabetic patients, suggesting that neither increased serum glucose (seen in both groups) or increased insulin (seen in nondiabetics) were sufficient to make a clinically significant change potassium removal (34).

Changes in plasma tonicity can affect the distribution of potassium between the intracellular and extracellular space. Administration of hypertonic saline or mannitol is sometimes used in the treatment of hypotension during dialysis. These agents would be expected to favor potassium removal during dialysis because the resultant increased tonicity would favor potassium movement into the extracellular space. There are no studies addressing whether there is any significant clinical benefit with this approach.

β-Adrenergic stimulation is known to shift potassium into cells and lower the extracellular concentration. Inhaled β stimulants have been reported to be effective in the acute treatment of hyperkalemia, so such therapy before dialysis may lower the total amount of potassium removed during the dialytic procedure. Allon and Shanklin (35) found that the cumulative dialytic potassium removal was significantly lower in patients who were treated with nebulized albuterol 30 minutes before the procedure as compared with patients in whom the albuterol treatment was omitted.

Alterations in serum potassium concentration during dialysis can conceivably have important effects on systemic hemodynamics. A decrease in serum potassium concentration during hemodialysis would be predicted to increase systemic vascular resistance. Hypokalemia has been shown to increase resistance in skeletal muscle, skin, and coronary vascular beds, possibly through effects on the electrogenic Na-K pump in the sarcolemmal membranes of vascular smooth muscle cells. In addition, decreased serum potassium concentration may enhance the sensitivity of the vasculature to endogenous pressor hormones (36).

Despite the potential for hypokalemia to increase systemic vascular resistance, Pogglitsch et al. (37) found the incidence of hypotensive episodes were, in fact, reduced when supplemental potassium was administered during the final 30 minutes of dialysis. One explanation for this seemingly paradoxical finding rests on the known interaction between hypokalemia and the autonomic nervous system. For example, hypokalemia has been found to be associated with dysautonomia in patients with hyperaldosteronism (38). It is reasonable to speculate that in patients with advanced kidney disease, who already have a propensity for autonomic insufficiency, a fall in plasma potassium may uncover or cause impairment in sympathetic responses (39).

In support of this suggestion, Henrich et al. (40) found that hypokalemic dialysis was accompanied by a fall in plasma catecholamine concentration as compared with dialysis in which serum potassium concentration was held constant. Moreover, despite similar reductions in blood pressure, the isokalemic dialysis group had a significant increase in heart rate after dialysis, whereas the hypokalemic group demonstrated no significant change. Further studies are needed to investigate the effects of fluctuations in serum potassium concentration during dialysis on the autonomic nervous system.

Changes in serum potassium concentration during dialysis may also influence systemic hemodynamics through effects on myocardial performance. Dialysis is associated with an increase in contractility, which can be attributed to an increase in ionized serum calcium. Increased ionized calcium is most closely related to improved ventricular contractility, but modifying effects of concomitant decreases in potassium may also be important. Haddy et al. (41) have demonstrated that the inotropic effect of increased serum calcium concentration is enhanced by simultaneous decreases in plasma potassium concentration. In this regard, Wizemann et al. (42) found that improvement in myocardial contractility during a series of isovolemic dialysis maneuvers was related to a simultaneous increase in plasma calcium and decrease in plasma potassium concentration. In the presence of an elevated plasma potassium concentration, a high plasma calcium concentration failed to exert a significant inotropic effect.

An increase in peripheral vascular resistance secondary to the development of hypokalemia could have potential detrimental effects on dialysis efficiency. This decrease in efficiency would result from decreased blood flow to urea-rich tissues such as skeletal muscle and in effect increase the amount of body wide recirculation. In support of this possibility, Dolson and Androgue (43) found that a dialysate potassium concentration of 1.0 mmol/L as compared with 3.0 mmol/L resulted in lower values for both the urea reduction ratio and Kt/V in 14 patients with ESKD. By contrast, Zehnder et al. (44) found no effect of dialysate potassium on dialysis adequacy. Although more studies are needed in this area, it is likely that any effect of a low dialysate potassium concentration to decrease dialysis adequacy is small in magnitude. In addition, increasing the dialysate potassium concentration to improve dialysis adequacy will increase the risk of hyperkalemia during the interdialytic period.

Most patients dialyzed with a fixed potassium dialysate tolerate the procedure well and do not suffer from complications of hypokalemia or hyperkalemia. Nevertheless, there are clinical conditions in which an individualized dialysate potassium concentration may be useful. Patients with underlying heart disease, particularly in the setting of digoxin therapy, are prone to arrhythmias, as hypokalemia develops toward the end of a typical treatment. Additionally, low dialysate potassium has been shown to unfavorably alter the QTc interval (a marker of risk of ventricular arrhythmias) (45).

Setting the dialysate potassium concentration to a higher value in any patient at risk for arrhythmias is not without risk. In an analysis of more than 80,000 maintenance hemodialysis patients, predialysis serum potassium values between 4.6 and 5.3 mEq/L were associated with the greatest survival, whereas values <4.0 or ≥5.6 mEq/L were associated with increased mortality. Use of a higher dialysate potassium concentration was associated with increased mortality in patients with predialysis potassium values ≥5.0 mEq/L (46). A separate case-control study found the use of a low potassium dialysate (<2.0 mEq/L) as an independent risk factor for the specific occurrence of in-center sudden cardiac arrest. Patients with cardiac arrest who were on low potassium dialysate were noted to have lower predialysis serum potassium than the control patients on low potassium dialysate (47). Altogether, when considering the risk for cardiac death or mortality, predialysis serum potassium should help guide the decision of the dialysate potassium with caution to avoid excessively high or low serum potassium levels. The use of variable dialysate potassium levels during a single treatment results in less QTc abnormalities compared to fixed levels, but it is uncertain if this would translate into overall better outcomes (48).

With these considerations in mind, Redaelli et al. (49) have studied the effects of modeling the dialysate potassium concentration in such a way as to minimize the initial rapid decline in the plasma potassium concentration (**FIGURE 2.2**). Patients with frequent intradialytic premature ventricular complexes were dialyzed using a dialysate with a fixed (2.5 mEq/L) potassium or one with an exponentially declining potassium (from 3.9 to 2.5 mEq/L), which maintained a constant blood to dialysate potassium gradient of 1.5 mEq/L throughout the procedure. In the fixed dialysate group, the blood to dialysate potassium gradient decreased over the

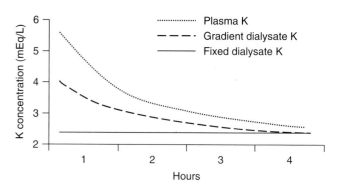

FIGURE 2.2 Hypothetical representation of the plasma-to-dialysate K gradient over time comparing a fixed versus a ramped K dialysate. The decline in the plasma K concentration is most rapid in the early stages of the hemodialysis procedure particularly when utilizing a fixed dialysate K. This more rapid decline is due to the initially large concentration gradient between the plasma and dialysate. The rapid decline can be attenuated by utilizing a ramped K dialysate, which acts to minimize the initial and thereafter maintain a constant plasma-to-dialysate K concentration gradient.

treatment from 3.0 to 1.4 mEq/L. The variable potassium dialysate decreased premature ventricular complexes, a finding most evident during the first hour of the procedure. The total drop in the serum potassium concentration was no different between the fixed and variable potassium dialysates.

In summary, because of kinetics of potassium movement from the intracellular to the extracellular space, one can expect only up to 70 to 90 mEq of potassium to be removed during a typical dialysis session. As a result, one should not overestimate the effectiveness of the dialytic procedure in the treatment of severe hyperkalemia. The total amount removed will exhibit considerable variability and will be influenced by changes in acid–base status, changes in tonicity, changes in glucose and insulin concentration, and catecholamine activity. Given the tendency for the plasma potassium to rise in the immediate postdialysis time period, the most efficient way to remove excess potassium stores would be to prescribe 2- to 3-hour periods of dialysis separated by several hours. Studies examining the hemodynamic effect of potassium fluxes during hemodialysis are limited. More importantly, deliberate alterations in dialysate potassium concentration to affect hemodynamic stability would not be without risk. Use of low potassium dialysate concentration may contribute to arrhythmias, especially in those patients with underlying coronary artery disease or those taking digoxin. On the other hand, use of dialysate with high potassium concentration may predispose patients to predialysis hyperkalemia. In patients who are at high risk for arrhythmias on dialysis, modeling the dialysate potassium concentration to maintain a constant blood to dialysate potassium gradient throughout the procedure may be of clinical benefit (**FIGURE 2.2**).

Dialysate Buffer

Acetate Buffer

The early use of bicarbonate as the base in dialysis solutions required a cumbersome system in which CO_2 was continuously bubbled through the dialysate to lower pH to prevent the precipitation of calcium and magnesium salts. As a result, in the early 1960s, acetate became the standard dialysate buffer used to correct uremic acidosis and to offset the diffusive losses of bicarbonate during hemodialysis. Over the next several years, reports began to accumulate linking routine use of acetate with cardiovascular instability and hypotension during dialysis. In particular, critically ill patients undergoing acute hemodialysis, especially with the use of large surface area dialyzers, were found to exhibit vascular instability when exposed to acetate in dialysis fluid. Given these observations, bicarbonate-containing dialysate began to reemerge as the principal dialysate buffer especially as advances in biotechnology made the use of bicarbonate dialysate less expensive and less cumbersome to use. Because acetate is still used as the principal dialysate buffer in some centers, the following paragraphs compare the clinical effects of acetate and bicarbonate dialysate.

During a routine dialysis in which acetate is used as the buffer, there are large fluxes of both acetate and bicarbonate across the dialyzer with little overall net gain in base. Because the acetate dialysate lacks bicarbonate, there is diffusion of actual bicarbonate from the blood into the dialysate. In addition, potential bicarbonate is lost from the blood in the form of organic anions such as citrate, lactate, pyruvate, β-hydroxy-butyrate, and acetoacetate because these anions diffuse across the dialyzer and into the dialysate (50). The pH of blood exiting the dialysis cartridge does not fall because CO_2 diffuses from the blood as well. Despite this large efflux of potential and actual bicarbonate from the body, there is a net gain of alkali because of the greater influx of acetate as it diffuses from the dialysate into the blood. Acetate is normally metabolized in muscle to acetyl coenzyme A (CoA). Acetyl CoA is then metabolized in the Krebs cycle to CO_2 and water with formation of one bicarbonate molecule for each molecule of acetate metabolized. The metabolism of acetate to carbon dioxide can contribute up to 40% of the total energy expenditure during dialysis (51). In addition, acetate-containing dialysate is associated with significant increases in the plasma concentration of ketone bodies. The accelerated ketogenesis and the extra caloric burden seen with acetate dialysate does not appear to be associated with an impairment in glucose utilization or change in plasma insulin during the procedure.

Chronic hemodialysis patients metabolize acetate at a reduced rate as compared with control patients (39). Decreased rates of metabolism of acetate to bicarbonate can potentially result in accumulation of acetate. This accumulation of acetate is magnified with use of dialyzers with large surface areas that allow for transfer of acetate to the plasma compartment at rates greater than a patient's ability to metabolize it. The consequent increase in blood concentration of acetate has been associated with nausea, vomiting, fatigue, and, more importantly, hemodynamic instability.

There are a number of mechanisms by which acetate might predispose to vascular instability (**TABLE 2.3**). Acetate, possibly by its

TABLE 2.3	**Mechanisms by which Acetate Buffer Contributes to Hemodynamic Instability**

- Directly decreases peripheral vascular resistance (in ~10% of patients)
- Stimulates release of the vasodilator compound, interleukin 1
- Induction of metabolic acidosis through bicarbonate loss through the dialyzer
- Associated with arterial hypoxemia and increases in oxygen consumption
- Possible myocardial effects of acetate

conversion to adenosine, has vasodilatory properties that can directly decrease peripheral vascular resistance. In addition, acetate might increase venous capacity leading to a decrease in cardiac filling (52). These vasodilatory effects of acetate are further augmented through the release of interleukin-1. Interleukin-1 has vasodilatory properties and its activity is increased from 8 to 12 times normal by standard acetate hemodialysis (53).

In addition to direct vasodilatory properties, incomplete acetate oxidation can lead to acid–base changes that can adversely affect hemodynamics. Metabolism of acetate to bicarbonate in an amount less than the diffusive losses of bicarbonate through the dialyzer will result in a decreased concentration of serum bicarbonate. A decrease in serum bicarbonate concentration can result in mild metabolic acidosis that may take 2 to 3 hours after dialysis to correct. Such loss of bicarbonate through the dialyzer contributes to vascular instability in addition to any direct vascular effects of acetate.

Arterial hypoxemia occurs with the use of acetate dialysate and may also contribute to vascular instability. During acetate dialysis, there is diffusive loss of soluble carbon dioxide from blood to dialysate. In an attempt to maintain normal blood carbon dioxide concentration, pulmonary hypoventilation occurs resulting in hypoxemia. In addition, metabolism of acetate leads to an increase in oxygen consumption further exacerbating any decrease in oxygenation. In susceptible individuals, acetate may provoke subendocardial ischemia by deleteriously affecting myocardial oxygen balance (54).

Despite the association of acetate with a higher frequency of symptoms in some studies, there is a poor correlation between symptoms and signs and blood acetate concentration. In an attempt to reconcile this discrepancy, Vinay et al. (55) studied a large population of dialysis patients and concluded that true acetate intolerance only occurred in about 10% of the dialysis population. The patients found intolerant were unable to metabolize acetate optimally and were predominately female. Because muscle is the primary site of metabolism of acetate, a reduced muscle mass often found in females might account for the reduced metabolism of acetate. Similarly, malnourished and elderly patients may be more predisposed to acetate intolerance by such a mechanism.

During conventional hemodialysis with acetate, the vasoconstrictive response to hypovolemia is masked by the vasodilatory tendency induced by the diffusive nature of the therapy. It is unclear, however, whether inability to vasoconstrict during conventional hemodialysis is related to use of acetate or rather a fall in serum osmolality. In this regard, several studies have found that vascular instability with acetate dialysis is generally improved with use of a higher Na dialysate concentration. In addition, substitution of bicarbonate for acetate as the base constituent in the dialysate has been purported to markedly improve symptoms on dialysis. It has been difficult to prove, however, whether bicarbonate dialysate can independently further improve hemodynamic and symptomatic tolerance to hemodialysis especially when a higher dialysate osmolality is used. Wehle et al. (56) found no added benefit of bicarbonate over acetate particularly if dialysate Na was increased to 145 mEq/L. Henrich et al. (57) in a comparative study of acetate and bicarbonate dialysis using a dialysate Na concentration of 140 mEq/L demonstrated strikingly similar hemodynamic responses. In a later study, Velez et al. (58) noted that with high Na dialysates (141 mEq/L), no detectable differences between bicarbonate and acetate were found with respect to cardiac output, mean blood pressure, or orthostatic tolerance to standing after dialysis. With use of a dialysate Na of 130 mEq/L, however, bicarbonate dialysate was associated with greater stability of blood pressure on standing after dialysis.

Controversy exists as to the overall effects of acetate and bicarbonate buffers on ventricular performance. Administration of sodium acetate as a bolus injection in dogs results in marked decreases in myocardial contractile force and blood pressure (59). However, if given as a continuous infusion, no definite depression of myocardial function is observed. Aizawa et al. (60) compared the effects of acetate and bicarbonate hemodialysis on cardiac function using phonocardiography. Left ventricular function was depressed to a greater extent with acetate than after bicarbonate dialysis.

The negative inotropic effect attributed to acetate has been contested by other reports in which sodium acetate was found to increase ventricular performance. Nitenberg et al. (61) using angiographic techniques studied left ventricular function in seven patients with plasma acetate concentrations comparable to that found during sodium acetate hemodialysis. An increase in cardiac index, ejection fraction, and maximum velocity of circumferential fiber (VCF) shortening not attributable to alterations in heart rate, preload, or afterload was demonstrated after sodium acetate infusion. Mansell et al. (62) noted that patients who developed hyperacetatemia during regular dialysis were still able to maintain an increased cardiac output. Schick et al. (63) studied nine patients in a double-blind, crossover manner and demonstrated improvement of left ventricular mean VCF of equal magnitude with both acetate and bicarbonate hemodialysis. Ruder et al. (64) performed a double-blind, crossover study of 36 patients comparing acetate and bicarbonate hemodialysis with respect to baseline left ventricular function. In patients with depressed VCF, hemodialysis with either buffer resulted in improvement of ventricular function with mean VCF significantly higher after bicarbonate dialysis as compared with acetate. In patients with normal VCF, only bicarbonate dialysis produced significantly better ventricular function. In contrast, Leunissen et al. (65,66) found increases in VCF in patients with normal left ventricular function with either acetate or bicarbonate dialysis. In patients with compromised left ventricular function, only bicarbonate dialysis resulted in significant increase in VCF.

The disparity of results in studies of effects of dialysate composition on cardiac function may in part results from failure to distinguish effects of volume removal. In this regard, Nixon et al. (67) demonstrated that dialysis with acetate with or without volume removal produced an increase in contractility. Mehta et al. (68) performed isovolemic dialysis and found that mean VCF improved to the same extent with both acetate and bicarbonate dialysis. Anderson et al. (69) studied left ventricular performance with two-dimensional echocardiography in five patients under three different cardiac filling volumes before and after a standard isovolemic hemodialysis. Cardiac performance as assessed by VCF improved comparably with acetate or bicarbonate under conditions of increased or decreased preloads.

In summary, many years of experience with acetate as the principal buffer in dialysate has not borne out concerns that acetate would be associated with long-term adverse consequences. In most chronic stable dialysis patients, cardiac function is improved with acetate or bicarbonate-containing dialysate. Under conditions in which a dialysate Na of more than 140 mEq/L is used, bicarbonate offers no apparent hemodynamic advantage over acetate. By contrast, use of a bicarbonate bath may provide more hemodynamic stability than acetate under conditions of a low Na dialysate

concentration (less than 135 mEq/L) or in patients who are truly acetate intolerant. In addition, bicarbonate-containing dialysate improves platelet function to a greater extent than acetate and may be less arrhythmogenic in susceptible patients. In either case, it should be pointed out that as high-efficiency and especially high-flux dialysis becomes more widely used, acetate-containing dialysate will become a thing of the past. The increased clearance seen with these procedures would allow the rate of influx of acetate to exceed the maximal rate of metabolism such that acid–base balance could not be maintained.

Bicarbonate Buffer

Bicarbonate is now the principal buffer used in dialysate. Producing bicarbonate dialysate requires a specifically designed system that mixes a bicarbonate concentrate and an acid concentrate with purified water. The acid concentrate contains a small amount of either lactic or acetic acid and all the calcium and magnesium. The exclusion of these cations from the bicarbonate concentrate prevents the precipitation of magnesium and calcium carbonate that would otherwise occur in the setting of a high bicarbonate concentration. During the mixing procedure, the acid in the acid concentrate will react with an equimolar amount of bicarbonate to generate carbonic acid and carbon dioxide. The generation of carbon dioxide causes the pH of the final solution to fall to approximately 7.0 to 7.4. This more acidic pH as well as the lower concentrations of calcium and magnesium in the final mixture allow for these ions to remain in solution. The final concentration of bicarbonate in the dialysate is generally fixed in the range of 33 to 38 mmol/L (**FIGURE 2.3**).

The use of a bicarbonate dialysate is associated with a number of potential complications (70). The liquid bicarbonate concentrate can be responsible for microbial contamination of the final dialysate largely because the bicarbonate concentrate is an excellent bacterial growth medium. This complication can be minimized by short storage time as well as filtration of the concentrate during the production procedure. Use of a bicarbonate cartridge can further minimize this complication. This device allows for the bicarbonate concentrate to be produced on-line by passing water through a column containing powdered bicarbonate. The concentrate is produced and proportioned immediately before mixing with the acid concentrate.

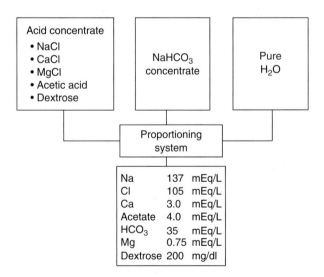

FIGURE 2.3 Components of the dialysate circuit in which bicarbonate serves as the buffer source.

Hypoxemia may occur during bicarbonate dialysis when high concentrations of bicarbonate are used. This complication appears to be the result of suppressed ventilation secondary to the increase in pH and serum bicarbonate concentration. In addition, excessively high levels of bicarbonate in the dialysate may result in acute metabolic alkalosis causing mental confusion, lethargy, weakness, and cramps.

The factors that determine bicarbonate requirements in hemodialysis patients include acid production during the interdialytic period, the removal of organic anions during the hemodialysis procedure, and the buffer deficit of the body. Because these factors are likely to vary from patient to patient, there is increasing interest in individualizing the dialysate bicarbonate concentration. The optimal level of dialysate bicarbonate would be a concentration low enough to prevent significant alkalosis in the postdialytic period and yet be high enough to prevent predialysis acidosis.

Maintaining a predialysis total CO_2 concentration of greater than 23 mmol/L can be achieved in most patients by individually adjusting the dialysate bicarbonate concentration. Oettinger and Oliver (71) found that 75% of patients exceeded this level with a dialysate bicarbonate concentration of 42 mmol/L. Use of this high bicarbonate dialysate did not result in progressive alkalemia, even in patients beginning the study with a normal predialysis total CO_2 using a standard bicarbonate dialysate concentration of 36 mmol/L. In addition, the high bicarbonate dialysate did not cause hypoxia or hypercarbia or alter the predialysis calcium, ionized calcium, or phosphorus.

Using high bicarbonate dialysate may improve nutrition, bone metabolism, and hemodynamic stability. Graham et al. (72) examined protein turnover in a group of chronic dialysis patients in whom dialysate bicarbonate concentration was increased from 35 to 40 mmol/L; supplemental oral bicarbonate therapy was given to two patients whose predialysis total CO_2 (tCO_2) concentration did not exceed 23 mmol/L. The mean tCO_2 concentration increased from 18.5 to 24.8 mmol/L during the high bicarbonate dialysate. Correction of the acidosis was associated with a significant decrease in protein degradation as suggested by leucine kinetic studies. In a similarly designed study, these investigators found an increase in the sensitivity of the parathyroid glands to calcium in patients using a dialysate bicarbonate concentration of 35 or 40 mmol/L (73). With regard to hemodynamics, increasing the bicarbonate concentration to 32 mmol/L is associated with a reduced incidence of both symptomatic and asymptomatic hypotension when compared to a bath bicarbonate concentration of 26 mmol/L (74).

Another strategy that may be effective in improving the acidosis of chronic dialysis patients is to use citric acid in place of acetic acid in the acid concentrate. In a recent study of 22 patients, use of citric acid decreased the number of patients with a predialysis bicarbonate concentration less than 23 mEq/L from 14 to 7 (75). Use of the citric acid dialysate was also associated with an increased delivered dose of dialysis, an effect postulated to be due to improved membrane permeability resulting from citrate's local anticoagulant effect. Improved membrane permeability with greater diffusive flux of bicarbonate from dialysate to blood or metabolism of citrate to bicarbonate in liver and muscle is the most likely explanation for the improvement in bicarbonate concentration.

Despite the positive effects of high bicarbonate dialysate concentrations listed above, it is unclear what specific serum bicarbonate or dialysate bicarbonate to target. Some epidemiologic data show that mild predialysis acidosis (serum bicarbonate 19 to 22 mEq/L) can be tolerated without an increase in mortality or

hospitalization, while more severe acidosis (serum bicarbonate less than 17 mEq/L) should be avoided (76), but another large study adjusting for markers related to inflammation and malnutrition shows that, in fact, metabolic acidosis (serum bicarbonate <22 mEq/L) predicts increased mortality (77). While replicating the finding that acidosis is associated with higher mortality, another observational study identified that higher prescribed dialysate bicarbonate concentrations were associated with increased mortality (78). Major limitations of these studies include their observational nature. Consequently, it is important to correct overt metabolic acidosis in hemodialysis patients, but caution is advised in raising the predialysis serum bicarbonate too high.

Dialysate Magnesium

The usual concentration of magnesium in the dialysate is 0.5 to 1.0 mEq/L and is only rarely manipulated. In an attempt to minimize the development of hypercalcemia associated with the use of calcium-containing phosphate binders and vitamin D, there has been interest in using magnesium-containing compounds as a phosphate binder. The use of oral magnesium requires the use of a low magnesium dialysate concentration to avoid the development of hypermagnesemia. Depending on which magnesium salt is used, this strategy has had variable success (79).

Use of oral $Mg(OH)_3$ in association with a magnesium-free dialysate had little or no effect on phosphate and increased mean serum magnesium to 4.3 mg/dL. In addition, diarrhea was a frequent side effect. More favorable results have been reported with oral $MgCO_3$. O'Donovan et al. (80) reported good control of the serum phosphorus level using oral $MgCO_3$ and a magnesium-free dialysate. On this regimen, diarrhea was mild and transient and the serum concentration of magnesium did not change. More recently, Kelber et al. (81) examined the feasibility of using a magnesium-free dialysate in the setting of high-efficiency dialysis. Despite the use of oral $MgCO_3$, patients developed severe muscle cramping that was immediately relieved by adding magnesium back to the dialysate. It was determined that measured magnesium removal exceeded the estimated predialysis extracellular fluid magnesium pool. By contrast, a dialysate magnesium of 0.6 mg/dL in combination with oral $MgCO_3$ was well tolerated.

Use of this later regimen was then examined in a prospective randomized crossover study (82). Patients were studied while taking $MgCO_3$ and one-half the usual dose of $CaCO_3$ along with a dialysate magnesium of 0.6 mg/dL and again while ingesting $CaCO_3$ given in the usual dose with a dialysate magnesium of 1.8 mg/dL. There was no difference in the serum concentrations of phosphorus, calcium, or magnesium between the two phases of the study. In addition, the $MgCO_3$-low $CaCO_3$ regimen permitted a greater amount of intravenous calcitriol to be used without the development of hypercalcemia. It was concluded that use of oral $MgCO_3$ as a phosphate binder and a low dialysate magnesium concentration may be a useful strategy in patients who develop hypercalcemia during treatment with calcitriol and $CaCO_3$.

Dialysate Calcium

The calcium concentration in the dialysate can be varied extensively according to the individual needs of the patient (TABLE 2.4). The most common concentrations used are 1.25, 1.5, and 1.75 mmol/L corresponding to 2.5, 3.0, 3.5 mEq/L and 5.0, 6.0, 7.0 mg/dL, respectively. In earlier times, a higher end dialysate calcium concentration (typically 3.5 mEq/L) was widely used to provide a net flux

TABLE 2.4	Considerations when Individualizing Components of the Dialysate	
Dialysate Component	**Advantage**	**Disadvantage**
Na: Increased	More hemodynamic stability Less cramping	Dipsogenic effect, increased interdialytic weight gain, chronic hypertension
Decreased (rarely used)	Less interdialytic weight gain	Intradialytic hypotension and cramping more common
Ca: Increased	Suppression of PTH; promotes hemodynamic stability	Hypercalcemia with vitamin D and Ca containing phosphate binders
Decreased	Permits greater use of vitamin D and calcium-containing phosphate binders	Potential for negative calcium balance, stimulation of PTH, slight decrease in hemodynamic stability
K: Increased	Less arrhythmias in setting of digoxin or coronary heart disease; less rebound hypertension	Limited by hyperkalemia
Decreased (ramped dialysate K ideal, prevents rapid initial decline in plasma K)	Greater dietary intake of K with less hyperkalemia, improvement in myocardial contractility	Increased arrhythmias; may exacerbate autonomic insufficiency
HCO_3: Increased	Corrects chronic acidosis, thereby benefits nutrition and bone metabolism	Postdialysis metabolic alkalosis
Decreased	Less metabolic alkalosis	Potential for chronic acidosis
Mg: Increased	Less arrhythmias, hemodynamic benefit	Hypermagnesemia
Decreased	Permits use of Mg-containing phosphate binders	Hypomagnesemia
PO_4 (rarely added to dialysate)	Treats or prevents hypophosphatemia in malnourished, chronic disease state, overdose setting, daily dialysis	Hyperphosphatemia

PTH, parathyroid hormone.

of calcium into the patient. The substitution of calcium for aluminum phosphate binders and the wider use of high doses of intravenous $1,25 (OH)_2$ vitamin D made the likelihood of hypercalcemia more common leading to a progressive lowering of the dialysate calcium concentration. For example, using a dialysate calcium concentration of 2.5 mEq/L, Slatopolsky et al. (83) was able to control the serum phosphorus in 21 patients with calcium carbonate at an average daily dose of 10.5 g with no instances of hypercalcemia. Despite the enthusiasm for use of low calcium dialysate, some recent studies have emphasized that such an approach requires careful monitoring to ensure that the patient does not develop negative calcium balance or worsening secondary hyperparathyroidism. Argiles et al. (84) found that serum immunoreactive parathyroid hormone (iPTH) levels increased significantly in patients treated with a 2.5 mEq/L dialysate calcium bath compared with a control group of patients dialyzed with a dialysate calcium of 3.0 mEq/L. This increase in iPTH occurred despite 2.4-fold more oral $CaCO_3$ ingested in the low dialysate calcium group. Although the increase in oral calcium intake was not sufficient to prevent the stimulation in iPTH, subsequent treatment with $1,25 (OH)_2$ vitamin D was effective in reversing the rise in iPTH levels.

Similar results were reported by Fernandez et al. (85) in a group of patients sequentially dialyzed against a 3.5 mEq/L and then 2.5 mEq/L calcium bath. While on the low calcium dialysate, there was a significant increase in both serum iPTH as well as serum alkaline phosphatase levels. These changes occurred despite the fact that oral calcium carbonate was administered at doses ranging from 3 to 6 g/day while on the low calcium dialysate. As determined by clearance studies, the authors suggested that the low calcium dialysate resulted in negative calcium balance that, in turn, contributed to the worsening hyperparathyroidism. Furthermore,

the maintenance of a normal serum calcium concentration noted in the study occurred at the expense of PTH-induced calcium mobilization from bone. Using measurements of total and ionized calcium in serum as well as in spent dialysate, Argiles et al. (86) have confirmed that a 2.5 mEq/L calcium dialysate is associated with negative calcium balance. Based on the potential of a 2.5 mEq/L dialysate calcium to cause negative calcium balance and to worsen secondary hyperparathyroidism, these authors now use a dialysate calcium of at least 3.0 mEq/L in most chronic dialysis patients (87).

The potential effect of a low dialysate calcium concentration to stimulate PTH release may have utility in patients with low bone turnover. Adynamic bone disease is becoming progressively more common in patients on maintenance hemodialysis. In patients clinically diagnosed with this entity, use of a dialysate calcium concentration of 1.25 mmol/L was found to increase serum PTH and total alkaline phosphatase to a greater extent than a dialysate calcium concentration of 1.75 mmol/L (88). The authors concluded that a low dialysate calcium concentration may be a therapeutic option in patients with this form of metabolic bone disease.

Another variable to consider in choosing a dialysate calcium concentration is the effect on hemodynamic stability during the dialysis procedure. Higher dialysate calcium concentrations may minimize intradialytic hypotension in patients with ejection fraction of less than 40% as well as other patients prone to intradialytic hypotension (89,90). In patients prone to intradialytic hypotension who are at risk for hypercalcemia, dialysate calcium profiling can be used as a strategy to improve hemodynamic stability and yet minimize the potential for hypercalcemia (91). In one study, patients were dialyzed for 4 hours in which the dialysate calcium concentration was set low (1.25 mmol/L) for the first 2 hours and then increased to 1.75 mmol/L for the last 2 hours (92). Use of the varying dialysate calcium concentration was associated with greater hemodynamic stability as compared with a fixed dialysate calcium concentration of either 1.25 or 1.5 mmol/L. This hemodynamic benefit was accomplished via an increase in cardiac output. At the end of 3 weeks, there was no difference in the predialysis ionized calcium concentration between the three groups.

Changes in serum calcium concentration may influence blood pressure through alterations in either systemic vascular resistance or the determinants of cardiac output or both. In an attempt to determine the physiologic mechanisms for calcium-induced changes in systemic arterial pressure, Fellner et al. (93) studied hemodynamic variables that determine arterial blood pressure as a function of changes in dialysate calcium concentration. Eight patients underwent hemodialysis three times within a single week with dialysate calcium concentrations of 1.0 mEq/L, 3.5 mEq/L, or 5.0 mEq/L. As in previous studies, changes in blood calcium concentration correlated directly with blood pressure. In addition, higher levels of calcium augmented left ventricular stroke volume and cardiac output while leaving total vascular resistance unchanged. It was concluded that alterations in blood calcium concentration affected blood pressure primarily through changes in left ventricular output rather than in peripheral vascular tone, and these findings have been replicated in a subsequent crossover study (94).

In addition to changes in ionized calcium concentration, hemodialysis leads to alterations in several factors that could conceivably be responsible for the observed changes in ventricular function. Henrich et al. (95) performed a series of dialysis maneuvers to determine the contribution of dialyzable toxins, ionized calcium, and acidemia to left ventricular performance during routine hemodialysis. The dialysate of each maneuver was adjusted to produce three effects: (a) isovolemic dialysis in which neither ionized calcium nor bicarbonate was allowed to increase (this procedure tested the effects of uremic toxin removal), (b) isovolemic dialysis during which ionized calcium increased but bicarbonate was held constant, and (c) isovolemic dialysis in which bicarbonate increased but ionized calcium was kept constant. Echocardiographic studies showed that left ventricular end-diastolic and end-systolic volumes decreased and ejection fraction and VCF increased only in the procedure in which plasma ionized calcium increased. This study suggested that the rise in ionized calcium is a major element in the observed improvement in myocardial contractility. Similar findings were recently reported by Lang et al. (96). Using dialysates differing only in calcium concentration, myocardial contractility was shown to correlate directly with plasma-ionized calcium. The mechanism by which increases in ionized calcium seen during hemodialysis lead to enhanced ventricular function is not known.

Despite the favorable effects on hemodynamics, there is a concern that long-term use of a high dialysate calcium concentration may contribute to adverse effects on the cardiovascular system by promoting vascular calcification. A higher dialysate calcium concentration has been linked to progression of aortic calcification and increases in arterial stiffness (97,98).

A final consideration to undertake in the selection of dialysate calcium is the rare occurrence of arrhythmias including sudden cardiac death. One case-control study evaluating more than 43,000 prevalent hemodialysis patients over the course of 4 years identified low dialysate calcium (<2.5 mEq/dL) as an independent risk factor for the occurrence of in-clinic cardiac arrest (47). Further analysis established that a larger dialysate to serum calcium gradient had linear relationship with the risk for cardiac arrest (99). These retrospective studies should heighten the awareness

that independent of bone and mineral disease, there are some risks involved with excessively low dialysate calcium.

In summary, the dialysate calcium concentration has implications with regard to metabolic bone disease, hemodynamic stability, and long-term effects on vascular calcification. The most recent National Kidney Foundation Kidney Disease Outcome Quality Initiative (NKF-K/DOQI) guidelines recommend a dialysate calcium concentration of 1.25 mmol/L as being a useful compromise between optimization of bone health and reductions in cardiovascular risk (100). However, as with the other dialysate constituents, the calcium concentration should be individually tailored to the patient. In patients who are prone to intradialytic hypotension, a higher dialysate calcium concentration may be of benefit. On the other hand, the use of a lower calcium concentration in the dialysate will allow increased doses of 1,25 (OH)$_2$ vitamin D to be utilized to reduce circulating levels of PTH with less fear of inducing hypercalcemia. This issue may be of importance given recent data suggesting vitamin D improves survival in dialysis patients (101). Further research is needed to define the optimal mix of dialysate calcium concentration, dose of vitamin D, amount of calcium- and non–calcium-containing phosphate binder, and use of the calcimimetic agent cinacalcet.

Dialysate Phosphate

In patients with mild to moderate hyperphosphatemia, hemodialysis has been estimated to remove 250 to 325 mg/day of phosphorus when extrapolated to an average week (102). Because a diet that provides adequate protein may provide approximately 900 mg of phosphorus daily, it follows that dialysis cannot provide adequate control of phosphate by itself. Rather, management of hyperphosphatemia requires a combination of dietary restriction, oral phosphate binders, and dialysis.

The limited ability of dialysis to remove phosphorus is primarily related to the kinetics of phosphorus distribution within the body and not inadequate clearance across the dialyzer. In a typical dialysis session, the rate of phosphorus removal is greatest during the initial stages of the procedure and then progressively declines to a low constant level toward the end of the treatment (**FIGURE 2.4**). This decline

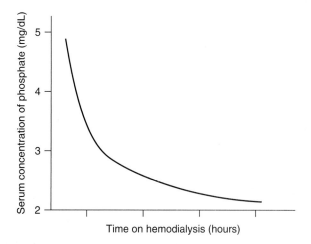

FIGURE 2.4 Plasma inorganic phosphate concentrations during a typical 4-hour dialysis procedure. The rate of phosphorus removal is greatest during the initial stages of the procedure and then progressively declines to a low constant level toward the end of the treatment. This decline is due to the decrease in plasma concentration and the slow efflux of phosphorus from the intracellular space and/or mobilization from bone stores.

is due to the decrease in plasma concentration and the slow efflux of phosphorus from the intracellular space and/or mobilization from bone stores. Although dialysis membranes differ with respect to plasma clearance of phosphate, it is the slow transfer of phosphorus to the extracellular space where it becomes accessible for dialytic removal that is the most important factor limiting phosphorus removal (103).

There are only a few situations in which one might consider adding phosphorus to the dialysate. Hypophosphatemia can be an occasional finding in the chronic dialysis patient who is malnourished and suffering from some chronic disease state. In such patients, adding phosphorus to the dialysate may be an effective means to treat hypophosphatemia without having to use a parenteral route of administration. The phosphate must be added to the bicarbonate component of a dual proportioning system to avoid the precipitation of calcium phosphate that would result from addition to the calcium-containing acid concentrate. Kaye et al. (104) described three hypophosphatemic dialysis patients who were treated by adding phosphorus to the dialysate in a single proportioning system. In these patients, phosphate was added to a bicarbonate concentrate that contained no calcium. To avoid hypocalcemia, calcium was infused into the venous drip chamber as a 10% $CaCl_2$ solution. A final phosphate concentration of 1 to 2 mmol/L was found effective in correcting the hypophosphatemia by the end of a 4-hour session.

Another situation in which addition of phosphate to the dialysate may be useful is in the setting of an overdose. In a patient with normal kidney function and a normal serum phosphate concentration, use of a phosphate-free dialysate will commonly result in hypophosphatemia. In most circumstances, the hypophosphatemia is of short duration and is of little clinical consequence. However, some intoxications may increase the risk for complications of hypophosphatemia such that addition of phosphate to the dialysate may be warranted.

Finally, hypophosphatemia has been noted in patients treated with prolonged daily nocturnal hemodialysis (105). In this setting, adding phosphate to the dialysate may prove useful as a means to normalize the serum phosphate concentration.

⬡ DIALYSATE COMPOSITION IN PERITONEAL DIALYSIS

Similar to the strategy in hemodialysis, the composition of the dialysis solution for peritoneal dialysis is designed to create favorable concentration gradients across the peritoneal membrane to achieve maximal removal of endogenous waste products, to maintain acid–base and electrolyte balance near normal, and to maintain the extracellular fluid volume constant. As with hemodialysis, the composition of the dialysate can be individually modified for ultrafiltration and clearance needs.

Osmotic Agents

The addition of a solute to render the dialysate hyperosmolar relative to plasma creates an osmotic gradient that results in the net movement of water into the peritoneal cavity. The degree of hypertonicity, the time that the fluid is allowed to dwell in the abdomen, and the hydraulic permeability of the peritoneal membrane determine the volume of fluid removed. Clinically, the magnitude of ultrafiltrate is determined by subtracting the volume of fluid instilled in the abdomen from the effluent volume.

In commercially available peritoneal dialysates, glucose is the most commonly used osmotic agent used to enhance ultrafiltration.

The concentrations available range from 1.36% glucose (1.5% dextrose) to 3.86% glucose (4.25% dextrose). Both the ultrafiltration rate and the time until osmotic equilibrium is reached are directly related to the glucose concentration used. Using 2-L exchanges with cycle times up to 6 hours, solutions containing 1.5% dextrose will generate 100 to 200 mL of net ultrafiltrate. Solutions containing 4.25% under the same conditions will generate up to 800 mL of net ultrafiltrate. By increasing the frequency of exchanges, this ultrafiltrate volume can be increased to as high as 1 L/h using the 4.25% solution. Over time, the osmolality of the dialysate declines as a result of water movement into the peritoneal cavity and absorption of dialysate glucose. By 4 hours of dwell using the 1.5% solution, the tonicity of the dialysate is essentially equal to that of plasma and the glucose concentration of the dialysate decreases to approximately one-half the original value.

The use of glucose as an osmotic agent is well recognized to have several deficiencies. The absorption of glucose contributes substantially to the caloric intake of patients on continuous peritoneal dialysis. This carbohydrate load over time is thought to contribute to progressive obesity, hypertriglyceridemia, and decreased nutrition as a result of loss of appetite and decreased protein intake. In addition, an increasing body of literature suggests that the high glucose concentrations and high osmolality of the currently available solutions adversely affect the function of the peritoneal membrane importantly contributing to technique failure over time.

Ultrafiltration failure resulting from increased permeability of small molecular weight solutes is one of the most frequent reasons patients are transferred from peritoneal to hemodialysis. This increase in permeability can be traced to an increase in the number of blood vessels in the peritoneal membrane effectively enlarging the vascular peritoneal surface area (106). High glucose concentrations have been linked to this process of neoangiogenesis through a variety of mechanisms to include stimulation of vascular endothelial growth factor and toxic effects of advanced glycosylation end products and glucose degradation products (107).

The bioincompatibility of glucose-containing solutions has prompted a search for alternative osmotic agents. Experimental and some clinical studies have been performed using substances such as fructose, sorbitol, xylitol, dextran, and gelatin. For one reason or another, these agents have either been proven unsafe or ineffective as an osmotic agent. Glycerol has received some interest as an osmotic agent particularly in patients with diabetes. This agent is not dependent on insulin for metabolism and may allow for better and easier glucose control in the diabetic population (108).

One of the most promising new peritoneal dialysis solutions uses glucose polymers as the osmotic agent (109). These compounds can be administered as a solution that is iso-osmolar to plasma because they generate an ultrafiltrate through the process of colloid osmosis. This process is based on the principle that water is transported from capillaries in the direction of impermeable large solutes rather than down an osmotic gradient as occurs with glucose-containing solutions. The icodextrin-based dialysis solution is a polymer of glucose that is now available in several countries. In a 6-hour dwell, the 7.5% icodextrin solution generates an ultrafiltrate volume that is higher than that generated by 1.5% dextrose despite having a lower osmolality (285 vs. 347 mOsm/kg). With prolonged dwell times of 8 to 12 hours, the icodextrin solution provides equivalent or higher ultrafiltrate volumes than that generated by the 4.25% dextrose solution (486 mOsm/kg). The ability to maintain a colloid osmotic pressure for prolonged periods of time makes this solution ideal for overnight dwells in patients on continuous ambulatory peritoneal dialysis (CAPD) as well as daytime dwells for those on automated peritoneal dialysis regimens.

In patients with ultrafiltration failure who would otherwise be transferred to hemodialysis, use of icodextrin has been shown to extend the time that patients remain on peritoneal dialysis by many months (110). In addition, use of icodextrin is associated with less weight gain, improved lipid control, and less hyperinsulinemia as compared with dextrose-containing solutions. It is likely that icodextrin will become the preferred agent for the long dwell in most peritoneal dialysis patients (111,112).

Because patients on peritoneal dialysis have a high incidence of protein-calorie malnutrition, in part, resulting from daily losses of protein and amino acids into the dialysate, studies have also examined the feasibility of using amino acids as a replacement for glucose as an osmotic agent. Use of amino acids should augment the amino acid intake and reduce the net amino acid losses of the patient potentially providing additional nutrition to the patient. The overall absorption of amino acids in various solutions ranges from 60% to 90% depending on the concentration used and the length of the dwell (92). One 2-L bag of 1.0% solution can provide at least 14 g of amino acids. Importantly, these solutions have no major impact on the transport characteristics of the peritoneal membrane and are as effective osmotic agents as glucose.

Initial studies using amino acid–containing solutions were unimpressive with regard to showing an improvement in nutritional parameters. Moreover, use of these solutions was associated with significant increases in the blood urea nitrogen concentration and development of metabolic acidosis. More recent studies have used amino acid–containing dialysates that have been altered to provide the optimal balance between essential and nonessential amino acids required for a chronic kidney disease patient (113,114). Kopple et al. (113) studied the effectiveness of the 1.1% amino acid solution (Nutrineal; Baxter Healthcare) in a group of patients who were clinically malnourished. The patients were fed a constant diet, and the number of amino acid exchanges per day was adjusted so that the total daily dietary protein plus dialysate amino acid intake would be 1.1 to 1.3 g/kg/day. Patients required one to two daily exchanges of the amino acid solution to achieve this goal. The amino acid dialysate was associated with positive nitrogen balance that remained significant throughout the study. In addition, there was net protein anabolism as directly demonstrated from radiolabeled N-glycine studies. Patients tolerated the treatment well; however, some patients developed mild metabolic acidemia.

This same solution has been examined in 15 stable CAPD patients in whom malnutrition was not an entry criterion (114). In this study,

one 2-L exchange of the 1.1% solution was performed at lunchtime to ensure the simultaneous uptake of sufficient carbohydrates. Previous experience with parenteral nutrition has shown that optimal utilization of amino acids occurs when there is combined uptake of nonprotein calories and amino acids. Over the 3 months of the study, there was a significant increase in the serum albumin concentration whether baseline malnutrition was present or not. Use of the dialysate in this manner did not result in acidosis although the blood urea nitrogen increased by 20%. Other studies have also confirmed that this 1.1% amino acid is effective in providing a nutritional benefit particularly in patients who are malnourished (115,116).

In summary, glucose remains the standard osmotic agent used in peritoneal dialysis solutions. In an attempt to develop a more physiologic solution, various new osmotic agents are now under investigation. It is likely that icodextrin will be used with greater frequency in peritoneal dialysis patients particularly as the osmotic agent for long dwell times. In patients with evidence of ultrafiltration failure, use of icodextrin may extend the time certain patients can remain on peritoneal dialysis before having to switch to hemodialysis. Amino acid containing solutions also show promise for patients with evidence of malnutrition. To limit the development of azotemia and acidosis, the use of these solutions will likely be confined to one exchange per day (**Table 2.5**).

Dialysate Buffer

The buffer present in most commercially available peritoneal dialysate solutions is lactate. In patients with normal hepatic function, lactate is rapidly converted to bicarbonate such that 1 mM of lactate absorbed generates 1 mM of bicarbonate. Even with the most vigorous peritoneal dialysis, there is no appreciable accumulation of circulating lactate. The rapid metabolism of lactate to bicarbonate maintains the high dialysate-to-plasma lactate gradient necessary for continued absorption. This absorption may be somewhat less with use of dialysate that contains higher concentrations of dextrose. Under these conditions, increased ultrafiltrate formation may dilute the concentration of lactate in the peritoneal cavity and therefore decrease the concentration gradient for diffusion. Lactate is normally provided as a racemic mixture of the dextro and levo isomers in approximately equal concentrations. There is some evidence that the natural isomer (l-lactate) is more rapidly absorbed than the D-isomer (D-lactate) (117).

The pH of commercially available peritoneal dialysis solutions is purposely made acidic by adding hydrochloric acid to prevent dextrose caramelization during the sterilization procedure. Once instilled into the abdomen, the pH of the solution rises to values

TABLE 2.5	Advantages and Disadvantages of New Peritoneal Dialysis Solutions	
Solution	**Advantage**	**Disadvantage**
Icodextrin	Sustained ultrafiltration in overnight dwell in CAPD, long dwell in APD, and during peritonitis, avoids effects of glucose absorption, isoosmotic	Skin reactions (less than 10%), maltose accumulation
Amino acids	Improve malnutrition	Azotemia and metabolic acidosis
Bicarbonate and bicarbonate/lactate buffer	Improved biocompatibility due to neutral pH, ↓ glucose degradation products	Two-chamber bags to separate Ca and Mg from bicarbonate
Glucose sterilized separately at lower pH	Improved biocompatibility, ↓ glucose degradation products	Two-chamber bag required

CAPD, continuous ambulatory peritoneal dialysis; APD, automated peritoneal dialysis; ↓, decrease.

greater than 7.0. The acidic nature and buffer composition of currently available solutions further contributes to the bioincompatibility of peritoneal dialysate (118).

To address this issue, neutral pH solutions buffered with bicarbonate or with a mixture of bicarbonate and lactate have been introduced into clinical practice. Up until recently, bicarbonate was not able to be used as the buffer in peritoneal dialysis solutions because calcium and magnesium would precipitate in the presence of bicarbonate in the setting of an alkaline pH. Omitting magnesium and calcium from the dialysate was not an option because patients undergoing chronic peritoneal dialysis would develop deficits of these divalent cations. These limitations have largely been overcome by the development of a two-chamber dialysate bag. One chamber contains the glucose and the electrolytes to include magnesium and calcium. The other chamber contains either bicarbonate alone or a bicarbonate-lactate mixture. The advantage of this setup is that glucose can be sterilized at a much lower pH as compared with a single-chamber bag, and as a result, the formation of glucose degradation products is markedly reduced. Mixing of the two components at the time of abdominal installation effectively raises the pH to a neutral value. Thus, the final solution has neutral pH, a low concentration of glucose degradation products, and contains bicarbonate.

In a trial of 106 patients, a pH neutral bicarbonate/lactate-based peritoneal dialysis solution was compared with the conventional acidic lactate buffered solution in which markers of peritoneal membrane integrity and inflammation were examined (119). At the end of 6 months, patients treated with the pH neutral solution had a significantly greater increase in the dialysate cancer antigen 125 (CA125) (a marker of viability and cell mass of the mesothelium). The same group also had a significantly greater decrease in dialysate hyaluronan (a marker of inflammation in the peritoneal cavity). The pH neutral solution is associated with less inflow pain, and no adverse effect has been demonstrated on peritoneal transport. Use of the pH neutral solution has also been shown to result in long-term improvement in peritoneal macrophage function as compared with conventional solutions (120). In addition to improved biocompatibility, the newer pH solutions have been linked to better preservation of residual renal function, less peritonitis, and in non-randomized trials, there is a suggestion these solutions may provide a survival benefit when compared to conventional solutions (121–125). More rigorous trials are needed to verify the extent these solutions are able to provide improved patient outcomes (126).

In summary, a great deal of progress has been made to improve the biocompatibility of peritoneal dialysis solutions. Both experimental and clinical studies demonstrate that these solutions are much better at preserving peritoneal membrane function. Because no one solution is ideal, it is likely that in the future, each patient will be prescribed a combination of fluids to meet specific individual needs. One can envision a daily regimen in a patient on CAPD consisting of one exchange of amino acids, two exchanges of bicarbonate/glucose, and an overnight exchange of icodextrin (127). Future studies will be required to determine the efficacy of various combinations.

Dialysate Sodium

The Na concentration in the ultrafiltrate during peritoneal dialysis is usually less than the extracellular fluid such that there is a tendency for water loss and the development of hypernatremia. Commercially available peritoneal dialysates have a Na concentration of 132 mEq/L to compensate for this tendency toward dehydration. This effect is most pronounced with increasing frequency of exchanges and with increasing dialysate glucose concentrations. Use of the more hypertonic solutions with frequent cycling can result in significant dehydration and hypernatremia. As a result of stimulated thirst, water intake and weight may increase resulting in a vicious cycle.

The use of a low Na dialysate does lead to net Na removal and can predispose to hypotension in patients with inadequate Na intake. In the occasional patient who is unable to increase dietary Na, the dialysate Na concentration can be raised to decrease the amount of Na removal so that extracellular fluid volume can be maintained.

Dialysate Potassium

Potassium is cleared by peritoneal dialysis at a rate similar to that of urea. With CAPD and 10 L of drainage per day, approximately 35 to 46 mEq of potassium is removed per day. Daily potassium intake is usually greater than this amount, yet significant hyperkalemia is uncommon in these patients. Presumably, potassium balance is maintained by increased colonic secretion of potassium as well as some residual kidney excretion. Given these considerations, potassium is not routinely added to the dialysate.

Maximal removal of potassium with peritoneal dialysis is approximately 10 mEq/h even in the setting of severe hyperkalemia. It should be noted that removal rates with Kayexalate enemas far exceed this value and may approach 30 mEq/hour. In patients undergoing frequent exchanges, hypokalemia may develop. In these instances, potassium can be added to the dialysate to achieve a final concentration of 2 to 3 mEq/L. This is particularly important in patients receiving digoxin because the development of hypokalemia can precipitate arrhythmias.

Dialysate Magnesium

Initially, the standard peritoneal dialysis solution contained 1.5 mEq/L magnesium. The concentration has since been lowered to 0.5 mEq/L to lessen the frequency of hypermagnesemia that was observed with the higher magnesium concentration. As discussed with hemodialysis, a lower dialysate magnesium concentration may allow use of magnesium salts as an additional calcium-free phosphate binder.

Dialysate Calcium

As discussed previously, patients with progressive chronic kidney disease have a tendency to develop hypocalcemia. To avoid negative calcium balance as well as potentially suppressing circulating PTH, commercially available peritoneal dialysis solutions evolved to contain a calcium concentration of 3.5 mEq/L (1.75 mmol/L) (128). This concentration is equal to or slightly greater than the ionized concentration in the serum of most patients. As a result, there is net calcium absorption in most patients when using a conventional dialysis regime. When ultrafiltration volume is high, as occurs with use of 4.25% dextrose concentration at high rates of exchange, net transfer of calcium can be reversed such that calcium balance becomes negative.

As the use of calcium-containing phosphate binders has increased, hypercalcemia has become a common problem when using the 3.5 mEq/L calcium dialysate. This complication has been particularly common in patients treated with peritoneal dialysis because these patients have a much greater incidence of adynamic bone disease as compared with hemodialysis patients (129). In fact, the continual positive calcium balance associated with the 3.5 mEq/L solution has been suggested as a contributing factor in the development of this lesion. The low bone turnover state typical of this disorder impairs the accrual of administered calcium contributing to the development of hypercalcemia. As a result, there has been increased interest in using a similar strategy as has been employed in hemodialysis, namely, lower the calcium content of the dialysate. This strategy can allow for increased usage of calcium-containing phosphate binders as well as more liberal use of 1,25 (OH)$_2$ vitamin D to effect decreases in the circulating level of PTH. In this manner, the development of hypercalcemia can be minimized.

A recent study examined the effects of a low dialysate calcium 1.0 mM as compared to a control calcium solution (1.62 mM) in 51 patients with biopsy proven adynamic bone disease. In this randomized trial lasting 16 months, use of the low calcium-containing solution was associated with both a significant reduction in episodes of hypercalcemia and increase in PTH levels compared to the control solution. Importantly, bone formation rates in the low calcium group all increased into the normal range, while no significant change was noted in the control group (130).

In summary, peritoneal dialysis solutions are widely available with a calcium concentration of either 1.25 or 1.75 mmol/L. The decision to use one concentration or the other should be made on an individual basis. Most patients can be treated with a dialysis solution that contains 1.75 mmol/L calcium. On the other hand, a low dialysate calcium solution offers a valuable therapeutic option to treat patients with increased doses of calcium-containing phosphate binders and calcitriol with a much lower incidence of hypercalcemia. A low calcium solution may also be of benefit in reversing adynamic bone disease. Close monitoring of patients is required when using a low calcium solution to ensure that secondary hyperparathyroidism is not exacerbated. This is particularly so in patients who are questionably compliant with their calcium-containing phosphate binders. Monitoring of bone mineralization is also indicated with long-term use of low calcium dialysate.

REFERENCES

1. Henrich W, Woodard T, McPhaul J. The chronic efficacy and safety of high sodium dialysate: double-blind, crossover study. *Am J Kidney Dis* 1982;2:349–353.
2. Bijaphala S, Bell A, Bennett C, et al. Comparison of high and low sodium bicarbonate and acetate dialysis in stable chronic hemodialysis. *Clin Nephrol* 1985;23:179–183.
3. Keshaviah P, Shapiro F. A critical examination of dialysis-induced hypotension. *Am J Kidney Dis* 1982;2:290–301.
4. Van Stone J, Meyer R, Murrin C, et al. Hemodialysis with glycerol dialysate. *Trans Am Soc Artif Intern Organs* 1979;25:354–356.
5. McCausland F, Prior L, Heher E, et al. Preservation of blood pressure stability with hypertonic mannitol during hemodialysis initiation. *Am J Nephrol* 2012;36:168–174.
6. Van Stone J, Bauer J, Carey J. The effect of dialysate sodium concentration on body fluid distribution during hemodialysis. *Trans Am Soc Artif Intern Organs* 1980;26:383–386.
7. Sarkar S, Wystrychowski G, Usvyat L, et al. Fluid dynamics during hemodialysis in relationship to sodium gradient between dialysate and plasma. *ASAIO J* 2007;53:339–342.
8. Schultze G, Maiga M, Neumayer H, et al. Prostaglandin E2 promotes hypotension on low sodium hemodialysis. *Nephron* 1984;37:250–256.
9. Dumler F, Grondin G, Levin N. Sequential high/low sodium hemodialysis: an alternative to ultrafiltration. *Trans Am Soc Artif Intern Organs* 1979;25:351–353.
10. Raja R, Kramer M, Barber K, et al. Sequential changes in dialysate sodium (DNa) during hemodialysis. *Trans Am Soc Artif Intern Organs* 1983;29:649–651.
11. Daugirdas J, Al-Kudsi R, Ing T, et al. A double-blind evaluation of sodium gradient hemodialysis. *Am J Nephrol* 1985;5:163–168.
12. Acchiardo S, Hayden A. Is Na+ modeling necessary in high flux dialysis? *ASAIO Trans* 1991;37:M135–M137.
13. Sadowski R, Allred E, Jabs K. Sodium modeling ameliorates intradialytic and interdialytic symptoms in young hemodialysis patients. *J Am Soc Nephrol* 1993;4:1192–1198.
14. Levin A, Goldstein M. The benefits and side effects of ramped hypertonic sodium dialysis. *J Am Soc Nephrol* 1996;7:242–246.
15. Sang G, Kovithavongs C, Ulan R, et al. Soidum ramping in hemodialysis: a study of beneficial and adverse effects. *Am J Kidney Dis* 1997;29:669–677.
16. Movilli E, Camerini C, Viola B, et al. Blood volume changes during three different profiles of dialysate sodium variation with similar intradialytic sodium balances in chronic hemodialyzed patients. *Am J Kidney Dis* 1997;30:58–63.
17. Sherman R. Intradialytic hypotension: an overview of recent, unresolves and overlooked issues. *Semin Dial* 2002;15:141–143.
18. Flanigan M. Role of sodium in hemodialysis. *Kidney Int* 2000;76: S72–S78.
19. Zhou Y, Liu H, Duan X, et al. Impact of sodium and ultrafiltration profiling on haemodialysis-related hypotension. *Nephrol Dial Transplant* 2006;21:3231–3237.
20. Paganini E, Sandy D, Moreno L, et al. The effect of sodium and ultrafiltration modelling on plasma volume changes and haemodynamic stability in intensive care patients receiving haemodialysis for acute renal failure: a prospective, stratified, randomized, cross-over study. *Nephrol Dial Transplant* 1996;11(Suppl 8):32–37.
21. Song J, Lee S, Suh C, et al. Time-averaged concentration of dialysate sodium relates with sodium load and interdialytic weight gain during sodium-profiling hemodialysis. *Am J Kidney Dis* 2002;40:291–301.
22. Flanigan M, Khairullah Q, Lim V. Dialysate sodium delivery can alter chronic blood pressure management. *Am J Kidney Dis* 1997;29: 383–391.
23. Thein H, Haloob I, Marshall M. Associations of a facility level decrease in dialysate sodium concentration with blood pressure and interdialytic weight gain. *Nephrol Dial Transplant* 2007;22:2630–2639.
24. Coli L, Ursino M, Dalmastri V, et al. A simple mathematical model applied to selection of the sodium profile during profiled haemodialysis. *Nephrol Dial Transplant* 1998;13:404–416.
25. Locatelli F, Andrulli S, Di Filippo S, et al. Effect of on-line conductivity plasma ultrafiltrate kinetic modeling on cardiovascular stability of hemodialysis patients. *Kidney Int* 1998;53:1052–1060.
26. Locatelli F, Manzoni C, Di Filippo S, et al. On-line monitoring and convective treatment modalities: short term advantages. *Nephrol Dial Transplant* 1999;14(Suppl 3):92–97.
27. Locatelli F, Covic A, Chazot C, et al. Optimal composition of the dialysate, with emphasis on its influence on blood pressure. *Nephrol Dial Transplant* 2004;19:785–796.
28. Waikar S, Curhan G, Brunelli S. Mortality associated with low serum sodium concentration in maintenance hemodialysis. *Am J Med* 2011; 124:77–84.
29. Hecking M, Karaboyas A, Saran R, et al. Predialysis serum sodium level, dialysate sodium, and mortality in maintenance hemodialysis patients: the Dialysis Outcomes and Practice Patterns Study (DOPPS). *Am J Kidney Dis* 2012;59:238–248.
30. Ketchersid T, Van Stone J. Dialysate potassium. *Semin Dial* 1991;4: 46–51.
31. Heguilén R, Sciurano C, Bellusci A, et al. The faster potassium-lowering effect of high dialysate bicarbonate concentrations in chronic haemodialysis patients. *Nephrol Dial Transplant* 2005;20:591–597.
32. Wiegand C, Davin T, Raij L, et al. Life threatening hypokalemia during hemodialysis. *Trans Am Soc Artif Intern Organs* 1979;25:416–418.
33. Sherman R, Hwang E, Bernholc A, et al. Variability in potassium removal by hemodialysis. *Am J Nephrol* 1986;6:284–288.
34. Raimann J, Kruse A, Thijssen S, et al. Metabolic effects of dialyzate glucose in chronic hemodialysis: results from a prospective, randomized crossover trial. *Nephrol Dial Transplant* 2012;27:1559–1568.

35. Allon M, Shanklin N. Effect of albuterol treatment on subsequent dialytic potassium removal. *Am J Kidney Dis* 1995;26:607–613.

36. Linas S. The role of potassium in the pathogenesis and treatment of hypertension. *Kidney Int* 1991;39:771–786.

37. Pogglitsch H, Holzer H, Waller J, et al. The cause of inadequate haemodynamic reactions during ultradiffusion. *Proc Eur Dial Transplant Assoc* 1978;15:245–252.

38. Biglieri E, McIlroy M. Abnormalities of renal function and circulatory reflexes in primary aldosteronism. *Circulation* 1966;33:78–86.

39. Henrich W. Hemodynamic instability during hemodialysis. *Kidney Int* 1986;30:605–612.

40. Henrich W, Katz F, Molinoff P, et al. Competitive effects of hypokalemia and volume depletion on plasma renin activity, aldosterone and catecholamine concentrations in hemodialysis patients. *Kidney Int* 1977;12:279–284.

41. Haddy F, Scott J, Emerson T, et al. Effects of generalized changes in plasma electrolyte concentration and osmolarity on blood pressure in the anesthetized dog. *Circ Res* 1969;24:I59–I74.

42. Wizemann V, Kramer W, Bechthold A, et al. Acute effects of dialysis on myocardial contractility: influence of cardiac status and calcium/potassium. *Contrib Nephrol* 1986;52:60–68.

43. Dolson G, Adrogue H. Low dialysate [K+] decreases efficiency of hemodialysis and increases urea rebound. *J Am Soc Nephrol* 1998;9:2124–2128.

44. Zehnder C, Gutzwiller J, Huber A, et al. Low-potassium and glucose-free dialysis maintains urea but enhances potassium removal. *Nephrol Dial Transplant* 2001;16:78–84.

45. Severi S, Grandi E, Pes C, et al. Calcium and potassium changes during haemodialysis alter ventricular repolarization duration: *in vivo* and *in silico* analysis. *Nephrol Dial Transplant* 2008;23:1378–1386.

46. Kovesdy C, Regidor D, Mehrotra R, et al. Serum and dialysate potassium concentrations and survival in hemodialysis patients. *Clin J Am Soc Nephron* 2007;2:999–1007.

47. Pun P, Lehrich R, Honeycutt E, et al. Modifiable risk factors associated with sudden cardiac arrest within hemodialysis clinics. *Kidney Int* 2011;79:218–227.

48. Buemi M, Aloisi E, Coppolino G, et al. The effect of two different protocols of potassium haemodiafiltration on QT dispersion. *Nephrol Dial Transplant* 2005;20:1148–1154.

49. Redaelli B, Locatelli F, Limido D, et al. Effect of a new model of hemodialysis potassium removal on the control of ventricular arrhythmias. *Kidney Int* 1996;50:609–617.

50. Gennari F. Acid-base balance in dialysis patients. *Kidney Int* 1985;28:678–688.

51. Skutches C, Sigler M, Teehan B, et al. Contribution of dialysate acetate to energy metabolism: metabolic implications. *Kidney Int* 1983;23:57–63.

52. Daugirdas J. Dialysis hypotension: a hemodynamic analysis. *Kidney Int* 1991;39:233–246.

53. Lonnemann G, Bingel M, Koch K, et al. Plasma interleukin-1 activity in humans undergoing hemodialysis with regenerated cellulosic membranes. *Lymphokine Res* 1987;6:63–70.

54. Wolff J, Pederson T, Rossen M, et al. Effects of acetate and bicarbonate dialysis on cardiac performance, transmural myocardial perfusion and acid-base balance. *Int J Artif Organs* 1986;9:105–110.

55. Vinay P, Prud'Homme M, Vinet B, et al. Acetate metabolism and bicarbonate generation during hemodialysis: 10 years of observation. *Kidney Int* 1987;31:1194–1204.

56. Wehle B, Asaba H, Castenfors J, et al. The influence of dialysis fluid composition on the blood pressure response during dialysis. *Clin Nephrol* 1978;10:62–66.

57. Henrich W, Woodard T, Meyer B, et al. High sodium bicarbonate and acetate hemodialysis: double-blind crossover comparison of hemodynamic and ventilatory effects. *Kidney Int* 1983;24:240–245.

58. Velez R, Woodard T, Henrich W. Acetate and bicarbonate hemodialysis in patients with and without autonomic dysfunction. *Kidney Int* 1984;26:59–65.

59. Kirkendol P, Devia C, Bower J, et al. A comparison of the cardiovascular effects of sodium acetate, sodium bicarbonate and other potential sources of fixed base in hemodialysate solutions. *Trans Am Soc Artif Intern Organs* 1977;23:399–405.

60. Aizawa Y, Ohmori T, Imai K, et al. Depressant action of acetate upon the human cardiovascular system. *Clin Nephrol* 1977;8:477–480.

61. Nitenberg A, Huyghebaert M, Blanchet F, et al. Analysis of increased myocardial contractility during sodium acetate infusion in humans. *Kidney Int* 1984;26:744–751.

62. Mansell M, Crowther A, Laker MF, et al. The effect of hyperlactatemia on cardiac output during regular hemodialysis. *Clin Nephrol* 1982;18:130–134.

63. Schick E, Idelson B, Liang C, et al. Comparison of the hemodynamic response to hemodialysis with acetate or bicarbonate. *Trans Am Soc Artif Intern Organs* 1983;29:25–28.

64. Ruder M, Alpert M, Van Stone J, et al. Comparative effects of acetate and bicarbonate hemodialysis on left ventricular function. *Kidney Int* 1985;27:768–773.

65. Leunissen K, Cheriex E, Janssen J, et al. Influence of left ventricular function on changes in plasma volume during acetate and bicarbonate dialysis. *Nephrol Dial Transplant* 1987;2:99–103.

66. Leunissen K, van Hooff J. Acetate or bicarbonate for haemodialysis? *Nephrol Dial Transplant* 1988;3:1–7.

67. Nixon J, Mitchell J, McPhaul J Jr, et al. Effect of hemodialysis on left ventricular function. *J Clin Invest* 1983;71:377–384.

68. Mehta B, Fischer D, Ahmad M, et al. Effects of acetate and bicarbonate hemodialysis on cardiac function in chronic dialysis patients. *Kidney Int* 1983;24:782–787.

69. Anderson L, Nixon J, Henrich W. Effects of acetate and bicarbonate dialysate on left ventricular performance. *Am J Kidney Dis* 1987;10:350–355.

70. Van Stone J. Bicarbonate dialysate: still more to learn. *Semin Dial* 1994;7:168–169.

71. Oettinger C, Oliver J. Normalization of uremic acidosis in hemodialysis patients with a high bicarbonate dialysate. *J Am Soc Nephrol* 1993;3:1804–1807.

72. Graham K, Reaich D, Channon S, et al. Correction of acidosis in hemodialysis decreases whole-body protein degradation. *J Am Soc Nephrol* 1997;8:632–637.

73. Graham K, Hoenich N, Tarbit M, et al. Correction of acidosis in hemodialysis patients increases the sensitivity of the parathyroid glands to calcium. *J Am Soc Nephrol* 1997;8:627–631.

74. Gabutti L, Ferrari N, Giudici G, et al. Unexpected haemodynamic instability associated with standard bicarbonate haemodialysis. *Nephrol Dial Transplant* 2003;18:2369–2376.

75. Ahmad S, Callan R, Cole J, et al. Dialysate made from chemicals using citric acid increases dialysis dose. *Am J Kidney Dis* 2000;35:493–499.

76. Bommer J, Locatelli F, Satayathum S, et al. Association of predialysis serum bicarbonate levels with risk of mortality and hospitalization in the Dialysis Outcomes and Practice Patterns Study (DOPPS). *Am J Kidney Dis* 2004;44:661–671.

77. Wu DY, Shinaberger CS, Regidor DL, et al. Association between serum bicarbonate and death in hemodialysis patients: is it better to be acidotic or alkalotic? *Clin J Am Soc Nephrol* 2006;1(1):70–78.

78. Tentori F, Karaboyas A, Robinson B, et al. Association of dialysate bicarbonate concentration with mortality in the Dialysis Outcomes and Practice Patterns Study (DOPPS). *Am J Kidney Dis* 2013;62:738–746.

79. Spiegel D. The role of magnesium binders in chronic kidney disease. *Semin Dial* 2007;20:333–336.

80. O'Donovan R, Baldwin D, Hammer M, et al. Substitution of aluminum salts by magnesium salts in control of dialysis hyperphosphataemia. *Lancet* 1986;1:880–882.

81. Kelber J, Slatopolsky E, Delmez J. Acute effects of different concentration of dialysate magnesium during high-efficiency dialysis. *Am J Kidney Dis* 1994;24:453–460.

82. Delmez J, Kelber J, Norwood K, et al. Magnesium carbonate as a phosphorus binder: a prospective, controlled, crossover study. *Kidney Int* 1996;49:163–167.

83. Slatopolsky E, Weerts C, Norwood K, et al. Long-term effects of calcium carbonate and 2.5 mEq/liter calcium dialysate on mineral metabolism. *Kidney Int* 1989;36:897–903.

84. Argiles A, Kerr P, Canaud B, et al. Calcium kinetics and the long-term effects of lowering dialysate calcium concentration. *Kidney Int* 1993;43:630–640.

85. Fernandez E, Borras M, Pais B, et al. Low-calcium dialysate stimulates parathormone secretion and its long-term use worsens secondary hyperparathyroidism. *J Am Soc Nephrol* 1995;6:132–135.

86. Argiles A, Mion C. Calcium balance and intact PTH variations during haemodiafiltration. *Nephrol Dial Transplant* 1995;10:2083–2089.

87. Argiles A, Mion C. Low-calcium dialysate worsens secondary hyperparathyroidism. *J Am Soc Nephrol* 1996;7:635–636.

88. Spasovski G, Gelev S, Masin-Spasovska J, et al. Improvement of bone and mineral parameters related to adynamic bone disease by diminishing dialysate calcium. *Bone* 2007;41:698–703.

89. Alappan R, Cruz D, Abu-Alfa A, et al. Treatment of severe intradialytic hypotension with the addition of high dialysate calcium concentration to midodrine and/or cool dialysate. *Am J Kidney Dis* 2001;37:294–299.

90. van der Sande F, Cheriex E, van Kiujk W, et al. Effect of dialysate calcium concentrations on intradialytic blood pressure course in cardiac-compromised patients. *Am J Kidney Dis* 1998;32:125–131.

91. Kyriazis J, Glotsos J, Bilirakis L, et al. Dialysate calcium profiling during hemodialysis: use and clinical implications. *Kidney Int* 2002;61: 276–287.

92. Faller B. Amino-acid based dialysis solutions. *Kidney Int* 1996;56: S81–S85.

93. Fellner S, Lang R, Neumann A, et al. Physiological mechanisms for calcium-induced changes in systemic arterial pressure in stable dialysis patients. *Hypertension* 1989;13:213–218.

94. Gabutti L, Bianchi G, Soldini D, et al. Haemodynamic consequences of changing bicarbonate and calcium concentrations in haemodialysis fluids. *Nephrol Dial Transplant* 2009;24:973–981.

95. Henrich W, Hunt J, Nixon J. Increased ionized calcium and left ventricular contractility during hemodialysis. *N Engl J Med* 1984;310:19–23.

96. Lang R, Fellner S, Neumann A, et al. Left ventricular contractility varies directly with blood ionized calcium. *Ann Intern Meds* 1988;108:524–529.

97. Yamada K, Fujimoto S, Nishiura R, et al. Risk factors of the progression of abdominal aortic calcification in patients on chronic haemodialysis. *Nephrol Dial Transplant* 2007;22:2032–2037.

98. Kyriazis J, Katsipi I, Stylianou K, et al. Arterial stiffness alterations during hemodialysis: the role of dialysate calcium. *Nephron Clin Pract* 2007;106:c34–c42.

99. Pun P, Horton J, Middleton J. Dialysate calcium concentration and the risk of sudden cardiac arrest in hemodialysis patients. *Clinical J Am Soc Nephrol* 2013;8:797–803.

100. Monge M, Shahapuni I, Oprisiu R, et al. Reappraisal of 2003 NKF-K/DOQI guidelines for management of hyperparathyroidism in chronic kidney disease patients. *Nat Clin Pract Nephrol* 2006;2:326–336.

101. Cheng S, Coyne D. Vitamin D and outcomes in chronic kidney disease. *Curr Opin Nephrol Hypertens* 2007;16:77–82.

102. DeSoi C, Umans J. Does the dialysis prescription influence phosphate removal? *Semin Dial* 1995;8:201–203.

103. Sam R, Vaseemuddin M, Leong W, et al. Composition and clinical use of hemodialysates. *Hemodial Int* 2006;10:15–28.

104. Kaye M, Vasilevsky M, Barber E. Correction of hypophosphatemia in patients on hemodialysis using a calcium-free dialysate with added phosphate. *Clin Nephrol* 1991;35:130–133.

105. Daugirdas J, Chertow G, Larive B, et al. Effects of frequent hemodialysis on measures of CKD mineral and bone disorder. *J Am Soc Nephrol* 2012;23:727–738.

106. Mateijsen M, van der Wal A, Hendriks P, et al. Vascular and interstitial changes in the peritoneum of CAPD patients with peritoneal sclerosis. *Perit Dial Int* 1999;19:517–525.

107. Davies S, Philips L, Naish P, et al. Peritoneal glucose exposure and changes in membrane solute transport with time on peritoneal dialysis. *J Am Soc Nephrol* 2001;12:1046–1051.

108. Matthys E, Dolkart R, Lameire N. Extended use of a glycerol-containing dialysate in diabetic CAPD patients. *Perit Dial Bull* 1987;7:10–15.

109. Vanholder R, Lameire N. Osmotic agents in peritoneal dialysis. *Kidney Int* 1996;56:S86–S91.

110. Krediet R, Mujais S. Use of icodextrin in high transport ultrafiltration failure. *Kidney Int* 2002;81:S53–S61.

111. Plum J, Gentile S, Verger C, et al. Efficacy and safety of a 7.5% icodextran peritoneal dialysis solution in patients treated with automated peritoneal dialysis. *Am J Kidney Dis* 2002;39:862–871.

112. Davies S, Brown E, Frandsen N, et al. Longitudinal membrane function in functionally anuric patients treated with APD: data from EAPOS on the effects of glucose and icodextrin prescription. *Kidney Int* 2005;67:1609–1615.

113. Kopple J, Bernard D, Messana J, et al. Treatment of malnourished CAPD patients with an amino acid based dialysate. *Kidney Int* 1995;47: 1148–1157.

114. Faller B, Aparicio M, Faict D, et al. Clinical evaluation of an optimized amino-acid solution for peritoneal dialysis. *Nephrol Dial Transplant* 1995;10:1432–1437.

115. Park M, Choi S, Song Y, et al. New insight of amino acid-based dialysis solutions. *Kidney Int* 2006;103:S110–S114.

116. Tijong H, Rietveld T, Wattimena J, et al. Peritoneal dialysis with solutions containing amino acids plus glucose promotes protein synthesis during oral feeding. *Clin J Am Soc Nephron* 2007;2:74–80.

117. Rubin J, Adair C, Johnson B, et al. Stereospecific lactate absorption during peritoneal dialysis. *Nephron* 1982;31:224–228.

118. Coles G. Towards a more physiologic solution for peritoneal dialysis. *Semin Dial* 1995;8:333–335.

119. Jones S, Holmes C, Krediet R, et al. Bicarbonate/lactate-based peritoneal dialysis solution increases cancer antigen 125 and decreases hyaluronic acid levels. *Kidney Int* 2001;59:1529–1538.

120. Jones S, Holmes C, Mackenzie R, et al. Continuous dialysis with bicarbonate/lactate-buffered peritoneal dialysis fluids results in a long-term improvement in ex vivo peritoneal macrophage function. *J Am Soc Nephrol* 2002;13(Suppl 1):97–103.

121. Montenegro J, Saracho R, Gallardo I, et al. Use of pure bicarbonate-buffered peritoneal dialysis fluid reduces the incidence of CAPD peritonitis. *Nephrol Dial Transplant* 2007;22:1703–1708.

122. Ahmad S, Sehmi J, Ahmad-Zakhi K, et al. Impact of new dialysis solutions on peritonitis rates. *Kidney Int* 2006;103:S63–S66.

123. Williams J, Topley N, Craig K, et al. The Euro-Balance Trial: the effect of a new biocompatible peritoneal dialysis fluid (balance) on the peritoneal membrane. *Kidney Int* 2004;66:408–418.

124. Lee H, Park H, Seo B, et al. Superior patient survival for continuous ambulatory peritoneal dialysis patients treated with a peritoneal dialysis fluid with neutral pH and low glucose degradation product concentration (balance). *Perit Dial Int* 2005;25:248–255.

125. Lee H, Choi H, Park H, et al. Changing prescribing practice in CAPD patients in Korea: increased utilization of low GDP solutions improves patient outcome. *Nephrol Dial Transplant* 2006;21:2893–2899.

126. Bargman J. New technologies in peritoneal dialysis. *Clin J Am Soc Nephrol* 2007;2:576–580.

127. Gokal R. Peritoneal dialysis in the 21st century: an analysis of current problems and future developments. *J Am Soc Nephrol* 2002;13: S104–S116.

128. McIntyre C. Update on peritoneal dialysis solutions. *Kidney Int* 2007;71:486–490.

129. Sherrard D, Hercz G, Pei Y, et al. The spectrum of bone disease in end-stage renal failure—an evolving disorder. *Kidney Int* 1993;43:436–442.

130. Haris A, Sherrard D, Hercz G. Reversal of adynamic bone disease by lowering of dialysate calcium. *Kidney Int* 2006;70:931–937

CHAPTER 3

Hemodialysis Vascular Access

Dirk M. Hentschel, Stephen J. Bander, and Steve Schwab

Hemodialysis sustains life in three general circumstances: poisoning, acute kidney injury with kidney failure, and end-stage kidney disease (ESKD). Successful hemodialysis in any of these circumstances requires access to large blood vessels capable of supporting rapid extracorporeal blood flow. Immediate and temporary access to the circulation in acute kidney injury and in poisoning is easily achieved by the percutaneous insertion of dual-lumen dialysis catheters into the femoral, internal jugular, or other large central veins.

The establishment and maintenance of vascular access in ESKD/ chronic kidney disease (CKD), however, provides a greater challenge. Adequate dialytic therapy requires reliable, long-term access to the circulation. Vascular access that is beset with complications exacts considerable morbidity and mortality. Reliable, long-term access to the circulation in ESKD is best achieved by the creation of an autogenous arteriovenous (AV) access [arteriovenous fistula (AVF)]. Less desirable but satisfactory is the placement of a non-autogenous prosthetic or biograft access [arteriovenous graft (AVG)].

When reading this chapter, one should not lose sight of the fact that careful preparation for autogenous access creation begins well before the need for hemodialysis and is often the single most important step that the nephrologist can take to ensure long-term, low-maintenance access to the circulation, as tunneled hemodialysis catheters (TCs), while used in the majority of patients for initiation of dialysis, can often lead to severe infections as well as central vein stenosis and occlusion.

Vascular access care in the United States falls into many hands. General, vascular, or transplant surgeons place AVFs, AVGs, and TCs and often perform endovascular procedures to treat access complications. Interventional radiologists are predominantly concerned with placement of TCs and the endovascular treatment of access complications such as stenoses and thromboses. More recently, nephrologists with training in endovascular or surgical

procedures have begun to provide access care to dialysis patients. Management of vascular access raises important questions regarding the quality of care that is delivered to patient with ESKD with so many physicians contributing. How good are we at doing what we are doing? Unfortunately, prospective randomized controlled studies in this field are rare, and we often rely on opinion and small retrospective trials. It remains the challenge to the practicing nephrologists to become knowledgeable conductors of hemodialysis care for their patients.

◆ BRIEF HISTORY OF VASCULAR ACCESS

The history of vascular access for hemodialysis is closely tied to the history of dialysis. In 1924, Georg Haas in Giessen, Germany, performed the first hemodialysis treatments in humans. It lasted for 15 minutes, and he used glass needles to access the radial artery and return blood into the cubital vein (1). In a total of 11 treatments in uremic patients until 1929, Haas used fractionated dialysis to clear approximately 400 mL of blood at a time. The artificial kidney was made up of three glass cylinders with U-shaped collodion tubes. Willem Kolff, a young physician from Kampen, The Netherlands, with the support of H. Berk in 1943 developed a "rotating drum kidney" with larger surface area of the filter made of a cellophane membrane. The first patient he dialyzed was a 29-year-old housemaid with CKD. She underwent 12 dialysis treatments, but the therapy had to be stopped as each cannula placement required a cut down to the artery and she ran out of access sites (2). In 1946, Kolff came to the United States and after a time in New York came to Boston, where he worked with John P. Merril and Carl Walter to construct the "Brigham Artificial Kidney."

The challenge of repetitive vascular access prevented dialysis from becoming a routine method for the treatment of chronic kidney insufficiency. This changed dramatically in the 1960s. Building on the idea of Nils Alwall (Lund, Sweden) to connect artery and vein with rubber tubing and a glass cannula, Quinton et al. (3) developed in Seattle an AV Teflon shunt. Their first patient, Clyde Shields, a Boeing machinist, survived for over 10 years after the insertion of his first Teflon AV shunt in March 1960. The tapered ends of two thin-walled Teflon cannulas were inserted into the radial artery and the adjacent cephalic vein in the distal forearm. While not on dialysis, the external ends were connected by a curved Teflon bypass tube, which was later replaced by a more flexible silicon rubber tubing. As with the availability of cellophane for the earliest artificial kidneys and heparin to maintain anticoagulation, the invention of Teflon and silicon allowed for new medical devices.

In 1966, Brescia et al. (4) (all New York) published their landmark account of 14 side-to-side anastomoses between the radial artery and the cephalic vein at the wrist, the native AVF was born. One year later, Sperling et al. (5) (Würzburg, Germany) presented 15 patients with end-to-end anastomoses, and in 1968, Lars Röhl et al. (6) (Heidelberg, Germany) presented results from 30 patients with radial-artery side-to-vein-end anastomoses. The different anastomosis techniques each fit specific anatomic needs and physiologic considerations. Another example is the Gracz fistula (7) presented in 1977, and modified by Klaus Konner (8), a proximal forearm fistula, that relies on the perforating vein from the superficial to the deep forearm venous system to limit blood flow in the fistula and prevent steal in patients with peripheral artery disease due to age, hypertension, or diabetes.

The Teflon shunt is an early example of an implanted medical device, partly internal, partly external. In 1961, Stanley Shaldon (London, United Kingdom) unable to find a surgeon to place the cannulae necessary for dialysis, inserted catheters into the femoral artery and vein with the Seldinger technique (9,10). Since then, catheters as a dialysis device have evolved to be placed with a cutaneous tunnel in which a Dacron cuff at the catheter's neck ensures secure placement and a relative seal against microorganisms.

Material sciences have continued to evolve the development of grafts for use in hemodialysis. In 1969, George Thomas (11) (Seattle) attached Dacron patches to the common femoral artery and vein, which were then connected with a silastic tube and brought to the surface of the anterior thigh. The Thomas shunt was soon replaced by the arrival of the expanded polytetrafluoroethylene (PTFE) graft, as LD Baker (12) (Phoenix) in 1976 presented first results in 72 hemodialysis patients. The PTFE graft has remained the graft material of choice, although grafts made of biologic material have been available since 1972 (13). More recent strategies are aiming at drug-eluting grafts to enhance the functional life of the access (14) and tissue-engineered blood vessels from autogenous fibroblasts and endothelial cells (15).

In parallel with the advances in surgical techniques and material science, the diagnostic armamentarium of physicians concerned with vascular access care has expanded dramatically. Most of this technology centers on minimally invasive imaging and endovascular procedures. Seldinger's idea of an endovascular guidewire over which diagnostic and therapeutic devices can be positioned is the basis for much of this development (9). In 1972 and 1973, Thelen et al. (16) and Staple (17) independently from each other described the angiographic retrograde imaging of AVFs in hemodialysis patients. David Ergun in 1979 first described a computerized fluoroscopy technique that revolutionized noninvasive cardiovascular imaging (18) and is now widely used in the diagnostic and

therapeutic evaluation of dialysis accesses. Dotter et al. (19) and Grüntzig et al. (20) advanced the use of catheter-guided balloon angioplasty, that in 1982 found its first documented use in hemodialysis AVFs and AVGs by Gordon et al. (21).

Providers of hemodialysis care into the 1990s were predominantly access surgeons with vascular, transplant, or general subspecialization and interventional radiologists. This left many of the growing number of dialysis patients in the United States without dedicated access care, and other types of procedures and patients often trumped their interventions. It was into this void that the nephrologists such as Steve Schwab and Gerald Beathard stepped by acquired expertise in dialysis access procedures, documenting equal or superior outcomes compared to established care (22–28), in turn creating interventional nephrology as a distinct clinical field.

⬢ VASCULAR ACCESS FOR ACUTE DIALYSIS

Nontunneled dual-lumen central venous catheters are the most available form of vascular access for acute dialytic therapy. Central venous catheters can be inserted at the bedside using the Seldinger technique with ultrasound guidance and may support extracorporeal blood-flow rates greater than 300 mL/min. Separation of the arterial and venous ports minimizes recirculation of blood. Central venous catheters may be used for conventional intermittent hemodialysis as well as continuous renal replacement therapies.

The National Kidney Foundation Dialysis Access Guidelines recommend nontunneled hemodialysis catheters for hemodialysis duration of less than 1 week in acute kidney injury because of the increased infection risk compared with tunneled hemodialysis catheters. Unlike time-limited and relative predictable episodes for intoxications requiring dialysis, recovery from acute kidney injury with need for dialysis is very difficult to predict. In fact, only a minority of patients recover renal function in less than 1 week (29). For this reason, we primarily place tunneled catheters in patients with acute kidney injury, unless the patient is too unstable for transport to the procedure suite or has other contraindications to insertion of a tunneled catheter.

Catheter Materials

Currently on the market available are polyurethane and silicone catheters. Polyurethane catheters are relatively rigid at room temperature allowing bedside insertion, and their softness at body temperature minimizes the risk of vein perforation during prolonged catheterization (30).

Although silicone is the softest and least thrombogenic material, its softness necessitates the use of a peel-away sheath or internal stylets for percutaneous insertion (31). Insertion of silicone catheters by internal or external jugular venotomy is an alternative approach.

Acute Catheter Insertion Sites

Dual-lumen hemodialysis catheters may be inserted into the femoral or internal jugular vein. Because subclavian vein catheter placement may lead to subclavian vein stenosis, subclavian vein catheters should not be placed in patients who will ultimately require fistula creation for chronic hemodialysis.

Femoral Vein

Cannulation of the femoral vein should be performed under ultrasound guidance; instructional videos for insertion technique have been published online (32). Femoral vein cannulation is an invaluable technique for patients with pulmonary edema because it may be performed with the patient in the semirecumbent position. The femoral vein is cannulated immediately below the inguinal ligament as with increasing distance from the inguinal ligament the femoral artery is found more frequently overlying the femoral vein such that attempts to puncture the femoral vein distally leads to higher complications (33). As in obese patients, the inguinal fold is often more distal than the inguinal ligament; its location has to be carefully determined by feeling for the bony landmarks, medially the pubic tubercle, laterally the anterior superior iliac spine. Usually the abdomen has to be moved cranially and taped in place for safe access to the vein. External rotation of the leg increases total and accessible femoral vein diameter and decreases surfaces depth (34). In patients with bleeding diathesis, the initial puncture can be performed using the 21G needle of a micropuncture kit and then increase the guidewire from 0.018 inches to the usually used 0.035 inches wire in the dialysis catheter kit.

The incidence of life-threatening complications is lower for femoral vein cannulation than for internal jugular vein cannulation. Complications of femoral vein cannulation include ileofemoral vein thrombosis, AVF, retroperitoneal hemorrhage from vein perforation, and hemorrhage from accidental puncture of the femoral artery. Using ultrasound guidance increases success of the procedure (risk of failure reduced by 90%) as well as shortens procedure time, while the risk of arterial puncture and hematoma formation are fourfold reduced (35). Patients with femoral vein catheters must remain at bed rest in the hospital. In intensive care unit (ICU) patients with body mass index <28.5, femoral vein catheter colonization rates are comparable or lower than internal jugular vein catheters, while slightly higher in more obese patients, but overall comparable (**FIGURE 3.1**) (36). This observation has been confirmed for nontunneled catheters used in the ICU in general (37) as well as in subsequent studies of dialysis catheters (38). Catheter infections appear to

be a random effect and not related to a threshold time beyond which a catheter has been in place as colonization of removed catheter in the same large randomized prospective study (36) was in fact higher for catheters removed within 5 days than those removed after 5 days.

The length of the femoral dialysis catheter is important and should be 24 cm or longer to place the catheter tip in the inferior vena cava as otherwise recirculation increases significantly (39).

Subclavian Vein

Subclavian vein catheterization may lead to subclavian vein stenosis, precluding fistula placement in the ipsilateral arm. As mentioned previously, subclavian vein catheters should not be placed in patients for whom chronic hemodialysis is anticipated. Recent guidelines discourage this technique regardless of anticipated duration of use.

Internal Jugular Vein

Ultrasound-guided insertion of internal jugular vein catheters is associated with high success and very low complications rates (35). Traditionally, due to relative stiffness of nontunneled hemodialysis catheters, the recommended target tip position for internal jugular vein catheters has been the superior vena cava to avoid atrial perforations. Typically 13- to 16-cm-long catheters are used for right-sided insertions, and 16 to 20 cm catheters for left-sided insertions. A recent randomized trial of longer, soft silicone nontunneled catheters targeting the right atrium for tip position documented improved dialyzer life span as well as increased dialysis dose for continuous renal replacement therapy in the ICU (40) without increasing atrial arrhythmias. Risk of local hematoma formation as well as vein thrombosis is higher for internal jugular than femoral vein catheters.

Duration of Temporary Catheter Use

Temporary catheters achieve lower blood-flow rates than other types of permanent vascular access. The 2006 update of the National Kidney Foundation/Kidney Disease Outcomes Quality Initiative (NKF/KDOQI) Clinical Practice Guidelines for Vascular Access (41) recommend limiting use of nontunneled internal jugular vein catheters to 1 week because of the high incidence of infection. Other risks include inadvertent removal, hemorrhage, air embolism, and patient discomfort, all of which are increased with temporary catheters (42). Plans should be made to convert all temporary catheters to a permanent access if use is expected to exceed 1 week (43). For most instances of acute kidney injury requiring renal replacement therapy, insertion of a tunneled hemodialysis catheter is preferred as the primary access modality (29). In some clinical settings where tunneled dialysis catheters are not available or too costly, nontunneled dialysis catheters have been used in conjunction with antibacterial ointments at the exit site for over 30 days with fewer than two infections per 1,000 catheter days (44), and nontunneled catheters may even be used to bridge the time until fistula maturation using antibiotic lock solutions (45). Given the stiffer nature of these temporary catheters, increased central vein stenoses seem likely, but data are lacking, and the use of nontunneled catheters beyond 1 to 2 weeks is strongly discouraged where tunneled catheters are available.

Complications of Central Vein Cannulation

Insertion Complications

Landmark-guided insertion complications become less likely as the operator gains experience (46). The incidence of serious insertion complications is higher for subclavian vein and internal jugular vein cannulation than for femoral vein cannulation (47). **TABLE 3.1** lists

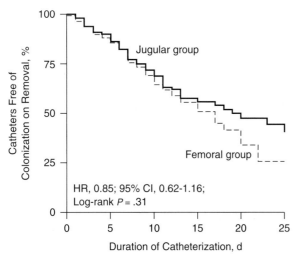

No. at risk

Femoral group	324	176	71	23	11
Jugular group	313	178	75	34	22

FIGURE 3.1 Colonization of catheter at time of removal in jugular and femoral vein insertion groups. [From Parienti JJ, Thirion M, Mégarbane B, et al. Femoral vs jugular venous catheterization and risk of nosocomial events in adults requiring acute renal replacement therapy: a randomized controlled trial. *JAMA* 2008;299(20):2413–2422.]

TABLE 3.1	**Acute Hemodialysis Catheter Insertion Complications**

Atrial and ventricular dysrhythmias
Arterial puncture
Hemothorax
Pneumothorax
Air embolism
Perforation of central vein or cardiac chamber
Pericardial tamponade

the most common insertion complications, which have markedly decreased with the transition from landmark techniques to ultrasound guidance.

Atrial arrhythmias may result from endocardial irritation by the guidewire or catheter but are generally of limited clinical significance (48). Ventricular arrhythmias occur in approximately 20% of patients but rarely require therapy (49).

Inadvertent arterial puncture is a common insertion complication. Manual pressure will prevent significant hematoma from femoral artery and carotid artery puncture, even in patients with bleeding diatheses (50). Although serious hemorrhage complicates less than 1% of subclavian vein catheterization attempts (42,51), we do not recommend attempts at subclavian vein catheterization in patients with coagulopathies or severe thrombocytopenia because of the difficulty of applying direct manual pressure to the subclavian artery.

To minimize the chance of fatal pneumothorax, two rules must be followed:

1. The operator should never attempt cannulation of the subclavian vein ipsilateral to the only healthy lung.
2. Even an unsuccessful attempt at subclavian or internal jugular cannulation may still lead to pneumothorax. A chest radiograph should be obtained before cannulation of the contralateral subclavian is attempted.

Perforations of the superior vena cava or cardiac chamber may lead to hemothorax, mediastinal hemorrhage, pericardial tamponade, and death (51). These complications are rare but are more likely following subclavian vein cannulation than following internal jugular vein cannulation, perhaps because of the curved path that a subclavian catheter must follow. To minimize the chance of perforation during insertion, the operator must never advance the catheter without protection by a J-tipped guidewire. A chest radiograph must be obtained following insertion to confirm that the catheter is within a central vein and exclude pneumothorax. If the catheter tip is in the right atrium, the catheter should be pulled back to prevent right atrial perforation. Prolonged catheterization may lead to erosion and perforation of the superior vena cava; pericardial tamponade should be considered in the hypotensive hemodialysis patient with a central venous dialysis catheter.

Air embolism rarely complicates central vein cannulation (51), but care should be taken to avoid accidental introduction of air through the introducer needle, dilator, or catheter.

Injuries to the brachial plexus (52), trachea (53), and recurrent laryngeal nerve (54) are rare complications of internal jugular vein cannulation.

Use of ultrasonographic guidance during catheter insertion decreases complications and should be used (55,56). Ultrasonographic confirmation of target vein patency before cannulation prevents futile attempts at cannulation of thrombosed veins. In addition, the

TABLE 3.2	**Prevention of Acute Hemodialysis Catheter Infection**

Skin disinfection with 2% aqueous chlorhexidine at the time of insertion
Sound sterile insertion technique using barriers, gowns, and masks
Skin disinfection with chlorhexidine or povidone-iodine solution at each hemodialysis treatment
Application of povidone-iodine ointment or mupirocin ointment to the catheter insertion site at each dressing change
Dry gauze dressings
Use of face shield or surgical mask by patients and nurses during connection and disconnection procedures
Limited duration of catheterization

introducer needle may be inserted under direct ultrasonographic visualization. Fewer needle passes are required for successful cannulation when the ultrasonographic device is used (35). Recent guidelines strongly encourage this technique.

Infection

The mechanism of infection is migration of bacteria from the patient's skin through the catheter insertion site and down the outer surface of the catheter or even more common contamination of the catheter lumen during hemodialysis (57). Rarely, infection is caused by infusion of infected solutions. The use of chlorhexidine-impregnated dressing at the exit site prevents catheter colonization as well as catheter-related bloodstream infections (58). Nontunneled catheter infection rates are higher for femoral than internal jugular and then subclavian vein catheters (59): 1.5, 3.6, and 4.6 infections per 1,000 catheter days in one recent large randomized controlled study (47) with the mean length of catheter use of 5 days.

Bacterial isolates associated with catheter colonization and catheter-related bacteremia (CRB) reflect the location of the catheter. While typical skin flora, such as *Staphylococcus epidermidis*, is most prevalent for any catheter site, gram-negative isolates are more common for femoral vein catheters (36).

Evidence of exit-site infection, even in the absence of systemic symptoms, should prompt catheter removal. Exit-site infection presages bacteremia, presumably because the absence of a cuff permits migration of bacteria along the tunnel and outer surface of the catheter.

Other preventive measures are listed in **TABLE 3.2**. Disinfection with 2% aqueous chlorhexidine at the time of insertion is preferred to disinfection with povidone-iodine or isopropyl alcohol (60,61). Careful attention to use of maximal sterile barrier precautions during catheter insertion or guidewire exchange is recommended (**TABLE 3.3**) (62). Hemodialysis catheters should not be used for infusions or blood sampling, but temporary catheter designs with

TABLE 3.3	**Maximal Sterile Barrier Precautions for Catheter Insertion and Exchange**

Large sterile sheet
Sterile gown
Sterile gloves
Hair cover
Face mask
New sterile gloves to handle new catheter for exchange

a third access port for blood sampling and infusions are available. After catheter placement and at the end of each hemodialysis treatment, the skin should be disinfected using chlorhexidine or povidone-iodine solution (63). An antimicrobial ointment, mupirocin or Polysporin, applied to the catheter exit site reduces infections (44,64,65), and antibiotic lock solutions such as a mixture of cefazolin (10 mg/mL), gentamicin (5 mg/mL), and heparin (10,000 U/mL) can reduce catheter associated infections (45) with catheter infection rate very similar to tunneled catheters over an initial 30- to 60-day period. Lastly, a dry gauze dressing or a semipermeable transparent dressing should be applied at each hemodialysis treatment rather than an occlusive dressing (66,67).

Adherence to the Centers for Disease Control and Prevention guidelines (68) for hand hygiene is low in both acute and chronic hemodialysis units (69). Aseptic technique during access handling, including use of a surgical mask for staff and patients, and adherence to hand hygiene guidelines decrease the risk for catheter-related infection (62).

A febrile hemodialysis patient with a central venous catheter should be presumed to have CRB unless there is strong evidence to the contrary. Rigors are especially suggestive of bacteremia. Blood cultures should be obtained, the catheter removed, and antibiotics administered. A new catheter may be placed once the patient defervesces. Antibiotic therapy should be continued for 2 to 3 weeks. In the event of metastatic infection (e.g., vertebral osteomyelitis or endocarditis), a longer course of antibiotic therapy will be required.

Catheter Thrombosis

Intracatheter thrombus impedes extracorporeal blood flow. Treatment consists of instilling reconstituted alteplase [recombinant human tissue plasminogen activator (tPA)] (or similar agent) in the affected catheter lumens for 30 to 120 minutes (70). This procedure may be repeated if necessary or tPA left in the catheter overnight. The slow leaking of tPA from the catheter may assist in lysing thrombus that may have formed around the catheter.

If catheter occlusion persists, catheter exchange may be performed using a J-tipped guidewire. We use a method where after careful cleaning of the skin and catheter, the sterile drape is applied such that the catheter ports are outside the sterile field. The catheter is then carefully retracted 2 to 4 cm, clamped just at the skin level, and cut 1 cm from the clamp. The guidewire is passed into the catheter while manually compressing the catheter. This approach uses a catheter segment that was inside the patient and reduces contamination from passing through and handling of the catheter ports which are difficult to sterilize effectively.

Extracatheter or mural thrombosis is a less frequent but more serious complication (71). Clinically symptomatic vessel thrombosis is most frequent with femoral vein catheters (47); however, the overall incidence is between 0.5% and 1.4%. Treatment of symptomatic central venous thrombosis should include systemic anticoagulation. If the catheter is still needed, it remains in its position but should be removed if not further necessary. In critically ill patients in the ICU, there is often a multitude of catheters, and possible cardiac device leads crowding the central veins, and removal of a catheter at one site and insertion into another may just lead to a second site of thrombosis.

Central Vein Stenosis

Subclavian vein stenosis may occur after placement of subclavian dialysis catheters (72–74), while central vein stenosis occurs less commonly after placement of internal jugular vein catheters (75–77). Arm edema is the presenting complaint of most central vein stenoses. As blood-flow rates in each of the subclavian veins is in the range of

100 to 250 mL/min, and 250 to 500 mL/min in the brachiocephalic veins, it is often only after the creation of an ipsilateral AV access with additional flow rates of 500 to 2,500 mL/min that clinical symptoms develop. This can be an immediate or a delayed occurrence, and in some cases, central vein stenoses develop and become apparent without prior cannulation of the central veins. Formation of venous collaterals can alleviate symptoms over time. While the exact pathogenesis of symptomatic central vein stenoses has not yet been determined conclusively, any form of vein injury and increased blood-flow rates seem to contribute and exacerbate each other.

VASCULAR ACCESS FOR CHRONIC HEMODIALYSIS

According to the most recent United States Renal Data System (USRDS) data collection, at the end of 2013, there were 466,607 prevalent dialysis patients in the United States, a 63.2% increase since 2000. The incidence of new dialysis patient in 2013 was 113,944, 24% larger than in 2000 (78); 90.8% of incident ESKD patient received hemodialysis, necessitating an autogenous AV access (AVF), a non-autogenous (prosthetic or biograft) AV access (AVG), or TC to provide access to high-volume blood flow. Successful hemodialysis procedures require adequate performance of any of these access options.

The ESKD population remains at less than 1% of the Medicare population but accounts for about 5.6% of Medicare spending in 2013. Costs for Medicare patient with an AVF are lower than for patients with a tunneled catheter or graft, and per person per year access event costs are also highest for graft, and higher for catheters than AVFs (USRDS 2010) (79). Creating and maintaining functional access for the large and growing number of dialysis patients poses economic challenges. One may speculate that these costs will rise out of proportion as diabetes and hypertension both affect the peripheral vasculature with potential detriment to long-term access options and increased vascular access complications. Vascular access remains the Achilles heel of chronic hemodialysis. Vascular access that is beset with complications is costly to both the patient and society; vascular access failure has been the most frequent cause of hospitalization for patients with ESKD/CKD; however, the availability of outpatient access centers has markedly reduced the need for admission. The primary AVF is the form of vascular access most likely to provide long-term complication-free vascular access. The importance of careful preparation for primary AVF placement months before the need for hemodialysis cannot be overemphasized.

Types of Permanent Vascular Access

There are three general types of long-term vascular access: tunneled hemodialysis catheters, autogenous AV accesses (AVF), and non-autogenous (prosthetic or biograft) AV accesses (AVG). The nomenclature for dialysis accesses follows the Society of Vascular Surgery (SVS) definitions. A tunneled catheter is named after the vessel it enters; for example, internal jugular vein tunneled hemodialysis catheter. For AVF site of use (forearm, upper arm, thigh, etc.), the originating artery and the connecting vein are used as well as an indication that this is an autogenous, transposed, or translocated access; for example, upper arm brachial-cephalic autogenous access for an AVF that connects the upper arm cephalic vein with the brachial artery (80).

Tunneled Cuffed Catheters

In 2013, more than 80% of patients initiating dialysis in the United States were using a tunneled hemodialysis catheter (78). The proportion of TC users decreased to 68.3% at 90 days and 20% at 1 year.

Overall mortality of patients using a tunneled catheter is higher than for those using an AVF or AVG for dialysis (81,82).

Subcutaneous ports connected to catheters were used for several years in the United States as part of the LifeSite Hemodialysis Access System (83–86). However, this device was removed from the market after several cases of skin breakdown and infection around the device access site.

Catheters for acute dialysis are made of the relatively rigid polyethylene, while TCs are made of silicone, polyurethane, or Carbothane (polyurethane/polycarbonate copolymers). Silicone catheters are very soft, require a larger wall thickness to prevent collapse, and are greatly weakened by iodine, and for these reasons are rarely used. Polyurethane has high material strength, which allows for thinner catheter walls and therefore thinner catheters with equal flow characteristics, and is also less thrombogenic than silicone (30). However, polyurethane is weakened by alcohol, which today is the preferred catheter cleansing solution. Carbothane combines the exceptional material advantages of polyurethane with even greater strength and tolerance of alcohol, iodine, and peroxide cleaning solutions (87).

For two decades, subclavian placement of dialysis catheters was the preferred route (88); however, this has now been abandoned, as venograms revealed the frequent presence of severe stenosis or venous occlusion at the site of subclavian cannulation. Internal and external jugular vein insertion is preferred over femoral, inferior vena cava, and transhepatic catheters. Subclavian vein insertion is only a last resort. More recently, inside-out placement of tunneled catheters, similar to cardiac lead placement, from the right atrial appendix through the anterior mediastinum (89) or the junction of brachiocephalic-subclavian vein (90) with percutaneous exit in the subclavian region has been demonstrated for patients with total occlusion of the chest central veins.

TC insertion can be achieved either be conversion of an existing nontunneled catheter (43) or by *de novo* insertion. Right-sided TC insertion is preferred as the catheter has a more direct passage into the right atrium with fewer wall contacts and better function (91). With each heartbeat, the catheter moves, and a left-sided TC will have two to three wall contact points, eliciting endothelial injury and potentially initiating a process of progressive central vein stenosis and occlusion. Tunneled catheters should be inserted using ultrasound and fluoroscopic guidance. Methods have been published for insertion of tunneled catheters without fluoroscopy (92), but success rates are lower, and the risk for major injury to large vascular structures as well as the pericardium through dilators and valved sheath is higher. We do not recommend insertion of tunneled catheters without real-time fluoroscopic guidance.

Technical details of the tunneled catheter insertion procedure are beyond the scope of this chapter. However, there are several procedural circumstances, knowledge of which aids the general nephrologist diagnosis and care of the patient with a TC.

The catheter should be sutured to skin at the wings of the catheter. Sutures that attach to the skin at the exit site irritate the skin and may facilitate exit site infections and protrusion of the catheter cuff. The cuff of the catheter should be positioned within 1 to 1.5 cm of the exit site to allow easy removal and exchange of the catheter while at the same time minimizing the length of the catheter segment that is colonized by skin flora between cuff and skin. Sutures that are tied circumferentially around the catheter body have the potential to constrict the catheter leading to dysfunction and facilitate cuff extrusion (**FIGURE 3.2**). This may present as an immediate catheter dysfunction on the day of insertion. The catheter cuff

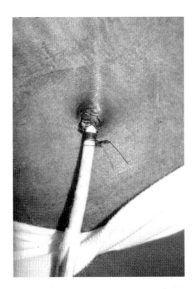

FIGURE 3.2 Catheter tunnel and exit sites: exit-site suture with skin irritation and exposed cuff.

should be fully attached after 3 to 4 weeks, and the wing sutures can be removed if they irritate the patient's skin.

The catheter tip should be positioned in the right atrium when the patient is recumbent during catheter insertion for a particular reason: TCs are encased in a fibrinous sheath in their course through the skin ("tunneled segment") as well as in the intravascular lumen. The only fix point for the catheter is the Dacron cuff which is fixed to the skin by invading skin cells and firmly connected to the fibrinous sheath of the tunneled segment. When sitting or standing, the tissue fixed to the cuff usually follows gravity to a more dependent location pulling up the catheter tip as much as the cuff moves downward. This effect is more pronounced in patients with voluminous breast tissue. The exit site should be in the lateral segment of clavicle and not more than 3 to 5 cm below its lower margin as elastic stretch of skin adds to catheter tip movement. Tunneled catheters support bidirectional 400 to 450 mL/min blood-flow rates (800 to 900 mL/min total volume moved). Recirculation is increased if these flow volumes are exchanged in the superior vena cava or the brachiocephalic veins rather than the right atrium. In addition, prolonged exposure of the relatively narrow brachiocephalic vein and superior vena cava to large blood-flow volumes leads to stenosis at the site of the catheter tips. This may be an effect of the mechanical injury by catheter tips, jet-like fluid propulsion or suction of the vessel wall, as well as presence of catheter-tethered thrombus. For all these reasons, catheter tip position in the right atrium is preferred.

Several catheter tip designs have been developed to reduce recirculation and allow high flow into the catheter tips: split tips, step tip, symmetric tip, and centrally angled tips. During episodes of catheter dysfunction (see the following texts for more in depth discussion), catheters are often used in reversed configuration, which increases recirculation in all but symmetric tip catheters. Colored dye video studies revealed that only symmetric tip catheters had negligible changes in recirculation when used in a reversed configuration (93). In patients with central vein stenosis or occlusion who are tunneled catheter–dependent, the available space for the catheter tip is shortened, and symmetric-tip catheters are more suitable to function in 2 to 3 cm shorter spaces.

Catheter diameter and length both influence venous and arterial pump pressure with a given blood flow; there is partial collapse of the arterial lumen and expansion of the venous lumen, such that the fraction of delivered flow in catheters decreases with increasing absolute flow rates (91,93). This effect is less pronounced in larger diameter catheters (#15.5 or #16 French vs. #14.5 French) and more pronounced in longer catheters, such as femoral vein or translumbar catheters.

Catheter Dysfunction

Catheter dysfunction can be categorized as early (within the first 4 weeks) and late (after 4 weeks) and, in addition, as static (the catheter has no or minimal aspiration but may be flushable) and dynamic (arterial or venous pressure alarms when blood-flow rates are increased beyond a threshold too low to deliver sufficient clearance, <200 mL/min).

Early dysfunction is usually related to tip position and other technical issues associated with the insertion of the catheter. Immediately after catheter insertion, circumferential sutures around the catheter and fixed at or around the exit site can—either in the context of procedural tissue edema or gravitational pull—constrict the catheter. This type of dysfunction can be treated by cutting the constricting suture and placing new sutures through the catheter wings. Posteroanterior and lateral chest x-ray images, if possible in recumbent and sitting position, are used to evaluate the catheter tip position and confirm that is in the right atrium and not outside vascular structures or in the azygous or hemiazygous vein. If the catheter tip position is not in a position consistent with the superior vena cava or right atrium, a chest computed tomography or fluoroscopic evaluation with contrast dye are necessary to determine location of the catheter and guide further treatment steps. Catheter tips that are retracted into the central veins usually present with early dynamic dysfunction, while catheter tips outside the vessel do not allow for fluid removal (early static).

Late static dysfunction is usually due to intracatheter formation of thrombus. Any fill solution in the catheter lumen very effectively leaks out of the catheter and blood mixes into the catheter (95) within hours after application due to the large diameter of the catheter and differences in viscosity between blood and typically used fill solutions. This type of endoluminal thrombus is very effectively treated by instilling 2 mg tPA into the catheter lumina (96).

Late dynamic dysfunction is usually seen in the context of a fibrinous sheath and catheter-associated thrombus (97). Guidewire-assisted exchange of the tunneled catheter with balloon disruption of the fibrinous sheath is very effective in treating this type of catheter dysfunction. An alternate strategy for sheath removal is stripping it with a gooseneck snare that is passed through a common femoral vein sheath into the right atrium. The snare encircles the catheter and strips away the fibrin sheath as it is retracted (**FIGURE 3.3**) (98).

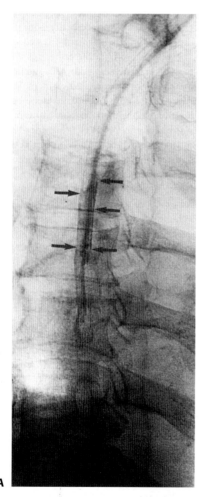 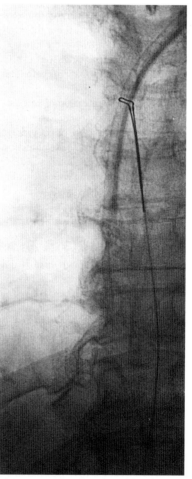

FIGURE 3.3 The catheter fibrinous sheath (arrows) is stripped by advancing a transfemoral snare over a guidewire placed through the catheter port and advanced into the inferior vena cava (**A**). The snare is repeatedly retracted with mild closing force around the catheter (**B**).

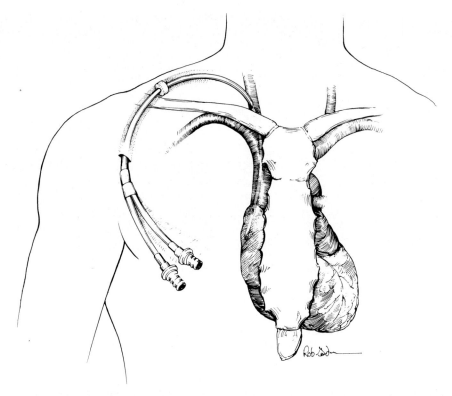

FIGURE 3.4 Cuffed double-lumen silastic catheter inserted through a subcutaneous tunnel into the right internal jugular vein. (From Schwab SJ, Buller GL, McCann RL, et al. Prospective evaluation of a Dacron cuffed hemodialysis catheter for prolonged use. *Am J Kidney Dis* 1988;11:166–169, with permission.)

Cuffed Tunneled Catheter Infection

There are four compartments in a tunneled catheter, each of which may become infected: the exit site, the subcutaneous tunnel, the intravascular segment of the catheter with its associated fibrinous sheath, and intra-atrial organized thrombus attached to the catheter (**FIGURE 3.4**). Indwelling catheters are seen to be colonized within 48 hours when the catheter surface is examined with electron microscopy (99). Infections during the first 10 days after catheter insertions are usually considered to come from the outer surface of the catheter (contamination during insertion procedure or migration along the catheter from the skin), while infections 30 days or more after insertion are considered to originate from the inner surface biofilm. Usually there is colonization of the biofilm prior to bacteremia and clinical symptoms (100).

Exit Site

Exit-site infections (**FIGURE 3.5**) are more common than CRB episodes, by some accounts 50% more, and over 90% are successfully treated with systemic antibiotics as well as local exit site (91). Prophylaxis of exit-site colonization to prevent infections has been evaluated. Johnson et al. (65) demonstrated that application of 2% mupirocin ointment to tunneled catheter exit sites significantly decreased rates of staphylococcal exit-site infections and bacteremias. A potential problem associated with mupirocin prophylaxis is the appearance of resistant staphylococcal strains (101,102). Using Polysporin ointment for tunneled catheter exit-site prophylaxis, Lok et al. (64) demonstrated decreased catheter-related infections and decreased mortality. A preliminary study has shown that application of antibacterial honey (MEDIHONEY) to catheter exit sites is as effective as mupirocin in decreasing catheter-related

infections (103). When choosing to apply ointments at the skin exit site, the carrier bases have to be compatible with the catheter material as otherwise focal deterioration may be caused (**FIGURE 3.6**). A dry gauze dressing or a semipermeable transparent dressing should be used to dress the catheter exit site (66,67). Occlusive dressings should be avoided; they trap any drainage and create a moist environment at the exit site. If the integrity of an exit site appears compromised without infection of the tunnel segment (see **FIGURE 3.5**), then the catheter can be exchanged with retunneling to a new

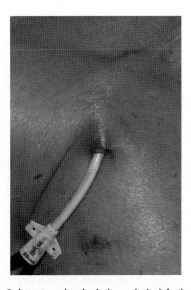

FIGURE 3.5 Catheter tunnel and exit sites: exit-site infection.

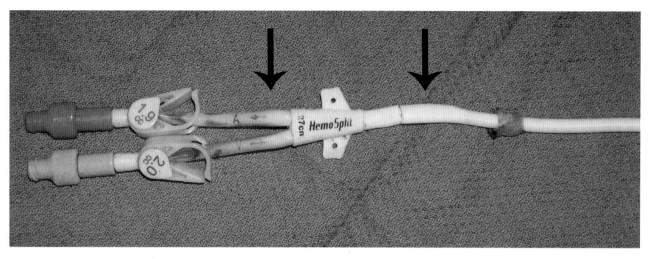

FIGURE 3.6 Catheter segments exposed repeatedly to antimicrobial ointment show dilatation and softening of the tunneled catheters (*arrows*).

exit site away from the infected area. This procedure requires a cut down on the catheter tunnel near the neck vein insertion site.

Catheter Tunnel

Infections of the tunneled catheter (**FIGURE 3.7**) require removal of the catheter and insertion of a new catheter, usually on the contralateral side as there often is some degree of cellulitis around the inflamed tunnel segment. As there is continuity of the skin tunnel into the endovascular fibrinous sheath, systemic antibiotics should be used for 2 to 3 weeks similar to a CRB. Blood culture and cultures of purulent material expressed during the catheter removal should be sent to narrow antibiotic treatment after initial coverage for gram-positive and gram-negative organisms. The choice of the initial combination depends on local patterns of drug resistance but usually includes vancomycin and a third- or fourth-generation cephalosporin.

Endovascular Segment and Fibrinous Sheath

Infection of the endovascular catheter segment is associated with CRB which is common in patients using a dialysis catheter, and the presence of a catheter is a major risk factor for bacteremia among hemodialysis patients (104,105). The relative risk for infection-related death is increased twofold to threefold among catheter-dependent hemodialysis patients compared to those using fistulas or grafts (106,107). The frequency of CRB reported in several large series ranges from 0.8 to 5.5 cases per 1,000 patient days or 0.9 to 2.0 episodes per patient-year (108,109). This wide range likely reflects differences in practice patterns as rates of bacteremia as low as 1/1,000 days at risk have been achieved with detailed catheter protocols (110). Infection is a common reason for catheter removal and morbidity in dialysis patients (108,110). Bacteremia can result in life-threatening complications, including septic shock, endocarditis, septic arthritis, osteomyelitis, or epidural abscess.

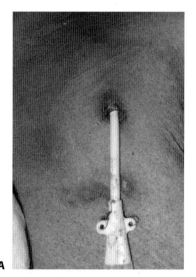 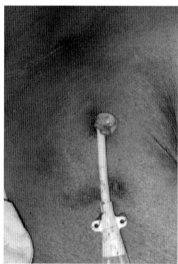

A
B

FIGURE 3.7 Catheter tunnel and exit sites: tunnel infection **(A)** revealing pus extrusion from exit site with massage along tunnel tract **(B)**. Note that cuff is not sealing the exit site any more.

Bacteremia should be suspected when a hemodialysis patient with a catheter develops fever and chills. Paired quantitative blood cultures from the peripheral blood and the catheter are the most accurate for diagnosing CRB (111). This is not routinely performed in outpatient units because of the difficulty in peripheral venous sticks in hemodialysis patients. In the absence of concurrent blood cultures from the catheter and a peripheral vein, a clinical diagnosis of CRB requires exclusion of alternate sources of infection (108). However, bacteremia will often lead to seeding of endovascular devices such that exchange of a tunneled catheter during successful treatment of bacteremia from a different source is reasonable, in particular for *Staphylococcus aureus*. Blood cultures should be obtained from the catheter 1 to 2 weeks after completion of antibiotics for non-CRB to ascertain that the catheter has not been colonized.

Catheter-Related Bacteremia Management

Empiric antibiotic treatment should be initiated immediately if CRB is suspected, without waiting for blood cultures to become positive (108). Gram-positive organisms, including a significant number of methicillin-resistant species, are isolated in the majority of CRBs. However, a substantial portion of bacteremia isolates are gram-negative organisms (108). Therefore, the optimal empiric antibiotic regimen for suspected CRB includes both vancomycin and an antibiotic with broad-spectrum gram-negative bacterial coverage, such as a third-generation cephalosporin. Antibiotic regimens should be adjusted once culture and sensitivity reports are available. Hospitalization is indicated if the patient is clinically septic or has evidence of metastatic complications such as endocarditis, osteomyelitis, epidural abscess, or septic arthritis. Aminoglycosides are excellent adjuncts for gram-positive infections treated with vancomycin as they are bacteriocidal rather than bacteriostatic. However, there are cumulative effects of aminoglycosides on hearing and balance such that lifetime exposure should be minimized (112). Continued bacteremia with hemodynamic instability despite sufficient treatment with appropriate antibiotics should prompt evaluation for catheter removal.

Treatment strategies for CRB that have been studied in hemodialysis catheter patients with regard to reemergence of the original organism after completion of antibiotics include (a) systemic antibiotics alone for 3 weeks, (b) systemic antibiotics plus a catheter lock solution, (c) systemic antibiotics plus catheter exchange (with or without disruption of a fibrinous sheath), and (d) catheter removal with delayed reinsertion (**TABLES 3.4 to 3.8**).

The overall success rate of antibiotics alone is only 50%, and we discourage this approach. Systemic antibiotics with catheter lock overall only succeed in just over 50% of catheter infections, but in some patients with coagulase-negative staphylococci infections, the success rate of approximately 77% may be sufficient if catheter exchange were to represent an undue burden. The utility of antibiotic lock therapy is believed to be treatment directed to the bacterial biofilms that form on the internal and external surfaces of catheters soon after insertion. These biofilms are thought to play a critical role in bacterial antimicrobial resistance and recalcitrant infections (113). Systemic antibiotics do not penetrate the biofilm well, and proteins in the biofilm provide adhesion sites for organisms to bind to, particularly *S. aureus*. Instillation of a concentrated antibiotic–anticoagulant solution into the catheter lumen (the antibiotic "lock") at concentrations significantly higher than those achievable in the blood may permit successful eradication of the infection while salvaging the catheter (114,115). Systemic antibiotics with exchange over guidewire, and as we perform it, with disruption of the fibrinous sheath during the procedure are as successful as removal and delayed reinsertion. Even for fungal infection, this approach is successful in over 80% of cases. A minority of about 10% of patients in the United States who use tunneled catheters long term is catheter dependent. Moving the catheter to a new site is often not possible, and exchange over a guidewire, frequently with treatment of an associated central vein stenoses or occlusions, preserves the only access option these patients rely on. Instillation of gentamicin (20 to 40 mg) into the catheter tunnel can be used as an adjunct during exchange. Guidewire exchange is the first recommendation for CRB by the Infectious Disease Society of America (116), and nephrologists will have to work within their institutions to create awareness for the special balance that needs to be struck between loss of access sites and catheter removals.

TABLE 3.4	**Success Rate Antibiotics Alone**				
Source	**Number of CRB Rx (number of all catheters)**	**Type of Study**	**Follow-up Interval (days)**	**Number of Cured**	**Cure Rate**
Moss et al. (90)	16	Retrospective	28	4	25%
Swartz et al. (241)	29	Retrospective		9	31%
Lund et al. (242)	32	Retrospective	180	7	22%
Marr et al. (243)	62	Retrospective	90	12	19%
Saad (244)	25	Retrospective	30	11	44%
Jean et al. (245)	56	Retrospective	90	29	52%
Mokrzycki et al. (121)	49	Prospective observational	90	36	73%
Troidle and Finkelstein (246)	34	Prospective observational	60	19	56%
Ashby et al. (247)	115	Prospective observational	180	76	66%
Total	418			203	49%

CRB, catheter-related bacteremia; Rx, prescription.

TABLE 3.5	Success Rate of Systemic Antibiotics plus Catheter Lock

Source	Number of CRB Rx (number of all catheters)	Type of Study	Follow-up Interval (days)	Number of Cured	Cure Rate
Capdevila et al. (248)	13	Retrospective		13	100%
Bailey et al. (249)	10	Retrospective	90	3	30%
Krishnasami et al. (115)	62	Retrospective	7	40	65%
Vardhan et al. (250)	26	Retrospective	7	16	62%
Poole et al. (114)	47	Prospective observational	150	33	70%
Maya et al. (251)	113	Retrospective	90	46	41%
Peterson et al. (252)	64	Retrospective	90	39	61%
Joshi and Hart (253)	46	Retrospective		27	59%
Total	381			217	57%

CRB, catheter-related bacteremia; Rx, prescription.

TABLE 3.6	Success Rate of Systemic Antibiotics plus Guidewire Exchange

Source	Number of CRB Rx (number of all catheters)	Type of Study	Follow-up Interval (days)	Number of Cured	Cure Rate
Shaffer (254)	13	Retrospective	>7	13	100%
Robinson et al. (255)	23	Retrospective	90	21	91%
Saad (244)	41	Retrospective	30	35	85%
Beathard (256)	49	Retrospective	45	49	100%
Mokrzycki et al. (121)	35	Prospective observational	90	34	97%
Troidle and Finkelstein (246)	31	Prospective observational	60	21	68%
Sychev et al. (257)	27	Retrospective	90	23	85%
Total	219			196	89%

CRB, catheter-related bacteremia; Rx, prescription.

TABLE 3.7	Removal and Delayed Reinsertion

Source	Number of CRB Rx (number of all catheters)	Type of Study	Follow-up Interval (days)	Number of Cured	Cure Rate
Beathard (256)	37	Retrospective	45	34	92%
Mokrzycki et al. (121)	35	Prospective observational	90	30	86%
Troidle and Finkelstein (246)	113	Prospective observational	60	99	88%
Sychev et al. (257)	13	Retrospective	90	11	85%
Total	198			174	88%

CRB, catheter-related bacteremia; Rx, prescription.

TABLE 3.8	**Success Rates by Treatment Strategy and Organism**					
Strategy/Organism	**Staphylococcus aureus**	**Coagulase-Negative Staphylococci**	**Enterococcus**	**GNR**	**Multiple Organisms**	**Fungus**
Antibiotics alone[a]	53% (25/47)	67% (84/126)		51% (41/80)	0% (0/10)	100% (1/1)
Antibiotics plus catheter lock[b]	40% (54/134)	77% (41/53)	59% (48/81)	66% (53/80)	37% (3/8)	0% (0/1)
Antibiotics plus guidewire exchange[c]	80% (16/20)	88% (29/33)	100% (1/1)	89% (40/45)	70% (7/10)	83% (24/29)
Antibiotics plus removal and delayed reinsertion[d]	87% (74/85)	89% (41/46)		88% (64/73)		85% (11/13)

[a]Swartz et al. (241), Marr et al. (243), Saad (244), Mokrzycki et al. (121), Troidle and Finkelstein (246), Ashby et al. (247).
[b]Capdevilla et al. (248), Bailey et al. (249), Krishnasami et al. (115), Poole et al. (114), Maya et al. (251), Peterson et al. (252), Joshi and Hart (253).
[c]Shaffer (254), Robinson et al. (255), Saad (244), Mokrzycki et al. (121), Troidle and Finkelstein (246), Langer et al. (258).
[d]Mokrzycki et al. (121), Troidle and Finkelstein (246).
GNR, Gram negative rods

Infection Prophylaxis for Cuffed Tunneled Catheters

Strategies to prevent CRB have been evaluated. Silver-coated tunneled dialysis catheters showed no difference in frequency of bacteremia compared to untreated catheters (117). Routine instillation in catheter lumens of antimicrobial solutions alone and in combination with anticoagulant or lytic solutions has been investigated. A gentamicin–citrate solution and a taurolidine solution have shown efficacy in decreasing incidence of bacteremias when used as interdialytic antibiotic lock solutions (118–120). These practices have not yet gained wide use but may hold promise for decreasing infection rates in the future. Several studies have shown that initiation of best practice techniques and staff education can improve outcomes for CRB, including decreased antibiotic treatment failure and decreased incidence of catheter infections (110,121,122). In a retrospective analysis of 872 patients during more than 476 patient catheter years, Sedlacek et al. (123) found that aspirin therapy, the 325-mg dose, was associated with a decrease in CRB caused by S. aureus. This effect was not seen with other antiplatelet agents, at a lower dose of aspirin, or for pathogens other than S. aureus. Tunnel dialysis catheters may also be heparin-coated based on studies in central venous catheters that documented a decreased rate of thrombosis and infection (124); however, clinical studies in dialysis populations did not show an effect on dysfunction and mixed effects on CRB rates (125,126).

Emerging Drug Resistance

Since 1996, five vancomycin-indeterminate Staphylococcus aureus (VISA) strains, vancomycin minimum inhibitory concentration (MIC) = 8 to 16 mg/L, have been identified worldwide. Vancomycin-resistant Staphylococcus aureus (VRSA), vancomycin MIC ≥32 mg/L, have been reported in the United States between 2002 and 2005 (127). Activity against these organisms is reported with new antimicrobials including ceftobiprole, quinupristin/dalfopristin, linezolid, and daptomycin. An older drug, trimethoprim-sulfamethoxazole, appears to be active against some of these organisms as well (128). Cases of resistance to linezolid and daptomycin have already been documented (129). Preventing transmission of antimicrobial-resistant microorganisms is of paramount importance in limiting the occurrence of these infections.

Autogenous and Prosthetic Arteriovenous Accesses

The creation of an AV access, either by direct anastomosis or by insertion of a prosthetic or biologic graft connecting an inflow artery with an outflow vein, fundamentally changes the existing flow and pressure states of the involved vasculature. Normal brachial artery blood flow is about 30 to 50 mL/min, while radial artery flow is as low as 10 to 15 mL/min. After anastomosis to a suitable graft or vein, flow rates in a 2-mm-diameter radial artery may increase to 800 mL/min. The associated shear stress will lead to arterial remodeling and over time to a larger diameter artery. The larger artery again will allow for higher flow rates at similar blood pressures. Arterial blood-flow wave forms change from triphasic before access creation to biphasic. The access vein experiences very similar changes in blood-flow volume, from less than 10 mL/min in a forearm cephalic vein to 400 to 800 mL/min within several weeks after access creation. Continuous flow changes to pulsatile flow near the anastomosis, which becomes less pulsatile with increasing distance from the anastomosis and addition of collaterals to the outflow network. Veins similarly remodel outward if exposed to the right shear stress and intra-access pressures, remodel little with low flows and pressures, and may form a stenosis with shear stress and intra-access pressures too high. The exact relationship between the different components of the vessel wall and the physiologic stimuli related to blood flow (shear stress and pressure) is currently not fully understood on the molecular level.

Stenoses at the inflow or outflow side of an access affect flow volume as well as intra-access pressures and thereby the biology of the involved vasculature. Recurrent outflow stenoses cause prolonged exposure to elevated intra-access pressures. Healing of needle insertion sites under elevated pressure leads to apposition of additional cell layers and connective tissue, which clinically manifests as aneurysm at the needle insertions sites. Over time, the skin thins and consists mostly of scar tissue. In this state, the reduced elasticity predisposes for prolonged bleeding after needle removal as well as scabbing and eventually ulceration of the overlying skin which may manifest as a terminal bleeding event.

While access stenoses can be treated with angioplasty, stents, or surgical revision, they are highly stenoses and are highly recurrent (outflow more so than inflow), such that this is properly referred to as *chronic access disease.*

Maturation of an autogenous access is defined by its usability for repeated needle insertion and removal. This requires a certain thickening of the vessel wall that is a result of shear stress and pressure-induced remodeling. Augmentation of the access vessel is necessary to avoid penetrating needle insertions and may be weak if there is an inflow stenosis or collaterals in or right after the needle insertion segment. Increased intra-access pressures (pulsatility) may lead to early infiltration and prolonged bleeding and can be found with high inflow (mismatch with access outflow) or an outflow stenosis.

Physical Examination of Vascular Access

Dialysis units may call to refer a patient for a variety of specific complaints:

- "Needles are pulling clots."—There may indeed be thrombus forming in a needle insertion segment, but this is rare. More commonly, needle tip position is such that the tip or the back hole is not fully within the access lumen; thrombus forms in the adjacent tissue from blood leaking from the needle. This is primarily a sign of difficulty with needle insertion. Most commonly, augmentation of the access vessel is impaired, either due to a collateral or an anastomotic or juxta-anastomotic inflow stenosis. An alternative is the presence of a very small vein diameter as the length of a dialysis needle bevel is about 4 mm such that the tip can easily cause injury of the posterior wall.
- "Vessel collapses," "access spasms"—During the first needle insertions into an access or a new segment of an access, there may be spasm of the vein at the needle insertion site. Typically, this resolves over the course of 20 to 30 minutes. However, intermittent collapse of the inflow vessel during the entire dialysis treatment may be a sign of access flows near or below dialysis pump speed. This can be seen with a true inflow stenosis or when a needle with the tape holding it in place compresses a flow-regulating inflow narrowing in a way that otherwise sufficient blood flows are reduced to or below pump speed. This can be exacerbated by periods of low systemic blood pressures which also affect access flows.
- "Long bleeding," "bleeding on a nondialysis day"—Bleeding from an access in such fashion is due to increased intra-access pressures, skin deterioration, anticoagulation, or a combination of the three. Other signs of a stenosis such as changes in pulsatility and location of a thrill should be determined.

The physical examination is instrumental in guiding imaging evaluation as well as correlating observed angiographic abnormalities with clinical dysfunction to counter the "oculo-manual" reflex for intervention. Each dialysis access presents with unique features as a result of smallest inflow diameter (flow-limiting/regulating segment), blood pressure, outflow capacity, and presence of collaterals. To capture all (patho-)physiologic components of a given access by physical examination, we suggest to evaluate the following five categories: pulsatility, flow murmur/bruit, thrill, augmentation, collapse of access against gravity (**TABLE 3.9**). Repeated examinations and correlation of physical findings with angiographic features as well as flow measurements will lead to useful mastery of this skill. Collapse of access against gravity can usually not be examined in prosthetic accesses, except if there are well-established needle insertion segment where the surface layer of PTFE has rarified over time (needle insertion aneurysm).

Pulsatility describes the force of access expansion during systole and the degree of softening during diastole. Very high blood pressures will suggest increased pulsatility, but the access softens remarkably during diastole. An outflow stenosis will lead to increased pulsatility and reduced softening during diastole. An inflow stenosis will blunt the systolic component and create the impression of an "empty" access during diastole, unless there is a coexisting outflow stenosis. Pressure measurements in the body of accesses (needle insertion segment) with "normal" pulsatility typically are in the 20 to 25 mm Hg range for forearm accesses and 25 to 30 mm Hg for upper arm accesses.

The audible **flow murmur** can be characterized by pitch and continuity. A change in pitch toward higher frequency is typical at the site of a stenosis due to accelerated flow velocity at this site. A discontinuous flow murmur indicates that during diastole, flow is so low that no audible shear force is created. This is the sign of a severe inflow or outflow stenosis. Typically, the stenotic inflow murmur is faint (like a whistle), while the stenotic outflow murmur can be coarse and loud (akin to a wood saw).

A **thrill** is palpable through the skin when the vessel is close enough to the surface and the flow high enough in relation to the diameter of the vessel to create vibration of the vessel wall. A thrill can be the sign of a well-developed access, usual in the inflow segment, dissipating as the access vessel branches and takes a deeper course. It is usually continuous with slight pronunciation during systole. In contrast, a discontinuous thrill can be found with severe stenosis. An isolated thrill is also found focally immediately after a stenosis. The differentiation from a "healthy" thrill can be made by documenting a change in pulsatility at the site of the focal thrill, increased retrograde (inflow side), and decreased antegrade (outflow).

Augmentation is the firming up and enlargement of the body of the access (where needles are inserted) with occlusion of the outflow. Without proper augmentation, needle insertion will be complicated by perforating injuries and hematomas. An inflow stenosis will impair augmentation as will side branches and collaterals between the occluding finger/tourniquet and the inflow. The location of side branches can be elucidated by moving the occluding finger closer toward the anastomosis until augmentation is achieved. With several collaterals, this may be a staged phenomenon.

Collapse of the access with arm elevation (against gravity) is a measure of inflow and outflow capacity match or mismatch. A forearm access typically displays complete collapse, while upper arm

TABLE 3.9	**Physical Examination of Dysfunctional Accesses**			
Type of Access	**Arteriovenous Graft**	**Radial-Cephalic**	**Brachial-Cephalic**	**Brachial-Basilic/Brachial**
Site of typical stenosis	**venous anastomotic**	**anastomotic/juxta-anastomotic**	**cephalic arch**	**basilic swing point**
Pulsatility	Increased	Decreased	Increased	Increased
Thrill	Only systolic or absent	Poststenotic only	Only systolic or absent	Only systolic or absent
Bruit	Discontinuous	Continuous, faint	Discontinuous	Discontinuous
Augmentation	Any (strong without occlusion)	Weak	Any (strong without occlusion)	Any (strong without occlusion)
Collapse with gravity	None	Complete (occasionally without gravity)	None	None

accesses typically show only partial collapse. Outflow stenoses or very high inflow will decrease the degree of collapse; banding of an upper arm access or a natural flow-limiting stenosis may lead to complete collapse of an upper arm access.

Enlarged needle insertion sites (and any sites of suspected skin thinning) are best examined while occluding the inflow: The completely empty access allows palpation of firm, layered thrombus inside aneurysms as well as better appreciation of the thickness of the overlying skin by rolling it between thumb and index finger.

Diagnostic imaging includes use of ultrasound as well as angiography using iodinated contrast agents or CO_2 gas. Ultrasound can accurately determine the depth of an access, demonstrate intraluminal thrombus, and provide estimates of access flow by measuring flow in the inflow artery. Angiography provides patterns of flow distribution, unmasking relevant side branches and stenoses. During angiography, access flows can be directly measured using special endovascular catheters based on a modified Fick's equation.

Guided by physical examination, angiographic studies and interventions can be performed with minimal contrast volume (5 to 10 mL), which typically does not jeopardize renal function even in patients with advanced CKD. We dilute contrast 1:1 with normal saline for central venous imaging and 1:3 with normal saline for peripheral images and perform pullback angiograms from central to peripheral (the usual access entry site). Diluted contrast allows for better appreciation of vascular details otherwise hidden by dense contrast.

Decisions to intervene on a given access have to be based on a sum of clinical findings, physical examination, and requirements for dialysis. For instance, a pre-ESKD patient with a stable inflow stenosis and relatively low flows may be best served with observation rather than recurrent interventions. Care systems have to be created to allow treatment of these access issues immediately before or at initiation of dialysis.

Natural History of Access Function and Dysfunction

First described by Brescia et al. (4) in 1961, the autogenous AV access remains the best form of long-term vascular access. AVFs are the preferred type of dialysis access because they are associated with the lowest morbidity and mortality, have excellent long-term patency, and require the fewest number of interventions to maintain patency. This is in particular true for forearm autogenous accesses (130). It is for these reasons that the NKF/KDOQI guidelines have set a goal of 65% of all hemodialysis patients having a functional AVF which we are soon approaching. The Fistula First Breakthrough Initiative also seeks to increase the use of AVFs for access while simultaneously decreasing the use of central venous catheters. In the United States, without dedicated programs to detect access dysfunction early and treat it appropriately, maturation failure is high (131). Even with interventions, some autogenous accesses do worse than others, require more interventions to function adequately, and still have higher failure rates (132), but accesses with low flow or maturing accesses seem to benefit from interventions (133). Once mature, native fistulas have excellent long-term patency rates and rarely become infected. The authors have seen primary AVFs provide adequate vascular access for 20 years.

The three dominant types of fistulas used in dialysis are the forearm radial-cephalic autogenous access, the upper arm brachial-cephalic or proximal radial-cephalic autogenous access, and the upper arm transposed brachial-basilic access.

Radial-cephalic forearm access is the preferred access if there is an appropriate cephalic vein and associated radial artery. The radial artery ideally will be without calcifications; however, even calcified radial arteries with 2-mm diameter may deliver 600 to 800 mL/min blood flow. The cephalic vein usually branches near the elbow with outflow toward the upper arm basilic, brachial, and cephalic veins, ensuring low intra-access pressures. If only one outflow is available in the upper arm, basilic/brachial is preferred over upper arm cephalic vein outflow as the cephalic arch has a tendency to develop stenoses over time. Maturation of the access to usability is most commonly impaired by juxta-anastomotic stenoses in the swing segment of the cephalic vein as well as lack of augmentation in the setting of multiple collateral veins. We prefer side-branch ligation over coil embolization as the veins are typically very superficial and easy to reach, and the foreign body sensation of a coil in the forearm can be limiting.

The upper arm brachial-cephalic, or proximal radial-cephalic, access is created in the antecubital area where the cephalic vein is mobilized for an end-to-side anastomosis to the brachial artery. A similar anastomosis can be fashioned using the proximal radial artery which aids in limiting flow and preventing steal. In some instances, a Gracz or Konner access (134) can be created by connecting the perforans branch to the deep venous system for an anastomosis with the proximal radial artery. Accesses utilizing the upper arm cephalic vein very often develop a chronically recurrent cephalic arch stenosis and less frequently also in the cephalic vein swing segment. Stenoses of the cephalic arch can be effectively treated with cephalic arch stent grafts (135).

An upper arm brachial-basilic superficialized access can be created as a two-stage or a single-stage procedure. A single-stage procedure involves mobilization of the upper arm basilic vein including a forearm branch after an incision from axillary to elbow, tunneling of the vein in a curve toward the anterior aspect of the arm with anastomotic area to the brachial artery near the elbow. Instead of tunneling, the vein can just be lifted within the skin flap. Ideally, the vein should come to rest away from the scar of the incision to allow easy palpation and needle insertion. In the two-stage procedure, a forearm branch of the basilic vein below the elbow is anastomosed to the proximal segment of a forearm artery or the brachial artery. This allows the vein to remodel and once there is wall thickening as well as increase in diameter, which is usually after 6 to 8 weeks, when the formal transposition can be done. Tunneling the vein to a new site of anastomosis with the brachial artery has often the best anatomic results. The vein can usually be cannulated 4 to 6 weeks after transposition. Typical sites for stenoses in this access are the "swing" point of the basilic vein as well as the inflow segment. Two-stage accesses appear to mature more frequently.

Other autogenous accesses that can be done are a superior femoral–saphenous vein access in the thigh, but the longevity of type of access over time has not been as good as upper (fore-)arm accesses. A superficial femoral-superficial femoral transposition thigh access is very similar to a basilic vein transposition in the arm and may have very high flows due to the larger vessels involved.

Non-autogenous accesses typically use expanded PTFE (ePTFE) (prosthetic) and less frequently bovine carotid artery, cryoveins, or tissue-engineered tubes with human cells (biograft). They are placed in the forearm in either a loop (brachial or proximal radial artery to cubital median, basilic, brachial, or cephalic vein) or straight (distal radial artery to vein) configuration. Within 3 to 4 weeks, fibrous tissue secures the graft in its subdermal tunnel and helps achieve hemostasis at needle puncture sites. Over time, the PTFE graft material wears out at site of repeated needle puncture.

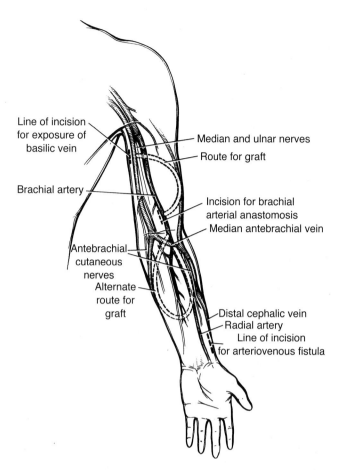

Line of incision for exposure of basilic vein

Median and ulnar nerves

Route for graft

Brachial artery

Incision for brachial arterial anastomosis

Median antebrachial vein

Antebrachial cutaneous nerves

Alternate route for graft

Distal cephalic vein

Radial artery

Line of incision for arteriovenous fistula

FIGURE 3.8 Looped forearm graft and upper arm graft. (From Stickel DL. Renal dialysis access procedures. In: Sabiston DC Jr, ed. *Atlas of General Surgery*. Philadelphia, PA: WB Saunders, 1994:90–98, with permission.)

More recently, early cannulation ePTFE grafts have become available that allow cannulation within days after placement, thereby reducing the need for tunneled catheters.

Grafts can be placed in many sites—after exhausting autogenous options and typical placement sites in the upper extremities, chest wall (axillary artery to axillary vein and axillary artery to jugular vein), or thigh (femoral artery to femoral vein), grafts are possible. FIGURE 3.8 depicts a looped forearm graft and an upper arm graft.

Very predictably, grafts develop stenoses at the venous anastomosis or in the immediate outflow vein. Access flows in grafts are related to their length and diameter and tend to be higher early on than an AVF with similar inflow, while the autogenous access has higher flow after many years of use. Although PTFE will withstand numerous thrombectomies and revisions, PTFE grafts are more prone to thrombosis and infection than are primary AVFs. By 3 years, many grafts have been lost to thrombosis or infection.

Preparation of the Patient for Permanent Vascular Access Placement

The role of careful planning for a successful AV access cannot be overemphasized. Studies consistently show that native fistula accesses have the best 4- to 5-year patency rates and require the fewest interventions compared to other access types (82,136). Epidemiologic studies have shown that greater use of fistulas is associated with reduced mortality and morbidity (137–140). Access

failure was the most frequent cause of hospitalization for patients with stage 5 CKD, based on data from the USRDS (1995) (141). Increased patient care cost is associated with graft use secondary to the increased number of procedures needed to maintain patency of grafts compared to fistulas (142). The clear superiority of fistula as the permanent vascular access for dialysis has led to national quality improvement projects, such as Fistula First (http://www.fistula-first.org), with the goal of maximizing the creation of fistulas. The Centers for Medicare and Medicaid Services has set a target of 65% fistula prevalence by 2009 (143,144). Early referral to nephrologists for evaluation and access planning is of primary importance in increasing fistula placement. Careful protection of the central and upper extremity venous and arterial system preserves vessels for fistula creation. Preoperative physical examination by an experienced individual, in combination with upper extremity vascular mapping, increases the number of functional fistulas placed (145–148).

The radial cephalic autogenous access at the wrist of the non-dominant arm is the preferred form of vascular access for the chronic hemodialysis patient, and the primary care physician must be instructed that the patient's morbidity on chronic hemodialysis will largely be determined by the adequacy of his or her vascular access (139). Patients should be taught to protect the vasculature of both arms; they should not permit placement of radial artery catheters and cephalic vein catheters. If possible, venipuncture should be avoided altogether except for the back of the hands. Peritoneal dialysis patients and patients with a kidney transplant should similarly preserve venous real estate in this fashion.

A history of subclavian vein catheter placement or current or previous transvenous pacemaker placement ipsilateral to the planned access site should prompt preoperative imaging to exclude central vein stenosis or occlusion; the presence of an untreatable central vein lesion requires careful access planning with anticipatory access flow reduction (149). Prior use of upper extremity peripherally inserted central venous catheters and central venous catheters (150) is associated with a high incidence (11% to 85%) of upper extremity stenosis and thrombosis (151–154) which leads to loss of potential sites for upper extremity fistulas. A history of severe congestive heart failure, peripheral vascular disease, or prior vascular surgery may limit surgical options.

Examination of the patient's upper extremity arterial and venous systems is important. Assessment of the arterial system includes bilateral blood pressure measurements, characterization of the peripheral pulses coupled with an Allen test of radial and ulnar flow. Insufficient arterial flow will preclude use of an extremity for AV access. Venous system evaluation includes assessment of bilateral arm size compatibility, examination for collateral veins or arm edema, and scrutiny of the patient's arm, neck, and chest wall for evidence of prior central venous cannulation or surgery (41).

Preoperative vascular mapping, the evaluation of arterial and venous vessels in the upper extremity, should be performed on all patients before placement of an AV access. Doppler ultrasound is the preferred method for preoperative vascular mapping (146–148). Vascular mapping of the arterial system includes pulse examination, differential blood pressure measurement, assessment of the palmar arch for patency, arterial diameter assessed by using Doppler ultrasound, and identification of arterial calcification. Venous system mapping comprises venous diameter assessment by Doppler ultrasonography, identification of vein continuity with proximal central veins, and the absence of venous obstruction (145). Venography or magnetic resonance angiography may also be used if central venous stenosis is suspected (155).

Controversy exists about the vessel diameter required to maximize successful maturation of the AV access. In general, studies support a minimum arterial diameter of 2.0 mm and minimum venous diameter of 2.5 mm by Doppler ultrasonography for the successful creation of a fistula. However, smaller vessel diameters have been used successfully to create fistulas. Surgical experience and individual vascular characteristics, such as the ability of the vessels to dilate postoperatively, may influence successful fistula maturation (145,156).

Access creation should begin distally. With enough time predialysis, even small appearing arteries and veins can mature into useable accesses. The increase venous flow of any radial-cephalic autogenous access will increase the success of access creation more proximally, as veins are partially matured.

There is discussion if a forearm loop graft should be inserted prior to an upper arm transposed brachial-basilic autogenous access. The more distal option should be preferred if the graft placement does not make impossible later transposition of the basilic vein.

In those patients in whom neither radial-cephalic nor brachial-cephalic primary fistula creation is possible, a transposed brachial-basilic autogenous access should be placed in the nondominant arm. The transposed brachial-basilic vein fistula is preferred but has several disadvantages compared to other fistulas (157–159). The transposition procedure may create significant arm swelling and patient pain, it is associated with a greater incidence of steal, and it is a technically more challenging surgery, especially in obese individuals. In some instances, a failing forearm graft can be converted to a more proximal fistula (41).

Vascular Access Patency

The chief marker of vascular access adequacy and patency is access blood flow. Low blood flow limits hemodialysis delivery resulting in underdialysis that is associated with increased morbidity and mortality (160). Of equal import, low access blood-flow rates can be associated with stenosis predisposing to access thrombosis and access loss.

Vascular access blood flow depends on the type, the location, and the age of the access. Initial blood-flow rates in primary AVFs are only 200 to 300 mL/min (161,162) but increase to greater than 600 mL/min as the venous drainage system dilates within 4 to 6 weeks (163). Blood-flow rates in non-autogenous accesses are high initially (164,165) but may fall with time because of progressive intimal and fibromuscular hyperplasia in the venous outflow system. Investigators have demonstrated that grafts with blood-flow rates less than 600 mL/min are more likely to clot than grafts with blood-flow rates greater than 600 mL/min (166,167). Grafts constructed using more proximal arteries have higher blood-flow rates (161,164) and may have higher patency rates.

The cumulative patency rate is defined as the percentage of accesses that remain patent at a given time regardless of the need for revision and thrombectomy. Cumulative patency rates for primary AVFs have been reported to be 60% to 70% at 1 year and 50% to 65% at 2 to 4 years (168,169). Cumulative patency rates for PTFE grafts have been reported to be 62% to 83% at 1 year and 50% to 77% at 2 years (166,169,170). Fifty percent or fewer of synthetic grafts are patent beyond 3 years. The lower cumulative patency rates for primary AVFs are due to early fistula failure; approximately one-fourth of these fistulas fail to mature. After correction for early failure, cumulative patency rates are at least as high as patency rates for PTFE grafts. In addition, native fistulas require fewer interventions to maintain patency than do synthetic fistulas.

Access Stenosis and Thrombosis

Stenosis usually precedes access thrombosis. There are three scenarios for stenosis, each with typical clinical signs and symptoms.

An inflow stenosis is usually characterized by decreasing augmentation to a point where staff may have difficulty with needle insertion. As the needle tip may not be perfectly inside the access conduit, "pulling clots" is a frequent comment, although the access has a palpable thrill and audible bruit. Blood flow may be reduced in absolute terms such that clearance is decreased and measurable recirculation can occur. While a prosthetic access may thrombose due to inflow stenosis, this is less common for an autogenous access. However, the last palpable segment of a low-flow AVF with inflow stenosis is between arterial anastomosis and the stenosis. Needle insertion into this space will often cause shutdown of the access by needle occlusion followed by access thrombosis when very tight tape has to be applied to stop the vigorously bleeding from the pressurized needle insertion site.

An outflow stenosis is characterized by much increase pulsatility of the access, prolonged bleeding from needle insertions sites, and enlargement of needle sites over time. Often, there is layered thrombus in the enlarged needle sites which can be dislodged inadvertently during needle insertion, embolizing into the stenosis to occlude the access. Access flows may be relatively high such that clearance is not yet affected. Particularly in graft, tight tape to control bleeding after needle removal can lead to complete luminal occlusion and then access thrombosis when the patient leaves the tape in place for 24 to 48 hours to avoid rebleeding.

More difficult to detect by clinical signs is the combination of balanced inflow and outflow stenoses: As the outflow stenosis progresses so does the inflow stenosis, with very little increase in pulsatility and postneedle removal bleeding. Only a full examination of the access evaluating continuity of the flow murmur/bruit and location of a thrill will identify this combination that frequently progresses to thrombosis before detection by dialysis unit staff.

Thrombosis is the leading cause of access loss. Thrombosis within 1 month of access creation is likely due to technical errors or to premature cannulation. After the first month, the thrombosis rate is 0.5 to 0.8 episodes per patient-year. Prosthetic accesses thrombose much more frequently than do autogenous accesses.

Approximately 90% of graft thromboses are associated with stenoses of the venous outflow tract (22,169,171,172). These lesions are characterized by intimal and fibromuscular hyperplasia (169,173). Most venous stenoses develop at or within 2 to 3 cm of the vein graft anastomosis (174). The remainder develops in more proximal veins, in central veins, or in the graft itself. Most accesses have more than one stenotic lesion at any one time (175). Arterial disease is now known to be more common than previously thought. Asif et al. (176) found in a multicenter trial that one-third of patients referred to interventional facilities for clinical evidence of venous stenosis or thrombosis had documented inflow arterial stenosis. Subclavian vein stenoses are associated with previous subclavian vein catheterization and with transvenous pacemaker placement (22,73,77). Intragraft stenoses are reported to result from pseudointimal hyperplasia (173) and fibroblastic ingrowth through needle puncture sites.

A minority of graft thromboses occurs in the absence of an identifiable anatomic lesion. Hypotension, intravascular volume depletion, and graft compression during sleep may decrease graft flow and lead to graft thrombosis. Excessive graft compression by patients or dialysis staff attempting to achieve hemostasis following dialysis may lead to graft thrombosis; complete and accurate treatment records may allow the identification and retraining of those individuals who apply excessive pressure.

Prospective Strategies for Maintaining Arteriovenous Access Patency

Prospective Identification of Access Stenoses

As venous outflow stenoses evolve, intra-access pressure increases and access blood flow decreases. Conversely, inflow stenoses lead to decreased intra-access pressures and decreased access flows. Eventually, the access may fail; approximately 90% of access thromboses are associated with venous stenoses (169,171). Prospective monitoring and surveillance of hemodialysis accesses for hemodynamically significant stenoses is advocated by the NKF/KDOQI Clinical Practice Guidelines for Vascular Access update in 2006 (41). A variety of techniques can be utilized to prospectively monitor for access stenosis (**TABLE 3.10**). It has not been conclusively proven that monitoring and surveillance programs prolong access survival, but a substantial body of evidence supports this conclusion. Access stenoses develop in the great majority of accesses over time; if detected and corrected in a planned and coordinated manner, underdialysis will be minimized and thrombotic events decreased (177). Every hemodialysis unit should institute a vascular access management team whose functions include identification of accesses at risk for dysfunction, tracking access complication rates and instituting protocols to maximize access longevity (178). A number of access monitoring and surveillance methods are available including the following: sequential access flow, sequential dynamic or static pressures, recirculation measurements, and physical examination. The most appropriate monitoring techniques differ, in some cases, for grafts and fistulas.

The goal of an access monitoring and surveillance program is detection of asymptomatic but hemodynamically significant access stenoses. Detection of stenoses and referral for appropriate intervention is key to protecting each dose of dialysis and preventing thrombosis. Hemodynamically significant stenosis is defined as a

decrease of greater than 50% of normal vessel diameter and a hemodynamic or clinical abnormality such as abnormal recirculation values, elevated venous pressures, decreased blood flow, a swollen extremity, an unexplained reduction in Kt/V, or inability to achieve prescribed blood-flow rate secondary to elevated negative arterial prepump pressures (177).

Clinical Monitoring and Physical Examination

For both fistulas and grafts, systematic monitoring includes a monthly physical examination by a qualified individual (179). Inspection of the access for swelling and palpation for a pulse and a thrill along the entire length of the graft or fistula vein should be performed (180). A fistula that does not at least partially collapse with arm elevation may have an outflow stenosis. In addition, downstream stenosis can produce an overall dilation of the fistula vein. Visual inspection will reveal new occurrences or changes in character of aneurysms. A low-pitched bruit over an access system and its draining veins should be continuous in systole and diastole. An isolated systolic (discontinuous) bruit or intensification of a bruit suggests stenosis (181). Clinical monitoring of access function is also important. Prolonged bleeding after needle removal is a late manifestation of access dysfunction. Arm edema is a common indicator of subclavian stenosis. Difficulty with needle placement can be an indicator of intragraft stenosis. An unexplained decrease in the amount of hemodialysis delivered is typically a very late signal indicating the presence of venous stenosis. Arterial inflow stenosis should be suspected if prepump arterial pressures more negative than -250 mm Hg are required to achieve the target blood-flow rate.

Access Blood Flow

Sequential measurement of access blood flow is a widely available method for the prospective monitoring of vascular accesses. Doppler ultrasonographic evaluation, magnetic resonance, and ultrasound dilution are the techniques that have been most extensively studied (41). Unfortunately, these techniques require special equipment and are not in widespread use. Each technique used for access flow measurement has specific limitations. The sequential measurement and systematic trend analysis of data is key to detecting stenosis and referring patients in a timely manner for intervention.

Direct measurement of access blood flow is performed by Doppler ultrasonography or magnetic resonance imaging. Doppler flow is predictive of access patency. Shackleton et al. (167) reported that, in synthetic grafts, Doppler flow less than 450 mL/min had a sensitivity of 83% and a specificity of 75% for the development of thrombosis within 2 to 6 weeks. Rittgers et al. (164) reported a mean blood flow of 307 mL/min in synthetic grafts that clotted within 2 weeks and a mean blood flow of 849 mL/min in synthetic grafts that remained patent. The expense and interobserver variability of Doppler blood-flow measurements have precluded its widespread use. In addition, Doppler measurements cannot be performed during the hemodialysis treatment because the needles prevent proper measurement. Magnetic resonance provides accurate measurements of access flow but is expensive (182).

Indirect techniques to measure access blood flow are ultrasound dilution, conductance dilution, or thermal dilution. A detailed description of the ultrasound dilution technique (183,184) is beyond the scope of this chapter. In brief, the hemodialysis blood lines are reversed. The blood pump is set at a rate of 300 mL/min, and ultrafiltration is turned off. A bolus of isotonic saline is then injected into the venous port. Because the velocity of ultrasound in blood is

---

TABLE 3.10	**Methods for the Prospective Identification of Venous Stenoses**

Physical examination and clinical assessment (difficulty with needle placement, prolonged bleeding following hemodialysis)

Venous dialysis pressure

    Dynamic venous dialysis pressure

    Static venous dialysis pressure

Access recirculation

    Urea recirculation

    Direct measurements of access recirculation (blood temperature monitoring method, saline dilution method, ultrasound dilution method)

Access blood flow

    Doppler ultrasonography

    Magnetic resonance

    Ultrasound dilution

    Conductance dilution

    Thermal dilution

determined primarily by the blood protein concentration, the isotonic saline will dilute blood protein and change the sound velocity in proportion to the concentration of injected saline in the blood. An ultrasonographic flow sensor on the arterial line measures blood flow in the tubing by a transit-time method and simultaneously detects saline dilution of the blood by measuring the velocity of an ultrasonographic beam. These measurements permit calculation of access blood flow. This technique yields accurate measurements and may be performed during the hemodialysis treatment.

A recent study demonstrated the utility of surveillance of access blood flow by the ultrasound dilution technique (185). Access blood-flow measurements were performed monthly. If access blood flow was less than 600 mL/min or if access blood flow fell by 20% and was less than 1,000 mL/min, fistulography was performed. All patients who agreed to fistulography were found to have significant access stenoses. Percutaneous transluminal angioplasty (PTA) increased access flow by 20% in 80% of the patients. The thrombosis rate for patients in this study was lower than that for historical controls. Of the 10 episodes of thrombosis that occurred during the study period, 8 occurred in patients who did not keep appointments for fistulography or who refused surgical revision after unsuccessful PTA.

Several common errors occur when using any indirect measurement of flow. The dialysis machine blood pump must be accurately calibrated before flow measurement, and this is frequently not done by busy staff. Access recirculation must be able to be separately calculated from cardiopulmonary recirculation, and this is unavailable with high-efficiency dialysis. Access flow is a function of the ratio of systemic to access resistance. Systemic resistance typically drops as a dialysis session progresses as a function of decreases in cardiac output or blood pressure related to ultrafiltration/hypotension (186). To minimize these errors, protocols should be instituted for monthly flow measurements which include calibration of blood pumps, measurement of flow within the first 90 minutes of a hemodialysis session, and use of the mean value of two separate determinations performed at a single treatment. All measurements of flow, except the ionic dialysance technique, require some disruption or modification of the hemodialysis treatment to obtain data (41). Flow data should be generated monthly for assessment. Systematic analysis of the trend of values in individual accesses is more valuable in detecting dysfunction than an individual reading.

Intra-access Dialysis Pressure

Measurement of dynamic venous dialysis pressure is the least expensive method for the prospective detection of venous stenoses. However, dynamic venous dialysis pressure is affected by factors other than venous stenosis, rendering it the least reliable method for detecting venous stenoses. Because needle gauge and extracorporeal blood-flow rate affect dynamic venous dialysis pressure, these factors must be held constant. It is recommended that dynamic venous dialysis pressure be measured through 15G needles at the beginning of a dialysis session and at blood flows of 50 to 225 mL/min because at higher blood flows, much of the resistance to flow is from the needle, and not the vascular access. In addition, different hemodialysis machines have different pressure monitors and different types and lengths of tubing. Each hemodialysis unit, then, must establish its own threshold pressure. Threshold dynamic venous dialysis pressures range from 125 to 150 mm Hg (41). These variables have led to wide differences among hemodialysis units in their ability to use this technique. The measurement of dynamic venous dialysis pressure is less sensitive and specific than measurement of access blood flow and is very prone to operator error. Indeed, some hemodialysis units have been unable to use this technique.

Elevated static venous dialysis pressures are highly predictive of the presence of venous stenoses. Besarab et al. (187) measured static venous dialysis pressure by inserting a stopcock-transducer system between the venous needle and the venous blood line. Static venous dialysis pressure was measured every 3 to 4 months. Fistulography was performed if static venous dialysis pressure/systolic blood pressure was equal to 0.4, and angioplasty was performed if stenoses resulted in a luminal diameter reduction greater than 50%. As this protocol evolved, the angioplasty rate at their institution increased 13-fold, the thrombosis rate decreased 70%, and the access replacement rate decreased 79%. The measurement of static venous dialysis pressure in this manner requires special equipment. Simplified techniques may allow widespread application of this approach. A static intra-access pressure surveillance protocol is detailed in the most recent NKF/KDOQI Clinical Practice Guidelines for Vascular Access (41). An inexpensive device to measure intra-access pressure has recently been demonstrated and allows in particular home hemodialysis patients to self-monitor their access (188).

Access stenoses do not all occur at the venous outflow tract, and frequently, multiple stenoses exist in a single access. Access pressures are affected by the type of access and location of stenoses. For instance, the intra-access pressure can remain in the normal range if stenosis is present between the needles, or it may actually decrease if inflow stenosis is present. Venous outflow from a native AVF can occur from multiple collateral veins making intra-access pressure ratios lower than those in synthetic grafts. All of these factors make a single measurement of intra-access pressure or intra-access pressure to systemic pressure ratio less valuable than serial measurements. Tracking sustained pressure changes over time is the most effective way to monitor access dysfunction when using intra-access pressures (189). The NKF/KDOQI 2006 Clinical Practice Guidelines characterize intra-access pressure to systemic pressure ratios which can be used to guide practitioners for referral for intervention. Pressures should be monitored at least twice a month.

A computerized algorithm has been developed that uses an empirical formula to calculate an equivalent intra-access pressure based on the dynamic venous pressure values stored in the machine during a hemodialysis session (190). During a single treatment, the dialysis machine records numerous measurements of dynamic venous pressure simultaneously with a mean arterial pressure. An average equivalent ratio of the intra-access pressure (calculated from the dynamic venous pressure readings) to the systemic pressure is calculated. The average values can be trended with each treatment. When the ratios consistently trend upward and exceed 0.55, the access is at risk for clotting. This technique has been commercialized and can provide monthly reports and trend analysis. These measurements are made during each dialysis treatment.

Urea Recirculation

Hemodialysis access recirculation occurs when dialyzed blood returning through the venous needle reenters the extracorporeal circuit through the arterial needle. Reentry of dialyzed blood into the extracorporeal circuit reduces solute concentration gradients across the dialysis membrane and thereby reduces the efficiency of dialysis. A high degree of access recirculation indicates low-access blood flow and heralds access thrombosis. Access recirculation will not be present until flow falls to the range of 350 to 500 mL/min. In this blood-flow range, fistulas can maintain patency, but grafts are at imminent risk for thrombosis. For this reason, recirculation is not recommended as a routine surveillance system to detect stenosis in grafts (41).

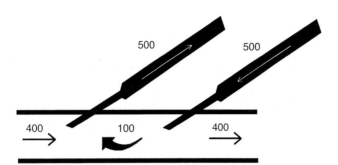

FIGURE 3.9 Access recirculation is 20% because extracorporeal blood flow exceeds access blood flow. (From Depner TA. Techniques for prospective identification of venous stenosis. *Adv Ren Replace Ther* 1994;1:119–130, with permission.)

Recirculation is usually caused by a venous stenosis that decreases access blood flow or by reversed needles. When the access blood-flow rate is lower than that demanded by the blood pump, reentry of dialyzed blood into the extracorporeal circuit is necessary to meet the demand of the blood pump (**FIGURE 3.9**). Less commonly, recirculation results from arterial stenosis.

Access recirculation is calculated from the following formula (**EQUATION 3.1**):

$$\text{Percentage recirculation} = [\text{Systemic (BUN)} - \text{Arterial blood line (BUN)}] / [\text{Systemic (BUN)} - \text{Venous blood line (BUN)}] \times 100 \quad (3.1)$$

Where, ideally, the systemic blood urea nitrogen (BUN) concentration is equal to the BUN concentration in the blood entering the fistula. One can see that access recirculation exists whenever the concentration of urea in arterial line blood is lower than the concentration of urea in systemic blood, indicating reentry of dialyzed blood into the arterial line.

The chief source of error in the determination of access recirculation lies with the determination of the systemic urea concentration. The systemic urea concentration is assumed to be equal to the urea concentration in blood entering the access. Traditionally, systemic blood has been sampled from a peripheral vein in the contralateral arm ("three-needle method"). This method has been found to be inadequate because of two phenomena: AV disequilibrium and venovenous disequilibrium.

The first phenomenon that renders the three-needle sampling method inadequate is AV disequilibrium (or cardiopulmonary recirculation) (191–194). Dialyzed blood (with a low urea concentration) returns to the central veins, dilutes blood returning from the systemic circulation (with a high urea concentration), and reduces the urea concentration in central venous blood (**FIGURE 3.10**). The urea concentration in blood leaving the left heart and entering the hemodialysis access will be lower than the urea concentration in peripheral venous blood. Use of the peripheral vein BUN in the recirculation formula, then, will result in overestimation of access recirculation. The degree of AV disequilibrium increases with increasing extraction of urea by the dialyzer, with increasing extracorporeal blood-flow rate, and with decreasing cardiac output. With increasing extracorporeal blood-flow rate or with decreasing cardiac output, a greater proportion of the cardiac output courses through the dialyzer, increasing the dilution of peripheral venous blood by dialyzed blood.

The second phenomenon that accounts for the different urea concentrations in peripheral venous blood and in blood entering

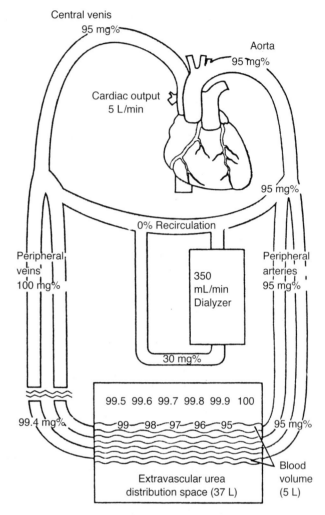

FIGURE 3.10 Arteriovenous recirculation. Dialyzed blood bypasses the systemic circulation, dilutes blood returning from the body, and decreases the concentration of urea in central venous blood. Because the concentration of urea in blood leaving the left heart and entering the access will be lower than the concentration of urea in peripheral venous blood, use of the peripheral vein blood urea nitrogen (BUN) in the recirculation formula will lead to overestimation of access recirculation. In this case, access recirculation is absent, but the percentage of urea recirculation using the peripheral vein method is (100 − 95) / (100 − 30) × 100 or 7%. (From Sherman RA. Recirculation revisited. *Semin Dial* 1991;4:221–223, with permission.)

the access is venovenous disequilibrium (191–194). Perfusion of the arm contralateral to the hemodialysis access is low during hemodialysis; urea removal in that limb is diminished in comparison to well-perfused compartments. As a result, the urea concentration is higher in the veins of the contralateral arm than in central venous blood and in blood entering the access. This difference increases with time. Again, use of the peripheral vein BUN concentration in the recirculation formula will result in overestimation of access recirculation.

Fortunately, there is an alternative to the three-needle method. Sherman and Levy (191) have devised the method described in **TABLE 3.11**. In this two-needle method, the extracorporeal blood-flow rate is decreased to 120 mL/min for 10 seconds to clear the arterial line of recirculated blood. Systemic blood is then sampled from the arterial line after the blood pump is shut off. This technique

TABLE 3.11	**Protocol for the Measurement of Urea Recirculation**

Turn off ultrafiltration 30 min after the initiation of hemodialysis.

Draw arterial (A) blood line and venous (V) blood line samples.

Immediately decrease extracorporeal blood-flow rate to 120 mL/min.

Turn blood pump off exactly 10 s after decreasing blood-flow rate.

Clamp arterial line immediately above port.

Draw systemic (S) sample from arterial line port.

Measure blood urea nitrogen (BUN) in the three samples.

Percentage recirculation = $(S - A) / (S - V) \times 100$

Adapted from National Kidney Foundation. *NKF-K/DOQI Clinical practice guidelines for vascular access.* New York, NY: National Kidney Foundation, 2001:48, with permission.

reduces but does not eliminate the effect of AV disequilibrium; systemic blood obtained in this manner will more closely approximate blood entering the hemodialysis access.

The threshold urea recirculation value that should prompt one to request fistulography is not known. Because access recirculation should not occur unless the access blood-flow rate is less than the extracorporeal blood-flow rate demanded by the blood pump (195), any degree of access recirculation is abnormal. Indeed, the blood temperature monitoring method and the saline dilution method have demonstrated that recirculation is absent in well-functioning fistulas (196,197). These techniques directly measure access recirculation and do not require urea measurements; the effects of AV and venovenous disequilibrium are completely eliminated.

Unfortunately, threshold values of urea recirculation have been determined using the three-needle (peripheral vein) method, which overestimates access recirculation (198,199). When the recommended two-needle method is used, urea recirculation values greater than 10% should prompt further investigation. When values exceed 20%, the possibility of reversed needle placement should be considered before fistulography is requested. The blood temperature monitoring method and the saline dilution method provide more accurate measurements of recirculation and are preferred to urea-based methods for measuring recirculation. If recirculation exceeds 5% when measured by these techniques, fistulography should be requested (41).

Treatment of Access Stenoses and Thrombosis

PTA is effective for the treatment of venous stenoses of both autogenous and non-autogenous accesses. The importance of prospective detection of venous stenosis cannot be overemphasized; patency rates are far higher for stenotic accesses angioplastied before thrombosis than for accesses angioplastied at the time of thrombolysis (172,200).

Angioplasty is well tolerated by patients; hospitalization is not required, and hemodialysis may be performed immediately after the procedure. Venous stenoses may also be corrected by surgical revision. This approach, however, usually requires hospitalization and, by use of jump grafts, sacrifices a segment of vein and eliminates a potential vascular access site. Studies comparing PTA with surgical revision have yielded conflicting results (201,202), and one approach cannot be recommended over the other.

PTA is effective for the treatment of venous anastomotic stenoses (**FIGURE 3.11**), inflow stenosis, central vein stenoses (**FIGURE 3.12**), and intragraft stenoses. In addition, PTA may correct multiple

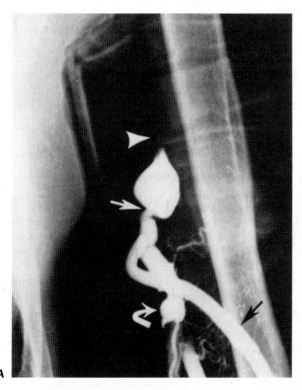
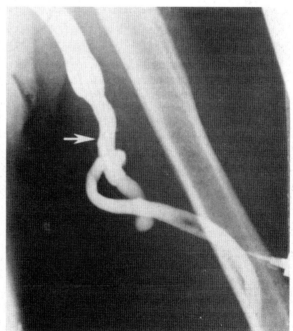

FIGURE 3.11 Stenosis at vein-graft anastomosis **(A)** before and **(B)** after percutaneous transluminal angioplasty. (From Schwab SJ, Saeed M, Sussman SK, et al. Transluminal angioplasty of venous stenoses in polytetrafluoroethylene vascular access grafts. *Kidney Int* 1987;32:395–398, with permission.)

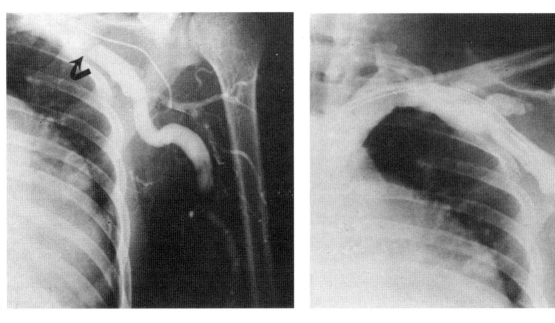

FIGURE 3.12 Subclavian vein stenosis **(A)** before and **(B)** after percutaneous transluminal angioplasty. (From Schwab SJ, Quarles LD, Middleton JP, et al. Hemodialysis-associated subclavian vein stenosis. *Kidney Int* 1988;33:1156–1159, with permission.)

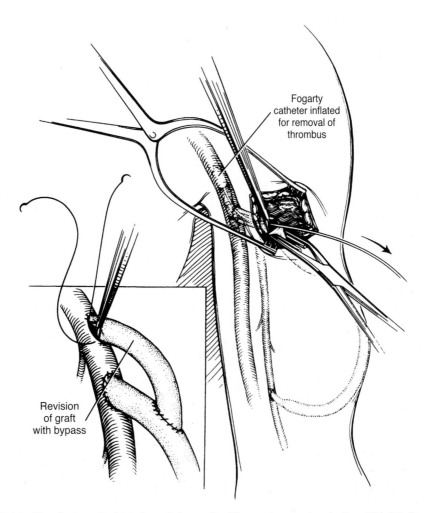

FIGURE 3.13 Thrombectomy of polytetrafluoroethylene graft and bypass of venous stenosis. (From Stickel DL. Renal dialysis access procedures. In: Sabiston DC Jr, ed. *Atlas of General Surgery*. Philadelphia, PA: WB Saunders, 1994:90–98, with permission.)

venous stenoses, long (6 to 40 cm) venous stenoses, and complete venous occlusions. Initial technical success is achieved in 82% to 94% of cases. In a large and carefully studied series, a successful treatment was defined as one that maintained graft patency and did not need to be repeated; success rates (unassisted patency rates) were 61% at 6 months and 38% at 1 year. Success rates for repeat treatments were no different than success rates for initial treatments. Other investigators have achieved similar results (174,201,203–208). Conversely, several small randomized trials have questioned the durability of PTA as a therapeutic method (209,210).

Self-expandable endovascular stents and more recently stent grafts, placed percutaneously, have been used in conjunction with PTA for the treatment of graft venous anastomotic stenoses (211) and appear superior to just angioplasty alone (211). Drug-eluting balloons have first been used (212) with promising results, albeit at a very high cost.

Once thrombosis occurs, surgical thrombectomy, pharmacomechanical thrombolysis, or mechanical thrombectomy may be employed. No matter which technique is performed, correction of the venous stenosis should be performed to maintain access patency. All thrombectomies are associated with micropulmonary emboli. Autogenous accesses with higher thrombus burden are more likely to cause clinically apparent pulmonary emboli. Palder et al. (169) demonstrated that surgical thrombectomy combined with bypass of the venous stenosis (**FIGURE 3.13**) produced significantly longer patency than did simple thrombectomy or patch angioplasty. It has been reported that surgical thrombectomy coupled with PTA is as effective as surgical thrombectomy coupled with surgical revision (213).

Success rates for thrombectomy of prosthetic access are usually >90%, while those for autogenous accesses are >70% to 80%. Large aneurysms with very large thrombus burden limit the feasibility and safety of the endovascular approach; however, mini-incision and sheath-hole thrombectomies have expanded the range of accesses that can be approached with a modified endovascular technique. One approach cannot be recommended over the others; instead, the decision as to whether an individual patient should be treated by surgical thrombectomy or by a nonsurgical technique should be guided by the expertise of the treating institution's vascular surgeons and interventional radiologist or nephrologist.

In pharmacomechanical thrombolysis (pulse-spray thrombolysis) (172,214), angiography is performed to determine the extent of the clot and to visualize the graft and draining veins. Two catheters with closely spaced side holes are inserted into the midportion of the graft in a crossed manner (**FIGURE 3.14**). A thrombolytic agent is "sprayed" into the clot under high pressure, and thrombolysis is achieved by both pharmacologic and mechanical means. An angioplasty balloon is then used to macerate residual clots and to dilate the venous stenosis. This technique is now rarely used.

The technique of mechanical thrombolysis uses a variety of devices to macerate thrombus and then aspirate or remove otherwise organized thrombus from the vascular lumen (24,214–216). These techniques may be performed in 1 to 2 hours, and the access may be used immediately for dialysis. Angioscopic observation has demonstrated that endovascular techniques utilizing wall-contact devices during thrombectomy leave less detectable material than other techniques (217). Surgical thrombectomy and revision may yield

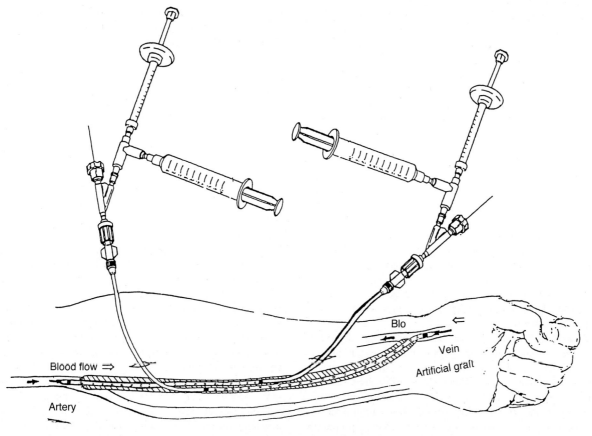

FIGURE 3.14 Pulse-spray thrombolysis. (From AngioDynamics Inc., Glens Falls, New York, with permission.)

a similar patency rate (218,219), but surgical treatment generally entails delays, hospitalization, and extension of the access up the extremity.

A recent analysis of graft thrombus obtained during thrombectomy revealed colonization in one-third of cases (220).

Other Arteriovenous Access Complications

Infection of Arteriovenous Accesses

Vascular access infection is a serious and, in some cases, life-threatening problem.

Autogenous access infections are uncommon; they are usually localized and can usually be treated successfully with antibiotic therapy (169). However, because these are endovascular infections, it has been recommended that they should be treated as subacute bacterial endocarditis—with 6 weeks of antibiotic therapy.

Synthetic fistula infections are not uncommon; they are the second most common cause of fistula loss (169,221,222). Gram-positive cocci—S. aureus and, less commonly, S. epidermidis and streptococcal species—are the culprits in most cases. Gram-negative bacteria account for approximately 15% of episodes of bacteremia in hemodialysis patients (223–226).

Some risk factors for graft infection are beyond the nephrologist's control. Intravenous drug use (169), dermatitis overlying the graft, and poor personal hygiene (223,227) predispose patients to graft infection. Femoral grafts have a high infection rate (228) most likely because of the proximity of the graft to the perineum. Nevertheless, preventive measures should be undertaken. We strongly believe that patients should wash the skin overlying their grafts with soap and water before each hemodialysis treatment. This practice may decrease the likelihood of inadvertent introduction of bacteria into the bloodstream during graft cannulation. Monitoring of graft cannulation and infection records may allow one to identify hemodialysis staff who employ poor needle insertion technique.

Fever, chills, and rigors are the typical presenting complaints of the bacteremic hemodialysis patient. Physical evidence of graft infection is often absent. The febrile hemodialysis patient with a synthetic fistula should be presumed to have graft-associated bacteremia unless the history, physical examination, and initial investigations provide strong evidence to the contrary. Blood cultures should be obtained. Initial antibiotic therapy should be effective against gram-positive organisms (including Enterococcus) and gram-negative organisms. At our institution, we administer loading doses of vancomycin and an aminoglycoside. Appropriate gram-negative coverage can also be provided by a third-generation cephalosporin, such as ceftazidime, dosed immediately upon the completion of dialysis. Because methicillin-resistant S. aureus (MRSA) and coagulase-negative staphylococci are common culprits, a β-lactam antibiotic should not be used as an empiric agent. The antibiotic regimen can be simplified if blood cultures yield a culprit. If staphylococci are isolated that are susceptible to β-lactam antibiotics, a β-lactam should be substituted for vancomycin unless the patient has a β-lactam allergy.

Patients with gram-positive bacteremia who defervesce promptly in response to antibiotic therapy and whose grafts have no associated pustule or abscess can often be successfully treated with intravenous antibiotics alone. However, extensive graft infection may be present even when the physical examination is unremarkable. If fever or bacteremia persists, strong consideration should be given to graft excision. Staphylococcal bacteremia has a propensity to lead to metastatic infection; endocarditis, osteomyelitis, septic

pulmonary emboli, empyema, septic arthritis, and meningitis have been reported. Persistent fever or bacteremia should also prompt one to search for evidence of metastatic infection. In hemodialysis patients with S. aureus bacteremia, this search should include transesophageal echocardiography to exclude infective endocarditis. If fever and bacteremia promptly remit and if there is no evidence of metastatic infection, a 3-week course of antibiotic should suffice. Otherwise, a 6-week or longer course of antibiotic therapy is required. Regardless of the length of therapy, blood cultures should be obtained after completion of therapy to ensure that the infection has been eradicated. Gram-negative infections less commonly lead to metastatic infection, and a 2- to 3-week course of antibiotic therapy should suffice.

Evaluation by the vascular surgeon is mandatory if a pustule or abscess overlies the graft. Localized infection of the graft may be treated by simple incision and drainage or by partial graft excision and bypass grafting. Extensive infection necessitates total graft excision. Grafts placed within the past month must be completely excised even if the infection is thought to be localized; because these grafts are incompletely incorporated into surrounding tissue, the infection is unlikely to be localized (41). Finally, it should be noted that bleeding through an area of eroded skin overlying a synthetic graft may be the initial manifestation of graft infection. "Herald bleeding" mandates evaluation by the vascular surgeon.

Vascular Access–Related Heart Failure

If fistula blood flow exceeds 20% of cardiac output, high-output congestive heart failure may develop in patients with ventricular dysfunction (229). Reduction of fistula blood flow by banding or interposition of a tapered synthetic segment may reduce symptoms (230–232). Reduction of access flows may be of particular importance in kidney transplant patients. While overt progressive heart failure is uncommon, other consequences of prolonged high cardiac output such as pulmonary hypertension and cardiac hypertrophy are more frequent. For these reasons and enlarging dialysis, access should prompt evaluation of access flows. Access flows greater than 1,500 mL/min with signs of increase intra-access pressures (pulsatility) should prompt dedicated observation if cardiac function or skin integrity are compromised.

Fistula takedown should be performed in refractory cases. In the authors' experience, although possible, this occurs rarely.

Hand Ischemia

Hand ischemia following fistula placement may be due to arterial insufficiency or venous hypertension. Arterial insufficiency results from direct shunting of arterial blood through the low-resistance fistula and from vascular steal, in which blood flows retrograde from the palmar arch through the radial artery into the fistula. Symptoms of hand ischemia usually decrease in the weeks following fistula construction, but close observation is warranted. If symptoms are severe (coldness or loss of motor function), fistula blood flow may be reduced by banding or by interposition of a tapered synthetic graft (230–232). If symptoms persist, or if hand viability is ever threatened, the radial artery distal to the anastomosis may be ligated. For brachial-cephalic autogenous accesses, a distal revascularization and interval ligation (DRIL) procedure may be performed in addition to banding. Proximalization of the inflow is another alternative if access flows are already low.

Venous hypertension may occur after side-to-side anastomosis of the radial artery and cephalic vein. In the presence of a proximal venous stenosis or occlusion, there may be retrograde blood flow through the fistula and arterialization of the distal venous system; the pressure in the venous system of the hand will approach arterial pressure. Treatment consists of ligation of the distal vein and correction of the venous stenosis.

Aneurysms and Pseudoaneurysms

True aneurysms occur very commonly in native fistulas and generally cause no problems. Surgical intervention is required only if the aneurysm compromises the arterial anastomosis or shows rapid expansion raising a danger of dissection or rupture.

Pseudoaneurysms of synthetic grafts appear as progressive damage to the graft material leads to inability to seal needle puncture sites. Pseudoaneurysms may rapidly expand or may threaten the viability of the overlying skin. Surgical intervention should be considered in these circumstances to prevent hemorrhage. Surgical treatment consists of excision of the involved graft segment and placement of an interposition graft.

Central Vein Stenosis

Even remote history of a tunneled catheter may over time lead to symptomatic central venous stenosis. Asymptomatic (no arm swelling) central venous stenosis should not be treated as recurrence is more severe after angioplasty. We know little about different types of central venous stenosis. However, some respond to angioplasty, while others recur rapidly. Some of these then respond well to placement of a noncovered stent, while others quickly require placement of stent graft.

A special situation is the external compression of the subclavian vein between the clavicle and the first rib that can be treated with resection of the first rib or the medial clavicle.

In some patients, there is compression of the left brachiocephalic vein between sternum and an enlarged aortic arch. This condition can respond to stent placement but as this is not a stenosis of the vessel, it should be left alone unless symptomatic.

Buttonholes

Buttonholes may be established to allow use of an access with limited length of the needle insertion segment. However, buttonholes are associated with an increased risk of local and systemic infection (233). Clinically, buttonholes mask the presence of outflow stenosis as bleeding is minimized. In this setting (impending), blowout of a buttonhole may occur (**FIGURE 3.15**), which requires surgical resection and repair of the underlying vessel. Often, there is infection of the buttonhole tract and resection is complicated.

Instead of creating buttonholes, an implantable needle guide may be used to assist in creating a tract (234).

More frequent needle insertion with daily dialysis adds strain to the needle insertion sites (235). We therefore recommend use of two sets of buttonholes in patients who dialyze more frequent than every other day.

Other Methods for the Prevention of Access Thrombosis

Prophylactic use of anticoagulation to extend access survival has been evaluated. Two randomized controlled trials, one with low-dose warfarin and the other with clopidogrel in combination with aspirin, have not demonstrated a decrease in thrombotic events or prolonged graft survival. Both studies were associated with statistically significant bleeding complications in the treated populations (236,237). A prospective, randomized trial suggested that dipyridamole decreases the thrombosis rate in patients with new PTFE grafts but that aspirin does not (238). Dipyridamole was not found to be beneficial in patients with previously thrombosed grafts. Fish oil, by inhibiting cyclooxygenase or preventing intimal hyperplasia, may prove to be useful. In a small randomized study, fish oil at a dose of 4,000 mg daily was found to increase the patency rate for newly constructed synthetic grafts (239). Angiotensin-converting enzyme (ACE) inhibitors also hold promise. In animal models, angiotensin II induces smooth muscle proliferation, and ACE inhibitors prevent myointimal proliferation. In a retrospective analysis of synthetic graft survival, it was found that ACE inhibitor therapy was associated with a higher access survival rate (240).

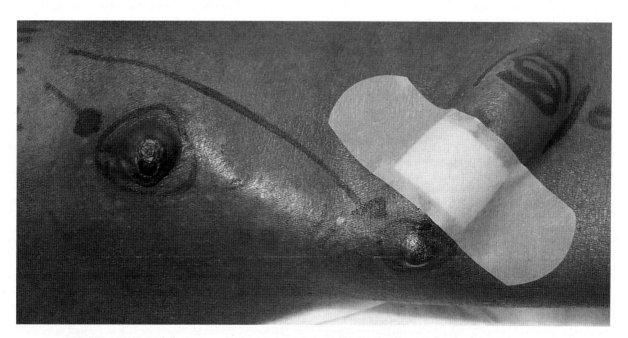

FIGURE 3.15 Buttonholes in pressurized access, presented with bleeding from buttonhole.

SUMMARY

Double-lumen central venous catheters are the preferred form of vascular access for acute hemodialysis. Insertion complications become less likely when ultrasonographic guidance is used and as the operator gains experience. Several measures may be undertaken that will reduce the likelihood of catheter-related infection. Catheter thrombosis remains a major problem but may be managed by instillation of lytic agents into the catheter lumens or by replacement of the catheter over a guidewire. Because of the association of subclavian vein catheterization with subsequent development of subclavian vein stenosis, subclavian vein catheters should be avoided.

Because autogenous arterial venous accesses are most likely to provide long-term complication-free access, they remain the preferred form of chronic vascular access. Careful planning months before the anticipated need for hemodialysis will maximize the chance for successful access creation and minimize catheter dialysis time. If an autogenous access cannot be created, a PTFE graft should be placed. The use of cuffed catheters as permanent vascular access is discouraged. Once permanent vascular access is established, maintenance of its patency presents a continual challenge to the nephrologist, dialysis staff, vascular surgeon, and interventional nephrologist/radiologist.

Thrombosis is the leading cause of vascular access loss, and venous stenoses are the leading cause of vascular access thrombosis. Prospective detection and correction of venous stenoses appears important to prolong access patency. Institution of a vascular access team whose role is the regular evaluation of access flow in combination with the physical examination is needed to preserve access function.

REFERENCES

1. Haas G. Versuche der Blutauswaschung am Lebenden mit Hilfe der Dialyse. *Klin Wochenschr* 1925;4:13–14.
2. International Society of Nephrology. ISN video legacy project: interview with Dr. Willem J. Kolff. http://cybernephrology.ualberta.ca/isn/vlp/trans/kolff.htm. Accessed September 30, 2007.
3. Quinton W, Dillard D, Scribner BH. Cannulation of blood vessels for prolonged hemodialysis. *Trans Am Soc Artif Intern Organs* 1960;6:104–113.
4. Brescia M, Cimino JE, Appel K, et al. Chronic hemodialysis using venipuncture and a surgically created arteriovenous fistula. *N Eng J Med* 1966;275:1089–1092.
5. Sperling M, Kleinschmidt W, Wilhelm A, et al. Subcutaneous arteriovenous shunt for intermittent hemodialysis treatment [in German]. *Dtsch Med Wochenschr* 1967;92(10):425–426.
6. Röhl L, Franz HE, Möhring K, et al. Direct arteriovenous fistula for hemodialysis. *Scand J Urol Nephrol* 1968;2(3):191–195.
7. Gracz KC, Ing TS, Soung LS, et al. Proximal forearm fistula for maintenance hemodialysis. *Kidney Int* 1977;11(1):71–75.
8. Konner K. Primary vascular access in diabetic patients: an audit. *Nephrol Dial Transplant* 2000;15(9):1317–1325.
9. Seldinger SI. Catheter replacement of the needle in percutaneous arteriography: a new technique. *Acta Radiol* 1953;39:368–376.
10. Shaldon S, Chiandussi L, Higgs B. Haemodialysis by percutaneous catheterization of the femoral artery and vein with regional heparinization. *Lancet* 1961;2:857–859.
11. Thomas GI. A large-vessel applique A-V shunt for hemodialysis. *Trans Am Soc Artif Intern Organs* 1969;15:288–292.
12. Baker LD Jr, Johnson JM, Goldfarb D. Expanded polytetrafluoroethylene (PTFE) subcutaneous arteriovenous conduit: an improved vascular access for chronic hemodialysis. *Trans Am Soc Artif Intern Organs* 1976;22:382–387.
13. Chinitz JL, Tokoyama T, Bower R, et al. Self-sealing prosthesis for arteriovenous fistula in man. *Trans Am Soc Artif Intern Organs* 1972;18:452–457.
14. Fleser PS, Nuthakki VK, Malinzak LE, et al. Nitric oxide-releasing biopolymers inhibit thrombus formation in a sheep model of arteriovenous bridge grafts. *J Vasc Surg* 2004;40(4):803–811.
15. L'Heureux N, McAllister T, de la Fuente L. Tissue-engineered blood vessel for adult arterial revascularization. *N Eng J Med* 2007;357(14):1451–1453.
16. Thelen M, Frotscher U, Frommhold H, et al. Angiographic demonstration of arteriovenous shunts in dialysis patients [in German]. *Fortschr Geb Rontgenstr Nuklearmed* 1972;117(4):438–444.
17. Staple TW. Retrograde venography of subcutaneous arteriovenous fistulas created surgically for hemodialysis. *Radiology* 1973;106(1):223–224.
18. Ergun DL, Mistretta CA, Kruger RA, et al. A hybrid computerized fluoroscopy technique for noninvasive cardiovascular imaging. *Radiology* 1979;132(3):739–742.
19. Dotter CT, Judkins MP, Rösch J. Nonoperative treatment of arterial occlusive disease: a radiologically facilitated technique. *Radiol Clin North Am* 1967;5(3):531–542.
20. Grüntzig A, Bollinger A, Brunner U, et al. Dotter's percutaneous recanalization in chronic arterial occlusions—a nonsurgical catheter technic [in German]. *Schweiz Med Wochenschr* 1973;103(23):825–831.
21. Gordon DH, Glanz S, Butt KM, et al. Treatment of stenotic lesions in dialysis access fistulas and shunts by transluminal angioplasty. *Radiology* 1982;143(1):53–58.
22. Beathard GA. Percutaneous transvenous angioplasty in the treatment of vascular access stenosis. *Kidney Int* 1992;42(6):1390–1397.
23. Beathard GA. Gianturco self-expanding stent in the treatment of stenosis in dialysis access grafts. *Kidney Int* 1993;43(4):872–877.
24. Beathard GA. Mechanical versus pharmacomechanical thrombolysis for the treatment of thrombosed dialysis access grafts. *Kidney Int* 1994;45(5):1401–1406.
25. Kovalik EC, Newman GE, Suhocki P, et al. Correction of central venous stenoses: use of angioplasty and vascular Wallstents. *Kidney Int* 1994;45(4):1177–1181.
26. Newman GE, Saeed M, Himmelstein S, et al. Total central vein obstruction: resolution with angioplasty and fibrinolysis. *Kidney Int* 1991;39(4):761–764.
27. Schwab SJ, Buller GL, McCann RL, et al. Prospective evaluation of a Dacron cuffed hemodialysis catheter for prolonged use. *Am J Kidney Dis* 1988;11(2):166–169.
28. Schwab SJ, Saeed M, Sussman SK, et al. Transluminal angioplasty of venous stenoses in polytetrafluoroethylene vascular access grafts. *Kidney Int* 1987;32(3):395–398.
29. Coryell L, Lott JP, Stavropoulos SW, et al. The case for primary placement of tunneled hemodialysis catheters in acute kidney injury. *J Vasc Interv Radiol* 2009;20(12):1578–1581; quiz 1582.
30. Gravenstein N, Blackshear RH. In vitro evaluation of relative perforating potential of central venous catheters: comparison of materials, selected models, number of lumens, and angles of incidence to simulated membrane. *J Clin Monit* 1991;7(1):1–6.
31. Cohen AM, Wood WC. Simplified technique for placement of long term central venous silicone catheters. *Surg Gynecol Obstet* 1982;154(5):721–724.
32. Tsui JY, Collins AB, White DW, et al. Videos in clinical medicine. Placement of a femoral venous catheter. *N Engl J Med* 2008;358(26):e30.
33. Hughes P, Scott C, Bodenham A. Ultrasonography of the femoral vessels in the groin: implications for vascular access. *Anaesthesia* 2000;55(12):1198–1202.
34. Read H, Holdgate A, Watkins S. Simple external rotation of the leg increases the size and accessibility of the femoral vein. *Emerg Med Australas* 2012;24(4):408–413.
35. Rabindranath KS, Kumar E, Shail R, et al. Use of real-time ultrasound guidance for the placement of hemodialysis catheters: a systematic review and meta-analysis of randomized controlled trials. *Am J Kidney Dis* 2011;58(6):964–970.
36. Parienti JJ, Thirion M, Mégarbane B, et al. Femoral vs jugular venous catheterization and risk of nosocomial events in adults requiring

acute renal replacement therapy: a randomized controlled trial. *JAMA* 2008;299(20):2413–2422.

37. Marik PE, Flemmer M, Harrison W. The risk of catheter-related bloodstream infection with femoral venous catheters as compared to subclavian and internal jugular venous catheters: a systematic review of the literature and meta-analysis. *Crit Care Med* 2012;40(8):2479–2485.

38. Chua HR, Schneider AG, Sherry NL, et al. Initial and extended use of femoral versus nonfemoral double-lumen vascular catheters and catheter-related infection during continuous renal replacement therapy. *Am J Kidney Dis* 2014;64(6):909–917.

39. Kelber J, Delmez JA, Windus DW. Factors affecting delivery of high-efficiency dialysis using temporary vascular access. *Am J Kidney Dis* 1993;22(1):24–29.

40. Morgan D, Ho K, Murray C, et al. A randomized trial of catheters of different lengths to achieve right atrium versus superior vena cava placement for continuous renal replacement therapy. *Am J Kidney Dis* 2012;60(2):272–279.

41. Vascular Access Work Group. Clinical practice guidelines for vascular access. *Am J Kidney Dis* 2006;48(suppl 1):S248–S273.

42. Vanholder V, Hoenich N, Ringoir S. Morbidity and mortality of central venous catheter hemodialysis: a review of 10 years' experience. *Nephron* 1987;47(4):274–279.

43. Falk A, Prabhuram N, Parthasarathy S. Conversion of temporary hemodialysis catheters to permanent hemodialysis catheters: a retrospective study of catheter exchange versus classic de novo placement. *Semin Dial* 2005;18(5):425–430.

44. Sesso R, Barbosa D, Leme IL, et al. *Staphylococcus aureus* prophylaxis in hemodialysis patients using central venous catheter: effect of mupirocin ointment. *J Am Soc Nephrol* 1998;9(6):1085–1092.

45. Kim SH, Song KI, Chang JW, et al. Prevention of uncuffed hemodialysis catheter-related bacteremia using an antibiotic lock technique: a prospective, randomized clinical trial. *Kidney Int* 2006;69(1):161–164.

46. Sznajder JI, Zveibil FR, Bitterman H, et al. Central vein catheterization. Failure and complication rates by three percutaneous approaches. *Arch Intern Med* 1986;146(2):259–261.

47. Parienti JJ, Mongardon N, Mégarbane B, et al. Intravascular complications of central venous catheterization by insertion site. *N Engl J Med* 2015;373(13):1220–1229.

48. Stuart RK, Shikora SA, Akerman P, et al. Incidence of arrhythmia with central venous catheter insertion and exchange. *JPEN J Parenter Enteral Nutr* 1990;14(2):152–155.

49. Brothers TE, Von Moll LK, Niederhuber JE, et al. Experience with subcutaneous infusion ports in three hundred patients. *Surg Gynecol Obstet* 1988;166(4):295–301.

50. Goldfarb G, Lebrec D. Percutaneous cannulation of the internal jugular vein in patients with coagulopathies: an experience based on 1,000 attempts. *Anesthesiology* 1982;56(4):321–323.

51. Vanherweghem JL, Cabolet P, Dhaene M, et al. Complications related to subclavian catheters for hemodialysis. Report and review. *Am J Nephrol* 1986;6(5):339–345.

52. Briscoe CE, Bushman JA, McDonald WI. Extensive neurological damage after cannulation of internal jugular vein. *Br Med J* 1974;1(5903):314.

53. Blitt CD, Wright WA. An unusual complication of percutaneous internal jugular vein cannulation, puncture of an endotracheal tube cuff. *Anesthesiology* 1974;40(3):306–307.

54. Butsch JL, Butsch WL, Da Rosa JF. Bilateral vocal cord paralysis. A complication of percutaneous cannulation of the internal jugular veins. *Arch Surg* 1976;111(7):828.

55. Jaques PF, Mauro MA, Keefe B. US guidance for vascular access. Technical note. *J Vasc Interv Radiol* 1992;3(2):427–430.

56. Troianos CA, Jobes DR, Ellison N. Ultrasound-guided cannulation of the internal jugular vein. A prospective, randomized study. *Anesth Analg* 1991;72(6):823–826.

57. Cheesbrough JS, Finch RG, Burden RP. A prospective study of the mechanisms of infection associated with hemodialysis catheters. *J Infect Dis* 1986;154(4):579–589.

58. Safdar N, O'Horo JC, Ghufran A, et al. Chlorhexidine-impregnated dressing for prevention of catheter-related bloodstream infection: a meta-analysis. *Crit Care Med* 2014;42(7):1703–1713.

59. Weijmer MC, Vervloet MG, ter Wee PM. Compared to tunnelled cuffed haemodialysis catheters, temporary untunnelled catheters are associated with more complications already within 2 weeks of use. *Nephrol Dial Transplant* 2004;19(3):670–677.

60. Maki DG, Ringer M, Alvarado CJ. Prospective randomised trial of povidone-iodine, alcohol, and chlorhexidine for prevention of infection associated with central venous and arterial catheters. *Lancet* 1991;338(8763):339–343.

61. Chaiyakunapruk N, Veenstra DL, Lipsky BA, et al. Chlorhexidine compared with povidone-iodine solution for vascular catheter-site care: a meta-analysis. *Ann Intern Med* 2002;136(11):792–801.

62. O'Grady NP, Alexander M, Dellinger EP, et al. Guidelines for the prevention of intravascular catheter-related infections. *Am J Infect Control* 2002;30(8):476–489.

63. Levin A, Mason AJ, Jindal KK, et al. Prevention of hemodialysis subclavian vein catheter infections by topical povidone-iodine. *Kidney Int* 1991;40(5):934–938.

64. Lok CE, Stanley KE, Hux JE, et al. Hemodialysis infection prevention with polysporin ointment. *J Am Soc Nephrol* 2003;14(1):169–179.

65. Johnson DW, MacGinley R, Kay TD, et al. A randomized controlled trial of topical exit site mupirocin application in patients with tunnelled, cuffed haemodialysis catheters. *Nephrol Dial Transplant* 2002;17(10):1802–1807.

66. Maki DG, Stolz SS, Wheeler S, et al. A prospective, randomized trial of gauze and two polyurethane dressings for site care of pulmonary artery catheters: implications for catheter management. *Crit Care Med* 1994;22(11):1729–1737.

67. Conly JM, Grieves K, Peters B. A prospective, randomized study comparing transparent and dry gauze dressings for central venous catheters. *J Infect Dis* 1989;159(2):310–319.

68. Centers for Disease Control and Prevention. Guideline for Hand Hygiene in Health-Care Settings. Recommendations of the Healthcare Infection Control Practices Advisory Committee and the HICPAC/SHEA/APIC/IDSA Hand Hygiene Task Force. Society for Healthcare Epidemiology of America/Association for Professionals in Infection Control/Infectious Diseases Society of America. *MMWR Recomm Rep* 2002;51(RR-16):1–45, quiz CE1–4.

69. Arenas MD, Sánchez-Payá J, Barril G, et al. A multicentric survey of the practice of hand hygiene in haemodialysis units: factors affecting compliance. *Nephrol Dial Transplant* 2005;20(6):1164–1171.

70. Zacharias JM, Weatherston CP, Spewak CR, et al. Alteplase versus urokinase for occluded hemodialysis catheters. *Ann Pharmacother* 2003;37(1):27–33.

71. Brismar B, Hårdstedt C, Jacobson S. Diagnosis of thrombosis by catheter phlebography after prolonged central venous catheterization. *Ann Surg* 1981;194(6):779–783.

72. Fant GF, Dennis VW, Quarles LF. Late vascular complications of the subclavian dialysis catheter. *Am J Kidney Dis* 1986;7(3):225–228.

73. Davis D, Petersen J, Feldman R, et al. Subclavian venous stenosis. A complication of subclavian dialysis. *JAMA* 1984;252(24):3404–3406.

74. Barrett N, Spencer S, McIvor J, et al. Subclavian stenosis: a major complication of subclavian dialysis catheters. *Nephrol Dial Transplant* 1988;3(4):423–425.

75. Schillinger F, Schillinger D, Montagnac R, et al. Post catheterisation vein stenosis in haemodialysis: comparative angiographic study of 50 subclavian and 50 internal jugular accesses. *Nephrol Dial Transplant* 1991;6(10):722–724.

76. Cimochowski GE, Worley E, Rutherford WE, et al. Superiority of the internal jugular over the subclavian access for temporary dialysis. *Nephron* 1990;54(2):154–161.

77. Schwab SJ, Quarles LD, Middleton JP, et al. Hemodialysis-associated subclavian vein stenosis. *Kidney Int* 1988;33(6):1156–1159.

78. United States Renal Data System. The 2015 USRDS Annual Report. http://www.usrds.org/adr.aspx. Accessed September 30, 2015.

79. U.S. Renal Data System. *USRDS 2010 Annual Data Report: Epidemiology of Kidney Disease in the United States.* Bethesda, MD: National Institutes of Health, National Institute of Diabetes and Digestive and Kidney Diseases, 2010.

80. Sidawy AN, Gray R, Besarab A, et al. Recommended standards for reports dealing with arteriovenous hemodialysis accesses. *J Vasc Surg* 2002;35(3):603–610.

81. Rehman R, Schmidt RJ, Moss AH. Ethical and legal obligation to avoid long-term tunneled catheter access. *Clin J Am Soc Nephrol* 2009;4(2):456–460.

82. Pisoni RL, Young EW, Dykstra DM, et al. Vascular access use in Europe and the United States: results from the DOPPS. *Kidney Int* 2002;61(1):305–316.

83. Beathard GA, Posen GA. Initial clinical results with the LifeSite Hemodialysis Access System. *Kidney Int* 2000;58(5):2221–2227.

84. Rayan SS, Terramani TT, Weiss VJ, et al. The LifeSite Hemodialysis Access System in patients with limited access. *J Vasc Surg* 2003;38(4):714–718.

85. Ross JR. Successful treatment of a LifeSite Hemodialysis Access System pocket infection with large-volume kanamycin solution irrigation. *Adv Ren Replace Ther* 2003;10(3):248–253.

86. Schwab SJ, Weiss MA, Rushton F, et al. Multicenter clinical trial results with the LifeSite hemodialysis access system. *Kidney Int* 2002;62(3):1026–1033.

87. Ash SR. Fluid mechanics and clinical success of central venous catheters for dialysis—answers to simple but persisting problems. *Semin Dial* 2007;20(3):237–256.

88. Erben J, Kvasnicka J, Bastecký J, et al. Long-term experience with the technique of subclavian and femoral vein cannulation in hemodialysis. *Artif Organs* 1979;3(3):241–244.

89. Elayi CS, Allen CL, Leung S, et al. Inside-out access: a new method of lead placement for patients with central venous occlusions. *Heart Rhythm* 2011;8(6):851–857.

90. Matsuura J, Dietrich A, Steuben S, et al. Mediastinal approach to the placement of tunneled hemodialysis catheters in patients with central vein occlusion in an outpatient access center. *J Vasc Access* 2011;12(3):258–261.

91. Moss AH, Vasilakis C, Holley JL, et al. Use of a silicone dual-lumen catheter with a Dacron cuff as a long-term vascular access for hemodialysis patients. *Am J Kidney Dis* 1990;16(3):211–215.

92. Yevzlin AS, Song GU, Sanchez RJ, et al. Fluoroscopically guided vs modified traditional placement of tunneled hemodialysis catheters: clinical outcomes and cost analysis. *J Vasc Access* 2007;8(4):245–251.

93. Vesely TM, Ravenscroft A. Hemodialysis catheter tip design: observations on fluid flow and recirculation. *J Vasc Access* 2016;17(1):29–39.

94. Suhocki PV, Conlon PJ Jr, Knelson MH, et al. Silastic cuffed catheters for hemodialysis vascular access: thrombolytic and mechanical correction of malfunction. *Am J Kidney Dis* 1996;28(3):379–386.

95. Polaschegg HD. Loss of catheter locking solution caused by fluid density. *ASAIO J* 2005;51(3):230–235.

96. Ponec D, Irwin D, Haire WD, et al. Recombinant tissue plasminogen activator (alteplase) for restoration of flow in occluded central venous access devices: a double-blind placebo-controlled trial—the Cardiovascular Thrombolytic to Open Occluded Lines (COOL) efficacy trial. *J Vasc Interv Radiol* 2001;12(8):951–955.

97. Alomari AI, Falk A. The natural history of tunneled hemodialysis catheters removed or exchanged: a single-institution experience. *J Vasc Interv Radiol* 2007;18(2):227–235.

98. Crain MR, Mewissen MW, Ostrowski GJ, et al. Fibrin sleeve stripping for salvage of failing hemodialysis catheters: technique and initial results. *Radiology* 1996;198(1):41–44.

99. Raad I, Costerton W, Sabharwal U, et al. Ultrastructural analysis of indwelling vascular catheters: a quantitative relationship between luminal colonization and duration of placement. *J Infect Dis* 1993;168(2):400–407.

100. Rodriguez-Aranda A, Alcazar JM, Sanz F, et al. Endoluminal colonization as a risk factor for coagulase-negative staphylococcal catheter-related bloodstream infections in haemodialysis patients. *Nephrol Dial Transplant* 2011;26(3):948–955.

101. Cookson BD. Mupirocin resistance in staphylococci. *J Antimicrob Chemother* 1990;25(4):497–501.

102. Hill RL, Casewell MW. Nasal carriage of MRSA: the role of mupirocin and outlook for resistance. *Drugs Exp Clin Res* 1990;16(8):397–402.

103. Johnson DW, van Eps C, Mudge DW, et al. Randomized, controlled trial of topical exit-site application of honey (Medihoney) versus mupirocin for the prevention of catheter-associated infections in hemodialysis patients. *J Am Soc Nephrol* 2005;16(5):1456–1462.

104. Al-Solaiman Y, Estrada E, Allon M. The spectrum of infections in catheter-dependent hemodialysis patients. *Clin J Am Soc Nephrol* 2011;6(9):2247–2252.

105. Hoen B, Paul-Dauphin A, Hestin D, et al. EPIBACDIAL: a multicenter prospective study of risk factors for bacteremia in chronic hemodialysis patients. *J Am Soc Nephrol* 1998;9(5):869–876.

106. Allon M, Depner TA, Radeva M, et al. Impact of dialysis dose and membrane on infection-related hospitalization and death: results of the HEMO Study. *J Am Soc Nephrol* 2003;14(7):1863–1870.

107. Pastan S, Soucie JM, McClellan WM. Vascular access and increased risk of death among hemodialysis patients. *Kidney Int* 2002;62(2):620–626.

108. Allon M. Dialysis catheter-related bacteremia: treatment and prophylaxis. *Am J Kidney Dis* 2004;44(5):779–791.

109. Silva TN, de Marchi D, Mendes ML, et al. Approach to prophylactic measures for central venous catheter-related infections in hemodialysis: a critical review. *Hemodial Int* 2014;18(1):15–23.

110. Beathard GA. Catheter management protocol for catheter-related bacteremia prophylaxis. *Semin Dial* 2003;6(5):403–405.

111. Safdar N, Fine JP, Maki DG. Meta-analysis: methods for diagnosing intravascular device-related bloodstream infection. *Ann Intern Med* 2005;142(6):451–466.

112. Gailiunas P Jr, Dominguez-Moreno M, Lazarus M, et al. Vestibular toxicity of gentamicin. Incidence in patients receiving long-term hemodialysis therapy. *Arch Intern Med* 1978;138(11):1621–1624.

113. Lewis K. Riddle of biofilm resistance. *Antimicrob Agents Chemother* 2001;45(4):999–1007.

114. Poole CV, Carlton D, Bimbo L, et al. Treatment of catheter-related bacteraemia with an antibiotic lock protocol: effect of bacterial pathogen. *Nephrol Dial Transplant* 2004;19(5):1237–1244.

115. Krishnasami Z, Carlton D, Bimbo L, et al. Management of hemodialysis catheter-related bacteremia with an adjunctive antibiotic lock solution. *Kidney Int* 2002;61(3):1136–1142.

116. Mermel LA, Allon M, Bouza E, et al. Clinical practice guidelines for the diagnosis and management of intravascular catheter-related infection: 2009 Update by the Infectious Diseases Society of America. *Clin Infect Dis* 2009;49(1):1–45.

117. Trerotola SO, Johnson MS, Shah H, et al. Tunneled hemodialysis catheters: use of a silver-coated catheter for prevention of infection—a randomized study. *Radiology* 1998;207(2):491–496.

118. Allon M. Prophylaxis against dialysis catheter-related bacteremia with a novel antimicrobial lock solution. *Clin Infect Dis* 2003;36(12):1539–1544.

119. Dogra GK, Herson H, Hutchison B, et al. Prevention of tunneled hemodialysis catheter-related infections using catheter-restricted filling with gentamicin and citrate: a randomized controlled study. *J Am Soc Nephrol* 2002;13(8):2133–2139.

120. Betjes MG, van Agteren M. Prevention of dialysis catheter-related sepsis with a citrate-taurolidine-containing lock solution. *Nephrol Dial Transplant* 2004;19(6):1546–1551.

121. Mokrzycki MH, Zhang M, Golestaneh L, et al. An interventional controlled trial comparing 2 management models for the treatment of tunneled cuffed catheter bacteremia: a collaborative team model versus usual physician-managed care. *Am J Kidney Dis* 2006;48(4):587–595.

122. Warren DK, Cosgrove SE, Diekema DJ, et al. A multicenter intervention to prevent catheter-associated bloodstream infections. *Infect Control Hosp Epidemiol* 2006;27(7):662–669.

123. Sedlacek M, Gemery JM, Cheung AL, et al. Aspirin treatment is associated with a significantly decreased risk of *Staphylococcus aureus* bacteremia in hemodialysis patients with tunneled catheters. *Am J Kidney Dis* 2007;49(3):401–408.

124. Long DA, Coulthard MG. Effect of heparin-bonded central venous catheters on the incidence of catheter-related thrombosis and infection in children and adults. *Anaesth Intensive Care* 2006;34(4):481–484.

125. Jain G, Allon M, Saddekni S, et al. Does heparin coating improve patency or reduce infection of tunneled dialysis catheters? *Clin J Am Soc Nephrol* 2009;4(11):1787–1790.

126. Clark TW, Jacobs D, Charles HW, et al. Comparison of heparin-coated and conventional split-tip hemodialysis catheters. *Cardiovasc Intervent Radiol* 2009;32(4):703–706.

127. Appelbaum PC. MRSA—the tip of the iceberg. *Clin Microbiol Infect* 2006;12(suppl 2):3–10.

128. McDonald LC, Hageman JC. Vancomycin intermediate and resistant *Staphylococcus aureus*. What the nephrologist needs to know. *Nephrol News Issues* 2004;18(11):63–64, 66–67, 71–72 passim.

129. Pai AB, Pai MP. Optimizing antimicrobial therapy for gram-positive bloodstream infections in patients on hemodialysis. *Adv Chronic Kidney Dis* 2006;13(3):259–270.

130. Rodriguez JA, Armadans L, Ferrer E, et al. The function of permanent vascular access. *Nephrol Dial Transplant* 2000;15(3):402–408.

131. Dember LM, Beck GJ, Allon M, et al. Effect of clopidogrel on early failure of arteriovenous fistulas for hemodialysis: a randomized controlled trial. *JAMA* 2008;299(18):2164–2171.

132. Lee T, Ullah A, Allon M, et al. Decreased cumulative access survival in arteriovenous fistulas requiring interventions to promote maturation. *Clin J Am Soc Nephrol* 2011;6(3):575–581.

133. Chan KE, Pflederer TA, Steele DJ, et al. Access survival amongst hemodialysis patients referred for preventive angiography and percutaneous transluminal angioplasty. *Clin J Am Soc Nephrol* 2011;6(11):2669–2680.

134. Konner K, Hulbert-Shearon TE, Roys EC, et al. Tailoring the initial vascular access for dialysis patients. *Kidney Int* 2002;62(1):329–338.

135. Shemesh D, Goldin I, Zaghal I, et al. Angioplasty with stent graft versus bare stent for recurrent cephalic arch stenosis in autogenous arteriovenous access for hemodialysis: a prospective randomized clinical trial. *J Vasc Surg* 2008;48(6):1524–1531, 1531.e1–1532.e2.

136. Kaufman JL. The decline of the autogenous hemodialysis access site. *Semin Dial* 1995;8(2):59–61.

137. Polkinghorne KR, McDonald SP, Atkins RC, et al. Vascular access and all-cause mortality: a propensity score analysis. *J Am Soc Nephrol* 2004;15(2):477–486.

138. Woods JD, Port FK. The impact of vascular access for haemodialysis on patient morbidity and mortality. *Nephrol Dial Transplant* 1997;12(4):657–659.

139. Pisoni RL, Arrington CJ, Albert JM, et al. Facility hemodialysis vascular access use and mortality in countries participating in DOPPS: an instrumental variable analysis. *Am J Kidney Dis* 2009;53(3):475–491.

140. Xue JL, Dahl D, Ebben JP, et al. The association of initial hemodialysis access type with mortality outcomes in elderly Medicare ESRD patients. *Am J Kidney Dis* 2003;42(5):1013–1019.

141. United States Renal Data System. *USRDS 1995 Annual Data Report.* Bethesda, MD: National Institutes of Health, National Institute of Diabetes and Digestive and Kidney Diseases, 1995. https://www.usrds.org/atlas95.aspx. Accessed June 15, 2016.

142. Feldman HI, Kobrin S, Wasserstein A. Hemodialysis vascular access morbidity. *J Am Soc Nephrol* 1996;7(4):523–535.

143. National Kidney Foundation. KDOQI Clinical Practice Guideline for Hemodialysis Adequacy: 2015 update. *Am J Kidney Dis* 2015;66(5):884–930.

144. Beasley C, Rowland J, Spergel L. Fistula first: an update for renal providers. *Nephrol News Issues* 2004;18(11):88, 90.

145. Silva MB Jr, Hobson RW II, Pappas PJ, et al. A strategy for increasing use of autogenous hemodialysis access procedures: impact of preoperative non-invasive evaluation. *J Vasc Surg* 1998;27(2):302–307; discussion 307–308.

146. Ascher E, Gade P, Hingorani A, et al. Changes in the practice of angioaccess surgery: impact of dialysis outcome and quality initiative recommendations. *J Vasc Surg* 2000;31(1 pt 1):84–92.

147. Allon M, Lockhart ME, Lilly RZ, et al. Effect of preoperative sonographic mapping on vascular access outcomes in hemodialysis patients. *Kidney Int* 2001;60(5):2013–2020.

148. Gibson KD, Caps MT, Kohler TR, et al. Assessment of a policy to reduce placement of prosthetic hemodialysis access. *Kidney Int* 2001;59(6):2335–2345.

149. Jennings WC, Maliska CM, Blebea J, et al. Creating arteriovenous fistulas in patients with chronic central venous obstruction. *J Vasc Access* 2016;17(3):239–242.

150. Gonsalves CF, Eschelman DJ, Sullivan KL, et al. Incidence of central vein stenosis and occlusion following upper extremity PICC and port placement. *Cardiovasc Intervent Radiol* 2003;26(2):123–127.

151. Trerotola SO, Stavropoulos SW, Mondschein JI, et al. Triple-lumen peripherally inserted central catheter in patients in the critical care unit: prospective evaluation. *Radiology* 2010;256(1):312–320.

152. Allen AW, Megargell JL, Brown DB, et al. Venous thrombosis associated with the placement of peripherally inserted central catheters. *J Vasc Interv Radiol* 2000;11(10):1309–1314.

153. Abdullah BJ, Mohammad N, Sangkar JV, et al. Incidence of upper limb venous thrombosis associated with peripherally inserted central catheters (PICC). *Br J Radiol* 2005;78(931):596–600.

154. Martin C, Viviand X, Saux P, et al. Upper-extremity deep vein thrombosis after central venous catheterization via the axillary vein. *Crit Care Med* 1999;27(12):2626–2629.

155. Smits JH, Bos C, Elgersma OE, et al. Hemodialysis access imaging: comparison of flow-interrupted contrast-enhanced MR angiography and digital subtraction angiography. *Radiology* 2002;225(3):829–834.

156. Mendes RR, Farber MA, Marston WA, et al. Prediction of wrist arteriovenous fistula maturation with preoperative vein mapping with ultrasonography. *J Vasc Surg* 2002;36(3):460–463.

157. Segal JH, Kayler LK, Henke P, et al. Vascular access outcomes using the transposed basilic vein arteriovenous fistula. *Am J Kidney Dis* 2003;42(1):151–157.

158. Hossny A. Brachiobasilic arteriovenous fistula: different surgical techniques and their effects on fistula patency and dialysis-related complications. *J Vasc Surg* 2003;37(4):821–826.

159. Zielinski CM, Mittal SK, Anderson P, et al. Delayed superficialization of brachiobasilic fistula: technique and initial experience. *Arch Surg* 2001;136(8):929–932.

160. Hakim RM, Breyer J, Ismail N, et al. Effects of dose of dialysis on morbidity and mortality. *Am J Kidney Dis* 1994;23(5):661–669.

161. Anderson CB, Etheredge EE, Harter HR, et al. Blood flow measurements in arteriovenous dialysis fistulas. *Surgery* 1977;81(4):459–461.

162. Anderson CB, Etheredge EE, Harter HR, et al. Local blood flow characteristics of arteriovenous fistulas in the forearm for dialysis. *Surg Gynecol Obstet* 1977;144(4):531–533.

163. Allon M, Greene T, Dember LM, et al. Association between preoperative vascular function and postoperative arteriovenous fistula development [published online ahead of print May 9, 2016]. *J Am Soc Nephrol.*

164. Rittgers SE, Garcia-Valdez C, McCormick JT, et al. Noninvasive blood flow measurement in expanded polytetrafluoroethylene grafts for hemodialysis access. *J Vasc Surg* 1986;3(4):635–642.

165. Burdick JF, Scott W, Cosimi AB. Experience with Dacron graft arteriovenous fistulas for dialysis access. *Ann Surg* 1978;187(3):262–266.

166. Strauch BS, O'Connell RS, Geoly KL, et al. Forecasting thrombosis of vascular access with Doppler color flow imaging. *Am J Kidney Dis* 1992;19(6):554–557.

167. Shackleton CR, Taylor DC, Buckley AR, et al. Predicting failure in polytetrafluoroethylene vascular access grafts for hemodialysis: a pilot study. *Can J Surg* 1987;30(6):442–444.

168. Kherlakian GM, Roedersheimer LR, Arbaugh JJ, et al. Comparison of autogenous fistula versus expanded polytetrafluoroethylene graft fistula for angioaccess in hemodialysis. *Am J Surg* 1986;152(2):238–243.

169. Palder SB, Kirkman RL, Whittemore AD, et al. Vascular access for hemodialysis. Patency rates and results of revision. *Ann Surg* 1985;202(2):235–239.

170. Winsett OE, Wolma FJ. Complications of vascular access for hemodialysis. *South Med J* 1985;78(5):513–517.

171. Etheredge EE, Haid SD, Maeser MN, et al. Salvage operations for malfunctioning polytetrafluoroethylene hemodialysis access grafts. *Surgery* 1983;94(3):464–470.

172. Beathard GA. The treatment of vascular access graft dysfunction: a nephrologist's view and experience. *Adv Ren Replace Ther* 1994;1(2): 131–147.

173. Bone GE, Pomajzi MJ. Management of dialysis fistula thrombosis. *Am J Surg* 1979;138(6):901–906.

174. Schwab SJ, Raymond JR, Saeed M, et al. Prevention of hemodialysis fistula thrombosis. Early detection of venous stenoses. *Kidney Int* 1989;36(4):707–711.

175. Lilly RZ, Carlton D, Barker J, et al. Predictors of arteriovenous graft patency after radiologic intervention in hemodialysis patients. *Am J Kidney Dis* 2001;37(5):945–953.

176. Asif A, Gadalean FN, Merrill D, et al. Inflow stenosis in arteriovenous fistulas and grafts: a multicenter, prospective study. *Kidney Int* 2005;67(5):1986–1992.

177. Lok CE, Bhola C, Croxford R, et al. Reducing vascular access morbidity: a comparative trial of two vascular access monitoring strategies. *Nephrol Dial Transplant* 2003;18(6):1174–1180.

178. Allon M, Bailey R, Ballard R, et al. A multidisciplinary approach to hemodialysis access: prospective evaluation. *Kidney Int* 1998;53(2):473–479.

179. Besarab A, Lubkowski T, Frinak S, et al. Detection of access strictures and outlet stenoses in vascular accesses. Which test is best? *ASAIO J* 1997;43(5):M543–M547.

180. Campos RP, Do Nascimento MM, Chula DC, et al. Stenosis in hemodialysis arteriovenous fistula: evaluation and treatment. *Hemodial Int* 2006;10(2):152–161.

181. Trerotola SO, Scheel PJ Jr, Powe NR, et al. Screening for dialysis access graft malfunction: comparison of physical examination with US. *J Vasc Interv Radiol* 1996;7(1):15–20.

182. Oudenhoven LF, Pattynama PM, de Roos A et al. Magnetic resonance, a new method for measuring blood flow in hemodialysis fistulae. *Kidney Int* 1994;45(3):884–889.

183. Krivitski NM. Theory and validation of access flow measurement by dilution technique during hemodialysis. *Kidney Int* 1995;48(1):244–250.

184. Depner TA, Krivitski NM. Clinical measurement of blood flow in hemodialysis access fistulae and grafts by ultrasound dilution. *ASAIO J* 1995;41(3):M745–M749.

185. Schwab SJ, Oliver MJ, Suhocki P, et al. Hemodialysis arteriovenous access: detection of stenosis and response to treatment by vascular access blood flow. *Kidney Int* 2001;59(1):358–362.

186. Pandeya S, Lindsay RM. The relationship between cardiac output and access flow during hemodialysis. *ASAIO J* 1999;45(3):135–138.

187. Besarab A, Sullivan KL, Ross RP, et al. Utility of intra-access pressure monitoring in detecting and correcting venous outlet stenoses prior to thrombosis. *Kidney Int* 1995;47(5):1364–1373.

188. Ash SR, Dhamija R, Zaroura MY, et al. The StenTec gauge for measuring static intra-access pressure ratio (P(Ia Ratio)) of fistulas and grafts. *Semin Dial* 2012;25(4):474–481.

189. Spergel LM, Holland JE, Fadem SZ, et al. Static intra-access pressure ratio does not correlate with access blood flow. *Kidney Int* 2004;66(4): 1512–1516.

190. Frinak S, Zasuwa G, Dunfee T, et al. Dynamic venous access pressure ratio test for hemodialysis access monitoring. *Am J Kidney Dis* 2002;40(4):760–768.

191. Sherman RA, Levy SS. Rate-related recirculation: the effect of altering blood flow on dialyzer recirculation. *Am J Kidney Dis* 1991;17(2):170–173.

192. Sherman RA. The measurement of dialysis access recirculation. *Am J Kidney Dis* 1993;22(4):616–621.

193. Depner TA, Rizwan S, Cheer AY, et al. High venous urea concentrations in the opposite arm. A consequence of hemodialysis-induced compartment disequilibrium. *ASAIO Trans* 1991;37(3):M141–M143.

194. Schneditz D, Polaschegg HD, Levin NW, et al. Cardiopulmonary recirculation in dialysis. An underrecognized phenomenon. *ASAIO J* 1992;38(3):M194–M196.

195. Besarab A, Sherman R. The relationship of recirculation to access blood flow. *Am J Kidney Dis* 1997;29(2):223–229.

196. Tattersall JE, Farrington K, Raniga PD, et al. Haemodialysis recirculation detected by the three-sample method is an artefact. *Nephrol Dial Transplant* 1993;8(1):60–63.

197. Depner TA, Krivitski NM, MacGibbon D. Hemodialysis access recirculation measured by ultrasound dilution. *ASAIO J* 1995;41(3):M749–M753.

198. Windus DW, Audrain J, Vanderson R, et al. Optimization of high-efficiency hemodialysis by detection and correction of fistula dysfunction. *Kidney Int* 1990;38(2):337–441.

199. Collins DM, Lambert MB, Middleton JP, et al. Fistula dysfunction: effect on rapid hemodialysis. *Kidney Int* 1992;41(5):1292–1296.

200. Katz SG, Kohl RD. The percutaneous treatment of angioaccess graft complications. *Am J Surg* 1995;170(3):238–242.

201. Brooks JL, Sigley RD, May KJ Jr, et al. Transluminal angioplasty versus surgical repair for stenosis of hemodialysis grafts. A randomized study. *Am J Surg* 1987;153(6):530–531.

202. Dapunt O, Feurstein M, Rendl KH, et al. Transluminal angioplasty versus conventional operation in the treatment of haemodialysis fistula stenosis: results from a 5-year study. *Br J Surg* 1987;74(11): 1004–1005.

203. Kanterman RY, Vesely TM, Pilgram TK, et al. Dialysis access grafts: anatomic location of venous stenosis and results of angioplasty. *Radiology* 1995;195(1):135–139.

204. Glanz S, Gordon D, Butt KM, et al. Dialysis access fistulas: treatment of stenoses by transluminal angioplasty. *Radiology* 1984;152(3): 637–642.

205. Glanz S, Gordon DH, Butt KM, et al. The role of percutaneous angioplasty in the management of chronic hemodialysis fistulas. *Ann Surg* 1987;206(6):777–781.

206. Mori Y, Horikawa K, Sato K, et al. Stenotic lesions in vascular access: treatment with transluminal angioplasty using high-pressure balloons. *Intern Med* 1994;33(5):284–287.

207. Gmelin E, Winterhoff R, Rinast E. Insufficient hemodialysis access fistulas: late results of treatment with percutaneous balloon angioplasty. *Radiology* 1989;171(3):657–660.

208. Turmel-Rodrigues L, Pengloan J, Blanchier D, et al. Insufficient dialysis shunts: improved long-term patency rates with close hemodynamic monitoring, repeated percutaneous balloon angioplasty, and stent placement. *Radiology* 1993;187(1):273–278.

209. Ram SJ, Work J, Caldito GC, et al. A randomized controlled trial of blood flow and stenosis surveillance of hemodialysis grafts. *Kidney Int* 2003;64(1):272–280.

210. Moist LM, Churchill DN, House AA, et al. Regular monitoring of access flow compared with monitoring of venous pressure fails to improve graft survival. *J Am Soc Nephrol* 2003;14(10):2645–2653.

211. Haskal ZJ, Trerotola S, Dolmatch B, et al. Stent graft versus balloon angioplasty for failing dialysis-access grafts. *N Engl J Med* 2010;362(6):494–503.

212. Kitrou PM, Katsanos K, Spiliopoulos S, et al. Drug-eluting versus plain balloon angioplasty for the treatment of failing dialysis access: final results and cost-effectiveness analysis from a prospective randomized controlled trial (NCT01174472). *Eur J Radiol* 2015;84(3):418–423.

213. Schwartz CI, McBrayer CV, Sloan JH, et al. Thrombosed dialysis grafts: comparison of treatment with transluminal angioplasty and surgical revision. *Radiology* 1995;194(2):337–341.

214. Valji K, Bookstein JJ, Roberts AC, et al. Pharmacomechanical thrombolysis and angioplasty in the management of clotted hemodialysis grafts: early and late clinical results. *Radiology* 1991;178(1):243–247.

215. Trerotola SO, Lund GB, Scheel PJ Jr, et al. Thrombosed dialysis access grafts: percutaneous mechanical declotting without urokinase. *Radiology* 1994;191(3):721–726.

216. Middlebrook MR, Amygdalos MA, Soulen MC, et al. Thrombosed hemodialysis grafts: percutaneous mechanical balloon declotting versus thrombolysis. *Radiology* 1995;196(1):73–77.

217. Vesely TM, Hovsepian DM, Darcy MD, et al. Angioscopic observations after percutaneous thrombectomy of thrombosed hemodialysis grafts. *J Vasc Interv Radiol* 2000;11(8):971–977.

218. Summers S, Drazan K, Gomes A, et al. Urokinase therapy for thrombosed hemodialysis access grafts. *Surg Gynecol Obstet* 1993;176(6): 534–538.

219. Beathard GA. Thrombolysis versus surgery for the treatment of thrombosed dialysis access grafts. *J Am Soc Nephrol* 1995;6(6):1619–1624.

220. Beathard GA. Bacterial colonization of thrombosed dialysis arteriovenous grafts. *Semin Dial* 2015;28(4):446–449.

221. Bhat DJ, Tellis VA, Kohlberg WI, et al. Management of sepsis involving expanded polytetrafluoroethylene grafts for hemodialysis access. *Surgery* 1980;87(4):445–450.

222. Munda R, First MR, Alexander JW, et al. Polytetrafluoroethylene graft survival in hemodialysis. *JAMA* 1983;249(2):219–222.

223. Kaplowitz LG, Comstock JA, Landwehr DM, et al. A prospective study of infections in hemodialysis patients: patient hygiene and other risk factors for infection. *Infect Control Hosp Epidemiol* 1988;9(12):534–541.

224. Dobkin JF, Miller MH, Steigbigel NH. Septicemia in patients on chronic hemodialysis. *Ann Intern Med* 1978;88(1):28–33.

225. Keane WF, Shapiro FL, Raij L. Incidence and type of infections occurring in 445 chronic hemodialysis patients. *Trans Am Soc Artif Intern Organs* 1977;23:41–47.

226. Higgins RM. Infections in a renal unit. *Q J Med* 1989;70(261):41–51.

227. Kaplowitz LG, Comstock JA, Landwehr DM, et al. Prospective study of microbial colonization of the nose and skin and infection of the vascular access site in hemodialysis patients. *J Clin Microbiol* 1988;26(7):1257–1262.

228. Morgan AP, Knight DC, Tilney NL, et al. Femoral triangle sepsis in dialysis patients: frequency, management, and outcome. *Ann Surg* 1980;191(4):460–464.

229. Anderson CB, Codd JR, Graff RA, et al. Cardiac failure and upper extremity arteriovenous dialysis fistulas. Case reports and a review of the literature. *Arch Intern Med* 1976;136(3):292–297.

230. Rivers SP, Scher LA, Veith FJ. Correction of steal syndrome secondary to hemodialysis access fistulas: a simplified quantitative technique. *Surgery* 1992;112(3):593–597.

231. West JC, Bertsch DJ, Peterson SL, et al. Arterial insufficiency in hemodialysis access procedures: correction by "banding" technique. *Transplant Proc* 1991;23(2):1838–1840.

232. Kirkman RL. Technique for flow reduction in dialysis access fistulas. *Surg Gynecol Obstet* 1991;172(3):231–233.

233. Wong B, Muneer M, Wiebe N, et al. Buttonhole versus rope-ladder cannulation of arteriovenous fistulas for hemodialysis: a systematic review. *Am J Kidney Dis* 2014;64(6):918–936.

234. Hill AA, Vasudevan T, Young NP, et al. Use of an implantable needle guide to access difficult or impossible to cannulate arteriovenous fistulae using the buttonhole technique. *J Vasc Access* 2013;14(2):164–169.

235. Lok CE, Sontrop JM, Faratro R, et al. Frequent hemodialysis fistula infectious complications. *Nephron Extra* 2014;4(3):159–167.

236. Kaufman JS, O'Connor TZ, Zhang JH, et al. Randomized controlled trial of clopidogrel plus aspirin to prevent hemodialysis access graft thrombosis. *J Am Soc Nephrol* 2003;14(9):2313–2321.

237. Crowther MA, Clase CM, Margetts PJ, et al. Low-intensity warfarin is ineffective for the prevention of PTFE graft failure in patients on hemodialysis: a randomized controlled trial. *J Am Soc Nephrol* 2002;13(9):2331–2337.

238. Sreedhara R, Himmelfarb J, Lazarus JM, et al. Anti-platelet therapy in graft thrombosis: results of a prospective, randomized, double-blind study. *Kidney Int* 1994;45(5):1477–1483.

239. Schmitz PG, McCloud LK, Reikes ST, et al. Prophylaxis of hemodialysis graft thrombosis with fish oil: double-blind, randomized, prospective trial. *J Am Soc Nephrol* 2002;13(1):184–190.

240. Gradzki R, Dhingra RK, Port FK, et al. Use of ACE inhibitors is associated with prolonged survival of arteriovenous grafts. *Am J Kidney Dis* 2001;38(6):1240–1244.

241. Swartz RD, Messana JM, Boyer CJ, et al. Successful use of cuffed central venous hemodialysis catheters inserted percutaneously. *J Am Soc Nephrol* 1994;4(9):1719–1725.

242. Lund GB, Trerotola SO, Scheel PF Jr, et al. Outcome of tunneled hemodialysis catheters placed by radiologists. *Radiology* 1996;198(2):467–472.

243. Marr KA, Sexton DJ, Conlon PJ, et al. Catheter-related bacteremia and outcome of attempted catheter salvage in patients undergoing hemodialysis. *Ann Intern Med* 1997;127(4):275–280.

244. Saad TF. Bacteremia associated with tunneled, cuffed hemodialysis catheters. *Am J Kidney Dis* 1999;34(6):1114–1124.

245. Jean G, Charra B, Chazot C, et al. Risk factor analysis for long-term tunneled dialysis catheter-related bacteremias. *Nephron* 2002;91(3):399–405.

246. Troidle L, Finkelstein FO. Catheter-related bacteremia in hemodialysis patients: the role of the central venous catheter in prevention and therapy. *Int J Artif Organs* 2008;31(9):827–833.

247. Ashby DR, Power A, Singh S, et al. Bacteremia associated with tunneled hemodialysis catheters: outcome after attempted salvage. *Clin J Am Soc Nephrol* 2009;4(10):1601–1605.

248. Capdevila JA, Segarra A, Planes AM, et al. Successful treatment of haemodialysis catheter-related sepsis without catheter removal. *Nephrol Dial Transplant* 1993;8(3):231–234.

249. Bailey E, Berry N, Cheesbrough JS. Antimicrobial lock therapy for catheter-related bacteraemia among patients on maintenance haemodialysis. *J Antimicrob Chemother* 2002;50(4):615–617.

250. Vardhan A, Davies J, Daryanani I, et al. Treatment of haemodialysis catheter-related infections. *Nephrol Dial Transplant* 2002;17(6):1149–1150.

251. Maya ID, Carlton D, Estrada E, et al. Treatment of dialysis catheter-related *Staphylococcus aureus* bacteremia with an antibiotic lock: a quality improvement report. *Am J Kidney Dis* 2007;50(2):289–295.

252. Peterson WJ, Maya ID, Carlton D, et al. Treatment of dialysis catheter-related Enterococcus bacteremia with an antibiotic lock: a quality improvement report. *Am J Kidney Dis* 2009;53(1):107–111.

253. Joshi AJ, Hart PD. Antibiotic catheter locks in the treatment of tunneled hemodialysis catheter-related blood stream infection. *Semin Dial* 2013;26(2):223–226.

254. Shaffer D. Catheter-related sepsis complicating long-term, tunnelled central venous dialysis catheters: management by guidewire exchange. *Am J Kidney Dis* 1995;25(4):593–596.

255. Robinson D, Suhocki P, Schwab SJ. Treatment of infected tunneled venous access hemodialysis catheters with guidewire exchange. *Kidney Int* 1998;53(6):1792–1794.

256. Beathard GA. Management of bacteremia associated with tunneled-cuffed hemodialysis catheters. *J Am Soc Nephrol* 1999;10(5):1045–1049.

257. Sychev D, Maya ID, Allon M. Clinical outcomes of dialysis catheter-related candidemia in hemodialysis patients. *Clin J Am Soc Nephrol* 2009;4(6):1102–1105.

258. Langer JM, Cohen RM, Berns JS, et al. Staphylococcus-infected tunneled dialysis catheters: is over-the-wire exchange an appropriate management option? *Cardiovasc Intervent Radiol* 2011;34(6):1230–1235.

CHAPTER 4

Anticoagulation Strategies during Hemodialysis Procedures

William J. Dahms, Jr.

Since the inception of the chronic hemodialysis procedure in the 1960s, anticoagulation has remained an important component of adequate treatment management. Traditionally, the challenging task of preventing clotting of the extracorporeal circuit without placing the patient at increased risk for bleeding complications has been managed using unfractionated heparin. However, the recently increased applications of continuous renal replacement therapies (CRRTs) to treat kidney disease have expanded the eligible dialysis patient population. These patients are often critically ill, and many of them have contraindications to heparin use. This chapter reviews some of the approaches to anticoagulation for dialysis procedures. The use of unfractionated heparin as well as low molecular weight heparin (LMWH) will be discussed, as will some of the newer alternative anticoagulant strategies available to nephrologists.

 ## COAGULATION IN DIALYSIS PATIENTS

There remains no universally accepted algorithm for anticoagulation in dialysis patients. This may be due in part to individual patient factors that influence abnormal hemostasis in end-stage kidney disease (ESKD). Although the uremic state tends to cause a bleeding diathesis, dialysis patients have been shown to exhibit hypercoagulable tendencies as well. Some evidence of a thrombotic susceptibility in patients with ESKD includes increased plasma concentrations of fibrinogen (1–3), increased factor VII activity (2,4), and increased fibrinolytic activity (1,3,5). Pulmonary emboli are more common in dialysis patients versus age-matched controls (6), and the anticoagulant proteins C and S have been shown to be deficient in this population (3,7,8).

In addition to patient factors, dialysis procedures themselves invariably induce nonphysiologic levels of turbulent blood flows with high shear stress, which can activate platelets. The exposure of blood to the artificial surfaces of dialysis tubing has also been shown to be thrombogenic, especially in the arterial and venous bubble traps where blood flow can be slower or even static at times (9).

The type of membrane selected for the dialysis procedure may impact thrombogenicity. Several studies have shown that membranes composed of regenerated cellulose (cuprophane) lead to more activation of coagulation compared with membranes composed of newer materials such as polyacrylonitrile or polysulfone (10–13). The results of two studies suggest that polysulfone membranes have minimal effects on coagulation activation as measured by thrombin–antithrombin complex levels and platelet activation (10,14). The process of dialysis membrane sterilization may affect anticoagulation. This was suggested after significant thrombocytopenia was noted following the introduction of dialyzers that has been sterilized using electron beam technology (15).

The presence of an arteriovenous (AV) access is yet another predisposing factor toward turbulent blood flow, platelet activation, and thrombosis (7). The risk for access thrombosis is greater in polytetrafluoroethylene (PTFE) grafts compared to native AV fistulae (16), and conditions such as systemic lupus erythematosus (SLE) may exacerbate the tendency to thrombose the access (17).

With the interplay of all of the aforementioned clinical entities, adequate anticoagulation should be viewed as essential to the hemodialysis procedure.

 ## UNFRACTIONATED HEPARIN

The anionic glycosaminoglycans present in unfractionated heparin prevent clotting of blood by the inhibition of serine proteases (18). Because heparin used for hemodialysis is a mixture of components, heparin formulations are standardized in terms of international units (IU), using a United States Pharmacopeia (USP) standard heparin as a reference. The therapeutic window for adequate anticoagulation without excessive bleeding using heparin is narrow. As such, measurement of the anticoagulant effects of heparin would be optimal. Unfortunately, the measurement of blood heparin levels is not practical. Historically, assays such as the activated clotting time (ACT) and the whole blood partial thromboplastin time (WBPTT) have been used to measure the anticoagulability of heparin. Both these tests use whole blood and can produce results in minutes, making them desirable for clinical use. Following enactment of the Clinical Laboratory Improvement Amendments (CLIA) of 1988, automated clotting time measurement systems replaced the manually performed WBPTT as the means of monitoring anticoagulation during hemodialysis in the United States (19). This law requires that any laboratory testing of human specimens be performed in a certified laboratory that incorporates quality control, proficiency testing, and calibration verification in its testing program.

Such procedures are associated with increased overhead costs and are difficult to incorporate into everyday use in a busy hemodialysis center. Indeed, many dialysis units in the United States have abandoned the testing of blood for clotting parameters and moved toward developing heparin-dosing algorithms. One such strategy has been developed based on a nonlinear mixed effects population kinetic model that was designed to estimate heparin-loading doses and infusion rates (20,21). In this equation, the loading dose of heparin is derived as follows (**EQUATION 4.1**):

$$\text{Loading dose (IU)} = 1,600 + 10 \times \quad (4.1)$$
$$(\text{Wgt} - 76) - 300 \times \text{Fd} - 100 \times \text{Fs}$$

In this equation, Wgt is the patient's weight (kg), Fd indicates the presence (Fd = 1) or absence (Fd = 0) of diabetes, and Fs indicates that the patient is (Fs = 1) or is not (Fs = 0) a smoker. The proposed infusion rate based on this model was 1,750 IU/h. Using these parameters to predict heparin-loading doses and infusion

rates, one study noted a significant improvement in dialyzer reuse rates with no decrease in the delivered dose of dialysis (19).

Data from Ward et al. (22) demonstrate that the sensitivity to heparin in nonuremic hemodialysis patients correlates with body weight. Low et al. (23) suggested an initial heparin-loading dose of 20 to 25 IU/kg was sufficient to maintain adequate anticoagulation during dialysis based on measured WBPTT. In 2002, the European Renal Association (24) published guidelines for anticoagulation in hemodialysis patients. Their recommendations include a loading dose of approximately 50 IU/kg followed by a continuous infusion rate of 800 to 1,500 IU/h. This approach of giving a loading dose followed by a continuous infusion of heparin offers the nephrologist the ability to titrate dosing to the lowest possible amount to prevent clotting of the circuit while avoiding excessive bleeding risk. The heparin infusion is then titrated off over the last 30 minutes of the dialysis session to allow for clotting time to decrease and to avoid bleeding when the access needles are withdrawn.

An alternative anticoagulation strategy uses intermittent heparin dosing. An initial loading dose of heparin is administered, followed by one or more additional bolus doses during dialysis. Intermittent dosing is simple and eliminates the need for an infusion pump and syringe. However, this approach results in periods of over- and under-anticoagulation compared to the loading dose and constant infusion method (25). Furthermore, the use of intermittent dosing is time-consuming and requires the constant attention of dialysis personnel to ensure that timely heparin boluses are given. **FIGURE 4.1** illustrates the anticoagulation profiles obtained with a continuous infusion versus intermittent bolus dosing of heparin after the initial loading dose is given.

Invariably, nephrologists will encounter patients who are at a high risk for bleeding complications. These patients include, but are not limited to, those who have recently had or will be undergoing surgery, those with a history of gastrointestinal bleeding, those with a history of hemorrhagic stroke, and those with severe

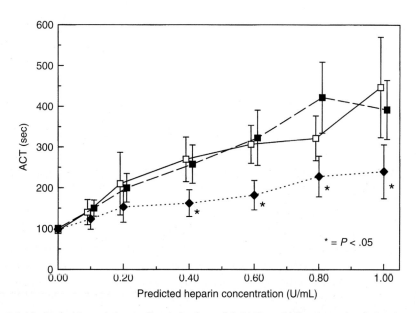

FIGURE 4.1 Idealized anticoagulation profiles during hemodialysis. The solid line shows the clotting time profile obtained with a loading dose and constant infusion of heparin; the broken line shows the profile obtained with a loading dose and midtreatment bolus of heparin. (From Ward RA. Heparinization for routine hemodialysis. *Adv Ren Replace Ther* 1995;2:362–370, with permission.)

liver disease. In these cases, low-dose heparin use has been shown to be an effective strategy for anticoagulation (26–28). Low-dose heparinization is achieved using a smaller bolus dose of 10 to 25 IU/kg. Maintenance heparin can then be given either as an infusion at a rate of 11 to 22 IU/kg/h or through small intermittent boluses. However, with low doses of heparin, increases in clotting time have been observed to vary by ±50% from day to day in individual patients who are given the same dose of heparin (29). Taking this into account, low-dose heparin should be reserved for select cases and performed with the understanding that minimizing the bleeding risk may result in increased clotting of the extracorporeal circuit on some occasions.

In addition to the inherent bleeding risks associated with its use, heparin therapy has other associated side effects including worsening of osteoporosis and dyslipidemia, allergic reactions such as pruritus, and thrombocytopenia. Hyperkalemia may be seen due to inhibition of aldosterone synthase (30), although this is seldom an issue for patients with ESKD. The development of heparin-induced thrombocytopenia (HIT), a rare but life-threatening immune-mediated disorder, requires absolute heparin avoidance during dialysis.

◆ LOW MOLECULAR WEIGHT HEPARIN

LMWH preparations are made from depolymerized fractions of heparin. These smaller saccharide chains have a molecular weight of 4 to 8 kDa and inhibit factor Xa up to threefold more when compared to unfractionated heparin, with less affinity for thrombin inhibition (9). For these reasons, monitoring the effect of LMWH requires the measurement of antifactor Xa activity as the activated partial thromboplastin time (aPTT) and ACT are not reliable (31,32). LMWH preparations have been extensively studied during dialysis in patients with ESKD. The longer half-life of LMWH allows these preparations to be given as a single predialysis dose, usually based on body weight (33–36). However, should the dialysis session be scheduled for greater than 4 hours, additional LMWH may need to be given either as a bolus or through continuous infusion (37,38). TABLE 4.1 illustrates the commonly used dosages of LMWH during hemodialysis.

Some authors advocate the use of LMWH as the preferred agent for anticoagulation in patients with ESKD (24). The appeal of single bolus dosing is one potential advantage offered compared to unfractionated heparin. Indeed, in one study, scanning electron microscopy was used to demonstrate that membrane-associated clotting during dialysis was less after treatment with LMWH compared to unfractionated heparin (43). Among the other purported benefits of LMWH include a reduction in the need for blood transfusions (44) and less of a tendency toward hyperkalemia (45).

There has been some debate in the literature about the effect of LMWH on the lipid profiles of dialysis patients. Several studies have demonstrated improvement in the total cholesterol (46–51) and triglyceride levels (46,49–51) in dialysis patients after switching from unfractionated heparin to LMWH. These studies included both diabetic and nondiabetic subjects, and the period of study ranged from 6 months to 4 years. Another study examined the effect of LMWH on lipid profiles in prevalent dialysis patients who had been previously receiving unfractionated heparin. Over 1 year, improvements were noted in total cholesterol, triglyceride, and Apo B concentrations. After the first 12 months, patients were randomly chosen to either continue with LMWH or revert to unfractionated heparin. Although the improvement in lipid profiles continued in the LMWH group, the unfractionated heparin group sustained no further benefit (52).

In contrast, a multicenter trial examining 153 patients on LMWH and 153 patients on unfractionated heparin failed to demonstrate any significant differences in lipid profiles between the two groups except for higher high-density lipoprotein (HDL) cholesterol levels in the heparin group (53). A smaller study by the same authors showed an improvement in lipid profiles after switching 24 incident dialysis patients from LMWH to unfractionated heparin after the first 6 months of treatment (54). These latter two studies suggest that it may be premature to assume that a benefit in lipid profiles is assured when using LMWH.

One factor that has precluded the routine use of LMWH during dialysis procedures is the concern for excess bleeding in patients with kidney disease. A meta-analysis investigating the safety of LWMH in patients with ESKD found no significant difference in bleeding events or extracorporeal circuit clotting when compared to unfractionated heparin (55). Other studies, however, have raised concerns. Brophy et al. (56) used the measurement of thrombin generation time in a prospective *ex vivo* study to demonstrate that the anticoagulant effect of enoxaparin was enhanced in patients with ESKD. These data suggested that even at similar levels of antifactor Xa activity, the effect of enoxaparin in ESKD remains unpredictable and could subject patients with ESKD to bleeding complications. Other clinically significant events such as retroperitoneal hemorrhage, gastrointestinal bleeding, intracranial bleeding, and hemorrhagic pericardial effusion have been described in patients with chronic kidney disease (CKD) stages 4 or 5 who were treated with fixed doses of LMWH (57). Additional concern when using

TABLE 4.1	**Common Dosing of Alternative Anticoagulants During Hemodialysis**		
Medication	**Category**	**Dose**	**Reference**
Enoxaparin	LMWH	100 anti-Xa-IU/kg administered as bolus dose	36
Dalteparin	LMWH	70 anti-Xa-IU/kg administered as bolus dose	35
Tinzaparin	LMWH	2,000–4,500 anti-Xa-IU, adjust dose based on clot visibility and postdialysis bleeding	9,34
Lepirudin	DTI	0.1–0.15 mg/kg bolus before dialysis session 0.005–0.01 mg/kg/h infusion for CRRT	9,39
Argatroban	DTI	250 μg/kg bolus predialysis, followed by either a repeat bolus of 250 μg/kg midsession or continuous infusion of 2 μg/kg/min; dose reduction required with hepatic insufficiency	40
Danaparoid sodium	Heparinoid	35 units/kg bolus predialysis	41,42

LMWH, low molecular weight heparin; DTI, direct thrombin inhibitor; IU, international units; CRRT, continuous renal replacement therapy.

LMWH preparations is that they are only partially reversible using protamine. The package inserts of the three major LMWH preparations commonly used in the United States (enoxaparin, dalteparin, and tinzaparin) state that these agents should be used with caution in patients with a creatinine clearance less than 30 mL/min. These facts, combined with the lack of readily available antifactor Xa level monitoring, suggest that patient safety concerns may outweigh the other purported advantages of using LMWH for chronic dialysis procedures.

◆ ALTERNATIVE ANTICOAGULATION STRATEGIES

Perhaps no other clinical diagnosis has focused more attention on the need for alternative anticoagulant agents than HIT. HIT is a life-threatening disorder resulting from antibodies formed against complexes of platelet factor 4 (PF4) and heparin (39). HIT has been classified into type I and type II, with type II being the most clinically significant entity. In type II HIT, platelet counts usually decline by 40% to 50% from baseline approximately 5 to 10 days after heparin exposure. Clotting of both the venous and arterial circulation can be seen, with 50% of patients developing clot formation of some kind within 30 days on average (58). Both unfractionated and LMWH have been shown to cause HIT, although the association with LMWH appears to be smaller.

The frequency of HIT in the population with ESKD has been reported to range anywhere from 0% to 12% (39,58). If the diagnosis of HIT is suspected, antibody testing should be used for confirmation, given the potential life-long implications and cost associated with treatment. Treatment of HIT includes absolute heparin avoidance, including all heparin flushes, ointments, and catheter lock solutions. In addition to these precautions, systemic anticoagulation is recommended in patients with HIT to prevent thrombotic complications.

Some alternative anticoagulation strategies that can be used in clinical situations such as HIT as well as in patients who are at high risk for bleeding will now be discussed. **TABLE 4.1** provides the usual dosing schemes for many of these agents during hemodialysis.

Direct Thrombin Inhibitors

Direct thrombin inhibitors prevent thrombin generation by binding to the active site on the thrombin molecule, thereby blocking the conversion of soluble fibrinogen to insoluble fibrin. The three direct thrombin inhibitors approved for use by the U.S. Food and Drug Administration (FDA) are recombinant hirudin, argatroban, and bivalirudin.

A natural derivative from the saliva of the *Hirudo medicinalis* leech species, hirudin, was actually the first anticoagulant used for dialysis procedures in the early 1920s before giving way to heparin (59). The primary route of excretion of hirudin is through kidney elimination. Therefore, its half-life is markedly prolonged in patients with kidney disease. Lepirudin, a form of recombinant hirudin, has been studied in patients with kidney disease including patients undergoing CRRT (60,61). Especially in cases of anuria, the dosing requirements for hirudin are small (60); however, meticulous monitoring of the aPTT levels should be undertaken. In patients on CRRT, lepirudin can be dosed through continuous infusion at 0.005 to 0.01 mg/kg/h, whereas for chronic dialysis, a bolus dose of 0.15 mg/kg can be given before the session (39).

Dosing should be carefully adjusted to achieve an aPTT of 1.5 to 2 times normal without exceeding 100 seconds in order to minimize bleeding risk. The reader should also keep in mind that the aPTT does not increase linearly with lepirudin blood levels (62). Therefore, aPTT times that are elevated above the goal range may reflect excessively high levels of blood lepirudin. These situations are all the more dangerous considering that there is no specific antidote to lepirudin. The formation of antihirudin antibodies that can occur in up to 40% of patients who receive lepirudin for more than 5 days and may enhance its anticoagulant effect is another factor to consider when using this agent (63).

Argatroban is a synthetic derivative of L-arginine that was first studied during hemodialysis procedures in the mid-1980s (64). The appeal of this agent for use in patients with kidney disease stems from the fact that it is metabolized and secreted by the liver. A retrospective review of 47 patients with HIT showed that argatroban was a safe and effective anticoagulant for both chronic dialysis and CRRT (40). In a prospective, randomized, three-way crossover study in patients with prevalent ESKD, argatroban was shown to be safe and effective for chronic dialysis (65). Of the three argatroban dosing strategies used in this study, there were no significant differences in achieved urea reduction ratio, thrombotic, or bleeding events. The clearance of argatroban through the dialysis membrane was also found to be insignificant. Using the methods employed in this study, a 250 μg/kg bolus of argatroban with a repeat 250 μg/kg bolus given midway through the session should achieve adequate anticoagulation. An alternative strategy would be to use an initial bolus of 250 μg/kg of argatroban followed by a continuous infusion of 2 μg/kg/min. Hospitalized patients who are already receiving an argatroban infusion for other reasons can be safely dialyzed without interruption of therapy. Given the hepatic metabolism of argatroban, liver function testing is imperative before using this agent. In cases of hepatic insufficiency, the dosing of argatroban should be reduced to 0.5 μg/kg/min through continuous infusion, and careful monitoring of the aPTT should be performed (39). In general, the aPTT has been found to correlate well with plasma argatroban levels (66), and the goal of therapy should be to achieve an aPTT of 1.5 to 3 times normal. The concern of antibody production against argatroban has not been reported.

Bivalirudin is a semisynthetic 20 amino acid derivative of hirudin. Its primary mode of elimination is through intracellular hydrolysis, with only 20% urinary excretion (67). Similar to lepirudin, the half-life of bivalirudin is prolonged in patients with impaired kidney function. With normal kidney function, the elimination half-life is 25 minutes, and is prolonged to 3.5 hours in dialysis patients (67). Although promising as an alternative anticoagulant to treat HIT, there are little published data regarding the use of bivalirudin in dialysis patients. Currently, the FDA has approved this agent only for use in conjunction with percutaneous coronary intervention.

Danaparoid

Danaparoid sodium is a heparinoid composed primarily of the nonheparin glycosaminoglycan heparan sulfate. Danaparoid exerts its anticoagulant effect by inhibition of factor Xa. Although not currently on the market in the United States, there is considerable experience treating HIT patients with danaparoid in Canada, Europe, and Australia. Danaparoid is considered to be a safe alternative agent to use in patients with HIT despite a 3.2% rate of cross-reactivity with heparin (68). A survey of 81 dialysis units in the United Kingdom revealed that 36% of patients with ESKD who tested positive for HIT were treated using danaparoid (69). Danaparoid is reported to allow successful dialysis without clotting or bleeding complications when administered as a single predialysis dose of 35 U/kg (41,42). Given that kidney excretion is the primary route of danaparoid elimination, monitoring of antifactor Xa levels should be performed before each dialysis session with a goal level of 0.5 to 0.8 IU/mL. Even with dose adjustment, these patients must be considered at risk for bleeding complications.

Regional Citrate Anticoagulation

Regional anticoagulation with citrate has been demonstrated to be an effective alternative for use of heparin. Trisodium citrate infusion into the blood entering the dialyzer chelates calcium and prevents coagulation. Anticoagulation is reversed, and ionized calcium levels restored, through a combination of citrate loss into the dialysate and infusion of calcium into the venous blood line or calcium influx from the dialysate. Multiple protocols have been described for citrate anticoagulation (70–73). The simplest method involves infusion of concentrated trisodium citrate solution into the arterial blood line, coupled with the use of dialysate containing normal levels of calcium and magnesium (71,73). The citrate infusion rate is adjusted to provide a 25% to 75% increase in ACT at the entry to the dialyzer (71–73). Other methods use calcium- and magnesium-free dialysate and reinfuse calcium into the venous blood line (70,74). A prospective study in dialysis patients who required heparin free treatment after recent surgery demonstrated that regional citrate anticoagulation was superior to the use of a heparin-coated polyacrylonitrile membrane in terms of clotting phenomena that necessitated termination of the dialysis session (75). Citrate anticoagulation may be useful in patients with heparin allergy, but problems with hypocalcemia, hypernatremia, and metabolic alkalosis render this technique more cumbersome than routine heparin anticoagulation (76,77). The dialysate bicarbonate concentration should be reduced to 25 to 30 mM to guard against metabolic alkalosis, which may develop if the bicarbonate generated from citrate metabolism is added to the normal influx of bicarbonate from the dialysate (78). In extreme cases, failure to adequately correct ionized calcium levels has been reported to result in electrolyte imbalance and cardiac arrest (79), and an ability to monitor ionized calcium concentrations during hemodialysis is considered essential for patient safety. One large but uncontrolled trial reported a 99.6% success rate using a regional citrate anticoagulation protocol in 1,009 high-flux dialysis procedures in 59 outpatients with ESKD (80). However, for the abovementioned safety concerns, regional anticoagulation using a citrate protocol is typically reserved for hospitalized patients who are at high risk for bleeding complications. Regional citrate anticoagulation by itself is insufficient to treat patients with HIT given the need for systemic anticoagulation.

Oral Anticoagulation

In general, oral anticoagulation is a poor choice for treating patients with ESKD. There are ample data that suggest warfarin may enhance the process of vascular calcification (81). Furthermore, no studies have conclusively demonstrated a benefit of warfarin on clotting profiles during hemodialysis. In studies looking at both tunneled, cuffed dialysis catheters (82) and PTFE grafts (83), minidose warfarin was no better than placebo at maintaining access patency. As expected, the rates of adverse bleeding events were higher in patients treated with warfarin. Another smaller study used a randomized, crossover design to investigate the efficacy of LMWH

versus no anticoagulation in 10 patients with ESKD treated with warfarin [international normalized ratio (INR) 2.0–3.0]. The patients who received no additional anticoagulation had significantly greater clotting of the dialyzer when compared to the LMWH group (84). Taken as a whole, these data suggest that oral warfarin should be reserved for those patients with ESKD who have a defined hypercoagulable state or for those with other compelling indications for continuous anticoagulation such as a mechanical heart valve. A recent retrospective cohort study of incident hemodialysis patients with atrial fibrillation actually suggested an increased risk for new stroke in patients taking warfarin (85). These data seem to be in accordance with some of the more recent studies recognizing advanced chronic kidney disease and ESKD as risk factors for increased bleeding when using oral anticoagulation. In particular, the Hypertension, Abnormal renal/liver function, Stroke, Bleeding history or predisposition, Labile international normalized ration, Eldery (>65 years), Drugs/alcohol concomitantly (HAS-BLED) scoring system defines an increased risk of 1 year major bleeding events in anyone with a history of kidney transplant, ESKD, or a serum creatinine value of greater than 2.6 mg/dL receiving oral anticoagulation for atrial fibrillation (86).

Antiplatelet Agents

The Dialysis Access Consortium Study Group has investigated the use of antiplatelet agents specifically to enhance the patency and reduce the failure rate of the arteriovenous access in hemodialysis patients. One study found that clopidogrel had a modest, but statistically significant, effect in reducing the rate of fistula thrombosis at 6 weeks after access creation (87). Unfortunately, clopidogrel therapy did not result in a significant increase in the proportion of fistulas that were suitable for dialysis compared to placebo (defined as the ability to sustain a blood pump speed of 300 mL/min or greater in 8 out of 12 dialysis treatments). Another randomized controlled trial examined the effect of dipyridamole plus aspirin given twice daily on the ability to maintain patency in newly created arteriovenous grafts (88). In this study, the treatment group exhibited a modest but significant increase in the incidence of primary unassisted graft patency at 1 year. In both studies, treatment with antiplatelet therapy did not result in significant adverse events, including major bleeding, compared to placebo.

Hemodialysis without Anticoagulation

Dialysis procedures can be successfully performed without the use of anticoagulation. This may be necessary in patients with an active bleeding diathesis (e.g., intracranial hemorrhage). In such cases, membranes with the lowest thrombogenicity (e.g., polysulfone) should be used. To minimize the chances for clotting, treatment times should be ideally limited to 2 to 3 hours and blood flows should be attempted at least as fast as 250 mL/min. Rinsing of the extracorporeal circuit with 25 to 150 mL of saline through the arterial port is another technique, which can aid in the prevention of circuit clotting (89,90).

◆ FACTORS PREVENTING ADEQUATE ANTICOAGULATION

Both dialyzer clotting and excessive bleeding can occur in patients with ESKD who have apparently stable heparin prescriptions. These situations can usually be traced to either patient-related issues or technical problems in therapy delivery.

Patient-Related Issues

Comorbid conditions such as infections, intercurrent illnesses, or underlying disease exacerbations [systemic lupus erythematosus (SLE), chronic obstructive pulmonary disease (COPD), congestive heart failure (CHF)] may change a patient's coagulation status. Intercurrent illnesses have been shown to affect the elimination rate of heparin (91). In cases of infection or disease exacerbations, vigilance should be maintained to ensure proper anticoagulation is maintained. These conditions often require a temporary increase in the heparin dosage to prevent extracorporeal circuit clotting.

Heparin can physically interact with a number of drugs (92); however, with the possible exception of nitroglycerin (93,94), there is little evidence that drugs alter the anticoagulant effect of heparin. Smoking increases the elimination rate of heparin (95), and a history of smoking was found to be a significant covariate in population pharmacodynamic models of heparin dosing in hemodialysis patients (21).

Patients treated with erythropoietin require more heparin to prevent dialyzer clotting (96,97). Whether this fact is a reflection of the induction of higher hematocrit concentrations or a result of some reversal of the uremic bleeding tendency is a matter of speculation. In either case, patients receiving erythropoietin-stimulating agents may require higher doses of anticoagulants to achieve successful dialysis.

Technical Problems in Therapy Delivery

As summarized in TABLE 4.2, there are many factors that can potentially go wrong during any given hemodialysis session, thereby leading to either dialyzer clotting or excessive bleeding. These situations should be investigated before attributing the problem to a faulty anticoagulation prescription.

Errors in the administration of heparin are a common problem. After administration of the heparin-loading dose into the access needle, sufficient saline must be used to ensure that the complete heparin dose enters the circulation. Three to 5 minutes are required for the heparin to distribute in the plasma before extracorporeal circulation is commenced. Failure to follow these steps results in clotting as unheparinized blood enters the dialyzer during the first minutes of dialysis. Once administered, the loading dose begins to be eliminated. If the constant infusion of heparin is not started immediately, this elimination will result in a steadily decreasing clotting time.

A number of factors may prevent the timely administration of the infused heparin. The line from the heparin syringe to the blood

line must be primed with heparin during the setup for dialysis to avoid infusing either saline or air during the first 30 minutes of dialysis. In addition, clamps should not be left on the line. Some heparin pumps have a maximum operating pressure. Beyond this pressure, they will not infuse accurately. Post–blood-pump pressures greater than 400 mm Hg should be avoided, particularly when high blood-flow rates are used in conjunction with high hematocrits and small-bore access needles.

Care must be taken to eliminate all air bubbles from the dialyzer during the priming process and to avoid excessive turbulence in the drip chambers during dialysis. Blood–air interfaces predispose to clotting, particularly if they are associated with turbulence and foam formation (12,98–100).

Recirculation in the vascular access may cause clotted dialyzers in the presence of apparently adequate clotting times. As blood passes through the dialyzer, ultrafiltration causes hemoconcentration. Blood of increased hematocrit then returns to the access. Recirculation results in some of this blood being returned to the dialyzer where it is concentrated further. In this manner, the hematocrit of the blood in the dialyzer progressively increases above systemic levels. In extreme circumstances, such as when the arterial access needle is inadvertently placed downstream of the venous needle and ultrafiltration rates are high, the hematocrit in the dialyzer will reach very high levels (greater than 60%), and the dialyzer will clot.

Prolonged bleeding from the access needle sites after dialysis is often blamed on excessive anticoagulation. Although the level of anticoagulation may play a role in this bleeding, mechanical problems related to venipuncture are also frequently a factor. In particular, failure to rotate needle sites with a synthetic graft will lead to destruction of the graft material and make it very difficult to stop bleeding, regardless of the level of heparin. Continued episodes of bleeding after needle withdrawal should also prompt the clinician to search for possible outflow stenosis of the AV access.

SUMMARY

Anticoagulation remains an invaluable ingredient in producing a successful hemodialysis prescription. This goal can best be achieved by a loading dose and constant infusion of heparin using one of the available weight-based nomograms when pharmacodynamic modeling is not readily available. The nephrologist's goal should be to maintain the lowest possible dose of heparin in order to prevent extracorporeal circuit clotting and minimize the risk of bleeding complications. Given the wide patient-to-patient variability, individualization of heparin dosing is required and periodic adjustments will often have to be made. In cases where heparin is contraindicated, the nephrologist now has several different treatment options including the direct thrombin inhibitors and regional citrate anticoagulation, although further studies will be needed before instituting these agents on a wider scale. Finally, both patient-related factors and technical problems with anticoagulant delivery should be investigated when problems arise with dialysis anticoagulation.

TABLE 4.2	**Problems in Therapy Delivery that May Result in Inadequate Anticoagulation or Failure to Prevent Clotting or Bleeding**

Errors in administration of the heparin dose
Heparin doses drawn up incorrectly
Insufficient time allowed for loading dose to distribute
Failure to deliver the prescribed constant infusion of heparin
Problems associated with the blood circuit
Failure to adequately prime the dialyzer
Excessive turbulence in the arterial drip chamber
Excessive recirculation
Failure to rotate needle sites

From Ward RA. Heparinization for routine hemodialysis. *Adv Renal Replace Ther* 1995;2:362–370, with permission.

REFERENCES

1. Nakamura Y, Chida Y, Tomura S. Enhanced coagulation-fibrinolysis in patients on regular hemodialysis treatment. *Nephron* 1991;58: 201–204.
2. Gris JC, Branger B, Vécina F, et al. Increased cardiovascular risk factors and features of endothelial activation and dysfunction in dialyzed uremic patients. *Kidney Int* 1994;46:807–813.

3. Vaziri ND, Gonzales EC, Wang J, et al. Blood coagulation, fibrinolytic, and inhibitory proteins in end-stage renal disease: effect of hemodialysis. *Am J Kidney Dis* 1994;23:828–835.

4. Kario K, Matsuo T, Yamada T, et al. Factor VII hyperactivity in chronic dialysis patients. *Thromb Res* 1992;67:105–113.

5. Mezzano D, Tagle R, Panes O, et al. Hemostatic disorder of uremia: the platelet defect, main determinant of the prolonged bleeding time, is correlated with indices of activation of coagulation and fibrinolysis. *Thromb Haemost* 1996;76:312–321.

6. Tveit DP, Hypolite IO, Hshieh P, et al. Chronic dialysis patients have high risk for pulmonary embolism. *Am J Kidney Dis* 2002;39:1011–1017.

7. Nampoory MR, Das KC, Johny KV, et al. Hypercoagulability, a serious problem in patients with ESRD on maintenance hemodialysis, and its correction after kidney transplantation. *Am J Kidney Dis* 2003;42:797–805.

8. Kushiya F, Wada H, Sakakura M, et al. Atherosclerotic and hemostatic abnormalities in patients undergoing hemodialysis. *Clin Appl Thromb Hemost* 2003;9:53–60.

9. Fischer KG. Essentials of anticoagulation in hemodialysis. *Hemodial Int* 2007;11:178–189.

10. Ishii Y, Yano S, Kanai H, et al. Evaluation of blood coagulation-fibrinolysis system in patients receiving chronic hemodialysis. *Nephron* 1996;73:407–412.

11. Seyfert UT, Helmling E, Hauck W, et al. Comparison of blood biocompatibility during haemodialysis with cuprophane and polyacrylonitrile membranes. *Nephrol Dial Transplant* 1991;6:428–434.

12. Sperschneider H, Deppisch R, Beck W, et al. Impact of membrane choice and blood flow pattern on coagulation and heparin requirement—potential consequences on lipid concentrations. *Nephrol Dial Transplant* 1997;12:2638–2646.

13. Wright MJ, Woodrow G, Umpleby S, et al. Low thrombogenicity of polyethylene glycol-grafted cellulose membranes does not influence heparin requirements in hemodialysis. *Am J Kidney Dis* 1999;34:36–42.

14. Mujais SK, Schmidt B, Hacker H, et al. Synthetic modification of PAN membrane: biocompatibility and functional characterization. *Nephrol Dial Transplant* 1995;10(Suppl 3):46–51.

15. Kiaii M, Djurdjev O, Farah M, et al. Use of electron-beam sterilized hemodialysis membranes and risk of thrombocytopenia. *JAMA* 2011;306(15):1679–1687.

16. Culp K, Flangan M, Taylor L, et al. Vascular access thrombosis in new hemodialysis patients. *Am J Kidney Dis* 1995;26:341–346.

17. Shafi ST, Gupta M. Risk of vascular access thrombosis in patients with systemic lupus erythematosus on hemodialysis. *J Vasc Access* 2007;8(2):103–108.

18. Rosenberg RD, Bauer KA. The heparin-antithrombin system: a natural anticoagulant mechanism. In: Colman RW, Hirsh J, Marder VJ, et al. eds. *Hemostasis and Thrombosis: Basic Principles and Clinical Practice*. 3rd ed. Philadelphia, PA: JB Lippincott, 1994:837–860.

19. Ouseph R, Brier ME, Ward RA. Improved dialyzer reuse after use of a population pharmacodynamic model to determine heparin doses. *Am J Kidney Dis* 2000;35:89–94.

20. Jannett TC, Wise MG, Shanklin NH, et al. Adaptive control of anticoagulation during hemodialysis. *Kidney Int* 1994;45:912–915.

21. Smith BP, Ward RA, Brier ME. Prediction of anticoagulation during hemodialysis by population kinetics and an artificial neural network. *Artif Organs* 1998;22:731–739.

22. Ward RA, et al. Precise heparinization for hemodialysis of nonuremic subjects. *ASAIO J* 1980;3:147–152.

23. Low CL, Bailie G, Morgan S, et al. Effect of a sliding scale protocol for heparin on the ability to maintain whole blood activated partial thromboplastin times within a desired range in hemodialysis patients. *Clin Nephrol* 1996;45:120–124.

24. European Best Practice Guidelines Expert Group on Hemodialysis. Section V. Chronic intermittent haemodialysis and prevention of clotting in the extracorporeal system. *Nephrol Dial Transplant* 2002;17(Suppl 7):63–71.

25. Ward RA. Heparinization for routine hemodialysis. *Adv Ren Replace Ther* 1995;2:362–370.

26. Swartz RD, Port FK. Preventing hemorrhage in high-risk hemodialysis: regional versus low-dose heparin. *Kidney Int* 1979;16:513–518.

27. Swartz RD. Hemorrhage during high-risk hemodialysis using controlled heparinization. *Nephron* 1981;28:65–69.

28. Ward DM, Mehta RL. Extracorporeal management of acute renal failure patients at high-risk of bleeding. *Kidney Int* 1993;41:S237–S244.

29. Ward RA. Effects of haemodialysis on coagulation and platelets: are we measuring membrane biocompatibility? *Nephrol Dial Transplant* 1995;10(Suppl 10):12–17.

30. Oster JR, Singer I, Fishman LM. Heparin-induced aldosterone suppression and hyperkalemia. *Am J Med* 1995;98:575–586.

31. Greiber S, Weber U, Galle J, et al. Activated clotting time is not a sensitive parameter to monitor anticoagulation with low molecular weight heparin in haemodialysis. *Nephron* 1997;76:15–19.

32. Frank RD, Brandenburg VM, Lanzmich R, et al. Factor Xa-activated whole blood clotting time (Xa-ACT) for bedside monitoring of dalteparin anticoagulation during hemodialysis. *Nephrol Dial Transplant* 2004;19:1552–1558.

33. Grau E, Sigüenza F, Maduell F, et al. Low molecular weight heparin (CY-216) versus unfractionated heparin in chronic hemodialysis. *Nephron* 1992;62:13–17.

34. Simpson HK, Baird J, Allison M, et al. Long-term use of the low molecular weight heparin tinzaparin in haemodialysis. *Haemostasis* 1996;26:90–97.

35. Sagedal S, Hartmann A, Sundstrøm K, et al. A single dose of dalteparin effectively prevents clotting during haemodialysis. *Nephrol Dial Transplant* 1999;14:1943–1947.

36. Saltissi D, Morgan C, Westhuyzen J, et al. Comparison of low-molecular-weight heparin (enoxaparin sodium) and standard unfractionated heparin for haemodialysis anticoagulation. *Nephrol Dial Transplant* 1999;14:2698–2703.

37. Lai KN, Ho K, Li M, et al. Use of single dose low-molecular-weight heparin in long hemodialysis. *Int J Artif Organs* 1998;21:196–200.

38. Van Hoof A, Schurgers M, Boelaert J, et al. Low-molecular-weight heparin dosage in haemodialysis. *Nephrol Dial Transplant* 1987;2:193–194.

39. Arepally GM, Ortel TL. Heparin-induced thrombocytopenia. *N Engl J Med* 2006;355:809–817.

40. Reddy BV, Grossman EJ, Trevino SA, et al. Argatroban anticoagulation in patients with heparin-induced thrombocytopenia requiring renal replacement therapy. *Ann Pharmacother* 2005;39:1601–1605.

41. Henny CP, ten Cate H, Surachno S, et al. The effectiveness of a low molecular weight heparinoid in chronic intermittent hemodialysis. *Thromb Haemost* 1985;54:460–462.

42. Polkinghorne KR, McMahon LP, Becker GJ. Pharmacokinetic studies of dalteparin (Fragmin), enoxaparin (Clexane), and danaparoid sodium (Orgaran) in stable chronic hemodialysis patients. *Am J Kidney Dis* 2002;40:990–995.

43. O'Shea SI, Ortel TL, Kovalik EC. Alternative methods of anticoagulation for dialysis-dependent patients with heparin-induced thrombocytopenia. *Semin Dial* 2003;16:61–67.

44. Hofbauer R, Moser D, Frass M, et al. Effect of anticoagulation on blood membrane interactions during hemodialysis. *Kidney Int* 1999;56:1578–1583.

45. Schrader J, Stribbe W, Armstrong VW, et al. Comparison of low molecular weight heparin to standard heparin in hemodialysis/hemofiltration. *Kidney Int* 1988;33:890–896.

46. Bambauer R, Rückr S, Weber U, et al. Comparison of low molecular weight heparin and standard heparin in hemodialysis. *ASAIO Trans* 1990;36:M646–M649.

47. Hottelart C, Achard JM, Moriniere P, et al. Heparin-induced hyperkalemia in chronic hemodialysis patients: comparison of low molecular weight and unfractionated heparin. *Artif Organs* 1998;22:614–617.

48. Deuber HJ, Schulz W. Reduced lipid concentrations during four years of dialysis with low molecular weight heparin. *Kidney Int* 1991;40:496–500.

49. Akiba T, Tachibana K, Ozawa K, et al. Long-term use of low molecular weight heparin ameliorates hyperlipidemia in patients on hemodialysis. *ASAIO J* 1992;38:M326–M330.

50. Schmitt Y, Schneider H. Low-molecular-weight heparin (LMWH): influence on blood lipids in patients on chronic hemodialysis. *Nephrol Dial Transplant* 1993;8:438–442.

51. Vlassopoulos D, Noussias C, Hadjipetrou A, et al. Long-term effect of low molecular weight heparin on serum lipids in hypertriglyceridemic chronic hemodialysis patients. *J Nephrol* 1997;10:111–114.

52. Yang C, Wu T, Huang C. Low molecular weight heparin reduces tri-glyceride, VLDL and cholesterol/HDL levels in hyperlipidemic diabetic patients on hemodialysis. *Am J Nephrol* 1998;18:384–390.

53. Kronenberg F, König P, Neyer U, et al. Influence of various heparin preparations on lipoproteins in hemodialysis patients: a multicentre study. *Thromb Haemost* 1995;74:1025–1028.

54. Kronenberg F, König P, Lhotta K, et al. Low molecular weight heparin does not necessarily reduce lipids and lipoproteins in hemodialysis patients. *Clin Nephrol* 1995;43:399–404.

55. Lim W, Cook DJ, Crowther MA. Safety and efficacy of low molecular weight heparins for hemodialysis in patients with end-stage renal failure: a meta-analysis of randomized trials. *J Am Soc Nephrol* 2004;15:3192–3206.

56. Brophy DF, Martin EJ, Gehr TW, et al. Enhanced anticoagulant activity of enoxaparin in patients with ESRD as measured by thrombin generation time. *Am J Kidney Dis* 2004;44:270–277.

57. Farooq V, Hegarty J, Chandrasekar T, et al. Serious adverse incidents with the usage of low molecular weight heparins in patients with chronic kidney disease. *Am J Kidney Dis* 2004;43:531–537.

58. Warkentin TE, Kelton JG. A 14-year study of heparin-induced thrombocytopenia. *Am J Med* 1996;101:502–507.

59. Fagette P. Hemodialysis 1912-1945: no medical technology before its time: part II. *ASAIO J* 1999;45:379–391.

60. Fischer KG. Hirudin in renal insufficiency. *Semin Thromb Hemost* 2002;28:467–482.

61. Fischer KG, van de Loo A, Böhler J. Recombinant hirudin (lepirudin) as anticoagulant in intensive care patients treated with continuous hemodialysis. *Kidney Int Suppl* 1999;56(Suppl 72):S46–S50.

62. Hafner G, Roser M, Nauck M. Methods for the monitoring of direct thrombin inhibitors. *Semin Thromb Hemost* 2002;28:425–430.

63. Eichler P, Friesen HJ, Lubenow N, et al. Antihirudin antibodies in patients with heparin-induced thrombocytopenia treated with lepirudin: incidence, effects on aPTT, and clinical relevance. *Blood* 2000;96:2373–2378.

64. Matsuo T, Nakao K, Yamada T, et al. Effect of a new anticoagulant (MD 805) on platelet activation in the hemodialysis circuit. *Thromb Res* 1986;41:33–41.

65. Murray PT, Reddy BV, Grossman EJ, et al. A prospective comparison of three argatroban treatment regimens during hemodialysis in end-stage renal disease. *Kidney Int* 2004;66:2446–2453.

66. Hursting MJ, Alford KL, Becker JC, et al. Novastan (brand of arga-troban): a small-molecule, direct thrombin inhibitor. *Semin Thromb Hemost* 1997;23:503–516.

67. Nawarskas JJ, Anderson JR. Bivalirudin: a new approach to anticoagulation. *Heart Dis* 2001;3:131–137.

68. Magnani HN, Gallus A. Heparin-induced thrombocytopenia (HIT). A report of 1,478 clinical outcomes of patients treated with danaparoid (Orgaran) from 1982 to mid-2004. *Thromb Haemost* 2006;95:967–981.

69. Hutchison CA, Dasgupta I. National survey of heparin-induced thrombocytopenia in the haemodialysis population of the UK population. *Nephrol Dial Transplant* 2007;22:1680–1684.

70. Pinnick RV, Wiegmann TB, Diederich DA. Regional citrate anticoagulation for hemodialysis in the patient at high risk for bleeding. *N Engl J Med* 1983;308:258–261.

71. von Brecht JH, Flanigan MJ, Freeman RM, et al. Regional anticoagulation: hemodialysis with hypertonic trisodium citrate. *Am J Kidney Dis* 1986;8:196–201.

72. Flanigan MJ, Pillsbury L, Sadewasser G, et al. Regional hemodialysis anticoagulation: hypertonic tri-sodium citrate or anticoagulant citrate dextrose-A. *Am J Kidney Dis* 1996;27:519–524.

73. Evenepoel P, Maes B, Vanwalleghem J, et al. Regional citrate anticoagulation for hemodialysis using a conventional calcium-containing dialysate. *Am J Kidney Dis* 2002;39:315–323.

74. Apsner R, Buchmayer H, Lang T, et al. Simplified citrate anticoagulation for high-flux hemodialysis. *Am J Kidney Dis* 2001;38:979–987.

75. Evenepoel P, Dejagere T, Verhamme P, et al. Heparin-coated polyacrylonitrile membrane versus regional citrate anticoagulation: a prospective randomized study of 2 anticoagulation strategies in patients at risk of bleeding. *Am J Kidney Dis* 2007;49:642–649.

76. Kelleher SP, Schulman G. Severe metabolic alkalosis complicating regional citrate hemodialysis. *Am J Kidney Dis* 1987;9:235–236.

77. Silverstein FJ, Oster JR, Perez GO, et al. Metabolic alkalosis induced by regional citrate hemodialysis. *ASAIO Trans* 1989;35:22–25.

78. van der Meulen J, Janssen MJ, Langendijk PN, et al. Citrate anticoagulation and dialysate with reduced buffer content in chronic hemodialysis. *Clin Nephrol* 1992;37:36–41.

79. Charney DI, Salmond R. Cardiac arrest after hypertonic citrate anticoagulation for chronic hemodialysis. *ASAIO Trans* 1990;36: M217–M219.

80. Apsner R, Buchmayer H, Gruber D, et al. Citrate for long-term hemodialysis: prospective study of 1,009 consecutive high-flux treatments in 59 patients. *Am J Kidney Dis* 2005;45:557–564.

81. Reynolds JL, Joannides AJ, Skepper JN, et al. Human vascular smooth muscle cells undergo vesicle-mediated calcification in response to changes in extracellular calcium and phosphate concentrations: a potential mechanism for accelerated vascular calcification in ESRD. *J Am Soc Nephrol* 2004;15:2857–2867.

82. Mokrzycki MH, Jean-Jerome K, Rush H, et al. A randomized trial of minidose warfarin for the prevention of late malfunction in tunneled, cuffed hemodialysis catheters. *Kidney Int* 2001;59:1935–1942.

83. Crowther MA, Clase CM, Margetts PJ, et al. Low-intensity warfarin is ineffective for the prevention of PTFE graft failure in patients on hemodialysis: a randomized controlled trial. *J Am Soc Nephrol* 2002;13:2331–2337.

84. Ziai F, Benesch T, Kodras K, et al. The effect of oral anticoagulation on clotting during hemodialysis. *Kidney Int* 2005;68:862–866.

85. Chan KE, Lazarus JM, Thadhani R, et al. Warfarin use associates with increased risk for stroke in hemodialysis patients with atrial fibrillation. *J Am Soc Nephrol* 2009;20:2223–2233.

86. Pisters R, Lane DA, Nieuwlaat R, et al. A novel user-friendly score (HAS-BLED) to assess 1-year risk of major bleeding in patients with atrial fibrillation: the Euro Heart Survey. *Chest* 2010;138(5): 1093–1100.

87. Dember LM, Beck GJ, Allon M, et al. Effect of clopidogrel on early failure of arteriovenous fistulas for hemodialysis. *JAMA* 2008;299: 2164–2171.

88. Dixon BS, Beck GJ, Vazquez MA, et al. Effect of dipyridamole plus aspirin on hemodialysis graft patency. *N Engl J Med* 2009;360:2191–2201.

89. Sanders PW, Taylor H, Curtis JJ. Hemodialysis without anticoagulation. *Am J Kidney Dis* 1985;5:32–35.

90. Schwab SJ, Onoranto JJ, Shahar LR, et al. Hemodialysis without anticoagulation. One-year prospective trial in hospitalized patients at risk for bleeding. *Am J Med* 1987;83:405–410.

91. Hirsh J, van Aken WG, Gallus AS, et al. Heparin kinetics in venous thrombosis and pulmonary embolism. *Circulation* 1976;53:691–695.

92. Colburn WA. Pharmacologic implications of heparin interactions with other drugs. *Drug Metab Rev* 1976;5:281–293.

93. Pizzulli L, Nitsch J, Lüderitz B. Inhibition of the heparin effect by nitroglycerin. *Dtsch Med Wochenschr* 1988;113:1837–1840.

94. Bode V, Welzel D, Franz G, et al. Absence of drug interaction between heparin and nitroglycerin. Randomized placebo-controlled crossover study. *Arch Intern Med* 1990;150:2117–2119.

95. Cipolle RJ, Seifert RD, Neilan BA, et al. Heparin kinetics: variables related to disposition and dosage. *Clin Pharmacol Ther* 1981;29: 387–393.

96. Spinowitz BS, Arslanian J, Charytan C, et al. Impact of epoetin beta on dialyzer clearance and heparin requirements. *Am J Kidney Dis* 1991; 18:668–673.

97. Veys N, Vanholder R, De Cuyper K, et al. Influence of erythropoietin on dialyzer reuse, heparin need, and urea kinetics in maintenance hemodialysis patients. *Am J Kidney Dis* 1994;23:52–59.

98. Ward RA, Schmidt B, Gurland HJ. Low-dose heparinization can be used with DEAE-cellulose hemodialysis membranes. *ASAIO Trans* 1990;36:M321–M324.

99. Osada H, Ward CA, Duffin J, et al. Microbubble elimination during priming improves biocompatibility of membrane oxygenators. *Am J Physiol* 1978;234:H646–H652.

100. Keller F, Seemann J, Preuschof L, et al. Risk factors of system clotting in heparin-free haemodialysis. *Nephrol Dial Transplant* 1990;5:802–807.

CHAPTER 5

Measuring Hemodialysis Using Solute Kinetic Models

Andrew I. Chin and Thomas A. Depner

 HISTORICAL PERSPECTIVE

Hemodialysis was first successfully applied during the 1940s to support life in patients with acute kidney injury (1). Soon after, it was clear that life could be prolonged where previously death from uremia was certain. This seemingly miraculous therapy, touted by some as the most effective medical therapy introduced during the last century, was first deliberately used to manage end-stage chronic kidney disease (CKD5) in 1960 (2). It soon became clear that periodic dialysis treatments could sustain life indefinitely, but for the early pioneering patients, the frequency and intensity of treatments were limited by equipment availability and by adverse reactions. In addition, during these early development years, limited membrane permeability and patient intolerance of high blood flows necessitated prolonged treatments often for 8 to 10 hours. As maintenance dialysis was applied to larger numbers of patients, three treatments per week appeared to restore health, whereas two treatments per week regardless of treatment duration were inadequate in anephric patients.

Important developments in the next few decades led to further changes in long-term hemodialysis administration. In the late 1970s, the National Cooperative Dialysis Study (NCDS), sponsored by the National Institutes of Health (NIH), showed that a minimum small solute clearance per dialysis was required for thrice-weekly dialysis (3–5). This heralded a shift in emphasis of hemodialysis adequacy determination from blood solute levels to solute clearance (6). Tolerance of hemodialysis improved as more permeable and biocompatible synthetic membranes became available, as bicarbonate was substituted for acetate in the dialysate, as fluid removal was stabilized by using balance chambers and redundant conductivity monitors, and as severe anemia was reversed by treatment with recombinant erythropoietin (7–9). Notably, improvements in

membrane biocompatibility and solute flux allowed shorter dialysis treatments to become feasible, a goal sought by many, especially the patients (10,11). The next major NIH-funded study of hemodialysis patients, the Hemodialysis (HEMO) study, showed that the previously accepted minimum dose standard is also the optimum dose for patients dialyzed three times weekly (12). One can conclude from this study that a minimum dose, based on small solute kinetics, is still required, but increasing the dose further would not provide any significant benefit to the patient whose life is already compromised by the demands of hemodialysis. More recently, the Frequent Hemodialysis Network trial examined the benefits of more frequent in-center hemodialysis as well as nocturnal hemodialysis compared to conventional thrice-weekly treatments (13,14). Analysis of data from those studies has given us improved methods to estimate small solute clearance at higher dialysis frequencies.

Today, the lives of more than 2 million patients across the globe are supported by long-term hemodialysis (15), which is a tribute to technique refinements that have improved patient tolerance of the treatments. In the United States, where the incident and prevalence rates remain high, concerns have been raised by clinical providers as well as governmental regulatory agencies about the unacceptably high mortality rate of hemodialysis patients compared to the general population and to hemodialysis patients in other countries where hemodialysis is also the predominant form of renal replacement therapy (16,17). Under such scrutiny, the dose and adequacy of dialysis continue to be a focus and benchmark of dialysis excellence (18–21). As a result, the practice of quantifying dialysis by measuring solute clearance has long since moved from the realm of scientific curiosity to acceptance by the dialysis community and a mandated requirement by dialysis sponsors. At present, a variety of options for long-term hemodialysis exists, including frequent home hemodialysis, short frequent in-center dialysis, and long nocturnal dialysis. With such an array of modalities, measuring the "dose" of dialysis is more important than ever to ensure optimal patient care.

This chapter reviews what is known about mathematical models of solute kinetics currently used to measure hemodialysis, including how to implement them and how to interpret the patient-specific parameters generated by the models. Definitions of the symbols used throughout this chapter and their common units of measurement are displayed in **TABLE 5.1**.

UREA, A MARKER FOR CLEARANCE AND PROTEIN CATABOLISM

The properties that qualify urea as an indicator of dialysis efficiency and adequacy are listed in **TABLE 5.2**. Perhaps because of its low toxic potency, urea accumulates in the blood and tissues of patients with kidney disease to levels higher than any other organic solute. Its rate of production, dictated by net protein catabolism, is constant (zero order kinetics), independent of urea levels in the patient. Its ease of diffusion, most likely because of its small size and relative electrical neutrality, promotes swift movement across extracorporeal dialysis membranes. It also moves easily across most *in vivo* membranes, including erythrocyte membranes, along highly conserved pathways for facilitated transport (22–28). Because of these properties, measurement of urea transport across dialysis membranes is a sensitive index of small solute clearance, a fundamental goal of dialysis.

Urea generation correlates closely with protein catabolism, which, in steady-state, stable patients, reflects protein intake, a measure that can provide assistance with dietary management. A relatively precise relationship between urea generation and protein catabolism was found several years ago in two separate metabolic studies, each in a small number of CKD5 and CKD3 to CKD4 patients (29,30). Both studies showed essentially the same result (**EQUATION 5.1**):

$$nPCR = 5,420 \times G / V + 0.17 \qquad (5.1)$$

where nPCR is the net normalized protein catabolic rate (g/kg/d) (29), G is the urea nitrogen generation rate (mg/min), and V is the urea distribution volume (mL). Protein catabolism is expressed per kilogram of lean or normalized body weight. The latter is derived from V, assuming that V is 58% of body weight.

Total protein catabolism exceeds net nPCR, often by several fold (31). Protein breakdown releases free amino acids that are mostly reincorporated into new protein. This anabolic resynthesis of protein is a large fraction of the total catabolic rate, the difference representing a smaller net rate of nitrogen loss from irreversible breakdown of amino acids to urea (32). Therefore, nPCR, determined from urea modeling, is a measure of *net protein catabolism*. Net protein catabolism is equal to protein intake in patients who are in stable nitrogen balance.

Single blood urea levels are difficult to interpret. In a patient not on dialysis, elevated urea levels may well correspond to the syndrome of kidney disease with all of its manifestations. Paradoxically, dialysis patients with low urea levels as a result of low urea generation rates have poorer outcomes (33). Reduced protein-derived urea generation results from poor nutritional intake that is usually due to suppression of the appetite. Appetite suppression is associated with either inadequate dialysis or with comorbid diseases such as infection or cardiovascular disease, the leading cause of death in dialysis patients (3,4,34–36). Low urea levels achieved by adequate

dialysis are beneficial, while low levels due to poor nutrition and decreased protein intake are associated with higher morbidity and mortality. The studies of pregnancy in women on hemodialysis support this notion—pregnancy outcomes are improved in women with lower blood urea levels as achieved by hemodialysis (37–39).

Attempts to demonstrate a direct toxic effect of urea have led to the conclusion that urea is at best a mild toxin (40–42), levels of which serve only to mirror other easily dialyzed solutes that are more toxic and responsible for the uremic syndrome (43). Alternatively, an indirect effect of urea such as carbamylation of protein may mediate its toxicity (44–47). However, posttranslational carbamylation of proteins requires time to develop in the presence of high urea concentrations and, conversely, to reverse after lowering the urea concentration. Therefore, the immediate benefits of dialysis that are observed clinically are difficult to explain on this basis. Evidence that carbamylated albumin levels associate with adverse outcomes in a cohort of diabetic hemodialysis patients suggests that long-term effects of protein modification by urea may warrant further investigation (48).

An inescapable conclusion from these observations, and one that guides the clinical application of urea modeling today, is that urea is a poor marker of uremia but its clearance is a good marker of dialysis. Measurements of urea concentration before and following dialysis, when combined with an appropriate model of urea kinetics, provide vital clinical information about both the adequacy of dialysis and the nutritional status of the patient.

FACTORS THAT DETERMINE THE REQUIREMENT FOR DIALYSIS

Several of the patient-specific factors listed in **TABLE 5.3** determine how much dialysis is needed. These include the patient's size, residual native kidney urea clearance, fluid gain between dialyses, and perhaps in the rare case of pregnancy (37,38,49,50). If adequate dialysis is provided, moderate increases in urea generation do not affect the need for dialysis but instead reflect improved protein nutrition (see section "Protein Catabolism"). Although solute compartmentalization (see section "Multi-Compartment Kinetic Model") affects the delivery of dialysis, the effect is predictable as explained in the subsequent text, and relatively constant from patient to patient and from time to time, so periodic adjustments are not necessary.

Protein Catabolism

Adjusting the dose to the urea generation rate has been considered less important in recent years because patients on average receive higher doses of dialysis (19). Higher doses cause mean urea concentrations to fall below the ceiling that was originally suggested by the NCDS, so an additional adjustment for urea generation is less critical and is usually unnecessary. In addition, increasing evidence suggests that nutrition has a strong influence on patient outcome, so the emphasis has shifted from restricting protein to encouraging more protein and caloric intake (51–53). The United States multi-centered Modification of Diet in Renal Disease (MDRD) study also raised concerns about protein restriction adversely influencing survival of patients in stages 3 and 4 of CKD (54,55).

Several investigators have reported a correlation between nPCR and the dose of dialysis expressed as Kt/V, suggesting that increasing the dose of dialysis will improve the appetite (56–59). This conclusion is subject to error for several reasons. First, if the dose of

TABLE 5.1 Symbols Used in This Chapter

Symbol	Unit of Measurement	Definition
avC_0	mg/mL	Average predialysis concentration
B	mL/min	Fluid gain (loss) between (during) dialyses
BUN	mg/mL, mg/dL	Blood urea nitrogen concentration
BW	Any units	Body weight
C	mg/mL	Concentration (e.g., of urea or urea N)
CAPD		Continuous ambulatory peritoneal dialysis
C_{Av}	mg/mL	Average concentration
C_0	mg/mL	Initial (predialysis) concentration
C_1	mg/mL	Concentration in the proximal compartment
C_2	mg/mL	Concentration in the remote compartment
C_D	mg/mL	Concentration in the dialysate
C_E	mg/mL	Postdialysis concentration after equilibration
C_i	mg/mL	Concentration (or conductivity) in blood entering the dialyzer
C_0	mg/mL	Concentration (or conductivity) in blood exiting the dialyzer
C_S	mg/mL	Concentration in systemic blood
C_T	mg/mL	Concentration at time T
D	mL/min	Dialysance
e		Natural logarithm base (2.718)
EKR	mL/min	Continuous equivalent of intermittent clearance
F_{CPR}	Fraction	Fractional cardiopulmonary recirculation
G	mg/min	Urea generation rate
K	mL/min	Total urea clearance
k	min^{-1}	Solute elimination (rate) constant
κ	min	Coefficient to allow addition of K_R to Kt/V
K_0A	mL/min	Dialyzer mass transfer area coefficient
Kt/V	Fraction per dialysis	Fractional clearance index for urea
spKt/V, eKt/V, stdKt/V, nKt/V		Variants of Kt/V (see text)
K_C	mL/min	Intercompartment mass transfer area coefficient
K_D	mL/min	Dialyzer urea clearance
K_R	mL/min	Residual (native kidney) urea clearance
nPCR	g/kg/d	Protein catabolic rate normalized to V
N		Number of treatments per week
Q_{AC}	mL/min	Access device blood flow
Q_B	mL/min	Dialyzer blood flow
Q_D	mL/min	Dialysate flow
Q_F	mL/min	Ultrafiltration rate during dialysis
Q_S	mL/min	Systemic blood flow (C_0 minus access flow)
R	Fraction per dialysis	Postdialysis BUN/predialysis BUN
RG	mg	Correction factor for K_R and urea generation
t	min or hours	Time
t_d	min or hours	Dialysis treatment time
t_i	min or hours	Time interval between two dialyses
TAC	mg/mL, mg/dL	Time-averaged concentration of BUN
U_F	L per dialysis	Ultrafiltrate volume
URR	Fraction per dialysis	Urea reduction ratio $(C_1C_2)/C_1$
V_0	mL, L	Predialysis volume of urea distribution
V, V_D, V_T	mL, L	Postdialysis volume of urea distribution
ΔV	mL, L	Change in V during and between dialyses
V_1	mL, L	Volume of the proximal (dialyzed) compartment
V_2	mL, L	Volume of the remote compartment
W	kg	Patient weight
ΔWt	Fraction per dialysis	Fractional weight loss during dialysis

TABLE 5.2	Properties of Urea Relevant to Kinetic Modeling

Most abundant of organic solutes that accumulate in patients with kidney disease

Distribution volume is total body water

Easily dialyzed

    Molecular weight = 60 Da

    Chemical formula $CO(NH_2)_2$

    Polar, water soluble

    Uncharged

    Not bound to serum or tissue proteins

Source

    Produced by the liver

    End product of protein amino acid catabolism

Transport

    Passive diffusion *in vitro* and *in vivo*

    Facilitated diffusion *in vivo*

    Relatively nontoxic

dialysis is not strictly controlled by urea modeling, physicians may simply give more dialysis to patients with high protein intake, creating a correlation that reflects a physician response to appetite rather than *vice versa*. Second, both nPCR and Kt/V are determined from the same set of blood urea nitrogen (BUN) values (see subsequent text); therefore, an artifactual mathematical correlation due to coupling is expected, the magnitude of which depends on the BUN measurement error (60,61). Third, observational studies of the curvilinear relationship between Kt/V and protein catabolism rate (PCR) are confounded by inclusion of very low doses. This causes a false exaggeration of the effect of increasing Kt/V above the range where the relationship reaches a plateau (58,62).

The above errors are important to avoid when interpreting nPCR. However, since appetite suppression is a well-known

TABLE 5.3	Variables that Impact the Hemodialysis Prescription

Patient variables

    Urea distribution volume, equated to total body water (V)

    Urea generation rate from net protein catabolism (G and PCR)

    Residual (native kidney) urea clearance (K_R)

    Fluid accumulation (ΔV)

    Solute compartmentalization (K_C)

Dialysis variables

    Dialyzer clearance components

    Model of dialyzer and its urea mass transfer area coefficient (K_oA)

    Blood flow (Q_B)

    Dialysate flow (Q_D)

    Ultrafiltration rate (Q_F)

    Treatment time (t_d)

    Schedule or frequency of dialysis (N)

PCR, protein catabolism rate.

consequence of uremia and dialysis reverses uremia, we can expect that dialysis will improve the appetite in patients with overt uremia (63). The HEMO study showed no improvement in nutrition after increasing the dose above the current optimal target in patients dialyzed three times weekly (64,65). While some uncontrolled studies have suggested that increasing the frequency of hemodialysis to four to six per week may improve the appetite in some patients (66), the analysis of the Frequent Hemodialysis Network data did not show significant improvements in lean body mass or nutritional parameters in patients receiving six times a week in-center treatment or those on nocturnal dialysis (67).

Residual Native Kidney Clearance

Seemingly insignificant levels of residual native kidney urea clearance (e.g., 1 or 2 mL/min) can markedly decrease the need for dialysis, but most nephrologists do not compensate for residual function (K_R) by prescribing a lower dialysis dose. Reasons for omitting this practice include the patient inconvenience and provider cost associated with collecting, measuring, analyzing urine, and calculating K_R. Those opposed to the regular evaluation of residual urea clearance have also pointed to the potential negative psychological effect on the patient from stepwise increases in the dialysis treatment time as K_R inevitably declines. It should also be noted that at the present time, regulatory agencies ignore the inclusion of K_R in total clearance and require submission of delivered Kt/V (or urea reduction ratio) as the only accepted clearance measure when dialysis clinic adequacy is monitored. Therefore, a nephrologist who does incorporate K_R in his or her dialysis prescriptions may place the dialysis clinic at risk for financial penalties. However, K_R has a strong influence on patient mortality, both for peritoneal dialysis and for hemodialysis (68–70), so K_R not only affects the required dialysis dose but it also has prognostic significance. In addition to an equivalent clearance of small solutes, residual renal function has other benefits that include removal of poorly dialyzable toxins (71,72). Since dialysis compromises a patient's quality of life, and the primary goal of kidney replacement is improving the quality of life, adjusting the dose in patients with significant K_R is worth considering. Acknowledging this benefit, the most recent Kidney Disease Outcomes Quality Initiative (KDOQI) 2015 guidelines have reemphasized the recommendation to adjust the dialysis prescription in patients who have substantial residual renal function, assuming K_R is periodically updated. Methods for incorporating K_R to create an expression of total depurative function are published in the KDOQI guidelines (73) and are briefly described later in the chapter (see section "How to Add K_R to Kt/V").

Body Size

Body size is an obvious modulator of dialysis need, but the precise denominator to use as an index of size is debated (74–76). Numerous isotope studies in animals and normal humans have shown that the urea distribution volume (V) is equivalent to total body water, which is proportionate to lean body mass (77–79). As discussed in the subsequent text, V is a mathematically convenient denominator, but it may not be appropriate, especially because body surface area (SA) has been used for several decades to normalize native creatinine or inulin clearances (80,81). Because outcome patterns in women and smaller patients differ from that of larger patients (82–84), and most metabolic functions vary with SA, not lean body mass, several investigators have attempted to convert V to SA by adjusting for body height using time-tested formulas for SA (85–87).

The concentrations of uremic toxins in body fluids are thought to modulate toxicity and therefore the need for dialysis (88), but for first-order processes, the concentration is a function of generation and removal and does not depend on the space of distribution. For a patient whose clearance (K) is constant, and whose toxin generation rate (G) is equal to the removal rate, changes in the volume of distribution (V) have no effect on concentration in the steady state (C = G/K). For example, an increase in V from edema formation or a decline in V from muscle loss would not affect steady-state concentrations if all else remain constant. It is unlikely that edema fluid is a source of uremic toxins, and analysis of outcomes suggests that muscle is also an unlikely source (89,90). Instead, individual solute generation rates modulate toxin concentrations and are therefore the most logical size variables to which the dose should be normalized. Unfortunately, the critical toxic compounds have not been identified, so the precise relationship between their generation rates and body size remains speculative (43).

Use of V as a normalizing denominator for the dialysis dose has also been questioned because observational studies have shown that V independently predicts and correlates positively with survival (91–94). Patients with lower body mass tend to have both a higher Kt/V and a higher mortality risk. African Americans with CKD5 tend to have a higher body mass and both a lower Kt/V and a lower mortality risk (95,96). These opposing effects of V confound the relationship between the V-normalized dose of dialysis and patient outcomes. Adjustment for the independent beneficial effect of V on survival creates an even steeper relationship between the survival benefit of increased dialysis dose (74). Larger patients likely have higher solute generation rates and require more clearance than smaller patients to achieve the same blood concentration. One possible explanation for the higher risk of mortality in smaller dialysis patients is use of V instead of SA, as noted earlier, which may overcorrect for body size, leading to inappropriately lower doses in smaller patients. *Post hoc* analysis of the HEMO study data suggested that women, who are generally smaller in body size, may benefit from the higher targeted Kt/V (97), lending some credence to the idea of underdosed dialysis in this subgroup. The higher risk of mortality may also result from the higher prevalence of malnutrition in smaller dialysis patients. While malnutrition alone portends a poor prognosis in the dialysis patient, it can also result from comorbid conditions including inflammatory states that may independently affect survival (98).

TABLE 5.3 also lists fluid accumulation between dialyses as a component of the dialysis prescription. Although it increases the requirement for fluid removal during each treatment, fluid accumulation actually decreases the need for dialysis both because of a dilution effect and because removing fluid during hemodialysis increases the efficiency of solute removal (99). See section "Effect of Fluid Gain" later in the chapter.

Hematocrit

Solutes other than urea do not always distribute in erythrocytes and transport out of the erythrocyte can be delayed as blood traverses the dialyzer within 10 to 30 seconds. As the red cell mass usually makes up 30% to 40% of a patient's blood volume, distribution and transport of solutes in erythrocytes can have a significant effect on clearance. Red cell urea transporters are very robust, causing near instantaneous equilibration, so the presence of erythrocytes has little effect on urea clearance (22–28). However, creatinine equilibrates slowly and phosphorus apparently does not move

at all across erythrocyte membranes during transit through the dialyzer (100,101). This in part explains the difference between *in vitro* and *in vivo* clearances, an effect that should be kept in mind when developing and applying kinetic models for solutes other than urea.

TARGETING THE AMOUNT OF DIALYSIS

How to Measure Dialysis; How Much Is Enough?

The NCDS showed not only that higher urea levels are not tolerated but also that morbidity and mortality are inversely correlated with protein catabolism (4,102). Because the urea level is directly correlated with urea generation from net protein catabolism, factoring one for the other is the essence of a clearance (see subsequent text). A later mechanistic analysis of the data showed that providing a size-adjusted minimum clearance of urea per dialysis (Kt/V) would assure the best outcome (3). The subsequent HEMO trial showed that further increases in this dose parameter were met with no further improvement in morbidity or mortality, so the minimum dose for three dialyses per week also turned out to be the optimum dose (12). Some observational studies have shown that markedly prolonging the treatment time (e.g., doubling or tripling t_d) on a thrice-weekly schedule may improve survival and intermediary cardiac outcomes (103–105). Analysis of the Dialysis Outcomes and Practice Patterns Study (DOPPS) observational data also suggested that in patients dialyzed three times weekly, incremental increases in treatment time are associated with a lower relative risk of death (106,107). However, no randomized clinical trials have been conducted to test this hypothesis.

The relationships among time-averaged BUN, Kt/V, and nPCR are shown in **FIGURE 5.1**. The "safe zone" is shown below the heavy line representing the isopleth for a single pool Kt/V of 1.2 per dialysis. The curvilinear surface represents the mathematical relationship among the three variables time-averaged concentration of BUN (TAC), nPCR, and Kt/V, for patients dialyzed three times weekly. Note that only two of the three variables are required to find a point on the surface plot, which means that the three variables are mathematically interdependent and that arguments favoring one as more accurate than another are trivial. Note also that the depicted Kt/V values are specific for dialysis given three times weekly. For twice-weekly dialysis or another schedule, the Kt/V axis must be changed.

The NCDS showed that to achieve optimal patient outcome, one must guarantee that the dose of dialysis (delivered Kt/V) is constant and relatively independent of the BUN (3,6). These findings reflect the failure of the serum urea concentration as an indicator of both dialysis adequacy and uremia (63). This should not be surprising to nephrologists, who have long held a double-standard interpretation of the BUN in patients who do not yet require dialysis. The BUN has been considered important to measure, but when the patient is symptomatic and the BUN is low, it is ignored (102). Some patients have died a uremic death with a BUN as low as 50 mg/dL. Clearly, dialyzable toxins other than urea account for a major part if not all of the uremic syndrome, so control of the BUN is not enough to guarantee adequate dialysis (40–42,88,108).

A safety net, expressed as Kt/V, guarantees the average patient will receive a minimum amount of dialysis, relatively independent of BUN levels and protein catabolism. However, patients' need for dialysis may differ, so if the patient is not improving or is failing for unknown reasons, it behooves the nephrologist to increase the dose of dialysis unless he or she is confident that the dose is already well

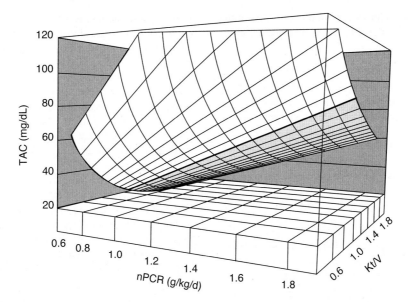

FIGURE 5.1 The mathematical relationships among normalized protein catabolic rate (nPCR), time-averaged concentration (TAC), and Kt/V form a curvilinear plane in three dimensions. Lines running diagonally across the plane are Kt/V isopleths; the line at Kt/V = 1.2 represents the currently accepted minimum standard, and the region of the plane below this is the "safe" domain. Data were derived from the single compartment model; all scales are linear.

above the level currently considered a safe minimum and that the patient's symptoms are not related to uremia. This recommendation acknowledges our current inability to define the uremic state more precisely (63), our ignorance of factors that may mediate individual requirements for dialysis, and our concerns about the contribution of protein catabolism to uremia (109–113).

Interpreting Kt/V: Limitations

The term *Kt/V* describes the *fractional clearance* of urea during a single hemodialysis or the fractional volume cleared. As such, this is a term without units. The fraction can be greater than 1 because blood flow circulates from patient to dialyzer, which allows the body water compartment to be dialyzed more than once during a single treatment. Modeled Kt/V is a measure of the amount or dose of dialysis received by the patient. It correlates with outcome, but the correlation is nonlinear, as demonstrated by the NCDS and other outcome studies (3,4,114). Part of the reason for this nonlinearity is the curvilinear relationship between solute removal and Kt/V as shown in **FIGURE 5.2**. Because dialysis is a self-limiting process driven by diffusion, the amount of solute removed diminishes exponentially as the amount of dialysis is increased linearly. In other words, doubling Kt/V does not double the amount of solute removed and may accomplish very little if the critical solutes have already fallen to low levels or disequilibrium prevents further solute removal. This self-limiting or self-defeating aspect of intermittent hemodialysis is important to recognize when expressing the dose as Kt/V. Once the dose reaches the minimum standard for adequacy, increasing per dialysis Kt/V further does not necessarily improve outcome (12). Kt/V is not a direct measure of outcome or the effectiveness of the dose but is simply a method of assuring dialysis adequacy in the absence of knowledge about the critical toxins removed. As will be emphasized later, Kt/V should not be viewed as a parameter of the dialysis machine but rather as the patient response to a particular dialysis prescription.

SINGLE-COMPARTMENT KINETIC MODEL

Clearance, a Better Measure of Dialysis

The clearance concept is intuitive, but its precise definition, origin, and application often escape nephrologists and even physiologists. It is probably best understood as a measure of the elimination process unencumbered by other variables, including the solute concentration. The solute removal rate is itself a measure of elimination, but for both filtration and dialysis, the rate is a linear function of (proportional to) the concentration. Expressing the elimination process as a clearance takes the effects of both the elimination rate and the concentration out of the rate term:

$$\text{Clearance} = (\text{removal rate}) / \text{concentration}$$

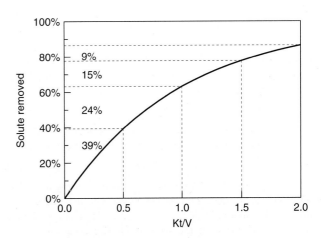

FIGURE 5.2 For each increment in Kt/V, the removal rate falls and will ultimately extinguish. Further increases in Kt/V beyond the plateau for this particular solute afford no benefit to the patient.

For dialysis, if the index solute is present on both sides of the membrane, diffusion is proportional to the solute gradient, so we define "dialysance":

Dialysance = (removal rate) / concentration gradient

When the removal rate is a linear function of concentration, the process is called *first order*, meaning that the removal rate is proportional to the first power of the concentration. In comparison, for zero order processes, the removal rate is constant, independent of the concentration, for example, urea generation by the liver. For both the native kidney, which uses convective clearance, and hemodialysis with diffusion-centered clearance, a generalized equation for a first-order process is (**Equation 5.2**):

$$dC / dt = -kC \qquad (5.2)$$

where C is the solute concentration at any time (t) and k is the elimination constant expressed as a fraction per unit of time. Rearranging **Equation 5.2**, and multiplying by the volume of solute distribution (V), clearance is defined as (**Equation 5.3**):

$$(dCV / dt) / C = -kV \qquad (5.3)$$

where dCV/dt is the solute removal rate and kV is the clearance. Because the removal rate divided by concentration is a flow, clearance is often described as the flow equivalent to complete removal of the solute. This definition is intuitive, but it bypasses the previous steps in the derivation of the clearance concept. Clearance is a useful expression only for first-order processes like diffusion and convection. We do not calculate the urinary clearance of sodium, for example, a non–first-order process.

Because removal of urea by the dialyzer is a first-order process, the rate of removal can be expressed mathematically using **Equation 5.2**. Integration over a period of time yields a familiar expression that describes the removal of drugs by a single exponential process (**Equation 5.4**) (115):

$$C = C_0 e^{-kt} \qquad (5.4)$$

where C_0 is the initial urea concentration and e is the base for natural logarithms (2.718). The rate of elimination falls with time because the concentration falls with time; that is, the process eventually extinguishes itself. However, the fractional rate of change in concentration, (dC/C)/dt, is constant (−k) and can be determined simply by measuring two timed concentrations, C_0 and C (**Equation 5.5**):

$$k = [\ln(C_0 / C)] / t \qquad (5.5)$$

where t is the time interval between measurements of C_0 and C and ln is the natural logarithm. When the fractional removal rate (k) is multiplied by the urea volume of distribution (V), the result is a clearance (K) (**Equation 5.6**):

$$K = kV \text{ or } k = K / V \qquad (5.6)$$

By substituting **Equation 5.6** into **Equation 5.5** and rearranging, another familiar expression appears (**Equation 5.7**):

$$Kt/V = \ln(C_0 / C) \qquad (5.7)$$

This equation shows that the log ratio of the starting urea concentration (C_0) to the ending concentration (C) can be used as an index of the amount of dialysis delivered during a single dialysis treatment, circumventing the necessity for measuring each of the three components of the expression Kt/V. **Figure 5.3** shows the relationship between time and C expressed as BUN on a linear scale to the left and on a logarithmic scale to the right (116). The slope

of the logarithmic line is −k or −K/V. Note that this simplified graphic analysis of urea kinetics gives the *ratio* of clearance to urea volume (K/V). To resolve K, V must be determined independently and *vice versa*. Note also that the absolute values for C_0 and C are not important; their relative values determine Kt/V. For example, if the BUN falls from 150 to 75 mg/dL or from 50 to 25 mg/dL during dialysis, Kt/V is the same. Because Kt/V is determined from BUN measurements in the patient, it is a patient-specific parameter, not a machine parameter; Kt/V is a measure of response to dialysis rather than a measure of the amount of dialysis prescribed (117).

Urea generation in milligrams per minute is derived from the change in urea concentration between dialyses in milligrams per milliliter multiplied by the urea volume in milliliters and divided by the time interval in minutes. Because the normalized protein catabolic rate is factored for patient volume (**Equation 5.1**), net protein catabolism can be determined from the changes in BUN between dialyses, provided there is no residual renal function or change in volume (**Equation 5.8**) (117,118):

$$nPCR = 5{,}420 \, [(C'_0 - C_T) / t_i] + 0.17 \qquad (5.8)$$

where nPCR is the normalized protein catabolic rate (gram per kilogram body weight per day), C'_0 is the second predialysis BUN (mg/mL), C_T is the postdialysis BUN (mg/mL), and t_i is the time interval between dialyses (min). It is important to note that the simplifications included in **Equations 5.4** through **5.8** help illustrate fundamental relationships but preclude their use in the clinical setting. These equations should not be used to model urea kinetics in patients because they fail to include several important patient variables already mentioned, the most important of which are native kidney urea clearance and the change in body fluid content during and between dialyses. Both factors lower the predialysis BUN and reduce the required change in BUN during dialysis, complicating the computation of nPCR. A third parameter that has a slight but significant effect on Kt/V and V is the amount of urea generated during dialysis. A more precise mathematical expression of urea

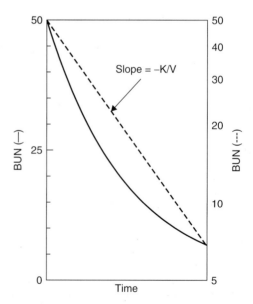

FIGURE 5.3 Blood urea nitrogen (BUN) concentrations fall logarithmically during hemodialysis treatments (**left axis**). The slope of the log decline (**right axis**) is −K/V. (Adapted from Depner TA. Quantification of dialysis. Urea modeling: the basics. *Semin Dial* 1991;4:179–184, with permission.)

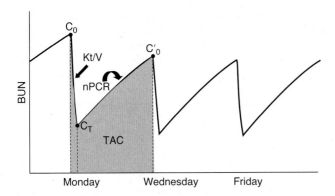

FIGURE 5.4 Weekly blood urea nitrogen (BUN) profile generated by the single-pool model. Kt/V is derived from the fall in BUN during dialysis, normalized protein catabolic rate (nPCR) from the rise between dialyses, and time-averaged BUN (TAC) from the shaded area under the curve. The rise from C_T to C'_0 is nonlinear when fluid is gained and/or when significant residual function exists.

concentrations during dialysis includes these additional three parameters (**EQUATION 5.9**):

$$d(VC) / dt = G - (K_D + K_R)C \qquad (5.9)$$

where V is the volume of urea distribution, G is the urea generation rate (presumed constant), K_D is the dialyzer urea clearance, and K_R is the patient's native kidney (residual) urea clearance. Integration of **EQUATION 5.9** gives a better, although more complex, expression of urea concentration during and between dialyses (**EQUATION 5.10**) (99,119):

$$C = C_0 \left(\frac{V_0 + Bt}{V_0}\right)^{-\frac{K+B}{B}} + \left(\frac{G}{K+B}\right)\left(1 - \frac{V_0 + Bt}{V_0}\right)^{-\frac{K+B}{B}} \qquad (5.10)$$

where V_0 is the volume of urea distribution before dialysis, K during dialysis is the sum of $K_D + K_R$, K between dialyses is K_R, and B is the rate of fluid gain between or during dialyses (a negative value during dialysis). **EQUATION 5.10** can be used to predict a urea concentration profile during and between dialyses such as that shown in **FIGURE 5.4**. It is the fundamental equation used for single pool urea kinetic modeling, but in this case, it is used in reverse, that is, values for K/V and G are fit to measured values of C and C_0 using an iterative computer-generated process. Kt/V is derived primarily from the fall in BUN during a single dialysis, and nPCR is determined primarily from the rise in BUN between dialyses, as indicated in **FIGURE 5.4**. The typical dialysis schedule, three treatments every 7 days, is asymmetric, with 2- and 3-day intervals between treatments. Most models can adjust for this or for any schedule.

Two–Blood Urea Nitrogen Method

When nPCR is determined from a postdialysis BUN and a subsequent predialysis BUN, only the difference between these two values enters into the calculation (**EQUATION 5.8**); their absolute values are ignored (116). Absolute values are also ignored for the calculation of Kt/V, which is derived mainly from the ratio of predialysis to postdialysis BUN (**EQUATION 5.7**). If the absolute values of the predialysis and postdialysis BUN are also included in the calculations, the third BUN measurement can be eliminated as shown in the subsequent text (99,102,120). This simplifies the urea modeling process without detracting from its accuracy.

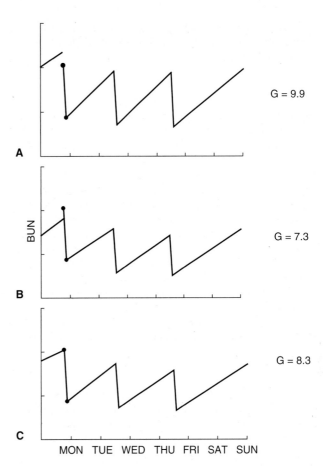

FIGURE 5.5 The two–blood urea nitrogen (BUN) method approximates G using a trial-and-error approach. **A:** G is set too high, predicting an inordinately high predialysis BUN 1 week later. **B:** G is set too low. The computer reproduces the BUN/time profile using different values for G until the calculated predialysis BUN 1 week later matches the measured BUN (as in **C**). (From Depner TA, Cheer AY. Modeling urea kinetics with two versus three BUN measurements. A critical comparison. *ASAIO J* 1989;35:499–502, with permission.)

The technique for resolving G from only two-BUN measurements is shown in **FIGURE 5.5**. The method requires a weekly steady state of nitrogen balance—that is, a constant dialysis prescription and a constant dietary nitrogen intake from day to day for at least a week. We assume these parameters to be true, realizing the likelihood of wide protein intake variation from day to day in most people. Paradoxically, the two-BUN technique for measuring nPCR is less influenced by a dietary binge than is the three-BUN method, because the absolute value of the predialysis BUN (the major determinant of nPCR) is determined by more than a single interdialysis interval (120). The two-BUN method also offers the patient less opportunity to influence the result by altering his or her diet during the interval between the second and third blood samplings. However, even when nPCR is carefully measured, the variance is at least twice that of Kt/V.

How to Implement Modeling with Two–Blood Urea Nitrogens

The single-compartment, variable-volume model is the most commonly applied clinical tool for quantifying hemodialysis. Two of the modeling assumptions, single-pool distribution during dialysis and absence of rebound, cause errors that are offsetting (see section

"Comparison with the Single-Compartment Model" later in the chapter), so the final calculations of V and Kt/V closely match those of more complex models (121).

The only two unknown variables in **EQUATION 5.10** are G and V; K is measurable and is required to start the modeling process. As shown in the subsequent text, the value chosen for K need not be precisely accurate to determine Kt/V. To start the modeling process, arbitrary values for G and V are chosen and the predialysis BUN is substituted for C_0 in **EQUATION 5.10**. V is then adjusted until the calculated value for C matches the measured postdialysis BUN using a repetitive (iterative) approach. Then K_D is set to zero, the postdialysis BUN is substituted for C_0 in **EQUATION 5.10**, and G is adjusted until C matches the predialysis BUN, using the technique described in **FIGURE 5.5** for two-BUN modeling. The iterations are then repeated with the new values for G and V. The accuracy of V and G will depend on the accuracy of the chosen value for K, but K/V and G/V will be affected little by inaccuracies in K or V. nPCR can be calculated from G/V using **EQUATION 5.1**, and Kt/V is the product of K and t for the modeled dialysis divided by V. K between dialyses consists of K_R only. Care should be taken to adjust B for asymmetric interdialysis intervals. Any schedule of dialysis treatments can be used, and the entire process takes less than a second of computer time.

The Prescribed Dose

Determinants of dialyzer clearance include the flow rates of blood and dialysate and properties of the membrane, primarily its SA, permeability, and geometry. Similar to the clearance concept, these encumbering variables can be removed from the expression of dialyzer function by defining the dialyzer mass transfer coefficient (**EQUATION 5.11**) (122):

$$K_0A = \frac{Q_B \cdot Q_D}{Q_B - Q_D} \ln\left[\frac{Q_D(Q_B - K_D)}{Q_B(Q_D - K_D)}\right] \qquad (5.11)$$

where K_0A is the mass transfer area coefficient, Q_B is the blood flow rate, Q_D is the dialysate flow rate, K_D is the dialyzer clearance, and

"ln" is the natural logarithm. The mass transfer area coefficient, sometimes called the dialyzer intrinsic clearance, is also expressed as a flow and is considered the maximum clearance possible at infinite flow rates for the particular dialyzer model and solute. A rearrangement of **EQUATION 5.11** has practical value for determining the prescribed dialyzer clearance from the machine settings of blood and dialysate flow and is a vital input parameter during the kinetic modeling process described in the subsequent text:

$$K_D = Q_B\left[\frac{e^{K_0A\left(\frac{Q_D - Q_B}{Q_DQ_B}\right)} - 1}{e^{K_0A\left(\frac{Q_D - Q_B}{Q_DQ_B}\right)} - \frac{Q_B}{Q_D}}\right] \qquad (5.12)$$

The dialysis center controls the dose by manipulating the dialysis variables listed in **TABLE 5.3** and then calculating the dialyzer clearance using **EQUATION 5.12**. Although it is helpful to be able to measure each of these parameters precisely, standard urea kinetic modeling allows a retrospective estimate of the amount of dialysis delivered to the patient without the need for measuring the prescribed dialyzer clearance, flow rates, or even treatment time. This closes the loop of quality control by allowing a comparison between the amount of dialysis prescribed and that actually delivered (123). Discrepancies between the two can help to detect equipment failures including poorly calibrated or nonoccluding blood pumps, failure of dialysate pumps, problems with reuse devices, and vascular access recirculation.

Effect of Fluid Gain between and Consequent Ultrafiltration during Hemodialysis

Ultrafiltration during standard hemodialysis, as currently practiced, adds a small increment to urea clearance or Kt/V. However, the fluid gains between treatments serve to dilute solute levels (**FIGURE 5.6**), potentially mitigating their toxicity. This effect and the additional clearance due to the ultrafiltration itself are incorporated in the

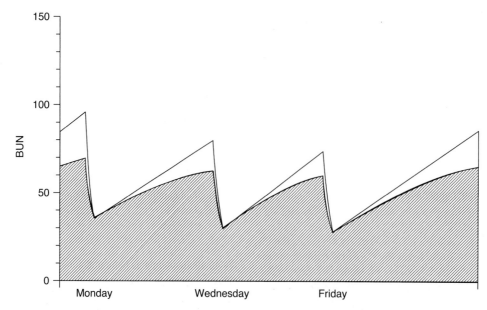

FIGURE 5.6 Effect of weight gain between dialyses. The upper profile of weekly steady-state urea concentrations represents a patient who gains no weight and requires no ultrafiltration during dialysis. The lower profile shows the effect of net fluid accumulation at 3 mL/min in the same patient. BUN, blood urea nitrogen.

formal modeling equation ("B" in **EQUATION 5.10**) and are most clearly seen when comparing urea reduction ratio values with Kt/V at differing levels of ultrafiltration (see section "The Urea Reduction Ratio" later in the chapter).

To add the small effect of ultrafiltration to the *prescribed* clearance during hemodialysis, an addition term must be added to K_D (**EQUATION 5.13**):

$$\text{Total Prescribed K} = K_D + Q_F (1 - K_D / Q_B) \qquad (5.13)$$

where K_D is the dialyzer clearance in the absence of ultrafiltration, Q_B is the dialyzer blood inflow rate, and Q_F is the ultrafiltration rate (mL/min). As the extraction ratio approaches 1, meaning that the clearance approaches the blood flow rate, the effect of Q_F diminishes and eventually extinguishes, because removal of solute across the dialyzer cannot exceed 100%.

Primary Hemofiltration Therapy

The same hollow fiber device used for hemodialysis can be used to filter the blood, eliminating the need for dialysate and providing clearance by convection akin to native kidney function. However, filtered electrolytes and fluid must be replaced, necessitating simultaneous infusion of a sterile physiologic salt solution in large volumes. To achieve adequate solute removal, primary hemofiltration and hemodiafiltration therapy require filtration rates that are much higher than required for standard hemodialysis. Filtration also follows the laws of first-order kinetics, so we can use the same mathematical model developed for hemodialysis to predict blood levels and measure the patient response to the dialysis treatment as Kt/V. The model makes no assumptions about how the urea was removed, only that the process was first order. The patient's blood circulates between the filter and the patient just as it does for dialysis, and concurrent replacement of filtrate causes a rapid decline in solute concentration during treatment that diminishes the effect over time, similar to hemodialysis. The major determinants of the modeled clearance are the predialysis and postdialysis BUN. Some authorities see hemofiltration as a trend for the future because it mimics the native kidney and has potential for removing larger molecular weight (MW) solutes more efficiently (124). However, outcomes data have not fully supported an advantage to hemofiltration versus hemodialysis (125–129). Of interest, delayed diffusion within the patient, one of the limitations to effective hemodialysis, also appears to limit the effectiveness of hemofiltration (127). Therefore, diffusion plays a significant physiologic role, whether the extracorporeal removal process is diffusive or convective.

How to Add K_R to Kt/V

Considering that the dialyzer urea clearance is usually an order of magnitude higher than the urea clearance achieved by two normal kidneys, the much-reduced clearance (K_R) contributed by the patient's impaired kidneys adds little to total urea clearance during dialysis; its major effect is seen between treatments where it serves to attenuate the rise in BUN as shown in **FIGURE 5.7**. In addition, the continuous nature of K_R makes it more efficient than intermittent hemodialyzer clearance, so simple addition of the two clearances is not possible. Two methods, both of which require formal urea kinetic modeling, have been used to generate a total clearance or total Kt/V that incorporates the effects of both clearances.

The first and oldest technique is based on and assumption of equivalent values for either the time-averaged concentration of BUN concentration (TAC) or the average predialysis BUN (avC_0) (102). Any of the previously described models can be used to generate

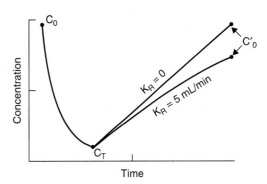

FIGURE 5.7 Effect of residual native kidney clearance (K_R). Dialyzable solute concentrations rise less steeply (*lower curve*) in a patient with significant K_R compared to the rise between dialyses in a patient with zero K_R (*upper line*).

TAC or avC_0 from the predialysis and postdialysis BUN while K_R is included in the model. K_R is then removed from the model to calculate the delivered K_D that is required to produce the same TAC or avC_0 in the patient with identical G and V_D. In the absence of K_R, K_D must be increased to maintain the same TAC or avC_0. The new value for Kt/V represents the total effect of both clearances. This approach is equivalent to inflating K_R to a level that mimics the relatively inefficient effect of intermittent dialysis before adding the two clearances. A simplified method that does not require the second set of iterations has been published (99,102) and is discussed in a later section (with details in **EQUATION 5.33** and **TABLE 5.5**). Also, see section "A Simplified Method for Incorporating K_R".

The second method takes the opposite approach by deflating the dialyzer clearance to a continuous equivalent clearance before adding the two. This method is described later in the section "A Continuous Equivalent Dose."

A major barrier that discourages addition of K_R to Kt/V is the inconvenience and expense of a timed urine collection. Non–urea-based methods of estimating K_R may eliminate these barriers. The nuclear medicine isotope determination of kidney function used in patients with relatively preserved glomerular filtration has proven to be inaccurate in more advanced CKD (130). Determining K_R in dialysis patients, using serum cystatin C levels when weekly or standard Kt/V is also known, has shown some promise (131,132). Recent KDOQI guidelines (73) have placed more emphasis on adjusting the dialysis prescription to patient K_R, and we may see more research in this area.

MULTIPLE-COMPARTMENT KINETIC MODEL

As the intensity of hemodialysis is increased and time is shortened, the potential for development of solute concentration gradients, called *solute disequilibrium*, increases. Evidence that disequilibrium develops during hemodialysis derives mainly from the rebound in solute concentration following dialysis (121,133). Even urea, which is a highly diffusible solute, has an easily detected rebound, indicating that the simple, single-compartment model has shortcomings. **FIGURE 5.8** shows a series of BUN measurements in a patient undergoing high-flux hemodialysis. The dashed line, representing the best fit of a single-compartment model, misses the data points by a significant margin, especially early into and immediately following the treatment. Two kinds of solute disequilibrium have been described: diffusion-dependent disequilibrium and flow-dependent disequilibrium; both reduce the effectiveness of hemodialysis.

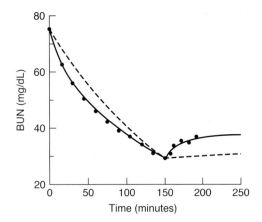

FIGURE 5.8 A two-compartment model (*solid line*) accurately predicts the measured blood urea nitrogen (BUN) values (*solid dots*) in a patient during and following high-intensity hemodialysis. A single-compartment variable-volume model (*dashed line*) overestimates the BUN during dialysis and fails to predict the rebound postdialysis. (From Depner TA. Refining the model of urea kinetics: compartment effects. *Semin Dial* 1992;5:147–154, with permission.)

Diffusion-Dependent Disequilibrium and the Two-Compartment Model

To improve the agreement of modeled predictions with the actual data, an additional compartment can be added as shown in **FIGURE 5.9** (121,134). Cell membrane resistance to diffusion is the physiologic correlate to this mathematical model of hemodialysis urea kinetics, which is patterned after the extracellular/intracellular separation of body water compartments (134). The dialyzed compartment, V_1, is separated from a remote compartment, V_2, by a resistance to diffusion, represented as K_C, the intercompartment mass transfer area coefficient. K_C is a solute-specific permeability

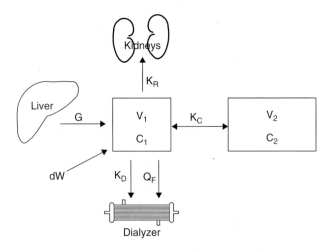

FIGURE 5.9 The two-compartment variable volume model of mass balance shows solute distributed in two compartments, V_1 and V_2. Solute moves by diffusion between compartments, driven by dialyzer removal. The rate of intercompartment diffusion is expressed as K_C, a mass transfer area coefficient. K_R is residual native kidney clearance of urea; K_D is dialyzer clearance; Q_F is ultrafiltration during dialysis; and dW is fluid gain between dialyses. (Adapted from Depner TA. *Prescribing Hemodialysis: A Guide to Urea Modeling*. Boston, MA: Kluwer Academic, 1991, with permission.)

factor that correlates positively with SA (e.g., cell membrane area) and inversely with resistance to diffusion between compartments. Addition of the second compartment requires modification of **EQUATION 5.9**:

$$d(V_1C_1) / dt = G - C_1(K_D + K_R) - K_C(C_1 - C_2) \quad (5.14)$$

$$d(V_2C_2) / dt = K_C(C_1 - C_2) \quad (5.15)$$

where V_1 is the proximal (dialyzed) compartment volume, V_2 is the remote compartment volume, C_1 is the urea nitrogen concentration in V_1, and C_2 is the urea nitrogen concentration in V_2. Several assumptions are usually made to reduce the complexity of this model. Because urea is generated by the liver and then diffuses into the blood, G is applied only to the dialyzed compartment. Salt and water intake in the interval between treatments causes V_1 to expand and then to shrink during dialysis, but the size of V_2 is assumed to be constant at all times, like the intracellular space.

In contrast to **EQUATION 5.9**, **EQUATIONS 5.14** and **5.15** are not easily solved when V_1 is allowed to vary during and between dialyses. Several solutions have been reported, most of which involve numerical approximations that require a high-speed computer to resolve the four unknown variables, V_1, V_2, G, and K_C (135–139). When this model is applied to clinical data, a better fit between measured and predicted values is observed, as shown in **FIGURE 5.8**. For urea, the ratio V_2:V_1 is usually close to 2 when fitted by this two-compartment modeling technique, which adds support to the intracellular/extracellular basis of the model, with the primary resistance to diffusion at the cell membrane.

Flow-Dependent Disequilibrium

In 1990, another type of disequilibrium was found within the blood compartment during high-flux treatments that could not be explained by the classic model (140). Urea concentration differences averaging 10 mg/dL and as high as 20 mg/dL were found in blood drawn simultaneously from both arms in a series of patients undergoing hemodialysis. The concentration gradient slowly dissipated over a 20- to 30-minute period after dialysis was stopped (140).

To explain the observed dialysis-induced intravascular concentration gradients, another model of hemodialysis urea kinetics was proposed, as shown in **FIGURE 5.10** (117). When the transit of blood through a particular circuit is delayed (e.g., by cutaneous vasoconstriction in a cold environment or during episodes of hypotension), urea removal from the affected organ is delayed. This causes urea concentrations to fall more rapidly in the central well-perfused compartment (reducing dialyzer efficiency), while higher urea concentrations persist in more peripheral, less well-perfused compartments. Viewed from the most peripheral compartment, flow through the remainder of the body consists of a series of parallel circuits as shown in **FIGURE 5.10**, each of which could be considered a path for recirculation of dialyzed blood. Later studies of the early response to dialysis, the response to exercise and ultrafiltration during dialysis, and measurements of cardiopulmonary recirculation using thermal and ultrasound dilution techniques confirmed the existence of blood flow–related solute disequilibrium (141–145). This convective type of resistance to dialysis has been quantified and is much better understood today. Diffusion-dependent disequilibrium is highly dependent on the nature of the solute as well as the membrane, but in contrast, flow-related disequilibrium, as described by the model, should not be affected by the molecular size of the solute.

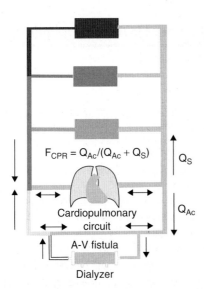

FIGURE 5.10 Flow-related disequilibrium. Solute disequilibrium within the blood compartment is explained by this model of multiple parallel circuits, each with a different blood flow/tissue volume. Blood leaving the heart is distributed to all tissue compartments at the same solute concentration, whereas solute concentrations in the blood leaving each compartment are different. The fraction of dialyzer venous blood that reenters the dialyzer by passing through the heart and lungs (F_{CPR}) is called *cardiopulmonary recirculation*. Q_{Ac}, access blood flow; Q_S, systemic blood flow.

Cardiopulmonary Recirculation

A specific subtype of flow-dependent disequilibrium, probably accounting quantitatively for more than half of hemodialysis-induced convective disequilibrium, has been called *cardiopulmonary recirculation* (143). Cardiopulmonary recirculation represents the fraction of blood returning from the dialyzer that is rapidly returned to the dialyzer through the heart and lungs. It is found only during dialysis conducted through peripheral arteriovenous (AV) shunts (**FIGURE 5.10**) and, accordingly, is absent during dialysis through central venous catheters in patients lacking a peripheral AV access. The recirculation fraction is simply the ratio of access flow to cardiac output (**EQUATION 5.16**):

$$F_{CPR} = \frac{Q_{AC}}{Q_{AC} + Q_S} \tag{5.16}$$

where F_{CPR} is the recirculation fraction (fraction of blood entering the dialyzer that has recirculated through the heart and lungs), Q_{Ac} is access blood flow, and Q_S is systemic blood flow (cardiac output minus Q_{Ac}). Part of the deviation from single-pool kinetics shown in **FIGURE 5.8** can be attributed to cardiopulmonary recirculation, which reduces urea concentrations entering the dialyzer to levels below that returning from the systemic circuit (**EQUATION 5.17**) (143):

$$\frac{C_i}{C_s} = \frac{Q_s}{Q_s + K_d} \tag{5.17}$$

where C_i is the urea concentration in blood entering the dialyzer and C_S is the urea concentration in blood returning from the systemic circuit. The reduced concentration C_i can be substituted for C_0 in **EQUATION 5.10** or for C_1 in **EQUATION 5.14**. Because the magnitude of this effect is predictable, based on estimates

of cardiac output and dialyzer clearance, even simpler single-compartment models can incorporate a correction for cardiopulmonary recirculation.

How to Implement Multiple-Compartment Modeling

More than two BUN measurements are required for formal two-compartment modeling. The best time points for obtaining these are midway during dialysis and midway during and at the end of the rebound phase. Numerical solutions to **EQUATIONS 5.14** and **5.15** are used in place of **EQUATION 5.10**. Urea concentrations in each compartment are computed at small time intervals, and then adjustments are made in V_1, V_2, G, and K_C, similar to the single-pool technique, until the computed profile fits the measured data points. C_1 in **EQUATION 5.14** can be adjusted for cardiopulmonary recirculation using **EQUATION 5.17** as shown earlier. A high-speed computer is required for this type of modeling.

Schneditz presented an analogous model (with an analytical solution) from flow considerations alone, a pure convectional model based on differences in regional organ perfusion during hemodialysis (146). Although the pattern of fall in BUN is slightly different, the rebound is indistinguishable from predictions of the classic diffusional model. The effect of flow disequilibrium on the concentration pattern and removal of other solutes has not been measured so it is not yet possible to determine the relative roles of these two radically different models.

Comparison with the Single-Compartment Model

Although the single-compartment variable-volume model fails to estimate intradialysis and postdialysis urea concentrations (**FIGURE 5.8**), it predicts V and, therefore, Kt/V with reasonable accuracy (121,136). The reason for this unexpected performance is the offsetting direction of errors in the numerator and the denominator of the equation for V. If G and ultrafiltration are ignored, V can be calculated during dialysis as the amount of urea removed divided by the change in urea concentration (**EQUATION 5.18**):

$$V = \frac{K_D \int_{t=0}^{t=T} C\,dt}{C_0 - C_E} \tag{5.18}$$

where C_0 is the predialysis BUN and C_E is the equilibrated postdialysis BUN.

The amount of urea removed during a single dialysis is the product of K_D and the area under the time versus BUN curve (numerator of **EQUATION 5.18**). **FIGURE 5.11** shows the error in that calculation as the shaded area between the two-compartment prediction and the single-compartment prediction of urea nitrogen concentrations. The error in the denominator is the difference between the immediate postdialysis BUN (C_T) and the equilibrated BUN (C_E). For the usual 3- to 4-hour dialysis with Kt/V = 1.2 to 1.3, the errors are of similar magnitude and offset each other (136,147). The result is a fairly accurate prediction of V by the single-compartment model, depending to some extent on the rate of ultrafiltration during dialysis. However, urea generation (G) and net protein catabolism (nPCR) are slightly but consistently overestimated by the single-compartment model because there is no compensating error.

Multiple-compartment modeling is not required for routine clinical application but should be used when an accurate profile of

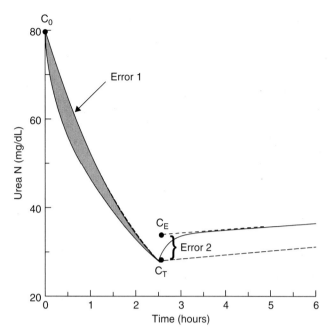

FIGURE 5.11 Balanced errors. The upper boundary of the shaded area shows the single-compartment prediction of blood urea nitrogen (BUN) during hemodialysis. The lower boundary is the two-compartment model line (compare with **FIGURE 5.8**). C_E is the equilibrated BUN extrapolated to the postdialysis time. The single-compartment model overestimates the BUN during dialysis and consequently overestimates the amount of urea removed shown as the shaded area (error 1) and in the numerator of **EQUATION 5.18**. It also underestimates the equilibrated BUN (C_T) causing a false over-estimate of the change in concentration (error 2) in the denominator of **EQUATION 5.18**.

TABLE 5.4	**Urea Clearances Defined**

Residual clearance

Clearance by the patient's native kidneys, often negligible or absent

    Contributes little to total clearance during dialysis

    Major effect on urea kinetics occurs between dialyses

Dialyzer clearance

Instantaneous: measured across the dialyzer from simultaneous inlet and outlet BUN

Modeled: integrated from predialysis and immediate postdialysis blood samples

    Average dialyzer clearance for an entire dialysis

    Not affected by urea disequilibrium

Patient clearance

Also called *whole body clearance*

    Derived from the predialysis and equilibrated postdialysis BUN

    Always lower than *dialyzer clearance*: difference due to urea disequilibrium

    Includes the contribution from *residual clearance*

Continuous equivalent of intermittent clearance

Derived from G/TAC^a or G/avC$_0$

    Always lower than *dialyzer clearance* or *patient clearance*

    Allows comparison of different schedules including continuous treatment

BUN, blood urea nitrogen.
^{a}G/TAC is the (urea generation rate) / (time-average concentration).

BUN during and immediately after dialysis is required, when an accurate measure of G is required, and when modeling the kinetics of solutes other than urea.

eKt/V and the Effect of Treatment Time

Both single-compartment and multiple-compartment models over-estimate the amount of dialysis *received* by the patient. The "K" in Kt/V is the effective *dialyzer* clearance of urea (**TABLE 5.4**). More important for the therapeutic effect is the *patient's* clearance, often termed the *whole body* clearance, defined in **TABLE 5.4**. For patients with significant urea disequilibrium, whole body clearance is significantly less than dialyzer clearance because some of the patient's urea is compartmentalized and only slowly released to the dialyzer. Whole body Kt/V, often called *eKt/V*, can be resolved by applying the single-compartment model to the *equilibrated* post-dialysis BUN instead of the *immediate* postdialysis BUN (136). Two-compartment models can be used to determine both the ef-fective dialyzer clearance and the patient's whole body clearance because these models predict both the immediate postdialysis BUN and the equilibrated postdialysis BUN.

Because urea modeling is used to tailor the dialysis dose to the individual patient's needs, concern has been raised about patients who may rebound more than others and may be underdialyzed because the single-compartment model fails to consider rebound. Studies both prior to and during the HEMO study (see subsequent text) found that rebound is highly predictable and that such outliers

may not actually exist (148,149). Based on BUN measurements up to 60 minutes postdialysis in several patient cohorts, eKt/V was estimated best by a simple equation, called the *rate equation*, that predicts rebound from the intensity or rate of solute removal during dialysis (**EQUATIONS 5.19** and **5.20**) (149,150):

$$eKt/V = spKt/V - 0.6K/V + 0.03 \quad (5.19)$$

$$eKt/V = spKt/V(1 - 0.6/t_d) + 0.03 \quad (5.20)$$

where K/V is the fractional clearance per hour and t_d is measured in hours. **EQUATION 5.20**, which is equivalent to **EQUATION 5.19**, shows that eKt/V relates to spKt/V as a function of treatment time (t_d) or intensity of dialysis (K/V). Although empirically de-rived, these equations can be predicted from current knowledge about the genesis of rebound from solute gradients in the patient. An alternative, perhaps more accurate rate equation based on retro-spective analysis of the HEMO study data from equilibrated blood samples may also be used to estimate eKt/V (**EQUATION 5.21**) (151):

$$eKt/V = spKt/V - 0.40 (K/V) \quad (5.21)$$

The magnitude of these gradients is increased by more in-tense dialysis where intensity is measured as the fractional rate of solute removal (K/V in **EQUATION 5.19** and **5.21**). Assuming that the same dose is given, the intensity of dialysis must increase when treatment time is shortened. Subsequent equations based on treatment time have been developed, all of which predict the effect shown in **FIGURE 5.12** as a reduction in eKt/V with short treatment times despite a constant spKt/V (152,153). The clinical lesson here is that as eKt/V is a better measure of patient clearance than spKt/V, shortening the treatment time also short-changes the patient.

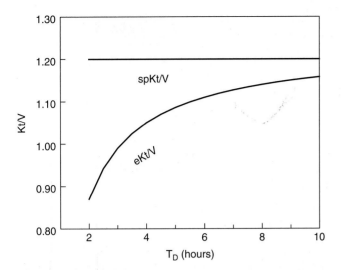

FIGURE 5.12 If spKt/V is set constant (*upper line*), eKt/V falls as treatment time (t_D) is reduced (**EQUATION 5.20**). This shows that dialysis becomes less efficient as t_D is shortened.

Conversely, increasing the treatment time improves the efficiency of solute removal, as shown in **FIGURE 5.12**, and may have other benefits that are not apparent when applying current models of solute kinetics. Serum concentrations of solutes like phosphate and potassium that deviate significantly from simple first-order kinetics can be predicted by applying more complex mathematical models (154,155). Both predicted and measured removal rates of inorganic phosphate are markedly affected by both treatment time and frequency (155–158). Phosphate is considered an indirect uremic toxin, and observational outcome studies have suggested a benefit from markedly prolonging t_d at a fixed dialysis frequency. In a comparison study to short daily hemodialysis, long nocturnal hemodialysis removed almost twice as much phosphorus per week, and many patients were able to discontinue their phosphate binders (159).

◆ DIALYSATE METHODS

Measuring patient clearance and eKt/V from dialysate collections is analogous to measuring native kidney clearance by collecting urine, except that the blood concentration changes rapidly during the measurement (160–163). Blood sampling can be avoided if equilibrated dialysate samples are taken predialysis, and the previously described models of solute clearance can be used to integrate and predict the intradialysis solute concentrations needed for the clearance measurement. Other advantages of the dialysate method include elimination of the needs for measuring several parameters including ultrafiltration, solute disequilibrium, and blood and plasma water content. Dialysate pumps are less prone to error than blood pumps and can be calibrated volumetrically during treatments. Dialysate is also readily available in large quantities for measurement. The disadvantages of dialysate methods include the cumbersome task of collecting large quantities of dialysate, the requirement for precise analytical methods due to low solute concentrations, and an inherent susceptibility to error when calculating urea clearance due to a requisite subtraction of two large numbers to obtain the desired measurement (164). Bacterial contamination of dialysate can also lead to urea degradation and erroneous dialysate urea concentrations (165). Many of these disadvantages

can be circumvented by multiple sampling techniques (160,162), but the method then becomes more cumbersome. As an alternative, applying the rate equation to blood side measurements, as described earlier, gives more precise and reproducible values for eKt/V (164).

To calculate urea eKt/V using the dialysate method, four critical measurements are required: C_0, V, C_D, and Q_D. The predialysis BUN (C_0) can be determined by sampling dialysate after equilibrating the dialysate compartment with the blood compartment by recirculating the dialysate. This has the advantage of giving the true blood water concentration automatically adjusted for the Gibbs-Donnan effect. The patient's urea volume (V) requires measurement of the equilibrated postdialysis BUN (C_E), but it requires only one accurate measurement. Once determined, V will not deviate significantly from month to month unless the patient's weight and/or nutritional status changes (**EQUATION 5.22**):

$$V = \frac{Q_D C_D t - \Delta V C_0 - RG}{C_0 - C_E} \tag{5.22}$$

where Q_D is total dialysate flow including Q_F, C_D is the dialysate urea nitrogen concentration, ΔV is the fluid lost during dialysis, and RG is a correction for K_R and urea generation. RG is the amount of urea generated during the dialysis minus the amount removed by the patient's native kidneys (**EQUATION 5.23**):

$$RG = t(G - K_R C_{Av}) \tag{5.23}$$

RG usually contributes very little in conventional three times weekly dialysis and in most patients can be ignored. If included, C_{Av} can be approximated as the log mean $C = (C_0 - C_E) / \ln(C_0 / C_E)$. Total body urea content at the start of dialysis is $C_0(V + \Delta V)$. The amount of urea removed is $Q_D C_D t$.

When solute removal is measured directly, the total effect of a single dialysis can be expressed as the solute removal index (SRI) (166,167). SRI is the fractional solute removal, the amount removed divided by the initial total body content (**EQUATION 5.24**):

$$SRI = \frac{Q_D C_D t}{C_0(V + \Delta V)} \tag{5.24}$$

Although SRI is a fraction of the initial solute content, the fraction may be greater than 1 because of ongoing solute generation during dialysis. For urea, a direct mathematical relationship between Kt/V and SRI may be demonstrated from **EQUATION 5.7** (**EQUATIONS 5.25 and 5.26**):

$$eKt/V = -\ln(1 - SRI) \tag{5.25}$$

$$SRI = (1 - e^{-eKt/V}) \tag{5.26}$$

EQUATION 5.7 can be used here instead of the more complex equations that include G, Q_F, and two compartment adjustments, because the amount of urea removed ($Q_D C_D t$) is measured directly; it includes the contribution of ultrafiltration and requires no correction for G or solute disequilibrium. SRI is easier to conceptualize and has been considered by some to be a better index of small solute removal and a better overall measure of dialysis than Kt/V. Unfortunately, there are no standards of adequacy for SRI. Until such standards are available, SRI can be converted to eKt/V using **EQUATION 5.25** with the understanding that "eK" represents whole body clearance as discussed earlier. Because whole body clearance is always lower than dialyzer clearance, eKt/V determined from **EQUATION 5.25** is lower than Kt/V estimated from one- or two-compartment modeling (168).

Dialysate Conductivity Methods

Measurements of dialysance using simple conductivity probes placed in the dialysate inlet and outlet lines are increasingly used to monitor the delivered dialysis dose (169–171). This inexpensive and noninvasive technique, termed the *ionic dialysance* method, can be automated to provide real-time measurements during each dialysis. Dialysate electrolytes (mostly sodium and its anions) are small molecules with clearances across dialyzer membranes roughly equivalent to that of urea. Therefore, changes in dialysate electrical conductivity can be used to reflect urea diffusion across the membrane. To create a significant electrolyte gradient between blood and dialysate, the dialysate concentration is abruptly increased for a few minutes by altering dialysate/water proportioning. The resulting change in conductivity from dialysate inlet to outlet reflects movement of electrolytes, mostly sodium, into the patient (**EQUATION 5.27**) (172):

$$D = (Q_D + Q_F)\left[1 - \frac{(Co_1 - Co_2)}{(Ci_1 - Ci_2)}\right] \qquad (5.27)$$

where Co and Ci are dialysate outlet and inlet conductivities (mS/cm), D is dialysance (mL/min), Q_D is dialysate flow, Q_F is ultrafiltration flow, and subscripts 1 and 2 indicate measurements before and after the step-up in conductivity. Several short measurements of conductivity (ionic) dialysance can be averaged over the course of a treatment to improve the measurement precision. If V is estimated and updated periodically, the actual delivered spKt/V can be calculated in real time for each treatment. Ionic dialysance closely correlates with standard blood and dialysate-side measurements of urea clearance but is approximately 5% lower (169,173). **FIGURE 5.13** shows the correlation and slight difference between ionic dialysance and urea clearance by single pool modeling (174). Addition of a step-down in conductivity (decrease in dialysate sodium from baseline) can eliminate this difference (175). Corrections for cardiopulmonary recirculation have also been suggested (175). The conductivity method has several advantages including on-line and more frequent determinations of delivered dose, decreased cost, and elimination of invasive blood sampling. Limitations to use of dialysate conductivity as a substitute for Kt/V derived from urea modeling include the need for an independent measure of V, no accounting for urea generation during the dialysis treatment, and convective clearance from ultrafiltration is not included. The problem with V is difficult to rectify, as the various anthropometric methods for calculating V all appear to substantially overestimate V as compared with V derived from urea modeling, and the difference is unpredictable (82). SA may be a better denominator for clearances measured using conductivity methods.

⬣ THE DIALYSIS SCHEDULE: MORE FREQUENT IS MORE EFFICIENT

The patient's own tissues present a barrier to intermittent dialysis that is greater than had been anticipated in the past. Even for urea, one of the most diffusible solutes, resistance to removal can be easily demonstrated as multiple concentration gradients that develop within the patient during both standard and high-efficiency dialysis. Increasing the frequency tends to diminish this effect and allows more efficient removal of solute. This phenomenon is illustrated in **FIGURE 5.14** as a reduced requirement for weekly Kt/V to maintain the same TAC. Increasing the frequency improves the efficiency of dialysis by reducing the amplitude of oscillations in solute concentration and by diminishing patient-dependent disequilibrium (176–178). Advances in dialysis technology have improved the dialyzer and dialyzer membranes but not the resistance to diffusion in patients.

Frequent dialysis schedules include short daily treatments with standard blood and dialysate flow rates and long nocturnal treatments using lower flow regimens. Both techniques are reported to improve extracellular volume control, blood pressure, and left ventricular mass (13,14,179). Nocturnal hemodialysis, when performed six to seven nights per week, may better reduce the concentrations of protein-bound, sequestered, and larger MW solutes, including phosphorus and β_2-microglobulin (159,177,180). The NIH-sponsored Frequent Hemodialysis Network trial showed better outcomes with more frequent hemodialysis treatments but

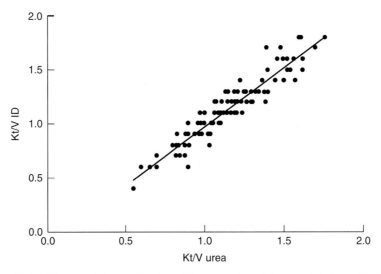

FIGURE 5.13 Modeled Kt versus Kt from on-line ionic dialysance measured during a single hemodialysis treatment in 37 in-center patients. The correlation is good ($R^2 = 0.76$) but the ionic dialysance method consistently underestimated the modeled value. [From McIntyre CW, Lambie SH, Taal MW, et al. Assessment of haemodialysis adequacy by ionic dialysance: intra-patient variability of delivered treatment. *Nephol Dial Transplant*, 2003;18(3):559–562.]

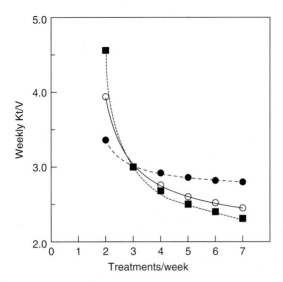

FIGURE 5.14 Kt/V required to achieve the same time-averaged concentration (TAC). As the frequency of hemodialysis treatments increases, the efficiency of each treatment increases. The vertical axis shows the total weekly dose (Kt/V) required to maintain the average blood urea nitrogen (TAC) constant. ● = prediction of the single-compartment model. ○ = two-compartment model predictions for urea (K_C = 500 mL/min). ■ = a theoretical molecule with K_C = 200 mL/min. (Adapted from Depner TA. Quantifying hemodialysis and peritoneal dialysis: examination of the peak concentration hypothesis. *Semin Dial* 1994;7:315–317, with permission.)

not to the extent shown in previous observational studies where confounding by selection bias was difficult to eliminate (13,14).

Application of urea modeling to quantify the dose becomes problematic because dialyzer spKt/V does not reflect patient clearance and a summation of daily Kt/V values to give a weekly Kt/V does not account for the improved efficiency of daily dialysis. Several methods have been proposed to measure the dose when dialysis is performed at different frequencies and intensities.

A Continuous Equivalent Dose

Adhering to the concept of small solute clearance as the best current measure of dialysis dose and adequacy, a continuous equivalent clearance for patients dialyzed intermittently can be defined as the weekly removal rate divided by the average solute concentration (TAC). For patients in a weekly steady state of nitrogen balance, the urea removal rate should equal the urea generation rate (G). Both G and TAC are readily measured from standard kinetic modeling, so an equivalent kidney clearance (EKR) is easily calculated (**EQUATION 5.28**) (99,181):

$$EKR = G / TAC \qquad (5.28)$$

Mathematically, it can be shown that the EKR for the KDOQI guideline specifying a minimum dialysis Kt/V of 1.2 per dialysis thrice weekly is approximately 3.0 volumes per week. This value does not compare favorably with the accepted continuous peritoneal dialysis guideline of 1.7 volumes per week (182). Two explanations have been given for this discrepancy, each of which forms the basis for another continuous equivalent index of intermittent hemodialysis, called "standard Kt/V" and "normalized Kt/V."

Standard Kt/V

Standard Kt/V (stdKt/V) invokes peak serum urea concentrations as the target of therapy with the presumption that peak levels

determine toxicity more so than trough or average levels (183). This method also requires calculation of G and utilizes the mean predialysis BUN, as opposed to TAC, as the denominator in the expression of steady-state clearance (**EQUATION 5.28**). Substituting the average peak urea concentration as the denominator of the clearance expression yields the "standard clearance" from which standard Kt/V is derived (**EQUATION 5.29**) (183):

$$Standard\ K = G / avC_0 \qquad (5.29)$$

Because spKt/V and its derivative, eKt/V, can be approximated with simplified formulas (**EQUATIONS 5.19**, to **5.21** and section "Explicit Equations" later in the chapter), another simplified formula has been developed, based on a fixed volume model and a symmetric week, to calculate stdKt/V from spKt/V and eKt/V (**EQUATION 5.30**) (152,183):

$$_{std}Kt/V = \frac{10,080 \dfrac{1 - e^{-eKt/V}}{t}}{\dfrac{1 - e^{-eKt/V}}{_{sp}Kt/V} + \dfrac{10,080}{Nt} - 1} \qquad (5.30)$$

where N is the number of treatment and 10,080 is the number of minutes in a week. This formula has been extended to include the effects of fluid accumulation/removal and residual native kidney clearance (184).

Estimating spKt/V at Higher Dialysis Frequencies

EQUATION 5.30 is based on eKt/V which is derived from spKt/V. If the simplified Daugirdas formula is used to calculate spKt/V from pre- and post-BUN values in patients dialyzed more frequently, significant errors occur especially at higher frequencies. A recent modification of the Daugirdas formula corrects this error (185).

Normalized Kt/V

The rationale for a *normalized Kt/V* is based on evidence that although urea is a good indicator solute for dialyzer clearance, it is not a good indicator for whole body patient clearance (88,89,186,187). Other toxins diffuse less readily among body compartments, creating a steeper dependency of effective clearance on dialysis frequency (176,186,188). Substituting another solute with dialyzer clearance similar to urea but lower K_C than urea yields a *normalized clearance* from which *normalized Kt/V* (nKt/V) is derived (**EQUATION 5.31**) (176,189,190):

$$Normalized\ K = G / TAC_X \qquad (5.31)$$

where TAC_X is the time-averaged concentration of another compound with lower K_C than urea.

Calculation of normalized Kt/V is based on the observation that disequilibrium for many small dialyzable solutes is greater than urea disequilibrium. The bottom tracing of **FIGURE 5.14** shows that solutes with low K_C (**EQUATION 5.14**) have a steeper decline in the clearance required to maintain a constant TAC when dialysis frequency varies over a range from one to seven treatments per week (176). Solutes exhibiting higher concentration gradients among body compartments are affected more by changes in frequency than urea. When a lower K_C value is entered into the two-compartment model, greater benefit is seen when frequency increases from three per week to six per week (190). The blood concentrations of solutes with low K_C values fall more than urea as frequency increases. This approach requires a formal two-compartment, variable-volume mathematical model that is not practical for current use in the dialysis clinic, but it demonstrates a fundamental principle that may be useful if the technique can be simplified.

Both standard and normalized clearance are lower than EKR, and when applied to the minimum KDOQI guideline of 1.2 per dialysis thrice weekly, both agree well with the recognized minimum value for weekly urea clearance in continuous ambulatory peritoneal dialysis (CAPD) patients (191). Calculated values for stdKt/V and nKt/V are similar, and both require calculation of G, usually from formal urea modeling. For intermittently dialyzed patients, these continuous equivalent clearances are always lower than the measured dialyzer clearance (spKt/V) and lower than the modeled patient clearance (eKt/V). The difference reflects the inefficiency of intermittent compared to continuous dialysis. **FIGURE 5.14** shows that infrequent dialysis requires a higher weekly clearance to achieve the same TAC as daily therapy.

Standards for continuous equivalent clearances do not change with dialysis frequency, so measures of intermittent hemodialysis can be directly compared to measures of CAPD and to functioning native kidneys. For patients maintained with hemodialysis who have residual native kidney function, the urea clearances may simply be added to stdKt/V, as both are considered continuous clearances. This universal applicability to patients before starting dialysis and after starting any mode of dialysis or transplantation is an attractive feature.

Limitations of Blood-Side Modeling as Frequency Increases

It is important to consider that blood-based methods of dose quantification lose some of their power when applied to more frequent prolonged treatments because the difference between the predialysis and postdialysis urea concentration is reduced leading to greater errors in the calculation of their ratio. As the frequency increases approaching continuous dialysis, blood-side modeling is no longer possible. Measuring the dose of more frequent hemodialysis may require measurement of cross-dialyzer clearances or dialysate methods, similar to measurements of continuous peritoneal dialysis.

⬡ SIMPLIFIED APPROACHES TO QUANTIFYING DIALYSIS

Because the relationships among time, solute removal, and clearance are logarithmic and influenced by multiple variables, the mathematical expressions of urea kinetics are often complex. Inclusion of all the pertinent variables using formal modeling requires computer software. To circumvent these complexities and to provide tools for quick "bedside" estimates, simplified approaches to urea modeling have been proposed (111,150,152,184,192–197).

Explicit Equations

Explicit solvable equations eliminate the need for stepwise iterative approximations of Kt/V and nPCR by ignoring the lesser variables. **EQUATION 5.7** is a simplified formula that ignores ultrafiltration, urea generation, and disequilibrium during dialysis. A more accurate formula, derived empirically by Daugirdas (198), is shown here in **EQUATION 5.32**:

$$Kt/V = -\ln(R - 0.03) + (4 - 3.5R)U_F / W \quad (5.32)$$

where R is the ratio of postdialysis/predialysis BUN, U_F is the total ultrafiltrate volume in liters per dialysis, and W is the patient's weight in kilograms. **EQUATION 5.32** approximates the contributions of urea generation and ultrafiltration during dialysis in the first and second terms, respectively. It requires use of

a scientific calculator or log table, but no iterative programming is required.

The protein catabolic rate is more difficult to resolve with explicit formulas because the dialysis schedule, residual clearance, and fluid gain play significant roles (195,199). **EQUATION 5.8** is an example of an explicit equation that ignores fluid gain and residual clearance, but it requires a third BUN measurement. To include the latter variables, and reduce the requirement to two BUN measurements, equations have been derived for hemodialysis given three times and two times weekly, with and without residual clearance (200).

The Urea Reduction Ratio

The urea reduction ratio (URR) is the fractional fall in BUN during a single dialysis (111,193,197) and is mathematically related to Kt/V. The denominator is the predialysis BUN, and the numerator is the difference between the predialysis and postdialysis BUN values. Unfortunately, URR does not account for the effects of ultrafiltration or urea generation during dialysis, both of which allow significant amounts of urea removal with little change in urea concentration (**FIGURE 5.15**). As an example, a dialysis treatment where 4 L of ultrafiltration is removed from a patient with a predialysis weight of 100 kg, the volume removal may augment Kt/V by almost 0.1, whereas URR may be unchanged compared to a treatment where no ultrafiltration was performed. Because urea generation matches urea removal in patients with continuous kidney function or in patient undergoing continuous dialysis (e.g., CAPD), URR is zero and cannot be used to measure depurative function. However, because it is simple to calculate, URR is widely used to quantify intermittent therapies like hemodialysis and assess its adequacy. If standards are set conservatively (high) in centers where URR is the only measure of dialysis, patients should be protected from underdialysis and are better managed than patients in whom no yardstick of dialysis is regularly applied. However, most the time and effort required to obtain and analyze blood samples for formal modeling is also

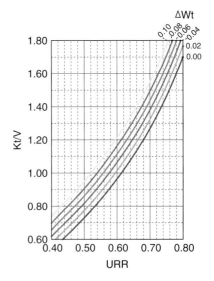

FIGURE 5.15 The logarithmic relationship between the urea reduction ratio (URR) and Kt/V derived from formal urea modeling. This relationship is significantly affected by fluid removal during dialysis. ΔWt is the change in weight during dialysis expressed as a fraction of the postdialysis weight. (From Depner TA. Estimation of Kt/V from URR for varying levels of weight loss: a bedside graphic aid. *Semin Dial* 1993;6:242, with permission.)

required for measurement of URR, so measuring Kt/V should take little additional resources.

A Simplified Method for Incorporating K_R

The first approach described in the previous section, "How to Add K_R to Kt/V," requires multiple additional iterations of the urea kinetic model to achieve an equivalent TAC or avC_0, with and without K_R in the model. Because this method has the effect of inflating K_R before adding it to K_D, a simplified equation can be generated to approximate this inflation. The magnitude of the inflation is expressed in the coefficient (κ) (EQUATION 5.33):

$$\text{Total Kt/V} = K_D t/V + \kappa K_R/V \qquad (5.33)$$

The coefficient (κ) also represents the time during which K_R is active, including the long interval between treatments. Values for κ can be approximated by applying a formal model of urea kinetics and using average values for G, V_D, and Q_F as the coefficient is insensitive to these parameters. The values for κ shown in TABLE 5.5 were generated from the single pool model for two to seven dialysis treatments per week (99,102).

A Comparison of Simplified Methods to Formal Modeling

The simplified formulas and graphics mentioned earlier are helpful instructional tools and allow quick estimates when a computer is not immediately available. For routine application in a clinic, however, little is gained by shortcutting formal urea modeling. The most time-consuming and expensive aspects of urea modeling are collecting the blood samples, blood analysis, and entry of data into the computer. Computers allow just about any dialysis clinic to obtain formal kinetic modeling data. In the present era of electronic medical records, the comparison of values to previous analyses, transmission of results to nephrologists, and quality control functions of the dialysis medical director takes but an instant. The terms *quick* and *bedside*, sometimes applied to simplified formulas, are misleading because the time lag between sampling the blood and return of data from the laboratory is ignored. A major goal of urea modeling is to individualize therapy; ignoring critical variables such as a volume change during dialysis, or assuming a mean value for all patients, defeats this purpose.

TABLE 5.5	Values for κ Depend on the Frequency of Dialysis and the Targeted Blood Urea Nitrogen		
		BUN Target	
Frequency	t_i Unadjusted	Time-Averaged[a]	Average Predialysis[a]
2	5040	6500	9500
3	3360	4000	5500
4	2520	2850	3700
5	2016	2200	2700
6	1680	1780	2100
7	1440	1500	1700

[a]The underlined numbers have been published. The remaining numbers were derived from urea kinetic modeling.
Depner TA. *Prescribing Hemodialysis: A Guide to Urea Modeling.* Boston, MA: Kluwer Academic Publishers, 1991; Gotch FA. Kinetic modeling in hemodialysis. In: Nissenson AR, Fine RN, Gentile DE, eds. *Clinical Dialysis.* Norwalk, CT: Appleton and Lange, 1995:156–188.

PRACTICE GUIDELINES AND STANDARDS

The Hemodialysis Study

The NCDS was the first randomized trial of dialysis dose, but as time passed and both the patients and the practice of dialysis changed, another NIH-sponsored clinical trial, the HEMO study, was instituted to evaluate potential benefits from further increases in the dialysis dose as depicted in FIGURE 5.16 (201). The method chosen to quantify and control the dose of hemodialysis in this study was formal urea modeling. The equilibrated Kt/V (eKt/V) that accounts for urea disequilibrium and is considered a more accurate reflection of true patient clearance was used to quantify the dialysis dose. The simple rate equation described in the preceding text was used to convert measured spKt/V to eKt/V, eliminating the need for a second postdialysis blood sample. The rate equation was validated before the HEMO study, and in the HEMO pilot study, eKt/V from the rate equation correlated well with eKt/V determined from dialysate collections (148). Patients were randomized to receive either a "standard" dose of dialysis (target eKt/V of 1.05 per treatment) or a "high" dose (target eKt/V of 1.45 per treatment). The two randomized prescriptions were tightly controlled by study investigators so that midway through the study, less than 4% of patients who received the "standard" dose of dialysis fell below the current minimum recommended spKt/V of 1.20.

No significant difference in morbidity or mortality between treatment groups was found at the conclusion of the study. Women who received the higher dialysis dose had a slightly lower risk of death and hospitalization of borderline significance compared to controls, whereas men showed no response to the higher dose. The HEMO study provides strong evidence that the minimum thrice-weekly hemodialysis dose recommended by KDOQI and other standard-setting organizations is also the optimal dose (19,202). Although the study showed no benefit from the higher dose when administered thrice weekly, the results are not inconsistent with reports from uncontrolled studies of improved outcomes after increases in dialysis frequency. Although the delivered high Kt/V averaged 36% higher than the control dose in this study, the separation, when expressed as standard or normalized Kt/V, was only about 17%. On the practical side, it appears that providers have reached a limit to delivering dialysis thrice weekly. Large increases in the weekly effective Kt/V are theoretically possible, as discussed in the preceding text, by increasing the frequency, by applying continuous dialysis, or by markedly prolonging the treatment time. In the Frequent Hemodialysis Network trial, the mean number of treatments per week of the frequent hemodialysis cohort was about 5.2 and the dialysis achieved stdKt/V was 3.54, compared with the conventional group's stdKt/V of 2.49 (203). Increases in dialyzer clearance or short increases in treatment time have less impact when the treatment is given infrequently.

Comparison of the Current Minimum Dialysis Dose with Native Kidney Clearance

The minimum single pool Kt/V of 1.2 volumes per dialysis thrice weekly, established by the latest KDOQI consensus (73), means that more than 100% of total body water is cleared during each treatment. However, this cannot be interpreted to mean that all solute is removed because the blood compartment continuously circulates through the patient and the dialyzer. A better reflection of urea removal is found in the URR, but as shown in FIGURE 5.15, URR is confounded by fluid gain between and loss during dialysis,

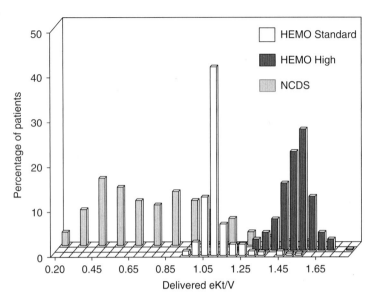

FIGURE 5.16 Distribution of patients in two major clinical trials of dialysis dose, expressed as a function of eKt/V shown on the x-axis. The highest delivered doses in the National Cooperative Dialysis Study (NCDS) were slightly below the lowest doses delivered to patients in the Hemodialysis (HEMO) study.

and it loses its meaning for frequent and continuous dialysis. Standard Kt/V, which is a continuous equivalent urea clearance based on comparisons of outcomes in peritoneal dialysis patients versus hemodialyzed patients, is probably a better reflection of the effectiveness of hemodialysis. The tentative minimum dose, expressed as standard Kt/V, is 2.0 volumes per week, which can be converted to milliliters per minute in a patient with an average of 30 L of water (**EQUATION 5.34**):

$$\frac{2.0 \text{ volumes/wk} \times 30,000 \text{ mL/volume}}{10,080 \text{ min/wk}} = 6.0 \text{ mL/min} \qquad (5.34)$$

Current KDOQI guidelines recommend that dialysis be started, in those who have had a discussion about all options with a nephrologist, when signs or symptoms associated with uremia are noted (73). A particular threshold of glomerular filtration rate at which to start long-term dialysis is no longer advised. During the transition to hemodialysis, native kidney clearance continues to play a role, augmenting solute removal and thereby helping to protect the patient from uremic consequences. However, when the patient loses K_R entirely, the minimum replacement dose may fall below the recommended threshold. Also, when comparing dialyzer with native kidney clearance, other solutes should be considered, many of which are more toxic than urea, do not undergo tubular reabsorption, and have dialyzer clearances that may be significantly lower than that of urea (187). This would explain the high serum creatinine concentration in anephric but well-dialyzed patients, which is often higher than the creatinine concentration in the same patient when hemodialysis treatments were initiated. This paradox is difficult to explain, especially in view of the HEMO study finding of no benefit from increasing the dose further. Part of the explanation may reside in the nonlinear relationship between the intermittent dialysis dose and the effective continuous clearance as discussed earlier. Another possible explanation is that the marked reduction in toxin levels at the end of dialysis is sufficient to allow recovery from the uremic consequences of high predialysis concentrations, an effect that lasts until the next dialysis.

Protein-Bound Solutes

Solute binding to serum or tissue macromolecules increases the apparent volume of distribution of the unbound molecule, often to levels well in excess of total body weight. Only the free fraction is available for diffusion across either tissue membranes or dialyzer membranes. This seriously limits the effectiveness of hemodialysis, which for highly bound solutes may be totally ineffective as a removal instrument (204). Unfortunately, many protein-bound solutes have been identified in uremic serum, binding mostly to serum albumin. Albumin is a transport protein that should be considered part of the kidney excretory system because the native kidney has the capacity to effectively remove its bound solutes (205–210). Kinetic modeling of serum protein-bound solutes shows a significant effect of dialysate flow and membrane SA, and little additional effect of hemofiltration compared to hemodialysis (211). Additions of sorbent to both hemodialysate and peritoneal dialysate have shown promising augmentation of removal (212). Clinical benefit of targeting the removal of these poorly dialyzed solutes remains to be seen.

◆ PITFALLS OF UREA MODELING

When urea modeling produces unexpected results, a troubleshooting routine should be initiated. The most common sources of error are listed in **TABLE 5.6**. A frequent source of error and probably the greatest source of scatter in the data generated by single-compartment modeling is the postdialysis BUN. Current consensus favors drawing the blood specimen at the immediate end of dialysis (see section "Comparison with the Single-Compartment Model" and **FIGURE 5.11**) while taking precautions against dilution of the blood urea due to access recirculation (213,214). To prevent an error from access recirculation, the specimen should be drawn approximately 10 seconds after slowing the blood pump to approximately 100 mL/min. If the delay is longer than 15 seconds, substantial rebound will occur due to cardiopulmonary recirculation. Special attention should be paid to the distance between the end of the arterial needle and the sampling port in the arterial (inflow) blood line.

TABLE 5.6	Pitfalls of Urea Modeling

1. Errors that affect the delivery or adequacy of dialysis

Predialysis BUN: most reliable of the two measurements

- Avoid any delay (even 30 s) after starting the blood pump.
- Avoid dilution from saline or heparin.

Postdialysis BUN: most subject to error

- Avoid local recirculation.
- Consider urea rebound from cardiopulmonary recirculation and other sources of disequilibrium.

2. Errors that affect the assessment of equipment function

Clearance errors: clearance is almost always overestimated

- Blood flow errors

Low prepump pressure (219)

Poor flow calibration

Poor pump segment occlusion

- Failure to correct for serum and whole blood water content
- Loss of surface area from reuse or clotting
- Inflated manufacturer's *in vitro* clearances
- Recirculation (refer to above)

Timing errors: wall clock syndrome (220)

Volume errors: patients may not conform to the anthropometric formulas

3. Errors that affect the measurement of nPCR

Predialysis and postdialysis BUN errors (see above)

Residual clearance errors

BUN, blood urea nitrogen; nPCR, normalized protein catabolic rate.

The volume between these two points should be replaced at least twice during the slow blood flow interval.

Another common source of error is found in deviations of the dialyzer clearance from predictions by EQUATION 5.12. These errors usually result from selection of a value for K_0A that was measured *in vitro* (215). Clearances from blood can be significantly lower than clearances measured *in vitro* by the dialyzer manufacturer using saline solutions, due to coating of the membrane by blood products and solute transport in erythrocytes. This error can be avoided by calculating K_0A from cross-dialyzer BUN measurements *in vivo*, using EQUATION 5.11, before applying EQUATION 5.12. Dialysate flow has been found to influence K_0A *in vitro* but the effect seems to be attenuated *in vivo* (216,217). These errors in K_0A affect only the prescribed dose; they have little or no effect on the delivered dose determined from urea modeling. More detailed discussions of the pitfalls of urea modeling can be found in other references (19,218–220).

Despite the mathematical complexities outlined earlier, the implementation of urea modeling is relatively simple. For instance, the most popular methods for assessing dialysis adequacy require only two BUN measurements. As a consequence, potential errors that might result from measuring more complex functions, such as dialyzer clearance, K_0A, or urea distribution volume, are minimized. Efforts to maintain or improve the reliability of the tests of dialysis adequacy should therefore focus on sampling techniques and accuracy of laboratory measurements. On the other hand, when urea modeling is used to evaluate equipment function, to determine, for example, why the prescribed amount of dialysis does not match that

delivered, accurate estimates of dialyzer clearance, urea volume, and dialysis duration are required. TABLE 5.6 separates the pitfalls of urea modeling into these two major categories, those impacting on adequacy assessment caused by errors in BUN measurement and those affecting assessment of equipment function caused by errors in the prescription or in V.

SUMMARY

It is fortunate and gratifying that an empirically derived treatment such as hemodialysis is so successful in reversing the life-threatening effects of uremia, but since the cause of uremia is inadequate native kidney function, the amount of dialysis substituted should be quantified to assure adequate replacement. What defines adequate versus optimal is less clear as increased frequencies and durations of treatment become more widely available and accepted. Nonetheless, because the major effect of dialysis is small solute removal, it seems reasonable to continue using a readily dialyzable and easily measured solute such as urea as a yardstick. Relative urea removal, expressed as a relative volume cleared, is the essence of the clearance concept.

Carefully controlled studies have shown that the clearance obtained from urea kinetic modeling of the up and down swings in urea concentration found in intermittently treated patients predicts outcome and therefore can be used to judge the adequacy of each treatment. Urea kinetic modeling is a mathematical simulation of urea flux, based on measurements of concentrations before and after intermittent hemodialysis, which allows calculation of urea clearance during dialysis and urea generation between treatments. Established and proven clinical techniques for quantifying dialysis permit tailoring of prescriptions to each patient's need. The goals of urea modeling are first to maintain a uniform quantity of treatment in all patients and second to identify potential problems that impair dialysis efficiency in each patient. The parameters Kt/V (and derivatives eKt/V, stdKt/V) and nPCR obtained from single- or multiple-compartment modeling help dialysis caregivers focus on patients whose prescriptions, including their dialysis schedule, time on dialysis, dialyzer clearance, and dietary protein, need adjustment.

Nephrologists today have accepted the need for measuring dialysis and have dropped the focus on BUN alone because it is a potentially misleading indicator of adequacy. Regulatory agencies have also included quantification of dialysis as a marker of clinical care quality. A consensus has been reached about the minimum dose, expressed as a clearance normalized to body size and treatment time (Kt/V). Several methods have been developed to measure Kt/V and new insights and methods continue to appear that may simplify this measurement in the future. As more patients are treated with frequent in-center hemodialysis, home hemodialysis and long nocturnal dialysis, the utilization of stdKt/V may expand. Inclusion of solute disequilibrium, residual kidney clearance, and recirculation has helped to sharpen the accuracy and usefulness of urea kinetic modeling, and standards are now available and accepted as benchmarks of routine dialysis care.

REFERENCES

1. Kolff WJ, Berk HTJ, ter Welle M, et al. The artificial kidney, a dialyzer with a great area. *Acta Med Scand* 1944;117:121–128.
2. Scribner BH, Caner JEZ, Buri R, et al. The treatment of chronic uremia by means of intermittent dialysis: a preliminary report. *Trans Am Soc Artif Intern Organs* 1960;6:114–119.

3. Gotch FA, Sargent JA. A mechanistic analysis of the National Cooperative Dialysis Study (NCDS). *Kidney Int* 1985;28(3):526–534.

4. Laird NM, Berkey CS, Lowrie EG. Modeling success or failure of dialysis therapy: the National Cooperative Dialysis Study. *Kidney Int* 1983; 23(Suppl 13):101–106.

5. Lowrie EG, Sargent JA. Clinical example of pharmacokinetic and metabolic modeling: quantitative and individualized prescription of dialysis therapy. *Kidney Int* 1980;18(Suppl 10):S11–S16.

6. Lowrie EG, Laird NM, Parker TF, et al. Effect of the hemodialysis prescription on patient morbidity: report from the National Cooperative Dialysis Study. *N Engl J Med* 1981;305(20):1176–1181.

7. Eschbach JW, Egrie JC, Downing MR, et al. Correction of the anemia of end-stage renal disease with recombinant human erythropoietin: results of a combined phase I and II clinical trial. *N Engl J Med* 1987;316: 73–78.

8. Roy T, Ahrenholz P, Falkenhagen D, et al. Volumetrically controlled ultrafiltration. Current experiences and future prospects. *Int J Artif Organs* 1982;5(3):131–135.

9. Schmidt R, Herrera R, Holtz M, et al. Technic and indication for controlled ultrafiltration [in German]. *Z Gesamte Inn Med* 1980;35(16): S55–S58.

10. Hakim RM, Pontzer M, Tilton D, et al. Effects of acetate and bicarbonate dialysate in stable chronic dialysis patients. *Kidney Int* 1985;28: 535–540.

11. Keshaviah P, Collins A. Rapid high-efficiency bicarbonate hemodialysis. *ASAIO Trans* 1986;32(1):17–23.

12. Eknoyan G, Beck GJ, Cheung AK, et al. Effect of dialysis dose and membrane flux in maintenance hemodialysis. *N Engl J Med* 2002; 347(25):2010–2019.

13. Chertow GM, Levin NW, Beck GJ, et al. In-center hemodialysis six times per week versus three times per week. *N Engl J Med* 2010;363(24): 2287–2300.

14. Rocco MV, Lockridge RS Jr, Beck GJ, et al. The effects of frequent nocturnal home hemodialysis: the Frequent Hemodialysis Network Nocturnal Trial. *Kidney Int* 2011;80(10):1080–1091.

15. Liyanage T, Ninomiya T, Jha V, et al. Worldwide access to treatment for end-stage kidney disease: a systematic review. *Lancet* 2015; 385(9981):1975–1982.

16. United States Renal Data System. *USRDS 2012 Annual Data Report: Atlas of Chronic Kidney Disease and End-Stage Renal Disease in the United States.* Bethesda, MD: National Institutes of Health, National Institute of Diabetes and Digestive and Kidney Diseases, 2012.

17. Goodkin DA, Bragg-Gresham JL, Koenig KG, et al. Association of comorbid conditions and mortality in hemodialysis patients in Europe, Japan, and the United States: the Dialysis Outcomes and Practice Patterns Study (DOPPS). *J Am Soc Nephrol* 2003;14(12): 3270–3277.

18. Grangé S, Hanoy M, Le Roy F, et al. Monitoring of hemodialysis quality-of-care indicators: why is it important? *BMC Nephrol* 2013;14:109.

19. Hemodialysis Adequacy 2006 Work Group. Clinical practice guidelines for hemodialysis adequacy, update 2006. *Am J Kidney Dis* 2006;48(Suppl 1): S2–S90.

20. Hull AR, Parker TF. Proceedings from the morbidity, mortality and prescription of dialysis symposium: introduction and summary. *Am J Kidney Dis* 1990;15:375–383.

21. Kopple JD, Hakim RM, Held PJ, et al. The National Kidney Foundation. Recommendations for reducing the high morbidity and mortality of United States maintenance dialysis patients. *Am J Kidney Dis* 1994; 24:968–973.

22. Bagnasco SM. The erythrocyte urea transporter UT-B. *J Membr Biol* 2006;212(2):133–138.

23. Hunter FL. Facilitated diffusion in human erythrocytes. *Biochim Biophys Acta* 1970;211:216–221.

24. Macey RI, Farmer REL. Inhibition of water and solute permeability in human red cells. *Biochim Biophys Acta* 1970;211:104–106.

25. Mayrand RR, Levitt DG. Urea and ethylene glycol facilitated transport system in the human red cell membrane. *J Gen Physiol* 1983;81: 221–237.

26. Sands JM, Timmer RT, Gunn RB. Urea transporters in kidney and erythrocytes. *Am J Physiol* 1997;273(3 Pt 2):F321–F339.

27. Shayakul C, Hediger MA. The SLC14 gene family of urea transporters. *Pflugers Arch* 2004;447(5):603–609.

28. Yousef LW, Macey RI. A method to distinguish between pore and carrier kinetics applied to urea transport across the erythrocyte membrane. *Biochim Biophys Acta* 1989;984:281–288.

29. Borah MF, Schoenfeld PY, Gotch FA, et al. Nitrogen balance during intermittent dialysis therapy of uremia. *Kidney Int* 1978;14:491–500.

30. Cottini EP, Gallina DK, Dominguez JM. Urea excretion in adult humans with varying degrees of kidney malfunction fed milk, egg, or an amino acid mixture: assessment of nitrogen balance. *J Nutr* 1973;103:11–21.

31. Mitch WE. Nutritional therapy and the progression of renal insufficiency. In: Mitch WE, Klahr S, eds. *Nutrition and the Kidney.* Boston, MA: Little, Brown and Company, 1988:154–179.

32. Lim VS, Bier DM, Flanigan MJ, et al. The effect of hemodialysis on protein metabolism. A Leucine Kinetic Study. *J Clin Invest* 1993;91(6): 2429–2436.

33. Teraoka S, Toma H, Nihei H, et al. Current status of renal replacement therapy in Japan. *Am J Kidney Dis* 1995;25:151–164.

34. Anderstam B, Mamoun AH, Sodersten P, et al. Middle-sized molecule fractions isolated from uremic ultrafiltrate and normal urine inhibit ingestive behavior in the rat. *J Am Soc Nephrol* 1996;7:2453–2460.

35. Foley RN. Clinical epidemiology of cardiac disease in dialysis patients: left ventricular hypertrophy, ischemic heart disease, and cardiac failure. *Semin Dial* 2003;16(2):111–117.

36. Lopes AA, Elder SJ, Ginsberg N, et al. Lack of appetite in haemodialysis patients—associations with patient characteristics, indicators of nutritional status and outcomes in the international DOPPS. *Nephrol Dial Transplant* 2007;22(12):3538–3546.

37. Asamiya Y, Otsubo S, Matsuda Y, et al. The importance of low blood urea nitrogen levels in pregnant patients undergoing hemodialysis to optimize birth weight and gestational age. *Kidney Int* 2009;75(11): 1217–1222.

38. Barua M, Hladunewich M, Keunen J, et al. Successful pregnancies on nocturnal home hemodialysis. *Clin J Am Soc Nephrol* 2008;3(2): 392–396.

39. Hladunewich MA, Hou S, Odutayo A, et al. Intensive hemodialysis associates with improved pregnancy outcomes: a Canadian and United States cohort comparison. *J Am Soc Nephrol* 2014;25(5):1103–1109.

40. Bergstrom J, Furst P. Uraemic toxins. In: Drukker W, Parsons FM, Maher JF, eds. *Replacement of Renal Function by Dialysis.* Boston, MA: Martinus Nijhoff, 1983:354–390.

41. Johnson WJ, Hagge WW, Wagoner RD, et al. Effects of urea loading in patients with far-advanced renal failure. *Mayo Clin Proc* 1972;47:21–29.

42. Merrill JP, Legrain M, Hoigne R. Observations on the role of urea in uremia. *Am J Med* 1953;14:519–520.

43. Cohen G, Glorieux G, Thornalley P, et al. Review on uraemic toxins III: recommendations for handling uraemic retention solutes *in vitro* towards a standardized approach for research on uraemia. *Nephrol Dial Transplant* 2007;22(12):3381–3390.

44. Davenport A, Jones S, Goel S, et al. Carbamylated hemoglobin: a potential marker for the adequacy of hemodialysis therapy in end-stage renal failure. *Kidney Int* 1996;50:1344–1351.

45. Fluckiger R, Harmon W, Meier W, et al. Hemoglobin carbamylation in uremia. *N Engl J Med* 1981;304:823–827.

46. Kwan JT, Carr EC, Neal AD, et al. Carbamylated haemoglobin, urea kinetic modelling and adequacy of dialysis in haemodialysis patients. *Nephrol Dial Transplant* 1991;6:38–43.

47. Smith WGJ, Holden M, Benton M, et al. Carbamylated haemoglobin in chronic renal failure. *Clin Chim Acta* 1988;178:297–304.

48. Drechsler C, Kalim S, Wenger JB, et al. Protein carbamylation is associated with heart failure and mortality in diabetic patients with end-stage renal disease. *Kidney Int* 2015;87(6):1201–1208.

49. Gipson D, Katz LA, Stehman-Breen C. Principles of dialysis: special issues in women. *Semin Nephrol* 1999;19(2):140–147.

50. Hou S. Pregnancy in women requiring dialysis for renal failure. *Am J Kidney Dis* 1987;9(4):368–373.

51. Bergstrom J. Why are dialysis patients malnourished? *Am J Kidney Dis* 1995;26:229–241.

52. Hakim RM, Levin N. Malnutrition in hemodialysis patients. *Am J Kidney Dis* 1993;21:125–137.

53. Ikizler TA, Greene JH, Wingard RL, et al. Spontaneous dietary protein intake during progression of chronic renal failure. *J Am Soc Nephrol* 1995;6:1386–1391.

54. Levey AS, Greene T, Beck GJ, et al. Modification of Diet in Renal Disease Study Group. Dietary protein restriction and the progression of chronic renal disease: what have all of the results of the MDRD study shown? *J Am Soc Nephrol* 1999;10(11):2426–2439.

55. Walser M. Does prolonged protein restriction preceding dialysis lead to protein malnutrition at the onset of dialysis? *Kidney Int* 1993;44:1139–1144.

56. Hakim RM, Breyer J, Ismail N, et al. Effects of dose of dialysis on morbidity and mortality. *Am J Kidney Dis* 1994;23:661–669.

57. Lindsay RM, Spanner E, Heidenheim RP, et al. Which comes first, Kt/V or PCR—chicken or egg? *Kidney Int Suppl* 1992;38:S32–S36.

58. Nolph KD. Small solute clearances and clinical outcomes in CAPD [editorial; comment]. *Perit Dial Int* 1992;12:343–345.

59. Ronco C, Bosch JP, Lew SQ, et al. Adequacy of continuous ambulatory peritoneal dialysis: comparison with other dialysis techniques. *Kidney Int Suppl* 1994;48:18–24.

60. Greene T, Depner TA, Daugirdas JT. Mathematical coupling and the association between Kt/V and PCRn. *Semin Dial* 1999;12(Suppl 1):S20–S28.

61. Uehlinger DE. Another look at the relationship between protein intake and dialysis dose. *J Am Soc Nephrol* 1996;7(1):166–168.

62. Gotch FA, Levin NW, Port FK, et al. Clinical outcome relative to the dose of dialysis is not what you think: the fallacy of the mean. *Am J Kidney Dis* 1997;30(1):1–15.

63. Meyer TW, Hostetter TH. Uremia. *N Engl J Med* 2007;357(13):1316–1325.

64. Burrowes JD, Larive B, Chertow GM, et al. Self-reported appetite, hospitalization and death in haemodialysis patients: findings from the Hemodialysis (HEMO) Study. *Nephrol Dial Transplant* 2005;20(12):2765–2774.

65. Dwyer JT, Larive B, Leung J, et al. Are nutritional status indicators associated with mortality in the Hemodialysis (HEMO) Study? *Kidney Int* 2005;68(4):1766–1776.

66. Schulman G. The dose of dialysis in hemodialysis patients: impact on nutrition. *Semin Dial* 2004;17(6):479–488.

67. Kaysen GA, Greene T, Larive B, et al. The effect of frequent hemodialysis on nutrition and body composition: frequent Hemodialysis Network Trial. *Kidney Int* 2012;82(1):90–99.

68. Termorshuizen F, Dekker FW, van Manen JG, et al. Relative contribution of residual renal function and different measures of adequacy to survival in hemodialysis patients: an analysis of the Netherlands Cooperative Study on the Adequacy of Dialysis (NECOSAD)-2. *J Am Soc Nephrol* 2004;15(4):1061–1070.

69. Bargman JM, Thorpe KE, Churchill DN. Relative contribution of residual renal function and peritoneal clearance to adequacy of dialysis: a reanalysis of the CANUSA study. *J Am Soc Nephrol* 2001;12(10):2158–2162.

70. Termorshuizen F, Korevaar JC, Dekker FW, et al. The relative importance of residual renal function compared with peritoneal clearance for patient survival and quality of life: an analysis of the Netherlands Cooperative Study on the Adequacy of Dialysis (NECOSAD)-2. *Am J Kidney Dis* 2003;41(6):1293–1302.

71. Meyer TW, Peattie JW, Miller JD, et al. Increasing the clearance of protein-bound solutes by addition of a sorbent to the dialysate. *J Am Soc Nephrol* 2007;18(3):868–874.

72. Sirich TL, Funk BA, Plummer NS, et al. Prominent accumulation in hemodialysis patients of solutes normally cleared by tubular secretion. *J Am Soc Nephrol* 2014;25(3):615–622.

73. National Kidney Foundation. K/DOQI clinical practice guideline and practice recommendations for hemodialysis adequacy: 2015 update. *Am J Kidney Dis* 2015;66:884–930.

74. Chertow GM, Owen WF, Lazarus JM, et al. Exploring the reverse J-shaped curve between urea reduction ratio and mortality. *Kidney Int* 1999;56(5):1872–1878.

75. Sherman RA. Quantitating peritoneal dialysis: the problem with V. *Semin Dial* 1996;9:381–383.

76. Tzamaloukas AH, Murata GH, Piraino B, et al. The relation between body size and normalized small solute clearances in continuous ambulatory peritoneal dialysis. *J Am Soc Nephrol* 1999;10(7):1575–1581.

77. Bowsher DJ, Avram MJ, Frederiksen MC, et al. Urea distribution kinetics analyzed by simultaneous injection of urea and inulin: demonstration that transcapillary exchange is rate limiting. *J Pharmacol Exp Ther* 1984;230(2):269–274.

78. Edelman IS, Leibman J. Anatomy of body water and electrolytes. *Am J Med* 1959;51:256–277.

79. San Pietro A, Rittenberg D. A study of the rate of protein synthesis in humans. I. Measurement of the urea pool and urea space. *J Biol Chem* 1953;201:445–452.

80. Levey AS. Measurement of renal function in chronic renal disease [clinical conference]. *Kidney Int* 1990;38:167–184.

81. Singer MA. Of mice and men and elephants: metabolic rate sets glomerular filtration rate. *Am J Kidney Dis* 2001;37(1):164–178.

82. Daugirdas JT, Greene T, Depner TA, et al. Anthropometrically estimated total body water volumes are larger than modeled urea volume in chronic hemodialysis patients: effects of age, race, and gender. *Kidney Int* 2003;64(3):1108–1119.

83. Depner T, Daugirdas J, Greene T, et al. Dialysis dose and the effect of gender and body size on outcome in the HEMO Study. *Kidney Int* 2004;65(4):1386–1394.

84. Lowrie EG, Li Z, Ofsthun N, et al. Body size, dialysis dose and death risk relationships among hemodialysis patients. *Kidney Int* 2002;62(5):1891–1897.

85. DuBois D, DuBois EF. A formula to estimate the approximate surface area if the height and weight be known. *Arch Intern Med* 1916;17:863–871.

86. Hume R, Weyers E. Relationship between total body water and surface area in normal and obese subjects. *J Clin Pathol* 1971;24:234–238.

87. Lowrie EG, Li Z, Ofsthun N, et al. The online measurement of hemodialysis dose (Kt): clinical outcome as a function of body surface area. *Kidney Int* 2005;68(3):1344–1354.

88. Cohen G, Glorieux G, Thornalley P, et al. Review on uraemic toxins III: recommendations for handling uraemic retention solutes *in vitro* towards a standardized approach for research on uraemia. *Nephrol Dial Transplant* 2007;22:3381–3390.

89. Depner TA. Uremic toxicity: urea and beyond. *Semin Dial* 2001;14(4):246–251.

90. Levin N, Gotch F. An hypothesis to account for the inverse relationship of relative risk of mortality to urea distribution volume in dialysis patients [abstract]. *J Am Soc Nephrol* 2002;13(9).

91. Kopple JD, Zhu X, Lew NL, et al. Body weight-for-height relationships predict mortality in maintenance hemodialysis patients. *Kidney Int* 1999;56(3):1136–1148.

92. Lowrie EG, Chertow GM, Lew NL, et al. The urea {clearance × dialysis time} product (Kt) as an outcome-based measure of hemodialysis dose. *Kidney Int* 1999;56(2):729–737.

93. Port FK, Ashby VB, Dhingra RK, et al. Dialysis dose and body mass index are strongly associated with survival in hemodialysis patients. *J Am Soc Nephrol* 2002;13(4):1061–1066.

94. Wolfe RA, Ashby VB, Daugirdas JT, et al. Body size, dose of hemodialysis, and mortality. *Am J Kidney Dis* 2000;35(1):80–88.

95. Owen WF Jr, Chertow GM, Lazarus JM, et al. Dose of hemodialysis and survival: differences by race and sex. *JAMA* 1998;280(20):1764–1768.

96. United States Renal Data System. *USRDS 2014 Annual Data Report: Atlas of Chronic Kidney Disease and End-Stage Renal Disease in the United States.* Bethesda, MD: National Institute of Health, National Institute of Diabetes and Digestive and Kidney Diseases, 2014.

97. Port FK, Wolfe RA, Hulbert-Shearon TE, et al. High dialysis dose is associated with lower mortality among women but not among men. *Am J Kidney Dis* 2004;43(6):1014–1023.

98. Kaysen GA, Stevenson FT, Depner TA. Determinants of albumin concentration in hemodialysis patients. *Am J Kidney Dis* 1997;29(5):658–668.

99. Depner TA. *Prescribing Hemodialysis: A Guide to Urea Modeling.* Boston, MA: Kluwer Academic Publishers, 1991.

100. Descombes E, Perriard F, Fellay G. Diffusion kinetics of urea, creatinine and uric acid in blood during hemodialysis. Clinical implications. *Clin Nephrol* 1993;40(5):286–295.

101. Gotch FA, Panlilio F, Sergeyeva O, et al. Effective diffusion volume flow rates (Qe) for urea, creatinine, and inorganic phosphorous (Qeu, Qecr, QeiP) during hemodialysis. *Semin Dial* 2003;16(6):474–476.

102. Gotch FA. Kinetic modeling in hemodialysis. In: Nissenson AR, Fine RN, Gentile DE, eds. *Clinical Dialysis.* 3rd ed. Norwalk, CT: Appleton and Lange, 1995:156–188.

103. Charra B, Chazot C, Jean G, et al. Long 3 × 8 hr dialysis: a three-decade summary. *J Nephrol* 2003;16(Suppl 7):S64–S69.

104. Weinreich T, De los Rios T, Gauly A, et al. Effects of an increase in time versus frequency on cardiovascular parameters in chronic hemodialysis patients. *Clin Nephrol* 2006;66(6):433–439.

105. Brunelli SM, Chertow GM, Ankers ED, et al. Shorter dialysis times are associated with higher mortality among incident hemodialysis patients. *Kidney Int* 2010;77(7):630–636.

106. Saran R, Bragg-Gresham JL, Levin NW, et al. Longer treatment time and slower ultrafiltration in hemodialysis: associations with reduced mortality in the DOPPS. *Kidney Int* 2006;69(7):1222–1228.

107. Flythe JE, Curhan GC, Brunelli SM. Shorter length dialysis sessions are associated with increased mortality, independent of body weight. *Kidney Int* 2013;83(1):104–113.

108. Vanholder R, Schoots A, Cramers C, et al. Hippuric acid as a marker. *Adv Exp Med Biol* 1987;223:59–67.

109. Giordano C, DePascale C, Esposito R, et al. Loss of large amounts of amino acids in hemodialysis. *Biochemie Applicata* 1968;15:373.

110. Giovannetti S, Maggiore Q. A low nitrogen diet with proteins of high biological value for severe chronic uraemia. *Lancet* 1964;1:1000–1001.

111. Lowrie EG, Teehan BP. Principles of prescribing dialysis therapy: implementing recommendations from the National Cooperative Dialysis Study. *Kidney Int* 1983;23(Suppl 13):S113–S122.

112. Richet G. Early history of uremia. *Kidney Int* 1988;33:1013–1015.

113. Schreiner GE, Maher JF. *Uremia: Biochemistry, Pathogenesis and Treatment.* Springfield, IL: Charles C Thomas Publishers, 1961.

114. Owen WF Jr, Lew NL, Liu Y, et al. The urea reduction ratio and serum albumin concentration as predictors of mortality in patients undergoing hemodialysis. *N Engl J Med* 1993;329:1001–1006.

115. Gibaldi M, Perrier D. *Pharmacokinetics.* New York, NY: Marcel Dekker Inc, 1982.

116. Depner TA. Hemodialysis urea modeling: the basics. *Semin Dial* 1991; 4:179–184.

117. Depner TA. Standards for dialysis adequacy. *Semin Dial* 1991;4: 245–252.

118. Hakim RM, Depner TA, Parker TF. In depth review: adequacy of hemodialysis [see comments]. *Am J Kidney Dis* 1992;20:107–123.

119. Sargent JA, Lowrie EG. Which mathematical model to study uremic toxicity—National Cooperative Dialysis Study. *Clin Nephrol* 1982; 17:303–314.

120. Depner TA, Cheer AY. Modeling urea kinetics with two versus three BUN measurements. A critical comparison. *ASAIO J* 1989;35:499–502.

121. Depner TA. Multicompartment models. In: Depner TA, ed. *Prescribing Hemodialysis: A Guide to Urea Modeling.* Boston, MA: Kluwer Academic Publishers, 1991:91–126.

122. Michaels AS. Operating parameters and performance criteria for hemodialyzers and other membrane-separation devices. *Trans Am Soc Artif Intern Organs* 1966;12:387–392.

123. Delmez JA, Windus DW. St. Louis Nephrology Study Group. Hemodialysis prescription and delivery in a metropolitan community. *Kidney Int* 1992;41:1023–1028.

124. Canaud B, Bragg-Gresham JL, Marshall MR, et al. Mortality risk for patients receiving hemodiafiltration versus hemodialysis: European results from the DOPPS. *Kidney Int* 2006;69(11):2087–2093.

125. Rabindranath KS, Strippoli GF, Daly C, et al. Haemodiafiltration, haemofiltration and haemodialysis for end-stage kidney disease. *Cochrane Database Syst Rev* 2006;(4):CD006258.

126. Rabindranath KS, Strippoli GF, Roderick P, et al. Comparison of hemodialysis, hemofiltration, and acetate-free biofiltration for ESRD: systematic review. *Am J Kidney Dis* 2005;45(3):437–447.

127. Ward RA, Schmidt B, Hullin J, et al. A comparison of on-line hemodiafiltration and high-flux hemodialysis: a prospective clinical study. *J Am Soc Nephrol* 2000;11(12):2344–2350.

128. Wang AY, Ninomiya T, Al-Kahwa A, et al. Effect of hemodiafiltration or hemofiltration compared with hemodialysis on mortality and cardiovascular disease in chronic kidney failure: a systematic review and meta-analysis of randomized trials. *Am J Kidney Dis* 2014;63(6): 968–978.

129. Grooteman MP, van den Dorpel MA, Bots ML, et al. Effect of online hemodiafiltration on all-cause mortality and cardiovascular outcomes. *J Am Soc Nephrol* 2012;23(6):1087–1096.

130. LaFrance ND, Drew HH, Walser M. Radioisotopic measurement of glomerular filtration rate in severe chronic renal failure. *J Nucl Med* 1988;29(12):1927–1930.

131. Hoek FJ, Korevaar JC, Dekker FW, et al. Estimation of residual glomerular filtration rate in dialysis patients from the plasma cystatin C level. *Nephrol Dial Transplant* 2007;22(6):1633–1638.

132. Huang SH, Filler G, Lindsay RM. Residual renal function calculated from serum cystatin C measurements and knowledge of the weekly standard Kt/V urea. *Perit Dial Int* 2012;32(1):102–104.

133. Pedrini LA, Zereik S, Rasmy S. Causes, kinetics and clinical implications of post-hemodialysis urea rebound. *Kidney Int* 1988;34:817–824.

134. Sargent JA, Gotch FA. Principles and biophysics of dialysis. In: Maher JF, ed. *Replacement of Renal Function by Dialysis.* Dordrecht, The Netherlands: Kluwer Academic Publishers, 1989:87–143.

135. Burgelman M, Vanholder R, Fostier H, et al. Estimation of parameters in a two-pool urea kinetic model for hemodialysis. *Med Eng Phys* 1997;19:69–76.

136. Depner TA. Refining the model of urea kinetics: compartment effects. *Semin Dial* 1992;5:147–154.

137. Evans JH, Smye SW, Brocklebank JT. Mathematical modelling of haemodialysis in children. *Pediatr Nephrol* 1992;6:349–353.

138. Grandi F, Avanzolini G, Cappello A. Analytic solution of the variable-volume double-pool urea kinetics model applied to parameter estimation in hemodialysis. *Comput Biol Med* 1995;25:505–518.

139. Heineken FG, Evans MC, Keen ML, et al. Intercompartmental fluid shifts in hemodialysis patients. *Biotechnol Progr* 1987;3:69–73.

140. Depner TA, Rizwan S, Cheer AY, et al. High venous urea concentrations in the opposite arm. A consequence of hemodialysis-induced compartment disequilibrium. *ASAIO J* 1991;37(3):141–143.

141. Depner TA, Krivitski NM, MacGibbon D. Hemodialysis access recirculation measured by ultrasound dilution. *ASAIO J* 1995;41: M749–M753.

142. Kong CH, Tattersall JE, Greenwood RN, et al. The effect of exercise during haemodialysis on solute removal. *Nephrol Dial Transplant* 1999;14(12):2927–2931.

143. Schneditz D, Kaufman AM, Polaschegg HD, et al. Cardiopulmonary recirculation during hemodialysis. *Kidney Int* 1992;42:1450–1456.

144. Schneditz D, Zaluska WT, Morris AT, et al. Effect of ultrafiltration on peripheral urea sequestration in haemodialysis patients. *Nephrol Dial Transplant* 2001;16(5):994–998.

145. Sombolos K, Natse T, Zoumbaridis N, et al. Urea concentration gradients during conventional hemodialysis. *Am J Kidney Dis* 1996;27: 673–679.

146. Schneditz D, Daugirdas JT. Formal analytical solution to a regional blood flow and diffusion based urea kinetic model. *ASAIO J* 1994; 40:M667–M673.

147. Daugirdas JT, Smye SW. Effect of a two compartment distribution on apparent urea distribution volume. *Kidney Int* 1997;51:1270–1273.

148. Daugirdas JT, Depner TA, Gotch FA, et al. Comparison of methods to predict equilibrated Kt/V in the HEMO Pilot Study. *Kidney Int* 1997; 52(5):1395–1405.

149. Daugirdas JT, Schneditz D. Overestimation of hemodialysis dose depends on dialysis efficiency by regional blood flow but not by conventional two pool urea kinetic analysis. *ASAIO J* 1995;41:M719–M724.

150. Daugirdas JT. Simplified equations for monitoring Kt/V, PCRn, eKt/V, and ePCRn. *Adv Ren Replace Ther* 1995;2:295–304.

151. Daugirdas JT, Greene T, Depner TA, et al; and the Hemodialysis Study Group. Factors that affect postdialysis rebound in serum urea concentration, including the rate of dialysis: results from the HEMO Study. *J Am Soc Nephrol* 2004;15(1):194–203.

152. Leypoldt JK, Jaber BL, Zimmerman DL. Predicting treatment dose for novel therapies using urea standard Kt/V. *Semin Dial* 2004;17(2):142–145.

153. Tattersall JE, DeTakats D, Chamney P, et al. The post-hemodialysis rebound: predicting and quantifying its effect on Kt/V. *Kidney Int* 1996;50:2094–2102.

154. DeSoi CA, Umans JG. Phosphate kinetics during high-flux hemodialysis. *J Am Soc Nephrol* 1993;4:1214–1218.

155. Spalding EM, Chamney PW, Farrington K. Phosphate kinetics during hemodialysis: evidence for biphasic regulation. *Kidney Int* 2002;61(2):655–667.

156. Achinger SG, Ayus JC. The role of daily dialysis in the control of hyperphosphatemia. *Kidney Int Suppl* 2005(95):S28–S32.

157. Kooienga L. Phosphorus balance with daily dialysis. *Semin Dial* 2007; 20(4):342–345.

158. Kuhlmann MK. Management of hyperphosphatemia. *Hemodial Int* 2006;10(4):338–345.

159. Al-Hejaili F, Kortas C, Leitch R, et al. Nocturnal but not short hours quotidian hemodialysis requires an elevated dialysate calcium concentration. *J Am Soc Nephrol* 2003;14(9):2322–2328.

160. Depner TA, Keshaviah PR, Ebben JP, et al. Multicenter clinical validation of an on-line monitor of dialysis adequacy. *J Am Soc Nephrol* 1996;7:464–471.

161. Ellis P, Malchesky PS, Magnusson MO, et al. Comparison of two methods of kinetic modeling. *Trans Am Soc Artif Intern Organs* 1984; 30:60–64.

162. Garred LJ. Dialysate-based kinetic modeling. *Adv Ren Replace Ther* 1995;2:305–318.

163. Malchesky PS, Ellis P, Nosse C, et al. Direct quantification of dialysis. *Dial Transpl* 1982;11:42–44.

164. Depner TA, Greene T, Gotch FA, et al. Hemodialysis Study Group. Imprecision of the hemodialysis dose when measured directly from urea removal. *Kidney Int* 1999;55(2):635–647.

165. Depner TA, Stanfel LA, Jarrard EA, et al. Impaired plasma phenytoin binding in uremia. Effect of in vitro acidification and anion-exchange resin. *Nephron* 1980;25(5):231–237.

166. Keshaviah P. The solute removal index—a unified basis for comparing disparate therapies [editorial]. *Perit Dial Int* 1995;15:101–104.

167. Keshaviah P, Star RA. A new approach to dialysis quantification: an adequacy index based on solute removal. *Semin Dial* 1994;7:85–90.

168. Flanigan MJ, Fangman J, Lim VS. Quantitating hemodialysis: a comparison of three kinetic models [see comments]. *Am J Kidney Dis* 1991; 17:295–302.

169. Mercadal L, Petitclerc T, Jaudon MC, et al. Is ionic dialysance a valid parameter for quantification of dialysis efficiency? *Artif Organs* 1998; 22(12):1005–1009.

170. Petitclerc T, Goux N, Reynier AL, et al. A model for non-invasive estimation of in vivo dialyzer performances and patient's conductivity during hemodialysis. *Int J Artif Organs* 1993;16:585–591.

171. Polaschegg HD. On-line dialyser clearance using conductivity. *Pediatr Nephrol* 1995;9(Suppl):S9–S11.

172. Petitclerc T, Bene B, Jacobs C, et al. Non-invasive monitoring of effective dialysis dose delivered to the haemodialysis patient. *Nephrol Dial Transplant* 1995;10:212–216.

173. Moret K, Beerenhout CH, van den Wall Bake AW, et al. Ionic dialysance and the assessment of Kt/V: the influence of different estimates of V on method agreement. *Nephrol Dial Transplant* 2007;22(8):2276–2282.

174. McIntyre CW, Lambie SH, Taal MW, et al. Assessment of haemodialysis adequacy by ionic dialysance: intra-patient variability of delivered treatment. *Nephrol Dial Transplant* 2003;18(3):559–563.

175. Gotch FA, Panlilio FM, Buyaki RA, et al. Mechanisms determining the ratio of conductivity clearance to urea clearance. *Kidney Int Suppl* 2004;66(89):S3–S24.

176. Depner TA. Quantifying hemodialysis and peritoneal dialysis: examination of the peak concentration hypothesis. *Semin Dial* 1994; 7(5):315–317.

177. Locatelli F, Buoncristiani U, Canaud B, et al. Dialysis dose and frequency. *Nephrol Dial Transplant* 2005;20(2):285–296.

178. Suri R, Depner TA, Blake PG, et al. Adequacy of quotidian hemodialysis. *Am J Kidney Dis* 2003;42(Suppl 1):42–48.

179. Culleton BF, Walsh M, Klarenbach SW, et al. Effect of frequent nocturnal hemodialysis versus conventional hemodialysis on left ventricular mass and quality of life: a randomized controlled trial. *JAMA* 2007;298(11):1291–1299.

180. Mucsi I, Hercz G, Uldall R, et al. Control of serum phosphate without any phosphate binders in patients treated with nocturnal hemodialysis. *Kidney Int* 1998;53:1399–1404.

181. Casino FG, Lopez T. The equivalent renal urea clearance: a new parameter to assess dialysis dose. *Nephrol Dial Transplant* 1996;11(8): 1574–1581.

182. National Kidney Foundation. K/DOQI clinical practice guidelines and clinical practice recommendations for 2006 updates: hemodialysis adequacy, peritoneal dialysis adequacy, and vascular access. *Am J Kidney Dis* 2006;48(Suppl 1):S1–S322.

183. Gotch FA. The current place of urea kinetic modelling with respect to different dialysis modalities. *Nephrol Dial Transpl* 1998;13(Suppl 6):10–14.

184. Daugirdas JT, Depner TA, Greene T, et al. Standard Kt/Vurea: a method of calculation that includes effects of fluid removal and residual kidney clearance. *Kidney Int* 2010;77(7):637–644.

185. Daugirdas JT, Leypoldt JK, Akonur A, et al. Improved equation for estimating single-pool Kt/V at higher dialysis frequencies. *Nephrol Dial Transplant* 2013;28(8):2156–2160.

186. Eloot S, Torremans A, De SR, et al. Complex compartmental behavior of small water-soluble uremic retention solutes: evaluation by direct measurements in plasma and erythrocytes. *Am J Kidney Dis* 2007; 50(2):279–288.

187. Eloot S, Torremans A, De SR, et al. Kinetic behavior of urea is different from that of other water-soluble compounds: the case of the guanidino compounds. *Kidney Int* 2005;67(4):1566–1575.

188. Ward RA, Greene T, Hartmann B, et al. Resistance to intercompartmental mass transfer limits β2-microglobulin removal by post-dilution hemodiafiltration. *Kidney Int* 2006;69(8):1431–1437.

189. Depner TA. Benefits of more frequent dialysis: lower TAC at the same Kt/V. *Nephrol Dial Transplant* 1998;13:20–24.

190. Depner TA, Bhat A. Quantifying daily hemodialysis. *Semin Dial* 2004; 17(2):79–84.

191. Depner TA. Why daily hemodialysis is better: solute kinetics. *Semin Dial* 1999;12(6):462–471.

192. Daugirdas JT. The post: pre-dialysis plasma urea nitrogen ratio to estimate K.t/V and NPCR: mathematical modeling [see comments]. *Int J Artif Organs* 1989;12:411–419.

193. Jindal KK, Manuel A, Goldstein MB. Percent reduction in blood urea concentration during hemodialysis (PRU): a simple and accurate method to estimate Kt/V urea. *Trans Am Soc Artif Intern Organs* 1987;33:286–288.

194. Daugirdas JT, Depner TA. A nomogram approach to hemodialysis urea modeling. *Am J Kidney Dis* 1994;23:33–40.

195. Depner TA, Daugirdas JT. Equations for normalized protein catabolic rate based on two-point modeling of hemodialysis urea kinetics. *J Am Soc Nephrol* 1996;7(5):780–785.

196. Garred LJ, Barichello DL, DiGiuseppe B, et al. Simple Kt/V formulas based on urea mass balance theory. *ASAIO J* 1994;40:997–1004.

197. Lowrie EG, Lew NL. The urea reduction ratio (URR): a simple method for evaluating hemodialysis treatment. *Contemp Dial Nephrol* 1991;12:11–20.

198. Daugirdas JT. Second generation logarithmic estimates of single-pool variable volume Kt/V: an analysis of error. *J Am Soc Nephrol* 1993; 4:1205–1213.

199. Garred LJ, Barichello DL, Canaud BC, et al. Simple equations for protein catabolic rate determination from predialysis and postdialysis BUN. *ASAIO J* 1995;41:889–895.

200. Depner TA. Quantifying hemodialysis. *Am J Nephrol* 1996;16(1):17–28.
201. Eknoyan G, Levey AS, Beck GJ, et al. The hemodialysis (HEMO) study: rationale for selection of interventions. *Semin Dial* 1996;9(1):24–33.
202. European Best Practice Guidelines Expert Group on Hemodialysis, European Renal Association. Section II. Haemodialysis adequacy. *Nephrol Dial Transplant* 2002;17(Suppl 7):16–31.
203. Chertow GM, Levin NW, Beck GJ, et al. In-center hemodialysis six times per week versus three times per week. *N Engl J Med* 2010;363(24):2287–2300.
204. Depner T, Himmelfarb J. Uremic retention solutes: the free and the bound. *J Am Soc Nephrol* 2007;18:675–676.
205. Bammens B, Evenepoel P, Keuleers H, et al. Free serum concentrations of the protein-bound retention solute p-cresol predict mortality in hemodialysis patients. *Kidney Int* 2006;69(6):1081–1087.
206. Bammens B, Evenepoel P, Verbeke K, et al. Removal of middle molecules and protein-bound solutes by peritoneal dialysis and relation with uremic symptoms. *Kidney Int* 2003;64(6):2238–2243.
207. Depner TA. Suppression of tubular anion transport by an inhibitor of serum protein binding in uremia. *Kidney Int* 1981;20:511–518.
208. Gulyassy PF, Bottini AT, Jarrard EA, et al. Isolation of inhibitors of ligand: albumin binding from uremic body fluids and normal urine. *Kidney Int* 1983;24(Suppl 16):S238–S242.
209. Gulyassy PF, Bottini AT, Stanfel LA, et al. Isolation and chemical identification of inhibitors of plasma ligand binding. *Kidney Int* 1986;30:391–398.
210. Tavares-Almeida I, Gulyassy PF, Depner TA, et al. Aromatic amino acid metabolites as potential protein binding inhibitors in human uremic plasma. *Biochem Pharmacol* 1985;34:2431–2438.
211. Meyer TW, Leeper EC, Bartlett DW, et al. Increasing dialysate flow and dialyzer mass transfer area coefficient to increase the clearance of protein-bound solutes. *J Am Soc Nephrol* 2004;15(7):1927–1935.
212. Pham NM, Recht NS, Hostetter TH, et al. Removal of the protein-bound solutes indican and p-cresol sulfate by peritoneal dialysis. *Clin J Am Soc Nephrol* 2008;3(1):85–90.
213. Depner TA. Assessing adequacy of hemodialysis: urea modeling. *Kidney Int* 1994;45:1522–1535.
214. Sherman RA, Matera JJ, Novik L, et al. Recirculation reassessed: the impact of blood flow rate and the low-flow method reevaluated. *Am J Kidney Dis* 1994;23:846–848.
215. Depner TA, Greene T, Daugirdas JT, et al. Dialyzer performance in the HEMO Study: in vivo K0A and true blood flow determined from a model of cross-dialyzer urea extraction. *ASAIO J* 2004;50(1):85–93.
216. Leypoldt JK, Cheung AK, Agodoa LY, et al. Hemodialyzer mass transfer-area coefficients for urea increase at high dialysate flow rates. The Hemodialysis (HEMO) Study. *Kidney Int* 1997;51(6):2013–2017.
217. Leypoldt JK, Kamerath CD, Gilson JF, et al. Dialyzer clearances and mass transfer-area coefficients for small solutes at low dialysate flow rates. *ASAIO J* 2006;52(4):404–409.
218. Depner TA. Pitfalls in quantitating hemodialysis. *Semin Dial* 1993;6:127–133.
219. Depner TA, Rizwan S, Stasi TA. Pressure effects on roller pump blood flow during hemodialysis. *ASAIO J* 1990;36:M456–M459.
220. Gotch FA, Keen ML. Care of the patient on hemodialysis. In: Cogan MG, Garovoy MR, eds. *Introduction to Dialysis*. New York, NY: Churchill Livingstone, 1985:73–143.

CHAPTER 6

Hemodialysis Adequacy and the Timing of Dialysis Initiation

Sharmeela Saha and Jay B. Wish

Since the advent of chronic renal replacement therapy in the 1960s, nephrologists have investigated various means of determining the appropriate delivery of dialysis. A review of the relevant literature reveals a considerable evolution during this period, and a discernible trend toward a consensus on what parameters determine adequacy continues to emerge. The concept of adequate dialysis has shifted from the minimum amount of dialysis needed to sustain life into a more complete expression of the amount of dialysis that will be beneficial for optimal patient survival while balancing available resources for maximal efficiency. Hence, adequate dialysis is now closer to "optimal dialysis."

Despite this increase in the overall size of the end-stage kidney disease (ESKD) population, there has been a markedly slower increase in the number of nephrologists (1). With this imbalance in the number patients to physicians, as well as the financial constraints related to the provision of dialysis therapy, it is necessary to define just what constitutes "adequate" dialysis therapy in order to streamline therapies and establish appropriate clinical guidelines for practice. At the end of 2012, there were 636,905 patients in the United States receiving treatment for ESKD, and over 450,000 of these patients were being treated with dialysis, whereas 186,303 had a functioning kidney transplant; 88,638 ESKD patients died during the year (2,3). Adjusted rates of all-cause mortality are 6.1 to 7.8 times greater for dialysis patients than for individuals in the general age–matched Medicare population. Mortality rates rise with age, reaching 287 per 1,000 patient-years for dialysis patients aged 65 and older, as compared to 62.3 for transplant patients and 47.4 for the general Medicare population of the same age (3).

Costs of dialysis treatments have continued to rise. Health care expenditures on the dialysis population are significant. Among hemodialysis patients prevalent in 2012, 35.2% of discharges from an all-cause hospitalization were followed by a rehospitalization within 30 days, and total Medicare paid claims in 2012 were $28.6 billion (3). Payers, including the Centers for Medicare and Medicaid Services (CMS) and private insurers, are increasingly demanding the demonstration of cost-effective care as a primary criterion in contracting with health care providers such as dialysis facilities. The quality of care provided continues to be a source of scrutiny and economic strain. A pivotal aspect of the quality of this care is the "adequacy" of dialysis provided.

Beginning in the early 1970s, with the implementation of "Medicare entitlement" relating to payment for dialysis services, CMS has systematically collected facility-specific data regarding the provision of dialysis care. To assist in the collection and monitoring of this patient-specific information, 18 regional ESKD networks were created. One goal of these networks is to establish an oversight system for the provision of dialysis care. Since 1991, the ESKD networks have also been involved in *Continuous Quality Improvement* (CQI) projects. Such activities allow individual providers within each network to examine their own practices, define areas for improvement, and develop plans to address the barriers to improvement. One such CQI initiative has been the monitoring and improvement in the adequacy of hemodialysis treatment.

This chapter reviews the key literature in an attempt to define adequate dialysis: how to prescribe it, how to deliver it, how to monitor it, and how to incorporate it into a cycle of CQI to achieve better patient outcomes. This discussion may touch on many aspects of hemodialysis that impact on adequacy, including membrane characteristics, dialysis modality selection, dialysate composition, intradialytic events, vascular assess function, and other important topics that are discussed in better detail elsewhere in this book.

After more than 50 years of providing dialysis therapy, our understanding of hemodialysis adequacy is still evolving. Nephrologists, health care payers, nephrology journals, national collaborative meetings and research funders such as the National Institutes of Health (NIH) continue to devote significant attention and resources to this subject. While the results of clinical trials and observational studies provide a framework for our understanding of the goals of dialytic therapy, ongoing basic and clinical investigations as well as monitoring of dialysis registries will undoubtedly lead to refinement of practice guidelines for prescribing and monitoring hemodialysis adequacy.

HISTORICAL PERSPECTIVE

Until 1974, nephrologists frequently prescribed hemodialysis regimens based on clinical judgment, often paying more attention to fluid balance than to the need to remove metabolic waste products. Amelioration of uremic signs and symptoms was the goal of the latter, but this was invariably subjective. The pathogenesis of the uremic syndrome was not clearly understood, although the paradigm that dialysis clears the blood of a responsible metabolic waste product(s) provided the framework of therapy (4). Multiple toxins have been proposed (**TABLE 6.1**) (5,6), some being linked to specific manifestations of the uremic syndrome; yet, the correlation of uremic symptoms to blood levels of these substances has not been clearly demonstrated. Even today, the true nature of the uremic syndrome remains incompletely understood.

Although it is inherently not a very toxic molecule (7), urea, a 60-Da solute widely distributed in total body water, has been used as the surrogate for other uremic toxins because of its size, abundance, ease of measurement, and dialyzability. This has often led to confusion by nephrologists and non-nephrologists, believing that the blood urea nitrogen (BUN) level causes uremic signs and symptoms and that dialysis is essential for BUN levels above 100 mg/dL. Historically, the clearance of urea has formed the cornerstone of measuring the efficacy and, by inference, the adequacy of dialysis therapy.

Poor outcomes, despite intensive dialysis treatments and "adequate" urea removal, led researchers familiar with solute kinetics to theorize that larger molecules with molecular weights of 500 to 5,000 Da, "middle molecules," may be responsible for the uremic syndrome (8). The smaller pores of standard cellulosic membranes of the 1960s and 1970s were able to clear urea, but urea clearance often failed to accurately predict patient outcomes. Despite the removal of urea by these membranes, many patients continued to experience symptoms attributable to the lack of removal of some undefined toxic metabolite (9,10). Furthermore, peritoneal dialysis (PD) patients seemed to fare better than hemodialysis patients despite increased levels of BUN and, by inference, less dialysis. This was ascribed to the larger pore size of the peritoneal membrane as compared to cellulosic hemodialysis membranes and the removal of some larger, ill-defined, middle molecule(s). These observations evolved into what is now known as the *middle molecule hypothesis* (8,11).

In 1974 under the guidance of the NIH, a consensus conference was held to discuss the nature of the uremic syndrome, as well the development of a clinically useful and meaningful marker of dialysis therapy. During this conference, various aspects of dialysis care were examined including the nature and pathogenesis of the uremic syndrome, quantification of dialysis therapy, nutritional status, renal osteodystrophy, as well as several other abnormalities commonly observed in hemodialysis patients.

The stage was set to test whether the clearance of urea or the as-yet-unidentified middle molecule correlated better with outcomes in hemodialysis patients. With the sponsorship of the

TABLE 6.1	Uremic Solutes with Potential Toxicity
Urea	Middle molecules
Guanidines	Ammonia
Methylguanidine	Alkaloids
Guanidine	Trace metals
β-Guanidinopropionic acid	Uric acid
Guanidinosuccinic acid	Cyclic AMP
γ-Guanidinobutyric acid	Amino acids
Taurocyamine	Myoinositol
Creatinine	Mannitol
Creatine	Oxalate
Arginic acid	Glucuronate
Homoarginine	Glycols
N-α-acetylarginine	Lysozyme
Phenols	Hormones
O-cresol	Parathormone
P-cresol	Natriuretic factor
Benzyl alcohol	Glucagon
Phenol	Growth hormone
Tyrosine	Gastrin
Phenolic acids	Xanthine
P-hydroxyphenylacetic acid	Hypoxanthine
β-(m-hydroxyphenyl)-hydracrilic acid	Furanpropionic acid
Hippurates	Amines
P-(OH) hippuric acid	Putrescine
O-(OH) hippuric acid	Spermine
Hippuric acid	Spermidine
Benzoates	Dimethylamine
Polypeptides	Polyamines
β$_2$-Microglobulin	Endorphins
Indoles	Pseudouridine
Indol-3-acetic acid	Potassium
Indoxy sulfate	Phosphorus
5-Hydroxyindol acetic acid	Calcium
Indol-3-acrylic acid	Sodium
5-Hydroxytryptophol	Water
N-acetyltryptophan	Cyanides
Tryptophan	

AMP, adenosine monophosphate.
Adapted from Vanholder RC, Ringoir SM. Adequacy of dialysis: a critical analysis. *Kidney Int* 1992;42:540–558.

NIH, a multicenter prospective randomized study was designed and implemented to target BUN levels by varying dialysate and blood flows while affecting the clearance of hypothetical middle molecules by varying the dialysis duration. This landmark study is known as the *National Cooperative Dialysis Study* (NCDS) (12–14).

National Cooperative Dialysis Study

A total of 160 patients were randomized into four groups, with each group targeting either a low or high BUN level (50 mg/dL vs. 100 mg/dL average) measured over a time-averaged period ["time-averaged concentration (TAC) urea"] and a short or long dialysis time (3 ± 0.5 hours vs. 4.5 to 5.0 hours). After a follow-up

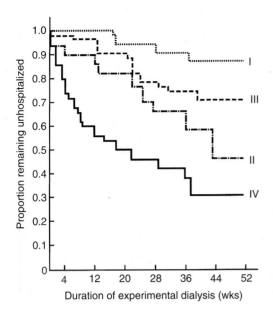

FIGURE 6.1 Proportion of patients in the NCDS remaining unhospitalized, shown as a function of time in the four study groups. The proportion was lower in the high-BUN groups (II and IV) than in the low-BUN groups (I and III). (Reprinted with permission from Lowrie EG, Laird NM, Parker TF, et al. Effect of hemodialysis prescription on patient morbidity: report from the National Cooperative Dialysis Study. *N Engl J Med* 1981;305:1176–1181.)

of 6 months, medical dropouts and hospitalization rates were measured. Subsequently, 12-month mortality rates were measured in follow-up studies (12–14). The results demonstrated that patients dialyzed with high BUNs and short times clearly had poor outcomes, with up to a 70% hospitalization rate (**FIGURE 6.1**) (15). Overall, this initial analysis of the data suggested that BUN was the major factor leading to morbidity. As a result of the findings of this study, for several years after the publication of this study, many nephrologists focused on control of BUN and did not consider the dose of dialysis when prescribing and delivering dialysis therapy (16).

Despite a number of aspects of the NCDS that persist as controversial, it was the largest multicenter trial for determining dialysis adequacy prior to the Hemodialysis (HEMO) study. Its enduring lesson, which was not learned until subsequent analyses of the NCDS data were published over several years following the study, is that quantifying and providing an adequate delivered dose of dialysis is of utmost importance for a positive impact on outcome. The NCDS also validated the importance of small molecule clearance, which forms the basis of current standards of adequacy (17).

The enormous contribution of the NCDS and its subsequent reanalysis to the current thinking regarding hemodialysis therapy cannot be overstated. Several weaknesses of the NCDS, however, preclude our applying the results universally into clinical practice. These issues point out the need for caution in the interpretation of the NCDS results, and a review of these should help place the study in proper perspective.

Age of the National Cooperative Dialysis Study Cohort

The NCDS study population had an average age range of 18 to 70 years with a mean age of 51 ± 12.9 years (12–14). The dialysis population has since grown older, and the elderly population have

different causes of ESKD (18), have varied and more comorbid conditions (19), and have been shown to die sooner regardless of dialysis prescription (20). In fact, after a mean age of 59 years, each year of advancing age has been associated with an approximately 3% increase in the odds ratio for death (20). Elderly patients generally have poorer nutrition, less opportunity for social rehabilitation, and less physical activity. They also have a greater chance of being demented and unable to influence their own treatment, let alone follow prescribed therapy (21,22). All of these factors highlight the changing demographics of the "typical" American dialysis patient and limit the application of the NCDS in determining how to dialyze an aging population.

Comorbid Conditions

Patients who had advanced atherosclerotic cardiovascular disease, pulmonary disease, recurrent infections, cancer, or other significant comorbid conditions were excluded from the NCDS to achieve the expected follow-up period of 1 to 3 years (12–14). However, comorbidity with multiple conditions has increased among patients with ESKD from 1976 to the present (23). Interestingly, a survey of the primary causes of death of dialysis patients highlights cardiovascular disease as the leading cause of death among dialysis patients. Internationally, this pattern of acceptance of older patients with increasing numbers and severity of comorbid illness also holds true (24). Thus, the application of the NCDS data to patients with multiple comorbidities is questionable.

Diabetes Mellitus

Patients with diabetes were excluded from the NCDS. Diabetic nephropathy is the single most common cause of ESKD in the United States (25). The effect of diabetes on survival has been suggested in a report by Collins et al. (19), where higher doses of dialysis may be beneficial in diabetic patients. The application of the NCDS data to a diabetic population is limited.

Duration of Dialysis

The patients entering the NCDS had a mean duration of dialysis of 4.3 hours, while the range studied was 2.5 to 5.5 hours (12–14). There are no data points below 2.5 hours and few data points below 3 hours. As a result of the NCDS findings, duration of dialysis was not considered as important as the BUN. In response to this, manufacturers of dialysis membranes began developing ways to achieve better urea clearance with shorter dialysis duration, as the dialysis facilities preferred to treat more patients for shorter time periods to maximize the efficiency of the facility and personnel (25,26).

It is predictable that as time for diffusion (i.e., dialysis) is shortened, there will be a point at which highly diffusible substances such as urea cease to predict adequate removal of other uremic waste products and an increase in morbidity, if not mortality, may result. Consequently, the role of duration of dialysis as an independent determinant of adequacy is being revisited. Studies have demonstrated a decreased survival in patients with dialysis time shorter than 3.5 hours (26,27). The NCDS data also revealed a trend toward increased morbidity with shorter dialysis times, although it was not as strong a correlation as with high BUN levels (15).

While the NCDS data do not address how to weigh the independent effect of dialysis duration in setting of current high-efficiency and high-flux dialysis membrane technology, observational outcomes have demonstrated the independence of dialysis treatment duration as a predictor of improved mortality rates. In fact, a few dialysis cohort studies have demonstrated that treatment time and dialysis dose are independent predictors of survival. In an Australian and New Zealand cohort, a dialysis time of 4.5 to 5 hours together with a Kt/V (a measure of dialysis dose, see subsequent text) of 1.3 to 1.4 was associated with better overall survival (28). Based on the lack of a statistical interaction between dialysis dose (Kt/V) and session length, the authors further suggest that the optimal "dialysis dose" may be a combination of a Kt/V of more than 1.3 and a treatment time greater than or equal to 4.5 hours, although they do concede that the retrospective nature of their patient cohort limits their ability to imply causation. The association between these "standard" doses of dialysis combined with a longer individual treatment has also been demonstrated by Saran et al. (29) in a large multinational observational cohort of patients. Importantly though, this analysis clearly demonstrated a mathematical interaction between higher Kt/V and longer session length and further demonstrated that an ultrafiltration rate greater than 10 mL/kg/h was associated with higher risk of both intradialytic hypotension and, more importantly, short-term patient mortality (29). On the other extreme of duration of dialysis treatment, the Centre de Rein Artificiel in Tassin, France, has reported excellent 10-year survival rates, as well as unparalleled anemia and hypertension control in their patient population. The directors of this unit attribute their success primarily to the technique of prolonged daily dialysis treatments (30,31). This form of dialysis therapy, so-called prolonged hemodialysis (PHD), does offer several documented advantages to the prevalent form of in-center, three times per week therapy practiced in the United States. However, the findings of the HEMO study (discussed in further detail in subsequent text) point out that simply increasing the delivered dose of dialysis may not lead to improved outcomes among hemodialysis patients (32). As a modification of daily therapy, the same group from Tassin has proposed thrice-weekly long nocturnal dialysis as a form of therapy that may be more acceptable to a larger number of patients with potentially equivalent outcomes (33). Therefore, in order to achieve patient outcomes similar to those in Tassin, what may be required is a fundamental rethinking of how to deliver dialysis therapy and whether treatment settings other than "in-center" would facilitate improved patient outcomes.

Dialyzer Membrane

The NCDS was performed using purely cellulosic membranes that have been replaced with newer, large-pore, high-flux, and more biocompatible membranes. Applicability of dialysis prescription in the NCDS to current synthetic membranes may be limited.

Quantity of Dialysis

The retrospectively computed dialysis dose (Kt/V, to be discussed later in this chapter) for the NCDS cohort in groups I and III, with target BUN levels of 50 mg/dL on average, was between 0.9 and 1.3 (12). Given that no groups in the NCDS received a greater dialysis dose, it is difficult to determine from the NCDS alone whether this dose is adequate, and impossible to determine whether this dose is optimal.

In another study using urea reduction ratio (URR) to quantify dialysis dose, it was demonstrated that patients receiving a URR of 60% or more had a lower mortality than patients receiving the NCDS URR of 50% or more (20). The HEMO study confirmed that doses of dialysis significantly greater [a single-pool Kt/V (SKt/V) of 1.71] than those currently recommended by the National Kidney

Foundation's Kidney Disease Outcomes Quality Initiative (NKF-KDOQI) guideline (i.e., a single pool or spKt/V of 1.2) failed to provide additional survival benefit in a representative group of hemodialysis patients on a three times per week treatment regimen. Specifically what was shown in the HEMO study was that with a "standard dose" of dialysis (achieved spKt/V of 1.32), the overall mortality was 17.1%. In the "high-dose" group (achieved spKt/V of 1.71), the mortality was 16.2%, a nonsignificant difference. Reviewing these findings, it is notable that these excellent clearance rates were achieved with mean dialysis times of 190 ± 23 minutes (standard dose) and 219 ± 23 minutes (high-dose group) (34). This finding speaks to the ability of modern dialysis technology to deliver adequate clearance of small molecules with only a modest increase in dialysis time.

Duration of the Study

The patients in the NCDS were studied for approximately 48 weeks, and most of the data were analyzed at 26 weeks (12). This may not have been enough longitudinal follow-up (19), especially as mortality actually increased approximately 1 year after the study was terminated (27,35). The report by Eknoyan et al. (34) from the HEMO study suggests that in a subgroup of female patients, a higher dose of dialysis may lead to a decrease in the risk of death and hospitalization, but this benefit of increased dose of dialysis did not appear for almost 3 years. Also in a separate subgroup of patients who had been on dialysis greater than 3.5 years at the start of the trial, the use of a high-flux dialysis filter appeared to reduce the risk of death (32,36). Also in the NCDS era, techniques such as ultrafiltration control, bicarbonate dialysate, and variable dialysate sodium programming were not in widespread use. Furthermore, the NCDS outcome measured was morbidity, not mortality (15), as is more commonly used in contemporary studies.

Nutrition

Notwithstanding the previously held misconception that a low BUN is always good, it was shown in the NCDS that the protein catabolic rate (PCR), which is computed to represent dietary protein intake, is a strong and independent predictor of poor outcome (13). This became evident despite the NCDS protocol, which was designed to provide patients with a constant protein intake of 1.1 ± 0.3 g/d/kg body weight. In the final analysis, the actual PCR range was more in the range of 0.6 to 1.5 g/d/kg body weight. Within this range, a strong negative correlation between the PCR and probability of failure (i.e., morbidity such as hospitalization) became evident, as demonstrated graphically in **FIGURE 6.2**. This relationship of increasing probability of failure, with declines in PCR, held true irrespective of randomization to the low BUN (50 mg/dL) or long duration (4.5 hours) dialysis groups. **FIGURE 6.2** shows how patients with very low PCR (0.6 g/d/kg body weight) will have at least a 35% probability of failure despite 4.5-hour dialysis treatment and a low (40 mg/dL) TAC urea. Conversely, a patient with a high PCR (1.2 g/d/kg body weight) will have less than a 15% probability of failure, even with a higher TAC urea of 60 mg/dL and the same dialysis duration.

Subsequent studies have demonstrated how nutrition affects survival in dialysis patients when serum albumin is used as a marker for prognosis. Lowrie (37) reported this with his National Medical Care [now Fresenius Medical Care (FMC)] database in 1990 and again in 1994 (38), which demonstrated a marked increase in mortality as the serum albumin falls. This albumin–mortality

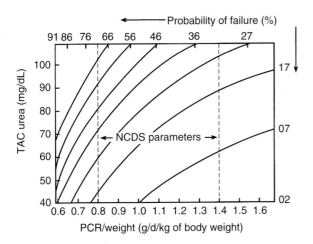

FIGURE 6.2 A comparison of time-averaged concentration (TAC) urea, protein catabolic rate (PCR), and probability of mortality for 4.5-hour dialysis in the NCDS. [Reprinted with permission from Lowrie EG, Laird NM, et al. The National Dialysis Cooperative Study. *Kidney Int* 1983;23(Suppl 13):S1–S122.]

relationship has also been noted by Owen et al. in 1993 (20), as well as several other authors.

Several authors and investigators have given increasing attention to the role that overall nutritional status plays in the survival of dialysis patients, as well as the relationship between adequacy of dialysis, nutritional status, and patient survival. Specifically, in a secondary analysis of the HEMO study, poor nutritional status predicted a high risk for mortality regardless of the targeted (or achieved) dialysis adequacy. In addition to albumin levels, other biochemical indices such as serum creatinine, total cholesterol, anthropometry [i.e., a low body mass index (BMI)] and Karnofsky functional index were each independently associated with higher risk for death. The association of most of these markers with outcome was nonlinear; with the risk of mortality increasing more steeply at lower levels, suggesting that as dialysis patients become progressively malnourished, the risk of short-term mortality escalates. Consistent with these reports, Chertow et al. (39) showed that decreasing serum prealbumin level is associated with all-cause hospitalization and increased mortality independent of dialysis dose. These findings reinforce the need for longitudinally monitoring both nutritional status and adequacy of therapy in all dialysis patients.

Another aspect of this nutrition–mortality relationship that has been explored by Chertow et al. (40) is the complexity of the relationship between dialysis dose, as measured by urea removal, and mortality. One of the most important aspects of the NCDS study came not from the study itself but rather from a reanalysis of the data several years later by Gotch and Sargent (12). In this mechanistic analysis of the data, a method of quantifying dialysis treatment by means of a dynamic rather than the static measure of urea removal was developed and verified as a valid measure of dialysis dose. However, even with the use of this dynamic measure, a complex relationship between dialysis dose and mortality is evident. Subsequently, several authors have independently noted a "reverse J"–shaped relationship between the dose of hemodialysis, as measured by either URR, or Kt/V (both terms are defined in subsequent text). What is meant by "reverse J" is that with both extreme low and high values of urea removal, as measured by URR

or Kt/V, there is an unexpected increase in the relative mortality of patients (41,42).

This complexity of the dose–mortality relationship has led some authors to propose that urea distribution volume, V, is a surrogate marker for nutritional fitness. As such, urea distribution volume may possess survival characteristics of its own (40,43–45). Technologic advances have also allowed for the continuous and near instantaneous measurement of ionic or online dialysis clearance and the calculation of a "real-time" Kt/V (46). The advantages of this method include no requirement for blood sampling and that it can be used with each dialysis treatment to predict the delivered Kt/V in real time before the treatment is finished. Among the disadvantages of this technique, however, is that in order to calculate Kt/V, time on dialysis and V must be determined accurately. The latter is a potential problem if anthropometric formulas are used to estimate V because these formulas are estimates that often differ significantly from the true value. Based on these potential shortcomings as well as the lack of outcomes data using this technique, most guidelines for adequacy continue to recommend blood side monitoring of dialysis dose.

The fine balance between trying to delay progression of kidney disease versus inducing malnutrition and the consequent adverse effects on mortality has created substantial confusion and variation in clinical practice, especially with regard to the appropriate timing of initiation of chronic dialysis therapy. Although the Modification of Diet in Renal Disease (MDRD) study (47) had provided some support for the hypothesis that dietary protein restriction slows the progression of kidney disease, studies have raised concern regarding the effects of pre-ESKD dietary protein restriction on patient mortality after ESKD supervenes. Kopple et al. (48) have concluded that 0.8 g/d/kg body weight of protein is safe for at least 2 to 3 years but recommend that additional indices of nutritional status such as serum transferrin, body weight, urine creatinine, and caloric intake be monitored regularly. The NIH Consensus in 1994 (49) recommended an initial diet of 0.7 to 0.8 g/d/kg body weight in pre-ESKD patients but cautioned to regularly assess for signs of malnutrition. Should such signs become evident, an increase of protein intake to 1 to 1.2 g/d/kg body weight as well as increased caloric intake is recommended. It is notable that decline in protein and energy intake and in indices of nutritional status have been documented in patients with a glomerular filtration rate (GFR) below about 50 mL/min when ingesting uncontrolled diets, suggesting that prescription of this level of protein restriction outside of a clinical trials setting may lead to ingestion of inadequate energy and insufficient protein. Lowrie and Lew (37) have demonstrated a strong correlation between higher serum creatinine levels and improved survival in hemodialysis patients, reflecting better muscle mass, which is likely a marker for nutritional status and may be independent of dialysis dose. All these studies compliment the NCDS and are reflections of the changing emphasis on nutrition in dialysis patients (50–53).

The earlier-noted controversy is further compounded when chronic kidney disease (CKD) patients progress to ESKD and are confronted by a multitude of factors affecting nutrition, such as anorexia due to uremia or underdialysis, the inconvenience of thrice-weekly dialysis schedules, comorbid conditions such as diabetic gastroparesis, hormonal factors, depression, and frequent hospitalizations (54). Indeed, more than one-third of dialysis patients report a poor or very poor appetite, and low self-reported appetite is associated with lower dietary energy and protein intakes, poorer nutritional status, higher comorbidity, and lower quality of life. Secondary analysis of the HEMO study indicated that low self-reported appetite is independently associated with increased hospitalizations, but the association of appetite with death in this study was confounded by comorbidity (55,56). In addition, depression is believed to be the most common psychiatric disorder in patients with ESKD, with previous studies reporting up to 25% of prevalent dialysis patients having a Beck Depression Inventory score in the moderate range of depression (57). Given the prevalence and associations between depression, treatment adherence, malnutrition, and mortality, it is clear that screening for mental health issues is an important part of the care of dialysis patients.

TIMING OF DIALYSIS INITIATION

In 2012, over 90% of new patients (98,954) began ESKD therapy with hemodialysis, 9,175 with PD, and 2,803 received a preemptive kidney transplant (these data exclude patients with missing demographic information). Use of PD and preemptive kidney transplant were relatively more common in younger age groups. Use of home dialysis therapies among incident ESKD patients has increased notably in recent years (3).

The appropriate timing of initiation of chronic dialysis therapy is also closely tied to nutritional markers in dialysis patients. This relationship has been demonstrated in a number of observational studies in which spontaneous dietary protein restriction was observed with declining GFRs (58,59). Concern regarding the long-term consequences of such dietary restriction as well as the long-term effects of long-standing uremic toxicity has prompted several groups to investigate the appropriate timing of initiation of dialysis therapy. Initially, multiple investigators showed that earlier initiation of dialysis therapy led to prolonged duration of life, increased potential for rehabilitation, and decreases in hospitalization (60–62). The Canada–United States of America (CANUSA) study likewise showed that for patients with weekly creatinine clearances less than 38 L/wk, 12- and 24-month survival was 82% and 74%, respectively. However, in a group of patients with creatinine clearance greater than 38 L/wk, 94.7% of patients survived 12 months and 90.8% of patients survived 24 months (63). While the CANUSA results demonstrate the survival benefit of residual renal function among PD patients, the role of diuretics and residual renal function was investigated among an international cohort of subjects through the Dialysis Outcomes and Practice Patterns Study (DOPPS). In this cohort of subjects, both diuretic use and residual renal function were positively associated with improvements in all-cause as well as cardiac mortality, potentially related to lower interdialytic weight gain and a reduced incidence of intradialytic hypotension. Other authors have postulated, however, that the benefits of residual renal function may be related to improved clearance of uremic toxins with a molecular weight higher than urea and other "small uremic molecules" (64,65). Prompted by these studies, as well as expert opinion, the NKF-KDOQI guidelines advise the initiation of dialysis therapy of some type when the weekly kidney (residual) Kt/V falls below a level of 2.0 (an approximate creatinine clearance of 9 to 14 mL/min/1.73 m^2). Clinical considerations that dialysis may not need to be imminently initiated were (a) stable or increasing edema-free body weight or (b) complete absence of clinical signs or symptoms attributable to uremia (66).

Despite these convincing arguments that earlier initiation of dialysis leads to improvements in patient outcomes, the relationship is still debated. The DOPPS, which compares a large cohort of American dialysis patients to groups of patients from Europe (France, Germany, Great Britain, Italy, Spain) and Japan, has shown that despite earlier initiation of dialysis among the American cohort of patients, the survival of this group of patients was actually worse than those of Europe and Japan. Even after consideration of potential confounding factors such as coexistent comorbidities and nutritional status as measured by serum albumin level, this increase in mortality persisted (67). The Netherlands Cooperative Study on the Adequacy of Dialysis phase-2 (NECOSAD-2) is a large multicenter study in the Netherlands. In this prospective analysis, patient's health-related quality of life (HRQOL) was measured by means of the Kidney Disease and Quality of Life Short Form repeatedly over the first year of dialysis therapy. Of 237 patients who had measurements of residual renal function measured between 0 and 4 weeks prior to the initiation of dialysis therapy, 38% were classified as late starters based on the NKF-KDOQI guidelines. At baseline, the HRQOL for this group of patients was statistically lower in the realms of physical role functioning, bodily pain, and vitality than those patients who initiated timely dialysis per the NKF-KDOQI guidelines. However, after a follow-up of 12 months, the differences among groups disappeared (68). Another study examined the effects of lead-time bias in perceived increased longevity with an earlier start of dialysis, that is, a perceived prolongation of survival due to longer monitoring of those patients who initiated dialysis at an earlier time in their disease process. In order to overcome the potential effects of lead-time bias, these authors assembled their cohort of patients on the basis of a residual creatinine clearance of 20 mL/min. Early and late start of hemodialysis was defined by a creatinine clearance cutoff of 8.0 mL/min. This analysis clearly showed that lead-time bias is a real phenomenon in dialysis patients and that by monitoring patients from a defined starting point that predates the initiation of dialysis, there was no difference in 10-year survival among the two groups of patients (69). Together, these studies underscore the need to individualize the timing of initiation of chronic dialysis therapy.

Initiating Dialysis Early and Late Study

Another trial examining the relationship of the timing of dialysis initiation is the Initiating Dialysis Early and Late (IDEAL) study. Published in August 2010, the IDEAL study was a randomized controlled trial of early versus late initiation of dialysis (70). Thirty-two centers in Australia and New Zealand examined whether the timing of maintenance dialysis initiation influenced survival in patients with CKD. Patients at least 18 years old with progressive CKD and an estimated glomerular filtration rate (eGFR) between 10.0 and 15.0 mL/min/1.73 m^2 of body surface area (BSA) (calculated with the use of the Cockcroft–Gault equation) were randomly assigned to planned initiation of dialysis when the eGFR was 10.0 to 14.0 mL/min (early start) or when the eGFR was 5.0 to 7.0 mL/min (late start). Between July 2000 and November 2008, 828 patients underwent randomization, and the mean age was 60.4 years. The primary outcome was death from any cause. Important to note that 75.9% of the patients in the late-start group initiated dialysis when the eGFR was above the target of 7.0 mL/min due to the development of symptoms. The decision to start was at the discretion of the patient's nephrologist. The mean duration of follow-up was 3.64 years in the early-start group as compared to 3.57 years in the late-start group.

The study found that early initiation was not associated with an improvement in survival, the primary outcome, or in several secondary clinical outcomes such as cardiovascular or infectious events. The median time from randomization to initiation of dialysis was 1.8 months in the early-start group and 7.40 months in the late-start group. The mean eGFR, using Cockcroft–Gault equation, was 12.0 mL/min in the early-start group and 9.8 mL/min in the late-start group. In the early-start group, 18.6% started dialysis with eGFR of less than 10.0 mL/min. This population was also unique when compared to the dialysis patients in the United States because PD was the initial method in 195 patients in the early-start group and 171 patients in the late-start group. Baseline characteristics were similar between the early- and late-start groups. The authors conclude that early initiation of dialysis had no significant effect on the rate of death or on the secondary clinical outcomes. Although there was only a 2.2 mL/min difference in actual achieved eGFR in the study, there was a 6-month time difference in time to dialysis initiation between the two groups, and 6 months off hemodialysis is a recognizable opportunity as well as a substantial financial cost savings without a change in survival.

A 6-month delay in initiation of dialysis seems beneficial, but one has to acknowledge that patients need to be very carefully monitored in the interim. The previously cited NECOSAD study clearly shows that HRQOL at the time of initiation of dialysis is significantly lower in those patients who are maintained off of dialysis therapy. Given this and the often subtle symptoms of uremic toxicity, patients with impending dialysis needs will require close monitoring in order to avoid untoward effects of uremia and to make the transition to dialysis therapy as smooth as possible. The decision when to initiate renal replacement therapy should be based on the patient's overall clinical status, not just the GFR, but when the GFR falls below 15 mL/min, the patient should be followed even more closely for signs and symptoms of uremia, and placement of dialysis vascular access for those choosing hemodialysis should certainly be completed at that level of kidney function.

There is not a consensus regarding the modality with which to initiate renal replacement therapy. In an article by Kalantar-Zadeh et al. (71) published in 2014, the authors propose further investigation to compare twice-weekly hemodialysis versus thrice-weekly hemodialysis in the initiation of renal replacement therapy in patients with ESKD. It is well established that mortality in incident dialysis patients and that the loss of residual renal function is higher in patients on hemodialysis therapy than PD. Erythropoiesis-stimulating agent (ESA) use is higher as well during the first months of dialysis therapy. In the Frequent Hemodialysis Network (FHN) nocturnal trial, there was a more rapid loss of residual renal function in the nocturnal hemodialysis group compared to the standard group (72). In a Taiwanese study, patients on twice-weekly hemodialysis had a slower decline in residual renal function as compared to the thrice-weekly group (73). To date, there are no randomized controlled trials to evaluate if there is a survival advantage with twice-weekly dialysis at initiation. A major confounder in the past in retrospective analyses has been insufficient data regarding baseline and/or subsequent residual renal function. The impetus for twice-weekly dialysis may include theoretical preservation of residual renal function, less frequent cannulations, and possibly complications of arteriovenous access as well as patient quality of life with less time spent on dialysis. However, some concerns include prolonging the interdialytic interval, which may increase the incidence of hyperkalemia, volume overload, and sudden death. In their 2014 publication, Kalantar-Zadeh et al. (71) have proposed 10 criteria including, but not limited to, urine output greater than 500 mL/day, potassium usually less than 5.5 mg/dL, phosphorus commonly

below 5.5 mg/dL, and hemoglobin greater than 8 g/dL to ascertain eligible candidates for twice-weekly hemodialysis therapy. They do not specify a particular GFR among the designated 10 criteria. The residual renal function needs to be reassessed monthly along with typical hemodialysis adequacy parameters. The validity of these proposals should be tested in clinical trials. These authors also advocate PD first before hemodialysis, highlighting the benefit of preservation of residual renal function (71).

The choice of an incremental dialysis prescription will require periodic measurement of urine output and endogenous kidney function, which can be an eGFR based on the average of creatinine and urea clearances on an interdialytic urine collection, or a weekly Kt/V for urea based on the predialysis BUN. The dialysis dose will need to be increased as endogenous kidney function inevitably declines. Because hemodialysis is an intermittent therapy compared to the continuous nature of residual renal function, the dialysis Kt/V cannot be simply added to the endogenous Kt/V to obtain the total weekly Kt/V as can be done for PD patients. The use of an "equivalent" Kt/V transformation is required, which is also required to calculate the "equivalent" Kt/V of hemodialysis therapies administered more or less frequently than three times per week. In this context, it is important to recall that the target Kt/V of greater than 1.2 for hemodialysis applies only to thrice-weekly therapy.

O'Hare et al. (74) have reviewed the epidemiologic trends in the timing and the clinical context of dialysis initiation based on reviewing United States Department of Veterans Affairs data in fiscal years 2000 to 2009 (72). In 2000 to 2004, as compared to 2005 to 2009, the mean eGFR at dialysis start increased from 9.8 ± 5.8 to 11.0 ± 5.5 mL/min/1.73 m^2 ($p <0.001$), and after stratification by illness acuity and a number of symptoms, there was still a significant increase in mean eGFR at initiation over time for all subgroups. The upward trend of eGFR at time of initiation appears to reflect changes in timing of initiation rather than variation in the clinical context or changing indications. The reason for the uptrending eGFR at initiation is unclear, but there are numerous speculations including, but not limited to, the adaptation of more liberal KDOQI guidelines allowing for dialysis initiation at higher levels of eGFR.

Although there are trends and general guidelines, the approach to dialysis initiation must be individualized. Bargman (75) describes an interesting patient interaction which highlights the many nuances of dialysis initiation and modality selection. Effective predialysis education is essential to allow for a smooth transition, and decisions such as whether to even pursue dialysis versus nondialysis supportive care are paramount. In a prospective observational study published in 2015, authors found that elderly patients with advanced CKD managed *via* a nondialysis pathway that included conservative and at times palliative kidney supportive care survived a median of 16 months with a 53% 1-year survival from the time of referral to a kidney supportive care clinic with mean eGFR of 16 mL/min/1.73 m^2 (76).

When dialysis is selected, the initial question should be in-center versus home therapies. Patients who start dialysis in a nonemergent setting may be candidates for incremental dialysis which could mean fewer sessions of hemodialysis per week or fewer hours per session or both; in the realm of PD, this could translate into just a couple of exchanges per day. Incremental dialysis could potentially ease patients into the transition from a patient with CKD to someone who relies on renal replacement therapy. There is potentially a practical benefit to early-start dialysis in that technical aspects such as malfunctioning PD catheters or needle infiltration of a fistula could be addressed in less dire situations than late-start dialysis. It has also been suggested that the institution of PD is associated with a slowing decline of residual renal function (75). The 2015 KDOQI adequacy update suggests that the decision to initiate maintenance dialysis should rely on a clinical assessment of signs and symptoms rather than a certain level of kidney function (17). The time to initiate dialysis is truly a collaborative process among the patient, medical staff, and any caretakers, and the plan of care should be individualized to allow for the best experience.

● DIALYSIS QUANTIFICATION

The most important contribution of the NCDS is the concept that the delivered dose of dialysis can and should be quantified. With urea as the marker for most small molecular weight uremic toxins, the NCDS targeted the dose of dialysis by maintaining a certain TAC urea or midweek predialysis BUN, with the caveat that protein nutrition must be maintained. It is important to note, however, that in this study, which forms the basis for our current measurement and monitoring of hemodialysis therapy, the currently accepted measure of hemodialysis dose, Kt/V, was neither monitored nor was a specific Kt/V "target" measured. Rather, the lasting impact of the NCDS came from a mathematical analysis of the data approximately 5 years after the completion of the study by Gotch and Sargent (12). The conceptual shift that resulted from this analysis moved physicians prescribing dialytic therapies from viewing urea not from a static model (single midweek or averaged blood levels) but from a kinetic model (the change in urea during the course of a hemodialysis procedure). The most familiar kinetic urea model today is Kt/V, which is the paradigm that evolved from analysis of the data consisting of the actual delivered dose of dialysis from the patients in the NCDS (12).

K is the dialyzer urea clearance in milliliters per minute.

t is the time (i.e., duration) of the dialysis therapy in minutes.

V is representative of the volume of distribution of urea (approximately equal to total body water).

This expression attempts to express the dose of dialysis as fractional urea clearance and is analogous to the effects of normal body clearance mechanisms on the blood level of an administered drug.

Measuring the Dose of Hemodialysis

Many methods have been proposed to measure the dose of dialysis a patient receives. The square meter hour hypothesis and dialysis index intended to address this issue (8) but did not take into consideration the volume of distribution of solute (e.g., urea). Teschan in the 1970s proposed a target dialytic clearance of 3,000 mL/wk/L of body water (20). This took into consideration urea distribution volume and, at a regimen of three dialysis treatments per week, a target of 1,000 mL/dialysis/L body water translating to the dialysis index of 1, which was used as the reference point. Certainly, other terms have been devised such as probability of failure in the NCDS (14), URR (20), and, as discussed earlier, the Kt/V (12). The latter two are currently the methods of choice for most institutions. In a large cohort of incident dialysis patients representative of the U.S. hemodialysis population, the overall predictive ability of URR, spKt/V, double pool or equilibrated Kt/V (dpKt/V), and Kt are all essentially the same (77).

Urea Reduction Ratio

The URR is an approximation of the fraction of BUN removed in a single dialysis session. The numerator is the difference between the pre- and postdialysis BUN, and the denominator is the predialysis BUN (**EQUATION 6.1**):

$$\text{URR} = \text{Predialysis BUN} - \text{Postdialysis BUN} \div \quad (6.1)$$
$$\text{Predialysis BUN}$$

The URR has the advantage of simplicity and has been used extensively to measure hemodialysis adequacy in large patient populations, including the FMC data set reported by Lowrie and Lew, (37) Lowrie (38), and Owen et al. (20) and the ESRD Core Indicators Project reported by the Health Care Financing Administration (now the Centers for Medicare & Medicaid Services or CMS) (78).

However, the URR has several very important shortcomings. Most importantly, like the static TAC urea used in the NCDS, the URR cannot be used to assess the patient's nutritional status, which is an independent predictor of outcome perhaps more powerful than the dose of dialysis (20,54). Although URR correlates well with spKt/V in population studies, significant variability in correlation in individual patients occurs because URR fails to include both the contraction in extracellular volume and the urea generation that typically occurs during routine hemodialysis. Despite these shortcomings, however, when outcomes are correlated with either URR or Kt/V, no difference in "predictability" is detectable. The reason for this lack of a better correlation with Kt/V may result from the narrow range of doses achieved during hemodialysis and the curvilinear relationship between the two parameters. When dose of kidney replacement therapy increases, especially when treatment is given daily, URR approaches zero. URR also is zero in continuously dialyzed patients or patients with normal kidney function. Other disadvantages of URR include the inability to adjust the prescription accurately when the value is off target (by adjusting K or t), inability to add the effect of residual kidney function, and inability to troubleshoot by comparing prescribed with delivered dose.

Kt/V

Kt/V has become the preferred method for measuring delivered dialysis dose because it more accurately reflects urea removal than does URR, it can be used to assess the patient's nutritional status by permitting calculation of the normalized protein catabolic rate (nPCR), and it can be used to modify the dialysis prescription for a patient who has residual renal function. The 2015 KDOQI adequacy guideline highlights how to properly obtain the urea Kt/V and advocates a monthly assessment; however, it also mentions that the URR should not be used routinely as it does not incorporate residual renal function nor does it account for the change in urea volume or urea generation during the course of the hemodialysis treatment (17).

Formal Urea Kinetic Modeling

Formal urea kinetic modeling (UKM) is the most accurate method for determining Kt/V and requires the use of a computer capable of solving differential equations to compute the following variables:

V, the volume of distribution of urea, which is approximately equivalent to total body water

K, by extrapolating a K_oA value for the dialyzer that can be applied within a range of blood and dialysate flows

G, the urea generation rate, from which the nPCR can be computed

Once the K and V are determined, one can arithmetically compute the t (time) required to deliver a target Kt/V. For example, if the target Kt/V is 1.4 and formal UKM has determined that K is

250 mL/min and V is 40 L, then the time required to deliver the target Kt/V of 1.4 would be $(40/0.25) \times 1.4 = 224$ minutes.

The use of the formal iterative UKM model of determining V has been shown to be more accurate that anthropomorphic formulas proposed by Hume and Weyers (79) and Watson et al. (80) because these formulas were derived from analysis of healthy individuals and are probably not applicable to patients with ESKD. Chertow et al. (81,82) has developed an ESKD population–specific equation for calculating total body water based on bioelectrical impedance monitoring. Although determination of V by this method, which utilizes several readily available patient-specific anthropometric parameters, is fairly simple, whether or not it leads to significant differences in the ability to predict patient outcomes is subject to speculation.

Daugirdas II

Although formal UKM is preferred by the Renal Physicians Association (RPA) and NKF-KDOQI clinical practice guidelines for the reasons outlined in the preceding text, its computational complexity has been a barrier to its widespread adoption. Many facilities have chosen instead to employ the more user-friendly second-generation natural logarithm formula for Kt/V proposed by Daugirdas (83), commonly known as Daugirdas II, which takes into account urea removed via ultrafiltration as well as urea generation during the dialysis treatment (**EQUATION 6.2**):

$$Kt/V = -\ln (R - 0.008 \times t) + (4 - 3.5 \times R) \times UF / W \quad (6.2)$$

where:

ln is the natural logarithm.
R is the postdialysis BUN/predialysis BUN.
t is the duration of the dialysis session in hours.
UF is the ultrafiltration volume in liters.
W is the patient's postdialysis weight in kilograms.

The Daugirdas II formula has been shown to approximate the formal UKM-derived result over the full range of single-pool, variable-volume Kt/V values (83–85) and has been endorsed by the NKF-KDOQI clinical practice guideline as the dialysis adequacy measurement of choice for providers unable or unwilling to perform formal UKM.

Surface Area Normalized Kt/V

Daugirdas et al. (86) have noted the inconsistency that eGFR is scaled to BSA in millimeters per minute per 1.73 m^2, but adequacy of dialysis is scaled to urea distribution volume (V). Because the V/BSA ratio is higher in men than in women, scaling the dialysis dose based on BSA instead of V would result in relatively higher Kt for women at the same level of V. Because V scales to weight while BSA scales to 0.425 power of weight, scaling the dialysis dose to BSA would also result in relatively higher Kt for smaller patients of either sex. Kt/BSA has been proposed but would require more accurate estimates of Kt than are readily available in most facilities. An alternative proposed by Daugirdas et al. (86) would be to measure Kt/V but then to rescale it to BSA based on a neutral correction when the V calculated by the Watson formula (Vant) (see section "Formal Urea Kinetic Modeling") equals 35 L in males. The net result is that the "surface area normalized" (SAN) Kt/V = Kt/V multiplied by Vant/$(3.271 \times Vant^{2/3})$, and in females, multiplied again by 0.91. For a woman with Vant = 35 L, the target Kt/V would be at least 1.2/0.91 = 1.32. For a man with Vant = 25 L, the target Kt/V would be at least 1.34. The net effect is to increase the

minimum required dialysis dose for smaller patients and women of all body sizes and to decrease the minimum required dialysis dose for larger male patients.

Ramirez et al. (87) discuss dialysis dose scaled to BSA and how the surface area–based dialysis dose results in different dose–mortality relationships than the ubiquitous volume-based dosing and that women and smaller patients may be underdialyzed using volume-based dosing. Daugirdas (88) eloquently discusses the scope of Kt/V and dialysis dosing, again highlighting that limiting calculations to total body water, that is, traditional assessments of volume may result in lower doses of dialysis for women and smaller patients. The predictive value of using SAN Kt/V on patient outcomes has yet to be tested in large populations.

Postdialysis Blood Urea Nitrogen Sampling

A number of technical issues involved in measuring dialysis adequacy have raised a great deal of controversy. The foremost is the timing and methodology for drawing the postdialysis BUN sample. This procedure is particularly important because inconsistency will tend to overestimate the dose of dialysis delivered.

Following the conclusion of a hemodialysis treatment, the BUN precipitously rises due to three factors: vascular access recirculation, cardiopulmonary recirculation, and compartmental disequilibrium (**FIGURE 6.3**) (89).

Vascular Access Recirculation

The first BUN rise after a hemodialysis treatment, which occurs within 10 to 20 seconds, is due to vascular access recirculation, if present. Vascular access recirculation occurs when the blood-flow rate through the extracorporeal circuit exceeds the arterial blood flow into the access, making the retrograde flow of blood back through the arterial circuit inevitable. Access recirculation is often the result of downstream venous stenoses at the prosthetic graft venous anastomosis or the subclavian vein.

The effects of access recirculation on the postdialysis BUN disappear within 10 to 20 seconds of the conclusion of the hemodialysis treatment. The importance of access recirculation and improper postdialysis blood drawing technique in the overestimation of dialysis adequacy has been demonstrated in a study of patients with

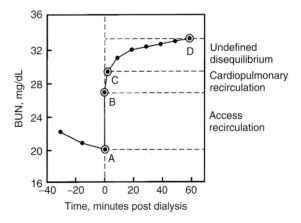

FIGURE 6.3 A typical example of urea rebound, with over half secondary to access recirculation (A, B), 15% from cardiopulmonary recirculation (B, C), and the remainder due to the resolution of perfusion and/or compartmental disequilibrium. (Reprinted with permission from Depner T. Assessing the adequacy of hemodialysis: urea modeling. *Kidney Int* 1994;45:1522–1535.)

well-functioning peripheral access, in which deliberately failing to follow a "slow flow" sampling technique was associated with an overestimation of dialysis adequacy of up to 40% (90). However, if the blood pump is turned down to 50 to 100 mL/min, it is extremely unlikely that access recirculation will occur, as arterial inflow into the graft or fistula invariably exceeds this rate. Therefore, the NKF-KDOQI clinical practice guideline for hemodialysis adequacy recommends that the blood pump be slowed to 50 to 100 mL/min for at least 15 seconds prior to drawing the postdialysis BUN sample from the arterial port closest to the patient (66).

Cardiopulmonary Recirculation

The second component of the rise in BUN immediately after the conclusion of the hemodialysis treatment is cardiopulmonary recirculation, which is completed in 2 to 3 minutes. Cardiopulmonary recirculation refers to that small portion of blood that returns to the patient through the venous limb of the extracorporeal circuit and then circulates through the heart, lungs, and back to the arterial limb of the extracorporeal circuit without passing through any urea-rich tissues.

Cardiopulmonary recirculation typically accounts for only 15% of urea rebound following the conclusion of the hemodialysis treatment and does not occur when venous catheters are used for angioaccess.

Compartmental Disequilibrium

The third component of urea rebound, due to compartment disequilibrium, is not complete until at least 30 minutes after the conclusion of the hemodialysis treatment.

Originally, this phase was thought to represent the resolution of disequilibrium between intra- and extracellular urea: Extracellular urea is removed effectively during the hemodialysis treatment, and then urea is released from the intracellular to the extracellular compartment at the conclusion of the treatment due to the gradient between the two pools.

It has been suggested that the compartment disequilibrium that occurs during a hemodialysis treatment is not between intracellular and extracellular fluid but between high blood flow vascular beds (such as the kidney, lungs, brain, and other viscera) where relatively little urea is generated, and lower blood flow vascular beds (such as muscle, skin, and bone) where the majority of urea is generated and which are more subject to vasoconstriction during hemodialysis (91). Once the hemodialysis treatment has concluded and blood flow increases to these organs, sequestered urea is "washed out" and the BUN concentration rebounds.

Adherence to the NKF-KDOQI practice guidelines for postdialysis blood draw and the use of formal UKM or the Daugirdas II formula will yield an spKt/V that eliminates the effects of access recirculation but not of cardiopulmonary recirculation or of urea disequilibrium. The NKF-KDOQI hemodialysis workgroup made their recommendations based on the small contribution of cardiopulmonary recirculation to urea rebound and the impracticality of detaining patients for 30 minutes after the conclusion of the hemodialysis treatment to draw the postdialysis BUN.

Equilibrated Kt/V

The magnitude of disequilibrium and urea rebound is proportional to the efficiency of the hemodialysis treatment, which can be described as Kt/V. In other words, the more efficient (shorter t for a given Kt/V) the hemodialysis treatment, the lower the BUN

measured immediately after the hemodialysis treatment, and the more the Kt/V based on this BUN will overestimate the equilibrated Kt/V (eKt/V).

Daugirdas and Schneditz (92) have developed a relatively simple formula to estimate the eKt/V, based on the "single-pool" postdialysis BUN sample (drawn as described in preceding text at the conclusion of the hemodialysis treatment) and the treatment time (**EQUATION 6.3**):

$$eKt/V = spKt/V - 0.6 \times spKt/V/h + 0.03 \qquad (6.3)$$

where spKt/V is the single-pool Kt/V calculated from the Daugirdas II formula.

This formula, which obviates the need to draw a 30-minute postdialysis BUN to calculate eKt/V, was able to predict the eKt/V (based on actual 30-minute postdialysis BUN) better than models that use online dialysate urea monitoring (93) or intradialysis BUN measurement according to the Smye et al. (94) technique. The Smye technique is based on the fact that urea rebound disequilibrium (the degree to which the equilibrated postdialysis BUN exceeds the single-pool postdialysis BUN) will equal urea inbound disequilibrium (the degree to which measured BUN during the hemodialysis treatment is less than that predicted by its pharmacokinetics, based on dialyzer clearance and volume of distribution).

⬡ HEMODIALYSIS DOSE AND OUTCOME

The survival of patients on hemodialysis tends to be better than that of lung cancer patients but is worse than the statistics for both colon and prostate cancer patients (38). It is significant that the mortality rate of ESKD patients in the United States is greater than that of their counterparts in other countries, notably those in Europe and in Japan (95). Analysts have tried to explain these data in terms of patient differences, especially with regard to age and comorbidity (19), nutritional status (20,37), incomplete data in the registry (96), and less than adequate dialysis dose delivery (19).

Numerous publications have demonstrated that the delivered dose of hemodialysis is a significant predictor of patient outcome (18). The HEMO trial convincingly demonstrated that above an spKt/V of 1.4, there is no longer a continuous decline in mortality. Moreover, augmentation of middle molecule clearance (as measured by β_2-microglobulin clearance) with the use of "high-flux" membranes failed to confer survival benefits in this large and well-designed study of contemporary hemodialysis practice patterns (32,34).

Renal Physicians Association's Clinical Practice Guideline

The high prevalence of low hemodialysis dose as well as the relatively high mortality among hemodialysis patients in the United States prompted the 1993 publication of the RPA's *Clinical Practice Guideline on Adequacy of Hemodialysis* (97). The RPA guideline was the first clinical practice guideline addressing the care of the patient with ESKD, and its dissemination likely contributed to the decline in patients with URR less than 0.65 between 1993 and 1996 (98).

The RPA guideline recommended a minimum Kt/V of 1.2, based on a probabilistic model to assess how variation in the hemodialysis prescription affected quality-adjusted life expectancy (QALE). The RPA guideline noted that, although QALE increased with raising Kt/V above 1.2, the significant increase in costs required to achieve this higher dose of dialysis must be considered. The RPA guideline's final recommendation reflected a balance of concerns regarding decreasing incremental QALE and marginal cost-effectiveness.

For facilities using URR rather than Kt/V, a minimum value of 0.65 was recommended.

National Kidney Foundation's Kidney Disease Outcomes Quality Initiative Clinical Practice Guideline

The first NKF Dialysis Outcomes Quality Initiative (DOQI, subsequently renamed KDOQI) clinical practice guideline on hemodialysis adequacy was published in 1997, revised in 2001, again in 2006 (66), and most recently revisited in 2015 (17). The updated 2015 guideline has maintained the standard of a target spKt/V of 1.4 per hemodialysis session for patients receiving three times per week hemodialysis and a minimum delivered spKt/V of 1.2. The update highlights that residual native kidney function (Kru) may allow for lower doses of dialysis; however, Kru must be measured regularly to ascertain significant residual renal function is present and whether the dialysis dose may need to be adjusted to account for a decrease in residual renal function.

Standard Kt/V (stdKt/V) is the weekly urea generation rate factored by the average predialysis serum urea concentration during the week and allows for the inclusion of more frequent treatments or continuous dialysis treatments, such as PD or residual renal function. For alternative hemodialysis schedules, the recent guideline suggests a target stdKt/V of 2.3 volumes per week with minimum delivered dose of 2.1. Kru of 3 mL/min is equivalent to a stdKt/V of about 1.0 volume per week, and if residual renal function is not accounted for, then PCR will be underestimated. The guideline advocates a quarterly assessment of Kru at a minimum; however, if there has been a change in urine volume, a repeat assessment of Kru should occur earlier. Furthermore, those patients whose dialysis prescription is altered due to significant Kru, it is important to monitor urine volume monthly.

The 2015 update also recommends a minimum of 3 hours per session for patients with low residual renal function and that longer treatment times may be indicated in certain patients such as those having difficulty to achieve their dry weight. With regard to ultrafiltration rate, there is no set recommended value; however, the guideline suggests balancing blood pressure control, solute clearance, intradialytic symptoms, and hemodynamic stability. Finally, the 2015 guideline also recommends using biocompatible membranes for intermittent hemodialysis.

National Institutes of Health HEMO Study

The lower mortality rates reported for hemodialysis patients outside the United States and the extremely low mortality rates reported from Tassin, France, where patients undergo 24 m^2 hours of dialysis weekly (18,31), raise several nagging questions:

1. Is dialysis duration an independent factor in dialysis adequacy (a return to the middle molecule hypothesis)?
2. Are shorter dialysis treatments to achieve a comparable (i.e., more efficient) Kt/V associated with adverse outcomes because they increase urea disequilibrium and therefore underestimate the equilibrated dose of dialysis delivered (which can be corrected for by using a double-pool eKt/V target)? Or is the adverse outcome due to other factors, such as cardiovascular instability or rapid transcellular molecule fluxes?
3. Is there any cost-effective benefit to increasing the dose of dialysis above that recommended by the RPA and NKF-KDOQI guidelines?

In an attempt to answer these types of question, NIH sponsored and completed the HEMO study, a multicenter, prospective, randomized trial designed to assess the effects of hemodialysis dose (i.e., small molecule clearance) and flux (i.e., middle molecule clearance) (34) on morbidity and mortality.

The sweep of this study was comparable to the NCDS but with turn of the millennium technology. Like the NCDS, the HEMO study had four arms in a 2 × 2 matrix:

1. Arm 1: standard urea clearance (URR about 0.67, spKt/V about 1.25, eKt/V about 1.05) and a high-efficiency polysulfone dialysis membrane
2. Arm 2: higher urea clearance (URR about 0.75, spKt/V about 1.65, eKt/V about 1.45) and a high-efficiency membrane
3. Arm 3: Standard urea clearance and a high-flux polysulfone dialysis membrane
4. Arm 4: Higher urea clearance and a high-flux membrane

The main outcome measure of the HEMO trial was again mortality but with several important secondary outcomes were also monitored, specifically cardiac hospitalizations or deaths, infection-related hospitalizations or deaths, declines in albumin, and all-cause hospitalizations. These main and secondary outcomes correspond to the main causes of morbidity and mortality within the U.S. hemodialysis population.

The results of the HEMO trial confirm that the minimum dose of hemodialysis recommended by the aforementioned guidelines is safe. Higher doses of dialysis and the use of high-flux membranes offer no specific morbidity or mortality advantage to the groups receiving these treatments (**FIGURES 6.4** and **6.5**). Therefore, in the context of conventional three times per week hemodialysis, neither the high-flux nor high-dose interventions substantially improved patient outcome compared to low-flux and standard-dose levels. However, certain secondary results from the trial are consistent with the hypothesis of subtle effects that may be magnified by more intensive therapies that extend beyond the limits of conventional three times per week dialysis. Specifically the use of high-flux dialysis membranes (with improved clearance of β_2-microglobulin) in subgroups composed of women and patients who had been on dialysis more than 3.5 years on entry to the trial showed a trend toward decreased morbidity, hospitalizations, and mortality (34).

◆ BARRIERS TO ADEQUATE HEMODIALYSIS

The discussion of hemodialysis adequacy must not obscure the fact that other parameters such as nutrition and patient-assessed functional health status have been shown to have an even stronger correlation with patient outcomes. Accordingly, appropriate care of the hemodialysis patient should not be focused on any single indicator such as dialysis dose. However, the clinician has more direct control over dialysis dose than over some of the other factors affecting outcomes, so it may constitute the greatest opportunity for physician behavior to influence patient survival.

Underprescription

Since the 1993 publication of the RPA guideline recommending a minimum URR of 0.65 or Kt/V of 1.2, a discernible trend toward improvements in the delivery of adequate dialysis to U.S. patients with ESKD has been demonstrated in a variety of databases including the ESKD Clinical Performance Measures (CPM) Project, the United States Renal Data System (USRDS), and the DOPPS. According to data from the DOPPS website (which is updated every 4 months), 95% of hemodialysis patients in the DOPPS stratified weighted sample (representative of the United States as

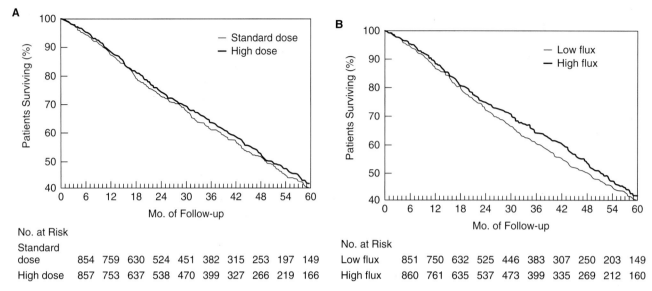

No. at Risk

Standard dose	854	759	630	524	451	382	315	253	197	149
High dose	857	753	637	538	470	399	327	266	219	166

No. at Risk

Low flux	851	750	632	525	446	383	307	250	203	149
High flux	860	761	635	537	473	399	335	269	212	160

FIGURE 6.4 Survival curves for the treatment groups in the HEMO study. After adjustment for the baseline factors, mortality in the high-dose group was 4% lower (95% confidence interval, −10 to 16; $p = 0.53$) than that in the standard-dose group (Panel A), and mortality in the high-flux group was 8% lower (95% confidence interval, −5 to 19; $p = 0.23$) than that in the low-flux group (Panel B). [Reprinted with permission from Eknoyan G, Beck GJ, Cheung AK, et al. Effect of dialysis dose and membrane flux in maintenance hemodialysis. *N Engl J Med* 2002;347(25):2010–2019.]

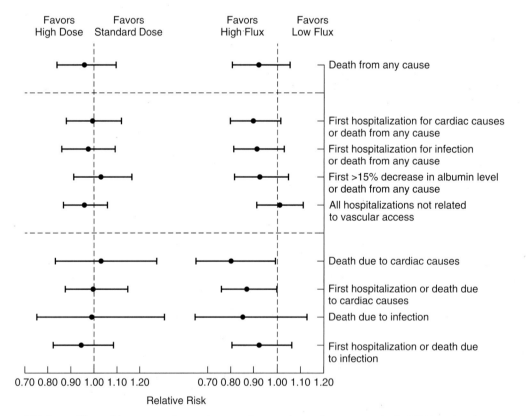

FIGURE 6.5 Effects of the treatment interventions on primary and secondary outcomes in the HEMO study. Values are shown as relative risks and 95% confidence intervals associated with assignment to the high-dose group as compared with assignment to the standard-dose group and assignment to the high-flux group as compared with assignment to the low-flux group. Analyses were stratified according to clinical center and adjusted for baseline age, sex, race, duration of dialysis, presence or absence of diabetes, score for coexisting conditions excluding diabetes, serum albumin level, and the interaction of albumin level with time from randomization. Percentage risk reductions for the high-dose and high-flux groups given in the text are obtained by subtraction of the relative risk from 1 followed by multiplication by 100. [Reprinted with permission from Eknoyan G, Beck GJ, Cheung AK, et al. Effect of dialysis dose and membrane flux in maintenance hemodialysis. *N Engl J Med* 2002;347(25):2010–2019.]

a whole) had Kt/V more than 1.2 in 2014 (99). However, despite continued improvements, still some patients do not meet minimum adequacy standards. More disturbing, however, the use of central venous catheters remains unacceptably high, with almost 20% of prevalent U.S. hemodialysis being dialyzed with a chronic venous catheter (99). Underprescription remains a significant problem, accounting for 55% of underdialyzed patients reported by Delmez and Windus (100) and 14% of all patients reported by Sehgal et al. (101).

As might be expected, underprescription of dialysis (Kt/V) is most likely to occur in a patient with a large urea volume of distribution (V), in whom the dialysis variables (Kt) have not been increased in proportion to patient size (102). The relationship between patient size and the likelihood of underprescription of dialysis therapy was also explored by Leon and Sehgal (103) in a group of dialysis patients drawn randomly from 22 chronic dialysis units in northeast Ohio. Using a Kt/V criterion of 1.3 as "adequate" dialysis, they found that 15% of patients were underdialyzed. Prescribed Kt (that portion of dialysis therapy which is modifiable by the prescribing physician) was strongly associated with patient volume, V. However, for every 10 L increment of V, Kt was only increased by a factor of 8.3, rather than 13 L, which would be required to maintain a Kt/V of 1.3. Due to this reduction in prescription, as patient size increased, the proportion of patients with a low prescription also increased from 2% of patients with V less than 35 L to 42% of patients with V 50 L or more (77).

Inadequate Vascular Access

The second most important barrier to achieving the target delivered hemodialysis dose is inadequate vascular access, which decreases the efficiency of dialysis due to both inadequate blood flow and access recirculation. Coyne et al. (104) found that among 146 patients with a decline in Kt/V over a 3-month period, 24% were due to decreased blood-flow rates and 25% were due to recirculation. Sehgal et al. (101) found 11% of his prevalent sample of 722 patients to be using catheters and that catheter use decreases the delivered Kt/V by 0.2. In patients with catheters, shortening of treatment time together with a higher likelihood of access recirculation help explain why minimum adequacy targets are still being missed.

Shortened Treatment Time

Patient noncompliance with treatment time was observed in 3% of the treatments reported by Sehgal et al. (101) in which adequacy was measured and accounted for 18% of the declines in Kt/V reported by Coyne et al. (104). Patient noncompliance reduced Kt/V by a factor of 0.1 in the Sehgal study, which is less significant than underprescription (0.5) or catheter use (0.2). Skipped hemodialysis treatments are obviously an issue in total dialysis dose but would not be reflected by a decreased Kt/V or URR because no blood would be drawn from an absent patient. In a survival analysis of skipped treatments and dialysis prescription noncompliance, Leggat et al. (105) demonstrated an approximate 10% increase in the risk of death for each hemodialysis session that is missed. In this analysis, the authors also found that approximately 8.5% of patients skipped hemodialysis treatments at least once per month and that 20% shortened treatment times.

Clotting

Clotting during hemodialysis occurred in 1% of the treatments reported by Sehgal et al. (101) in a study that measured adequacy, resulting in a decrease on Kt/V of 0.3. As a general rule, the treatment duration was not extended to compensate for the "down"

time of changing the extracorporeal circuit. Also notable is that the overall efficiency of the dialysis procedure decreased due to loss of dialyzer surface area to clotting. Adequate anticoagulation is obviously the most effective method to overcome this barrier to adequacy, but clearly, there are patients whose bleeding risk precludes this approach. Further investigation is needed to determine the best course of action for this small subset of patients.

Other Variables

TABLES 6.2 and **6.3**, adapted from Parker (106), illustrate the plethora of variables that may confound the provision of an adequate dialysis dose. It is clearly not an exact science, and a normal distribution of delivered dialysis from a given prescribed dialysis dose will lead to a significant fraction of patients receiving less than the prescribed dose (107). Therefore, for 90% of patients to receive a delivered Kt/V of 1.2 or more, the NKF-KDOQI guideline recommends a prescribed Kt/V of 1.3 or more (URR 0.70 or more) (66).

⬡ CONTEMPORARY TRIALS OF INCREASED DIALYSIS

Frequent Hemodialysis Network Daily Trial

Another landmark trial in dialysis adequacy research is the large multicenter randomized FHN trial which included two studies. In the first reported study, published in *The New England Journal of Medicine* in 2010, patients were randomly assigned to hemodialysis

TABLE 6.2	**Reasons for Compromised Urea Clearance**

Patient-related reasons

Decreased effective time on dialysis (breakdown on **TABLE 6.3**)
Decreased blood-flow rates (BFR)
1. Access clotting
2. Use of catheters
3. Inadequate flow through vascular access
Recirculation
1. Use of catheters
2. Inadequate access for prescribed BFR
3. Stenosis/clotting of access

Staff-related reasons

Decreased effective time (see **TABLE 6.3**)
Decreased BFR
  1. Less than prescribed
  2. Difficult cannulation
Decreased dialysate flow rate
  1. Less than prescribed
  2. Inappropriately set
Dialyzer
  1. Inadequate quality of control of "reuse"

Mechanical problems

Dialyzer clotting during reuse
Blood pump calibration error
Dialysate pump calibration error
Inaccurate estimation of dialyzer performance by the manufacturer
Variability in blood tubing

Modified and adapted from Parker TF. Trends and concepts in the prescription and delivery of dialysis in the United States. *Semin Nephrol* 1992;12(3):271.

TABLE 6.3	**Reasons for Decreased Effective Time on Dialysis**

Patient-related reasons

Late start (patient tardy)
Early signoff
1. With consent (i.e., symptoms)
2. Against advice (i.e., social)
Medical complications (e.g., hypotension)
"No show"

Staff-related reasons

Late start (staff tardy)
Wrong patient taken off
Time calculated incorrectly
Time on/off read incorrectly
Clinical deficiencies (e.g., no time registered)
Premature discontinuation for unit convenience
1. Scheduling conflicts
2. Emergencies
Incorrect assumptions of continuous treatment time
(e.g., failure to account for interruptions of treatment like
repositioning needles or accidental removal)
Inaccurate assessment of effective time by using variable
time pieces

Mechanical reasons

Clotting of dialyzer
Dialyzer leaks
Machine malfunction

Modified and adapted from Parker TF. Trends and concepts in the prescription and delivery of dialysis in the United States. *Semin Nephrol* 1992;12(3):271.

six times per week (frequent, $n = 125$) or three times per week (conventional, $n = 120$) for a period of 12 months (108). The two coprimary composite outcomes were death or change in left ventricular (LV) mass [from baseline to 12 months, assessed by magnetic resonance imaging (MRI)] and death or change in physical health composite (PHC) score of the RAND 36-Item Health Survey.

Patients in the frequent group averaged 5.2 sessions per week, and their weekly stdKt/V urea was 3.54 versus 2.49 in conventional group. Frequent hemodialysis was associated with benefits in the coprimary composite outcomes, but frequent group patients were also more likely to undergo vascular access interventions. Frequent hemodialysis was associated with beneficial changes for death or increase in LV mass (hazard ratio 0.61) and for death and decrease in physical heath score (hazard ratio 0.70). For time to first access intervention, frequent dialysis was associated with hazard ratio for 1.71 and for multiple interventions hazard ratio was 1.35 for frequent group (**FIGURE 6.6**).

In this multicenter, prospective randomized parallel-group trial, a total of 78% of the patients who were assigned to frequent arm attended at least 80% of the prescribed sessions. Adherence was high in the daily trial but not in the nocturnal trial discussed later. FHN daily trial has some limitations, including small sample size was not sufficient to determine the effects of frequent in-center hemodialysis on death, cause-specific death, hospitalization, or other events. The rate of death was low in both groups, and therefore, the treatment effect was mostly supported by the intermediate outcomes, 12-month change in LV mass or PHC score. FHN daily trial excluded patients whose expected survival was less than

6 months and patients who residual renal function was more than 3 mL/min/1.73 m². Although overall positive for its coprimary outcome, the FHN daily trial was again not powered to definitively assess the effects of frequent dialysis on mortality. The trial has not established frequent dialysis as the standard of care but does continue to raise the ongoing discussion about adequacy and the ever elusive ideal hemodialysis prescription.

Frequent Hemodialysis Network Nocturnal Trial

The nocturnal study of FHN compared daily nocturnal (6 to 8 hours) home hemodialysis to conventional thrice-weekly home hemodialysis (72). Eighty-seven patients were randomized to thrice-weekly conventional hemodialysis or to nocturnal hemodialysis six times per week. The frequent nocturnal arm had a 1.82-fold higher mean weekly stdKt/V urea, 1.74-fold higher average number of treatments per week, 2.45-fold higher average weekly treatment time, and 1.23-fold higher total weekly ultrafiltration. No significant effect of nocturnal hemodialysis for either of the two coprimary outcomes, death or LV mass, or death or RAND PHC (**FIGURE 6.7**). The nocturnal patients had improvement in hyperphosphatemia, but there was a trend for increased vascular access events (**FIGURE 6.8**).

The main limitations of the trial were the small sample size and lower adherence in the frequent arm. Patients in the frequent nocturnal arm had lower adherence (72.7%) than the patients in the conventional arm (97.6%). The study acknowledges that one would need a sample size of 275 patients to obtain 80% power to detect a mean effect on LV mass of 10 g. Another cofounding factor was that only 87.3% of the patients randomized completed the 12 months of follow-up and has actual measurements of both coprimary outcomes. Also, about a quarter of the patients in the frequent arm performed less than five dialysis treatments per week.

Other important differences include that the patients were younger (52.8 years old), had more residual renal function, and were less likely to be African American (26.4%) as compared to the average patients receiving chronic hemodialysis therapy. The residual renal function criterion for the nocturnal trial was greater than 10 mL/min/1.73 m² as the average of the urea and creatinine clearances compared to the cutoff of 3 mL/min/1.73 m² in the daily trial. Recruitment was challenging as the initial protocol was randomizing to in-center versus home hemodialysis, and eligible patients preferred to be dialyzed at home. Recruitment improved somewhat after the choice was between two types of home dialysis rather than home versus in-center. In conclusion, frequent nocturnal hemodialysis as compared to three times per week hemodialysis did not result in significant benefits in the coprimary outcomes of death/LV mass or death/PHC. PHC improved in both groups most likely secondary to the effect of home hemodialysis.

Time to Reduce Mortality in End-Stage Renal Disease Trial

The TiME Trial is a cluster-randomized, parallel-group pragmatic ongoing clinical trial to determine whether dialysis facility implementation of a minimum session length of 4.25 hours three times per week versus usual care has benefits on mortality, hospitalizations, and HRQOL (109). The primary outcome measure is time to death; a secondary outcome measure is hospitalization rate, and the maximum duration of follow-up is 3 years.

A Death or Change in LV Mass

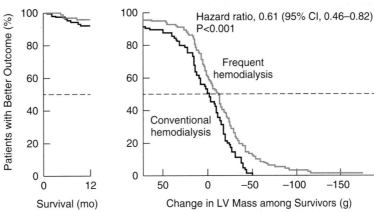

B Death or Change in PHC Score

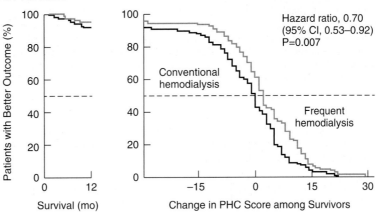

C Main Secondary Outcomes

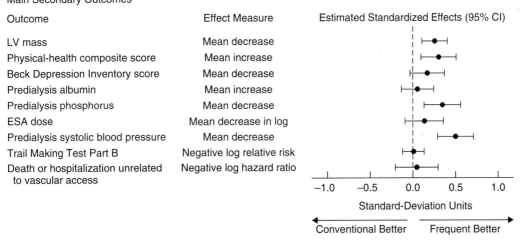

FIGURE 6.6 Coprimary composite outcomes and main secondary outcomes in the Frequent Hemodialysis Network daily trial. Kaplan–Meier curves are shown for the composite outcomes of death or change in left ventricular (LV) mass (Panel A) and death or change in the physical health composite (PHC) score from the RAND 36-Item Health Survey (Panel B). The standardized effect sizes for the main secondary outcomes are shown in Panel C. [Reprinted with permission from Chertow GM, Levin NW, Beck GJ, et al. In-center hemodialysis six times per week versus three times per week. *N Engl J Med* 2010;363(24):2287–2300.]

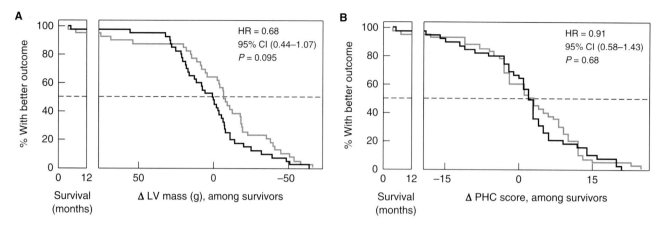

FIGURE 6.7 Mortality/LV mass composite and mortality/PHC composite results in the Frequent Hemodialysis Network nocturnal trial. Kaplan–Meier curves (conventional arm, black; frequent nocturnal arm, red) for the death/LV mass composite **(A)** and the death/PHC composite **(B)**. For any given value of the composite outcome indicated on the horizontal axis (time of death on the left, change in either LV mass or PHC among survivors on the right), the Kaplan–Meier curves indicate the proportion of patients in the respective treatment groups with an equal or more favorable outcome. The horizontal distance between the Kaplan–Meier curves at the 50% value on the vertical axis indicates the median composite outcome results. CI, confidence interval; HR, hazard ratio; LV, left ventricular; PHC, physical health composite. [Reprinted with permission from Rocco MV, Lockridge RS Jr, Beck GJ, et al. The effects of frequent nocturnal home hemodialysis: the Frequent Hemodialysis Network Nocturnal Trial. *Kidney Int* 2011;80(10):1080–1091.]

The hypothesis is that the risk of death will be lower in the facilities randomized to the intervention group. Another outcome measure is quality of life, assessed with a Health-Related Quality of Life questionnaire. The estimated study completion date is September 2017. The inclusion criteria include ESKD patients over 18 years of age that are on hemodialysis three times per week who have started maintenance dialysis within the prior 120 days. Exclusion criteria are unwillingness to participate or inability to provide consent for dialysis. The nephrology community is anxiously awaiting the results of this pertinent trial with its primary outcome measure, time to death, and the critical variable, dialysis treatment time.

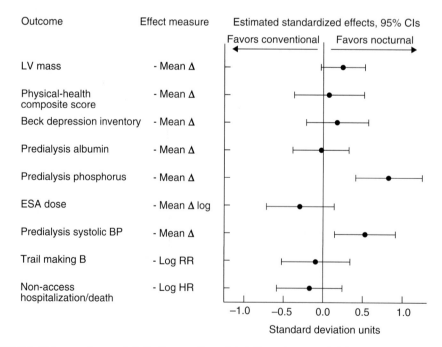

FIGURE 6.8 Main secondary results in the Frequent Hemodialysis Network nocturnal trial. BP, blood pressure; CI, confidence interval; ESA, erythropoiesis-stimulating agent; HR, hazard ratio; LV, left ventricular. [Reprinted with permission from Rocco MV, Lockridge RS Jr, Beck GJ, et al. The effects of frequent nocturnal home hemodialysis: the Frequent Hemodialysis Network Nocturnal Trial. *Kidney Int* 2011;80(10):1080–1091.]

CONCLUSION

Looking forward, it seems that we should, first and foremost, evaluate the patient while evaluating the adequacy of dialysis. Understanding the interaction of the multiple factors that affect overall survival and quality of life will heighten our awareness of specific issues that need to be addressed. We must evaluate nutritional status, physical activity, comorbid conditions, fluid and electrolyte balance, social and home conditions, and find specific barriers to adequate hemodialysis. We must aim for Kt/V of 1.3 or more (URR 70% or more) with a delivered Kt/V of 1.2 or more measured monthly, along with other laboratory values within target ranges. Although one-third of the declines in Kt/V reported by Coyne et al. (104) could not be explained and returned spontaneously to adequate levels, the majority were real and therefore should be investigated and corrected.

Increasing recognition of the underprescription of hemodialysis is still challenging. Facilities constantly reshuffle station allocation and turnover to meet the needs of patients as well as the care team. Increased patient education to improve buy-in of longer treatment times when appropriate needs to occur at the facility level but can and should use the materials and media that have been developed regionally and nationally for this purpose. Peer education by other patients through local, regional, or national patient advocacy groups can also prove to be highly effective in increasing patients' participation in their care. An exploration of the patient's home, family, and socioeconomic situation can provide valuable insights that help to break down barriers to patient partnership.

In the last four decades, we still focus on urea as primarily responsible for the uremic syndrome and as our main marker for dialysis adequacy. Although urea is a good surrogate marker, identifying the responsible toxins and then removing them more efficiently remains a formidable challenge. The continued disparity in mortality rates between the United States and Europe points out the need for continued investigation regarding the most appropriate methods of delivering renal replacement therapy as well as the best indicators for measurement of dialysis adequacy.

The NIH's HEMO study helps to clarify some of these issues and provides guidance in applying hemodialysis technology to achieve the best patient outcomes. We must deal with the fact that 5% of patients in the DOPPS random sample did not have today's target Kt/V of 1.2 or more and that a larger percentage of incident dialysis patients are classified as overweight or obese, with up to 20% of these patients failing to meet adequacy targets. With contemporary trials such as the FHN studies and TiME, we continue to pursue how to better the care and lives of our patients. We must also consider the kind of dialysis that best suits our patients, including home and incremental therapies. We have the quality improvement tools to identify the barriers to adequate hemodialysis in each of our facilities and the human capital to overcome them.

REFERENCES

1. Kletke PR, Marder WD. The supply of renal physicians: an analysis of data from the American Medical Association Physician Masterfile. *Am J Kidney Dis* 1991;18(3):384–391.
2. Collins AJ, Foley RN, Chavers B, et al. United States Renal Data System 2011 Annual Data Report: atlas of chronic kidney disease & end-stage renal disease in the United States. *Am J Kidney Dis* 2012;59(1 Suppl 1): A7, e1–e420.
3. Collins AJ, Foley RN, Chavers B, et al. US Renal Data System 2013 Annual Data Report. *Am J Kidney Dis* 2014;63(1 Suppl):A7.
4. Wolf AV, Remp DG, Kiley JE, et al. Artificial kidney function, kinetics of hemodialysis. *J Clin Invest* 1951;30(10):1062–1070.
5. Vanholder RC, Ringoir SM. Adequacy of dialysis: a critical analysis. *Kidney Int* 1992;42(3):540–558.
6. Vanholder R, De Smet R, Glorieux G, et al. Review on uremic toxins: classification, concentration, and interindividual variability. *Kidney Int* 2003;63(5):1934–1943.
7. Luke RG. Uremia and the BUN. *N Engl J Med* 1981;305(20):1213–1215.
8. Babb AL, Ahmad S, Bergstrom J, et al. The middle molecule hypothesis in perspective. *Am J Kidney Dis* 1981;1(1):46–50.
9. Ginn HE. Neurobehavioral dysfunction in uremia. *Kidney Int Suppl* 1975;8(Suppl 1):217–221.
10. Ginn HE, Teschan PE, Walker PJ, et al. Neurotoxicity in uremia. *Kidney Int Suppl* 1975;8:357–360.
11. Vanholder R, Eloot S, Van Biesen W. Do we need new indicators of dialysis adequacy based on middle-molecule removal? *Nat Clin Pract Nephrol* 2008;4(4):174–175.
12. Gotch FA, Sargent JA. A mechanistic analysis of the National Cooperative Dialysis Study (NCDS). *Kidney Int* 1985;28(3):526–534.
13. Lowrie EG, Laird NM, Henry RR. Protocol for the National Cooperative Dialysis Study. *Kidney Int Suppl* 1983;23(Suppl 13):S11–S18.
14. Lowrie EG. History and organization of the National Cooperative Dialysis Study. *Kidney Int Suppl* 1983;13:S1–S7.
15. Lowrie EG, Laird NM, Parker TF, et al. Effect of the hemodialysis prescription of patient morbidity: report from the National Cooperative Dialysis Study. *N Engl J Med* 1981;305(20):1176–1181.
16. Depner TA. Optimizing the treatment of the dialysis patient: a painful lesson. *Semin Nephrol* 1997;17(4):285–297.
17. National Kidney Foundation. KDOQI clinical practice guidelines for hemodialysis adequacy: 2015 update. *Am J Kidney Dis* 2015;66(5): 884–930.
18. Charra B, Calemard E, Ruffet M, et al. Survival as an index of adequacy of dialysis. *Kidney Int* 1992;41(5):1286–1291.
19. Collins AJ, Ma JZ, Umen A, et al. Urea index and other predictors of hemodialysis patient survival. *Am J Kidney Dis* 1994;23(2):272–282.
20. Owen WF Jr, Lew NL, Liu Y, et al. The urea reduction ratio and serum albumin concentration as predictors of mortality in patients undergoing hemodialysis. *N Engl J Med* 1993;329(14):1001–1006.
21. Sehgal AR, Grey SF, DeOreo PB, et al. Prevalence, recognition, and implications of mental impairment among hemodialysis patients. *Am J Kidney Dis* 1997;30(1):41–49.
22. Muto Y, Murase M. Metabolic encephalopathy in the aged. *Nihon Naika Gakkai Zasshi* 1990;79(4):468–474.
23. Keane WF, Collins AJ. Influence of co-morbidity on mortality and morbidity in patients treated with hemodialysis. *Am J Kidney Dis* 1994;24(6):1010–1018.
24. Krishnan M, Lok CE, Jassal SV. Epidemiology and demographic aspects of treated end-stage renal disease in the elderly. *Semin Dial* 2002;15(2):79–83.
25. Berger EE, Lowrie EG. Mortality and the length of dialysis. *JAMA* 1991;265(7):909–910.
26. Bennett WM. Divided loyalties: relationships between nephrologists and industry. *Am J Kidney Dis* 2001;37(1):210–221.
27. Held PJ, Levin NW, Bovbjerg RR, et al. Mortality and duration of hemodialysis treatment. *JAMA* 1991;265(7):871–875.
28. Marshall MR, Byrne BG, Kerr PG, et al. Associations of hemodialysis dose and session length with mortality risk in Australian and New Zealand patients. *Kidney Int* 2006;69(7):1229–1236.
29. Saran R, Bragg-Gresham JL, Levin NW, et al. Longer treatment time and slower ultrafiltration in hemodialysis: associations with reduced mortality in the DOPPS. *Kidney Int* 2006;69(7):1222–1228.
30. Charra B, Calemard M, Laurent G. Importance of treatment time and blood pressure control in achieving long-term survival on dialysis. *Am J Nephrol* 1996;16(1):35–44.
31. Raj DS, Charra B, Pierratos A, et al. In search of ideal hemodialysis: is prolonged frequent dialysis the answer? *Am J Kidney Dis* 1999;34(4):597–610.
32. Mitka M. How to reduce mortality in hemodialysis patients still a puzzle. *JAMA* 2002;287(20):2643–2644.

33. Charra B. Is there a magic in long nocturnal dialysis? *Contrib Nephrol* 2005;149:100–106.

34. Eknoyan G, Beck GJ, Cheung AK, et al. Effect of dialysis dose and membrane flux in maintenance hemodialysis. *N Engl J Med* 2002; 347(25):2010–2019.

35. Hakim RM. Assessing the adequacy of dialysis. *Kidney Int* 1990; 37(2):822–832.

36. Rocco MV, Cheung AK, Greene T, et al. The HEMO Study: applicability and generalizability. *Nephrol Dial Transplant* 2005;20(2):278–284.

37. Lowrie EG, Lew NL. Death risk in hemodialysis patients: the predictive value of commonly measured variables and an evaluation of death rate differences between facilities. *Am J Kidney Dis* 1990;15(5): 458–482.

38. Lowrie EG. Chronic dialysis treatment: clinical outcome and related processes of care. *Am J Kidney Dis* 1994;24(2):255–266.

39. Chertow GM, Goldstein-Fuchs DJ, Lazarus JM, et al. Prealbumin, mortality, and cause-specific hospitalization in hemodialysis patients. *Kidney Int* 2005;68(6):2794–2800.

40. Chertow GM, Owen WF, Lazarus JM, et al. Exploring the reverse J-shaped curve between urea reduction ratio and mortality. *Kidney Int* 1999;56(5):1872–1878.

41. Owen WF Jr, Chertow GM, Lazarus JM, et al. Dose of hemodialysis and survival: differences by race and sex. *JAMA* 1998;280(20): 1764–1768.

42. Held PJ, Port FK, Wolfe RA, et al. The dose of hemodialysis and patient mortality. *Kidney Int* 1996;50(2):550–556.

43. Sternby J. Significance of distribution volume in dialysis quantification. *Semin Dial* 2001;14(4):278–283.

44. Owen WF Jr, Coladonato J, Szczech L, et al. Explaining counter-intuitive clinical outcomes predicted by Kt/V. *Semin Dial* 2001;14(4):268–270.

45. Sarkar SR, Kotanko P, Heymsfeld SB, et al. Quest for V: body composition could determine dialysis dose. *Semin Dial* 2007;20(5):379–382.

46. Lowrie EG, Li Z, Ofsthun NJ, et al. Evaluating a new method to judge dialysis treatment using online measurements of ionic clearance. *Kidney Int* 2006;70(1):211–217.

47. Klahr S, Levey AS, Beck GJ, et al. The effects of dietary protein restriction and blood-pressure control on the progression of chronic renal disease. Modification of Diet in Renal Disease Study Group. *N Engl J Med* 1994;330(13):877–884.

48. Kopple JD, Levey AS, Greene T, et al. Effect of dietary protein restriction on nutritional status in the Modification of Diet in Renal Disease Study. *Kidney Int* 1997;52(3):778–791.

49. Consensus Development Conference Panel. Morbidity and mortality of renal dialysis: an NIH consensus conference statement. *Ann Intern Med* 1994;121(1):62–70.

50. Port FK, Ashby VB, Dhingra RK, et al. Dialysis dose and body mass index are strongly associated with survival in hemodialysis patients. *J Am Soc Nephrol* 2002;13(4):1061–1066.

51. Bergstrom J. Nutrition and mortality in hemodialysis. *J Am Soc Nephrol* 1995;6(5):1329–1341.

52. Leavey SF, Strawderman RL, Jones CA, et al. Simple nutritional indicators as independent predictors of mortality in hemodialysis patients. *Am J Kidney Dis* 1998;31(6):997–1006.

53. Mitch WE. Malnutrition: a frequent misdiagnosis for hemodialysis patients. *J Clin Invest* 2002;110(4):437–439.

54. Hakim RM, Levin N. Malnutrition in hemodialysis patients. *Am J Kidney Dis* 1993;21(2):125–137.

55. Burrowes JD, Larive B, Chertow GM, et al. Self-reported appetite, hospitalization and death in haemodialysis patients: findings from the Hemodialysis (HEMO) Study. *Nephrol Dial Transplant* 2005;20(12):2765–2774.

56. Bossola M, Tazza L, Giungi S, et al. Anorexia in hemodialysis patients: an update. *Kidney Int* 2006;70(3):417–422.

57. Cohen SD, Norris L, Acquaviva K, et al. Screening, diagnosis, and treatment of depression in patients with end-stage renal disease. *Clin J Am Soc Nephrol* 2007;2(6):1332–1342.

58. Pollock CA, Ibels LS, Zhu FY, et al. Protein intake in renal disease. *J Am Soc Nephrol* 1997;8(5):777–783.

59. Ikizler TA, Greene JH, Wingard RL, et al. Spontaneous dietary protein intake during progression of chronic renal failure. *J Am Soc Nephrol* 1995;6(5):1386–1391.

60. Bonomini V, Albertazzi A, Vangelista A, et al. Residual renal function and effective rehabilitation in chronic dialysis. *Nephron* 1976;16(2): 89–102.

61. Bonomini V, Feletti C, Scolari MP, et al. Benefits of early initiation of dialysis. *Kidney Int Suppl* 1985;17:S57–S59.

62. Tattersall J, Greenwood R, Farrington K. Urea kinetics and when to commence dialysis. *Am J Nephrol* 1995;15(4):283–289.

63. Churchill DN, Thorpe KE, Vonesh EF, et al. Canada-USA (CANUSA) Peritoneal Dialysis Study Group. Lower probability of patient survival with continuous peritoneal dialysis in the United States compared with Canada. *J Am Soc Nephrol* 1997;8(6):965–971.

64. Fry AC, Singh DK, Chandna SM, et al. Relative importance of residual renal function and convection in determining β-2-microglobulin levels in high-flux haemodialysis and on-line haemodiafiltration. *Blood Purif* 2007;25(3):295–302.

65. Chandna SM, Farrington K. Residual renal function: considerations on its importance and preservation in dialysis patients. *Semin Dial* 2004;17(3):196–201.

66. Hemodialysis Adequacy 2006 Work Group. Clinical practice guidelines for hemodialysis adequacy, update 2006. *Am J Kidney Dis* 2006; 48(Suppl 1):S2–S90.

67. Goodkin DA, Mapes DL, Held PJ. The dialysis outcomes and practice patterns study (DOPPS): how can we improve the care of hemodialysis patients? *Semin Dial* 2001;14(3):157–159.

68. Korevaar JC, Jansen MA, Dekker FW, et al. National Kidney Foundation-Dialysis Outcomes Quality Initiative. Evaluation of DOQI guidelines: early start of dialysis treatment is not associated with better health-related quality of life. *Am J Kidney Dis* 2002;39(1):108–115.

69. Traynor JP, Simpson K, Geddes CC, et al. Early initiation of dialysis fails to prolong survival in patients with end-stage renal failure. *J Am Soc Nephrol* 2002;13(8):2125–2132.

70. Cooper BA, Branley P, Bulfone L, et al. The Initiating Dialysis Early and Late (IDEAL) study: study rationale and design. *Perit Dial Int* 2004;24(2):176–181.

71. Kalantar-Zadeh K, Unruh M, Zager PG, et al. Twice-weekly and incremental hemodialysis treatment for initiation of kidney replacement therapy. *Am J Kidney Dis* 2014;64(2):181–186.

72. Rocco MV, Lockridge RS Jr, Beck GJ, et al. The effects of frequent nocturnal home hemodialysis: the Frequent Hemodialysis Network Nocturnal Trial. *Kidney Int* 2011;80(10):1080–1091.

73. Lin YF, Huang JW, Wu MS, et al. Comparison of residual renal function in patients undergoing twice-weekly versus three-times-weekly haemodialysis. *Nephrology* 2009;14(1):59–64.

74. O'Hare AM, Wong SP, Yu MK, et al. Trends in the timing and clinical context of maintenance dialysis initiation. *J Am Soc Nephrol* 2015;26(8):1975–1981.

75. Bargman JM. Timing of initiation of RRT and modality selection. *Clin J Am Soc Nephrol* 2015;10(6):1072–1077.

76. Brown MA, Collett GK, Josland EA, et al. CKD in elderly patients managed without dialysis: survival, symptoms, and quality of life. *Clin J Am Soc Nephrol* 2015;10(2):260–268.

77. O'Connor AS, Leon JB, Sehgal AR. The relative predictive ability of four different measures of hemodialysis dose. *Am J Kidney Dis* 2002;40(6):1289–1294.

78. McClellan WM, Frankenfield DL, Frederick PR, et al. Can dialysis therapy be improved? A report from the ESRD Core Indicators Project. *Am J Kidney Dis* 1999;34(6):1075–1082.

79. Hume R, Weyers E. Relationship between total body water and surface area in normal and obese subjects. *J Clin Pathol* 1971;24(3): 234–238.

80. Watson PE, Watson ID, Batt RD. Total body water volumes for adult males and females estimated from simple anthropometric measurements. *Am J Clin Nutr* 1980;33(1):27–39.

81. Chertow GM, Lazarus JM, Lew NL, et al. Bioimpedance norms for the hemodialysis population. *Kidney Int* 1997;52(6):1617–1621.

82. Chertow GM, Lazarus JM, Lew NL, et al. Development of a population-specific regression equation to estimate total body water in hemodialysis patients. *Kidney Int* 1997;51(5):1578–1582.

83. Daugirdas JT. Second generation logarithmic estimates of single-pool variable volume Kt/V: an analysis of error. *J Am Soc Nephrol* 1993; 4(5):1205–1213.

84. Flanigan MJ, Fangman J, Lim VS. Quantitating hemodialysis: a comparison of three kinetic models. *Am J Kidney Dis* 1991;17(3): 295–302.

85. Bankhead MM, Toto RD, Star RA. Accuracy of urea removal estimated by kinetic models. *Kidney Int* 1995;48(3):785–793.

86. Daugirdas JT, Depner TA, Greene T, et al. Surface-area-normalized Kt/V: a method of rescaling dialysis dose to body surface area-implications for different-size patients by gender. *Semin Dial* 2008; 21(5):415–421.

87. Ramirez SP, Kapke A, Port FK, et al. Dialysis dose scaled to body surface area and size-adjusted, sex-specific patient mortality. *Clin J Am Soc Nephrol* 2012;7(12):1977–1987.

88. Daugirdas JT. Dialysis dosing for chronic hemodialysis: beyond Kt/V. *Semin Dial* 2014;27(2):98–107.

89. Depner TA. Assessing adequacy of hemodialysis: urea modeling. *Kidney Int* 1994;45(5):1522–1535.

90. Daugirdas JT, Burke MS, Balter P, et al. Screening for extreme postdialysis urea rebound using the Smye method: patients with access recirculation identified when a slow flow method is not used to draw the postdialysis blood. *Am J Kidney Dis* 1996;28(5):727–731.

91. Alquist M, Thysell H, Ungerstedt U, et al. Development of a urea concentration gradient between muscle interstitium and plasma during hemodialysis. *Int J Artif Organs* 1999;22(12):811–815.

92. Daugirdas JT, Schneditz D. Overestimation of hemodialysis dose depends on dialysis efficiency by regional blood flow but not by conventional two pool urea kinetic analysis. *ASAIO J* 1995;41(3): M719–M724.

93. Daugirdas JT, Depner TA, Gotch FA, et al. Comparison of methods to predict equilibrated Kt/V in the HEMO Pilot Study. *Kidney Int* 1997;52(5):1395–1405.

94. Smye SW, Dunderdale E, Brownridge G, et al. Estimation of treatment dose in high-efficiency haemodialysis. *Nephron* 1994;67(1):24–29.

95. Held PJ, Brunner F, Odaka M, et al. Five-year survival for end-stage renal disease patients in the United States, Europe, and Japan, 1982 to 1987. *Am J Kidney Dis* 1990;15(5):451–457.

96. Wolfe RA, Ashby VB, Daugirdas JT, et al. Body size, dose of hemodialysis, and mortality. *Am J Kidney Dis* 2000;35(1):80–88.

97. Renal Physicians Association. *Clinical Practice Guideline in Adequacy of Hemodialysis*. Dubuque, IA: Kendall Hunt Publishing; 1996.

98. Helgerson SD, McClellan WM, Frederick PR, et al. Improvement in adequacy of delivered dialysis for adult in-center hemodialysis patients in the United States, 1993 to 1995. *Am J Kidney Dis* 1997;29(6):851–861.

99. DOPPS practice monitor. http://www.dopps.org/dpm/DPMSlideBrowser .aspx?type=Topic&id=4. Accessed May 16, 2016.

100. Delmez JA, Windus DW. The St. Louis Nephrology Study Group. Hemodialysis prescription and delivery in a metropolitan community. *Kidney Int* 1992;41(4):1023–1028.

101. Sehgal AR, Snow RJ, Singer ME, et al. Barriers to adequate delivery of hemodialysis. *Am J Kidney Dis* 1998;31(4):593–601.

102. Port FK, Wolfe RA. Optimizing the dialysis dose with consideration of patient size. *Blood Purif* 2000;18(4):295–297.

103. Leon JB, Sehgal AR. Identifying patients at risk for hemodialysis underprescription. *Am J Nephrol* 2001;21:200–207.

104. Coyne DW, Delmez J, Spence G, et al. Impaired delivery of hemodialysis prescriptions: an analysis of causes and an approach to evaluation. *J Am Soc Nephrol* 1997;8(8):1315–1318.

105. Leggat JE Jr, Orzol SM, Hulbert-Shearon TE, et al. Noncompliance in hemodialysis: predictors and survival analysis. *Am J Kidney Dis* 1998;32(1):139–145.

106. Parker TF III. Technical advances in hemodialysis therapy. *Semin Dial* 2000;13(6):372–377.

107. Gotch FA, Levin NW, Port FK, et al. Clinical outcome relative to the dose of dialysis is not what you think: the fallacy of the mean. *Am J Kidney Dis* 1997;30(1):1–15.

108. Chertow GM, Levin NW, Beck GJ, et al. In-center hemodialysis six times per week versus three times per week. *N Engl J Med* 2010; 363(24):2287–2300.

109. Dember L. UH3 Project: Time to Reduce Mortality in End-Stage Renal Disease (TiME). https://www.nihcollaboratory.org/demonstration-projects /Pages/TiME.aspx. Accessed May 16, 2016.

CHAPTER 7

High-Efficiency and High-Flux Hemodialysis

Thomas A. Golper, Rafia Chaudhry, Iheanyichukwu Ogu, and Gerald Schulman

For a glossary of abbreviations, please see **TABLE 7.1**. In the era of the previous editions of this book, high-efficiency hemodialysis (HEHD) was a prevalent and popular form of in-center hemodialysis (HD), for reasons discussed below. As dialysis sciences progressed in informing us about solute kinetics, ultrafiltration tolerance, and new techniques, it became increasingly more evident that the utilization of HEHD as originally conceived would decrease. However, since it is still being practiced under certain circumstances, we describe the technique and how best to perform it. On the other hand, high-flux hemodialysis (HFHD) is the most prevalent form of HD in the United States currently, and we suspect that this represents >90% of all treatments. When HEHD utilizes a high-flux membrane as described below, that is termed high-efficiency, high-flux hemodialysis (HEHFHD). The year 2001 was the last year that the United States Renal Data System (USRDS) Annual Data Report described HD in a manner where the efficiency and/or flux was reported (1), again emphasizing the overwhelming trend toward HFHD. Furthermore, as the dialysis population aged and was burdened by ever more comorbidities, treatment times (TTs) increased such that the concept of "efficiency" became somewhat less relevant.

DEFINITIONS: HIGH-EFFICIENCY, HIGH-FLUX, AND PERMEABILITY

It is important to conceptualize and understand the basics of high-efficiency (HE) and high-flux (HF) dialyzer devices in order to compare the uses, differences, and technical needs of each. **TABLE 7.2** provides a comparison of the various characteristics of conventional, HE, and HF dialyzers. The definitions of HE and HF procedures were formed primarily from the historical development of HD and the technical needs of each treatment. The primary

TABLE 7.1	Glossary of Abbreviations
HD	hemodialysis
HE	high-efficiency
HF	high-flux
β_2-MG	β_2-microglobulin
DRA	dialysis-related amyloidosis
IDWG	interdialytic weight gain
IDH	intradialytic hypotension
KoA	mass transfer area coefficient
KUF	ultrafiltration coefficient
PR	pyrogenic reaction
Qb	blood-flow rate
Qd	dialysate flow rate
RR	relative risk
TMP	transmembrane pressure
TT	treatment time
UF	ultrafiltration
UFR	ultrafiltration rate
USRDS	United States Renal Data System

operating characteristics of HD are blood-flow rate (Qb), dialysate flow rate (Qd), duration and frequency of treatment, and dialyzer characteristics such as membrane surface area and composition, which affects solute dialysance and water permeability. By convention, "small" molecular weight solutes are <500 Da, "middle" molecular weight solutes are 500 to 5,000 Da, and "large" molecular

114

TABLE 7.2	**Comparison of Conventional, High-Efficiency, and High-Flux Dialyzers**		
Characteristics	**Conventional**	**High Efficiency**	**High Flux**
KoA$_{urea}$	<450 mL/min	>450 mL/min	>450 mL/min
Urea clearance	<200 mL/min	>200 mL/min	>200 mL/min
KUF	<15 mL/h/mm Hg	Variable	>15 mL/h/mm Hg
β$_2$-MG clearance	<10 mL/min	Variable	>20 mL/min

KoA$_{urea}$, mass transfer area coefficient of urea; KUF, ultrafiltration coefficient; β$_2$-MG, β$_2$-microglobulin.

weight solutes are >5,000 Da. Herein, we use urea as the surrogate molecule for "small" solutes and its clearance to define small molecular weight solute clearance. The term *efficiency* has been used with reference to the small solute or urea clearance. *Flux* refers to membrane hydraulic (water) permeability. Solute transfer across the membrane is calculated as the urea mass transfer area coefficient (KoA$_{urea}$), the theoretical maximum urea clearance at infinite Qb and Qd, and is an intrinsic characteristic of the membrane thickness, composition, and surface area. Obviously Qb and Qd are not infinite, but the greater they are, the greater the clearance. In typical HD, urea clearance is much more highly dependent on Qb than on Qd. However, possibly because of internal filtration/convection, dialyzers with higher flux membranes demonstrate a greater dependence on Qd than dialyzers with low-flux membranes (2). In any case, if 100% of a solute is extracted across the dialyzer, the clearance is equal to the Qb. If the dialysate is 100% saturated with the solute, the clearance is equal to the Qd. So clearance can never exceed either the Qb or the Qd. Thus, for practical purposes, the "efficiency" of a dialyzer is dependent on its surface area, membrane solute permeability, and the operational conditions. Once the KoA$_{urea}$ for a given dialyzer is known, the urea clearance under any given Qb or Qd can be calculated or located on a nomogram (3) and used to compare dialyzers. HEHD is achieved primarily by increasing surface area, Qb, and Qd. By most conventions, HE dialyzers have a KoA$_{urea}$ >450 mL/min, which translates to *in vivo* urea clearance rates >200 mL/min at Qb 300 mL/min and Qd

500 mL/min. This can then be extrapolated to say that dialyzers can be compared and classified based on urea clearance at a fixed Qb and Qd (**TABLE 7.2**).

FIGURE 7.1 demonstrates the differences in urea clearances between higher efficiency dialyzers (higher KoA, upper curve) and lower efficiency dialyzers (lower KoA, lower curve) at varying Qb. In lower efficiency dialyzers, urea clearance tends to plateau at lower Qb. By contrast, urea clearance in higher efficiency dialyzers continues to rise with higher Qb and does not plateau until Qb exceeds 400 mL/min. Therefore, an access that can deliver such a Qb is important to take full advantage of HE dialyzers.

"Flux" refers to the hydraulic (water) permeability of the dialyzer membrane and can be quantified by the ultrafiltration coefficient (KUF) and sometimes additionally by β$_2$-microglobulin (β$_2$-MG) clearance. β$_2$-MG is an 11.8-kDa molecule implicated in the development of dialysis-related amyloidosis (DRA) and is used as a surrogate representation for large molecules. KUF is defined as the ultrafiltration rate (UFR) divided by the transmembrane pressure (TMP) and the units are milliliters per hour per millimeter of Hg of applied TMP (mL/h/mm Hg). **TABLE 7.3** lists technical specifications of selected dialyzers commonly in use by the two largest dialysis provider groups in the United States, as examples of how to use the concepts described above.

As mentioned, another way to define flux relates to membrane permeability defined by the clearance of substances with a molecular weight greater than 10 kDa. This definition owes its origin to the

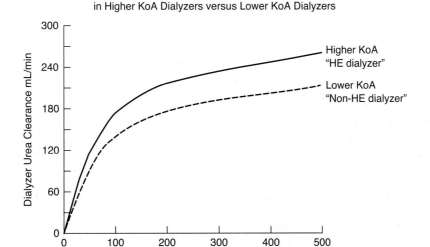

FIGURE 7.1 Dialyzer urea clearance as a function of blood-flow rate comparing a higher efficiency dialyzer with a greater urea mass transfer area coefficient (KoA) to a dialyzer with a lower KoA and lower efficiency.

TABLE 7.3	Specifications of Commonly Utilized Dialyzers in the United States			
Manufacturer/Model	**KoA (mL/min)**	**KUF (mL/h/mm Hg)**	**Surface Area (m²)**	**Material Type**
Fresenius Optiflux F160NR	1,064	50	1.5	Polysulfone
Fresenius Optiflux F180NR	1,239	60	1.8	Polysulfone
Fresenius Optiflux F200NR	1,317	62	2.0	Polysulfone
Fresenius Optiflux F250NR	1,808	107	2.5	Advanced polysulfone
Gambro Polyflux Revaclear	1,190	50	1.4	Polyarylethersulfone, polyvinylpyrrolidone
Gambro Polyflux Revaclear Max	1,495	60	1.8	Polyarylethersulfone, polyvinylpyrrolidone

KoA, mass transfer area coefficient; KUF, ultrafiltration coefficient.
Gambro Revaclear Polyflux Catalog, http://www.gambro.com/PageFiles/7915/306150161_2_RevaclearSpecs-lo.pdf?epslanguage=en, Fresenius Optiflux Dialyzers Catalog. Accessed July 20, 2015.

Hemodialysis (HEMO) trial, where HF membranes were defined by KUF >14 mL/h/mm Hg with a mean β_2-MG clearance >20 mL/min (4). The first application of HEHD was characterized by high urea clearance, using cellulosic large surface area membranes, and high KUF in the range of 10 to 20 (5). The high KUF was largely the consequence of the membrane surface area. Cellulosic materials were utilized because of their great tensile strength, which was needed because of the high applied TMP. As membrane synthesis became less costly, the cellulosic membranes were replaced with HF synthetic materials, which had greater KUF, and required less TMP to achieve the same UFR. Hence, dialyzer membranes should ideally be compared under equal operating conditions on the basis of KOA_{urea}, KUF, β_2-MG clearance, and surface area, as well as other factors not discussed here such as extracorporeal blood commitment, biocompatibility, and reuse potential.

⬡ TECHNICAL ASPECTS

With the increased popularity of HEHFHD in the United States, standard requirements and features must be met in the current dialysis machines and facilities. Precise ultrafiltration control is a standard feature in most currently available dialysis machines, achieved with varying methods. This section is intended to help clinicians ask specific questions of manufacturers and dialysis providers to investigate which systems are best for a particular facility.

Ultrafiltration Control Systems

Precise ultrafiltration (UF) control is mandatory because of the high KUF of these dialyzers, which actually began as hemofiltration cartridges with KUF of >100 mL/h/mm Hg. Control of fluid balance was best achieved with sophisticated computerized UF controllers to match UF and reinfusion of fluid, thereby maintaining hemodynamic stability. This historical perspective is important, since the outgrowth of HE and HF treatments came from the clinical comparison of HEHD and hemofiltration during a short TT therapy. The initial UF control systems applied during the era of hemofiltration were the forerunners of the systems applied today. The original microprocessor-based hemofiltration equipment, produced by Gambro Healthcare (Lakewood, Colorado), utilized a sophisticated strain gauge attached to a load cell that measured the rate of weight change from the 35-L containers used to collect ultrafiltrate and provide reinfusion fluid. This was, in fact, the first true volumetric UF control system. But this system was not directly applicable to an on-line, single-pass dialysis system in which approximately 100 to

160 L of fluid had to be accurately measured. Further improvements in the UF control systems for hemofiltration led to a continuous on-line system that used electromagnetic flow sensors to measure dialysate inflow and outflow. This system was microprocessor controlled and had no mechanical flow components. This is classified as the first microprocessor-based electronic UF control system and is still used in some HD machines. A secondary application of these microprocessor-based electronic UF control systems centered on the development of a bearingless rotor placed in a centrifugal flow path, which spun a ring where the optical characteristics were sensed through a fiber-optic network that then determined flow rates. Instead of being electromagnetically based, they are a combination of mechanical and electronic sensing. Typical examples of this type of equipment were produced by Baxter Healthcare Corporation (Deerfield, Illinois) in their 1550 dialysis machines.

The third major type of UF control system, developed in the early 1980s, utilized a mechanical-based system to control the very high KUF of hemofilters (100 to 200 mL/h/mm Hg) and hemodiafilters. These so-called volumetric control systems are based on the creation of a closed inflow and outflow loop by multiple-valve isolation systems, with a secondary UF pump that removed fluid from the relatively closed circuit at a fixed rate. The closed-circuit system matched dialysis inflow and outflow by bellows displacement pumps as the UF control pump generated the appropriate TMP needed to limit UF during the dialysis treatment. Examples of this type of equipment were the Cobe Century III (Cobe Renal Intensive Care Division of Gambro Healthcare, Lakewood, Colorado), the Fresenius series of HD machines (Fresenius Medical Care, Lexington, Massachusetts), the System 1000 by Althin Medical, Inc (Miami, Florida), the Toray UF control system (Houston, Texas), and the Italian Bellco machine (Bellco S.P.A., Saluggia, Vercelli, Italy). The UF control achieved by these mechanical bellows systems was compatible with both HE and HF dialyzers. Some of these systems may still be available on secondary markets. The current mainstream equipment that meets these requirements include the Fresenius 2008K/K² machine series.

Bicarbonate Dialysate

Bicarbonate dialysate has become the predominant buffer in the era of HEHFHD. When acetate was the buffering system in the 1980s, the use of more efficient dialyzers with KoA_{urea} >450 mL/min was associated with more frequent intradialytic symptoms and complications. Because of their more rapid diffusion of small solutes, HE dialyzers allowed acetate from the dialysate to accumulate in the patient faster than it could be metabolized (6). High levels of acetate can have a negative inotrope effect and can be vasodilatory peripherally, thus contributing to hypotension (7,8). In addition, acetate dialysate has a low partial pressure of carbon dioxide, which leads to net carbon dioxide removal. By removing the respiratory drive of carbon dioxide, patients were found to hypoventilate, and hypoxemia was a common problem that may have contributed to acetate intolerance (9). Thus, use of acetate contributed to hypoxemia, decreased cardiac output, and hypotension (10). These complications helped to usher in bicarbonate as the dialysate buffer of choice while using the new HE dialyzers.

Bicarbonate dialysis is not without its own complications and technical difficulties. In contrast to acetate dialysate, which is prepared from a single concentrate that inhibits bacterial growth, bicarbonate dialysate must be prepared from two concentrates to prevent precipitation when stored as concentrate containing calcium and magnesium. One of these concentrates is pH neutral and supports bacterial growth, which can lead to contamination. Solutions are buffered to pH of 5.2 to 5.5 to delay bacterial growth during storage.

SOLUTE CLEARANCE

Defining Uremic Toxins

While many "uremic toxins" remain unidentified and unmeasured, the current measurable solutes have been divided based on molecular weight, as mentioned above. While some small molecular weight substances are easily removed and measurable, there are significant implications of the presence of middle molecules on both morbidity and mortality, including their impact on cardiovascular morbidity. To date, there has been suggestion of approximately 40 groups or categories of middle molecules that may have been identified; these are often thought to be proinflammatory (11).

Diffusive removal capacity of middle molecules is dependent on molecular weight, protein binding, properties of the membrane including porosity and surface area, and molecular kinetic behavior of the middle molecule including compartmental distribution (12). Furthermore, middle molecular removal is directly dependent on increased convective clearance strategies, the latter especially important for protein-bound solutes. HF dialyzers thus may confer additional benefits due to their porosity for middle and large molecular weight toxins, for example, β_2-MG. Several studies have revealed significantly decreased plasma β_2-MG levels in patients undergoing HF therapies (13–16). In a prospective, multicenter study of 380 patients randomized to four different dialysis techniques for 24 months, Locatelli et al. (16) demonstrated substantial reductions in pretreatment β_2-MG levels in patients receiving HD (23% reduction) or hemodiafiltration (16% reduction) using HF polysulfone membranes. In contrast, there were no changes in β_2-MG levels in the patients assigned to cuprophane and low-flux polysulfone HD (13). These results support the hypothesis that removal, as a consequence of membrane flux, may have a greater impact on β_2-MG levels than a lower rate of generation due to biocompatibility. Although a direct relationship between predialysis β_2-MG levels and DRA has not been established, Küchle et al. (17) noted a significantly lower incidence of carpal tunnel syndrome and/or osteoarticular lesions among 20 long-term dialysis patients randomized to HF polysulfone membranes versus low-flux cuprophane membranes after an 8-year follow-up. These findings could have important clinical implications, given the significant morbidity related to DRA in long-term dialysis patients.

Middle molecular removal is thus greatly time-dependent in part due to the rebound effect and mobilization from the multicompartmental distribution (4,12). Hence, clearance may be improved by increasing dialysis frequency or increasing session duration. This is clearly demonstrated by almost doubling of β_2-MG clearance with increased dialysis time from 4 to 8 hours, despite a similar Kt/V_{urea} (12,18). While the primary analysis of the HEMO study demonstrated no significant effect of membrane flux on mortality, a subanalysis of the HEMO study demonstrates an inverse relationship between mortality and β_2-MG clearance (19). Predialysis β_2-MG concentrations fell over the course of the study in the HF arm patients far more than those in the low-flux arm. Similarly, in the Membrane Permeability Outcome (MPO) study, HF dialysis resulted in statistically significant lower β_2-MG accumulation over a period of 36 months when compared to low-flux group (20). The MPO study further demonstrated a significant survival benefit with the use of HF dialysis membranes in the subgroup of patients with serum albumin ≤4, a relative risk (RR) reduction of 37% after adjusting for confounders.

As dialysis technology evolved, the required "adequacy goals" were achieved in less time. Hence, dialysis session duration was decreased. Incentives for the facility to shorten session duration were the ability to accommodate more patients per day, spreading costs over more patients, and for patients, less time at the facility. Shorter TTs used increased dialysate quantities with increased Qd, but this cost balanced out with the decreased time. And while increased Qb up to 400 mL/min may improve small molecular clearance, it translates into decreased middle molecular clearance due to decreased session time. We fully agree with Vanholder et al. (21) that the small solute definition of "adequacy" of HD, the concept of Kt/V_{urea} is too simple to explain or define the complexities of uremia and modern dialysis techniques.

POTENTIAL BENEFITS

Subgroup analysis of the HEMO study concluded an insignificant trend favoring mortality benefit for large-pore, HFHD membranes in achieving the 1.3 Kt/V goal (4,19). However, these were not necessarily HEHD treatments. Similarly, the MPO study noted superiority for HF dialysis in certain subsets (20). In any case, the emphasis should remain that removal of middle and large molecular weight substances is predominantly time-dependent, and even with the currently available HF dialyzers, clearance of these substances will be greater with longer therapies.

LIMITATIONS

There remains a concern regarding the risk associated with large pore size and the transfer of impurities from the dialysate to the patient. Hence, a very regular control and check for dialysis impurities must be in place and is advocated strongly by European Best Practice Guidelines (22) and Association for the Advancement of Medical Instrumentation (23).

Contaminated dialysate can lead to both short- and long-term complications. Acute pyrogenic reactions (PR) from bacterial contamination or endotoxin exposure may occur in 1 of 10,000 dialysis sessions, and approximately 20% of all dialysis centers report more than one PR per year (24). Less obvious reactions to contaminated dialysate include cytokine release that can contribute to hypotension, sedation, and anorexia. Chronic complications are less well understood or documented. Chronic inflammation due to contaminated dialysate may contribute to the pathogenesis β_2-MG amyloidosis, catabolic loss of muscle proteins, erythropoietin-resistant anemia, and atherosclerotic cardiovascular disease (25–28).

Historically, it has been thought that HE—and more so, HF—dialyzers are more permeable to endotoxin fragments and therefore lead to more PR. Many investigators have demonstrated that bacterial products can diffuse across dialysis membranes (29,30). It follows that the larger surface areas, permeability, and Qd used in HE–HF dialysis would lead to greater potential diffusion of bacterial products across the membrane. However, *in vitro* studies have demonstrated that cellulosic low-flux membranes are actually more permeable to endotoxin fragments than synthetic HF membranes, which have high pyrogen-adsorbing capacity (31). This perceived benefit may be countered *in vivo* by endotoxin transfer across HF membranes due to backfiltration. They concluded that in contrast to cellulosic membranes, some synthetic membranes do not permit transfer of lipopolysaccharide and attenuate cytokine induction on the blood side of the dialyzer by removal of activated complement factors. Bicarbonate dialysate and HF membranes have been associated with a higher risk of PR (32). Some studies have shown that the practice of reuse, in which water comes into direct contact with the blood compartment, may be of more importance than membrane type (29). Gordon et al. (33) showed no statistical difference in PR rates by treatment modality (conventional, HE, and HF). Despite this controversy, it is accepted that dialysis membranes are permeable to bacterial products, although not uniformly, and important short-term and long-term effects of contaminated dialysate are likely.

⬡ ULTRAFILTRATION

UF is performed during dialysis to remove volume accumulated during the interdialytic period which on the average patient on thrice-weekly dialysis ranges between 1 and 4 kg. Actually, the interdialytic weight gain (IDWG) is assumed to be water and treated as such, but this assumption can lead to problems in some circumstances. For this discussion, the IDWG will be assumed to be acquired fluid volume between the dialysis sessions. As discussed earlier, HEHFHD utilizes operating conditions, KoA_{urea}, and KUF and requires ultrafiltration controllers, such that fluid removal at dialysis is quite accurate. Recent observational studies have informed us as to the safety of how much and how rapid the fluid accumulated can be withdrawn at dialysis. Thus, the concept of fast dialysis, which is why HEHD was developed in the first place, starts to become obsolete.

Potential Benefits of High-Flux Hemodialysis

As mentioned earlier, HF can be defined by KUF or by β_2-MG clearance. HF membranes confer additional benefits due to their porosity for middle and large molecular weight toxins. For example, decreased plasma β_2-MG levels are noted in patients undergoing HFHD (16,17,34). Since HEHFHD has some similarities to hemodiafiltration with regard to solute removal of all sizes, a review of that literature is relevant here. In the Dialysis Outcome and Practice Patterns Study (DOPPS), a survival benefit was observed only in hemodiafiltration patients who were treated with high convective volumes (replacements of >15 L per treatment) (35). For optimal efficiency, the use of large convective volumes has been recommended. Other potential benefits of HF membranes include a reduction in erythropoietin resistance, delay in loss of residual renal function, improved lipid profiles, specifically increased high-density

lipoprotein (HDL) cholesterol and lowered triglyceride levels, as well as removal of advanced glycosylation end products, which have been implicated in the pathogenesis of atherosclerosis and DRA (36–45). Furthermore, the use of ultrafiltration with HF dialyzers improved convective clearance of urea (as most of these membranes are also HE) and thus enhanced the shortening of dialysis period, a key motivating force behind its use.

Concerns and Implications

UF which is necessary to maintain volume control can at the same time dangerously promote nonphysiologic fluid shifts and hemodynamic instability. During dialysis, fluid is removed directly from the vascular space. When dialytic removal outpaces redistribution (refilling) from other compartments, circulating volume is reduced and transient myocardial ischemia and intradialytic hypotension (IDH) can result (46). This effect is amplified by limitation in cardiac reserve and autonomic dysfunction, both of which are common among HD patients. Previous research has demonstrated that transient ischemia during dialysis can result in "myocardial stunning" (regional wall motion abnormalities) and associated compromises in cardiac contractility, systolic function, and survival. Ventricular dysfunction in dialysis patients can be particularly hazardous as it has been linked to greater hemodynamic instability during dialysis, which can result in a vicious cycle of further myocardial stunning and cardiac decline (46,47).

In current practice, HD TT is determined by indices of small molecule (i.e., urea) clearance; UFR is adjusted to allow for necessary removal of IDWG within this fixed short TT (47). Excessive IDWG has been shown to be an independent predictor of mortality in a number of observational studies (47,48). Lee et al. (49) showed that increased IDWG percentage is a significant independent predictor of major adverse cardiac and cerebrovascular event in HD patients. Patients with excessive IDWG tend to receive a high UFR within this fixed TT, potentially resulting in increased frequency of IDH. IDH in turn could result in altered sensorium, myocardial ischemia and infarction, blindness, and even stroke (48). Flythe et al. (47) studied three categories of UFR: <10 mL/h/kg, 10 to 13 mL/h/kg, and >13 mL/h/kg, and noted that higher UFR in HD patients are associated with a greater risk of all-cause and cardiovascular death.

The rate-limiting factor for short HD is generally related to patient tolerance of UF, specifically, the ability to correct IDWG while maintaining cardiovascular stability as discussed below. Many factors contributed to this fixed short HD TT, including patient preference for less time on dialysis, economic incentives, availability of HEHF therapies, and results of the National Cooperative Dialysis Study (50). The study utilized short (2.5 to 3.5 hours) and long (4.5 to 5.5 hours) treatment groups for both high blood urea nitrogen (BUN) patient groups and low BUN patient groups. The actual mean TTs achieved were 3.2 and 4.5 hours. Patients in the high BUN and shorter treatment group were hospitalized more frequently than other groups, but this was determined to not be statistically significant ($p < 0.06$), and the final analysis suggested that TT was only marginally important. Although shorter TT did not demonstrate meaningful differences in serum biochemistries other than phosphorous levels, weight gains were typically higher, blood pressure control more difficult, and episodes of IDH more frequent. Although these results were not statistically significant, their potential clinical importance was not emphasized. The rather small sample size ($n = 151$) and the premature stopping of the National Cooperative Dialysis Study may have contributed to the failure to demonstrate a clinically significant difference between the long and short treatment arms.

There are two options to minimize UFR in current clinical practice: (a) limit fluid intake (i.e., IDWG) and/or (b) allow more time for fluid removal (i.e., extended dialysis time). Experience and published data demonstrate that interventions aimed at reducing patient's IDWG are often ineffective (47).

There is concern that with short TTs, suboptimal volume removal due to intradialytic symptoms may contribute to the high incidence or persistence of hypertension and ultimately to cardiovascular mortality, which underlies approximately 50% of the deaths in the dialysis population (48). The prevalence of hypertension has been reported in 50% to 80% of chronic HD patients in the United States, and there have been reports of increased antihypertensive medication requirements and a higher prevalence of left ventricular hypertrophy in patients dialyzed for shorter times (51–54). Thus, caution must be exercised when selecting patients for short therapies. A number of investigators describe favorable experiences with short dialysis in patients without excessive IDWG (55,56). For instance, a prospective study by Dumler et al. (55) found no changes in pre- or postdialysis blood pressures in a group of patients dialyzed less than 3 hours compared with conventional TT of between 3 and 4 hours when IDWG <4 kg. Likewise, shorter TTs were not associated with an increase in intradialytic complications, and the frequency of nausea, vomiting, headaches, and back pain was decreased. However, centers incorporating unconventionally long TT observed that most patients were able to discontinue antihypertensive medications (57,58). Extended HD was also associated with near normalization of left ventricular mass and improvement in left ventricular systolic function (48,59). The experience from the centers performing slow nocturnal dialysis and Tassin, France, have repeatedly emphasized the importance of TT, reporting consistently excellent results, especially with respect to blood pressure control, reduced erythropoietin requirements, fluid management, reduced frequency of IDH, and improved quality of life (48,57). The Netherlands Cooperative Study on the Adequacy of Dialysis recently reported the association between excessive UF and mortality, independent of delivered Kt/V (60). Saran et al. (48) examined the relationship between TT and UFR with patient outcome in DOPPS in an international, prospective cohort study of HD patients and facilities. Europe and Japan had significantly longer average TT than the United States. Kt/V increased concomitantly with TT in all three regions with the largest absolute difference observed in Japan. TT >240 minutes was independently associated with significantly lower RR of mortality. Every 30 minutes longer on HD was associated with a 7% lower RR; the reduction with longer TT was greatest in Japan. UFR >10 mL/h/kg was associated with 30% higher odds of IDH and a higher risk of mortality. However, there was no significant trend in mortality with lower categories of UFR. It is uncertain whether, for a given value of Kt/V, short HEHFHD provides the same total therapy as standard or longer TT. Observational data has suggested that any level of Kt/V is associated with a lower RR of mortality when TT is lengthened (61). Furthermore, at higher levels of Kt/V, a longer TT was found to be even more beneficial than the same TT for a lower level of Kt/V. These findings imply a synergistic relationship between TT and Kt/V with respect to mortality risk (48).

The removal of middle and large molecular weight substances is predominantly time-dependent, and even with the currently available HF dialyzers, clearance of these substances will be greater with longer therapies. There are also reports of improved phosphorus control without the use of binders as well as better control of anemia with concomitant decreases in erythropoietin requirements when long TT are employed (58,59,62). Recent data from the Australia and New Zealand Dialysis and Transplant Registry indicate that TT >270 minutes may be associated with a lower RR of mortality and duration of <210 minutes may be associated with a higher mortality risk (61). Short HD is attractive because it offers the potential for reduced labor costs as well as patient and staff convenience. However, the same requirements for adequacy must apply to these shortened treatments as with conventional HD: to ensure effective solute removal and volume control without compromising patient well-being. At present, most studies evaluating the adverse effects of shortened TT on morbidity and mortality are limited by confounding issues, such as delivery of inadequate small solute clearance, inconsistencies among membrane characteristics with regard to efficiency, flux, and biocompatibility, as well as lack of long-term follow-up. Data in support of extended TT sessions are accumulating and suggest that these modalities may offer significant advantages over conventional therapies. Thus, longer TT may be beneficial in several ways: improved tolerability of the treatment (primarily the result of slower UFR), better removal of larger sized uremic toxins, better control of blood pressure, and better volume management. These mechanisms may in turn reduce cardiovascular morbidity and mortality (48).

There are numerous issues facing nephrologists practicing in today's climate: economic pressures, personnel shortage, patient education, and cultural differences. Because there are no randomized trials evaluating TT and outcome (the TIME trial is underway), we continue to define dialysis adequacy by complicated mathematical equations that are inherently flawed, allowing us to drive time on dialysis toward zero as long as small solute dialyzer clearance continues to increase.

Nevertheless, using an individualized approach to dialysis prescription is generally well tolerated when individual patient characteristics regarding cardiovascular stability, blood pressure, and IDWG are considered. We reiterate our agreement with the argument against the defining of adequate dialysis by the use of Kt/V_{urea} as articulated by Vanholder et al. (21).

High IDWG, volume expansion, the economic barriers to long duration HD, and the inherent unphysiology of thrice-weekly HD all predispose patient to the necessity of higher UFR with increased frequency of IDH and increased risk of death (48). We and many others believe that UFR should factor more prominently into the determination of dialytic TT. Such an approach might involve session-length titration on a nearly session-to-session basis based on observed IDWG with some floor level determined by consideration of urea clearance (47). In particular, John Burkart, as chief medical officer of an intermediate-sized dialysis provider, has implemented a policy that the dialysis duration accomplishes the Kt/V_{urea} goal as well as limiting the UFR to no more than 13 mL/kg/h. If in that duration the IDWG is not removed, the session length is increased, or an extra dialysis session is performed. We strongly endorse this initiative and approach.

CONCLUSION

While we have described the performance of HEHD, we did so predominantly for historical reasons. In general, we do not recommend that approach to chronic maintenance HD. On the other hand, when the treatments are not shortened, HFHD has many advantages. Using small molecule clearance such as Kt/V_{urea} as the definition of dialysis adequacy is an egregious error in our opinion and we have described why. Setting dialysis time by the tolerance of ultrafiltration seems critically important and a limit of 13 mL/kg/h is prudent. We fully agree with Vanholder et al. (21) and strongly urge the dialysis community and regulatory bodies to appreciate the scientific evidence and change the way we define the adequacy of HD.

ACKNOWLEDGMENTS

We thank the following people who helped with this chapter: Edith Simmons, Blake Weathersby, Fred Arndt, Steve Clyne (from previous editions), and Cailtin Sulham.

REFERENCES

1. United States Renal Data System. *USRDS 2001 Annual Data Report: Atlas of End-Stage Renal Disease in the United States.* Bethesda, MD: National Institutes of Health, National Institute of Diabetes and Digestive and Kidney Diseases, 2001.
2. Leypoldt JK, Cheung AK. Increases in mass transfer-area coefficients and urea Kt/V with increasing dialysate flow rate are greater for high flux dialyzers. *Am J Kidney Dis* 2001;38(3):575–579.
3. Daugirdas JT. Physiologic principles and urea kinetic modeling. In: Daugirdas JT, Blake PG, Ing TS, eds. *Handbook of Dialysis.* 3rd ed. Philadelphia, PA: Lippincott Williams & Wilkins, 2001:670–676.
4. Eknoyan G, Beck GJ, Cheung AK, et al. Effect of dialysis dose and membrane flux in maintenance hemodialysis. *N Engl J Med* 2002;347: 2010–2019.
5. Barth, RH. Pros and cons of short, high efficiency and high flux dialysis. In: Winchester JF, Jacobs C, Kjellstrand C, et al, eds. *Replacement of Renal Function by Dialysis.* 4th ed. Dordrecht, The Netherlands: Kluwer Academic Publishers, 1996:418–454.
6. Gonzalez FM, Pearson JE, Garbus SB, et al. On the effects of acetate during hemodialysis. *Trans Am Soc Artif Intern Organs* 1974;20A: 169–174.
7. Vincent J-L, Vanherweghem J-L, Degaute J-P, et al. Acetate-induced myocardial depression during hemodialysis for acute renal failure. *Kidney Int* 1982;22:653–657.
8. Henrich WL, Woodard TD, Meyer BD, et al. High sodium bicarbonate and acetate hemodialysis: double-blind crossover comparison of hemodynamic and ventilatory effects. *Kidney Int* 1983;24:240–245.
9. Kaiser BA, Potter DE, Bryant RE, et al. Acid-base changes and acetate metabolism during routine and high-efficiency hemodialysis in children. *Kidney Int* 1981;19:70–79.
10. Novello AC, Kjellstrand CM. Is bicarbonate dialysis better than acetate dialysis? *ASAIO J* 1983;6:103–107.
11. Weissinger EM, Kaiser T, Meert N, et al. Proteomics: a novel tool to unravel the patho-physiology of uraemia. *Nephrol Dial Transplant* 2004;19:3068–3077.
12. Vanholder R, Glorieux G, Biesen WV. Advantages of new hemodialysis membranes and equipment. *Nephron Clin Pract* 2010;114:c165–c172.
13. Schiffl H, Lang S, Fischer R. Ultrapure dialysis fluid slows loss of residual renal function in new dialysis patients. *Nephrol Dial Transplant* 2002;17:1814–1818.
14. Canaud BJM, Mion C. Water treatment for contemporary hemodialysis. In: Winchester JF, Jacobs C, Kjellstrand C, et al, eds. *Replacement of Renal Function by Dialysis.* 4th ed. Dordrecht: Kluwer Academic Publishers, 1996:231–255.
15. Lonnemann G. The quality of dialysate: an integrated approach. *Kidney Int* 2000;58:S112–S119.
16. Locatelli F, Mastrangelo F, Redaelli B, et al. Effects of different membranes and dialysis technologies on patient treatment tolerance and nutritional parameters. The Italian Cooperative Dialysis Study Group. *Kidney Int* 1996;50:1293–1302.
17. Küchle C, Fricke H, Held E, et al. High-flux hemodialysis postpones clinical manifestation of dialysis-related amyloidosis. *Am J Nephrol* 1996;16:484–488.
18. Eloot S, Van Biesen W, Dhondt A, et al. Impact of hemodialysis duration on the removal of uremic retention solute. *Kid Int* 2008;73:765–770.
19. Cheung AK, Levin NW, Greene T, et al. Effect of high-flux hemodialysis on clinical outcomes: results of the HEMO study. *J Am Soc Nephrol* 2003;14:3251–3263.
20. Locatelli F, Martin-Malo A, Hannedouche T, et al; and the Membrane Permeability Outcome (MPO) Study Group. Effect of membrane permeability on survival of hemodialysis patients. *J Am Soc Nephrol* 2009;20:645–654.
21. Vanholder R, Glorieux G, Eloot S. Once upon a time in dialysis: the last days of Kt/V? *Kid Int* 2015;88:460–465. doi:10.1038/ki.2015.155.
22. European Best Demonstrated Practice Guidelines for Haemodialysis (Part 1). Section IV. Dialysis fluid purity. *Nephrol Dial Transplant* 2002;17(Suppl 7):45–62.
23. Association for the Advancement of Medical Instrumentation. *American National Standard: Dialysate for Hemodialysis.* Arlington, VA: Association for the Advancement of Medical Instrumentation, 2004. http://www.therenalnetwork.org/home/resources/CfC/AAMI_RD520408.pdf. Accessed July 20, 2015.
24. Brunet P, Berland Y. Water quality and complications of haemodialysis. *Nephrol Dial Transplant* 2000;15:578–580.
25. Baz M, Durand C, Ragon A, et al. Using ultrapure water in hemodialysis delays carpal tunnel syndrome. *Int J Artif Organs* 1991;14:681–685.
26. Bistrian BR, McCowen KC, Chan S. Protein-energy malnutrition in dialysis patients. *Am J Kidney Dis* 1999;33:172–175.
27. Mattila KJ, Valtonen VV, Nieminen MS, et al. Role of infection as a risk factor for atherosclerosis, myocardial infarction, and stroke. *Clin Infect Dis* 1998;26:719–734.
28. Pereira BJG, Snodgrass BR, Hogan PJ, et al. Diffusive and convective transfer of cytokine-inducing bacterial products across hemodialysis membranes. *Kidney Int* 1995;47:603–610.
29. Bommer J, Becker KP, Urbaschek R. Potential transfer of endotoxin across high-flux polysulfone membranes. *J Am Soc Nephrol* 1996;7:883–888.
30. Lonnemann G, Behme TC, Lenzner B, et al. Permeability of dialyzer membranes to TNF alpha-inducing substances derived from water bacteria. *Kidney Int* 1992;42:61–68.
31. Schindler R, Ertl T, Beck W, et al. Reduced cytokine induction and removal of complement products with synthetic hemodialysis membranes. *Blood Purif* 2006;24(2):203–211.
32. Alter MJ, Favero MS, Moyer LA, et al. National surveillance of dialysis-associated diseases in the United States, 1989. *ASAIO Trans* 1991;37: 97–109.
33. Gordon SM, Oettinger CW, Bland LA, et al. Pyrogenic reactions in patients receiving conventional, high-efficiency, or high-flux hemodialysis treatments with bicarbonate dialysate containing high concentrations of bacteria and endotoxin. *J Am Soc Nephrol* 1992;2:1436–1444.
34. Koda Y, Nishi S, Miyazaki S, et al. Switch from conventional to high-flux membrane reduces the risk of carpal tunnel syndrome and mortality of hemodialysis patients. *Kidney Int* 1997;52(4):1096–1101.
35. Penne EL, van der Weerd NC, Blankestijn PJ, et al. Role of residual kidney function and convective volume on change in beta2-microglobulin levels in hemodiaflltration patients. *Clin J Am Soc Nephrol* 2010;5(1):80–86.
36. Hornberger JC, Chernew M, Petersen J, et al. A multivariate analysis of mortality and hospital admissions with high-flux dialysis. *J Am Soc Nephrol* 1992;3(6):1227–1237.
37. Hakim RM, Held PJ, Stannard DC, et al. Effect of dialysis membrane on mortality of chronic hemodialysis patients. *Kidney Int* 1996;50: 566–570.
38. Bloembergen WE, Hakim RM, Stannard DC, et al. Relationship of dialysis membrane and cause-specific mortality. *Am J Kidney Dis* 1999; 33:1–10.
39. Gutierrez A, Alvestrand A, Wahren J, et al. Effect of in vivo contact between blood and dialysis membranes on protein catabolism in humans. *Kidney Int* 1990;38:487–494.

40. Parker TF III, Wingard RL, Husni L, et al. Effect of the membrane biocompatibility on nutritional parameters in chronic hemodialysis patients. *Kidney Int* 1996;49(2):551–556.

41. Kobayashi H, Ono T, Yamamoto N, et al. Removal of high molecular weight substances with large pore size membrane (BK-F). *Kidney Dial* 1993;34(Suppl):154–157.

42. Locatelli F, Del Vecchio L, Andrulli S. The modality of dialysis treatment: does it influence response to erythropoietin treatment? *Nephrol Dial Transplant* 2001;16:1971–1974.

43. Seres DS, Strain GW, Hashim SA, et al. Improvement of plasma lipoprotein profiles during high-flux dialysis. *J Am Soc Nephrol* 1993;3(7): 1409–1415.

44. Blankestijn PJ, Vos PF, Rabelink TJ, et al. High-flux dialysis membranes improve lipid profile in chronic hemodialysis patients. *J Am Soc Nephrol* 1995;5(9):1703–1708.

45. Josephson MA, Fellner SK, Dasgupta A. Improved lipid profiles in patients undergoing high-flux hemodialysis. *Am J Kidney Dis* 1992;20(4):361–366.

46. Burton JO, Jefferies HJ, Selby NM, et al. Hemodialysis-induced cardiac injury: determinants and associated outcomes. *Clin J Am Soc Nephrol* 2009;4(5):914–920.

47. Flythe JE, Kimmel SE, Brunelli SM. Rapid fluid removal during dialysis is associated with cardiovascular morbidity and mortality. *Kidney Int* 2011;79:250–257.

48. Saran R, Bragg-Gresham JL, Levin NW, et al. Longer treatment time and slower ultrafiltration in hemodialysis: associations with reduced mortality in the DOPPS. *Kidney Int* 2006;69:1222–1228.

49. Lee MJ, Doh FM, Kim CH, et al. Interdialytic weight gain and cardiovascular outcome in incident hemodialysis patients. *Am J Nephrol* 2014;39:427–435.

50. Lowrie EG, Laird NM, Parker TF, et al. Effect of the hemodialysis prescription on patient morbidity: report from the National Cooperative Dialysis Study. *N Engl J Med* 1981;305:1176–1181.

51. Salem MM. Hypertension in the hemodialysis population: a survey of 649 patients. *Am J Kidney Dis* 1995;26:461–468.

52. Mailloux LU, Haley WE. Hypertension in the ESRD patient: pathophysiology, therapy, outcomes, and future directions. *Am J Kidney Dis* 1998;32(5):705–719.

53. Mittal SK, Kowalski E, Trenkle J, et al. Prevalence of hypertension in a hemodialysis population. *Clin Nephrol* 1999;51(2):77–82.

54. Wizemann V, Kramer W. Short-term dialysis—long-term complications. Ten years experience with short-duration renal replacement therapy. *Blood Purif* 1987;5(4):193–201.

55. Dumler F, Stalla K, Mohini R, et al. Clinical experience with short-time hemodialysis. *Am J Kidney Dis* 1992;19(1):49–56.

56. Velasquez MT, von Albertini B, Lew SQ, et al. Equal levels of blood pressure control in ESRD patients receiving high-efficiency hemodialysis and conventional hemodialysis. *Am J Kidney Dis* 1998;31(4):618–623.

57. Charra B, Calemard M, Laurent G. Importance of treatment time and blood pressure control in achieving long-term survival on dialysis. *Am J Nephrol* 1996;16(1):35–44.

58. Pierratos A. Nocturnal home haemodialysis: an update on a 5-year experience. *Nephrol Dial Transplant* 1999;14(12):2835–2840.

59. Culleton BF, Walsh M, Klarenbach SW, et al. Effect of frequent nocturnal hemodialysis vs conventional hemodialysis on left ventricular mass and quality of life: a randomized controlled trial. *JAMA* 2007;298:1291–1299.

60. Termorshuizen F, Dekker FW, van Manen JG, et al. Relative contribution of residual renal function and different measures of adequacy to survival in hemodialysis patients: an analysis of the Netherlands Cooperative Study on the Adequacy of Dialysis (NECOSAD)-2. *J Am Soc Nephrol* 2004;15:1061–1070.

61. Marshall MR, Byrne BG, Kerr PG, et al. Associations of hemodialysis dose and session length with mortality risk in Australian and New Zealand patients. *Kidney Int* 2006;69(7):1229–1236.

62. Vos PF, Zilch O, Kooistra MP. Clinical outcome of daily dialysis. *Am J Kidney Dis* 2001;37(1 Suppl 2):S99–S102.

CHAPTER 8

Long and Daily Hemodialysis

Andreas Pierratos

Despite improvements in the technical aspects of dialysis treatments and some recent clinical improvements, the outcomes of patients with end-stage kidney disease (ESKD) are poor (1). Furthermore, the cost of dialysis continues to increase rapidly due to the increasing number of patients requiring treatment.

In an effort to alter these statistics and their financial impact, several approaches have been considered and studied. These apply to the following:

Dialysis dose: studied initially in the National Cooperative Dialysis Study (NCDS) (2) and then the Hemodialysis (HEMO) and Adequacy of Peritoneal Dialysis in Mexico (ADEMEX) study (3)

Dialysis technology: improved hemodialysis machines, bicarbonate dialysis, better quality membranes, ultrapure dialysate, and so on

Dialysis schedules: Frequent hemodialysis, long hemodialysis, as well as various combinations of the two. The main forms include short daily hemodialysis, long intermittent hemodialysis, and daily nocturnal hemodialysis.

Methods of blood depuration: peritoneal dialysis (PD), the convective techniques (hemofiltration and hemodiafiltration), and the use of sorbents either as complete replacement of dialysis or as adjunct to other methods

Location of the treatment: Locations include hospitals, freestanding units, or home.

Method of delivery: Full care, assisted care, and self-care. Assistance is provided by nurses and technicians, paid helpers, or relatives.

Focus: a shift to address the comorbidities rather than dialysis itself

Finances: Different methods of cost reimbursement such as bundling of ancillary treatment payments with the dialysis fee or use of a capitated system of reimbursement have been employed (4).

In this chapter, the alternative dialysis schedules, specifically long and/or frequent hemodialysis, will be addressed. In addition, aspects of the location of the treatment as well as cost will be also discussed.

 HISTORICAL PERSPECTIVE

In the early days of hemodialysis, long (8-hour) dialysis was necessary as the dialysis technique was inefficient (5–7). Improving patient well-being with more than one or two dialysis sessions per week led to the adoption of the current standard of the thrice-weekly dialysis regimen. Improvement in the dialysis efficiency led to shorter hemodialysis sessions.

Perseverance with the original long (8-hour) thrice-weekly regimen in Tassin, France, and some other centers for more than 30 years, was associated with impressive patient outcomes and supported the notion that *long* dialysis was beneficial irrespective of the dialysis dose (8), an idea not clearly supported by the NCDS study (9). Long overnight hemodialysis (nocturnal hemodialysis) three times a week at home is credited to Shaldon (10). Long intermittent hemodialysis is financially attractive in comparison to daily hemodialysis, and therefore, recently, there has been an increased interest in its utilization at home or in the dialysis centers (11,12).

Home hemodialysis was necessary in the early dialysis days as it was less costly. More than 70% of dialyses in Seattle in the late 1960s was performed at home (5). Payment for dialysis with public funds, availability of hemodialysis close to the patients' home, inception of continuous ambulatory peritoneal dialysis (CAPD), and acceptance of dialysis for sicker patients unable to be trained led to the decline of home hemodialysis. Regional or national differences in the dialysis modality distribution are often striking and can be explained by financial, geographic, and cultural factors. For example, despite some decline, home hemodialysis has been more popular in Australia and New Zealand (13). The high incidence of CAPD technique failure and reports of improved outcomes with long and/or frequent hemodialysis rekindled the interest in home hemodialysis, although there is a recent resurgence of PD in the United States (14).

The use of *daily* hemodialysis was reported in the 1960s first by DePalma (15,16) followed by others. Despite better patient satisfaction, blood pressure (BP) control, and anemia improvement, the initial attempts failed due to financial constraints. The published positive outcomes from the use of short daily hemodialysis by a small number of centers in Italy led by Buoncristiani and others (17–19), the advent of quotidian nocturnal hemodialysis (20), as well as interest by industry inspired renewed focus on daily hemodialysis.

Although *nocturnal* hemodialysis thrice weekly at home was used by Shaldon (10), the combination of long and frequent hemodialysis was reported by Uldall in 1994 (21).

Moreover, interest in alternative dialysis schedules was rekindled by the failure of both HEMO (3) and ADEMEX (22) studies to show a decrease in patient mortality rates by increasing the dose in either hemodialysis or PD, respectively.

More detailed historical aspects of home and frequent dialysis regimens are described elsewhere (5). Although most of the studies on daily and long hemodialysis were cohort studies, randomized controlled trials (RCTs) have been recently published. These include the Alberta trial on nocturnal hemodialysis (23) and the Frequent Hemodialysis Network (FHN) trials sponsored by the National Institutes of Health (NIH) (24,25).

Dialysis Prescription/Technical Aspects

Short, daily hemodialysis is characterized by dialysis performed for 1.5 to 3.0 hours, 5 to 7 days per week. There are calls for at least 3-hour short daily hemodialysis as it is characterized by better phosphate control (26). High blood and dialysate flows are used, aiming for the highest dialysis dose possible. Dialysate composition is similar to conventional hemodialysis. It is done either in the dialysis facility or at home.

Daily (*quotidian*) *nocturnal* hemodialysis is performed 5 to 7 days per week (typically 6) during night sleep at home for an average of 8 hours. It is done by the patient or by a helper. Similarly, *intermittent nocturnal* hemodialysis occurs thrice weekly at the facility or at home (usually every other night). Facility-based nocturnal hemodialysis is typically performed by the dialysis staff. Blood flow is low on long hemodialysis (as a rule 200 to 300 mL/min and as low as 100 mL/min in children), whereas a typical dialysate flow is 300 mL/min. Lower dialysate volume is used by the NxStage machine. In the case of the daily nocturnal hemodialysis, the dialysate contains lower bicarbonate [typical: 30 mEq (mmol)/L] and higher calcium concentration [typical: 3.0 to 3.5 mEq (1.5 to 1.75 mmol)/L] than conventional hemodialysis (**TABLE 8.1**). A less significant deviation from the usual concentrate composition of the conventional hemodialysis is followed in the intermittent form. In more than 50% of patients on quotidian and less than 20% on the intermittent form, the dialysate contains a sodium phosphate additive (e.g., Fleet Enema 30 to 135 mL/4.5 L acid or bicarbonate concentrate) which corresponds to a final phosphate concentration of 1 to 3 mg/dL (0.3 to 0.9 mmol/L) (11,27,28). A higher calcium and phosphate concentration than described in the preceding text has been used during the so-called "hungry bone syndrome."

Although all hemodialysis machines are acceptable for each of the stated regimens, several manufacturers have modified existing machines to be patient-friendly for use at home, and new machines aiming for the short daily or the long hemodialysis market have been produced. Some of the advantages include ease of use, portability, less reliance on water quality, and so on.

Anticoagulation during hemodialysis is similar irrespective of regimen. Danaparoid or argatroban have been used in cases of heparin-induced thrombocytopenia. Low molecular weight heparin has been employed for both as well as for longer dialysis. Tinzaparin has been used during nocturnal hemodialysis (29).

Water treatment at home is accomplished through the use of standard reverse osmosis systems with a carbon tank or the use of deionizer columns. The former provides for less expensive operation, and the latter is less noisy, more relevant to nightly hemodialysis. Occasionally, a water softener prior to water purification

TABLE 8.1	**Typical Initial Dialysis Prescriptions for Alternative Dialysis Schedules**		
	Short Daily	**Long Intermittent**	**Daily Nocturnal**
Q_b	350–400	200–300	200–300
Q_d	700–800	300	300
Na	140	140	140[a]
K	1–2	2	2
Bicarbonate	40	35	30
Ca	2.5	3.0	3.5
Phosphate as sodium phosphate—Fleet Enema (mL/4-L jug)	0	0[b]	40[c]
Mg	0.5 mEq (0.25 mmol)/L	1 mEq (0.5 mmol)/L	1.5 mEq (0.75 mmol)/L

[a]Consider lower dialysate Na if a high dose of sodium phosphate (Na_3PO_4) is added (>80 mL Fleet Enema) into the dialysate and significant fluid gains or difficulty to control hypertension are encountered.

[b]Initially, discontinue phosphate binders if serum phosphate is <4.5 mg/dL (1.5 mmol/L) or if on low dose of phosphate binders.

[c]Do not add Fleet Enema initially if the prehemodialysis serum phosphate is high [>6 mg/dL (2 mmol/L)] despite the use of high dose of phosphate binders while on conventional hemodialysis. Stop phosphate binders in all patients.

system has also been employed. The use of "ultrapure" dialysate is encouraged, although most of the published experience did not include the use of this enhancement.

Although dialyzer reuse has been practiced on home hemodialysis, it has been abandoned with the decrease in the cost of dialyzers (30). Remote monitoring of patients on nocturnal hemodialysis has been practiced by some centers (31–33), but it is considered optional. If BP monitoring without a cuff inflation and decrease in the cost of remote monitoring are achieved, remote monitoring could be attractive (33).

Dialysis Access

All types of accesses including permanent central venous catheters, arteriovenous (AV) fistulas, and grafts can be used with long or frequent hemodialysis either in-center or at home. Although fewer complications were reported in observational studies (34–36), the FHN trial reported increased incidence of vascular complications on daily hemodialysis (37). Lower access survival was also reported on long frequent home hemodialysis compared to long less frequent home dialysis (38). Dialysis catheter survival as well as infection rates were reported to be better on nocturnal hemodialysis when compared to conventional hemodialysis (39,40), but the infection rates were higher than when using AV accesses (41). Safety issues are very important for unattended nocturnal hemodialysis (42). The use of preperforated catheter caps during the dialysis procedure is highly recommended (InterLink, Tego) (**FIGURE 8.1**) (43). They prevent air emboli and bleeding from the "arterial limb" in the case of accidental disconnection.

The so-called "buttonhole" technique has been used for fistula but not graft cannulation (44). Prospective studies on the outcomes when used at home are missing (44–48). Using this technique, the dialysis needle (usually "blunt," noncutting) is inserted through the same cannulation track. A "buttonhole" is established using regular sharp needles for about 1 week. The use of the buttonhole technique

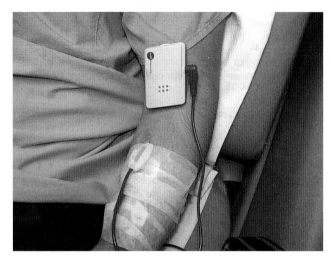

FIGURE 8.2 The "enuresis" moisture alarm.

has been associated with significantly higher rate of bacteremias. The putative advantages including less pain, familiarity with the site, and predictability of cannulation success have not been proved in RCTs. If used, attention should be given to proper technique and antisepsis during the "buttonhole" cannulation. Careful removal of the scab prior to the cannulation and local application of a small amount of antibiotic cream (e.g., mupirocin) after the completion of dialysis on the "buttonhole" has been advocated (47). Caution regarding the use of the buttonhole technique has been expressed by several authors (43,49). Proper secure taping of the dialysis needle is important for nocturnal hemodialysis. A single-needle system is preferable for long hemodialysis as it requires fewer cannulations and is safer in the case of accidental needle disconnection. The lower blood flow provided by the single-needle system is not a limitation for long hemodialysis. A moisture sensor taped on top of the needle insertion site is useful to awaken the patient in the event of blood extravasation during the dialysis procedure (31). An inexpensive nondisposable "enuresis alarm" is used by most centers in the interim until a dedicated product is developed (**FIGURE 8.2**). Commercially available sensors specifically designed for dialysis are available (50). Several inexpensive moisture sensors placed strategically on the floor in the vicinity of the dialysis machine alert the patient in case of either blood or dialysate leak (31).

⬢ THEORY/KINETICS

Small Molecule Removal

The use of Kt/V urea and urea reduction rate (URR) based on the NCDS study became popular as a measure of dialysis dose (51). These parameters are inadequate, however, in explaining the differences in outcomes between various modalities, between different schedules, or related to the presence of residual kidney function. The relatively positive clinical outcomes of patients on CAPD when compared to hemodialysis, despite the lower Kt/V offered by this method (weekly Kt/V 1.7 to 2.0 vs. 3.2, respectively), has been ascribed to the continuous nature of this treatment (52). Continuous (or frequent) dialysis can provide hemodynamic stability and therefore better cardiovascular tolerance and reduced fluctuation of physiologic parameters (53); better removal of larger molecules, which is time-dependent; and decreased exposure to the toxic peak

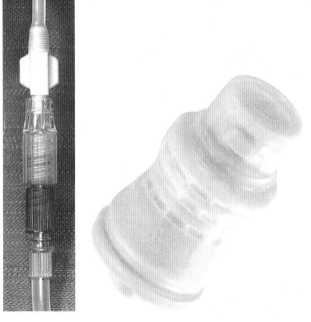

FIGURE 8.1 The Interlink and Tego venous catheter caps.

levels of solutes which characterize intermittent dialysis. The most popular measure incorporating this effect of the dialysis frequency is the standard Kt/V (stdKt/V) proposed by Gotch (54,55). Similar weekly stdKt/V values offered by different regimens are expected to lead to similar clinical outcomes. Its calculation is based on the midweek predialysis serum blood urea nitrogen (BUN) (or the continuous BUN level in the case of native kidney function or CAPD). An stdKt/V of 2.0 corresponds to the Kidney Disease Outcomes Quality Initiative (KDOQI) dose guideline levels.

The usefulness of the stdKt/V in predicting clinical outcomes needs to be established. The use of stdKt/V increases the perceived value of high dialysis frequency, but this dose measure is not affected significantly by the increased dialysis length, as long intermittent dialysis has a smaller effect on the predialysis BUN levels. Therefore, based on this concept, the outcomes of long intermittent dialysis are expected to be inferior to the outcomes of short daily hemodialysis, which has not been established and may not be accurate. A single-pool Kt/V (spKt/V) of only about 0.53 is required daily to maintain the same weekly stdKt/V delivered by thrice-weekly hemodialysis when adhering to the KDOQI guideline dose of a spKt/V of 1.2 per dialysis session. Maintenance of the same length of weekly dialysis after the conversion to the daily regimen provides an stdKt/V of 2.5 to 3 (56). The spKt/V offered by daily nocturnal hemodialysis is much higher at about 1.8 to 2.5 per treatment, whereas the stdKt/V is 4 to 6 for the six times per week regimen (57). This concept of stdKt/V is utilized by the proponents of the NxStage machine. The prescription includes usually lower dialysate volume (about 25 L) with weekly stdKt/V similar to PD to achieve financial feasibility of daily hemodialysis.

Middle Molecule Removal

The evidence that higher larger molecule weight solute removal correlates with better clinical outcomes is supported by some studies (58–60). Patient outcomes correlated well with the length of dialysis, surrogate of middle molecule removal, in two studies from the Australian/New Zealand (61) and Dialysis Outcomes and Practice Pattern Study (DOPPS) registries (62).

As predicted, middle molecule removal is increased mainly by longer dialysis and less significantly by short daily hemodialysis. This was shown by mathematical modeling (63) as well as in clinical studies. Weekly β_2-microglobulin removal increased fourfold from 127 to 585 mg after the conversion from conventional to quotidian nocturnal hemodialysis. Serum predialysis β_2-microglobulin levels decreased from 27.2 to 13.7 mg/dL in 9 months (64). Advanced glycation end-product (AGE) levels decreased on daily hemodialysis (65) as did the levels of protein-bound solutes such as indole-3-acetic and acid indoxyl sulfate (66).

Phosphate Removal

Hyperphosphatemia has been considered a significant risk factor for both kidney osteodystrophy as well as cardiovascular disease and has been correlated to patient mortality (67). Despite the adequate phosphate clearance during dialysis, phosphate removal is limited by the slow intercompartmental movement of phosphate, resulting in low serum phosphate both during and in rebound posthemodialysis (68). The most significant parameter affecting phosphate removal is the length of dialysis. The effect of the dialysis regimens on phosphate control is therefore predictable. Short daily hemodialysis increases phosphate removal because phosphate removal is higher during the early part of dialysis when the blood to dialysate gradient is highest. This has been confirmed by measuring phosphate in spent dialysate (26,69). However, a 2-hour short daily hemodialysis has only a modest effect on serum phosphate as phosphate intake often increases with improving appetite. Significant improvement in phosphate control was found in studies when the dialysis time was extended to 3 hours (26,70). Daily nocturnal hemodialysis is effective in phosphate removal not only leading to elimination of the need for phosphate binders and unrestricted diet but even necessitating the addition of phosphate into the dialysate in order to avoid hypophosphatemia in 75% of the patients (**TABLE 8.1**) (31,71). The effect of intermittent nocturnal hemodialysis on phosphate removal is also significant, but some patients still needing binders while for others a phosphate additive into the dialysate is necessary (11). In this modality, the predialysis phosphate can be high while the posthemodialysis value can be in the hypophosphatemic range. The effectiveness of long intermittent hemodialysis in phosphate removal is higher than that of short daily hemodialysis (**TABLE 8.2**). The improvement in phosphate control was confirmed in the FHN in both daily and nocturnal trials (70) as well as the Alberta trial (72).

Patient Selection/Training and Utilization of the Alternative Dialysis Schedules

Patient selection and method utilization are affected by several factors. They include the local availability of the modality, finances, medical indications/contraindications, dialysis team biases, and patient/family choice. In turn, availability of the method depends on local expertise and financial factors.

The type of patients who is treated using the alternative dialysis schedules tend to follow a bimodal distribution. This includes patients who experience "technique failure" in their current modality and for whom an alternative dialysis method is used as a "rescue" treatment (73,74). Alternatively, other patients opt for these dialysis modalities motivated by a desire to improve their quality of life (QOL). The former group of patients tends to be switched either to short daily hemodialysis or intermittent nocturnal hemodialysis in the dialysis facility or daily nocturnal hemodialysis at home. Usual reasons for this "rescue" treatment include significant hemodynamic instability, cardiovascular disease, refractory hypertension, intra- and interdialytic symptoms, ascites, malnutrition, "failure to thrive," or large body size. The second group tends to include younger patients who are more likely to dialyze at home. In the absence of comorbidities, it is often difficult to convince prevalent dialysis patients to convert to the alternative dialysis schedules especially in the form of home hemodialysis. Incident compared to prevalent dialysis patients are the more likely to elect to do home hemodialysis irrespective of the regimen. Interestingly, only 56% of the patients on conventional hemodialysis questioned would agree to come to the dialysis facility daily even if the benefits of the method were established (75). Conversely, it has been rare that patients who started on daily hemodialysis revert back to thrice-weekly hemodialysis. The age of patients opting for home hemodialysis is on average 10 years older than in center hemodialysis.

Contraindications for home hemodialysis include patient inability or lack of motivation to be trained in the absence of a suitable helper. Other contraindications include inadequate housing or difficulty with oral communication (including difficulty communicating in the prevalent language) necessary in case of an emergency in

TABLE 8.2	**Comparison of the Alternative Schedule Hemodialysis Regimens with Conventional Hemodialysis Based on Preliminary or Confirmed Evidence**			
	Conventional Hemodialysis	**Short Daily (Same Total Weekly Duration)**	**Intermittent Long (or Nocturnal)**	**Daily Nocturnal**
Small molecule clearance using conventional kinetics (eKt/V)	+	+	+ +	+ + + +
Small molecule clearance using dose measure favoring frequency (e.g., stdKt/V)	+	+ + +	+ +	+ + + +
Middle molecule clearance	+	+ +	+ + +	+ + + +
Middle molecule clearance using stdKt/V	+	+ + +	+ + +	+ + + +
Phosphate control	±	+(>3h++)	+ + +	+ + + +
Improved BP control with fewer or no medications	+	+ + +	+ + +	+ + + +
Regression of LVH	−	+ + +	+ + ?	+ + +
Improved endothelial function	−	?	?	+ + +
Decrease in sympathetic nervous system activity	−	+ +	?	+ + +
HR variability	−	+ +	?	+ +
Quality of life	+	+ + +	+ + +	+ + (?)
Dietetic freedom	−	+ +	+ + +	+ + + +
Nutrition	+	+ +	+ +	+ +
Anemia control/ESA dose	−	+ + ?	+ + ?	+ + ?
Sleep apnea improvement	−	?	?	+ + +
Patient survival	+	+ + +	+ + +	+ + + (?)

BP, blood pressure; LVH, left ventricular hypertrophy; HR, heart rate; ESA, erythropoiesis-stimulating agent; −, none; ±, negligible; +, very low; ++, low; +++, medium; ++++, high; +(+), variable between + and ++; ?, no data; ++(?), weak or conflicting data.

the absence of a helper at home. The presence of significant hemodynamic instability is an indication for daily nocturnal hemodialysis. Allergy to heparin is a relative contraindication to home nocturnal hemodialysis. Of course, alternative anticoagulants such as danaparoid or argatroban can be used.

Training for home hemodialysis typically lasts for 4 to 6 weeks and is usually done while on thrice-weekly hemodialysis. Self-care dialysis can be used as an interim phase as it allows for a longer training period. Beyond the basic aspects, the training usually includes blood sampling and spinning for laboratory tests, blood cultures, as well as infusion of intravenous antibiotics and iron preparations. In view of the hemodynamic stability offered by these regimens, the presence of a home helper has not been considered obligatory at least for the long form of dialysis, although it has been required in certain jurisdictions. Monthly laboratory tests and clinic visits every 2 to 3 months are the usual practice.

 OUTCOMES

Health Economics and Quality of Life

Health Economics

The cost of dialysis can be viewed from the multiple stakeholders' perspectives. Stakeholders include the society at large, payers, dialysis facilities, members of the dialysis team affecting the patient's decision (including health providers), patients themselves, and patients' families. The cost/benefit ratio to the several stakeholders affects the utilization of the method. Dialysis costs are very high, challenging society's willingness to pay. (**TABLE 8.3**)

Some of the important fiscal elements of the alternative dialysis schemes, which contribute to the financial picture, are as follows:

a. Home dialysis is associated with increased capital costs (one machine per patient) but decreased labor costs.

b. Daily dialysis incurs high consumable costs (daily regimen).

c. In-center short hemodialysis may decrease the patient capacity of the dialysis unit due to frequent machine preparation with possible time lost, which consequently affects revenue (76).

d. Long dialysis potentially increases quality with negligible increase in consumable cost ("better bang for the buck").

e. Savings from the putative improved patient outcomes can be derived from both decreased hospitalization rate and length, as well as lower medication utilization.

f. Higher cost to the payer is incurred from possible increased patient survival.

g. Societal, patient, and patient's family benefit can be derived from the improvement of the vocational rehabilitation of the patient with lower utilization of societal services.

h. Possible decreased use of injectables on the alternative dialysis schedule regimens can harm (no bundling) or benefit the dialysis provider's finances (with bundling).

i. Increased cost of dialysis burdens the dialysis provider, whereas decreased hospitalization rates benefit the payer. In a capitated system, it benefits the provider.

TABLE 8.3	Relative Cost of Hemodialysis (HD) Modalities from Different Stakeholder Perspectives[a]				
	Intermittent Thrice-Weekly HD	Long Intermittent HD In-center	Short Daily HD In-center (Half-Time, Double Frequency)	Short Daily HD at Home	Daily Nocturnal HD at Home
Real estate (dialysis unit)	+++	+ (uses existing facilities)	+++	−	−
Capital (excluding real estate)	++	± (uses existing machines)	++	++++	++++
Consumables	++	++	++++	++++	++++
Labor	+++	++(++)[b]	++++	−	−
Transportation cost	++	++	++++	±	±
Payor's perspective in a developed country (including hospitalization/medication cost but not total life cost)	+++++	++(+)	+++	++	++
Payor's perspective in a developing country	++++	++[c]	+++(+)[c]	+++(+)	+++(+)
Provider's perspective (no bundling) (excluding real estate cost)	+++	+++(+)	++++	+++(+)	+++(+)
Provider's perspective (with bundling) (excluding real estate cost)	+++	++(+)	+++(+)	+++	+++
Provider's perspective (capitated) (excluding real estate cost)	++++	++(+)	+++	++	++
Societal perspective	++++(+)	+++	+++	+(+)	+(+)

−, none; ±, negligible; +, very low; ++, low; +++, medium; ++++, high; +(+), variable between + and ++.
[a]Author's assumptions when no data.
[b]Depends on the nurse/technician-to-patient ratio. It needs to decrease by 50% to break even as the length of dialysis is double.
[c]Lower labor cost but usually higher consumable cost than in developed countries.

j. Increased cost of home utilities (water and electricity) from home hemodialysis is usually incurred by the patient.
k. Transportation cost reduction, by using home hemodialysis, benefit the patient or the publically supported transit system.

The differential cost and benefit allocation among the stakeholders as it is dictated by the structure of the system is *critically* important for the adoption of these regimens. At the international level, the *consumable/labor cost ratio* in different countries also has a major impact on the potential adoption of these methods irrespective of the clinical benefits. In a country with high consumable to labor cost ratio daily hemodialysis is not financially attractive.

Several published studies have addressed the costs of quotidian home hemodialysis (77–79). These studies are either retrospective (80,81) or prospective (78,82–84), and although they are controlled, they are not randomized with the exception of the Alberta study (78). All these studies showed that although the cost of capital and consumables increases on daily (short and nocturnal), the decrease in labor cost offsets the increased expense as long as the treatment is delivered at home. In-center daily hemodialysis is clearly more expensive. Although in a retrospective analysis the decrease in hospitalization offsets the increased cost of the in-center short daily hemodialysis (80), this may apply only to patients with increased morbidity who require frequent hospital admissions (73).

It is reasonable to speculate that home intermittent nocturnal hemodialysis is the least expensive of the alternative schedule modalities. There are no studies published on the cost of in-center

intermittent hemodialysis. In this modality, although the cost of consumables is probably similar to conventional hemodialysis, the labor cost has not been quantitated in a published study. Higher labor cost related to the longer dialysis could be offset by the lower staff to patient ratio related to the hemodynamic stability of the patients.

Several studies suggested that daily hemodialysis is associated with fewer hospital admissions and reduced costs for hospitalization, as well as lower cost of medications including erythropoiesis-stimulating agent (ESA), cardiovascular medications, and phosphate binders (on nocturnal hemodialysis) (77,83,85). In all of the studies, the total cost of health care for in-center conventional hemodialysis was higher than for quotidian hemodialysis, with cost savings estimated to be between $5,000 and $10,000 per patient-year (80,82–85). Importantly, home programs were less expensive even when patient-specific savings (such as reductions in hospitalization) were excluded. These results need to be confirmed in more properly designed studies.

Quality of Life

Several approaches to the measurement of the QOL on the alternative dialysis schedules have been adopted. They include dialysis-independent measures, dialysis-dependent measures, and utility scores. Although most studies were not randomized, two RCTs have been published.

Improvements in QOL have been reported on several elements of Kidney Disease Quality of Life (KDQOL) (73,80,86–89).

Patient testimonials has been very positive (90). Minutes to recovery after a hemodialysis session were shorter after daily hemodialysis (91).

Utility scores calculating quality-adjusted life years (QALYs) were published in both short daily and nocturnal hemodialysis (89,92). The utility instruments used included the willingness to pay, time trade-off, standard gamble technique (92), and Health Utility Index tool (83). Daily nocturnal hemodialysis was an economically "dominant" modality as it improved QOL while it decreased cost (92,93). There were no negative effects on QOL measures after the conversion from conventional to in-center intermittent nocturnal hemodialysis (94). The daily hemodialysis arm of the FHN trial demonstrated a significant improvement of the composite end point of death and physical component of the KDQOL (24). The nocturnal arm of the study failed to show improvement in the similar index (25). The Alberta study did not find improvement in the QOL in the patients randomized to nocturnal hemodialysis using the EuroQol five dimensions questionnaire (EQ-5D) index scores ($p = 0.06$) but showed improvement using the visual analog of the same index as well as several kidney disease-specific subscores (95).

Cognitive Function

There is some evidence, in one observational study, of improvement in the cognitive function of patients after their conversion to quotidian nocturnal hemodialysis (96). Improvement in cognitive function, as well as electroencephalogram (EEG) tracing, was also seen on short daily hemodialysis (97). Self-reported general mental health improved on daily hemodialysis in the FHN trial, but the depressive symptoms did not change significantly (98). The FHN trial did not show any improvement in cognition on frequent dialysis (99).

Cardiovascular Effects

Blood pressure, left ventricular geometry, and left ventricular function. Improved BP control has been reported consistently in all forms of alternative dialysis schedules (15,100). This includes short daily hemodialysis (19,73,86,101,102), long intermittent hemodialysis (103,104), and daily nocturnal hemodialysis (105,106). The antihypertensive medication dose was decreased, and medications were often discontinued. This is usually achieved by decreasing the postdialysis weight (dry weight), which is well tolerated on the alternative dialysis regimens. The beneficial effects on BP were confirmed in the Alberta (72) and FHN (24,107) RCTs. Although salt restriction has been advocated for intermittent nocturnal hemodialysis (108), no such restrictions are usually imposed on daily nocturnal hemodialysis patients (27).

Regression of cardiac hypertrophy have been reported on both short daily and quotidian nocturnal hemodialysis (102,105). These effects have been correlated with a decrease in extracellular fluid volume on short daily hemodialysis (102), but this has not been the case on quotidian nocturnal hemodialysis (106) where extracellular volume, as measured by bioelectrical impedance, remained unchanged (105). Regression of left ventricular mass (LVM) was also demonstrated in the Alberta RCT on daily nocturnal hemodialysis. The FHN RCT also confirmed the regression in LVM in the daily arm but showed only a similar trend in the nocturnal arm, likely related to the lower power of this arm of the trial. A more pronounced effect of frequent hemodialysis on LVM was evident among patients with left ventricular hypertrophy (LVH) at baseline. Changes in LVM were associated with changes in BP (109). In the case of intermittent long hemodialysis, although lack of regression of LVH was reported in older studies (110), such a regression was noted

in more recent studies (111–113). LV function improved in six patients with LV ejection fraction $<40\%$ after conversion to quotidian nocturnal hemodialysis, with the ejection fraction increasing from 28% to 41% (114).

The exercise capacity as measured by the oxygen consumption ($\dot{V}O_2$ max) was found to improve upon conversion from conventional to nocturnal hemodialysis (115).

Endothelial function, autonomic nervous system. The mechanism of the improvement in BP and regression of LVH has been studied further. There is evidence that quotidian nocturnal hemodialysis is associated with vasodilatation, decrease in sympathetic tone, and improvement in endothelial function.

Using echocardiographic techniques, it was found that the calculated peripheral vascular resistance decreased 1 month after conversion to quotidian nocturnal hemodialysis, as did the serum norepinephrine levels (116). Both the endothelium-dependent (postischemia) as well as independent (response to nitroglycerin) vasodilatation improved (116). The number of the endothelial progenitor cell (EPC) number in the blood increased and function improved (117). Low number and function of the EPC have been associated with increased cardiovascular risk in the non-ESKD populations (118). These abnormalities are highly prevalent in the ESKD population (119). Baroreceptor function as expressed by the heart rate response to changes in BP improved as did arterial compliance (120). Lastly, there was an increase in heart rate variability during sleep, consistent with a decrease in the sympathetic/parasympathetic tone ratio (121). The FHN study also detected beneficial effects of daily hemodialysis in the form of increased vagal modulation and increased beat-to-beat variation (122). Decreased heart rate variability is common in the ESKD population and is associated with poorer cardiovascular outcomes in the general as well as the ESKD population (123,124).

Vascular calcifications. Early evidence suggest that coronary artery calcification score, as measured by helical computed tomographic (CT) scan, did not progress significantly 1 year after conversion from conventional to nocturnal hemodialysis (125). Decrease in vascular calcification was reported on intermittent nocturnal hemodialysis (126). Longer follow-up and controlled studies are needed for confirmation.

Anemia Control/Erythropoiesis-Stimulating Agent Dose

Increase in hemoglobin and decrease in the ESA dose have been described in some of the observational studies on the alternative dialysis schedules (73,86,127). Despite an increase in hemoglobin in the daily hemodialysis group in the FHN daily and nocturnal trials, more frequent hemodialysis did not have a significant or clinically important effect on anemia management (128).

Nutrition

After the conversion to short daily hemodialysis, most patients report increase in appetite and well-being. Patients on nocturnal hemodialysis are on an unrestricted diet, although diet is liberal on both short daily and intermittent nocturnal hemodialysis. Several observational studies have reported increases in serum albumin, prealbumin, cholesterol, and body weight (104,129,130). Serum amino acid pattern improved on daily nocturnal hemodialysis (131). Serum albumin posthemodialysis is usually lower than the predialysis value in the daily nocturnal regimen, likely as a result of increased vascular refilling in the recumbent position (132). The FHN trial, using bioimpedance measures, found that frequent in-center hemodialysis did not increase serum albumin or body cellular mass, whereas frequent nocturnal hemodialysis yielded no net effect on parameters of nutritional status or body composition (133). In the Alberta study, there was a nonstatistically significant increase in serum albumin and dietetic intake of some nutrients (134).

Mineral Metabolism

Calcium balance is of significant importance. Calcium balance is positive on conventional hemodialysis if the patients are on calcium-containing phosphate binders (135). This may contribute to vascular and extraosseous calcifications. In the absence of treatment with calcium-based phosphate binders, calcium balance depends on the calcium absorption from the gastrointestinal (GI) tract and the dialysis-related calcium losses. Negative calcium balance can lead to elevated parathyroid hormone (PTH) and alkaline phosphatase levels as well as decreasing bone density (136). The need for high dialysate calcium levels or oral calcium supplements depends on the length of dialysis (longer dialysis requires lower gradient for the same total flux), dietary calcium, and treatment with vitamin D analogs. Quotidian nocturnal hemodialysis requires higher dialysate calcium compared to the other regimens to maintain calcium balance. A dialysate calcium of at least 3 mEq/L (1.5 mmol) is necessary in the case of nocturnal hemodialysis (137), which may have to be increased to as high as 4.5 mEq (2.25 mmol)/L in cases of bone repair, following surgical or medical parathyroidectomy (as when on calcimimetics), or pregnancy (138). High-dialysate calcium can be either fixed [usually 3.5 mEq (1.75 mmol)/L] or variable following the needs of the patient, as dictated by serum levels of calcium pre- and posthemodialysis, and PTH. This can be achieved by adding calcium chloride powder into the "acid" or bicarbonate concentrate [7 mL of powder increases dialysate calcium concentration by 0.5 mEq (0.125 mmol)/L]. Calcium and phosphate precipitation does not take place in the presence of low pH in the "acid" concentrate. It should be expected that in order for the calcium balance to be maintained, the posthemodialysis calcium could even be in the hypercalcemic range. This should be avoided, if possible, in the presence of vascular calcifications.

PTH has been reported to decrease in both short and nocturnal hemodialysis (26,126,136). This is mainly a function of dialysate calcium. PTH can be changed by adjusting dialysate calcium. The PTH target on short daily or nocturnal hemodialysis has not been established. Until this happens, KDOQI guidelines regarding the target PTH should be followed. Increased levels of serum alkaline phosphatase, in the presence of high PTH levels, warrants an increase in dialysate calcium in the absence of hypercalcemia.

As described in the preceding text, phosphate removal increases and hyperphosphatemia improves on daily and long dialysis schedules, although the improvement on short daily hemodialysis is seen when the length of dialysis is increased to 3 hours (26). This was confirmed during the Alberta (139) and FHN trials (70). The need for phosphate binders decreases with the weekly dialysis duration. About 20% of patients on every other night hemodialysis, and 75% of the patients on quotidian nocturnal hemodialysis need phosphate addition into the dialysate usually in the form of sodium phosphate (see preceding text). The dose of both calcium and phosphate additive is adjusted based on serum values of calcium and phosphate.

The improvement in phosphate control and the improved ability to achieve PTH targets leads to improvement or normalization of the Ca × P product (in all patients in the case of daily nocturnal hemodialysis) (126,140). This led to resolution of extraosseous calcification in one patient (141).

Sleep

Sleep disturbances are highly prevalent in the population with ESKD (142). They present in a multitude of forms including sleep apnea, insomnia, restless leg syndrome, periodic limb movements, and daytime sleepiness. Sleep apnea mainly in the obstructive form affects patients at all stages of kidney disease including chronic kidney disease (CKD), dialysis, and transplantation (143–146). Conventional hemodialysis and PD do not offer significant benefit.

Nocturnal hemodialysis was found to improve obstructive sleep apnea (OSA) (147) associated with improvement in nocturnal oxygen saturation. Daytime sleepiness and periodic limb movement were not affected (148). The mechanism for the improvement is unclear, but it may be related to enhanced chemoresponsiveness to CO_2 on nocturnal hemodialysis (149). Other possibilities include improvement (decrease) of the pharyngeal collapsibility or decrease in the pharyngeal edema (150,151). Nocturnal rostral fluid shift during the night is associated with the severity of OSA in ESKD (152). This can be ameliorated by nightly dialysis (both PD and hemodialysis) (147,153).

Patient Hospitalization/Survival

The impressive patient survival rates on intermittent long hemodialysis reported by the Tassin group (85% over 5 years) may have been partially related to the patient selection criteria (8,154). Two studies based on the national databases of Australia and New Zealand, and data from the DOPPS, found an association between length of dialysis and patient survival over and above the effect of dialysis dose (61,62). Consistent with these studies, decreased hospitalization and a survival advantage on in-center intermittent nocturnal hemodialysis as compared to conventional hemodialysis has also been reported (155). Although the overall hospitalization rate was not different, cardiovascular disease-related admissions were fewer in the short daily group using the NxStage machine versus thrice-weekly dialysis controls, whereas infection-related admissions were higher. Patient survival rates were slightly better as well (156,157). Patient survival rate using mostly long intermittent dialysis at home (usually every other night) was reported (38). The survival rate of patients on in-center daily hemodialysis was lower than the thrice-weekly dialysis population likely related to the high comorbidity rate in this population, which has likely led to the adoption of this expensive regimen (74). Conversely, the survival of patients on home intensive hemodialysis was higher than the in-center thrice-weekly dialysis population (158). Other observational studies also reported similar results favoring frequent dialysis (19,159). The patient survival rates on daily nocturnal hemodialysis were comparable to the U.S. cadaveric transplantation survival rates (84.5% vs. 86.2% over 5 years) (160), but treatment failure/death was higher in the daily nocturnal hemodialysis group when compared to the Canadian transplantation population (161). In a recent study, 1,116 daily hemodialysis patients from the United States Renal Data System (USRDS) database were matched by propensity scores to 2,784 contemporaneous patients on PD and 3,173 patients on conventional hemodialysis. The composite hospitalization rate was lower on daily hemodialysis than PD [Hazard Ratio (HR) 0.73] or conventional hemodialysis (HR 0.68) (162). The HR for switching to in-center hemodialysis for PD versus Daily Hemo Dialysis (DHD) was 3.4 (<0.001). In a recently published study, the survival of patients on nocturnal hemodialysis was lower than the home hemodialysis control in the nocturnal arm of the FHN trial (163). The deaths took place mainly during the year after the completion of the study. The results were unexpected and contradict the data from the observational studies. It should be noted that the survival rate of the control group was surprisingly low, the sample size was small, and there was a high rate of hemodialysis prescription change after the completion of the study. A similar analysis of patients on the daily arm of the FHN trial followed over a median of 3.6 years revealed that the relative mortality hazard for frequent versus conventional hemodialysis was 0.54 (95% confidence interval, 0.31 to 0.93), suggesting that daily hemodialysis may benefit patients with ESKD (164).

In summary, there is evidence suggestive of improved hospitalization and patient survival rates on frequent and/or long hemodialysis, but they are based on observational studies. There was an unexpected higher mortality in the nocturnal hemodialysis group than the controls in the FHN trial mainly during the year after the completion of the trial, whereas the mortality of patients on daily hemodialysis was lower than the controls.

Daily Hemo(dia)filtration

Convective techniques have been used for several decades. Their utilization is higher in Europe with little adoption in North America (165,166). The main advantage of convection is the enhanced large molecular solute removal. Clinical outcomes include improved intra- and interdialytic tolerance, improved QOL, better hypertension control, and evidence for improved patient survival (165,167,168).

Despite the enhanced middle molecule removal exemplified by β_2-microglobulin, the thrice-weekly hemodiafiltration does not have a significant effect on predialysis levels of β_2-microglobulin. Daily hemofiltration and hemodiafiltration have been used; the former in the home setting (169) and the latter in the in-center setting (170). The outcomes were similar. The results on short daily hemodialysis had the added advantage of the improved middle molecule removal offered by the convective techniques. They included improved BP and hyperphosphatemia control as well as improvement in several elements of QOL measures. There was a regression of cardiac hypertrophy. Predialysis β_2-microglobulin levels decreased.

Pediatric Daily Hemodialysis

Quotidian nocturnal hemodialysis as well as daily hemodiafiltration have also been used in children. There have been reports of improved well-being, nutrition, and school attendance as well as growth (171–174).

Obstacles for the Alternative Schedules/Modality Choice

Despite the favorable literature on the alternative dialysis regimens, their adoption has been slow. The main reasons for the slow change have roots in several areas:

Reimbursement structure. Although there is evidence that the cost of daily hemodialysis at home, when seen from the payer's perspective, can be lower than the in-center hemodialysis, the savings in most jurisdictions do not benefit the dialysis providers which incur the added expense of the daily treatments.

Lack of training and experience/inertia. Most of the physicians, nurses, and dialysis centers have limited or no expertise with daily or home hemodialysis. This, in the absence of other incentives, fosters inertia.

Limited adaptation of hemodialysis machines for home dialysis. Despite some remarkable progress toward more patient-friendly hemodialysis machines for use at home, the difficulty in training patients for home hemodialysis is a significant obstacle in the adoption of the alternative regimens. Most experts do not expect more than 20% to 25% of the patients to be able to perform home hemodialysis using current technology.

Lack of dialysis industry incentives. Under the current reimbursement structure, there is limited incentive for the dialysis industry to pursue the alternative dialysis modalities. This may change as new dialysis machines are produced, the cost of daily hemodialysis decreases to meet the current reimbursement rates, or if there is an adjustment of either the dialysis reimbursement rates or structure. The contribution of the industry to the adoption of the alternative dialysis techniques and wider adoption of home hemodialysis is pivotal. This may be changing. Recently, several new machines have been produced, and others will be available in the next few years.

If daily hemodialysis is not available due to insufficient funding, overnight hemodialysis every other night or three times a week at home or in the dialysis facility should be considered. Assuming there is accessibility to daily hemodialysis and until the methods (short vs. nocturnal) are more formally compared, the choice of modality should be based on patient choice, medical indications, and local expertise. Daily nocturnal hemodialysis is the closest to the normal kidney function, offers better hemodynamic stability, excellent phosphate control, and improves sleep apnea. These advantages are to be weighed against the potential for deficiency syndromes (no evidence yet), long exposure to dialysis membranes, and safety concerns at night. Daily convective therapies are also attractive, but more experience is needed before they are widely adopted especially in the home setting.

Randomized Controlled Trials

Two RCTs on daily hemodialysis have been published. Most of the outcomes have already been incorporated in this chapter but will be summarized below.

The Alberta trial (2007): Fifty-two patients from two centers in Alberta, Canada, were randomized to receive home nocturnal hemodialysis six or three times weekly for 6 months. Primary outcomes were change in LVM and QOL.

Results: Nocturnal hemodialysis significantly decreased LVM, improved selected kidney disease-specific domains, but not the overall QOL. It improved BP control and hyperphosphatemia but not anemia control.

The FHN trial (sponsored by NIH) (2011): The trial included two arms: the daily in-center trial—245 patients from 11 regional centers in the United States and Canada randomized to 12 months of six times per week or three times per week hemodialysis and the nocturnal trial—87 (out of 250 initially planned) patients from eight regional centers randomized to 12 months of six times per week home nocturnal or three times per week home conventional hemodialysis. The primary outcomes of both trials were death/LVM composite score and death/PHC (physical health component of KDQOL) composite score.

Results: The daily trial was associated with significant improvement of the death/LVM outcome, but the nocturnal trial was associated by only a similar trend. The daily trial showed an improvement in the death/primary health composite (PHC) outcome but not the nocturnal trial. Both trials showed improved BP as well as phosphate control; the latter was more pronounced in the nocturnal trial. There was some improvement in the autonomic nervous system parameters. Frequent dialysis did not improve anemia control, cognitive function, albumin, or body cell mass. Frequent dialysis was associated with more vascular access complications and nocturnal hemodialysis with a more rapid decline in residual kidney function. There were an increased number of deaths during the year after the completion of the study on nocturnal hemodialysis. It is unclear if the negative results of the nocturnal trial were related to method itself or the low patient enrolment rate, the looser enrolment criteria [higher glomerular filtration rate (GFR) up to 11 mL/min], or the high percentage of enrolled incident rather than prevalent patients, when compared to the daily trial (164). The survival rate of patients on daily hemodialysis was higher than the controls, suggesting that daily hemodialysis should be considered for selected patients (165).

CONCLUSION

There are significant benefits ascribed to long as well as frequent dialysis. Out of these, BP improvement, regression of LVH, phosphate control, and QOL improvements (only partially in nocturnal hemodialysis) were confirmed by RCTs. The rest of the benefits were shown only in observational studies, where usually patient served as their own controls. Although until recently, hospitalization and survival benefits of frequent or long hemodialysis were based on observational studies, the recently published results of the FHN trial showed increased mortality rates after the completion of the study in the nocturnal hemodialysis patient group but decreased mortality rates in the daily hemodialysis patient group compared to controls.

The financial benefits using long intermittent dialysis in-center or at home are firmer, although daily hemodialysis in-center is more expensive. Daily home/nocturnal hemodialysis may be financially beneficial in countries with high labor/consumable price ratio especially for patients who are expected to be on dialysis for longer than 1 year.

REFERENCES

1. United States Renal Data System. Chapter 3: morbidity and mortality in patients with CKD. https://www.usrds.org/2015/view/v1_03.aspx. Accessed May 19, 2016.
2. Gotch FA, Sargent JA. A mechanistic analysis of the National Cooperative Dialysis Study (NCDS). *Kidney Int* 1985;28(3):526–534.
3. Eknoyan G, Beck GJ, Cheung AK, et al. Effect of dialysis dose and membrane flux in maintenance hemodialysis. *N Engl J Med* 2002; 347(25):2010–2019.
4. Golper TA, Guest S, Glickman JD, et al. Home dialysis in the new USA bundled payment plan: implications and impact. *Perit Dial Int* 2011; 31(1):12–16.
5. Blagg CR. The early history of dialysis for chronic renal failure in the United States: a view from Seattle. *Am J Kidney Dis* 2007;49(3):482–496.
6. Blagg CR. A brief history of home hemodialysis. *Adv Ren Replace Ther* 1996;3(2):99–105.
7. Blagg CR, Ing TS, Berry D, et al. The history and rationale of daily and nightly hemodialysis. *Contrib Nephrol* 2004;145:1–9.
8. Charra B, Calemard E, Ruffet M, et al. Survival as an index of adequacy of dialysis. *Kidney Int* 1992;41(5):1286–1291.
9. Chertow GM, Kurella M, Lowrie EG. The tortoise and hare on hemodialysis: does slow and steady win the race? *Kidney Int* 2006;70(1):24–25.
10. Shaldon S. Independence in maintenance haemodialysis. *Lancet* 1968; 1(7541):520.
11. Mahadevan K, Pellicano R, Reid A, et al. Comparison of biochemical, haematological and volume parameters in two treatment schedules of nocturnal home haemodialysis. *Nephrology* 2006;11(5):413–418.
12. Lacson E Jr, Xu J, Suri RS, et al. Survival with three-times weekly in-center nocturnal versus conventional hemodialysis. *J Am Soc Nephrol* 2012; 23(4):687–695.
13. MacGregor MS, Agar JWM, Blagg CR. Home haemodialysis— international trends and variation. *Nephrol Dial Transplant* 2006;21(7): 1934–1945.
14. Neumann ME. PD takes a big jump in 2014, while HHD shows progress. *Nephrol News Issues* 2014;28(10):14, 17, 34.
15. DePalma JR, Pecker EA, Maxwell MH. A new automatic coil dialyser system for 'daily' dialysis. *Proc EDTA* 1969;6:26–34.
16. DePalma JR, Pecker EA, Maxwell MH. A new automatic coil dialyser system for 'daily' dialysis. *Semin Dial* 1999;12:410–418.
17. Buoncristiani U, Giombini L, Cozzari M, et al. Daily recycled bicarbonate dialysis with polyacrylonitrile. *Trans Am Soc Artif Intern Organs* 1983;29:669–672.
18. Buoncristiani U. Fifteen years of clinical experience with daily haemodialysis. *Nephrol Dial Transplant* 1998;13(Suppl 6):148–151.
19. Woods JD, Port FK, Orzol S, et al. Clinical and biochemical correlates of starting "daily" hemodialysis. *Kidney Int* 1999;55(6):2467–2476.
20. Pierratos A, Ouwendyk M, Francoeur R, et al. Nocturnal hemodialysis: three-year experience. *J Am Soc Nephrol* 1998;9(5):859–868.
21. Uldall PR, Francoeur R, Ouwendyk M. Simplified nocturnal home hemodialysis (SNHHD). A new approach to renal replacement therapy. *J Am Soc Nephrol* 1994;5:428.
22. Paniagua R, Amato D, Vonesh E, et al. Effects of increased peritoneal clearances on mortality rates in peritoneal dialysis: ADEMEX, a prospective, randomized, controlled trial. *J Am Soc Nephrol* 2002;13(5):1307–1320.
23. Culleton BF, Walsh M, Klarenbach SW, et al. Effect of frequent nocturnal hemodialysis vs conventional hemodialysis on left ventricular mass and quality of life: a randomized controlled trial. *JAMA* 2007;298(11): 1291–1299.
24. Chertow GM, Levin NW, Beck GJ, et al. In-center hemodialysis six times per week versus three times per week. *N Engl J Med* 2010;363(24): 2287–2300.
25. Rocco MV, Lockridge RS Jr, Beck GJ, et al. The effects of frequent nocturnal home hemodialysis: the Frequent Hemodialysis Network Nocturnal Trial. *Kidney Int* 2011;80:1080–1091.
26. Ayus JC, Achinger SG, Mizani MR, et al. Phosphorus balance and mineral metabolism with 3 h daily hemodialysis. *Kidney Int* 2007;71(4):336–342.
27. Pierratos A. Daily nocturnal home hemodialysis. *Kidney Int* 2004;65(5): 1975–1986.
28. Su WS, Lekas P, Carlisle EJ, et al. Management of hypophosphatemia in nocturnal hemodialysis with phosphate-containing enema: a technical study. *Hemodial Int* 2011;15(2):219–225.
29. Bell R, Nolin L, Pichette V, et al. Efficacy and safety of tinzaparin anticoagulation of the extracorporeal circuit with a single bolus administration in nocturnal home hemodialysis. *Nephrol Dial Transplant* 2014;29:218.
30. Pierratos A, Francoeur R, Ouwendyk M. Delayed dialyzer reprocessing for home hemodialysis. *Home Hemodial Int* 2000;4:51–54.
31. Pierratos A. Nocturnal home haemodialysis: an update on a 5-year experience. *Nephrol Dial Transplant* 1999;14(12):2835–2840.
32. Hoy CD. Remote monitoring of daily nocturnal hemodialysis. *Hemodialysis Int* 2001;4:8–12.
33. Diaz-Buxo JA, Schlaeper C, VanValkenburgh D. Evolution of home hemodialysis monitoring systems. *Hemodial Int* 2003;7(4):353–355.
34. Quintaliani G, Buoncristiani U, Fagugli R, et al. Survival of vascular access during daily and three times a week hemodialysis. *Clin Nephrol* 2000;53(5):372–377.
35. Kjellstrand CM, Blagg CR, Twardowski ZJ, et al. Blood access and daily hemodialysis: clinical experience and review of the literature. *ASAIO J* 2003;49(6):645–649.
36. Piccoli GB, Bermond F, Mezza E, et al. Vascular access survival and morbidity on daily dialysis: a comparative analysis of home and limited care haemodialysis. *Nephrol Dial Transplant* 2004;19(8):2084–2094.

37. Suri RS, Larive B, Sherer S, et al. Risk of vascular access complications with frequent hemodialysis. *J Am Soc Nephrol* 2013;24(3):498–505.

38. Jun M, Jardine MJ, Gray N, et al. Outcomes of extended-hours hemodialysis performed predominantly at home. *Am J Kidney Dis* 2013; 61(2):247–253.

39. Perl J, Lok CE, Chan CT. Central venous catheter outcomes in nocturnal hemodialysis. *Kidney Int* 2006;70(7):1348–1354.

40. Pipkin M, Craft V, Spencer M, et al. Six years of experience with nightly home hemodialysis access. *Hemodial Int* 2004;8(4):349–353.

41. Hayes WN, Tennankore K, Battistella M, et al. Vascular access-related infection in nocturnal home hemodialysis. *Hemodial Int* 2014;18: 481–487.

42. Wong B, Zimmerman D, Reintjes F, et al. Procedure-related serious adverse events among home hemodialysis patients: a quality assurance perspective. *Am J Kidney Dis* 2014;63:251–258.

43. Mustafa RA, Zimmerman D, Rioux JP, et al. Vascular access for intensive maintenance hemodialysis: a systematic review for a Canadian Society of Nephrology clinical practice guideline. *Am J Kidney Dis* 2013; 62(1):112–131.

44. Twardowski Z, Kubara H. Different sites versus constant sites of needle insertion into arteriovenous fistulas for treatment by repeated dialysis. *Dial Transpl* 1979;8:978–980.

45. Marticorena RM, Hunter J, Macleod S, et al. The salvage of aneurysmal fistulae utilizing a modified buttonhole cannulation technique and multiple cannulators. *Hemodial Int* 2006;10(2):193–200.

46. Ball LK, Treat L, Riffle V, et al. A multi-center perspective of the buttonhole technique in the Pacific Northwest. *Nephrol Nurs J* 2007;34(2): 234–241.

47. Nesrallah GE, Cuerden M, Wong JH, et al. Staphylococcus aureus bacteremia and buttonhole cannulation: long-term safety and efficacy of mupirocin prophylaxis. *Clin J Am Soc Nephrol* 2010;5(6):1047–1053.

48. MacRae JM, Ahmed SB, Hemmelgarn BR. Arteriovenous fistula survival and needling technique: long-term results from a randomized buttonhole trial. *Am J Kidney Dis* 2014;63(4):636–642.

49. Lok CE, Sontrop JM, Faratro R, et al. Frequent hemodialysis fistula infectious complications. *Nephron Extra* 2014;4(3):159–167.

50. Redsense Medical. www.redsensemedical.com/index.php/product. Accessed September 19, 2016.

51. Lowrie EG, Laird NM, Parker TF, et al. Effect of the hemodialysis prescription of patient morbidity: report from the National Cooperative Dialysis Study. *N Engl J Med* 1981;305(20):1176–1181.

52. Fenton SS, Schaubel DE, Desmeules M, et al. Hemodialysis versus peritoneal dialysis: a comparison of adjusted mortality rates. *Am J Kidney Dis* 1997;30(3):334–342.

53. Kjellstrand CM, Evans RL, Petersen RJ, et al. The "unphysiology" of dialysis: a major cause of dialysis side effects? *Hemodial Int* 2004;8(1): 24–29.

54. Gotch FA. The current place of urea kinetic modelling with respect to different dialysis modalities. *Nephrol Dial Transplant* 1998;13(Suppl 6): 10–14.

55. Gotch FA. Modeling the dose of home dialysis. *Home Hemodial Int* 1998;2:37–40.

56. Suri RS, Depner T, Lindsay RM. Dialysis prescription and dose monitoring in frequent hemodialysis. *Contrib Nephrol* 2004;145:75–88.

57. Suri R, Depner TA, Blake PG, et al. Adequacy of quotidian hemodialysis. *Am J Kidney Dis* 2003;42(1 Suppl):42–48.

58. Leypoldt JK, Cheung AK, Carroll CE, et al. Effect of dialysis membranes and middle molecule removal on chronic hemodialysis patient survival. *Am J Kidney Dis* 1999;33(2):349–355.

59. Cheung AK, Sarnak MJ, Yan G, et al. Cardiac diseases in maintenance hemodialysis patients: results of the HEMO Study. *Kidney Int* 2004; 65(6):2380–2389.

60. Cheung AK, Rocco MV, Yan G, et al. Serum beta-2 microglobulin levels predict mortality in dialysis patients: results of the HEMO Study. *J Am Soc Nephrol* 2006;17(2):546–555.

61. Marshall MR, Byrne BG, Kerr PG, et al. Associations of hemodialysis dose and session length with mortality risk in Australian and New Zealand patients. *Kidney Int* 2006;69(7):1229–1236.

62. Saran R, Bragg-Gresham JL, Levin NW, et al. Longer treatment time and slower ultrafiltration in hemodialysis: associations with reduced mortality in the DOPPS. *Kidney Int* 2006;69(7):1222–1228.

63. Clark WR, Leypoldt JK, Henderson LW, et al. Quantifying the effect of changes in the hemodialysis prescription on effective solute removal with a mathematical model. *J Am Soc Nephrol* 1999;10(3):601–609.

64. Raj DSC, Ouwendyk M, Francoeur R, et al. Beta(2)-microglobulin kinetics in nocturnal haemodialysis. *Nephrol Dial Transplant* 2000; 15(1):58–64.

65. Fagugli RM, Vanholder R, De Smet R, et al. Advanced glycation end products: specific fluorescence changes of pentosidine-like compounds during short daily hemodialysis. *Int J Artif Organs* 2001;24(5):256–262.

66. Fagugli RM, De Smet R, Buoncristiani U, et al. Behavior of non-protein-bound and protein-bound uremic solutes during daily hemodialysis. *Am J Kidney Dis* 2002;40(2):339–347.

67. Block GA, Klassen PS, Lazarus JM, et al. Mineral metabolism, mortality, and morbidity in maintenance hemodialysis. *J Am Soc Nephrol* 2004;15(8):2208–2218.

68. DeSoi CA, Umans JG. Phosphate kinetics during high-flux hemodialysis. *J Am Soc Nephrol* 1993;4(5):1214–1218.

69. Galland R, Traeger J, Delawari E, et al. Optimal control of phosphatemia by short daily hemodialysis. *Hemodial Int* 2003;7(1):73–104.

70. Daugirdas JT, Chertow GM, Larive B, et al. Effects of frequent hemodialysis on measures of CKD mineral and bone disorder. *J Am Soc Nephrol* 2012;23(4):727–738.

71. Mucsi I, Hercz G, Uldall R, et al. Control of serum phosphate without any phosphate binders in patients treated with nocturnal hemodialysis. *Kidney Int* 1998;53(5):1399–1404.

72. Culleton BF, Walsh M, Klarenbach SW, et al. Effect of frequent nocturnal hemodialysis vs conventional hemodialysis on left ventricular mass and quality of life: a randomized controlled trial. *JAMA* 2007;298(11): 1291–1299.

73. Ting GO, Kjellstrand C, Freitas T, et al. Long-term study of high-comorbidity ESRD patients converted from conventional to short daily hemodialysis. *Am J Kidney Dis* 2003;42(5):1020–1035.

74. Suri RS, Lindsay RM, Bieber BA, et al. A multinational cohort study of in-center daily hemodialysis and patient survival. *Kidney Int* 2013; 83:300–307.

75. Halpern SD, Berns JS, Israni AK. Willingness of patients to switch from conventional to daily hemodialysis: looking before we leap. *Am J Med* 2004;116(9):606–612.

76. Ting G, Carrie B, Freitas T, et al. Global ESRD costs associated with a short daily hemodialysis program in the United States. *Home Hemodial Int* 1999;3:41–44.

77. Walker R, Marshall MR, Morton RL, et al. The cost-effectiveness of contemporary home haemodialysis modalities compared with facility haemodialysis: a systematic review of full economic evaluations. *Nephrology* 2014;19(8):459–470.

78. Klarenbach S, Tonelli M, Pauly R, et al. Economic evaluation of frequent home nocturnal hemodialysis based on a randomized controlled trial. *J Am Soc Nephrol* 2014;25(3):587–594.

79. Klarenbach SW, Tonelli M, Chui B, et al. Economic evaluation of dialysis therapies. *Nat Rev Nephrol* 2014;10(11):644–652.

80. Mohr PE, Neumann PJ, Franco SJ, et al. The case for daily dialysis: its impact on costs and quality of life. *Am J Kidney Dis* 2001;37(4): 777–789.

81. Komenda P, Copland M, Makwana J, et al. The cost of starting and maintaining a large home hemodialysis program. *Kidney Int* 2010;77(11):1039–1045.

82. McFarlane PA, Pierratos A, Redelmeier DA. Cost savings of home nocturnal versus conventional in-center hemodialysis. *Kidney Int* 2002;62(6):2216–2222.

83. Kroeker A, Clark WF, Heidenheim AP, et al. An operating cost comparison between conventional and home quotidian hemodialysis. *Am J Kidney Dis* 2003;42(1 Suppl):49–55.

84. Agar JW, Knight RJ, Simmonds RE, et al. Nocturnal haemodialysis: an Australian cost comparison with conventional satellite haemodialysis. *Nephrology* 2005;10(6):557–570.

85. McFarlane PA. Reducing hemodialysis costs: conventional and quotidian home hemodialysis in Canada. *Semin Dial* 2004;17(2):118–124.

86. Kooistra MP, Vos J, Koomans HA, et al. Daily home haemodialysis in The Netherlands: effects on metabolic control, haemodynamics, and quality of life. *Nephrol Dial Transplant* 1998;13(11):2853–2860.

87. McPhatter LL, Lockridge RSJ, Albert J, et al. Nightly home hemodialysis: improvement in nutrition and quality of life. *Adv Ren Replace Ther* 1999;6(4):358–365.

88. Heidenheim AP, Muirhead N, Moist L, et al. Patient quality of life on quotidian hemodialysis. *Am J Kidney Dis* 2003;42(1 Suppl):36–41.

89. Buoncristiani U, Cairo G, Giombini L, et al. Dramatic improvement of clinical-metabolic parameters and quality of life with daily dialysis. *Int J Artif Organs* 1989;12:133–136.

90. Levenspiel B. My experience with daily dialysis. *ASAIO J* 2001;47(5):469.

91. Lindsay RM, Heidenheim PA, Nesrallah G, et al. Minutes to recovery after a hemodialysis session: a simple health-related quality of life question that is reliable, valid, and sensitive to change. *Clin J Am Soc Nephrol* 2006;1(5):952–959.

92. McFarlane PA, Bayoumi AM, Pierratos A, et al. The quality of life and cost utility of home nocturnal and conventional in-center hemodialysis. *Kidney Int* 2003;64(3):1004–1011.

93. McFarlane PA, Bayoumi AM, Pierratos A, et al. The impact of home nocturnal hemodialysis on end-stage renal disease therapies: a decision analysis. *Kidney Int* 2006;69(5):798–805.

94. Troidle L, Hotchkiss M, Finkelstein F. A thrice weekly in-center nocturnal hemodialysis program. *Adv Chronic Kidney Dis* 2007;14(3):244–248.

95. Manns BJ, Walsh MW, Culleton BF, et al. Nocturnal hemodialysis does not improve overall measures of quality of life compared to conventional hemodialysis. *Kidney Int* 2009;75(5):542–549.

96. Jassal SV, Devins GM, Chan CT, et al. Improvements in cognition in patients converting from thrice weekly hemodialysis to nocturnal hemodialysis: a longitudinal pilot study. *Kidney Int* 2006;70(5):956–962.

97. Vos PF, Zilch O, Jennekens-Schinkel A, et al. Effect of short daily home haemodialysis on quality of life, cognitive functioning and the electroencephalogram. *Nephrol Dial Transplant* 2006;21(9):2529–2535.

98. Unruh ML, Larive B, Chertow GM, et al. Effects of 6-times-weekly versus 3-times-weekly hemodialysis on depressive symptoms and self-reported mental health: Frequent Hemodialysis Network (FHN) trials. *Am J Kidney Dis* 2013;61(5):748–758.

99. Kurella TM, Unruh ML, Nissenson AR, et al. Effect of more frequent hemodialysis on cognitive function in the frequent hemodialysis network trials. *Am J Kidney Dis* 2013;61(2):228–237.

100. Twardowski ZJ. Effect of long-term increase in the frequency and/or prolongation of dialysis duration on certain clinical manifestations and results of laboratory investigations in patients with chronic renal failure. *Acta Med Pol* 1975;16:31–44.

101. Buoncristiani U, Quintaliani G, Cozzari M, et al. Daily dialysis: long-term clinical metabolic results. *Kidney Int* 1988;24:S137–S140.

102. Fagugli RM, Reboldi G, Quintaliani G, et al. Short daily hemodialysis: blood pressure control and left ventricular mass reduction in hypertensive hemodialysis patients. *Am J Kidney Dis* 2001;38(2):371–376.

103. Charra B, Calemard M, Laurent G. Importance of treatment time and blood pressure control in achieving long-term survival on dialysis. *Am J Nephrol* 1996;16(1):35–44.

104. Laurent G, Charra B. The results of an 8 h thrice weekly haemodialysis schedule. *Nephrol Dial Transplant* 1998;13(Suppl 6):125–131.

105. Chan CT, Floras JS, Miller JA, et al. Regression of left ventricular hypertrophy after conversion to nocturnal hemodialysis. *Kidney Int* 2002;61(6):2235–2239.

106. Nesrallah G, Suri R, Moist L, et al. Volume control and blood pressure management in patients undergoing quotidian hemodialysis. *Am J Kidney Dis* 2003;42(1 Suppl):13–17.

107. Kotanko P, Garg AX, Depner T, et al. Effects of frequent hemodialysis on blood pressure: results from the randomized frequent hemodialysis network trials. *Hemodial Int* 2015;19:386–401.

108. Charra B, Chazot C. The neglect of sodium restriction in dialysis patients: a short review. *Hemodial Int* 2003;7(4):342–347.

109. Chan CT, Greene T, Chertow GM, et al. Determinants of left ventricular mass in patients on hemodialysis: Frequent Hemodialysis Network (FHN) trials. *Circ Cardiovasc Imaging* 2012;5(2):251–261.

110. Covic A, Goldsmith DJ, Georgescu G, et al. Echocardiographic findings in long-term, long-hour hemodialysis patients. *Clin Nephrol* 1996;45(2):104–110.

111. Weinreich T, De los Rios T, Gauly A, et al. Effects of an increase in time vs. frequency on cardiovascular parameters in chronic hemodialysis patients. *Clin Nephrol* 2006;66(6):433–439.

112. Fagugli RM, Pasini P, Pasticci F, et al. Effects of short daily hemodialysis and extended standard hemodialysis on blood pressure and cardiac hypertrophy: a comparative study. *J Nephrol* 2006;19(1):77–83.

113. Wald R, Yan AT, Perl J, et al. Regression of left ventricular mass following conversion from conventional hemodialysis to thrice weekly in-centre nocturnal hemodialysis. *BMC Nephrol* 2012;13:3.

114. Chan C, Floras JS, Miller JA, et al. Improvement in ejection fraction by nocturnal haemodialysis in end-stage renal failure patients with coexisting heart failure. *Nephrol Dial Transplant* 2002;17(8):1518–1521.

115. Chan CT, Notarius CF, Merlocco AC, et al. Improvement in exercise duration and capacity after conversion to nocturnal home haemodialysis. *Nephrol Dial Transplant* 2007;22:3285–3291.

116. Chan CT, Harvey PJ, Picton P, et al. Short-term blood pressure, noradrenergic, and vascular effects of nocturnal home hemodialysis. *Hypertension* 2003;42(5):925–931.

117. Chan CT, Li SH, Verma S. Nocturnal hemodialysis is associated with restoration of impaired endothelial progenitor cell biology in end-stage renal disease. *Am J Physiol Renal Physiol* 2005;289(4):F679–F684.

118. Hill JM, Zalos G, Halcox JPJ, et al. Circulating endothelial progenitor cells, vascular function, and cardiovascular risk. *N Engl J Med* 2003;348(7):593–600.

119. de Groot K, Hermann Bahlmann F, Sowa J, et al. Uremia causes endothelial progenitor cell deficiency. *Kidney Int* 2004;66(2):641–646.

120. Chan CT, Jain V, Picton P, et al. Nocturnal hemodialysis increases arterial baroreflex sensitivity and compliance and normalizes blood pressure of hypertensive patients with end-stage renal disease. *Kidney Int* 2005;68(1):338–344.

121. Chan CT, Hanly P, Gabor J, et al. Impact of nocturnal hemodialysis on the variability of heart rate and duration of hypoxemia during sleep. *Kidney Int* 2004;65(2):661–665.

122. Chan CT, Chertow GM, Daugirdas JT, et al. Effects of daily hemodialysis on heart rate variability: results from the Frequent Hemodialysis Network (FHN) Daily Trial. *Nephrol Dial Transplant* 2014;29(1):168–178.

123. Tsuji H, Larson MG, Venditti FJ Jr, et al. Impact of reduced heart rate variability on risk for cardiac events. The Framingham Heart Study. *Circulation* 1996;94(11):2850–2855.

124. Fukuta H, Hayano J, Ishihara S, et al. Prognostic value of heart rate variability in patients with end-stage renal disease on chronic haemodialysis. *Nephrol Dial Transplant* 2003;18(2):318–325.

125. Yuen D, Pierratos A, Richardson RM, et al. The natural history of coronary calcification progression in a cohort of nocturnal haemodialysis patients. *Nephrol Dial Transplant* 2006;21(5):1407–1412.

126. Van Eps CL, Jeffries JK, Anderson JA, et al. Mineral metabolism, bone histomorphometry and vascular calcification in alternate night nocturnal haemodialysis. *Nephrology* 2007;12(3):224–233.

127. Schwartz DI, Pierratos A, Richardson RM, et al. Impact of nocturnal home hemodialysis on anemia management in patients with end-stage renal disease. *Clin Nephrol* 2005;63(3):202–208.

128. Ornt DB, Larive B, Rastogi A, et al. Impact of frequent hemodialysis on anemia management: results from the Frequent Hemodialysis Network (FHN) trials. *Nephrol Dial Transplant* 2013;28(7):1888–1898.

129. Galland R, Traeger J, Arkouche W, et al. Short daily hemodialysis rapidly improves nutritional status in hemodialysis patients. *Kidney Int* 2001;60(4):1555–1560.

130. Spanner E, Suri R, Heidenheim AP, et al. The impact of quotidian hemodialysis on nutrition. *Am J Kidney Dis* 2003;42(1 Suppl):30–35.

131. Raj DS, Ouwendyk M, Francoeur R, et al. Plasma amino acid profile on nocturnal hemodialysis. *Blood Purif* 2000;18(2):97–102.

132. Agar JW, Pierratos A. Changes in hemoglobin and albumin concentration during nocturnal home hemodialysis. *Hemodial Int* 2007; 11(3):303–308.

133. Kaysen GA, Greene T, Larive B, et al. The effect of frequent hemodialysis on nutrition and body composition: frequent Hemodialysis Network Trial. *Kidney Int* 2012;82(1):90–99.

134. Schorr M, Manns BJ, Culleton B, et al. The effect of nocturnal and conventional hemodialysis on markers of nutritional status: results from a randomized trial. *J Ren Nutr* 2011;21:271–276.

135. Gotch F, Kotanko P, Handelman G, et al. A kinetic model of calcium mass balance during dialysis therapy. *Blood Purif* 2007;25(1): 139–149.

136. Toussaint N, Boddington J, Simmonds R, et al. Calcium phosphate metabolism and bone mineral density with nocturnal hemodialysis. *Hemodial Int* 2006;10(3):280–286.

137. Al Hejaili F, Kortas C, Leitch R, et al. Nocturnal but not short hours quotidian hemodialysis requires an elevated dialysate calcium concentration. *J Am Soc Nephrol* 2003;14(9):2322–2328.

138. Gangji AS, Windrim R, Gandhi S, et al. Successful pregnancy with nocturnal hemodialysis. *Am J Kidney Dis* 2004;44(5):912–916.

139. Walsh M, Manns BJ, Klarenbach S, et al. The effects of nocturnal compared with conventional hemodialysis on mineral metabolism: a randomized-controlled trial. *Hemodial Int* 2010;14(2):174–181.

140. Lindsay RM, Alhejaili F, Nesrallah G, et al. Calcium and phosphate balance with quotidian hemodialysis. *Am J Kidney Dis* 2003;42(1): S24–S29.

141. Kim SJ, Goldstein M, Szabo T, et al. Resolution of massive uremic tumoral calcinosis with daily nocturnal home hemodialysis. *Am J Kidney Dis* 2003;41(3):E12.

142. Kimmel PL, Miller G, Mendelson WB. Sleep apnea syndrome in chronic renal disease. *Am J Med* 1989;(3):308–314.

143. Unruh ML, Sanders MH, Redline S, et al. Sleep apnea in patients on conventional thrice-weekly hemodialysis: comparison with matched controls from the sleep heart health study. *J Am Soc Nephrol* 2006;17(12):3503–3509.

144. Parker KP, Bliwise DL, Bailey JL, et al. Polysomnographic measures of nocturnal sleep in patients on chronic, intermittent daytime haemodialysis vs those with chronic kidney disease. *Nephrol Dial Transplant* 2005;20:1422–1488.

145. Holley JL, Nespor S, Rault R. A comparison of reported sleep disorders in patients on chronic hemodialysis and continuous peritoneal dialysis. *Am J Kidney Dis* 1992;19(2):156–161.

146. Beecroft JM, Zaltzman J, Prasad R, et al. Impact of kidney transplantation on sleep apnoea in patients with end-stage renal disease. *Nephrol Dial Transplant* 2007;22:3028–3033

147. Hanly PJ, Pierratos A. Improvement of sleep apnea in patients with chronic renal failure who undergo nocturnal hemodialysis. *N Engl J Med* 2001;344(2):102–107.

148. Hanly PJ, Gabor JY, Chan C, et al. Daytime sleepiness in patients with CRF: impact of nocturnal hemodialysis. *Am J Kidney Dis* 2003;41(2):403–410.

149. Beecroft J, Duffin J, Pierratos A, et al. Enhanced chemo-responsiveness in patients with sleep apnoea and end-stage renal disease. *Eur Respir J* 2006;28(1):151–158.

150. Beecroft JM, Hoffstein V, Pierratos A, et al. Pharyngeal narrowing in end-stage renal disease: implications for obstructive sleep apnoea. *Eur Respir J* 2007;30(5):965–971.

151. Chiu KL, Ryan CM, Shiota S, et al. Fluid shift by lower body positive pressure increases pharyngeal resistance in healthy subjects. *Am J Respir Crit Care Med* 2006;174(12):1378–1383.

152. Elias RM, Chan CT, Paul N, et al. Relationship of pharyngeal water content and jugular volume with severity of obstructive sleep apnea in renal failure. *Nephrol Dial Transplant* 2013;28(4):937–944.

153. Tang SC, Lam B, Ku PP, et al. Alleviation of sleep apnea in patients with chronic renal failure by nocturnal cycler-assisted peritoneal dialysis compared with conventional continuous ambulatory peritoneal dialysis. *J Am Soc Nephrol* 2006;17:2607–2616.

154. Charra B, Calemard E, Cuche M, et al. Control of hypertension and prolonged survival on maintenance hemodialysis. *Nephron* 1983;33(2): 96–99.

155. Lacson E Jr, Wang W, Lester K, et al. Outcomes associated with in-center nocturnal hemodialysis from a large multicenter program. *Clin J Am Soc Nephrol* 2010;5(2):220–226.

156. Weinhandl ED, Nieman KM, Gilbertson DT, et al. Hospitalization in daily home hemodialysis and matched thrice-weekly in-center hemodialysis patients. *Am J Kidney Dis* 2015;65(1):98–108.

157. Weinhandl ED, Liu J, Gilbertson DT, et al. Survival in daily home hemodialysis and matched thrice-weekly in-center hemodialysis patients. *J Am Soc Nephrol* 2012;23(5):895–904.

158. Nesrallah GE, Lindsay RM, Cuerden MS, et al. Intensive hemodialysis associates with improved survival compared with conventional hemodialysis. *J Am Soc Nephrol* 2012;23(4):696–705.

159. Blagg CR, Kjellstrand CM, Ting GO, et al. Comparison of survival between short-daily hemodialysis and conventional hemodialysis using the standardized mortality ratio. *Hemodial Int* 2006;10(4):371–374.

160. Pauly RP, Gill JS, Rose CL, et al. Survival among nocturnal home haemodialysis patients compared to kidney transplant recipients. *Nephrol Dial Transplant* 2009;24(9):2915–2919.

161. Tennankore KK, Kim SJ, Baer HJ, et al. Survival and hospitalization for intensive home hemodialysis compared with kidney transplantation. *J Am Soc Nephrol* 2014;25(9):2113–2120.

162. Suri RS, Li L, Nesrallah GE. The risk of hospitalization and modality failure with home dialysis. *Kidney Int* 2015;88:360–368.

163. Rocco MV, Daugirdas JT, Greene T, et al. Long-term effects of frequent nocturnal hemodialysis on mortality: the Frequent Hemodialysis Network (FHN) nocturnal trial. *Am J Kidney Dis* 2015;66(3):459–468.

164. Chertow GM, Levin NW, Beck GJ, et al. Long-term effects of frequent in-center hemodialysis [published online ahead of print October 14, 2015]. *J Am Soc Nephrol*. doi:10.1681/ASN.2015040426.

165. Canaud B, Bragg-Gresham JL, Marshall MR, et al. Mortality risk for patients receiving hemodiafiltration versus hemodialysis: European results from the DOPPS. *Kidney Int* 2006;69(11):2087–2093.

166. Friedman EA. Birth and agony of hemofiltration. *Am J Kidney Dis* 2005;45(3):603–606.

167. Maduell F, Moreso F, Pons M, et al. High-efficiency postdilution on-line hemodiafiltration reduces all-cause mortality in hemodialysis patients. *J Am Soc Nephrol* 2013;24(3):487–497.

168. Wang AY, Ninomiya T, Al-Kahwa A, et al. Effect of hemodiafiltration or hemofiltration compared with hemodialysis on mortality and cardiovascular disease in chronic kidney failure: a systematic review and meta-analysis of randomized trials. *Am J Kidney Dis* 2014;63(6):968–978.

169. Jaber BL, Zimmerman DL, Teehan GS, et al. Daily hemofiltration for end-stage renal disease: a feasibility and efficacy trial. *Blood Purif* 2004;22(6):481–489.

170. Maduell F, Navarro V, Torregrosa E, et al. Change from three times a week on-line hemodiafiltration to short daily on-line hemodiafiltration. *Kidney Int* 2003;64(1):305–313.

171. Warady BA, Fischbach M, Geary D, et al. Frequent hemodialysis in children. *Adv Chronic Kidney Dis* 2007;14(3):297–303.

172. Geary DF, Piva E, Tyrrell J, et al. Home nocturnal hemodialysis in children. *J Pediatr* 2005;147(3):383–387.

173. Fischbach M, Terzic J, Laugel V, et al. Daily on-line haemodiafiltration: a pilot trial in children. *Nephrol Dial Transplant* 2004;19(9):2360–2367.

174. Fischbach M, Terzic J, Menouer S, et al. Daily on line haemodiafiltration promotes catch-up growth in children on chronic dialysis. *Nephrol Dial Transplant* 2010;25(3):867–873.

CHAPTER 9

Home Hemodialysis

Brent W. Miller

Hemodialysis performed in the patient's home has been a safe and effective form of dialysis therapy for over 40 years (1). The dialysis principles discussed in the previous chapters apply equally to therapy in the patient's home, but the logistics of delivering care in the home and involving the patient in every aspect of his or her therapy necessitate a different approach than conventional center-based hemodialysis.

Similar to peritoneal dialysis, many reports outline benefits of various forms of home hemodialysis; however, the overwhelming majority are uncontrolled, observational and retrospective analyses. For example, a recent attempted review comparing home hemodialysis and center-based hemodialysis found only one short-term randomized controlled trial involving nine patients and concluded no definitive relative statements could be made contrasting the medical risks and benefits of the two modalities (2). Thus, this chapter focuses on the principles and practical points specific to home hemodialysis.

HISTORY

The concept of an outpatient hemodialysis center in the United States was not fully developed until the mid-1970s when legislation granted coverage for hemodialysis to most citizens regardless of age (3). This led to a rapid expansion of center-based dialysis culminating in the 2000s with thrice-weekly, center-based outpatient hemodialysis being the therapy of choice of greater than 90% of end-stage kidney disease (ESKD) patients. Prior to this event and the subsequent development of widespread, successful outpatient peritoneal dialysis in the 1980s, a large proportion of hemodialysis was performed in the patient's home, usually by a family member or close friend (**FIGURE 9.1**). Some staff-assisted home hemodialysis has been done, but the associated labor costs have made this impractical for the majority of patients.

TECHNICAL CONCERNS

Machine

Almost any dialysis machine can and has been utilized in the patient's home. Several dialysis machines have been studied for safety and efficacy in the home and approved for home use by the U.S. Food and Drug Administration (**TABLE 9.1**) (4,5). The NxStage System One utilizes a cartridge-based extracorporeal circuit and dialysate of up to 60 L with lactate as a buffer. Its maximum dialysate flow is 300 mL/min (**FIGURE 9.2**). The Fresenius 2008K@home is based on a traditional hemodialysis machine requiring water treatment similar to traditional hemodialysis and bicarbonate as a buffer (**FIGURE 9.3**). Four other hemodialysis machines designed specifically for home hemodialysis are under development: The Tablo hemodialysis machine from Outset Medical with an integrated patient interface and production of dialysate from tap water, the PAK hemodialysis machine from Fresenius Medical, a sorbent-based hemodialysis system, the Vivia hemodialysis machine from Baxter Healthcare and the Quanta SC+ from Quanta.

The choice of a machine is important for the home dialysis program. Machines will differ in their cost, maintenance, physical footprint, portability within and outside the home, plumbing and electrical requirements, training time, set-up and breakdown time, and water and dialysate preparation. While it is feasible and sometimes helpful to use multiple hemodialysis machines within a home program, this will introduce more required training, knowledge, and experience of the entire staff.

Water

Successful dialysis starts with the production of water free from microbiological and chemical contaminants that can harm the patient (6,7). While water production in the outpatient unit is similar

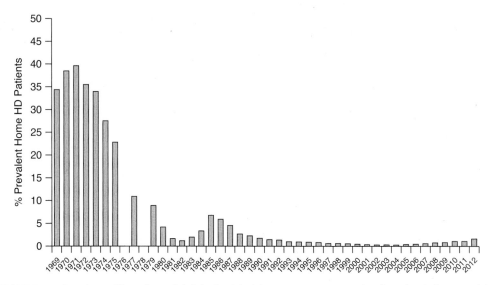

FIGURE 9.1 Prevalence of home hemodialysis in the United States 1969–2012. Data taken from the Final Report of the National Dialysis Registry, 1976, the Bureau of Health Insurance (BHI), and United States Renal Data System (USRDS) 2014. (Adapted with permission from Advanced Renal Education Program, Fresenius Medical Corporation of North America.)

in each unit, each patient's home installation will be unique. Furthermore, while the cost of providing water and dialysate in the outpatient unit is usually less than 2% of the overall cost of the treatment, it is a major cost in the home hemodialysis treatment and also entails some cost to the patient for additional water usage and plumbing. The Centers for Medicare and Medicaid Services (CMS) has applied water quality and testing standards developed by the Association for the Advancement of Medical Instrumentation (AAMI) since 1987. These standards are updated approximately every 5 years (8). The water quality of both the outpatient unit and the patient's home is ultimately the responsibility of the medical director of the dialysis facility. These general principles of water treatment for hemodialysis are covered in Chapter 8.

In the home environment, the water system will be unique in every installation while adhering to the same AAMI standards. The source water should be tested to see if it meets the minimum standards of the Safe Water Drinking Act (9). If the source water does not meet these standards, then the product water should undergo an AAMI analysis to ensure the contaminants have been removed by the water treatment system. Numerous water supplies in the United States have elevated levels in the source water of elements such as iron, manganese, sulfates, copper, lead, aluminum, and others that

will need to be tested in this way. Furthermore, occasional contamination of municipal water supplies such as the Elk River accident with 4-methyl cyclohexane methanol in West Virginia in 2014 can endanger the home hemodialysis patient (10). Most water treatment systems will adequately remove these contaminants; however, the poor source water quality may lead to early exhaustion of components of the treatment system at substantial cost and inconvenience. In this circumstance, installation of a second system between the source water and the water treatment system will often alleviate the problem.

Dialysate

Dialysate can be provided in a patient's home in a number of methods: bagged dialysate delivered to the patient's home similar to peritoneal dialysis, dialysate prepared in the patient's home prior to dialysis, or in-line dialysate from an appropriate water source mixed at the machine. Cost, convenience, storage, installation, and maintenance all factor in the type of dialysate to utilize.

Bagged dialysate similar to peritoneal dialysis has the advantage of providing a sterile, ultrapure dialysate to the patient. However, limitations accompany this advantage. Practical considerations of delivery, storage, cost, and logistics generally limit this method to

TABLE 9.1	Comparison of Common Settings of the Two Current Home Dialysis Systems Approved by the U.S. Food and Drug Administration Specifically for Home Dialysis Use	
	NxStage System One	**Fresenius 2008K@home**
Dialysate delivery	Bagged sterile fluid or batched dialysate production	In-line reverse osmosis machine or de-ionized water tanks
Maximum dialysate flow	200–300 mL/min	800 mL/min
Typical Q_D/Q_B	0.3–0.5	1.5–2.0
Dialysate buffer	Lactate 40 or 45 mEq/L	Bicarbonate (variable)
Dialysate potassium	1 or 2 mEq/L	1–3 mEq/L
Dialysate sodium	140 mEq/L	130–140 mEq/L
Dialysate calcium	3 mEq/L	2–3.5 mEq/L

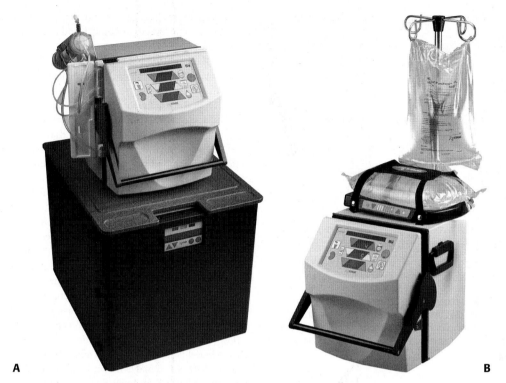

A

B

FIGURE 9.2 Current NxStage home hemodialysis system. **A:** Complete system with dialysis cartridge, machine, and water treatment system together. **B:** NxStage System One with premixed, bagged fluid as dialysate. (Images used with permission of NxStage Medical, Inc.)

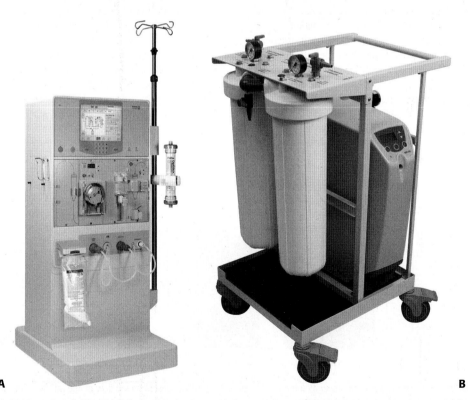

A

B

FIGURE 9.3 Conventional home hemodialysis system with the Fresenius 2008K@home **(A)** and a reverse osmosis system that can be connected to the patient's home water supply **(B)**. (Photographs used with permission and provided courtesy of Fresenius Medical Care.)

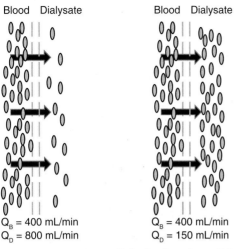

Blood Dialysate   Blood Dialysate

Q_B = 400 mL/min Q_B = 400 mL/min
Q_D = 800 mL/min Q_D = 150 mL/min

A. Conventional hemodialysis   B. Low-volume hemodialysis
(30–48 L/h)   (8–12 L/h)

FIGURE 9.4 As Q_D/Q_B is changed from conventional hemodialysis **(A)** to low-volume hemodialysis **(B)**, dialysate saturation increases dramatically. Thus, small molecule clearance for the same period of time is not directly proportional to the decrease in dialysate volume particularly as Q_D exceeds 350 mL/min.

approximately 30 L of dialysate yielding a single pool urea Kt/V of approximately 0.7 in the typical 80-kg adult; thus, in the absence of significant residual renal function, more than three times a week dialysis will be needed to obtain what is currently considered "adequate" hemodialysis based on small molecule clearance. Second, lactate is typically the base in bagged dialysate fluid for both stability and microbiological concerns. Lactate showed improvement in tolerability over acetate as a hemodialysis buffer before the widespread introduction of bicarbonate-based buffer (11). Yet, in hemodialysis with a lactate buffer, serum lactate levels will be increased slightly, but patients with significant liver dysfunction, higher volumes of dialysate, and/

or poorly controlled diabetes may not tolerate lactate as defined by a serum lactate level of >5 mEq/L and transient symptoms of muscle cramping, lower blood pressure, nausea, headache, or weakness. Lastly, the production of bagged dialysate offers a limited number of dialysate baths negating one of the benefits of home hemodialysis—optimizing the dialysis prescription for the individual.

Replicating dialysate production similar to the outpatient unit or the acute care setting in the hospital also has limitations. Typically, either a reverse osmosis (RO) machine or a deionized (DI) water system must be installed in the patient's home. The RO machine adds another machine to install, maintain, and monitor. The DI system usually requires an outside vendor to change the tanks and regenerate the beads in addition to plumbing installation delivering the water to the machine in the home.

Several systems that produce water and dialysate in novel methods in the home are being developed. These include the use of sorbent, distillation, and miniaturization of the dialysate production.

Home dialysis regimens often use lower dialysate flows (<500 mL/min) and total dialysate volumes (<60 L) necessitating a change in standard chemical components of the dialysate bath, particularly small molecules such as potassium (12). Some have termed this *low-volume dialysis*, but no consistent term has been applied (**FIGURE 9.4**). Whereas a conventional hemodialysis treatment may use a blood flow of 400 mL/min and a dialysate flow of 600 mL/min, home dialysis treatments may use a dialysate flow much lower such as 200 mL/min. As dialysate flow is decreased relative to blood flow, the dialysate effluent will be more highly saturated (**FIGURE 9.5**). To remove the same amount of solute over the same time, the starting gradient in the dialyzer must be higher (13,14). For example, a potassium bath of 2 mEq/L for a 3-hour conventional, high-efficiency hemodialysis treatment with a dialysate flow of 600 mL/min (108 total L of dialysate with approximately 20% solute saturation) will need to be changed to 1 mEq/L for the 3-hour home hemodialysis treatment at 200 mL/min (36 total L of dialysate with approximately 80% solute saturation).

Finally, it is important to note that as dialysate flow is increased relative to blood flow, the incremental amount of small molecule clearance rapidly decreases particularly as dialysate flow moves

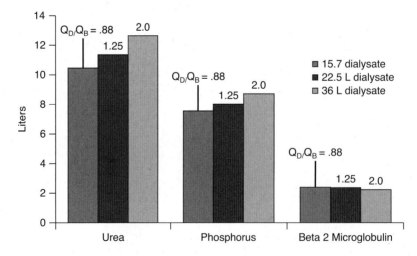

FIGURE 9.5 Removal of solutes over 45 minutes of hemodialysis with a constant blood flow of 400 ml/min with varying dialysate volumes. Note that: 1) dialysate saturation of all solutes decreases as Q_D/Q_B increases and 2) solute removal does not increase for the large molecule as dialysate volume is increased over a constant time. (Adapted from Bhimani JP, Ouseph R, Ward RA. Effect of increasing dialysate flow rate on diffusive mass transfer or urea, phosphate and β2-microglobulin during clinical haemodialysis. *Nephrol Dial Transplant* 2010;25:3990–3995.)

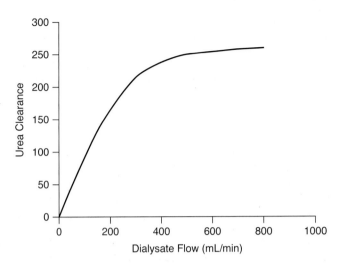

FIGURE 9.6 Estimated urea clearance as a function of dialysate flow with a fixed blood flow of 400 mL/min based on historical observations. Note that the efficiency (amount removed/dialysate utilized) of urea clearance begins to decline significantly after approximately 350 mL/min and precipitously after approximately 500 mL/min. Thus, significant urea clearance can be achieved with dialysate flows of <200 mL/min or approximately 30 L in a 3-hour hemodialysis treatment.

TABLE 9.2	**Patient-Centered Outcomes for Potential Home Hemodialysis Patients**

Control over treatment schedule
Removal of frequent travel to dialysis center
Substantial involvement in care
More frequent dialysis
Ability to travel with dialysis equipment
More time with family and friends
Better blood pressure control
Improved appetite
Improved physical activity

above approximately 350 mL/min (**FIGURE 9.6**). Because of the incremental cost of additional water and dialysate preparation, several dialysis providers have reduced their conventional dialysate flow to a maximum of 500 mL/min and suggested even 400 mL/min.

One of the more common home dialysis machines, the Nx-Stage System One, utilizes a fixed dialysate flow to blood flow ratio ("the flow fraction" or Q_D/Q_B), typically less than 0.5, in order to saturate the relatively small amount of dialysate. Adjusting the "flow fraction" down will increase the saturation of the dialysate or the efficiency of the dialysis treatment, while increasing the flow fraction will decrease the efficiency of the treatment. Similarly, the Fresenius 2008K@home machine can utilize a fixed Q_D/Q_B of 1.5 or 2.0 ("autoflow").

◆ CLINICAL CONCERNS

Patient Selection

Not every patient is willing or capable to perform hemodialysis at home. Placing a patient who is unwilling to follow treatment protocols at home raises additional safety concerns. Furthermore, training patients for home hemodialysis is a time-consuming, labor-intensive, and expensive process. If patients fail at home shortly after training, both nursing morale and the financial performance of the home dialysis program suffer.

However, choosing patients whom in some physician's eyes seem to be the perfect candidate for home therapy—less comorbid illnesses, employed, extensive social support networks, younger age, well-educated, and so on—does not necessarily ensure success. First, that "ideal" candidate rarely exists. Second, many of those patients are doing well with their current therapy and may not see a substantial improvement with home therapy. Lastly, the patient whom may benefit the most from home hemodialysis and succeed at home hemodialysis is not well-defined and not always obvious to the physician.

In lieu of studies or trials that evaluate this question, a simplified approach generally works. First, why does the patient want to perform home hemodialysis or, alternatively, why is the physician recommending home hemodialysis? Is the specified expectation or reason a measurable outcome that can be evaluated in a reasonable time frame (**TABLE 9.2**)? Second, what type of support at home does the patient have? *Support* should not be confused with *effort* by family members, friends, or care partners in the home. Patients should be encouraged to perform as much of the dialysis treatment as possible and be involved in their care as much as possible. Kidney failure and dialysis is a long and difficult journey, and encouragement and support are critical to the success, particularly at home. Having a spouse, family member, or friend actually *performing the dialysis treatment* is not crucial to success for every patient. In fact, the additional stress on the "care partner" may lead to modality failure despite the improvement of the patient clinically. Lastly, while it seems that the amount of support would correlate with success at home, some data suggests that success is more likely to occur where the patient's expectation of support matches what is actually received rather than the absolute quantity delivered (15).

To help delineate these issues, it is helpful for the patient to meet with the treatment team (nurse, social worker, nephrologist, financial representative) to discuss these issues before training. Having additional small meetings with the patient and family separated may allow previously unvoiced concerns to be discussed. These concerns may be as simple as "I don't want my home to become a medical facility" or "will this interfere with our intimacy?" or as complex as "I have a demanding 40-hr job and now you are asking me to learn and perform dialysis on my spouse after work . . . ."

Prescription Management

Kinetic modeling and solute clearance are discussed at length in Chapters 6 and 7. Although those concepts remain the same for hemodialysis at home, the change in location of the dialysis treatment unshackles the nephrologist and the patient from the logistics and rigid thrice-weekly schedule of the typical outpatient dialysis center. Thus, multiple options for dialysis including varying schedules, different frequencies, and longer times as discussed in the preceding chapter are obtainable. For the patient, tailoring a dialysis schedule to a particular lifestyle is also possible and likely a major motivation for performing dialysis in the home even if the medical outcomes are equivalent. This motivation should not be discounted when considering the prescription. For example, the patient may want to perform dialysis at night after work during the week and early in the morning on the weekend.

While the relative risks and benefits remain to be studied definitively in controlled trials, optimizing solute clearance at home by increasing the dialysis frequency or length as discussed in preceding chapter is easily obtainable in the patient's home. Certain patients, such as those with a longer life expectancy or transplant sensitization, may desire a prescription that optimizes larger solute clearance, lowers ultrafiltration rates, controls plasma phosphorus, and may lower utilization of erythropoiesis stimulating agents.

Several studies suggest that a dialysis frequency greater than 3 times per week may be preferable for many patients. Several analyses of large databases, most recently in 2011 with United States Renal Data System (USRDS), demonstrated markedly increased all-cause mortality and cardiovascular hospital admission rate related to the long interdialytic interval in thrice-weekly hemodialysis (16). A randomized, 1-year trial of thrice-weekly hemodialysis versus six times weekly hemodialysis in 247 patients demonstrated an improvement in the combined end point of mortality and left ventricular hypertrophy (17). Conversely, a longitudinal follow-up of the 87 patients from the Frequent Hemodialysis Network study of nocturnal hemodialysis suggested a potential lower survival with more frequent, home nocturnal hemodialysis (18). However, this study has several limitations including a conventional arm that provided longer dialysis than is typically performed, a large number of both incident patients and patients with significant residual function, and a large number of patients from one of the study centers. Analysis of loss of residual renal function in the study was higher in the nocturnal arm; thus, one potential conclusion is that intensive dialysis regimens should be reserved for anuric or oliguric patients (19).

The nephrologist should also consider potential changes to the prescription that will enhance the stability and safety of the treatment in the home environment in addition to optimizing the solute removal (**TABLE 9.3**).

Training

The different types of adult learning are usually not topics in medical training; however, knowledge and application of learning principles is key to the success of a home hemodialysis program. While this may be more important for the nurse trainer to utilize, the nephrologist should review training materials and techniques to ensure successful training of all patients. Additionally, training is often thought of as the intense, initial phase. But it is important that ongoing training and retraining are regularly incorporated into the home hemodialysis program.

TABLE 9.3	**Changes in Home Hemodialysis Prescription That May Optimize Stability and/or Safety**

Careful adjustment of the estimated "dry weight" during the training period
Limitation of ultrafiltration rate
Avoidance of long interdialytic intervals
Lower blood flow
Lower dialysate temperature
Longer dialysis times
Use of single needle for access
Avoidance of large meals during treatment
Use of bicarbonate-based buffer

The dialysis treatment itself is usually incorporated into the patient training time. Most nephrologists have patients train in an outpatient facility, but occasionally, home-based training in a stable patient can be accomplished. Training usually takes 4 to 6 weeks depending upon the intensity, type of machine, and learning ability of the patient. Most nephrologists check urea kinetics and electrolytes after 1 week and make further adjustments to the prescription so that the patient is on a final, stable prescription before being sent home. Patients who increase the frequency of their dialysis schedule will often need a change in the estimated dry weight, decreased antihypertensive medications, and a higher potassium bath.

Patient Burnout

The improvement in dialysis patient survival and the increasing length of kidney transplantation waiting times often means that a patient will experience multiple dialysis modalities. It is important not to view either a temporary or permanent change from home hemodialysis to another dialysis modality as a "failure" and engage the patients and their families in discussions about the impact of performing dialysis has on their life, how they are coping with the impact, and whether a change is needed. Currently, approximately 4% of patients on hemodialysis stop each month. About half is due to kidney transplantation and death, and the remaining transfer to center-based dialysis for a variety of reasons.

Ongoing involvement of the multidisciplinary team with frank, open discussions of the burden of the therapy and its effects, social isolation, and changes in family dynamics may preclude a significant problem.

When a patient or family member expresses negative concerns about the burden of therapy, temporary placement in an outpatient center should be offered. This may entail a few self-care treatments in the home training area or alternatively a longer intermission of conventional hemodialysis in an outpatient setting. Additionally, there may be certain situations that necessitate a respite from the home setting: changes in vascular access, temporary or permanent loss of a care partner, illness, or electrical and water problems in the home. The routine flux of patients in and out of the home program should be expected and planned.

Vascular Access

Vascular access is discussed at length in Chapter 4. For the home hemodialysis patient, several additional concerns need consideration: patient training, technique, ergonomics, safety, management of potential infection, and clinical monitoring of the vascular access. All types of vascular access utilized in center-based dialysis have been successfully utilized in patients at home. The type of access should not be a deterrent to a patient dialyzing at home.

Currently, approximately half of home hemodialysis patients cannulate themselves and half have care partners performing cannulation. Rarely is fear of cannulation an insurmountable obstacle to home hemodialysis training. Since all dialysis patients may be taught self-care in their therapy, it is often helpful to begin cannulation training before starting home hemodialysis training (unless the patient is new to hemodialysis).

For the patient with the arteriovenous fistula (AVF), either the rotating site ("rope-ladder") or single-site ("buttonhole) method of cannulation can be chosen. The pros and cons of the single-site approach are discussed in Chapter 4. Although many practitioners believe the self-cannulator has less discomfort and easier needle insertion, this has not been adequately studied and the infectious risk appears higher as currently practiced (20–22).

The sites of cannulation should be chosen with careful collaboration between the training nurse and the patient. The patient should give significant input to the ergonomics of cannulation and decannulation, while the nurse should choose the safest sites. For example, the nonmedical person choosing a site to insert a needle may inappropriately see the top of an aneurysmal dilatation as the easiest site to be successful. Removal of the needle also demands careful attention especially for the self-cannulator. The synchrony of safe needle removal, placement in an appropriate waste container, pressure, and hemostasis is often more technically difficult than needle insertion. Another ergonomic factor for the self-cannulator at home is the insertion and subsequent removal of both arterial and venous needles in a proximal or upward direction in both AVF and arteriovenous graft (AVG).

Similar to peritoneal dialysis, aseptic technique cannot be emphasized, monitored, and retrained enough. Aseptic technique is often a foreign concept to the new home hemodialysis patient. Several antibacterial agents are available to utilize in the event of a significant local skin reaction to one (**TABLE 9.4**). Whether or not to utilize an antibiotic cream or ointment after hemostasis, particularly of single-site or "buttonhole" cannulation, remains unresolved (22).

Unlike peritoneal dialysis, the signs and symptoms of an access infection in a home hemodialysis patient can be subtle. The threshold for a clinical evaluation, potential blood cultures, and possible preemptive antibiotics should be low. How and where to perform these should be determined prior to the end of patient training for each patient so no delay will occur when a potential problem develops. With a documented access infection, the patient's aseptic technique should be reviewed, observed, and adjusted as needed. Similarly, the home hemodialysis program should monitor the rate of bloodstream infections carefully. Since the 2016 CMS national standard is approximately 0.27 bloodstream infections per 1,000 patient-days, a home hemodialysis program of 10 patients should not see more than one bloodstream infection per year and ideally not more than one bloodstream infection every 3 years (23).

Changes in the vascular access should be noted for possible intervention. An unexplained decline in urea kinetics would be one measure. Reports from patients of changes in blood flow, increased venous pressure during dialysis, or a change in bleeding after pulling needles may indicate a problem with the access. One of the advantages of home dialysis is that a full exam of the access can occur monthly by the physician without needles in place and a complete range of motion of the limb. Assessing the appearance, thrill, bruit, augmentation, temperature, and location of the cannulation sites is easy to do in the home patient during a clinic visit by both the nurse and physician.

TABLE 9.4	Antibacterial Agents for Home Hemodialysis Vascular Access

Povidone-iodine solution
Chlorhexidine gluconate 2% and isopropyl alcohol 70%
Chlorhexidine gluconate 0.5% and isopropyl alcohol 70%
Sodium hypochlorite 0.114%
Alcohol

SAFETY CONSIDERATIONS

Home hemodialysis as currently practiced has an excellent safety record (24). In one review of two home hemodialysis programs, only seven serious events were noted over 500 patient-years, and most of those events were operator errors that could be prevented by a combination of technology and education. However, several specific topics merit discussion.

Hypotension

Some have estimated that intradialytic hypotension, defined as the need to stop ultrafiltration and administer saline intravenously, occurs in up to 20% of conventional hemodialysis treatments. Hypotension in the home environment poses a clear safety risk and must be minimized. The most common cause of intradialytic hypotension in the home environment is incorrect calculation or entry of the ultrafiltration volume. Some of the strategies to reduce hypotension in the outpatient center also are available in the home such as limiting the ultrafiltration rate to approximately 10 mL/kg/h, decreasing the dialysate temperature, and avoiding antihypertensive medications prior to the dialysis treatment.

Bleeding

Miscannulation of AVF or AVG should be reported promptly to the home dialysis nurse to determine the cause such as incorrect location, angle, depth, or advancement of the needle. Infiltration of blood into a misplaced venous needle can cause significant blood loss, pain, and impair the future function of the access. Venous dislodgment of a needle with the arterial needle still in place with the blood pump engaged can lead to life-threatening blood loss quickly, particularly if the patient is performing a nocturnal hemodialysis treatment while sleeping. Fortunately, this is a rare event, but moisture detectors placed near the venous needle can help prevent this from occurring.

Air Embolism

Hemodialysis technology has advanced so that air embolism during a hemodialysis treatment is extraordinarily rare. Air embolism now occurs during manipulation of the vascular access either prior to or after the dialysis treatment. Careful training and emphasis is needed in this regard; a patient death from air embolism during manipulation of a central venous catheter following a home dialysis treatment occurred at the University of Iowa in the 87-patient Frequent Hemodialysis Network trial (25; P. W. Eggers, written communication, March 2008).

Leaks

The placement of large quantities of water in close proximity to electrical equipment and a patient requires several safeguards. Prior to installation, the home should be inspected so that ground fault circuit interrupter outlets are utilized and appropriate pans and moisture detectors are installed underneath the equipment.

Outpatient Follow-up

One of the most surprising aspects of home hemodialysis is the effort the provider must provide after successful training. Most nephrologists perform a face-to-face encounter monthly with their home hemodialysis patients. This often works best if a multidisciplinary approach including the dialysis nurse, dialysis social worker, and renal dietitian are included in this visit. Treatment logs for the month are reviewed for problems. Most patients draw their monthly blood work themselves and bring it to the center for analysis. Full medical waste containers can be exchanged for empty containers. While many supplies may be delivered to the patients' homes, it is often more cost-effective to have the patient pick up smaller supplies such as needles, gauze pads, syringes, and so on at this visit.

As with all forms of dialysis, problems will occur that require medical attention. A clear communication strategy should be in place for the patient. Technical problems with the machine should be routed to either the biomedical technician of the dialysis center or the technical support staff of the dialysis machine manufacturer. Medical problems should be routed to the home dialysis nurse or nephrologist on call. Many home dialysis programs will post this contact information physically on the dialysis machine for patient ease.

Future Advances

In the United States, only 2% of ESKD patients utilize home hemodialysis at present. One of the impediments to more patients choosing this therapy is the slow pace of technologic advancements applied to home hemodialysis. One can understand the lack of incentive in developing innovative medical devices for a small proportion of a relatively small number of people in a low-margin, capitated fiscal environment; however, the inflexibility and fixed labor and capital costs of center-based hemodialysis, the lengthening of transplant waiting times, and the continued high failure rate of peritoneal dialysis may eventually add motivation for new approaches to home hemodialysis.

◆ REFERENCES

1. Blagg CR, Hickman RO, Eschbach JW, et al. Home hemodialysis: six years' experience. *N Engl J Med* 1970;283:1126–1131.
2. Palmer SC, Palmer AR, Craig JC, et al. Home versus in-centre haemodialysis for end-stage kidney disease. *Cochrane Database Syst Rev* 2014;(11):CD009535.
3. Eggers PW. Medicare's end stage renal disease program. *Health Care Financ Rev* 2000;22:55–60.
4. U.S. Food and Drug Administration. 510(k) summary K070049. http://www.accessdata.fda.gov/cdrh_docs/pdf7/K070049.pdf. Published February 3, 2011. Accessed July 11, 2015.
5. U.S. Food and Drug Administration. 510(k) summary K050525. http://www.accessdata.fda.gov/cdrh_docs/pdf5/K050525.pdf. Published June 24, 2005. Accessed July 11, 2015.
6. Hoenich N, Ward RA. Maintaining water quality for hemodialysis. http://www.uptodate.com/contents/maintaining-water-quality-for-hemodialysis. Accessed August 30, 2015.
7. Ahmad S. Essentials of water treatment in hemodialysis. *Hemodial Int* 2005;9:127–134.
8. Association for the Advancement of Medical Instrumentation. *Water for Hemodialysis and Related Therapies ANSI/AAMI 13959/2014.* Arlington, VA: Association for the Advancement of Medical Instrumentation, 2014.
9. United States Environmental Protection Agency. Drinking water contaminants—standards and regulations. http://www.epa.gov/safewater/contaminants/index.html#mcls. Accessed July 13, 2015.
10. Centers for Disease Control and Prevention. 2014 West Virginia chemical release. http://emergency.cdc.gov/chemical/MCHM/westvirginia2014/. Accessed August 12, 2015.
11. Dalal S, Yu AW, Gupta DK, et al. L-lactate high efficiency hemodialysis: hemodynamics, blood gas changes, potassium/phosphorus and symptoms. *Kidney Int* 1990;38:896–903.
12. Pierratos A, Ouwendyk M, Francoeur R, et al. Nocturnal hemodialysis: three-year experience. *J Am Soc Nephrol* 1998;9:859–868.
13. Eloot S, Van Biesen W, Dhondt A, et al. Impact of hemodialysis duration on the removal of uremic retention solutes. *Kidney Int* 2008;73:765–770.
14. Basile C, Libutti P, Di Turo AL, et al. Removal of uraemic retention solutes in standard bicarbonate haemodialysis and long-hour slow-flow bicarbonate hemodialysis. *Nephrol Dial Transplant* 2011;26:1296–1303.
15. Thong MSY, Kaptein AA, Krediet RT, et al. Social support predicts survival in dialysis patients. *Nephrol Dial Transplant* 2007;22:845–850.
16. Foley RN, Gilbertson DT, Murray T, et al. Long interdialytic interval and mortality among patients receiving hemodialysis. *N Engl J Med* 2011;365:1099–1107.
17. FHN Trial Group. In-center hemodialysis six times per week versus three times per week. *N Engl J Med* 2010;363:2287–2300.
18. Rocco MV, Daugirdas JT, Greene T, et al. Long-term effects of frequent nocturnal hemodialysis on mortality: the Frequent Hemodialysis Network (FHN) Nocturnal Trial. *Am J Kidney Dis* 2015;66:459–468.
19. Daugirdas JT, Greene T, Rocco MV, et al. Effect of frequent hemodialysis on residual kidney function. *Kidney Int* 2013;83:949–958.
20. Lok CE, Sontrop JM, Faratro R, et al. Frequent hemodialysis fistula infectious complications. *Nephron Extra* 2014;4:159–167.
21. MacRae JM, Ahmed SB, Hemmelgarn BR, et al. Arteriovenous fistula survival and needling technique: long-term results from a randomized buttonhole trial. *Am J Kidney Dis* 2014;63:636–642.
22. Nesrallah GE, Cuerden M, Wong JH, et al. Staphylococcus aureus bacteremia and buttonhole cannulation: long-term safety and efficacy of mupirocin prophylaxis. *Clin J Am Soc Nephrol* 2010;5:1047–1053.
23. Centers for Medicare and Medicaid Services. ESRD QIP Payment Year 2016: final rule. https://www.cms.gov. Accessed July 17, 2015.
24. Wong B, Zimmerman D, Reintjes F, et al. Procedure-related serious adverse events among home hemodialysis patients: a quality assurance perspective. *Am J Kidney Dis* 2014;63:251–258.
25. Rocco MV, Lockridge RS Jr, Beck GJ, et al. The effects of frequent nocturnal home hemodialysis: the Frequent Hemodialysis Network Nocturnal Trial. *Kidney Int* 2011;80:1080–1091.

CHAPTER **10**

Continuous Dialysis Therapeutic Techniques

Piyush Mathur, Celina Cepeda, and Ravindra L. Mehta

Acute kidney injury (AKI) is a frequent complication in critically ill patients and reflects a broad spectrum of clinical presentations ranging from mild to severe injury that may result in permanent and complete loss of renal function. AKI represents a significant risk factor for adverse outcomes and has been associated with mortality greater than 50% (1). The underlying mechanisms of AKI include a decrease in the kidney's ability to excrete nitrogenous waste, manage electrolytes, regulate intravascular volume, and regulate acid–base status (2,3). Depending on the severity of AKI, dialysis is often required to support renal function. Over the last two decades, significant advances have been made in the availability of different dialysis methods for replacement of renal function. Renal replacement therapy (RRT) can be provided as hemodialysis, hemofiltration, or a combination thereof and as intermittent, or as continuous therapy. Intermittent hemodialysis remains the mainstay of RRT in most part of the world, and modifications in duration and operational characteristics of the therapy have resulted in development of prolonged intermittent renal replacement therapy (PIRRT) also termed slow low-efficiency dialysis (SLED). The most common form of continuous therapies is peritoneal dialysis (PD), which is not as commonly used to manage AKI. Continuous renal replacement therapies (CRRTs) encompass several methods of hemofiltration and hemodialysis and are increasingly utilized for managing patients with AKI in the intensive care unit (ICU) setting (4,5). In this chapter, we provide a description of CRRT techniques, an outline of the key areas of application, and a summary of the results with these therapies.

MODALITIES OF CONTINUOUS RENAL REPLACEMENT THERAPY–TECHNICAL CONSIDERATIONS

Terminology

Continuous therapies encompass a variety of modalities that vary in the terminology. Recently, an international group of experts has developed the Acute Dialysis Quality Initiative (ADQI) (6) and has proposed adopting previously developed standardized terms for these therapies. The basic goal was to link the nomenclature to the operational characteristics of the different techniques (7). Each letter in the acronym represents a specific characteristic related to the duration, driving force, and operational features. The letter C is used in all the terms to describe the continuous nature. The letters AV or VV in the terminology identify the technique's driving force, that is, the mean arterial pressure (MAP) for arteriovenous (AV) circuits and external pumps for venovenous (VV) circuits. Solute removal in these techniques is achieved by either convection, diffusion, or a combination of both these methods. Therefore, the letters UF, H, HD, and HDF identify the technique's operational characteristics:

Convective techniques, including ultrafiltration (UF) and hemofiltration (H), depend on solute removal by solvent drag (8).

Diffusion-based techniques, similar to intermittent hemodialysis (IHD), are based on the principle of a solute gradient between the blood and the dialysate (9).

TABLE 10.1	Modalities of Continuous Renal Replacement Therapy			
	SCUF	**CVVH**	**CVVHD**	**CVVHDF**
Vascular access	VV	VV	VV	VV
Average blood flow (mL/min)	100	100–200	100–200	100–200
Dialysate flow (mL/min)	0	0	10–30	10–30
Replacement fluid (L/d)	0	21.6	0	16.8
Ultrafiltrate (mL/min)	2–8	10–30	2–4	10–30
Anticoagulation	Yes/no	Yes/no	Yes/no	Yes/no
Clearance mechanism	C	C	D	C + D
Urea clearance (L/d)	1.7	16.7	21.7	30

SCUF, slow continuous ultrafiltration; CVVH, continuous venovenous hemofiltration; CVVHD, continuous venovenous hemodialysis; CVVHDF, continuous venovenous hemodiafiltration; VV, venovenous.

Hemodiafiltration (HDF) processes use both diffusion and convection in the same technique. In this instance, both dialysate and a replacement solution are used, and both small and middle molecules can be removed easily (10).

The only exception to this nomenclature system is the acronym SCUF (slow continuous ultrafiltration), which designates UF alone without any fluid replacement.

TYPES OF CONTINUOUS RENAL REPLACEMENT THERAPY MODALITIES

As discussed in section "Terminology", the predominant mechanism of achieving clearance defines the modality of CRRT.

Simple diffusion: continuous venovenous hemodialysis (CVVHD)
Convection: continuous venovenous hemofiltration (CVVH)
Combination of both [continuous venovenous hemodiafiltration (CVVHDF)] (TABLE 10.1 and FIGURE 10.1)

MACHINES AND COMPONENTS OF CONTINUOUS RENAL REPLACEMENT THERAPY

Modern CRRT machines are designed specifically for acute dialysis and are equipped with a friendly user interface to perform SCUF, CVVH, CVVHD, and CVVHDF. These new machines utilize preset disposables, have integrated safety alarms, fluid balancing controls, and connected blood modules that are controlled with sophisticated microprocessors in the machine. The ease of setting wide range of blood, dialysate/replacement flows as well use of highly permeable membranes and pressure sensing systems has improved clearances of large molecules and efficiency of the treatment (11).

VASCULAR ACCESS AND CIRCUIT FOR CONTINUOUS RENAL REPLACEMENT THERAPY

A well-functioning vascular access is a prerequisite for successful CRRT. Several options now exist for access and can be selected based on individual patient requirements, local availability of the various catheters, and unit expertise. AV fistulas and grafts are generally not recommended for CRRT due to the risk for needle displacement and high risk for injury to the access that may make it unusable in the future. If an AV fistula or graft is to be utilized,

it should be for a very limited time and preferably cannulated with plastic angiocatheters to minimize risk of complications.

Temporary or tunnelled cuffed hemodialysis (HD) catheters are currently used as vascular access for CRRT. Temporary catheters are generally inserted at bedside ideally under ultrasound guidance (USG) by modified Seldinger technique into internal jugular (IJ), femoral, or subclavian veins using stringent sterile precautions. Although tunneled, cuffed, double-lumen silastic catheters are the preferred access for short- and intermediate-term use in chronic dialysis patients, they are generally not the initial choice for CRRT as they are more difficult to place (12). However, if CRRT continues for longer than a week, ideally a tunnelled catheter should be placed for improving blood flow and reducing the risk of infections.

ADQI recommends use of USG for catheter placement as its use has been reported to reduce the failure and complication rates of central venous catheter insertion in level II and III studies. A single-center study (13) and meta-analysis (14) showed that USG reduces placement failure, complications, and need for multiple attempts.

Optimal site for catheterization in any given patient is determined by the risks of thrombosis and infection, ease of placement, and adequacy of function. The right IJ vein is preferred for temporary catheter, given its more direct route to superior vena cava. The left jugular vein has a more circuitous route to the right atrium, and this can lead to inadequate blood flow in patients with frequent neck movements. Femoral veins should be used as second choice for CRRT, given their ease of accessibility. Subclavian veins cannulation is discouraged, as it may lead to stenosis of the vessel and may interfere with the functioning of an AV fistula or graft that maybe required in the future (15).

Most clinicians do not consider catheter location to be a determinant of risk of infection, as results of various studies are conflicting. A recent meta-analysis has not shown any difference in the rate of catheter-related bloodstream (CRB) infections between the three sites (16). Another prospective study showed that frequency of catheter-related bacteremia was similar in jugular and femoral cannulation. The main risk factors for development of CRB were duration of catheter use and the number of performed dialyses (17). A prospective study by Oliver et al. (18) in 218 patients concluded that IJ catheters may be left in place for up to 3 weeks without a high risk of bacteremia, but femoral catheters in bed-bound patients should be removed after 1 week. Other characteristics, which may influence infection rates, include the catheter material and antimicrobial coating or impregnation. Polyurethane catheters are preferred for CRRT. A prospective randomized study showed that use of polyurethane HD catheters impregnated with minocycline and rifampin

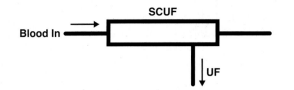

Qb = 100–200 ml/min, Qf = 2–8 ml/min

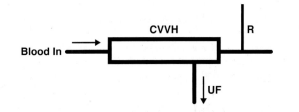

Qb = 100–200 mL/min, Qf = 10–30 mL/min, K = 20–50 L/d

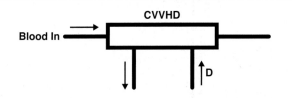

Qb = 100–200 mL/min, Qf = 2–4 mL/min, Qd = 10–30 mL/min, K = 20–50 L/d

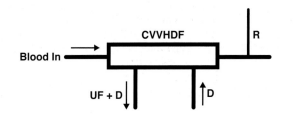

Qb = 100–200 mL/min, Qf = 10–30 mL/min, Qd = 10–30 mL/min, K = 20–50 L/d

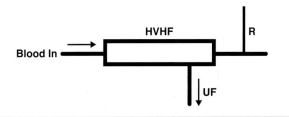

Qb = 200–300 mL/min, Qf = 50–1000 mL/min, K = 60–120 L/day

FIGURE 10.1 Modalities of continuous renal replacement therapies (CRRTs). Commonly available modalities in intensive care unit (ICU). SCUF, slow continuous ultrafiltration; Qb, blood flow; Qf, ultrafiltration rate; CVVH, continuous venovenous hemofiltration; R, replacement; UF, ultrafiltration; K, clearance; CVVHD, continuous venovenous hemodialysis; D, dialysate; Qd, dialysate flow; CVVHDF, continuous venovenous hemodiafiltration; HVHF, high-volume hemofiltration. [Adapted from Cerdá J, Ronco C. Modalities of continuous renal replacement therapy: technical and clinical considerations. *Semin Dial* 2009;22(2):114–122.]

decreases the risk of catheter-related infection (19). Another prospective study proved the efficacy of catheter-restricted filling using an antibiotic lock solution in preventing CRB (20). But toxicity, allergic reaction, and bacterial resistance are the concerns associated with antibiotics limiting their widespread use. Recently, trisodium citrate (TSC) has been advocated as a catheter lock solution because of its antimicrobial properties and local anticoagulation. In a multicenter, double-blind, randomized controlled trial (RCT); TSC 30% was compared with unfractionated heparin 5,000 U/mL for prevention of catheter-related infections, thrombosis, and bleeding complications. The study was stopped prematurely because of a difference in catheter-related bacteremia ($p < 0.01$) (21). After this trial, many studies have shown safety and superiority of TSC over heparin (22,23).

Besides infection, catheter malfunction due to thrombosis, kinking of catheter, fibrin sheath around catheter tip is another complication associated with CRRT. Instillation of heparin into both lumens prevents formation of intraluminal thrombus. However, in a completely occluded catheter by thrombus, recombinant tissue plasminogen activator (rtPA)/alteplase can be instilled to reestablish blood flow. In a study by Daeihagh et al. (24), tissue plasminogen activator (tPA) used in a dose of 2 mg with median dwell time of 24 hours appears to be as effective as urokinase for reestablishing adequate blood-flow rates through HD catheters that are thrombosed or have low blood-flow rates. tPA was effective in establishing adequate blood-flow rates (≥ 200 mL/min) during the next dialysis session in 87.5% cases. Another study also showed that Reteplase installation in dysfunctional HD catheters with dwell until the next HD session was effective in restoring catheter function in 87% of episodes. A dose of 1 U appears to be as effective as 4 and 6 U (25). Fibrin sheaths that form outside the catheter are resistant to thrombolytics and may require mechanical brushing or stripping (26).

⬡ ANTICOAGULATION FOR CONTINUOUS RENAL REPLACEMENT THERAPY

As in other extracorporeal circuits, anticoagulation is essential to prevent the activation of clotting mechanisms within the circuit (27,28) and is necessary for effective delivery of CRRT. The choice of anticoagulant should be based on multiple factors, including (a) the access site; (b) the nature and geometry of the membrane; (c) whether enhancements for UF, such as predilution, are used; and (d) the clinical status of the patient and preexisting coagulation abnormalities. The ideal anticoagulant should provide optimal antithrombotic activity with minimal bleeding complications and negligible systemic side effects. It should be inexpensive, have a short half-life, and be easily reversed (29). Adequate anticoagulation ensures efficacy of the filter in fluid and solute removal, overall filter longevity, and optimum patient management. When the anticoagulation is insufficient, filtration performance deteriorates and the filter may eventually clot (30), contributing to blood loss. Excessive anticoagulation, on the other hand, may result in bleeding complications, which have been reported to occur in 5% to 26% of treatments (31).

Several methods of anticoagulation are now available, and the key features of the most common methods are summarized in **TABLE 10.2**.

Unfractionated Heparin

Unfractionated heparin (UFH) continues to be the most commonly used anticoagulant. It catalyses the inactivation of thrombin, factor Xa and factor IXa by antithrombin. The main advantage of UFH is the large experience, the short biologic half-life (90 minutes but can

TABLE 10.2	**Anticoagulation Methods**				
Method	**Initial Dose**	**Maintenance Dose**	**Advantage**	**Disadvantage**	**Monitoring**
Heparin	30 U/kg bolus	5–10 U/kg/h	Standard method Easy to use Inexpensive	Bleeding risk Thrombocytopenia	aPTT 1.5–2 times of normal
LMWH Nadroparin/ dalteparin Enoxaparin	15–25 IU/kg 0.15 mg/kg	5–10 IU/kg/h 0.05 mg/kg/h	Decreased risk of bleeding Higher anti-Xa/anti-IIa Lesser HIT	Poor reversibility with protamine Expensive Monitoring not easily available	Factor Xa levels; maintained between 0.1 and 0.41 U/mL
Regional citrate	4% trisodium citrate 150–180 mL/h	100–180 mL/h 3%–7% of BFR, Ca replaced by central line	No bleeding No thrombocytopenia Improved filter efficacy Longevity	Complex; needs Ca monitoring; alkalosis	ACT: 200–250 maintain ionized calcium 0.96–1.2 mmol/L
Heparinoids (Danaparoid)	750–2,500 U	1–2 U/kg/h	Decreased HIT	Bleeding risk Cross-reactivity with heparin/PF4 Prolonged half-life in renal failure No antidote	Anti-Xa level between 0.25 and 0.35 IU/mL
Thrombin antagonist Hirudin Argatroban	250 μg/kg	0.005–0.01 mg/kg/h OR 0.002 g/kg bolus doses 0.5–2 μg/kg/min	Can be used in patients with HIT Hepatic excretion, so no dose modification in renal failure	Renal excretion: prolonged half-life No antidote	Ecarin clotting test (ECT): not easily available Target: 80–100 s aPTT 1–1.5 times normal
Platelet inhibiting agents Prostacyclin		2–8 ng/kg/min infusion prefilter	Better circuit life	Hypotension Expensive Usually needs UFH coadministration	Not required aPTT when UFH used
Nafamostat		0.1 mg/kg/h	No heparin	Anaphylaxis Agranulocytosis hyperkalemia	ACT

aPTT, activated partial thromboplastin time; LMWH, low molecular weight heparin; HIT, heparin-induced thrombocytopenia; BFR, blood-flow rate; ACT, activated clotting time; PF4, platelet factor 4; UFH, unfractionated heparin.

increase up to 3 hours in presence of renal insufficiency), the availability of an efficient inhibitor, and the possibility to monitor its effect with routine laboratory tests. Limitations of UFH includes time- and dose-dependent unpredictable pharmacokinetics, resulting in considerable inter- and intrapatient variability (32), resistance to heparin due to reduced level of antithrombin III in renal insufficiency, high incidence of bleeding, and heparin-induced thrombocytopenia (HIT) (33–36). Dosing of heparin and target activated partial thromboplastin time (aPTT) varies in different units with the aim of maintain aPTT 1.5 to 2 times of normal. UFH is usually administered as a bolus of 30 IU/kg (2,000 to 5,000 IU), followed by a continuous infusion of 5 to 10 IU/kg/h into arterial limb of the dialysis circuit. Circuit survival time ranges from 20 to 40 hours. In view of the potential side effects of heparin, alternative methods of anticoagulation have been investigated, including regional heparin/protamine, low molecular weight heparins, heparinoids, thrombin antagonists (hirudin and argatroban), regional citrate, prostanoids, and nafamostat, with regional citrate anticoagulation (RCA) gaining wider acceptance with the development of simplified and safer protocols.

Low Molecular Weight Heparin

Recently, low molecular weight heparins (LMWHs) have been shown to be safe and effective drugs for anticoagulation of CRRT circuit (37–40).

These agents have higher anti-Xa/anti-IIa activity than UFH (32), less protein binding, more predictable pharmacokinetics, and lesser incidence of HIT (41). The LMWHs are potent agents with renal excretion, have an increased half-life compared with UFH, poor reversibility with protamine because of stronger anti-Xa effect, more expensive than UFH, and also require specialist laboratory monitoring. Nadroparin, dalteparin in a dose of 15 to 25 IU/kg as bolus followed by 5 to 10 IU/kg/h (39–40), and enoxaparin as 0.15 mg/kg and a maintenance infusion starting at 0.05 mg/kg/h are the agents used in various studies (38).

Regional Citrate

Citrate ($C_6H_7O_7$) is a small negatively charged molecule with a molecular weight of 191 Da. The use of citrate as anticoagulant in HD was first described by Morita et al. (42) in 1961 and in CRRT circuit by Mehta et al. in 1990 (43). Since then, various studies have shown better filter life and less bleeding with citrate in varied patient population including severe sepsis, liver failure, cardiac surgery, and both adults as well as pediatric patients population (36,44–61). In a prospective randomized multicenter trial by Hetzel et al. (62), citrate was found to have less systemic anticoagulation, a lower risk of bleeding, and a longer hemofilter patency. Some studies have shown evidence of improved biocompatibility by decreasing thrombogenicity and low polymorphonuclear cell degranulation (63–65), while effects of citrate on complement activation are not uniform (66–68). A recent study by Schilder et al. (69) has not shown any difference in mortality and renal outcome between RCA and UFH, but citrate was superior in terms of safety, efficacy, and costs.

Citrate is infused into the blood at the beginning of the extracorporeal circuit which chelates ionized calcium and provides anticoagulation in the circuit. Optimal regional anticoagulation occurs when the ionized calcium in the postfilter circuit is kept below 0.35 mmol/L. Calcium-citrate complex which is formed in the circuit is freely filtered and is lost in effluent, so calcium is infused systemically to replace the lost calcium to keep the ionized calcium within normal limits and infusion is titrated accordingly. Citrate which enters the body is metabolized by tricarboxylic acid pathway in liver, kidney, and skeletal muscles, and each citrate molecule yields three bicarbonate molecules, thereby avoiding systemic anticoagulation.

Patients with severe liver failure and lactic acidosis may have difficulty in metabolizing citrate and may develop citrate toxicity, which is characterized by increased total to ionized calcium ratio, metabolic acidosis, and high anion gap (55,70–73). Other complications which may occur during RCA are hypernatremia particularly with hypertonic sodium citrate and metabolic alkalosis when too much citrate enters the circulation (43); therefore, frequent monitoring of electrolytes, acid–base status, and ionized calcium is required.

Various protocols for RCA have been described in literature (36,44–60). The ideal CRRT protocol should provide volume control, metabolic (acid–base and electrolyte) control, and adequate solute clearance, without significant complications related to bleeding or clotting. **TABLE 10.3** shows CRRT prescription and citrate protocol at University of California, San Diego (UCSD). **FIGURE 10.2** shows CRRT circuit using RCA.

TABLE 10.3 Continuous Renal Replacement Therapy Prescription and Regional Citrate Protocol at University of California, San Diego

Modality	CVVHDF	Allows combination of diffusive and convective clearance. Consequently, UF rates can be limited and do not require high blood-flow rates for filtration fraction (FF).
Membrane	M 100	0.9 m² AN69 polyacrylonitrile membrane adequate for clearances required
Blood-flow rate	100 mL/min	Not constrained by access, adequate flow for maintaining filtration fraction <25%
Effluent volume	2.2 L/h	Allows small solute clearance of approximately 37 mL/min, adequate clearance to compensate for catabolic state and for reduction due to partial predilution
Dialysate flow rate	1 L/h	Slower than blood-flow rate with complete saturation of dialysate for small solutes; diffusive clearance = 16.7 mL/min
Predilution fluid	0.5 L/h	Administered prefilter, prepump dilutes blood entering the filter with filtration fraction of 25%.
Postfilter replacement fluid	0.7 L/h	Administered postfilter in venous circuit; volume greater than all anticipated intake to allow fixed effluent volume and clearance. Volume adjusted hourly to achieve desired fluid balance.
Anticoagulation	4% trisodium citrate	At access exit through three-way stopcock to chelate ionized calcium and prevent clotting; rate 160–200 mL/h adjusted to maintain postfilter ionized calcium 0.25–0.4 mmol/L; provides base from conversion of citrate to bicarbonate
	0.1 mEq/mL calcium chloride	Replaces calcium removed across filter, administered through separate central line at initial flow rate of 40–60 mL/h and adjusted to maintain peripheral ionized calcium of 1.12–1.32 mmol/L
Dialysate fluid composition	0.45% saline + 40 mEq of Na as NaHCO₃ or NaCl + Mg 2.0 mEq/L + 2–5 mEq/L KCl + 0.1% dextrose	Low sodium (117 mEq/L) allows removal of sodium load in trisodium citrate (Na = 420 mmol/L, citrate 140 mmol/L), varying amounts of bicarbonate added to provide extra base for correction of acidosis and compensate for bicarbonate loss across filter, no calcium allows removal of citrate-calcium chelate.
Predilution fluid composition	0.9% saline	Isotonic for diluting blood
Postfilter fluid composition	0.9% saline, 0.45% saline + 75 mEq/L of sodium bicarbonate, sterile water + 150 mEq/L of sodium bicarbonate	Normal saline adequate to maintain normal sodium levels. Additional bicarbonate added to solutions depending on acid–base status and bicarbonate requirement
Monitoring	Serum electrolytes and blood gases; Postfilter ionized calcium; Peripheral ionized calcium; UF/plasma urea nitrogen; Fluid balance	Initially every 12 hours then every 24 hours: Adjust solutions composition. Postfilter ionized calcium every 12 hours: Adjust citrate flow rates. Peripheral ionized calcium every 12 hours: Adjust CaCl₂ drip. UF/plasma urea nitrogen every 12 hours: Assess filter efficacy and allow preemptive change in filter if ratio <0.6. Fluid balance: Set goals every 24 hours and monitor and adjust fluid balance by varying amount of replacement solution hourly to achieve target balance desired.

CVVHDF, continuous venovenous hemodiafiltration; UF, ultrafiltration.

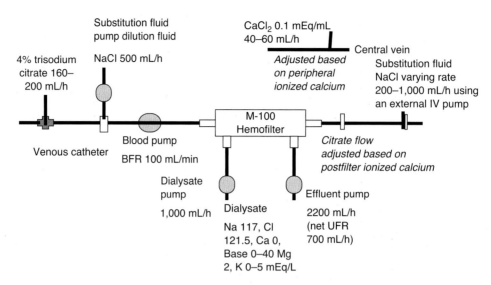

FIGURE 10.2 Continuous renal replacement therapy (CRRT) circuit using regional citrate anticoagulation with the Gambro PRISMA machine and M-100 filter.

Other methods for anticoagulation in CRRT include regional heparin/protamine (37,74), heparinoids (75), thrombin antagonists [hirudin (76–78) and argatroban (79–83)], and platelet-inhibiting agents (prostacyclin and nafamostat) (84–91). Each of these techniques has unique advantages and disadvantages, and anticoagulation for CRRT should be adapted to the patient's characteristics and institution's experience. Doses, advantages, and disadvantages of these agents are summarized in TABLE 10.2.

CONTINUOUS RENAL REPLACEMENT THERAPY SOLUTIONS

All CRRT other than SCUF and CVVHD require the use of replacement fluids to compensate for the ultrafiltrate removed. HD and HDF techniques in addition use a dialysate. The composition of these solutions can be varied extensively to achieve specific metabolic goals (92). Commercially prepared sterile fluids are now available as premixed dialysis and replacement solutions for CRRT. Fluid can also be manufactured at the level of pharmacy/hospital, but manufacturing or customization is labor intensive,

more expensive, have short shelf life, and is prone for human error (93,94).

TABLE 10.4 shows the composition of the most commonly used solutions for replacement and dialysate.

A consequence of all CRRT methods is the ongoing loss of bicarbonate and electrolytes across the filter generally equivalent to the plasma concentration of these solutes times the total effluent (UF and dialysate) flow rates (9). Bicarbonate losses can be replaced by addition of sodium bicarbonate or other base (e.g., lactate, acetate, citrate) to replacement solution administered intravenously, addition of base to the dialysate, or by a combination of these techniques (95). One of the major advantages of CRRT is that the composition of replacement fluid and dialysate can be modified to achieve any specific change in plasma composition.

Fluid Composition

Alkali

The choice of alkali depends on the clinical situation and availability. Both lactate and bicarbonate can correct metabolic acidosis as lactate is metabolized to bicarbonate by the liver.

TABLE 10.4 Continuous Renal Replacement Therapy Solutions

	1.5% Dianeal	Hemosol AG 4D	Hemosol LG 4D	Baxter	UCSD Citrate	PrismaSate BK0/3.5	PrismaSate BK2/0
Na (mEq/L)	132	140	140	140	117	140	140
K (mEq/L)	–	4	4	2	4	0	2
Cl (mEq/L)	96	119	109.5	117	121	109.5	108
Lactate (mEq/L)	35	–	40	30	–	3	3
Acetate (mEq/L)	–	30	–	–	–	–	–
Bicarb (mEq/L)	–	–	–	–	Variable	32	32
Ca (mEq/L)	3.5	3.5	4	3.5	–	3.5	0
Mg (mEq/L)	1.5	1.5	1.5	1.5	1.5	1	1
Dextrose (g/dL)	1.5	0.8	0.11	0.1–2.5	0.1–0.5	0	0.11

UCSD, University of California, San Diego.

Lactate-Based Solutions

Available lactate concentrations range from 28 to 49 mM. When base solutions other than bicarbonate are used, replacement of buffer stores depends on the metabolic rate for conversion to bicarbonate. In the absence of lactic acidosis, endogenous lactate clearance does not appear to be impaired. However, the filter clearance of lactate accounts for only 2.4% of overall lactate clearance (96). Lactate levels are generally higher with lactate solutions and might confuse the interpretation of blood lactate levels. Whether this hyperlactatemia is associated with morbidity is not clear. Potential concerns are hemodynamic compromise (96) or increased urea generation (97). Additionally, the ability to convert lactate to bicarbonate might be impaired in the setting of hypotension and multiorgan failure and could contribute to the deleterious effects of lactate accumulation (97). Hyperlactatemia can become pronounced during high-volume CRRT. "Lactate intolerance" is arbitrarily defined as a 5 mmol/L or more rise in serum lactate levels during CRRT.

Bicarbonate-Based Solutions

Bicarbonate concentrations are typically 22 to 35 mM and are preferred in patients with lactic acidosis and/or liver failure (98). One practical issue with the use of bicarbonate-based solutions is that it is difficult to store premixed bicarbonate solutions. A study by Kanagasundaram et al. (99) concluded that sustained bacterial contamination of bicarbonate-based CVVHD is common and could relate to the completeness of dialysate circuit change. Another factor to consider is that premixed solution containing calcium and bicarbonate shows evidence of microprecipitation of calcium carbonate crystals. Although some centers have developed nonsterile bicarbonate solution for CRRT, this practice is not recommended (99,100).

The combination of citrate anticoagulation and bicarbonate-containing solutions has been used effectively to manage complex acid–base disorders (43–59). At our center in UCSD, the hospital pharmacy prepared customized solutions for CRRT. Standard formulation at UCSD uses 1 L of 0.45% saline, to which is added 40 mL of 23% saline (yielding a sodium concentration of 117 mEq/L and a chloride concentration of 121.5 mEq/L), 1.5 mEq/L of magnesium, and 0 to 5 mEq/L of potassium. We use a dialysate dextrose concentration of 0.1% (43). In some circumstances, we add bicarbonate to the dialysate, substituting the 23% NaCl with NaHCO₃ so that the final concentration of sodium is 117 mEq/L. More recently, secondary to nationwide drug shortages of bicarbonate, we switched to commercial calcium dialysate and replacement fluids and have not found any difference in filter performance.

ADQI recommends that lactate is an effective buffer in most CRRT patients. Bicarbonate is preferred in patients with lactic acidosis and/or liver failure and in high-volume H. When citrate is used as anticoagulant, no other buffer should be administered, but monitoring of pH is required.

Electrolytes

The replacement fluid and/or dialysate should contain electrolytes in concentrations aiming for physiologic levels and taking into account preexisting deficits or excesses and all inputs and losses. Customized solutions will be required in patients with some electrolyte imbalances, but these fluids should be used with caution, as accidental alteration is infusion rates can lead to significant electrolyte derangements. Therefore, frequent monitoring of serum electrolytes is imperative during CRRT. Most commercially available solutions do not contain phosphate but prolonged use of CRRT is associated with hypophosphatemia. Several methods are used to manage this problem including enteral feed with high phosphorus concentrations, intravenous supplementation with sodium phosphate (101). Recently, the U.S. Food and Drug Administration (FDA) approved Phoxillum Renal Replacement Solutions (BK4/2.5 and B22K4/0) as a replacement solution for CRRT to correct electrolyte and acid–base imbalances. The drug can also be used in the case of drug poisoning when CRRT is used to remove dialyzable substances. This product from Baxter is the only FDA-approved premixed solution including phosphate in a 5-L bag. (See more at http://www.pharmacytimes.com/product-news/fda-approves-new-solution-for-continuous-renal-replacement-therapy)

MODALITIES OF CONTINUOUS RENAL REPLACEMENT THERAPY–CLINICAL CONSIDERATIONS

Principles of Continuous Renal Replacement Therapy

Solute removal in CRRT can be obtained by convection, diffusion, or both. Each component of the therapy can be precisely controlled, and by use of high-flux membrane filters, removal of middle and high molecules can be maximized.

Diffusion

Diffusion is movement of solutes across concentration gradient through semipermeable membrane and depends upon

Concentration gradient (Cs)
Surface area of membrane (A)
Thickness of membrane (Mt)
Diffusion coefficient of the solute (D)
Temperature of solution (T)

The gradient is affected by the dialysate infusion rate (Q_d) and blood-flow rate (Q_b). The dialysate runs countercurrent to the blood, so faster Q_b allows for greater gradient. This is the same technique used in IHD, but Q_d are much slower than Q_b so there is complete saturation of the dialysate. Therefore, the Q_d is the rate-limiting factor for solute removal, but it allows for enhanced clearance. The smaller the size/weight of the solute and the greater the gradient, the more efficiently solute clearance occurs.

Diffusion Flux of a Given Solute Sd = (Cs / Mt) D · T · A

Convection

Convective techniques (UF and H) rely on what is known as "solvent drag," whereby dissolved molecules are dragged along with ultrafiltrated plasma water across a semipermeable membrane driven by a transmembrane pressure gradient (TMP) in response to a hydrostatic or osmotic force. The process of forcing a liquid against a membrane is called ultrafiltration; the fluid collected after it passes through a membrane is the ultrafiltrate. This can be described by the following equation (**EQUATION 10.1**):

$$Uf = Kf \cdot TMP \qquad (10.1)$$

Kf = coefficient of hydraulic permeability

$$TMP = (Pb - Puf) - \pi \qquad (10.2)$$

where Pb is hydrostatic pressure of blood, Puf is the hydrostatic pressure of the ultrafiltrate or dialysate, and π is the oncotic pressure of plasma proteins (**EQUATION 10.2**).

The convective clearance (Cx) of a solute x will therefore depend on the following (**Equation 10.3**):

$$Cx = Jf \cdot Cs \cdot S \qquad (10.3)$$

Jf = amount of ultrafiltration
Cs = concentration of solute in plasma water
S = sieving characteristics of membrane

Sieving coefficient (S) is the ratio of solute concentration in filtrate to solute concentration in plasma and is regulated by the reflection coefficient of the membrane (S = 1 − σ). A solute with an SC of 1 means that it can pass freely through a filter; if the SC is 0, then a solute cannot pass through the filter at all. Protein-bound solutes or those that exceed the molecular weight cutoff (generally 20,000 Da for polysulfone and polyacrylonitrile membranes) have sieving coefficients less than 1.

Solute Clearances

In all forms of CRRT, the "effluent" from the filter represents the end product of the filtration process and comprises the ultrafiltrate in CVVH, the spent dialysate in CVVHD, and the combination of the ultrafiltrate and spent dialysate in CVVHDF. Consequently, filter clearance (UF × V/P) for most CRRT circuits is equal to Qef (the effluent flow rate = V) × SC (UF/P) for most small and middle molecules and is directly proportional to the amount of effluent volume. Blood-side clearances often do not match the filter clearances, as membrane adsorption modifies the amount of solute in the ultrafiltrate. Consequently, for some solutes [such as tumor necrosis factor-α (TNF-α)] that are adsorbed by membranes, SC can be low, but overall blood clearance can be greater than filter clearance.

CRRT vary in their ability to remove small and middle molecules. For small-sized solutes (e.g., urea nitrogen, creatinine, phosphates), filter clearances were directly proportional to the effluent volume and did not vary significantly with convective or diffusive removal across a spectrum of effluent volumes (0.5 to 4.5 L/h). In contrast, β2-microglobulin removal was influenced by the membrane type and the amount of convective clearance (102).

Clearance of molecules in CRRT circuits also depends on the site of replacement solution administration either pre- or postfilter.

In postdilution CVVH (purely convective therapy), primary determinants of solute clearances are ultrafiltration rate (Qef), sieving coefficient of membrane (S). Therefore, clearance in milliliters per minute (K) equals to product of ultrafiltration rate and sieving coefficient (**Equation 10.4**).

$$K = Qef \cdot S \qquad (10.4)$$

For small molecules, as S approaches unity, clearance equals the UF rate in postdilution.

Removal of ultrafiltrate across the filter concentrates the cellular elements and proteins in the blood emerging from the filter and is directly proportional to the ratio of ultrafiltrate to plasma flow rate (filtration fraction = FF). Plasma flow rate in turn depends upon blood flow (Qb) and patient hematocrit (Hct). Therefore, in postdilution CVVH (**Equation 10.5**):

$$FF = Qef / Qb (1 − Hct) \qquad (10.5)$$

Previous studies have demonstrated that FF >20% contributes to reduced filter performance and filter clotting. Consequently, if UF rates are increased, the blood-flow rate should be increased to maintain FF less than 20%. As higher blood flows are usually difficult to reach with the temporary dialysis catheters and poor hemodynamics among these patients, achieving higher doses are difficult to do in postdilution mode.

Predilution fluid replacement reduces the FF and reduces the solute concentration in the blood entering the filter. Thus, it is useful in preventing clotting of the extracorporeal circuit and to extend filter life. The effective small-solute clearance (K) for predilutional H is equal to Qef × (Qb/[Qb + Qr]), where Qb and Qr represent blood and replacement fluid rates. Clearance in predilution H is less than in postdilutional H for the same Qef. However, because of the dilution of blood entering the filter, much higher filtration fractions (larger Qef and Qr) are feasible in predilutional H (103).

In convective removal, the only way to increase solute clearances is to increase the amount of ultrafiltrate generated and consequently increase the volume of replacement fluid given. A study by Brunet et al. (104) showed that convection is effective than diffusion in removing middle molecular weight solutes during CRRT and that high convective fluxes should be applied if the goal is to remove middle molecules more efficiently.

◆ CONTINUOUS RENAL REPLACEMENT THERAPY–APPLICATIONS

Fluid Management in Continuous Renal Replacement Therapy

Volume management is an integral component of the care of critically ill patients to maintain hemodynamic stability and optimize organ function. The dynamic nature of critical illness often necessitates volume resuscitation and contributes to fluid overload particularly in the presence of altered renal function. Diuretics are commonly used as an initial therapy to increase urine output; however, they have limited effectiveness due to underlying AKI and other factors contributing to diuretic resistance. In this setting, successful volume management with CRRT depends on an accurate assessment of fluid status, an adequate comprehension of the principles of fluid management with UF, and clear treatment goals. In the Beginning and Ending Supportive Therapy (BEST) for the Kidney study (105), fluid overload was present in 36.7%, while oliguria and anuria was present in 70.2% of patients. Fluid overload increases complications associated with acute lung injury, acute respiratory distress syndrome (106–108), tissue healing, gut, and cerebral edema (109). Emerging data overwhelmingly suggest that fluid overload is associated with adverse outcomes (110–112).

CRRT techniques have three inherent characteristics that make them highly effective and versatile methods for fluid control (113) (a) the use of highly permeable membranes, (b) the infusion of various replacement solutions, and (c) the continuous nature of the techniques. Adjustments in the UF and replacement fluid rates allow CRRT techniques to serve as fluid regulatory systems that can maintain fluid balance without compromising the system's ability to maintain metabolic balance. A major distinction for these methods is the ability to dissociate solute removal (e.g., sodium) from fluid balance. As an example, by varying the composition of the replacement fluid or dialysate, solute balance can be altered while overall fluid balance can be kept even, negative, or positive (113). Fluid removal in CRRT is achieved by formation of an ultrafiltrate. The UF rate used depends on two factors: the type of technique and the fluid balance requirements of the patient. In convective techniques (CVVH), the UF rate can vary from 0.5 to 12.0 L/h, although most centers use a range of 1.0 to 3.0 L/h. When dialysate is used (CVVHDF), almost all the current machines limit UF rate to a maximum of 2 L/h.

Bouchard and Mehta (114) describe three techniques for achieving fluid balance with CRRT (**Table 10.5**). The level 1 technique is to vary the net ultrafiltration rate (Quf) to meet the

TABLE 10.5	**Continuous Renal Replacement Therapy (CRRT) Fluid Balance Techniques**		
Variable	**Level 1**	**Level 2**	**Level 3**
Intake	Variable	Variable	Variable
Non-CRRT output	Variable	Variable	Variable
Ultrafiltration rate	Variable to achieve fluid balance	Fixed to achieve target effluent volume	Fixed to achieve target effluent volume
Substitution fluid rate	Fixed $\leq Q_{uf}$	Postdilution replacement varies to achieve −, zero, or + fluid balance.	Postdilution replacement varies to achieve −, zero, or + fluid balance.
Fluid balance	Achieved by varying Q_{uf}	Achieved by adjusting amount of substitution fluid	Targets the hourly fluid balance to achieve a predefined hemodynamic parameter
Key difference	Output varies to accommodate changes in intake and fluid balance goals.	Output is fixed to achieve desired solute clearance and allow flexibility in accommodating varying intake.	Output is fixed to achieve desired solute clearance and allow flexibility in accommodating varying intake.
Examples	SCUF, CVVHD	CVVH, CVVHDF	CVVH, CVVHDF
Advantages			
Patient factors	Strategy similar to fluid removal in intermittent dialysis	Solute clearance is constant. Allows variation in intake. Individualizes prescription.	Solute clearance is constant. Allows variation in intake. Individualizes prescription.
CRRT factors	Fluid balance calculations can be deferred to longer intervals (every 8–12 h).	Clearance requirements dissociated from fluid balance. Deceases interactions with CRRT pump to adjust UFR. Regimen simplified for caregiver.	Clearance requirements dissociated from fluid balance. Deceases interactions with CRRT pump to adjust UFR. Regimen simplified for caregiver.
Disadvantages			
Patient factors	Patient assumed to be in static state. Similar to ESKD prescription. Intake may fluctuate. Fluid boluses not accounted for. Commonly over- or undershoot. Fluctuations in solute clearance, especially when dependent on convection.	Requires hourly calculations for amount of fluid replacement to be given. Potential for fluid imbalances if balance sheet not used.	Requires hourly calculations for amount of fluid replacement to be given. Potential for fluid imbalances if balance sheet not used. Requires scale be made for hemodynamic parameter targets.
CRRT factors	Requires frequent interactions with CRRT pump to adjust UFR. Underutilizes CRRT for fluid removal only.	Requires use of external pump to achieve fluid regulation.	Requires use of external pump to achieve fluid regulation.

SCUF, slow continuous ultrafiltration; CVVHD, continuous venovenous hemodialysis; CVVH, continuous venovenous hemofiltration; CVVHDF, continuous venovenous hemodiafiltration; UFR, ultrafiltration rate; ESKD, end-stage kidney disease.
Data from Bouchard J, Mehta RL. Volume management in continuous renal replacement therapy. *Semin Dial* 2009;22(2):146–150.

anticipated fluid balance needs over 8 to 24 hours; the net ultrafiltrate is the difference between the total ultrafiltrate (the plasma water removed) and the total replacement (the fluid given to the patient). As an example, a patient may have a total anticipated fluid intake of 3 L with a desired 1-L net loss over 24 hours; the Q_{uf} would be set at −170 mL/h (3 L + 1 L/24 h). This may not be the best technique to use, as there may be unanticipated changes in clinical status and fluid needs, leading to a different net ultrafiltrate that is different from the desired fluid balance. Also, effluent volume and treatment dose will vary, as net Q_{uf} are not steady with this method.

The level 2 method of maintaining fluid balance is to vary the amount of postdilution replacement fluid administered; the net ultrafiltrate stays the same and exceeds the anticipated hourly intake. With this technique, the postdilution fluid is not given through the CRRT pump but through a separate pump. A patient can be maintained in negative fluid balance by decreasing the amount of postdilution fluid received to be less than the total output, in positive fluid balance by increasing postdilution replacement to be greater than all output, or in even balance by having equal postdilution replacement and total output. This method allows for variation in intake and a predetermined convective clearance, as net ultrafiltrate does not vary as in the first technique.

The level 3 technique is similar to the second, but fluid balance is tailored to achieve a targeted hemodynamic parameter every hour. Predefined targets are set for parameters, such as central venous pressure (CVP), MAP, or pulmonary arterial wedge pressure, and scales are prescribed to achieve these targets. For example, if the CVP is to be maintained between 8 and 12 mm Hg, when this is achieved, the scale would determine that net fluid balance be set to zero. If the CVP is above target, the scale would call for fluid removal; if CVP is below target, then fluid would be added. This technique allows for greater flexibility and maximally utilizes CRRT as a fluid regulatory device.

DRUG CLEARANCE AND DOSING IN CONTINUOUS RENAL REPLACEMENT THERAPY

Some drugs are removed significantly by CRRTs, and a substitutional dose is required to prevent underdosing of the substance. Doses used in IHD cannot be directly applied to these patients, and drug pharmacokinetics is different than those in patients with normal renal function. Dose amount and frequency can be calculated from knowledge of the basic pharmacokinetic factors relating to distribution and elimination of a drug within the body, along with knowledge of the desired drug concentration in plasma.

A fundamental concept in pharmacokinetics is drug clearance, that is, elimination of drugs from the body, analogous to the concept of creatinine clearance. Clearance can conceptually be considered to be a function of both distribution and elimination. In the simplest pharmacokinetic model,

$$Clearance = V \cdot K \qquad (10.6)$$

V is the volume of distribution, and K is the elimination constant (**EQUATION 10.6**). V is the volume of fluid in which the dose is initially diluted, and thus, the higher the V, the lower the initial concentration. K is the elimination constant, which is inversely proportional to the half-life, the period of time that must elapse to reach a 50% decrease in plasma concentration. When the half-life is short, K is high and plasma concentrations decline rapidly. Thus, both a high V and a high K result in relatively low plasma concentrations and a high clearance. It is possible to predict elimination of a given drug by CRRT from the knowledge of the relative contributions of the various mechanisms of clearance to total clearances (**EQUATION 10.7**).

$$Cl\,(T) = Cl\,(R) + Cl\,(HB) + Cl\,(EC) \qquad (10.7)$$

where Cl (T) is total clearance, Cl (R) is renal clearance, Cl (HB) is hepatobiliary clearance, and Cl (EC) is extracorporeal clearance via CRRT. If there is high nonrenal clearance via hepatobiliary route, then extracorporeal clearance is usually nonsignificant. The same applies to situations where renal clearances remain important despite need of CRRT. **FIGURE 10.3** shows drug metabolism in its simplest form.

Depending on the mode of CRRT, the combined dialysate and ultrafiltrate flow rates have been recommended as a rough estimate of creatinine clearance. During CVVH, solute elimination Cl (H) is through convection and depends upon ultrafiltration rate (Qf) and sieving coefficient (S), whereas CVVHD utilizes diffusion gradients through countercurrent dialysate flow, and drug removal depends on dialysate and blood-flow rates. CVVHDF utilizes both diffusive and convective solute transports and can require a large amount of fluid to replace losses during UF.

The pharmacokinetics of drug removal in critically ill patients receiving CRRT is very complex, with multiple variables affecting clearance and both patient- and CRRT technique–related factors should be considered for drug dosing in CRRT. In general, factors which affects drug dosing are bioavailability, volume of distribution, protein binding, lipid solubility, drug metabolism, loading and maintenance dose, and dialysis-related factors like molecular weight of drug, type of dialyzer, mode of CRRT, and various flow rates. These variables make generalized dosing recommendations difficult. Drug–protein complexes have a larger molecular weight; therefore, antibiotics/drugs with low protein binding capacity in serum are removed by CRRT more readily. Similarly, drugs that penetrate and bind to tissues have a larger volume of distribution, reducing the quantity removed during CRRT. Sepsis itself increases the volume of distribution, extends drug half-life, and alters the protein binding capacity of many antimicrobials. CRRT mechanical factors may also affect drug clearance. Increasing the blood or dialysate flow rate can change the transmembrane pressure and increase drug clearance (115). The dialysate concentration may also affect drug removal in H. Lastly, the membrane pore size is directly proportional to the degree of drug removal by CRRT, often expressed as a sieving coefficient. Generally, biosynthetic membranes have larger pores, which result in higher drug clearance rates especially for drugs of middle molecular weight size like vancomycin (MW = 1,450 Da) or daptomycin (MW = 1,620 Da) (116,117). Other CRRT technique-related factors that influence drug clearance are placement of replacement fluid (pre- vs. postfilter) and filter age. Prefilter replacement fluid dilutes the blood that is presented to hemodialyzer and decreases the amount of drug that is cleared. Uchino et al. (118) demonstrated that vancomycin clearance was lowest when all fluids were given prefilter and almost 25% higher when fluids were given postfilter. Similarly, other factor that is less studied is hemodiafilter age (119). The sieving coefficient for a drug is highest at commencement of CRRT and declines with time because of building up of protein layer on membrane and decline in number unclotted hollow fibers. Mode of CRRT also impacts drug clearance, particularly at larger dialysate/ultrafiltrate flow rates, and with higher molecular weight drugs. The drug clearance at any given dialysate/ultrafiltrate flow rate is:

$$CVVH > CVVHDF > CVVHD$$

These patient, drug, and mechanical variables significantly diminish the utility of routine pharmacokinetic calculations for determining antimicrobial dosing during CRRT.

TABLE 10.6 summarizes various factors effecting drug clearances; **TABLE 10.7** summarizes antibiotic dosing in CRRT.

MOBILIZATION DURING CONTINUOUS RENAL REPLACEMENT THERAPY

Research has shown that early mobilization is a safe and effective practice in the ICU, although there are many barriers making mobilization difficult. Despite studies demonstrating benefit, patients with femoral vascular catheters placed for CRRT are frequently restricted from mobilization. The mobility barriers for patients undergoing CRRT include risk to the HD catheter that is accessed and attached to an extracorporeal circuit at all times, along with potential to disrupt flow, leading to clotting of the circuit and interruption of therapy. In addition, other barriers to consider include

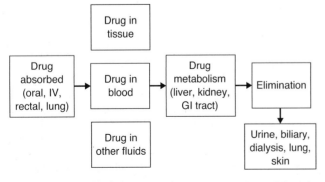

FIGURE 10.3 Drug metabolism in body. For any given drug and dose, the plasma concentration of the drug will rise and fall according to the rates of three processes: absorption, distribution, and elimination.

TABLE 10.6	**Factors Affecting Drug Clearance in Continuous Renal Replacement Therapy**

Drug- and Patient-Related	Dialysis-Related
Bioavailability	Molecular weight of drug
Volume of distribution	Type of dialyzer
Protein binding and lipid solubility	Mode of CRRT
Drug metabolism	Flow rates
Elimination route	
Loading and maintenance dose	

CRRT, continuous renal replacement therapy.

disease severity, cognitive state and ability to follow commands, adequate staff to assist, and equipment that is needed for the mobilization. Wang et al. (120) studied mobilization of 33 patients in ICU undergoing CRRT with different vascular access. In their study, patients underwent one of three levels of mobilization intervention as appropriate: (a) passive bed exercises, (b) sitting on the bed edge, or (c) standing and/or marching. They found that mobilization during RRT via a vascular catheter in patients who are critically ill is safe and no episodes of filter occlusion or failure occurred during any of the interventions. Also, catheter dislodgment, hematoma, bleeding, and nursing workloads between the intervention shift and the following shift were no different from nonintervention group. Brownback et al. (121) also reported successful mobilization of patient on CRRT. However, large multicenter studies are warranted to confirm the benefits of mobilization during CRRT.

TABLE 10.7	**Antibiotic Dosing on Continuous Renal Replacement Therapy**	
Drug	**CVVH**	**CVVHD/CVVHDF**
Amphotericin B formulation		
Deoxycholate	0.4–1.0 mg/kg q24h	0.4–1.0 mg/kg q24h
Lipid complex	3–5 mg/kg q24h	3–5 mg/kg q24h
Liposomal	3–5 mg/kg q24h	3–5 mg/kg q24h
Acyclovir	5–7.5 mg/kg q24h	5–7.5 mg/kg q24h
Ampicillin-sulbactam	3 g q12h	3 g q8h
Amikacin	10 mg/kg load and then 7.5 mg/kg q24–48 h	
Aztreonam	1–2 g q12h	2 g q12h
Cefazolin	1–2 g q12h	2 g q12h
Cefepime	1–2 g q12h	2 g q12h
Cefotaxime	1–2 g q12h	2 g q12h
Ceftazidime	1–2 g q12h	2 g q12h
Ceftriaxone	2 g q12–24h	2 g q12–24h
Cefuroxime	1.5 g q8–12h	1.5 g q8h
Clindamycin	600–900 mg q8h	600–900 mg q8h
Ciprofloxacin	200 mg q12h	200–400 mg q12h
Colistin	2.5 mg/kg q48h	2.5 mg/kg q48h
Daptomycin	4 or 6 mg/kg q48h	4 or 6 mg/kg q48h
Fluconazole	200–400 mg q24h	400–800 mg q24h
Imipenem-cilastatin	250 mg q6h or 500 mg q8h	250 mg q6h, 500 mg q8h, or 500 mg q6h
Levofloxacin	250 mg q24h	250 mg q24h
Linezolid	600 mg q12h	600 mg q12h
Meropenem	1 g q12h	1 g q12h
Moxifloxacin	400 mg q24h	400 mg q24h
Nafcillin or oxacillin	2 g q4–6h	2 g q4–6h
Piperacillin-tazobactam	2.25 g q6h	2.25–3.375 g q6h
Ticarcillin-clavulanate	2 g q6–8h	3.1 g q6h
TMP/SMX	2.5 mg/kg TMP q8h (consider higher doses with CVVHDF)	
Vancomycin	1 g q48h	1 g q24h
Voriconazole	4 mg/kg PO q12h	4 mg/kg PO q12h

All dosages are administered intravenously, unless otherwise indicated. The recommendations assume an ultrafiltration rate of 1 L/h, a dialysate flow rate of 1 L/h, and no residual renal function. CVVH, continuous venovenous hemofiltration; CVVHD, continuous venovenous hemodialysis; CVVHDF, continuous venovenous hemodiafiltration; TMP/SMX, trimethoprim/sulfamethoxazole.

COMPLICATIONS DURING CONTINUOUS RENAL REPLACEMENT THERAPY

CRRT is commonly used in critically ill patients with AKI. Clinicians must be aware of the complications associated with CRRT, particularly at higher doses. **TABLE 10.8** summarizes the common complications associated with the use of CRRT.

Vascular Access

Complications of vascular access, including infection and vascular injury, are a common concern with CRRT. These complications are reported to occur in 5% to 19% of patients, depending on the access site selected. Arterial puncture, hematoma, hemothorax, and pneumothorax are the most common complications reported. AV fistulas, aneurysms, thrombus formation, pericardial tamponade, air embolism due to increased negative pressure, and retroperitoneal hemorrhage have also been described. Another concern is catheter-related infection, and all measures should be taken to reduce it. These include stringent sterile placement technique, catheter care, avoidance of the femoral site, use of antibiotic coated catheters, and use of antimicrobial locking solutions. Lastly, clinician should also keep in mind recirculation of blood through double-lumen catheters, which may affect delivered dose by hemoconcentrating the blood and premature filter clotting.

Extracorporeal Circuit

Hypothermia is common with CRRT. This occurs because replacement fluids and dialysate are not warmed leading to cooling of core temperature secondary to extracorporeal radiant heat exchange

which occurs in 5% to 50% of patients. This may result in heat loss of 750 kcal/d, thereby increasing the patient's daily energy requirement. Thermal loss may also mask fever, delaying recognition of infection, thereby delaying administration of antibiotics. The newer CRRT machines have warming devices to prevent heat loss. Extracorporeal circuit/filter membrane may activate inflammatory-immune mediators including various cytokines which may increase protein breakdown and energy expenditure. Rarely, anaphylactoid reactions due to bradykinin activation, particularly with use of angiotensin-converting enzyme (ACE) inhibitors have been described.

Hematologic

CRRT needs either systemic or regional anticoagulation to prevent filter clotting. These critically ill patients have multiple factors which make them prone for increased risk of bleeding, particularly with heparin which is used as systemic anticoagulant. The use of heparin can also lead to HIT. CRRT also reduces number of platelets and impairs platelet aggregation. Some hemolysis also occurs because of shearing forces through the circuit or roller pump. Other causes of hemolysis include electrolyte abnormalities—hypophosphatemia, hyponatremia, and hypokalemia.

Electrolytes and Acid–Base Disturbances

Hypophosphatemia and hypomagnesemia are the commonest electrolyte disturbances associated with CRRT. Phosphate clearance is significantly high due to larger filter pore size and ongoing intercompartmental mass transfer. Hypophosphatemia is associated with higher doses and if severe enough can lead to decreases in cardiac output and blood pressure, rhabdomyolysis, respiratory muscle weakness, and granulocyte dysfunction with increased infection rates. Commercially available replacement fluids do not typically contain phosphate or magnesium, so these electrolytes need to be replaced separately. Sodium and acid–base disturbances can also occur during CRRT and should be monitored 6 to 8 hourly.

Nutritional Losses

Most critically ill patients on CRRT are hypercatabolic and in addition lose nutrients across dialysis membrane. Several factors including insulin resistance, release of inflammatory mediators, infection, metabolic acidosis, and so forth affects protein breakdown. Amino acid loss in patients on CRRT is estimated to be 10 to 20 g/d depending on UF volume, and patients should receive increased daily protein or amino acid intake to about 1.5 to 2.5 g/kg/d; of note, carbohydrates should be given at 5 to 7 g/kg/d and lipids at 1.2 to 1.5 g/kg/d (122–124). Larger molecules like albumin are also lost particularly with increased filter age. Water-soluble vitamins, micronutrients, and trace elements are also lost during CRRT and should be replaced during prolonged therapy.

THERAPEUTIC GOALS, INTENSITY, AND OUTCOMES OF CONTINUOUS RENAL REPLACEMENT THERAPY

The CRRT prescription ideally is targeted to match the therapeutic potential of the technique to specific goals for the patient. The broad goals for treating AKI with dialysis are to (a) maintain fluid and electrolyte, acid–base, and solute homeostasis; (b) prevent further insults to the kidney; (c) promote healing and renal recovery; and (d) permit other support measures (e.g., nutrition) to proceed without limitation. CRRT techniques differ in their operational characteristics and their ability to provide renal support, and these differences should be

TABLE 10.8	Complications during Continuous Renal Replacement Therapy
Vascular access	Bleeding
	Thrombosis
	Hemothorax
	Pneumothorax
	Hematoma
	AV fistula
	Aneurysm
	Infection
Extracorporeal	Hypothermia
	Air embolism
	Reduced filter life
	Anaphylaxis and immune activation
Electrolyte and acid–base disturbances	Hypophosphatemia
	Hypomagnesemia
	Hypocalcemia
	Hypokalemia
	Hypo- and hypernatremia
	Metabolic acidosis
	Metabolic alkalosis
Hematologic	HIT
	Hemolysis
Nutritional losses	Loss of amino acids/proteins, vitamins, and trace minerals

AV, arteriovenous; HIT, heparin-induced thrombocytopenia.

considered in the dialysis decision. For instance, CRRT techniques can be successfully utilized for fluid regulation, selective replacement of specific electrolytes, for example, bicarbonate, without the addition of sodium or fluid, or to add substances to the blood.

Dosing and intensity of CRRT are generally defined in terms of solute clearance and is traditionally assessed by measuring clearance of urea. For a small uncharged molecule such as urea, clearance during continuous H is essentially equal to the UF rate because the filter membrane negligibly impedes the passage of urea. Thus, in the simplest way, effluent volume (derived from blood-based kinetics) is thought to represent clearance and is used to prescribe and measure dose in CRRT. This would require that filter permeability stays the same over time; filter permeability is equal to effluent fluid urea nitrogen (FUN)/blood urea nitrogen (BUN), which should equal to one.

Most studies considered the prescribed dose as the effluent rate represented by milliliter per kilogram per hour and reported this volume as a surrogate of solute removal. Because filter fouling can reduce the efficacy of solute clearance, the actual delivered dose may be substantially lower than the observed effluent rate. Claure-Del Granado et al. (125) in their study concluded that effluent volume significantly overestimates delivered dose of small solutes in CRRT. Much of this variation in dose may be accounted for by the use of standard doses of CRRT unadjusted for weight, and it is far from clear whether estimates of ideal body weight, premorbid weight, "dry" weight, or actual body weight should be used (126,127). This greatly confounds the interpretation of observational data on CRRT dose since weight is likely to have a complex causal relationship with outcome.

To assess adequacy of CRRT, solute clearance should be measured rather than estimated by the effluent volume. Prescribed urea nitrogen clearance (K) in milliliter per minute can be calculated by effluent rate from following equation (**Equation 10.8**):

$$K = Q_d + Q_{uf} \qquad (10.8)$$

where Q_d = dialysate flow rate in milliliter per minute and Q_{uf} = total ultrafiltration volume in milliliter per minute which is equal to replacement fluid rate (Q_r) plus net fluid removal rate (Q_{net}). Therefore, prescribed urea nitrogen clearance (K) is (**Equation 10.9**):

$$K \text{ prescribed} = Q_d + Q_r + Q_{net}$$
$$\text{(effluent volume rate)} \qquad (10.9)$$

Delivered K is derived from the ratio of mass removal rate to blood concentration. This is based on the principle that the effluent represents the end product of filtration and compromises the sum of the net fluid removal rate (Q_{net}), the spent dialysate (Q_d), and the replacement fluid rate (Q_r) in combined therapies like CVVHDF. Because urea nitrogen is a small molecular solute, the ratio of the concentration of effluent FUN to BUN is generally 1. Clearance is then (**Equation 10.10**):

$$K \text{ delivered} = FUN \text{ (mg/dL)} /$$
$$BUN \text{ (mg/dL)} \times \text{effluent volume rate} \qquad (10.10)$$

Various trials have assessed relationship between intensity of CRRT and outcomes of AKI. In the first of these, Ronco et al. randomly assigned 425 critically ill patients with AKI treated using continuous venovenous hemofiltration(CVVHF) at a single center to ultrafiltration rates of 20, 35, or 45 mL/kg/h (128). Survival 15 days after discontinuation of CRRT was significantly better in the highest and intermediate dose arms in comparison with the lowest dose arm (58% and 57% vs. 41%, respectively; $p <0.001$). On the other hand, in contrast to above study and Saudan et al. study (129), two studies (130,131) that included 200 and 106 patients, respectively, failed

to demonstrate any beneficial effects of increased CRRT intensity on patient survival or renal recovery. Disparity in these results and consequent uncertainty about the optimum dosing of CRRT in the ICU led to the initiation of the Acute Renal Failure Trial Network (ATN) and Randomized Evaluation of Normal versus Augmented Level Replacement Therapy (RENAL) studies. The Veterans Affairs/National Institutes of Health Acute Renal Failure Trial Network (ARFTN) (132) performed a large, multicenter study comparing standard-dose CVVHDF of 20 mL/kg/h to high-intensity CVVHDF of 35 mL/kg/h in critically ill AKI patients; it demonstrated no significant difference in 60-day all-cause mortality, rate of recovery of renal function, and duration of RRT. The Randomized Evaluation of Normal versus Augmented Level (RENAL) Renal Replacement Therapy Study (133) was another large, multicenter study comparing CVVHDF effluent flow of 40 mL/kg/h to 25 mL/kg/h to see if there was a difference in 90-day mortality and continued need for RRT in ICU patients with AKI; there was no significant difference in either outcome between the two groups. The ATN and RENAL studies have now established an upper limit of intensity for CRRT, but CRRT dose should be prescribed on the basis of patient body weight to the established effluent flow rate target of 20 to 25 mL/kg of body weight per hour. DOse REsponse Multicentre International collaborative initiative (DO-RE-MI) study (126) was sought to evaluate the relationship between RRT dose and outcome. This was a prospective multicenter observational study in 30 ICUs in eight countries from June 2005 to December 2007. Dose was categorized into more intensive [CRRT ≥35 mL/kg/h, intermittent renal replacement therapy (IRRT) ≥6 sessions per week] or less intensive (CRRT <35 mL/kg/h, IRRT <6 sessions per week). Study concluded that no evidence for a survival benefit afforded by higher dose RRT and actual delivered dose of RRT in AKI patients is frequently smaller than the prescribed dose. Recently, in a single-center, prospective, randomized controlled study (CONVINT), Schefold et al. (134) compared effect of two major RRT strategies (IHD and CVVH) on mortality and renal-related outcome measures. They concluded that intermittent and continuous RRTs may be considered equivalent approaches for critically ill patients with dialysis-dependent AKI.

Patient outcomes after starting CRRT are influenced greatly by underlying disease and comorbidities and indication for initiation, among other clinical criteria. In 2013, Schneider et al. (135) conducted a systematic review and meta-analysis of the literature at the time to analyze data on dialysis dependence among critically ill survivors of an episode of AKI that required acute RRT; patients who initially received IRRT were compared to those who initially received CRRT. Seven RCTs and 16 observational studies were identified. Pooling all studies together demonstrated that IRRT was associated with 17 times increased risk of dialysis dependence compared to CRRT. This increased risk was present even when subgroups were analyzed (RCTs pooled and observational studies pooled separately); however, the increased risk was not statistically significant among RCTs.

Allegretti et al. (136) analyzed a prospective cohort of ICU patients started on CRRT with AKI at a single center to examine renal recovery and in-hospital and postdischarge mortality. They found only 25% of AKI patients were dialysis-free at the end of the follow-up period (4 years of rolling postdischarge data). While in the hospital, mortality was about 61%; after discharge, about 28% of patients died. The total rate of renal recovery was 93% by the end of the study period.

More recently, Wald et al. (137) performed a retrospective cohort study matching 1:1 CRRT and IRRT patients in the ICU with AKI. Only those patients that survived past 90 days after RRT initiation were followed for a median duration of 3 years. It was found

TABLE 10.9	Factors Affecting Dose Delivery in Continuous Renal Replacement Therapy

Filter clotting/type of anticoagulation
Decreased sieving coefficient
Secondary membrane formation
Concentration polarization
Changing catabolic rate/urea generation in AKI and critically ill patients
Catheter-related problems (type of catheter, site of placement, hygiene, etc.)
Circuit down-time (routine filter changes)
Time off for diagnostic procedures and therapeutic interventions

AKI, acute kidney injury.

that chronic dialysis risk was lower in those patients who received CRRT versus IRRT [hazard ratio 0.75, 95% confidence interval (CI) 0.65 to 0.87]. These results confirmed the findings of Schneider's review and meta-analysis.

Data for children regarding mortality has been gathered from the Prospective Pediatric Continuous Renal Replacement Therapy (ppCRRT). Overall mortality was 42%. Survival was lowest for patients who had fluid overload and electrolyte imbalances at CRRT initiation. Children weighing over 10 kg and those older than 1 year of age had better overall survival.

Other reviews and observational studies have shown worse outcomes seem to be associated with greater burden of illness, multiple organ involvement, and hemodynamic instability. Also, infant survival has been consistent between about 35% and 45%, and infants less than 3 kg have worse survival around 24% compared to infants over 3 kg (41%) as reported by Symons et al. (138) in 2003. **TABLE 10.9** summarizes various factors which can affect dose delivery in CRRT.

CONTINUOUS RENAL REPLACEMENT THERAPY IN SPECIAL SITUATIONS

Continuous Renal Replacement Therapy in Sepsis and Multisystem Organ Failure

Severe sepsis and septic shock are the primary causes of multiple organ dysfunction syndrome (MODS) and is associated with AKI in 5% to 50% of the patients. The sequence of events leading to septic shock and MODS is initiated by endotoxins or other structural components of microorganisms that cause inappropriate inflammatory response through the cells responsible for immunity and release of inflammatory mediators such as cytokines, active products of complement, arachidonic acid metabolites, nitric oxide, oxygen reactive substances, proteases, and so forth. CRRT is often used with the concept of modulating immune response in sepsis. With the intention of influencing circulating levels of inflammatory mediators, several modifications of CRRT have been developed over the last years. These include high-volume H, high-adsorption H, use of high cut-off (HCO) membranes, and hybrid systems like coupled plasma filtration absorbance.

Small experimental and human clinical studies have suggested that high-volume hemofiltration (HVHF) may improve hemodynamic profile and mortality. High-flux H (Qf = 60 mL/kg/h) performed by Servillo et al. (139) in their study demonstrated interleukin-6 (IL-6) mRNA reduction after 12 hours of treatment and a progressive increase after 24, 48, and 72 hours. In the Impact of High-volume Veno-venous Continuous Hemofiltration in the Early Management of Septic Shock

Patients With Acute Renal Failure (IVOIRE) trial (140), there was no evidence that HVHF at 70 mL/kg/h, when compared with contemporary standard-volume hemofiltration (SVHF) at 35 mL/kg/h, leads to a reduction of 28-day mortality or contributes to early improvements in hemodynamic profile or organ function. HVHF, as applied in this trial, cannot be recommended for treatment of septic shock complicated by AKI. Recently, Clark et al. (141) did systematic review and meta-analysis which included four trials and found that there was no difference in primary outcome of 28-day mortality and secondary end points like recovery of kidney function, lengths of ICU and hospital stays, vasopressor dose reduction, and adverse events. They concluded that presently insufficient evidence exists of a therapeutic benefit for routine use of HVHF for septic AKI.

With respect to immunomodulation, the use of HCO membranes has also been considered. High-permeability hemofilters are characterized by an increased pore size which facilitates the filtration of inflammatory mediators. Pilot trials in septic patients with AKI demonstrated immunomodulation by altering neutrophil phagocytosis as well as mononuclear cell function *ex vivo* (142,143). Atan et al. (144) measured proapoptotic or pronecrotic activity using annexin V-FITC and showed significant drop in proapoptotic activity across the filter for the CVVH-HCO group ($p = 0.043$) but not for the CVVH-Std group.

CONTINUOUS RENAL REPLACEMENT THERAPY IN HEART FAILURE

The cardiorenal interaction is a dynamic, bidirectional interplay wherein acute decompensated heart failure (ADHF) patients often develop AKI and volume overload. Congestive heart failure (CHF) and chronic kidney disease (CKD) share common risk factor like hypertension, atherosclerosis, and diabetes mellitus for the development of each disease. Analysis of Acute Decompensated Heart Failure National Registry (ADHERE) (145) database found that 30% of the patients hospitalized with heart failure have renal insufficiency. Not only is the comorbidity of CKD at hospitalization for heart failure is common but development of AKI with worsening renal function is also common and has significant implications for patient outcomes.

Improved understandings of the pathophysiology of ADHF and renal dysfunction and limitations of conventional therapy have led clinicians to employ different forms of extracorporeal therapy to treat this difficult clinical syndrome. Intermittent isolated UF (IUF), SCUF, and CVVH have been used as modes of extracorporeal therapy to treat ADHF.

Currently, there is minimal data supporting the use of IUF in management of heart failure and is associated with hemodynamic instability (146). In comparison to IUF, studies have demonstrated benefits of SCUF in the treatment of ADHF. UF versus usual care for hospitalized patients with heart failure: The Relief for Acutely Fluid-Overloaded Patients with Decompensated Congestive Heart Failure (RAPID-CHF) trial offered more insight into potential benefits of SCUF over usual care. This trial showed early application of UF for patients with CHF was feasible, well tolerated, and resulted in significant weight loss and fluid removal. Safety and efficacy of SCUF was demonstrated in ultrafiltration versus intravenous diuretics for patients hospitalized for acute decompensated heart failure (UNLOAD) study (147). This study was designed to compare the safety and efficacy of venovenous UF and standard intravenous diuretic therapy for hypervolemic heart failure (HF) patients and concluded that UF safely produces greater weight and fluid loss than intravenous diuretics, reduces 90-day resource utilization for HF, and is an effective alternative therapy.

IUF and SCUF share a common principle that the extracorporeal blood circuit only changes in the form of fluid removal via a pressure gradient and the fluid removed is isotonic with minimal solute clearance. CVVH, however, not only removes fluid but also provides a means to correct metabolic derangements like acidosis and electrolyte disturbances. Correction of hypocalcemia via CVVH may improve cardiac function in ADHF as cardiac myocytes depends on intracellular calcium for effective function (148). Recent evidence suggests that myocardial depressant factors like IL-8 and anti-monocyte chemoattractant protein-1, which have adverse effect on cardiac function are effectively removed via H (149,150). Despite of above potential benefits, robust clinical data to use CVVH as first-line therapy for ADHF is required.

CONTINUOUS RENAL REPLACEMENT THERAPY IN ACUTE BRAIN INJURY

AKI occurs in 8% to 23% of patients with acute brain injury (ABI) and is an independent predictor of poor outcome in these patients (151,152). The patient with an ABI requiring RRT presents a major problem in that conventional IHD may exacerbate the injury by compromising cerebral perfusion pressure (CPP), either after a reduction in cerebral perfusion or because of increased cerebral edema. To maximize full potential neurologic recovery in patients requiring renal dialytic support, it is important that treatments do not themselves cause further cerebral ischemia. The goal for ABI and increased intracranial pressure (ICP) patients is to maintain CPP >60 mm Hg; this is done by ensuring MAP stays up, as CPP = MAP − ICP. With IHD, intradialytic hypotension is common, leading to decreased MAP and CPP and increased ICP by compensatory cerebral vasodilation. This may result in infarction or secondary injury. Also, dialysis disequilibrium results when solutes are removed quickly causing shifts in intracellular fluid; worsening cerebral edema and further increases in ICP ensue.

CRRT should be the first option in these patients because it is associated with less increase in ICP compared with intermittent therapies (153). Using computed tomography (CT) scans to measure brain density, Ronco et al. (154) showed an increase of brain water content after IHD, whereas no such changes were observed after CRRT. CRRT is also associated with better maintenance of cerebral blood flow autoregulation after traumatic brain injury (155). The disadvantage of CRRT is that anticoagulation may be required, and anticoagulants with systemic effects may provoke intracerebral hemorrhage, either at the site of damage or around the ICP monitoring device. RCA is therefore the preferred mode of anticoagulation in these patients. Also, citrate may provide some neuroprotection by attenuating hypoxic neuronal injury through its effects on astrocytes and oxidative phosphorylation (156). Kidney Disease: Improving Global Outcomes (KDIGO) suggests CRRT, rather than intermittent RRT, for AKI patients with ABI or other causes of increased ICP pressure or generalized brain edema.

SUMMARY

CRRT is now the leading form of RRT for AKI in ICUs worldwide and is widely accepted as the most appropriate therapy for vasopressor-dependent patients who require RRT for AKI in the ICU. However, practice variation in the application of CRRT remains considerable owing to the absence of clear evidence-based guidelines. Presently, CRRT has many applications and its use can be adapted to fit different situations beyond the classic renal indications. In the near future, technical developments in extracorporeal devices will lead to the creation of multiple organ support therapies, so that comprehensive replacement or at least support can be provided to multiple organs simultaneously. Such machines ideally will be able to automatically detect both "traditional" (urea) and "inflammatory" (cytokines) solutes in plasma of critically ill patients in order to automatically (or semiautomatically) tailor the therapy toward the "perfect blood purification" system (**FIGURE 10.4**).

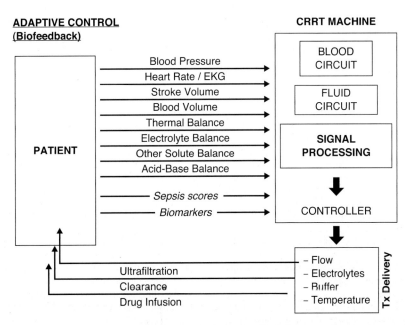

FIGURE 10.4 The "ideal" future renal replacement technology. The "ideal" future renal replacement technology will couple renal replacement therapy intensity (treatment delivery) with different biofeedback systems to tailor dose and ultrafiltration rate to the complex needs of the individual critically ill patient. EKG, electrocardiogram; Tx, treatment. (Adapted from Ronco C, Ricci Z, De Backer D, et al. Renal replacement therapy in acute kidney injury: controversy and consensus. *Crit Care* 2015;19:146.)

REFERENCES

1. Case J, Khan S, Khalid R, et al. Epidemiology of acute kidney injury in the intensive care unit. *Crit Care Res Pract* 2013;2013:479730.
2. Chertow GM, Burdick E, Honour M, et al. Acute kidney injury, mortality, length of stay, and costs in hospitalized patients. *J Am Soc Nephrol* 2005;16(11):3365–3370.
3. Hoste EA, Schurgers M. Epidemiology of acute kidney injury: how big is the problem? *Crit Care Med* 2008;36(4 Suppl):S146–S151.
4. Mehta RL. Continuous renal replacement therapy in the critically ill patient. *Kidney Int* 2005;67(2):781–795.
5. Ronco C, Brendolan A, Bellomo R. Continuous renal replacement techniques. *Contrib Nephrol* 2001;(132):236–251.
6. Ronco C, Kellum J, Mehta RL. Acute dialysis quality initiative. *Blood Purif* 2001;19(2):222–226.
7. Bellomo RRC, Mehta RL. Nomenclature for continuous renal replacement therapies. *Am J Kidney Dis* 1996;28(5):S32–S37.
8. Henderson L. Hemofiltration: from the origin to the new wave. *Am J Kidney Dis* 1996;28(5):S100–S104.
9. Sigler MH. Transport characteristics of the slow therapies: implications for achieving adequacy of dialysis in acute renal failure. *Adv Ren Replace Ther* 1997;4(1):68–80.
10. Sigler MH, Teehan BP. Solute transport in continuous hemodialysis: a new treatment for acute renal failure. *Kidney Int* 1987;32(4):562–571.
11. Ronco C, Ricci Z, De Backer D, et al. Renal replacement therapy in acute kidney injury: controversy and consensus. *Crit Care* 2015;19:146.
12. Hemodialysis Adequacy 2006 Work Group. Clinical practice guidelines for hemodialysis adequacy, update 2006. *Am J Kidney Dis* 2006;48 (Suppl 1):S2–S90.
13. Prabhu MV, Juneja D, Gopal PB, et al. Ultrasound-guided femoral dialysis access placement: a single-center randomized trial. *Clin J Am Soc Nephrol* 2010;5(2):235–239.
14. Randolph AG, Cook DJ, Gonzales CA, et al. Ultrasound guidance for placement of central venous catheters: a meta-analysis of the literature. *Crit Care Med* 1996;24(12):2053–2058.
15. Cimochowski GE, Worley E, Rutherford WE, et al. Superiority of the internal jugular over the subclavian access for temporary dialysis. *Nephron* 1990;54(2):154–161.
16. Marik PE, Flemmer M, Harrison W. The risk of catheter-related bloodstream infection with femoral venous catheters as compared to subclavian and internal jugular venous catheters: a systematic review of the literature and meta-analysis. *Crit Care Med* 2012;40(8):2479–2785.
17. Naumovic RT, Jovanovic DB, Djukanovic LJ. Temporary vascular catheters for hemodialysis: a 3-year prospective study. *Int J Artif Organs* 2004;27(10):848–854.
18. Oliver MJ, Callery SM, Thorpe KE, et al. Risk of bacteremia from temporary hemodialysis catheters by site of insertion and duration of use: a prospective study. *Kidney Int* 2000;58(6):2543–2545.
19. Chatzinikolaou I, Finkel K, Hanna H, et al. Antibiotic-coated hemodialysis catheters for the prevention of vascular catheter-related infections: a prospective, randomized study. *Am J Med* 2003;115(5):352–357.
20. Kim SH, Song KI, Chang JW, et al. Prevention of uncuffed hemodialysis catheter-related bacteremia using an antibiotic lock technique: a prospective, randomized clinical trial. *Kidney Int* 2006;69(1):161–164.
21. Weijmer MC, van den Dorpel MA, Van de Ven PJ, et al. Randomized, clinical trial comparison of trisodium citrate 30% and heparin as catheter-locking solution in hemodialysis patients. *J Am Soc Nephrol* 2005;16(9):2769–2777.
22. Bevilacqua JL, Gomes JG, Santos VF, et al. Comparison of trisodium citrate and heparin as catheter-locking solution in hemodialysis patients. *J Bras Nefrol* 2011;33(1):86–92.
23. Pierce DA, Rocco MV. Trisodium citrate: an alternative to unfractionated heparin for hemodialysis catheter dwells. *Pharmacotherapy* 2010;30(11):1150–1158.
24. Daeihagh P, Jordan J, Chen J, et al. Efficacy of tissue plasminogen activator administration on patency of hemodialysis access catheters. *Am J Kidney Dis* 2000;36(1):75–79.

25. Hilleman DE, Dunlay RW, Packard KA. Reteplase for dysfunctional hemodialysis catheter clearance. *Pharmacotherapy* 2003;23(2):137–141.
26. Vijayan A. Vascular access for continuous renal replacement therapy. *Semin Dial* 2009;22(2):133–136.
27. Webb AR, Mythen MG, Jacobson D, et al. Maintaining blood flow in the extracorporeal circuit: haemostasis and anticoagulation. *Intensive Care Med* 1995;21(1):84–93.
28. Mehta RL. Anticoagulation during continuous renal replacement therapy. *ASAIO J* 1994;40(4):931–935.
29. Tolwani AJ, Wille KM. Anticoagulation for continuous renal replacement therapy. *Semin Dial* 2009;22(2):141–145.
30. Martin PY, Chevrolet JC, Suter P, et al. Anticoagulation in patients treated by continuous venovenous hemofiltration: a retrospective study. *Am J Kidney Dis* 1994;24:806–812.
31. Ward DM, Mehta RL. Extracorporeal management of acute renal failure patients at high risk of bleeding. *Kidney Int Suppl* 1993;41:S237–S244.
32. Hirsh J, Warkentin TE, Raschke R, et al. Heparin and low-molecular-weight heparin: mechanisms of action, pharmacokinetics, dosing considerations, monitoring, efficacy, and safety. *Chest* 1998;114(5 Suppl):489S–510S.
33. van de Wetering J, Westendorp RG, van der Hoeven JG, et al. Heparin use in continuous renal replacement procedures: the struggle between filter coagulation and patient hemorrhage. *J Am Soc Nephrol* 1996;7(1):145–150.
34. Schneider T, Heuer B, Deller A, et al. Continuous haemofiltration with r-hirudin (lepirudin) as anticoagulant in a patient with heparin induced thrombocytopenia (HIT II). *Wien Klin Wochenschr* 2000;112(12):552–555.
35. Tillman J. Heparin versus citrate for anticoagulation in critically ill patients treated with continuous renal replacement therapy. *Nurs Crit Care* 2009;14(4):191–199.
36. Wu MY, Hsu YH, Bai CH, et al. Regional citrate versus heparin anticoagulation for continuous renal replacement therapy: a meta-analysis of randomized controlled trials. *Am J Kidney Dis* 2012;59(6):810–818.
37. van der Voort PH, Gerritsen RT, Kuiper MA, et al. Filter run time in CVVH: pre- versus post-dilution and nadroparin versus regional heparin-protamine anticoagulation. *Blood Purif* 2005;23(3):175–180.
38. Joannidis M, Kountchev J, Rauchenzauner M, et al. Enoxaparin vs. unfractionated heparin for anticoagulation during continuous veno-venous hemofiltration: a randomized controlled crossover study. *Intensive Care Med* 2007;33(9):1571–1579.
39. de Pont AC, Oudemans-van Straaten HM, Roozendaal KJ, et al. Nadroparin versus dalteparin anticoagulation in high-volume, continuous venovenous hemofiltration: a double-blind, randomized, crossover study. *Crit Care Med* 2000;28(2):421–425.
40. Reeves JH, Cumming AR, Gallagher L, et al. A controlled trial of low-molecular-weight heparin (dalteparin) versus unfractionated heparin as anticoagulant during continuous venovenous hemodialysis with filtration. *Crit Care Med* 1999;27(10):2224–2228.
41. Junqueira DR, Perini E, Penholati RR, et al. Unfractionated heparin versus low molecular weight heparin for avoiding heparin-induced thrombocytopenia in postoperative patients. *Cochrane Database Syst Rev* 2012;(9):CD007557.
42. Morita Y, Johnson R, Dorn R, et al. Regional anticoagulation during hemodialysis using citrate. *Am J Med Sci* 1961;242:32–43.
43. Mehta RL, McDonald BR, Aguilar MM, et al. Regional citrate anticoagulation for continuous arteriovenous hemodialysis in critically ill patients. *Kidney Int* 1990;38(5):976–981.
44. Palsson R, Niles JL. Regional citrate anticoagulation in continuous venovenous hemofiltration in critically ill patients with a high risk of bleeding. *Kidney Int* 1999;55(5):1991–1997.
45. Tolwani AJ, Campbell RC, Schenk MB, et al. Simplified citrate anticoagulation for continuous renal replacement therapy. *Kidney Int* 2001;60(1):370–374.
46. Frank RD. Citrate anticoagulation in acute renal replacement therapy: method of choice. *Med Klin Intensivmed Notfmed* 2014;109(5):336–341.

47. Liao YJ, Zhang L, Zeng XX, et al. Citrate versus unfractionated heparin for anticoagulation in continuous renal replacement therapy. *Chin Med J (Engl)* 2013;126(7):1344–1349.

48. Morabito S, Pistolesi V, Tritapepe L, et al. Regional citrate anticoagulation in CVVH: a new protocol combining citrate solution with a phosphate-containing replacement fluid. *Hemodial Int* 2013;17(2):313–320.

49. Oudemans-van Straaten HM, Ostermann M. Bench-to-bedside review: citrate for continuous renal replacement therapy, from science to practice. *Crit Care* 2012;16(6):249.

50. Soltysiak J, Warzywoda A, Kociński B, et al. Citrate anticoagulation for continuous renal replacement therapy in small children. *Pediatr Nephrol* 2014;29(3):469–475.

51. Tolwani A, Wille KM. Advances in continuous renal replacement therapy: citrate anticoagulation update. *Blood Purif* 2012;34(2):88–93.

52. Chadha V, Garg U, Warady BA, et al. Citrate clearance in children receiving continuous venovenous renal replacement therapy. *Pediatr Nephrol* 2002;17(10):819–824.

53. Tolwani AJ, Prendergast MB, Speer RR, et al. A practical citrate anticoagulation continuous venovenous hemodiafiltration protocol for metabolic control and high solute clearance. *Clin J Am Soc Nephrol* 2006;1(1):79–87.

54. Morgera S, Scholle C, Melzer C, et al. A simple, safe, and effective citrate anticoagulation protocol for the genius dialysis system in acute renal failure. *Nephron Clin Pract* 2004;98(1):c35–c40.

55. Morgera S, Scholle C, Voss G, et al. Metabolic complications during regional citrate anticoagulation in continuous venovenous hemodialysis: single-center experience. *Nephron Clin Pract* 2004;97(4):c131–c136.

56. Morabito S, Pistolesi V, Tritapepe L, et al. Regional citrate anticoagulation in cardiac surgery patients at high risk of bleeding: a continuous veno-venous hemofiltration protocol with a low concentration citrate solution. *Crit Care* 2012;16(3):R111.

57. Durão MS, Monte JC, Batista MC, et al. The use of regional citrate anticoagulation for continuous venovenous hemodiafiltration in acute kidney injury. *Crit Care Med* 2008;36(11):3024–3029.

58. Cointault O, Kamar N, Bories P, et al. Regional citrate anticoagulation in continuous venovenous haemodiafiltration using commercial solutions. *Nephrol Dial Transplant* 2004;19(1):171–178.

59. Kutsogiannis DJ, Mayers I, Chin WD, et al. Regional citrate anticoagulation in continuous venovenous hemodiafiltration. *Am J Kidney Dis* 2000;35(5):802–811.

60. Tobe SW, Aujla P, Walele AA, et al. A novel regional citrate anticoagulation protocol for CRRT using only commercially available solutions. *J Crit Care* 2003;18(2):121–129.

61. Park JS, Kim GH, Kang CM, et al. Regional anticoagulation with citrate is superior to systemic anticoagulation with heparin in critically ill patients undergoing continuous venovenous hemodiafiltration. *Korean J Intern Med* 2011;26(1):68–75.

62. Hetzel GR, Schmitz M, Wissing H, et al. Regional citrate versus systemic heparin for anticoagulation in critically ill patients on continuous venovenous haemofiltration: a prospective randomized multicentre trial. *Nephrol Dial Transplant* 2011;26(1):232–239.

63. Bos JC, Grooteman MP, van Houte AJ, et al. Low polymorphonuclear cell degranulation during citrate anticoagulation: a comparison between citrate and heparin dialysis. *Nephrol Dial Transplant* 1997;12(7):1387–1393.

64. Hofbauer R, Moser D, Frass M, et al. Effect of anticoagulation on blood membrane interactions during hemodialysis. *Kidney Int* 1999;56(4):1578–1583.

65. Polanská K, Opatrný K Jr, Rokyta R Jr, et al. Effect of regional citrate anticoagulation on thrombogenicity and biocompatibility during CV-VHDF. *Ren Fail* 2006;28(2):107–118.

66. Gabutti L, Ferrari N, Mombelli G, et al. The favorable effect of regional citrate anticoagulation on interleukin-1beta release is dissociated from both coagulation and complement activation. *J Nephrol* 2004;17(6):819–825.

67. Dhondt A, Vanholder R, Tielemans C, et al. Effect of regional citrate anticoagulation on leukopenia, complement activation, and expression of leukocyte surface molecules during hemodialysis with unmodified cellulose membranes. *Nephron* 2000;85(4):334–342.

68. Böhler J, Schollmeyer P, Dressel B, et al. Reduction of granulocyte activation during hemodialysis with regional citrate anticoagulation: dissociation of complement activation and neutropenia from neutrophil degranulation. *J Am Soc Nephrol* 1996;7(2):234–241.

69. Schilder L, Nurmohamed SA, Bosch FH, et al. Citrate anticoagulation versus systemic heparinisation in continuous venovenous hemofiltration in critically ill patients with acute kidney injury: a multi-center randomized clinical trial. *Crit Care* 2014;18(4):472.

70. Kramer L, Bauer E, Joukhadar C, et al. Citrate pharmacokinetics and metabolism in cirrhotic and noncirrhotic critically ill patients. *Crit Care Med* 2003;31(10):2450–2455.

71. Meier-Kriesche HU, Gitomer J, Finkel K, et al. Increased total to ionized calcium ratio during continuous venovenous hemodialysis with regional citrate anticoagulation. *Crit Care Med* 2001;29(4):748–752.

72. Egi M, Naka T, Bellomo R, et al. The acid-base effect of changing citrate solution for regional anticoagulation during continuous veno-venous hemofiltration. *Int J Artif Organs* 2008;31(3):228–236.

73. Bakker AJ, Boerma EC, Keidel H, et al. Detection of citrate overdose in critically ill patients on citrate-anticoagulated venovenous haemofiltration: use of ionised and total/ionised calcium. *Clin Chem Lab Med* 2006;44(8):962–966.

74. Biancofiore G, Esposito M, Bindi L, et al. Regional filter heparinization for continuous veno-venous hemofiltration in liver transplant recipients. *Minerva Anestesiol* 2003;69(6):527–538.

75. Lindhoff-Last E, Betz C, Bauersachs R. Use of a low-molecular-weight heparinoid (danaparoid sodium) for continuous renal replacement therapy in intensive care patients. *Clin Appl Thromb Hemost* 2001;7(4):300–304.

76. Fischer KG, van de Loo A, Böhler J. Recombinant hirudin (lepirudin) as anticoagulant in intensive care patients treated with continuous hemodialysis. *Kidney Int Suppl* 1999;(72):S46–S50.

77. Vargas Hein O, von Heymann C, Lipps M, et al. Hirudin versus heparin for anticoagulation in continuous renal replacement therapy. *Intensive Care Med* 2001;27(4):673–679.

78. Gajra A, Vajpayee N, Smith A, et al. Lepirudin for anticoagulation in patients with heparin-induced thrombocytopenia treated with continuous renal replacement therapy. *Am J Hematol* 2007;82(5):391–393.

79. Murray PT, Reddy BV, Grossman EJ, et al. A prospective comparison of three argatroban treatment regimens during hemodialysis in end-stage renal disease. *Kidney Int* 2004;66(6):2446–2453.

80. Reddy BV, Grossman EJ, Trevino SA, et al. Argatroban anticoagulation in patients with heparin-induced thrombocytopenia requiring renal replacement therapy. *Ann Pharmacother* 2005;39(10):1601–1605.

81. Tang IY, Cox DS, Patel K, et al. Argatroban and renal replacement therapy in patients with heparin-induced thrombocytopenia. *Ann Pharmacother* 2005;39(2):231–236.

82. Link A, Girndt M, Selejan S, Argatroban for anticoagulation in continuous renal replacement therapy. *Crit Care Med* 2009;37(1):105–10.

83. Sun X, Chen Y, Xiao Q, et al. Effects of argatroban as an anticoagulant for intermittent veno-venous hemofiltration (IVVH) in patients at high risk of bleeding. *Nephrol Dial Transplant* 2011;26(9):2954–2959.

84. Lee YK, Lee HW, Choi KH, et al. Ability of nafamostat mesilate to prolong filter patency during continuous renal replacement therapy in patients at high risk of bleeding: a randomized controlled study. *PLoS One* 2014;9(10):e108737.

85. Kozek-Langenecker SA, Kettner SC, Oismueller C, et al. Anticoagulation with prostaglandin E1 and unfractionated heparin during continuous venovenous hemofiltration. *Crit Care Med* 1998;26(7):1208–1212.

86. Kozek-Langenecker SA, Spiss CK, Gamsjäger T, Anticoagulation with prostaglandins and unfractionated heparin during continuous venovenous haemofiltration: a randomized controlled trial. *Wien Klin Wochenschr* 2002;114(3):96–101.

87. Fiaccadori E, Maggiore U, Rotelli C, et al. Continuous haemofiltration in acute renal failure with prostacyclin as the sole anti-haemostatic agent. *Intensive Care Med* 2002;28(5):586–593.

88. Hwang SD, Hyun YK, Moon SJ, et al. Nafamostat mesilate for anticoagulation in continuous renal replacement therapy. *Int J Artif Organs* 2013;36(3):208–216.

89. Balik M, Waldauf P, Plášil P, et al. Prostacyclin versus citrate in continuous haemodiafiltration: an observational study in patients with high risk of bleeding. *Blood Purif* 2005;23(4):325–329.

90. Baek NN, Jang HR, Huh W, et al. The role of nafamostat mesylate in continuous renal replacement therapy among patients at high risk of bleeding. *Ren Fail* 2012;34(3):279–285.

91. Maruyama Y, Yoshida H, Uchino S, et al. Nafamostat mesilate as an anticoagulant during continuous veno-venous hemodialysis: a three-year retrospective cohort study. *Int J Artif Organs* 2011;34(7): 571–576.

92. Davenport A. Dialysate and substitution fluids for patients treated by continuous forms of renal replacement therapy. *Contrib Nephrol* 2001(132):313–322.

93. Barletta JF, Barletta GM, Brophy PD, et al. Medication errors and patient complications with continuous renal replacement therapy. *Pediatr Nephrol* 2006;21(6):842–845.

94. Johnston RV, Boiteau P, Charlebois K, et al. Responding to tragic error: lessons from Foothills Medical Centre. *CMAJ* 2004;170(11): 1659–1660.

95. Mehta RL. Continuous renal replacement therapies in the acute renal failure setting: current concepts. *Adv Ren Replace Ther* 1997;4(2 Suppl 1):81–92.

96. Heering P, Ivens K, Thümer O, et al. The use of different buffers during continuous hemofiltration in critically ill patients with acute renal failure. *Intensive Care Med* 1999;25(11):1244–1251.

97. Hilton PJ, Taylor J, Forni LG, et al. Bicarbonate-based haemofiltration in the management of acute renal failure with lactic acidosis. *QJM* 1998;91(4):279–283.

98. Agarwal B, Kovari F, Saha R, et al. Do bicarbonate-based solutions for continuous renal replacement therapy offer better control of metabolic acidosis than lactate-containing fluids? *Nephron Clin Pract* 2011;118(4):c392–c398.

99. Kanagasundaram NS, Larive AB, Paganini EP. A preliminary survey of bacterial contamination of the dialysate circuit in continuous veno-venous hemodialysis. *Clin Nephrol* 2003;59(1):47–55.

100. Leblanc M, Moreno L, Robinson OP, et al. Bicarbonate dialysate for continuous renal replacement therapy in intensive care unit patients with acute renal failure. *Am J Kidney Dis* 1995;26(6):910–917.

101. Troyanov S, Geadah D, Ghannoum M, et al. Phosphate addition to hemodiafiltration solutions during continuous renal replacement therapy. *Intensive Care Med* 2004;30(8):1662–1665.

102. Troyanov S, Cardinal J, Geadah D, et al. Solute clearances during continuous venovenous haemofiltration at various ultrafiltration flow rates using Multiflow-100 and HF1000 filters. *Nephrol Dial Transplant* 2003;18(5):961–966.

103. Garred L, Leblanc M, Canaud B. Urea kinetic modeling for CRRT. *Am J Kidney Dis* 1997;30(5 Suppl 4):S2–S9.

104. Brunet S, Leblanc M, Geadah D, et al. Diffusive and convective solute clearances during continuous renal replacement therapy at various dialysate and ultrafiltration flow rates. *Am J Kidney Dis* 1999;34(3): 486–492.

105. Uchino S, Bellomo R, Morimatsu H, et al. Continuous renal replacement therapy: a worldwide practice survey. The beginning and ending supportive therapy for the kidney (B.E.S.T. kidney) investigators. *Intensive Care Med* 2007;33(9):1563–1570.

106. Sakr Y, Vincent JL, Reinhart K, et al. High tidal volume and positive fluid balance are associated with worse outcome in acute lung injury. *Chest* 2005;128(5):3098–3108.

107. Humphrey H, Hall J, Sznajder I, et al. Improved survival in ARDS patients associated with a reduction in pulmonary capillary wedge pressure. *Chest* 1990;97(5):1176–1180.

108. Schuller D, Mitchell JP, Calandrino FS, et al. Fluid balance during pulmonary edema. Is fluid gain a marker or a cause of poor outcome? *Chest* 1991;100(4):1068–1075.

109. Brandstrup B, Tønnesen H, Beier-Holgersen R, et al. Effects of intravenous fluid restriction on postoperative complications: comparison of two perioperative fluid regimens: a randomized assessor-blinded multicenter trial. *Ann Surg* 2003;238(5):641–648.

110. Heung M, Wolfgram DF, Kommareddi M, et al. Fluid overload at initiation of renal replacement therapy is associated with lack of renal recovery in patients with acute kidney injury. *Nephrol Dial Transplant* 2012;27(3):956–961.

111. Schiffl H, Lang SM. Oliguria, fluid overload and recovery of renal function from acute renal failure requiring renal replacement therapy. *Nephrol Dial Transplant* 2011;26(12):4151.

112. Vincent JL, Sakr Y, Sprung CL, et al. Sepsis in European intensive care units: results of the SOAP study. *Crit Care Med* 2006;34(2): 344–353.

113. Mehta RL. Fluid management in CRRT. *Contrib Nephrol* 2001;(132): 335–348.

114. Bouchard J, Mehta RL. Volume management in continuous renal replacement therapy. *Semin Dial* 2009;22(2):146–150

115. Mueller BA, Pasko DA, Sowinski KM. Higher renal replacement therapy dose delivery influences on drug therapy. *Artif Organs* 2003;27(9);808–814.

116. Joy MS, Matzke GR, Frye RF, et al. Determinants of vancomycin clearance by continuous venovenous hemofiltration and continuous venovenous hemodialysis. *Am J Kidney Dis* 1998;31(6):1019–1027.

117. Churchwell MD, Pasko DA, Mueller BA. Daptomycin clearance during modeled continuous renal replacement therapy. *Blood Purif* 2006;24(5–6):548–554.

118. Uchino S, Cole L, Morimatsu H, et al. Clearance of vancomycin during high-volume haemofiltration: impact of pre-dilution. *Intensive Care Med* 2002;28(11):1664–1667.

119. Pasko DA, Churchwell MD, Salama NN, et al. Longitudinal hemodiafilter performance in modeled continuous renal replacement therapy. *Blood Purif* 2011;32(2):82–88.

120. Wang YT, Haines TP, Ritchie P, et al. Early mobilization on continuous renal replacement therapy is safe and may improve filter life. *Crit Care* 2014;18(4):R161.

121. Brownback CA, Fletcher P, Pierce LN, et al. Early mobility activities during continuous renal replacement therapy. *Am J Crit Care* 2014;23(4):348–352.

122. Joannes-Boyau O, Rapaport S, Bazin R, et al. Impact of high volume hemofiltration on hemodynamic disturbance and outcome during septic shock. *ASAIO J* 2004;50(1):102–109.

123. Scheinkestel CD, Adams F, Mahony L, et al. Impact of increasing parenteral protein loads on amino acid levels and balance in critically ill anuric patients on continuous renal replacement therapy. *Nutrition* 2003;19(9):733–740.

124. Umber A, Wolley MJ, Golper TA, et al. Amino acid losses during sustained low efficiency dialysis in critically ill patients with acute kidney injury. *Clin Nephrol* 2014;81(2):93–99.

125. Claure-Del Granado R, Macedo E, Chertow GM, et al. Effluent volume in continuous renal replacement therapy overestimates the delivered dose of dialysis. *Clin J Am Soc Nephrol* 2011;6(3):467–475.

126. Vesconi S, Cruz DN, Fumagalli R, et al. Delivered dose of renal replacement therapy and mortality in critically ill patients with acute kidney injury. *Crit Care* 2009;13(2):R57.

127. Lameire N, Van Biesen W, Vanholder R. Dose of dialysis in the intensive care unit: is the venom in the dose or in the clinical experience? *Crit Care* 2009;13(3):155.

128. Abichandani R, Pereira BJ. Effects of different doses in continuous veno-venous haemofiltration on outcomes of acute renal failure: a prospective randomised trial, by Ronco C, Bellomo R, Homel P, Brendolan A, Dan M, Piccinni P, and La Greca G. Lancet 355:26-30, 2000. *Semin Dial* 2001;14(3):233–234.

129. Saudan P, Niederberger M, De Seigneux S, et al. Adding a dialysis dose to continuous hemofiltration increases survival in patients with acute renal failure. *Kidney Int* 2006;70(7):1312–1317.

130. Tolwani AJ, Campbell RC, Stofan BS, et al. Standard versus high-dose CVVHDF for ICU-related acute renal failure. *J Am Soc Nephrol* 2008;19(6):1233–1238.

131. Bouman CS, Oudemans-Van Straaten HM, Tijssen JG, et al. Effects of early high-volume continuous venovenous hemofiltration on survival and recovery of renal function in intensive care patients with

acute renal failure: a prospective, randomized trial. *Crit Care Med* 2002;30(10):2205–2211.

132. Palevsky PM, Zhang JH, O'Connor TZ, et al. Intensity of renal support in critically ill patients with acute kidney injury. *N Engl J Med* 2008;359(1):7–20.

133. Bellomo R, Cass A, Cole L, et al. Intensity of continuous renal-replacement therapy in critically ill patients. *N Engl J Med* 2009;361(17):1627–1638.

134. Schefold JC, von Haehling S, Pschowski R, et al. The effect of continuous versus intermittent renal replacement therapy on the outcome of critically ill patients with acute renal failure (CONVINT): a prospective randomized controlled trial. *Crit Care* 2014;18(1):R11.

135. Schneider AG, Bellomo R, Bagshaw SM, et al. Choice of renal replacement therapy modality and dialysis dependence after acute kidney injury: a systematic review and meta-analysis. *Intensive Care Med* 2013;39(6):987–997.

136. Allegretti AS, Steele DJ, David-Kasdan JA, et al. Continuous renal replacement therapy outcomes in acute kidney injury and end-stage renal disease: a cohort study. *Crit Care* 2013;17:R109.

137. Wald R, Shariff SZ, Adhikari NK, et al. The association between renal replacement therapy modality and long-term outcomes among critically ill adults with acute kidney injury: a retrospective cohort study. *Crit Care Med* 2014;42(4):868–877.

138. Symons JM, Brophy PD, Gregory MJ, et al. Continuous renal replacement therapy in children up to 10 kg. Am *J Kidney Dis* 2003;41:984–989.

139. Servillo G, Vargas M, Pastore A, et al. Immunomodulatory effect of continuous venovenous hemofiltration during sepsis: preliminary data. *Biomed Res Int* 2013;2013:6.

140. Joannes-Boyau O, Honoré PM, Perez P, et al. High-volume versus standard-volume haemofiltration for septic shock patients with acute kidney injury (IVOIRE study): a multicentre randomized controlled trial. *Intensive Care Med* 2013;39(9):1535–1546.

141. Clark E, Molnar AO, Joannes-Boyau O, et al. High-volume hemofiltration for septic acute kidney injury: a systematic review and meta-analysis. *Crit Care* 2014;18(1):R7.

142. Morgera S, Haase M, Rocktäschel J, et al. Intermittent high-permeability hemofiltration modulates inflammatory response in septic patients with multiorgan failure. *Nephron Clin Pract* 2003;94(3):c75–c80.

143. Morgera S, Rocktäschel J, Haase M, et al. Intermittent high permeability hemofiltration in septic patients with acute renal failure. *Intensive Care Med* 2003;29(11):1989–1995.

144. Atan R, Virzi GM, Peck L, et al. High cut-off hemofiltration versus standard hemofiltration: a pilot assessment of effects on indices of apoptosis. *Blood Purif* 2014;37(4):296–303.

145. Adams KF Jr, Fonarow GC, Emerman CL, et al. Characteristics and outcomes of patients hospitalized for heart failure in the United States: rationale, design, and preliminary observations from the first 100,000 cases in the Acute Decompensated Heart Failure National Registry (ADHERE). *Am Heart J* 2005;149(2):209–216.

146. Ronco C, Ricci Z, Bellomo R, et al. Extracorporeal ultrafiltration for the treatment of overhydration and congestive heart failure. *Cardiology* 2001;96(3–4):155–168.

147. Costanzo MR, Guglin ME, Saltzberg MT, et al. Ultrafiltration versus intravenous diuretics for patients hospitalized for acute decompensated heart failure. *J Am Coll Cardiol* 2007;49(6):675–683.

148. Wong CK, Pun KK, Cheng CH, et al. Hypocalcemic heart failure in end-stage renal disease. *Am J Nephrol* 1990;10(2):167–170.

149. Morgera S, Slowinski T, Melzer C, et al. Renal replacement therapy with high-cutoff hemofilters: impact of convection and diffusion on cytokine clearances and protein status. *Am J Kidney Dis* 2004;43(3):444–453.

150. Blake P, Hasegawa Y, Khosla MC, et al. Isolation of "myocardial depressant factor(s)" from the ultrafiltrate of heart failure patients with acute renal failure. *ASAIO J* 1996;42(5):M911–M915.

151. Zacharia BE, Ducruet AF, Hickman ZL, et al. Renal dysfunction as an independent predictor of outcome after aneurysmal subarachnoid hemorrhage: a single-center cohort study. *Stroke* 2009;40(7):2375–2381.

152. Corral L, Javierre CF, Ventura JL, et al. Impact of non-neurological complications in severe traumatic brain injury outcome. *Crit Care* 2012;16(2):R44.

153. Davenport A, Will EJ, Davison AM. Early changes in intracranial pressure during haemofiltration treatment in patients with grade 4 hepatic encephalopathy and acute oliguric renal failure. *Nephrol Dial Transplant* 1990;5(3):192–198.

154. Ronco C, Bellomo R, Brendolan A, et al. Brain density changes during renal replacement in critically ill patients with acute renal failure. Continuous hemofiltration versus intermittent hemodialysis. *J Nephrol* 1999;12(3):173–178.

155. Ko SB, Choi HA, Gilmore E, et al. Pearls & Oysters: the effects of renal replacement therapy on cerebral autoregulation. *Neurology* 2012;78(6):e36–e8.

156. Kelleher JA, Chan TY, Chan PH, et al. Protection of astrocytes by fructose 1,6-bisphosphate and citrate ameliorates neuronal injury under hypoxic conditions. *Brain Res* 1996;726(1–2):167–173.

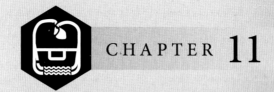

CHAPTER **11**

Renal Replacement Therapy–Wearable and Implantable Therapies

Edward R. Gould and William H. Fissell

Prior to the advent of dialysis, kidney disease was a death sentence. The introduction and widespread use of the semipermeable membrane for semiselective removal of small solutes changed that. This use of the semipermeable membrane in this fashion was initially described by Thomas Graham in 1861—who also coined the term "dialysis." He described diffusion of crystalloids through a membrane of vegetable parchment (1). However, it would be another century before dialysis was implemented as a human medical treatment.

After disappointing results in Germany in the early 1920s, the first successful dialysis treatment for acute kidney injury is attributed to Willem Kolff of the Netherlands in 1944–1945. In the subsequent decade, Dr. Nils Alwall (2) modified his dialysis apparatus to include higher pressure rigid dialyzers. This development allowed for volume removal through the application of a pressure across the dialysis membrane.

The final necessary technology was the development of vascular access that was reliable and relatively safe for outpatient use, first by Scribner, Quinton, and Dillard. These technologies allowed the introduction of outpatient chronic hemodialysis. Since their introduction, renal replacement therapies have moved from the intensive care unit, where they temporized the critically ill with kidney disease, to the clinic where nearly 400,000 Americans receive life-sustaining therapy for their end-stage kidney disease (ESKD) at a cost of over $40 billion a year, according to 2009 data (3).

As the first therapy designed to replace a failed organ, dialysis provides a durable treatment option for an otherwise fatal diagnosis. That, however, does not mean that the patients receiving routine outpatient dialysis are the same as their counterparts who are otherwise healthy. Indeed, the burden of dialysis extends well beyond simply the actuarial expense. Dialysis patients are at increased risk

of cardiovascular death, they suffer from reproductive irregularities, and they have the socioeconomic consequences of the time spent on dialysis. These burdens have led to renewed interest in modernizing and mobilizing the dialysis technologies to help mitigate these repercussions and, ideally, improving the clinical outcomes of patients on dialysis.

BASIC PRINCIPLES

Dialysis practices vary around the world, but in the United States, it is generally performed three times weekly in an outpatient unit using an extracorporeal circuit that includes a semipermeable membrane. Given that the specific toxins responsible for uremia remain imperfectly defined, there has never been a full understanding of the best metric for effective dialysis. Reliance on measures of small and middle molecular clearance has given us the ability to develop dialysis membranes that have become increasingly effective and provides a starting point for the evaluation of newer artificial dialysis systems. A comparison of the various physiologic functions as performed by native kidneys, conventional dialysis, and newer implantable options is outlined in **TABLE 11.1**.

Small Molecule Clearance

Small molecules have long been the target of dialysis assessment, with a focus particularly on urea which serves as a small molecular weight marker for the variety of other uremic toxins that accumulate in ESKD. While often treated collectively, these molecules behave differently according to their molecular characteristics, interactions with the dialysis membrane and, most importantly, their kinetic behaviors between and within various body compartments. The differences in urea and phosphorus clearance are illustrative of the variance in clearance.

TABLE 11.1	Comparison of Native Kidneys, Hemodialysis, and Implantable Artificial Kidney		
Physiologic Function	**Native Kidney**	**Conventional Dialysis**	**Miniaturized RAD**
Toxin clearance	High-volume convective ultra-filtration, followed by active tubular electrolyte, water, organic anion, and small protein reabsorption from the ultrafiltrate with fine tuning by subsequent cellular secretion	Predominantly diffusive clearance of small water-soluble solutes from plasma water to dialysate, with some convective clearance of middle-sized molecules depending upon dialyzer flux and design	High-volume convective ultrafil-tration by silicon nanoporous membrane, followed by selective reabsorption of elec-trolytes and water by tubule cell bioreactor or synthetic "tubular"-like membrane
Volume homeostasis	Active distant and intrarenal neu-rohumoral feedback systems controlling glomerular blood flow, perfusion pressure, filtra-tion, and tubular reabsorption	Ultrafiltration volume determined clinically by assessment of dry weight and ultrafiltration rate by dialysis session time	Computerized synthesis of physiologic data and patient-entered weight data to control balance between ultrafiltration and reabsorp-tion rates
Calcium–phosphorus metabolism	Calcium and phosphorus are filtered by the glomerulus and differentially reabsorbed by the tubule under hormonal and phosphatonin control and tubular flow rate	As dialysis does not adequately remove sufficient phosphate, patients are re-quired to avoid phosphate-rich food-stuffs and require phosphate-binding medications. Additional active vita-min D sterols are required. Dialysate calcium is adjusted to maintain serum calcium concentration.	Calcium and phosphorus are filtered by the silicon nanoporous membrane, some calcium and phos-phate is reabsorbed, and any deficiencies will be supple-mented by oral medications.
Potassium regulation	Potassium is filtered by the glomerulus, then reabsorbed by the tubule, and then se-creted under hormone control, and exchanged to maintain acid–base homeostasis.	Patients require a potassium-restricted diet, and then dialysate potassium is adjusted to maintain a target predial-ysis concentration.	Patient will self-monitor blood potassium at home by fin-gerstick blood sampling, and adjust diet and, if necessary, adjust ion exchange resin dose accordingly.
Red blood cell mass	Kidney tubular cells in kidney interstitium cells secrete eryth-ropoietin in an oxygen delivery–dependent fashion regulated by hypoxia inhibitory factor (HIF).	Require exogenous erythropoiesis-stimulating agents or HIF receptor blockers. Iron supplementation is required for blood lost in dialyzer.	Require exogenous erythropoiesis-stimulating agents or HIF receptor blockers.
Acid–base balance	The kidney reabsorbs bicarbonate and excretes acid by an ammonium-based buffering system and hydrogen ion exchange for other cations.	Patients adhere to a protein-restricted diet to reduce acid generation, and dialysate bicarbonate concentration is adjusted to control pH.	A kidney tubular cell bioreactor will excrete some acid, but oral bicarbonate will be nec-essary to completely buffer dietary acid load.

RAD, renal assist device.
The healthy kidney (left) accomplishes critical physiology functions to maintain homeostasis: waste removal, fluid balance, electrolyte, and acid–base regulation. Hemodialysis (center) uses a combination of the procedure and drugs to approximate the same functions. The implantable artificial kidney uses a combination of technology and biology to free the patient from dialysis.

Urea

Having a molecular weight of approximately 60 Da and a large vol-ume of distribution, urea is an endogenously produced molecule that is generated as a product of protein degradation. Protein me-tabolism leads to the endogenous production of urea at a rate of approximately 10 to 13 mg/min. Dialysis is able to remove small solutes, like urea, in direct proportion to their concentration in the blood. Typically, a single compartment model for urea removal is used to estimate the clearance of urea (**Equation 11.1**):

$$U_{final} = U_{initial} \times e^{-\frac{Kt}{V}} \qquad (11.1)$$

In this model, U_{final} and $U_{initial}$ represent the urea concentration at the beginning and the end of the hemodialysis session, respectively. Here, K is the instantaneous clearance, a parameter that is governed by the membrane characteristics, and the dialysis flow rate, though

is predominately limited by the blood flow rate. Time is represented by t, and V represents the volume of distribution. The targeted urea removal for a given dialysis session is typically a single-pool Kt/V of 1.2 to 1.4. A Kt/V of one equates to the clearance of 1.0 volume of distribution. The targeted Kt/V of 1.2 to 1.4 allows for slightly greater clearance and to account for urea rebound from the unmod-eled peripheral compartment. It is possible to further quantify urea removal by solving for the following (**Equation 11.2**):

$$U_{removed} = \int_0^T K \times U_{initial} \times e^{-\frac{Kt}{V}} \qquad (11.2)$$

Given that the urea generation between dialysis sessions is ap-proximately 28 to 43 g, we can then determine what the expected ini-tial urea concentration is in these patients in order for urea removal to match urea production. As noted above, K is primarily limited by dialysis blood flow, so if we assume that K = 350 to 400 mL/min, we can see that predialysis blood urea nitrogen (BUN) must rise to 70 mg/dL or higher in order to remove the urea at its production rate of 10 mg/min or greater. Indeed, in practice, it is understood that patients who do not reach this threshold in their azotemia—barring significant residual renal function—are typically suffering from being undernourished and do not have adequate protein intake. This has been found, through observational assessment of other clinical metrics, to be strongly associated with mortality in these patients.

Phosphorus

Phosphorus is another small molecule, like urea, that is able to pass through the dialysis membrane but does so slightly less ably than the slightly larger creatinine. The difference in behaviors is largely attributable to the negative charge carried by phosphorous in combination with the water of hydration. However, unlike urea, which mobilizes relatively quickly from the peripheral compartment for dialytic clearance and approaches a one-compartment kinetic model, phosphorus is better described with two-compartment modeling and probably a multicompartment model. Phosphorus concentrations very quickly fall to a low level in the plasma compartment during dialysis but mobilize slowly from peripheral tissues and achieve a concentration postdialysis that approaches initial starting concentration.

To explore this more fully, the average dialysis patient, who is pursuing the desired 1 to 1.2 g/kg/day of protein, consumes approximately 780 to 1,450 mg of phosphorus daily, of which approximately 60% to 80% is absorbed in the gastrointestinal tract. Four-hour dialysis treatments are only able to remove approximately 1,000 mg of phosphorus per treatment, which is sufficient to maintain normal phosphorus levels in only a minority of patients. As a consequence, most dialysis patients are put on oral phosphorus binders which can reduce gastrointestinal absorption to approximately 40% or 400 to 650 mg daily.

In contrast to intermittent dialysis, continuous renal replacement therapies (CRRTs) provide significant phosphorous clearance. In these patients, the slow mobilization from peripheral tissues allows phosphorous to be removed by the dialysis modality. If critically ill patients are left on continuous therapy for any length of time, their limited oral intake often leads to profound hypophosphatemia and requires supplemental phosphorus.

Middle Molecule Clearance

Middle molecular weight molecules include those that range from approximately 2 kDa ($\sim$20 times the size of creatinine) to 45 kDa. The most commonly studied middle molecule is β_2-microglobulin. It is a component of the major histocompatibility complex and in normal physiology is shed from the cell surface during regular cell turnover and then is eliminated, almost exclusively, by the kidney [4]. Despite being readily able to pass through the kidney filtration barrier, it is relatively poorly cleared by traditional hemodialysis filters. Even so-called "high-flux" dialyzers have β_2-microglobulin clearances that are only one-tenth to one-fifth that of urea [5]. If serum concentrations are sufficiently high, β_2-microglobulin can go on to polymerize and coalesce in amyloid plaques that have been found in nearly every major organ system. Common manifestations include nerve entrapment syndromes like carpal tunnel syndrome and joint disease, but it has been implicated in cardiovascular disease and neurologic plaques as well in ESKD patients [6–8].

The clearance of these middle molecules is largely a consequence of the dialysis membrane "cut-off" or pore size maximum, although it is important to recognize that even in an idealized membrane, pore size is not completely uniform, and solute transport does not abruptly stop at some given or defined molecular size. That is to say that there are pores that vary around a certain mean. In order to effectively facilitate transport of these middle molecules, while avoiding transport of so-called large molecules, like albumin with a molecular weight of 66.5 kDa, the manufacturer must engineer a pore size sufficient to span the size of interest but to tail off before larger serum proteins are given passage.

Salt and Water Management

The native kidneys are wonderfully adept at managing extracellular fluid volume and osmolality within very finely regulated margins. That regulation is the product of interwoven and overlapping neurohormonal feedback loops that allow for accommodation of widely varying intake. In patients who are dependent on dialysis, those hormonal signals that would normally influence kidney sodium handling go unanswered and salt and water removal are driven mechanically through modulation of the dialysis concentrations and ultrafiltration (UF) rates set at the bedside.

The average fluid intake in adults is approximately 1.5 L/day; an additional 350 to 400 mL/day of water is generated through the metabolism of carbohydrates. This "intake" is balanced in adults by fecal losses averaging 100 mL/day, insensible losses of about 400 to 600 mL/day, and urinary output. In balance, using the above values—which vary widely between individuals—that leaves approximately 1.3 L/day of water that must be excreted by the kidneys in order to stay in steady state. From a dialysis perspective, this means that three weekly sessions of intermittent hemodialysis must remove approximately 9 L of water per week that must be removed in dialysis-dependent patients who lack residual renal function. Thrice-weekly dialysis, then, requires 3 L be removed per treatment which, depending on the size of the patient, can be both physiologically taxing and technically challenging. The physiologic stresses, in particular, have been suggested as the primary driver behind increased cardiovascular mortality, with high UF rates showing correlation negative outcomes [9–11].

Sodium management is also intimately tied to the dialysis gradients established across the semipermeable membrane. Sodium balance is generally achieved by dialyzing patients against a dialysis bath containing 140 mmol/L of sodium, matching the serum concentration. Higher sodium baths tend to lead to higher interdialytic weight gain and higher blood pressures. Lower sodium dialysate baths on thrice-weekly hemodialysis tend to lead to intradialytic hypotension [12]. There is some preliminary data on using lower sodium dialysate solutions with nocturnal or frequent dialysis to maintain slight negative sodium balance, but the long-term effects of this technique remain unknown [13]. Obviously, in developing an artificial kidney, implantable, wearable, or otherwise "portable," all of these clearances need to be collectively considered.

Wearable Dialysis Options

The first dialysis performed to treat chronic kidney disease (CKD) was performed in Seattle in March of 1960 [14]. Since that time, a quest has been underway to balance the medical and mechanical demands of dialysis with the patients' desires to live full and productive lives. It is important to realize that in the 1970s, just as the U.S. Congress was preparing to grant nearly universal health coverage to Americans with ESKD, most patients who were dependent on chronic dialysis were performing the procedure in their own homes [15] and were largely homebound. At that time, there was an interest in developing portable kidney replacement options to help liberate these patients from their homes; literature published during that era investigates the theoretical possibility of portable dialysis (16–19). However, as Medicare reimbursement allowed for a rapid growth in the CKD patient population, an extensive network of dialysis clinics was developed, which eliminated the homebound nature of the therapy by not only allowing for movement to and from treatments but also allowing for travel accommodations as needed.

Recently, however, interest in portable therapies has resumed as observational data accumulates indicating that longer dialysis sessions may be beneficial with respect to patient outcomes (20). While incompletely understood, these longer sessions likely have less negative physiologic impact through slow UF. The improved solute control—as evidenced by the superior phosphorus management seen in these patients—may also lend itself to improved outcomes. Collectively, these observations have led to renewed interest in possible slow continuous dialysis using wearable or implantable systems, which are compared with conventional hemodialysis in TABLE 11.2, although these systems have their attendant challenges.

First among these challenges is the necessity of vascular access. Hemodialysis depends on reliable vascular access facilitating an unimpeded supply from and return to patients' circulation (21). Significant data has shown the superiority of arteriovenous fistulae or grafts to catheter access. Fistula or graft access requires needle access and secure connections. Indeed, the risk of accidental venous needle disconnect is great, given the high throughput of blood. In standard dialysis treatments, with a blood flow rate of 400 mL/min, exsanguination could occur in less than 15 minutes. In a dialysis unit, safety is ensured by stabilizing the involved limb and maintaining direct visualization through the duration of treatment. With a wearable system, the fundamental driving impetus for which is mobility to better suit patient lifestyles, this vascular might not necessarily be so stable. Indeed a dislodged line could quickly become disastrous. While catheters may provide additional stability, they have been linked to increased infectious risk and indeed may be related to ongoing inflammatory activation (22,23), and possible association with cardiovascular and other disease states (11).

The volume of required dialysate is another logistical challenge. In order to maintain the electrochemical gradients required to provide dialysis in the limited time allotted for traditional thrice-weekly dialysis, mandate that the dialysis flow rates exceed the blood flow with maximal dialysis achieved with countercurrent flows.

In conventional thrice-weekly dialysis, the dialysis flow rates—typically in excess of 600 mL/min—lead to the use of approximately 200 L of dialysate per treatment. Other therapies that have allowed for less intensive but more frequent dialysis have limited the amount of dialysis needed at home, with six times weekly dialysis requiring lower dialysate flows and thus only 30 to 50 L of dialysate per treatment. One novel strategy that has been used to regenerate fresh dialysate form waste dialysate is the application of solute sorbent materials to the circuit.

Solute removal devices that utilize sorbent materials have been in commercial production for decades. Initially developed by National Aeronautics and Space Administration (NASA) for water purification on manned spaceflight missions, these solute removal devices have since been adapted for use in dialysis systems (24). The REDY system, standing for REcirculation of DialYsate, was introduced commercially in the 1970s and remains available for use. The sorbent materials are able to remove various elements of spent dialysate in several steps to regenerate usable dialysate solutions. It is worth reviewing the details of this process briefly.

Spent dialysate, of course, contains metabolic toxins that need to be removed if that dialysate is meant to be reused. These include urea, potassium, phosphorus, and a variety of organic acids. By moving that dialysate through several steps, one can remove not only those known toxins but presumably many other metabolites that are removed by dialysis. In these systems, the dialysate is first exposed to urease, which cleaves the urea to carbon dioxide and ammonia. The newly formed ammonia scavenges free protons to form NH_4^+ given that the pK_a of the ammonia–ammonium system (NH_3/NH_4^+) of around 9, it favors a protonated form in dialysate with a neutral pH. This is the first step in excreting dietary acid. The dialysate then moves through a cation exchange resin and then an anion exchange resin to remove potassium and ammonium, and then phosphorus and sulfate, respectively. Other cationic and anionic solutes removed by dialysis are also eliminated in these columns, including calcium and magnesium. Lastly, the dialysate moves through an activated charcoal filter to remove organic solutes. Typically, because of the removal of calcium and magnesium by the cationic resin and removal of bicarbonate by the anionic resin, these must be replaced to some extent before returning the dialysate for use as well (24,25).

These sorbent systems have become an important element among the wearable dialysis options currently being explored for wider market.

TABLE 11.2	Comparison of Conventional Hemodialysis, Wearable Artificial Kidney, and Implantable Artificial Kidney		
	Conventional Hemodialysis	**Wearable Artificial Kidney**	**Implantable Artificial Kidney**
Access	Arteriovenous graft/fistula or dialysis catheter	Catheter	Permanent grafts to vasculature
Blood flow rates	High: typically 300–400 mL/min	Low: 50–100 mL/min	200–300 mL/min
Dialysis membrane	Commercial high flux dialyzers	Same	Silicon nanopore membrane
Dialysate	Large volumes of prepared dialysate	Small volumes of dialysate that are continuously regenerated	None
Treatment length	3–4 h thrice weekly	6–10 h daily	Continuous
Small molecule clearance	~200 L/wk	~200 L/wk	25 mL/min
Phosphorus clearance	Limited by intercompartmental kinetics	Limited by blood and dialysate flow	Limited by filtration rate and solute size

Peritoneal Dialysis

Peritoneal dialysis (PD) can be described as the first "wearable" dialysis option. It only requires intermittent exchanges of peritoneal dialysate and allows patients to fit their treatment to their lives, contrary to the more rigid schedules demanded by in-center hemodialysis. PD also has drawbacks, including a significant commitment on the part of the patient with potentially many hours per week devoted to treatments, as well a large storage area and reserve for PD fluid is required. As early as 1976, Raja (25) reported the use of the REDY system to recycle spent PD fluid for reuse.

Presently, a commercially available option for PD patients is being developed by the Singapore-based Automated Wearable Artificial Kidney (AWAK) Technologies. Their device uses urease, zirconium oxide, and zirconium phosphate along with activated charcoal to facilitate peritoneal dialysate regeneration as described above. Unlike in standard hemodialysis, PD requires an osmotic gradient to facilitate water removal in these patients. The AWAK system, then, not only replaces the adsorbed salts after purification but also replaces glucose in the solution to maintain that gradient.

Another distinct difference between the standard PD routine and the AWAK system is the use of tidal dialysis. While typically, patients will infuse large volumes with long dwells, tidal dialysis allows for small volumes, with short dwells and almost continuous exchange. According to the published literature on these systems, approximately 4 L/hr is exchanged in patients using their systems (26) with achieved clearances that are superior to standard PD. Whether there is any improvement in observed patient outcomes like mortality, using this modality remain to be tested.

Ronco describes a similar device, the Vicenza Wearable Artificial Kidney for Peritoneal Dialysis (ViWAK) that also utilizes a specialized PD catheter with an inflow and outflow lumen—the Ronco catheter—and a small wearable cartridge containing the sorbent materials. The initial morning dwell is done manually by the patient, and after approximately 2 hours, when approximately 50% dialysate/plasma equilibrium has been achieved, recirculation is activated for the ensuing 10 hours or so, at a rate of 20 mL/min. Again, this allows for high daily clearances, and a weekly clearance >100 L/wk (27,28).

Hemodialysis

Just as there have been advances using these sorbent regenerated dialysis models in hemodialysis, so too have advances been made in so-called continuous ambulatory hemodialysis with two major current extracorporeal hemodialysis options being explored. The Wearable Artificial Kidney, or WAK, was trialed in Vincenza, Italy, in the mid-2000s and recently (2015) completed an initial human trial in the United States. As noted previously, while we are accustomed to high blood flow rates when patients are receiving extracorporeal kidney support, these are a mandate not of the modality but of the short treatment time offered to our outpatients. Indeed, the device currently being explored was described by Gura first in 2005 using off-the-shelf dialyzer membranes. The dialysate is circulated through a miniaturized system using the REDY components that reconstitutes the dialysate and then a series of syringes add the additional salts to the solution; heparin is added to the blood circuit. The entire device weighs approximately 5 kg.

The earliest clinical studies of this device were on patients requiring additional UF that could be provided by routine dialysis (29). This was followed by experimental use in a small cohort of ESKD patients. Blood flow rates of 50 mL/min were achieved and total urea clearances of approximately 22 mL/min. Unfortunately, access indeed proved to be a hurdle with two of the eight patients experiencing catheter thrombosis and at least one episode of needle dislodgment during treatment, although safety measures prevented significant blood loss and treatment continued after needle replacement (30). As with traditional CRRT options, phosphate and β_2-microglobulin clearances were much higher than they are on thrice-weekly dialysis, again supporting the idea that mobilization from peripheral compartments is the fundamental problem in achieving higher clearances on dialysis (31).

The Netherlands-based Nanodialysis Company has developed a slightly different approach that deviates from the REDY sorbent design described above. Instead of using disposable cartridges, a regenerable sodium polystyrene-based cartridge is used for cation exchange. With this device, the sodium polystyrene resin allows for displacement of sodium ions for cations in the dialysate that need to be expunged (potassium, ammonium, etc.). After a certain "lifetime," the polystyrene is bathed again in a high concentration sodium bath, which displaces those cations that accumulated during dialysate exposure (32). In addition to reusable cation exchangers, they have also opted to use an electrochemical reaction to eliminate urea from the dialysate. With electrodes placed into the system, an electrical current oxidizes the spent urea into nitrogen, hydrogen, and carbon dioxide. This allows for less risk of urease failure or worse yet, urease breakthrough, but trades out that problem for the issues associated with gas production and heavy metal use with risk of metal ionization into the dialysate (33).

Implantable Renal Replacement Systems

Indeed, the pinnacle of this field's aspiration is to achieve a bioengineered implantable device that would overcome the concerns associated with both infection and with access failure while providing adequate dialytic clearance to manage the metabolic consequences of ESKD. While wearable therapies emphasize the use of regenerable dialysate solutions and have minimized the concerns associated with dialyzer exchange simply because of accessibility, these parts would pose inherent issues to implantable devices as intermittent replacement would be necessary. While the membrane is likely a requisite piece of an implantable strategy and its lifespan will determine the frequency of exchange, successful strategies will likely forego the use of dialysis.

Recellularization

Great interest has arisen around the prospect of rejuvenating a failed kidney by either reawakening its own cellular apparatus, or by replacing or repurposing other cell types to provide kidney function on an implanted engineered device. Both of these prospective treatment techniques share common features that lend themselves to review here.

While many different researchers have developed basic science techniques to harvest, grow, and influence differentiation of kidney tissues, those that have demonstrated the most promise include somatic cell nuclear transfer, and recellularizing organ matrices for implantation.

Somatic cell nuclear transfer involves generation of syngeneic donor tissue for a variety of uses. The tissues are generated by harvesting the nuclei of a somatic cell and then implanting that into an enucleated oocyte. The resulting embryonic or fetal tissue is then harvested for use (34). In the case of the kidney, those cells could

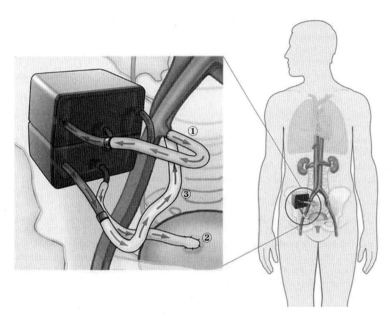

FIGURE 11.1 Schematic of implantable artificial kidney. Left, a two-stage implanted device is perfused from the iliac artery via a polytetrafluoroethylene (PTFE) vascular graft (*number 1*). The HemoCartridge filters approximately 20 to 30 mL/min from the flowing blood. Both filtrate and postfilter blood flow to a bioreactor of living human kidney cells, which return valuable fluids and electrolytes to the blood, and concentrates toxins in the ultrafiltrate, which then flows to the bladder (*number 2*). Purified blood returns to the patient's veins (*number 3*). (Courtesy of Shuvo Roy.)

theoretically be used to replace lost kidney tissues. More recent work has focused on using dedifferentiation signaling to change terminally differentiated cells of the host to return to pluripotency and then deliver these to the organ of interest (35). While promising, with tissues showing some histology consistent with kidney tissues, neither of these techniques have yet shown full reconstitution of the nephron.

Alternatively, some researchers have devised ways to use the matrix of an existing decellularized kidney as the structure of the kidney and then adding cellular elements in the hopes of recreating complete kidney architecture. This has the benefit of providing the superstructure necessary for nephron and vascular scaffolding. The earliest work in this area was on cardiac tissue with recapitulation of myocyte architecture and appropriate contractile orientations (36). However, the kidney architecture is significantly more complex and the process of recellularizing a bit more intensive. In 2013, Song et al. (37) published work wherein a decellularized rat kidney was seeded with human umbilical vein endothelial cells from the arterial circulation and neonatal rat kidney cells were seeded from the lower genitourinary tract. Histologically, structures similar to glomeruli and tubules were seen, though in vitro testing of the implants that were inferior to matched cadaveric kidneys with less stringent filtration specificity (37).

Implantable Devices

An alternate approach has been to develop a bioengineered device that could be implanted to permanently manage ESKD. Current concepts, being pioneered by Fissell and Roy, would involve two functional elements, similar to those in a native kidney—the first component would be akin to the glomerulus, generating a large volume filtrate. The filtrate would proceed on to the bioreactor which would function much like the tubular portion of the nephron does, modifying that filtrate through secretion and reabsorption to

optimize the waste product outflow. A schematic of one possible design is seen in **FIGURE 11.1**.

Implantable Filter

Modern dialyzers, composed of hollow-fiber tubes composed of cellulosic materials, are far too bulky and have a propensity for detrimental filtration changes over time due to thrombosis and coagulation activation to be used for implantation. Instead, Roy has taken advantage of silicon micromachining to manufacture silicon chips that have very specific and controlled pore sizes (38). These can then be used in an implantable manifold to facilitate filtration. While silicon has been challenging to use in biologic models due to protein adsorption with its intended risk for pore preservation, these chips, when coated with hydrated polymers, have shown to resist this process and have reasonable half-lives (39,40). Thus far, results from *in vitro* and *in vivo* tests of the filtration apparatus have been promising.

Bioreactor

The bioreactor would then serve to modify the generated ultrafiltrate from the silicon chip by exposing it to bioengineered cell cultures. The same group that has bioengineered the silicon nanopore membrane have explored a variety of facets for bioreactor implementation, including exploring growth substrates, and tubular behaviors according to adjacent fluid mechanics (41–43) but have not yet published *in vivo* studies of a complete apparatus.

◆ REFERENCES

1. Jacobs C. Renal replacement therapy by hemodialysis: an overview. *Nephrol Ther* 2009;5(4):306–312.
2. Alwall N. On the artificial kidney, I: apparatus for dialysis of the blood in vivo. *Acta Med Scand* 1947;128(4):317–325.

3. United States Renal Data System. Costs of ESRD. In: *2011 USRDS Annual Data Report: Volume 2. Atlas of End-stage Renal Disease in the United States.* Ann Arbor, MI: National Institutes of Health, National Institute of Diabetes and Digestive and Kidney Diseases, 2011:281–290.

4. Thomas G, Jaber BL. Convective therapies for removal of middle molecular weight uremic toxins in end-stage renal disease: a review of the evidence. *Semin Dial* 2009;22(6):610–614.

5. Schmidt JJ, Hafer C, Clajus C, et al. New high-cutoff dialyzer allows improved middle molecule clearance without an increase in albumin loss: a clinical crossover comparison in extended dialysis. *Blood Purif* 2012;34(3–4):246–252.

6. Cheung CL, Lam KS, Cheung BM. Serum beta-2 microglobulin concentration predicts cardiovascular and all-cause mortality. *Int J Cardiol* 2013;168(5):4811–4813.

7. Sedighi O, Abediankenari S, Omranifar B. Association between plasma Beta-2 microglobulin level and cardiac performance in patients with chronic kidney disease. *Nephrourol Mon* 2015;7(1):e23563.

8. Mazanec K, McClure J, Bartley CJ, et al. Systemic amyloidosis of beta 2 microglobulin type. *J Clin Pathol* 1992;45(9):832–833.

9. Flythe JE, Kimmel SE, Brunelli SM. Rapid fluid removal during dialysis is associated with cardiovascular morbidity and mortality. *Kidney Int* 2011;79(2):250–257.

10. Flythe JE, Curhan GC, Brunelli SM. Disentangling the ultrafiltration rate-mortality association: the respective roles of session length and weight gain. *Clin J Am Soc Nephrol* 2013;8(7):1151–1161.

11. Burton JO, Jefferies HJ, Selby NM, et al. Hemodialysis-induced cardiac injury: determinants and associated outcomes. *Clin J Am Soc Nephrol* 2009;4(5):914–920.

12. Santos SF, Peixoto AJ. Revisiting the dialysate sodium prescription as a tool for better blood pressure and interdialytic weight gain management in hemodialysis patients. *Clin J Am Soc Nephrol* 2008;3(2):522–530.

13. Thomson BK, Huang SH, Lindsay RM. The choice of dialysate sodium is influenced by hemodialysis frequency and duration: what should it be and for what modality? *Semin Dial* 2015;28(2):180–185.

14. Blagg CR. The early history of dialysis for chronic renal failure in the United States: a view from Seattle. *Am J Kidney Dis* 2007;49(3):482–496.

15. Blagg CR, Mailloux LU. Introduction: the case for home hemodialysis. *Adv Ren Replace Ther* 1996;3(2):96–98.

16. Friedman EA, Galonsky RS, Hessert RL, et al. Mobilizing hemodialysis. *J Dial* 1977;1(8):797–803.

17. Briefel GR, Galonsky RS, Hutshisson JT, et al. Field trial of compact travel dialysis system. *J Dial* 1976;1(1):57–66.

18. Briefel GR, Hutchisson JT, Galonsky RS, et al. Compact, travel hemodialysis system. *Proc Clin Dial Transplant Forum* 1975;5:61–64.

19. Dharnidharka SG, Kirkham R, Kolff WJ. Toward a wearable artificial kidney using ultrafiltrate as dialysate. *Trans Am Soc Artif Intern Organs* 1973;19:92–97.

20. Pauly RP. Survival comparison between intensive hemodialysis and transplantation in the context of the existing literature surrounding nocturnal and short-daily hemodialysis. *Nephrol Dial Transplant* 2013;28(1):44–47.

21. Fissell WH, Roy S, Davenport A. Achieving more frequent and longer dialysis for the majority: wearable dialysis and implantable artificial kidney devices. *Kidney Int* 2013;84(2):256–264.

22. Sabry AA, Elshafey EM, Alsaran K, et al. The level of C-reactive protein in chronic hemodialysis patients: a comparative study between patients with noninfected catheters and arteriovenous fistula in two large Gulf hemodialysis centers. *Hemodial Int* 2014;18(3):674–679.

23. Banerjee T, Kim SJ, Astor B, et al. Vascular access type, inflammatory markers, and mortality in incident hemodialysis patients: the Choices for Healthy Outcomes in Caring for End-Stage Renal Disease (CHOICE) Study. *Am J Kidney Dis* 2014;64(6):954–961.

24. Agar JW. Review: understanding sorbent dialysis systems. *Nephrology (Carlton)* 2010;15(4):406–411.

25. Raja RM, Kramer MS, Rosenbaum JL. Recirculation peritoneal dialysis with sorbent Redy cartridge. *Nephron* 1976;16(2):134–142.

26. Lee DB, Martin R. Automated Wearable Artificial Kidney (AWAK): a peritoneal dialysis approach in proceedings of the World Congress on Medical Physics and Biomedical Engineering. Paper presented at: 11th International Congress of the IUPESM; September 2009; Munich, Germany.

27. Ronco C, Fecondini L. The Vicenza wearable artificial kidney for peritoneal dialysis (ViWAK PD). *Blood Purif* 2007;25(4):383–388.

28. Amerling R, Winchester JF, Ronco C. Continuous flow peritoneal dialysis: update 2012. *Contrib Nephrol* 2012;178:205–215.

29. Gura V, Ronco C, Nalesso F, et al. A wearable hemofilter for continuous ambulatory ultrafiltration. *Kidney Int* 2008;73(4):497–502.

30. Davenport A. Portable or wearable peritoneal devices—the next step forward for peritoneal dialysis? *Adv Perit Dial* 2012;28:97–101.

31. Gura V, Davenport A, Beizai M, et al. Beta2-microglobulin and phosphate clearances using a wearable artificial kidney: a pilot study. *Am J Kidney Dis* 2009;54(1):104–111.

32. Wester M, Simonis F, Gerritsen KG, et al. A regenerable potassium and phosphate sorbent system to enhance dialysis efficacy and device portability: an in vitro study. *Nephrol Dial Transplant* 2013;28(9):2364–2371.

33. Wester M, Simonis F, Lachkar N, et al. Removal of urea in a wearable dialysis device: a reappraisal of electro-oxidation. *Artif Organs* 2014;38(12):998–1006.

34. Lanza RP, Chung HY, Yoo JJ, et al. Generation of histocompatible tissues using nuclear transplantation. *Nat Biotechnol* 2002;20(7):689–696.

35. Takasato M, Vanslambrouck JM, Little MH. Reprogramming somatic cells to a kidney fate. *Semin Nephrol* 2014;34(4):462–480.

36. Ott HC, Matthiesen TS, Goh SK, et al. Perfusion-decellularized matrix: using nature's platform to engineer a bioartificial heart. *Nat Med* 2008;14(2):213–221.

37. Song JJ, Guyette JP, Gilpin SE, et al. Regeneration and experimental orthotopic transplantation of a bioengineered kidney. *Nat Med* 2013;19(5):646–651.

38. Fissell WH, Dubnisheva A, Eldridge AN, et al. High-performance silicon nanopore hemofiltration membranes. *J Memb Sci* 2009;326(1):58–63.

39. Li Y, Liu CM, Yang JY, et al. Anti-biofouling properties of amphiphilic phosphorylcholine polymer films. *Colloids Surf B Biointerfaces* 2011;85(2):125–130.

40. Melvin ME, Fissell WH, Roy S, et al. Silicon induces minimal thromboinflammatory response during 28-day intravascular implant testing. *ASAIO J* 2010;56(4):344–348.

41. Fissell WH, Manley S, Westover A, et al. Differentiated growth of human renal tubule cells on thin-film and nanostructured materials. *ASAIO J* 2006;52(3):221–227.

42. Humes HD, Fissell WH, Weitzel WF, et al. Metabolic replacement of kidney function in uremic animals with a bioartificial kidney containing human cells. *Am J Kidney Dis* 2002;39(5):1078–1087.

43. Fissell WH, Roy S. The implantable artificial kidney. *Semin Dial* 2009;22(6):665–670.

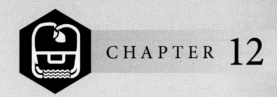

CHAPTER 12

Adequacy of Peritoneal Dialysis

John M. Burkart

Chronic dialysis is certainly a remarkable medical success story, extending the lives of some patients with kidney failure for more than 20 years (1). This success routinely occurs despite the finding that typical urea clearances for patients on renal replacement therapies (RRTs) and in particular peritoneal dialysis (PD) are only approximately one-tenth that of the normal kidney (70 L urea clearance/wk on PD vs. 750 L/wk for normal kidney function) (**TABLE 12.1**) and the fact that dialysis itself replaces only some of the typical functions of the normal human kidney. For instance, it does a fair job or replacing some of the filtration functions of the normal kidney (removal of urea and creatinine, etc.), but dialysis typically does not correct anemia and renal osteodystrophy without additional medications. Furthermore, dialysis does not replace other poorly recognized systemic metabolic functions mainly by the proximal tubules typically present in health. Despite the success of current RRTs, there is room for improvement. Mortality rates in the United States have historically been in the range of 10% to 25% per annum (2), on average, 10 times higher than that of age- and sex-matched controls in the healthy population (3).

Some have suggested that this increased rate of mortality in dialysis patients is due to inadequacies in the prescribed dose of dialysis (4,5). However, it is acknowledged that there is more to "adequacy" of dialysis than what any single yardstick for "dialysis dose" can measure. In an attempt to improve patient outcomes, both National and International Medical Societies have developed guidelines intended to standardize medical care, help practicing nephrologists, identify research needs, and ultimately improve clinical outcomes. For PD, the first of these was the National Kidney Foundation (NKF)-sponsored Dialysis Outcomes Quality Initiative (DOQI) clinical practice guidelines for adequacy of PD (6). These have subsequently been revised twice (7,8).

This chapter discusses adequacy for PD in terms of total solute clearance, volume control, and other issues related to the PD prescription. Although it focuses on small solute clearance issues, it is acknowledged that the optimal treatment of a patient with end-stage kidney disease (ESKD) must additionally address blood pressure (BP) and volume control, treatment of acidosis, anemia, prevention of metabolic bone disease, and perhaps treatment/prevention of a chronic inflammatory state. These particular issues are discussed in other sections of this text.

WHAT YARDSTICK FOR ADEQUACY OF DIALYSIS SHOULD WE USE?

Some of the clinical manifestations of uremia or "underdialysis" are readily apparent to the clinician and/or the patient (9). These include decreased appetite, metallic taste, nausea, vomiting, pericarditis, pleuritis, and encephalopathy. Not so readily evident as a manifestation of "underdialysis," is the presence of hypertension (10), lipid abnormalities (11), and peripheral neuropathy (12). In addition, patients often underreport their symptoms. Therefore, in addition to the clinical assessment of the patient, it would be clinically helpful if nephrologists had a reliable and easily measured laboratory parameter that can be obtained during the course of chronic kidney disease (CKD) and when a patient is on dialysis that predicts the presence of uremic complications and patient outcome. There is no documented single substance that has been shown to be the "uremic" toxin. Undoubtedly, the clinical manifestations of the uremic syndrome are the result of the synergistic effect of multiple retained solutes across a broad spectrum of molecular weights. It is because retained levels (body burden) of these solutes that the uremic syndrome occurs. Therefore, because there is no single

TABLE 12.1	Solute Removal by Dialysis and the Natural Kidney			
	Natural Solute Kidney	**Hemodialysis—Standard Flux**	**Hemodialysis—High Flux**	**CAPD**
Urea L/wk	750	130	130	70
Vitamin B_{12} L/wk	1,200	30	60	40
Inulin L/wk	1,200	10	40	20
β_2-Microglobulin	1,000	0	300	250

CAPD, continuous ambulatory peritoneal dialysis.
From Keshaviah P. Adequacy of CAPD: a quantitative approach. *Kidney Int* 1992;42 (Suppl 28):S160–S164.

"uremic" toxin, one must rely on "surrogate" markers for "adequacy of dialysis." Current commonly used surrogates include clearances or serum levels of urea nitrogen, creatinine, phosphorous, or β_2-microglobulin. At present, if a physician was going to pick one yardstick as a measure of dialysis dose, it would be a urea-based surrogate (Kt/V_{urea}).

There are historical data which suggests that the outcome for patients on both hemodialysis (HD) (13) and PD (14) was related to total small solute clearance and to surrogates of nutritional status such as dietary protein intake (DPI), body mass, and serum albumin levels. It was not uncommon to observe an improvement in overall patient well-being and nutritional intake after small solute clearance was increased. There appeared to be a relationship between protein intake, solute clearance, and the manifestations of uremia or nutritional status that were likely to be different in each patient but, in the absence of significant comorbid disease, tended to correlate positively with solute clearance (15). As a result, in the initial clinical practice guidelines for "adequacy of PD," the recommended standard "yardsticks" for dose of PD included urea clearance normalized to its volume of distribution (Kt/V_{urea}) and creatinine clearance (Ccr) normalized to 1.73 m^2. However, as will be discussed in subsequent text, contemporary data may suggest that one may also need to refocus on other known "yardsticks" of renal replacement therapy such as sodium removal, volume control, phosphate, and β_2-microglobulin clearance. Our historical small solute marker, Kt/V_{urea}, should just be the starting point of an adequacy of dialysis evaluation.

Correlation between Solute Clearance and Risk of Death

Steady-state serum levels of various solutes are related to their generation and removal rates. To guide dosing of dialysis, one needs to monitor serum levels and measure the amount of the surrogate solutes removed from the body. However, serum levels alone may be misleading. Take blood urea nitrogen (BUN) levels for instance. These levels are related to generation (dietary intake) and removal (native kidney function and/or dialysis). If a patient is underdialyzed, he or she may not eat well. In this case, the BUN level may look as expected or low, suggesting adequate dialysis, but the patient's dialysis dose could be low and the cause of under-eating—uremia. Similarly, if one was malnourished, one may have a low muscle mass and serum creatinine levels may look low, suggesting adequate dialysis when in fact, the low creatinine was a reflection of low production (low muscle mass) not adequate dialysis. As a result, it was felt that a surrogate for adequate dialysis should be something other than simply looking at blood levels of these two solutes. Consequently, current guidelines for "adequacy of PD" recommend obtaining a 24-hour collection of both urine and peritoneal effluent for analysis of total removal for a particular solute (K_{renal} + $K_{peritoneal}$ = $K_{rp \; or \; total}$). Urea and Ccr are obtained and then normalized to

volume of distribution (urea) and body surface area (BSA) (creatinine) to calculate weekly Kt/V_{urea} and weekly Ccr/1.73 m^2. Historically, to determine total solute removal (kidney and dialysis), it was recommended that when making these calculations, the residual kidney and peritoneal clearances was added together 1:1. This was initially based on the assumption that the potential beneficial effect on patient outcome from 1 unit of residual kidney and 1 unit of peritoneal clearances was equal. However, it is now recognized that this is not the case. Specifically, if one were to look at the benefit in terms of small solute removal only, the residual kidney component seems to be superior to that of RRTs (see subsequent text). However, because the most recent prospective randomized controlled trials (PRCTs) that have evaluated the relationship between relative risk of death and solute removal (in terms of Kt/V_{urea}) were conducted using total solute clearance adding kidney and peritoneal in a 1:1 way, current NKF Kidney Disease Outcomes Quality Initiative (KDOQI) and other guidelines still make this recommendation.

Why Small Solute Clearance as the Adequacy Surrogate?

If one was to look quantitatively at urinary solutes, you would see that urea is one of the most plentiful solutes in the urine in health. Furthermore, it is well documented clinically that in patients with advanced stages of kidney disease, some uremic symptoms are related to protein intake. It would therefore make some sense to use some index related to urea as a potential marker for dialysis dose. Multiple retrospective cohort studies, all differing in methodology and the number of patients enrolled, have examined the relationship between patient outcomes in terms of relative risk of death or morbidity and its relationship to total small solute clearance, the significance of which has been reviewed elsewhere (16,17). Historical studies tended to conclude that outcomes such as relative risk of death and hospitalizations were in some way related to total small solute clearance. These studies and more contemporary, but contradictory, PRCTs are briefly reviewed in subsequent text.

Kt/V Data

Current recommendation for PD adequacy is to target a total [PD and residual renal function (RRF)] Kt/V_{urea} of at least 1.7 per week. What are these recommendations based on?

Historical Publications

Original theoretic constructs for continuous ambulatory peritoneal dialysis (CAPD) predicted that an anephric 70-kg patient [total body water (TBW) or V = 42 L] would remain in positive nitrogen balance when prescribed five, 2-L PD exchanges per day (18). Studies using *univariate* analysis of observational data correlating outcomes with small solute clearance suggested the following: In patients with RRF, to optimize clinical outcomes, one should maintain a total weekly Kt/V_{urea} target of more than 1.5 in one (19) and more than 2.0 in another (20). A study in anuric patients suggested that patients with a Kt/V of greater than 1.89 did best (21).

Studies using the statistically more correct *multivariate* analysis of observational data to determine the predictive value of Kt/V_{urea} on survival found the following: a survival advantage in patients with a weekly Kt/V_{urea} greater than 1.89 in one study (22), and, in another study of *prevalent* PD patients [mean baseline glomerular filtration rate (GFR) 1.73 mL/min] followed up for up to 3 years, the best survival was noted in patients with a total Kt/V_{urea} of at least 1.96 with no incremental improvement in survival with higher small solute clearances (23). While the Canada–United States of America (CANUSA) study (14), a prospective, multicenter, observational cohort study of *incident* patients in North America and Canada (mean baseline GFR 3.8 mL/min), predicted that over the range of solute clearance studied every 0.1 unit increase in Kt/V would be associated with a 6% decrease in the relative risk of death. The same effect was predicted for Ccr, and there was no evidence of a plateau effect. In the original analysis, RRF was not evaluated as an independent predictor of relative risk of death.

Although in 1995, the CANUSA study provided the best historical evidence that survival on PD is related to total solute clearance, it is important to remember two points. First of all, it was not a PRCT, and secondly, the results were based on theoretic constructs and two very important assumptions: (a) Total solute clearance remained stable over time and (b) 1 unit or mL/min of clearance due to RRF is equal to 1 unit or mL/min of clearance due to PD. In actual fact, the total solute clearance decreased over time as RRF decreased with no corresponding increase in the peritoneal component. Therefore, because the peritoneal component of total solute clearance tended not to change over the course of the study, one interpretation of CANUSA would be to say that the more RRF the patient has, the better the predicted outcome (24). This was in fact confirmed with a residual renal centric reanalysis of the CANUSA data (25). Similar outcome data from CANUSA correlating patient outcome with small solute clearance in terms of Ccr are available. In some publications, total weekly $Ccr/1.73 \text{ m}^2$ was more predictive of all-cause outcomes than total weekly Kt/V_{urea}. As will be seen, this was likely due to the residual kidney component of the total solute clearance.

On the basis of historical observational studies published before 1996, and the possible association between solute clearance and DPI (reviewed in subsequent text), the original NKF-DOQI working group on adequacy of PD recommended the following total solute clearance goals for CAPD: a total weekly Kt/V_{urea} of more than 2.0 per week and a total weekly Ccr of more than $60 \text{ L}/1.73 \text{ m}^2/\text{wk}$. For continuous cyclic peritoneal dialysis (CCPD) and for nightly intermittent peritoneal dialysis (NIPD), slightly higher total weekly Kt/V_{urea} and total weekly $Ccr/1.73 \text{ m}^2$ were recommended (6). It was acknowledged that the CAPD targets were only marginally evidence-based and that there were no prospective randomized studies to support those recommendations. The original guidelines have subsequently been replaced. It was also acknowledged that targets for CCPD and NIPD were opinion-based with little to no outcome data for the recommendations. Subsequently, other medical societies recommended targeting a total weekly Kt/V_{urea} of 2.0 (Canada guidelines) (26) and 1.7 (UK guidelines) (27) for all PD therapies.

Contemporary Observational Studies

Contemporary studies have further examined the effect of increasing peritoneal clearance on survival. There are three studies from a group in China. Szeto et al. (28) retrospectively reviewed their experience in 168 prevalent CAPD patients followed up for 1 year. Outcomes for patients with a total Kt/V_{urea} of more than 1.7 per week (baseline mean total Kt/V_{urea} 2.03 ± 0.25 for patients with RRF, and a baseline mean total Kt/V_{urea} was 1.93 ± 0.18 for patients without RRF) were compared to those for patients with a total Kt/V_{urea} of less than 1.7 per week (mean total Kt/V_{urea} was 1.38 ± 0.22). Overall mortality at 1 year was 8.3%; however, although there was no statistically significant difference between the groups, 9 out of 14 deaths occurred in the anuric patients with a weekly Kt/V_{urea} of less than 1.7 per week. On the basis of this, one might infer that a weekly peritoneal Kt/V_{urea} of less than 1.7 in an anuric patient may be associated with an increased relative risk of death in the long term if these trends continued. In another study, these authors showed an association between outcome and total solute clearance, mainly due to the residual kidney component (29). In contrast, in an evaluation of 140 prevalent anuric patients, followed up for a mean of $22.0 + 11.9$ months, they found a positive correlation between peritoneal clearance and survival (30). In these patients, the mean baseline peritoneal Kt/V_{urea} was 1.72 ± 0.31 per week and 42% were prescribed three 2-L exchanges per day [patients whose prescription was modified if there were ultrafiltration (UF) problems]. Each 0.1 unit decrease in Kt/V was associated with a 6% increase in mortality, similar to that predicted by CANUSA.

These data in Asian patients suggest that once a certain minimal peritoneal small solute clearance is achieved (perhaps a peritoneal Kt/V_{urea} greater than 1.7 to 1.8 per week) and the patient is on 24 per day of peritoneal clearance, that further incremental increases in small solute clearance in the range that was studied result in little increase in short-term outcome.

Davies et al. (31,32) found an association between total solute clearance and survival, and as in other studies, this was all due to variations in residual renal clearance, not peritoneal. In a study of 122 anuric Canadian patients, Bhaskaran et al. (33) reported that the best survival, representing a 58% reduction in mortality, was found in the group of patients with a Kt/V_{urea} greater than 1.8/wk (Ccr greater than $50 \text{ L}/1.73 \text{ m}^2/\text{wk}$). There was no demonstrable incremental improvement for higher weekly clearances. However, the 95% confidence interval (CI) of the study was 0.26 to 1.13, reflecting the low statistical power achieved in this study in a relatively small number of patients.

Contemporary Prospective Randomized Trials

There are three prospective, randomized trials that evaluated the effect of an increase in peritoneal clearance on survival. In the smaller of the three studies, Mak et al. (34) prospectively evaluated the effect of an increase in dialysis dose in a controlled trial in 82 CAPD patients. Baseline, all patients were prescribed three 2-L exchanges per day. They were then randomized to continue this regimen (mean Kt/V_{urea} of 1.67 per week) or increase their PD prescription to four 2-L exchanges per day (mean Kt/V_{urea} 2.02 per week) and were followed up for 1 year. Over short-term follow-up (1 year), there was a difference in hospitalization rates. However, hospitalization rates increased in the control group and decreased in the intervention group, so this may be misleading.

A provocative prospective, randomized, interventional study evaluating the effect of an increase in peritoneal solute clearance compared to continuing on "standard therapy" in 965 CAPD patients in Mexico, the "adequacy of peritoneal dialysis in Mexico (ADEMEX)" study, found no beneficial effect on relative risk of death for the intervention group patients who had a statistically significant increase in their peritoneal solute clearance (35). All patients had 24 h/d of peritoneal dwell, and at baseline, all were on four 2-L exchanges per day, and RRF was similar in the two groups. Averaged total solute clearances over the course of that study were total Kt/V_{urea}, 1.80 $\pm$ 0.02 in controls versus 2.27 $\pm$ 0.02 in the interventional group, whereas peritoneal-only Kt/V_{urea} was 1.62 $\pm$ 0.01 in controls versus 2.13 $\pm$ 0.01 in the intervention group. Corresponding Ccr values in L/wk/1.73 m^2 were 54.1 $\pm$ 1.0 versus 62.9 $\pm$ 0.7 and 46.1 $\pm$ 0.45 versus 56.9 $\pm$ 0.48, respectively. The distribution of prescriptions in the interventional group was 10 L/d in 37%, 11 L/d in 20%, 12 L/d in 21%, 12.5 L/d in 8%, and 15 L/d in 14%. Quality of life was also assessed in the ADEMEX trial. There were no significant differences between the two groups at any point in time for physical composite summary score, mental composite summary score, or kidney disease component summary (36). Interestingly, in a subgroup analysis of anuric patients, there was also no benefit to an increase in peritoneal clearance. Therefore, in the ADEMEX study, neither survival nor the quality of life was benefited by higher small molecule clearances.

As noted in the observational studies cited in preceding text, RRF was the main predictor of mortality, with an 11% increase in mortality for each 10 L/wk/1.73 m^2 decrease in weekly kidney Ccr and a 6% increase in mortality for each 0.1 unit decrease in weekly kidney Kt/V_{urea}. In this study, although there was a statistically significant increase in peritoneal UF volume increased in the intervention group (0.97 $\pm$ 0.05 L/d vs. 0.84 $\pm$ 0.03 L/d, $p < 0.05$), there was no demonstrable improvement in outcome with increasing peritoneal UF.

The results of the ADEMEX trial are consistent with a subsequent randomized trial done in Hong Kong comparing three total Kt/V_{urea} groups (1.5 to 1.7, 1.7 to 2.0, and more than 2.0) in CAPD patients (37). Again, despite the statistically significant differences in solute clearances, there were no differences in 2-year patient survival in the three groups. All patients at the start of the study had residual kidney Kt/V_{urea} of 1.0 or less, ensuring minimal residual kidney function. Baseline residual GFR was 2.38, 2.48, and 2.64 mL/min (representing kidney Kt/V_{urea} of 0.44, 0.46, and 0.49, respectively) in the three groups, not statistically different. Average body mass index (BMI) was 22 kg/m^2, somewhat smaller than the patients in the ADEMEX trial and the typical patient in the United States. Before randomization, the usual prescription was three 2-L exchanges per day in contrast to the "standard" prescription of four 2-L exchanges per day in the control arm of the ADEMEX trial. Dialysis adequacy was assessed every 6 months and based on the results, during the course of the 2-year follow-up in the Hong Kong study, the PD prescription was adjusted up or down, as RRF changed, to stay within the randomized total Kt/V_{urea} category. By the end of the study, residual kidney Kt/V_{urea} was at or less than 0.1 in all three categories. This is an important distinction between the Hong Kong study and the ADEMEX study. In ADEMEX, the control group consisted of a group of patients who continued on the current "standard" therapy, whereas in the Hong Kong study, some patients randomized to the low-dose arm actually had their dialysis prescription reduced.

In summary, these data suggest that for the average patient on standard CAPD (24 h/d of peritoneal dwell time), once small solute clearance is above a certain minimal amount, further increases in small solute clearance in range easily obtained clinically with current technologies result in no demonstrable incremental increase in patient outcome. These studies did not examine a lower "dose" of PD, and therefore, the absolute minimal total delivered solute clearance in terms of Kt/V_{urea} has not been established. However,

available evidence suggests that the weekly minimal delivered total solute clearance in terms of Kt/V_{urea} should be more than 1.7 per week. This is consistent with observational data in anuric patients (38). The data *do not* say that the recommended minimal prescribed total weekly small solute clearances goals should be lowered for all patients. They *do suggest* that nephrologists should be more comfortable with individualizing their prescriptions and, that if a patient is not at goal but is eating well and feeling well, that there is no reason to have to transfer the patient to HD due to inadequate dialysis. The data suggest that one also needs to consider focusing on additional "yardsticks" of adequacy of dialysis. These studies were by design relatively short term (2 years of follow-up) and did not look at differences in middle molecule clearance or volume control, other possible markers for "adequacy" of dialysis.

Creatinine Clearance Data

Current guidelines do not recommend using Ccr as the adequacy yardstick. Why not? Most of the studies reviewed earlier that examined the predictive value of total Kt/V_{urea} on outcome also evaluated the effect of total Ccr/1.73 m^2. In the CANUSA study, total Ccr predicted not only death but also technique survival and hospitalization (14). Analysis of those observational cohort data suggested that a total weekly Ccr of more than 70 L/1.73 m^2 would predict a 78% 2-year patient survival. Other studies suggested that the minimal total weekly target should be more than 58 L/1.73 m^2 (23) or more than 50 L/1.73 m^2 (2,39), whereas anuric patients did best if their clearance was more than 50 L/1.73 m^2 (33). In the ADEMEX study, there was no difference in outcome between the control group (mean total Ccr of 54 L/1.73 m^2/wk) versus the intervention group (mean total Ccr of 62.9 L/1.73 m^2/wk) (35). The Hong Kong study (36) was not analyzed in terms of Ccr.

These data suggest that as with Kt/V_{urea}, once above a certain minimal total weekly Ccr, further increases in dialysis dose were not associated with further improvement in the relative risk of death for patients as a group.

⬢ SUMMARY OF CURRENT RECOMMENDED ACCEPTABLE TOTAL SOLUTE CLEARANCE TARGETS FOR PERITONEAL DIALYSIS

In response to the ADEMEX and Hong Kong trial data, original (late 1990s) guidelines for the adequacy of PD were revised by multiple societies and national guideline committees. Before reviewing these recommendations, it is important to remember the following caveats: First of all, it is possible that the influence of solute clearance on outcome may vary in different ethnic populations. In the United States Renal Data System (USRDS) experience, African Americans and Asians on HD tend to have a lower relative risk of death than whites, presumably with the same solute clearance. Reasons for this are unclear. Perhaps this is due to differences in protein intake. Second, patients in Mexico and Hong Kong have different DPIs than patients in North America or Europe. Third, there may be differences in compliance between countries and ethnic groups. Fourth, there may be unrecognized factors or differences in comorbid diseases (40). Fifth, the ranges of solute clearances examined may not have been sufficiently different to have been able to show a clinically significant difference in survival. More data are clearly needed.

The International Society for Peritoneal Dialysis (ISPD) commissioned a work group with representation from North America, Asia, Australia, and Europe to formulate recommendations for the delivery of adequate PD, taking into account the more recent studies cited in this chapter (41). With respect to small solute removal, it was recommended that the total (renal and peritoneal) weekly Kt/V_{urea} should be greater than 1.7/wk. If using RRF as part of the total, for simplification, the renal and peritoneal Kt/V_{urea} can be added together in a 1:1 manner, although it was acknowledged that the contribution of renal and peritoneal clearances are likely very different from each other. Although it was felt that a separate recommendation for Ccr was not necessary, it was suggested that in patients on cycler a weekly minimum clearance of 45 L/1.73 m^2 should be reached. (The reason for adding a Ccr target for the patients on cycler is because of the temptation to prescribe multiple rapid cycles overnight and a dry day—a prescription that could increase the removal of urea but compromise removal of the more slowly transported, larger uremic toxins.) PD should be carried out 24 hours a day except in special circumstances because of the time dependence for the transport of larger molecular weight toxins. Although a daily UF target was not specified, it was emphasized that maintenance of euvolemia is an important part of adequate dialysis, and attention must be given to urine and UF volume. Within the confines of financial and adherence realities and limitations, the dose of PD should be increased as a trial in any patient who is not doing well because of underdialysis or for uncertain reasons.

The NKF in the United States published similar recommendations in 2006 (8), stating that the minimal delivered total solute clearance should be a Kt/V_{urea} of 1.7 per week. The work group did not see any benefit in adding Ccr solute recommendations nor did they see any data suggesting that the minimal targets needed to be different for patients on CAPD or NIPD or CCPD. Guidelines on protecting RRF and maintaining euvolemia were also added.

The Australian guidelines formulated by a work group Caring for Australians with Renal Impairment (CARI) published on the Internet in 2005 recommends that the weekly total Kt/V_{urea} be greater than or equal to 1.6 and that the Ccr be no less than 60 L/wk in high and high-average transporters, and 50 L/wk in low and low-average transporters (www.cari.org.au). The renal association from the United Kingdom has similar recommendations (1.7 and 50 L/wk) and also recommends that if UF does not exceed 750 mL/d in an anuric patient, consideration be given to a change in therapy (www.renal.org). The European Best Practice Guidelines published in 2005 have the same target Kt/V_{urea}, while also recommending a Ccr of at least 45 L/wk/1.73 m^2 for those patients on cycler and a UF goal of 1 L/d for anuric patients (42).

◆ IMPORTANCE OF RESIDUAL RENAL FUNCTION

Of course, it is well recognized that in an anuric patient, there is a survival benefit associated with doing dialysis. The question is how much or are we just limited in how much we can provide given our current technologies. In contrast to the conflicting data about the benefit of increasing peritoneal clearance on survival, studies have consistently shown that the presence of residual renal clearance is associated with a decrease in the relative risk of death both for patients on PD and for patients on HD (43).

Reanalysis of the CANUSA data (25) suggested that for each 5 L/wk/1.73 m^2 increase in GFR, there was a 12% decrease in the relative risk of death. There was no demonstrable benefit from peritoneal clearance. Estimates of net fluid removal suggested that a 250 mL/d increment in urine volume was associated with a 36%

decrease in the relative risk of death, whereas net peritoneal UF and total fluid removed were not predictive of outcome. In the ADEMEX study reviewed earlier, RRF, not peritoneal, was a predictor of mortality, with an 11% increase in mortality for each 10 L/wk/1.73 m^2 decrease in weekly kidney Ccr and a 6% increase in mortality for each 0.1 unit decrease in weekly kidney Kt/V_{urea} clearance. An evaluation of 673 patients followed up for 1 year reported that decreasing renal clearance, not peritoneal clearance, was statistically associated with an increased mortality rate (44). Similar findings were reported in a review of 873 patients selected for evaluation in the 2000 Health Care Financing Administration Clinical Practice Management project database (45). Other smaller observational studies have also replicated these findings (46–48).

Reasons for these observations are unclear. Some plausible hypotheses for these findings are as follows: (a) Although 1 unit of residual renal clearance may be the same as 1 unit of peritoneal clearance when measured in terms of Kt/V_{urea}, this may not be true for other solutes. For instance, as will be discussed later, if a patient has a residual kidney Kt/V_{urea} of 2.0, his or her residual kidney Ccr is likely to be approximately 120 L/wk. In contrast, an anuric patient with a peritoneal Kt/V_{urea} of 2.0/wk will likely have a peritoneal Ccr of approximately 55 L/wk (**FIGURE 12.1**). This difference may be even more pronounced for middle molecular weight solutes such as β$_2$-microglobulin. (b) As one increases peritoneal Kt/V_{urea}, there may not be a corresponding increase in clearance of larger solutes such as β$_2$-microglobulin, whereas with residual renal clearance, as Kt/V_{urea} increases, the clearance of other solutes may increase to the same degree. In fact, even with advanced CKD and severe reductions in GFR, there is relatively more removal of middle molecules than small solutes when compared to the removal by PD (49). It is well recognized that β$_2$-microglobulin levels are lowest in patients with RRF (50–52). It has been shown that increasing instilled volume is likely to relieve clinical signs and symptoms of uremia (53), although the major effect is to increase small solute, not middle molecular weight solute clearances (**FIGURE 12.2**). It is known that once on 24 h/d of peritoneal dwell time, maneuvers that result in a further increase in small solute clearance tend to have little influence on the clearance of other solutes (54,55). Perhaps alternative PD therapies such as those associated with continuous flow

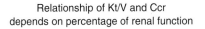

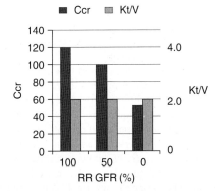

FIGURE 12.1 Relationship between creatinine clearance and Kt/V based on percentage of total clearance that is residual renal (*dark bars*) versus peritoneal (*light bars*). Ccr, creatinine clearance; RR GFR, residual renal glomerular filtration rate.

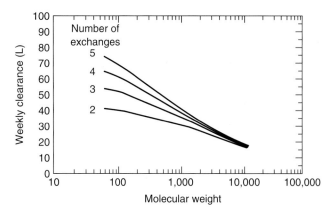

FIGURE 12.2 Effect of increasing number of peritoneal dialysis exchanges on removal of various solutes. The influence of the number of continuous ambulatory peritoneal dialysis exchanges on the weekly solute clearance for a range of solute molecular weights derived from a computerized model of peritoneal transport. [From Keshaviah P. Adequacy of CAPD: a quantitative approach. *Kidney Int* 1992;42(Suppl 38):S160–S164.]

technologies, which appear to offer an increase in β_2-microglobulin clearance over standard technologies, will be beneficial (56). (c) Residual renal clearance may allow better control of BP and volume than what is typically achieved in anuric PD patients. (d) It may be that intrinsically healthier patients keep their RRF longer, and they have better survival because they are healthier and not because of anything that the kidneys are contributing. (e) It is important to remember that the effect of dialysis is always a constant balance between benefit and toxicity. Is it possible that one can increase the toxicity of the therapy when increasing instilled volume or when attempting to increase UF with current therapies? When using 2.5-L exchanges versus 2.0-L exchanges, there is increased glucose absorption from the peritoneal cavity. (f) There may be unrecognized intrinsic "anti-inflammatory" effect of functioning renal parenchyma (perhaps by the proximal tubules) that has been described in the general nondialysis population, which may also apply to RRF in those on dialysis. Studies in the general population have shown that loss of kidney function is associated with an increased risk of cardiovascular (CV) death, in a way that cannot be fully explained by "conventional" risk factors (57).

Interestingly, neither a prospective multicenter study in The Netherlands (47) nor data from the ADEMEX study (35) was able to show an association between dose of PD and benefit in quality of life. In these studies, however, there was a correlation between the amount of RRF and quality of life.

Because of the observational cohort data reviewed in the preceding text, it is important to preserve RRF when possible. One should avoid the use of nephrotoxins (such as NSAIDs, intravenous contrast dye, prolonged aminoglycoside use) whenever possible. In an open label controlled trial of 60 patients on CAPD randomized to ramipril 5 mg daily versus no additional treatment, residual Glomerular Filtration Rate (rGFR) at 1 year (primary outcome) was higher among those randomized to receive ramipril (adjusted GFR: 1.72 vs. 0.64 mL/min). There also was less likelihood of anuria (58). Similarly, in a prospective randomized trial of 34 CAPD patients randomized to valsartan (40 to 80 mg/d; *n* = 18) or no additional treatment (*n* = 16), better preservation of residual Ccr and urine volume were observed after 2 years in the valsartan group (59).

Hence, the last KDOQI guidelines recommended "use of ACE inhibitors or angiotensin II inhibitors in PD patients who need an antihypertensive medication and that there use be considered for renal protection among normotensive patients."

IMPACT OF NUTRITIONAL STATUS ON PATIENT OUTCOME

It is well known that nausea, vomiting, and appetite suppression are symptoms of uremia and patients with uremia tend to have decreased DPI (60). Furthermore, spontaneous DPI decreases as residual kidney GFR decreases to less than 50 to 25 mL/min (61). These tendencies may be exacerbated during the period before the initiation of dialysis when many patients are not only anorexic but also acidotic and often treated with low-protein "kidney protective" diets. Consequently, patients may exhibit signs of protein malnutrition when they present for dialysis. A more "timely" start of dialysis may prevent this.

As a result of these observations, the working hypothesis has been that underdialysis or uremia leads to a decreased appetite, malnutrition, and decreased albumin synthesis. However, cross-sectional studies have provided contradictory results regarding the potential association between nutrition and dialysis dose (15,62–65). Some investigators believe that this relationship is simply mathematical coupling of data (66). Prospective studies, however, have demonstrated that in appropriate cohorts of patients, increasing the dose of dialysis tended to result in an increase in normalized protein equivalent of nitrogen appearance (nPNA) values, an increase in energy intake (31), and increase in percent lean body mass (LBM). These findings are in accordance with the observation that the relationship between dose of dialysis and protein intake seems to level off at a weekly Kt/V_{urea} level greater than approximately 1.9 (67,68) and are the basis for the clinical recommendation that suggests that a malnourished dialysis patient may be malnourished because of "underdialysis."

Studies in both ESRD (69–73) and non-ESRD (74) patients have shown that one of the most important predictors of a patient's relative risk of death is the patient's underlying nutritional status. In HD patients, as the serum albumin decreases from the reference value of 4.5 to 4.0 g/dL to an albumin of less than 2.5 g/dL, the risk of death increased to 18 times that of the reference group (68). Malnutrition is also a significant risk factor for mortality and hospitalizations in chronic PD patients (75,76). Estimates of malnutrition in chronic PD patients ranges from 40% to 76%, with the variability in prevalence due to differing definitions of malnutrition as well as differences in the patient population studied (77–79). There are few studies that provide data on longitudinal changes in nutritional parameters. A prospective study performed in 118 patients who were started on PD found that mean serum albumin levels increased by approximately 0.2 g/dL over 24 months, nPNA declined by approximately 0.1 g/kg/24 h, whereas BMI and body fat were essentially unchanged (80).

The link between malnutrition and poor clinical outcome was not established using serum albumin alone as a marker for nutritional status. Other surrogates for nutritional status such as loss of muscle mass as indicated by lower serum creatinine levels, lower creatinine generation rates, or total body nitrogen levels as well as low serum albumin levels, low prealbumin levels, and subjective global assessment (SGA) score are all good predictors of morbidity and mortality.

These data suggest that death risk is related to nutritional status, a parameter that may be influenced by a patient's total small solute clearance. However, it is important to remember that nutritional status is dependent not only on the prevention of or treatment of uremia but also on many non–ESRD-related factors (comorbid diseases, depression, gastroparesis, etc.). It is now noted that malnutrition can be reflective of poor nutritional intake, inflammation (81–83), or both (84,85). Serum albumin levels are known to be an acute phase reactant, decreasing in the face of inflammation. C-reactive protein (CRP) levels are abnormally high in most PD patients, and there is a direct association between elevated CRP levels and increased rates of mortality (86,87) and CV disease (88–90).

The International Society for Renal Nutrition and Metabolism (ISRNM) published standardized criteria for the diagnosis of protein-energy wasting in 2008. Those criteria define a serum albumin concentration of less than 3.8 g/dL, not an uncommon finding in a PD patient, as consistent with protein-energy wasting (91). Using the plasma albumin concentration, creatinine production, or other nutritional parameters, historical publications have estimated that 40% to 66% of PD patients in the United States are malnourished (75,77), whereas in a more recent cohort study using the ISRNM definition of protein-energy wasting (serum albumin of <3.8 g/dL), it was noted that 63% of PD patients compared to 55% of HD patients were malnourished (92). The ISRNM has suggested that there are four categories of protein-energy wasting. These are (a) evidence of biochemical abnormalities, (b) reduced body mass, (c) reduced muscle mass, and (d) unintentionally low dietary caloric intake.

Dialysis itself is associated with unique metabolic and nutritional problems that may cause one of the four conditions listed by the ISRNM. As mentioned earlier, they could be "underdialyzed" which may suppress appetite. It has been noted that PD patients often have a decreased appetite and early satiety (93,94). Perhaps, this is due to the presence of dialysate in abdomen which imparts a feeling of fullness, perhaps related to the continuous infusion of glucose which may suppress appetite. PD patients typically lose 5 to 15 g of protein and 2 to 4 g of amino acids per day in their dialysate (95). These losses amount to a net loss equivalent to 0.2-g protein/kg/d and tend to be higher in rapid transporters than in low transporters (96). They also are increased during episodes of peritonitis (97), at times doubling even after a mild episode. Although peritoneal losses of protein may correlate with serum albumin levels, they do not seem to correlate with other surrogates for nutritional status of chronic PD patients (98). The PD fluids may cause a chronic inflammatory state. Finally, one must remember, many new dialysis patients still have significant urine volumes and may have proteinuria causing a low albumin.

MEASUREMENTS OF NUTRITIONAL STATUS

Of the readily available measures of nutritional status, serum albumin levels, protein equivalent of nitrogen appearance (PNA), and SGA scores have traditionally been used.

Serum Albumin Levels

Serum albumin levels, in part a reflection of visceral protein storage, predict patient outcome in populations with ESKD, no matter if obtained at the initiation of therapy (14,99) over the duration of dialysis (100) or measured at a stable period while on dialysis (101,102). Different assays for serum albumin give markedly different results (103). The Bromocresol green assay is preferred. Using this, the mean serum albumin level in 1,202 PD patients in late 1994/early 1995 was 3.5 g/dL (104). In an individual PD patient,

TABLE 12.2	Causes of Hypoalbuminemia

Dilutional (volume overload)
Decreased synthesis
Increased body losses
  Urine
  Dialysate
Chronic inflammatory states

the significance of an isolated serum albumin level must be viewed with caution. An isolated low level does not necessarily predict a high risk of death or malnutrition. Levels must be followed up over time and interpreted in context of other patient-related issues such as trends in the level, transport type, solute clearance, comorbid diseases, and so on.

We now have a better understanding of the causes of hypoalbuminemia. They are multifactorial (TABLE 12.2). When evaluating an individual patient, all causes must be considered, including the possibility that a chronic inflammatory state exists. Evolving data suggests that ESKD or perhaps the treatment of ESKD represents a chronic inflammatory state. During PD, the peritoneal cavity is repeatedly exposed to unphysiologic fluids (105,106), which may (107) or may not (108) induce a chronic inflammatory state.

Dietary Protein Intake

Most (95%) nitrogen intake in humans is in the form of protein. Therefore, when the patient is in a steady state (not catabolic or anabolic), total nitrogen excretion multiplied by 6.25 (there are approximately 6.25 g of protein per gram of nitrogen) is thought to be an estimation of a person's DPI (109). Estimated DPI is calculated from urea nitrogen appearance (UNA) in dialysate and urine. Multiple equations have been derived, some of which have been validated in CAPD (not NIPD) patients (PNA = PCR + protein losses) (TABLE 12.3). These estimations were initially called the *protein catabolic rate (PCR)*. However, PCR actually represents the amount of protein catabolism exceeding synthesis required to generate an amount of nitrogen that is excreted. PCR is actually a net catabolic equivalent. Therefore, because these calculations are based on nitrogen appearance, the term is more appropriately called the *PNA*.

TABLE 12.3	Commonly Used Formulas for Calculating Dietary Protein Intake

Formula for Calculating PNA	
Randerson I	PNA = 10.76 (UNA / 1.44 + 1.46), where UNA is in g/d
Randerson II	PNA = 10.76 (UNA + 1.46), where UNA is in mg/min
Modified Borah	PNA = 9.35 G_{un} + 0.294 V + protein losses
Teehan	PNA = 6.25 (UN_{loss} + 1.81 + 0.031 BW)
Kjeldahl	PNA = 6.25 × N. loss
Bergstrom	PNA = 19 + 7.62 × UNA

PNA, protein equivalent of nitrogen appearance; UNA, urea nitrogen appearance; BW, body weight.
Modified from Kopple JD, Jones MR, Keshaviah PK, et al. A proposed glossary for dialysis kinetics. *Am J Kidney Dis* 1995;26:963–981; Keshaviah P, Nolph K. Protein catabolic rate calculations in CAPD patients. *ASAIO Trans* 1991;37:M400–M402.

Keshaviah and Nolph (110) have compared these formulas and recommended the Randerson equation (111), where PNA = 10.76 (UNA + 1.46), and UNA is in milligram per minute, or PNA = 10.76 (UNA / 1.44 + 1.46), and UNA is in gram per day. These equations assume that the patient is in a steady state where UNA = urea nitrogen output which equals urea generation. The Randerson equation also assumes that the average daily protein loss in the dialysate is 7.3 g/d. In dialysis patients with substantial urinary or dialysate protein losses, these direct protein losses must be added to the equation to yield a true PNA. Most societies had historically recommended monitoring a patient's estimated DPI over time to assure adequate nutritional status. This was not recommended in the most recent KDOQI guideline for adequacy of PD. If used, a baseline PNA should be obtained during training. These should then be recalculated every 4 to 6 months using the same 24-hour dialysate and urine collections used to monitor solute clearances. Decreasing values would then suggest a decreasing protein intake. One cause for this may be a suboptimal total solute clearance.

For comparison purposes, it is recommended that PNA be normalized for patient size (nPNA). The weight to use for that normalization is contested. Depending on what weight is used in calculating nPNA, there may or may not be a statistical relationship between clinical evidence of malnutrition and nPNA values below target. The PNA normalized by actual weight tends to be high or may appear to be increasing over time in malnourished individuals who are losing body weight if normalized (divided) by a smaller malnourished weight when compared to the patient's baseline weight (112). This fact is important not only for evaluating patient to patient comparisons but more importantly when comparing serial measurements in an individual patient. The DOQI working group and others have recommended using standard weight or V/0.58 for normalization (113). In this case, the weight used for normalization does not change over time so that nPNA is more likely to reflect actual changes in DPI. Although most guidelines recommend monitoring estimated nPNA over time, looking for changes, it has been suggested that in cross-sectional analysis that the absolute amount of protein intake, not nPNA, correlated best with outcome and signs of malnutrition.

Data from the Centers for Medicare & Medicaid Services–Clinical Performance Measures (CMS–CPM) project for the year 2000 found that in chronic PD patients, the mean nPNA was 0.95 ± 0.31 g/kg/d, their normalized creatinine appearance rate was 17 ± 6.5 mg/kg/d, and the mean percentage of LBM was 64% ± 17% of actual body weight (ABW) (114).

There is some controversy as to what amount of DPI, in terms of grams of protein per kilogram of body weight, is needed to maintain positive nitrogen balance in PD patients. Early studies suggested that a DPI of at least 1.2 g/kg/d was needed to maintain nitrogen balance (115,116), a value considerably higher than that recommended for normal individuals. The 2001 NKF Clinical Practice DOQI guidelines recently recommended a DPI for chronic PD patients of 1.2 to 1.3 g/kg/d (117). Cross-sectional studies by Bergstrom and Lindholm (64) and Nolph (118) suggest that their patients who show no signs of malnutrition seem to eat less (0.99, 0.88 g protein/kg/d, respectively). The results are likely due to variations in the patient populations studied, historical dietary patterns, and amounts of RRF present. Therefore, several investigators have proposed that the daily protein intake in these patients should be in the range of 0.9 to 1.1 g/kg/d (119,120). It is interesting to note that the 2006 KDOQI guidelines do not have a guideline for protein intake due to the fact that there are no recent PRCTs that have evaluated the effect of increasing protein intake on relative risk of death.

Patients undergoing chronic PD should target a total daily energy intake of at least 35 kcal/kg/d for patients who are younger than 60 years and 30 kcal/kg for patients 60 years or older (117,121,122). This includes both dietary intake and the energy intake derived from glucose absorbed from the peritoneal dialysate. Many patients will typically eat less (122,123). Food supplements, enteral tube feedings, and both intradialytic and total parenteral nutrition have been used to treat malnutrition (124). Percutaneous endoscopic gastrostomy tubes should be used cautiously, however, as their use has been associated with a high rate of peritonitis. In addition, bicarbonate supplementation can result in improvements in weight and BMI (125). It is important to note however that for many PD patients, the dialysate glucose that is absorbed is a significant portion of their total caloric intake.

Subjective Global Assessment Score

One instrument that assesses nutritional status, the SGA score (126) has been modified for PD and was shown to be a valid estimate of nutritional status in PD patients (127). In the CANUSA study, a modified SGA using a 7-point scale addressing four items (weight change, anorexia, subcutaneous tissue, and muscle mass) predicted outcome (14). On multivariate analysis, poorer SGA scores were associated with a higher relative risk of death. It is recommended that this simple test be obtained sequentially (twice a year) in PD patients to evaluate nutritional status. If a decline is noted, evaluate for comorbid diseases and consider a suboptimal total solute clearance as the cause.

Possible Interventions for Suspected Malnutrition

Possible interventions when albumin is low include increasing the dialysis dose if "underdialysis" is suspected; restricting dietary sodium intake, water intake, or consider use of diuretics to increase urine volume and minimize use of hypertonic glucose if satiety from glucose is suspected (remember that the absorbed glucose is actually a source of calories); treating any poor dentation that is present; and if available, considering use of alternative dialysate solutions such as amino acid solutions. Initial observations suggest that use of amino acid–containing fluids can lead to an elevation in the plasma albumin concentration and improvement in other biochemical parameters of nutritional status (128,129); however, data are conflicting as to if this can be sustained without side effects if more than one exchange per day are used. Consensus exists that if used only once a day, they are generally safe and are associated with daily protein and amino acid gains that exceed daily amino acid losses although they may not significantly improve albumin concentrations (130).

◆ MAJOR DETERMINANTS OF TOTAL SOLUTE CLEARANCE

Small solute clearance is typically measured in terms of urea kinetics (Kt/V_{urea}) and $Ccr/1.73$ m^2. Guidelines (reviewed earlier) recommend attaining certain minimal "total" (peritoneal and residual kidney) clearances per week.

Residual Renal Function

Creatinine and urea are used as surrogate markers for small molecular weight clearance. When calculating the Ccr due to RRF, it is important to remember that at very low GFRs or Ccrs, much of the creatinine in the urine is due to proximal tubular secretion rather than actual glomerular filtration. As a result, traditional measurements of Ccr (24-hour collection) can significantly overestimate the true GFR. If using creatinine kinetics as the surrogate, it is recommended that the sum of the measured urea clearance and Ccr divided by 2 be used to approximate underlying residual kidney GFR. This amount in liters per day is then added to the daily peritoneal Ccr to determine total daily Ccr. The clearance of most other small molecular weight substances such as urea by the kidney only involves glomerular filtration and little to no tubular secretion. Therefore, if one is measuring dialysis dose using urea kinetics, no adjustment for tubular secretion is needed.

Each 1 mL/min of corrected residual kidney Ccr (measured as GFR) adds approximately 10 L/wk/1.73 m² of Ccr for the average patient with a BSA of 1.73 m². Similarly, each 1 mL/min of residual renal urea clearance adds approximately 0.25 Kt/V_{urea} units to the total weekly Kt/V_{urea} urea for a 70-kg male. At the initiation of dialysis, residual kidney function often represents a significant amount of the recommended minimal solute clearances. In one report, the residual kidney component represented 39% of total clearance (131), while representing 25% of the total in another review (132). If a patient starts PD with a residual kidney Ccr of 5 mL/min (not an unusual scenario), the corrected kidney CCr (GFR) may be approximately 4 mL/min, adding approximately 40 L/wk of Ccr to overall solute clearance, whereas the residual kidney urea clearance might be approximately 3 mL/min (a weekly RRF Kt/V_{urea} of about 0.75 for a 70-kg male). In this instance, a patient may only need to do one or two exchanges per day at the start of dialysis.

Some have suggested that RRF is better preserved with PD than with HD (123–136). It is acknowledged that residual renal clearance is an important supplement to that provided by dialysis and is an important predictor of outcome. As RRF decreases, total clearance expressed as Kt/V_{urea} or Ccr will decrease unless replaced by an increase in the peritoneal component. Tattersall et al. (137,138) have shown that it was possible to compensate for declining RRF and maintain minimal solute clearance goals by increasing dialysis dose as residual kidney function declines. This is a common practice in PD units where "incremental dialysis" is prescribed and dialysis dose increased over time as RRF decreases.

Peritoneal Membrane Transport Characteristics

The first step in tailoring an individual patient's PD prescription is to know that patient's peritoneal membrane transport characteristics. Unlike HD, where the physician has a wide menu of dialyzers to choose from for each individual patient, PD patients are "born" with their membrane. At present, there is no clinically proven way to favorably change membrane transport or predict transport type before beginning PD.

The peritoneal equilibration test (PET) (139) is the standard way to characterize peritoneal membrane transport properties of an individual patient. It is a standardized test in which, after an overnight dwell, 2 L of 2.5% dextrose dialysate is instilled (time 0) and allowed to dwell for 4 hours. Dialysate urea, glucose, sodium, and creatinine are measured at time 0, and after 2 and 4 hours of dwell time. Serum values are drawn after 2 hours. Dialysate is drained after 4 hours of dwell, and drain volume (DV) is measured. Dialysate to plasma (D/P) ratios of creatinine and urea are determined after 2 and 4 hours of dwell, as is the ratio of dialysate glucose at a particular drain time to the initial dialysate glucose concentration

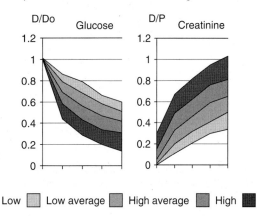

Peritoneal equilibration test :
comparison of D/P creatinine and D/Do glucose values

FIGURE 12.3 Dialysate to plasma (D/P) ratio urea and dialysate glucose at time of sampling to dialysate glucose at time zero ratios for glucose during typical 4-hour dwell with 2.5% dextrose. D/Do, dialysate glucose concentration. (Modified from Twardowski ZJ, Nolph KD, Khanna R, et al. Peritoneal equilibration test. *Perit Dial Bull* 1987;7:138–147; Twardowski ZJ, Khanna R, Nolph KD. Peritoneal dialysis modifications to avoid CAPD dropouts. In: Khanna R, Nolph KD, Prowant BF, et al, eds. *Advances in Continuous Ambulatory Peritoneal Dialysis*. Proceedings of the Seventh Annual CAPD Conference, Kansas City, Missouri, February 1987. Toronto, Canada: Peritoneal Dialysis Bulletin, 1987:171–178.)

(D/Do) (**FIGURE 12.3**). On the basis of published data, the patient's peritoneal membrane type is then characterized as high, high average, low average, and low. In a review of 806 patients, 10.4% were found to be high transporters, 53.1% high average, 30.9% low average, and 5.6% low transporters (140). Once characterized, the PD prescription that would best match the patient's transport characteristics can be then chosen.

These D/P ratios can be calculated for any solute. By doing so, one can appreciate the difference in expected clearances for various sized solutes. For instance, as noted in **FIGURE 12.4** urea (molecular weight: 60 Da) is transported faster than creatinine (molecular

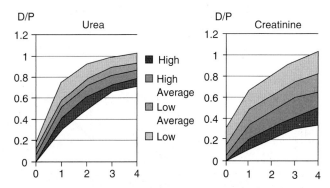

FIGURE 12.4 Dialysate to plasma (D/P) ratios for creatinine and urea. D/P ratios for urea and creatinine during the standard peritoneal equilibration test. Exact values at 2 and 4 hours are shown. (Modified from Twardowski ZJ, Nolph KD, Khanna R, et al. Peritoneal equilibration test. *Perit Dial Bull* 1987;7:138–147; Twardowski ZJ, Khanna R, Nolph KD. Peritoneal dialysis modifications to avoid CAPD dropouts. In: Khanna R, Nolph KD, Prowant BF, et al, eds. *Advances in Continuous Ambulatory Peritoneal Dialysis*. Proceedings of the Seventh Annual CAPD Conference, Kansas City, Missouri, February 1987. Toronto, Canada: Peritoneal Dialysis Bulletin, 1987:171–178.)

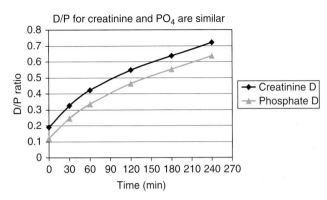

FIGURE 12.5 Theoretic constructs for dialysate to plasma (D/P) ratios of creatinine and phosphorous (PO₄) during a peritoneal dialysis dwell.

weight: 112 Da). Most patients are greater than 90% equilibrated for urea after a 4-hour dwell, whereas for creatinine, the average patient is only 65% equilibrated at 4 hours. As noted in the figure, these differences are even more marked for low transporters and is clinically most noted when using a therapy that utilizes multiple short dwells (CCPD, NIPD). Phosphate has a larger molecular weight than creatinine but is similar in size, so creatinine removal can be used as a surrogate for phosphate removal (**FIGURE 12.5**).

Solute removal by PD is related to the concentration of the solute in question in the dialysate (D/P ratio) and the dialysate DV. Patients with small DVs tend to have lower clearances. UF during a dwell is related to crystalloid (glucose, amino acid) or colloid (icodextrin)-induced osmotic forces. It is important to point out that rapid transporters of creatinine/urea also tend to be rapid absorbers of dialysate glucose. Once the osmotic glucose gradient is mitigated by absorption, UF ceases and lymphatic absorption of fluid predominates (**FIGURE 12.6**). Therefore, in rapid transporters, although the D/P ratios of urea and creatinine at 4 hours or longer dwells tend to be close to unity, their DVs tend to be small and hence their solute removal is less than optimal due to the small DVs

(141). In fact, during the long overnight dwell of CAPD (9 hours) or during the long daytime dwell of classic CCPD (15 hours), rapid transporters may have DVs that are actually less than the *instilled* volume. For these patients, short dwell times are needed to reduce or minimize fluid reabsorption and optimize clearances. In patients who are low transporters, intraperitoneal glucose is slowly absorbed; hence, peak UF occurs later during the dwell and net UF can be obtained even after prolonged dwells. In these patients, the D/P ratio increases almost linearly during the dwell. It is not until 8 to 10 hours that the D/P ratio reaches unity.

To put these differences in perspective, one can appreciate that after only a 2-hour dwell time, a rapid transporter likely will have achieved 2 L of Ccr, whereas the Ccr in a low transport individual may be only 1 L or less, despite a larger DV (**FIGURE 12.7**). It may take the low transporter up to 7 or 8 hours of dwell time to achieve the same clearance that a rapid transporter achieves after only a 2-hour dwell. These differences must be taken into account when attempting to tailor an individual patient's PD prescription.

Peritoneal membrane transport tends to remain stable over time. Rippe and Krediet (142) reviewed 9 cross-sectional and 16 longitudinal studies of peritoneal transport. In 14 out of 25 studies, there tended to be no change in peritoneal transport over time on PD; in the other 11 out of 25 studies, there was a slight increase in low/medium molecular weight solute transport over time. Others found no change in peritoneal transport in 23 patients followed up for at least 7 years (143), especially in patients with low peritonitis rates (144). In contrast, there was a tendency toward increase in small solute transport and loss of UF, especially in patients with frequent peritonitis (145,146). Others have noted that up to 30.9% of patients developed UF failure (change in transport) after 6 years on PD (147). These data emphasize the importance of monitoring membrane transport (usually with PET testing) over time to optimize solute clearance, DVs, BP, and UF, while minimizing hypertonic glucose use. If peritoneal transport type changes, the patient's prescription may need to be altered.

The PET is the most practical and widely used method to classify peritoneal transport; however, there are also other ways. In

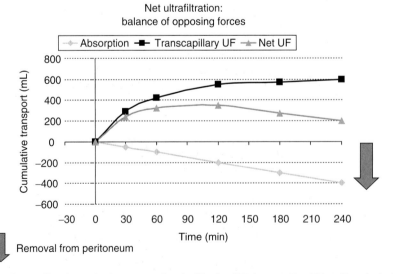

FIGURE 12.6 Time profiles of opposing forces governing ultrafiltration (UF) (transcapillary UF) and lymphatic absorption. *Diamond*, lymphatic absorption; *square*, transcapillary ultrafiltration; *triangle*, net ultrafiltration. (Modified from Mactier RA, Khanna R, Twardowski ZJ, et al. Contribution of lymphatic absorption to loss of ultrafiltration and solute clearances on continuous ambulatory peritoneal dialysis. *J Clin Invest* 1987;80:1311–1316.)

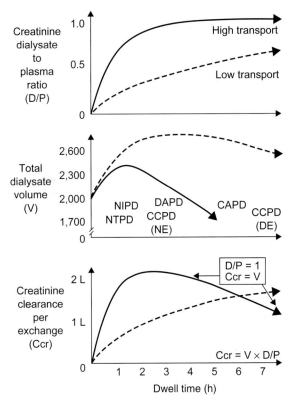

FIGURE 12.7 Comparison of idealized curves for solute and water transport during an exchange in patients with low and high transport characteristics. Idealized curves of creatinine and water transport during an exchange with 2 L of 2.5% glucose dialysis solutions in patients with extremely low and high transport characteristics. NIPD, nightly intermittent peritoneal dialysis; DAPD, daytime ambulatory peritoneal dialysis; CAPD, continuous ambulatory peritoneal dialysis; NTPD, nightly tidal peritoneal dialysis; NE, nightly exchange; DE, daytime exchange; CCPD, continuous cyclic peritoneal dialysis. [From Twardowski ZJ. Nightly peritoneal dialysis (Why? who? how? and when?). *ASAIO Trans* 1990;36:8–16.]

these other tests, instead of using D/P ratios, these tests use mass transfer area coefficients (MTACs) (148,149), which are more precise and more succinctly define transport. The MTACs define transport independent of UF (convection-related solute removal) and hence in theory are not influenced by dwell volume or glucose concentration. The practical use of MTAC for modeling a PD prescription requires additional laboratory measurements and computer models but once obtained, MTAC can be easily used in the clinical setting (150). The standard peritoneal permeability analysis is another less often used test to follow transport and UF characteristics (151). The test not only determines transport characteristics but also better evaluates lymphatic reabsorption. If one does a PET using 4.25% dextrose dwell rather than the classic 2.5% dextrose dwell to maximize UF, one is better able to determine actual UF properties of the membrane the amount of sodium sieving and can better differentiate the causes of UF failure (152,153).

Normalization and Influence of Body Size on Solute Clearance

Removal of the same absolute amount of solute from a 55-kg elderly woman as from an 80-kg muscular man may not result in the same control of uremia. These patients likely have different metabolic rates and protein intakes. Therefore, the absolute amount of daily solute

removed or cleared must be normalized for differences in body size (traditionally when using urea as a surrogate, it is normalized by V or volume of distribution for Kt/V$_{urea}$ and by BSA for Ccr/1.73 m^2).

Kt/V$_{urea}$ is normalized by V, whereas Ccr in L/wk/1.73 m^2 by BSA. For recommended formulas, see **TABLE 12.4**. TBW (V) can be estimated as a fixed percentage of body weight, or more accurately, by using anthropometric formulas based on sex, age, height, and weight such as the Watson et al. (154) or Hume and Weyers (155) formulas in adults. These equations provide unrealistic estimates for V in patients whose weights are markedly different than normal body weight (NBW). BSA is usually calculated using the formula by Dubois and Dubois (156).

In a review of 806 patients with PD, the median BSA was 1.85 m^2 (not 1.73 m^2), the 25th percentile was 1.71 m^2, and the 75th percentile was 2.0m^2 (140), whereas data from the CMS–CPM project for the year 2000 found that chronic patients with PD had a mean body weight of 76 ± 19 kg and BMI of 27.5 ± 6.4 kg/m^2 (109). Despite the finding that most PD patients are larger than the "standard" BSA of 1.73 m^2, a review of the predicted clearances for Kt/V$_{urea}$ for an average transporter over a broad range of BSA suggests that if one was able to individualize therapy (increased instilled volumes, daytime exchange for CCPD, nightly exchange device), one should be able to achieve the recommended acceptable target total Kt/V$_{urea}$ clearances for most patients on PD (157). On the basis of the patient's body size, one can predict whether or not an individual patient who is an average transporter would meet NKF-DOQI targets for small solute clearance using four 2-L exchanges/d once they were anuric (158–160) and also what instilled volume/prescription would be needed to achieve the small solute clearance targets. Only anuric patients who are low transporters and who have large BSAs (greater than 1.8 m^2) would not be likely to achieve these targets.

For malnourished patients whose weight is more than 10% below than their ideal weight, the NKF-DOQI guidelines recommend adjusting total solute clearance targets by the ratio of ideal/actual weight. In this case, a relatively higher target solute removal to promote anabolism and an increased protein intake is targeted. Jones (161) noted that when ABW was used for normalization, there was no difference in total solute clearance (Kt/V or Ccr) between patients who were well nourished and those who were malnourished. However, when calculated V and BSA were determined using desired body weight (dBW), there was a statistically significant difference between the groups for both weekly Kt/V$_{urea}$ (1.68 ± 0.46 vs. 1.40 ± 0.41, p <0.05) and for Ccr in liters per 1.73 m^2 per week (52.5 ± 10.3 vs. 41.6 ± 19.0, p <0.01).

It is noted that large patients (BMI greater than 27.5) on PD tend to do as well as or better than patients who are within 10% of their ideal weight (162). If one uses actual weight versus ideal weight, there is a marked difference in adequacy calculations (**TABLE 12.5**). Some have managed their patients, adjusting the PD prescription based on Kt/V urea and Ccr/1.73 m^2, where the normalization calculations were done using ideal weight when calculating V or BSA found no difference in survival for patients whose actual weights were more than 10% above their ideal weight when compared to those whose weights were within 10% of ideal weight (34). Currently, it is still unclear what weight to use when calculating Kt/V or Ccr in obese individuals. However, it is clear that many obese patients do very well on PD and if clearances are individualized, most are able to achieve target. Unfortunately, this often results in transfer from PD to HD because the adequacy number is not above target despite fact that the NKF-DOQI guidelines suggested to attempt to reach recommended targets. If one cannot, look at

TABLE 12.4	Equations for Normalization (Calculating V for Kt/V or BSA for Creatinine Clearance)

Formula for Estimating BSA

For all formulas, weight (Wt) is in kilogram and height (Ht) is in centimeter:

DuBois and Dubois method:	$BSA\ (m^2) = 0.007184 \times Wt^{0.425} \times Ht^{0.725}$
Gehan and George method:	$BSA\ (m^2) = 0.235 \times Wt^{0.51456} \times Ht^{0.42246}$
Haycock method:	$BSA\ (m^2) = 0.024265 \times Wt^{0.5378} \times Ht^{0.3964}$

Formulas for Estimating V

Watson Method		
For men:	V (L)	$= 2.447 + 0.3362 \times Wt\ (kg) + 0.1074 \times Ht\ (cm) - 0.09516 \times Age\ (yr)$
For women:	V	$= 2.097 + 0.2466 \times Wt + 0.1069 \times Ht$
Hume Method		
For men:	V (L)	$= -14.012934 + 0.296785 \times Wt + 0.194786 \times Ht$
For women:	V	$= -35.270121 + 0.183809 \times Wt + 0.344547 \times Ht$
Mellits-Cheek Method for Children		
For boys:	V (L)	$= -1.927 + 0.465 \times Wt\ (kg) + 0.045 \times Ht\ (cm)$, when height is ≤ 132.7 cm
	V	$= -31.993 + 0.406 \times Wt + 0.209 \times Ht$, when height is ≥ 132.7 cm
For girls:	V	$= 0.076 + 0.507 \times Wt + 0.013 \times Ht$, when height is < 110.8 cm
	V	$= -10.313 + 0.252 \times Wt\ 0.154 \times Ht$, when height is ≥ 110.8 cm

BSA, body surface area.

Data from Dubois D, Dubois EF. A formula to estimate the approximate surface area if height and weight be known. *Arch Intern Med* 1916;17:863–871; Gehan E, George SL. Estimation of human body surface area from height and weight. *Cancer Chemother Rep* 1970;54(Pt 1):225–235; Haycock GB, Chir B, Schwartz GJ, et al. Geometric method for measuring body surface area: a height-weight formula validated in infants, children and adults. *J Pediatr* 1978;93:62–66; Watson PE, Watson ID, Batt RD. Total body water volumes for adult males and females estimated from simple anthropometric measurements. *Am J Clin Nutr* 1980;33:27–39; Hume R, Weyers E. Relationship between total body water and surface area in normal and obese subjects. *J Clin Pathol* 1971;24:234–238; Mellits ED, Cheek DB. The assessment of body water and fatness from infancy to adulthood. *Monographs Soc Res Child Dev* 1970;35:12–26.

the individual and decide how they are doing clinically before one automatically transfer the patient to HD.

SPECIAL CONSIDERATIONS

Rapid Transporters

Rapid transporters tend to optimize both solute clearance and UF after a short dwell time (approximately 2 hours) and, therefore, are likely to do well on short dwell therapies such as NIPD, with or without one or two 2- to 4-hour daytime dwells. One would predict that they would easily reach total small solute clearance goals for Kt/V$_{urea}$ and Ccr, at times reaching that goal while only doing nightly dwells. Despite this relative ease in the ability to achieve recommended minimal total solute clearance goals, some (163–165) but not all (35,166–168) studies have suggested that after controlling for urea

TABLE 12.5	Adequacy Calculations: What Weight Should You Use?		
BW Ratio	**<0.9**	**0.9–1.1**	**>1.1**
Percentage	19	33	48
BWa/BWd	0.82	1.01	1.37
Kt/Va	1.95	2.08	1.94
Kt/Vd	1.74	2.08	2.25
Ccra (L/wk)	68.1	71.5	64.1
Ccrd (L/wk)	62.6	71.7	72.4

BW, body weight; a, actual; d, desired; Ccr, creatinine clearance.

From Satko SG, Burkart JM. Frequency and causes of discrepancy between Kt/V and creatinine. *Perit Dial Int* 1997;17:S23.

clearance rapid transporters tended to have a higher relative risk of death. In the CANUSA study, patients with a 4-hour D/P creatinine of greater than 0.65 (high) were compared to those with a 4-hour D/P creatinine of less than 0.65 (low). The 2-year probability for technique survival was 79% among low transporters compared to 71% for high transporters. The probability of 2-year patient survival was 82% among low transporters versus 72% for high transporters with a relative risk of death of 2.18 for high versus low transporters. Heaf (165) noted increased morbidity in rapid transporters.

The reason(s) for this possible increased relative risk while on CAPD are unclear and may be related to malnutrition (169), increased protein losses in the DV (170–172), or overt or subtle volume overload. This volume overload may lead to increased BP and/or increased left ventricular hypertrophy (LVH) with its associated increased risks of death. Furthermore, to optimize UF, these patients will likely increase their percentage of glucose in fluids, leading to better UF but increased glucose absorption with its associated side effects. A meta-analysis of studies published between 1987 and end of December 2005 that correlated membrane transport and relative risk of death was conducted. Twenty studies were identified, 19 of which were pooled to generate a summary mortality relative risk of 1.15 for every 0.1 increase in the D/P creatinine (95% CI 1.07 to 1.23; $p < 0.001$) (173). They concluded that higher peritoneal membrane status is associated with a higher mortality risk (increased mortality risk of 21.9%, 45.7%, and 77.3% in low-average, high-average, and high transporters, respectively) as compared to low transport status. Note that these historical data tend to be mainly from patients on CAPD. They do not include more contemporary advances in therapy such as newer innovations in automated peritoneal dialysis (APD) therapy and alternative PD solutions designed for better UF such as icodextrin.

Contemporary data has evaluated the death risk for rapid transporters on APD.

Studies that have evaluated a greater proportion of patients on cycler therapy demonstrated a lower mortality risk for a given increase in D/P creatinine compared to studies that mainly enrolled CAPD patients. This is consistent with the reported observational finding that in patients all given the same CAPD prescription, those with high transport status were more likely to be hypertensive (100% vs. 0%) and have LVH (100% vs. 33%) than the low transporters on the same prescription (3 × 1.36% G daytime dwells and 1 × 3.86% G overnight) (174). In these patients, when prescription was altered to increase UF, their BP improved. When these observations were noted, more attention was paid to individualizing the PD prescription for patients with high peritoneal membrane transport. With such maneuvers, it has been shown that patients with high membrane transport can be managed on PD without the increased mortality risk demonstrated in historical studies (175) (**Figure 12.8**). Current data would suggest that patients who are baseline high transporters are not at increased relative risk of death as long as their prescription is managed appropriately.

Acid–Base Metabolism

An essential component of providing "optimal" dialysis is correction of acidosis. Chronic acidosis has a detrimental effect on protein, carbohydrate, and bone metabolism. In patients with CAPD, body base balance is self-regulated by feedback between plasma bicarbonate levels and bicarbonate gain/loss (176). Dialysis must provide sufficient replenishment of buffers to compensate for the daily acid load. Lactate (concentration 35 to 40 mmol/L) is the standard buffer in PD fluids. Lactate is converted to pyruvate and oxygenated or used in gluconeogenesis with the consumption of H+ and the generation of bicarbonate (177). With lactate-containing buffer solutions, buffer balance is governed by the relative amounts of

H+ generation, bicarbonate loss, lactate absorption, and lactate metabolism (178–180). Newer bicarbonate-based solutions are in use in some countries but mainly for their "biocompatibility" properties and not to better treat acidosis (181). Most patients with CAPD have stable mean plasma bicarbonate levels of approximately 25.6 mmol/L using a dialysate lactate of 35 mmol/L, although some patients with CAPD remain mildly acidotic. Increasing dialysate lactate results in a higher serum bicarbonate level (182).

Control of acidosis is important to prevent protein catabolism (183–185); however, two studies have found no correlation between serum albumin levels and bicarbonate concentration (186,187). A recent survey of serum bicarbonate levels in patients with PD showed that only consumption of the phosphate binder sevelamer hydrochloride was associated with a decline in serum bicarbonate concentration (188).

Which Is the Preferred Target–Kt/V or Creatinine Clearance?

Both total Kt/V_{urea} and total Ccr/1.73 m^2 can be used to monitor solute clearance. There are no data to suggest that one index is better than the other. Of course, these solutes are just surrogates for small solute removal; other solutes could be used, but there are currently no data to correlate relative risk of death with the removal of other solutes. Although these two yardsticks do not fall on the same linear scale, the two values usually correlate (189).

If one uses residual kidney and peritoneal clearance of these solutes, it is important to remember the following caveats: Residual renal clearance of a solute is the result of glomerular filtration and tubular manipulation of that filtrate. Ccr by the kidneys is due to glomerular filtration and proximal tubular secretion, especially in advanced stages of kidney insufficiency where the absolute amount tubular creatinine secretion can increase by as much as 30% accounting for up to 35% of total urinary creatinine (190). In contrast, with urea,

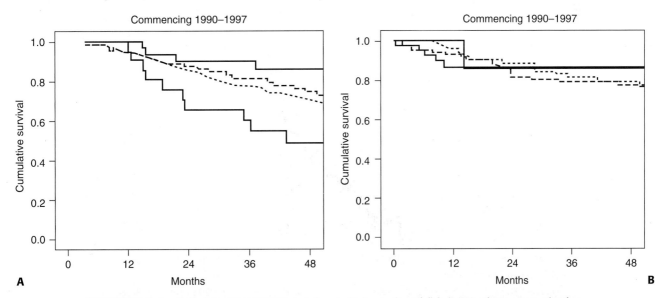

FIGURE 12.8 Correlation between transport type and survival in two peritoneal dialysis (PD) cohorts commencing therapy during different years. Survival on PD [patients censored at transplant or transfer to hemodialysis (HD)] according to transport category at start of treatment comparing two cohorts commencing therapy between **(A)** 1990 to 1997, n = 320, and **(B)** 1998 to 2005, n = 300. Low (*solid line*), low average (*dotted line*), high average (*dashed line*), and high (*solid bold line*). In the first cohort, transport category was significantly (p = 0.0009) associated with survival, whereas in the more recent cohort, transport type was not associated with survival. (From Davies SJ. Mitigating peritoneal membrane characteristics in modern peritoneal dialysis therapy. *Kidney Int* 2006;70:S76–S83.)

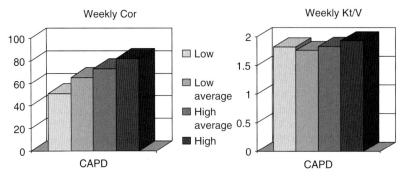

FIGURE 12.9 Representative total weekly Kt/V$_{urea}$ and Ccr/1.73 m^2 for an average 70-kg male, who is an average transporter with various amounts of residual renal function contributing to total solute clearance (100%, 50%, 0%). Ccr, creatinine clearance; BSA, body surface area; CAPD, continuous ambulatory peritoneal dialysis. (Modified from Blake P, Burkart JM, Churchill DN, et al. Recommended clinical practices for maximizing PD clearances. *Perit Dial Int* 1996;16:448–456.)

there is glomerular filtration but also tubular reabsorption. Therefore, in advanced stages of kidney disease, residual renal clearance of creatinine will be relatively greater than that for urea. Peritoneal clearance is predominantly diffusion-driven. (There is also a component of convective clearance due to UF, but this contribution is relatively smaller than that due to diffusion.) Therefore, because urea is a smaller molecular weight solute than creatinine, the numerical value for peritoneal clearance of urea tends to be relatively greater than that for Ccr. This difference is most pronounced in patients who are low transporters (**FIGURE 12.9**).

Peritoneal membrane transport characteristics may also explain this discrepancy. The diffusive clearance for urea is relatively greater than that for creatinine. During the typical dwells associated with CAPD, the D/P ratio for urea tends to reach unity (equilibration between blood and dialysate) in all patients, whereas the D/P for creatinine tends to reach unity only in high transporters. Therefore, the urea clearance/dwell tends to be greater than that for creatinine. This is most pronounced in low transporters.

The guidelines do not differentiate between genders. The patient's weight has a different effect on normalization (V or BSA) for male or female and for Ccr versus Kt/V. In patients with similar BSA, instilled volume, transport type, and gender all have a significant effect on Kt/V calculations but not on Ccr calculations. The mathematical relationship between BSA and V is not fixed. It is disturbed by both gender and obesity. Furthermore, the actual V is different if "obesity" is due to a change in body fat versus a change in body water (overhydration) (191) and if the patient has had an amputation (192). Therefore, in the average anuric patient on 5- to 2-L exchanges per day with average peritoneal transport characteristics, peritoneal Ccr will be 73% of urea clearance (193). Therefore, in an anuric average transporter with a weekly peritoneal Kt/V of 2.0, the expected Ccr is approximately 55 L/1.73 m^2/wk in males and 47 L/1.73 m^2/wk in females. Similarly, for NIPD patients with average transport, the peritoneal Ccr will be 64% of urea. Therefore, for an anuric average transporter on NIPD, with a weekly Kt/V of 2.2, the expected weekly Ccr will be 53 L/1.73 m^2 in males and 45 L/1.73 m^2 in females (**TABLE 12.6**).

TABLE 12.6	Creatinine Clearance (L) at Kt/V of 2.2 in Nightly Intermittent Peritoneal Dialysis (NIPD) and 2.0 in Continuous Ambulatory Peritoneal Dialysis (CAPD)			
	NIPD		**CAPD**	
Transport Category	**Females**	**Males**	**Females**	**Males**
Minimal value	32.90	38.80	30.70	36.30
Low transporters	33.70	39.80	35.70	41.60
Mean ± SD	34.30	40.50	39.40	46.50
Low-average transporters	40.00	47.20	43.20	51.00
Mean	44.70	52.70	46.70	55.10
High-average transporters	48.00	56.60	50.10	59.10
Mean + SD	50.80	59.90	53.20	62.80[a]
High transporters	55.60	65.60	58.10	68.50[a]
Maximal value	59.40	70.00[a]	62.70[a]	73.90[a]

Assumptions: Total body water in males = 41.7 L; total body water in females = 32.1 L; body surface area in males = 1.92 m^2; body surface area in females = 1.74 m^2; NIPD (nocturnal intermittent peritoneal dialysis): hourly 2-L exchanges. CAPD (continuous ambulatory peritoneal dialysis): five 2-L exchanges. SD, standard deviation.
[a]Values are above the Dialysis Outcomes Quality Initiative guidelines for creatinine clearance at recommended Kt/V.
From Twardowski ZJ. Relationships between creatinine clearances and Kt/V in peritoneal dialysis patients: a critique of the DOQI document. *Perit Dial Int* 1998;18:252–255.

There are no clinical outcome data to support the use of one solute clearance yardstick (Ccr or Kt/V) over the other. Most of the published outcome data is related to Kt/V_{urea}. NKF-DOQI guidelines and others (194) have historically suggested that one should always strive to at least have Kt/V_{urea} above target, stating that there was no additional benefit to using Ccr. As reviewed earlier, current guidelines use Kt/V_{urea} as the "dose surrogate."

VOLUME AND BLOOD PRESSURE CONTROL ISSUES

CV disease continues to be the leading cause of death in patients with ESKD. There is a high prevalence of LVH and congestive heart failure (CHF) in patients initiating dialysis. The prevalence of LVH is higher in the elderly population and is increasing yearly (195). It is well known that predisposing factors for the development of LVH include volume overload and hypertension.

Multiple observational studies have compared BP and volume status in PD and HD patients. Counterintuitive to what would be expected in a PD patient where there is an opportunity for daily control of extracellular volume, PD patients tend to be volume expanded (**FIGURE 12.10**). Using bioimpedance measurements (BIA) to determine intracellular and extracellular fluid spaces, it was noted that both TBW and extracellular fluid volume (Vecf) were actually greater in PD patients than both before and after dialysis values in chronic HD patients and baseline values of healthy controls (196). Furthermore, the ratio of Vecf/TBW positively correlated with systolic BP and negatively correlated with serum albumin levels. Others have shown that CAPD patients have an increase in mean pulmonary artery pressure when compared to HD patients. In that study, pulmonary artery pressures were measured pretransplant in both PD and HD patients and found to be a mean of 22 + 7 mm Hg in 56 CAPD patients and 16.3 + 7.2 mm Hg in 296 HD patients ($p < 0.01$) (197). In another study, it was shown that CAPD patients ($n = 28$) had a considerable fall in "dry weight" (66.6 + 2.3 kg on PD vs. 62.4 + 2.4 kg on HD, $p < 0.05$) after transfer to HD (3). This was associated with no change in systolic BP but a significant improvement in diastolic BP. These observations

suggest that PD patients tend to be chronically plasma volume overloaded.

Uncontrolled hypertension due to volume overload is thought to contribute to higher left ventricular mass in CAPD patients (198). Some have demonstrated that long-term PD patients were more likely to have LVH than long-term HD patients (199). In that study, 51 CAPD patients were compared to a group of 201 HD patients. LVH was more severe in CAPD patients than in HD patients ($p < 0.0001$), and CAPD patients were more likely to need antihypertensive medications (65% vs. 38%, $p < 0.001$) despite CAPD patients being younger. Note this study was done in CAPD patients, and it is uncertain if individualization of prescription and use of APD would alter the results. Hypertension is a common finding in the PD patient with reported prevalence in PD populations of between 29% and 88% (104,200,201) (**FIGURE 12.11**). Conventional wisdom would suggest that hypertension in patients with ESKD is in part related to volume expansion and presumably excess total body sodium. As will be discussed, due to "sodium sieving" across aquaporins, it is important to remember that with PD, not all of the UF volume is always sodium replete. In fact, the UF volumes of the short dwells of APD when using dextrose-based solutions may be up to 50% sodium-free.

Interestingly in HD patients, it has been noted that with chronic expansion of extracellular space, BP increases slowly over weeks to months (202). Short-term expansion of extracellular space tended not to have a major effect on BP and slow reduction in dry weight was associated with a gradual decrease in BP (203). This suggests that acute volume expansion *per se* may not be the only mechanism that causes hypertension in patients with ESKD, rather the increase in peripheral vascular resistance associated with chronic volume expansion (a situation not uncommon in a PD patient) may play a key role, and therefore, close attention to dry weight and patient's BP needs to be addressed in every PD patient.

The relationship between BP control and risk of death in patients with ESKD is controversial. Some observational studies suggest that in fact, there seems to be a reverse epidemiology, where in contrast to what is noted in the general population, the lower the systolic BP, the higher the relative risk of death in patients with

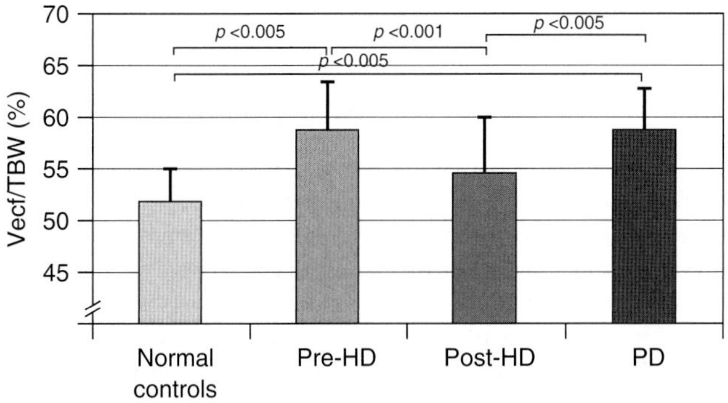

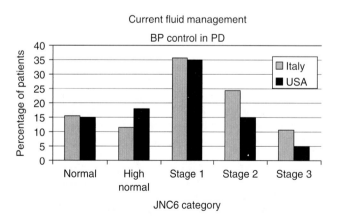

FIGURE 12.10 Volume status in peritoneal dialysis (PD) and hemodialysis (HD) (both pre- and postdialysis). Ratio of Vecf/TBW in HD patients (measured pre- and postdialysis, in PD patients and in healthy subjects. Measurements were performed after 20 minutes in the supine position using multifrequency bioimpedance. Vecf, volume of extracellular fluid; TBW, total body water. (From Plum J, Shoenicke G, Kleophas W, et al. Comparison of body fluid distribution between chronic hemodialysis and peritoneal dialysis patients as assessed by biophysical and biochemical methods. *Nephrol Dial Transplant* 2001;16:2378–2385.)

FIGURE 12.11 Blood pressure (BP) control in peritoneal dialysis (PD) patients. BP control in PD patients in Italy and the United States per Joint National Commission recommendations version 6. (Modified from Frankenfield DL, Prowant BF, Flanigan MJ, et al. Trends in clinical indicators of care for adult peritoneal dialysis patients in the United States from 1995 to 1997. *Kidney Int* 1999;55:1998–2010; Cocchi R, Degli Esposti E, Fabbri A, et al. Prevalence of hypertension in patients on peritoneal dialysis: results of an Italian multicentre study. *Nephrol Dial Transplant* 1999;14:1536–1540.)

ESKD (204,205). Others have shown a "U"-shaped curve, wherein patients with both the lowest and highest postdialysis systolic BP have an increased relative risk of death (206). This observation could be due to the fact that in the population with ESKD, it is a "selective" cohort and in fact patients with the lowest BP may have comorbidities (CHF, malnutrition) that contribute to this increased risk; alternatively, this finding may be related to the HD procedure itself. If due to the HD procedure itself, PD patients would not have this reverse epidemiologic observation. In a prospective observational study of 125 PD patients where the mean BP was 131.2 ± 17.4/83.4 ± 9.8 mm Hg, BP was found to be an independent predictor of mortality—no reverse epidemiology was seen. Hypertensive patients (not defined) had a significantly worse 3-year survival than normotensives (60.5% vs. 92.1%, respectively; $p = 0.0001$). Similarly, total ($p = 0.001$) and CV ($p < 0.01$) hospitalizations were significantly worse in hypertensive patients (207). This study did not define a BP target. To examine the association between BP control and various clinical outcomes, 1,053 random PD patients from the USRDS Dialysis Morbidity and Mortality Study (DMMS) wave 2 study were evaluated (208). Using a Cox model and adjusting for covariates and a mean follow-up of only 23 months, these authors found that the two lowest BP categories (systolic BP less than 100 mm Hg and systolic BP 101 to 110 mm Hg) were associated with an increased all-cause and CV-related mortality. They did not find a similar association for diastolic BP. This study could not evaluate for the development of comorbidities during follow-up (new-onset CHF), nor were they able to adjust for differences in confounding factors between groups or over time. Higher systolic BP was associated with shorter duration hospitalization. They concluded that based on their data, aggressive treatment of hypertension should be done with caution in the PD population and again did not establish a BP target. In the European Automated Peritoneal Dialysis Outcomes Study (EAPOS), there was no significant relationship between BP and survival when examined as a continuous variable [relative risk (RR) 0.99/mm Hg, $p = 0.188$]. When evaluated by tertiles, there was no significant difference by category ($p = 0.23$), although there was a tendency toward an earlier death in the lowest BP tertile (209).

As a result of these studies, a specific "target" BP for PD patients cannot be recommended. In fact, there have been no prospective randomized trials done in an attempt to identify what BP should be targeted in an attempt to improve an individual patient's outcome as there has been in the general population. Furthermore, there is little evidence to show which antihypertensive would be "best" to use in the PD patient for BP control. However, because there are data to suggest using an angiotensin-converting enzyme (ACE) or adrenergic receptor binder (ARB) for CV protection, preservation of RRF (58,59,210), or stabilization of peritoneal membrane transport characteristics, it is recommended that one consider giving preference to using these agents. The 2006 NKF-DOQI guidelines did not give a target BP but recommended that one should try to control BP with less aggressive approaches than used in the general population and that one should consider use of an ACE or an ARB. They further recommended that "one should optimize volume status because of the detrimental effect of volume overload on CHF, LVH, and BP control," stating, "Each facility should implement a program that monitors and reviews peritoneal dialysate DVs, RRF and BP control on a monthly basis, and that some of the therapies one should consider to optimize extracellular water and blood volume include but are not limited to restricting dietary sodium intake, use

of diuretics in patients with RRF and optimization of peritoneal UF volume and sodium removal" (8).

How Does One Achieve Euvolemia in Peritoneal Dialysis?

A rational approach to fluid management in PD has been reviewed elsewhere (211,212). In the reevaluation of the CANUSA study, it was shown that residual kidney volume, not peritoneal UF, was predictive of outcome (25). In another study, both fluid and sodium removal were independent predictors of death (207). The survival rate increased linearly with both fluid and sodium removal. Elevated systolic BP correlated positively with risk of death and negatively with salt and water removal. In a cohort of anuric APD patients, all obtaining a certain minimal small solute clearance, peritoneal UF not small solute clearance was predictive of outcome (213). Some have shown that aggressive interventions directed at controlling blood volume using salt restriction and, if needed, alterations of the PD prescription to improve UF can result in control of BP in most patients without the need to use antihypertensive medications (214). More data relating to the effect of fluid removal on outcome are needed; however, these preliminary data do underscore the clinical significance of including BP and volume control as part of adequacy of any dialysis therapy. As with small solute clearance issues, what is not as clear is if the same volume removed by PD alone is as predictive as that removed by the native kidney.

As with any other solute, achievement of a steady state is related to removing the same amount of solute that is either ingested or produced/generated during a specified time. So if one is interested in controlling BP and volume in patients on PD, then obtaining the desired steady state for sodium and TBW are key to success. It is important therefore not to forget dietary restrictions if indicated. Although historically one tended to be less restrictive of sodium intake in a PD patient, one should always consider dietary sodium restriction as an intervention. One also needs to consider all the ways that sodium and water are removed. Again, remember the importance of urine volume and use of diuretic when possible. One should also be cognizant of how sodium and water are removed with PD and how they cross from the blood side to the dialysate. It is best to picture the pathways as a series of pores, some of which are functional aquaporins similar to what are found in the kidney. These aquaporins only allow the passage of water, whereas other "pores"—the so-called small and large pores—allow passage of water and any solute in that water fits through the pore (convective removal) as well of passage of a solute down concentration gradients (diffusion) independent of any water movement. Both of these processes (diffusion and convection) and both of these pathways (pores and aquaporins) are important factors when considering BP and volume control in PD patients. During a typical glucose dwell, water moves from the blood side to dialysate via small pores, large pores, and aquaporins. Given the fact that glucose is also absorbed via small and large pores and therefore exerts very little osmotic gradient across those pores and that aquaporins only allow passage of water, it turns out that about 50% of the UF volume during a dextrose dwell is sodium-free or "free water." If the dwell time is long enough, sodium can catch up to that free water by diffusion and if long enough, all the UF will be sodium replete. In contrast with icodextrin, the gradient is the same across all pores (small and large and aquaporins). In this case, because greater than 95% of the pore surface area are the small and large pores, the UF with icodextrin is essentially sodium replete. These differences are important when managing a PD patient and trying to control BP and volume.

TABLE 12.7	Likely Pathways for Peritoneal Fluid and Solute Removal	
Glucose-Based Solutions	**Icodextrin-Based Solutions**	
Crystalloid-induced osmosis	Colloid-induced osmosis	
Water transport through	Water transport through	
Small and ultrasmall pores	Small pores predominantly	
Small solute movement	Small solute transport	
By diffusion through small pores	By diffusion through small pores	
By convection through small pores	By convection through small pores	
Macromolecule movement	Macromolecule movement	
Across large pores and into lymphatics	Across large pores and into lymphatics	
Osmotic agent (glucose)	Osmotic agent (icodextrin)	
Rapidly absorbed by diffusion	Slowly absorbed into lymphatics	
Across small and large pores		

Classic PD solutions contain glucose as the osmotic agent. Glucose is readily absorbed from the peritoneal cavity, and as it is, the osmotic concentration of the intraperitoneal dialysate approaches that of blood. When there no longer is an osmotic gradient for crystalloid-induced UF, lymphatic reabsorption of fluid predominates and the intraperitoneal and eventual DV decreases. As a result, during the long dwell (overnight) in CAPD or during the long daytime dwell of APD, this phenomenon is likely to occur. Up to 30% of CAPD patients actually absorb fluid during their overnight dwell if using 1.5% dextrose PD solutions. Increasing the percentage of dextrose from 1.5% to 2.5% or 4.25% decreases the percentage of patients with negative net UF to approximately 20% and 5%, respectively, whereas if on APD therapies, 80% of patients may have fluid adsorption during the "long" daytime dwell if using 2.5% dextrose versus 20% of patients using 4.25% dextrose (211). This means that in an anuric patient on APD, the remaining night dwells must first remove this "absorbed" fluid before removing any fluids taken by mouth during the day to maintain fluid balance. However, as discussed earlier, this approach of increasing all the UF during the night results in UF volumes that may be up to 50% sodium-free or "free water." If overnight dwell times are short and multiple dwells are done, this "free water" volume minimally may elevate serum sodium causing thirst when patient wakes up. Because of the known effect of hypertension and volume overload on left ventricular function and risk of death, it is important to focus on maintaining positive UF during the long dwell. This can be done by increasing the tonicity of the dialysate; modifying the dwell time, at times by breaking up the dwell; and by doing two dwells during that same time period or by just doing one short dwell with some dry time. Having dry time may solve the UF problem and maintain small solute clearance but will likely compromise peritoneal middle molecular weight clearance. If available, an alternative would be to use other osmotic agents which result in more sustained UF during the long dwell.

Polyglucose (icodextrin) is a macromolecule and can be used as an alternative osmotic agent (215). It is a mixture of high molecular weight, water-soluble, glucose polymers isolated by fractionation of hydrolyzed starch ranging in molecular weight from 13,000 to 19,000 Da. It is very slowly absorbed from the peritoneal cavity by direct absorption into the peritoneal lymphatics, not by diffusion because it is too large to move across small pores. Because of the slow absorption, there is sustained UF even during long dwells of

up to 15 hours. The differences between expected UF with the different solutions are especially apparent in patients who are high and high-average transporters. This UF is achieved while using isotonic solutions (216). The reason one can obtain sustained UF with icodextrin solutions is because the force driving the UF is due to colloid osmotic differences between the peritoneal cavity and blood. These colloid osmotic forces are due to the difference between the number of large molecular weight solutes between the two compartments (polyglucose vs. albumin). The clinical differences in UF profiles between dextrose solutions and polyglucose in CAPD and APD have been reviewed elsewhere (217–220). **TABLE 12.7** outlines the reason for these differences, and **FIGURE 12.12** illustrates the UF profiles of typically available dialysis fluids. Also an important consideration when using icodextrin is that, because >95% of the UF volume comes across small or large pores and NOT the aquaporins, all of the UF volume with icodextrin contains sodium in contrast to what happens initially in the dwell with dextrose solutions.

Although not available in the United States, lowering dialysate sodium allows for more diffusive removal of sodium independent of convective sodium removal. Although not currently available

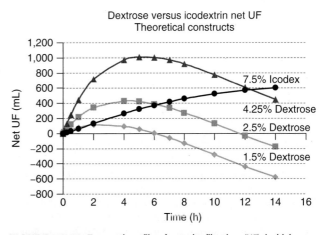

FIGURE 12.12 Temporal profile of net ultrafiltration (UF) in high-average transport patients with use of 1.5% dextrose (*diamonds*), 2.5% dextrose (*squares*), 4.25% dextrose (*triangles*), or 7.5% icodextrin (*circles*) solutions. [From Mujias S, Vonesh E. Profiling of peritoneal ultrafiltration. *Kidney Int* 2002;62(Suppl 81):S17–S22.]

in the United States, many investigators have evaluated the use of low sodium solutions. Ahearn and Nolph (221) found that using 7% dextrose dialysis solutions with sodium concentration of 100 to 130 mmol/L compared to 140 mmol/L resulted in increased sodium removal/exchange. In another study, the authors have shown that one could increase total sodium removal without any change in UF volume by lowering dialysate sodium. Nine anuric patients were studied in a crossover trial in patients on APD. A dialysate sodium of 132 mmol/L was compared to one with a sodium concentration of 126 mmol/L. On the lower sodium solution, daily sodium removal increased to 94 mmol/L of UF compared to 32 mmol/L while on standard dialysate sodium solutions. Four patients experienced an improvement in BP, and three were able to discontinue BP medicines. There was no significant change in UF or body weight during the study (222). In another study, the effects of ultralow sodium dialysis solutions (Na 102 mmol/L) were compared to baseline (when at least one exchange was 3.86% glucose/4.25% dextrose and one exchange with icodextrin) in five anuric PD patients (223). The better sodium removal (80 + 14 mEq vs. 56 + 15.9 mEq/d, $p < 0.05$), the better BP control (mean BP 98 + 5.5 mm Hg vs. 109 + 7.6 mm Hg, p + 0.046) with the ultralow sodium solutions. Clearly, these solutions may work, but current data is limited and more studies are needed. Generally, if dialysate sodium is lowered, one would need to increase dialysate glucose to maintain UF. For a further review of low sodium dialysate solutions, see Khandelwal et al. (224).

HOW TO MONITOR DIALYSIS DOSE?

The most accurate way to measure dialysis dose is to measure the total amount of the solute in question cleared from the body during a specific time interval. In practice, for patients on PD, this means that 24-hour collections of dialysate and urine (if included in dose calculations) should be obtained. Total solute clearance is then calculated. An alternative would be to estimate the daily clearance either mathematically or with the use of computer-assisted kinetic modeling programs. However, although the estimations do tend to correlate with the actual clearance measured from 24-hour collections, there is a high degree of discordance (225,226). Therefore, the gold standard for measurement of dialysis dose is to obtain 24-hour collections of both urine and dialysate to document the actual amount of solute removed. These studies should be obtained at baseline and then every 4 months and within 1 month of any prescription change. If RRF is included, then the RRF component should be measured every 2 months—as it is the most likely component of the two to change—and that value is then added to the prior 24-hour dialysate collection. The 2006 NKF-DOQI guidelines recommend that one only uses residual kidney component if (for simplicity) urine volume is more than 100 mL/d.

PET is obtained to characterize the patient's peritoneal membrane transport characteristics, not to determine clearance or any other clinical outcome. The two tests (24-hour collections and PET) are complementary to each other and are routinely used together for developing a patient's dialysis prescription and for problem solving. Several studies have documented that an individual patient's peritoneal membrane tends to be stable over time (227). However, in some patients, it may change. Therefore, peritoneal transport should be monitored to optimize clearance and UF. The PET is the most practical way to do this, and originally, it was recommended that it be obtained twice a year. It has been shown that over time, if there tends to be any change in transport characteristics, the D/P ratios were likely to increase slightly, associated with

TABLE 12.8	Usefulness of 24-Hour Collections of Dialysis and Urine Collection	
Creatinine Kinetics		**Urea Kinetics**
Creatinine clearance[D]		Urea clearance[D]
Creatinine clearance[U]		Urea clearance[U]
Total creatinine clearance[D+U]		Total urea clearance[D+U]
Creatinine production[D+U]		PNA[D+U]
Lean body mass[D+U]		Urea generation[D+U]
D/P creatinine[D]		
Ratio of measured to predicted creatinine generation		
Creatinine and Urea Kinetics		*24° Urine*
Estimated GFR (modified creatinine clearance)		Drain volume—UF rates

D, dialysis only; U, urine only; PNA, protein equivalent of nitrogen appearance; D/P, dialysis to plasma ratio; GFR, glomerular filtration rate; UF, ultrafiltration. From Burkart JM, Schreiber M, Korbet S, et al. Solute clearance approach to adequacy of peritoneal dialysis. *Perit Dial Int* 1996;16:457–470.

a small decrease in UF. Alternatively, one can estimate D/P values for PET from D/P values on 24-hour dialysate collections (*Dialysis Adequacy and Transport Test*, or DATT) when followed sequentially in an individual patient (228). Because of the stability over time, current recommendations are to obtain a baseline PET approximately 1 month after starting dialysis and only repeat the PET when clinically indicated (such as unexplained inadequate dialysis, unexplained volume overload, failure to thrive). Dialysate collections over 24 hours can also be used to calculate LBM, creatinine generation rates, and estimate protein intake (**TABLE 12.8**).

NONCOMPLIANCE

Noncompliance with a medical regimen is not uncommon and is a real issue for PD as documented by patient questionnaires (229) and by looking at patient home inventories (230). Because PD is a home therapy, it is not easy to document the degree of noncompliance with a patient's prescription. In contrast, the degree of noncompliance with the dialysis prescription itself is easily documented in in-center HD populations (5,231). Historic publications have suggested that a value above unity for the ratio of measured to predicted creatinine production may be an indication of recent periods of noncompliance (232–234). These authors speculated that if the patient had been noncompliant before obtaining the 24-hour dialysate and urine collection but was compliant on the day of collection, then a "washout" effect would occur. In such a case, the creatinine production would be higher than would be predicted from standard equations, resulting in an elevated ratio of measured to predicted creatinine production. From these studies, it has been estimated that only 78% of the prescribed therapy is actually delivered. Others have shown that the index is *not* a good indicator of patient compliance (235,236). Perhaps sequential rather than individual ratios will be helpful. At the moment, there is no recommended test as a measurement of compliance other than index of suspicion based on how the patient is doing and clinical studies. In the United States, most patients use an automated device to do their PD, most of which have a card to record actual prescription history; therefore, compliance can be evaluated this way. Interestingly, noncompliance may be more of an issue in the United States than in other countries such as Canada.

To minimize noncompliance, one should be sure to design PD prescriptions with the patients' lifestyle needs and abilities in mind. To do five manual exchanges per day is not realistic for most patients. Automated therapies may be. Education and importance of compliance with prescription should be emphasized.

PRESCRIPTION DIALYSIS

Timing of Initiation

The NKF-DOQI guidelines (8) and Obrador et al. (237) have highlighted the need to treat patients throughout all the stages of CKD as a continuum. The traditional indications for initiation of dialysis such as pericarditis, encephalopathy, refractory hyperkalemia, nausea, vomiting, and volume overload raise little controversy. Weight loss and signs of malnutrition are other more subtle, "relative" indications for initiation. Interestingly, as opposed to ESKD when minimal target values for weekly total solute clearance have been established (i.e., Kt/V_{urea} greater than 1.7), minimal values for solute clearance by RRF alone have not been established. This seems paradoxical. There are data to suggest that patients are starting dialysis with a higher serum creatinine, but this is likely a surrogate for number of comorbidities and sickness, not an indication that patients are starting dialysis in a healthier state. At the moment, the timing of when to start dialysis should not be driven by a number— eGFR, Ccr, serum creatinine. Rather, a constellation of clinical signs and symptoms along with input from the patient.

Initial Prescription

When a patient presents with near-ESKD or ESKD, and PD is elected, two alternatives for writing the initial prescription exist. For those patients with minimal RRF, the initial prescription should consist of a "full dose" of PD dialysis to meet minimal total solute clearance goals. If the patient has a significant amount of RRF (defined by the 2006 NKF-KDOQI guidelines as a residual urine volume of more than 100 mL/d and a residual kidney Kt/V_{urea} of less than 1.7 per week) less dialysis is needed. In this, an "incremental" approach to the dosage of PD can be used (238,239).

In both instances, the initial prescription is based on the patient's body size and amount of RRF (both potentially known variables at initiation of dialysis). At initiation, peritoneal transport is not known. Initial prescriptions are based on the assumption that the patient's peritoneal transport is average. Once stable on PD, a PET can be obtained (usually after 1 month) determining an individual patient's transport type, so that his or her prescription can be more appropriately tailored. During training, transport type can be predicted from DV during a timed (4-hour) dwell with 2.5% glucose and compared to those predicted by PET.

Pitfalls in Prescribing Peritoneal Dialysis

There are some common pitfalls in prescribing the peritoneal component of total solute clearance. The following is a brief summary of some of these and should be considered whenever a patient appears underdialyzed.

For patients on standard CAPD, these include (a) inappropriate dwell times (a rapid transporter would do better with short dwells), (b) failure to increase dialysis dose to compensate for loss of RRF, (c) inappropriate instilled volume or dialysis "dumping" (patient may only infuse 2 L of a 2.5-L bag) (240), (d) multiple rapid exchanges and one very long dwell (patient may do three exchanges between 9 AM and 5 PM and a long dwell from 5 PM to 9 AM (241), (e) inappropriate selection of dialysate osmotic agent for long dwells which may not maximize UF and consequently clearance, and (f) noncompliance.

Other problems are specific for those patients on cycler or APD therapy; these would include the following: (a) The drain time may be inappropriately long (more than 20 minutes), thereby increasing the time the patient must be connected to the cycler, perhaps limiting the number of exchanges a patient would tolerate and spending more time in fill and dwell than needed. (b) Inappropriately short dwell times may also be prescribed, making the therapy less effective for the average patient where length of dwell is crucial. (c) Failure to augment total dialysis dose with a daytime dwell ("wet" day vs. "dry" day) could also result in underdialysis. APD patients are typically on the cycler for 9 to 10 hours per night. Therefore, the daytime dwell is long (15 to 14 hours). During this long dwell (longer than the long nighttime dwell for typical CAPD patients), diffusion stops and reabsorption often begins, minimizing clearance. (d) Failure to consider using a midday exchange to augment clearances. Use of a mid day exchange is an effective way to optimize both clearance and UF in these patients. (e) Failure to consider use of alternative osmotic agents such as icodextrin, which maintain UF during long dwells (242). These optimize both clearance and UF without hypertonic glucose. (f) Poor selection of dialysate glucose may not allow maximization of UF with subsequent reabsorption of fluid and solutes. (g) Noncompliance.

When changing from standard CAPD (long dwells) to cycler therapy (short dwells), it is important to remember the difference in transport rates of urea and creatinine and the effect that this change will have on the patient's overall clearance. These differences and their relevance for CAPD, CCPD, NIPD, and other modifications are reviewed by Twardowski (243). Transport of urea into the dialysate tends to occur faster than for creatinine. Therefore, if total solute clearance targets are measured using urea kinetics, keeping Kt/V constant going from long to short dwells may decrease Ccr. In contrast, if Ccr is the total solute clearance target, keeping Ccr constant when changing from long to short dwells will keep Kt/V constant or even increase it. This concept has been termed *horizontal modeling* (244). Knowledge of the individual patient's peritoneal transport characteristics and familiarity with the differences in dialysis needs for rapid versus slow transporters is imperative to avoid problems or confusion.

Adjusting Dialysis Dose

When determining an individual patient's prescription, one should aim for a total solute clearance that is not only above target but also allow for other indices of adequate dialysis such as quality of life issues, BP control, volume control, and DPI. If during routine monitoring or clinical evaluation of the patient the delivered dose of dialysis needs to be altered, this can easily be done in a scientific manner if one knows the patient's present transport characteristics (PET), the present total clearance of urea or creatinine, and one understands the relationship between dialysis clearance, DV, and dwell time based on the measured D/P ratios. In general, when the goal is to increase total solute clearance, it is best to increase dwell volume, not number of exchanges. Increasing the number of exchanges decreases dwell time/exchange, making the therapy less effective for the average patient.

It is important that these relationships are understood because increasing the total instilled volume per day does not always result in an increase in clearance. For instance, in a patient who is a low transporter and in whom clearance is critically dependent on dwell time, changing from standard CAPD (infused volume—8 L) to a form of cycler therapy using 2-hour dwells where the infused volume may be as high as 10 to 14 L may not always result in an overall increase in that patient's clearance.

Once familiar with these relationships, to adjust the dialysate prescription, one would need to know the D/P ratios at the anticipated dwell time and the patient's DV for that dwell time. By altering dwell time, you change the D/P ratio and the DV. By altering instilled volume, you will also affect total DV and therefore clearance. In general, just increasing the instilled volume without changing dwell time will result in an increase in solute clearance.

Another means to tailor a dialysis prescription would be with the use of computer-assisted kinetic modeling programs (245,246), which allows for ease in adjusting a patient's dialysis prescription. Baseline PET data, DVs, and patient weights are needed for input data. Use of these programs usually allows one to set targets for solute clearance, glucose absorption, and anticipated DPI. These computer simulations then give you a menu of prescriptions that should achieve these targets, and you can choose the one that would best suit the patient's lifestyle.

Tidal PD is a form of automated dialysis in which, after an initial dialysate fill, only a portion of the dialysate is drained from the peritoneum and is replaced with fresh dialysate after each cycle. This leaves most dialysate in constant contact with the peritoneal membrane. A typical tidal dialysis prescription would usually require 23 to 28 L of instilled volume, but preliminary studies suggest that tidal dialysis may be approximately 20% more efficient than nightly PD at dialysate flow rates of approximately 3.5 L/h (247) and are therefore not cost effective and very seldom used in clinical practice.

SUMMARY

The delivered dose of dialysis does have an influence on certain patient outcomes. When considering adequacy of dialysis, one must not only maintain a minimal total solute clearance but also monitor other parameters such as overall clinical assessment, BP, and volume control, treatment of anemia, osteodystrophy, and other comorbid diseases. Periods of inadequate dialysis can result in subtle symptoms of uremia that are insidious in onset and may not be reversible. These can influence outcome in a negative way. To prevent this symptomatology and provide as close to optimal dialysis as possible, it is important to monitor dialysis dose so that changes in dialysis prescription can be made proactively rather than reactively. There does appear to be a "minimal" dose of dialysis measured in terms of small solute clearance that one should obtain to optimize outcomes (near a Kt/V_{urea} of 1.7/wk). When tailoring PD prescriptions, it is important that the prescribed dialysis dose be targeted to at least achieve these minimal doses. What is still unknown is if one was to achieve markedly higher small solute clearances with PD would this result in an incremental improvement in outcome. Preliminary data would suggest no, but it is important to remember that these maneuvers did not concomitantly increase or improve other "adequacy" parameters such as middle molecular weight solute clearance or volume control. Further studies, which specifically address these issues, are needed.

REFERENCES

1. Lundin PA III. Prolonged survival on hemodialysis. In: Maher JF, ed. *Replacement of Renal Function*. 3rd ed. Dordrecht, The Netherlands: Kluwer Academic Publishers, 1989:1133–1140.
2. Held PJ, Brunner F, Odaka M, et al. Five-year survival for end stage renal disease patients in the United States, Europe and Japan 1982–1987. *Am J Kidney Dis* 1990;5:451–457.
3. Lamiere N, Vanholder RC, Van Loo A, et al. Cardiovascular disease in peritoneal dialysis patients: the size of the problem. *Kidney Int* 1996;50(Suppl 56):S28–S36.
4. Sargent JA. Shortfalls in the delivery of dialysis. *Am J Kidney Dis* 1990;15:500–510.
5. Parker TF, Husni L. Delivering the prescribed dialysis. *Semin Dial* 1993;6:13–15.
6. Peritoneal Dialysis Adequacy Work Group of the National Kidney Foundation. Dialysis Outcomes Quality Initiative (DOQI): clinical practice guidelines. *Am J Kidney Dis* 1997;30(Suppl 2)S67–S136.
7. National Kidney Foundation Dialysis Quality Initiative. NKFK/DOQI clinical practice guidelines for peritoneal dialysis adequacy: update 2000. *Am J Kidney Dis* 2000;37(Suppl 1):S65–S136.
8. National Kidney Foundation. KDOQI clinical practice guidelines and clinical practice recommendations for 2006 updates: hemodialysis adequacy, peritoneal dialysis adequacy and vascular access. *Am J Kidney Dis* 2006;48(Suppl 1):S1–S322.
9. May RC, Kelly RA, Mitch WE. Pathophysiology of uremia. In: Brenner BM, Rector FC, eds. *The Kidney*. Philadelphia, PA: WB Saunders, 1991:1997–2018.
10. Luik AJ, Kooman JP, Leunissen KML. Hypertension in haemodialysis patients: is it only hypervolaemia? *Nephrol Dial Transplant* 1997;12:1557–1560.
11. Bagdade JD, Porte D, Bierman EL. Hypertriglyceridemia: a metabolic consequence of chronic renal failure. *N Engl J Med* 1968;279:181–185.
12. Neilsen VK. The peripheral nerve function in chronic renal failure. VII. Longitudinal course during terminal renal failure and regular hemodialysis. *Acta Med Scand* 1974;195:155.
13. Lowrie EG, Laird NM, Parker TF, et al. Effect of the hemodialysis prescription on patient morbidity. *N Engl J Med* 1981;305:1176–1181.
14. Churchill DN, Taylor DW, Keshaviah PR. Adequacy of dialysis and nutrition in continuous peritoneal dialysis: association with clinical outcomes. *J Am Soc Nephrol* 1996;7:198–207.
15. Lindsay RM, Spanner E. A hypothesis: the protein catabolic rate is dependent upon the type and amount of treatment in dialyzed uremic patients. *Am J Kidney Dis* 1989;13(5):382–389.
16. Churchill DN. Adequacy of peritoneal dialysis: how much do we need? *Kidney Int* 1994;46(Suppl 48):S2–S6.
17. Burkart JM, Schreiber M, Korbet S, et al. Solute clearance approach to adequacy of peritoneal dialysis. *Perit Dial Int* 1996;16:457–470.
18. Popovich RP, Moncrief JW. Kinetic modeling of peritoneal transport. *Contrib Nephrol* 1979;17:59–72.
19. Blake PG, Balaskas E, Blake R, et al. Urea kinetic modeling has limited relevance in assessing adequacy of dialysis in CAPD. In: Khanna R, Nolph KD, Prowant BF, et al, eds. *Advances in Peritoneal Dialysis*. Toronto, Canada: Peritoneal Dialysis Bulletin, 1992:65–70.
20. De Alvaro F, Bajo MA, Alvarez-Ude F, et al. Adequacy of peritoneal dialysis: does Kt/V have the same predictive value as for HD? A multicenter study. In: Khanna R, Nolph KD, Prowant BF, et al, eds. *Advances in Peritoneal Dialysis*. Toronto, Canada: Peritoneal Dialysis Bulletin, 1992:93–97.
21. Lameire NH, Vanholder R, Veyt D, et al. A longitudinal, five year survey of urea kinetic parameters in CAPD patients. *Kidney Int* 1992;42:426–432.
22. Teehan BP, Schleifer CR, Brown JM, et al. Urea kinetic analysis and clinical outcome on CAPD. A five year longitudinal study. In: Khanna R, Nolph KD, Prowant BF, et al, eds. *Advances in Peritoneal Dialysis*. Toronto, Canada: Peritoneal Dialysis Bulletin, 1990:181–185.
23. Maiorca R, Brunori G, Zubani R, et al. Predictive value of dialysis adequacy and nutritional indices for morbidity and mortality in CAPD and HD patients. A longitudinal study. *Nephrol Dial Transplant* 1995;10:2295–2305.
24. Churchill DN. Implications of the Canada-USA (CANUSA) study of the adequacy of dialysis on peritoneal dialysis schedule. *Nephrol Dial Transplant* 1998;13(Suppl 6):158–163.
25. Bargman J, Thorpe K, Churchill D. Relative contribution of residual renal function and peritoneal clearance to adequacy of dialysis: a re-analysis of the CANUSA study. *J Am Soc Nephrol* 2001;12:2158–2162.
26. Blake PG, Bargman JN, Bick J, et al. Guidelines for adequacy and nutrition in peritoneal dialysis. *J Am Soc Nephrol* 1999;10(Suppl 13):S311–S321.

27. Renal Association and Royal College of Physicians of London. *Treatment of Adult Patients with Renal Failure: Recommended Standards and Audit Measures.* London, United Kingdom: Royal College of Physicians, 1997.

28. Szeto CC, Wong TY, Chow KM, et al. The impact of increasing the daytime dialysis exchange frequency on peritoneal dialysis adequacy and nutritional status of Chinese anuric patients. *Perit Dial Int* 2002;22(2):197–203.

29. Szeto CC, Wong TY, Leung CB, et al. Importance of dialysis adequacy in mortality and morbidity of Chinese CAPD patients. *Kidney Int* 2000;58:400–407.

30. Szeto CC, Wong TY, Chow KM, et al. Impact of dialysis adequacy on the mortality and morbidity of anuric Chinese patients receiving continuous ambulatory peritoneal dialysis. *J Am Soc Nephrol* 2001;12:355–360.

31. Davies SJ, Phillips L, Griffiths AM, et al. Analysis of the effects of increasing delivered dialysis treatment to malnourished peritoneal dialysis patients. *Kidney Int* 2000;57:1743–1754.

32. Davies SJ, Phillips L, Russell GI. Peritoneal solute transport predicts survival on CAPD independently of residual renal function. *Nephrol Dial Transplant* 1998;13:962–968.

33. Bhaskaran S, Schaubel DE, Jassal V, et al. The effect of small solute clearance on survival of anuric peritoneal dialysis patients. *Perit Dial Int* 2000;20:181–187.

34. Mak SK, Wong PN, Lo KY, et al. Randomized prospective study of the effect of increased dialytic dose on nutritional and clinical outcome in continuous ambulatory peritoneal dialysis patients. *Am J Kidney Dis* 2000;36:105–114.

35. Paniagua R, Amato D, Vonesh E, et al. Effects of increased peritoneal clearances on mortality rates in peritoneal dialysis: ADEMEX, a prospective, randomized, controlled trial. *J Am Soc Nephrol* 2002;13(5):1307–1320.

36. Paniagua R, Amato D, Vonesh E, et al. Mexican Nephrology Collaborative Study Group. Health-related quality of life predicts outcomes but is not affected by peritoneal clearance: the ADEMEX trial. *Kidney Int* 2005;67:1093–1104.

37. Lo WK, Ho YW, Li CS, et al. Effect of Kt/V on survival and clinical outcome in CAPD patients in a randomized prospective study. *Kidney Int* 2003;64:649–656.

38. Lo WK, Lui SL, Chan TM, et al. Minimal and optimal peritoneal Kt/V targets: results of an anuric peritoneal dialysis patient's survival analysis. *Kidney Int* 2005;67:2032–2038.

39. Genestier S, Hedelin G, Schaffer P, et al. Prognostic factors in CAPD patients: a retrospective study of a 10 year period. *Nephrol Dial Transplant* 1995;10:1905–1911.

40. Collins AJ, Hanson G, Umen A, et al. Changing risk factor demographics endstage renal disease patients entering hemodialysis and the impact on long-term mortality. *Am J Kidney Dis* 1990;15:422–432.

41. Lo WK, Bargman JM, Burkart J, et al. ISPD Adequacy Work Group. Guidelines on targets for solute and fluid removal in adult patients on chronic peritoneal dialysis. *Perit Dial Int* 2006;26(5):520–522.

42. Dombros N, Dratwa M, Feriani M, et al; and the EBPG Expert Group on Peritoneal Dialysis. European best practice guidelines. *Nephrol Dial Transplant* 2005;20(Suppl 9).

43. Shemin D, Bostom AG, Laliberty P, et al. Residual renal function and mortality risk in hemodialysis patients. *Am J Kidney Dis* 2001;38:85–90.

44. Diaz-Buxo JA, Lowrie EG, Lew NL, et al. Associate of mortality among peritoneal dialysis patients with special reference to peritoneal transport rates and solute clearance. *Am J Kidney Dis* 2000;33:523–534.

45. Rocco M, Soucie JM, Pastan S, et al. Peritoneal dialysis adequacy and risk of death. *Kidney Int* 2000;58:446–457.

46. Jager KJ, Merkus MP, Dekker FW, et al. Mortality and technique failure in patients starting chronic peritoneal dialysis: results of the Netherlands cooperative study on the adequacy of dialysis. *Kidney Int* 1999;55:1476–1485.

47. Temorshuizen F, Korevaar JC, Dekker FW, et al. The relative importance of residual renal function compared with peritoneal clearance for patient survival and quality of life: an analysis of the Netherlands Cooperative Stud on the Adequacy of Dialysis (NECOSAD)-2. *Am J Kidney Dis* 2003;41:1293–1302.

48. Merkus MP, Jager KJ, Dekker FW, et al. Physical symptoms and quality of life in patients on chronic dialysis: results of The Netherlands Cooperative Study on Adequacy of Dialysis (NECOSAD). *Nephrol Dial Transplant* 1999;14:1163–1170.

49. Bammens B, Evenepoel P, Verbeke K, et al. Removal of middle molecules and protein-bound solutes by peritoneal dialysis and relation with uremic symptoms. *Kidney Int* 2003;64(6):2238–2243.

50. Kagan A, Elimalech E, Lemer Z, et al. Residual renal function affects lipid profile in patients undergoing continuous ambulatory peritoneal dialysis. *Perit Dial Int* 1997;17(3):243–249.

51. López-Menchero R, Miguel A, García-Ramón R, et al. Importance of residual renal function in continuous ambulatory peritoneal dialysis: its influence on different parameters of renal replacement treatment. *Nephron* 1999;83(3):219–225.

52. Bammens B, Evenepoel P, Verbeke K, et al. Time profiles of peritoneal and renal clearances of different uremic solutes in incident peritoneal dialysis patients. *Am J Kidney Dis* 2005;46(3):512–519.

53. Keshaviah P. Adequacy of CAPD: a quantitative approach. *Kidney Int* 1992;42(Suppl 38):S160–S164.

54. Kim DJ, Do JH, Huh W, et al. Dissociation between clearances of small and middle molecules in incremental peritoneal dialysis. *Perit Dial Int* 2001;21:462–466.

55. Brophy DF, Sowinski KM, Kraus MA, et al. Small and middle molecular weight solute clearance in nocturnal intermittent peritoneal dialysis. *Perit Dial Int* 1999;19:534–539.

56. Leypoldt JK, Burkart JM. Small solute and middle molecule clearances during continuous flow peritoneal dialysis. *Adv Perit Dial* 2002;18:26–31.

57. Sarnak MJ, Levey AS, Schoolwerth AC, et al. American Heart Association councils on kidney in cardiovascular disease, high blood pressure research, clinical cardiology, and epidemiology and prevention—kidney disease as a risk factor for development of cardiovascular disease: a statement from the American Heart Association Councils on Kidney in Cardiovascular Disease, High Blood Pressure Research, Clinical Cardiology, and Epidemiology and Prevention. *Circulation* 2003;108(17):2154–2169.

58. Li PK, Chow KM, Wong TYH, et al. Effects of an angiotensin-converting enzyme inhibitor on residual renal function in patients receiving peritoneal dialysis. A randomized, controlled study. *Ann Intern Med* 2003;139:105–112.

59. Suzuki H, Kanno Y, Sugahara S, et al. Effects of angiotensin II blocker, valsartan on residual renal function in patients on CAPD. *Am J Kid Disease* 2004;43(6):1056–1064.

60. Gilbert R, Goyal RK. The gastrointestinal system. In: Eknoyan G, Knochel JP, eds. *The Systemic Consequences of Renal Failure.* New York, NY: Grune & Stratton, 1984:133.

61. Ikizler TA, Wingard RL, Hakim RM. Malnutrition in peritoneal dialysis patients: etiologic factors and treatment options. *Perit Dial Int* 1995;15:S63–S66.

62. Wang AY, Sea MM, Ip R, et al. Independent effects of residual renal function and dialysis adequacy on actual dietary protein, calorie, and other nutrient intake in patients on continuous ambulatory peritoneal dialysis. *J Am Soc Nephrol* 2001;12:2450–2457.

63. Lo WK, Tong KL, Li SC, et al. Relationship between adequacy of dialysis and nutritional status, and their impact on patient survival on CAPD in Hong Kong. *Perit Dial Int* 2001;21:441–447.

64. Bergstrom J, Lindholm B. Nutrition and adequacy of dialysis how do hemodialysis and CAPD compare? *Kidney Int* 1993;43(Suppl 40):S39–S50.

65. Gotch FA. The application of urea kinetic modeling to CAPD. In: La Greca G, Ronco C, Feriani M, et al, eds. *Peritoneal Dialysis: Proceedings of the Fourth International Course on Peritoneal Dialysis.* Milan, Italy: Wichtig Editore, 1991:47.

66. Harty JC, Farragher B, Boulton H, et al. Is the correlation between normalized protein catabolic rate and Kt/V due to mathematic coupling? *J Am Soc Nephrol* 1993;4:407.

67. Ronco C, Bosch JP, Lew SQ, et al. Adequacy of continuous ambulatory peritoneal dialysis: comparison with other dialysis techniques. *Kidney Int* 1994;46(Suppl 48):S18–S24.

68. Lindsay RM, Spanner E, Heidenheim P, et al. Which comes first, Kt/V or PCR—chicken or egg? *Kidney Int* 1992;42:S32.

69. Agadoa LYC, Held PJ, Port FK, eds. Survival probabilities and causes of death. In: *USRDS Annual Data Report 1991*. 2nd ed. Bethesda, MD: National Institutes of Health, National Institute of Diabetes and Digestive and Kidney Diseases, 1991:31–40.

70. Lowrie EG, Lew NL. Death risk in hemodialysis patients: the predictive value of commonly measured variables and an evaluation of death rate differences between facilities. *Am J Kidney Dis* 1990;15:458–482.

71. Degoulet P, Legrain M, Reach I, et al. Mortality risk factors in patients treated by chronic hemodialysis. *Nephron* 1982;31:103–110.

72. Kupin W, et al. Protein catabolic rate (PCR) as predictor of survival in chronic hemodialysis patients. *J Ren Nutr* 1986;10:15–17.

73. Acchiardo SR, Moore LW, Latour PA. Malnutrition as main factor in morbidity and mortality of hemodialysis patients. *Kidney Int* 1983;24(Suppl 15):S199–S203.

74. Harris T, Cook EF, Garrison R, et al. Body mass index and mortality among nonsmoking older persons. The Framingham Heart Study. *JAMA* 1988;259:1520–1524.

75. Marckmann P. Nutritional status of patients on hemodialysis and peritoneal dialysis. *Clin Nephrol* 1988;29:75–78.

76. Chung SH, Lindholm B, Lee HB. Influence of initial nutritional status on continuous ambulatory peritoneal dialysis patient survival. *Perit Dial Int* 2000;20:19–26.

77. Young GA, Kopple JD, Lindholm B, et al. Nutritional assessment of CAPD patients: an international study. *Am J Kidney Dis* 1991;17:462–471.

78. Tan SH, Lee EJ, Tay ME, et al. Protein nutrition status of adult patients starting chronic ambulatory peritoneal dialysis. *Adv Perit Dial* 2000;16:291–293.

79. Passadakis P, Thodis E, Vargemezis V, et al. Nutrition in diabetic patients undergoing continuous ambulatory peritoneal dialysis. *Perit Dial Int* 1999;19(Suppl 2):S248–S254.

80. Jager KJ, Merkus MP, Huisman RM, et al. Nutritional status over time in hemodialysis and peritoneal dialysis. *J Am Soc Nephrol* 2001;12(6):1272–1279.

81. Bergstrom J, Heimburger O, Lindholm B, et al. Elevated serum C-reactive protein is a strong predictor of increased mortality and low serum albumin in hemodialysis (HD) patients. *J Am Soc Nephrol* 1995;6:573.

82. Han DS, Lee SW, Kang SW, et al. Factors affecting low values of serum albumin in CAPD patients. In: Khanna R, ed. *Advances in Peritoneal Dialysis*, Vol. 12. Toronto, Canada: Peritoneal Dialysis Publications, 1996:288–292.

83. Yeun JY, Kaysen GA. Active phase proteins and peritoneal dialysate albumin loss are the main determinants of serum albumin in peritoneal dialysis patients. *Am J Kidney Dis* 1997;30:923–927.

84. Kaysen GA, Stevenson FT, Depner T. Determinants of albumin concentration in hemodialysis patients. *Am J Kidney Dis* 1997;29:658–668.

85. Kaysen GA, Rathore V, Shearer GC, et al. Mechanism of hypoalbuminemia in hemodialysis patients. *Kidney Int* 1995;48:510–516.

86. Haubitz M, Brunkhorst R. C-reactive protein and chronic *Chlamydia pneumoniae* infection-long term predictors for cardiovascular disease survival in patients on peritoneal dialysis. *Nephrol Dial Transplant* 2001;16:809–815.

87. Noh H, Lee SW, Kang SW, et al. Serum C-reactive protein: a predictor of mortality in continuous ambulatory peritoneal dialysis patients. *Perit Dial Int* 1998;18(4):387–394.

88. Ducloux D, Bresson-Vautrin C, Kribs M, et al. C-reactive protein and cardiovascular disease in peritoneal dialysis patients. *Kidney Int* 2002;62(4):1417–1422.

89. Kim SB, Min WK, Lee SK, et al. Persistent elevation of C-reactive protein and ischemic heart disease in patients with continuous ambulatory peritoneal dialysis. *Am J Kidney Dis* 2002;39(2):342–346.

90. Herzig KA, Purdie DM, Chang W, et al. Is C-reactive protein a useful predictor of outcome in peritoneal dialysis patients? *J Am Soc Nephrol* 2001;12(4):814–821.

91. Fouque D, Kalantar-Zadeh K, Kopple J, et al. A proposed nomenclature and diagnostic criteria for protein-energy wasting in acute and chronic kidney disease. *Kidney Int* 2008;73:391–398.

92. Mehrotra R, Duong U, Jiwakanon S, et al. Serum albumin as a predictor of mortality in peritoneal dialysis: comparisons with hemodialysis. *Am J Kidney Dis* 2011;58:418–428.

93. Hylander B, Barkeling B, Rossner S. What contributes to poor appetite in CAPD patients? *Perit Dial Int* 1991;11(Suppl 1):117.

94. Hylander B, Barkeling B, Rossner S. Appetite and eating behavior—a comparison between CAPD patients, HD patients, and healthy controls. *Perit Dial Int* 1992;12(Suppl 1):137A.

95. Lindholm B, Bergstrom J. Nutritional management of patients undergoing peritoneal dialysis. In: Nolph KD, ed. *Peritoneal Dialysis*. 3rd ed. Boston, MA: Kluwer Academic Publishers, 1989:230–260.

96. Burkart JM, Jordan J, Rocco MV. Cross sectional analysis of D/P creatinine ratios versus serum albumin values in NIPD patients. *Perit Dial Int*. 1994;14(Suppl 1):S18.

97. Bannister DK, Archiardo SR, Moore LW. Nutritional effects of peritonitis in continuous ambulatory peritoneal dialysis (CAPD) patients. *J Am Diet Assoc* 1987;87:53–56.

98. Ates K, Oztemel A, Nergizoglu G, et al. Peritoneal protein losses do not have a significant impact on nutritional status in CAPD patients. *Perit Dial Int* 2001;21(5):519–522.

99. McCusker FM, Teehan BP, Thorpe K, et al. How much peritoneal dialysis is required for the maintenance of a good nutritional state? *Kidney Int* 1996;50:S56–S61.

100. Blake PG, Flowerdew G, Blake RM, et al. Serum albumin in patients on continuous ambulatory peritoneal dialysis—predictors and correlations with outcomes. *J Am Soc Nephrol* 1993;3:1501–1507.

101. Spiegel DM, Anderson M, Campbell U, et al. Serum albumin: a marker for morbidity in peritoneal dialysis patients. *Am J Kidney Dis* 1993;21:26–30.

102. Rocco MV, Burkart JM. Lack of correlation between efficacy number and traditional measures of peritoneal dialysis adequacy. *J Am Soc Nephrol* 1992;3:417.

103. Koomen GCM, van Straalen JP, Boeschoten EW, et al. Comparison between dye binding methods and nephelometry for the measurement of albumin in plasma of dialysis patients. *Perit Dial Int* 1992;12(Suppl 1):S133.

104. Rocco MV, Flanigan MJ, Beaver S, et al. Report from the 1995 core indicators for peritoneal dialysis study group. *Am J Kidney Dis* 1997;30:165–173.

105. Liberek T, Topley N, Jörres A, et al. Peritoneal dialysis fluid inhibition of phagocyte function: effects of osmolality and glucose concentration. *J Am Soc Nephrol* 1993;3:1508–1515.

106. Dawnay A. Advanced glycation end products in peritoneal dialysis. *Perit Dial Int* 1996;16:S50–S53.

107. Beelen RHJ, van der Meulen J, Verbrugh HA, et al. CAPD, a permanent state of peritonitis: a study on peroxidase activity. In: Maher JF, Winchester JF, eds. *Frontiers in Peritoneal Dialysis*. New York, NY: Field & Rich, 1986:524–530.

108. Dobbie JW. Durability of the peritoneal membrane. *Perit Dial Int* 1995;15:S87–S92.

109. Kopple JD, Jones MR, Keshaviah PK, et al. A proposed glossary for dialysis kinetics. *Am J Kidney Dis* 1995;26:963–981.

110. Keshaviah P, Nolph K. Protein catabolic rate calculations in CAPD patients. *ASAIO Trans* 1991;37:M400–M402.

111. Randerson DH, Chapman GV, Farrell PC. Amino acid and dietary status in CAPD patients. In: Atkins RC, Farrell PC, Thompson N, eds. *Peritoneal Dialysis*. Edinburgh, Scotland: Churchill Livingstone, 1981:171–191.

112. Harty JC, Boulton H, Curwell J, et al. The normalized protein catabolic rate is a flawed marker of nutrition in CAPD patients. *Kidney Int* 1994;45:103–109.

113. Nolph KD, Moore HL, Prowant B, et al. Cross sectional assessment of weekly urea and creatinine clearances and indices of nutrition in continuous ambulatory peritoneal dialysis patients. *Perit Dial Int* 1993;13:178–183.

114. Health Care Financing Administration. *2000 Annual Report, End Stage Renal Disease Clinical Performance Measures Project*. Baltimore, MD: Department of Health and Human Services, Health Care Financing Administration, Office of Clinical Standards and Quality, 2000.

115. Blumenkrantz MJ, Kopple JD, Moran JK, et al. Metabolic balance studies and dietary protein requirements in patients undergoing continuous ambulatory peritoneal dialysis. *Kidney Int* 1982;21:849–861.

116. Diamond SM, Henrich WL. Nutrition and peritoneal dialysis. In: Mitch WE, Klahr S, eds. *Nutrition and the Kidney*. Boston, MA: Little, Brown and Company, 1988:198–223.

117. National Kidney Foundation. *NKF-K/DOQI Clinical Practice Guidelines for Nutrition in Chronic Renal Failure*. New York, NY: National Kidney Foundation, 2001.

118. Nolph KD. What's new in peritoneal dialysis—an overview. *Kidney Int* 1992;42(Suppl 38):S148–S152.

119. Lim VS, Flanigan MJ. Protein intake in patients with renal failure: comments on the current NKF-DOQI guidelines for nutrition in chronic renal failure. *Semin Dial* 2001;14:150–152.

120. Uribarri J, Levin NW, Delmez J, et al. Association of acidosis and nutritional parameters in hemodialysis patients. *Am J Kidney Dis* 1999;34:493–499.

121. Lindholm B, Bergstrom J. Nutritional requirements of peritoneal dialysis. In: Gokal R, Nolph KD, eds. *Textbook of Peritoneal Dialysis*. Dordrecht, The Netherlands: Kluwer Academic Publishers, 1994:443–472.

122. Grzegorzewska AE, Dobrowolska-Zachwieja A, Chmurak A. Nutritional intake during continuous ambulatory peritoneal dialysis. *Adv Perit Dial* 1997;13:150–154.

123. Fernstorm A, Hylander B, Rossner S. Energy intake in patients on continuous ambulatory peritoneal dialysis and haemodialysis. *J Intern Med* 1996;240:211–218.

124. Kopple JD. Therapeutic approaches to malnutrition in chronic dialysis patients: the different modalities of nutritional support. *Am J Kidney Dis* 1999;33:180–185.

125. Pickering WP, Price SR, Bircher G, et al. Nutrition in CAPD: serum bicarbonate and the ubiquitin-proteasome system in muscle. *Kidney Int* 2002;61:1286–1292.

126. Detsky AS, McLaughlin JR, Baker JP, et al. What is subjective global assessment of nutritional status. *JPEN J Parenter Enteral Nutr* 1987; 11:8–13.

127. Enia G, Sicuso C, Alati G, et al. Subjective global assessment of nutrition in dialysis patients. *Nephrol Dial Transplant* 1993;8:1094–1098.

128. Kopple JD, Bernard D, Messana J, et al. Treatment of malnourished CAPD patients with an amino acid based dialysate. *Kidney Int* 1995; 47:1148.

129. Jones M, Hagen T, Boyle CA, et al. Treatment of malnutrition with 1.1% amino acid peritoneal dialysis solution: results of a multicenter outpatient study. *Am J Kidney Dis* 1998;32:761.

130. Jones MR, Gehr TW, Burkart JM, et al. Replacement of amino acid and protein losses with 1% amino acid peritoneal dialysis solution. *Perit Dial Int* 1998;18:210–216.

131. Lutes R, Perlmutter J, Holley JL, et al. Loss of residual renal function in patients on peritoneal dialysis. In: Khanna R, Nolph KD, Prowant BF, et al, eds. *Advances in Peritoneal Dialysis*, Vol. 9. Toronto, Canada: Peritoneal Dialysis Publications, 1993:165–168.

132. Gotch FA, Gentile DE, Schoenfeld P. CAPD prescription in current clinical practice. In: Khanna R, Nolph KD, Prowant BF, et al, eds. *Advances in Peritoneal Dialysis*, Vol. 9. Toronto, Canada: Peritoneal Dialysis Publications, 1993:69–72.

133. Rottembourg J, Issad B, Gallego JL, et al. Evolution of residual renal functions in patients undergoing maintenance hemodialysis or continuous ambulatory peritoneal dialysis. *Proc EDTA* 1993;19:397–403.

134. Cancarini GC, Brunori G, Camerini C, et al. Renal function recovery and maintenance of residual diuresis in CAPD and hemodialysis. *Perit Dial Bull* 1986;5:77–79.

135. Lysaght MJ, Vonesh EF, Gotch F, et al. The influence of dialysis treatment modality on the decline of remaining renal function. *ASAIO Trans* 1991;37:598–604.

136. Hallet M, Owen J, Becker G, et al. Maintenance of residual renal function: CAPD versus HD [abstract]. *Perit Dial Int* 1992;12(Suppl 1):124.

137. Tattersall JE, Doyle S, Greenwood RN, et al. Maintaining adequacy in CAPD by individualizing the dialysis prescription. *Nephrol Dial Transplant* 1994;9:749–752.

138. Page DE, Cheung V. Role still exists for cycler therapy in anuric patients with a low-transport membrane. *Adv Perit Dial* 2001;17:114–116.

139. Twardowski ZJ. Clinical value of standardized equilibration tests in CAPD patients. *Blood Purif* 1989;7:95–108.

140. Blake P, Burkart JM, Churchill DN, et al. Recommended clinical practices for maximizing peritoneal dialysis clearances. *Perit Dial Int* 1996;16:448–456.

141. Twardowski ZJ. Nightly peritoneal dialysis (why? who? how? and when?). *ASAIO Trans* 1990;36:8–16.

142. Rippe B, Krediet R. Peritoneal physiology-transport of solutes. In: Gokal R, Nolph KD, eds. *Textbook of Peritoneal Dialysis*. Dordrecht, The Netherlands: Kluwer Academic Publishers, 1994:69–113.

143. Faller B, Lameire N. Evolution of clinical parameters and peritoneal function in a cohort of CAPD patients followed over 7 years. *Nephrol Dial Transplant* 1994;9:280–286.

144. Selgas R, Fernandez-Reyes MJ, Bosque E, et al. Functional longevity of the human peritoneum: how long is continuous peritoneal dialysis possible? Results of a prospective medium long-term study. *Am J Kidney Dis* 1994;23:64–73.

145. Selgas R, Bajo MA, del Peso G, et al. Preserving the peritoneal dialysis membrane in long-term peritoneal dialysis patients. *Semin Dial* 1995;8:326–332.

146. Selgas R, Bajo MA, Paiva A, et al. Stability of the peritoneal membrane in long-term peritoneal dialysis patients. *Adv Ren Replace Ther* 1998;5:168–178.

147. Heimburger O, Waniewski J, Werynski A, et al. Peritoneal transport characteristics in CAPD patients with permanent loss of ultrafiltration. *Kidney Int* 1990;38:495–506.

148. Garred LJ, Canaud B, Farrell PC. A simple kinetic model for assessing peritoneal mass transfer in chronic ambulatory peritoneal dialysis. *ASAIO J* 1983;3:131–137.

149. Popovich RP, Moncrief SW. Transport kinetics. In: Nolph KD, ed. *Peritoneal Dialysis*. 2nd ed. Boston, MA: Martinus Nijhoff, 1985:115–158.

150. Vonesh EF, Lysaght MJ, Moran J. Kinetic modeling as a prescription aid in peritoneal dialysis. *Blood Purif* 1991;9:246–270.

151. Krediet RT, Struijk DG, Koomen GCM, et al. Peritoneal fluid kinetics during CAPD measured with intraperitoneal dextran 70. *ASAIO Trans* 1991;37:662–667.

152. Pannakeet MM, Imholz AL, Struijk DG, et al. The standard peritoneal permeability analysis: a tool for the assessment of peritoneal permeability characteristics in CAPD patients. *Kidney Int* 1995;48:866–875.

153. Pride ET, Gustafson J, Graham A, et al. Comparison of a 2.5% and a 4.25% dextrose peritoneal equilibration test. *Perit Dial Int* 2002;22:365–370.

154. Watson PE, Watson ID, Batt RD. Total body water volumes for adult males and females estimated from simple anthropometric measurements. *Am J Clin Nutr* 1980;33:27–39.

155. Hume R, Weyers E. Relationship between total body water and surface area in normal and obese subjects. *J Clin Pathol* 1971;24:234–238.

156. Dubois D, Dubois EF. A formula to estimate the approximate surface area if height and weight be known. *Arch Intern Med* 1916;17:863–871.

157. Blake PG. Targets in CAPD and APD prescription. *Perit Dial Int* 1996;16:S143–S146.

158. Jensen RA, Nolph KD, Moore HL, et al. Weight limitations for adequate therapy using commonly performed CAPD and NIPD regimens. *Semin Dial* 1994;7:61–64.

159. Nolph KD. Has peritoneal dialysis peaked? The impact of the CANUSA study. *ASAIO Trans* 1996;42:136–138.

160. Rocco MV. Body surface area limitations in achieving adequate therapy in peritoneal dialysis patients. *Perit Dial Int* 1996;16:617–622.

161. Jones MR. Etiology of severe malnutrition: results of an international cross-sectional study in continuous ambulatory peritoneal dialysis patients. *Am J Kidney Dis* 1994;23:412–420.

162. Johnson DW, Herzing KA, Purdie DM, et al. Is obesity a favorable prognostic factor in peritoneal dialysis patients? *Perit Dial Int* 2000;20: 715–721.

163. Churchill DN, Thorpe KE, Nolph KD, et al. Increased peritoneal transport is associated with decreased CAPD technique and patient survival. *J Am Soc Nephrol* 1997;8:189A.

164. Davies SJ, Phillips L, Russell GI. Peritoneal solute transfer is an independent predictor of survival on CAPD. *J Am Soc Nephrol* 1996;7:1443.

165. Heaf J. CAPD adequacy and dialysis morbidity: detrimental effect of a high peritoneal equilibrium rate. *Ren Fail* 1995;17:575–587.

166. Harty JC, Boulton H, Venning M, et al. Is peritoneal permeability an adverse risk factor for malnutrition in CAPD patients? *Miner Electrolyte Metab* 1996;22:97–101.

167. Blake P. What is the problem with high transporters? *Perit Dial Int* 1997;17:317–320.

168. Park HC, Kang SW, Choi KH, et al. Clinical outcome in continuous ambulatory peritoneal dialysis is not influenced by high peritoneal transport status. *Perit Dial Int* 2001;21(Suppl 3):S80–S85.

169. Nolph KD, Moore HL, Prowant B, et al. Continuous ambulatory peritoneal dialysis with a high flux membrane: a preliminary report. *ASAIO J* 1993;39:M566–M568.

170. Burkart JM. Effect of peritoneal dialysis prescription and peritoneal membrane transport characteristics on nutritional status. *Perit Dial Int* 1995;15:S20–S35.

171. Kagan A, Bar-Khayim Y, Schafe Z, et al. Heterogeneity in peritoneal transport during continuous ambulatory peritoneal dialysis and its impact on ultrafiltration, loss of macromolecules and plasma level of proteins, lipids and lipoproteins. *Nephron* 1993;63:32–42.

172. Struijk DG, Krediet RT, Koomen GC, et al. Functional characteristics of the peritoneal membrane in long term continuous ambulatory peritoneal dialysis. *Nephron* 1991;59:213–220.

173. Brimble KS, Walker M, Margettes PJ, et al. Meta-analysis: peritoneal membrane transport, mortality and technique failure in peritoneal dialysis. *J Am Soc Nephrol* 2006;17:2591–2598.

174. Tonbul Z, Altintepe L, Sozlu C, et al. The association of peritoneal transport properties with 24-hour blood pressure levels in CAPD. *Perit Dial Int* 2003;23:46–52.

175. Davies SJ. Mitigating peritoneal membrane characteristics in modern peritoneal dialysis therapy. *Kidney Int* 2006;70:S76–S83.

176. Feriani M. Adequacy of acid base correction in continuous ambulatory peritoneal dialysis patients. *Perit Dial Int* 1994;14:S133–S138.

177. Feriani M, Ronco Ck, La Greca G. Acid-base balance with different CAPD solutions. *Perit Dial Int* 1996;16:S126–S129.

178. La Greca G, Biasioli S, Chiaramonte S, et al. Acid-base balance on peritoneal dialysis. *Clin Nephrol* 1981;16:1–7.

179. Uribarri J, Buquing J, Oh MS. Acid-base balance in chronic peritoneal dialysis patients. *Kidney Int* 1995;47:269–273.

180. Graham KA, Reaich D, Goodship THJ. Acid-base regulation in peritoneal dialysis. *Kidney Int* 1994;46(Suppl 48):S47–S50.

181. Topley N. *In vitro* biocompatibility of bicarbonate-based peritoneal dialysis solutions. *Perit Dial Inter* 1997;17:42–47.

182. Walls J, Pickering W. Does metabolic acidosis have clinically important consequences in dialysis patients? *Semin Dial* 1998;11:18–19.

183. Bailey JL, Mitch WE. Does metabolic acidosis have clinically important consequences in dialysis patients? *Semin Dial* 1998;11:23–24.

184. Graham KA, Reaich D, Channon SM, et al. Correction of acidosis in CAPD decreases whole body protein degradation. *Kidney Int* 1996;49:1396–1400.

185. Löfberg E, Gutierrez A, Anderstam B, et al. Effect of bicarbonate on muscle protein in patients receiving hemodialysis. *Am J Kidney Dis* 2006;48(3):419–429.

186. Lowrie EG, Lew NL. Commonly measured laboratory variables in hemodialysis patients: relationships among them and to death risk. *Semin Nephrol* 1992;12:276–283.

187. Bergstrom J. Why are dialysis patients malnourished? *Am J Kidney Dis* 1995;26:229–241.

188. Kasimatis E, Maksich D, Jassal V, et al. Oreopoulos DG Predictive factors of low HCO3-levels in peritoneal dialysis patients. *Clin Nephrol* 2005;63(4):290–296.

189. Acchiardo SR, Kraus AP, Kaufman PA, et al. Evaluation of CAPD prescription. In: Khanna R, Nolph KD, Prowant BF, et al, eds. *Advances in Peritoneal Dialysis*, Vol. 7. Toronto, Canada: Peritoneal Dialysis Bulletin, 1991:47–50.

190. Doolan PD, Alpen EL, Theil GB. A clinical appraisal of the plasma concentration and endogenous clearance of creatinine. *Am J Med* 1962;32:65–79.

191. Tzamaloukas AH. Effect of edema on urea kinetic studies in peritoneal dialysis. *Perit Dial Int* 1994;14:398–400.

192. Tzamaloukas AH, Saddler MC, Murphy G, et al. Volume of distribution and fractional clearance of urea in amputees on continuous ambulatory peritoneal dialysis. *Perit Dial Int* 1994;14:356–361.

193. Twardowski ZJ. Relationships between creatinine clearances and Kt/V in peritoneal dialysis patients: a critique of the DOQI document. *Perit Dial Int* 1998;18:252–255.

194. Nolph KD. Is total creatinine clearance a poor index of adequacy in CAPD patients with residual renal function? *Perit Dial Int* 1997;17: 232–233.

195. Foley RN, Parfrey PS, Harnett JD, et al. Clinical and echocardiographic disease in patients starting end stage renal disease therapy. *Kidney Int* 1995;47:186–192.

196. Plum J, Shoenicke G, Kleophas W, et al. Comparison of body fluid distribution between chronic hemodialysis and peritoneal dialysis patients as assessed by biophysical and biochemical methods. *Nephrol Dial Transplant* 2001;16:2378–2385.

197. Rottembourg J. Residual renal function and recovery of renal function in patients treated with CAPD. *Kidney Int* 1993;43(Suppl 40): S106–S110.

198. Koc M, Toprak A, Tezcan H, et al. Uncontrolled hypertension due to volume overload contributes to higher left ventricular mass index in CAPD patients. *Nephrol Dial Transplant* 2002;17:1661–1666.

199. Enia G, Mallamaci F, Benedetto FA, et al. Long term CAPD patients are volume expanded and display more left ventricular hypertrophy than hemodialysis patients. *Nephrol Dial Transplant* 2001;16:1459–1464.

200. Cocchi R, Degli Esposti E, Fabbri A, et al. Prevalence of hypertension in patients on peritoneal dialysis: results of an Italian multicenter study. *Nephrol Dial Transplant* 1999;14:1536–1540.

201. Frankenfield DL, Prowant BF, Flanigan MJ, et al. Trends in clinical indicators of care for adult peritoneal dialysis patients in the United States from 1995 to 1997. *Kidney Int* 1999;55:1998–2010.

202. Luik AJ, Charra B, Katzarski K, et al. Blood pressure control and hemodynamic changes in patients on long time dialysis treatment. *Blood Purif* 1998;16:197–209.

203. Katzarsjki KS, Charra B, Luik AJ, et al. Fluid state and blood pressure control in patients treated with long and short hemodialysis. *Nephrol Dial Transplant* 1999;14(2):369–375.

204. Klassen PS, Lowrie EG, Reddan DN, et al. Association between pulse pressure and mortality in patients undergoing maintenance hemodialysis. *J Am Med Assoc* 2002;287:1548–1555.

205. Port FK, Hulbert-Shearon TE, Wolfe RA, et al. Predialysis blood pressure and mortality risk in a national sample of maintenance hemodialysis patients. *Am J Kidney Dis* 1999;33:507–517.

206. Zager PG, Nikolic J, Broen RH, et al. "U" curve association of blood pressure and mortality in hemodialysis patients. *Kidney Int* 1998;54: 561–569.

207. Ates K, Nergizoglu G, Keven K, et al. Effect of fluid and sodium removal on mortality in peritoneal dialysis patients. *Kidney Int* 2001;60:767–776.

208. Goldfarb-Rumyantzev AS, Baird BC, Leypoldt JK, et al. The association between BP and mortality in patients on chronic peritoneal dialysis. *Nephrol Dial Transplant* 2005;20:1693–1701.

209. Davies SJ, Brown EA, Reigel W, et al. The EAPOS Group. What is the link between poor ultrafiltration and increased mortality in anuric patients on automated peritoneal dialysis? Analysis of data from EAPOS. *Perit Dial Int* 2006;26(4):458–465.

210. Moist L, Port F, Orzol S, et al. Predictors of loss of residual renal function among new dialysis patients. *J Am Soc Nephrol* 2000;11:556–564.

211. Alfa Abu, Burkart J, Piranio B, et al. Approach to fluid management in peritoneal dialysis: a practical algorithm. *Kidney Int* 2002;62 (Suppl 81):S8–S16.

212. Mujais S, Nolph K, Gokal R, et al. Evaluation and management of ultrafiltration problems in peritoneal dialysis. International Society for Peritoneal Dialysis Ad Hoc Committee on Ultrafiltration Management in Peritoneal Dialysis. *Perit Dial Int* 2000;20(Suppl 4):S5–S21.

213. Brown EA, Davies SJ, Rutherford P, et al. Ultrafiltration and not solute clearance or solute transport status predicts outcomes at 2 years for APD in anuric patients. *J Am Soc Nephrol* 2002;13:70.

214. Gunal AI, Duman S, Orzol SM, et al. Strict volume control normalizes hypertension in peritoneal dialysis patients. *Am J Kidney Dis* 2001;37:588–593.

215. Moberly JB, Mujais S, Gehr T, et al. Pharmacokinetics of icodextrin in peritoneal dialysis patients. *Kidney Int* 2002;62(S81):S23–S33.

216. Mujias S, Vonesh E. Profiling of peritoneal ultrafiltration. *Kidney Int* 2002;62(S81):S17–S22.

217. Mistry CD, Gokal R, Peers E. MIDA Study Group: a randomized multicenter clinical trial comparing iso-osmolar icodextrin with hyperosmolar glucose solutions in CAPD. *Kidney Int* 1994;46:496–503.

218. Gokal R, Mistry CD, Peers E. United Kingdom multicenter study of icodextrin in continuous ambulatory peritoneal dialysis (MIDAS). *Perit Dial Int* 1994;14(Suppl 2):S22–S27.

219. Plum J, Gentile S, Verger C, et al. Efficacy and safety of a 7.5% icodextrin peritoneal dialysis solution in patients treated with automated peritoneal dialysis. *Am J Kidney Dis* 2002;39:862–871.

220. Woodrow G, Stables G, Oldroyd B, et al. Comparison of icodextrin and glucose solutions for the daytime dwell in automated peritoneal dialysis. *Nephrol Dial Transplant* 1999;14:1530–1535.

221. Ahearn DJ, Nolph KD. Controlled sodium removal with peritoneal dialysis. *Trans Am Soc Artif Intern Organs* 1972;18:423–428, 440.

222. Freida PH, Issad B. Impact of a low sodium dialysate on usual parameters of cardiovascular outcome of anuric patients during APD [abstract]. *Perit Dial Int* 1998; 18(Suppl 2):S2.

223. Vrtovsnik F, Hufnagel G, Michel C, et al. Long term effects of ultralow sodium dialysate on water and sodium balance in peritoneal dialysis patients with ultrafiltration failure. *J Am Soc Nephrol* 2002;13:206A.

224. Khandelwal M, Kothari J, Krishnan M, et al. Volume expansion and sodium balance in peritoneal dialysis patients. Part II: newer insights in management. *Adv Perit Dial* 2003;19:44.

225. Burkart JM, Jordan JR, Rocco MV. Assessment of dialysis dose by measured clearance versus extrapolated data. *Perit Dial Int* 1993;13:184–188.

226. Misra M, Reaveley DA, Ashworth J, et al. Six-month prospective crossover study to determine the effects of 1.1% amino acid dialysate on lipid metabolism in patients on continuous ambulatory peritoneal dialysis. *Perit Dial Int* 1997;17:279–286.

227. Blake PG, Abraham G, Sombolos K, et al. Changes in peritoneal membrane transport rates in patients on long term CAPD. In: Khanna R, Nolph KD, Prowant BF, et al, eds. *Advances in Peritoneal Dialysis*, Vol. 15. Toronto, Canada: Peritoneal Dialysis International, 1989:3–7.

228. Rocco MV, Jordan JR, Burkart JM. 24-hour dialysate collection for determination of peritoneal membrane transport characteristics: longitudinal follow-up data for the dialysis adequacy and transport test. *Perit Dial Int* 1996;16:590–593.

229. Blake PG, Korbet SM, Blake R, et al. A multicenter study of noncompliance with continuous ambulatory peritoneal dialysis exchanges in US and Canadian patients. *Am J Kid Dis* 2000;35(3):506–514.

230. Bernardini J, Piraino B. Measuring compliance with prescribed exchanges in CAPD and CCPD patients. *Perit Dial Int* 1997;17:338–342.

231. Rocco MV, Burkart JB. Prevalence of missed treatments and early signoffs in hemodialysis patients. *J Am Soc Nephrol* 1993;4:1178–1183.

232. Keen ML, Lipps BJ, Gotch FA. The measured creatinine generation rate in CAPD suggests that only 78% of prescribed dialysis is delivered. In: Khanna R, Nolph KD, Prowant BF, et al, eds. *Advances in Peritoneal Dialysis*. Toronto, Canada: Peritoneal Publications Inc, 1993:73–75.

233. Warren PJ, Brandes JC. Compliance with the peritoneal dialysis prescription is poor. *J Am Soc Nephrol* 1994;4:1627–1629.

234. Nolph KD, Twardowski ZJ, Khanna R, et al. Predicted and measured daily creatinine production in CAPD: identifying noncompliance. *Perit Dial Int* 1995;15:22–25.

235. Burkart JM, Bleyer AJ, Jordan JR, et al. An elevated ratio of measured to predicted creatinine production in CAPD patients is not a sensitive predictor of noncompliance with the dialysis prescription. *Perit Dial Int* 1996;16:142–146.

236. Blake PG, Spanner E, McMurray S, et al. Comparison of measured and predicted creatinine excretion is an unreliable index of compliance in PD patients. *Perit Dial Int* 1996;16:147–153.

237. Obrador GT, Arora P, Kausz AT, et al. Pre-end stage renal disease care in the United States: a state of disrepair. *J Am Soc Nephrol* 1998;9: S44–S54.

238. Mehrotra R, Nolph KD, Gotch F. Early initiation of chronic dialysis: role of incremental dialysis. *Perit Dial Int* 1997;17:497–508.

239. Nolph KD. Rationale for early incremental dialysis with continuous ambulatory peritoneal dialysis. *Nephrol Dial Transplant* 1998;13:117–119.

240. Caruana RJ, Smith KL, Hess CP, et al. Dialysate dumping: a novel cause of inadequate dialysis in continuous ambulatory peritoneal dialysis patients. *Perit Dial Int* 1989;9:319–320.

241. Sevick MA, Levine DW, Burkart JW, et al. Measurement of CAPD adherence using a novel approach. *Perit Dial Int* 1999;19:23–30.

242. Mistry CD, Mallick NP, Gokal R. Ultrafiltration with an isosmotic solution during long peritoneal dialysis exchanges. *Lancet* 1987;2: 178–182.

243. Twardowski ZJ. Influence of different automated peritoneal dialysis schedules on solute and water removal. *Nephrol Dial Transplant* 1998;13(Suppl 6):103–111.

244. Nolph KD, Twardowski ZJ, Keshaviah PR. Weekly clearances of urea and creatinine on CAPD and NIPD. *Perit Dial Int* 1992;12:298–303.

245. Vonesh EF, Keshaviah PR. Applications in kinetic modeling using PD Adequest®. *Perit Dial Int* 1997;17:S119–S125.

246. Gotch FA, Lipps BJ, Pack PD. A urea kinetic modeling computer program for peritoneal dialysis. *Perit Dial Int* 1997;17:S126–S130.

247. Twardowski ZJ. New approaches to intermittent peritoneal dialysis therapies. In: Nolph KD, ed. *Peritoneal Dialysis*. 3rd ed. Boston, MA: Kluwer Academic Publishers, 1990:133–151.

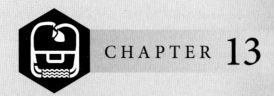

CHAPTER 13

Causes, Diagnosis, and Treatment of Peritoneal Membrane Failure

Shweta Bansal and Isaac Teitelbaum

Over the last several decades, peritoneal dialysis (PD) has become an established alternative to hemodialysis (HD) for the treatment of end-stage kidney disease (ESKD), and the number of patients and PD programs have grown rapidly recently with implementation of bundle payment programs. A number of studies, including the most recent ones, have confirmed its equivalent dialysis adequacy, somewhat better mortality and fluid balance status, at least for the first 4 to 5 years of renal replacement therapy (1,2). The success of PD as a long-term therapeutic option in the treatment of ESKD depends on the efficient removal of both solute and fluid. The ability to provide "adequate" dialysis (see Chapter 12) is a function of patient compliance, residual renal function (RRF), the transport characteristics of the peritoneal membrane, and the capacity to deliver a required dialysate flow rate in a manner that is tolerable to the patient. Therefore, alterations in any of these factors, not only in the characteristics of the peritoneal membrane, can significantly influence the efficiency of PD (TABLE 13.1) leading to "inadequate" dialysis and perceived "failure" of PD as a technique.

TABLE 13.1	Factors Influencing Peritoneal Dialysis Efficiency

Residual renal function
Patient compliance
Peritoneal membrane characteristics
   Permeability
   Effective surface area
Lymphatic absorption
Dialysate volume/osmolarity/flow
Effective blood flow

From Twardowski ZJ. The fast peritoneal equilibration test. *Semin Dial* 1990;3:141–142.

Owing to improved technology and the decline in peritonitis rates, ultrafiltration failure (UFF)/membrane failure has now become one of the major factors leading to technique failure in PD patients. Typically, alterations in peritoneal membrane function have a disproportionately greater effect on fluid removal than solute removal and therefore the most overwhelming cases of membrane failure are due to inability to achieve adequate ultrafiltration (UF), whereas the inability to achieve adequate solute removal is relatively uncommon. In most patients maintained on PD for 4 or more years, peritoneal clearance of small solutes is stable or increases, whereas net UF has been shown to decrease by as much as 40% from baseline (3–5).

Although UFF can occur in any stage of PD, it develops over time, and is, therefore, especially important in long-term PD. The exact prevalence of UFF in patients treated with PD is not known. Heimbürger et al. (6) demonstrated the cumulative risk for permanent loss of net UF capacity to be 2.6% at 1 year, 9.5% at 3 years, and in excess of 30% for those patients on continuous ambulatory peritoneal dialysis (CAPD) for 6 years or more. Similarly, in a Japanese long-term study, dropout because of UFF was as high as 51% after 6 years (7). Over an 18-month period, Davies et al. (8) observed UFF in 14% of their patients. Inadequate dialysis including UFF was responsible for transfer to HD in 18% of the patients in one series, whereas infection was responsible for 28% of the transfers (9). All the studies were based on clinical signs of UFF and not on a standardized test.

The definition of UFF had been under discussion over the past years. Some applied a clinical definition: the inability to remain at a certain dry weight and the use of more than two hypertonic (3.86%) bags per day had been considered as UFF (10–12). Others used a definition based on a standardized exchange and considered UFF to be present, for instance, when there was negative net UF with a

1.36% glucose dwell (13,14). In 2000, the International Society for Peritoneal Dialysis (ISPD) committee on UFF advised performing a standardized test with 3.86% glucose and considered a net UF of less than 400 mL after a 4-hour dwell as UFF (15). A cross-sectional study in a small number of PD patients, using the 400 mL/4 h on 3.86% glucose definition, reported a prevalence of 23% (14). Smit et al. (16) reported prevalence of 36% in 55 patients after a median period of 61 months.

Although the inability to achieve adequate solute and fluid removal is often attributed to a "failure" of the peritoneal membrane, it must be remembered that this is but one of several factors that affect the efficiency of PD (Table 13.1). It is therefore critical that nephrologists consider and understand these issues when evaluating patients with signs and symptoms of UFF. In this chapter, we review the factors that influence UF efficiency and present an approach to evaluating and treating these patients in clinical practice.

SOLUTE AND FLUID TRANSPORT IN PERITONEAL DIALYSIS

The Peritoneal Membrane

Solute and fluid transport in PD results from the development of concentration and pressure (hydrostatic and osmotic) gradients between blood and dialysate across the semipermeable peritoneal "membrane." Therefore, the physical characteristics (surface area and permeability) of the peritoneal membrane become major determinants in solute and fluid transport. The physical features of HD membranes are known by design; however, these properties are unknown for the peritoneal membrane and have largely been determined indirectly based on conceptual models and mathematical analyses. From these efforts, our concept of the transport physiology of the peritoneal membrane is evolving.

Originally, peritoneal transport properties were based on a "membrane model" in which the peritoneum was simply viewed as a single membrane comprising capillary wall, interstitium, and mesothelium. In this model, a concentration gradient exists from the capillary lumen on one side of the membrane to the peritoneal cavity on the other (17). More recently, the concept of a "distributed model" was proposed to better explain the observed transport properties of the peritoneum. Here, the capillaries are viewed as "distributed" throughout the interstitium, resulting in varying distances between capillary lumens and the peritoneal cavity (18). The contribution of a given capillary depends on the proximity of that capillary to the dialysate interface.

The "anatomic" surface area of the peritoneal membrane correlates best with body surface area (BSA) and is estimated to range from 1.7 to 2.0 m^2 (19). However, it is the "effective" surface area of the peritoneal membrane that is important in determining solute and fluid transport in PD. The effective peritoneal surface area is defined as that area of peritoneal membrane perfused by capillaries that comes into contact with dialysate and contributes to solute and fluid transport (20–22). The effective peritoneal surface area therefore depends not only on the volume of dialysate used but also on the effective peritoneal blood flow (that portion of the peritoneal microcirculation that actually comes into contact with dialysate and participates in solute and fluid transport). The largest portion (47%) of the overall small solute diffusive transport is across the peritoneal membrane associated with hollow viscera. However, as much as 43% of diffusive transport during PD occurs across the peritoneum associated with the liver (abdominal wall 6% and diaphragm 4%) (23).

The permeability of the peritoneal membrane is determined by the resistances created by the capillary wall, interstitium, and mesothelium. Of these, the capillary wall is the most important and the mesothelium the least important as barriers to transport. On the basis of the three-pore model of the peritoneal membrane, initially derived from a computer model for peritoneal transport mechanisms, solute and water transport occurs through three different pore types located in the capillary endothelium (24). "Large pores" are believed to correspond to interendothelial gaps (radius 12 to 15 nm) and are responsible for transport of macromolecules (e.g., albumin) across the membrane. Large pores account for less than 1% of the effective pore area for small solute diffusion, and, to a minor extent, they account for UF through fluid convection. "Small pores" (radius 4 nm) represent intercellular endothelial clefts and account for approximately 90% of total pore area. They are the primary route for the diffusive and convective transport of small molecular weight solutes (e.g., urea, creatinine, and electrolytes). More than 50% of glucose-induced UF occurs through small pores. It is through back diffusion across these pores that glucose absorption from the peritoneal cavity also occurs. However, small pores are essentially impermeable to macromolecules such as proteins. The third pore type is a water-selective, intracellular, so-called ultrasmall pore (radius less than 0.5 nm). The "ultrasmall pore" is the only pore type that is molecularly defined and corresponds to aquaporin 1 (AQP-1). The AQP-1 channel is located in endothelial and mesothelial cells (MCs) of the peritoneal wall. Although these pores comprise only 1% to 2% of the total pore area, they contribute up to 40% of the ultrafiltrate (25). Because the ultrafiltrate generated by the ultrasmall pores is solute-free, the concentration of solutes in the ultrafiltrate is less than that in the plasma, a phenomenon called *solute sieving*, usually referred as *sodium sieving* (see section "Convective Transport" in subsequent text).

Although the three-pore model has proven successful for modeling purposes in several physiologic and pathophysiologic conditions and for various osmotic agents, it does not take into account of the distributed nature of the peritoneal capillaries and also of the influence of the peritoneal tissue interstitium as explained in the distributed model (18). The pore-matrix model explains the complex nature of distributed peritoneal barrier by incorporating the concepts from these two models (26). As mentioned in three-pore model, small and large pores have not been found to be distinct anatomic entity. Rather, these are interendothelial spaces filled with a luminal glycocalyx that restricts passage of solutes and sets up alternative pressure forces. Large pores have a very sparse glycocalyx that permits transport of macromolecules, while small pores have a denser glycocalyx that are more restrictive. In addition to the aquaporins and glycocalyx-filled pores, the integrated cellular-interstitial matrix also makes the peritoneal barrier. According to this model, the distributed geometry of the capillary bed yields a substantial decrease in the effective reflection coefficient for crystalloid osmotic agents compared with their reflection coefficient in the capillary wall.

Solute Transport

Diffusive Transport

In PD, solute removal results from a combination of diffusive and convective transport. Diffusion, the primary mechanism for small solute removal, results from the concentration gradient between blood and dialysate created across the peritoneal membrane by the instillation of dialysate into the peritoneal cavity. The rate of diffusion for a solute (J_s) depends on the product of the peritoneal membrane solute permeability (P_s), effective peritoneal surface area (A), and the magnitude of the plasma to dialysate concentration (DC) gradient for that solute (**EQUATION 13.1**):

$$J_s = P_s \times A \times DC \qquad (13.1)$$

The intrinsic permeability of the peritoneal membrane for a given solute is relatively constant and is determined by its molecular weight. The peritoneal membrane is therefore highly permeable to low molecular weight solutes such as urea and creatinine but has a low permeability to high molecular weight solutes such as β_2-microglobulin and other large proteins.

Increasing the effective peritoneal surface area, by increasing the intraperitoneal volume of dialysate, can significantly improve the rate of diffusive transport for small solutes (**FIGURE 13.1**) (4). Keshaviah et al. (27) demonstrated that transport rates for urea, creatinine, and glucose doubled as infused volumes of dialysate were increased from 0.5 to 2.5 L. The infused volume producing the maximal diffusive transport rate for a given patient increased with increasing BSA, being 2.5 L for an average-sized person (BSA 1.7 m²) and 3 to 3.5 L for a person with a BSA of more than 2 m². The improved transport with larger volumes is felt to result from an increase in contact between dialysate and peritoneum, thereby increasing the effective peritoneal surface area by recruiting more peritoneal membrane. Beyond these maximal volumes, little to no improvement in diffusive transport is attained as the effective peritoneal surface area is completely exposed to dialysate and any further increases in volume results in "pooling" of dialysate.

Maintaining a maximal concentration gradient also enhances the rate of diffusive transport. This is dependent on the effective peritoneal blood flow as well as dialysate flow. The concentration gradient (ΔC) across the peritoneum is maximal early in the dwell cycle but decreases over time as solute diffuses from blood to dialysate. As the gradient decreases, the rate of diffusion decreases. Increasing the dialysate flow rate (shorter dwell times) and/or volume (increased exchange volumes) enhances the gradient, and therefore, the rate of diffusion can be increased (**FIGURE 13.1**). Diffusion

ceases when the concentration gradient between blood and dialysate no longer exists. Smaller molecules cross the peritoneal membrane more easily, equilibrate faster, and are influenced more by dialysate flow rates than are larger molecules (28,29).

It has generally been accepted that effective peritoneal blood flow is not a rate-limiting factor for the diffusive transport of small molecular weight solutes, as estimates of peritoneal blood flows are more than two to three times that estimated for the transport rates of small solutes like urea (17,18,30,31). However, given the large contribution of the liver-to-sinusoid transport and the fact that the liver may be more permeable to small solutes than other vascular beds in the abdomen, the rate of transport across the sinusoids may be so rapid that blood flow could be a limiting factor for this vascular bed (23). The major contribution of the liver to small solute clearance may account, in part, for the increased solute transport observed in the supine position or with increased dwell volumes as these maneuvers increase the contact of dialysate with the liver (23,29,32,33).

Convective Transport

Solute removal also occurs through convection. As osmotic forces cause water to move across the peritoneal membrane and into the peritoneal cavity, frictional forces between the solvent (water) and solutes (e.g., Na^+, urea) result in these solutes being convectively carried along with water. This is referred to as *solvent drag*. Because the peritoneal membrane provides greater resistance to solutes than to water (particularly by way of fluid transport across ultrasmall or transcellular pores), the concentration of solutes in the ultrafiltrate is less than that in plasma; this is referred to as *solute sieving*. The sieving coefficient for a given solute is the ratio of the solute concentration in the ultrafiltrate to that in the plasma. The rate of solute transport by convection (J_s) is therefore related not only to the transcapillary ultrafiltrate rate or water flux (J_w) but also to the serum concentration (C_s) and sieving coefficient (S) for that solute (**EQUATION 13.2**);

$$J_s = J_w \times C_s \times S \qquad (13.2)$$

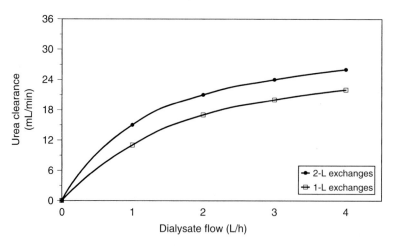

FIGURE 13.1 Effect of dialysate flow rate and volume on small molecular weight solute clearance. With an increase in dialysate flow clearances increase, but at a given flow rate, the clearances are even better with the use of larger fill volumes. This results from an increase in diffusive transport due to the increase in effective peritoneal surface area with larger fill volumes. *Open circle*, 2-L volumes; *open square*, 1-L volumes. (Modified with permission from Robson M, Oreopoulos DG, Izatt S, et al. Influence of exchange volume and dialysate flow rate on solute clearance in peritoneal dialysis. *Kidney Int* 1978;14:486–490.)

Because the rate of UF decreases over the time course of a dwell (see section "Fluid Transport" in subsequent text), the relative contribution of convective transport to overall solute removal also decreases during the same time period. The percentage of total solute transfer that is provided by convective as compared with diffusive transport increases significantly as the molecular size increases. It may be responsible for as little as 10% of total urea transport but may be responsible for more than 80% of protein transport (34,35).

Fluid Transport (Ultrafiltration)

Ultrafiltration occurs primarily through osmosis, as a consequence of the osmotic gradient created between the peritoneal blood compartment and the intraperitoneal dialysate compartment. This is achieved by utilizing hyperosmolar dialysate created by the addition of an osmotically active substance, usually dextrose, to the solution. The rate of transcapillary UF or water flux (J_w) is dependent on the peritoneal membrane hydraulic permeability (L_p) and effective surface area (A), as well as the transmembrane osmotic ($\Delta\pi$) and hydrostatic pressure gradients (ΔP) (EQUATION 13.3):

$$J_w = L_p \times A\ (\Delta\pi + \Delta P) \tag{13.3}$$

Transcapillary UF is highest at the beginning of a peritoneal exchange when the osmotic gradient is greatest. As a result of dilution of glucose by the ultrafiltrate and glucose absorption from the peritoneal cavity, as the osmotic gradient decreases over time, the rate of UF declines. The transcapillary UF rate (and therefore net UF—see later) can be increased by either the use of larger dialysate volumes (which decreases the rate of dilution) or more hypertonic solutions (which increases the osmotic gradient) or both (FIGURE 13.2).

Factors that lead to an increase in peritoneal membrane permeability or effective surface area (e.g., peritonitis) increase solute transport (e.g., glucose absorption), resulting in a more rapid decline in the osmotic gradient and therefore decrease the rate of UF (36).

Lymphatic absorption (LA) of fluid from the abdominal cavity opposes the effects of transcapillary UF. As shown in FIGURE 13.3, the combined effects of these two forces determine the ultimate drain volume or net ultrafiltration (net UF) (EQUATION 13.4):

$$\text{Net UF} = \text{TCUF} - \text{LA} \tag{13.4}$$

LA rates appear to be constant, regardless of the initial volume or tonicity of the dialysate instilled, and have been estimated to average from 1 to 1.5 mL/min (22,37,38). As long as the rate of transcapillary UF is greater than the rate of LA, intra-abdominal fluid volume or net UF increases above the initial fill volume (38,39). Peak intraperitoneal volume (net UF) is reached when the rate of transcapillary UF equals the rate of LA (FIGURE 13.4). This actually precedes the point in time at which osmotic equilibration of dialysate and plasma occurs. However, once the LA rate exceeds the rate of UF, a net absorption of fluid from the peritoneal cavity occurs, causing a decline in the intraperitoneal volume (declining net UF). Net UF can be increased by measures that increase the transcapillary UF rate (hypertonic dextrose solutions and/or increasing dialysate volume, as noted earlier), or by taking advantage of the time of peak UF (decrease the dwell time) (FIGURES 13.2 and 13.3). In addition to decreasing net UF, absorption of peritoneal fluid by lymphatic uptake impairs overall solute removal by partially negating the effects of both diffusive and convective transport.

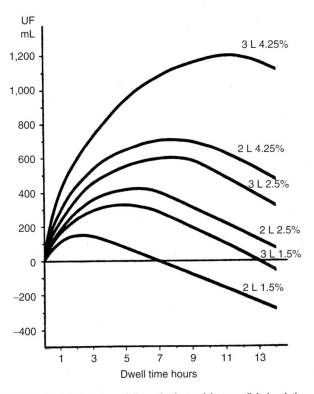

FIGURE 13.2 Effect of osmolality and volume of dextrose dialysis solutions on net ultrafiltration (UF). (Reproduced with permission from Twardowski Z, Khanna R, Nolph KD. Osmotic agents and ultrafiltration in peritoneal dialysis. *Nephron* 1986;42:93–101.)

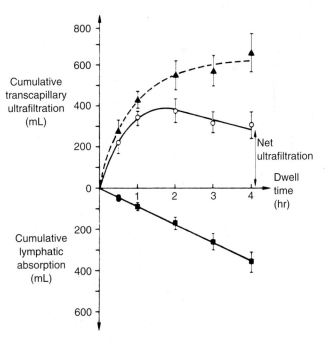

FIGURE 13.3 Net ultrafiltration (*open circle*) is a result of the additive effects of transcapillary ultrafiltration (*solid triangle*) and the negative effects of lymphatic absorption (*solid square*). Net ultrafiltration actually decreases as lymphatic absorption rate exceeds transcapillary ultrafiltration. (Solution used is 2.5% dextrose.) (Reproduced with permission from Mactier RA, Khanna R, Twardowski Z, et al. Contribution of lymphatic absorption to loss of ultrafiltration and solute clearances in continuous ambulatory peritoneal dialysis. *J Clin Invest* 1987;80:1311–1316.)

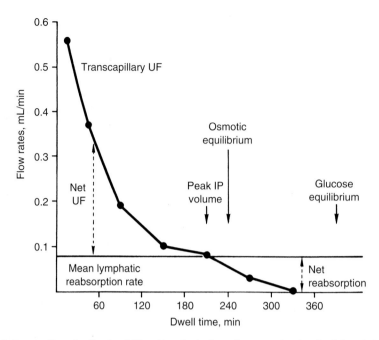

FIGURE 13.4 Transcapillary ultrafiltration (UF) and lymphatic absorption rates related to dwell time during an exchange using 2 L of 1.5% dextrose. Peak intraperitoneal volume occurs when the rate of transcapillary UF equals the rate of lymphatic absorption of fluid from the peritoneal cavity. This precedes osmotic equilibrium (there is still an osmolar gradient, although markedly attenuated because of the combined effects of dilution by ultrafiltrate and absorption of glucose from dialysate to blood) and glucose equilibration. IP, intraperitoneal pressure. (Reproduced with permission from Nolph KD, Mactier R, Khanna R. The kinetics of ultrafiltration during peritoneal dialysis: the role of lymphatics. *Kidney Int* 1987;32:219–226.)

◆ EVALUATION OF PERITONEAL MEMBRANE FUNCTION

Unlike HD membranes, the solute and fluid transport characteristics (surface area and permeability) of the peritoneal membrane in a given patient are unknown. Because of the alterations in transport parameters during the course of PD, regular follow-up is necessary to assess the delivered dialysis dose and, if needed, to characterize the functional status of the membrane. As a result, several indirect methods of evaluating the transport properties of the peritoneal membrane have been established. These protocols usually require that a PD exchange be performed with a specified dialysate volume and dextrose concentrations, assessing solute concentrations in serum and dialysate at specific points in time during a set dwell period, as well as determining the final drain volume. Through the information derived from these studies, a patient's transport characteristics can be established. This is most often done by determining either the dialysate to plasma (D/P) ratio—best standardized by the peritoneal equilibration test (PET) (40) or the peritoneal membrane mass transfer area coefficient (MTAC) (35,41,42) for various solutes. Because the D/P ratio of a given solute (the measure of transport utilized in the PET) depends upon both diffusive and convective transport, the MTAC was introduced to separate those influences on solute transfer from membrane function alone. From a practical perspective, information on peritoneal membrane function that is gained by the MTAC adds little to that of the PET and the MTAC is therefore not commonly utilized in clinical practice (43).

Peritoneal Equilibration Test

We are all indebted to Twardowski for his seminal observation of the variability of small solute transport rate and UF capacity within the PD population when he initially described the PET (44). This test semiquantitatively measures the peritoneal membrane transfer rates for solutes (usually urea and creatinine), based on the ratio of their concentration in D/P ratio at specific times (t) during the dialysate dwell, and for glucose, based on the ratio of dialysate glucose at dwell times t to dialysate glucose at 0 dwell time (D_t/D_0). The procedure for performing PET is outlined in **TABLE 13.2**.

In determining the D/P creatinine ratio, it must be appreciated that high glucose levels will falsely elevate creatinine measurements when determined by the picric acid method. As a result, creatinine levels must be corrected for the glucose level using a correction factor (**EQUATION 13.5**):

$$\text{Corrected Creatinine (mg/dL)} = \text{Creatinine (mg/dL)} \quad (13.5)$$
$$- [\text{Glucose (mg/dL)} \times \text{Correction factor}]$$

The correction factor in our laboratory is 0.00053, but this may differ from one laboratory to another, depending upon the analyzer used. Enzymatic methods for determining creatinine are not altered by glucose concentration and therefore do not require the use of a correction factor.

From 103 PETs performed in 86 patients on PD from 0.1 to 84 months at the time of the PET, Twardowski (40) categorized patients according to transport rates (based on the relationship of ±1 standard deviation from the mean) as low, low average, high average, and high (**FIGURES 13.5** and **13.6**). The PET results have been found to be highly reproducible, varying by less than 3% in repeated studies (8,45). The PET provides a valuable tool for categorizing and monitoring changes in peritoneal membrane transport (solute transport). Although the standard PET is also useful in assessing UF (water transport), it is limited by the fact that the use of a 2.5% exchange does not create a maximal osmotic gradient (15)

TABLE 13.2	**Standard Peritoneal Equilibration Test (PET)**[a]

1. An 8- to 12-h exchange with 4.25% dialysate precedes the test exchange.
2. Drain pretest exchange over 20 min in the vertical position (sending a sample for creatinine and glucose will allow for the determination of residual volume).
3. Infuse 2 L of 2.5%[a] dextrose dialysate over 10 min with patient supine.
4. After each volume of 400 mL is infused, have patient roll from side to side.
5. At the completion of the infusion, or 0 dwell time, and at 120 min dwell time, 200 mL of dialysate is drained, 10 mL is taken, and the remaining 190 mL is reinfused.
6. The patient is otherwise ambulatory during the dwell period.
7. At 120 min dwell time, a serum sample is obtained.
8. At 240 min dwell time, with the patient in the vertical position, the dialysate is drained over 20 min, the volume is measured, and a final sample is obtained.
9. All samples are sent for glucose and creatinine concentrations[b].

[a]The modified PET uses a 4.25% exchange.
[b]Sodium concentration may also be assessed when pursuing an abnormality in transcapillary ultrafiltration (type I ultrafiltration failure or an abnormality in transcellular pore function) versus an increase in lymphatic absorption rate. In this case, an additional dialysate sample at 60 minutes may also be helpful.
Twardowski ZJ. Peritoneal equilibration test. *Perit Dial Bull* 1987;7:138–147; Twardowski ZJ. Clinical value of standardized equilibration tests in CAPD patients. *Blood Purif* 1989;7:95–108.

(see section "Modified Peritoneal Equilibration Test" in subsequent text where 4.25% exchange is used). Nonetheless, information from the PET, in conjunction with clearance studies, aids in choosing an appropriate dialysis technique, developing a PD prescription, as well as following peritoneal membrane function (46). Because of the labor-intensive and time-consuming requirements of the standard PET, a "fast PET" was devised (47) (**TABLE 13.3**). The fast PET

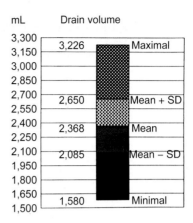

FIGURE 13.6 Drain volumes after standardized 4-hour dwell time test exchanges (PET), *n* = 94. Patients with high solute transport rates usually have low drain volumes, and *vice versa*. SD, standard deviation. (Reproduced with permission from Twardowski ZJ. Clinical value of standardized equilibration tests in CAPD patients. *Blood Purif* 1989;7:95–108.)

allows assessment of net UF and categorization of solute transport status using only the 4-hour D/P creatinine ratio (**FIGURE 13.5**) and glucose concentration (**TABLE 13.4**). The reproducibility of the fast PET results has also been shown to be quite good with coefficients of variation of less than 5% for the D/P creatinine and drain volumes (48). Transport category determinations obtained utilizing the results of the fast PET have been shown to correlate extremely well with those obtained by the standard PET method (49). One can therefore accurately follow up patients using the more labor-efficient fast PET. One disadvantage of the fast PET is that intermediate evaluation points at 1-, 2-, or 3-hour dwell times are not obtained; this may pose a problem when using this test for planning or altering dialysis prescriptions that use shorter dwell times such as continuous cyclic peritoneal dialysis (CCPD) regimens. Therefore, its primary value is as a tool for evaluating changes in membrane permeability over time.

Factors Influencing the Accuracy of Peritoneal Equilibration Test

The accuracy and reproducibility of the PET depend on its being performed exactly as outlined in **TABLE 13.2**. Any alteration in the method (e.g., dialysate volume) could significantly alter the results. For example, a larger instilled volume of dialysate may delay equilibration and lead to a lower D/P ratio and *vice versa*. Although using a more hypertonic exchange (4.25%) compared to 2.5% exchange

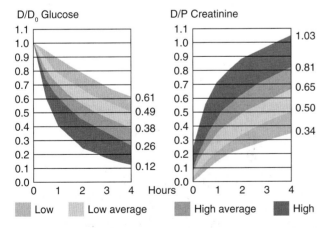

FIGURE 13.5 Results of 103 peritoneal equilibration tests (PETs) done in 86 patients. Areas shaded in different patterns portray results representing peritoneal transport rates that are high, high average, low average, and low. Creatinine concentrations in dialysate and plasma are corrected for glucose (see text). D/D_0, dialysate glucose concentration; D/P, dialysate to plasma. The numbers to the right separate the categories. (Reproduced with permission from Twardowski ZJ. Clinical value of standardized equilibration tests in CAPD patients. *Blood Purif* 1989;7:95–108.)

TABLE 13.3	**Fast Peritoneal Equilibration Test (PET)**

1. Steps 1, 2, and 3 of the standard PET are performed by the patient at home.
2. The exact time the infusion ended is noted by the patient.
3. The patient comes to the clinic at 240 min dwell time; in the vertical position, the dialysate is drained over 20 min.
4. The drained dialysate amount is measured and a sample is obtained.
5. A serum sample is obtained at 240 min dwell time.
6. All samples are sent for glucose and creatinine concentrations.

From Twardowski ZJ. The fast peritoneal equilibration test. *Semin Dial* 1990;3:141–142.

TABLE 13.4	Dialysate Glucose Concentrations at 4 Hours Using the Fast Peritoneal Equilibration Test (PET)	
Permeability	**Dialysate Glucose Concentration (mg/dL)**	
High	230–501	
High average	502–723	
Low average	724–944	
Low	945–1,214	

From Twardowski ZJ. The fast peritoneal equilibration test. *Semin Dial* 1990;3:141–142.

has been shown to significantly change the D/D_0 glucose and drain volume, the effect on D/P ratios for creatinine and designated transport category has been insignificant (50).

TABLE 13.5 outlines common errors in performing the PET. One additional note of caution is the use of the PET in patients with serum glucose concentrations of more than 300 mg/dL, as this can lead to unreliable results (47). Hyperglycemia decreases the D/P glucose (osmotic) gradient, thereby reducing the transcapillary UF rate as well as the rate of diffusion of glucose. This results in drain volumes that are less than expected and D/D_0 glucose concentrations that are higher than expected based on the patient's 4-hour D/P creatinine transport categorization. Finally, peritoneal surface area is larger relative to body weight in infants and children as compared with adults, and correlates more closely to BSA. Therefore, when performing the PET in infants and children, an exchange volume of 1,100 to 1,200 mL/m^2 BSA is recommended. This allows the use of the same transport categories defined for adults (40,43) to be applied to infants and children (51–53).

Modified Peritoneal Equilibration Test

Although standardized and highly reproducible, the use of standard PET may not be optimal in determining UFF because the osmotic gradient created by the use of a 2.5% exchange is modest and does not test maximal UF, as would be seen using a 4.25% exchange. The large drained volume with a 4.25% exchange makes the result less subject to measurement errors and more sensitive to detect clinically significant UFF. Therefore, it has been recommended that a modification of the standard PET be made and that a 4.25% exchange be used rather than a 2.5% exchange. The use of a 4.25% exchange does not result in any significant difference in MTAC or D/P creatinine (D/P_{Creat}) transport group characterization compared with that determined using a 2.5% exchange (50). The "modified PET" is currently considered the procedure of choice in the evaluation of UFF (water transport) and can be used to define peritoneal membrane function (solute transport) as well (14,15,54,55).

TABLE 13.5	Common Errors in Performing the Peritoneal Equilibration Test (PET)

Incomplete drainage of the overnight exchange
Incomplete final drainage of the PET exchange
Poor mixing of the dialysate during PET
Allowing fresh dialysate to flow into the drain bag
Errors in calculation

Miniperitoneal Equilibration Test

During a hypertonic dwell, approximately 60% of total UF is dependent on transport through small pores [ultrafiltration through small pores (UFSP)], which is coupled to the transport of small solutes, whereas approximately 40% of UF occurs through aquaporins resulting in the transcellular transport of free water without solutes (56–58). Estimation of free water transport can help in determining whether the cause of apparent UFF is due to decreased osmotic conductance in response to glucose or to a deficiency of aquaporins. A semiquantitative assessment of free water transport may be obtained by performing a 3.86% PET and examining either the D/P sodium concentration ratio (D/P_{Na}) or the magnitude of the dip in D/P_{Na} (15). However, even after correction for sodium diffusion (59), D/P_{Na} and the dip in D/P_{Na} are only approximate estimates of free water transport. Another indirect method to estimate free water transport is the comparison of net UF obtained during two modified PETs (standard peritoneal permeability analysis) performed with a PD solution with a glucose concentration of 1.36% or of 3.86% (54), but this method is complicated, time consuming, and not easily applicable in everyday clinical practice. In addition, it cannot properly quantify free water transport because the difference in net UF during a 1.36% or 3.86% test is the sum of the contribution of free water transport and of UFSP during the 3.86% test.

La Milia et al. (60) suggested another method with the consideration that during the first hour of a 3.86% exchange the free water transport is maximal—as glucose in the dialysate is at its highest concentration and diffusive sodium transport is very low—because of low plasma to dialysate sodium gradient. Therefore, if one shortens the duration of the 3.86% PET from 4 to 1 hour, UF through the large pores and reabsorption through lymphatics are both low (61); sodium transport is due mainly to convective transport through small pores. It is then possible to estimate UFSP as the sodium removal divided by the plasma water sodium concentration; free water transport is easily calculated by subtracting UFSP from total UF. This is referred to as the *3.86% mini-PET*. The values of D/P_{Creat} during the 3.86% PET and the 3.86% mini-PET were well correlated (**FIGURE 13.7**). Computer simulations by Venturoli and Rippe (62) showed that the La Milia method leads to reliable results and is easy to use in common practice. Furthermore, the

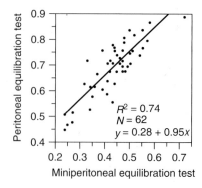

FIGURE 13.7 Linear correlation between the values of D/P (dialysate to plasma) creatinine during the 3.86% peritoneal equilibration test and the 3.86% miniperitoneal equilibration test. [From La Milia V, Di Filippo S, Crepaldi M, et al. Mini-peritoneal equilibration test: a simple and fast method to assess free water and small solute transport across the peritoneal membrane. *Kidney Int* 2005;68(2):840–846.]

free water transport calculated by this method was correlated to vascular AQP-1 expression (25). The mini-PET is a promising new tool, but its utility in the follow-up of prevalent patients' needs to be explored.

Alternative Methods for Evaluating Peritoneal Membrane Function

A number of authors have offered alternative approaches to evaluating and monitoring peritoneal transport. These are all variations on the principles of the PET but are felt to offer either greater accuracy or ease than the standard PET. These include the standardized peritoneal permeability analysis (SPA), a modification of the PET using 1.5% dextrose to which dextran is added (63); the dialysis adequacy and transport test (DATT), which utilizes the D/P creatinine and urea ratios established by the 24-hour dialysate collection available from clearance studies (64); and the peritoneal permeability and surface area (PSA) index, which separates the contribution of diffusive and convective transport to the D/P ratio (65). But their complexity, accuracy, or reproducibility make them inferior substitutes for the PET, and they are not commonly used in clinical practice.

⬡ DIAGNOSTIC APPROACH, DIFFERENTIAL DIAGNOSIS, AND TREATMENT OF THE PATIENT WITH ULTRAFILTRATION FAILURE

UFF is suspected clinically when patients cannot maintain an edema-free state or their target weight despite frequent use of hypertonic exchanges and dietary restriction. The observed increase in solute transport with time on dialysis explains, in part, the more frequent occurrence of signs and symptoms of UFF rather than that of inadequate solute removal (TABLE 13.6) (66–68). However, a change in peritoneal membrane function is only one of a number of possible factors that must be considered in a patient with suspected evidence of UFF (TABLE 13.1). A diagnostic approach (FIGURE 13.8) directed to the patient with possible UFF is therefore particularly germane.

When a patient presents with signs or symptoms of fluid overload, it is important to obtain a good medical history and to perform a thorough physical examination (FIGURE 13.8). Issues such as compliance with diet and dialysis are obviously critical, and a significant reduction in urine output may identify another potential reason for this problem. In addition, knowing the time frame over which the fluid accumulation occurred may be extremely helpful; patients with membrane failure as well as those with increased LA usually develop symptoms of UFF gradually, whereas those with mechanical problems (malpositioned catheter or dialysate leak) have a more acute presentation. When the

dialysate flow is described as positional, this suggests a malpositioned catheter. Findings of edema localized to the abdomen or inguinal area can be important clinical clues to the presence of a peritoneal leak.

At the time of the initial evaluation of a patient with fluid overload, a quick "fill and drain" with 2 L of dialysate is beneficial to directly observe the nature and rate of inflow and outflow. Usually, the inflow rate for dialysate is approximately 1,700 mL over 10 minutes and the outflow rate is similar. The presence of fibrin clots may explain abnormalities with flow that reduce the efficiency of drainage and volume removal and can often be resolved with intraperitoneal heparin. If incomplete drainage or positional drainage is observed, a flat-plate radiograph of the abdomen should be performed to determine catheter position and to assess the degree of stool in the bowel as the distension of bowel loops because feces is the single most common cause of poor catheter drainage (FIGURE 13.9). When a peritoneal leak is suspected by clinical examination, computed tomography or magnetic resonance imaging (MRI) of the abdomen—even without contrast—will often confirm its presence (FIGURES 13.10 and 13.11). It is extremely important to communicate to the radiologist the purpose of any radiographic procedure used in assessing problems with PD, as well as to review the radiograph(s) personally.

When the etiology of fluid overload is not apparent after the initial clinical assessment and mechanical causes have been ruled out, the use of the modified PET is recommended as the best way to evaluate patients suspected of having UFF (15). The modified PET allows one to construct a logical approach to the differential diagnosis and treatment of this common problem (FIGURE 13.8).

⬡ FLUID OVERLOAD WITHOUT ULTRAFILTRATION FAILURE

When a patient presents with unexplained fluid overload without UFF (drain volume greater than or equal to 2,400 mL), the possibility of noncompliance with diet or dialysis prescription must be entertained (FIGURE 13.8). In addition, the unrecognized and therefore uncompensated loss of RRF is a common cause for signs and symptoms of inadequate fluid removal, particularly in high-transport patients.

Patient Compliance

Noncompliance with the dialysis prescription and/or diet is a common problem that is often difficult to diagnose, as it is almost totally dependent on the patient's willingness to be honest. Estimates of the rate of noncompliance with the dialysis prescription range from 13% to 78% (69–71). Unfortunately, the methods presently used in documenting dialysis noncompliance such as comparing measured to calculated creatinine production are highly inaccurate (70). An estimate of dialysate use can be obtained through the shipping records of the dialysate supply company and therefore may allow an objective parameter by which to judge a patient's compliance. Although difficult to resolve, education and positive reinforcement may help improve this problem in a motivated patient.

Residual Renal Function

At the initiation of chronic dialysis, most patients still have RRF that may contribute as much as 30% to the overall maintenance of solute and fluid balance (72). Outcome studies in PD patients have clearly demonstrated a significant survival benefit with preservation

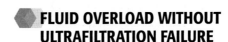

TABLE 13.6	Signs and Symptoms of Inadequate Dialysis

Ultrafiltration failure
  Increasing hypertension or edema
  Increasing requirement for hypertonic exchanges
Solute removal failure
  Increasing creatinine
  Increasing or decreasing blood urea nitrogen
  Worsening anemia or neuropathy
  Anorexia, nausea, vomiting, lethargy, insomnia

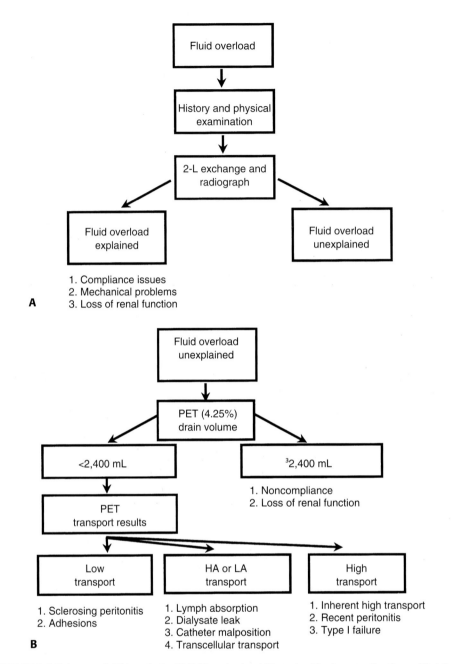

FIGURE 13.8 Initial approach **(A)** to patients with fluid overload and **(B)** an algorithm incorporating the modified (4.25%) peritoneal equilibration test (PET) to further evaluate those patients in whom the cause of fluid overload remains unexplained after the initial assessment. HA, high average; LA, low average.

of RRF (73). The potential benefits include better clearance of middle and larger molecular weight toxins, better volume and blood pressure control, decreased inflammation, improved appetite and nutritional status, relative preservation of kidney endocrine functions, and improved phosphate control and quality of life. However, RRF [glomerular filtration rate (GFR)] continues to decline on dialysis, which is associated with a significant decrease in urine volume. As a result, measures to preserve RRF are an important target in the treatment of patients receiving dialysis. Aggressive measures taken before initiation of dialysis to preserve kidney function, such as avoidance of nephrotoxic insults including intravenous contrast, antibiotics (e.g., aminoglycosides), and prevention of hypotensive

episodes, should continue to be addressed once dialysis has been initiated. Randomized trials have shown that use of an angiotensin-converting enzyme (ACE) inhibitor or angiotensin receptor blocker reduces the rate of decline in RRF and possibly delays the development of complete anuria in patients performing PD, although these trials were of small size (74,75). Another intervention which may be useful for preservation of RRF has been the use of biocompatible PD solution. Several trials comparing biocompatible solutions based on (a) neutral pH with low glucose degradation product (GDP) (balANZ trial), (b) 1.1% amino acids, or (c) 7.5% icodextrin with conventional dextrose-based dialysate recently have been shown to decrease the rate of decline in RRF, with a

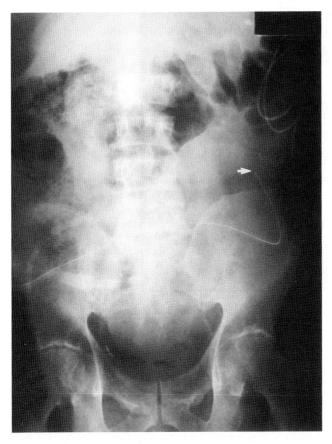

FIGURE 13.9 Plain roentgenogram (flat plate) of the abdomen demonstrating malpositioned catheter. Catheter tip can be seen in left upper abdomen (*arrow*).

smaller decline in urine volume or longer time to the development of anuria (76–79). To closely monitor for changes in kidney function, the ISPD recommends that 24-hour urine volumes and clearances be assessed regularly and at an appropriate frequency (every 1 to 2 months if practicable, otherwise no less frequently than every 4 to 6 months) so that the PD prescription can be adjusted in a timely manner (evidence level C). If there is a decrease in urine volume or a change in blood chemistries suggesting a decline in RRF, it should be measured sooner (80).

⬡ FLUID OVERLOAD WITH ULTRAFILTRATION FAILURE

A drain volume of less than 2,400 mL following a 4-hour 4.25% exchange defines the patient with UFF. UFF occurs when the balance between the transcapillary UF and LA rates has been altered, resulting in a decrease in drain volume (**FIGURE 13.8**). Clinically, this is identified by the need for more hypertonic exchanges to resolve signs of volume overload. These changes can be the result of (a) an increase in surface area/permeability leading to greater glucose absorption and a more rapid dissipation of the osmolar gradient (type I UFF), (b) a decrease in the osmotic conductance of glucose that leads to inadequate water removal (type II UFF), (c) a severe decrease in effective peritoneal surface area/permeability that significantly restricts the transport of both solute and fluid (type III UFF), (d) an increase in LA (type IV UFF), or (e) an increase in residual volume that leads to a more rapid loss of osmotic gradient by dilution (4). Therefore, a number of factors, in addition to changes in the peritoneal membrane, must be considered in the differential diagnosis of patients with UFF (**TABLE 13.7**). The PET allows an important assessment of both water and solute transport, which aids in the evaluation of UFF.

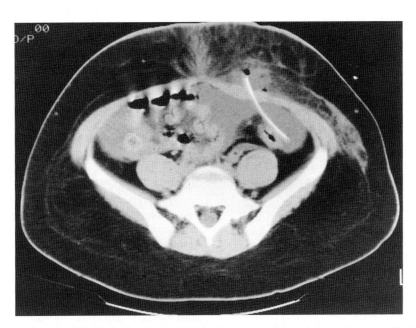

FIGURE 13.10 Computed tomographic scan of abdomen without intraperitoneal contrast in a patient with ultrafiltration failure and abdominal wall edema. Increased markings, representing fluid, can be seen within the anterior and left lateral subcutaneous tissues adjacent to the Tenckhoff catheter and indicate a dialysate leak.

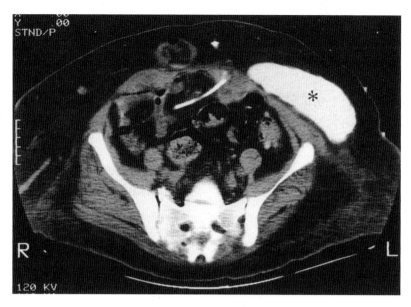

FIGURE 13.11 Computed tomographic scan of abdomen in patient with ultrafiltration failure and abdominal wall swelling. Radiocontrast material has been injected into dialysate to facilitate tracking. A large collection of contrast material can be seen in the anterior abdominal wall and subcutaneous tissues (*), indicating a dialysate leak.

TABLE 13.7	Factors Resulting in Ultrafiltration Failure

I. Peritoneal membrane function
   A. Increased effective surface area/permeability
      1. Peritonitis
      2. Type I ultrafiltration failure[a]
   B. Decreased osmotic conductance to glucose
      1. Type II ultrafiltration failure[b]
   C. Decreased effective surface area/permeability
      1. Type III ultrafiltration failure[c]
         a. Sclerosing peritonitis
         b. Adhesion
II. Lymphatic absorption
   A. Increased
      1. Primary increase (type IV ultrafiltration failure[d])
      2. Secondary increase (dialysate leak)
III. Dialysate volume/osmolarity/flow
   A. Increased residual volume (diluting osmotic gradient)
      1. Malpositioned catheter
      2. Loculations from adhesions
IV. Peritoneal blood flow
   A. Decreased
      1. Vascular disease

[a]The term applied to ultrafiltration failure when unexplained changes in membrane properties result in high solute transport. This has also been referred to as *type I membrane failure*.
[b]The term applied to ultrafiltration failure when changes in function of ultrasmall pore (aquaporins) cause decrease in osmotic conductance of glucose and leads to inadequate water removal.
[c]The term applied to ultrafiltration failure when changes in membrane properties result in decreased water and (low) solute transport as seen with sclerosing peritonitis or severe abdominal adhesions. This has also been referred to as *type III membrane failure*.
[d]The term applied to ultrafiltration failure as a result of a primary increase in lymphatic absorption.

Patients with High Solute Transport (D/P Creatinine Greater Than 0.81)

Patients with a low drain volume (less than 2,400 mL/4 h with a 4.25%/3.86% modified PET) and a D/P creatinine greater than 0.81 likely represent the largest group of patients with inadequate filtration due to peritoneal membrane characteristics. These patients tend to have good low molecular weight solute transport but have poor UF during standard CAPD or CCPD using glucose-containing dialysate, due to rapid absorption of glucose and dissipation of the osmotic gradient. If their dwell times are mismatched for their membrane transport characteristics, they often appear to have inadequate UF as they lose RRF and no longer have urine flow to supplement net daily peritoneal fluid removal. This clinical picture may develop over the course of months to years (so-called type I UFF), may be the consequence of a recent episode of peritonitis, or may be intrinsic to a particular patient's peritoneal membrane.

Type I Ultrafiltration Failure

This is the most common cause of UFF and is due to large effective peritoneal surface area with subsequent hyperpermeability of the membrane. Unfortunately, the development of slowly increasing hyperpermeability is a typical feature of chronic PD. The pathomorphologic cause of type I UFF is probably both fibrosis and, especially, angiogenesis, resulting in a large effective surface area (**FIGURE 13.12**). The avascular submesothelial fibrotic layer results in decreased osmotic pressure toward the endothelial exchange area of the capillaries. Additionally, by angiogenesis, an increased number of perfused capillaries under the fibrotic matrix rapidly dissipate the glucose-driven osmotic pressure. In an excellent animal model, an adenovirus-mediated gene transfer of angiostatin, a highly potent inhibitor of angiogenesis, resulted in higher UF by suppressing angiogenesis. An inverse correlation was found

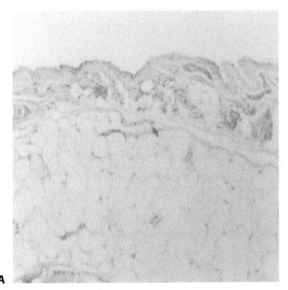

A

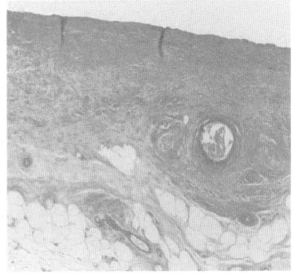

B

FIGURE 13.12 **(A)** Peritoneal histomorphology at the beginning of peritoneal dialysis (PD) and **(B)** after 6 years of PD, with submesothelial fibrosis, increased numbers of vessels, and vasculopathy. [From Fusshoeller A. Histomorphological and functional changes of the peritoneal membrane during long-term peritoneal dialysis. *Pediatr Nephrol* 2008;23(1):19–25.]

between the number of vessels and UF, underlining the important role of increased effective peritoneal surface area by angiogenesis in decreasing UF (81).

Hyperpermeability is a predictor of higher mortality in long-term PD patients (80). In 1998, the single-center Stoke PD study (83,84) and the multicenter Canada–United States of America (CANUSA) study (85), both prospective cohorts adequately powered to look at mortality, demonstrated that high transport was associated with worse patient and technique survival independent of other important predictors, such as age, comorbidities, and RRF. Later analysis from the Australian and New Zealand Dialysis and Transplant (ANZDATA) registry, by far the largest study published to date, also reported the association of high transport rates with increased mortality and technique failure (86). Moreover, further analyses of these studies exhibited that relationship between high transport and survival was confined to CAPD and not apparent in CCPD patients (87). Similarly, ANZDATA reported a high transport-modality interaction supporting higher mortality in CAPD patients. These analyses clearly suggest that excess mortality associated with high permeability is related to impaired ultrafiltration, which is better managed by CCPD.

Etiology and Pathogenesis

Recently, much work has been done to identify the mechanisms that are involved in the pathogenesis of peritoneal membrane failure during long-term PD (**FIGURE 13.13**). The major studied factors contributing to morphologic and functional alterations of the peritoneal membrane have been uremia, peritonitis, and the nonphysiologic nature of dialysis fluids. In uremia circulating nitric oxide (NO), advanced glycation end-products (AGEs), vascular endothelial growth factor (VEGF), and inflammatory cytokines [interleukin (IL)-1β, tumor necrosis factor alpha (TNF-α), and IL-6] are all significantly increased (88). The increase in effective peritoneal surface area is strongly related to VEGF and NO. The peritoneal expression of VEGF has been reported to correlate with the permeability

of the peritoneal membrane and the degree of angiogenesis (89). In addition, during chronic PD, endothelial nitric oxide synthase (eNOS) is significantly upregulated, which may contribute to an increase in vascular density and endothelial area (90). Data from the peritoneal biopsy registry confirmed that uremia *per se* leads to thickening of the submesothelial zone and mild vasculopathy (91).

To provide a stable peritoneal solution with a practicable shelf life, the pH of the solution is kept moderately acidic at approximately 5.2. This prevents the formation of GDPs. Moreover, standard peritoneal dialysate is buffered with lactate rather than bicarbonate as the latter has the potential to react with calcium and form calcium carbonate precipitate. Given the acid pH (but not sufficiently acidic to halt completely the formation of GDPs), high lactate and absent bicarbonate, peritoneal dialysate is not completely physiologic or "biocompatible." In an international peritoneal biopsy registry, more than 130 biopsies of long-term PD patients were compared with healthy controls and uremic patients not undergoing PD to evaluate the role of PD fluid as a cause for functional and morphologic alteration of the peritoneal membrane (91). In uremic patients, the submesothelial zone was three times thicker than in healthy individuals, and, in PD patients, it was even five times as thick. Both the thickness of the submesothelial zone and the degree of obliterating vasculopathy correlated directly with the duration of PD (**FIGURE 13.14**). The number of vessels (angiogenesis) was increased, especially in patients with clinical UFF and in patients with severe fibrosis. Patients on high-volume automatic peritoneal dialysis (APD) tended to have even more peritoneal fibrosis after shorter times on PD, which underlines the effect of cumulative glucose exposition. Glucose is a proinflammatory agent and has an additional profibrotic effect, especially through transforming growth factor (TGF)-1β stimulation and activation of protein kinase C. Glucose further stimulates the production of reactive oxygen species (ROS) causing oxidative stress and induces local angiotensin II production (92), which can also promote fibrosis through TGF-1β and fibronectin. GDPs and AGEs (AGEs form when GDPs link with

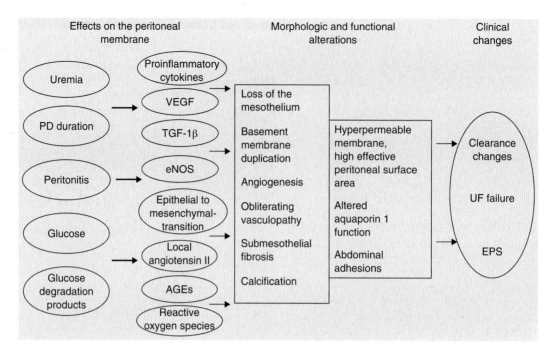

FIGURE 13.13 Effects of long-term peritoneal dialysis (PD) on the peritoneal membrane, and the subsequent morphologic, functional, and clinical consequences. VEGF, vascular endothelial growth factor; TGF, transforming growth factor; eNOS, endothelial nitric oxide synthase; AGE, advanced glycation end-product; UF, ultrafiltration; EPS, encapsulating peritoneal sclerosis. [From Fusshoeller A. Histomorphological and functional changes of the peritoneal membrane during long-term peritoneal dialysis. *Pediatr Nephrol* 2008;23(1):19–25.]

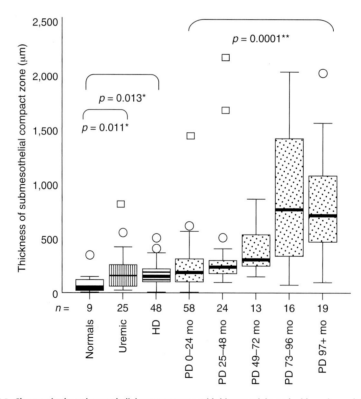

FIGURE 13.14 Changes in the submesothelial compact zone with biopsy origin and with peritoneal dialysis (PD) duration. The thickness of the submesothelial compact zone (in micrometers) was measured in biopsies from normal individuals, uremic patients, patients undergoing hemodialysis (HD), and patients undergoing PD, grouped according to the duration of dialysis. Data are presented as box plots, with the boxes representing the interquartile range (IQR). Lines extend from the box to the highest and lowest values, excluding outliers. The median value is represented by the thick line across each box. *, statistical comparisons made using the Mann-Whitney U test; **, statistical comparison made using Kruskal-Wallis one-way analysis of variance; ○ outliers; □ extremes. [From Williams JD, Craig KJ, Topley N, et al. Morphologic changes in the peritoneal membrane of patients with renal disease. *J Am Soc Nephrol* 2002;13(2):470–479.]

proteins) are potent proinflammatory agents and strong inducers of angiogenesis through VEGF (93). Through stimulation of plasminogen activator inhibitor (PAI)-1, additional fibrosis is promoted (94). Peritoneal AGE depositions correlate directly with the degree of fibrosis, the increase in effective peritoneal surface area, and functionally with the decline in UF. Diabetic rats have been shown to have a much higher density of small blood vessels in their peritoneum than nondiabetic rats (95). This neovascularization resembles that seen in proliferative diabetic retinopathy. However, among the small number of biopsies from diabetic patients represented in the peritoneal biopsy registry, there did not seem to be an increased incidence of vasculopathy (91).

Classically, resident stromal fibroblasts and inflammatory cells have been considered the main cells responsible for structural and functional peritoneal alterations, whereas MCs have been considered mere victims of peritoneal injury. However, recently, it has been shown that MCs also play an active role in peritoneal membrane alteration. It has been demonstrated that soon after PD is initiated, peritoneal MCs show a progressive loss of epithelial phenotype and acquire myofibroblast-like characteristics by an epithelial-mesenchymal transition (EMT) (96). MCs that have undergone an EMT acquire higher migratory and invasive capacities, which allow these cells to invade the submesothelial stroma, where they contribute to peritoneal fibrosis and angiogenesis and ultimately lead to peritoneal membrane failure (96–98). The myofibroblastic conversion of MCs has been confirmed in an *in vivo* animal model based on the injection of an adenovirus vector that transferred active TGF-β1 in rat peritoneum (99). In these studies, EMT appears as the central point in the early pathogenesis of peritoneal damage associated with PD. All the factors described earlier such as inflammation, uremia, and glucose stimulate the MCs to undergo EMT. MCs that have undergone EMT produce higher amounts of extracellular matrix component, including fibronectin and collagen I (98), and display less fibrinolytic capacity as a result of unbalanced ratio between tissue plasminogen activator and PAI-1 (100). The transdifferentiated MCs are also an important source of VEGF in PD patients; in fact, mesenchymal conversion of these cells appears to be the mechanism underlying upregulation of VEGF in PD (98). This suggests a direct and active role of MCs not only in fibrosis but also in peritoneal angiogenesis. Previous studies remained inconclusive regarding an association between markers of chronic inflammation and membrane transport failure (16,101,102); however, the most recent analysis of Global Fluid study, a multinational, multicenter, prospective, combined incident and prevalent cohort study ($n = 959$ patients) with up to 8 years of follow-up, reports that local subclinical intraperitoneal inflammation, as determined by dialysate IL-6 concentration, is the most significant known predictor of peritoneal solute transport rate (PTSR). Nonetheless, association of higher PTSR with worse survival remained independent of inflammation (103). The relevance of membrane inflammation is yet to be determined.

Treatment

Discontinuing PD and resting the peritoneum for at least 4 weeks by a temporary transfer to HD has been associated with significant improvement in UF capacity and normalization of solute transport characteristics in more than 81% of patients (104,105). A latest study reports that peritoneal rest enabled patients with UFF to continue on PD for a median time of 23 months (range, 13 to

46 months), although this beneficial effect was not be seen in patients with more than 6 months of UFF (106). This discontinuation of PD is felt to allow time for repair and remesothelialization of the damaged peritoneal membrane. Cancer antigen 125 (CA125) is a high molecular weight glycoprotein that is secreted by MCs. The level in PD fluid is considered a marker of MC mass (107). A decrease in CA125 levels in the absence of peritonitis has been seen before the development of type I membrane failure. Serial evaluations of CA125 may therefore provide a means by which to monitor mesothelial mass, allowing for peritoneal resting before the development of type I membrane failure. More research is required, however, to determine the best method for measuring CA125 and to establish normal values.

In most patients with type I UFF, especially those previously managed on standard CAPD, a change in the PD prescription to a regimen that takes advantage of shorter dwell times [e.g., nightly intermittent peritoneal dialysis (NIPD) and CCPD] may improve UF. Recent experience with the glucose polymer solution icodextrin 7.5% has proved beneficial in enhancing UF due to a modest oncotic pressure gradient that is sustained because of its relatively slow absorption and metabolism during the dwell period. This more than counterbalances Starling's forces (108,109), and it enables a slow but linear UF combined with almost complete prevention of fluid reabsorption during the long daytime dwell of CCPD or nighttime dwell of CAPD. Some patients cannot be maintained with these measures, fail PD, and require a transfer to HD for better volume control. The peritoneal catheter may be left in place and the PET may be repeated after a peritoneal rest period of 1 to 2 months. If solute transfer and UF normalize, PD may be reinitiated. If the patient's peritoneal membrane remains hyperpermeable, the transfer should be considered permanent and the PD catheter should be removed. An additional concern for patients with type I UFF is the fact that some patients have been reported to progress to type II UFF or sclerosing peritonitis (see subsequent text) (110).

Prevention

As alterations in membrane characteristics are a major cause of UFF, their prevention has been much emphasized. Davies et al. (111) reported stable peritoneal permeability and better volume control in long-term PD patients using icodextrin in contrast to increasing hyperpermeability in "no-icodextrin" patients. They examined the longitudinal changes in membrane function and divided the patients according to baseline glucose concentration of dialysate and reported decreased UF capacity even during the short study period of 24 months, more marked and with earlier onset in patients using greater than or equal to 2.27% solution, least apparent in the patients using icodextrin from the start of the study (111). Systemic review of 11 randomized controlled trials confirmed the previously described observation and demonstrated that use of icodextrin resulted in significant reduction in episodes of uncontrolled fluid overload and improvement in peritoneal ultrafiltration without any complications (79). New biocompatible, double-chamber dialysates, which have normal pH, low GDP, and are buffered with bicarbonate rather than lactate, demonstrate reduced inflow pain, improved correction of acidosis (112,113), and a survival benefit (114). Recent analysis of balANZ trial revealed that patients who performed PD with the neutral pH, lactate buffered, and low GDP solution initially had a higher rate of peritoneal membrane transport. This rate remained stable over the 2-year observation compared to a progressive increase in peritoneal membrane permeability with conventional solutions (115). Long-term histomorphologic and functional data are lacking so far.

Another possibility for reducing GDP formation in PD solutions is sterilization by filtration. *In vitro* studies showed a significant increase in cell viability, equivalent to that of control cells, following exposure to filter-sterilized PD fluids (116). To date, only a few reports regarding the utilization of filter-sterilized PD solutions have been published, and they date some years back (117,118). Another approach to reducing glucose-related toxicity is the replacement of glucose with other osmotic agents. The use of amino acids (not yet available in the United States) is relatively well established for this purpose. Exposure of human peritoneal MCs to amino acid–based solutions resulted in better preservation of ultrastructure, viability, and protein synthesis compared with conventional glucose-based PD fluids (119). Animal studies with amino acid–based PD fluids showed reduced activation of the peritoneal immune system as well as reduced peritoneal neoangiogenesis, fibrosis, and damage to MCs (120). Although not well studied, some data suggest that these solutions may also have a protective effect on the peritoneal membrane in humans (77,121). There have been no serious side effects seen and no differences in UF, dialysis efficiency (Kt/V) (122), mortality, hospital duration, or serial C-reactive protein levels (123) compared to the particular controls. Yet, no impact on long-term technique survival has been reported to date. Upregulation of renin-angiotensin-aldosterone system (RAAS) in response to acute inflammation and chronic exposure bioincompatible PD solution play an important role in the morphologic alteration of peritoneal membrane. Beneficial effects of ACE inhibitors on the development of these alterations have been reported in experimental models (124,125) and were also shown in few retrospective controlled trials of patients on PD treated with 2 years of ACE inhibitors/angiotensin receptor blockers (ARBs) (126,127).

Recent Peritonitis

Acute peritonitis is associated with an enormous intraperitoneal network of pro- and anti-inflammatory cytokines and a complex interaction of peritoneal cell lines (128). A rapid and reversible increase in the effective peritoneal surface area occurs, most likely under the influence of NO, proinflammatory cytokines (IL-1β, TNF-α, IL-6), and prostaglandins (129). This results in an increase in the D/P creatinine, a proportionate decrease in the D/D_0 glucose, and a significant reduction in net UF as compared with baseline (130). As a result, patients frequently become fluid overloaded, requiring a change in their dialysis prescription to improve UF. This may be achieved by an increase in the hypertonicity or number of hypertonic exchanges, the use of icodextrin, or a regimen that utilizes shorter dwell times [e.g., NIPD and daytime ambulatory peritoneal dialysis (DAPD)]. Fortunately, these membrane permeability changes are generally transient and patients are usually able to resume their previous PD prescription within a month of the peritonitis episode. Similar to acute peritonitis, recurrent peritonitis is also reported to affect peritoneal structure and function in PD. Again, hyperpermeability of the membrane and morphologic changes such as submesothelial fibrosis and angiogenesis are typical and important results of recurrent infectious episodes and may lead to type I UFF (131). It seems that the increased intraperitoneal release of IL-1β–stimulated TGF-β plays an important role in the

development of fibrosis. Additionally, IL-1β, IL-6, and TNF-α are also strong stimulators of angiogenesis.

Recovery of peritonitis may not be associated with significant remesothelialization of the peritoneum until 6 weeks or more have elapsed, although clinical recovery of peritonitis may occur within days (132). Therefore, the PET should be delayed for at least 4 weeks after an episode of peritonitis as it may otherwise not be representative of a patient's true peritoneal transport characteristics.

Inherent High Transporter

Ten percent of patients starting PD display this transport profile. When patients originally defined as high transporters present with volume overload, it may be the result of a loss of RRF. When this occurs, a change in the dialysis regimen (similar to that for type I membrane failure) and strict dietary restrictions are required. If there has been no loss of RRF, an evaluation for mechanical problems as well as compliance issues must be pursued.

Patients with Average Solute Transport (D/P Creatinine 0.5 to 0.81)

A low drain volume coupled with either high-average or low-average transport (D/P creatinine 0.5 to 0.81) can result from mechanical problems (e.g., a peritoneal leak or malpositioned catheter), a decrease in transcellular water transport, or an increase in LA (**FIGURE 13.8B**).

Dialysate Leak

Dialysate leaks from the intra-abdominal cavity to extra-abdominal tissues, usually the abdominal wall, result in a decrease in UF drain volume. Although the reason drain volume is lowered is obvious, the fluid leaked into the interstitium is subsequently removed by the lymphatic system and therefore technically falls into the category of UFF secondary to increased lymphatic flow. An extraperitoneal dialysate leak is frequently accompanied by an abdominal wall hernia, history of multiple abdominal surgeries, or a patent processus vaginalis (133). Some systemic conditions of ESKDs, including uremia, obesity, transperitoneal protein loss, and anemia, also contribute to these problems.

Extraperitoneal leakage of dialysate may occur at the catheter site as well as from tears in the peritoneum within hernia sacs (134,135). Edema localized to the abdominal wall, upper thigh, or genitalia is usually evident. Most reports indicate that the incidence of dialysis leakage is somewhat more than 5% in PD patients (133,136); patients with ESKD due to cystic kidney diseases are especially prone to the development of abdominal wall defects (133). Diagnosis may be confirmed by utilizing an appropriate radiographic technique. These include intraperitoneal infusion of radiographic contrast through the catheter followed by plain roentgenogram or computed tomography (137) (**TABLES 13.8 and 13.9; FIGURES 13.10 and 13.11**), or intraperitoneal infusion of a radioisotope evaluated with peritoneal scintigraphy or MRI

TABLE 13.8	Peritoneography

Take flat-plate radiogram of the abdomen.
Place 100–200 mL of nonionic contrast in dialysate (2-L bag).
Infuse 1 L of the dialysate into the supine patient.
Have the patient change positions for mixing.
Repeat flat-plate radiogram of the abdomen.

TABLE 13.9	**Peritoneal Computed Tomography (CT)**

Take plain CT of abdomen.
Place 100–200 mL of nonionic contrast in dialysate (2-L bag).
Infuse 1 or 2 L of the dialysate into the supine patient.
Have the patient change positions for mixing.
Repeat CT of abdomen.

without contrast (the dialysate itself functions as contrast material) (138,139). Peritoneal membrane function is not compromised in patients with dialysate leaks. Therefore, peritoneal transport as evaluated by the PET is not changed compared with a patient's baseline study.

Treatment of peritoneal leaks is aimed at repairing the defect in the peritoneum. Leaks associated with hernias usually require surgical repair of the hernia. Temporary transfer to HD for several weeks until adequate healing has occurred has been standard in the past, but a recent report from Shah et al. illustrates that this is not mandatory (140). Leaks that occur in the absence of a hernia usually represent a tear in the parietal peritoneum. These patients frequently have a history of multiple abdominal surgeries, pregnancies, recent corticosteroid usage, or abdominal straining (coughing, Valsalva maneuver). These patients may heal with nothing more than a period of several weeks without a daytime dwell (i.e., NIPD).

Catheter Malposition

Mechanical problems, such as a malpositioned catheter (**FIGURE 13.9**), resulted in UFF in 7% of patients in one center (8). Although this may occur because of improper initial catheter placement, it often results from the migration of catheters originally in good position due to entanglement by omentum, or it may be due to adhesions from previous surgery (141). A malpositioned catheter does not drain the peritoneal cavity effectively and leads to an increase in residual volume. A normal residual volume (R) is approximately 200 to 250 mL (40) and can be determined from information obtained during the PET using the following equation (**EQUATION 13.6**):

$$R = Vin (S3 - S2) / (S1 - S3) \qquad (13.6)$$

where Vin = instillation volume, S1 = solute concentration (urea or creatinine) in the pretest drain, S2 = solute concentration of the instilled fluid (0 for urea or creatinine), and S3 = solute concentration immediately following instillation (40). An increase in residual volume dilutes the glucose concentration in the freshly instilled dialysate. This decreases the osmotic gradient and thereby reduces the rate of transcapillary UF without any significant effect on solute transport. Net UF is decreased and the D/P ratio remains essentially unchanged.

An increase in the calculated residual volume should raise the suspicion of a malpositioned catheter. However, the presence of this problem is often clinically apparent and the diagnosis is easily made with the aid of simple radiographic techniques (**FIGURE 13.9**) as PD catheters have radiopaque material embedded within them. Either open or laparoscopic repositioning of the catheter tip can be done; however, recurrence is common and may require replacing or repositioning the straight Tenckhoff catheter through a new exit site, decreasing the angle (or bend) between the exit site and tunnel. This maneuver tends to force the path of the catheter caudad into the pelvis and may prevent recurrent migration. Success with nonsurgical manipulation of catheter position through the usage of a

stiff guide wire and fluoroscopy has been reported (142) but should be attempted only as a last resort. Unfortunately, despite catheter repositioning with various procedures, recurrent malpositioning may occur in up to two-thirds of patients utilizing the straight Tenckhoff catheter. If this occurs, the use of a catheter with a fixed swan neck is now recommended, as malposition recurrence with this catheter appears to be rare (143). Use of "front-loaded" catheters (that have a 5- to 12-g weight on the distal end) has also been reported to decrease migration; these catheters are not presently available in the United States (144).

Insertion of the dialysis catheter under direct laparoscopic visualization offers a number of advantages which prevent subsequent malpositioning of the catheter. The operator can ensure that the catheter tip is placed deep in pelvis, adhesions can be lysed, and redundant omentum can be tacked to the upper interior abdominal wall. Furthermore, the portion of the catheter that traverses the rectus sheath can be tunneled superoinferiorly so that the catheter has a "built-in" directionality into the pelvis, thereby decreasing the chances of its migrating into the middle or upper abdomen (145).

Decreased Transcellular Water Transport (Type II Ultrafiltration Failure)

In a group of patients with UFF, there is no associated increase in solute transport (for creatinine or glucose), residual volume, or LA rate (146,147). However, in all these patients, the normal drop in dialysate sodium concentration (**FIGURE 13.15**) is lost (i.e., no sieving is noted) due to a selective defect in peritoneal free water transport through the AQP-1 channel (ultrasmall pore). AQP-1–mediated UF is responsible for 40% to 50% of the effective transcapillary UF and is thought to decline with the duration of PD causing this selective defect in water transport. Yet, in immunohistochemical studies, no evidence was found for reduced expression of AQP-1 channels in long-term PD patients, even in those having reduced AQP-1–mediated free water transport (148). Fusshoeller et al. (113) reported a structurally modified AQP-1 form, found in the effluent of long-term PD patients, that increased in number over time on PD. Therefore, it seems that a functional alteration of AQP-1 channels, rather than a decrease of their expression, is responsible for less free water removal in long-term PD. The underlying mechanism is not clear, but a glycation- or NO-mediated process is most likely to be causative. In an animal model of acute peritonitis, the increase in nitric oxide synthase (NOS) activity correlated significantly with the decrease in AQP-1–mediated water transport, favoring an NO-related phenomenon (149). However, in a more recent human study in which AQP-1–mediated water transport was calculated more adequately, no effect of AQP-1–mediated water transport could be discerned during acute peritonitis (150). At present, a specific treatment that enhances AQP-1–mediated water transport is not available. However, corticosteroids have been shown to upregulate the expression of AQP-1 in the peritoneal capillaries in the rats. In the same context, an increase in the sodium sieving and ultrasmall pore ultrafiltration volume was noted in PD patients shortly after living donor kidney transplantation and treatment with high-dose methylprednisone (151). More recently, an AQP-1 agonist has been developed that has been shown to improve water transport across the peritoneal membrane in an animal model (152). These two therapies open potential therapeutic avenues to treat type II UFF.

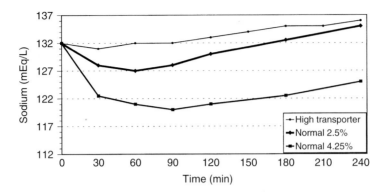

FIGURE 13.15 Dialysate sodium concentration over 4 hours using 2-L dialysate volumes in normal patients with 2.5% and 4.25% glucose concentrations and in high transporters (or patients with impaired transcellular pore transport) with ultrafiltration failure using 2 L of dialysate with 2.5% glucose concentration. The normal drop in sodium concentration is essentially lost in patients with markedly attenuated transcapillary ultrafiltration (high-transport patients or patients with impaired transcellular pore transport). [Data from Heimbürger O, Waniewski J, Werynski A, et al. Peritoneal transport in CAPD patients with permanent loss of ultrafiltration capacity. *Kidney Int* 1990;38(3):495–506; Heimbürger O, Waniewski J, Werynski A, et al. A quantitative description of solute and fluid transport during peritoneal dialysis. *Kidney Int* 1992;41(5):1320–1332; Monquil MC, Imholz AL, Struijk DG, et al. Does impaired transcellular water transport contribute to net ultrafiltration failure during CAPD? *Perit Dial Int* 1995;15(1):42–48.]

Increased Lymphatic Flow (Type IV Ultrafiltration Failure)

LA of peritoneal fluid negatively influences the overall removal of water (decreases net UF) and solute (partially negating the effect of diffusive and convective solute transport). Because the absorption of peritoneal fluid by lymphatics does not alter the concentration of solutes in the dialysate, the D/P ratio remains unchanged with increased lymphatic flow, although net UF can be significantly decreased. In a recent study, 30 of the 53 patients (57%) had UFF associated with a high LA, often in combination with other causes (153). An analysis of 20 patients on PD for more than 4 years showed that high LA was a cause of UFF in 6 of the 20, in 2 as the only cause, and in 4 in combination with other causes (16).

The mean value of the LA rate in PD patients during their first 2 years of PD treatment, as measured with intraperitoneal dextran 70, averages 1.52 mL/min (95% confidence interval of 0.30 to 2.50) when a 2-L exchange is used (153). The day-to-day intraindividual coefficient of variation averages 20%, the main part of which is due to biologic and not methodologic variation (154). The LA rate is influenced by instilled dialysate volume. Compared to 2 L, lower values are found with 1.5 L (153) and higher values with 3 L (155). It is likely that the effects of the instilled volume on LA are due to alteration in intra-abdominal pressure. Intraperitoneal (IP) pressure is 10 to 20 cm H_2O 2 hours after a 2-L exchange utilizing a 4.25% dextrose solution but may vary from 5 to 25 cm H_2O. A correlation between IP and net UF has been reported, with each increase of 1 cm H_2O pressure associated with a decrease in net UF of 74 mL over a 2-hour dwell (156). Increased intra-abdominal pressure causes a decline in net UF primarily not only by the increase in LA rate (1.9 mL/min vs. 1.0 mL/min) but also by a slight decrease in transcapillary UF rate (1.73 mL/min vs. 2.0 mL/min) (22). This may be more of an issue in patients who require larger dwell volumes to obtain adequate solute clearance. No relationship is present between the LA rate and BSA (154,157), or the tonicity of the dialysate (158). Also, the osmotic agent used has no influence. This has been shown for amino acids (159), icodextrin (57), and glycerol (160). Contrary to prior studies (37,63),

a latest study did not show any influence of patient position on LA rate, despite a higher IP pressure in the upright position compared to recumbency (154). This may be due to reduced contact area between the subdiaphragmatic lymphatics and dialysate in the upright position.

Pathogenesis

Michels et al. found significant correlations between the LA rate and MTACs of low molecular weight solutes (161). The explanation is speculative, but it may be that the presence of a large vascular peritoneal surface area, as suggested by high MTACs, is associated with a large lymphatic surface area as lymphatic vessels often accompany blood vessels. A recent study has shed light on the role of lymphangiogenesis in the UFF. It demonstrates that peritoneal tissue from patients with UFF contained more lymphatic vessels than tissue from patients without UFF. In the animal model, this enhanced lymphangiogenesis was mediated by increased VEGF-C expression induced by high TGF-β in the dialysate (162). Although, the effect of duration of PD on the LA rate has remained controversial (161,163). A deficiency in the dialysate content of surface active phospholipids (SAPLs) has also been attributed for increased LA rate. However, many trials in which peritoneal surfactant was replenished by adding exogenous SAPL to dialysate produced mixed results. The spectrum of outcomes ranged from totally negative (164,165) to increased UF (166,167). The range of compositions and their varying sources of SAPL, combined with a lack of physicochemical experience in formulation, accounted for much of the variation in the results (168). As demonstrated by Di Paolo et al. (167), a positive outcome was confirmed only in cases where UF had been previously diminished. This occurred without a change in solute transport, indicating that the increase in UF is secondary to a decrease in LA. Chen et al. (169) suggested that exogenously administered SAPL imparts semipermeability to the peritoneal mesothelium. Although able to demonstrate this in an *in vitro* model, they could not prove conclusively that addition of SAPL does the same to peritoneal mesothelium *in vivo*.

Diagnosis

Measurement of LA rate is uncommon in clinical practice because of the complexity of the procedure. Therefore, UFF secondary to increased LA becomes a diagnosis of exclusion. Icodextrin gets absorbed from the peritoneal cavity almost exclusively by lymphatics and ordinarily achieve good UF outcome even in patients with rapid transport rate. Failure to achieve UF with icodextrin over an 8- to 10-hour dwell may serve as an indirect evidence for excessive reabsorption.

The oral administration of bethanechol chloride, 0.27 mg/kg/d up to 50 mg, in four divided doses before each exchange has been demonstrated to result in an 18% increase in net UF in patients with type III UFF. Bethanechol chloride is similar to phosphatidylcholine in having cholinergic properties. An increase in cholinergic tone appears to contract the subdiaphragmatic lymphatic stomata, thereby reducing lymph flow (170).

Experience with larger numbers of patients is necessary to confirm the benefits of these therapies. These oral preparations appear to be well tolerated and may provide an option for the management of the patient with UFF presumed to be secondary to high LA. Certainly this therapy, if successful, may obviate the need for an increased exposure to hypertonic dialysate exchanges and their potential long-term deleterious effects.

Patients with Low Solute Transport (D/P Creatinine Less Than 0.5)

A much less common cause for UFF is that associated with low solute transport (D/P creatinine less than 0.5) (**FIGURE 13.8B**), which often stems from conditions leading to a severe reduction in effective peritoneal membrane surface area and permeability (type III UFF) (4,63,146). Therefore, signs and symptoms of both fluid overload and inadequate solute removal can be present (**TABLE 13.6**). This is observed in patients who have sclerosis of the peritoneal membrane (sclerosing peritonitis) as well as in patients with extensive intra-abdominal adhesions.

Encapsulating Peritoneal Sclerosis

Encapsulating peritoneal sclerosis (EPS) is recognized as being the most serious complication of PD; it is most often associated with an extended duration of PD. An *ad hoc* committee of the ISPD defines EPS as: "A clinical syndrome with persistent, intermittent or recurrent presence of intestinal obstruction with or without the existence of inflammation parameters and the existence of peritoneal thickening, sclerosis, calcifications and encapsulation (**FIGURE 13.16**) confirmed by macroscopic inspection or radiological findings" (171). Most data on EPS comes from Japan (where, due to the unavailability of kidney transplantation, treatment with PD for more than 10 years is common) and Australia. The most recent overall EPS incidence is reported to be 2.5% in Japan (172), 0.7% in Australia (173), and 3.3% in a single-center study in United Kingdom (174).

The diagnosis of EPS is suspected clinically when PD patients with peritoneal deterioration complain of gastrointestinal symptoms of insidious nature. Progressive peritoneal sclerosis, with the formation of intra-abdominal adhesions, leads to signs and symptoms of intestinal obstruction and strangulation. The transmural extension of the sclerosing process results in encapsulation of bowel, transforming the peritoneum into a "leathery cocoon." Peritoneal biopsy is the ultimate diagnostic tool, but various imaging techniques are the key tools for early diagnosis of EPS. Computed tomography (CT) is considered a valid and reliable tool for the diagnosis of EPS. Based on CT findings, Tarzi et al. (175) have developed a scoring system including peritoneal calcification (0 to 4) and thickening (0 to 4), bowel wall thickening (0 to 4), dilatation (0 to 4) and tethering (0 to 3), and loculation of ascites (0 to 3). They report a median total score of 9 of 22 (range 2 to 16)

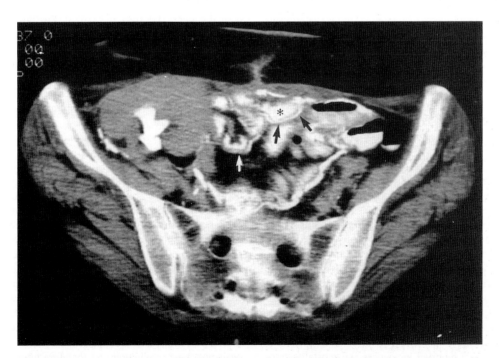

FIGURE 13.16 Computed tomographic scan of abdomen after oral contrast in a patient with sclerosing peritonitis demonstrating intestinal intraluminal coral contrast (*) and a diffusely thickened and calcified peritoneum (*arrows*).

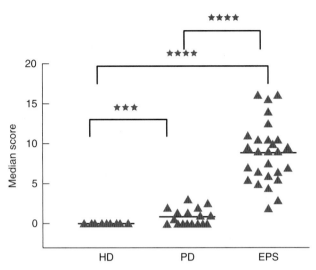

FIGURE 13.17 Ligand: computed tomographic scan scores for encapsulating peritoneal sclerosis (EPS) patients, hemodialysis (HD) and peritoneal dialysis (PD) controls (sum of scores for each parameter out of a maximum of 22). ***$p < 0.0001$, ****$p < 0.00001$. Wilcoxon rank-sum test. Horizontal lines indicates median score. Each triangle represents individual patient. [From Tarzi RM, Lim A, Moser S, et al. Assessing the validity of an abdominal CT scoring system in the diagnosis of encapsulating peritoneal sclerosis. *Clin J Am Soc Nephrol* 2008;3(6):1702–1710.]

in EPS patients with good interrater agreement (**FIGURE 13.17**). However, in this study, CT scan results neither correlated with the clinical outcome nor helped as a screening tool for EPS as the scans were frequently normal even a few months before the fulminant illness (175).

Abdominal ultrasonographic examination may demonstrate haustration of the ileum, fixed and rigid bowel loops with ineffective peristaltic contractions, clear-cut separation between the loops involved in the sclerotic process and loops that are still free, dilated fixed loops matted together and tethered posteriorly, intraperitoneal echogenic strands, trilaminar appearance of the bowel wall, and an echogenic "sandwich" appearance of the membrane (176,177). Early diagnosis, before the development of irreversible fibrosis and encapsulation, is critical in the prevention and treatment of EPS. Unfortunately, there is as yet no reliable noninvasive method by which to screen and thereby diagnose patients during the preclinical and potentially "reversible" phase of this condition.

The causes of EPS are diverse. In one report, only 9.4% of all EPS cases occurred in PD patients (178). That is to say, non–dialysis-related causes are common and include idiopathic (primary), abdominal tuberculosis (179,180), use of the β-blocker practolol (181), ventriculoperitoneal and peritoneovenous shunts (182,183), liver transplantation (184), and recurrent peritonitis. The pathogenesis of PD-related EPS, however, still remains uncertain, although a widely accepted hypothesis is the "two-hit theory," where the first hit is chronic peritoneal membrane injury from long-standing PD followed by a second hit such as an episode of peritonitis, genetic predisposition, and/or acute cessation of PD, leading to EPS (**FIGURE 13.18**). Prolonged PD duration constitutes the single most significant risk factor for EPS. Kawanishi and Moriishi (172) reported incidences and mortality rates for EPS for patients who had undergone PD for 3, 5, 8, 10, 15, and more than 15 years, respectively (**TABLE 13.10**). As discussed

earlier regarding type I UFF, chronic exposure to high concentration of glucose, GDPs, and AGEs may cause remodeling and fibrosis of the peritoneal membrane. The second factor most widely linked to an increased risk of EPS is peritonitis—especially if it is severe, recurrent, or nonresolving in nature (171). Patients with EPS have early loss of UF capacity and sodium sieving supporting the role of previously described factors in the pathogenesis of EPS (185). Preliminary studies have shown that AGE receptor (186) and eNOS gene polymorphisms (187) may play a role in the susceptibility to EPS. Increased T-cell activation has also recently been implicated in pathophysiology of excessive fibrosis as patients with EPS demonstrated increased serum-soluble CD25 (sCD25) concentration and intraperitoneal production of sCD25 (188).

Treatment of EPS is very difficult. In patients with milder or earlier forms of sclerosis, treatment with a period of peritoneal resting with transfer to HD may be of benefit (171). With regard to pharmacologic treatment, most reports in the literature advocate the use of corticosteroids as the immunosuppressive agent (189). Azathioprine, mycophenolate, and sirolimus have been tried with some success in case reports (190). However, once this condition becomes encapsulating, improvement is unlikely to occur. The subsequent gastrointestinal manifestations of obstruction and poor motility lead to malnutrition, requiring aggressive intravenous hyperalimentation. In patients with bowel obstruction, intervention with surgical viscerolysis may be required; however, this is generally associated with a high mortality (greater than 75%), often from sepsis (135,136).

Small-scale, noncontrolled studies indicate a positive effect of tamoxifen on peritoneal sclerosis (191–194). The results of the large Dutch multicenter retrospective study supports the use of tamoxifen in patients with EPS. Survival in tamoxifen-treated patients, adjusted for calendar time, age, use of corticosteroids, presence of functioning transplantation, use of parental nutrition, and center influences, was longer in comparison to not treated patients (HR 0.39, $p = 0.056$) (**FIGURE 13.19**) (195). This antiestrogen agent acts by inhibiting protein kinase C, a mediator of cell proliferation. It has been used to treat retroperitoneal fibrosis, a condition that has some similarities to sclerosing peritonitis (144). Although data on the use of immunosuppression or tamoxifen are limited, the experience with these agents is encouraging and at least provides an option in the treatment of this highly fatal disease.

Earlier, there were reports of improved survival after kidney transplantation (196–198). However, a recent analysis reported transplantation as a risk factor for the development of EPS because most patients with EPS underwent kidney transplantation at some point in time (199). This suggestion was strengthened by the fact that, in some patients, EPS developed shortly after kidney transplantation. It remains unclear at this point whether transplantation is beneficial or not and whether the transplantation procedure itself or the concomitant medications are responsible for the development of EPS. Cessation of peritoneal lavage after transplantation could lead to diminished clearance of fibrin and may therefore contribute to peritoneal fibrosis. Also, the known profibrotic effects of calcineurin inhibitors (CNIs) may have an effect to promote development of EPS (200,201). On the other hand, discontinuation of PD, and immunosuppression, by their inhibitory effects on lymphokine production and therefore fibroblast activity, may be responsible for the improvement in patients receiving kidney transplantation.

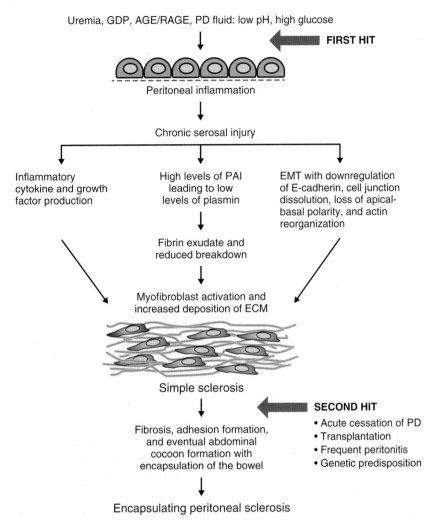

FIGURE 13.18 Proposed pathogenesis of encapsulating peritoneal sclerosis: "two-hit" theory. GDP, glucose degradation product; AGE, advanced glycation end-products; RAGE, receptors for advanced glycation end-products; PD, peritoneal dialysis; PAI, plasminogen activator inhibitor; EMT, epithelial to mesenchymal transdifferentiation; ECM, extracellular matrix. (From Augustine T, Brown PW, Davies SD, et al. Encapsulating peritoneal sclerosis: clinical significance and implications. *Nephron Clin Pract* 2009;111:149–154.)

Abdominal Adhesions

Recurrent or severe peritonitis, catastrophic intra-abdominal events, or complicated abdominal surgery may lead to the development of extensive intra-abdominal adhesions (145). Adhesions limit dialysate flow throughout the abdominal cavity and decrease

TABLE 13.10	The Incidence and Mortality Rate for Encapsulating Peritoneal Sclerosis (EPS) with Increasing Duration of Peritoneal Dialysis (PD)		
PD Duration (yr)	**Incidence Rate (%)**	**Mortality Rate (%)**	
3	0	0	
5	0.7	0	
8	2.1	8.3	
10	5.9	28.6	
15	5.8	61.5	
>15	17.2	100	

the effective surface area of the peritoneum, thereby compromising both solute transport and UF. The diagnosis can be made by radiographic techniques that utilize the intraperitoneal infusion of a radiographic contrast material through the dialysis catheter with plain roentgenographic or computed tomographic visualization, or with the intraperitoneal infusion of a radioisotope and peritoneal scintigraphy (137,202,203). If adhesions are present, peritoneal fluid will not distribute equally throughout the abdominal cavity despite changes in patient position or posture (**FIGURE 13.20**). Surgical lysis of adhesions may result in an improvement of dialysate flow and distribution; however, if adhesions are extensive, this procedure may not increase the peritoneal membrane surface area sufficiently to provide adequate solute transport for PD.

Compromised Peritoneal Blood Flow

Although a severe reduction in effective peritoneal blood flow or vascular permeability could theoretically compromise both fluid and solute removal, this must be an extremely rare cause of UFF as we have seen no reports to date. A significant decrease in the peritoneal clearance of urea and creatinine has been observed in

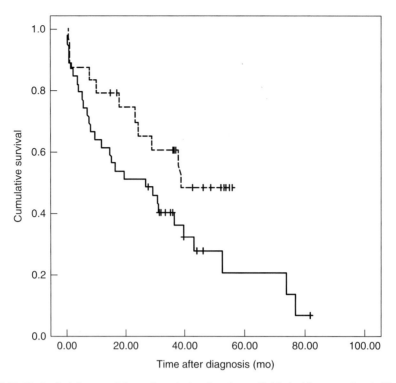

FIGURE 13.19 Survival of encapsulating peritoneal sclerosis patients with (*dashed line*, n = 24) and without (*solid line*, n = 39) treatment with tamoxifen. Time after diagnosis means times in months after EPS diagnosis. The *p* value was 0.077 on univariate analysis. +, censored in analysis. [Data from Korte MR, Fieren MW, Sampimon DE, et al. Tamoxifen is associated with lower mortality of encapsulating peritoneal sclerosis: results of the Dutch Multicentre EPS Study. *Nephrol Dial Transplant* 2011;26(2):691–697.]

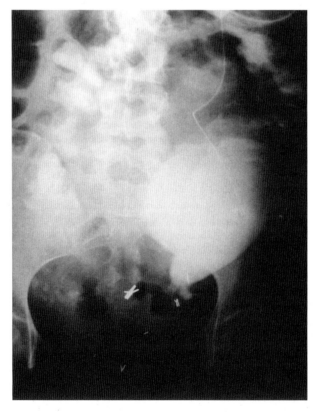

FIGURE 13.20 Plain roentgenogram (flat plate) of the abdomen in a patient with ultrafiltration failure. Before the radiographic examination, 2 L of dialysate containing 100 mL of nonionic radiocontrast were infused into the abdomen. Adhesions in the left lower quadrant of the abdomen result in a loculation of dialysate. This limits flow throughout the abdominal cavity and causes a decrease in the effective peritoneal surface area.

a few patients with systemic vascular disease (e.g., systemic lupus erythematosus, vasculitis, scleroderma, or malignant hypertension), but this was not associated with UFF (204–206).

 CONCLUSION

The potential for UFF increases as patients are successfully maintained on PD for longer periods of time. As a result, assessment of peritoneal membrane function (PET) and RRF should be done on a regular and frequent basis. UFF is usually attributed to changes in the function of the peritoneal membrane that occur with increasing frequency as time on dialysis is prolonged. However, one must recognize that a number of other factors, including loss of RRF, can significantly impact on the efficiency of this therapy and must be considered when faced with a volume-overloaded (or inadequately dialyzed) patient. Although the initial office evaluation may identify the cause of this problem in many cases, the modified PET (using a 4.25% exchange with UFF defined by a 4-hour drain volume of less than 2,400 mL) becomes an essential tool to further assist in the workup of those patients in whom the etiology of volume overload remains unexplained. With the valuable information provided by the PET and the diagnostic algorithm we provide, a logical approach to the assessment of patients with UFF can be developed. Once the appropriate diagnosis is defined, a therapeutic approach can be devised.

 REFERENCES

1. Fenton SS, Schaubel DE, Desmeules M, et al. Hemodialysis versus peritoneal dialysis: a comparison of adjusted mortality rates. *Am J Kidney Dis* 1997;30(3):334–342.
2. Lukowsky LR, Mehrotra R, Kheifets L, et al. Comparing mortality of peritoneal and hemodialysis patients in the first 2 years of dialysis therapy: a marginal structural model analysis. *Clin J Am Soc Nephrol* 2013;8:619–628.
3. Davies SJ, Bryan J, Phillips L, et al. Longitudinal changes in peritoneal kinetics: the effects of peritoneal dialysis and peritonitis. *Nephrol Dial Transplant* 1996;11(3):498–506.
4. Struijk DG, Krediet RT, Koomen GC, et al. A prospective study of peritoneal transport in CAPD patients. *Kidney Int* 1994;45(6):1739–1744.
5. Selgas R, Fernandez-Reyes MJ, Bosque E, et al. Functional longevity of the human peritoneum: how long is continuous peritoneal dialysis possible? Results of a prospective medium long-term study. *Am J Kidney Dis* 1994;23(1):64–73.
6. Heimbürger O, Waniewski J, Werynski A, et al. Peritoneal transport in CAPD patients with permanent loss of ultrafiltration capacity. *Kidney Int* 1990;38(3):495–506.
7. Kawaguchi Y, Hasegawa T, Nakayama M, et al. Issues affecting the longevity of the continuous peritoneal dialysis therapy. *Kidney Int Suppl* 1997;62:S105–S107.
8. Davies SJ, Brown B, Bryan J, et al. Clinical evaluation of the peritoneal equilibration test: a population-based study. *Nephrol Dial Transplant* 1993;8(1):64–70.
9. Mujais S, Story K. Peritoneal dialysis in the US: evaluation of outcomes in contemporary cohorts. *Kidney Int* 2006;73(Suppl 103):S21–S26.
10. Slingeneyer A, Canaud B, Mion C. Permanent loss of ultrafiltration capacity of the peritoneum in long-term peritoneal dialysis: an epidemiological study. *Nephron* 1983;33(2):133–138.
11. Gokal R, Jakubowski C, King J, et al. Outcome in patients on continuous ambulatory peritoneal dialysis and haemodialysis: 4-year analysis of a prospective multicentre study. *Lancet* 1987;2(8568):1105–1109.
12. Coles GA, Williams JD. The management of ultrafiltration failure in peritoneal dialysis. *Kidney Int Suppl* 1994;48:S14–S17.
13. Krediet RT, Imholz AL, Struijk DG, et al. Ultrafiltration failure in continuous ambulatory peritoneal dialysis. *Perit Dial Int* 1993;13 (Suppl 2):S59–S66.
14. Ho-dac-Pannekeet MM, Atasever B, Struijk DG, et al. Analysis of ultrafiltration failure in peritoneal dialysis patients by means of standard peritoneal permeability analysis. *Perit Dial Int* 1997;17(2):144–150.
15. Mujais S, Nolph K, Gokal R, et al. International Society for Peritoneal Dialysis Ad Hoc Committee on Ultrafiltration Management in Peritoneal Dialysis. Evaluation and management of ultrafiltration problems in peritoneal dialysis. *Perit Dial Int* 2000;20(Suppl 4):S5–S21.
16. Smit W, Schouten N, van den Berg N, et al. Analysis of the prevalence and causes of ultrafiltration failure during long-term peritoneal dialysis: a cross-sectional study. *Perit Dial Int* 2004;24(6):562–570.
17. Nolph KD, Popovich RP, Ghods AJ, et al. Determinants of low clearances of small solutes during peritoneal dialysis. *Kidney Int* 1978;13(2):117–123.
18. Flessner MF. Peritoneal transport physiology: insights from basic research. *J Am Soc Nephrol* 1991;2(2):122–135.
19. Wegner G. Chirurgische bemerkingen uber die peritoneal hole, mit besonderer berucksichti der ovariotomie [in German]. *Arch Klin Chir* 1877;20:51–59.
20. Nolph KD. Clinical implications of membrane transport characteristics on the adequacy of fluid and solute removal. *Perit Dial Int* 1994;14(Suppl 3):S78–S81.
21. Krediet RT, Struijk DG, Boeschoten EW, et al. The time course of peritoneal transport kinetics in continuous ambulatory peritoneal dialysis patients who develop sclerosing peritonitis. *Am J Kidney Dis* 1989;13(4):299–307.
22. Imholz AL, Koomen GC, Struijk DG, et al. Effect of an increased intraperitoneal pressure on fluid and solute transport during CAPD. *Kidney Int* 1993;44(5):1078–1085.
23. Flessner MF, Dedrick RL. Role of the liver in small-solute transport during peritoneal dialysis. *J Am Soc Nephrol* 1994;5(1):116–120.
24. Rippe B, Stelin G, Haraldsson B. Computer simulations of peritoneal fluid transport in CAPD. *Kidney Int* 1991;40(2):315–325.
25. Schoenicke G, Diamant R, Donner A, et al. Histochemical distribution and expression of aquaporin 1 in the peritoneum of patients undergoing peritoneal dialysis: relation to peritoneal transport. *Am J Kidney Dis* 2004;44(1):146–154.
26. Flessner MF. Peritoneal ultrafiltration: physiology and failure. *Contrib Nephrol* 2009;163:7–14.
27. Keshaviah P, Emerson PF, Vonesh EF, et al. Relationship between body size, fill volume, and mass transfer area coefficient in peritoneal dialysis. *J Am Soc Nephrol* 1994;4(10):1820–1826.
28. Nolph KD, Twardowski ZJ, Popovich RP, et al. Equilibration of peritoneal dialysis solutions during long-dwell exchanges. *J Lab Clin Med* 1979;93(2):246–256.
29. Robson M, Oreopoulos DG, Izatt S, et al. Influence of exchange volume and dialysate flow rate on solute clearance in peritoneal dialysis. *Kidney Int* 1978;14(5):486–490.
30. Ronco C, Feriani M, Chiaramonte S, et al. Pathophysiology of ultrafiltration in peritoneal dialysis. *Perit Dial Int* 1990;10(2):119–126.
31. Grzegorzewska AE, Moore HL, Nolph KD, et al. Ultrafiltration and effective peritoneal blood flow during peritoneal dialysis in the rat. *Kidney Int* 1991;39(4):608–617.
32. Imholz AL, Koomen GC, Struijk DG, et al. Residual volume measurements in CAPD patients with exogenous and endogenous solutes. *Adv Perit Dial* 1992;8:33–38.
33. Mactier R. Influence of dwell time, osmolarity, and volume of exchanges on solute mass transfer and ultrafiltration in peritoneal dialysis. *Semin Dial* 1988;1:40–49.
34. Heimbürger O, Waniewski J, Werynski A, et al. A quantitative description of solute and fluid transport during peritoneal dialysis. *Kidney Int* 1992;41(5):1320–1332.
35. Pyle WK. *Mass Transfer in Peritoneal Dialysis* [dissertation]. Austin, TX: University of Texas, 1981.
36. Leypoldt JK. Evaluation of peritoneal membrane permeability. *Adv Ren Replace Ther* 1995;2(3):265–273.
37. Abensur H, Romäo Júnior JE, Prado EB, et al. Use of dextran 70 to estimate peritoneal lymphatic absorption rate in CAPD. *Adv Perit Dial* 1992;8:3–6.

38. Mactier RA, Khanna R, Twardowski Z, et al. Contribution of lymphatic absorption to loss of ultrafiltration and solute clearances in continuous ambulatory peritoneal dialysis. *J Clin Invest* 1987;80(5):1311–1316.

39. Nolph KD, Mactier R, Khanna R, et al. The kinetics of ultrafiltration during peritoneal dialysis: the role of lymphatics. *Kidney Int* 1987;32(2):219–226.

40. Twardowski Z. Peritoneal equilibration test. *Perit Dial Bull* 1987;7:138–147.

41. Garred L. A simple kinetic model for assessing peritoneal mass transfer in continuous ambulatory peritoneal dialysis. *ASAIO J* 1983;6:131–137.

42. Hiatt MP, Pyle WK, Moncrief JW, et al. A comparison of the relative efficacy of CAPD and hemodialysis in the control of solute concentration. *Artif Organs* 1980;4(1):37–43.

43. Twardowski ZJ. Clinical value of standardized equilibration tests in CAPD patients. *Blood Purif* 1989;7(2–3):95–108.

44. Twardowski ZJ. Peritoneal dialysis glossary III. *Perit Dial Int* 1990;10(2):173–175.

45. Lo WK, Brendolan A, Prowant BF, et al. Changes in the peritoneal equilibration test in selected chronic peritoneal dialysis patients. *J Am Soc Nephrol* 1994;4(7):1466–1474.

46. Twardowski ZJ, Nolph KD, Khanna R. Limitations of the peritoneal equilibration test. *Nephrol Dial Transplant* 1995;10(11):2160–2161.

47. Twardowski Z. The fast peritoneal equilibration test. *Semin Dial* 1990;3:141–142.

48. Enia G, Curatola G, Panuccio V, et al. The reproducibility of the fast peritoneal equilibration test. *Perit Dial Int* 1995;15(8):382–384.

49. Adcock A, Fox K, Walker P, et al. Clinical experience and comparative analysis of the standard and fast peritoneal equilibration tests (PET). *Adv Perit Dial* 1992;8:59–61.

50. Pride ET, Gustafson J, Graham A, et al. Comparison of a 2.5% and a 4.25% dextrose peritoneal equilibration test. *Perit Dial Int* 2002;22(3):365–370.

51. Warady BA, Alexander SR, Hossli S, et al. Peritoneal membrane transport function in children receiving long-term dialysis. *J Am Soc Nephrol* 1996;7(11):2385–2391.

52. Bouts AH, Davin JC, Groothoff JW, et al. Standard peritoneal permeability analysis in children. *J Am Soc Nephrol* 2000;11(5):943–950.

53. Kohaut EC, Waldo FB, Benfield MR. The effect of changes in dialysate volume on glucose and urea equilibration. *Perit Dial Int* 1994;14(3):236–239.

54. Smit W, Langedijk MJ, Schouten N, et al. A comparison between 1.36% and 3.86% glucose dialysis solution for the assessment of peritoneal membrane function. *Perit Dial Int* 2000;20(6):734–741.

55. Rippe B. How to measure ultrafiltration failure: 2.27% or 3.86% glucose? *Perit Dial Int* 1997;17(2):125–128.

56. Rippe B, Stelin G. Simulations of peritoneal solute transport during CAPD. Application of two-pore formalism. *Kidney Int* 1989;35(5):1234–1244.

57. Ho-dac-Pannekeet MM, Schouten N, Langendijk MJ, et al. Peritoneal transport characteristics with glucose polymer based dialysate. *Kidney Int* 1996;50(3):979–986.

58. Carlsson O, Nielsen S, Zakaria ER, et al. In vivo inhibition of transcellular water channels (aquaporin-1) during acute peritoneal dialysis in rats. *Am J Physiol* 1996;271(6 Pt 2):H2254–H2262.

59. Zweers MM, Imholz AL, Struijk DG, et al. Correction of sodium sieving for diffusion from the circulation. *Adv Perit Dial* 1999;15:65–72.

60. La Milia V, Di Filippo S, Crepaldi M, et al. Mini-peritoneal equilibration test: a simple and fast method to assess free water and small solute transport across the peritoneal membrane. *Kidney Int* 2005;68(2):840–846.

61. Rippe B, Venturoli D, Simonsen O, et al. Fluid and electrolyte transport across the peritoneal membrane during CAPD according to the three-pore model. *Perit Dial Int* 2004;24(1):10–27.

62. Venturoli D, Rippe B. Validation by computer simulation of two indirect methods for quantification of free water transport in peritoneal dialysis. *Perit Dial Int* 2005;25(1):77–84.

63. Pannekeet MM, Imholz AL, Struijk DG, et al. The standard peritoneal permeability analysis: a tool for the assessment of peritoneal permeability characteristics in CAPD patients. *Kidney Int* 1995;48(3):866–875.

64. Rocco MV, Jordan JR, Burkart JM. Determination of peritoneal transport characteristics with 24-hour dialysate collections: dialysis adequacy and transport test. *J Am Soc Nephrol* 1994;5(6):1333–1338.

65. Sherman RA. The peritoneal permeability and surface area index. *Perit Dial Int* 1994;14(3):240–242.

66. Blake PG, Abraham G, Sombolos K, et al. Changes in peritoneal membrane transport rates in patients on long term CAPD. *Adv Perit Dial* 1989;5:3–7.

67. Passlick-Deetjen J, Chlebowski H, Koch M, et al. Changes of peritoneal membrane function during long-term CAPD. *Adv Perit Dial* 1990;6:35–43.

68. Hallett MD, Charlton B, Farrell PC. Is the peritoneal membrane durable indefinitely? *Adv Perit Dial* 1990;6:197–201.

69. Warren PJ, Brandes JC. Compliance with the peritoneal dialysis prescription is poor. *J Am Soc Nephrol* 1994;4(8):1627–1629.

70. Brandes JC. Do we have an objective method to determine compliance with the peritoneal dialysis prescription? *Perit Dial Int* 1996;16(2):114–115.

71. Blake PG, Korbet SM, Blake R, et al. A multicenter study of noncompliance with continuous ambulatory peritoneal dialysis exchanges in US and Canadian patients. *Am J Kidney Dis* 2000;35(3):506–514.

72. Canada-USA (CANUSA) Peritoneal Dialysis Study Group. Adequacy of dialysis and nutrition in continuous peritoneal dialysis: association with clinical outcomes. *J Am Soc Nephrol* 1996;7(2):198–207.

73. Bargman JM, Thorpe KE, Churchill DN. Relative contribution of residual renal function and peritoneal clearance to adequacy of dialysis: a reanalysis of the CANUSA study. *J Am Soc Nephrol* 2001;12(10):2158–2162.

74. Li PK, Chow KM, Wong TY, et al. Effects of an angiotensin-converting enzyme inhibitor on residual renal function in patients receiving peritoneal dialysis. A randomized, controlled study. *Ann Intern Med* 2003;139(2):105–112.

75. Suzuki H, Kanno Y, Sugahara S, et al. Effects of an angiotensin II receptor blocker, valsartan, on residual renal function in patients on CAPD. *Am J Kidney Dis* 2004;43(6):1056–1064.

76. Johnson DW, Brown FG, Clarke M, et al. Effects of biocompatible versus standard fluid on peritoneal dialysis outcomes. *J Am Soc Nephrol* 2012;23(6):1097–1107.

77. Lui SL, Yung S, Yim A, et al. A combination of biocompatible peritoneal dialysis solutions and residual renal function, peritoneal transport, and inflammation markers: a randomized clinical trial. *Am J Kidney Dis* 2012;60(6):966–975.

78. Kim S, Oh KH, Oh J, et al. Biocompatible peritoneal dialysis solution preserves residual renal function. *Am J Nephrol* 2012;36(4):305–316.

79. Cho Y, Johnson DW, Badve S, et al. Impact of icodextrin on clinical outcomes in peritoneal dialysis: a systematic review of randomized controlled trials. *Nephrol Dial Transplant* 2013;28(7):1899–1907.

80. Lo WK, Bargman JM, Burkart J, et al. Guideline on targets for solute and fluid removal in adult patients on chronic peritoneal dialysis. *Perit Dial Int* 2006;26(5):520–522.

81. Margetts PJ, Gyorffy S, Kolb M, et al. Antiangiogenic and antifibrotic gene therapy in a chronic infusion model of peritoneal dialysis in rats. *J Am Soc Nephrol* 2002;13(3):721–728.

82. Brimble KS, Walker M, Margetts PJ, et al. Meta-analysis: peritoneal membrane transport, mortality, and technique failure in peritoneal dialysis. *J Am Soc Nephrol* 2006;17(9):2591–2598.

83. Davies SJ, Phillips L, Griffiths AM, et al. What really happens to people on long-term peritoneal dialysis? *Kidney Int* 1998;54(6):2207–2217.

84. Davies SJ, Phillips L, Russell GI. Peritoneal solute transport predicts survival on CAPD independently of residual renal function. *Nephrol Dial Transplant* 1998;13(4):962–968.

85. Churchill DN, Thorpe KE, Nolph KD, et al. The Canada-USA (CANUSA) Peritoneal Dialysis Study Group. Increased peritoneal membrane transport is associated with decreased patient and technique survival for continuous peritoneal dialysis patients. *J Am Soc Nephrol* 1998;9(7):1285–1292.

86. Rumpsfeld M, McDonald SP, Johnson DW. Higher peritoneal transport status is associated with higher mortality and technique failure in the Australian and New Zealand peritoneal dialysis patient populations. *J Am Soc Nephrol* 2006;17(1):271–278.

87. Brimble KS, Walker M, Margetts PJ, et al. Meta-analysis: peritoneal membrane transport, mortality, technique failure in peritoneal dialysis. *J Am Soc Nephrol.* 2006;17(9):2591–2598.

88. Mortier S, De Vriese AS, Lameire N. Recent concepts in the molecular biology of the peritoneal membrane–implications for more biocompatible dialysis solutions. *Blood Purif* 2003;21(1):14–23.

89. Szeto CC, Wong TY, Lai KB, et al. The role of vascular endothelial growth factor in peritoneal hyperpermeability during CAPD-related peritonitis. *Perit Dial Int* 2002;22(2):265–267.

90. Combet S, Miyata T, Moulin P, et al. Vascular proliferation and enhanced expression of endothelial nitric oxide synthase in human peritoneum exposed to long-term peritoneal dialysis. *J Am Soc Nephrol* 2000;11(4):717–728.

91. Williams JD, Craig KJ, Topley N, et al. Morphologic changes in the peritoneal membrane of patients with renal disease. *J Am Soc Nephrol* 2002;13(2):470–479.

92. Noh H, Kim JS, Han KH, et al. Oxidative stress during peritoneal dialysis: implications in functional and structural changes in the membrane. *Kidney Int* 2006;69(11):2022–2028.

93. Sitter T, Sauter M. Impact of glucose in peritoneal dialysis: saint or sinner? *Perit Dial Int* 2005;25(5):415–425.

94. Goffin E, Devuyst O. Phenotype and genotype: perspectives for peritoneal dialysis patients. *Nephrol Dial Transplant* 2006;21(11):3018–3022.

95. De Vriese AS, Stoenoiu MS, Elger M, et al. Diabetes-induced microvascular dysfunction in the hydronephrotic kidney: role of nitric oxide. *Kidney Int* 2001;60(1):202–210.

96. Yáñez-Mó M, Lara-Pezzi E, Selgas R, et al. Peritoneal dialysis and epithelial-to-mesenchymal transition of mesothelial cells. *N Engl J Med* 2003;348(5):403–413.

97. Jiménez-Heffernan JA, Aguilera A, Aroeira LS, et al. Immunohistochemical characterization of fibroblast subpopulations in normal peritoneal tissue and in peritoneal dialysis-induced fibrosis. *Virchows Arch* 2004;444(3):247–256.

98. Aroeira LS, Aguilera A, Selgas R, et al. Mesenchymal conversion of mesothelial cells as a mechanism responsible for high solute transport rate in peritoneal dialysis: role of vascular endothelial growth factor. *Am J Kidney Dis* 2005;46(5):938–948.

99. Margetts PJ, Bonniaud P, Liu L, et al. Transient overexpression of TGF-β-1 induces epithelial mesenchymal transition in the rodent peritoneum. *J Am Soc Nephrol* 2005;16(2):425–436.

100. Rougier JP, Guia S, Hagège J, et al. PAI-1 secretion and matrix deposition in human peritoneal mesothelial cell cultures: transcriptional regulation by TGF-β-1. *Kidney Int* 1998;54(1):87–98.

101. Chung SH, Heimbürger O, Stenvinkel P, et al. Association between inflammation and changes in residual renal function and peritoneal transport rate during the first year of dialysis. *Nephrol Dial Transplant* 2001;16(11):2240–2245.

102. Wang T, Heimbürger O, Cheng HH, et al. Does a high peritoneal transport rate reflect a state of chronic inflammation? *Perit Dial Int* 1999;19(1):17–22.

103. Lambie M, Chess J, Donovan KL, et al. Independent effects of systemic and peritoneal inflammation on peritoneal dialysis survival. *J Am Soc Nephrol* 2013;24(12):2071–2080.

104. Miranda B, Selgas R, Celadilla O, et al. Peritoneal resting and heparinization as an effective treatment for ultrafiltration failure in patients on CAPD. *Contrib Nephrol* 1991;89:199–204.

105. de Alvaro F, Castro MJ, Dapena F, et al. Peritoneal resting is beneficial in peritoneal hyperpermeability and ultrafiltration failure. *Adv Perit Dial* 1993;9:56–61.

106. De Sousa E, Del Peso G, Alvarez L, et al. Peritoneal resting with heparinized lavage reverses peritoneal type I membrane failure. A comparative study of the resting effects on normal membranes. *Perit Dial Int* 2014;34(7):698–705.

107. Krediet RT. Dialysate cancer antigen 125 concentration as marker of peritoneal membrane status in patients treated with chronic peritoneal dialysis. *Perit Dial Int* 2001;21(6):560–567.

108. Plum J, Gentile S, Verger C, et al. Efficacy and safety of a 7.5% icodextrin peritoneal dialysis solution in patients treated with automated peritoneal dialysis. *Am J Kidney Dis* 2002;39(4):862–871.

109. Wolfson M, Piraino B, Hamburger RJ, et al. A randomized controlled trial to evaluate the efficacy and safety of icodextrin in peritoneal dialysis. *Am J Kidney Dis* 2002;40(5):1055–1065.

110. Huarte-Loza E, Selgas R, Carmona AR, et al. Peritoneal membrane failure as a determinant of the CAPD future. An epidemiological, functional and pathological study. *Contrib Nephrol* 1987;57:219–229.

111. Davies SJ, Brown EA, Frandsen NE, et al. Longitudinal membrane function in functionally anuric patients treated with APD: data from EAPOS on the effects of glucose and icodextrin prescription. *Kidney Int* 2005;67(4):1609–1615.

112. Haas S, Schmitt CP, Arbeiter K, et al. Improved acidosis correction and recovery of mesothelial cell mass with neutral-pH bicarbonate dialysis solution among children undergoing automated peritoneal dialysis. *J Am Soc Nephrol* 2003;14(10):2632–2638.

113. Fusshoeller A, Plail M, Grabensee B, et al. Biocompatibility pattern of a bicarbonate/lactate-buffered peritoneal dialysis fluid in APD: a prospective, randomized study. *Nephrol Dial Transplant* 2004;19(8):2101–2106.

114. Lee HY, Choi HY, Park HC, et al. Changing prescribing practice in CAPD patients in Korea: increased utilization of low GDP solutions improves patient outcome. *Nephrol Dial Transplant* 2006;21(10):2893–2899.

115. Johnson DW, Brown FG, Clarke M, et al. The effect of low glucose degradation product, neutral pH versus standard peritoneal dialysis solutions on peritoneal membrane function: the balANZ trial. *Nephrol Dial Transplant* 2012;27(12):4445–4453.

116. Witowski J, Bender TO, Gahl GM, et al. Glucose degradation products and peritoneal membrane function. *Perit Dial Int* 2001;21(2):201–205.

117. Ing TS, Yu AW, Thompson KD, et al. Peritoneal dialysis using conventional, lactate-containing solution sterilized by ultrafiltration. *Int J Artif Organs* 1992;15(11):658–660.

118. Yu AW, Manahan FJ, Filkins JP, et al. Peritoneal dialysis using bicarbonate-containing solution sterilized by ultrafiltration. *Int J Artif Organs* 1991;14(8):463–465.

119. Chan TM, Leung JK, Sun Y, et al. Different effects of amino acid-based and glucose-based dialysate from peritoneal dialysis patients on mesothelial cell ultrastructure and function. *Nephrol Dial Transplant* 2003;18(6):1086–1094.

120. Zareie M, van Lambalgen AA, ter Wee PM, et al. Better preservation of the peritoneum in rats exposed to amino acid-based peritoneal dialysis fluid. *Perit Dial Int* 2005;25(1):58–67.

121. Yung S, Lui SL, Ng CK, et al. Impact of a low-glucose peritoneal dialysis regimen on fibrosis and inflammation biomarkers. *Perit Dial Int* 2015;35(2):147–158.

122. le Poole CY, van Ittersum FJ, Weijmer MC, et al. Clinical effects of a peritoneal dialysis regimen low in glucose in new peritoneal dialysis patients: a randomized crossover study. *Adv Perit Dial* 2004;20:170–176.

123. Li FK, Chan LY, Woo JC, et al. A 3-year, prospective, randomized, controlled study on amino acid dialysate in patients on CAPD. *Am J Kidney Dis* 2003;42(1):173–183.

124. Duman S, Günal AI, Sen S, et al. Does enalapril prevent peritoneal fibrosis induced by hypertonic (3.86%) peritoneal dialysis solution? *Perit Dial Int* 2001;21(2):219–224.

125. van Westrhenen R. Lisinopril protects against the development of fibrosis during chronic peritoneal exposure to dialysis fluid [abstract]. *Perit Dial Int* 2004;24(Suppl 2):S10.

126. Kolesnyk I, Dekker FW, Noordzij M, et al. Impact of ACE inhibitors and AII receptor blockers on peritoneal membrane transport characteristics in long-term peritoneal dialysis patients. *Perit Dial Int* 2007;27(4):446–453.

127. Kolesnyk I, Noordzij M, Dekker FW, et al. A positive effect of AII inhibitors on peritoneal membrane function in long-term PD patients. *Nephrol Dial Transplant* 2009;24(1):272–277.

128. Horton JK, Davies M, Topley N, et al. Activation of the inflammatory response of neutrophils by Tamm-Horsfall glycoprotein. *Kidney Int* 1990;37(2):717–726.

129. Albrektsen GE, Widerøe TE, Nilsen TI, et al. Transperitoneal water transport before, during, and after episodes with infectious peritonitis in patients treated with CAPD. *Am J Kidney Dis* 2004;43(3):485–491.

130. Panasiuk E. Characteristics of peritoneum after peritonitis in CAPD patients. *Adv Perit Dial* 1988;4:42–45.

131. Davies SJ, Phillips L, Griffiths AM, et al. Impact of peritoneal membrane function on long-term clinical outcome in peritoneal dialysis patients. *Perit Dial Int* 1999;19(Suppl 2):S91–S94.

132. Dobbie JW. Morphology of the peritoneum in CAPD. *Blood Purif* 1989;7(2–3):74–85.

133. Van Dijk CM, Ledesma SG, Teitelbaum I. Patient characteristics associated with defects of the peritoneal cavity boundary. *Perit Dial Int* 2005;25(4):367–373.

134. Kopecky RT, Frymoyer PA, Witanowski LS, et al. Complications of continuous ambulatory peritoneal dialysis: diagnostic value of peritoneal scintigraphy. *Am J Kidney Dis* 1987;10(2):123–132.

135. Perez-Fontan M. Rupture of hernia sac as cause of massive subcutaneous dialysis leak in CAPD: diagnostic value of peritoneography. *Dial Transplant* 1986;10:123–132.

136. Leblanc M, Ouimet D, Pichette V. Dialysate leaks in peritoneal dialysis. *Semin Dial* 2001;14(1):50–54.

137. Twardowski Z. Computerized tomography CT in the diagnosis of subcutaneous leak sites during continuous ambulatory peritoneal dialysis (CAPD). *Perit Dial Bull* 1984;4:163–166.

138. Juergensen PH, Rizvi H, Caride VJ, et al. Value of scintigraphy in chronic peritoneal dialysis patients. *Kidney Int* 1999;55(3):1111–1119.

139. Tokmak H, Mudun A, Türkmen C, et al. The role of peritoneal scintigraphy in the detection of continuous ambulatory peritoneal dialysis complications. *Ren Fail* 2006;28(8):709–713.

140. Shah H, Chu M, Bargman JM. Perioperative management of peritoneal dialysis patients undergoing hernia surgery without the use of interim hemodialysis. *Perit Dial Int* 2006;26(6):684–687.

141. Schleifer C. Migration of peritoneal catheters: personal experience and survey of 72 other units. *Perit Dial Bull* 1987;1987:189–193.

142. Moss JS, Minda SA, Newman GE, et al. Malpositioned peritoneal dialysis catheters: a critical reappraisal of correction by stiff-wire manipulation. *Am J Kidney Dis* 1990;15(4):305–308.

143. Crabtree JH. Selected best demonstrated practices in peritoneal dialysis access. *Kidney Int Suppl* 2006;70(103):S27–S37.

144. Di Paolo N, Petrini G, Garosi G, et al. A new self-locating peritoneal catheter. *Perit Dial Int* 1996;16(6):623–627.

145. Bargman JM. New technologies in peritoneal dialysis. *Clin J Am Soc Nephrol* 2007;2(3):576–580.

146. Monquil MC, Imholz AL, Struijk DG, et al. Does impaired transcellular water transport contribute to net ultrafiltration failure during CAPD? *Perit Dial Int* 1995;15(1):42–48.

147. Dobbie JW, Krediet RT, Twardowski ZJ, et al. A 39-year-old man with loss of ultrafiltration. *Perit Dial Int* 1994;14(4):384–394.

148. Goffin E, Combet S, Jamar F, et al. Expression of aquaporin-1 in a long-term peritoneal dialysis patient with impaired transcellular water transport. *Am J Kidney Dis* 1999;33(2):383–388.

149. Combet S, Van Landschoot M, Moulin P, et al. Regulation of aquaporin-1 and nitric oxide synthase isoforms in a rat model of acute peritonitis. *J Am Soc Nephrol* 1999;10(10):2185–2196.

150. Smit W, van den Berg N, Schouten N, et al. Free-water transport in fast transport status: a comparison between CAPD peritonitis and long-term PD. *Kidney Int* 2004;65(1):298–303.

151. de Arteaga J, Ledesma F, Garay G, et al. High-dose steroid treatment increases free water transport in peritoneal dialysis patients. *Nephrol Dial Transplant* 2011;26(12):4142–4145.

152. Yool AJ, Morelle J, Cnops Y, et al. AqF026 is a pharmacologic agonist of the water channel aquaporin-1. *J Am Soc Nephrol* 2013;24(7):1045–1052.

153. Smit W, van Dijk P, Langedijk MJ, et al. Peritoneal function and assessment of reference values using a 3.86% glucose solution. *Perit Dial Int* 2003;23(5):440–449.

154. Imholz AL, Koomen GC, Voorn WJ, et al. Day-to-day variability of fluid and solute transport in upright and recumbent positions during CAPD. *Nephrol Dial Transplant* 1998;13(1):146–153.

155. Krediet RT, Boeschoten EW, Struijk DG, et al. Differences in the peritoneal transport of water, solutes and proteins between dialysis with two- and with three-litre exchanges. *Nephrol Dial Transplant* 1988;3(2):198–204.

156. Durand PY, Chanliau J, Gamberoni J, et al. Intraperitoneal pressure, peritoneal permeability and volume of ultrafiltration in CAPD. *Adv Perit Dial* 1992;8:22–25.

157. Chan PC, Wu PG, Tam SC, et al. Factors affecting lymphatic absorption in Chinese patients on continuous ambulatory peritoneal dialysis (CAPD). *Perit Dial Int* 1991;11(2):147–151.

158. Imholz AL, Koomen GC, Struijk DG, et al. Effect of dialysate osmolarity on the transport of low-molecular weight solutes and proteins during CAPD. *Kidney Int* 1993;43(6):1339–1346.

159. Douma CE, de Waart DR, Struijk DG, et al. Effect of amino acid based dialysate on peritoneal blood flow and permeability in stable CAPD patients: a potential role for nitric oxide? *Clin Nephrol* 1996;45(5):295–302.

160. Smit W, de Waart DR, Struijk DG, et al. Peritoneal transport characteristics with glycerol-based dialysate in peritoneal dialysis. *Perit Dial Int* 2000;20(5):557–565.

161. Michels WM, Zweers MM, Smit W, et al. Does lymphatic absorption change with the duration of peritoneal dialysis? *Perit Dial Int* 2004;24(4):347–352.

162. Kinashi H, Ito Y, Mizuno M, et al. TGF-β1 promotes lymphangiogenesis during peritoneal fibrosis. *J Am Soc Nephrol* 2013;24(10):1627–1642.

163. Fusshöller A, zur Nieden S, Grabensee B, et al. Peritoneal fluid and solute transport: influence of treatment time, peritoneal dialysis modality, and peritonitis incidence. *J Am Soc Nephrol* 2002;13(4):1055–1060.

164. Querques M, Procaccini DA, Pappani A, et al. Influence of phosphatidylcholine on ultrafiltration and solute transfer in CAPD patients. *ASAIO Trans* 1990;36(3):M581–M583.

165. De Vecchi A, Castelnovo C, Guerra L, et al. Phosphatidylcholine administration in continuous ambulatory peritoneal dialysis (CAPD) patients with reduced ultrafiltration. *Perit Dial Int* 1989;9(3):207–210.

166. Krack G, Viglino G, Cavalli PL, et al. Intraperitoneal administration of phosphatidylcholine improves ultrafiltration in continuous ambulatory peritoneal dialysis patients. *Perit Dial Int* 1992;12(4):359–364.

167. Di Paolo N, Buoncristiani U, Capotondo L, et al. Phosphatidylcholine and peritoneal transport during peritoneal dialysis. *Nephron* 1986;44(4):365–370.

168. Hills BA. Role of surfactant in peritoneal dialysis. *Perit Dial Int* 2000;20(5):503–515.

169. Chen Y, Burke JR, Hills BA. Semipermeability imparted by surface-active phospholipid in peritoneal dialysis. *Perit Dial Int* 2002;22(3):380–385.

170. Baranowska-Daca E, Torneli J, Popovich RP, et al. Use of bethanechol chloride to increase available ultrafiltration in CAPD. *Adv Perit Dial* 1995;11:69–72.

171. Kawaguchi Y, Kawanishi H, Mujais S, et al. Encapsulating peritoneal sclerosis: definition, etiology, diagnosis, and treatment. International Society for Peritoneal Dialysis Ad Hoc Committee on Ultrafiltration Management in Peritoneal Dialysis. *Perit Dial Int* 2000;20(Suppl 4):S43–S55.

172. Kawanishi H, Moriishi M. Epidemiology of encapsulating peritoneal sclerosis in Japan. *Perit Dial Int* 2005;25(Suppl 4):S14–S18.

173. Rigby RJ, Hawley CM. Sclerosing peritonitis: the experience in Australia. *Nephrol Dial Transplant* 1998;13(1):154–159.

174. Summers AM, Clancy MJ, Syed F, et al. Single-center experience of encapsulating peritoneal sclerosis in patients on peritoneal dialysis for end-stage renal failure. *Kidney Int* 2005;68(5):2381–2388.

175. Tarzi RM, Lim A, Moser S, et al. Assessing the validity of an abdominal CT scoring system in the diagnosis of encapsulating peritoneal sclerosis. *Clin J Am Soc Nephrol* 2008;3(6):1702–1710.

176. Krestin GP, Kacl G, Hauser M, et al. Imaging diagnosis of sclerosing peritonitis and relation of radiologic signs to the extent of the disease. *Abdom Imaging* 1995;20(5):414–420.

177. Hollman AS, McMillan MA, Briggs JD, et al. Ultrasound changes in sclerosing peritonitis following continuous ambulatory peritoneal dialysis. *Clin Radiol* 1991;43(3):176–179.

178. Célicout B, Levard H, Hay J, et al. French Associations for Surgical Research. Sclerosing encapsulating peritonitis: early and late results of surgical management in 32 cases. *Dig Surg* 1998;15(6):697–702.

179. Kaushik R, Punia RP, Mohan H, et al. Tuberculous abdominal cocoon—a report of 6 cases and review of the literature. *World J Emerg Surg* 2006;1:18.

180. Lalloo S, Krishna D, Maharajh J. Case report: abdominal cocoon associated with tuberculous pelvic inflammatory disease. *Br J Radiol* 2002;75(890):174–176.

181. Eltringham WK, Espiner HJ, Windsor CW, et al. Sclerosing peritonitis due to practolol: a report on 9 cases and their surgical management. *Br J Surg* 1977;64(4):229–235.

182. Cudazzo E, Lucchini A, Puviani PP, et al. Sclerosing peritonitis. A complication of LeVeen peritoneovenous shunt. *Minerva Chir* 1999;54(11):809–812.

183. Stanley MM, Reyes CV, Greenlee HB, et al. Peritoneal fibrosis in cirrhotics treated with peritoneovenous shunting for ascites. An autopsy study with clinical correlations. *Dig Dis Sci* 1996;41(3):571–577.

184. Maguire D, Srinivasan P, O'Grady J, et al. Sclerosing encapsulating peritonitis after orthotopic liver transplantation. *Am J Surg* 2001;182(2):151–154.

185. Morelle J, Sow A, Hautem N, et al. Interstitial fibrosis restricts osmotic water transport in encapsulating peritoneal sclerosis. *J Am Soc Nephrol* 2015;26(10):2521–2533.

186. Numata M. A single nucleotide polymorphism (SNP) in the RAGE-429 T/C genotype may be related to encapsulating peritoneal sclerosis (EPS) in Japanese peritoneal dialysis (PD) patients [abstract]. *J Am Soc Nephrol* 2003;14:214A.

187. Wong TY, Szeto CC, Szeto CY, et al. Association of ENOS polymorphism with basal peritoneal membrane function in uremic patients. *Am J Kidney Dis* 2003;42(4):781–786.

188. Betjes MG, Habib MS, Struijk DG, et al. Encapsulating peritoneal sclerosis is associated with T-cell activation. *Nephrol Dial Transplant* 2015;30(9):1568–1576.

189. Kawaguchi Y, Saito A, Kawanishi H, et al. Recommendations on the management of encapsulating peritoneal sclerosis in Japan, 2005: diagnosis, predictive markers, treatment, and preventive measures. *Perit Dial Int* 2005;25(Suppl 4):S83–S95.

190. Balasubramaniam G, Brown EA, Davenport A, et al. The Pan-Thames EPS study: treatment and outcomes of encapsulating peritoneal sclerosis. *Nephrol Dial Transplant* 2009;24(10):3209–3215.

191. Allaria PM, Giangrande A, Gandini E, et al. Continuous ambulatory peritoneal dialysis and sclerosing encapsulating peritonitis: tamoxifen as a new therapeutic agent? *J Nephrol* 1999;12(6):395–397.

192. del Peso G, Bajo MA, Gil F, et al. Clinical experience with tamoxifen in peritoneal fibrosing syndromes. *Adv Perit Dial* 2003;19:32–35.

193. Eltoum MA, Wright S, Atchley J, et al. Four consecutive cases of peritoneal dialysis-related encapsulating peritoneal sclerosis treated successfully with tamoxifen. *Perit Dial Int* 2006;26(2):203–206.

194. Wong CF. Clinical experience with tamoxifen in encapsulating peritoneal sclerosis. *Perit Dial Int* 2006;26(2):183–184.

195. Korte MR, Fieren MW, Sampimon DE, et al. Tamoxifen is associated with lower mortality of encapsulating peritoneal sclerosis: results of the Dutch Multicentre EPS Study. *Nephrol Dial Transplant* 2011;26(2):691–697.

196. Bhandari S. Recovery of gastrointestinal function after renal transplantation in patients with sclerosing peritonitis secondary to continuous ambulatory peritoneal dialysis. *Am J Kidney Dis* 1996; 27(4):604.

197. Hawley CM, Wall DR, Johnson DW, et al. Recovery of gastrointestinal function after renal transplantation in a patient with sclerosing peritonitis secondary to continuous ambulatory peritoneal dialysis. *Am J Kidney Dis* 1995;26(4):658–661.

198. Bowers VD, Ackermann JR, Richardson W, et al. Sclerosing peritonitis. *Clin Transplant* 1994;8(4):369–372.

199. Korte MR, Yo M, Betjes MG, et al. Increasing incidence of severe encapsulating peritoneal sclerosis after kidney transplantation. *Nephrol Dial Transplant* 2007;22(8):2412–2414.

200. Khanna A, Plummer M, Bromberek C, et al. Expression of TGF-β and fibrogenic genes in transplant recipients with tacrolimus and cyclosporine nephrotoxicity. *Kidney Int* 2002;62(6):2257–2263.

201. Maluccio M, Sharma V, Lagman M, et al. Tacrolimus enhances TGF-β-1 expression and promotes tumor progression. *Transplantation* 2003;76(3):597–602.

202. Schultz S, Harmon TM, Nachtnebel KL. Computerized tomographic scanning with intraperitoneal contrast enhancement in a CAPD patient with localized edema. *Perit Dial Int* 1984;4:253–254.

203. Kopecky RT, Frymoyer PA, Witanowski LS, et al. Prospective peritoneal scintigraphy in patients beginning continuous ambulatory peritoneal dialysis. *Am J Kidney Dis* 1990;15(3):228–236.

204. Nolph KD, Stoltz ML, Maher JF. Altered peritoneal permeability in patients with systemic vasculitis. *Ann Intern Med* 1971;75(5): 753–755.

205. Brown ST, Ahearn DJ, Nolph KD. Reduced peritoneal clearances in scleroderma increased by intraperitoneal isoproterenol. *Ann Intern Med* 1973;78(6):891–894.

206. Copley JB, Smith BJ. Continuous ambulatory peritoneal dialysis and scleroderma. *Nephron* 1985;40(3):353–356.

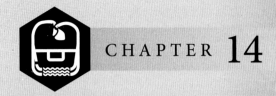

CHAPTER 14

Peritoneal Dialysis–Related Infections

William Salzer

Peritonitis remains the most frequent infection in patients receiving peritoneal dialysis (PD). PD has been used since the 1940s. In the early days, dialysis catheters were directly inserted into the peritoneum and were associated with very high rates of peritonitis. The Tenckhoff catheter was introduced in the late 1960s by Henry Tenckhoff. This catheter is inserted surgically and has a cuff in the subcutaneous tissue and an inner cuff where the catheter enters the peritoneum. Despite this, peritonitis rates averaged 6 episodes per patient-year. Subsequently, with improvements in equipment, techniques, and prevention strategies, peritonitis rates have decreased by 90%, such that the current International Society of Peritoneal Dialysis (ISPD) benchmark is 0.5 episodes per patient-year, or 1 episode every 2 years (1). The use of collapsible bags for peritoneal drain fluid, Y-sets for connecting, and fill-flush methods have probably contributed to reduced peritonitis rates. Also, the frequent use of automated continuous cycling peritoneal dialysis (CCPD) or automated peritoneal dialysis (APD) results in fewer connect and disconnect episodes, potentially reducing the opportunity for peritoneal fluid touch contamination which may reduce infection rates. Patient training is essential and each case of peritonitis should be investigated as to the cause and followed with patient retraining and review.

Despite best efforts, peritonitis continues to occur. PD peritonitis is fatal in about 4% but is a cofactor in mortality in about 16% of patients. Peritonitis with more virulent organisms such as *Staphylococcus aureus*, *Candida*, and *Pseudomonas* as well as repeated episodes of peritonitis results in damage to the peritoneal membrane and is the leading cause of technique failure of PD and permanent transfer to hemodialysis. Prompt diagnosis and treatment of peritonitis is the highest priority for the success of patients on PD.

PERITONEAL DIALYSIS PERITONITIS– PATHOGENESIS

Organisms that colonize the skin, *S. aureus* and coagulase-negative staphylococci (CNS), are the most frequent pathogens isolated in PD peritonitis, accounting for 50% or more of cases in most series (2,3). The most frequent cause of PD peritonitis is "touch contamination," which occurs when organisms are transferred from the hands of the patient or helper during connection or disconnection. Less common modes of infection are periluminal introduction of organisms from an exit-site or tunnel infection, transvisceral introduction of organisms from an intra-abdominal process, or rarely from hematogenous seeding. Once introduced into the peritoneum, the organisms encounter an environment that favors growth, with a high glucose content and few inflammatory cells initially. In the early stages of infection, the host immune response is inadequate to control the infection, with small numbers of peritoneal macrophages, very few neutrophils, and negligible quantities of host defense proteins such as immunoglobulins and complement. As the organisms proliferate, they produce toxins and other products that stimulate the resident macrophages to generate proinflammatory cytokines such as tumor necrosis factor (TNF), interleukin 1 (IL-1), interleukin 6 (IL-6), interleukin 8 (IL-8), which recruits inflammatory cells such as neutrophils, monocytes, and lymphocytes into the peritoneum. These cells and their products are responsible for the predominant symptoms of peritonitis—pain, cloudy effluent, and fever.

Factors that make the treatment of PD peritonitis more difficult are the characteristics of PD fluid and the presence of a foreign body, the catheter itself, in the peritoneum. Standard PD fluids are hyperosmolar and have a low pH, which may impair the function of neutrophils and macrophages. Although necessary to cure peritonitis, the constant exchange of PD fluid removes host phagocytic cells and host defense compounds from the peritoneum. Another factor that impairs host defense in PD peritonitis is the formation of biofilms. Biofilms are aggregates of organisms, adherent to a surface, usually embedded in an extracellular matrix composed of host compounds and products of the organism (4). Biofilms can form on infected PD catheters, particularly with infection by CNS species. Bacteria within the deeper portions of the biofilm do not divide as rapidly and therefore are far less susceptible to antibiotics and may persist despite clinical resolution of infection, providing a nidus for relapsing infection. Relapsing infection is often the result of biofilm formation and is an indication for catheter exchange.

Less common mechanisms of PD peritonitis include extraluminal spread from an exit-site or more often a tunnel infection producing a route for organisms to enter the peritoneum. These are usually clinically evident at the time of diagnosis of peritonitis. Peritonitis may arise from an intra-abdominal site, either a perforated viscus, focal intra-abdominal infection, transmural migration from the gut into the peritoneal cavity, or ascending infection from the female genital tract. The isolation of multiple enteric bacteria or the presence of particulate matter in the effluent suggests a perforated viscus and should prompt immediate imaging and surgical evaluation. Bacteremia or fungemia from an extraperitoneal site may also result in PD peritonitis.

⬡ EXIT-SITE INFECTION

Purulent drainage at the PD exit site, with or without erythema or induration, usually indicates an exit-site infection. Exit-site infection is a superficial infection that involves only the distal 2 cm or less of the catheter tunnel, which can spread proximally, resulting in a tunnel infection or frank peritonitis. The organisms that cause most exit-site infections are those that colonize the skin and exit site itself; *S. aureus*, CNS, *Candida*, and gram-negative enterics. Topical mupirocin or gentamicin cream applied to the exit site have been shown to reduce the incidence of exit-site infection overall (5,6) but increase the incidence of infection caused by antibiotic-resistant pathogens such as diphtheroids, *Candida*, and nontuberculous mycobacteria (NTM) (7).

Exit-site infection should be suspected if the patient develops purulent drainage around the catheter. Swelling, pain, and crust formation may also be present. Erythema, by itself is neither a sensitive nor a specific indicator of infection without other findings. Pericatheter drainage should be sent for Gram stain and culture. Do not culture the exit site in the absence of purulent drainage or other signs of infection because exit sites are rarely sterile and may be colonized by the same types of organisms that cause infection.

The goals of therapy are to prevent progression to a tunnel infection or peritonitis. Mild exit-site infections may be treated topically with chlorhexidine, dilute hydrogen peroxide, or gentamicin ophthalmic solution and close monitoring. In more severe infections, systemic therapy is indicated which can usually be administered orally. See **Table 14.1** for dosing of oral antibiotics in PD patients. Gram staining of the exudate may be helpful in directing initial antimicrobial therapy, and culture and sensitivity will direct definitive therapy. If gram-positive cocci are

TABLE 14.1	Oral Antibiotics Used in Exit-Site and Tunnel Infection
Amoxicillin	250–500 mg b.i.d.
Cephalexin	500 mg b.i.d. to t.i.d.
Ciprofloxacin	250 mg b.i.d.
Clarithromycin	500 mg loading dose, then 250 mg b.i.d. or q.d.
Dicloxacillin	500 mg q.i.d.
Erythromycin	500 mg q.i.d.
Flucloxacillin (or cloxacillin)	500 mg q.i.d.
Fluconazole	200 mg q.d. for 2 days, then 100 mg q.d.
Flucytosine	0.5–1 g/day titrated to response and serum trough levels (25–50 μg/mL)
Isoniazid	200–300 mg q.d.
Linezolid	400–600 mg b.i.d.
Metronidazole	400 mg t.i.d.
Moxifloxacin	400 mg daily
Ofloxacin	400 mg first day, then 200 mg q.d.
Pyrazinamide	25–35 mg/kg 3 times per week
Rifampicin	450 mg q.d. for <50 kg; 600 mg q.d. for >50 kg
Trimethoprim/ sulfamethoxazole	80/400 mg q.d.

b.i.d., 2 times per day; q.d., every day; t.i.d., 3 times per day; q.i.d., 4 times daily.
Reprinted from Li PK, Szeto C-C, Piraino B, et al. Peritoneal dialysis-related infections recommendations: 2010 update. *Perit Dial Int* 2010;30(4):393–423, with permission.

seen, therapy should be directed against staphylococcal species and empiric choices would be dependent on the incidence of methicillin-resistant staphylococci in your program. With a low incidence of methicillin resistance, oral therapy with dicloxacillin 500 mg po qid or cephalexin 500 mg bid to tid would be adequate. If methicillin resistance is a concern, oral therapy with trimethoprim/sulfamethoxazole (TMP/SMX) 80/400 mg po qd or clindamycin 300 mg po tid would be a better choice. Linezolid (400 to 600 mg po bid) is also an option but is much more expensive and may produce adverse effects with courses longer than 14 days (8,9). If gram-negative bacteria are seen on Gram stain, oral ciprofloxacin 250 mg po bid should be used pending culture and sensitivity results. If the Gram stain is unavailable or unrevealing, empiric therapy should cover both staphylococcal species and gram-negative bacteria including *Pseudomonas*. Use of topical antimicrobials for prevention can affect the types of organisms responsible for exit-site infection. In patients receiving topical mupirocin, gram-negative organisms are more likely, whereas topical gentamicin results in more frequent staphylococcal and fungal infection (7).

Upon receipt of culture and sensitivity results, therapy should be focused. For methicillin-susceptible staphylococcal species, oral therapy with cephalexin or dicloxacillin should be used. Streptococcal species should be treated with amoxicillin 250 to 500 mg po bid or cephalexin and with enterococci oral amoxicillin. "Community-acquired" strains of methicillin-resistant *Staphylococcus aureus* (MRSA) are often susceptible to TMP/SMX, clindamycin, doxycycline 100 mg po bid or minocycline 100 mg po bid and can be treated orally with these. Hospital-acquired strains maybe susceptible only to vancomycin and can be treated with vancomycin 15 to 30 mg/kg every 5 to 7 days administered intraperitoneally or oral linezolid if susceptible. For more difficult MRSA infections, rifampin 600 mg po daily may be added (1). Infection with gram-negative enterics should be treated with oral ciprofloxacin or possibly TMP/SMX depending on drug susceptibilities. Exit-site infections caused by *Pseudomonas aeruginosa* can be more difficult to treat and may relapse (10). If the isolate is susceptible, initial therapy with oral ciprofloxacin is appropriate. In the case of ciprofloxacin resistance, a slow response to oral ciprofloxacin or a relapsing infection, treatment with intraperitoneal tobramycin 0.6 mg/kg IP daily, cefepime 1 g IP qd, or meropenem 1 g IP qd should be added. Treatment for pseudomonal exit-site infection should be continued for at least 3 weeks or until the infection has resolved clinically. Nonpseudomonal exit-site infections should be treated for at least 2 weeks or until resolution.

The goal of treating exit-site infections is to prevent progression to a tunnel infection or peritonitis. An exit-site infection that is refractory to treatment or progresses to a tunnel infection or peritonitis requires catheter removal and replacement. The one exception is CNS infection, which in some cases can be successfully treated without catheter replacement. In the absence of peritonitis, catheter removal and replacement can be performed in a one-stage procedure, with catheter placement at a different site.

 TUNNEL INFECTION

Erythema, swelling, or pain along the catheter extending more than 2 cm proximal to the catheter–skin interface is indicative of a tunnel infection. These infections usually result from the spread of bacteria from the exit site along the subcutaneous portion of the catheter and pose a higher risk of peritonitis. Ultrasound of the subcutaneous track of the catheter may reveal pericatheter fluid or abscess formation. The most common pathogens causing tunnel infection are *S. aureus* and *Pseudomonas*. Gram stain and culture of material milked from the exit site should be obtained, and appropriate antibiotic therapy should be started. In most cases, antibiotic therapy alone is inadequate and catheter removal is necessary—particularly with infections caused by *S. aureus* or *Pseudomonas*.

PERITONEAL DIALYSIS PERITONITIS

Peritonitis–Diagnosis

Prompt recognition, diagnosis, and treatment of PD peritonitis is essential for patient safety and preservation of the peritoneal membrane. Peritonitis may follow an exit-site or tunnel infection or an intra-abdominal source but most often results from contamination of the external catheter connection by breaks in sterile technique, touch contamination. The earliest signs of peritonitis are cloudy dialysate effluent and/or abdominal pain, which may be accompanied by fever or nausea and vomiting. Patients using automated PD may be less likely to notice cloudy dialysate. The first drain is most likely to be cloudy. The degree of inflammation and severity of abdominal pain is dependent on the virulence of the infecting organism. *S. aureus*, gram-negative rods, and β-hemolytic streptococci generally produce more severe abdominal pain and are more likely to be associated with fever than CNS. Patients should be educated to be alert for these signs and symptoms and to notify their providers for prompt evaluation.

Diagnosis of peritonitis is made by examining the dialysis effluent. In patients with prominent systemic symptoms, blood cultures should be obtained as well (11). Effluent should be sent for cell counts, white blood cell (WBC) differential, Gram stain, and culture prior to administering antibiotics whenever possible. Dialysate WBC $>100/\mu L$ and $>50\%$ polymorphonuclear cells (PMNs) from a sample of fluid that has had a dwell of >2 hours is very suggestive of peritonitis. In patients receiving APD, fluid samples with <100 WBC but $>50\%$ PMNs usually have peritonitis. In a patient with a dry abdomen, 1 L of dialysate is infused, allowed to dwell for 1 to 2 hours, and then removed for cell counts and microbiologic studies.

Fluid specimens must be obtained for microbiologic studies before administering antimicrobials whenever possible to identify the infecting organisms and their drug susceptibilities to guide effective antimicrobial therapy. Five to 10 mL of fluid should be inoculated directly into aerobic and anaerobic blood culture bottles at the bedside. Use of BACTEC/Alert culture bottles may improve yield and reduce culture-negative cases (12). In addition, 50 mL of fluid should be centrifuged at 3,000 g for 15 minutes and the sediment resuspended in 3 to 5 mL of saline. The sediment should be examined with a Gram stain and inoculated into liquid blood culture bottles and solid bacterial media plates. Cultures are usually positive in 24 to 48 hours, but if liquid media cultures are negative at 3 days, they should be subcultured on solid media and examined for an additional 3 to 5 days. ISPD guidelines suggest a benchmark for culture negative peritonitis at $<20\%$ of cases. In the patient with negative cultures who fails to respond clinically to empiric antibiotic therapy by 3 days, repeat PD effluent sampling for cell counts and microbiologic studies should be performed. In addition to repeating routine bacteriologic studies, consideration of fastidious bacterial, mycobacterial, and fungal causes should be explored with additional microbiologic studies.

Initial Empiric Therapy for Peritonitis

Prompt initial empiric antimicrobial therapy is essential for optimal short- and long-term outcomes (**FIGURE 14.1**). A positive peritoneal fluid Gram stain can guide initial empiric therapy, focusing on gram-positive or gram-negative bacteria. If the Gram stain is negative, empiric antibiotic therapy, including coverage for both gram-positive and gram-negative bacteria should be started promptly. Antibiotics should be administered intraperitoneally, added to the dialysate. The choice of empiric therapy should be determined by the local prevalence of antimicrobial resistance in gram-positive and gram-negative bacterial causes of peritonitis. In most programs, gram-positive bacteria account for 50% or more of cases and gram-negative enterics 10% to 20%. Empiric coverage for gram positives with cefazolin 15 to 20 mg/kg IP qd or vancomycin 15 to 30 mg/kg IP every 5 to 7 days is recommended, with the choice dependent on the local incidence of methicillin-resistant staphylococcal species. Empiric coverage for gram-negative bacteria should include coverage for *P. aeruginosa*. Choices include ceftazidime 1 to 1.5 g IP qd, cefepime 1 g IP qd, gentamicin 0.6 mg/kg IP qd, or tobramycin 0.6 mg/kg IP

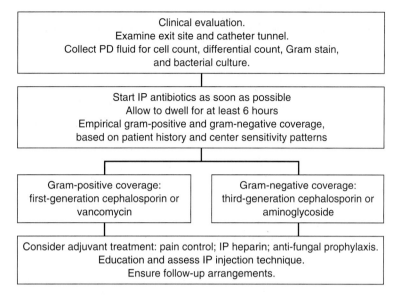

FIGURE 14.1 Initial management of peritonitis. IP, intraperitoneal. [Reprinted with permission from Li PK, Szeto C-C, Piraino B, et al. ISPD peritonitis recommendations: 2016 Update on Prevention and Treatment (published online ahead of print June 9, 2016). *Perit Dial Int.*]

qd, again depending on local antimicrobial resistance patterns. A recent episode of peritonitis or exit-site infection or recent antibiotic therapy may modify initial empiric antibiotic choices. Results of peritoneal fluid cultures and drug susceptibilities will direct definitive therapy for peritonitis.

Intraperitoneal Antibiotics for Peritonitis

Intraperitoneal administration of antibiotics is the recommended route of administration for the treatment of PD peritonitis for a number of reasons (13) (TABLE 14.2). IV access and continued IV administration is not necessary. Antibiotics added to the dialysate are delivered in high concentrations to the site of infection. The peritoneal membrane is permeable to most intraperitoneally administered antibiotics, resulting in therapeutic serum levels, which allows diffusion back into the peritoneum when the patient is not undergoing dialysis. If antibiotics are administered intermittently, the antibiotic containing fluid should dwell for at least 6 hours, usually with a daytime dwell in patients receiving APD. There is less data on the dosing and efficacy of IP antibiotics in patients receiving APD, particularly with β-lactam compounds, and some recommend converting to continuous ambulatory peritoneal dialysis (CAPD), if possible, during therapy for peritonitis. (14)

Peritonitis Treatment Course and Outcomes

Upon receiving the results of peritoneal fluid cultures and drug susceptibilities, antibiotic therapy should be focused on the infecting pathogen using the narrowest spectrum, least toxic agent. Duration of treatment is usually 14 to 21 days depending on the pathogen. Patient symptoms should be improving, and peritoneal effluent should be clear after 2 to 4 days of definitive treatment. In one study, effluent WBC of >1,000 on day 3 of treatment predicted failure of therapy (15). If the effluent does not clear after 5 days of culture-directed therapy, ISPD guidelines define this as

refractory peritonitis and recommend consideration of catheter removal. Catheter removal should also be considered for culture-negative cases if the effluent does not clear in 5 days. Failure of the effluent to clear after 5 days of appropriate empiric therapy should also raise suspicion for infections caused by fastidious bacterial pathogens, mycobacterial, or filamentous fungal causes. This should prompt repeat cultures for bacteria, fungal, and acid-fast bacteria.

Relapsing peritonitis is defined as a second episode of peritonitis caused by the same pathogen or as a culture negative case within 4 weeks after the end of treatment for the first episode. Recurrent peritonitis is a second episode occurring within 4 weeks of completion of therapy for a prior one, caused by a different organism (16,17). Repeat peritonitis is a second episode caused by the same organism as the first, more than 4 weeks after the completion of therapy. These three forms of peritonitis are associated with subsequent cases of peritonitis. ISPD guidelines suggest that removal and replacement of the PD catheter be considered to prevent damage to the peritoneal membrane and technique failure (1).

Catheter Management in Peritoneal Dialysis Peritonitis

Appropriate management of peritonitis, tunnel, and exit-site infections is focused on resolving the current infection, preventing subsequent infection, and preserving the peritoneal membrane. Patients with refractory exit-site and tunnel infections should have their catheters removed and replaced. Catheter removal and replacement simultaneously in a one-stage procedure is feasible in patients with refractory exit-site infections and in patients with relapsing CNS infection if the effluent has cleared on appropriate therapy. Patients with refractory infections caused by *S. aureus, Pseudomonas*, fungi, or mycobacteria should have their catheters removed in a timely fashion and suspend PD until their infections have resolved before catheter replacement.

Table 14.2	Intraperitoneal Antibiotic Dosing Recommendations for Treatment of Peritonitis	
	Intermittent (1 exchange daily)	**Continuous (all exchanges)**
Aminoglycosides		
Amikacin	2 mg/kg daily	LD 25 mg/L, MD 12 mg/L
Gentamicin	0.6 mg/kg daily	LD 8 mg/L, MD 4 mg/L
Netilmicin	0.6 mg/kg daily	MD 10 mg/L
Tobramycin	0.6 mg/kg daily	LD 3 mg/kg, MD 0.3 mg/kg
Cephalosporins		
Cefazolin	15–20 mg/kg daily	LD 500 mg/L, MD 125 mg/L
Cefepime	1,000 mg daily	LD 250–500 mg/L, MD 100–125 mg/L
Cefoperazone	no data	LD 500 mg/L, MD 62.5-125 mg/L
Cefotaxime	500–1,000 mg daily	no data
Ceftazidime	1,000–1,500 mg daily	LD 500 mg/L, MD 125 mg/L
Ceftriaxone	1,000 mg daily	no data
Penicillins		
Penicillin G	no data	LD 50,000 unit/L, MD 25,000 unit/L
Amoxicillin	no data	MD 150 mg/L
Ampicillin	no data	MD 125 mg/L
Ampicillin/Sulbactam	2 gm/1 gm every 12 hours	LD 750–100 mg/L, MD 100 mg/L
Piperacillin/Tazobactam	no data	LD 4 gm/0.5 gm, MD 1 gm/0.125 gm
Others		
Aztreonam	2 gm daily	LD 1,000 mg/L, MD 250 mg/L
Ciprofloxacin	no data	MD 50 mg/L
Clindamycin	no data	MD 600 mg/bag
Daptomycin	no data	LD 100 mg/L, MD 20 mg/L
Imipenem/Cilastatin	500 mg in alternate exchange	LD 250 mg/L, MD 50 mg/L
Ofloxacin	no data	LD 200 mg/L, MD 25 mg/L
Polymyxin B	no data	MD 300,000 unit (30 mg)/bag
Quinupristin/Dalfopristin	25 mg/L in alternate exchange[a]	no data
Meropenem	1 gm daily	no data
Teicoplanin	15 mg/kg every 5 days	LD 400 mg/bag, MD 20 mg/bag
Vancomycin	15–30 mg/kg every 5–7 days[b]	LD 30 mg/kg, MD 1.5 mg/kg/bag
Antifungals		
Fluconazole	IP 200 mg every 24 to 48 hours	no data
Voriconazole	IP 2.5 mg/kg daily	no data

LD, loading dose in mg; MD, maintenance dose in mg; IP, intraperitoneal; APD, automated peritoneal dialysis.
[a]Given in conjunction with 500 mg intravenous twice daily.
[b]Supplemental dose may be needed for APD patients.
Reprinted with permission from Li PK, Szeto C-C, Piraino B, et al. ISPD peritonitis recommendations: 2016 update on prevention and treatment (published online ahead of print June 9, 2016). *Perit Dial Int.*

⬡ ORGANISM-SPECIFIC TREATMENT AND MANAGEMENT OF PERITONEAL DIALYSIS PERITONITIS

Two to 3 days after obtaining peritoneal fluid, cultures are usually growing a pathogen (**FIGURES 14.2** and **14.3**). If the peritoneal Gram stain was positive on the initial sample or when cultures become positive, your microbiology laboratory will be able to identify the organism as gram-positive, gram-negative, or yeast and whether it is cocci or bacilli. Where available, polymerase chain reaction (PCR) (BioFire) or matrix-assisted laser desorption/ionization time-of-flight (MALDI-TOF) can rapidly identify the species of the infecting organism and also determine whether it contains resistance genes such as mecA for methicillin resistance, vancomycin resistance genes in enterococci, and carbapenem resistance in gram-negative bacilli. This information would allow focusing or changing antibiotic therapy.

Coagulase-Negative Staphylococcal Peritonitis

CNS are the most common cause of PD peritonitis in most series. These organisms are ubiquitous colonizers of human skin and are a group of species, one of which is *Staphylococcus epidermidis*, the commonest pathogen in PD peritonitis (18–21). Peritonitis caused by these organisms is almost always the result of touch contamination in the course of manipulating the catheter or connectors during dialysis. CNS species are not very virulent

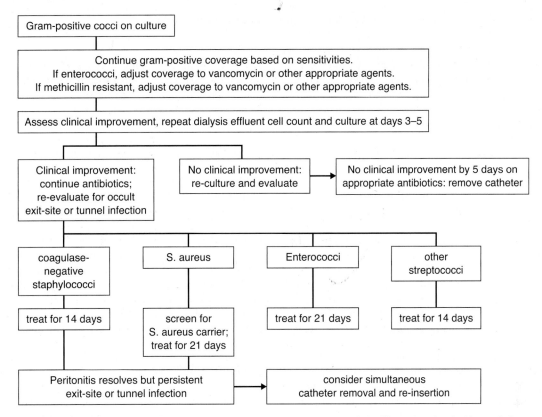

FIGURE 14.2 Management algorithm for gram-positive cocci identified in dialysis effluent. [Reprinted with permission from Li PK, Szeto C-C, Piraino B, et al. ISPD peritonitis recommendations: 2016 update on prevention and treatment (published online ahead of print June 9, 2016). *Perit Dial Int.*]

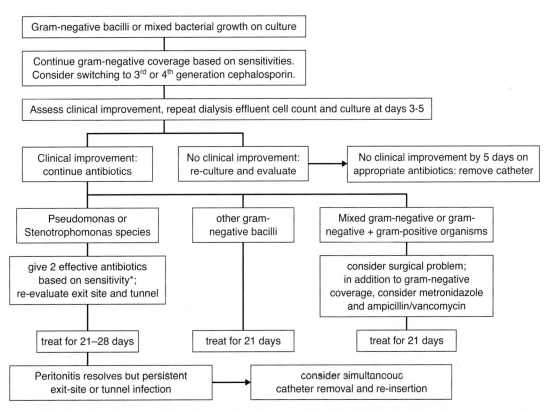

FIGURE 14.3 Management algorithm for gram-negative bacilli or mixed bacterial growth identified in dialysis effluent. *Trimethoprim/sulfamethoxazole is preferred for *Stenotrophomonas* species. [Reprinted with permission from Li PK, Szeto C-C, Piraino B, et al. ISPD peritonitis recommendations: 2016 update on prevention and treatment (published online ahead of print June 9, 2016). *Perit Dial Int.*]

organisms and usually produce a milder form of peritonitis with less pain, peritoneal inflammation, and fewer systemic symptoms. However, these organisms have a higher propensity to produce biofilms on catheters due to their production of "slime," an extracellular matrix of bacterial and host compounds (22). Organisms in biofilms are much more resistant to antimicrobials, being embedded in slime, impairing antibiotic access, and having reduced replication in the deeper levels of the complex. Probably because of biofilm production, CNS are frequent causes of relapsing and repeat cases of peritonitis (17). Relapsing or repeat peritonitis by these organisms requires catheter removal and replacement in most cases.

Initial empiric antibiotic therapy should always include antibiotic coverage for these organisms. If methicillin-resistant organisms are uncommon in your program, cefazolin can be used empirically; otherwise, vancomycin should be used for empiric therapy. In a series of 115 cases of CNS PD peritonitis cases from Brazil, 70% of their isolates were methicillin-resistant and initial therapy including vancomycin empirically improved outcomes (21). Upon receipt of culture and sensitivity results, methicillin-susceptible isolates can be treated with cefazolin, and methicillin-resistant strains with vancomycin. Intraperitoneal cefazolin is administered 15 to 20 mg/kg to one exchange a day, with a long dwell (>6 hours). There are some concerns about using cefazolin in patients receiving APD in that peritoneal drug levels may be inadequate during APD due to more rapid exchanges, with some authorities recommending conversion to CAPD during cefazolin therapy (1). However, the published experience suggests that these patients may receive therapy on APD, with one study showing equivalent cure rates in patients treated on APD or CAPD (22) and another study showing higher failure rates in those switched to CAPD during therapy (23). This is not a concern with vancomycin therapy, which is administered every third to fifth day intraperitoneally.

Clinical response is usually prompt, with resolution of symptoms and clearing of the effluent, with reduction in peritoneal WBC by 3 to 5 days. Patients with a good clinical response can be treated for 14 days. Failure to respond by 3 to 5 days should prompt reevaluation with repeat cultures and consideration of catheter removal, especially in the presence of an exit-site or tunnel infection. Relapsing or repeat episodes should also prompt considering catheter removal and replacement, which can be done as a one-stage procedure after treatment of peritonitis.

Staphylococcus aureus Peritonitis

In contrast to CNS species, *S. aureus* is a much more virulent organism, producing clinically more severe peritonitis with a significant risk of failure, morbidity, and mortality (24,25). The cause is often touch contamination but also may result from concurrent exit-site or tunnel infection. Initial empiric therapy should include cefazolin or vancomycin 15 to 30 mg/kg/d IP every 5 to 7 days, depending on the local prevalence of methicillin-resistant strains, followed by focused therapy based on the drug susceptibility of the infecting strain. ISPD guidelines recommend the addition of rifampin, 600 mg po qd for 7 days in addition to the primary antibiotic (1). Rifampin has synergistic activity on *S. aureus* and is active on bacteria adherent to the catheter and in biofilms. If rifampin is used, be aware of its induction of multiple drug metabolizing enzymes and its effect on concomitant medications.

S. aureus usually produces more clinically severe peritonitis, with pain, higher peritoneal effluent WBC, and systemic signs of infection such as fever and signs of sepsis. For methicillin-susceptible

strains, cefazolin 15 to 20 mg/kg IP qd or continuous dosing with cefazolin, a 500 mg/L IP loading dose followed by 125 mg/L IP with oral rifampin. Methicillin-resistant strains should be treated with an initial IP loading dose of vancomycin, 15 to 30 mg/kg up to 2 g, followed by 1 g IP every 3 to 7 days, based on serum vancomycin levels. Trough serum vancomycin levels of <15 μg/mL should prompt redosing with vancomycin. Patients who are intolerant of vancomycin or have vancomycin-resistant strains can be treated with daptomycin 100 mg/L IP loading dose and then 20 mg/L IP continuously, linezolid 300 to 600 mg po bid, or perhaps ceftaroline. Ceftaroline is a third-generation cephalosporin with good MRSA activity but has not been used in PD patients at this point (26). Oral rifampin 600 mg should be given as well. Patients with a good clinical response, with decreasing pain and clearing of the effluent should be treated with 21 days of therapy. Failure to respond after 5 days of appropriate antibiotic therapy, or the presence of an exit-site or tunnel infection, are indications for prompt catheter removal and converting to hemodialysis for 2 to 3 weeks before catheter replacement (1). MRSA peritonitis is associated with an increased risk of technique failure and permanent switching to hemodialysis (25).

Streptococcal Peritonitis

Streptococcal species are less common causes of PD peritonitis than staphylococcal species. Like staph species, the clinical presentation depends on virulence of the species, with β-hemolytic streptococci, Groups A, B, etc., resembling *S. aureus* and viridans streptococci more resembling the clinical features of CNS (27). The mode of infection is probably touch contamination in most cases, but viridans streptococci are inhabitants of the alimentary tract so a gastrointestinal (GI) source is possible. Initial empiric therapy with cefazolin 15 to 20 mg/kg/d IP or vancomycin 15 to 30 mg/kg IP every 3 to 7 days IP will cover all the β-hemolytic streptococci and most viridans streptococci, which have been shown to have increasing resistance to penicillins and cephalosporins (28). Results of cultures and sensitivities will allow focused therapy with a single agent. Continuous dosing with ampicillin 125 mg/L IP has been recommended for penicillin susceptible strains (1). Some studies have shown that ampicillin in solution begins to lose antimicrobial activity after of mixing, creating problems with patients on home therapy. A better choice may be cefazolin, which has good activity against these strains and is stable for 8 days at room temperature and 14 days refrigerated in solution (29).

β-Hemolytic streptococcal peritonitis presents like *S. aureus*, with significant abdominal pain, high peritoneal WBCs, and frequent fever and signs of sepsis. These organisms remain very susceptible to most β-lactam antibiotics and peritonitis usually responds promptly to appropriate antibiotic therapy, including cefazolin. Therapy should be continued for 14 days. Failure to respond promptly should raise questions about an exit-site or tunnel infection, or a concomitant skin and soft tissue infection or other focus.

Viridans streptococci, like CNS, include a large number of species and, like CNS, are not very virulent organisms. They are normal inhabitants of the alimentary tract, including the mouth and upper and lower GI tract and probably produce peritonitis through touch contamination, occasionally via the GI tract or hematogenously following invasive procedures involving mucosal surfaces without prophylactic antibiotics (30). Peritonitis caused by these organisms resembles CNS, with less severe abdominal pain, milder inflammatory changes on peritoneal fluid examination, and fewer systemic symptoms like fever (31). One study, however, identified an increased risk of recurrent and refractory peritonitis following an episode of viridans streptococci peritonitis (32). For penicillin-susceptible strains, continuous IP ampicillin has been recommended, but because of poor stability in solution, IP cefazolin might be a better choice. Penicillin-resistant strains with minimum inhibitory concentration (MIC) >4 μg/mL or relatively resistant strains with penicillin MICs >0.5 μg/mL should be treated with IP vancomycin. Therapy should be continued for 14 days.

The organism formerly known as *Streptococcus bovis* has been reclassified as *Streptococcus gallolyticus*. In a series of 20 patients with 23 episodes of peritonitis caused by *S. gallolyticus* reported by Yap et al. (33), some degree of penicillin resistance was common. Patients were successfully treated with cefazolin or vancomycin and an aminoglycoside for 14 days. *S. bovis/S. gallolyticus* bacteremia is classically associated with GI malignancies, particularly colon cancer. Ten of their 20 patients underwent diagnostic studies—colonoscopy or barium enema—and none were found to have colon cancer.

Enterococcal Peritonitis

Enterococcal species are normal inhabitants of the GI tract and are more common causes of peritonitis than streptococcal species in most series. The source of infection is usually touch contamination, but GI tract contamination also occurs and should be suspected if other enteric organisms are present. In fact, in some series, nearly half of enterococcal peritonitis cases were polymicrobial, and polymicrobial infections were associated with high rates of catheter loss and permanent transfer to hemodialysis (34,35). The clinical presentation of enterococcal peritonitis, without other organisms, is moderately severe in terms of pain and systemic symptoms. Cephalosporins have no activity against enterococci and aminoglycosides alone have very little so that empiric regimens containing cephalosporins or a cephalosporin and aminoglycoside have virtually no effect on enterococcal peritonitis. Vancomycin covers most enterococci, the exception being vancomycin-resistant enterococci (VRE).

Therapy of enterococcal peritonitis can be problematic, given that the organism is not susceptible to most commonly used antibiotics. *Enterococcus faecalis* is usually susceptible to ampicillin, penicillin, and piperacillin as well as vancomycin. Occasional strains of *E. faecalis* are resistant to vancomycin (VRE) but remain susceptible to penicillins. Ampicillin IP has been recommended as the drug of choice, but problems with stability in solution requires that it be reconstituted right before use. Piperacillin is stable in solution up to 8 days refrigerated, but there is little published experience in PD peritonitis. Vancomycin is commonly used and is recommended as the first choice in the 2016 ISPD guidelines, which also recommend the addition of IP aminoglycoside in "severe" cases of enterococcal peritonitis (1). *Enterococcus faecium* is inherently resistant to ampicillin and penicillin, making vancomycin the drug of choice. Most strains of VRE are *E. faecium*, which are resistant to all commonly used classes of antibiotics. Case reports and a few small series have reported successful treatment of VRE peritonitis with daptomycin. Daptomycin has most often been used IP with a loading dose of 100 mg/L for at least a 6-hour dwell and then 20 mg/L for APD or CAPD (36,37). Daptomycin has also been given at 7 mg/kg every 48 hours IP (38) and 5 mg/kg IV every 48 hours (39). Linezolid has also been used to treat VRE peritonitis. Because of presumed instability in dialysis fluids, linezolid has been given systemically, 600 mg IV every 12 hours (40,41). The bioavailability of linezolid given orally is 100%, so if the patient is taking po meds, po administration is certainly reasonable (42). Also be aware of the potential for hematologic and neurologic toxicities of linezolid with doses

of 600 mg bid for courses exceeding 10 days (8,9). Quinupristin/ dalfopristin has been used successfully treat *E. faecium* VRE peritonitis (43), but this compound has no activity on *E. faecalis*. The recommended duration of therapy for VRE peritonitis is 21 days. A suboptimal response to therapy should prompt consideration for catheter removal.

Corynebacterium Peritonitis

The genus *Corynebacterium* includes a number of species of small, gram-positive rods, often referred to as *diphtheroids*. These organisms, like CNS, are part of normal skin flora, of low pathogenicity, and usually produce infections related to implanted devices. In most case series, *Corynebacterium* account for less than 3% of peritonitis cases. This group of organisms is of low pathogenicity, and peritonitis resembles CNS clinically. Infection most likely occurs through touch contamination. Most *Corynebacterium* strains are susceptible to cefazolin. The notable exception is *Corynebacterium jeikeium*, which is resistant to β lactams and many other classes but is susceptible to vancomycin.

The optimal treatment of *Corynebacterium* peritonitis is not clear based on the two largest case series. A series of 27 patients reported from Hong Kong (44) found a better overall response and fewer recurrences after treatment with vancomycin for 2 to 3 weeks than with cephalosporins. In contrast, another series of 82 patients with *Corynebacterium* peritonitis found that 2 weeks of therapy with cefazolin was comparable to vancomycin or longer treatment courses (45). In both studies, recurrent peritonitis was frequent. One study also reported that in cases of refractory peritonitis, delaying catheter removal beyond 7 days resulted in 90% technique failure with permanent transfer to hemodialysis (45).

Gram-Negative (*Enterobacteriaceae*) Peritonitis

Gram-negative enteric bacteria, the family *Enterobacteriaceae*, are normal inhabitants of the gastrointestinal tract. The most common species causing PD peritonitis are *Escherichia coli*, *Klebsiella*, and *Enterobacter* species (46–48). The incidence of these organisms varies in different centers but usually accounts for 10% to 20% of PD peritonitis cases. Their relative percentage has increased over the past two decades, probably due to decreases in staphylococcus cases as a result of improved connective technologies and the use of mupirocin for exit-site prophylaxis. The mechanisms of infection are probably touch contamination but also exit-site and tunnel infections. Some infections may arise from an intra-abdominal source, constipation, or transmural migration of bacteria. Multiple species on Gram stains and culture suggest an intra-abdominal infection or perforated viscus. The clinical presentation is moderately severe, with fever in about one-third of cases.

Treatment of gram-negative enteric peritonitis is more complex than gram-positive bacteria, given the variety of species and differing antibiotic susceptibilities. Initial empiric therapy with a broad-spectrum cephalosporin IP, like cefepime or ceftazidime or an aminoglycoside, will cover most of these organisms. Results of culture and sensitivity will allow focused therapy. In a series of 210 patients with gram-negative enteric peritonitis, therapy with a single effective antibiotic was associated with a 39% failure rate and a high relapse and recurrence rate (46). Treatment with two effective agents improved response rates and decreased relapse. Depending on drug susceptibilities, a broad-spectrum β-lactam IP like cefepime or ceftazidime combined with either an aminoglycoside or a fluoroquinolone, ciprofloxacin or levofloxacin, would be reasonable choices.

Gram-negative enterics have a variety of potential resistance mechanisms (49). *Enterobacter*, *Serratia*, and *Citrobacter* species have a chromosomal β-lactamase enzyme, AmpC, which is derepressed when exposed to β-lactam antibiotics. Expression of AmpC results in resistance to cephalosporins and is not inhibited by β-lactamase inhibitors. The last decade has seen the emergence and spread of two novel resistance mechanisms. Extended spectrum β-lactamases (ESBLs) are plasmid mediated enzymes, first described in *Klebsiella pneumoniae*, but are present in many other gram-negative bacteria as well. Strains expressing ESBLs are resistant to all cephalosporins but remain susceptible to carbapenems and most β-lactam/β-lactamase inhibitors (50–52). Even more problematic is the emergence of carbapenem-resistant *Enterobacteriaceae* (CRE), also known as KPC—*Klebsiella pneumoniae* carbapenemase (53). These β-lactamase enzymes are carried on mobile genetic elements and induce resistance to all β-lactam antibiotics, including carbapenems. In addition, CRE strains are usually resistant to fluoroquinolones, variably resistant to aminoglycosides, and often only susceptible to polymyxin B and colistin. Colistin has been given systemically to treat PD peritonitis, 300 mg IV on day 1 and then 150 to 200 mg IV qd. There is little experience in the occurrence or treatment of CRE infections in PD peritonitis or the use of colistin or polymyxin B intraperitoneally (54).

Nonfermenting (Aerobic) Gram-Negative Rods– *Pseudomonas, Acinetobacter,* and *Stenotrophomonas*

Pseudomonas

Pseudomonas species are aerobic, nonfermenting gram-negative rods that are inherently resistant to many antibiotics. *Pseudomonas*, most often *P. aeruginosa*, usually accounts for less than 5% of peritonitis cases in most programs but was the causative agent in 13% of cases in a series from Hong Kong (55). Recent antibiotic therapy appears to predispose for *Pseudomonas* peritonitis. Catheter infection, either an exit-site or a tunnel infection, is often present and is an indication for catheter removal. Clinically, compared to other bacterial pathogens, pseudomonas peritonitis results in a twofold increased risk of catheter removal and permanent transfer to hemodialysis (56).

Treatment with two effective anti-pseudomonal antibiotics, based on drug susceptibility studies, appears to improve outcomes. Oral ciprofloxacin combined with IP cefepime, ceftazidime, piperacillin, aminoglycoside, meropenem, or imipenem appear to be the most efficacious combinations. In Szeto's (55) series, outcomes were better with cephalosporin versus aminoglycoside combinations. In patients with a good primary response, antibiotics should be continued for 3 weeks. In refractory cases or in the presence of a catheter infection, prompt catheter removal improves outcomes. Following catheter removal, transfer to hemodialysis with 2 weeks of parenteral anti-pseudomonal therapy is recommended prior to catheter replacement.

Acinetobacter

Acinetobacter species are nonfermenting aerobic, gram-negative rods that are frequent agents of health care–associated infection (57). Most human infections are caused by *Acinetobacter baumannii*, which is often multidrug-resistant. *Acinetobacter*, like *Pseudomonas*, is inherently resistant to many antibiotics, frequently develops resistance during therapy, and not infrequently requires treatment with colistin or polymyxin B because of resistance to all other classes of drugs. Interestingly, most *Acinetobacter* strains are susceptible to ampicillin/sulbactam due to susceptibility to the sulbactam component. In a series of seven patients with *Acinetobacter* peritonitis reported by Zhang (58), three patients with multidrug-resistant strains failed antibiotic therapy and transferred to hemodialysis. Peritonitis caused by *Acinetobacter* should probably treated like *Pseudomonas* with two effective drugs based on drug susceptibilities, for 3 weeks, with early catheter removal for refractory cases.

Stenotrophomonas maltophilia

Stenotrophomonas maltophilia is another aerobic gram-negative bacillus that causes health care–associated infections and is multidrug-resistant. This organism is inherently resistant to all carbapenems, possessing a chromosomal carbapenemase, most fluoroquinolones, aminoglycosides, and tetracyclines (59). It is most susceptible to TMP/SMX, ticarcillin/clavulanate (no longer available in the United States), tigecycline, and colistin and polymyxin. *Stenotrophomonas* is not a common cause of PD peritonitis, but in three small case series, failure with catheter loss occurred in about half of treated patients (60,61). The most effective therapy seems to be TMP/SMX combined with an additional effective drug for 3 to 4 weeks of therapy.

Polymicrobial Peritoneal Dialysis Peritonitis

Polymicrobial peritonitis is a case of peritonitis in which more than one organism is isolated in a single episode of peritonitis. This occurs in 10% or less of peritonitis episodes. The isolation of multiple species of organisms, particularly gram-negative enterics and anaerobic bacteria, in a patient with more severe abdominal pain and systemic signs of sepsis should raise concerns for a perforated viscus or other serious intra-abdominal infection and should prompt immediate surgical consultation. In most case series of polymicrobial peritonitis, these intra-abdominal catastrophes occur in fewer than 10% of patients with polymicrobial peritonitis (62–64).

In the majority of cases of polymicrobial peritonitis, the pathogenesis is probably similar to monomicrobial cases, the result of touch contamination or catheter-related infection. Outcomes seem to be best with mixed infection with gram-positive cocci. Isolation of gram-negative bacteria and particularly fungi is associated with higher rates of failure, catheter removal, and permanent transfer to hemodialysis.

Culture-Negative Peritonitis

Culture negative peritonitis is defined as clinical signs of peritonitis, cloudy dialysate with more than 100 WBC/µL, >50% PMNs, and with negative peritoneal fluid cultures after 3 days. PD guidelines suggest a benchmark of fewer than 20% culture-negative cases of peritonitis. A recent history of antibiotic use or initiating antibiotic therapy for peritonitis before obtaining peritoneal fluid cultures is common in these cases. It is thought that most of these cases are due to gram-positive bacteria through touch contamination based on the observation that most patients respond to standard empiric antibiotic regimens (65). If peritoneal fluid cultures remain negative after 3 days of therapy, peritoneal WBC and differential should be repeated. If the patient responds to empiric antibiotic therapy with clearing of the effluent, and persistent negative cultures, gram-negative coverage can be discontinued and cefazolin or vancomycin should be continued for 14 days.

If there is a lack of clinical response after 3 days of antibiotic therapy, peritoneal fluid WBC, differential, and cultures should be repeated. Possible causes in these patients include resistant bacteria, fastidious bacteria, mycobacterial infection, fungal infection (other than candida), or a noninfectious cause. In addition to routine bacterial cultures, peritoneal fluid should be sent for fungal and mycobacterial cultures and bacterial cultures should be held for a longer period of time and subcultured on enriched and specialized media. If there is no clinical improvement after 5 days of therapy, catheter removal should be considered.

Fungal Peritonitis

Fungal peritonitis usually accounts for less than 5% of cases in most centers, but some have higher rates (66). The clinical presentation resembles bacterial peritonitis with cloudy dialysate and abdominal pain. More than half of patients with fungal peritonitis will have a history of antibiotic therapy in the prior month, often for an episode of bacterial peritonitis (67). The presumed mechanism is that antibiotic therapy reduces the normal bacterial flora of the skin and GI tract, facilitating overgrowth or colonization by candida or other fungi. PD fluid studies are similar to bacterial infection with elevated WBC and neutrophilic predominance. Occasionally, eosinophils will be seen in PD effluent with infection by some filamentous fungi (molds). *Candida* species are responsible for 90% or more of fungal peritonitis cases; infection with molds is less common. On Gram stain, *Candida* species are seen as gram-positive, ovoid cells, about 5 μm in diameter. Mold species do not stain with Gram stain. Calcofluor white or Gomori methenamine silver stains will detect molds and yeasts if enough organisms are present in the specimen. β-D-Glucan is an important component of most fungal cell walls and is usually measured in the serum in patients with suspected fungal infections (68). It might be a useful adjunct in the diagnosis of suspected fungal peritonitis to measure serum and peritoneal fluid β-D-glucan levels—but to my knowledge, this has not been done. *Candida* species grow well on standard bacterial culture media, usually taking a day or two longer than bacteria. In contrast, molds require specialized fungal culture media and usually take longer to grow.

In the 20th century, *Candida albicans* was the predominant species in PD peritonitis and most other sites of candida infection. In the last 15 years, *C. albicans* now accounts for fewer than 50% of cases (69–71). Of the non-*C. albicans* species that have been appearing, *Candida krusei* is always resistant to fluconazole and *Candida glabrata* is often resistant. Upon identification of Candida on Gram stain or culture of PD fluid, initial therapy is usually with fluconazole 200 mg po on day 1 and then 50 to 100 mg po qd or 200 mg IP every 24 to 48 hours (**TABLE 14.3**) (1). Upon receipt of the species ID and drug susceptibility testing results, if fluconazole resistance is present, therapy may need to be changed to a broader spectrum agent. Itraconazole, voriconazole, posaconazole, and isavuconazole are broader spectrum azole drugs that have better activity on many non-*C. albicans* species and some molds as well. Of the broader spectrum azoles, voriconazole 2.5 mg/kg IP qd (72) or 200 mg po BID (73) has the best penetration into aqueous compartments and is a potential option for fluconazole-resistant strains. Echinocandin antifungal drugs have excellent activity against *Candida* species, but there is little experience in treating PD peritonitis. A possible concern is that echinocandins are large molecules that are highly protein-bound and do not penetrate other aqueous sites such as cerebrospinal fluid (CSF) and urine well. However, caspofungin 50 mg IV qd has been used successfully in combination with amphotericin B to treat a multiresistant *C. albicans* (74) and alone IV to treat trichosporon PD peritonitis cases (75). IP administration

Table 14.3	**Systemic Antibiotic Dosing Recommendations for Treatment of Peritonitis**
Drug	**Dosing**
Anti-bacterials	
Ciprofloxacin	oral 250 mg BD[a]
Colistin	IV 300 mg loading, then 150–200 mg daily[b]
Ertapenem	IV 500 mg daily
Levofloxacin	oral 250 mg daily
Linezolid	IV or oral 600 mg BD
Moxifloxacin	oral 400 mg daily
Rifampicin	450 mg daily for BW<50 kg; 600 mg daily for BW≥50 kg
Trimethoprim/ Sulfamethoxazole	oral 160 mg/800 mg BD
Anti-fungals	
Amphotericin	IV test dose 1 mg; starting dose 0.1 mg/kg/day over 6 hours; increased to target dose 0.75–1.0 mg/kg/day over 4 days
Caspofungin	IV 70 mg loading, then 50 mg daily
Fluconazole	oral 200 mg loading, then 50–100 mg daily
Flucytosine	oral 1 gm/day
Posaconazole	IV 400 mg every 12 hours
Voriconazole	oral 200 mg every 12 hours

BD, twice a day; IV, intravenous; BW, body weight.
[a]Ciprofloxacin 500 mg BD may be needed if residual glomerular filtration rate is above 5 mL/min.
[b]Expressed as colistin base activity (CBA).
Reprinted with permission from Li PK, Szeto C-C, Piraino B, et al. ISPD peritonitis recommendations: 2016 update on prevention and treatment (published online ahead of print June 9, 2016). *Perit Dial Int.*

has not been studied to my knowledge. Amphotericin B is active on most fungal species, including molds. Early attempts at using amphotericin IP failed because of severe irritant peritonitis, even at low doses. Amphotericin B given IV penetrates the peritoneal fluid poorly but has been used successfully to treat *Candida* peritonitis IV at a dose of 0.75 to 1 mg/kg/d along with po flucytosine (76). Flucytosine, 1 g po qd, is recommended to be used in combination with an azole or amphotericin B by the ISPD for the treatment of *Candida* peritonitis (1). If used, flucytosine serum levels should be measured, maintaining trough levels less than 25 to 50 μg/mL to avoid excessive levels and hematologic and GI toxicity. Most published series of *Candida* peritonitis (77) and ISPD guidelines (1) emphasize the importance of prompt catheter removal. Culture-directed antifungal therapy should be given for at least 2 weeks, followed by catheter replacement after 4 to 6 weeks (71).

Failure to remove the catheter in a timely fashion is reported to increase mortality and significantly increases the risk of technique failure in most series. However, Boer (78) reported eight patients with *Candida* peritonitis who were successfully treated with IP fluconazole, po flucytosine, and whose PD catheters were locked with 10 mL of 0.1 mg/mL of amphotericin B between CAPD exchanges. In a series of 13 patients reported by Wong et al. (76) who were treated with amphotericin B 0.75 to 1 mg/kg/d IV and oral flucyto-sine with their PD catheters in place until catheter replacement after about 4 weeks of treatment, 9 were able to continue PD.

Peritonitis caused by filamentous fungi (molds) is much less common than that caused by *Candida*. Infection caused by molds appears to be more common in tropical and subtropical climates (79). Antifungal treatment of mold infection is much more difficult. Fluconazole has no activity on molds. Itraconazole, voriconazole (72), posaconazole 400 mg IV bid (80), and more recently, isavuco-nazole are broader spectrum azoles that have activity on many common molds, but there is little reported clinical experience in using these agents to treat fungal peritonitis. Amphotericin B is active on many mold species (81). Treatment of mold infections is directed by the species identified and antifungal drug susceptibilities when available. Catheter removal is almost always necessary.

Mycobacterial Peritonitis

Tuberculous Peritonitis in Peritoneal Dialysis

Patients with chronic kidney disease (CKD) on dialysis have a much higher incidence of tuberculosis (TB), with some studies reporting rates that are 7 to 50 times greater than the general population (82). In a series of 790 CAPD patients in China, 38 cases of TB were diagnosed, yielding a prevalence of 4.8% and a case rate of 800/100,000 (83). In that series, more than half of the patients had extrapulmonary TB and 37 % had TB peritonitis. Almost all cases of TB peritonitis result from reactivation of latent tuberculous infection. In developed countries, many cases of TB arise in immigrants from countries with high incidences of TB (82) and are potentially preventable by screening for latent TB and administering preventive treatment.

The clinical presentation of TB peritonitis in a patient on PD resembles bacterial peritonitis (84). Abdominal pain, fever, and cloudy dialysate are usually evident, although the onset and progression of symptoms is often more subacute than most cases of bacterial infection. Peritoneal WBCs are similar to bacterial cases, with a few hundred to a few thousand WBCs that are predominantly PMNs in most cases (85). The usual clinical course is they are treated empirically for bacterial peritonitis and meet the clinical definition of refractory, culture-negative peritonitis because they do not respond. Cases of refractory peritonitis should prompt repeat cultures and studies for mycobacteria, fungi, and fastidious organisms. In most published series, the diagnostic yield of acid-fast bacilli (AFB) smears of peritoneal fluid in TB peritonitis in PD patients is less than 20% and the yield of peritoneal fluid cultures is around 30% (86). This is because the organisms are growing in granulomas in the peritoneal membrane rather than the fluid itself. Obtaining 50 to 150 mL of peritoneal fluid, centrifuging, and processing the pellet for cultures and smears can increase the yield. Traditionally, the most reliable diagnostic method has been peritoneal biopsy with histology and AFB cultures (87). More recent series in PD patients have reported peritoneal fluid cultures positive in 50% to 100% of patients. The widespread use of the BACTEC liquid culture media systems are probably responsible for the better yield on PD fluid cultures and also reduce the time to culture positivity to 10 to 14 days in most cases rather than 3 to 6 weeks with the traditional mycobacterial culture techniques (84). Another rapid and useful test for TB diagnosis is PCR. These rapid PCR tests were initially approved for direct testing of sputum samples but have been used successfully to detect TB in extrapulmonary specimens (88). The sensitivity of PCR in detecting TB in peritoneal fluid in TB peritonitis has been reported to be 50% or more, and a result is obtained in 2 hours. In summary, the

diagnosis of TB peritonitis is challenging but should be considered in the patient with refractory peritonitis with negative bacterial who fails to respond to appropriate empiric therapy.

Positive mycobacterial cultures should be sent for species identification to confirm TB versus NTM and drug susceptibility testing. Most referral laboratories can provide drug susceptibility results in about 2 weeks. Pending these results, therapy with four anti-TB drugs should be started. In patients with end-stage kidney disease (ESKD), the American Thoracic Society/Centers for Disease Control and Prevention/Infectious Diseases Society of America Guidelines recommend isoniazid (INH) 300 mg po qd or 900 mg po three times weekly, pyridoxine 50 mg po qd, rifampin 600 mg po qd or 600 mg po three times weekly, pyrazinamide 25 to 35 mg/kg three times a week, and ethambutol 15 to 25 mg/kg three times weekly (89). If the organism is fully susceptible, ethambutol may be stopped and pyrazinamide discontinued after 2 months. INH and rifampin are continued for a total of 6 months. However, these guidelines were recommended for patients on hemodialysis. The 2016 ISPD guidelines for the treatment of TB peritonitis in PD patients are slightly different (1). The use of ethambutol is discouraged because of the potential risk of optic neuritis, suggesting a fluoroquinolone, ofloxacin 200 mg po qd in its place. These guideline suggest using INH 300 mg po qd, pyridoxine 50 mg po qd, rifampin 600 mg po qd, pyrazinamide 25 to 35 mg/kg three times a week and ofloxacin. Ofloxacin and pyrazinamide are discontinued after 3 months, and INH and rifampin are continued for a total of 12 to 18 months of therapy. Lui et al. (90) reported a series of 10 CAPD patients with TB peritonitis. Two patients died during therapy, and two were converted to hemodialysis. The remaining six patients were successfully treated with INH rifampin and pyrazinamide for 9 to 12 months. In a subsequent publication, Lui et al. (83) treated 14 CAPD patients with TB peritonitis. Patients were treated for 12 to 15 months with INH, rifampin, ofloxacin, and pyrazinamide. Pyrazinamide was discontinued at 3 months, and the other drugs were continued for a total of 12 to 15 months. PD catheters were left in place during therapy. Nine patients were treated successfully, and the five deaths were not the result of TB infection itself. In summary, the optimal treatment of TB peritonitis in PD patients is not entirely clear regarding specific drugs and duration. The most prudent approach is to use standard antituberculous drugs in the regimens described earlier for about 12 months (91).

The vast majority of cases of TB peritonitis and other sites of infection are due to the reactivation of latent tuberculous infection. All dialysis programs should strongly consider screening patients for latent tuberculous infection as part of preparing for dialysis. This can be done with tuberculin skin testing or blood testing with an interferon-γ release assay (IGRA). Patients with chronic renal insufficiency have an increased risk of being anergic on skin testing and IGRA testing resulting in false-negative screening (92). Patients found to have latent tuberculous infection should be offered therapy for latent tuberculous infection and strongly encouraged to accept it. The standard regimen is INH 300 mg po qd with pyridoxine 50 mg po qd for 9 months. Identifying and treating latent TB infection will greatly reduce the risk of all forms of reactivation TB, including peritonitis.

Nontuberculous Mycobacterial Peritonitis and Exit-Site Infections in Peritoneal Dialysis Patients

NTM are a group of about 150 species, of which about half have been associated with human infections. These organisms are present in the environment, mostly in soil and water, and can cause human infections, but are not spread from person to person. In the past, NTM have been grouped according to Runyon classification, but more recently classified according to growth rates—rapid, intermediate, or slow-growing (92). Most reported cases of exit-site infections and peritonitis in PD patients have been caused by the rapid growers—*Mycobacterium abscessus*, *Mycobacterium chelonae*, and *Mycobacterium fortuitum* (93–99).

NTM have been reported to cause exit-site and tunnel infections as well as peritonitis in PD patients. Particularly with the rapid growing NTMs, exit-site infection is often present or precedes the diagnosis of peritonitis with these organisms. Recent antibiotic use, often for exit-site infection and the use of gentamicin cream for exit-site prophylaxis seem to be common predisposing factors for these infections (100,101). NTM exit-site infections are often described as culture-negative, chronic, and persistent. NTM peritonitis clinically resembles bacterial peritonitis, with fever, abdominal pain, cloudy dialysate, with a few hundred WBC that are usually >50% PMNs. Exit-site or peritoneal fluid sample Gram stains are usually negative but may show a few gram-positive rods, AFB smears are usually negative. The rapid growing NTMs will grow on most standard bacterial culture media but usually take about 5 days and are often misidentified as "diphtheroids." These patients are often classified as refractory bacterial peritonitis, which should prompt repeat PD fluid cultures for fastidious bacteria, AFB, and fungi.

Obtaining a positive culture is important to identify the species and obtain drug susceptibility studies, which vary according to the species and within species. The optimal treatment of NTM PD peritonitis is not well defined. Most published studies reporting the treatment of the rapid growing NTMs in PD infections have used culture and sensitivity directed therapy for 2 to 9 months for peritonitis. In most cases, the PD catheter was removed, but in some, in the absence of exit-site or tunnel infection, successful treatment was achieved with the catheter in place. Experience treating NTM PD peritonitis caused by other NTM is sparse and confined to isolated case reports.

PREVENTING PERITONITIS (102)

Reporting Monitoring Peritonitis Rates

ISPD guidelines recommend that each program monitor and report its peritonitis rates, expressed as number of episodes of peritonitis per patient year, the rates for individual organisms, and antibiotic susceptibility (1). The currently recommended benchmark rate is 0.5 episodes of peritonitis per patient-year, or 1 episode every 2 years, by 2016 ISPD guidelines. Relapsing episodes are only counted once. The rates of peritonitis for each individual pathogen should also be reported as episodes per patient-year rather than as percentage of cases.

Continuous Quality Improvement

ISPD guidelines also suggest that each program have a continuous quality improvement (CQI) committee to perform root cause analysis on each PD-related infection to determine if there were modifiable risk factors or potentially preventable causes (103,104).

Peritoneal Dialysis Catheter Placement

Several randomized controlled trials have shown that preoperative antibiotic prophylaxis with cefazolin, cefuroxime, or vancomycin prior to catheter placement reduces the incidence of early postop peritonitis (105). Several randomized controlled trials have compared postop infection rates in patients who underwent PD catheter

placement peritoneoscopically, laparoscopically, or via standard laparotomy placement and found very little difference in outcomes (1). Also, placement of the catheter via a midline or lateral incision did not affect peritonitis rates. Other studies have shown no significant difference in infection rates between swan-neck and Tenckhoff catheters or an advantage to a downward facing exit site (102,106,107).

Peritoneal Dialysis–Automated Peritoneal Dialysis versus Continuous Ambulatory Peritoneal Dialysis

At this point, there is no clear definitive evidence that patients using APD have fewer episodes of peritonitis than patients using CAPD. In patients using CAPD, however, the two-bag, Y-connector flush-and-fill technique appears to reduce the rate of peritonitis compared to other methods (1,102). There is also little evidence to suggest that the choice of dialysis solution affects peritonitis rates (1,102).

Peritoneal Dialysis Patient Training

Before the initiation of home PD, patients must be trained by a qualified staff member, usually a nurse (102,108). Training should include the concepts of PD, strict adherence to aseptic technique, connecting and deconnecting procedures, care of the exit site, and recognizing complications such as possible peritonitis and taking appropriate actions. The patients and helpers should demonstrate competence in these areas before attempting home PD. A home visit by a PD nurse after initiating home PD is often useful as well. Retraining at 6-month intervals may be helpful and is indicated after an episode of peritonitis or if there is any change in the patient's PD equipment.

Exit-Site Care

The patient must also be trained in exit-site care during these training sessions, in particular, handwashing and sterile technique when cleaning and dressing the exit site. Using sterile technique, the exit site should be gently cleansed with soap and water. Cleansing with dilute sodium hypochlorite may also reduce exit-site infections (1,102). Daily application of topical antimicrobial agents to the exit site has been shown to reduce exit-site infections and peritonitis. Daily topical mupirocin has been shown to reduce the incidence of *S. aureus* exit-site infections and peritonitis (5). Gentamicin cream applied daily to the exit site can reduce the *S. aureus* and *Pseudomonas* exit-site infections (6,109). Subsequent studies of gentamicin cream revealed increases in *S. aureus*, *Pseudomonas*, and *Enterobacteriaceae* exit-site infections (7) and increases in exit-site infections and peritonitis caused by rapid growing NTM (100,101).

Miscellaneous Sources of Peritonitis and Prophylaxis

Peritonitis may follow endoscopic or other invasive procedures involving the GI or genitourinary (GU) tract. Periprocedure prophylactic antibiotics have been shown to reduce the incidence of peritonitis after colonoscopy, sigmoidoscopy, cystoscopy, and hysteroscopy (1,110). The most commonly used prophylactic regimen has been ampicillin and gentamicin. Transient bacteremia during dental procedures occasionally results in peritonitis. Some authorities recommend the administration of a single dose of amoxicillin before invasive dental procedures as in endocarditis prophylaxis (111).

Finally, most cases of *Candida* peritonitis follow a course of antibiotics for peritonitis or other indications. A number of studies have shown that administering prophylactic oral nystatin (112) or fluconazole (113) concomitant with the antibiotic course can reduce the incidence or secondary *Candida* peritonitis in programs with more frequent episodes of *Candida* peritonitis.

◈ REFERENCES

1. Li PK, Szeto C-C, Piraino B, et al. ISPD peritonitis recommendations: 2016 update on prevention and treatment [published online ahead of print June 9, 2016]. *Perit Dial Int.*
2. Mujais S. Microbiology and outcomes of peritonitis in North America. *Kidney Int* 2006;70:S55–S62.
3. Ghali JR, Bannister KM, Brown FG, et al. Microbiology and outcomes of peritonitis in Australian peritoneal dialysis patients. *Perit Dial Int* 2011;31:651–662.
4. Hall-Stoodley L, Costerton JW, Stoodley P. Bacterial biofilms: from the natural environment to infectious diseases. *Nat Rev Microbiol* 2004;2:95–108.
5. Xu G, Tu W, Xu C. Mupirocin for preventing exit-site infection and peritonitis in patients undergoing peritoneal dialysis. *Nephrol Dial Transplant* 2009;25:587–592.
6. Chen SS, Sheeth H, Piraino B, et al. Long-term exit-site gentamicin prophylaxis and gentamicin resistance in a peritoneal dialysis program. *Perit Dial Int* 2016;36:387–389.
7. Pierce DA, Williamson JC, Mauck VS, et al. The effect on peritoneal dialysis pathogens of changing topical antibiotic prophylaxis. *Perit Dial Int* 2011;32:525–530.
8. Wu V-C, Wang Y-T, Wang C-Y, et al. High frequency of linezolid-associated thrombocytopenia and anemia among patients with end-stage renal disease. *Clin Infect Dis* 2006;42:66–72.
9. Gervasoni C, Bergia R, Cozzi V, et al. Is it time to revise linezolid doses in peritoneal dialysis patients? *J Antimicrob Chemother* 2015;70: 2918–2920.
10. Burkhalter F, Clemenger M, Haddoub SS, et al. *Pseudomonas* exit site infection: treatment outcomes with topical gentamicin in addition to systemic antibiotics. *Clin Kidney J* 2015;8:781–784.
11. Beiber SD, Anderson AE, Mehrota R. Diagnostic testing for peritonitis in patients undergoing peritoneal dialysis. *Semin Dial* 2014;27: 602–606.
12. Alfa MA, Degagne P, Olson N, et al. Improved detection of bacterial growth in continuous ambulatory peritoneal dialysis effluent by use of BacT/Alert FAN bottles. *J Clin Microbiol* 1997;35:862–866.
13. DeVin F, Rutherford P, Faict D. Intraperitoneal administration of drugs in peritoneal dialysis patients: a review of compatibility and guidance for clinical use. *Perit Dial Int* 2009;29:5–15.
14. Ballenger AE, Palmer SC, Wiggins KJ, et al. Treatment for peritoneal dialysis associated peritonitis. *Cochrane Database Syst Rev* 2014;(4):CD005284.
15. Chow KM, Szeto C-C, Cheung KKK, et al. Predictive value of dialysis cell counts in peritonitis complicating peritoneal dialysis. *Clin J Am Soc Nephrol* 2006;1:768–773.
16. Szeto C-C, Kwan BC-H, Chow K-M, et al. Recurrent and relapsing peritonitis: causative organisms and response to treatment. *Am J Kidney Dis* 2009;54:702–710.
17. Burke M, Hawley CM, Badve SV, et al. Relapsing and recurrent peritoneal dialysis-associated peritonitis: a multicenter registry study. *Am J Kidney Dis* 2011;58:429–436.
18. Fahim M, Hawley CM, McDonald SP, et al. Coagulase-negative staphylococcal peritonitis in Australian peritoneal dialysis patients: predictors, treatment, and outcome in 936 cases. *Nephrol Dial Transplant* 2010;25:3386–3392.
19. Kofteridis DP, Valachis A, Perakis K, et al. Peritoneal dialysis-associated peritonitis: clinical features and predictors of outcome. *Int J Infect Dis* 2010;14:e484–e493.
20. Camargo CH, de Lourdes M, Caramori JCT, et al. Peritoneal dialysis-related peritonitis due to coagulase-negative *Staphylococcus*: a review of 115 cases in a Brazilian center. *Clin J Am Soc Nephrol* 2014;9:1074–1081.
21. Von Eiff C, Peters G, Heilmann C. Pathogenesis of infections due to coagulase-negative staphylococci. *Lancet Infect Dis* 2002;2:677–685.
22. Ruger W, van Ittersum FJ, Comazzettos SE, et al. Similar peritonitis outcomes in CAPD and APD patients with dialysis modality continuation during peritonitis. *Perit Dial Int* 2011;31:39–47.
23. De Moraes TP, Olandoski M, Caramori JC, et al. Novel predictors of peritonitis-related outcomes in the BRAZPD cohort. *Perit Dial Int* 2012;34:179–187.
24. Szeto C-C, Chow K-M, Kwan BC-H, et al. *Staphylococcus aureus* complicates peritoneal dialysis: review of 245 consecutive cases. *Clin J Am Soc Nephrol* 2007;2:245–251.
25. Govindarajulu S, Hawley CM, McDonald SP, et al. Staphylococcus aureus peritonitis in Australian peritoneal dialysis patients: predictors, treatment and outcomes in 503 patients. *Perit Dial Int* 2010;30: 311–319.
26. Saravolatz LD, Stein GE, Johnson LB. Ceftaroline: a novel cephalosporin with activity against methicillin-resistant *Staphylococcus aureus*. *Clin Infect Dis* 2011;52:1156–1163.
27. Munoz de Bustillo E, Aguilera A, Jimenez C, et al. Streptococcal versus Staphylococcus epidermidis peritonitis in CAPD. *Perit Dial Int* 1997;17:392–395.
28. Knoll B, Tleyjeh IM, Steckelberg JM, et al. Infective endocarditis due to penicillin-resistant viridans group streptococci. *Clin Infect Dis* 2007;44:1585–1592.
29. Roberts DM, Fernando G, Singer RF, et al. Antibiotic stability in commercial peritoneal dialysis solutions: influence of formulation, storage, and duration. *Nephrol Dial Transplant* 2011;26:3344–3349.
30. Shukla A, Abreu Z, Bargman JM. Streptococcal PD peritonitis—a 10-year review of one centre's experience. *Nephrol Dial Transplant* 2006;21:3545–3549.
31. O'Shea S, Hawley CM, McDonald SP, et al. Streptococcal peritonitis in Australian peritoneal dialysis patients: predictors, treatment and outcomes in 287 cases. *BMC Nephrology* 2009;10:19.
32. Chao C-J, Lee S-Y, Yang W-S, et al. Viridans streptococci in peritoneal dialysis peritonitis: clinical courses and long-term outcomes. *Perit Dial Int* 2015;35:333–341.
33. Yap DYH, To KKW, Yip TPS, et al. Streptococcus bovis peritonitis complicating peritoneal dialysis—a review of 10 years' experience. *Perit Dial Int* 2012;32:55–59.
34. Edey M, Hawley CM, McDonald SP, et al. Enterococcal peritonitis in Australian peritoneal dialysis patients: predictors, treatment, and outcomes in 116 cases. *Nephrol Dial Transplant* 2010;25:1272–1278.
35. Yip T, Tsa K-C, Ng F, et al. Clinical course and outcomes of single organism enterococcus peritonitis in peritoneal dialysis patients. *Perit Dial Int* 2011;31:522–528.
36. Huen SC, Hall I, Topal J, et al. Successful use of intraperitoneal daptomycin in the treatment of vancomycin-resistant enterococcus peritonitis. *Am J Kidney Dis* 2009;54:538–541.
37. Gilmore JF, Kin M, LaSalvia MT, et al. Treatment of enterococcal peritonitis with intraperitoneal daptomycin in a vancomycin-allergic patient and a review of the literature. *Perit Dial Int* 2013;33:353–357.
38. Khadzhynov D, Joukhadar C, Peters H. Plasma and peritoneal dialysate levels during daptomycin therapy for peritonitis. *Am J Kidney Dis* 2009;53:911–912.
39. Bahte SK, Bertram A, Burkhardt O, et al. Therapeutic serum concentrations of daptomycin after intraperitoneal administration in a patient with peritoneal dialysis associated peritonitis. *J Antimicrob Chemother* 2010;65:1312–1314.
40. Yang JW, Kim YS, Choi SO, et al. Successful use of intravenous linezolid in CAPD patient with vancomycin-resistant enterococcal peritonitis. *Perit Dial Int* 2011;31:209–210.
41. Song IJ, Seo JW, Kwon YE, et al. Successful treatment of vancomycin-resistant enterococcus peritonitis using linezolid without catheter removal in a peritoneal dialysis patient. *Perit Dial Int* 2014;34:235–239.
42. Moellering RC. Linezolid: the first oxazolidinone antimicrobial. *Ann Intern Med* 2003;138:135–142.
43. Lynn WA, Clutterbuck E, Want S, et al. Treatment of CAPD-peritonitis due to glycopeptide-resistant Enterococcus faecium with quinupristin/dalfopristin. *Lancet* 1994;344:1025–1036.
44. Szeto C-C, Chow KM, Chung K-Y, et al. The clinical course of peritoneal dialysis-related peritonitis caused by Corynebacterium species. *Nephrol Dial Transplant* 2005;20:2793–2796.

45. Barraclough K, Hawley CM, McDonald SP, et al. Corynebacterium peritonitis in Australian peritoneal dialysis patients: predictors, treatment and outcomes in 82 cases. *Nephrol Dial Transplant* 2009;24: 3834–3839.

46. Szeto C-C, Chow VC-Y, Chow K-M, et al. Enterobacteriaceae peritonitis complicating peritoneal dialysis: a review of 210 consecutive cases. *Kidney Int* 2006;69:1245–1252.

47. Jarvis EM, Hawley CM, McDonald SP, et al. Predictors, treatment and outcomes of non-Pseudomonas gram-negative peritonitis. *Kidney Int* 2010;78:408–414.

48. Jain AK, Blake PG. Non-Pseudomonas gram-negative peritonitis. *Kidney Int* 2006;69:1107–1109.

49. Wong SSY, Ho P-L, Yuen K-Y. Evolution of antibiotic resistance mechanisms and their relevance to dialysis-related infections. *Perit Dial Int* 2007;27(suppl 2):S272–S280.

50. Yip T, Tse K-C, Lam M-F, et al. Risk factors and outcomes of extended-spectrum beta-lactamase-producing E. coli peritonitis in CAPD patients. *Perit Dial Int* 2006;26:191–197.

51. Bradford PA. Extended-spectrum beta-lactamases in the 21st century: characterization, epidemiology, and detection of this important resistance threat. *Clin Microbiol Rev* 2001;14:933–951.

52. Feng X, Yang X, Yi C, et al. *Escherichia coli* peritonitis in peritoneal dialysis: the prevalence, antibiotic resistance, and clinical outcomes in a south China dialysis center. *Perit Dial Int* 2014;34:308–316.

53. Gupta N, Limbago BM, Patel JB, et al. Carbapenem-resistant *Enterobacteriaceae*: epidemiology and prevention. *Clin Infect Dis* 2011;53: 60–67.

54. Mirkovic TD, Gvozdenovic L, Majstorvic-Strazmester G, et al. An experience with colistin applied in treatment of immunocompromised patients with peritonitis on peritoneal dialysis. *Vojnositeski Pregled* 2015;72:379–382.

55. Szeto C-C, Chow KM, Leung CB, et al. Clinical course of peritonitis due to *Pseudomonas* species complicating peritoneal dialysis: a review of 104 cases. *Kidney Int* 2001;59:2309–2315.

56. Siva B, Hawley CM, McDonald SP, et al. Pseudomonas peritonitis in Australia: predictors, treatment and outcomes in 191 cases. *Clin J Am Soc Nephrol* 2009;4:957–964.

57. Munoz-Price LS, Weinstein RA. Acinetobacter infection. *N Engl J Med* 2008;558:1271–1281.

58. Zhang W, Wu Y-G, Qi Z-M, et al. Peritoneal dialysis-related peritonitis with *Acinetobacter baumannii*: a review of seven cases. *Perit Dial Int* 2012;34:317–321.

59. Tzanetou K, Trianraphillis G, Tsoutsos D, et al. Stenotrophomonas maltophilia peritonitis in CAPD patients: susceptibility to antibiotics and treatment outcome: a report of five cases. *Perit Dial Int* 2004;24:401–424.

60. Szeto C-C, Li PKT, Leung CB, et al. Xanthomonas maltophilia peritonitis in uremic patients receiving continuous ambulatory peritoneal dialysis. *Am J Kidney Dis* 1997;29:91–95.

61. Taylor G, McKenzie M, Buchanan-Chell M, et al. Peritonitis due to *Stenotrophomonas maltophilia* in patients undergoing chromic peritoneal dialysis. *Perit Dial Int* 1999;19:259–262.

62. Kim GC, Korbet SM. Polymicrobial peritonitis in continuous ambulatory peritoneal dialysis patients. *Am J Kidney Dis* 2000;36:1000–1008.

63. Szeto C-C, Chow K-M, Wong TY-H, et al. Conservative management of polymicrobial peritonitis complicating peritoneal dialysis—a series of 140 consecutive cases. *Am J Med* 2002;113:728–733.

64. Barraclough K, Hawley CM, McDonald SP, et al. Polymicrobial peritonitis in peritoneal dialysis patients in Australia: predictors, treatment, and outcomes. *Am J Kidney Dis* 2010;55:121–131.

65. Fahim M, Hawley CM, McDonald SP, et al. Culture-negative peritonitis in peritoneal dialysis patients in Australia: predictors, treatment and outcomes in 435 patients. *Am J Kidney Dis* 2010;55:690–697.

66. Matuczkiewicz-Rowinska J. Update on fungal peritonitis and its treatment. *Perit Dial Int* 2009;29(suppl 2):S161–S165.

67. Prasad N, Gupta A. Fungal peritonitis in peritoneal dialysis patients. *Perit Dial Int* 2005;25:207–222.

68. Ostrosky L, Alexander BD, Kett DH, et al. Multi-center evaluation of the (1-3) beta-D-glucan assay as an aid to diagnosis of fungal infections in humans. *Clin Infect Dis* 2005;41:654–659.

69. Miles R, Hawley CM, McDonald SP, et al. Predictors and outcomes of fungal peritonitis in peritoneal dialysis patients. *Kidney Int* 2009;76: 622–628.

70. Levallois J, Nadeau-Fredette A-C, Labbe A-C, et al. Ten-year experience with fungal peritonitis in peritoneal dialysis patients: antifungal susceptibility patterns in a North-American center. *Int J Infect Dis* 2012;16:e41–e43.

71. Nadeau-Fredette A-C, Bargman JM. Characteristics and outcomes of fungal peritonitis in a modern North American cohort. *Perit Dial Int* 2015;35:78–84.

72. Roberts DM, Kauter G, Ray JE, et al. Intraperitoneal voriconazole in a patient with aspergillus peritoneal dialysis peritonitis. *Perit Dial Int* 2013;33:92–93.

73. Ulusoy S, Ozkan G, Tosun I, et al. Peritonitis due to Aspergillus nidulans and its effective treatment with voriconazole: the first case report. *Perit Dial Int* 2011;31:212–213.

74. Fourtounas C, Marangos M, Kalliakani P, et al. Treatment of peritoneal dialysis related fungal peritonitis with caspofungin plus amphotericin B combination therapy. *Nephrol Dial Transplant* 2006;21:236–237.

75. Madariaga MG, Tenorio A, Proia L. Trichosporon inkin peritonitis treated with caspofungin. *J Clin Microbiol* 2003;41:5827–5829.

76. Wong P-N, Lo K-Y, Tong GMW, et al. Treatment of fungal peritonitis with a combination of intravenous amphotericin B and oral flucytosine, and delayed catheter replacement in continuous ambulatory peritoneal dialysis. *Perit Dial Int* 2008;28:155–162.

77. Chang TI, Kim HW, Park JT, et al. Early catheter removal improves patient survival in peritoneal dialysis patients with fungal peritonitis: results of ninety-four episodes of fungal peritonitis at a single center. *Perit Dial Int* 2011;31:60–66.

78. Boer WH. Successful treatment of eight episodes of Candida peritonitis without catheter removal using intracatheter administration of amphotericin B. *Perit Dial Int* 2007;27:208–210.

79. Baer RA, Killen JP, Cho Y, et al. Non-candidal fungal peritonitis in far North Queensland: a case series. *Perit Dial Int* 2013;33:559–564.

80. Sedlacek M, Cotter JG, Suriawinata AA, et al. Mucormycosis peritonitis: more than 2 years of disease-free follow-up after posaconazole salvage therapy after failure of liposomal amphotericin B. *Am J Kidney Dis* 2008;51:302–306.

81. Serna JH, Wanger A, Dosekun AK. Successful treatment of Mucormycosis peritonitis with liposomal amphotericin B in a patient on long-term peritoneal dialysis. *Am J Kidney Dis* 2003;42:e14–e17.

82. Moore DAJ, Lightstone L, Javid B, et al. High rates of tuberculosis in end stage renal failure: the impact of international migration. *Emerg Infect Dis* 2002;8:77–78.

83. Lui SL, Tang S, Fuk L, et al. Tuberculosis infection in Chinese patients undergoing continuous peritoneal dialysis. *Am J Kidney Dis* 2001;38:1055–1060.

84. Chau TN, Leung VKS, Wong S, et al. Diagnostic challenges of tuberculosis in patients with and without end-stage renal disease. *Clin Infect Dis* 2007;45:e141–e146.

85. Talwani R, Horvath JA. Tuberculous peritonitis in patients undergoing continuous peritoneal dialysis: case report and review. *Clin Infect Dis* 2000;31:70–75.

86. Akpolat T. Tuberculous peritonitis. *Perit Dial Int* 2009;29:S166–S169.

87. Chow KM, Chow VCY, Hung LCT, et al. Tuberculosis peritonitis-associated mortality is high among patients waiting for the results of mycobacterial cultures of ascitic fluid. *Clin Infect Dis* 2002;35:409–413.

88. Vadwai V, Boehme C, Nabeta P, et al. Xpert MTB/RIF: a new pillar in diagnosis of extrapulmonary tuberculosis? *J Clin Microbiol* 2011;49:2540–2545.

89. American Thoracic Society, Centers for Disease Control and Prevention, Infectious Diseases Society of America. Treatment of tuberculosis. *MMWR Recomm Rep* 2003;52(RR-11):1–77.

90. Lui SL, Lo CY, Choy BY, et al. Optimal treatment and long-term outcome of tuberculous peritonitis complicating continuous ambulatory peritoneal dialysis. *Am J Kidney Dis* 1996;28:747–751.

91. Abraham G, Matthews M, Sekar L, et al. Tuberculous peritonitis in a cohort of continuous ambulatory dialysis patients. *Perit Dial Int* 2001;21(suppl 3):S202–S204.

92. Griffith DE, Askamit T, Brown-Elliott BA, et al. An official ATS/IDSA statement: diagnosis, treatment and presentation of nontuberculous mycobacterial diseases. *Am J Respir Crit Care Med* 2007;175:367–416.

93. White R, Abreo K, Flanagan R, et al. Nontuberculous mycobacterial infection in continuous ambulatory peritoneal dialysis patients. *Am J Kidney Dis* 1993;22:581–587.

94. Hakim A, Hisam N, Reuman PD. Environmental mycobacterial peritonitis complicating peritoneal dialysis: three cases and review. *Clin Infect Dis* 1993;16:426–431.

95. Rho M, Bia F, Brewster UC. Nontuberculous mycobacterial peritonitis in peritoneal dialysis patients. *Semin Dial* 2006;20:271–276.

96. Renaud CJ, Subramanian S, Tambyah PA, et al. The clinical course of rapidly growing nontuberculous mycobacterial peritoneal dialysis infections in Asians: a case series and literature review. *Nephrology* 2011;16:174–179.

97. Song Y, Wu J, Yan H, et al. Peritoneal dialysis-associated nontuberculous mycobacterium peritonitis: a systematic review of reported cases. *Nephrol Dial Transplant* 2012;27:1639–1644.

98. Jiang SH, Roberts DM, Clayton PA, et al. Non-tuberculous mycobacterial PD peritonitis in Australia. *Int Urol Nephrol* 2013;45:1423–1428.

99. Kunin M, Knecht A, Holtzman EJ. Mycobacterium chelonae peritonitis in peritoneal dialysis. Literature review. *Eur J Clin Microbiol Infect Dis* 2014;33:1267–1271.

100. Tse K-C, Lui S-L, Cheng VC-C, et al. A cluster of rapidly growing mycobacterial peritoneal dialysis catheter exit-site infections. *Am J Kidney Dis* 2007;50:E1–E5.

101. Lo M-W, Siu K-M, Wong Y-Y, et al. Atypical mycobacterial exit-site infection and peritonitis in peritoneal dialysis patients on prophylactic exit-site gentamicin cream. *Perit Dial Int* 2013;33:267–272.

102. Piraino B, Bernardini J, Brown E, et al. ISPD position statement on reducing the risks of peritoneal dialysis-related infections. *Perit Dial Int* 2011;31:614–630.

103. Qamar M, Sheth H, Bender FH, et al. Clinical outcomes in peritoneal dialysis: impact of continuous quality improvement initiatives. *Adv Perit Dial* 2009;25:76–79.

104. Cho Y, Johnson DW. Peritoneal dialysis-related peritonitis: towards improving evidence, practices and outcomes. *Am J Kidney Dis* 2014;64:279–289.

105. Strippoli GFM, Tong A, Johnson D, et al. Antimicrobial agents to prevent peritonitis in peritoneal dialysis: a systematic review of randomized controlled trials. *Am J Kidney Dis* 2004;44:591–603.

106. Lo W-K, Lui S-L, Li F-K, et al. A prospective randomized study on three different peritoneal dialysis catheters. *Perit Dial Int* 2003;23(suppl 1):S127–S131.

107. Flanigan M, Gokal R. Peritoneal catheters and exit site practices toward optimum peritoneal access: a review of current developments. *Perit Dial Int* 2005;25:132–139.

108. Figueiredo AE, Bernardini J, Bowes E, et al. ISPD guideline recommendations: a syllabus for teaching peritoneal dialysis patients and caregivers [published ahead of print February 25, 2016]. *Perit Dial Int.*

109. Fried L, Bernardini J, Piraino B. Iatrogenic peritonitis: the need for prophylaxis. *Perit Dial Int* 2000;20:243–245.

110. Yip T, Tse KC, Lam MF, et al. Risks and outcomes of peritonitis after flexible colonoscopy in CAPD patients. *Perit Dial Int* 2007;27:560–564.

111. Wilson W, Taubert KA, Gewitz M, et al. Prevention of infective endocarditis. Guidelines from the American Heart Association. *Circulation* 2007;116:1736–1754.

112. Wong P-N, Lo K-Y, Tong GMW, et al. Prevention of fungal peritonitis with nystatin prophylaxis in patients receiving CAPD. *Perit Dial Int* 2007;27:531–536.

113. Restrepo C, Chacon J, Manjarres G. Fungal peritonitis in peritoneal dialysis patients: successful prophylaxis with fluconazole as demonstrated by prospective randomized control trial. *Perit Dial Int* 2010;30:619–625.

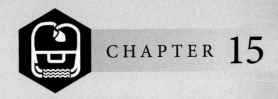

CHAPTER 15

Hypertension in Dialysis Patients

Arjun D. Sinha and Rajiv Agarwal

Hypertension is both a cause (1) and consequence of chronic kidney disease (CKD) across its spectrum of severity, up to and including end-stage kidney disease (ESKD). Despite steady improvement, mortality remains high in the dialysis population with a 5-year survival rate of only 40% (2), which is comparable to some advanced cancers (3). Cardiovascular events remain the leading cause of death in dialysis (4), with hypertension as an important contributor. Thus, the diagnosis and management of hypertension in dialysis is a vital topic to all dialysis patients and providers. This chapter will review the epidemiology, pathogenesis, diagnosis, prognosis, and treatment of hypertension in the dialysis population.

 EPIDEMIOLOGY

The diagnosis of hypertension is complicated in the hemodialysis (HD) patient due to the episodic nature of HD and the wide fluctuations in blood pressure (BP) that result, with BP typically highest before the HD session, lowest at the end of the HD session, and slowly rising during the interdialytic period (5). Therefore, the epidemiology of hypertension in HD can vary depending not only on the BP threshold employed but also on when and where BP is measured: in the HD clinic before or after dialysis (termed peridialytic BP) versus outside the dialysis unit using ambulatory BP monitoring (ABPM) or home BP monitoring during the interdialytic period. **TABLE 15.1** summarizes the various methods of assessing BP in HD.

Epidemiology Using Peridialytic Blood Pressure Measurements

Numerous observational studies have found a high prevalence of hypertension in HD ranging from 62% to 86% based on peridialytic BP measurements; notably, these studies employed varying

TABLE 15.1	Methods of Hemodialysis Blood Pressure Measurement	
Method	**Description**	**Comments**
Peridialytic BP	Measured both before and after HD	Easily available but highly variable
Intradialytic BP	Median of all BP measures during one HD run	Easily available but needs more study
Ambulatory BP	Measured every 20–30 min over 44 h between HD runs	Gold standard but cumbersome
Home BP	Measured twice daily at home	Correlates well to ambulatory BP and accessible by most patients

BP, blood pressure; HD, hemodialysis.

threshold BP values ranging from 140/90 mm Hg to 160/90 mm Hg and variously included antihypertensive drug use in their definitions of hypertension (6–9).

More recent analyses of randomized trials have found similar rates of hypertension in the HD population using peridialytic BP. The Hemodialysis (HEMO) study of the late 1990s was a landmark multicenter trial of HD dose and dialyzer flux on survival (10) that recruited clinically stable HD patients (11). An analysis of the baseline characteristics of the first 1,238 subjects randomized into the HEMO study found 72% of the cohort to be hypertensive, defined as peridialytic BP ≥140/90 mm Hg during the baseline

235

HD session (12). This high rate of hypertension was found despite 74% of the cohort receiving antihypertensive medications, with a median of 1.0 drug per subject.

A similarly high prevalence for hypertension was found when the BP data from another large randomized trial from the late 1990s was examined in detail (13). The original study was a double-blind and placebo-controlled clinical trial of sodium ferric gluconate that enrolled 2,535 clinically stable HD patients (14). With hypertension defined as pre-HD BP >150/85 mm Hg averaged over 1 week or the use of antihypertensive medications, an analysis of baseline data found a prevalence of 86% for hypertension in this cohort (13). Within the hypertensive subjects, only 30% were controlled, while 12% were not treated pharmacologically and 58% were treated but still uncontrolled (13), which is similar to previous reports (8).

Epidemiology Using Ambulatory Blood Pressure Measurements

A recent single-center study of 369 prevalent and clinically stable HD patients employed 44-hour interdialytic ABPM and found a prevalence for hypertension at 86% using a definition of hypertension as average ambulatory BP of ≥135/85 mm Hg or antihypertensive drug use (15); this prevalence is similar to prior small studies of ABPM in HD (16). In the cohort of 369 patients, hypertension was treated with medications in 89% of patients but was controlled adequately in only 38% of patients (15).

Thus, whether using peridialytic BP measurements or 44-hour ABPM, hypertension is common in the HD population with a prevalence ranging from 70% to 85%, and a majority of these affected patients have poor control of their hypertension.

Epidemiology in Peritoneal Dialysis Patients

It has been suggested that peritoneal dialysis (PD) controls hypertension better than HD; for example, a single-center study of 56 prevalent and clinically stable PD patients found that only 9% of the cohort was hypertensive with BP >140/90 mm Hg by standardized auscultation as compared to a hypertension prevalence of 56% in the same center's HD unit (17). Similarly, control of BP was compared in the retrospective Peritoneal Dialysis Core Indicators Study in the mid-1990s that found among the 926 PD patients with BP data, only 35% were hypertensive with BP >150/90 mm Hg, and the cohort having an average BP of 139/80 mm Hg as compared to a contemporaneous cohort of HD patients whose average pre-HD BP was 151/79 mm Hg and post-HD BP 137/74 mm Hg (18). A larger study using United States Renal Data System (USRDS) data from the Dialysis Morbidity and Mortality Wave 2 study in the late 1990s found that from 1,034 PD patients, only 54% had systolic BP (SBP) of >140 mm Hg while on a mean of 1.6 antihypertensive medications (19), as compared to the 70% to 85% prevalence of hypertension in HD.

However, the reduced prevalence of hypertension among PD patients is not a universal finding. A prospective study of 504 prevalent and clinically stable PD patients found a prevalence of 88% for hypertension defined as BP >140/90 mm Hg or use of antihypertensive medications, and among the hypertensive patients, only 16% were adequately controlled (20). Additionally, 24-hour ABPM was performed, and of the 414 adequate examinations, hypertension was present in 69% based on BP load >30%, with load defined as the percentage of ambulatory BP readings >140/90 mm Hg during the day or >120/80 mm Hg at night. Another study utilized ABPM to compare 22 HD patients versus 24 PD patients that were

well matched for major clinical characteristics and found no significant difference in either daytime or nighttime BP between the two groups (21). Thus, while some studies suggest that hypertension control is superior among PD patients versus HD patients, there is no conclusive evidence that this is the case.

 PATHOGENESIS

As both a cause and consequence of kidney disease, the pathogenesis of hypertension in CKD not only shares commonalities with the general hypertensive population but also has complicated causes that are unique to kidney disease and its treatment. TABLE 15.2 summarizes the major modifiable causes of hypertension in dialysis.

Risk Factors in Common with the General Population

Patients with CKD often carry a burden of preexisting primary hypertension prior to the recognition of their kidney disease. Additionally, risk factors in the general hypertensive population are similarly present in the CKD population including obesity, excessive salt intake, alcohol consumption, and physical inactivity. Two additional comorbidities contributing to hypertension are important to consider, namely, arterial stiffness and obstructive sleep apnea (OSA).

Arterial stiffness, measured as pulse wave velocity, is elevated in dialysis patients (22,23), and it has long been recognized as a risk factor for cardiovascular events in both the general hypertensive population (24) and in the dialysis population (25,26). It is in this setting that a study of 125 subjects on HD found increased pulse wave velocity to be significantly associated with increased 44-hour interdialytic ambulatory BP (27), as illustrated in FIGURE 15.1.

In the general population, OSA frequently coexists with hypertension (28–30), with hypopnea leading to hypoxemia and ultimately to sympathetic activation. OSA is strongly linked with resistant hypertension as the presence of OSA is a risk factor for resistant hypertension and the severity of OSA correlates with the severity of hypertension (31–33). Given this link, it is important to note that OSA is very common in the setting of CKD with the prevalence increasing with declining kidney function (34), culminating in a prevalence over 50% for those patients on dialysis (34,35). The association between OSA and resistant hypertension is similarly strong in ESKD as a recent cohort study of subjects with advanced CKD including 75 subjects on HD and 20 on PD found a sevenfold increased risk of resistant hypertension in those dialysis patients with severe OSA (36). Interestingly, there is a growing recognition that OSA itself is caused or exacerbated by volume overload that leads to parapharyngeal edema, which worsens at bedtime

TABLE 15.2	Major Treatable Causes of Hypertension in Dialysis
Cause	**Treatment**
Obstructive sleep apnea	Continuous positive airway pressure
Volume overload	Dry-weight reduction
Renin-angiotensin-aldosterone system	ACEI, ARB, and spironolactone
Sympathetic overactivity	β-Blockers, renal nerve ablation
Erythropoietin	Reduce dose

ACEI, angiotensin-converting enzyme inhibitor; ARB, angiotensin receptor blocker.

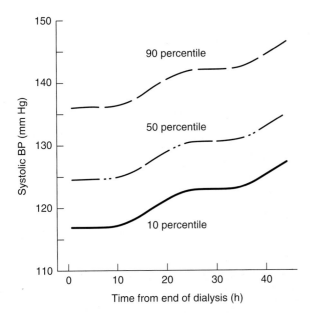

FIGURE 15.1 Impact of aortic pulse wave velocity on ambulatory blood pressure (BP) between two consecutive dialysis sessions in 125 subjects; 10th percentile of pulse wave velocity 4.1 m/s (*solid line*), 50th percentile 6.0 m/s (*dashed and dotted line*), and 90th percentile 10.6 m/s (*dashed line*). [Adapted from Agarwal R, Light RP. Arterial stiffness and interdialytic weight gain influence ambulatory blood pressure patterns in hemodialysis patients. *Am J Physiol Renal Physiol* 2008;294(2):F303–F308, with permission.]

in the recumbent position, both in patients without CKD (30) and in those with ESKD (37,38).

While most studies of continuous positive airway pressure (CPAP) for OSA in the non-CKD population find significant improvement in BP, this improvement is typically modest compared to medication (39), with CPAP use yielding a 1.7 mm Hg improvement in mean 24-hour ambulatory BP (40), so similarly modest improvements would be expected with CPAP treatment in ESKD.

Classical Mechanisms of Hypertension in Dialysis: Volume Overload and the Renin-Angiotensin-Aldosterone System

The two mechanisms classically felt to be responsible for hypertension in the "renoprival" state of ESKD are volume overload and an inappropriately activated renin-angiotensin-aldosterone system (RAAS) (41). Sodium loading has long been clinically recognized as a major and essential contributor to hypertension both in those with normal kidney function (42) and in the setting of kidney disease. As the glomerular filtration rate (GFR) declines, less sodium is filtered leading to sodium retention and to an expanded extracellular fluid volume. The increased plasma volume leads to increased cardiac output and then to increased total peripheral resistance, whereby normal kidney autoregulation would lead to a pressure natriuresis and normalization of BP (43); however, this natriuresis is incomplete or absent in advanced CKD and ESKD, and the increased total peripheral resistance persists. While ultrafiltration has been recognized as an effective means of BP control in ESKD for decades since the earliest days of chronic dialysis (44), only recently has a randomized clinical trial, the Dry-Weight Reduction in Hypertensive Hemodialysis Patients (DRIP) trial, confirmed this truism (45).

The other classically recognized contributor is an inappropriately activated RAAS (46), possibly provoked by kidney ischemia in patients with renovascular disease or by regional intrarenal ischemia due to kidney fibrosis. As expected, angiotensin-converting enzyme inhibitor (ACEI) therapy has been shown to be effective at reducing BP in dialysis patients (47,48).

Novel Mechanisms of Hypertension in Dialysis

In addition to the two classically recognized causes of hypertension in dialysis patients, several additional contributors have gained widespread acceptance including increased sympathetic nervous system activity, altered vascular endothelial function, and erythropoiesis-stimulating agents.

Sympathetic Nervous System Overactivity

Among the novel mechanisms of hypertension in advanced kidney disease, sympathetic overactivity is now widely recognized as a contributor. Increased catecholamine levels (49) and increased catecholamine sensitivity (50) in CKD were both demonstrated in the 1980s, and increased catecholamine levels have been shown to predict cardiovascular events and mortality in chronic HD patients (51). Unidentified uremic toxins were originally thought to provoke this sympathetic overactivity; however, Converse et al. (52) implicated the diseased kidneys themselves via experiments where they measured muscle sympathetic nerve activity in three groups of subjects: those on chronic HD with their native kidneys, those on chronic HD status post bilateral nephrectomy, and normal controls (52). They found increased sympathetic activity and higher BP in those chronic HD patients still with their native kidneys, but those subjects who were surgically anephric had sympathetic nerve activity and BP similar to the normal controls. Uremic toxins do not appear to be the cause of the increased kidney afferent nerve signals that increase sympathetic activity, as demonstrated by studies of patients who have had kidney transplantation and still retain their native kidneys (53), but kidney ischemia is a likely contributor (54). As further evidence, a pilot study of kidney denervation by endovascular radioablation with a before-after design performed in 12 chronic HD patients with resistant hypertension showed a significant improvement in BP (55); however, with a recent negative result from a large randomized clinical trial employing this technique in subjects without CKD, it may not be developed further (56).

Another unique contributor to sympathetic overactivity in ESKD is renalase, which was discovered only in the last 10 years (57). Renalase is a circulating monoamine oxidase enzyme that is produced primarily by the kidney that metabolizes circulating catecholamines and which is deficient in ESKD (58). As a novel mechanism contributing to hypertension in ESKD, it remains to be demonstrated via clinical trials what improvement in BP may be achieved by increasing levels of renalase in the dialysis population.

Altered Endothelial Function

Additional factors contribute to increased vasoconstriction in kidney disease, including altered endothelial cell function such that there is an imbalance in the levels of endothelial derived vasoconstrictors versus vasodilators. Nitric oxide is a potent vasodilator and is synthesized by endothelial nitric oxide synthase (eNOS) from L-arginine; however, a circulating inhibitor of eNOS has been identified in CKD patients, asymmetric dimethyl arginine (ADMA) (59). ADMA is a product of protein metabolism that is excreted into the urine by the healthy kidney, competitively inhibits eNOS, and causes local vasoconstriction on experimental infusion, and ADMA levels are elevated in ESKD (60). Elevated ADMA levels have also been shown to predict cardiovascular events and mortality in a cohort of 225 chronic HD patients (61). It remains to be demonstrated via interventional trials what improvement, if any, reductions in ADMA will make to hypertension in the dialysis population.

On the side of vasoconstriction are endothelins, which are released from the basolateral surface of endothelial cells and exert autocrine and paracrine functions that include mediating vasoconstriction via the endothelin-A receptor on vascular smooth muscle (62). Endothelin levels have been found to be elevated in various stages of CKD including ESKD (63,64). Endothelin receptor antagonists have shown efficacy for reducing BP in randomized controlled trials in primary (65) and resistant hypertension (66,67) as well as in diabetic nephropathy (68). However, some results have been mixed with divergent BP results between office and ABPM (67,68), and adverse events including edema have been frequent.

Erythropoiesis-Stimulating Agents

Conventional medications such as over-the-counter nonsteroidal anti-inflammatory drugs and decongestants can exacerbate hypertension; however, erythropoiesis-stimulating agents (ESAs) are commonly prescribed for the anemia of CKD, and resultant hypertension has been recognized since the early days of ESA use in ESKD (69). The incidence of hypertension provoked by ESA administration is associated with the ESA dose but is independent of red blood cell mass or viscosity (70,71). While the exact mechanism of how ESA use causes hypertension is unknown, the current evidence suggests that it is mediated via vasoconstrictor effects, likely through increased levels of endothelin-1 or increased vasoconstrictive response to that peptide (72–74).

Up to 30% of dialysis patients develop hypertension or require an adjustment in antihypertensive medications with ESA use (75,76), while the rise in BP with ESA use typically ranges from 5 to 8 mm Hg in SBP and 4 to 6 mm Hg in diastolic blood pressure (DBP) (77). The rise in BP with ESA administration is more likely in those with baseline hypertension (78) or a family history of hypertension (79). There is unfortunately a dearth of evidence to guide the prevention of ESA-induced hypertension but recommended strategies include changing to subcutaneous administration, reducing the goal hemoglobin level in those who are unresponsive to ESA therapy, minimizing the ESA dose by starting low and increasing slowly, and avoiding ESA use entirely (80).

⬢ DIAGNOSIS

ABPM is the accepted gold standard for diagnosing hypertension in the general population and in the ESKD population on dialysis (81–84). The use of ABPM permits the diagnosis of nocturnal hypertension, which is common in the ESKD population (85,86), and it is also superior to peridialytic BP measurements for correlating to end organ damage manifest as left ventricular hypertrophy (LVH) (87) and for predicting the outcome of mortality (88). The proper ABPM technique includes employing a validated monitor (89) to measure BP every 20 minutes during the day from 6 AM to 10 PM and then every 30 minutes at night from 10 PM to 6 AM (90). This prolonged interval of measurement permits observation of the full

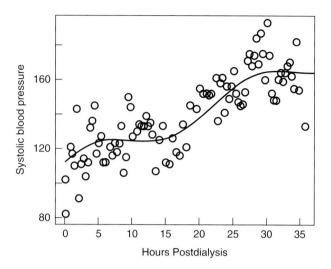

FIGURE 15.2 An example of observed interdialytic blood pressure (BP) values with fitted trended cosinar curve in an individual hemodialysis patient. [Adapted from Kelley K, Light RP, Agarwal R. Trended cosinor change model for analyzing hemodynamic rhythm patterns in hemodialysis patients. *Hypertension* 2007;50(1):143–150, with permission.]

change in BP during the interdialytic period, where SBP increases an average of 2.5 mm Hg every 10 hours (5,27), as depicted in **FIGURE 15.2**.

While ABPM is the gold standard method for diagnosing hypertension, it is also cumbersome to use especially over 44 continuous hours so it remains a research technique in ESKD. More convenient methods of routinely measuring BP and diagnosing hypertension must be employed in the dialysis population. Since BP changes both during the HD session and during the interdialytic interval, there remains uncertainty about how best to diagnose and manage hypertension in the HD population, and this uncertainty contributes to both under treatment (16,91) and to over treatment of hypertension (92). Further complicating matters, HD patients have significant seasonal BP variability with lower BP during the summer and higher during the winter (93), potentially due to temperature mediated vasodilation or sweat induced volume losses.

Classically, the peridialytic BP measures taken before and after an HD session have been used to diagnose and manage hypertension, and while there are no randomized clinical trials to guide goal BP recommendations in ESKD, long-standing professional guidelines have employed peridialytic BP values. The National Kidney Foundation Kidney Disease Outcomes Quality Initiative (NKF-KDOQI) guidelines recommend to target pre-HD BP <140/90 mm Hg and post-HD BP <130/80 mm Hg (94). Unfortunately, making treatment decisions based on peridialytic BP can be associated with adverse outcomes, as shown by a study of 11 HD units in London, England, that found those HD units with more patients reaching the post-HD BP goal had significantly more episodes of symptomatic hypotension requiring saline infusion (95). Peridialytic BP is highly variable such that the variability within a given patient over time is similar to the variability between patients (96), possibly due in part to these measurements often being made without attention to technique (97). While peridialytic BP does have a statistically significant relationship to gold standard interdialytic ABPM (98), a meta-analysis of 18 studies comparing peridialytic BP and interdialytic ABPM found very wide limits of agreement between the techniques such that peridialytic BP provides a very imprecise estimate of interdialytic BP (99). In the meta-analysis, the limits of agreement between pre-HD SBP and interdialytic ambulatory SBP ranged from +41.7 mm Hg to −25.2 mm Hg and the limits of agreement for post-HD SBP were similarly wide, which illustrates the reduced clinical utility of a diagnosis of hypertension or normotension based on peridialytic BP for an individual HD patient (99).

A readily available alternative to peridialytic BP is to use all the BP measurements made during a single midweek HD session to calculate a median BP, which is easier to calculate at the bedside compared to mean BP. A study of 150 chronic HD patients found that median intradialytic BP had the best reproducibility and was superior to either pre- or post-HD BP or their average for predicting 44-hour interdialytic ambulatory BP (100). In this study, median intradialytic SBP >140 mm Hg during a midweek HD session had an 80% sensitivity and specificity for diagnosing hypertension by gold standard ABPM (100). Median intradialytic BP has also been shown to change in response to interventional reduction in dry weight to reduce BP (101), adding further support for the clinical usefulness of this easily calculated measure.

After peridialytic BP and median intradialytic BP, home BP monitoring is the third alternative to the clinically inconvenient gold standard of ABPM. Home BP monitoring is the recommended method of both the American Heart Association (102) and the European Society of Hypertension (103) for the routine diagnosis and management of BP in the general hypertension population and its use is feasible and practical both in patients with CKD and ESKD (104,105). Importantly, home BP monitoring is superior to peridialytic BP measurements by *every* methodologic and clinical standard. This includes superior correlation with gold standard ABPM (106), week-to-week reproducibility (107), the ability to reflect BP changes from interventional probing of dry weight (107), correlation to the end-organ damage of LVH (87,108), and predicting outcomes including cardiovascular events (109) and mortality (109,110). **Table 15.3** summarizes the advantages of home BP monitoring.

Two small randomized trials have found home BP monitoring to be beneficial versus usual care for management of BP in HD patients. The first randomized 34 patients to home BP monitoring plus usual care versus usual care only over 12 weeks and found that the home BP group had significantly lower BP at the end of the study (111). A subsequent trial of 65 HD patients randomized participants to usual hypertension care based on pre-HD BP versus open label monthly home BP monitoring for 6 months (112). At the end of the trial, the home BP monitoring group had a significant reduction in ambulatory SBP both from baseline and versus the usual

TABLE 15.3	**Advantages of Home Blood Pressure Monitoring over Peridialytic Blood Pressure**

1. Predicts gold standard ambulatory BP
2. Reproducibility
3. Reflects changes in dry weight
4. Correlates to left ventricular hypertrophy
5. Predicts cardiovascular events
6. Predicts mortality
7. Randomized trial evidence for efficacy of BP control
8. Recommended by major professional societies

BP, blood pressure.

TABLE 15.4	**Suggested Method for Home Blood Pressure Monitoring**

1. Check both morning and evening.
2. Check for 4–7 consecutive days duration.
3. Check once monthly or more often if clinically unstable.
4. Goal home blood pressure ≤140/90 mm Hg.

care group, which had no change in ambulatory SBP from baseline. However, the primary endpoint of reduction in echocardiographic LVH was no different between groups, possibly due to lack of power and variability in the timing of the echocardiograms relative to the HD schedule (112).

As with ABPM, home BP increases between HD sessions, at an average rate of 4 mm Hg every 10 hours (113), so it is important to adequately sample home BP at spaced intervals between HD sessions. Randomized trials have used protocols of home BP monitoring performed twice daily over 4 to 7 days once per month (112,114), and we recommend a similar regimen for routine clinical use and decision making. Measurements performed more than once per month may be needed in more unstable patients including those recently discharged from the hospital. **Table 15.4** summarizes our suggested method of home BP monitoring.

There are no randomized trials comparing goal BP levels in the dialysis population using any of the available BP methods including peridialytic BP, intradialytic BP, home BP, or interdialytic ambulatory BP. However, the American Heart Association defines hypertension as home BP >135/85 mm Hg on average for the general population (102), so we advocate for an interdialytic home BP target of ≤140/90 mm Hg as a reasonable goal (80), which was the target used in a recent large randomized trial of BP control in HD (114). Notably, the results of the randomized controlled Systolic Blood Pressure Intervention Trial (SPRINT) were published in November 2015 showing improved cardiovascular outcomes in over 9,000 subjects randomized to office SBP target <120 mm Hg versus a conventional target of <140 mm Hg (115). While subjects with CKD were included in the trial, those with estimated GFR <20 mL/min/1.73 m^2 or ESKD were excluded so no direct conclusions can be drawn from the trial regarding the management of hypertension in the dialysis population.

Intradialytic Hypertension

The focus of diagnosis and treatment of hypertension in chronic HD is on interdialytic BP between HD sessions, but the case of intradialytic hypertension merits special mention. BP normally declines during the HD, but approximately 5% to 15% of chronic HD patients have a paradoxical rise in BP during the HD session (116). Intradialytic hypertension has been described variously, and there currently is no universally accepted definition. Definitions have included (a) a change in SBP or mean arterial pressure from pre-HD to post-HD greater than a given threshold ranging from >0 mm Hg to ≥10 mm Hg change (117,118), (b) a positive slope after regression of all intradialytic SBP values (119), or (c) BP increase during or immediately following HD resulting in post-HD BP >130/80 mm Hg (116).

Intradialytic hypertension has recently been recognized to be associated with worse outcomes. Inrig et al. (120) performed a secondary analysis of a randomized clinical trial including 443 prevalent HD subjects and found intradialytic hypertension to be significantly associated with greater mortality at 6 months (117). Similarly, in a subsequent observational study of a cohort of 1,748 incident HD patients, Inrig et al. (120) found 2-year survival to be significantly decreased for each 10 mm Hg increase in SBP from pre-HD to post-HD BP; however, this relationship was limited to those patients whose pre-HD SBP was <120 mm Hg. Most recently, a prospective cohort study of 115 prevalent HD patients found an average pre-HD to post-HD rise in SBP of >5 mm Hg to significantly predict both all-cause and cardiovascular mortality (121).

Intradialytic hypertension has been associated with interdialytic hypertension as measured by 44-hour ABPM (118,119), so it is not surprising that the same mechanisms implicated in causing interdialytic hypertension between HD sessions have also been implicated in causing intradialytic hypertension during the HD session (116), but the preponderance of evidence currently points to volume overload and endothelial dysfunction. Markers of volume overload such as increased cardiothoracic ratio has been associated with intradialytic hypertension (121), but most importantly, interventional trials have shown volume removal through dry-weight reduction improves intradialytic hypertension. An early study from the mid-1990s included seven patients with intradialytic hypertension and found them all to have marked cardiac dilation and to be very hypertensive with mean pre-HD BP 172/99 mm Hg despite medications (122). Dry weight was reduced in all subjects with an average weight loss of 6.7 kg that was associated with an improvement in pre-HD BP by 46/21 mm Hg despite discontinuation of all BP medications. More recently, a secondary analysis of the DRIP trial (45) regressed the intradialytic BP values for the 150 trial subjects and found that the quintile of subjects with the greatest reduction in dry weight, more than 0.94 kg reduction after the first 4 weeks of the trial, also had the most positive BP slope at baseline as they were the only quintile with intradialytic hypertension by this definition (119). Importantly, after subsequent lowering of dry weight, this same quintile had reduction in BP slopes at the finish of the trial, meaning their intradialytic hypertension had resolved such that their BP slopes were similar to the other subjects. Thus, intradialytic hypertension appears to be a marker of volume overload that is amenable to dry-weight reduction.

Endothelial dysfunction has also been identified as an important mediator as there is evidence both for a rise in endothelin-1 levels (123) and a decrease in nitric oxide during HD (124) in patients with intradialytic hypertension. The contribution of endothelial function was investigated in 25 HD patients recruited in an 8-week pilot study with a before-after design using carvedilol (125), which has been shown to block endothelin-1 release *in vitro* (126). Subjects were given carvedilol up to a dose of 50 mg twice a day, and while endothelin-1 levels were unchanged on carvedilol, flow-mediated dilation significantly improved (125). Of clinical importance, the frequency of intradialytic hypertension was significantly reduced from 77% of HD sessions down to 28% of sessions and average 44-hour interdialytic ambulatory SBP was also reduced from 155 mm Hg to 148 mm Hg with carvedilol treatment.

Thus, based on the available evidence, a renewed focus on addressing volume overload should be a priority for those patients with a paradoxical rise in BP on HD, and specifically targeting endothelial dysfunction with agents such as carvedilol can also be considered. The features of intradialytic hypertension are summarized in **TABLE 15.5**.

TABLE 15.5	Features of Intradialytic Hypertension

5%–15% prevalence
No single accepted definition
Associated with increased mortality
Associated with volume overload and endothelial dysfunction
Evidence for improvement with dry-weight reduction and
    carvedilol therapy

PROGNOSIS

Despite a strong and direct relationship between hypertension and both cardiovascular and all-cause mortality (127) and copious evidence of benefit for treatment of hypertension in the nondialysis population (128), the relationship between BP and outcomes in dialysis patients remains a topic of controversy (129,130). A variety of studies have found an association between peridialytic hypertension and strokes (131), heart failure (132), arrhythmias (133), cardiovascular events (134), and all-cause mortality (135). However, other studies suggest that peridialytic hypertension is protective and lower BP is associated with worse mortality (6,136–138), and the risk of normotensive BP is magnified when BP is considered as a time dependent covariate (136,138). This paradoxical relationship between BP and mortality has been termed the *reverse epidemiology* of hypertension (130) and has raised concern that treatment of hypertension may be harmful (139).

When examining the prognostic value of hypertension in dialysis, it is important to additionally consider the severity of comorbid illness as well as dialysis vintage. These interactions are illustrated by a retrospective cohort study of 2,770 prevalent PD patients where a fully adjusted analysis found higher SBP, DBP, mean arterial pressure, and pulse pressure, all to be associated with decreased mortality during the first year on dialysis (140). However, higher SBP and pulse pressure were associated with increased mortality for those patients on dialysis ≥6 years. Similar findings were shown in a cohort of 16,959 HD patients where SBP <120 mm Hg was associated with increased mortality within the first 2 years of starting dialysis, but SBP >150 mm Hg was associated with increased mortality among those that survived at least 3 years (141). These findings suggest lower BP may be an indicator of more severe illness in those patients new to dialysis who are likely to have advanced chronic but unstable systemic comorbidities that recently culminated in ESKD, whereas the survivors that have been on dialysis for at least 3 to 6 years have a more normal relationship between hypertension and outcomes because they are less acutely ill. This explanation is further bolstered by the subgroup in the PD cohort who were listed for transplant within 6 months of starting dialysis, as in this healthier subgroup higher SBP, DBP, mean arterial pressure, and pulse pressure were not associated with improved mortality during the first year of dialysis (140).

The technique of BP measurement also contributes to the controversial relationship between BP and outcomes as the reverse epidemiology of hypertension is primarily a phenomenon of peridialytic BP values. Ambulatory BP, however, has a strong relationship with mortality on HD, first demonstrated by Amar et al. (142) in a study of 57 HD patients. Alborzi et al. (110) have confirmed the relationship between ambulatory BP and mortality in a cohort of 150 HD patients, and in the same cohort, they also demonstrated home BP to have a similarly strong relationship with mortality. In an expanded cohort of 326 HD patients followed for a mean of 32 months, Agarwal (88) subsequently has shown increased mortality at the extremes of ambulatory and home BP and that mortality was best at a home SBP 120 to 130 mm Hg and ambulatory SBP 110 to 120 mm Hg, while peridialytic BP had no relationship with mortality in this cohort. Most recently, an analysis of the Chronic Renal Insufficiency Cohort (CRIC) study compared pre-HD SBP and out of HD unit SBP for prediction of mortality in the 403 subjects who started HD since the start of the study (143). There were 98 deaths over a mean follow-up of 2.7 years and pre-HD SBP showed a U-shaped relationship to mortality consistent with reverse epidemiology of hypertension. However, in the 326 subjects who had BP checked out of the HD unit in a standardized manner during a research visit, there was a significant and direct linear relationship between BP and mortality with hazard ratio 1.26 for every 10 mm Hg rise in SBP, which further emphasizes the importance of BP measurement technique when considering prognosis (143).

Thus, while there is concern for reverse epidemiology of hypertension when analyzing peridialytic BP, which would suggest that lowering BP would be harmful in HD patients, the evidence from ambulatory and home BP studies do not support those conclusions. Additionally and significantly, the evidence from two meta-analyses of randomized clinical trials of antihypertensive medication use in HD found cardiovascular benefit rather than harm with active treatment (144,145), so based on the available evidence, we strongly recommend to actively diagnose and treat hypertension in dialysis patients.

TREATMENT

Hypertension is common and poorly controlled in dialysis, and it often requires a combined approach to achieve adequate control of BP. The cornerstone of therapy is nonpharmacologic control of volume overload, but pharmacology therapy is frequently necessary, and invasive treatments have a long and recurrent history for the management of hypertension in dialysis patients.

Volume Control

The focus of nonpharmacologic treatment of hypertension on dialysis is to treat volume overload through complementary strategies, both to reduce sodium intake by dietary sodium restriction and individualization of the dialysate sodium while also augmenting sodium removal by dry-weight reduction, providing adequate time on dialysis, and considering frequent dialysis. **TABLE 15.6** summarizes the nonpharmacologic treatment of hypertension in dialysis. The archetype for this multipronged management of hypertension on dialysis is reported by Charra (146) from Tassin, France, where patients are dialyzed for extended hours on a low-sodium

TABLE 15.6	Complementary Components of Nonpharmacologic Treatment of Hypertension on Dialysis

1. Dry-weight reduction
2. Dietary sodium restriction
3. Dialysate sodium reduction
4. Adequate time on dialysis
5. Consideration of frequent dialysis

dialysate, and low-sodium diet is emphasized to such a degree that low-sodium bread is provided to the patients. They report excellent control of BP despite antihypertensive medication use at only 1% to 2% (147), as well as low mortality with a 5-year survival rate reported at 87% (148), which is more than twice the current reported 5-year survival rate in the United States (2). More recently, a trial of low-sodium diet and dry-weight reduction in 19 hypertensive HD patients with a before-after design found this combined strategy reduced echocardiographic LVH (149). Similar results have been reported in PD from a single center, where all 47 of the center's hypertensive patients had their antihypertensive medications withdrawn and BP was subsequently successfully controlled in 37 patients with a combination of strict low-sodium diet and added ultrafiltration (150). A consistent feature of all these examples is the multifaceted approach to volume control requiring not only reduction in dry weight but also strict attention to reducing dietary and dialysate sodium as well as maximizing the probability of successful dry-weight reduction by providing adequate time on dialysis.

Dry-Weight Reduction

Malignant hypertension was common in ESKD prior to the advent of chronic HD, and since those earliest days, ultrafiltration has been recognized as an effective means of BP control in ESKD (44), including for the very first chronic HD patient in the United States, Clyde Shields, under the care of Dr. Belding Scribner (151). Only recently has the randomized controlled DRIP trial of dry-weight reduction definitively confirmed those original observations (45). The DRIP trial recruited 150 chronic and stable HD patients with hypertension confirmed by 44-hour interdialytic ABPM despite being on an average of 2.6 antihypertensive medications who were then randomized in a two-to-one ratio to intervention versus usual care for the 8-week trial. All subjects had their antihypertensive medications and their prescribed time on HD kept stable, and all were visited by a study physician on each HD session during the trial. The intervention group received progressive reduction in dry weight by at least 0.2 kg each HD session until they had symptoms of hypovolemia. Compared to the control group at 8 weeks, the intervention group had 1 kg of weight reduction and average 44-hour interdialytic ambulatory BP improved by 6.6/3.3 mm Hg (45), as illustrated in **FIGURE 15.3**. Notably, by design, those in the intervention group necessarily had to have symptoms of hypovolemia before dry-weight reduction was stopped, but despite this requirement, there was no change in any domain of the Kidney Disease Quality of Life questionnaire during the trial. Additionally, it is important to note that the DRIP trial improved BP with additional ultrafiltration without extending time on HD, which is a finding supported by older observational studies that suggest BP can be improved without extending time on HD provided volume overload is successfully reduced (152).

Management of Dry Weight

Unfortunately, there is no single universally accepted definition of dry weight. We suggest a reasonable definition of dry weight to be the lowest tolerated post-HD weight achieved via gradual change in post-HD weight at which there are minimal signs or symptoms of either hypovolemia or hypervolemia (153). Thus, achieving and maintaining an adequately low dry weight is a hands-on and iterative process that requires attention to details beyond only the prescribed dry weight (154), including adherence to a low-sodium diet, minimization of dialysate sodium content, providing adequate time on HD, and consideration of more frequent dialysis.

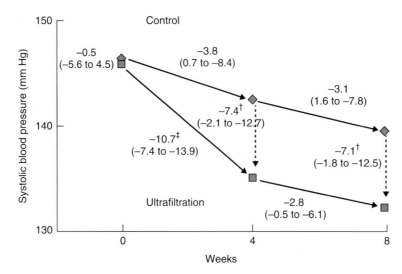

FIGURE 15.3 The effect of dry-weight reduction on interdialytic ambulatory systolic blood pressure (BP) in hypertensive hemodialysis patients. The mean systolic BPs are shown for the control and ultrafiltration groups. The mean changes in BP are shown for weeks 4 and 8 after randomization (*solid arrows*) as well as the mean differences in BPs (*dotted arrows*) between the two groups at each 4-week interval. The numbers next to the *dotted lines* connecting the data points are the mean changes in BP between groups at 4 and 8 weeks after randomization. The 95% confidence intervals are given in parentheses. †$p < 0.01$ and ‡ $p < 0.001$ indicate significant differences between groups or within groups. [Adapted from Agarwal R, Alborzi P, Satyan S, et al. Dry-weight reduction in hypertensive hemodialysis patients (DRIP): a randomized, controlled trial. *Hypertension* 2009;53(3):500–507, with permission.]

When deciding whether to adjust the dry weight prescription, the first step is the assessment for volume overload. Unfortunately, while the routine clinical exam performs well at detecting acute or massive volume overload, it performs poorly for detecting subtle and chronic volume overload (153). This is illustrated by a cross-sectional study of 150 chronic HD patients that found the presence of pedal edema to have no correlation with putative objective markers of volume overload including brain natriuretic peptide, echocardiographic inferior vena cava diameter, or relative plasma volume slope (155). As another example, it is important to consider that all the hypertensive subjects of the DRIP trial were at their clinical dry weight as determined by their primary nephrologist to start the trial, yet the subjects of the intervention group had their dry weight successfully reduced, which resulted in a clinically significant improvement in 44-hour ambulatory BP (45). This further highlights the difficulty in detecting subtle volume overload that if ameliorated by means of dry-weight reduction will result in improved BP.

A number of experimental objective measures of volume status have been studied including natriuretic peptides, inferior vena cava diameter, relative plasma volume monitoring, and bioelectrical impedance analysis (156). The latter two have the most supporting evidence with a secondary analysis of the DRIP trial showing that baseline relative plasma volume monitoring identified the most volume overloaded subjects, who subsequently had the largest average reduction in weight at 1.5 kg and the largest improvement in ambulatory SBP at 12.6 mm Hg (157). Most recently, a randomized trial of bioelectrical impedance analysis to guide dry weight management in a cohort of largely normotensive HD subjects found a significant improvement in LVH as well as improvement in peridialytic BP despite reductions in antihypertensive drug use for the intervention group (158).

However, these objective measures of volume status remain investigational and remain to be adequately validated. Therefore, the onus is on the treating nephrologist to have a high index of suspicion for occult volume overload. Signs that should prompt consideration for reduction in dry weight include uncontrolled hypertension, especially in those patients who are on multiple medications such as in the DRIP trial where subjects were on an average of 2.6 antihypertensive drugs at baseline (45). Numerous studies have shown that greater antihypertensive drug use is associated with worse control of hypertension (15,159), which is plausibly due to inadequately addressed volume overload which could be improved with reduction in dry weight. **TABLE 15.7** summarizes the clinical signs of volume overload.

Another sign to consider reduction in dry weight is a low interdialytic weight gain. This comes from the observation that interdialytic weight gain tends to rise when dry weight is reduced (160), as illustrated in **FIGURE 15.4**. Additionally, the secondary analysis of the DRIP trial that employed relative plasma volume monitoring found the flattest relative plasma volume slopes, corresponding to the most volume overload, in the group with the lowest ultrafiltration volume (157). This is not surprising considering the mechanism of relative plasma volume monitoring; however, the ultrafiltration volume generally equals the interdialytic weight gain, and, as noted in the preceding text, subsequent reduction in dry weight per the

TABLE 15.7	Clinical Signs of Volume Overload on Dialysis

1. Elevated interdialytic blood pressure by home or ambulatory monitoring
2. Multiple antihypertensive medications
3. Low interdialytic weight gain
4. Constellation of symptoms and signs such as peripheral edema, cardiomegaly, elevated jugular venous pressure, pulmonary congestion, pleural effusion

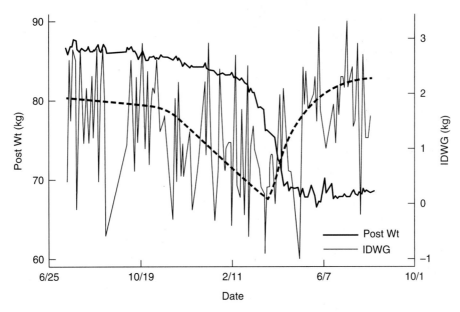

FIGURE 15.4 Relationship of dry weight to interdialytic weight gain. The subject participating in a clinical trial who previously had well-controlled BP measured at home was hospitalized for pneumonia, and on hospital discharge, home BP was poorly controlled despite increasing the number of antihypertensive medications. As shown, dry weight was reduced gradually over time. Over a few weeks, home BP was controlled to <140/90 mm Hg (not shown). The modeled *dotted line* overlying the interdialytic weight gain (IDWG) illustrates that reduction in dry weight was accompanied by increasing IDWG. [Reprinted from Sinha AD, Agarwal R. What are the causes of the ill effects of chronic hemodialysis? The fallacy of low interdialytic weight gain and low ultrafiltration rate: lower is not always better. *Semin Dial* 2014;27(1):11–13, with permission.]

trial protocol in the group with the lowest interdialytic weight gain resulted in the greatest weight loss at 1.5 kg and in the greatest reduction in 44-hour ambulatory SBP at 12.6 mm Hg compared to any of the other groups with higher interdialytic weight gains. Thus, low interdialytic weight gain may be a sign of occult volume overload, and low interdialytic weight gain should not be considered to be synonymous with euvolemia (161). As a purely practical matter, a low interdialytic weight gain also makes it easier to challenge the dry weight.

It is important to note that while volume overload is a major contributor to hypertension in ESKD and volume removal is the foundation of hypertension control in ESKD, hypertension and volume overload are not equivalent. The presence or absence of hypertension does not definitively rule volume overload either in or out. This is illustrated by a study of 500 HD patients using bioelectric impedance analysis that found 33% of the cohort to be euvolemic and normotensive based on peridialytic BP, while 10% were hypervolemic yet still normotensive, and 13% were euvolemic but still hypertensive (162). The distinction is even more important when outcomes are considered. Volume overload has been shown to be independently associated with mortality both when assessed by bioelectrical impedance analysis (163) and by relative plasma volume monitoring (164), even after adjusting for BP in both studies. Therefore, while the presence or absence of hypertension is an important finding to guide the clinical assessment of volume status in dialysis, the treating nephrologist must keep an open mind and look for other confirming signs.

We recommend to reduce dry weight gradually in decrements as small as 0.2 to 0.3 kg per HD session based on the recognition that even small changes in dry weight can improve BP, as the DRIP trial had only 1-kg reduction in the dry weight of the intervention

group yet found a large change in ambulatory SBP, and other trials of dry weight management have similarly found significant BP reduction with similar changes in dry weight of only 1 kg or less (165,166). An added benefit of making small and gradual changes in dry weight is that it builds a rapport with patients who are often reluctant to permit their dry weight to be lowered for fear of provoking symptoms such as cramping.

There are risks to challenging dry weight including increased risk of clotted vascular access (110), accelerated loss of residual renal function (150), and increased frequency of intradialytic hypotension, which has itself been associated with myocardial stunning (167) and increased mortality (168). As the DRIP trial lasted only 8 weeks, long-term randomized trials are needed to examine the balance between benefits and risks of dry-weight reduction.

Dietary Sodium Restriction

Despite recent observational evidence questioning the benefits of a low-sodium diet for the general population (169), there is ample randomized trial evidence supporting the efficacy of low-sodium diet to treat resistant hypertension in those without kidney disease (170), to treat hypertension in stage 3 to 4 CKD (171), and for reduction of proteinuria and albuminuria in diabetic nephropathy (172). In the HD patient, sodium intake provokes increased interdialytic weight gain (173) which also leads to increased ultrafiltration rates, both of which are associated with cardiovascular mortality (174,175). Restricting sodium intake reduces interdialytic weight gain, which will also practically improve the ability to achieve an adequately low dry weight with dialysis (176,177). However, in the dialysis patient, reducing dietary sodium intake should be followed by probing dry weight to improve control of hypertension. In the absence of probing dry weight, the full benefit of restricting dietary sodium intake may not be realized. The American Heart Association recommends <1,500 mg (equivalent to 65 mmol) daily intake (178), which is a reasonable prescription for dialysis patients (80). Notably, except for hyponatremia treatment, there is zero rational role for fluid restriction in dialysis patients (173,179).

Dialysate Sodium Reduction

In the earliest days of chronic HD, low dialysate sodium concentrations were used and sodium removal on HD was thus in part due to diffusion in addition to convective removal with ultrafiltration. As the efficiency of dialyzers improved and dialysis times were reduced, higher dialysate sodium concentrations became the norm to reduce hemodynamic instability, cramping, and symptoms of disequilibrium (180), and initial studies suggested that hypertension was not a complication (181). However, more recently, it has been recognized that higher dialysate sodium concentrations will reduce or reverse the diffusive removal of sodium on HD, which undermines the effective management of volume control (182). As an example of the impact of dialysate sodium concentration, in a pilot study that reduced dialysate sodium from 137.8 to 135.6 mmol/L stepwise over 7 weeks, net sodium removal was significantly increased from 383 mmol to 480 mmol per HD session (183).

Numerous studies have shown interdialytic weight gain to be directly related to dialysate sodium concentration with higher dialysate sodium leading to higher intradialytic weight gain (183–185). Increased interdialytic weight gain is additionally seen with sodium profiles, also called sodium ramping, where the dialysate sodium concentration generally starts high and then is gradually lowered during the HD session (184,186,187). While higher dialysate sodium concentrations are prescribed to promote hemodynamic stability, the resulting higher interdialytic weight gain can lead to higher ultrafiltration rates which lead to the very hemodynamic instability originally to be avoided. Additionally, more recent studies of higher dialysate sodium concentrations, whether constant or with a profile, have been associated with higher BP in some (186,187), but not all investigations (185).

An alternative to avoid the vicious cycle in the preceding text is to individualize the dialysate sodium prescription to the patient's pre-HD serum sodium. The importance of individualization is illustrated by a cross-sectional study of 1,084 HD patients that examined the difference between the individual dialysate sodium concentration and the patient's pre-HD serum sodium and found that this difference is directly related to interdialytic weight gain, with a higher dialysate sodium concentration relative to the pre-HD serum sodium being associated with greater weight gain (188). A single-blind crossover study of 27 HD patients illustrated one method of individualizing the dialysate sodium concentration by first dialyzing all patients with a standard 138 mmol/L sodium dialysate for 3 weeks and then on a dialysate sodium concentration set to 0.95 multiplied by the pre-HD serum sodium for 3 weeks (189). On the low-sodium dialysate prescription, significant reductions were seen in interdialytic weight gain by 0.6 kg, in the frequency of intradialytic hypotension, and in the pre-HD SBP in the hypertensive subjects. Based on these findings, it is reasonable to recommend that dialysate sodium be individualized to avoid being higher than the individual patient's pre-HD serum sodium and possibly as low as 0.95 multiplied by the serum sodium in hypertensive individuals or those with high interdialytic weight gain precluding the achievement of an adequately low dry weight.

A trial in 25 PD patients employed a before-after design to investigate the use of low-sodium dialysate over 2 months (190). All subjects had one exchange per day changed to a low-sodium solution, but 10 subjects had the dextrose concentration increased to compensate for reduced osmolality, while 15 subjects had no change to their dextrose concentration. The first group had significantly improved BP along with markers of improved volume overload, adding further evidence that reducing dialysate sodium is only useful if it is accompanied by adequate ultrafiltration.

Adequate Time on Dialysis

Despite reducing both dietary sodium intake and the dialysate sodium concentration to reduce interdialytic weight gain, attempts to reduce dry weight to improve BP will be unsuccessful in many patients due to intradialytic hypotension or symptoms on HD including cramping. In these patients, increasing the HD time can make ultrafiltration easier to tolerate, thus facilitating the achievement of an adequate dry weight. A secondary analysis of the DRIP trial recently showed shorter HD times to be associated both with higher BP and slower improvement in BP when dry weight is reduced (191). A randomized crossover trial of 38 HD patients evaluated time on HD by assigning subjects to 2 weeks of 4-hour versus 5-hour HD sessions and found significantly less intradialytic hypotension and post-HD orthostatic hypotension during the longer HD runs (192). An added salutary effect of longer HD time is that for a given amount of interdialytic weight gain, an increased HD time will lead to a lower ultrafiltration rate, which has been associated with mortality (175).

It is for all these reasons that the European Best Practice Guidelines recommend that HD should be delivered at least three times weekly for a total duration of at least 12 hours, unless substantial residual renal function remains (193). However, in the United States, a recent cohort study among 32,000 HD patients found that the average single HD session was only 217 minutes and that one-quarter of patients dialyzed less than 3 hours and 15 minutes per session (194). The lower average treatment times in the United States are likely due to the practice of reducing the prescribed time to achieve a minimum goal Kt/V; however, we recommend that this practice should be avoided on account of the potential harmful effects that shorter treatment time can have on volume status and hypertension (195).

Frequent Dialysis

An additional strategy to treat patients who cannot achieve an adequately low dry weight on a conventional three times weekly HD schedule is to consider a change in modality to more frequent dialysis. Observational studies have shown frequent HD to be associated with reductions in BP despite lower antihypertensive drug use (196,197), as well as with improvements in LVH (197). More recently, randomized trials have confirmed some of these findings with a trial of 52 patients that assigned subjects to either conventional three times weekly HD versus six nights weekly nocturnal HD for 6 months and found significantly improved BP, lower antihypertensive drug use, and improved LVH in the nocturnal HD group (198). Subsequently, the Frequent Hemodialysis Network (FHN) nocturnal trial recruited 87 HD patients and randomized them to three times weekly conventional HD versus six nights weekly nocturnal HD, and weekly average pre-HD BP significantly improved in the nocturnal HD group despite a reduction in antihypertensive medication use; however, the trends toward improvement in the primary endpoints including LVH were nonsignificant, possibly due to lack of power from difficulty with subject recruitment (199). The companion FHN trial of daily HD recruited 245 patients who were randomized to three times weekly conventional HD versus 6 days weekly HD for 12 months, and this trial did find significantly reduced hazard for both coprimary composite endpoints of death or increase in left ventricular mass and death or decrease in the physical health composite score (200). Both weekly average pre-HD SBP and the number of antihypertensive medications for the intervention group were reduced significantly as well. These improvements in BP and LVH are plausibly due to better control of volume (201), especially when it is recognized that the daily HD group had significantly more ultrafiltration per week at 10.58 L on average compared to 8.99 L for the control group (200).

Pharmacologic Treatment

Patients with ESKD are routinely excluded from drug trials, limiting the evidence base from which to make recommendations for antihypertensive drug therapy. Two meta-analyses of randomized trials employing antihypertensive drugs in dialysis have found significant improvements in the cardiovascular event rates associated with treatment (144,145), which was particularly pronounced in subjects with hypertension (145). However, the trials included in these meta-analyses were highly heterogeneous; most trials were not limited to hypertensive patients, and only two trials targeted a specific BP goal.

Despite the benefits from the use of antihypertensive medication in ESKD, it must be emphasized that greater use of antihypertensive medications is associated with worse control of hypertension (15,159), which is plausibly due to inadequately treated volume overload in those cases. Thus, the first step in treating hypertension in ESKD should always be to address volume overload. All classes of antihypertensive medications have roles in the treatment of hypertension in ESKD (202), as detailed in the following text.

Diuretics

While published evidence is lacking, diuretics are often used to address hypertension and volume overload in patients with significant residual renal function, which includes those new to HD and nonoliguric patients on PD. In the setting of advanced kidney disease, higher doses of diuretics will be necessary to be effective (203). However, in anuric patients, even doses of furosemide as high as 250 mg intravenously are ineffective (204). While some investigators have suggested that thiazide diuretics exert an antihypertensive vasodilator effect (205,206), the placebo-controlled administration of thiazides to anuric dialysis patients has been shown to have no effect on BP (207). Thus, the role for diuretics in the treatment of hypertension in dialysis is at best limited to the subset of patients with significant residual renal function.

β-Blockers

β-Adrenergic blocking agents have well-established benefits in the nondialysis population including in the setting of heart failure (208) and coronary artery disease (209). As cardiovascular events are the leading cause of death in ESKD and increased sympathetic nervous system overactivity is common (52), β-blockers are an attractive therapy in this population. A retrospective cohort study of PD patients found β-blocker use to be associated with a significantly reduced risk of new-onset heart failure or the composite endpoint of new onset heart failure and cardiac mortality (210). More provocatively, Cice et al. (211) recruited 114 HD patients with reduced left

ventricular ejection fraction <35% and randomized them to carvedilol versus placebo and reported significantly improved 2-year survival in the carvedilol group.

Despite these encouraging findings, enthusiasm for β-blockers as first-line pharmacologic treatment for hypertension in dialysis is tempered by the nondialysis experience where β-blockers are not recommended for initial monotherapy of hypertension (212,213); consequently, ACEI medications are often instead recommended for initial therapy of hypertension (214). While head-to-head studies of antihypertensives are few, a recent randomized controlled trial in HD comparing lisinopril to atenolol begins to address the question of which medication to prescribe first for hypertension in HD.

The Hypertension in Hemodialysis Patients Treated with Atenolol or Lisinopril (HDPAL) trial recruited 200 chronic HD patients with hypertension confirmed by 44-hour interdialytic ABPM and echocardiographic LVH and randomized them to lisinopril- or atenolol-based therapy for 12 months to determine which drug is superior for reduction of LVH (114). All patients were treated to target goal home BP ≤140/90 mm Hg checked monthly, first by maximizing the study drug and then by addition of other drugs, sodium restriction, and reduction in dry weight. The trial was terminated early by an independent data safety monitoring board for cardiovascular safety because of significantly more serious adverse cardiovascular events in the lisinopril group, which had 43 events in 28 subjects compared to only 20 events in 16 subjects in the atenolol group (incidence rate ratio 2.36, p = 0.001). Similarly, the combined serious adverse events of myocardial infarction, stroke, hospitalization for heart failure, or cardiovascular death occurred 23 times in 17 subjects in the lisinopril group compared to only 11 events in 10 subjects in the atenolol group (incidence rate ratio 2.29, p = 0.002). LVH improved in both groups, but no differences between drug groups were found.

While 44-hour ambulatory BP improved similarly in both groups measured at baseline, 3 months, 6 months, and 12 months, the monthly home BP was consistently lower in the atenolol group, as shown in **FIGURE 15.5**, despite significantly more antihypertensive medications and greater dry-weight reduction in the lisinopril group (114). Thus, atenolol appears to be superior to lisinopril in terms of cardiovascular event rates and BP reduction in this HD population. Based on the findings of this head-to-head clinical trial of atenolol versus lisinopril in HD patients, we recommend that β-blockers should be the first-line pharmacologic therapy for hypertension. **TABLE 15.8** summarizes the recommendations for pharmacologic therapy for hypertension in dialysis. Atenolol in particular may be practically useful as it can be dosed just three times per week after HD, as was the protocol in the HDPAL trial, and this schedule has been previously shown to significantly reduce 44-hour interdialytic ambulatory BP (215). Three times weekly dosing permits the possibility of directly observed administration of atenolol in the HD unit to improve compliance with the antihypertensive regimen.

Angiotensin-Converting Enzyme Inhibitors and Angiotensin Receptor Blockers

It cannot be concluded from the HDPAL trial that ACEI medications are harmful because there was no placebo-controlled group in the study (114). Indeed, ACEI and angiotensin receptor blocker (ARB) drugs are mainstays of therapy in predialysis CKD (128) and in cardiovascular disease (216,217). Both ACEI (47,48,218) and ARB medications (219) have been shown to improve BP in ESKD.

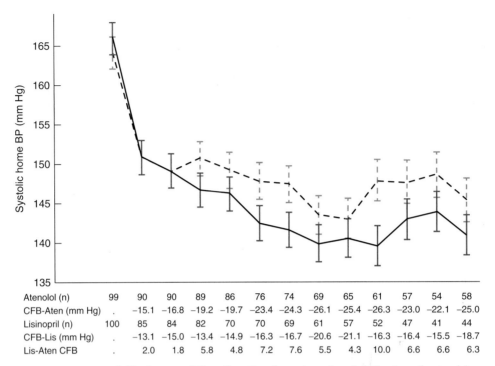

Atenolol (n)	99	90	90	89	86	76	74	69	65	61	57	54	58
CFB-Aten (mm Hg)	.	−15.1	−16.8	−19.2	−19.7	−23.4	−24.3	−26.1	−25.4	−26.3	−23.0	−22.1	−25.0
Lisinopril (n)	100	85	84	82	70	70	69	61	57	52	47	41	44
CFB-Lis (mm Hg)	.	−13.1	−15.0	−13.4	−14.9	−16.3	−16.7	−20.6	−21.1	−16.3	−16.4	−15.5	−18.7
Lis-Aten CFB	.	2.0	1.8	5.8	4.8	7.2	7.6	5.5	4.3	10.0	6.6	6.6	6.3

FIGURE 15.5 Home systolic blood pressure (BP) profiles at baseline and over time. *Solid line* shows the atenolol group, and the *dotted line* the lisinopril group; *vertical bars* represent standard error of mean. The table at the bottom of the figure shows the number of patients in each drug [atenolol (n), lisinopril (n)]; the change from baseline (CFB) and between group comparisons of the changes (lisinopril–atenolol CFB). Home BP monitoring was performed at baseline and at every month for the entire duration of the trial; the mean reduction in BP overall was reduced more with atenolol therapy [linear rate of change for atenolol was −1.5 mm Hg systolic per month and that for lisinodiol was 0.47 mm Hg flatter ($p = −0.037$)]. [Adapted from Agarwal R, Sinha AD, Pappas MK, et al. Hypertension in hemodialysis patients treated with atenolol or lisinopril: a randomized controlled trial. *Nephrol Dial Transplant* 2014;29(3):672–681, with permission.]

As with atenolol, both lisinopril (47) and trandolapril (218) have been shown to be effective at lowering BP when dosed only three times weekly after HD.

Three randomized clinical trials have examined ACEI or ARB therapy in HD patients with cardiovascular events as the

TABLE 15.8	**Suggested Approach to Pharmacologic Therapy for Hypertension in Dialysis**
Medication Class	**Comments**
β-Blockers	First-line therapy, superior to ACEI in a randomized trial
ACEI or ARB	Second-line therapy, superior to calcium channel blockers
Calcium channel blockers	Third-line therapy, effective even when volume overloaded
Centrally acting α agonists	Clonidine patch; guanfacine preferred since less sedation
Direct vasodilators	Minoxidil preferred to hydralazine since once daily
Mineralocorticoid receptor antagonists	Emerging evidence of efficacy and mortality benefit but definitive trials in progress.
Loop diuretics	Use limited only to those with substantial residual renal function

ACEI, angiotensin-converting enzyme inhibitor; ARB, angiotensin receptor blocker.

primary endpoint, and they warrant more detailed mention. The only randomized clinical trial investigating an ACEI and cardiovascular events in HD patients is the Fosinopril in Dialysis Study (FOSIDIAL) (48), which recruited 397 chronic HD patients with LVH who were followed for a 2-week run-in period on fosinopril, and those who tolerated the therapy were randomized to fosinopril or placebo and treated to goal peridialytic BP <160/90 mm Hg for 24 months (220). No benefit was found for fosinopril in decreasing cardiovascular events in this trial (48).

Two randomized controlled trials have investigated ARB use in HD and found a benefit for cardiovascular events. The first enrolled 80 HD patients who were randomized to candesartan or open label usual care for a planned 3 years (221). The trial was stopped early on account of an interim analysis that found significant and substantial benefit for candesartan for the primary endpoint of cardiovascular events as well as for mortality with zero deaths in the candesartan group and 18.9% mortality in the control group (221). The second trial included 360 HD patients randomized to open label ARB therapy with losartan, valsartan, or candesartan versus usual care with goal peridialytic SBP <150 mm Hg over 3 years (222). ARB treatment significantly reduced the primary endpoint of cardiovascular events with a 49% reduction in risk of cardiovascular events [hazard ratio (HR) = 0.51, $p = 0.002$].

In the setting of the divergent outcomes for the three randomized clinical trials using ACEI or ARB drugs in the preceding text, a recent meta-analysis examined the pooled results for cardiovascular events in the 837 total subjects in these three trials and found a trend toward benefit with a relative risk for cardiovascular events at 0.66, but this did not reach statistical significance (95% confidence interval 0.35 to 1.25, $p = 0.20$) (223). However, the intermediate endpoint of reduction of LVH did significantly favor ACEI or ARB treatment in this meta-analysis (223). Each trial had different definitions for cardiovascular events and not surprisingly significant heterogeneity was found. Similarly, a systematic review of ACEI and ARB therapy in PD patients included three randomized clinical trials and found no improvement in cardiovascular events for the intervention groups (224).

As ACEI and ARB therapy has been shown to delay progression of predialysis CKD (225), these agents may be effective at preserving residual renal function in dialysis patients, which is emerging as an important goal for both PD and HD patients (226). Two randomized controlled open label trials in PD, one investigating ramipril in 60 subjects (227) and the other studying valsartan in 34 subjects (228), both found active treatments reduced the rate of decline in GFR, while a meta-analysis pooled the difference between the intervention groups and the control groups at 12 months and found a clinically and statistically significant benefit of 0.9 mL/min/1.73 m² in favor of the intervention groups (224). In HD, however, a recent randomized placebo-controlled trial of irbesartan over 1 year in 82 nonoliguric HD patients found no benefit for irbesartan in decline of GFR or development of anuria (229).

The risk of hyperkalemia with ACEI or ARB use in dialysis appears low based on the evidence from the aforementioned randomized controlled trials in both HD (48,221,222) and PD (227). We recommend ACEI or ARB agents as a reasonable second choice after β-blockers for treatment of hypertension in dialysis based on their tolerability, the evidence of benefit in the nondialysis population, and the randomized trial evidence of benefit on intermediate endpoints such as reduction in LVH (223).

Calcium Channel Blockers

Amlodipine has been shown to be effective versus placebo in improving BP in a randomized trial of 251 hypertensive HD patients where the primary endpoint of cardiovascular events showed no improvement for active treatment (230). Calcium channel blockers have the practical benefits of being well tolerated and requiring only once a day dosing; however, ACEI or ARB therapy is preferred before calcium blockers based on head-to-head trials showing calcium channel blockers to be significantly inferior for regression of LVH (231,232).

Centrally Acting α Agonists

These medications are typically reserved only for those patients whose BP is uncontrolled on the combination of β-blocker, ACEI or ARB, plus calcium channel blocker. To minimize pill burden and dosing schedule, we recommend to avoid oral clonidine and to instead use the long-acting clonidine patch, which can be administered once a week at the dialysis unit as directly observed therapy. As the clonidine patch can be expensive, a cheaper alternative is oral guanfacine, dosed only once daily at bedtime to minimize the impact of dose-related drowsiness.

Vasodilators

Direct vasodilator agents are usually reserved as last-line therapy for hypertension in ESKD. However, hydralazine use is becoming more common based on trial evidence of benefit for heart failure in the African American population in combination with isosorbide dinitrate (233), but it is important to recognize that this combination of medications has not been studied specifically in ESKD. Furthermore, the pill burden and requirement of three times daily dosing of hydralazine makes it less attractive for use in ESKD. It is for that reason that we recommend minoxidil over hydralazine on account of its antihypertensive effectiveness with only once-daily dosing in the setting of CKD.

Mineralocorticoid Receptor Antagonists

Mineralocorticoid receptor antagonists have well-established roles in the nondialysis population for treatment of resistant hypertension (234) and heart failure (235,236). In the dialysis population, spironolactone has been shown to significantly reduce 24-hour ambulatory BP by 10.9/5.8 mm Hg in a randomized controlled double-blind trial of 76 hypertensive dialysis patients on HD or PD treated with spironolactone 25 to 50 mg daily versus placebo over 12 weeks (237). Recently, the Dialysis Outcomes Heart Failure Aldactone Study (DOHAS) clinical trial randomized 309 HD patients to spironolactone 25 mg daily versus open label usual care for 3 years and found both cardiovascular death and hospitalizations as well as all-cause mortality were significantly improved in the spironolactone group (238). Notably, spironolactone therapy was discontinued for hyperkalemia in only three patients during the trial. While the results of the DOHAS trial are very promising, they require confirmation in future blinded randomized trials to balance the risk of hyperkalemia with the potential benefits before routine use of spironolactone for hypertension in HD can be recommended.

Invasive Treatment

The history of invasive treatments for hypertension dates back at least to the 1930s when surgical sympathectomy was employed for essential hypertension (239). As efficacious oral antihypertensive agents with tolerable side effect profiles were discovered, surgery fell out of favor as a treatment for simple hypertension. However, in the early era of chronic HD in the 1960s and 1970s, it was recognized that a subset of patients with ESKD did not achieve adequate control of hypertension despite ultrafiltration on HD and the use of the antihypertensive medications available at the time (41). As high renin levels were common in these cases, bilateral nephrectomy was advocated as an effective means to reduce renin levels and BP, although it was recognized even then that other mechanisms likely were responsible for the improved BP after nephrectomy (41). With the introduction of ACEI drugs, bilateral nephrectomy too became much less common.

However, Converse et al. (52) demonstrated that sympathetic overactivity from kidney afferent nerves are a major source of hypertension in ESKD, and with the invention of a radiofrequency catheter-based approach to target the kidney nerves, there has been renewed interest in renal sympathectomy via the endovascular approach (54). A pilot study of kidney denervation by radiofrequency ablation was performed in 12 chronic HD patients with uncontrolled hypertension, and office BP was reduced in the 9 patients who had the procedure versus unchanged BP in those 3 patients whose atrophic kidney arteries precluded the endovascular denervation procedure (55). However, enthusiasm for kidney denervation must be tempered by the experience with kidney denervation in the resistant hypertension population without CKD where initial trials showed promise (240), but when a randomized, sham placebo-controlled, and blinded trial was performed, there was no BP reduction for the intervention (56). While ESKD patients are an ideal group who may benefit from this therapy, it remains to be seen whether the disappointing result from the randomized controlled trial of endovascular kidney denervation will preclude further development of this technique.

REFERENCES

1. Klag MJ, Whelton PK, Randall BL, et al. Blood pressure and end-stage renal disease in men. *N Engl J Med* 1996;334(1):13–18.
2. Saran R, Li Y, Robinson B, et al. US Renal Data System 2014 Annual Data Report: epidemiology of kidney disease in the United States. *Am J Kidney Dis* 2015;65(6 Suppl 1):A7.
3. O'Connell JB, Maggard MA, Ko CY. Colon cancer survival rates with the new American Joint Committee on Cancer sixth edition staging. *J Natl Cancer Inst* 2004;96(19):1420–1425.
4. United States Renal Data System. *USRDS 2013 Annual Data Report: Atlas of Chronic Kidney Disease and End-Stage Renal Disease in the United States.* Bethesda, MD: National Institutes of Health, National Institute of Diabetes and Digestive and Kidney Diseases, 2013.
5. Kelley K, Light RP, Agarwal R. Trended cosinor change model for analyzing hemodynamic rhythm patterns in hemodialysis patients. *Hypertension* 2007;50(1):143–150.
6. Salem MM. Hypertension in the hemodialysis population: a survey of 649 patients. *Am J Kidney Dis* 1995;26(3):461–468.
7. Mittal SK, Kowalski E, Trenkle J, et al. Prevalence of hypertension in a hemodialysis population. *Clin Nephrol* 1999;51(2):77–82.
8. Rahman M, Dixit A, Donley V, et al. Factors associated with inadequate blood pressure control in hypertensive hemodialysis patients. *Am J Kidney Dis* 1999;33(3):498–506.
9. Rahman M, Fu P, Sehgal AR, et al. Interdialytic weight gain, compliance with dialysis regimen, and age are independent predictors of blood pressure in hemodialysis patients. *Am J Kidney Dis* 2000;35(2):257–265.
10. Eknoyan G, Beck GJ, Cheung AK, et al. Effect of dialysis dose and membrane flux in maintenance hemodialysis. *N Engl J Med* 2002;347(25):2010–2019.
11. Greene T, Beck GJ, Gassman JJ, et al. Design and statistical issues of the Hemodialysis (HEMO) study. *Control Clin Trials* 2000;21(5):502–525.
12. Rocco MV, Yan G, Heyka RJ, et al. Risk factors for hypertension in chronic hemodialysis patients: baseline data from the HEMO study. *Am J Nephrol* 2001;21(4):280–288.
13. Agarwal R, Nissenson AR, Batlle D, et al. Prevalence, treatment, and control of hypertension in chronic hemodialysis patients in the United States. *Am J Med* 2003;115(4):291–297.
14. Michael B, Coyne DW, Fishbane S, et al. Sodium ferric gluconate complex in hemodialysis patients: adverse reactions compared to placebo and iron dextran. *Kidney Int* 2002;61(5):1830–1839.
15. Agarwal R. Epidemiology of interdialytic ambulatory hypertension and the role of volume excess. *Am J Nephrol* 2011;34(4):381–390.
16. Cheigh JS, Milite C, Sullivan JF, et al. Hypertension is not adequately controlled in hemodialysis patients. *Am J Kidney Dis* 1992;19(5):453–459.
17. Boudville NC, Cordy P, Millman K, et al. Blood pressure, volume, and sodium control in an automated peritoneal dialysis population. *Perit Dial Int* 2007;27(5):537–543.
18. Rocco MV, Flanigan MJ, Beaver S, et al. Report from the 1995 Core Indicators for Peritoneal Dialysis Study Group. *Am J Kidney Dis* 1997;30(2):165–173.
19. Goldfarb-Rumyantzev AS, Baird BC, Leypoldt JK, et al. The association between BP and mortality in patients on chronic peritoneal dialysis. *Nephrol Dial Transplant* 2005;20(8):1693–1701.
20. Cocchi R, Degli EE, Fabbri A, et al. Prevalence of hypertension in patients on peritoneal dialysis: results of an Italian multicentre study. *Nephrol Dial Transplant* 1999;14(6):1536–1540.
21. Tonbul Z, Altintepe L, Sozlu C, et al. Ambulatory blood pressure monitoring in haemodialysis and continuous ambulatory peritoneal dialysis (CAPD) patients. *J Hum Hypertens* 2002;16(8):585–589.
22. London GM, Marchais SJ, Safar ME, et al. Aortic and large artery compliance in end-stage renal failure. *Kidney Int* 1990;37(1):137–142.

23. Pannier B, Guerin AP, Marchais SJ, et al. Stiffness of capacitive and conduit arteries: prognostic significance for end-stage renal disease patients. *Hypertension* 2005;45(4):592–596.
24. Laurent S, Boutouyrie P, Asmar R, et al. Aortic stiffness is an independent predictor of all-cause and cardiovascular mortality in hypertensive patients. *Hypertension* 2001;37(5):1236–1241.
25. Blacher J, Guerin AP, Pannier B, et al. Impact of aortic stiffness on survival in end-stage renal disease. *Circulation* 1999;99(18):2434–2439.
26. Guerin AP, Blacher J, Pannier B, et al. Impact of aortic stiffness attenuation on survival of patients in end-stage renal failure. *Circulation* 2001;103(7):987–992.
27. Agarwal R, Light RP. Arterial stiffness and interdialytic weight gain influence ambulatory blood pressure patterns in hemodialysis patients. *Am J Physiol Renal Physiol* 2008;294(2):F303–F308.
28. Goodfriend TL, Calhoun DA. Resistant hypertension, obesity, sleep apnea, and aldosterone: theory and therapy. *Hypertension* 2004;43(3):518–524.
29. Drager LF, Diegues-Silva L, Diniz PM, et al. Obstructive sleep apnea, masked hypertension, and arterial stiffness in men. *Am J Hypertens* 2010;23(3):249–254.
30. Dudenbostel T, Calhoun DA. Resistant hypertension, obstructive sleep apnoea and aldosterone. *J Hum Hypertens* 2012;26(5):281–287.
31. Goncalves SC, Martinez D, Gus M, et al. Obstructive sleep apnea and resistant hypertension: a case-control study. *Chest* 2007;132(6):1858–1862.
32. Pedrosa RP, Drager LF, Gonzaga CC, et al. Obstructive sleep apnea: the most common secondary cause of hypertension associated with resistant hypertension. *Hypertension* 2011;58(5):811–817.
33. Ruttanaumpawan P, Nopmaneejumruslers C, Logan AG, et al. Association between refractory hypertension and obstructive sleep apnea. *J Hypertens* 2009;27(7):1439–1445.
34. Nicholl DD, Ahmed SB, Loewen AH, et al. Declining kidney function increases the prevalence of sleep apnea and nocturnal hypoxia. *Chest* 2012;141(6):1422–1430.
35. Forni Ogna V, Ogna A, Pruijm M, et al. Prevalence and diagnostic approach to sleep apnea in hemodialysis patients: a population study. *Biomed Res Int* 2015;2015:103686.
36. Abdel-Kader K, Dohar S, Shah N, et al. Resistant hypertension and obstructive sleep apnea in the setting of kidney disease. *J Hypertens* 2012;30(5):960–966.
37. Tada T, Kusano KF, Ogawa A, et al. The predictors of central and obstructive sleep apnoea in haemodialysis patients. *Nephrol Dial Transplant* 2007;22(4):1190–1197.
38. Park J, Campese VM. Resistant hypertension and obstructive sleep apnea in end-stage renal disease. *J Hypertens* 2012;30(5):880–881.
39. Pepin JL, Tamisier R, Barone-Rochette G, et al. Comparison of continuous positive airway pressure and valsartan in hypertensive patients with sleep apnea. *Am J Respir Crit Care Med* 2010;182(7):954–960.
40. Haentjens P, Van MA, Moscariello A, et al. The impact of continuous positive airway pressure on blood pressure in patients with obstructive sleep apnea syndrome: evidence from a meta-analysis of placebo-controlled randomized trials. *Arch Intern Med* 2007;167(8):757–764.
41. Lazarus JM, Hampers C, Merrill JP. Hypertension in chronic renal failure. Treatment with hemodialysis and nephrectomy. *Arch Intern Med* 1974;133(6):1059–1066.
42. Murphy RJ. The effect of "rice diet" on plasma volume and extracellular fluid space in hypertensive subjects. *J Clin Invest* 1950;29(7):912–917.
43. Guyton AC, Coleman TG, Cowley AV Jr, et al. Arterial pressure regulation. Overriding dominance of the kidneys in long-term regulation and in hypertension. *Am J Med* 1972;52(5):584–594.
44. Vertes V, Cangiano JL, Berman LB, et al. Hypertension in end-stage renal disease. *N Engl J Med* 1969;280(18):978–981.
45. Agarwal R, Alborzi P, Satyan S, et al. Dry-weight reduction in hypertensive hemodialysis patients (DRIP): a randomized, controlled trial. *Hypertension* 2009;53(3):500–507.
46. Schalekamp MA, Beevers DG, Briggs JD, et al. Hypertension in chronic renal failure. An abnormal relation between sodium and the renin-angiotensin system. *Am J Med* 1973;55(3):379–390.

47. Agarwal R, Lewis R, Davis JL, et al. Lisinopril therapy for hemodialysis hypertension: hemodynamic and endocrine responses. *Am J Kidney Dis* 2001;38(6):1245–1250.

48. Zannad F, Kessler M, Lehert P, et al. Prevention of cardiovascular events in end-stage renal disease: results of a randomized trial of fosinopril and implications for future studies. *Kidney Int* 2006;70(7):1318–1324.

49. Ishii M, Ikeda T, Takagi M, et al. Elevated plasma catecholamines in hypertensives with primary glomerular diseases. *Hypertension* 1983;5(4):545–551.

50. Beretta-Piccoli C, Weidmann P, Schiffl H, et al. Enhanced cardiovascular pressor reactivity to norepinephrine in mild renal parenchymal disease. *Kidney Int* 1982;22(3):297–303.

51. Zoccali C, Mallamaci F, Parlongo S, et al. Plasma norepinephrine predicts survival and incident cardiovascular events in patients with end-stage renal disease. *Circulation* 2002;105(11):1354–1359.

52. Converse RL Jr, Jacobsen TN, Toto RD, et al. Sympathetic overactivity in patients with chronic renal failure. *N Engl J Med* 1992;327(27):1912–1918.

53. Hausberg M, Kosch M, Harmelink P, et al. Sympathetic nerve activity in end-stage renal disease. *Circulation* 2002;106(15):1974–1979.

54. Schlaich MP, Socratous F, Hennebry S, et al. Sympathetic activation in chronic renal failure. *J Am Soc Nephrol* 2009;20(5):933–939.

55. Schlaich MP, Bart B, Hering D, et al. Feasibility of catheter-based renal nerve ablation and effects on sympathetic nerve activity and blood pressure in patients with end-stage renal disease. *Int J Cardiol* 2013;168(3):2214–2220.

56. Bhatt DL, Kandzari DE, O'Neill WW, et al. A controlled trial of renal denervation for resistant hypertension. *N Engl J Med* 2014;370(15):1393–1401.

57. Xu J, Li G, Wang P, et al. Renalase is a novel, soluble monoamine oxidase that regulates cardiac function and blood pressure. *J Clin Invest* 2005;115(5):1275–1280.

58. Desir GV. Renalase deficiency in chronic kidney disease, and its contribution to hypertension and cardiovascular disease. *Curr Opin Nephrol Hypertens* 2008;17(2):181–185.

59. Vallance P, Leone A, Calver A, et al. Accumulation of an endogenous inhibitor of nitric oxide synthesis in chronic renal failure. *Lancet* 1992;339(8793):572–575.

60. Vallance P, Leiper J. Cardiovascular biology of the asymmetric dimethylarginine: dimethylarginine dimethylaminohydrolase pathway. *Arterioscler Thromb Vasc Biol* 2004;24(6):1023–1030.

61. Zoccali C, Bode-Boger S, Mallamaci F, et al. Plasma concentration of asymmetrical dimethylarginine and mortality in patients with end-stage renal disease: a prospective study. *Lancet* 2001;358(9299):2113–2117.

62. Campese VM, Mitra N, Sandee D. Hypertension in renal parenchymal disease: why is it so resistant to treatment? *Kidney Int* 2006;69(6):967–973.

63. Koyama H, Tabata T, Nishzawa Y, et al. Plasma endothelin levels in patients with uraemia. *Lancet* 1989;1(8645):991–992.

64. Shichiri M, Hirata Y, Ando K, et al. Plasma endothelin levels in hypertension and chronic renal failure. *Hypertension* 1990;15(5):493–496.

65. Krum H, Viskoper RJ, Lacourciere Y, et al. The effect of an endothelin-receptor antagonist, bosentan, on blood pressure in patients with essential hypertension. Bosentan Hypertension Investigators. *N Engl J Med* 1998;338(12):784–790.

66. Weber MA, Black H, Bakris G, et al. A selective endothelin-receptor antagonist to reduce blood pressure in patients with treatment-resistant hypertension: a randomised, double-blind, placebo-controlled trial. *Lancet* 2009;374(9699):1423–1431.

67. Bakris GL, Lindholm LH, Black HR, et al. Divergent results using clinic and ambulatory blood pressures: report of a darusentan-resistant hypertension trial. *Hypertension* 2010;56(5):824–830.

68. de ZD, Coll B, Andress D, et al. The endothelin antagonist atrasentan lowers residual albuminuria in patients with type 2 diabetic nephropathy. *J Am Soc Nephrol* 2014;25(5):1083–1093.

69. Buckner FS, Eschbach JW, Haley NR, et al. Hypertension following erythropoietin therapy in anemic hemodialysis patients. *Am J Hypertens* 1990;3(12 Pt 1):947–955.

70. Abraham PA, Macres MG. Blood pressure in hemodialysis patients during amelioration of anemia with erythropoietin. *J Am Soc Nephrol* 1991;2(4):927–936.

71. Kaupke CJ, Kim S, Vaziri ND. Effect of erythrocyte mass on arterial blood pressure in dialysis patients receiving maintenance erythropoietin therapy. *J Am Soc Nephrol* 1994;4(11):1874–1878.

72. Carlini R, Obialo CI, Rothstein M. Intravenous erythropoietin (rHuEPO) administration increases plasma endothelin and blood pressure in hemodialysis patients. *Am J Hypertens* 1993;6(2):103–107.

73. Carlini RG, Dusso AS, Obialo CI, et al. Recombinant human erythropoietin (rHuEPO) increases endothelin-1 release by endothelial cells. *Kidney Int* 1993;43(5):1010–1014.

74. Bode-Boger SM, Boger RH, Kuhn M, et al. Recombinant human erythropoietin enhances vasoconstrictor tone via endothelin-1 and constrictor prostanoids. *Kidney Int* 1996;50(4):1255–1261.

75. Eschbach JW, Abdulhadi MH, Browne JK, et al. Recombinant human erythropoietin in anemic patients with end-stage renal disease. Results of a phase III multicenter clinical trial. *Ann Intern Med* 1989;111(12):992–1000.

76. Eschbach JW, Kelly MR, Haley NR, et al. Treatment of the anemia of progressive renal failure with recombinant human erythropoietin. *N Engl J Med* 1989;321(3):158–163.

77. Krapf R, Hulter HN. Arterial hypertension induced by erythropoietin and erythropoiesis-stimulating agents (ESA). *Clin J Am Soc Nephrol* 2009;4(2):470–480.

78. Lebel M, Kingma I, Grose JH, et al. Effect of recombinant human erythropoietin therapy on ambulatory blood pressure in normotensive and in untreated borderline hypertensive hemodialysis patients. *Am J Hypertens* 1995;8(6):545–551.

79. Ishimitsu T, Tsukada H, Ogawa Y, et al. Genetic predisposition to hypertension facilitates blood pressure elevation in hemodialysis patients treated with erythropoietin. *Am J Med* 1993;94(4):401–406.

80. Agarwal R, Flynn J, Pogue V, et al. Assessment and management of hypertension in patients on dialysis. *J Am Soc Nephrol* 2014;25(8):1630–1646.

81. Townsend RR, Ford V. Ambulatory blood pressure monitoring: coming of age in nephrology. *J Am Soc Nephrol* 1996;7(11):2279–2287.

82. Mansoor GA, White WB. Ambulatory blood pressure monitoring is a useful clinical tool in nephrology. *Am J Kidney Dis* 1997;30(5):591–605.

83. Peixoto AJ, Santos SF, Mendes RB, et al. Reproducibility of ambulatory blood pressure monitoring in hemodialysis patients. *Am J Kidney Dis* 2000;36(5):983–990.

84. Thompson AM, Pickering TG. The role of ambulatory blood pressure monitoring in chronic and end-stage renal disease. *Kidney Int* 2006;70(6):1000–1007.

85. Baumgart P, Walger P, Gemen S, et al. Blood pressure elevation during the night in chronic renal failure, hemodialysis and after renal transplantation. *Nephron* 1991;57(3):293–298.

86. Farmer CK, Goldsmith DJ, Cox J, et al. An investigation of the effect of advancing uraemia, renal replacement therapy and renal transplantation on blood pressure diurnal variability. *Nephrol Dial Transplant* 1997;12(11):2301–2307.

87. Agarwal R, Brim NJ, Mahenthiran J, et al. Out-of-hemodialysis-unit blood pressure is a superior determinant of left ventricular hypertrophy. *Hypertension* 2006;47(1):62–68.

88. Agarwal R. Blood pressure and mortality among hemodialysis patients. *Hypertension* 2010;55(3):762–768.

89. Peixoto AJ, Gray TA, Crowley ST. Validation of the SpaceLabs 90207 ambulatory blood pressure device for hemodialysis patients. *Blood Press Monit* 1999;4(5):217–221.

90. Agarwal R, Lewis RR. Prediction of hypertension in chronic hemodialysis patients. *Kidney Int* 2001;60(5):1982–1989.

91. Cannella G, Paoletti E, Ravera G, et al. Inadequate diagnosis and therapy of arterial hypertension as causes of left ventricular hypertrophy in uremic dialysis patients. *Kidney Int* 2000;58(1):260–268.

92. Bishu K, Gricz KM, Chewaka S, et al. Appropriateness of antihypertensive drug therapy in hemodialysis patients. *Clin J Am Soc Nephrol* 2006;1(4):820–824.

93. Argiles A, Mourad G, Mion C. Seasonal changes in blood pressure in patients with end-stage renal disease treated with hemodialysis. *N Engl J Med* 1998;339(19):1364–1370.

94. K/DOQI Workgroup. K/DOQI clinical practice guidelines for cardiovascular disease in dialysis patients. *Am J Kidney Dis* 2005; 45(4 Suppl 3):S1–S153.

95. Davenport A, Cox C, Thuraisingham R. Achieving blood pressure targets during dialysis improves control but increases intradialytic hypotension. *Kidney Int* 2008;73(6):759–764.

96. Rohrscheib MR, Myers OB, Servilla KS, et al. Age-related blood pressure patterns and blood pressure variability among hemodialysis patients. *Clin J Am Soc Nephrol* 2008;3(5):1407–1414.

97. Rahman M, Griffin V, Kumar A, et al. A comparison of standardized versus "usual" blood pressure measurements in hemodialysis patients. *Am J Kidney Dis* 2002;39(6):1226–1230.

98. Conion PJ, Walshe JJ, Heinle SK, et al. Predialysis systolic blood pressure correlates strongly with mean 24-hour systolic blood pressure and left ventricular mass in stable hemodialysis patients. *J Am Soc Nephrol* 1996;7(12):2658–2663.

99. Agarwal R, Peixoto AJ, Santos SF, et al. Pre- and postdialysis blood pressures are imprecise estimates of interdialytic ambulatory blood pressure. *Clin J Am Soc Nephrol* 2006;1(3):389–398.

100. Agarwal R, Metiku T, Tegegne GG, et al. Diagnosing hypertension by intradialytic blood pressure recordings. *Clin J Am Soc Nephrol* 2008;3(5):1364–1372.

101. Agarwal R, Light RP. Median intradialytic blood pressure can track changes evoked by probing dry-weight. *Clin J Am Soc Nephrol* 2010; 5(5):897–904.

102. Pickering TG, Miller NH, Ogedegbe G, et al. Call to action on use and reimbursement for home blood pressure monitoring: a joint scientific statement from the American Heart Association, American Society of Hypertension, and Preventive Cardiovascular Nurses Association. *Hypertension* 2008;52(1):10–29.

103. Parati G, Stergiou GS, Asmar R, et al. European Society of Hypertension guidelines for blood pressure monitoring at home: a summary report of the Second International Consensus Conference on Home Blood Pressure Monitoring. *J Hypertens* 2008;26(8):1505–1526.

104. Agarwal R. Role of home blood pressure monitoring in hemodialysis patients. *Am J Kidney Dis* 1999;33(4):682–687.

105. Agarwal R, Peixoto AJ, Santos SF, et al. Out-of-office blood pressure monitoring in chronic kidney disease. *Blood Press Monit* 2009;14(1):2–11.

106. Agarwal R, Andersen MJ, Bishu K, et al. Home blood pressure monitoring improves the diagnosis of hypertension in hemodialysis patients. *Kidney Int* 2006;69(5):900–906.

107. Agarwal R, Satyan S, Alborzi P, et al. Home blood pressure measurements for managing hypertension in hemodialysis patients. *Am J Nephrol* 2009;30(2):126–134.

108. Moriya H, Ohtake T, Kobayashi S. Aortic stiffness, left ventricular hypertrophy and weekly averaged blood pressure (WAB) in patients on haemodialysis. *Nephrol Dial Transplant* 2007;22(4):1198–1204.

109. Moriya H, Oka M, Maesato K, et al. Weekly averaged blood pressure is more important than a single-point blood pressure measurement in the risk stratification of dialysis patients. *Clin J Am Soc Nephrol* 2008;3(2):416–422.

110. Alborzi P, Patel N, Agarwal R. Home blood pressures are of greater prognostic value than hemodialysis unit recordings. *Clin J Am Soc Nephrol* 2007;2(6):1228–1234.

111. Kauric-Klein Z, Artinian N. Improving blood pressure control in hypertensive hemodialysis patients. *CANNT J* 2007;17(4):24–26.

112. da Silva GV, de Barros S, Abensur H, et al. Home blood pressure monitoring in blood pressure control among haemodialysis patients: an open randomized clinical trial. *Nephrol Dial Transplant* 2009;24(12):3805–3811.

113. Agarwal R, Light RP. Chronobiology of arterial hypertension in hemodialysis patients: implications for home blood pressure monitoring. *Am J Kidney Dis* 2009;54(4):693–701.

114. Agarwal R, Sinha AD, Pappas MK, et al. Hypertension in hemodialysis patients treated with atenolol or lisinopril: a randomized controlled trial. *Nephrol Dial Transplant* 2014;29(3):672–681.

115. Wright JT Jr, Williamson JD, Whelton PK, et al. A randomized trial of intensive versus standard blood-pressure control. *N Engl J Med* 2015;373(22):2103–2116.

116. Inrig JK. Intradialytic hypertension: a less-recognized cardiovascular complication of hemodialysis. *Am J Kidney Dis* 2010;55(3): 580–589.

117. Inrig JK, Oddone EZ, Hasselblad V, et al. Association of intradialytic blood pressure changes with hospitalization and mortality rates in prevalent ESRD patients. *Kidney Int* 2007;71(5):454–461.

118. Van Buren PN, Kim C, Toto R, et al. Intradialytic hypertension and the association with interdialytic ambulatory blood pressure. *Clin J Am Soc Nephrol* 2011;6(7):1684–1691.

119. Agarwal R, Light RP. Intradialytic hypertension is a marker of volume excess. *Nephrol Dial Transplant* 2010;25(10):3355–3361.

120. Inrig JK, Patel UD, Toto RD, et al. Association of blood pressure increases during hemodialysis with 2-year mortality in incident hemodialysis patients: a secondary analysis of the Dialysis Morbidity and Mortality Wave 2 Study. *Am J Kidney Dis* 2009;54(5):881–890.

121. Yang CY, Yang WC, Lin YP. Postdialysis blood pressure rise predicts long-term outcomes in chronic hemodialysis patients: a four-year prospective observational cohort study. *BMC Nephrol* 2012;13:12.

122. Cirit M, Akçiçek F, Terzioğlu E, et al. 'Paradoxical' rise in blood pressure during ultrafiltration in dialysis patients. *Nephrol Dial Transplant* 1995;10(8):1417–1420.

123. El-Shafey EM, El-Nagar GF, Selim MF. Is there a role for endothelin-1 in the hemodynamic changes during hemodialysis? *Clin Exp Nephrol* 2008;12(5):370–375.

124. Chou KJ, Lee PT, Chen CL, et al. Physiological changes during hemodialysis in patients with intradialysis hypertension. *Kidney Int* 2006;69(10):1833–1838.

125. Inrig JK, Van BP, Kim C, et al. Probing the mechanisms of intradialytic hypertension: a pilot study targeting endothelial cell dysfunction. *Clin J Am Soc Nephrol* 2012;7(8):1300–1309.

126. Saijonmaa O, Metsarinne K, Fyhrquist F. Carvedilol and its metabolites suppress endothelin-1 production in human endothelial cell culture. *Blood Press* 1997;6(1):24–28.

127. Lewington S, Clarke R, Qizilbash N, et al. Age-specific relevance of usual blood pressure to vascular mortality: a meta-analysis of individual data for one million adults in 61 prospective studies. *Lancet* 2002;360(9349):1903–1913.

128. James PA, Oparil S, Carter BL, et al. 2014 evidence-based guideline for the management of high blood pressure in adults: report from the panel members appointed to the Eighth Joint National Committee (JNC 8). *JAMA* 2014;311(5):507–520.

129. Dorhout Mees EJ. Hypertension in haemodialysis patients: who cares? *Nephrol Dial Transplant* 1999;14(1):28–30.

130. Kalantar-Zadeh K, Kilpatrick RD, McAllister CJ, et al. Reverse epidemiology of hypertension and cardiovascular death in the hemodialysis population: the 58th annual fall conference and scientific sessions. *Hypertension* 2005;45(4):811–817.

131. Kawamura M, Fijimoto S, Hisanaga S, et al. Incidence, outcome, and risk factors of cerebrovascular events in patients undergoing maintenance hemodialysis. *Am J Kidney Dis* 1998;31(6):991–996.

132. Foley RN, Parfrey PS, Harnett JD, et al. Impact of hypertension on cardiomyopathy, morbidity and mortality in end-stage renal disease. *Kidney Int* 1996;49(5):1379–1385.

133. De Lima JJ, Lopes HF, Grupi CJ, et al. Blood pressure influences the occurrence of complex ventricular arrhythmia in hemodialysis patients. *Hypertension* 1995;26(6 Pt 2):1200–1203.

134. Takeda A, Toda T, Fujii T, et al. Discordance of influence of hypertension on mortality and cardiovascular risk in hemodialysis patients. *Am J Kidney Dis* 2005;45(1):112–118.

135. Tomita J, Kimura G, Inoue T, et al. Role of systolic blood pressure in determining prognosis of hemodialyzed patients. *Am J Kidney Dis* 1995;25(3):405–412.

136. Zager PG, Nikolic J, Brown RH, et al. "U" curve association of blood pressure and mortality in hemodialysis patients. Medical Directors of Dialysis Clinic, Inc. *Kidney Int* 1998;54(2):561–569.

137. Port FK, Hulbert-Shearon TE, Wolfe RA, et al. Predialysis blood pressure and mortality risk in a national sample of maintenance hemodialysis patients. *Am J Kidney Dis* 1999;33(3):507–517.

138. Li Z, Lacson E Jr, Lowrie EG, et al. The epidemiology of systolic blood pressure and death risk in hemodialysis patients. *Am J Kidney Dis* 2006;48(4):606–615.

139. Lacson E Jr, Lazarus JM. The association between blood pressure and mortality in ESRD-not different from the general population? *Semin Dial* 2007;20(6):510–517.

140. Udayaraj UP, Steenkamp R, Caskey FJ, et al. Blood pressure and mortality risk on peritoneal dialysis. *Am J Kidney Dis* 2009;53(1):70–78.

141. Stidley CA, Hunt WC, Tentori F, et al. Changing relationship of blood pressure with mortality over time among hemodialysis patients. *J Am Soc Nephrol* 2006;17(2):513–520.

142. Amar J, Vernier I, Rossignol E, et al. Nocturnal blood pressure and 24-hour pulse pressure are potent indicators of mortality in hemodialysis patients. *Kidney Int* 2000;57(6):2485–2491.

143. Bansal N, McCulloch CE, Rahman M, et al. Blood pressure and risk of all-cause mortality in advanced chronic kidney disease and hemodialysis: the chronic renal insufficiency cohort study. *Hypertension* 2015;65(1):93–100.

144. Heerspink HJ, Ninomiya T, Zoungas S, et al. Effect of lowering blood pressure on cardiovascular events and mortality in patients on dialysis: a systematic review and meta-analysis of randomised controlled trials. *Lancet* 2009;373(9668):1009–1015.

145. Agarwal R, Sinha AD. Cardiovascular protection with antihypertensive drugs in dialysis patients: systematic review and meta-analysis. *Hypertension* 2009;53(5):860–866.

146. Charra B. Control of blood pressure in long slow hemodialysis. *Blood Purif* 1994;12(4–5):252–258.

147. Chazot C, Charra B, Laurent G, et al. Interdialysis blood pressure control by long haemodialysis sessions. *Nephrol Dial Transplant* 1995;10(6):831–837.

148. Charra B, Calemard E, Ruffet M, et al. Survival as an index of adequacy of dialysis. *Kidney Int* 1992;41(5):1286–1291.

149. Ozkahya M, Toz H, Qzerkan F, et al. Impact of volume control on left ventricular hypertrophy in dialysis patients. *J Nephrol* 2002;15(6):655–660.

150. Gunal AI, Duman S, Ozkahya M, et al. Strict volume control normalizes hypertension in peritoneal dialysis patients. *Am J Kidney Dis* 2001;37(3):588–593.

151. Scribner BH. A personalized history of chronic hemodialysis. *Am J Kidney Dis* 1990;16(6):511–519.

152. Katzarski KS, Charra B, Luik AJ, et al. Fluid state and blood pressure control in patients treated with long and short haemodialysis. *Nephrol Dial Transplant* 1999;14(2):369–375.

153. Sinha AD, Agarwal R. Can chronic volume overload be recognized and prevented in hemodialysis patients? *Semin Dial* 2009;22:480–482.

154. Agarwal R, Weir MR. Dry-weight: a concept revisited in an effort to avoid medication-directed approaches for blood pressure control in hemodialysis patients. *Clin J Am Soc Nephrol* 2010;5(7):1255–1260.

155. Agarwal R, Andersen MJ, Pratt JH. On the importance of pedal edema in hemodialysis patients. *Clin J Am Soc Nephrol* 2008;3(1):153–158.

156. Jaeger JQ, Mehta RL. Assessment of dry weight in hemodialysis: an overview. *J Am Soc Nephrol* 1999;10(2):392–403.

157. Sinha AD, Light RP, Agarwal R. Relative plasma volume monitoring during hemodialysis aids the assessment of dry weight. *Hypertension* 2010;55(2):305–311.

158. Hur E, Usta M, Toz H, et al. Effect of fluid management guided by bioimpedance spectroscopy on cardiovascular parameters in hemodialysis patients: a randomized controlled trial. *Am J Kidney Dis* 2013;61(6):957 965.

159. Grekas D, Bamichas G, Bacharaki D, et al. Hypertension in chronic hemodialysis patients: current view on pathophysiology and treatment. *Clin Nephrol* 2000;53(3):164–168.

160. Sinha AD, Agarwal R. What are the causes of the ill effects of chronic hemodialysis? The fallacy of low interdialytic weight gain and low ultrafiltration rate: lower is not always better. *Semin Dial* 2014;27(1):11–13.

161. Hecking M, Karaboyas A, Antlanger M, et al. Significance of interdialytic weight gain versus chronic volume overload: consensus opinion. *Am J Nephrol* 2013;38(1):78–90.

162. Wabel P, Moissl U, Chamney P, et al. Towards improved cardiovascular management: the necessity of combining blood pressure and fluid overload. *Nephrol Dial Transplant* 2008;23(9):2965–2971.

163. Wizemann V, Wabel P, Chamney P, et al. The mortality risk of overrhydration in haemodialysis patients. *Nephrol Dial Transplant* 2009;24(5):1574–1579.

164. Agarwal R. Hypervolemia is associated with increased mortality among hemodialysis patients. *Hypertension* 2010;56(3):512–517.

165. Zhu F, Kuhlmann MK, Sarkar S, et al. Adjustment of dry weight in hemodialysis patients using intradialytic continuous multifrequency bioimpedance of the calf. *Int J Artif Organs* 2004;27(2):104–109.

166. Zhou YL, Liu J, Sun F, et al. Calf bioimpedance ratio improves dry weight assessment and blood pressure control in hemodialysis patients. *Am J Nephrol* 2010;32(2):109–116.

167. Burton JO, Jefferies HJ, Selby NM, et al. Hemodialysis-induced cardiac injury: determinants and associated outcomes. *Clin J Am Soc Nephrol* 2009;4(5):914–920.

168. Shoji T, Tsubakihara Y, Fujii M, et al. Hemodialysis-associated hypotension as an independent risk factor for two-year mortality in hemodialysis patients. *Kidney Int* 2004;66(3):1212–1220.

169. O'Donnell M, Mente A, Rangarajan S, et al. Urinary sodium and potassium excretion, mortality, and cardiovascular events. *N Engl J Med* 2014;371(7):612–623.

170. Pimenta E, Gaddam KK, Oparil S, et al. Effects of dietary sodium reduction on blood pressure in subjects with resistant hypertension: results from a randomized trial. *Hypertension* 2009;54(3):475–481.

171. McMahon EJ, Bauer JD, Hawley CM, et al. A randomized trial of dietary sodium restriction in CKD. *J Am Soc Nephrol* 2013;24(12):2096–2103.

172. Suckling RJ, He FJ, Macgregor GA. Altered dietary salt intake for preventing and treating diabetic kidney disease. *Cochrane Database Syst Rev* 2010;(12):CD006763.

173. Ramdeen G, Tzamaloukas AH, Malhotra D, et al. Estimates of interdialytic sodium and water intake based on the balance principle: differences between nondiabetic and diabetic subjects on hemodialysis. *ASAIO J* 1998;44(6):812–817.

174. Kalantar-Zadeh K, Regidor DL, Kovesdy CP, et al. Fluid retention is associated with cardiovascular mortality in patients undergoing long-term hemodialysis. *Circulation* 2009;119(5):671–679.

175. Flythe JE, Kimmel SE, Brunelli SM. Rapid fluid removal during dialysis is associated with cardiovascular morbidity and mortality. *Kidney Int* 2011;79(2):250–257.

176. Krautzig S, Janssen U, Koch KM, et al. Dietary salt restriction and reduction of dialysate sodium to control hypertension in maintenance haemodialysis patients. *Nephrol Dial Transplant* 1998;13(3):552–553.

177. Charra B. Fluid balance, dry weight, and blood pressure in dialysis. *Hemodial Int* 2007;11(1):21–31.

178. Appel LJ, Frohlich ED, Hall JE, et al. The importance of population-wide sodium reduction as a means to prevent cardiovascular disease and stroke: a call to action from the American Heart Association. *Circulation* 2011;123(10):1138–1143.

179. Tomson CR. Advising dialysis patients to restrict fluid intake without restricting sodium intake is not based on evidence and is a waste of time. *Nephrol Dial Transplant* 2001;16(8):1538–1542.

180. Ogden DA. A double blind crossover comparison of high and low sodium dialysis. *Proc Clin Dial Transplant Forum* 1978;8:157–165.

181. Cybulsky AV, Matni A, Hollomby DJ. Effects of high sodium dialysate during maintenance hemodialysis. *Nephron* 1985;41(1):57–61.

182. Santos SF, Peixoto AJ. Revisiting the dialysate sodium prescription as a tool for better blood pressure and interdialytic weight gain management in hemodialysis patients. *Clin J Am Soc Nephrol* 2008;3(2):522–530.

183. Manlucu J, Gallo K, Heidenheim PA, et al. Lowering postdialysis plasma sodium (conductivity) to increase sodium removal in volume-expanded hemodialysis patients: a pilot study using a biofeedback software system. *Am J Kidney Dis* 2010;56(1):69–76.

184. Daugirdas JT, Al-Kudsi RR, Ing TS, et al. A double-blind evaluation of sodium gradient hemodialysis. *Am J Nephrol* 1985;5(3):163–168.

185. Barre PE, Brunelle G, Gascon-Barre M. A randomized double blind trial of dialysate sodiums of 145 mEq/L, 150 mEq/L, and 155 mEq/L. *ASAIO Trans* 1988;34(3):338–341.

186. Sang GL, Kovithavongs C, Ulan R, et al. Sodium ramping in hemodialysis: a study of beneficial and adverse effects. *Am J Kidney Dis* 1997;29(5):669–677.

187. Song JH, Lee SW, Suh CK, et al. Time-averaged concentration of dialysate sodium relates with sodium load and interdialytic weight gain during sodium-profiling hemodialysis. *Am J Kidney Dis* 2002;40(2):291–301.

188. Munoz MJ, Sun S, Chertow GM, et al. Dialysate sodium and sodium gradient in maintenance hemodialysis: a neglected sodium restriction approach? *Nephrol Dial Transplant* 2011;26(4):1281–1287.

189. de Paula FM, Peixoto AJ, Pinto LV, et al. Clinical consequences of an individualized dialysate sodium prescription in hemodialysis patients. *Kidney Int* 2004;66(3):1232–1238.

190. Davies S, Carlsson O, Simonsen O, et al. The effects of low-sodium peritoneal dialysis fluids on blood pressure, thirst and volume status. *Nephrol Dial Transplant* 2009;24(5):1609–1617.

191. Tandon T, Sinha AD, Agarwal R. Shorter delivered dialysis times associate with a higher and more difficult to treat blood pressure. *Nephrol Dial Transplant* 2013;28(6):1562–1568.

192. Brunet P, Saingra Y, Leonetti F, et al. Tolerance of haemodialysis: a randomized cross-over trial of 5-h versus 4-h treatment time. *Nephrol Dial Transplant* 1996;11(Suppl 8):46–51.

193. Tattersall J, Martin-Malo A, Pedrini L, et al. EBPG guideline on dialysis strategies. *Nephrol Dial Transplant* 2007;22(Suppl 2):ii5–ii21.

194. Foley RN, Gilbertson DT, Murray T, et al. Long interdialytic interval and mortality among patients receiving hemodialysis. *N Engl J Med* 2011;365(12):1099–1107.

195. Twardowski ZJ. Treatment time and ultrafiltration rate are more important in dialysis prescription than small molecule clearance. *Blood Purif* 2007;25(1):90–98.

196. Woods JD, Port FK, Orzol S, et al. Clinical and biochemical correlates of starting "daily" hemodialysis. *Kidney Int* 1999;55(6):2467–2476.

197. Chan CT, Floras JS, Miller JA, et al. Regression of left ventricular hypertrophy after conversion to nocturnal hemodialysis. *Kidney Int* 2002;61(6):2235–2239.

198. Culleton BF, Walsh M, Klarenbach SW, et al. Effect of frequent nocturnal hemodialysis vs conventional hemodialysis on left ventricular mass and quality of life: a randomized controlled trial. *JAMA* 2007;298(11):1291–1299.

199. Rocco MV, Lockridge RS Jr, Beck GJ, et al. The effects of frequent nocturnal home hemodialysis: the Frequent Hemodialysis Network Nocturnal Trial. *Kidney Int* 2011;80(10):1080–1091.

200. Chertow GM, Levin NW, Beck GJ, et al. In-center hemodialysis six times per week versus three times per week. *N Engl J Med* 2010;363(24):2287–2300.

201. Agarwal R. Frequent versus standard hemodialysis. *N Engl J Med* 2011;364(10):975–976.

202. Levin NW, Kotanko P, Eckardt KU, et al. Blood pressure in chronic kidney disease stage 5D-report from a Kidney Disease: Improving Global Outcomes controversies conference. *Kidney Int* 2010;77(4):273–284.

203. Brater DC. Diuretic therapy. *N Engl J Med* 1998;339(6):387–395.

204. Hayashi SY, Seeberger A, Lind B, et al. Acute effects of low and high intravenous doses of furosemide on myocardial function in anuric haemodialysis patients: a tissue Doppler study. *Nephrol Dial Transplant* 2008;23(4):1355–1361.

205. Pickkers P, Hughes AD, Russel FG, et al. Thiazide-induced vasodilation in humans is mediated by potassium channel activation. *Hypertension* 1998;32(6):1071–1076.

206. Eladari D, Chambrey R. Identification of a novel target of thiazide diuretics. *J Nephrol* 2011;24(4):391–394.

207. Bennett WM, McDonald WJ, Kuehnel E, et al. Do diuretics have antihypertensive properties independent of natriuresis? *Clin Pharmacol Ther* 1977;22(5 Pt 1):499–504.

208. Foody JM, Farrell MH, Krumholz HM. Beta-blocker therapy in heart failure: scientific review. *JAMA* 2002;287(7):883–889.

209. Teo KK, Yusuf S, Furberg CD. Effects of prophylactic antiarrhythmic drug therapy in acute myocardial infarction. An overview of results from randomized controlled trials. *JAMA* 1993;270(13):1589–1595.

210. Abbott KC, Trespalacios FC, Agodoa LY, et al. β-Blocker use in long-term dialysis patients: association with hospitalized heart failure and mortality. *Arch Intern Med* 2004;164(22):2465–2471.

211. Cice G, Ferrara L, D'Andrea A, et al. Carvedilol increases two-year survival in dialysis patients with dilated cardiomyopathy: a prospective, placebo-controlled trial. *J Am Coll Cardiol* 2003;41(9):1438–1444.

212. Mancia G, De BG, Dominiczak A, et al. 2007 Guidelines for the Management of Arterial Hypertension: the Task Force for the Management of Arterial Hypertension of the European Society of Hypertension (ESH) and of the European Society of Cardiology (ESC). *J Hypertens* 2007;25(6):1105–1187.

213. Wiysonge CS, Bradley HA, Volmink J, et al. Beta-blockers for hypertension. *Cochrane Database Syst Rev* 2012;(11):CD002003.

214. Denker MG, Cohen DL. Antihypertensive medications in end-stage renal disease. *Semin Dial* 2015;28(4):330–336.

215. Agarwal R. Supervised atenolol therapy in the management of hemodialysis hypertension. *Kidney Int* 1999;55(4):1528–1535.

216. Pfeffer MA, Braunwald E, Moye LA, et al. Effect of captopril on mortality and morbidity in patients with left ventricular dysfunction after myocardial infarction. Results of the survival and ventricular enlargement trial. The SAVE Investigators. *N Engl J Med* 1992;327(10):669–677.

217. Pfeffer MA, McMurray JJ, Velazquez EJ, et al. Valsartan, captopril, or both in myocardial infarction complicated by heart failure, left ventricular dysfunction, or both. *N Engl J Med* 2003;349(20):1893–1906.

218. Zheng S, Nath V, Coyne DW. ACE inhibitor-based, directly observed therapy for hypertension in hemodialysis patients. *Am J Nephrol* 2007;27(5):522–529.

219. Saracho R, Martin-Malo A, Martinez I, et al. Evaluation of the Losartan in Hemodialysis (ELHE) Study. *Kidney Int Suppl* 1998;68:S125–S129.

220. Zannad F, Kessler M, Grunfeld JP, et al. FOSIDIAL: a randomised placebo controlled trial of the effects of fosinopril on cardiovascular morbidity and mortality in haemodialysis patients. Study design and patients' baseline characteristics. *Fundam Clin Pharmacol* 2002;16(5):353–360.

221. Takahashi A, Takase H, Toriyama T, et al. Candesartan, an angiotensin II type-1 receptor blocker, reduces cardiovascular events in patients on chronic haemodialysis—a randomized study. *Nephrol Dial Transplant* 2006;21(9):2507–2512.

222. Suzuki H, Kanno Y, Sugahara S, et al. Effect of angiotensin receptor blockers on cardiovascular events in patients undergoing hemodialysis: an open-label randomized controlled trial. *Am J Kidney Dis* 2008;52(3):501–506.

223. Tai DJ, Lim TW, James MT, et al. Cardiovascular effects of angiotensin converting enzyme inhibition or angiotensin receptor blockade in hemodialysis: a meta-analysis. *Clin J Am Soc Nephrol* 2010;5(4):623–630.

224. Akbari A, Knoll G, Ferguson D, et al. Angiotensin-converting enzyme inhibitors and angiotensin receptor blockers in peritoneal dialysis: systematic review and meta-analysis of randomized controlled trials. *Perit Dial Int* 2009;29(5):554–561.

225. Jafar TH, Stark PC, Schmid CH, et al. Progression of chronic kidney disease: the role of blood pressure control, proteinuria, and angiotensin-converting enzyme inhibition: a patient-level meta-analysis. *Ann Intern Med* 2003;139(4):244–252.

226. Krediet RT. How to preserve residual renal function in patients with chronic kidney disease and on dialysis? *Nephrol Dial Transplant* 2006;21(Suppl 2):ii42–ii46.

227. Li PK, Chow KM, Wong TY, et al. Effects of an angiotensin-converting enzyme inhibitor on residual renal function in patients receiving peritoneal dialysis. A randomized, controlled study. *Ann Intern Med* 2003;139(2):105–112.

228. Suzuki H, Kanno Y, Sugahara S, et al. Effects of an angiotensin II receptor blocker, valsartan, on residual renal function in patients on CAPD. *Am J Kidney Dis* 2004;43(6):1056–1064.

229. Kjaergaard KD, Peters CD, Jespersen B, et al. Angiotensin blockade and progressive loss of kidney function in hemodialysis patients: a randomized controlled trial. *Am J Kidney Dis* 2014;64(6):892–901.

230. Tepel M, Hopfenmueller W, Scholze A, et al. Effect of amlodipine on cardiovascular events in hypertensive haemodialysis patients. *Nephrol Dial Transplant* 2008;23(11):3605–3612.

231. London GM, Pannier B, Guerin AP, et al. Cardiac hypertrophy, aortic compliance, peripheral resistance, and wave reflection in end-stage renal disease. Comparative effects of ACE inhibition and calcium channel blockade. *Circulation* 1994;90(6):2786–2796.

232. Shibasaki Y, Masaki H, Nishiue T, et al. Angiotensin II type 1 receptor antagonist, losartan, causes regression of left ventricular hypertrophy in end-stage renal disease. *Nephron* 2002;90(3):256–261.

233. Taylor AL, Ziesche S, Yancy C, et al. Combination of isosorbide dinitrate and hydralazine in blacks with heart failure. *N Engl J Med* 2004; 351(20):2049–2057.

234. Chapman N, Dobson J, Wilson S, et al. Effect of spironolactone on blood pressure in subjects with resistant hypertension. *Hypertension* 2007;49(4):839–845.

235. Pitt B, Zannad F, Remme WJ, et al. The effect of spironolactone on morbidity and mortality in patients with severe heart failure. Randomized Aldactone Evaluation Study Investigators. *N Engl J Med* 1999; 341(10):709–717.

236. Pitt B, Williams G, Remme W, et al. The EPHESUS trial: eplerenone in patients with heart failure due to systolic dysfunction complicating acute myocardial infarction. Eplerenone Post-AMI Heart Failure Efficacy and Survival Study. *Cardiovasc Drugs Ther* 2001;15(1):79–87.

237. Ni X, Zhang J, Zhang P, et al. Effects of spironolactone on dialysis patients with refractory hypertension: a randomized controlled study. *J Clin Hypertens (Greenwich)* 2014;16(9):658–663.

238. Matsumoto Y, Mori Y, Kageyama S, et al. Spironolactone reduces cardiovascular and cerebrovascular morbidity and mortality in hemodialysis patients. *J Am Coll Cardiol* 2014;63(6):528–536.

239. Allen EV. Sympathectomy for essential hypertension. *Circulation* 1952;6(1):131–140.

240. Krum H, Schlaich M, Whitbourn R, et al. Catheter-based renal sympathetic denervation for resistant hypertension: a multicentre safety and proof-of-principle cohort study. *Lancet* 2009;373(9671):1275–1281.

CHAPTER 16

Left Ventricular Dysfunction and Valvular Heart Disease in Dialysis Patients

Sean P. Martin, Sean W. Murphy, and Patrick S. Parfrey

Cardiovascular (CV) disease is the leading cause of mortality in patients with end-stage kidney disease (ESKD) and accounts for approximately one-half of all deaths (1–3). The prevalence of left ventricular (LV) disorders or ischemic heart disease (IHD) is extremely high in this population. Roughly 80% of patients starting maintenance dialysis therapy already have established left ventricular hypertrophy (LVH) or systolic dysfunction, disorders that are predictive of heart failure (HF), IHD, and death (4). Cohort studies have determined that the annual incidence of myocardial infarction (MI) or acute coronary syndrome requiring hospitalization among hemodialysis patients is 8%; the per annum risk of developing HF requiring hospitalization or treatment with ultrafiltration is 10% (5). United States Renal Data System (USRDS) registry data suggests that the cumulative probability of HF in incident hemodialysis patients is approximately 30% at 6 months, 56% at 2 years, and 66% by 3 years (2).

The high burden of cardiac disease associated with chronic kidney disease (CKD) is likely the end result of many etiologic factors. The prevalence of many "traditional" risk factors for heart disease, for example, diabetes and hypertension, is clearly higher among patients with kidney disease than in the general population. These same risk factors may be responsible for the development of CKD in many patients. This confounds analyses of CKD itself as an independent risk factor for CV disease, and currently, there is some debate as to whether or not this is the case. Regardless, several metabolic and hemodynamic disturbances that occur and progress in relation to declining kidney function do increase CV risk.

This chapter focuses on the pathogenesis, risk factors, and treatment of disorders of LV geometry and function in dialysis patients. The cardiomyopathy associated with uremia may manifest itself in many ways, including arrhythmia and dialysis-associated hypotension (**Figure 16.1**). These disorders, therefore, also are considered

in this chapter. IHD is discussed in detail elsewhere in this book, but it should be recognized that myocardial dysfunction and ischemic disease are closely associated and coexist in many patients.

LEFT VENTRICULAR HYPERTROPHY AND HEART FAILURE

Pathogenesis of Left Ventricular Disorders

Ventricular growth occurs in response to mechanical stresses, primarily volume or pressure overload (6). Volume overload results in addition of new sarcomeres in series, leading to increased cavity diameter (7). Larger diameter results in increased wall tension, a direct consequence of Laplace's law. This increase in wall tension stimulates the addition of new sarcomeres in parallel. Such remodeling thickens the ventricular wall, distributing the tension over a larger cross-sectional area of muscle and returning the tension in each individual fiber back toward normal. This combination of cavity enlargement and wall thickening is called *eccentric hypertrophy*. Pressure overload, on the other hand, increases wall tension by increasing intraventricular pressure, resulting directly in the parallel addition of new sarcomeres. Because sarcomeres are not added in series, isolated pressure overload leads to concentric hypertrophy, that is, wall thickening without cavity enlargement.

Both eccentric and concentric hypertrophy are initially compensatory and therefore beneficial. Dilatation permits an increase in stroke volume without an increase in the inotropic state of the myocardium and as such is an efficient adaptation to volume overload (8). It also permits the maintenance of a normal stroke volume and cardiac output in the presence of decreased contractility. Muscular hypertrophy returns the tension per unit muscle fiber back to normal, decreasing ventricular stress.

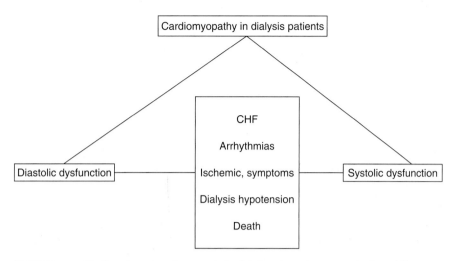

FIGURE 16.1 Manifestations of cardiomyopathy in dialysis patients. CHF, congestive heart failure.

If the stimuli for ventricular remodeling persist, however, LVH eventually becomes maladaptive. Hypertrophy is associated with progressive, deleterious changes in myocardial cells. Early in the evolution of LVH, abnormalities of cellular calcium handling lead to abnormal ventricular relaxation; combined with decreased passive compliance of a thickened ventricular wall, these changes may precipitate diastolic dysfunction (9). Decreased capillary density, impaired coronary reserves, and abnormal relaxation may decrease subendocardial perfusion, promoting ischemia (10). Frequent coexistence of coronary artery disease (CAD) may exacerbate the situation. Fibrosis of the cardiac interstitium also occurs and appears to be more marked in pressure than volume overload (11). In the late phases of chronic overload, oxidative stress is prominent and contributes to cellular dysfunction and demise (12). Together, these various processes lead to progressive cellular attrition, fibrosis, HF, and death. The results of the 2013 Chronic Renal Insufficiency Cohort (CRIC) study are consistent with the HF literature, whereby LVH is a precursor to systolic dysfunction (13). A subset of 190 patients from this longitudinal study had serial echocardiograms during advanced CKD [mean estimated glomerular filtration rate (eGFR) 16.9 mL/min/1.73 m^2] and ESKD. The majority (80%) of patients included had LVH at baseline, and the left ventricular mass index (LVMI) did not change significantly from advanced CKD to ESKD suggesting LVH is fixed by moderate to advanced stages of CKD. There was a significant decline in ejection fraction, however, from 53% to 50% ($p = 0.002$).

Many factors unique to patients with CKD appear to contribute to cardiac dysfunction. Anemia, salt and water overload, and arteriovenous (AV) fistulas in hemodialysis patients are common causes of volume overload. Hypertension is highly prevalent in patients with ESKD and is a major cause of pressure overload. These same factors promote arterial remodeling in the large and resistance arteries, characterized by diffuse arterial thickening and stiffening (arteriosclerosis), which can increase the effective load on the LV independently of mean arterial pressure (12,14).

Aside from hemodynamic factors, the uremic milieu may also lead to myocyte death. Although CAD is the major factor promoting ischemia and infarction, hyperparathyroidism increases susceptibility to ischemia through dysregulation of cellular energy metabolism (15). Poor nutrition, oxidative stress, and inadequate dialysis may all additionally promote myocyte death (6,16,17).

Diagnosis of Left Ventricular Disorders in Dialysis Patients

LV disorders can be asymptomatic or they may be manifested clinically as HF, arrhythmias, dialysis-associated hypotension, or ischemic symptoms. The diagnosis of HF is based on clinical symptoms and signs and can usually be made with an appropriate history and physical examination. HF typically presents as progressive fatigue and a decline in exercise tolerance or, alternatively, as a syndrome characterized by dyspnea, jugular venous distension, and bilateral lung crepitations and the characteristic chest x-ray appearance.

Some physicians attempt to distinguish HF from "volume overload" or circulatory congestion. This is a difficult task, as the clinical findings of both conditions are identical. The clinical context may be of some assistance, especially when fluid gains are known to be minimal based on the patient's dry weight. Even in this situation, diastolic dysfunction may be the underlying problem. In general, HF symptoms are not likely to occur in a patient with a perfectly normal heart. Physicians are well advised to consider all episodes of symptomatic HF as evidence of some degree of myocardial dysfunction and investigate them further.

Echocardiography is an important method for the assessment of LV structure and function (18–20). Although LV mass measurement using echocardiography is highly reproducible between observers, its measurement varies over the course of a hemodialysis session by as much as 25 g/m^2 (20). This occurs because LV internal diastolic diameter decreases as the patient's blood volume decreases, as a result of fluid withdrawal. A concomitant decrease in LV wall thickness is not observed. Consequently, the LVMI measured predialysis is higher than the postdialysis measurement, although the actual LV mass has not changed. Therefore, when possible, imaging should be carried out when the patient is close to dry weight.

Echocardiography provides relatively accurate measures of LV mass, cavity size, geometry, systolic function, and diastolic function. Systolic dysfunction is defined as an ejection fraction of less than 40%. It is often associated with LV dilatation (LV end-diastolic diameter greater than 5.6 cm), defined as LV cavity volume index of greater than 90 mL/m^2 (18). Concentric LVH is characterized by a thickened LV wall (greater than 1.2 cm during diastole) with normal cavity volume. LVMI is a calculated parameter that reflects the degree of hypertrophy. In non-CKD patients, the upper limits of normal are LVMI 130 g/m² for men and 102 g/m² for women (21). Although indexing LV mass to patient weight is the standard approach, it has been reported that LV mass indexed to patient height is more predictive of CV mortality in dialysis patients (22).

Cardiac magnetic resonance (CMR) imaging offers an alternative to echocardiography. It has been established as the most accurate noninvasive method of assessing ventricular dimensions in patients and is a useful tool in assessing cardiomyopathy in patients with ESKD (23–25). Compared to echocardiography, CMR has been shown to provide a more volume-independent measurement of the cardiac structure (26). In addition, echocardiography significantly overestimates LV mass relative to CMR in the presence of LVH and dilation, and this error is amplified in dialysis patients (27).

Other imaging techniques, such as nuclear medicine imaging of the LV using technetium-labeled red blood cells may be particularly useful in diagnosing areas of focal hypokinesis (usually resulting from ischemia). This method allows a more accurate estimate of global ejection fraction than does echocardiography alone.

Approximately half of patients presenting with a new diagnosis of HF have preserved ejection fraction (28). These patients have diastolic HF, and numerous society HF guidelines have consensus on the diagnostic criteria (28–32). The general criteria accepted by these guidelines include (a) clinical signs and symptoms typical of HF; (b) normal or only mildly reduced ejection fraction normal LV size and dimensions; (c) relevant structural heart disease including LVH, LA enlargement, and/or echo Doppler or catheterization evidence of diastolic dysfunction; and (d) a nonmyocardial cause of HF must be excluded. Overall, noninvasive measurements of diastolic function have low sensitivity, specificity, and predictive accuracy (33). The gold standard for diagnosis remains cardiac catheterization, which will directly demonstrate high LV filling pressures in the presence of normal ventricular volumes and contractility in these patients. Despite the limitations of echocardiography, however, it remains clinically useful and sufficient for diagnosis in most cases. An ejection fraction of greater than or equal to 50% is a more appropriate cutoff value to distinguish systolic from diastolic HF (34).

Because most dialysis patients have echocardiographic abnormalities at the beginning of ESKD treatment, it is a reasonable practice to perform M-mode and two-dimensional echocardiography on all patients at or before the start of ESKD therapy. This will provide baseline information for future comparisons, and the detection of LV disease at an earlier stage may allow more specific therapy to be employed in affected patients. Echocardiograms have the additional benefit of allowing detection of valve disease or a pericardial effusion, conditions that can potentially precipitate HF. Additionally, physicians may choose to give patients with significant myocardial dysfunction a somewhat different dialysis prescription than might otherwise be recommended. More frequent treatments or longer dialysis sessions may help the patient avoid symptomatic HF episodes. The Kidney Disease Outcomes Quality Initiative (KDOQI) guidelines for the management of CV disease in patients with CKD recommend repeating the echocardiogram when there is a change in the patient's clinical status and at 3-year intervals (35).

Outcome of Left Ventricular Disorders and Heart Failure

The presence of concentric LVH, LV dilation with normal contractility, and systolic dysfunction at baseline has been associated with progressively worse survival, independent of age, gender, diabetes, and IHD (36). All three abnormalities are also associated with increased risk for the development of HF (**FIGURES 16.2** and **16.3**). This relationship between LV mass and CV events in dialysis patients has been confirmed, as was the prognostic impact of the different types of hypertrophy (22,37).

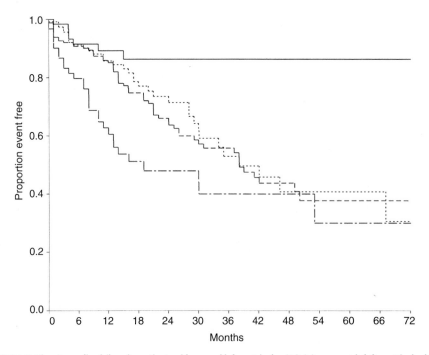

FIGURE 16.2 Time to cardiac failure for patients with normal left ventricular (LV) (–), concentric left ventricular hypertrophy (LVH) (––), LV dilation (– -), and systolic dysfunction (– - –) at inception of dialysis therapy. (Modified from Parfrey PS, Foley RN, Harnett JD, et al. Outcome and risk factors for left ventricular disorders in chronic uraemia. *Nephrol Dial Transplant* 1996;11:1277–1285. With permission from Oxford University Press.)

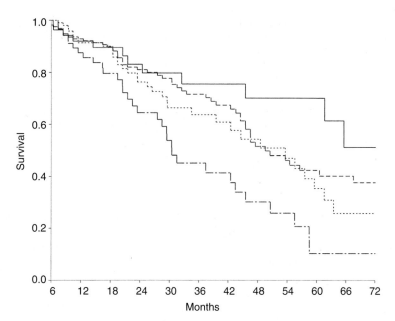

FIGURE 16.3 Survival for patients with normal left ventricular (LV) (–), concentric left ventricular hypertrophy (LVH) (––), LV dilation (– -), and systolic dysfunction (– - –) at inception of dialysis therapy. (Modified from Parfrey PS, Foley RN, Harnett JD, et al. Outcome and risk factors for left ventricular disorders in chronic uraemia. *Nephrol Dial Transplant* 1996;11:1277–1285. With permission from Oxford University Press.)

Symptomatic HF confers a poor prognosis for dialysis patients. In one cohort, the median survival of patients who had HF at or before initiation of ESKD therapy was 36 months compared with 62 months in subjects without baseline HF. This adverse prognosis was independent of age, diabetes, and IHD. Among patients who had HF at baseline, 56% developed recurrent HF and 44% remained failure-free during follow-up. Median survival in those with recurrent HF was 29 months, significantly less than in those without recurrence (45 months) (38). An analysis from the USRDS registry indicates that 1-year survival after treatment for HF is 68% for incident hemodialysis patients (2). It is interesting to note that HF has been consistently shown to be a strong independent risk factor for death, whereas the presence of IHD is not a significant risk factor for death independent of age, diabetes, and presence of HF (38). This suggests that the adverse impact of IHD exerts its effect through compromising LV pump function.

Risk Factors for Left Ventricular Disorders and Heart Failure

Independent predictors of HF at or before the time of ESKD therapy initiation include systolic dysfunction, older age, diabetes mellitus, and IHD. For patients without HF at baseline, predictors of the development of *de novo* HF include older age, systolic dysfunction, anemia, hypoalbuminemia, hypertension, and LVH (5,38). Numerous other risk factors, some unique to the dialysis patient, are known or suspected contributors to LV disorders. These include AV fistulas, disorders of divalent ion metabolism, chronic salt and water overload, altered oxidative stress, and chronic inflammation. The relative contribution of each of these risk factors in the pathogenesis of LVH has not been fully elucidated.

Nonmodifiable Risk Factor

Diabetes Mellitus

Diabetic patients without ESKD appear to be subject to a specific type of cardiomyopathy (39,40). Glycation of collagen may induce cross-linking of collagen fibers (41), and this may be a reason for large and small vessel diseases as well as myocardial dysfunction. In addition, LVH is more prevalent in hypertensive diabetic patients than in hypertensive nondiabetic patients (40,42).

In both the general and the dialysis population, diabetes is an independent risk factor for the development of HF and CAD (17,43,44). More than 50% of prevalent hemodialysis patients with a diagnosis of HF have diabetes (2). Some diabetic patients with ESKD have impairment of LV function despite normal coronary arteries, possibly resulting from the development of a diabetic cardiomyopathy as discussed earlier. Having said this, any analysis of the contribution of diabetes to the development of LV dysfunction in uremic patients is confounded by the very high prevalence of other risk factors, particularly hypertension.

The impact of diabetes was examined in a cohort study of dialysis patients who survived at least 6 months following the initiation of dialysis; 15% of these patients had insulin-dependent diabetes and 12% had non–insulin-dependent diabetes. On starting dialysis therapy, the prevalence of clinical manifestations of cardiac disease was significantly higher in diabetic patients compared with nondiabetic patients. Only 11% of diabetic patients had normal echocardiographic dimensions compared with 25% of nondiabetic patients, predominantly because of the prevalence of severe LVH (34% vs. 18%) (45). Older age, LVH, history of smoking, IHD, cardiac failure, and hypoalbuminemia were independently associated with mortality. Diabetes was a strong risk factor for the development of IHD but not for cardiac failure (45), suggesting that the excessive cardiac morbidity and mortality of diabetic patients may be mediated through ischemic disease rather than progression of cardiomyopathy while patients are on dialysis. Echocardiographic determination of LV size and function was a good predictor of survival. Diabetic patients receiving dialysis therapy with abnormal LV wall motion and abnormal LV internal diameter had the lowest mean survival (8 months), a mortality rate not matched by any subgroup defined by coronary anatomy, ventricular function, or clinical manifestation (46).

Ischemic Heart Disease

The risk factors and outcome for IHD are discussed elsewhere in this book. CAD is an important cause of systolic and diastolic dysfunction in the general population and in dialysis patients (17,47). Dialysis patients diagnosed with impaired LV systolic function should be evaluated for CAD.

Modifiable Risk Factors

Hypertension

The prevalence of hypertension is approximately 80% in hemodialysis patients, but it is closer to 50% in peritoneal dialysis patients (48). A cohort study of more than 2,500 adult hemodialysis patients reported that 86% had a systolic blood pressure (BP) greater than 150 mm Hg or a diastolic BP greater than 85 mm Hg; hypertension was controlled in only 30% of patients, and 12% were untreated (49).

The impact of hypertension was assessed in a cohort of 261 hemodialysis and 171 peritoneal dialysis patients. These patients were followed up prospectively for an average of 41 months per patient, and echocardiographic assessments were performed annually. The mean arterial BP level during dialysis therapy was 101 ± 11 mm Hg. When adjustments were made for age, diabetes, and IHD and hemoglobin (Hb) and serum albumin levels were measured serially, each 10 mm Hg rise in mean arterial BP was independently associated with the development of concentric LVH [odds ratio (OR) 1.48, $p = 0.02$], IHD (OR 1.39, $p = 0.05$), and de novo HF (OR 1.44, $p = 0.007$) (50). Hypertension was also associated with progressive concentric LVH in 596 incident hemodialysis patients without symptomatic cardiac disease or dilatation in a blinded, randomized controlled trial (51). Patients had echocardiograms within 18 months of starting dialysis and subsequently at 24, 48, and 96 weeks later. LVMI rose significantly during the study period from 114.2 g/m^2 at baseline to 128.2 kg/m^2 at week 96. High systolic BP was also associated with an increase in the composite outcome of CV events and death.

In the non–kidney disease population, reductions in BP are associated with regression of LVH. Although a similar effect in patients with ESKD seems highly likely, there is considerably less direct evidence that this is the case. In an attempt to determine the effect of BP lowering on LV size, while partially correcting anemia with erythropoietin, London et al. (52) enrolled 153 hemodialysis patients in a longitudinal study and followed them up for a mean of 54 months. The first step to control BP was achievement of dry weight. If this failed to achieve the target BP, an angiotensin-converting enzyme (ACE) inhibitor, calcium channel blocker, and then α-blocker was added as required. Predialysis BP decreased from 169/90 to 147/78 mm Hg, and Hb increased from 8.7 to 10.5 g/L. LVMI decreased from 174 to 162 g/m^2. The hazard ratio associated with a 10% LV mass decrease was 0.78 for all-cause mortality and 0.72 for CV mortality. The authors concluded that alteration of hemodynamic overload favorably influenced the natural history of LVH in hemodialysis by reducing LVH, an outcome that had a beneficial effect on survival.

Current guidelines for the treatment of hypertension in the general population do not recommend different target BP for patients with and without LVH (53,54). The optimal target BP for patients requiring dialysis is not at all clear. In this group, low BP has been repeatedly associated with increased mortality (55,56). It is likely that low BP is a marker for the presence of cardiac failure (and/or other comorbidity), confounding analyses of BP and death. This hypothesis is supported by an analysis in the general population (57). In the absence of specific trial data, a conservative target is a predialysis BP of 140/90 mm Hg or less, unless the patient develops symptomatic hypotension during or after dialysis. This should be achieved primarily by maintenance of an accurate dry weight, with antihypertensive therapy added if satisfactory results are not achieved.

Anemia

There is considerable epidemiologic evidence that persistent anemia in patients with CKD is a risk factor for cardiac disease; it has been associated with LV dilatation and LVH in both CKD and ESKD patients [relative risk (RR) for LVH progression, per 10 g/L drop, is 1.74 in CKD and 1.48 in dialysis] (17,54–58). It is also a risk factor for the development of de novo HF and death but is not associated with de novo IHD (58).

Recombinant human erythropoietin is indicated for the treatment of anemia in patients with ESKD. The optimal treatment target for Hb, however, is subject to debate. Recent 2012 Kidney Disease Improving Global Outcomes (KDIGO) guidelines recommend starting erythropoietin-stimulating agents (ESAs) when the Hb is between 9 and 10 g/dL to avoid the Hb falling below 9 g/dL. ESAs should not be used to maintain Hb concentration of Hb above 11.5 g/dL as multiple randomized controlled trials have suggested that higher Hb targets may be harmful (59). Potential harms include increased rates of mortality CV events (60,61) and cerebrovascular events (62).

Numerous uncontrolled studies in CKD and dialysis patients have assessed the treatment of anemia using ESAs with the effect on LVMI as an outcome. One hundred forty-six hemodialysis patients without symptomatic cardiac disease were randomized to normalization of Hb with erythropoietin or to partial correction of anemia. Two groups were studied, patients with preexisting LV dilatation and patients with concentric hypertrophy. In the former group, mean LV volume was high at baseline (approximately 120 mg/m^2) and a substantial minority had systolic dysfunction. Normalization of Hb failed to induce regression of LV dilatation. In the latter group, normalization of Hb failed to induce regression of LVH but it did prevent progressive LV dilatation (63).

Another randomized double blind trial involved of 596 hemodialysis patients without symptomatic cardiac disease and LV dilatation. Patients were allocated to lower (9.5 to 11.5 g/dL) and higher (13.5 to 14.5 g/dL) Hb targets using epoetin alpha. Both groups had increases in LV volume index (7.6% and 8.3%) and LVMI (16.8% vs. 14.2%). Thus, the investigators concluded that neither partial nor complete normalization of Hb has a beneficial effect on cardiac structure (62).

In contrast to these results, two studies showed favorable reductions in LVMI with correction of anemia. One study involved 230 patients and corrected Hb to 13.5 g/L for women and 14.5 g/L for men. A significant reduction in LVMI of -28 g/m^2 was observed (64). However, optimization of HF therapy during this study confounds the true effect of anemia correction alone. A lower Hb target of 10.5 g/dL was used in a study of 153 hemodialysis patients that received parallel treatment of hypertension and anemia. This study showed a regression in LVMI by 12 g/m^2 (52).

Whether treatment of anemia at an earlier stage of renal disease (e.g., in CKD) may be beneficial is still unclear. Small, uncontrolled studies have suggested that correction of anemia was associated with reductions in LVH (65,66). This has been contradicted by a trial in which 155 patients with CKD were randomized to a target Hb of 120 to 130 g/L versus 90 to 100 g/L. At the end of follow-up (2 years or the initiation of dialysis), there was no significant difference in changes in LVMI between the groups (67).

In order to further determine the impact of erythropoietin therapy on changes in the LVMI among CKD and ESKD patients, a meta-analysis of 15 studies, including those mentioned in the preceding text, involving 1,731 patients was performed. This study provided higher quality evidence that correction of severe anemia (Hb <10 g/dL) to a target of Hb ≤12 g/dL with recombinant erythropoietin resulted in significant reductions in LVMI [-32.7 g/m^2, 95% confidence interval (CI) -49.2 to 16.1, p <0.05] (68). This meta-analysis was limited, however, because the studies lacked control groups and the studies involved patients with both CKD and ESKD. Furthermore, patients in many of these studies may have benefited from parallel treatment of hypertension and HF.

Although some authors have advocated individualized targets for patients with ESKD, there has yet to be any outcome-based studies to demonstrate either the safety or efficacy of this approach. Currently, it is reasonable to follow the most recent KDIGO guidelines for treatment of anemia for all patients including those with cardiac disease (59). These recommendations have been made based on studies demonstrating improvement in quality of life and exercise tolerance at Hb levels of 11.0 to 12.0 g/dL. At the same time, the current body of evidence provides no evidence of mortality benefit and a suggestion of potential for harm when anemia is fully corrected.

Hypoalbuminemia

Low albumin is a powerful predictor of poor outcome in dialysis patients and has been associated with LV dilatation, de novo HF, and IHD (69). The mechanisms underlying this association are unclear. It may be a marker for malnutrition, inadequate dialysis, vitamin deficiency, or a chronic inflammatory state. To date, there is no real evidence as to the impact of the correction of any these factors on cardiac function.

Volume Overload

Sodium and water overload causes plasma volume expansion. Blood volume correlates directly with LV diameter in hemodialysis patients, as does the magnitude of weight changes between sessions (70,71). Despite these associations, it is difficult to clearly discern cause and effect. It is possible that salt and water retention is induced by preexisting systolic or diastolic dysfunction in some patients rather than predisposing to it.

Keeping the patient's dry weight optimal may minimize the degree of enlargement of the LV. It is interesting to note that LVH is more severe in long-term continuous ambulatory peritoneal dialysis (CAPD) patients than in hemodialysis patients (72). This finding is associated with evidence of more pronounced volume expansion, hypertension, and hypoalbuminemia.

In a retrospective study of 41 patients with symptomatic HF, the initiation of hemodialysis was associated with a significant decrease in LVMI by -24.3 ± 35.4 g/m^2 (p <0.001) after 9 months of treatment. The authors of this study concluded the decrease in LVMI could not be explained by a decrease in BP but by better volume control and relief of venous congestion (73).

Abnormal Calcium and Phosphate Metabolism

There is considerable experimental and clinical evidence that the hyperparathyroid state associated with uremia contributes to cardiomyopathy, LVH, LV fibrosis, atherosclerosis, myocardial ischemia, and vascular and cardiac calcification (74–76). Registry data indicate that hyperphosphatemia and raised calcium × phosphate product are independent predictors of mortality (77), especially death from CAD and sudden death (78).

The appropriate use of dietary modification, vitamin D analogs, and phosphate binders are recommended to achieve target levels for serum calcium of 8.4 to 9.5 mg/dL, for serum phosphorus of 2.7 to 4.6 mg/dL, for calcium × phosphate product of 55 mg/dL, and for intact parathyroid hormone (PTH) 150 to 300 pg/mL (79). The availability of aluminum- and calcium-free phosphorus binders has significantly changed the management of ESKD patients. Sevelamer hydrochloride is an effective, although costly, phosphorus binder that is not associated with hypercalcemia. Meta-analysis suggests a survival benefit for non–calcium-based phosphate binders compared to calcium-based binders, but the evidence is weak (80). Evidence from the randomized trial of cinacalcet versus placebo in hemodialysis patients with moderate to severe hyperparathyroidism reveals a clinical benefit in the prevention of CV events in patients aged ≥65 years or in the prevention of severe unremitting hyperparathyroidism in all patients (81,82).

The recent Paricalcitol Capsule Benefits in Renal Failure-Induced Cardiac Morbidity (PRIMO) trial was a randomized, placebo-controlled trial involving 227 patients who assessed the effects of activated vitamin D on LV mass over 48 weeks (83). Enrolled patients had stage 3 and 4 CKD along with mild to moderate LVH. Despite sufficient suppression of immunoreactive parathyroid hormone (iPTH), paricalcitol failed to reduce LVMI over a 48-week period.

Valve Disease

Acquired aortic stenosis may occur in a few patients and may induce concentric LVH (84). Calcification of the aortic valve has been observed in 28% to 55% of dialysis patients in various series, whereas hemodynamically important stenosis has been reported in 3% to 13%. Progression at times may be extremely rapid. The major factors predisposing to aortic valve calcification appear to be hyperparathyroidism, duration of dialysis, and degree of elevation of calcium × phosphate product (85).

In ESKD patients, intimal arterial disease, age, duration of dialysis, and inflammation all appear to be predictors for valve calcification. The prominent risk factor for mitral annular calcification was diabetes (86).

Mode and Quantity of End-Stage Kidney Disease Therapy

The question as to whether higher dosing targets for dialysis than those currently recommended will result in improvements in cardiac outcomes has been addressed in two randomized controlled trials, with conflicting results. The recently published Frequent Hemodialysis Network (FHN) daily trial was a multicenter, prospective, randomized parallel group trial that compared frequent, six times per week, in-center hemodialysis to conventional three times weekly dialysis (87). The two coprimary outcomes were death or change in LV mass, as assessed by CMR imaging. Two hundred forty-five patients were randomized, and frequent dialysis was associated with significant benefits in the coprimary outcome (HR 0.61, 95% CI 0.46

to 0.82). Stand-alone reduction in LV mass was assessed as a secondary outcome, and the adjusted mean LV mass decreased by 16.4 ± 2.9 g in the frequent hemodialysis group, as compared with 2.6 ± 3.2 g in the conventional group. By comparison, in the Hemodialysis (HEMO) study, 1,846 patients on thrice-weekly hemodialysis were randomized to either "standard" dose (target equilibrated K_t/V = 1.05) or "high" dose (target equilibrated K_t/V = 1.45). No difference in the primary outcome of all-cause mortality or any of the prespecified secondary outcomes was observed between the groups (88). Chertow et al. (87) note that the benefit observed in the FHN trial may have been due to an even greater between-group difference in urea clearance compared to the HEMO study.

A recent randomized, controlled, open-label, blinded endpoint study aimed to determine if cooled dialysate provided long-term cardiac protection using serial CMR imaging (89). This study group had previously demonstrated that cooled dialysate can reduce recurrent myocardial stunning during HD. Seventy-three patients were initially randomized to either a dialysate temperature of 37°C or individualized cooling at 0.5°C below body temperature for 12 months. The investigators found no difference in the primary outcome of ejection fraction. However, there was a significant reduction in LV mass in the intervention group (decreased by 15.6 g compared to control) and a significant reduction of −23.8 mL in LV-end diastolic volume in the intervention group. Furthermore, global LV systolic function was maintained in the experimental group but decreased in the control group (difference of −3.3%, 95% CI −6.5% to −0.2%). The investigators concluded that individualized cooled dialysate slowed the progression of hemodialysis-associated cardiomyopathy. The generalization of these findings is limited as only 44 participants completed the study and the experimental group had a larger baseline LV mass (157.9 ± 50.5 g vs. 140.3 ± 48.7 g).

Although some patients who are unable to tolerate the intradialytic volume expansion associated with intermittent hemodialysis may be more easily managed with peritoneal dialysis, there is no good evidence that either modality is associated with improved outcomes for patients with heart disease. Nocturnal hemodialysis has been associated with an improvement in many clinical parameters, including BP and regression of LVH (90,91). Whether the observed cardiac benefits are due to amelioration of hypertension, improvement in anemia, or higher dialysis dose is not clear.

Kidney transplantation is undoubtedly the best treatment for ESKD, and a good model of what happens to cardiac function when uremia is optimally treated. Following kidney transplantation, concentric LVH and LV dilatation improves, but the most striking observation is the improvement in systolic dysfunction (92). It is not known which adverse risk factors characteristic of the uremic state have been corrected to produce the improvement in LV contractility, but hypertension and AV fistulas usually persist posttransplantation.

Management of Left Ventricular Disorders and Heart Failure

Asymptomatic LV disease is usually detected with screening echocardiography. Aggressive treatment of risk factors, particularly hypertension, anemia, and IHD, is critical to prevent further myocardial dysfunction. Periodic echocardiography to assess the efficacy of such measures is prudent, and careful observation for clinical evidence of HF is required.

The initial step in the treatment of any patient with symptoms of HF should be a careful assessment for reversible precipitating or aggravating factors. Arrhythmias, uncontrolled hypertension, and use of drugs that may adversely affect cardiac performance (e.g., most calcium channel blockers, most antiarrhythmic agents, or nonsteroidal anti-inflammatory drugs) are examples. IHD may be associated with HF. This diagnosis is not always obvious, especially in diabetic patients who may not have typical symptoms.

For some patients with CKD, the appearance of HF symptoms refractory to standard treatment heralds the need for dialysis initiation. ESKD patients with severe HF will usually require hemofiltration for relief of their acute symptoms, and those on maintenance dialysis will require careful assessment of their target weights. The maintenance of a patient's true dry weight is of paramount importance in managing HF symptoms but may not be easily done in some cases. The occurrence of hypotension during dialysis, large interdialytic weight gains, and the possible overprescription of hemodynamically active drugs may need to be addressed. In difficult cases, ultrafiltration with simultaneous direct pressure monitoring using right heart catheterization may be helpful to define the optimal intravascular volume. HF unresponsive to changes in dry weight may be a complication of unsuspected IHD or valvular disease and should prompt further investigation.

Distinguishing systolic from diastolic dysfunction on clinical grounds is difficult, although the presence of hypertension with signs of HF is suggestive of hypertrophic disease with diastolic dysfunction. Systolic and diastolic dysfunction may coexist, and the relative contribution of each process may change with the evolution of LV disease in a given patient. Nonetheless, the clinical management of HF differs according to whether systolic or diastolic dysfunction predominates. An echocardiographic diagnosis of mainly diastolic disease could lead to changes in therapy, as discussed later. Consequently, an echocardiogram is an integral part of the evaluation of patients with HF.

A suggested approach to the treatment of LV disorders and HF is shown in **Figure 16.4**.

Pharmacotherapy

Patients who have LVH without HF benefit from control of hypertension, and this should be aggressively pursued. Although many classes of drugs have been shown to improve LVH, ACE inhibitors reduce LVH beyond their BP lowering effect (93).

Non–kidney disease patients with symptomatic HF resulting from systolic dysfunction are usually managed with a combination of renin-angiotensin system (RAS) blockade, β-receptor antagonists, diuretics, and/or digoxin.

Many well-designed trials in non-CKD patients have demonstrated that ACE inhibitors consistently improve symptoms, reduce morbidity, and improve survival in patients with symptomatic HF (94). Furthermore, current trial data suggests that angiotensin receptor blockers (AT_1 blockers) may be effective for the treatment of symptomatic HF in the general population, particularly for patients who do not tolerate ACE inhibitors (95,96). In dialysis patients, the Fosinopril in Dialysis (FOSIDIAL) trial was the largest trial to date to assess ACE inhibition in the reduction of coronary vascular events (97). In this randomized, double-blind study, 397 patients with ESKD and LVH were randomized to either fosinopril (n = 196) or placebo (n = 201). Although the study lacked statistical power due to a lower than predicted event rate, patients treated with fosinopril did appear to have a lower risk for coronary vascular events in the adjusted analysis. RAS blockade was also studied in multiple small studies. A trial of 30 hemodialysis patients randomized patients to losartan, enalapril, or amlodipine (98). LVMI was

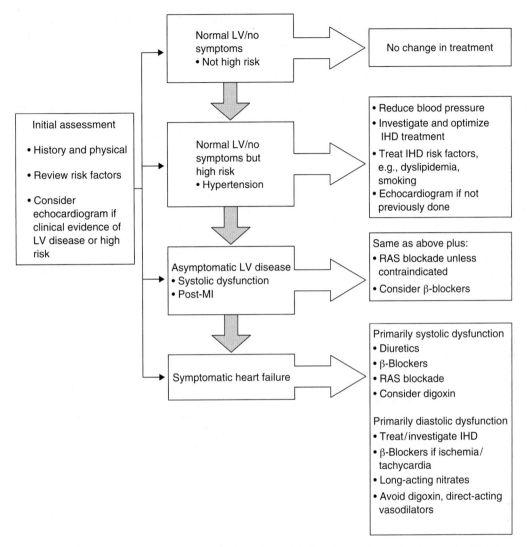

FIGURE 16.4 An approach to the treatment of left ventricular (LV) disorders and heart failure in patients with kidney disease. IHD, ischemic heart disease; MI, myocardial infarction; RAS, renin-angiotensin system.

measured before and after 6 months of treatment. Losartan treatment significantly reduced the LVMI by $-24.7 \pm 3.2\%$ compared to enalapril ($-11.4 \pm 4.1\%$) and amlodipine ($-10.5 \pm 5.2\%$). Extrapolation of these results to the general dialysis population is obvious limited due to the very small sample size. Another small study of 33 diabetic dialysis patients were randomized patients to enalapril 10 mg, losartan 100 mg, or combination therapy (99). At 1 year, there was a reduction of LVH in all groups, but dual blockade resulted in a further 28% reduction. The clinical benefit of combination ACE inhibitor and AT_1 blocker therapy is still unclear, however. For now, such combination therapy should be employed with caution in dialysis patients as emphasized in the Veterans Affairs Nephropathy in Diabetes (VA NEPHRON-D) trial involving CKD patients (100).

Although there is insufficient trial data on RAS blockade in the dialysis population, the overwhelming benefit seen in the general population makes it likely that patients with advanced CKD will benefit as well. Although there is a risk in that these drugs may predispose dialysis patients to hyperkalemia, ACE inhibitors and AT_1 blockers are generally considered safe as long as appropriate dose titration and monitoring are instituted. Current guidelines for the

general population recommend ACE inhibitors for patients who are either post-MI with an LV ejection fraction of less than 40% or who are asymptomatic with an LV ejection fraction of less than 35% (31,101). It is reasonable to apply these recommendations to dialysis patients when there is no specific contraindication.

β-Receptor antagonists are now a standard component in the management of LV systolic dysfunction. Improvements in mortality and/or hospitalization have been shown in patients with mild to moderate symptomatic congestive heart failure (CHF) treated with carvedilol, bisoprolol, or controlled-release metoprolol (102–105). Current guidelines for the general population suggest the routine use of β-receptor antagonists in clinically stable patients with LV ejection fraction less than 40% and mild to moderate HF symptoms who are on standard therapy, that is, diuretics, an ACE inhibitor, and digoxin (101). Such therapy should also be considered for asymptomatic patients with LV ejection fraction less than 40%, but the evidence supporting its use in this setting is not as strong. β-Receptor antagonists are not currently recommended for patients with severe symptomatic CHF. In one of the few randomized trials performed in dialysis patients, Cice et al. (106,107) have demonstrated that treatment of patients with dilated cardiomyopathy with carvedilol reduced 2-year mortality [51.7% in the carvedilol group compared with 73.2% in the placebo group ($p <0.01$)]. Carvedilol reduced CV deaths and hospital admissions. A recent open label randomized controlled trial compared atenolol to lisinopril in 200 maintenance hemodialysis patients with hypertension and LVH (108). Both groups had an improvement in LVMI at 12 months: -21.4 ± 5.7 g/m² with atenolol and -15.1 ± 6.2 g/m² in lisinopril, and this difference was nonsignificant. However, the trial was terminated early because the lisinopril group experienced an increase in all-cause serious events, all-cause hospitalization rates, hospitalizations for CHF, hypertension, and hyperkalemia. It is difficult to ascertain the cause of this significant difference in event rates, but the withdrawal of β-blockers in the lisinopril group may have been contributory. Overall, the investigators concluded that among predominantly black hemodialysis patients with hypertension (HTN) and LVH, β-blocker therapy may be superior to ACE inhibition. These studies, along with numerous observational data, suggest that β-receptor antagonists may be safely used in dialysis populations in the same manner recommended for the general population. However, the initiation of highly dialyzable β-blockers compared to lowly dialyzable β-blockers may be associated with a higher risk of death, possibly secondary to increased ventricular arrhythmias (109). Specific contraindications to β-blockers include reactive airway disease, sinus node dysfunction, and cardiac conduction abnormalities. As in the nondialysis population, these agents should be started in low doses with careful clinical reevaluation during the titration phase. β-Blockers with intrinsic sympathomimetic activity appear to be detrimental and should not be used in patients with HF.

Loop diuretics are widely used to maintain euvolemia in most patients with HF, but their effect may be negligible in patients requiring dialysis. Thiazide diuretics usually become ineffective with a glomerular filtration rate (GFR) less than 30 mL/min and are therefore not useful in patients with severe renal impairment. Aldosterone antagonists are similarly ineffective in patients with ESKD, and hyperkalemia can result when these drugs are combined with RAS blockade and β-receptor antagonists (110). They should be avoided in such patients.

Digoxin is useful in the treatment of patients with atrial fibrillation and HF. Although digoxin does not improve survival, nonuremic patients with symptomatic LV systolic dysfunction have less morbidity and improved exercise tolerance when given digoxin in conjunction with standard therapy, that is, diuretics and ACE inhibitors (111,112). The only data from a randomized trial concerning patients with CKD is the *post hoc* analyses of data from the Digoxin Intervention Group (DIG) trial. In this case, the efficacy of digoxin did not differ by level of GFR, ranging from patients with normal kidney function to those on dialysis (113). Digoxin should therefore be considered for dialysis patients with systolic dysfunction, given a reduction in dose appropriate to their level of renal impairment. Low dialysate potassium levels should be avoided for hemodialysis patients, as hypokalemia may predispose to arrhythmias in the presence of digoxin. Peritoneal dialysis patients will frequently require potassium supplementation to maintain normal levels. Digoxin should not be given to patients with primarily diastolic dysfunction, as the increased contractility could worsen diastolic impairment.

The treatment of diastolic dysfunction is less well defined. Attempts to eliminate the cause are generally the focus of therapy. This includes aggressive control of hypertension and IHD. Long-acting nitrates may be advantageous in some patients, and β-receptor antagonists are useful for treating IHD and tachycardia. Digoxin and direct vasodilators, such as prazosin, hydralazine, or minoxidil, are generally contraindicated in this setting (101).

⬡ CARDIAC ARRHYTHMIAS AND SUDDEN CARDIAC DEATH

Sudden cardiac death (SCD) and arrhythmias occur in hemodialysis patients who encounter stressors to a vulnerable myocardium (114) (**FIGURE 16.5**). These patients develop cardiomyopathy with diastolic and systolic dysfunction, fibrosis, and vascular disease. In addition, sympathetic over activity, inflammation, abnormalities in mineral metabolism, electrolyte shifts, hypervolemia/hypovolemia, and QT prolongation together predispose to arrhythmia and SCD. In the general population, CAD and LVH appear to be associated

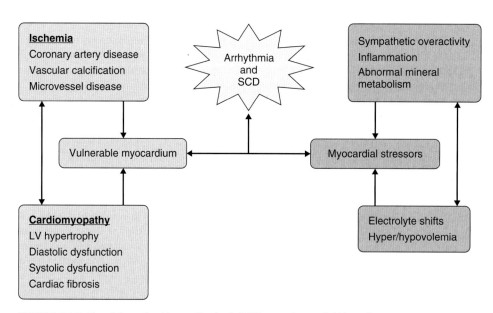

FIGURE 16.5 The etiology of sudden cardiac death (SCD) occurs in uremic kidney disease.

with an increased risk of arrhythmias (115,116). In patients with CAD, for each 10 mL/min decrement in eGFR, the risk of SCD increased by 11%. CAD is present in at least 38% of the prevalent dialysis population (117), and in these patients, the intra- and post-dialytic period is associated with a high frequency and lengthy persistence of ventricular arrhythmias (118). In other studies, CAD has been associated with a higher frequency of arrhythmias in some (119,120) but not all studies on patients receiving hemodialysis (121,122). While the association with LVH has not been well documented in ESKD, a 10-year cohort of 123 dialysis patients revealed that worsening of LVH is a strong predictor of sudden death (123). Furthermore, in the Deutsche Diabetes Dialyse Studie (4D) trial, the presence of LVH doubled the risk of SCD (124).

There are conflicting data about the effect of dialysis and various dialysis compositions and dialysis protocols on the occurrence of rhythm disturbances. Some studies show higher incidence of premature ventricular contractions (PVCs) during dialysis or immediately after dialysis (122,125,126), whereas in others, no differences could be observed (101,121). Other studies showed that a low dialysate potassium of <2 mEq/L was associated with a significantly increased risk for SCD (127,128).

In cross-sectional studies of patients with ESKD, the prevalence of atrial arrhythmias was between 68% and 88%, ventricular arrhythmias were present in 56% to 76% of patients, and PVCs were found in 14% to 21% (121,122,126). Older age, preexisting heart disease, LVH, and use of digitalis therapy were associated with higher prevalence and greater severity of cardiac arrhythmias (120).

Most PVCs observed are unifocal and below 30 per hour, but high-grade ventricular arrhythmias like multiple PVCs, ventricular couplets, and ventricular tachycardia have been found in 27% of 92 patients with 24-hour Holter monitoring (129). The finding of high-grade ventricular arrhythmias in the presence of IHD was associated with increased risk of cardiac mortality and sudden death (120,130). Whereas the dialysis method, membrane, and buffer used do not seem to have a direct effect on the incidence of arrhythmias (131), dialysis-associated hypotension seems to be an important factor in precipitating high-grade ventricular arrhythmias, irrespective of the type of dialysis (131,132).

Holter monitoring of cardiac rhythm of 21 peritoneal dialysis patients revealed a high frequency of atrial and/or ventricular premature beats (133). There were no differences in the type and frequency of the extrasystoles between the day on peritoneal dialysis and the day on which dialysis was deliberately withheld. It seems that, in contrast with HD, peritoneal dialysis is by itself not responsible for provoking or aggravating arrhythmias. The arrhythmias are more a reflection of the patient's age, underlying IHD, or an association with LVH (134,135).

A study in which 27 peritoneal dialysis patients were compared with 27 hemodialysis patients revealed that severe cardiac arrhythmias occurred in only 4% of CAPD and in 33% of the hemodialysis group (135). Patients in both groups were matched for age, sex, duration of treatment, and cause of CKD. The lower frequency of LVH, the maintenance of a relatively stable BP, the absence of sudden hypotensive events, and the significantly lower incidence of severe hyperkalemia in patients on peritoneal dialysis may explain the lower incidence of severe arrhythmias in patients with CAPD (136).

Digoxin use in hemodialysis patients has raised concern regarding precipitation of arrhythmias, especially in the immediate postdialysis period, when both hypokalemia and relative hypercalcemia may occur (119,120,137). Keller et al. (138) studied 55 patients in a crossover study of "on-and-off" digoxin and found no increase in incidence of arrhythmias when patients were on the drug.

Given the high prevalence of dysrhythmias in the dialysis population, it is worthwhile to perform a 12-lead electrocardiogram (ECG) in all patients at the time that treatment is initiated. The treatment of arrhythmias with pharmacologic agents is controversial, regardless of the patient population. Certain antiarrhythmics may increase the likelihood of sudden death (139). In kidney disease, pharmacokinetics are altered, and hemodialysis *per se* may have a major effect on antiarrhythmic drug levels. Most agents require significant dose adjustments, and some drugs, such as procainamide and dofetilide, are to be avoided in dialysis patients altogether (35). In general, management should first be directed at the underlying cardiac disease and the amelioration of any aspects of the dialysis procedure or uremic state that may be aggravating the situation. Only then should drug therapy be considered. It is our policy to be conservative in initiating treatment with antiarrhythmic drugs in dialysis patients.

⬡ DIALYSIS-ASSOCIATED HYPOTENSION

The hemodynamic response to hemodialysis depends on the amount and rate of fluid removal and the presence and nature of any underlying ventricular dysfunction. Fluid removal during hemodialysis leads to a decrease in plasma volume and a reduction in ejection fraction and diameter. Arterial hypotension may also result. The normal defense against such hypotension is mediated by the sympathetic nervous system that causes peripheral vasoconstriction, increasing systemic vascular resistance and heart rate with a resultant rise in cardiac output. In dialysis patients, this compensatory response may be defective if autonomic dysfunction is present.

The influence of the nature of the underlying cardiac disease on the occurrence of dialysis hypotension has not been well studied. Theoretically, hypotension also may occur if LV dysfunction does not allow a compensatory rise in cardiac output (140). In patients with diastolic dysfunction, there is a shift of the normal ejection fraction and pressure relationship (**FIGURE 16.6**). These individuals

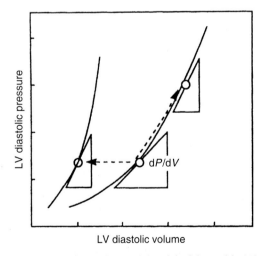

FIGURE 16.6 Compliance characteristics of the left ventricle (LV) during diastolic filling. In uremia, compliance is decreased with a leftward shift of the pressure–volume curve. (Reprinted with permission from Palmer BF, Henrich WL. The effect of dialysis on left ventricular contractility. In: Parfrey PS, Harnett JD, eds. *Cardiac Dysfunction in Chronic Uremia*. Boston, MA: Kluwer Academic Publishers, 1992.)

are more likely to develop decreased cardiac output and hypotension with smaller decreases in intravascular volume. Conversely, they are also more likely to develop HF with smaller increments in intravascular volume.

If the amount and rate of volume removal is too high, hypotension may result even in the presence of an intact autonomic nervous system and the absence of cardiac disease. Dialysis-associated hypotension is therefore often multifactorial. Indeed, it cannot entirely be explained by changes in volume status, because hypotension occurs more readily with conventional hemodialysis than with ultrafiltration, given identical fluid removal. The stability of plasma osmolality during ultrafiltration may be an important factor (141,142).

The most important means of preventing hypotensive episodes is the prescription of an accurate dry weight. Stepwise reduction of weight with clinical assessment at each stage is still the most common method of achieving this, but newer methods such as ultrasonic inferior vena cava measurement and bioelectric impedance determination are becoming more widely used. Cooling of the dialysate or sympathicomimetic agents such as midodrine are useful in selected patients (143). Sodium modeling during dialysis and reduction in ultrafiltration rates are also useful strategies to try (144). Overall, the prevention and treatment of hypotension are no different in patients with underlying cardiac disease than in those with normal hearts. The existence of underlying ventricular dysfunction should, however, alert the clinician that hypotension is more likely, particularly for patients with severe LVH.

CONCLUSION

LV dysfunction and HF is a common problem in patients with ESKD. Such disease may be asymptomatic and may contribute to arrhythmias or dialysis-associated hypotension. Our understanding of the optimal treatment of patients with ESKD is still evolving. In the absence of specific trial data, it is wise to consider treating this patient group in much the same way as the general population. Management is aimed at treating any reversible causes, optimizing salt and water balance, and ameliorating uremic anemia. RAS blockade is a cornerstone of treatment, and β-receptor antagonists should be considered. Digoxin may be useful in patients with systolic dysfunction even in the absence of atrial fibrillation, but it should be avoided in those patients with predominantly diastolic dysfunction. Prevention of LV disease through early and aggressive treatment of risk factors is likely the best way to reduce morbidity and mortality.

REFERENCES

1. Foley RN, Parfrey PS, Sarnak MJ. Epidemiology of cardiovascular disease in chronic renal disease. *J Am Soc Nephrol* 1998;9(Suppl 12):S16–S23.
2. United States Renal Data System. *USRDS 2007 Annual Data Report: Atlas of Chronic Kidney Disease and End-Stage Renal Disease in the United States.* Bethesda, MD: National Institutes of Health, National Institute of Diabetes and Digestive and Kidney Diseases, 2007.
3. Canadian Institute for Health Information. *2007 Annual Report—Treatment of End-Stage Organ Failure in Canada 1996 to 2005.* Ottawa, Canada: Canadian Institute for Health Information, 2007.
4. Foley RN, Parfrey PS, Harnett JD, et al. The prognostic importance of left ventricular geometry in uremic cardiomyopathy. *J Am Soc Nephrol* 1995;5(12):2024–2031.
5. Churchill DN, Taylor TW, Cook RJ, et al. Canadian Hemodialysis Morbidity Study. *Am J Kidney Dis* 1992;19(3):214–234.
6. London GM, Parfrey PS. Cardiac disease in chronic uremia: pathogenesis. *Adv Ren Replace Ther* 1997;4(3):194–211.
7. Grossman W, Jones D, McLaurin LP. Wall stress and patterns of hypertrophy in the human left ventricle. *J Clin Invest* 1975;56(1):56–64.
8. Grossman W. Cardiac hypertrophy: useful adaptation or pathologic process? *Am J Med* 1980;69(4):576–584.
9. Rozich JD, Smith B, Thomas JD, et al. Dialysis-induced alterations in left ventricular filling: mechanisms and clinical significance. *Am J Kidney Dis* 1991;17(3):277–285.
10. Hoffman JI. Transmural myocardial perfusion. *Prog Cardiovasc Dis* 1987;29(6):429–464.
11. Amann K, Ritz E. Cardiac disease in chronic uremia: pathophysiology. *Adv Ren Replace Ther* 1997;4(3):212–224.
12. London GM, Guerin AP, Marchais SJ, et al. Cardiac and arterial interactions in end-stage renal disease. *Kidney Int* 1996;50(2):600–608.
13. Bansal N, Keane M, Delafontaine P, et al. A longitudinal study of left ventricular function and structure from CKD to ESRD: the CRIC study. *Clin J Am Soc Nephrol* 2013;8(3):355–362.
14. London GM, Drueke TB. Atherosclerosis and arteriosclerosis in chronic renal failure. *Kidney Int* 1997;51(6):1678–1695.
15. Massry SG, Smogorzewski M. Mechanisms through which parathyroid hormone mediates its deleterious effects on organ function in uremia. *Semin Nephrol* 1994;14(3):219–231.
16. Rigatto C, Singal P. Oxidative stress in uremia: impact on cardiac disease in dialysis patients. *Semin Dial* 1999;12:91–96.
17. Parfrey PS, Foley RN, Harnett JD, et al. Outcome and risk factors for left ventricular disorders in chronic uraemia. *Nephrol Dial Transplant* 1996;11(7):1277–1285.
18. Pombo JF, Troy BL, Russell RO Jr. Left ventricular volumes and ejection fraction by echocardiography. *Circulation* 1971;43(4):480–490.
19. Devereux RB, Roman MJ. Ultrasonic techniques for the evaluation of hypertension. *Curr Opin Nephrol Hypertens* 1994;3(6):644–651.
20. Harnett JD, Murphy B, Collingwood P, et al. The reliability and validity of echocardiographic measurement of left ventricular mass index in hemodialysis patients. *Nephron* 1993;65(2):212–214.
21. Levy D, Savage DD, Garrison RJ, et al. Echocardiographic criteria for left ventricular hypertrophy: the Framingham Heart Study. *Am J Cardiol* 1987;59(9):956–960.
22. Zoccali C, Benedetto FA, Mallamaci F, et al. Prognostic impact of the indexation of left ventricular mass in patients undergoing dialysis. *J Am Soc Nephrol* 2001;12(12):2768–2774.
23. Mark PB, Johnston N, Groenning BA, et al. Redefinition of uremic cardiomyopathy by contrast-enhanced cardiac magnetic resonance imaging. *Kidney Int* 2006;69(10):1839–1845.
24. Stewart GA, Mark PB, Johnston N, et al. Determinants of hypertension and left ventricular function in end stage renal failure: a pilot study using cardiovascular magnetic resonance imaging. *Clin Physiol Funct Imaging* 2004;24(6):387–393.
25. Bellenger NG, Burgess MI, Ray SG, et al. Comparison of left ventricular ejection fraction and volumes in heart failure by echocardiography, radionuclide ventriculography and cardiovascular magnetic resonance. Are they interchangeable? *Eur Heart J* 2000;21(16):1387–1396.
26. Myerson SG, Bellenger NG, Pennell DJ. Assessment of left ventricular mass by cardiovascular magnetic resonance. *Hypertension* 2002;39(3):750–755.
27. Stewart GA, Foster J, Cowan M, et al. Echocardiography overestimates left ventricular mass in hemodialysis patients relative to magnetic resonance imaging. *Kidney Int* 1999;56(6):2248–2253.
28. Paulus WJ, Tschöpe C, Sanderson JE, et al. How to diagnose diastolic heart failure: a consensus statement on the diagnosis of heart failure with normal left ventricular ejection fraction by the Heart Failure and Echocardiography Associations of the European Society of Cardiology. *Eur Heart J* 2007;28:2539–2550.
29. Lindenfeld J, Albert NM, Boehmer JP, et al. HFSA 2010 Comprehensive Heart Failure Practice Guideline. *J Card Fail* 2010;16(6):e1–e194.
30. Hunt SA, Abraham WT, Chin MH, et al. 2009 focused update incorporated into the ACC/AHA 2005 Guidelines for the Diagnosis and Management of Heart Failure in Adults: a report of the American

College of Cardiology Foundation/American Heart Association Task Force on Practice Guidelines: developed in collaboration with the International Society for Heart and Lung Transplantation. *Circulation* 2009;119(14):e391–e479.

31. Arnold JM, Liu P, Demers C, et al. Canadian Cardiovascular Society consensus conference recommendations on heart failure 2006: diagnosis and management. *Can J Cardiol* 2006;22(1):23–45.

32. McMurray JJ, Adamopoulos S, Anker SD, et al. ESC Guidelines for the diagnosis and treatment of acute and chronic heart failure 2012: The Task Force for the Diagnosis and Treatment of Acute and Chronic Heart Failure 2012 of the European Society of Cardiology. Developed in collaboration with the Heart Failure Association (HFA) of the ESC. *Eur Heart J* 2012;33(14):1787–1847.

33. Murphy SW. Diastolic dysfunction. *Curr Treat Options Cardiovasc Med* 2004;6(1):61–68.

34. Zile MR. Heart failure with preserved ejection fraction: is this diastolic heart failure? *J Am Coll Cardiol* 2003;41(9):1519–1522.

35. National Kidney Foundation. K/DOQI clinical practice guidelines for cardiovascular disease in dialysis patients. *Am J Kidney Dis* 2005;45(4 Suppl 3):S1–153.

36. Foley RN, Parfrey PS, Harnett JD, et al. Clinical and echocardiographic disease in patients starting end-stage renal disease therapy. *Kidney Int* 1995;47(1):186–192.

37. Zoccali C, Benedetto FA, Mallamaci F, et al. Prognostic value of echocardiographic indicators of left ventricular systolic function in asymptomatic dialysis patients. *J Am Soc Nephrol* 2004;15(4):1029–1037.

38. Harnett JD, Foley RN, Kent GM, et al. Congestive heart failure in dialysis patients: prevalence, incidence, prognosis and risk factors. *Kidney Int* 1995;47(3):884–890.

39. Galderisi M, Anderson KM, Wilson PW, et al. Echocardiographic evidence for the existence of a distinct diabetic cardiomyopathy (the Framingham Heart Study). *Am J Cardiol* 1991;68(1):85–89.

40. Grossman E, Messerli FH. Diabetic and hypertensive heart disease. *Ann Intern Med* 1996;125(4):304–310.

41. Brownlee M, Cerami A, Vlassara H. Advanced glycosylation end products in tissue and the biochemical basis of diabetic complications. *N Engl J Med* 1988;318(20):1315–1321.

42. van Hoeven KH, Factor SM. A comparison of the pathological spectrum of hypertensive, diabetic, and hypertensive-diabetic heart disease. *Circulation* 1990;82(3):848–855.

43. Greaves SC, Gamble GD, Collins JF, et al. Determinants of left ventricular hypertrophy and systolic dysfunction in chronic renal failure. *Am J Kidney Dis* 1994;24(5):768–776.

44. Kannel WB, McGee DL. Diabetes and cardiovascular disease. The Framingham Study. *JAMA* 1979;241(19):2035–2038.

45. Foley RN, Culleton BF, Parfrey PS, et al. Cardiac disease in diabetic end-stage renal disease. *Diabetologia* 1997;40(11):1307–1312.

46. Weinrauch LA, D'Elia JA, Gleason RE, et al. Usefulness of left ventricular size and function in predicting survival in chronic dialysis patients with diabetes mellitus. *Am J Cardiol* 1992;70(3):300–303.

47. Saxon LA, Stevenson WG, Middlekauff HR, et al. Predicting death from progressive heart failure secondary to ischemic or idiopathic dilated cardiomyopathy. *Am J Cardiol* 1993;72(1):62–65.

48. Mailloux LU, Levey AS. Hypertension in patients with chronic renal disease. *Am J Kidney Dis* 1998;32(5 Suppl 3):S120–S141.

49. Agarwal R, Nissenson AR, Batlle D, et al. Prevalence, treatment, and control of hypertension in chronic hemodialysis patients in the United States. *Am J Med* 2003;115(4):291–297.

50. Foley RN, Parfrey PS, Harnett JD, et al. Impact of hypertension on cardiomyopathy, morbidity and mortality in end-stage renal disease. *Kidney Int* 1996;49(5):1379–1385.

51. Foley RN, Curtis BM, Randell EW, et al. Left ventricular hypertrophy in new hemodialysis patients without symptomatic cardiac disease. *Clin J Am Soc Nephrol* 2010;5(5):805–813.

52. London GM, Pannier B, Guerin AP, et al. Alterations of left ventricular hypertrophy in and survival of patients receiving hemodialysis: follow-up of an interventional study. *J Am Soc Nephrol* 2001;12(12):2759–2767.

53. James PA, Oparil S, Carter BL, et al. 2014 evidence-based guideline for the management of high blood pressure in adults: report from the panel members appointed to the Eighth Joint National Committee (JNC 8). *JAMA* 2014;311(5):507–520.

54. Hackam DG, Quinn RR, Ravani P, et al. The 2013 Canadian Hypertension Education Program recommendations for blood pressure measurement, diagnosis, assessment of risk, prevention, and treatment of hypertension. *Can J Cardiol* 2013;29(5):528–542.

55. Zager PG, Nikolic J, Brown RH, et al. "U" curve association of blood pressure and mortality in hemodialysis patients. Medical Directors of Dialysis Clinic, Inc. *Kidney Int* 1998;54(2):561–569.

56. Lowrie EG, Lew NL. Commonly measured laboratory variables in hemodialysis patients: relationships among them and to death risk. *Semin Nephrol* 1992;12(3):276–283.

57. Boutitie F, Gueyffier F, Pocock S, et al. J-shaped relationship between blood pressure and mortality in hypertensive patients: new insights from a meta-analysis of individual-patient data. *Ann Intern Med* 2002;136(6):438–448.

58. Foley RN, Parfrey PS, Harnett JD, et al. The impact of anemia on cardiomyopathy, morbidity, and mortality in end-stage renal disease. *Am J Kidney Dis* 1996;28(1):53–61.

59. Kidney Disease Improving Global Outcomes. KDIGO Clinical Practice Guidelines for Anemia in Chronic Kidney Disease. *Kidney Int Suppl* 2012;2(4):279–335.

60. Besarab A, Bolton WK, Browne JK, et al. The effects of normal as compared with low hematocrit values in patients with cardiac disease who are receiving hemodialysis and epoetin. *N Engl J Med* 1998;339(9):584–590.

61. Singh AK, Szczech L, Tang KL, et al. Correction of anemia with epoetin alfa in chronic kidney disease. *N Engl J Med* 2006;355(20):2085–2098.

62. Parfrey PS, Foley RN, Wittreich BH, et al. Double-blind comparison of full and partial anemia correction in incident hemodialysis patients without symptomatic heart disease. *J Am Soc Nephrol* 2005;16(7):2180–2189.

63. Foley RN, Parfrey PS, Morgan J, et al. Effect of hemoglobin levels in hemodialysis patients with asymptomatic cardiomyopathy. *Kidney Int* 2000;58(3):1325–1335.

64. Hampl H, Hennig L, Rosenberger C, et al. Optimized heart failure therapy and complete anemia correction on left-ventricular hypertrophy in nondiabetic and diabetic patients undergoing hemodialysis. *Kidney Blood Press Res* 2005;28(5–6):353–362.

65. Hayashi T, Suzuki A, Shoji T, et al. Cardiovascular effect of normalizing the hematocrit level during erythropoietin therapy in predialysis patients with chronic renal failure. *Am J Kidney Dis* 2000;35(2):250–256.

66. Portolés J, Torralbo A, Martin P, et al. Cardiovascular effects of recombinant human erythropoietin in predialysis patients. *Am J Kidney Dis* 1997;29(4):541–548.

67. Roger SD, McMahon LP, Clarkson A, et al. Effects of early and late intervention with epoetin alpha on left ventricular mass among patients with chronic kidney disease (stage 3 or 4): results of a randomized clinical trial. *J Am Soc Nephrol* 2004;15(1):148–156.

68. Parfrey PS, Lauve M, Latremouille-Viau D, et al. Erythropoietin therapy and left ventricular mass index in CKD and ESRD patients: a meta-analysis. *Clin J Am Soc Nephrol* 2009;4(4):755–762.

69. Foley RN, Parfrey PS, Harnett JD, et al. Hypoalbuminemia, cardiac morbidity, and mortality in end-stage renal disease. *J Am Soc Nephrol* 1996;7(5):728–736.

70. Chaignon M, Chen WT, Tarazi RC, et al. Effect of hemodialysis on blood volume distribution and cardiac output. *Hypertension* 1981;3(3):327–332.

71. London GM, Marchais SJ, Guerin AP, et al. Cardiovascular function in hemodialysis patients. *Adv Nephrol Necker Hosp* 1991;20:249–273.

72. Enia G, Mallamaci F, Benedetto FA, et al. Long-term CAPD patients are volume expanded and display more severe left ventricular hypertrophy than hemodialysis patients. *Nephrol Dial Transplant* 2001;16(7):1459–1464.

73. Ganda A, Weiner SD, Chudasama NL, et al. Echocardiographic changes following hemodialysis initiation in patients with advanced chronic

kidney disease and symptomatic heart failure with reduced ejection fraction. *Clin Nephrol* 2012;77(5):366–375.

74. Rostand SG, Drüeke TB. Parathyroid hormone, vitamin D, and cardiovascular disease in chronic renal failure. *Kidney Int* 1999;56(2):383–392.

75. Abdelfatah AB, Motte G, Ducloux D, et al. Determinants of mean arterial pressure and pulse pressure in chronic haemodialysis patients. *J Hum Hypertens* 2001;15(11):775–779.

76. Klassen PS, Lowrie EG, Reddan DN, et al. Association between pulse pressure and mortality in patients undergoing maintenance hemodialysis. *JAMA* 2002;287(12):1548–1555.

77. Block GA, Hulbert-Shearon TE, Levin NW, et al. Association of serum phosphorus and calcium x phosphate product with mortality risk in chronic hemodialysis patients: a national study. *Am J Kidney Dis* 1998;31(4):607–617.

78. Ganesh SK, Stack AG, Levin NW, et al. Association of elevated serum PO(4), Ca x PO(4) product, and parathyroid hormone with cardiac mortality risk in chronic hemodialysis patients. *J Am Soc Nephrol* 2001;12(10):2131–2138.

79. National Kidney Foundation. K/DOQI clinical practice guidelines for bone metabolism and disease in chronic kidney disease. *Am J Kidney Dis* 2003;42(4 Suppl 3):S1–S201.

80. Jamal SA, Vandermeer B, Raggi P, et al. Effect of calcium-based versus non-calcium-based phosphate binders on mortality in patients with chronic kidney disease: an updated systematic review and meta-analysis. *Lancet* 2013;382(9900):1268–1277.

81. Chertow GM, Block GA, Correa-Rotter R, et al. Effect of cinacalcet on cardiovascular disease in patients undergoing dialysis. *N Engl J Med* 2012;367(26):2482–2494.

82. Parfrey PS, Chertow GM, Block GA, et al. The clinical course of treated hyperparathyroidism among patients receiving hemodialysis and the effect of cinacalcet: the EVOLVE trial. *J Clin Endocrinol Metab* 2013;98(12):4834–4844.

83. Thadhani R, Appelbaum E, Pritchett Y, et al. Vitamin D therapy and cardiac structure and function in patients with chronic kidney disease: the PRIMO randomized controlled trial. *JAMA* 2012;307(7):674–684.

84. Raine AE. Acquired aortic stenosis in dialysis patients. *Nephron* 1994;68(2):159–168.

85. Rufino M, García S, Jiménez A, et al. Heart valve calcification and calcium x phosphorus product in hemodialysis patients: analysis of optimum values for its prevention. *Kidney Int* 2003;63(Suppl 85):S115–S118.

86. Leskinen Y, Paana T, Saha H, et al. Valvular calcification and its relationship to atherosclerosis in chronic kidney disease. *J Heart Valve Dis* 2009;18(4):429–438.

87. Chertow GM, Levin NM, Beck GJ, et al. In-center hemodialysis six times per week versus three times per week. *N Engl J Med* 2010;363(24):2287–2300.

88. Eknoyan G, Beck GJ, Cheung AK, et al. Effect of dialysis dose and membrane flux in maintenance hemodialysis. *N Engl J Med* 2002;347(25):2010–2019.

89. Odudu A, Eldehni MT, McCann GP, et al. Randomized controlled trial of individualized dialysate cooling for cardiac protection in hemodialysis patients. *Clin J Am Soc Nephrol* 2015;10(8):1408–1417.

90. Chan CT, Floras JS, Miller JA, et al. Regression of left ventricular hypertrophy after conversion to nocturnal hemodialysis. *Kidney Int* 2002;61(6):2235–2239.

91. Chan C, Floras JS, Miller JA, et al. Improvement in ejection fraction by nocturnal haemodialysis in end-stage renal failure patients with coexisting heart failure. *Nephrol Dial Transplant* 2002;17(8):1518–1521.

92. Parfrey PS, Harnett JD, Foley RN, et al. Impact of renal transplantation on uremic cardiomyopathy. *Transplantation* 1995;60(9):908–914.

93. Cruickshank JM, Lewis J, Moore V, et al. Reversibility of left ventricular hypertrophy by differing types of antihypertensive therapy. *J Hum Hypertens* 1992;6(2):85–90.

94. Garg R, Yusuf S. Overview of randomized trials of angiotensin-converting enzyme inhibitors on mortality and morbidity in patients with heart failure. Collaborative Group on ACE Inhibitor Trials. *JAMA* 1995;273(18):1450–1456.

95. Young JB, Dunlap ME, Pfeffer MA, et al. Mortality and morbidity reduction with Candesartan in patients with chronic heart failure and left ventricular systolic dysfunction: results of the CHARM low-left ventricular ejection fraction trials. *Circulation* 2004;110(17):2618–2626.

96. Cohn JN, Tognoni G. A randomized trial of the angiotensin-receptor blocker valsartan in chronic heart failure. *N Engl J Med* 2001;345(23):1667–1675.

97. Zannad F, Kessler M, Lehert P, et al. Prevention of cardiovascular events in end-stage renal disease: results of a randomized trial of fosinopril and implications for future studies. *Kidney Int* 2006;70(7):1318–1324.

98. Shibasaki Y, Masaki H, Nishiue T, et al. Angiotensin II type 1 receptor antagonist, losartan, causes regression of left ventricular hypertrophy in end-stage renal disease. *Nephron* 2002;90(3):256–261.

99. Suzuki H, Kanno Y, Kaneko K, et al. Comparison of the effects of angiotensin receptor antagonist, angiotensin converting enzyme inhibitor, and their combination on regression of left ventricular hypertrophy of diabetes type 2 patients on recent onset hemodialysis therapy. *Ther Apher Dial* 2004;8(4):320–327.

100. Fried LF, Emanuele N, Zhang JH, et al. Combined angiotensin inhibition for the treatment of diabetic nephropathy. *N Engl J Med* 2013;369(20):1892–1903.

101. Yancy CW, Jessup M, Bozkurt B, et al. 2013 ACCF/AHA guideline for the management of heart failure: a report of the American College of Cardiology Foundation/American Heart Association Task Force on Practice Guidelines. *J Am Coll Cardiol* 2013;62(16):e147–e239.

102. Cardiac Insufficiency Bisoprolol Study II Investigators and Committees. The Cardiac Insufficiency Bisoprolol Study II (CIBIS-II): a randomised trial. *Lancet* 1999;353(9146):9–13.

103. Metoprolol CR/XL Randomised Intervention Trial in Congestive Heart Failure Study Group. Effect of metoprolol CR/XL in chronic heart failure: Metoprolol CR/XL Randomised Intervention Trial in Congestive Heart Failure (MERIT-HF). *Lancet* 1999;353(9169):2001–2007.

104. Hjalmarson A, Goldstein S, Fagerber B, et al. Effects of controlled-release metoprolol on total mortality, hospitalizations, and well-being in patients with heart failure: the Metoprolol CR/XL Randomized Intervention Trial in congestive heart failure (MERIT-HF). MERIT-HF Study Group. *JAMA* 2000;283(10):1295–1302.

105. Packer M, Bristow MR, Cohn JN, et al. The effect of carvedilol on morbidity and mortality in patients with chronic heart failure. U.S. Carvedilol Heart Failure Study Group. *N Engl J Med* 1996;334(21):1349–1355.

106. Cice G, Ferrera L, D'Andrea A, et al. Carvedilol increases two-year survival in dialysis patients with dilated cardiomyopathy: a prospective, placebo-controlled trial. *J Am Coll Cardiol* 2003;41(9):1438–1444.

107. Cice G, Ferrara L, Di Benedetto, et al. Dilated cardiomyopathy in dialysis patients—beneficial effects of carvedilol: a double-blind, placebo-controlled trial. *J Am Coll Cardiol* 2001;37(2):407–411.

108. Agarwal R, Sinha AD, Pappas MK, et al. Hypertension in hemodialysis patients treated with atenolol or lisinopril: a randomized controlled trial. *Nephrol Dial Transplant* 2014;29(3):672–681.

109. Weir MA, Dixon SN, Fleet JL, et al. β-Blocker dialyzability and mortality in older patients receiving hemodialysis. *J Am Soc Nephrol* 2015;26(4):987–996.

110. Beizer JL. Rates of hyperkalemia after publication of the Randomized Aldactone Evaluation Study. *Consult Pharm* 2005;20(2):148–149.

111. Digitalis Investigation Group. The effect of digoxin on mortality and morbidity in patients with heart failure. *N Engl J Med* 1997;336(8):525–533.

112. Young JB, Gheorghiade M, Uretsky BF, et al. Superiority of "triple" drug therapy in heart failure: insights from the PROVED and RADIANCE trials. Prospective Randomized Study of ventricular function and efficacy of digoxin. Randomized assessment of digoxin and inhibitors of angiotensin-converting enzyme. *J Am Coll Cardiol* 1998;32(3):686–692.

113. Shlipak MG, Smith GL, Rathore SS, et al. Renal function, digoxin therapy, and heart failure outcomes: evidence from the digoxin intervention group trial. *J Am Soc Nephrol* 2004;15(8):2195–2203.

114. Kannel WB, Gagnon DR, Cupples LA. Epidemiology of sudden coronary death: population at risk. *Can J Cardiol* 1990;6:439–444.

115. Whitman IR, Feldman HI, Deo R. CKD and sudden cardiac death: epidemiology, mechanisms, and therapeutic approaches. *J Am Soc Nephrol* 2012;23:1929–1939.

116. Shamseddin MK, Parfrey PS. Sudden cardiac death in chronic kidney disease: epidemiology and prevention. *Nat Rev Nephrol* 2011;7: 145–154.

117. Stack AG, Bloembergen WE. Prevalence and clinical correlates of coronary artery disease among new dialysis patients in the United States: a cross-sectional study. *J Am Soc Nephrol* 2001;12(7):1516–1523.

118. Kitano Y, Kasuga H, Watanabe M, et al. Severe coronary stenosis is an important factor for induction and lengthy persistence of ventricular arrhythmias during and after hemodialysis. *Am J Kidney Dis* 2011;44(2):328–336.

119. Blumberg A, Haüsermann M, Strub B, et al. Cardiac arrhythmias in patients on maintenance hemodialysis. *Nephron* 1983;33(2):91–95.

120. D'Elia JA, Weinrauch LA, Gleason RE, et al. Application of the ambulatory 24-hour electrocardiogram in the prediction of cardiac death in dialysis patients. *Arch Intern Med* 1988;148(11):2381–2385.

121. Wizemann V, Kramer W, Thormann J, et al. Cardiac arrhythmias in patients on maintenance hemodialysis: causes and management. *Contrib Nephrol* 1986;52:42–53.

122. Gruppo Emodialisi e Patologie Cardiovasculari. Multicentre, cross-sectional study of ventricular arrhythmias in chronically haemodialysed patients. *Lancet* 1988;2(8606):305–309.

123. Paoletti E, Specchia C, Di Maio G, et al. The worsening of left ventricular hypertrophy is the strongest predictor of sudden cardiac death in haemodialysis patients: a 10 year survey. *Nephrol Dial Transplant* 2004;19(7):1829–1834.

124. Krane V, Winkler K, Drechsler C, et al. Effect of atorvastatin on inflammation and outcome in patients with type 2 diabetes mellitus on hemodialysis. *Kidney Int* 2008;74(11):1461–1467.

125. Burton JO, Korsheed S, Grundy BJ, et al. Hemodialysis-induced left ventricular dysfunction is associated with an increase in ventricular arrhythmias. *Ren Fail* 2008;30(7):701–709.

126. Kimura K, Tabei K, Asano Y, et al. Cardiac arrhythmias in hemodialysis patients. A study of incidence and contributory factors. *Nephron* 1989;53(3):201–207.

127. Karnik JA, Young BS, Lew NL, et al. Cardiac arrest and sudden death in dialysis units. *Kidney Int* 2001;60(1):350–357.

128. Pun PH, Lehrich RW, Honeycutt EF, et al. Modifiable risk factors associated with sudden cardiac arrest within hemodialysis clinics. *Kidney Int* 2011;79:218–227.

129. Niwa A, Taniguchi K, Ito H, et al. Echocardiographic and Holter findings in 321 uremic patients on maintenance hemodialysis. *Jpn Heart J* 1985;26(3): 403–411.

130. Sforzini S, Latini R, Mingardi G, et al. Ventricular arrhythmias and four-year mortality in haemodialysis patients. *Lancet* 1992;339(8787): 212–213.

131. Wizemann V, Kramer W, Funke T, et al. Dialysis-induced cardiac arrhythmias: fact or fiction? Importance of preexisting cardiac disease in the induction of arrhythmias during renal replacement therapy. *Nephron* 1985;39(4):356–360.

132. Quellhorst E, Scheunemann B, Hildebrand U. Hemofiltration—an improved method of treatment for chronic renal failure. *Contrib Nephrol* 1985;44:194–211.

133. Peer G, Korzets A, Hochhauzer E, et al. Cardiac arrhythmia during chronic ambulatory peritoneal dialysis. *Nephron* 1987;45(3):192–195.

134. McLenachan JM, Dargie HJ. Ventricular arrhythmias in hypertensive left ventricular hypertrophy. Relationship to coronary artery disease, left ventricular dysfunction, and myocardial fibrosis. *Am J Hypertens* 1990;3(10):735–740.

135. Canziani ME, Saragoça MA, Draibe SA, et al. Risk factors for the occurrence of cardiac arrhythmias in patients on continuous ambulatory peritoneal dialysis. *Perit Dial Int* 1993;13(Suppl 2):S409–S411.

136. Tzamaloukas AH, Avasthi PS. Temporal profile of serum potassium concentration in nondiabetic and diabetic outpatients on chronic dialysis. *Am J Nephrol* 1987;7(2):101–109.

137. Morrison G, Michelson EL, Brown S, et al. Mechanism and prevention of cardiac arrhythmias in chronic hemodialysis patients. *Kidney Int* 1980;17(6):811–819.

138. Keller F, Weinmann J, Schwarz A, et al. Effect of digitoxin on cardiac arrhythmias in hemodialysis patients. *Klin Wochenschr* 1987;65(22): 1081–1086.

139. Ruskin JN. The cardiac arrhythmia suppression trial (CAST). *N Engl J Med* 1989;321(6):386–388.

140. de Simone G. Left ventricular geometry and hypotension in end-stage renal disease: a mechanical perspective. *J Am Soc Nephrol* 2003;14(10): 2421–2427.

141. Henrich WL. Hemodynamic instability during hemodialysis. *Kidney Int* 1986;30(4):605–612.

142. Keshaviah P, Shapiro FL. A critical examination of dialysis-induced hypotension. *Am J Kidney Dis* 1982;2(2):290–301.

143. Perazella MA. Pharmacologic options available to treat symptomatic intradialytic hypotension. *Am J Kidney Dis* 2001;38(4 Suppl 4):S26–S36.

144. Mann H, Stiller S. Sodium modeling. *Kidney Int Suppl* 2000;76: S79–S88.

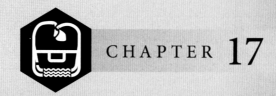

CHAPTER 17

Coronary Artery Disease and Sudden Cardiac Death in Patients with End-Stage Kidney Disease

Wajeh Y. Qunibi, L. Richard A. Lange, and William L. Henrich

The number of patients with end-stage kidney disease (ESKD) who are receiving maintenance dialysis in the United States continues to increase and is now approaching 500,000 (1). Unfortunately, these patients are at considerably higher risk of premature death than the general population. Cardiovascular disease (CVD) is the leading cause of death in dialysis patients, accounting for 42% of deaths; a rate that is 10 to 30 times higher than in patients in the general population (2,3). This relative risk (RR) is remarkably higher in younger dialysis patients, which can be several hundredfold higher than their age-matched counterparts in the general population (FIGURE 17.1) (4). Simply stated, the risk of death in a 30-year-old dialysis patient is similar to that of an 80-year-old patient in the general population. Coronary artery disease (CAD) affects 30% to 60% of patients with ESKD and has been (5–8) documented by angiographic studies in >50% of patients at the initiation of renal replacement therapy (9). Indeed, by the time they begin hemodialysis (HD), 73% of patients with angina and 54% of asymptomatic patients will have CAD (7). Of great concern is the high mortality rate of dialysis patients after a cardiovascular event. Approximately 20% of deaths from CVD have been attributed to acute myocardial infarction (MI) (10). Interestingly, dialysis patients who develop an acute MI are less likely to have ST-segment elevations and are more likely to suffer in-hospital cardiac arrest (11). In-hospital mortality after acute MI among patients on dialysis is approximately 30%; at 1 year, the mortality rate is 60% and at 5 years, the mortality rate increases to 90% (10) (FIGURE 17.2). Moreover, dialysis patients have more than a 10-fold increased risk for CAD-related death per 1,000 person-years than a patient with five Framingham risk factors (12). The large burden of CAD among patients with ESKD prompted the American Heart Association and the National Kidney Foundation to state that individuals with chronic kidney disease (CKD) are members of the "highest risk group" for subsequent cardiovascular events (13,14).

Thus, understanding both the risk factors for CAD as well as the most effective therapeutic modalities are critically important in reducing the burden and consequences of CAD in dialysis patients.

Some of the factors that contribute to the high prevalence of CAD in patients with ESKD include advancing age and diabetes. The average age of dialysis patients has increased steadily over the past two decades, such that currently their median age is 65 years (1). This older age group has the highest rate of cardiovascular-related deaths in the ESKD population (15). At the same time, even young HD patients have a high prevalence of CVD death: Among ESKD subjects aged 20 to 44 years, the incidence of CVD death is roughly 40 per 1,000 patient-years (15,16). Interestingly, the percentage of deaths that are cardiovascular in cause is similar in all age groups with ESKD (16), leading some investigators to suggest that atherosclerosis may be accelerated in this patient population (17). Also, diabetes mellitus is the leading cause of ESKD in the United States (1). CVD accounts for almost 75% of deaths of patients with diabetes, almost entirely as a result of CAD (18). In a recent study of new diabetic dialysis patients without cardiac symptoms or a known cardiac history, significant CAD was present in 83% (9). In many patients with diabetes mellitus and resultant ESKD, atherosclerosis is well established by the time dialysis is initiated so that many of them manifest ischemic heart disease (IHD), peripheral vascular disease, ischemic bowel disease, or cerebrovascular events shortly after dialysis is begun (19). Not surprisingly, therefore, diabetic patients with ESKD have an extremely high risk for cardiac death.

PATHOGENESIS OF ATHEROSCLEROSIS IN PATIENTS WITH END-STAGE KIDNEY DISEASE

The hypothesis that ESKD, in some way, might cause accelerated atherosclerosis was proposed more than 30 years ago by Lindner et al. (17) who reported a high incidence of MI in the Seattle

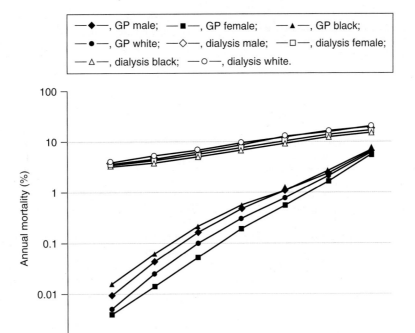

FIGURE 17.1 Cardiovascular mortality in general population [National Center for Health Statistics (NCHS)] compared to dialysis population [United States Renal Data System (USRDS)]. Data stratified by age, gender, and race. (Reprinted with permission from Foley RN, Parfrey PS, Sarnak MJ. Clinical epidemiology of cardiovascular disease in chronic renal disease. *Am J Kidney Dis* 1998;32:S112–S119.)

dialysis population. Of their 39 subjects undergoing HD for an average of 6.5 years, 23 (59%) died, 14 of which were attributed to complications of atherosclerosis (MI in 8, cerebrovascular accident in 3, and refractory congestive heart failure in 3). The incidence of these complications was several times higher than that noted in normal and hypertensive patients of similar age without ESKD.

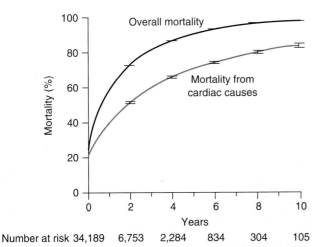

FIGURE 17.2 Estimated cumulative mortality after myocardial infarction among dialysis patients. (Reprinted with permission from Herzog CA, Ma JZ, Collins AJ. Poor long-term survival after acute myocardial infarction among patients on long-term dialysis. *N Engl J Med* 1998;339:799–805.)

Subsequent postmortem (20) and angiographic (21,22) studies confirmed that the prevalence of atherosclerotic CAD is increased in dialysis patients when compared with age-matched individuals with normal renal function. For example, in a postmortem examination of dialysis patients, Ansari et al. (20) found >50% luminal diameter narrowing of at least one epicardial coronary artery in 60% and at least some degree of atherosclerotic CAD in 86%.

Subsequent studies have shown that the high prevalence of atherosclerosis among patients on maintenance dialysis is the result of the high prevalence of both "traditional" and uremia-related risk factors (**TABLE 17.1**). Whether maintenance HD in itself promotes progression of atherosclerosis (due, e.g., to exposure to bioincompatible dialysis membranes and/or contaminated dialysis fluids) remains unclear. Long-term studies have shown no correlation between the duration of dialysis and the occurrence of cardiac events, a relation that might be expected if, in fact, dialysis itself promotes atherogenesis (23,24). Dialysis patients have a high prevalence of many of the Framingham risk factors for CAD. A cross-sectional comparison of 1,041 dialysis patients with the general population (via the National Health and Nutrition Examination Survey database) found a high prevalence of hypertension (96%), limited physical activity (80%), diabetes mellitus (54%), hypertriglyceridemia (36%), and electrocardiographic evidence of left ventricular hypertrophy (LVH) (22%) in those with ESKD (25). Even after adjusting for race, gender, and atherosclerotic vascular disease, these factors remained more common in ESKD patients (25). Apart from the increased prevalence of these "traditional" risk factors in patients with CKD (26,27), several uremia-related risk factors are thought to contribute to CAD in these patients (**TABLE 17.1**),

TABLE 17.1 Risk Factors for Cardiovascular Disease in Patients with End-Stage Renal Dysfunction	
Traditional CAD Risk Factors	**Uremia-Related Risk Factors**
• Older age • Male gender • Hypertension • Diabetes • Smoking • High serum LDL cholesterol • Low serum HDL cholesterol • Physical inactivity • Family history of premature coronary artery disease	• Uremic serum • Hyperphosphatemia • Calcium load • Elevated serum PTH levels • Dialysis vintage • Hyperhomocysteinemia • Anemia • Malnutrition • Chronic inflammation • Oxidative stress • Sympathetic overactivity • Increased asymmetric dimethylarginine (ADMA)

CAD, coronary artery disease; LDL, low-density lipoprotein; HDL, high-density lipoprotein; PTH, parathyroid hormone.
Reproduced with permission from Murphy SW, Parfrey PS. Screening for cardiovascular disease in dialysis patients. *Curr Opin Neph Hypert* 1996;5:532–540.

including hyperphosphatemia, oxidative stress, inflammation, and hyperhomocysteinemia. Finally, newly discovered risk factors for atherosclerosis in patients with ESKD may contribute, such as the accumulation of the endogenous inhibitor of nitric oxide (NO) synthase, asymmetric dimethylarginine (ADMA), which results in reduced NO synthesis (28,29).

An increased prevalence of atherosclerotic CAD is progressive over a range of reduced glomerular filtration rates (GFRs) even before the initiation of dialysis (30–33). In a landmark study of >1 million subjects, Go et al. (30) showed that the age-adjusted rate of cardiovascular events (i.e., MI, stroke, heart failure, and peripheral arterial disease) increased markedly below an estimated GFR of 60 mL/min/1.73 m². After adjustment for a variety of potentially confounding variables, a lower estimated GFR persisted as a graded, independent predictor of adverse outcomes, and this association was robust in those with or without diabetes. CKD patients with known CAD are at the highest risk for subsequent cardiovascular complications and death, with nearly 46% of subjects with an estimated GFR <45 mL/min/1.73 m² dead within 3 years of follow-up (31). In angiographic studies, patients with CKD were more likely to have severe three-vessel disease and left main disease as estimated GFR decreases (34,35). These findings may explain the high early risk of acute MI after the initiation of dialysis; in one study, 29% of infarctions occur within 1 year and 52% within 2 years of dialysis initiation (10).

 RISK FACTORS FOR ATHEROSCLEROSIS IN PATIENTS WITH END-STAGE KIDNEY DISEASE

The Role of Traditional Risk Factors for Coronary Artery Disease

The Choices for Healthy Outcomes in Caring for ESRD (CHOICE) study reported a prevalence of traditional risk factors for atherosclerotic CVD in incident dialysis patients (25). This population,

which was more likely to be older, African American, and male than the general United States adult population, had a high prevalence of hypertension (96%), low physical activity (80%), diabetes (54%), hypertriglyceridemia (36%), low high-density lipoprotein (HDL) cholesterol (33%), and LVH by electrocardiogram (ECG) criteria (22%). A high proportion of dialysis patients have multiple traditional risk factors such as older age, hypertension, and diabetes (36). Also, smoking seems to be more prevalent in dialysis patients with CAD than those without CAD (37,38).

Hypertension

Hypertension, defined as 1-week average predialysis systolic blood pressure (BP) measurements >150 mm Hg or diastolic BP >85 mm Hg or the use of antihypertensive medications, was documented in 86% of clinically stable adult HD patients (39). Among HD patients who were hypertensive, 58% were treated but had uncontrolled BP and only 30% had controlled BP (40,41). The independent determinants of poor control of BP were the use of antihypertensive drugs and an expanded extracellular volume state (42). It has been suggested that hypertension may be better controlled in peritoneal dialysis patients than in those on HD (43–45). However, 44-hour ambulatory BP monitoring showed no differences in daytime and nighttime BP (46). Hypertension is believed to be the predominant risk factor for atherosclerosis in this patient population (47–50). Hypertension in most dialysis patients is systolic (due to arterial stiffness), although an increased pulse pressure (also a reflection of arterial stiffness) is common in these subjects as well. Systolic pressure is more strongly associated with an increased risk of cardiovascular death than either pulse or diastolic pressures in this patient population (51). Interestingly, a U-shaped relation between systolic pressure and mortality is present in dialysis subjects, in that both lower and higher levels are associated with an increased mortality (**FIGURE 17.3**) (3,52).

Hypertension is usually present for years during the course of CKD before dialysis is initiated. Despite aggressive dialysis and antihypertensive therapy, BP is poorly controlled in about half of ESKD patients. The long duration of poorly controlled hypertension is an important contributor to the increased risk of CAD (53). The increased tensile and sheer stresses caused by hypertension induce endothelial cell injury and activation. This, in turn, is followed by secretion of vasoactive and growth-regulating factors which can elicit a series of cellular interactions that culminate in the appearance and progression of atherosclerosis (54). Aside from its role as a major risk factor for atherosclerosis, poorly controlled hypertension is associated with an increased likelihood of complex ventricular arrhythmias (55–57), and the hypertension-induced increase in left ventricular mass increases the morbidity and mortality of these arrhythmias, should they occur (57–59). Not surprisingly, a reduction of left ventricular mass (e.g., accomplished through an increase in hematocrit, effective antihypertensive therapy, sympathetic nervous system blockade, or improved control of intravascular volume) is associated with a reduced morbidity and mortality in ESKD patients (60–62). Interestingly, conversion from conventional to nocturnal daily dialysis has been reported to induce regression of LVH (63).

Diabetes Mellitus

Diabetes mellitus affects >11% of the adult population in the United States, and its prevalence continues to increase (64). Moreover, diabetes is associated with increased risk of CVD morbidity

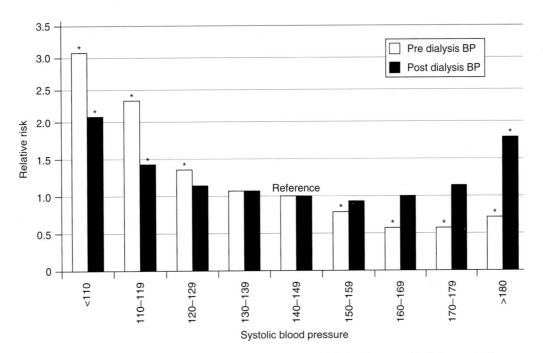

FIGURE 17.3 Mortality risk versus systolic blood pressure (BP) in hemodialysis patients. Asterisk (*) denotes significance. (Adapted with permission from Sarnak MJ, Levey AS, Schoolwerth AC, et al. Kidney disease as a risk factor for development of cardiovascular disease: a statement from the American Heart Association Councils on Kidney in Cardiovascular Disease, High Blood Pressure Research, Clinical Cardiology, and epidemiology and Prevention. *Circulation* 2003;108;2154–2169; and Zager PG, Nikolic J, Brown RH, et al. "U" curve association of blood pressure and mortality in hemodialysis patients. Medical Directors of Dialysis Clinic, Inc. *Kidney Int* 1998;54:561–569.)

and mortality in the general population (65,66). Diabetes mellitus is also the leading cause of ESKD in the United States, accounting for nearly 40% of cases (1). In dialysis patients, the presence of diabetes is an independent risk factor for IHD, heart failure, and all-cause mortality (1,26). The incidence of CAD in diabetic patients with nephropathy is 8 to 15 times higher than in diabetics without nephropathy (49,67). Furthermore, diabetic patients with ESKD have a cardiovascular mortality twice that of age-matched nondiabetic patients. In patients with diabetes mellitus in whom coronary angiography is performed routinely as a prelude to renal transplantation, significant CAD is noted in 25% to 50% (21,22,68). The prevalence of CAD in diabetic patients awaiting renal transplantation is particularly high in those older than 45 years (69). Moreover, these patients have worse long-term outcomes after coronary interventions than nondiabetic patients (70,71).

Although virtually all studies of CAD have defined "significant" coronary atherosclerosis as a luminal diameter narrowing >50% to 70%, the extent of luminal diameter narrowing and the occurrence of acute coronary events (unstable angina pectoris, MI, or sudden cardiac death) are not tightly coupled. Ambrose et al. (72) and Little et al. (73) showed that the extent of atherosclerotic coronary arterial narrowing often does not predict the risk of total or subtotal thrombotic coronary arterial occlusion, in that many acute ischemic events are caused by thrombotic occlusion of a coronary artery without a significant stenosis.

Glycemic control improves survival in diabetic patients on HD (74,75). Two studies in Japanese diabetic dialysis patients reported a higher risk of death in those with worse glycemic control (76,77). Furthermore, even mild degrees of hyperglycemia in nondiabetic dialysis populations are associated with reduced survival (78). In

short, effective glycemic control in dialysis patients is an important determinant of survival. The hemoglobin A1c assay (HbA1c) is the gold standard test for monitoring glycemic control in patients with diabetes mellitus. Unfortunately, its measurements may not be as reliable in ESKD subjects as in the general population. HbA1c levels may be falsely elevated or decreased in patients with ESKD. This may be due to a number of factors that contribute to shortened red blood cell survival such as uremia, recent transfusion, iron deficiency, erythropoietin-induced accelerated erythropoiesis, and metabolic acidosis. Moreover, the decreased time for glucose and erythrocytes to interact in patients with ESKD leads to lower HbA1c levels for any given level of glycemia compared to those with normal kidney function (79). In some assays such as agar gel electrophoresis, analytical interference from carbamylated hemoglobin formed in the presence of elevated concentrations of urea may lead to false elevations in the HbA1c level. By contrast, the Boronate-agarose affinity chromatography (80–82) and the thiobarbituric acid method (82,83) are more reliable in measuring HbA1c in patients with ESKD. However, other studies have reported that HbA1c significantly underestimates glycemic control in diabetic dialysis patients, whereas those of glycated albumin more accurately reflect this control (84). As a result, glycated albumin may be a more robust indicator of long-term glycemia than HbA1c in HD patients (84). Recent studies have shown that glycated albumin levels more accurately predict hospitalizations and patient survival in ESKD than HbA1c (85,86).

Hyperlipidemia

Dyslipidemia, defined as increased levels of serum cholesterol and triglycerides, is a well-established traditional risk factor for CAD

TABLE 17.2	Lists the Various Lipid Abnormalities in Nondialyzed Chronic Kidney Disease Patients and Dialysis Patients		
	CKD Stages 1–4	**Hemodialysis Patients**	**Peritoneal Dialysis Patients**
Triglycerides	Normal or high	High	Very high
Total cholesterol	High, normal, or low	Normal, low, or rarely high	Commonly high
LDL-cholesterol	High, normal or low	Normal, low or rarely high	Commonly high
HDL-cholesterol	Normal or low	Low	Low
VLDL	High	High	High
Small dense LDL-cholesterol	High	High	High
IDL cholesterol	High	High	High
Lp(a)	High	High	High

CKD, chronic kidney disease; LDL, low-density lipoprotein; HDL, high-density lipoprotein; VLDL, very low-density lipoprotein; IDL, intermediate dense lipoprotein; Lp(a), lipoprotein(a).

Reproduced with permission from Qunibi WY. Dyslipidemia in dialysis patients. *Semin Dial* 2015;28:345–353.

in the general population and in patients with mild to moderate CKD particularly those with nephrotic-range proteinuria (87). The pathogenic role of serum cholesterol as a risk factor in atherosclerotic CVD was confirmed by several randomized clinical trials which demonstrated that reductions in total and low-density lipoprotein (LDL) cholesterol levels, primarily with statins, is effective in reducing coronary artery events and mortality (88–91). Clinical trials have also shown that lipid-lowering therapy is effective in reducing the risk of atherosclerotic cardiovascular events in the nondialyzed CKD population (92,93). Serum lipid abnormalities are frequent in dialysis patients and are considered a major risk for CAD (87,94). These are characterized most often by elevated serum triglycerides and triglyceride-rich lipoproteins—such as very low-density lipoprotein (VLDL)—as well as low HDL cholesterol (**TABLE 17.2**) (87,95–99). The prevalence of dyslipidemia (defined as the presence of at least one abnormal lipid variable) in ESKD patients is approximately 67% (96). Peritoneal dialysis appears to be associated with a somewhat more atherogenic lipid profile than HD (96). The cause of kidney disease does not appear to influence the specific lipid abnormalities that are seen. The most common pattern, seen in 50% to 75% of patients on HD, is an elevated serum triglyceride concentration in conjunction with a normal LDL cholesterol concentration (87,95–99). This pattern is caused by diminished removal of triglyceride from the serum due to an acquired deficiency of lipoprotein lipase and hepatic triglyceride lipase. Apoprotein (apo) CII, an activator of lipoprotein lipase, is reduced in ESKD patients, whereas apo CIII, an inhibitor of lipoprotein lipase, is increased (24,97). The serum concentration of HDL is reduced substantially in many subjects with ESKD, probably because of a reduction in its synthesis and turnover (**TABLE 17.2**) (87,95,98,99). Rapoport et al. (98), for example, reported that dialysis patients had an average serum HDL cholesterol concentration of only 26 mg/dL, substantially lower than the average of 52 mg/dL in normal individuals.

Because hypertriglyceridemia is only weakly associated with CAD in patients with ESKD, it is likely that other more complex lipid abnormalities are important in promoting atherogenesis in these patients (87,97,100–102). Deficiencies of lipoprotein lipase and hepatic triglyceride lipase delay hydrolysis of triglycerides, allowing intestinal and hepatic triglyceride remnants to accumulate, thereby enriching the triglyceride content of VLDL, intermediate-density lipoprotein (IDL), and LDL cholesterol (**TABLE 17.2**) (102). Apo

A-IV and apo B-48, absent in the serum of normal individuals during fasting, are present in patients with ESKD (102), and prolonged exposure of vascular endothelium to these remnant lipoproteins may promote atherogenesis (101,102). The cholesterol content of VLDL is increased and that of HDL is decreased in patients with ESKD (95,97). This cholesterol-enriched form of VLDL, termed β-VLDL (because of its electrophoretic properties), may be more atherogenic than VLDL (**TABLE 17.2**). In addition, the apo E content of VLDL is increased in patients with ESKD, and this may allow VLDL to interact with LDL at apo B and apo E receptors (97). Finally, lipoprotein (a) [Lp(a)] concentrations are increased in patients with ESKD, independent of the cause of kidney disease (103). All these factors, combined with the decreased antiatherogenic defense mechanisms that accompany a decreased HDL, likely contribute to the development of atherosclerosis.

In patients with early stages of CKD, dyslipidemia contributes significantly to the pathogenesis of atherosclerotic CAD (14,94). This process was thought to be accelerated in HD patients as was initially described by Lindner et al. (17) in 1974. Subsequently, Lowrie and Lew (104) reported a U-shaped relationship between serum total cholesterol level and the risk for all-cause mortality in dialysis patients. Other large observational studies have confirmed the negative relationship between low serum total or LDL cholesterol and CVD in dialysis (105) and nondialyzed CKD patients (106). In one study, serum LDL cholesterol <70 mg/dL was strongly associated with all-cause mortality risk, but black patients displayed a more conventional association between high LDL cholesterol and increased death risk (105). The high risk associated with low cholesterol level was attributed to malnutrition-inflammation complex. To clarify this relationship further, Liu et al. (107) reported that hypercholesterolemia is an independent risk factor for all-cause and CVD mortality in a subgroup of ESKD patients without serologic evidence of inflammation or malnutrition. Given that statins reduce inflammation in addition to cholesterol level, these authors stated that their findings support the use of statins in preventing CVD in dialysis patients.

Oxidative Stress

The association between oxidative stress and atherosclerosis was recognized by Glavind et al. (108) in 1952. Since then, increased production of reactive oxygen species (ROS) in the vascular wall has been recognized as a characteristic feature of atherosclerosis (109).

This entity results from an imbalance between reactive oxygen and nitrogen species production and antioxidant defense mechanisms. Oxidative stress with or without endothelial dysfunction occurs commonly in dialysis patients and is thought to contribute to the pathogenesis of CVD (110–112). There has been mounting evidence that ESKD is associated with increased oxidation and impaired antioxidation systems (111–117). Oxidative stress may contribute to atherogenesis by multiple mechanisms that may or may not be linked to LDL oxidation (118) since ROS may mediate pathologic processes in the endothelium, smooth muscle cells, and inflammatory cells. Free oxygen radicals can rapidly react with and inactivate NO and enhance proatherogenic factors, such as leukocyte adherence to the endothelium, impaired vasorelaxation, and platelet aggregation (118).

Exogenous factors may contribute to the increased oxidant activity noted in ESKD patients. The use of incompatible dialysis membranes (cellulosic) may dramatically increase H_2O_2 release from activated granulocytes (119). This increase in ROS and activated neutrophils in close proximity to endothelial cells may contribute to endothelial cell injury. The chronic, cumulative exposure to cellulosic membranes may augment lipid peroxidation, thereby contributing to the generation of oxidized LDL (117,120). The use of cellulosic membranes may lead to an increased production of ROS by complement-dependent and complement-independent processes (119,121). In addition to the role of exogenous factors, a reduced concentration of endogenous antioxidants, such as vitamins C and E, has been reported in HD patients (122,123).

On the other hand, the antioxidant activity is significantly improved with HD to a level comparable to that of healthy controls, as shown by Nagasi et al. (121). In short, ESKD patients manifest diminished oxygen-scavenging activity, which is improved with dialysis. Some studies have shown a decrease in fatal cardiac events in nonkidney disease patients who consume large amounts of β-carotene or vitamin E (124,125). However, prospective, randomized trials in patients with ESKD have not observed a reduction in the incidence of fatal cardiac events with antioxidant dietary supplementation (126). Nonetheless, vitamin E may slow the progression of atherosclerosis in ESKD patients (127), and endothelium-dependent vasoreactivity may be improved by the combination of antioxidant and lipid-lowering therapy (128,129). In this regard, two randomized trials of antioxidants (N-acetylcysteine and vitamin E) in HD patients reported a decreased risk of cardiovascular events in patients randomized to the antioxidant arm (130,131). Given the small sample size of these studies, further trials are clearly required to confirm their results.

Advanced Glycosylation End Products

Advanced glycosylation end products (AGEs) are formed by a series of complex nonenzymatic reactions between glucose and the amino groups of proteins, peptides, and amino acids. Their serum concentrations are increased up to 10-fold in ESKD patients when compared to healthy subjects. They are not removed by dialysis (132–134). The levels of AGEs in nondiabetic patients undergoing dialysis may be even higher than diabetic nonuremic patients not requiring dialysis. This increase in AGEs levels is due to both an increase in AGE synthesis by oxidative or carbonyl stress and a decrease in AGE excretion by the kidney and the dialyzer (133). Strong evidence exists to suggest a role for AGE compounds in most diabetic vascular complications (134). In this regard, high levels of AGEs can inhibit the production of NO, thereby diminishing

vasodilation (134,135). This may result in an increase in BP as well as an increased risk of stroke and ischemic cardiac events.

Advanced glycation end product moieties may also modify lipid biomolecules, particularly LDL cholesterol, which contributes to the development of atherosclerosis (136). On the basis of data from experimental animals, Palinski et al. (137) suggested that AGEs are present in atherosclerotic lesions. Through all these mechanisms, it seems plausible that AGEs may potentiate atherosclerosis in ESKD patients (138). By contributing to the increased oxidative stress that exists in patients with ESKD, AGEs may contribute to the excessive CVD seen in this patient population. In this regard, tissue accumulation of AGEs, as estimated by skin autofluorescence, has been implicated as a risk predictor for cardiovascular mortality in patients with ESKD (139,140). In contrast, the relationship between serum AGEs and mortality in HD patients remains controversial with some studies reporting a strong relationship between serum AGEs levels and survival (141,142), whereas others did not (139,143,144).

Oxidized Low-Density Lipoproteins

As stated previously, dialysis patients are exposed to enhanced oxidative stress initiated by the generation of oxygen free radicals. Oxidation of LDL occurs *in vivo* and contributes to the development of atherosclerosis by causing endothelial cell injury and apoptosis (145). Cellular lipoxygenase and ROS are believed to induce LDL oxidation (146,147), which leads to a chemical rearrangement of fatty acid structure and subsequent fragmentation, resulting in aldehyde and ketone formation. These alterations favor the recognition of oxidized LDL by monocytes, which act as scavengers in the subendothelial space. Scavenger cells that take up oxidized LDL gradually become cholesterol enriched and form foam cells, the initial "building blocks" of atherosclerosis (148). Leukocyte-endothelial cell interaction further promotes the process of atherosclerosis by potentiating monocyte chemotaxis. In addition, oxidized LDL directly damages endothelial cells (137,149). One intriguing observation is that LDL oxidation can occur *in vivo* and generate antigenic epitopes (149), leading Salonen et al. (150) to propose that autoantibody formation against oxidized LDL may contribute to the progression of atherosclerosis. Other reactions, such as the carbamylation of LDL, may contribute to altered LDL clearance and influence the scavenger pathway in ESKD patients. An elevated urea nitrogen concentration can trigger condensation of cyanate with lipoprotein lysine residues, leading to reduced clearance and increased pathogenicity (151).

Oxidized LDL is present in chronic dialysis patients, and ESKD patients have an increase in plasma lipid peroxidation products (152–154). In fact, oxidized LDL is more than eightfold higher in chronic dialysis patients when compared with controls (155). In short, ESKD patients on dialysis have increased concentrations of oxidized LDL, which play an important role in accelerated atherogenesis.

Lipoprotein(a)

In CKD, there is accumulation of highly atherogenic lipoproteins such as chylomicron remnants, IDLs, oxidized LDL, small dense-LDL (sd-LDL), and Lp(a) (95). Lp(a) is an LDL-like lipoprotein consisting of apolipoprotein (a) that is covalently bound to an LDL particle. Lp(a) has been linked to atherogenesis in the general population and in ESKD patients (156). In patients with CKD, plasma Lp(a) levels are significantly influenced by the GFR. In patients with large (but not small) apo(a) isoforms, plasma Lp(a) levels begin to rise early in the course of kidney disease (157). This isoform-specific increase in plasma Lp(a) levels has also been observed in HD patients (158). Concomitant malnutrition and inflammation have been associated with high plasma Lp(a) levels in HD patients (159). Its atherogenicity may be related to its binding of apolipoprotein B and subsequent uptake by macrophages, forming foam cells. Lp(a) accumulates in atherosclerotic plaque, after which it undergoes further alterations, including oxidation, which may contribute to its atherogenicity (156). In addition, Lp(a) inhibits plasminogen activation and may stimulate vascular smooth muscle proliferation, each of which may further enhance atherosclerotic plaque formation (160). Lp(a) serum concentrations are typically two to three times higher in ESKD patients than in healthy controls (157,158), resulting largely from a decreased renal catabolism of Lp(a). Certain Lp(a) phenotypes may be particularly atherogenic, for example, the low molecular weight phenotype of Lp(a) may increase the risk of atherosclerosis in ESKD patients. Following successful renal transplantation, the plasma Lp(a) concentration decreases in HD patients with large apo(a) isoforms (161).

Malnutrition–Inflammation Complex Syndrome

Protein-energy malnutrition and inflammation, known as *malnutrition–inflammation complex syndrome* (MICS), have been implicated as a powerful predictor of death in dialysis patients (162,163). Hypoalbuminemia, a reliable indicator of the presence of MICS, is common in dialysis patients and correlates strongly with a poor outcome, including cardiovascular death (163). In one study, an increase in serum albumin above 3.8 g/dL was associated with improved survival, whereas a falling serum albumin over time correlated with increased cardiovascular death independent of demographic, clinical, or other laboratory variables (164). Malnutrition may contribute to atherosclerosis, in that an inverse relation between low serum albumin and elevated Lp(a) concentrations is present in chronic dialysis patients (159). Whether vascular reactivity is altered by poor nutrition is unknown, but Ritz et al. (165) suggested that malnourished patients have diminished NO production. Although the mechanisms underlying the increased CVD risk of hypoalbuminemia are unclear, it is possible that albumin may act as an oxidative product scavenger so that hypoalbuminemia renders the patient more vulnerable to atherogenesis. In diabetic subjects with ESKD, Koch et al. (166) demonstrated an association between lower skin fold thickness and mortality. Moreover, a low baseline body fat percentage and fat loss over time are independently associated with a higher mortality in dialysis patients even after adjustment for demographics and surrogates of muscle mass and inflammation (167). Also, inflammation is associated with an enhanced cardiovascular risk profile and an increased cardiovascular mortality in HD patients. Inflammation plays a key role in CAD and other manifestations of atherosclerosis (168). A number of plasma markers of inflammation such as high-sensitivity C-reactive protein (hs-CRP), serum amyloid A, and cytokines such as interleukin-6 (IL-6) and soluble intercellular adhesion molecule type 1 have been advocated as potential tools for predicting the risk of CAD events (169). Approximately half of HD patients exhibit an activated acute phase response characterized by increased concentrations of CRP and serum amyloid A (167). In addition, several changes in the atherogenic risk profile in HD patients, such as elevated Lp(a) and fibrinogen levels as well as decreased HDL cholesterol and apo A-I concentrations, are due, at least in part, to an activated acute phase response (170). Finally, the plasma IL-6 concentration, the major

mediator of the acute phase response, is elevated in ESKD patients and is considered to be a strong predictor of clinical outcome. Although hypertension, adiposity, insulin resistance, fluid overload, and persistent infections can be associated with elevated IL-6 levels, factors related to the dialysis procedure, such as bioincompatibility of dialyzer membranes and dialysis solutions, also may stimulate its production (171).

Role of Nontraditional Risk Factors for Coronary Artery Disease

Evidence from recent studies suggests that the underlying pathophysiology of CAD is different in patients with CKD when compared to the general population (172). A recent postmortem analysis of CAD showed that the ESKD group had significantly increased coronary arterial medial thickness, higher degree of plaque calcification, and reduced vessel lumen compared with CAD patients and normal renal function (173). Of interest, this study also reported that the frequency of both advanced atherosclerotic lesions and calcified lesions increased as the estimated glomerular filtration rate (eGFR) decreased. In another study that used intravascular ultrasound, which can detect coronary plaque composition, the eGFR was significantly associated with an increase in the percentage of lipid volume and a decrease in the percentage of fibrous volume in coronary lesions with mild to moderate stenosis: a change in composition that may contribute to coronary plaque vulnerability (174). Even after adjustment for coronary risk factors, a low eGFR was independently associated with this shift in coronary plaque composition. Thus, it appears that CKD may independently exacerbate the effects of other conventional CVD risk factors such as hypertension or anemia (175).

Cardiovascular Calcification

The Work Group of the Kidney Disease: Improving Global Outcomes (KDIGO) included cardiovascular calcification in the newly described systemic disorder "chronic kidney disease-mineral and bone disorder (CKD-MBD)" that occurs as a result of CKD (176). The kidney plays a central role in regulating mineral metabolism. Disturbances in mineral metabolism may occur in the course of CKD because of the inability of the failing kidneys to maintain the levels of serum phosphorus and calcium in the normal range. Vascular calcification develops early, and its prevalence increases as the GFR declines such that approximately 80% of incident dialysis patients have evidence of coronary artery calcification (CAC) (177–181) (see Chapter 24 on CKD-MBD).

Vascular calcification results from abnormal deposition of calcium phosphate salts into the vascular wall. This process, which affects coronary arteries and peripheral vessels, may also affect other cardiac structures including the cardiac valves and aorta. Vessels from healthy subjects do not usually calcify even after long-term exposure to supraphysiologic levels of phosphate and/or calcium *in vitro*, whereas vessels from subjects with CKD and dialysis calcify (182). However, calcification starts as early as CKD stage 2, as shown in an animal model of CKD (183) and accelerates with progressive loss of GFR particularly in patients with ESKD who are receiving dialysis. Vascular calcification in patients with CKD can be atherosclerotic, affecting the intima or medial with calcium phosphate deposition in the media of the vessel wall. It has been argued that medial calcification is a manifestation of accelerated atherosclerosis in patients with CKD (184). However, others argue that atherosclerotic and medial calcification are two distinct entities, with the latter developing more commonly in patients with CKD particularly those with diabetes mellitus (185). Clearly, both forms of calcification can occur concomitantly in patients with CKD.

Vascular calcification in patients with CKD was initially believed to be a passive, physicochemical process in which serum phosphate and calcium are deposited in the arterial wall. However, we now know that vascular calcification is an active, cell-mediated, and highly regulated process similar to bone formation with vascular smooth muscle cells (VSMC) playing a critical role. Just as in bone formation, vascular calcification results from either an imbalance between factors that promote calcification and those that act to inhibit calcification (177,179,186). Incubation of human aortic smooth muscle cells in high phosphate or calcium medium directly induces transformation of VSMC to an osteoblast-like cell (182). It is likely that calcium and phosphate have synergistic procalcification effects (187). Transformed VSMCs lose their contractile function and behave like bone-forming cells that lay down a collagen-1 rich extracellular matrix and form matrix vesicles rich in calcium and phosphate that pinch off from the plasma membrane and interact with the extracellular matrix. These vesicles are capable of initiating mineralization of the vascular wall just as they do so in bone (186). Increased calcium levels promote calcification further by inducing apoptosis of VSMC (182,188,189). Both matrix vesicles and apoptotic bodies serve as nucleation sites for hydroxyapatite, particularly in the presence of low calcification inhibitors such as matrix-Gla protein (MGP) and fetuin-A. Thus, unlike vessels from healthy individuals, vessels from predialysis and, to a much greater extent, dialysis patients have been primed to calcify (182). Susceptibility to calcification in CKD may be related both to a decrease in matrix vesicle calcification inhibitors such as fetuin-A and MGP and to degradation of the extracellular matrix by matrix metalloproteases (MMP), such as MMP-2 and MMP-9, which are upregulated in the arterial wall in CKD patients (186). The latter leads to overexpression of transforming growth factor (TGF)-β, which is thought to be involved in osteoblast differentiation and in enhancing VSMC calcification and arterial stiffness (186).

The cause of accelerated calcification in patients with ESKD is multifactorial and includes both the traditional CVD risk factors and uremia-related risk factors (177) (**Table 17.1**). High serum phosphate, even within the normal range, is associated with a greater risk of coronary calcification and cardiovascular mortality in patients with CKD (190,191). However, recent *in vitro* studies found calcium to be a stronger procalcification factor than phosphate. In one study in which arterial rings obtained during abdominal surgery from children with normal renal function, those with impaired renal function, and from those on dialysis were exposed to high phosphate or calcium media, calcium-induced calcification more potently than phosphate, but only in rings from patients with CKD or those on dialysis (182). This suggests that VSMC from healthy vessels have effective inhibitory mechanisms that prevent calcification, while those from subjects with CKD, particularly dialysis patients, become susceptible to calcification. Also, both high and low parathyroid hormone levels may increase the risk of vascular calcification (192). Some studies reported an independent association between circulating fibroblast growth factor (FGF)-23 levels with the progression of coronary calcifications (193,194), but more recent data indicate that FGF-23 is not involved in vascular calcification (195). On the other hand, klotho deficiency is a well-recognized factor in this process (196).

One of the factors that was suspected of enhancing vascular calcification in general, and CAC in particular, in dialysis and CKD

patients is the calcium load provided from use of calcium-based phosphate binders (CBPBs). While a number of clinical trials (197–199), epidemiologic studies (200,201), and meta-analysis (202) have shown increased risk of all-cause mortality or progression of cardiovascular calcification in CKD patients treated with CBPB, other clinical trials (203,204), epidemiologic studies (205), and meta-analysis (206) did not show a difference between calcium-based and non-CBPBs. In fact, a recent randomized, placebo-controlled pilot clinical trial by Block et al. (207) showed that therapy with both noncalcium and CBPBs resulted in progression of vascular calcification, albeit to a lesser degree in noncalcium phosphate binders. Thus, the effect of calcium load from use of CBPB on progression of cardiovascular calcification, while plausible, remains controversial (208). An important issue that needs to be investigated is whether slowing vascular calcification by any means, including phosphate binders, will translate into improvements in clinical outcomes. Two epidemiologic studies have in fact reported that use of any type of phosphate binder, possibly with the exception of aluminum-based binders, is independently associated with improved survival in dialysis patients compared with no use of binder at all (209,210). A third study in an incident United States Renal Data System (USRDS) cohort that started dialysis in 1996 to 1997, when only CBPBs were used in the United States, found no association between the use of these agents and mortality (211). The KDIGO work group stated that there were inconclusive data to indicate that any one binder has beneficial effects on mortality or other patient-centered outcomes when compared with any other binder (176). However, in patients with CKD stages 3 to 5D, the work group recommends restricting the dose of CBPBs and/or the dose of calcitriol or vitamin D analog in the presence of persistent or recurrent hypercalcemia, arterial calcification, or adynamic bone disease.

The clinical consequences of vascular calcification in patients with CKD are serious. Cardiovascular calcification increases the risk of cardiovascular events including MI, fatal arrhythmia, congestive heart failure, and valvular heart disease (212,213). Measurement of CAC by electron beam computed tomography (EBCT) can help in the evaluation of asymptomatic ESKD patients. Using this technique, several studies have shown a high prevalence of CAC and cardiac valve calcification in HD patients, even those who are young (172,197,198,203,214–218). In the Calcium Acetate Renagel Evaluation (CARE-2) study, we found mitral valve calcification in 55%, aortic valve calcification in 40%, and both in 27% (203). Unfortunately, there is no proven effective treatment for cardiovascular calcification in HD patients. In the ADVANCE (A Randomized Study to Evaluate the Effects of Cinacalcet plus Low-Dose Vitamin D on Vascular Calcification in Subjects with Chronic Kidney Disease Receiving Hemodialysis) Study, subjects with CAC scores ≥30 were randomized to cinacalcet (30 to 180 mg/d) plus low-dose calcitriol, or vitamin D analog (≤2 μg paricalcitol equivalent/ dialysis), or flexible vitamin D therapy for 52 weeks (219). The cinacalcet-treated patients had a trend toward lesser progression of calcification of four cardiac structures (coronaries, aorta, mitral, and aortic valves) despite the fact that all subjects received CBPBs. However, the effect was modest and statistically insignificant except for the aortic valve. The clinical significance of these findings is currently unclear but probably at best is likely to be minimal (219). Indeed, the Evaluation of Cinacalcet Hydrochloride Therapy to Lower Cardiovascular Events (EVOLVE) trial tested the hypothesis that cinacalcet, as compared with placebo, would reduce the risk of death and cardiovascular events in dialysis patients with secondary hyperparathyroidism (220). The trial enrolled 3,883 participants from many countries and followed them for up to 5 years. Patients in the cinacalcet group experienced a nonsignificant relative reduction in the primary outcome of only 7% compared to placebo (220). Thus, the trial does not provide clear evidence that treatment of HD patients with cinacalcet provides protection against cardiovascular events.

CLINICAL PRESENTATION OF CORONARY ARTERY DISEASE IN PATIENTS WITH END-STAGE KIDNEY DISEASE

Myocardial ischemia is caused by a relative imbalance of myocardial oxygen supply and demand. Most often, it occurs during transient increases in oxygen demand in the presence of atherosclerotic narrowing of one or more coronary arteries. Less often, it may be caused by (a) a transient primary fall in myocardial oxygen supply, such as that caused by coronary arterial vasospasm, or (b) an excessive augmentation of myocardial oxygen demand without any decrease in supply, such as that which may occur with severe aortic stenosis, a sustained supraventricular or ventricular tachyarrhythmia, or severe sustained systemic arterial hypertension. Myocardial ischemia is usually diagnosed when typical angina pectoris occurs during exertion, emotional excitement, or HD. Physical exertion or emotional excitement cause an increase in the three major determinants of myocardial oxygen demand (heart rate, left ventricular wall tension, and cardiac contractility). HD may induce myocardial ischemia by precipitating hypotension, thereby diminishing coronary arterial blood flow and myocardial oxygen supply, or by provoking tachycardia and/or increased cardiac contractility, thereby increasing myocardial oxygen demand. It is not surprising, therefore, that angina pectoris sometimes occurs during HD.

Chest pain, abnormal findings on physical examination, and electrocardiographic changes, the cardinal features of myocardial ischemia in the general population, may occur in patients with ESKD, but these patients are likely to manifest myocardial ischemia in an atypical fashion. For example, many subjects with ESKD have baseline electrocardiographic ST-T wave abnormalities (221), making the electrocardiographic diagnosis of ischemia difficult or impossible. Not uncommonly, dialysis patients with acute coronary events may be asymptomatic. Such "silent" (painless) ischemia is considered to be present when, in the absence of chest pain, (a) ST segment alterations of ischemia are noted during provocative testing or ambulatory electrocardiographic monitoring, (b) reversible myocardial perfusion defects appear with thallium imaging, or (c) reversible segmental wall motion abnormalities are noted by echocardiography. Although the pathogenesis of such silent ischemia is uncertain, three mechanisms have been proposed. *First*, some patients may have altered neural pathways, such that they cannot sense the pain of myocardial ischemia. Cardiac transplant recipients, in whom the heart is surgically denervated, and diabetic patients with generalized neuropathy are particularly likely to have such episodes. *Second*, patients with silent myocardial ischemia may have unusually high thresholds for pain and, therefore, do not sense painful stimuli as other individuals do. *Third*, differences in the duration and severity of ischemic episodes may explain why some of them occur without pain. Because chest pain is a relatively late manifestation of myocardial ischemia, short-lived episodes may interfere with myocardial relaxation and contraction, induce electrocardiographic and perfusion abnormalities, but resolve before chest pain appears.

The presence of silent myocardial ischemia provides helpful prognostic information. In asymptomatic patients without a cardiac history, silent ischemia identifies those at increased risk of a subsequent cardiac event, such as angina pectoris, MI, or sudden cardiac death. Patients with silent as well as painful ischemia or a previous MI are more likely to have an adverse outcome (i.e., MI, the need for coronary revascularization, or cardiac death) in comparison to those without silent ischemia. Although agents that are useful in treating painful ischemia are also effective in treating silent ischemia, the overall impact of therapy (medical or nonmedical) on prognosis is unknown.

DIAGNOSIS OF CORONARY ARTERY DISEASE IN END-STAGE KIDNEY DISEASE PATIENTS

In stable patients with ESKD, the occurrence of angina pectoris, pulmonary edema without major changes in intravascular volume, unexplained hypotension, or a marked change in exercise capacity may trigger an investigation of the presence of CAD. Because most deaths in dialysis patients are caused by CVD, two important assumptions have been used in order to justify screening these patients for CAD. *First*, dialysis patients have a high frequency of obstructive CAD, even in the absence of angina. In a recently reported cohort of stable asymptomatic HD patients, 41% had obstructive CAD, and almost 30% had stenosis in the proximal segments of at least one coronary artery (222). *Second*, it is hypothesized that early and aggressive intervention in subjects with asymptomatic CAD could prevent MI and cardiac death.

Despite the high prevalence of CAD in CKD patients, routine screening tests are not currently recommended for most patients in the absence of suggestive clinical symptoms and signs of CAD. Clinical practice guidelines have recommended that coronary angiography or noninvasive testing be performed based on the individual's estimated risk of CAD (223). Routine coronary angiography in new dialysis patients was proposed as a means of improving the detection and treatment of high-risk patients (222). Among diabetic patients with ESKD who are awaiting transplantation, CAD, symptomatic or asymptomatic, is associated with an increased incidence of allograft failure and mortality (22,47,224,225). Philipson et al. (224) performed coronary angiography in 53 diabetic transplant candidates, detecting significant CAD in 20 (38%). During an average follow-up of 1 year, mortality was 44% in those with and only 5% in those without CAD. Based on data such as these, transplant candidates with angina or evidence of previous MI typically undergo coronary angiography as a part of the pretransplant evaluation, and subsequent transplantation may be denied if CAD is extensive and not amenable to revascularization (224,225).

Patients with ESKD without angina or with atypical symptoms of CAD pose a difficult management problem because many of them, particularly if they are diabetic, have CAD (11). For example, Weinrauch et al. (22) reported that 41% of asymptomatic diabetic patients with ESKD awaiting transplantation had significant CAD, and their 2-year survival was only 22%, compared to 88% in those without CAD. Similar findings were reported by Braun et al. (47), who also noted that depressed left ventricular systolic performance was associated with a particularly guarded cardiovascular outcome (47,68,226). ESKD patients with diabetes, peripheral vascular disease, or previous MI are clearly at higher risk of CAD, major adverse coronary events, or both; as a result, they usually are referred for coronary angiography (222). Such an approach may not be justified in other patients with ESKD. Hence, noninvasive cardiac risk stratification is thought to offer a more appropriate alternative to routine diagnostic catheterization.

Levels of cardiac biomarkers may be chronically elevated in 80% to 90% of asymptomatic patients with ESKD who are receiving maintenance dialysis in the absence of myocardial ischemia, possibly because of myocardial apoptosis or silent microinfarction due to small vessel disease (227). However, serial serum cardiac troponin level elevation indicates acute myocardial damage. Serum concentration of troponin T (cTnT) was consistently found to be associated with all-cause mortality and cardiovascular events in patients with ESKD (228). Thus, elevated serum concentrations of troponin T may offer diagnostic and prognostic information in ESKD patients (228). The National Kidney Foundation Kidney Disease Outcomes Quality Initiative (K/DOQI) Clinical Practice Guidelines for Cardiovascular Disease in Dialysis endorse the use of the serum troponin concentration for risk stratification in dialysis patients (229).

Serum concentrations of troponin T and troponin I (cTnI) often are elevated in dialysis patients; increased concentrations of these biomarkers are predictive of subsequent death in these individuals (230–232). Measurement of cTnT may have a greater potential for its diagnostics and prognostic capabilities. However, cTnI remains more specific than cTnT in the diagnosis of acute MI (228). Of importance, troponin levels should be obtained just before dialysis, as the dialysis procedure can affect levels (233). Data from Zoccali et al. (234) and deFilippi et al. (35) suggest that ESKD patients with a cTnT >0.07 ng/mL are at a particularly high risk for underlying CAD and its associated adverse events. Other studies have found that cTnT is useful in predicting short-term prognosis in patients with a wide range of renal function (235–237). In addition to the relationship between cTnT and CAD, elevated cTnT levels have been linked to increased left ventricular mass in dialysis patients (238–240).

The increased risk of CAD in patients with ESKD may be mediated, at least in part, through chronic inflammation (241–247). Serum markers of inflammation, such as CRP, brain natriuretic peptide (BNP), and the endogenous inhibitor of NO synthase, ADMA, are elevated in patients with ESKD, and they identify those with a high cardiovascular risk (241). In addition, plasma IL-6 may be useful in predicting cardiovascular mortality in HD patients (244). A study from Pisa, Italy, of 757 HD patients prospectively followed for 30 months found that those with combined high levels of CRP and proinflammatory cytokines had an increased risk of cardiovascular and all-cause mortality (245). In addition, elevated serum concentrations of BNP and its inactive N-terminal fragment, Nt-proBNP, both surrogates of myocardial vulnerability, appear to predict cardiovascular events in this patient population (246,247). Finally, Zoccali et al. (248) suggested that raised plasma concentrations of ADMA in ESKD patients are associated with a 52% increased risk of death and a 34% increased risk of cardiovascular events in dialysis patients.

Screening for Coronary Artery Disease in Candidates for Renal Transplantation

Based on Medicare billing claims, it has been estimated that the cumulative incidence of MI is in the range of 8.7% to 16.7% by 3 years after kidney transplant listing and from 4.7% to 11.1% after kidney transplantation (249,250). Observational studies have also found a high frequency of cardiovascular events in the first months after kidney transplantation (249,251,252). Since most ischemic cardiac events in renal transplant recipients are related to preexisting CAD and occur during the first few months after transplantation (253–256), screening for the presence of CAD is an important component of the pretransplant evaluation. A recent study from Spain that screened 356 patients for CVD before inclusion in the renal transplant waiting list found significant CAD in 38% of patients. Among these, 82% had no cardiac symptoms (257). In asymptomatic patients, screening for CAD should be done if the results are expected to lead to changes in management that improve patients' outcomes. Moreover, screening should also be cost-effective, and its results may be used to deny transplantation to high-risk patients if they have short life expectancy. However, one study found that in selected high-risk patients, the overall 5-year survival after renal transplantation was superior to the expected 5-year survival with continued dialysis (258).

Evaluation should start with a thorough history and physical examination to identify active cardiac conditions before renal transplantation. In asymptomatic patients who are undergoing pretransplant evaluation, guidelines by the American College of Cardiology/American Heart Association (ACC/AHA) and NKF/KDOQI differ (259). While the NKF/KDOQI recommends noninvasive cardiac stress imaging in patients with diabetes mellitus out of concern for silent (asymptomatic) ischemia, the AHA/ACCF stated that "based on available data, routine noninvasive screening of patients with diabetes mellitus either for peritransplantation cardiac evaluation or for long-term care is not justified by existing evidence." However, the statement added that noninvasive stress testing may be considered in kidney transplantation candidates with no active cardiac conditions based on the presence of multiple CAD risk factors regardless of functional status (260). Relevant risk factors include diabetes mellitus, prior CVD, over 1 year on dialysis, left ventricle hypertrophy, age >60 years, smoking, hypertension, and dyslipidemia; the specific number of risk factors that should be used to prompt testing remains to be determined, but the committee considers >3 to be reasonable (260). The AHA/ACCF Scientific Statement emphasized the high variability in the sensitivity and specificity of radionuclide stress testing and dobutamine stress echocardiography (DSE) for the detection of significant CAD in patients with ESKD (260). In general, CKD patients may not able to undergo full exercise testing and their ST-segment response may not be specific for myocardial ischemia. Moreover, the sensitivity and specificity of noninvasive cardiac tests in CKD patients is lower than that in the general population (261). Radionuclide perfusion imaging is more sensitive but less specific than stress echocardiography for diagnosis of significant CAD in patients on renal replacement therapy (262).

Given that coronary angiography is expensive, invasive, and not risk-free, it is not an ideal screening procedure for all patients with ESKD who are being considered for transplantation. Among its potential deleterious effects, contrast-induced nephrotoxicity may cause further deterioration in patients with some degree of residual renal function. As a result, coronary angiography should be reserved for those who are likely to have significant CAD and may benefit from revascularization (263,264). The reader is directed to **FIGURE 17.4** for a suggested approach to the management of patients with ESKD and possible CAD (265). According to the American Society of Transplantation (223), patients with diabetes

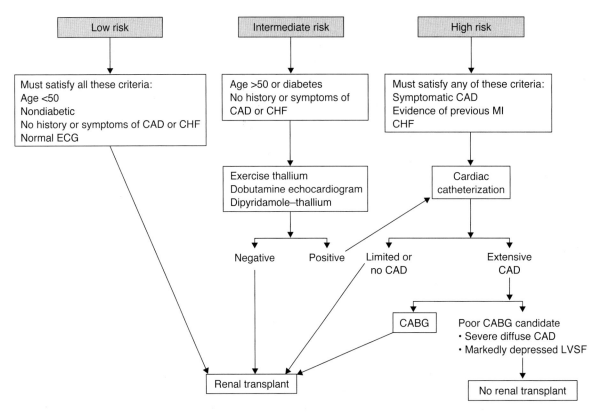

FIGURE 17.4 Proposed management strategy for end-stage kidney disease (ESKD) patients who are candidates for renal transplantation. CABG, coronary artery bypass grafting; CAD, coronary artery disease; CHF, congestive heart failure; ECG, electrocardiogram; LVSF, left ventricular systolic function; MI, myocardial infarction. (Modified and reproduced with permission from DeLemos JA, Hillis DL. Diagnosis and management of coronary artery disease in patients with end-stage renal disease on hemodialysis. *J Am Soc Nephrol* 1996;7:2044–2054.)

mellitus, a history of IHD, an abnormal ECG, or age >50 years are at high risk for CAD and should undergo noninvasive stress testing and, if abnormal, then one should proceed to coronary angiography (266). Also, patients with typical angina, previous MI (by history or ECG), or congestive heart failure should be considered high risk, and they should undergo cardiac catheterization to assess left ventricular systolic function and the presence and severity of CAD (267). Other noninvasive studies for the diagnosis of CAD are provided in Table 17.3 (268). Patients with congestive heart

failure are considered to be high risk because those with CAD and concomitant left ventricular systolic dysfunction have a particularly guarded prognosis and may derive a survival benefit with revascularization (268,269). Even after successful renal transplantation, left ventricular systolic dysfunction is a persistent risk factor for cardiac morbidity and mortality (270).

Several investigators have attempted to devise a strategy whereby low-risk patients, who can safely undergo renal transplantation without a preoperative cardiovascular evaluation, can be

TABLE 17.3	Sensitivity and Specificity of Noninvasive Testing for Coronary Artery Disease in Patients without or with End-Stage Kidney Disease			
	No Renal Disease (%)		**Renal Disease (%)**	
	Sensitivity	**Specificity**	**Sensitivity**	**Specificity**
Exercise ECG	50–85	85	QNS	QNS
Exercise thalium-201	82	91	76	62
Dipyridamole thallium	79	76	37–86	73–79
Adenosine thallium	83	76	QNS	QNS
Exercise echocardiogram	76–84	95	QNS	QNS
Dobutamine echocardiogram	72–89	85–95	69–96	95
Dipyridamole echocardiogram	52–60	95	QNS	QNS

ECG, electrocardiogram; QNS, quantity not sufficient.
Adapted with permission from Murphy SW, Parfrey PS. Screening for cardiovascular disease in dialysis patients. *Curr Opin Neph Hypert* 1996;5:532–540.

identified expeditiously, inexpensively, and noninvasively. Le et al. (264) prospectively enrolled 189 consecutive candidates for renal transplantation in a risk stratification program based on the presence of five risk variables: insulin-dependent diabetes mellitus, age >50 years, a history of angina, a history of congestive heart failure, and an abnormal ECG. Patients were considered to be low risk if they had none of these variables and high risk if any was present. Of the 189 subjects, 94 were considered low risk and 95 high risk. Over a follow-up period averaging almost 4 years, cardiac mortality was 17% in the high-risk subjects and only 1% in the low-risk individuals (264).

Other investigators have used a similar approach in diabetic patients with ESKD. In a retrospective study, analysis of the cardiac catheterization data of 97 asymptomatic type 1 and 2 diabetes mellitus kidney and kidney-pancreas transplant candidates revealed that 33% of type 1 and 48% of type 2 diabetic patients had significant CAD (271). By multivariate logistic regression analysis, a body mass index greater than 25, older age, and cigarette smoking were associated with CAD. African American patients, who comprised 30% of the sample, had a 71% lower risk of CAD compared with whites ($p = 0.03$) (271). Manske et al. (272) retrospectively identified several clinical variables that were associated with CAD in diabetic transplant candidates: age older than 45 years, more than 5 pack-year history of cigarette smoking, more than 25 years of diabetes mellitus, and nonspecific ST-T wave abnormalities on a resting ECG. In a small group of subjects studied prospectively, they showed that these variables provided a sensitivity of 97% and a negative predictive value of 96% for detecting angiographically significant CAD. Furthermore, they concluded that diabetic patients younger than 45 years with none of these variables could safely undergo renal transplantation without a preoperative cardiovascular assessment.

Most renal transplant candidates are at intermediate risk for CAD. This group includes older patients without symptoms of CAD, previous MI, or congestive heart failure, as well as most diabetic patients with no symptoms or atypical symptoms of CAD. In these subjects, noninvasive testing may be particularly useful in the pretransplant cardiac evaluation (273–275). Many patients with ESKD have electrocardiographic abnormalities at rest that make the ECG difficult or impossible to interpret during provocation (often because of LVH). Moreover, other patients, particularly those who are diabetic, fail to attain a sufficient heart rate during exercise to provide a reasonable predictive accuracy (22,134,276). As a result, provocative pharmacologic testing with concomitant cardiac imaging (using nuclear scintigraphy or echocardiography) has been used in an attempt to identify patients with underlying CAD.

Conflicting reports have appeared concerning the utility of thallium imaging with dipyridamole to identify CAD in patients with ESKD awaiting transplantation. On the one hand, Marwick et al. (277) and Boudreau et al. (278) concluded that such imaging was of little use in identifying angiographically significant CAD or in predicting cardiac prognosis in this patient population. Of Marwick and colleagues' (277) transplant candidates, thallium imaging with dipyridamole offered only fair specificity and poor sensitivity in identifying CAD. Importantly, five of the six individuals who died of cardiac causes over a mean follow-up of 2 years had normal thallium imaging studies. Of the 80 patients reported by Boudreau et al. (278), 36 had negative dipyridamole thallium studies, 6 (17%) of whom had significant angiographic CAD, giving a negative predictive value of only 83% (**TABLE 17.3**). In contrast, several reports

have concluded that thallium imaging with dipyridamole provides an effective noninvasive means of identifying transplant candidates with no chest pain or atypical chest pain who are at increased risk of having a subsequent cardiac event. Camp et al. (274) showed that 6 of 9 patients with dipyridamole-induced reversible perfusion abnormalities had a subsequent cardiovascular event, whereas none of 31 patients without reversible defects had a subsequent event. Other studies (226,279) have supported the contention that thallium imaging with dipyridamole can identify those at increased risk of an adverse cardiovascular outcome. In addition, a normal thallium imaging study appears to predict a very low likelihood of a subsequent cardiovascular event (226,264,274). The reasons that these dipyridamole-thallium data are disparate are not clear but may include differences in study design, definition of end points, interpretation of "positive" thallium images, and patient selection. In addition, most of these studies included only patients referred for noninvasive evaluation, and the differences in referral patterns between centers may explain some of the variability in results.

Two-dimensional echocardiography during the intravenous infusion of dobutamine (so-called dobutamine stress echocardiography) was evaluated in 97 patients (some diabetic, others not) with ESKD awaiting renal transplantation (275). In these patients, this technique had a sensitivity of 95% and a specificity of 86% for predicting cardiovascular complications or death during the subsequent year. Although the positive predictive value was poor (only 14%), the negative predictive value was excellent (97%) (**TABLE 17.3**). In a more recent study, renal transplant candidates had coronary angiography, DSE, and resting and exercise electrocardiography. Of the 125 patients, 36 (29%) had severe CAD, 55% were on dialysis, and 39% were diabetic. Stepwise logistic regression analysis identified an abnormal resting ECG and a positive stress echocardiogram result as independent predictors of severe CAD (280). Finally, a meta-analysis of 12 observational studies involving 913 patients was performed to determine the prognostic significance of myocardial perfusion studies on future MI and cardiac death in patients with ESKD assessed for kidney or kidney-pancreas transplantation (281). In comparison to patients with normal tests, those with evidence of inducible ischemia (reversible perfusion defects or new wall motion abnormalities) had a sixfold increased risk of MI and an almost fourfold increased risk of cardiac death. In addition, those with noninducible ischemia (fixed perfusion defects or wall motion abnormalities at rest) had a significantly higher risk of cardiac death (RR 4.7). Diabetic patients had a similar pattern of risk, with reversible perfusion defects alone strongly associated with MI (RR 9.3) and both fixed and reversible perfusion defects associated with cardiac death (RR 4.0 to 4.7). In an assessment of symptoms, electrocardiographic findings, thallium dipyridamole scintigraphic results, and resting echocardiographic results in 42 ESKD patients and 42 patients after renal transplantation, the presence of angina offered the best prognostic information (282), whereas the other variables lacked sensitivity and/or specificity in the identification of those with CAD.

In summary, all high-risk transplant candidates (those with symptoms of CAD, previous MI, or congestive heart failure) should undergo coronary angiography before renal transplantation. At the opposite extreme, young, nondiabetic patients without symptoms of CAD or previous MI comprise a low-risk group, and they do not require cardiac evaluation before transplantation. In addition, young diabetic patients, particularly nonsmokers who have had diabetes for less than 25 years and whose ECGs are normal, may not require cardiac evaluation before renal transplantation. Subjects in the intermediate risk group include older patients without symptomatic CAD. In preparation for transplantation, these individuals should undergo noninvasive evaluation (DSE or dipyridamole-thallium imaging), recognizing that neither procedure is perfect. Because most insulin-dependent diabetic patients older than 45 years have underlying CAD, we recommend that these individuals routinely undergo coronary angiography, even in the absence of angina or evidence of previous MI (**FIGURE 17.4**) (265,269,283).

MANAGEMENT OF CORONARY ARTERY DISEASE IN PATIENTS WITH END-STAGE RENAL DISEASE

Medical Management

Evidence-based recommendations for the medical management of CAD in patients with ESKD are hampered by the lack of data from randomized controlled trials because the studies which demonstrated that aspirin, β-blockers, angiotensin-converting enzyme (ACE) inhibitors, and lipid-lowering agents are efficacious in patients with CAD excluded patients with ESKD (284). Because of concern that these agents have limited efficacy and/or enhanced toxicity in subjects with ESKD, they often are underused in this patient population (12). Given that the etiology of CVD in ESKD is complex and may be different from that in the general population, randomized trials that evaluate the efficacy and safety of these drugs in patients with ESKD are still needed. Until such studies are performed, the medications noted previously should be used in patients with ESKD. In addition, correction of the hemoglobin concentration to 10 to 11 g/dL to improve oxygen-carrying capacity should be pursued with erythropoietin therapy and intravenous iron supplementation (285). Such an improvement in hemoglobin may allow the patient to participate in exercise training, which offers additional benefits (286,287). Adequate BP control is critically important in reducing the magnitude of LVH and myocardial oxygen demand, resulting in reduced angina frequency, ventricular irritability, and perhaps even mortality (287–289). Several studies have shown an independent association between measures of glycemic control and mortality in patients with or without diabetes (290). The role of glycemic control in diabetic ESKD was examined by Shurraw et al. (291) in 1,484 incident HD patients during a follow-up of up to 8 years. The authors found that increased serum glucose and HbA1c levels were not independently and directly associated with mortality and strict glycemic control may not benefit dialysis patients with or without diabetes mellitus (291). Other interventions such as smoking cessation, exercise, dietary salt reduction, weight loss, and control of hypertension should be tried, although clear evidence for these measures in ESKD patients is limited.

Several antianginal medications may be useful in dialysis patients with stable angina. Long-acting nitrates are effective orally or cutaneously in reducing angina frequency and severity, but their influence on survival is unknown. Twice-daily dosing with a nitrate-free period is recommended so that nitrate tolerance is minimized. The use of sublingual nitroglycerin may induce hypotension, particularly if the patient uses it during dialysis. Other drugs that are often prescribed in patients with ESKD and angina include β-blockers, which reduce heart rate, contractility, and left ventricular wall tension, and calcium channel blockers, which

induce coronary arterial vasodilation and simultaneously reduce the determinants of myocardial oxygen demand. These agents reduce angina frequency and the frequency of cardiovascular events in patients with painless myocardial ischemia (292). Some of these agents should be given with caution to patients with ESKD because they are excreted unchanged by the kidney. However, since the calcium channel blockers diltiazem, verapamil, and the dihydropyridines are metabolized by the liver, dosing adjustments are unnecessary in patients with ESKD.

For patients with known CAD with or without ESKD, low-dose aspirin is recommended. Unfortunately, the frequency of aspirin use in dialysis and CKD patients who have survived an MI is low in comparison to those without CKD: In one study, the rate of aspirin use was only 61% in dialysis patients compared to 89% in subjects with normal renal function (293). This reduced frequency of aspirin use is due, at least in part, to safety concerns because aspirin prolongs the bleeding time. Subgroup analyses of randomized trials have demonstrated convincing cardiovascular risk reduction from daily aspirin in individuals with estimated GFR <45 mL/min/1.73m^2, including dialysis patients, although the risk of bleeding is higher in these patients (294,295). In survivors of MI, aspirin reduces mortality irrespective of renal function. The efficacy of aspirin after MI was examined in 1,025 patients with ESKD and 145,740 controls (296). The benefit of aspirin treatment on 30-day mortality was similar in the two groups (**FIGURE 17.5**). In short, the routine use of aspirin after MI in all CKD patients could save one life for every five patients treated (296). To minimize bleeding risks, low-dose aspirin, 81 mg/d, is recommended.

Similarly, β-blockers are underutilized in survivors of MI with ESKD when compared to those without ESKD. In the above-mentioned study, β-blockers were prescribed in only 43% of dialysis patients (296), despite the fact that survivors of MI receiving dialysis had a 22% reduction in mortality with their use [RR 0.78, 95% confidence interval (CI) 0.60 to 0.99] (compared to a 30% reduction in those without ESKD). Apart from the beneficial effects of β-blockers on mortality following MI, they also reduced the incidence of new-onset heart failure (297,298). It should be recognized that some β-blockers are removed by HD ("high dialyzability"), while others

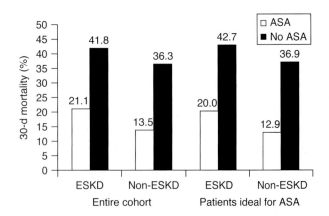

FIGURE 17.5 Thirty-day mortality following myocardial infarction in end-stage kidney disease (ESKD) patients. ASA, aspirin. (Reproduced with permission from Berger AK, Duval S, Krumholz HM. Aspirin, β-blocker, and angiotensin-converting enzyme inhibitor therapy in patients with end-stage renal disease and an acute myocardial infarction. *J Am Coll Cardiol* 2003;42:201–208.)

are not ("low dialyzability") (299). The high-dialyzability group includes atenolol, acebutolol, and metoprolol; these β-blockers should be administered after dialysis. The low-dialyzability group includes bisoprolol and propranolol.

Dyslipidemia is very common in patients with ESKD (87). Although statins are very effective in lowering total and LDL cholesterol concentrations in ESKD patients, their efficacy in reducing cardiovascular events and mortality in this patient population is uncertain. Some retrospective and small prospective studies showed that statins reduced cardiovascular and all-cause mortality (87), but the recently published Die Deutsche Diabetes-Dialyze (4D) study, a randomized comparison of placebo and atorvastatin in 1,255 diabetic patients on HD, showed no mortality benefit with statin therapy (300). Also, the Study to Evaluate the Use of Rosuvastatin in Subjects on Regular Hemodialysis: An Assessment of Survival and Cardiovascular Events (AURORA) trial which randomly assigned 2,776 patients on maintenance HD to either rosuvastatin or placebo found no effect of statin therapy on the combined primary end point of death from cardiovascular causes, nonfatal MI, and nonfatal stroke [hazard ratio (HR) 0.96, 95% CI 0.84 to 1.11] or on its individual components despite a 43% reduction in LDL cholesterol levels, and an 12% reduction in median hs-CRP levels (301). However, the Study of Heart and Renal Protection (SHARP) trial showed that reduction of LDL cholesterol with simvastatin plus ezetimibe reduced major atherosclerotic events by 17% but did not appear to reduce overall mortality (302). A review of the medical literature by an expert panel concluded that statin therapy is safe in patients with CKD, although the risk of myopathy may be increased when statins are used in combination with fibrates (303–305). A proposed schema for treatment of dyslipidemia in HD patients is shown in **FIGURE 17.6** (87). The KDIGO Work Group does not recommend a specific on-treatment LDL-C target and thus does not recommend adjusting the dose of statins based on LDL-C levels (306).

Finally, the beneficial effect of ACE inhibitors and/or angiotensin receptor blockers (ARBs) on reducing the risk of cardiovascular events and death in dialysis patients has not been well studied. ACE inhibitor therapy exerts a short-term survival benefit among patients with ESKD similar to that observed in patients not receiving dialysis. Berger et al. (296) reported that ACE inhibitor use was associated with a 16% absolute reduction in 30-day mortality in dialysis patients age 65 years and older presenting with clinical evidence of MI. In a small study, HD patients treated with an ACE inhibitor had a 52% RR reduction in 5-year mortality (307). Over an 8-year period, McCullough et al. (308) identified ESKD patients admitted to a coronary care unit. Of the 368 patients, 37% were given an ACE inhibitor during the hospital stay, and 63% were not; patient assignment was not random. The incidence of hypotension and arrhythmias was similar in the two groups. Those receiving an ACE inhibitor manifested a 37% reduction in mortality ($p = 0.0145$). In contrast, a prospective comparison of placebo and fosinopril in 400 HD patients with documented LVH demonstrated no mortality difference in the two groups (309).

Acute MI in patients with ESKD is associated with increased risk of morbidity and mortality. Among these patients, the overall proportion of ST-elevation MI (STEMI) was approximately 18% as compare to 40% in the general population with acute MI (11,310). Herzog et al. (11) hypothesized that the lower proportion of STEMI in patients with ESKD may be due to a greater prevalence of preexisting obstructive CAD and the resultant increase in coronary collateralization and myocardial ischemic preconditioning, thus reducing the likelihood of transmural ischemia in the setting of acute coronary occlusion.

Management and outcomes of STEMI in these patients has recently been examined. Gupta et al. (310) analyzed the 2003 to 2011 Nationwide Inpatient Sample databases to examine the temporal trends in STEMI, use of mechanical revascularization for STEMI,

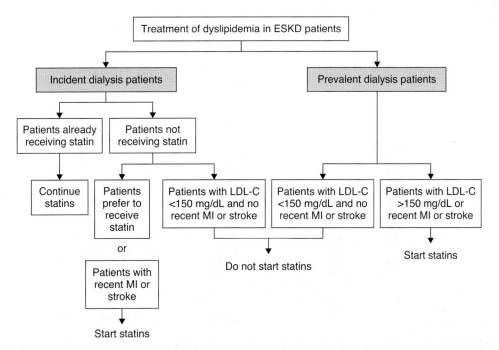

FIGURE 17.6 Schema for treatment of dyslipidemia in end-stage kidney disease (ESKD) patients. MI, myocardial infarction; LDL-C, low-density lipoprotein cholesterol. (Reproduced with permission from Qunibi WY. Dyslipidemia in dialysis patients. *Semin Dial* 2015;28:345–353.)

and in-hospital outcomes in patients with ESKD aged >18 years in the United States. From 2003 to 2011, the number of patients with ESKD admitted with the primary diagnosis of acute MI increased from 13,322 to 20,552, there was a decrease in the number of STEMI hospitalizations from 3,169 to 2,558 (p_{trend} <0.001). The overall incidence rate of cardiogenic shock in patients with ESKD and STEMI increased from 6.6% to 18.3% (p_{trend} <0.001). The use of percutaneous coronary intervention (PCI) for STEMI increased from 18.6% to 37.8% (p_{trend} <0.001), but there was no significant change in the use of coronary artery bypass grafting ($p = 0.32$). During the study period, in-hospital mortality increased from 22.3% to 25.3% [adjusted odds ratio (OR) (per year) 1.09, 95% CI 1.08 to 1.11; p_{trend} <0.001] (310).

Coronary Artery Revascularization

Percutaneous Coronary Intervention

In patients with CKD, particularly those with ESKD, atherosclerotic coronary artery lesions are more frequently proximal and longer in length and substantially more calcified than their counterparts with normal renal function. Thus, revascularization procedures in these patients may be more complicated than those with normal renal function. Unfortunately, there are limited data on outcomes of coronary artery revascularization in CKD patients. Moreover, dialysis patients are less likely than those with normal renal function to be referred for coronary revascularization (**FIGURE 17.7**) (311). However, the number of PCI in these patients has increased by almost 50% over the past decade (312). Earlier studies reported unfavorable outcomes with balloon angioplasty in patients with ESKD (313,314). However, recent experience with the use of coronary arterial stenting in dialysis patients has been shown to be associated with good outcomes. Le Feuvre et al. (315) reported comparable rates of procedural success (90% vs. 93%), in-hospital mortality (1% vs. 0%), stent thrombosis (0% vs. 0%), and STEMI (0% vs. 1%) in dialysis patients compared with those with normal renal function, respectively. In addition, the incidence of symptomatic restenosis within 1 year of the procedure (31% vs. 28%) and MI during that same time period (6% vs. 2%) was similar in the two groups. However, cardiac death occurred more commonly in the dialysis patients (11% vs. 2%, p <0.03).

In subjects with normal renal function, the likelihood of symptomatic restenosis following balloon angioplasty is about 35%; it is approximately 20% to 25% following implantation of a bare metal stent and <10% after deployment of a drug eluting stent. In patients with ESKD, the incidence of restenosis after balloon angioplasty is considerably higher (roughly 65% to 80%) (316,317). Although few data are available concerning the incidence of restenosis following insertion of a bare metal stent in subjects with ESKD, some reports have suggested that its incidence in these individuals is similar to that of those with normal renal function (318). The incidence of symptomatic restenosis in ESKD patients following implantation of a drug eluting stent is uncertain. A small nonrandomized study of 89 consecutive ESKD patients receiving drug eluting or bare metal stents and then followed for at least 9 months showed that target vessel revascularization was required in 1 (4%) of the former group and 17 (26%) of the latter group ($p = 0.036$) (319). During the period of observation, death, MI, or target vessel revascularization occurred in 8 (33%) of those receiving a drug eluting stent and in 39 (60%) of those in whom a bare metal stent was implanted ($p = 0.005$). In contradistinction, a small nonrandomized study from Japan compared the results of drug eluting stenting in 88 consecutive HD patients with bare metal stenting in 78 HD patients in whom stent implantation was accomplished in the preceding year (320). The primary end point of the comparison was angiographic restenosis (defined as 50% or greater diameter stenosis at the site of stenting 6 to 8 months after the procedure). The rate of angiographic restenosis was 22% in those receiving a drug eluting stent and 24% in those in whom a bare metal stent was implanted

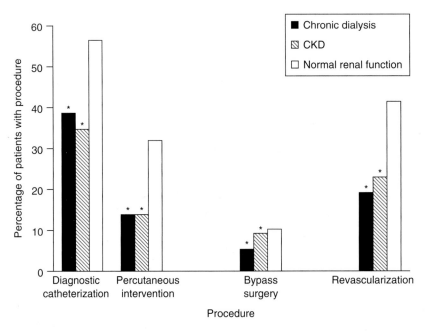

FIGURE 17.7 Rates of interventional procedures and revascularization in chronic kidney disease (CKD) and dialysis patients compared with individuals with normal renal function. *p <0.001. (Reproduced with permission from Charytan D, Mauri L, Agarwal A, et al. The use of invasive cardiac procedures after acute myocardial infarction in long-term dialysis patients. *Am Heart J* 2006;152:558–564.)

(320). Given that 80% of dialysis patients have calcified coronary arteries, a recent study from Japan found a higher risk of death and target lesion revascularization beyond 1 year of drug eluting stent placement for HD patients with calcified lesions versus those with noncalcified lesions (321). More research is needed concerning the relative efficacies of bare metal versus drug eluting stent use in subjects with ESKD.

Subjects with CKD, particularly ESKD patients on maintenance dialysis, have an increased risk of periprocedural and postprocedural morbidity and mortality during and after PCI when compared to those with normal renal function. In fact, the likelihood of adverse periprocedural and postprocedural events is related to the magnitude of preprocedural renal dysfunction. Best et al. (322) reviewed all adverse events that occurred in-hospital and within 1 year of PCI in 5,327 subjects undergoing balloon angioplasty (in 25% to 30%) or coronary stenting (in 65% to 70%) at the Mayo Clinic, after which they related these events to the estimated preprocedural creatinine clearance. Periprocedural in-hospital death occurred in 0.5% of those with a creatinine clearance greater than 70 mL/min, 0.7% of those with a clearance of 50 to 69 mL/min, 2.3% of those with a clearance of 30 to 49 mL/min, 7.1% of those with a clearance less than 30 mL/min, and 6.0% of those on dialysis. Similarly, death within 1 year of hospital discharge occurred in 1.5% of those with a creatinine clearance greater than 70 mL/min, 3.6% of those with a clearance of 50 to 69 mL/min, 7.8% of those with a clearance of 30 to 49 mL/min, 18.3% of those with a clearance less than 30 mL/min, and 19.9% of those on dialysis (322). Rubenstein et al. (323) reviewed the Massachusetts General Hospital experience in 3,334 patients undergoing PCI. Of these, 362 had a preprocedural serum creatinine greater than 1.5 mg/dL, whereas the other 2,972 had a creatinine less than 1.5 mg/dL. In comparison to those with a serum creatinine less than 1.5 mg/dL, those with a serum creatinine greater than 1.5 mg/dL had a lower rate of procedural success (90% vs. 93%, $p = 0.007$) and a markedly increased periprocedural mortality (10.8% vs. 1.1%, $p < 0.0001$). Similar data recently were reported by Gruberg et al. (324).

In summary, PCIs of all types (balloon angioplasty or coronary stenting) in patients with CKD are associated with substantial periprocedural and short-term postprocedural morbidity and mortality, particularly in subjects with ESKD. Mortality in this patient population remains high after successful PCI, probably due to a multiplicity of comorbid diseases. However, patients presenting with STEMI should undergo primary PCI with stenting, with the goal of performing the procedure within 90 minutes of presentation (door-to-balloon time) (325).

Coronary Artery Bypass Grafting

Data from several registries have consistently shown better long-term outcomes with coronary artery bypass grafting (CABG) compared to PCI in patients with ESKD, even though CABG in this patient population is associated with a high incidence of periprocedural complications. A retrospective study compared the outcomes of 279 dialysis patients with those of 15,271 patients with normal renal function who underwent a first CABG (326). After adjusting for age and comorbidities, the dialysis patients were 3.1 times more likely to die after CABG (9.6% vs. 3.1%), and they had an increased risk of postoperative mediastinitis (3.6% vs. 1.2%) and stroke (4.3% vs. 1.7%) (**FIGURE 17.8**). A follow-up study from the same database reported an 84% 5-year postoperative survival for patients with normal renal function and a 56% 5-year survival in those

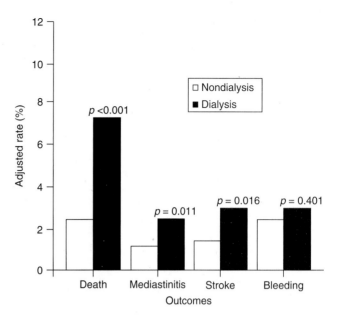

FIGURE 17.8 Adjusted adverse outcome rates after bypass surgery according to the presence or absence of dialysis-dependent kidney disease. Note the significantly higher adverse rates in end-stage kidney disease patients. (Reproduced with permission from Liu JY, Birkmeyer NJ, Sanders JH, et al. Risks of morbidity and mortality in dialysis patients undergoing coronary artery bypass surgery. Northern New England Cardiovascular Disease Study Group. *Circulation* 2000;24:2973–2977.)

with ESKD (327). The survivals of dialysis patients after coronary angioplasty, coronary arterial stenting, and CABG were reported from the USRDS database (71): 4,836 dialysis patients were treated with balloon angioplasty, 4,280 with stenting, and 6,668 with CABG. Those undergoing balloon angioplasty were more likely to require a repeat revascularization procedure than those in whom stenting was performed. Those who had CABG had the lowest rate of repeat revascularization procedures. Although the in-hospital mortality was higher (8.6%) in the CABG-treated patients than in those undergoing balloon angioplasty (6.4%) or stenting (4.1%), the 2-year survival was better in the CABG patients (56.4%) when compared with balloon angioplasty (48.2%) and coronary arterial stenting (48.4%) ($p < 0.0001$) (**FIGURE 17.9**). After adjustment for comorbidities, the RR for CABG [vs. percutaneous transluminal coronary angioplasty (PTCA)] was 0.80 (95% CI 0.76 to 0.84, $p < 0.0001$) for all-cause death and 0.72 (95% CI 0.67 to 0.77, $p < 0.0001$) for cardiac death.

The optimal revascularization strategy in patients with ESKD and CAD remains unknown. However, recent studies have highlighted the more favorable long-term survival benefit with CABG compared with PCI. In the Alberta Provincial Project for Outcomes Assessment in Coronary Heart Disease (APPROACH) study which captures information on all patients undergoing cardiac catheterization in Alberta, Canada, Hemmnelgarn et al. (328) compared survival in 662 dialysis patients and 750 nondialysis-dependent CKD patients with 40,374 non-CKD patients. In the nondialysis-dependent CKD group, they reported adjusted 8-year survival rates of 46% for CABG, 33% for PCI, and 30% with no revascularization ($p < 0.001$ for CABG vs. NR; $p = 0.48$ for PCI vs. NR). In the dialysis group, adjusted 8-year survival rates were 45% for CABG, 41% for PCI, and 30% with no revascularization ($p = 0.003$ for CABG vs. NR; $p = 0.03$ for PCI vs. NR). They concluded that CABG was

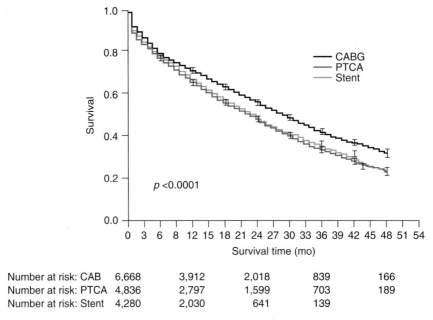

FIGURE 17.9 Survival of dialysis patients after coronary artery bypass grafting (CABG), percutaneous transluminal coronary angioplasty (PTCA), and stenting from the United States Renal Data System (USRDS). (Reprinted with permission Herzog CA, Ma JZ, Collins AJ. Comparative survival of dialysis patients in the United States after coronary angioplasty, coronary artery stenting, and coronary artery bypass surgery and impact of diabetes. *Circulation* 2002;106:2207–2211.)

associated with better survival than no revascularization in all categories of kidney function and that PCI was associated with a lower risk of death than no revascularization in the non-CKD patients and dialysis-dependent kidney disease patients but not in patients with nondialysis-dependent CKD. Accordingly, the presence of kidney disease or dependence on dialysis should not be a deterrent to revascularization, particularly with CABG (328). A recent meta-analysis of retrospective observational trials comparing CABG with PCI in ESKD patients with CAD showed that CABG was associated with a lower risk for late mortality (RR 0.90, 95% CI 0.87 to 0.93), MI (RR 0.64, 95% CI 0.61 to 0.68), repeat revascularization (RR 0.22, 95% CI 0.16 to 0.31), and cumulative events (RR 0.69, 95% CI 0.65 to 0.73), despite having a higher risk for early mortality (RR 1.98, 95% CI 1.51 to 2.60) (329). In another meta-analysis comparing CABG with PCI using 17 trials (N = 33,584) in the ESKD arm and 6 studies (N = 15,493) in the CKD arm, the authors

found significantly reduced early mortality with PCI with the OR of 2.08 (1.90 to 2.26, p <0.00001) and 2.55 (1.45 to 4.51, p = 0.001), respectively (330). However, they found decreased late mortality with the CABG when compared with PCI [OR 0.86 (0.83 to 0.89, p <0.000001) and 0.82 (0.76 to 0.88, p <0.00001)] in the ESKD and CKD arms, respectively. There was also a strong trend for decreased risk of stroke with PCI when compared with CABG in the ESKD and CKD populations (330). In summary, dialysis patients that require coronary revascularization appear to have a better long-term survival with CABG than after PCI.

Given that there are no randomized controlled trials comparing various interventions for coronary artery revascularization in patients with ESKD, it is difficult to make evidence-based decisions for the management of these patients. A summary of our recommendations for CABG in patients with ESKD is displayed in **TABLE 17.4**, which was adapted from the work of Fellner et al.

TABLE 17.4	General Recommendations for Coronary Bypass Surgery in Patients with End-Stage Kidney Disease		
Generally indicated	**Intermediate interactions**	**Not indicated**	
Limiting angina despite adequate medical therapy	Severe three-vessel disease	Asymptomatic and one- or two-vessel disease	
Left main disease of >50%	Symptomatic two-vessel disease with LV dysfunction	Stable angina with one-vessel disease	
Severe three-vessel disease (>70% narrowing) with LV dysfunction (ejection fraction <50%)	Symptomatic two-vessel disease with a normal LV function	Angina with no significant CAD	
Severe two- or three-vessel disease including a proximal left anterior descending artery	Symptomatic one-vessel disease		

Symptomatic can refer to clinical symptoms or an abnormal exercise stress test result. Asymptomatic refers to no symptoms or a negative stress test result.
LV, left ventricular; CAD, coronary artery disease.
Adapted and reproduced with permission from Fellner SK, Follman D, Dasgupta DS, et al. Ischemic heart disease in patients with end-stage renal disease. *Adv Ren Replace Ther* 1996;3:240–249.

(331). In general, the indications for CABG in ESKD patients are similar to those in subjects with normal renal function. *First*, individuals with limiting angina despite adequate medical therapy should be considered for bypass grafting to eliminate or to improve symptoms. *Second*, certain patient subgroups should be considered for bypass grafting to improve long-term survival, including those with (a) more than 50% luminal diameter narrowing of the left main coronary artery; (b) more than 70% luminal diameter narrowing of two or three major epicardial coronary arteries, in whom the proximal portion of the left anterior descending coronary artery is significantly narrowed; and (c) more than 70% luminal diameter narrowing of all three major epicardial coronary arteries in association with left ventricular systolic dysfunction (ejection fraction less than 0.50) (331). No data from prospectively performed, randomized trials have shown that CABG is superior to medical therapy in improving survival in subjects with ESKD and any of the three aforementioned arterial anatomic patterns. Subjects with no or mild symptoms obviously do not require bypass grafting for symptom relief. Those with less extensive CAD (involving one, two, or all three coronary arteries without involvement of the proximal portion of the left anterior descending coronary artery) do not manifest a better survival with CABG than with medical therapy.

Numerous reports have noted the high perioperative morbidity and mortality in patients with ESKD undergoing CABG (332–339). In all these reports, the perioperative mortality of ESKD subjects is 5% to 10% (in contrast to the 1% to 2% in patients with normal renal function). In addition, perioperative morbidity, such as stroke, mediastinitis, and excessive bleeding, occurs in as many as 20% of ESKD patients (326). Recently developed "off-pump" bypass grafting, with which surgical revascularization is accomplished on the beating heart without cardiopulmonary bypass, may be associated with less morbidity and mortality than the classic "on-pump" procedure (340), but adequately sized, randomized comparisons of on-pump and off-pump bypass grafting in patients with CKD have not yet been reported. Beckermann et al. (341) reviewed the experience in almost 4,000 subjects in the USRDS who underwent bypass graft surgery. Of these, on-pump surgery was performed in 3,382 and off-pump surgery in 540. Significantly less postoperative atrial fibrillation was noted in those undergoing off-pump CABG (37.5% on-pump vs. 4.8% off-pump, $p = 0.028$), and off-pump bypass grafting was associated with a 16% reduction in all-cause mortality ($p = 0.032$). Off-pump bypass grafting is still performed uncommonly in dialysis patients in the United States even though it may provide a lower risk of morbidity. The 5-year survival of ESKD patients undergoing bypass grafting (regardless of how it is performed) is only 50% (340–342).

◢ SUDDEN CARDIAC DEATH

Definition and Incidence of Sudden Cardiac Death in Patients with End-Stage Kidney Disease

In 2006, the American College of Cardiology/American Heart Association/Heart Rhythm Society (ACC/AHA/HRS) proposed the following definition of sudden cardiac death (SCD): "Sudden cardiac arrest is the sudden cessation of cardiac activity so that the victim becomes unresponsive, with no normal breathing and no signs of circulation. If corrective measures are not taken rapidly, this condition progresses to sudden death. Cardiac arrest should be used to signify an event as described above, that is reversed, usually

by CPR and/or defibrillation or cardioversion, or cardiac pacing. Sudden cardiac death should not be used to describe events that are not fatal" (343). SCD in dialysis patients has been defined as unexpected death from a cardiac cause within 1 to 24 hours after the last dialysis and/or onset of symptoms in a patient not known to have a potentially fatal condition (344,345).

SCD is now considered the leading cause of death in HD patients, accounting for up to 70% of deaths from CVD and 27% of all causes of mortality in this population (1,344,346). This represents about 20-fold higher risk that dialysis patients may experience SCD compared with the general population (1,347). Recent estimates from the USRDS suggest that the annual SCD rate among prevalent dialysis patients is 5.5% (348). Data from the Dialysis Outcomes and Practice Patterns Study (DOPPS) registry suggest that sudden death accounts for the highest proportion of HD deaths in the United States (33%) compared with other countries (349).

Pathophysiology of Sudden Cardiac Death in Patients with End-Stage Kidney Disease

Sudden Cardiac Death in Chronic Kidney Disease Patients versus the General Population

The biologic mechanisms and pathogenesis of SCD among the dialysis and CKD population have not been established but are clearly different from those in the general population. In the general population, up to 80% of SCD cases have post mortem evidence of CAD. By contrast, CAD is not as prevalent in dialysis patients who are victims of SCD (344). In one postmortem study of 93 dialysis patients who had sudden death, only 12% of cardiac sudden deaths that occurred within 24 hours of onset of symptoms were due to CAD (350). Similarly, LVH or poor left ventricular systolic function are strong predictors of SCD in the general population but may not be so in dialysis patients. In a multivariate analysis, Genovesi et al. (351) found LVH not to be associated with sudden death and also found no significant difference in the incidence of sudden death between patients with left ventricular ejection fraction <40% or >40%. However, a subgroup analysis of the 4D study showed that electrocardiographic evidence of LVH was associated with a higher rate of sudden death in diabetic HD patients (352). Two other studies in HD patients who experienced SCD found LVH in more than 70% of cases (353,354). Moreover, an increase in left ventricular mass index over time was found to be the most potent predictor of SCD in 10-year observational study of HD patients (355).

Thus, although patients with CKD share some of these risk factors, including atherosclerosis, with the general population, the presence of renal dysfunction *per se* increases the risk of SCD to an extent that cannot be simply explained by the severity of atherosclerotic CAD or known risk factors. Studies have shown that decreased renal function is an independent risk factor for SCD, and this risk is present from the early stages of CKD, increases as renal function declines, and reaches its peak in the dialysis population (**FIGURE 17.10**). In a retrospective longitudinal study encompassing 19,440 consecutive patients who underwent cardiac catheterization at a single academic institution, Pun et al. (356) reported 3.8 SCD events in 14,652 patients with estimated GFR ≥60 (stage 2 CKD or better) and 7.9 events in 4,788 patients with GFR <60 (stages 3 to 5 CKD). In an adjusted multivariate Cox proportional hazards model, the eGFR was independently associated with SCD (HR = 1.11 per 10 mL/min decline in the eGFR).

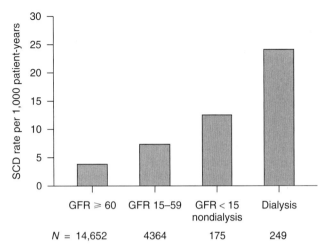

FIGURE 17.10 Rates of sudden cardiac death (SCD) by the baseline estimated glomerular filtration rate (eGFR) category. (Reproduced with permission from Pun PH, Smarz TR, Honeycutt EF, et al. Chronic kidney disease is associated with increased risk of sudden cardiac death among patients with coronary artery disease. *Kidney Int* 2009;6:652–658.)

Triggers for Sudden Cardiac Death Unique To Chronic Kidney Disease Patients

What could explain this unique predisposition of CKD patients to SCD since CAD does not seem to be the major culprit? A plausible explanation is that the myocardium is vulnerable to various arrhythmic triggers that are prevalent in CKD and dialysis patients, in part due to diffuse myocardial fibrosis. Studies of HD patients using magnetic resonance imaging (MRI) describe a diffuse pattern of myocardial fibrosis underlying LVH, and this pattern occurs in the absence of significant CAD (357–359). This myocardial fibrosis may result from various factors that are commonly encountered in CKD patients such as microvessel disease with capillary deficit (the so-called capillary/myocyte mismatch) (359), abnormal mineral metabolism (360), and recurrent myocardial ischemia from reduced myocardial perfusion during dialysis (**TABLE 17.5**) (361). In one study, 64% of patients had significant myocardial stunning during HD. Age, ultrafiltration volumes, intradialytic hypotension, and cTnT levels were independent determinants associated with myocardial stunning (361).

It is likely that many of the dialysis-associated factors may trigger serious cardiac arrhythmias, such as sustained ventricular tachycardia or ventricular fibrillation, similar to terminal events in the general population. For example, intermittent fluctuations of BP, fluid, and electrolytes during the dialysis cycle may pose a significant risk for SCD which seems to be more frequent in HD patients particularly following a long interdialytic interval. Bleyer et al. (353) reported a bimodal distribution of SCD in HD patients, with a 1.7-fold increased death risk occurring in the 12-hour period starting with the dialysis procedure and a threefold increased risk of death in the 12 hours before HD at the end of the weekend interval (*p* = 0.011) (**FIGURE 17.11**). They also reported that patients with SCD had a high prevalence of congestive heart failure and CAD. Only 40% of patients experiencing SCD were receiving β-blockers, and the prior monthly serum potassium value was less than 4 mEq/L in 25%. They suggested that every other day, HD could be beneficial in preventing SCD (353). Genovesi et al. (351) found that a serum potassium level >6.0 mEq/L was associated

TABLE 17.5	**Potential Risk Factors for Sudden Cardiac Death in Patients with End-Stage Kidney Disease**

Systemic diseases:
- Diabetes mellitus
- Systemic inflammation/malnutrition

Underlying cardiac disease
- Coronary artery disease
- Diastolic dysfunction
- Left ventricular hypertrophy
- Congestive heart failure
- Myocardial fibrosis

Lack of cardioprotective drugs
- β-Blockers

Electrolyte abnormalities
- Hypokalemia
- Hyperkalemia
- Hypocalcemia
- Hypomagnesemia
- Metabolic alkalosis

Dialysis-related risk factors
- Long interdialytic interval
- Low dialysate potassium concentration
- Low dialysate calcium concentration
- Rapid ultrafiltration
- High bicarbonate dialysate concentration leading to metabolic alkalosis
- Prolongation of the QTc interval during dialysis
- Air embolism

with a significant increase in risk of SCD in dialysis patients (HR 2.74, *p* = 0.009), while Paoletti et al. (355) could not reproduce this finding in their study of 123 patients followed up for 10 years. In a large observational study of 81,013 dialysis patients, Kovesdy et al. (362) reported that a predialysis serum potassium level of 4.6 to 5.3 mEq/L was associated with the lowest all-cause mortality. Thus, both hypokalemia and hyperkalemia may increase the risk of SCD in HD patients (363). Moreover, dialysis conducted with low potassium and/or calcium dialysate may increase the risk of SCD in

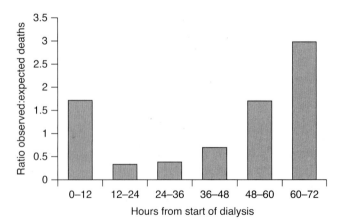

FIGURE 17.11 Ratio of actual to expected number of occurrences of sudden death for each 12 hour interval beginning with the start of hemodialysis. (Reproduced with permission from Bleyer AJ, Hartman J, Brannon PC, et al. Characteristics of sudden death in hemodialysis patients. *Kidney Int* 2006;69:2268–2273.)

these patients (363,364). Also, aggressive ultrafiltration may be associated with dialysis-associated hypotension and dialysis-induced myocardial "stunning" (361,365–367). In addition, higher dialysate bicarbonate concentrations and metabolic alkalosis have been associated with hypokalemia, hemodynamic instability, QTc interval prolongation, and increased mortality risk (368,369).

Other potential risk factors for SCD in dialysis patients have been the subject of recent investigations (TABLE 17.5). Diabetes mellitus is known to be associated with an independent risk of SCD likely due to arrhythmias caused by nocturnal hypoglycemia and QT interval prolongation. The presence of diabetes in dialysis patients is also associated with an increased risk of SCD (370). In the 4D, patients with an HbA1c level ≥8% had a twofold increased risk for SCD compared with those with an HbA1c level <6% (371). The role of inflammation and malnutrition in SCD was examined in the CHOICE cohort of 1,041 incident dialysis patients (372). In this study, SCD was responsible for 22% of all mortality over a median 2.5 years of follow-up. Using Cox proportional hazards, they found that the highest tertiles of serum levels of hs-CRP and IL-6 were each associated with twice the adjusted risk of SCD compared to their lowest tertiles. Decreased serum albumin was associated with a 1.35 times increased risk for SCD in the lowest compared to the highest tertiles independent of traditional cardiovascular risk factors (372). Interestingly, a recent study identified 5,117 pairs of patients who came from the same family from a sample of 647,457 dialysis patients and matched each to a control subject from the same population and found that genetically related family members who did not cohabitate had an OR of 1.88 (95% CI 1.25 to 2.84) for cardiac arrest compared with their phenotypically matched unrelated controls (373). Genetically related family members who lived together in the same environment had an OR of 1.66 (95% CI 1.20 to 2.28). Spouses, who were genetically unrelated but lived together in the same environment, had an OR of 0.95 (95% CI 0.60 to 1.59) for cardiac arrest. The authors suggested that the risk of cardiac arrest in patients on dialysis may be attributable to inherited factors (373).

Nature of Terminal Arrhythmia in Sudden Cardiac Death of Chronic Kidney Disease Patients

The terminal arrhythmias associated with SCD in CKD and dialysis patients are not well defined. Some studies suggested that ventricular tachyarrhythmia is the common final pathway for SCD (374), while other studies found bradycardia, asystole, and pulseless electrical activity more common (375). Wan et al. (374) described the characteristics of sudden cardiac arrest (SCA) and post-SCA survival in 75 HD patients who experienced at least one SCA event using a wearable cardioverter defibrillator (WCD) between 2004 and 2011. Sixty-six (79%) SCA events were due to ventricular tachycardia or ventricular fibrillation, and 18 (21%) were due to asystole. Most SCA episodes occurred during the daytime. Of these, 70% occurred during dialysis sessions. Acute 24-hour survival was 71% for all SCA events; 30-day and 1-year survival were 51% and 31%, respectively. Monday was the day where most arrhythmias occurred (*n* = 31), followed by Tuesday, Thursday, and Saturday with 19 each; Wednesday had the least number of SCA events (*n* = 6) (FIGURE 17.12). The distribution was statistically significant (*p* = 0.001). Women had a better post-SCA survival than men (HR = 2.41, 95% CI 1.09 to 5.36, *p* = 0.03). In an animal model of CKD, Hsueh et al. (376) found that cardiac ion channel and calcium handling are abnormal, leading to increased vulnerability to early after-depolarization, triggered activity, and ventricular arrhythmias.

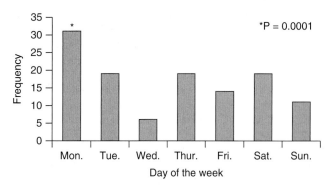

FIGURE 17.12 Timing of arrhythmia episodes by day of the week (*N* = 119). *p <0.001. (Reproduced with permission Wan C, Herzog CA, Zareba W, et al. Sudden cardiac arrest in hemodialysis patients with wearable cardioverter defibrillator. *Ann Noninvasive Electrocardiol* 2014;19:247–257.)

Prevention of Sudden Cardiac Death in Dialysis Patients

There are no randomized clinical trials of interventions to reduce SCD in dialysis patients, and thus, current recommendations are based on existing evidence from observational studies as well as on demographic, comorbid, clinical, and behavioral risk factors (377). In order to prevent or minimize the occurrence of SCD, an understanding of its pathogenesis among dialysis patients is required. An important observation is that the first month after initiation of HD appears to be a period of increased risk of SCD (378,379). However, the risk seems to increase with longer dialysis vintage for both HD and peritoneal dialysis patients alike (380). This is particularly true for dialysis patients who have large interdialytic weight gains, extremes of serum potassium level, or abnormal mineral metabolism and nutrition (363,381). For all CKD patients, victims of SCD are commonly diabetic and have a history of arrhythmias and preexisting heart disease (356,382).

Some risk factors for SCD may be modifiable. Shastri et al. (383) used baseline clinical characteristics to identify predictors associated with various causes of death in the Hemodialysis (HEMO) Study and to develop a prediction model for SCD using a competing risk approach. During a median follow-up of 2.5 years, SCD was recorded in 22% of patients. They found age, diabetes, peripheral vascular disease, IHD, serum creatinine, and alkaline phosphatase to be independent predictors of SCD. However, the primary predictors for SCD in their study were diabetes and IHD. Traditional risk factors such as smoking, hypertension, cholesterol level, and obesity were not associated with SCD. Unfortunately, no data on dialysis prescription, dialysis bath, or arrhythmias, factors that increase risk for SCD, were readily available. It is not clear yet whether identifying predictors for SCD may lead to different interventions in a particular patient. As an example, it is unclear whether tighter glycemic control will reduce the risk for SCD in this population. On the other hand, IHD may trigger arrhythmias and its treatment may decrease the risk of SCD, although this has not been clearly shown in dialysis patients. The use of β-blockers has been shown to reduce SCD after MI in the general population but not in dialysis patients. However, their use in HD patients has been shown in some studies to reduce overall mortality and mortality after cardiac arrest, with a nonsignificant reduction in SCD (384,385). Medications that are known to lower cardiovascular risk in the general population such as lipid-lowering agents and the renin-angiotensin-aldosterone blockers have not been shown to reduce cardiovascular risk in CKD or dialysis patients or at best to have minimal effect (386).

Given that the dialysis prescription may have adverse effects in HD patients, it is imperative that large fluctuation in fluid and electrolytes be avoided in order to reduce the risk of SCD. Thus, dialysate potassium level <2.0 mEq/L and/or dialysate calcium <2.0 mEq/L should be avoided (387). In one study, the use of a dialysate potassium modeling to maintain a constant serum-to-dialysate potassium gradient during the procedure was shown to reduce the incidence of premature ventricular contractions during dialysis (388). Also, the use of lower dialysate sodium concentration may help reduce interdialytic weight gain and large ultrafiltration targets (389). Other maneuvers that may be beneficial include the use of dialysate cooling as well as more frequent or long slow dialysis. In a small randomized crossover study of 11 patients comparing left ventricular regional wall motion abnormalities, reducing dialysate temperature by 2°C below body temperature was associated with reduced dialysis-induced myocardial wall motion abnormalities which are known risks for cardiac death (390).

The Role of Implantable Cardiac Defibrillators

The benefits of implantable cardiac defibrillators (ICDs) for prevention of SCD in patients with ESKD remain unclear. This is because CKD and dialysis patients have been excluded from major clinical trials which showed reduction in SCD with ICDs in the general population. As of now, no clinical trials have been published assessing the efficacy and safety of ICDs for prevention of SCD in dialysis patients. A recent meta-analysis of three randomized trials of primary prevention in patients with symptomatic heart failure and left ventricular ejection fraction <35% used data from the Multicenter Automatic Defibrillator Implantation Trial I (MADIT-I), MADIT-II, and the Sudden Cardiac Death in Heart Failure Trial (SCD-HeFT) (391). The investigators found that the mortality reduction associated with the ICD is significantly impacted by the baseline renal function, with decreasing benefit as eGFR declines. The study documented no survival benefit for ICDs in patients with eGFR <60 mL/min/1.73 m^2 (adjusted HR 0.8, 95% CI 0.4 to 1.5) compared to usual care. In contradistinction, a significant survival benefit was observed for patients with eGFR >60 mL/min/1.73 m^2 (adjusted HR 0.49, CI 0.24 to 0.95) (391) (**FIGURE 17.13**). In fact, several studies have reported increased complication rates and mortality in CKD patients treated with ICDs (392–395). These complications include bacteremia, central venous stenosis, access malfunction, and others. A recent retrospective cohort study of 9,528 HD patients who received ICDs from 1994 to 2006 found a high annual mortality rate of 45%, and that most deaths were attributed to arrhythmias (396). The rate of infection was also high with annual rates of bacteremia of 52% and device infection in 4%. In that study, the authors noted that almost all ICDs used in the 1990s was for secondary prevention, while half the patients received ICDs for apparent primary prevention in 2006. Patients receiving ICDs for secondary prevention had an overall 14% (95% CI 9% to 19%) lower mortality risk compared with propensity-matched controls, but these benefits seemed to be restricted to the early postimplantation time (396). Based on the above discussion, ICDs have not been shown to afford a significant benefit among U.S. dialysis patients who received an implantable defibrillator, even after a MI. However, the ICD2 trial, a prospective randomized controlled study designed to evaluate the efficacy and safety of prophylactic ICD therapy in reducing SCD in 200 dialysis patients aged 55 to 80 years over a 4-year period, is currently underway (397). Given that the initiation of HD is characterized by a marked increase in the rate of SCD, particularly in the first 3 months after HD initiation, a new trial entitled "WED-HED" (Wearable External Defibrillator in Hemodialysis patients), has been initiated to test the efficacy of wearable external defibrillators in preventing SCD in incident HD patients (398). Until further studies become available, a rational approach to identify HD patients at high risk for SCD and to target these patients for focused attention on their dialysis-related risk factors. Timely changes in the dialysis prescription and/or medications may help in attenuating or preventing SCD in this vulnerable population.

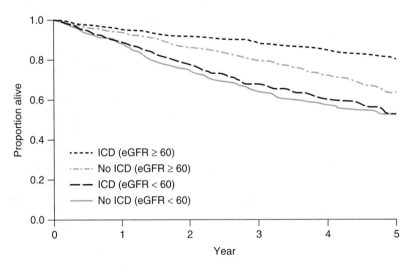

FIGURE 17.13 Kaplan-Meier survival curves in implantable cardiac defibrillators (ICDs) recipients versus nonrecipients according to estimated glomerular filtration rate (eGFR). Unadjusted hazard ratio (HR) for mortality benefit of ICD. (Reproduced with permission from Pun PH, Al-Khatib SM, Han JY, et al. Implantable cardioverter-defibrillators for primary prevention of sudden cardiac death in CKD: a meta-analysis of patient-level data from 3 randomized trials. *Am J Kidney Dis* 2014;64:32–39.)

REFERENCES

1. United States Renal Data System. *USRDS 2013 Annual Data Report: Atlas of End-Stage Renal Disease in the United States.* Bethesda, MD: National Institutes of Health, National Institute of Diabetes and Digestive and Kidney Diseases, 2013.
2. Herzog CA, Asinger RW, Berger AK, et al. Cardiovascular disease in chronic kidney disease. A clinical update from Kidney Disease: Improving Global Outcomes (KDIGO). *Kidney Int* 2011;80:572–586.
3. Sarnak MJ, Levey AS, Schoolwerth AC, et al. Kidney disease as a risk factor for development of cardiovascular disease: a statement from the American Heart Association Councils on Kidney in Cardiovascular Disease, High Blood Pressure Research, Clinical Cardiology, and epidemiology and Prevention. *Circulation* 2003;108;2154–2169.
4. Foley RN, Parfrey PS, Sarnak MJ. Clinical epidemiology of cardiovascular disease in chronic renal disease. *Am J Kidney Dis* 1998;32: S112–S119.
5. Charytan D, Kuntz RE, Mauri L, et al. Distribution of coronary artery disease and relation to mortality in asymptomatic hemodialysis patients. *Am J Kidney Dis* 2007;49:409–416.
6. Kumar N, Baker CSR, Chan K, et al. Cardiac survival after pre-emptive coronary angiography in transplant patients and those awaiting transplantation. *Clin J Am Soc Nephrol* 2011;6:1912–1919.
7. Joki N, Hase H, Takahashi Y, et al. Angiographical severity of coronary atherosclerosis predicts death in the first year of hemodialysis. *Int Urol Nephrol* 2003;35:289–297.
8. Coll B, Betriu A, Martínez-Alonso M, et al. Cardiovascular risk factors underestimate atherosclerotic burden in chronic kidney disease: usefulness of non-invasive tests in cardiovascular assessment. *Nephrol Dial Transplant* 2010;25:3017–3025.
9. Ohtake T, Kobayashi S, Moriya H, et al. High prevalence of occult coronary artery stenosis in patients with chronic kidney disease at the initiation of renal replacement therapy: an angiographic examination. *J Am Soc Nephrol* 2005;16:1141–1148.
10. Herzog CA, Ma JZ, Collins AJ. Poor long-term survival after acute myocardial infarction among patients on long-term dialysis. *N Engl J Med* 1998;339:799–805.
11. Herzog CA, Littrell K, Arko C, et al. Clinical characteristics of dialysis patients with acute myocardial infarction in the United States: a collaborative project of the United States Renal Data System and the National Registry of Myocardial Infarction. *Circulation* 2007;116:1465–1472.
12. McCullough PA. Cardiorenal risk: an important clinical intersection. *Rev Cardiovasc Med* 2002;3:71–76.
13. Sarnak MJ, Levey AS, Schoolwerth AC, et al. Kidney disease as a risk factor for the development of cardiovascular disease: a statement from the American Heart Association Councils on Kidney in Cardiovascular Disease, High Blood Pressure Research, Clinical Cardiology, and Epidemiology and Prevention. *Hypertension* 2003;42:1050–1065.
14. National Kidney Foundation. K/DOQI clinical practice guidelines for managing dyslipidemia in chronic kidney disease. *Am J Kidney Dis* 2003;41(Suppl 3):S1–S92.
15. Becker BN, Himmelfarb J, Henrich WL, et al. Reassessing the cardiac risk profile in chronic hemodialysis patients: a hypothesis on the role of oxidant stress and other non-traditional cardiac risk factors. *J Am Soc Nephrol* 1997;8:475–486.
16. Held P, Levin N, Port F. Cardiac disease in chronic uremia: an overview. In: Parfrey PS, Harnett JD, eds. *Cardiac Dysfunction in Chronic Uremia.* Boston, MA: Kluwer Academic Publishers, 1992:3–17.
17. Lindner A, Charra B, Sherrard DJ, et al. Accelerated atherosclerosis in prolonged maintenance hemodialysis. *N Engl J Med* 1974;290: 697–701.
18. Berry J, Keebler ME, McGuire DK. Diabetes mellitus and cardiovascular disease. *Herz* 2004;29:456–462.
19. Rostand SG, Brunzell JD, Cannon RO III, et al. Cardiovascular complications in renal failure. *J Am Soc Nephrol* 1991;2:1053–1062.
20. Ansari A, Kaupke CJ, Vaziri ND, et al. Cardiac pathology in patients with end-stage renal disease maintained on hemodialysis. *Int J Artif Organs* 1993;16:31–36.
21. Rostand S, Kirk KA, Rutsky EA. The epidemiology of coronary artery disease in patients on maintenance hemodialysis: implications for management. *Contrib Nephrol* 1986;52:34–41.
22. Weinrauch L, D'elia JA, Healy RW, et al. Asymptomatic coronary artery disease: angiography in diabetic patients before renal transplantation. *Ann Intern Med* 1978;88:346–348.
23. Nicholls A, Catto GR, Edward N, et al. Accelerated atherosclerosis in long-term dialysis and renal-transplant patients: fact or fiction? *Lancet* 1980;1:276–278.
24. Ritz E, Wiecek A, Gnasso A, et al. Is atherogenesis accelerated in uremia? *Contrib Nephrol* 1986;52:1–9.
25. Longenecker JC, Coresh J, Powe NR, et al. Traditional cardiovascular disease risk factors in dialysis patients compared with the general population: the CHOICE study. *J Am Soc Nephrol* 2002;13:1918–1927.
26. Cheung AK, Sarnak MJ, Yan G. Atherosclerotic cardiovascular disease risks in chronic hemodialysis patients. *Kidney Int* 2000;58:353–362.
27. Uhlig K, Levey AS, Sarnak MJ. Traditional cardiac risk factors in individuals with chronic kidney disease. *Semin Dial* 2003;16(2):118–127.
28. Mallamaci F, Zoccali C, Tripepi G, et al. Hyperhomocysteinemia predicts cardiovascular outcomes in hemodialysis patients. *Kidney Int* 2002;61:609–614.
29. Zoccali C, Benedetto FA, Maas R, et al. Asymmetric dimethylarginine, C-reactive protein, and carotid intima-media thickness in end-stage renal disease. *J Am Soc Nephrol* 2002;13:490–496.
30. Go AS, Chertow GM, Fan D, et al. Chronic kidney disease and the risks of death, cardiovascular events, and hospitalization. *N Engl J Med* 2004;351:1296–1305.
31. Anavekar NS, McMurray JJV, Velazquez EJ, et al. Relation between renal dysfunction and cardiovascular outcomes after myocardial infarction. *N Engl J Med* 2004;351:1285–1295.
32. Amann K, Ritz C, Adamczak M, et al. Why is coronary heart disease of uraemic patients so frequent and so devastating? *Nephrol Dial Transplant* 2003;18:631–640.
33. Hase H, Tsunoda T, Tanaka Y, et al. Risk factors for de novo acute cardiac events in patients initiating hemodialysis with no previous cardiac symptom. *Kidney Int* 2006;70:1142–1148.
34. Chonchol M, Whittle J, Desbien A, et al. Chronic kidney disease is associated with angiographic coronary artery disease. *Am J Nephrol* 2008;28:354–360.
35. deFilippi C, Wasserman S, Rosanio S, et al. Cardiac troponin T and C-reactive protein for predicting prognosis, coronary atherosclerosis, and cardiomyopathy in patients undergoing long-term hemodialysis. *JAMA* 2003;290:353–359.
36. Xue JL, Frazier ET, Herzog CA, et al. Association of heart disease with diabetes and hypertension in patients with ESRD. *Am J Kidney Dis* 2005;45:316–323.
37. Di Benedetto A, Marcelli D, D'Andrea A, et al. Risk factors and underlying cardiovascular diseases in incident ESRD patients. *J Nephrol* 2005;18:592–598.
38. Shah DS, Polkinghorne KR, Pellicano R, et al. Are traditional risk factors valid for assessing cardiovascular risk in end-stage renal failure patients? *Nephrology (Carlton)* 2008;13:667–671.
39. Agarwal R, Nissenson AR, Batlle D, et al. Prevalence, treatment, and control of hypertension in chronic hemodialysis patients in the United States. *Am J Med* 2003;115:291–297.
40. Salem MM. Hypertension in the hemodialysis population: a survey of 649 patients. *Am J Kidney Dis* 1995;26:461–468.
41. Rocco MV, Yan G, Heyka RJ, et al. Risk factors for hypertension in chronic hemodialysis patients: baseline data from the HEMO study. *Am J Nephrol* 2001;21:280–288.
42. Agarwal R, Flynn J, Pogue V, et al. Assessment and management of hypertension in patients on dialysis. *J Am Soc Nephrol* 2014;25(8):1630–1646.
43. Velasquez MT, Lew SQ, von Albertini B, et al. Control of hypertension is better during hemodialysis than during continuous ambulatory peritoneal dialysis in ESRD patients. *Clin Nephrol* 1997;48:341–345.
44. Rocco MV, Flanigan MJ, Beaver S, et al. Report from the 1995 Core Indicators for Peritoneal Dialysis Study Group: report from the 1995 Core Indicators for Peritoneal Dialysis Study Group. *Am J Kidney Dis* 1997;30:165–173.

45. Weiler EWJ, Saldanha LF, Khalil-Manesh F, et al. Relationship of Na-K-ATPase inhibitors to blood-pressure regulation in continuous ambulatory peritoneal dialysis and hemodialysis. *J Am Soc Nephrol* 1996;7:454–463.

46. Tonbul Z, Altintepe L, Sözlü C, et al. Ambulatory blood pressure monitoring in haemodialysis and continuous ambulatory peritoneal dialysis (CAPD) patients. *J Hum Hypertens* 2002;16:585–589.

47. Braun W, Phillips DF, Vidt DG, et al. Coronary artery disease in 100 diabetics with end-stage renal failure. *Transplant Proc* 1984;16:603–607.

48. Manske C, Wilson RF, Wang Y, et al. Prevalence of, and risk factors for, angiographically determined coronary artery disease in type 1-diabetic patients with nephropathy. *Arch Intern Med* 1992;152:2450–2455.

49. Jensen T, Borch-Johnsen K, Kofoed-Enevoldsen A, et al. Coronary heart disease in young type 1 (insulin-dependent) diabetic patients with and without diabetic nephropathy: incidence and risk factors. *Diabetologia* 1987;30:144–148.

50. Port FK, Hulbert-Shearon TE, Wolfe RA, et al. Predialysis blood pressure and mortality risk in a national sample of maintenance hemodialysis patients. *Am J Kidney Dis* 1999;33:507–517.

51. Agarwal R. Systolic hypertension in hemodialysis patients. *Semin Dial* 2003;16:208–213.

52. Zager PG, Nikolic J, Brown RH, et al. "U" curve association of blood pressure and mortality in hemodialysis patients. Medical Directors of Dialysis Clinic, Inc. *Kidney Int* 1998;54:561–569.

53. Foley RN. Cardiac disease in chronic uremia: can it explain the reverse epidemiology of hypertension and survival in dialysis patients? *Semin Dial* 2004;17:275–278.

54. Ross R. The pathogenesis of atherosclerosis—an update. *N Engl J Med* 1986;314:488–500.

55. DeLima JJG, Lopes HF, Grupi CJ, et al. Blood pressure influences the occurrence of complex ventricular arrhythmia in hemodialysis patients. *Hypertension* 1995;26:1200–1203.

56. Morales MA, Gremigni C, Dattolo P, et al. Signal-averaged ECG abnormalities in hemodialysis patients. *Nephrol Dial Transplant* 1998;13:668–673.

57. Meier P, Vogt P, Blanc E. Ventricular arrhythmias and sudden cardiac death in end-stage renal disease patients on chronic hemodialysis. *Nephron* 2001;87:199–214.

58. Verdeccia P, Carini G, Circo A, et al. Left ventricular mass and cardiovascular morbidity in essential hypertension: the MAVI study. *J Am Coll Cardiol* 2001;38:1829–1835.

59. Foley RN, Parfrey PS, Kent GM, et al. Serial change in echocardiographic parameters and cardiac failure in end-stage renal disease. *J Am Soc Nephrol* 2000;11:912–916.

60. Harnett JD, Kent GM, Foley RN, et al. Cardiac function and hematocrit level. *Am J Kidney Dis* 1995;25:S3–S7.

61. Kestenbaum B, Gillen DL, Sherrard DJ, et al. Calcium channel blocker use and mortality among patients with end-stage renal disease. *Kidney Int* 2002;61:2157–2164.

62. Cice G, Ferrara L, Di Benedetto A, et al. Dilated cardiomyopathy in dialysis patients—beneficial effects of carvedilol: a double-blind, placebo-controlled trial. *J Am Coll Cardiol* 2001;37:407–411.

63. Chan CT, Floras JS, Miller JA, et al. Regression of left ventricular hypertrophy after conversion to nocturnal hemodialysis. *Kidney Int* 2002;61:2235–2239.

64. Centers for Disease Control and Prevention. National Diabetes Fact Sheet: National Estimates and General Information on Diabetes and Prediabetes in the United States, 2011. http://www.cdc.gov/diabetes/pubs/pdf/ndfs_2011.pdf. Accessed January 3, 2014.

65. Seshasai SRK, Kaptoge S, Thompson A, et al. Diabetes mellitus, fasting glucose, and risk of cause-specific death. *N Engl J Med* 2011;364(9):829–841.

66. Fox CS, Matsushita K, Woodward M, et al. Associations of kidney disease measures with mortality and end-stage renal disease in individuals with and without diabetes: a meta-analysis. *Lancet* 2012;380(9854):1662–1673.

67. Krolewski A, Kosinski EJ, Warram JH, et al. Magnitude and determinants of coronary artery disease in juvenile-onset, insulin-dependent diabetes mellitus. *Am J Cardiol* 1987;59:750–755.

68. Braun W, Phillips D, Vidt DG, et al. Coronary arteriography and coronary artery disease in 99 diabetic and nondiabetic patients on chronic hemodialysis or renal transplantation programs. *Transplant Proc* 1981;13:128–135.

69. Manske C. Coronary artery disease in diabetic patients with nephropathy. *Am J Hypertens* 1993;6(Suppl):S367–S374.

70. Le Feuvre C, Borentain M, Beygui F, et al. Comparison of short- and long-term outcomes of coronary angioplasty in patients with and without diabetes mellitus and with and without hemodialysis. *Am J Cardiol* 2003;92:721–725.

71. Herzog CA, Ma JZ, Collins AJ. Comparative survival of dialysis patients in the United States after coronary angioplasty, coronary artery stenting, and coronary artery bypass surgery and impact of diabetes. *Circulation* 2002;106:2207–2211.

72. Ambrose J, Tannenbaum MA, Alexopoulos D, et al. Angiographic progression of coronary artery disease and the development of myocardial infarction. *J Am Coll Cardiol* 1988;12:56–62.

73. Little W, Constantinescu M, Applegate RJ, et al. Can coronary angiography predict the site of a subsequent myocardial infarction in patients with mild-to-moderate coronary artery disease? *Circulation* 1988;78:1157–1166.

74. Oomichi T, Emoto M, Tabata T, et al. Impact of glycemic control on survival of diabetic patients on chronic regular hemodialysis: a 7-year observational study. *Diabetes Care* 2006;29:1496–1500.

75. Kalantar-Zadeh K, Kopple JD, Regidor DL et al. A1C and survival in maintenance hemodialysis patients. *Diabetes Care* 2007;30:1049–1055.

76. Wu MS, Yu CC, Wu CH, et al. Pre-dialysis glycemic control is an independent predictor of mortality in type II diabetic patients on continuous ambulatory peritoneal dialysis. *Perit Dial Int* 1999;19(Suppl 2):S179–S183.

77. Morioka T, Emoto M, Tabata T, et al. Glycemic control is a predictor of survival for diabetic patients on hemodialysis. *Diab Care* 2001;24:909–913.

78. Lin-Tan DT, Lin JL, Wang LH, et al. Fasting glucose levels in predicting 1-year all-cause mortality in patients who do not have diabetes and are on maintenance hemodialysis. *J Am Soc Nephrol* 2007;18:2385–2391.

79. Robinson TW, Freedman BI. Assessing glycemic control in diabetic patients with severe nephropathy. *J Ren Nutr* 2013;23:199.

80. Scott MG, Hoffmann JW, Meltzer VN, et al. Effects of azotemia on results of the boronate-agarose affinity and ion-exchange methods for glycated hemoglobin. *Clin Chem* 1984;30:896.

81. Bruns DE, Lobo PI, Savory J, et al. Specific affinity-chromatographic measurement of glycated hemoglobins in uremic patients. *Clin Chem* 1984;30:569–571.

82. Paisey R, Banks R, Holton R, et al. Glycosylated haemoglobin in uraemia. *Diabet Med* 1986;3:445–448.

83. Freedman BI, Shenoy RN, Planer JA, et al. Comparison of glycated albumin and hemoglobin A1c concentrations in diabetic subjects on peritoneal and hemodialysis. *Perit Dial Int* 2010;30:72–79.

84. Peacock TP, Shihabi ZK, Bleyer AJ, et al. Comparison of glycated albumin and hemoglobin A_{1c} levels in diabetic subjects on hemodialysis. *Kidney Int* 2008;73:1062–1068.

85. Freedman BI, Andries L, Shihabi ZK, et al. Glycated albumin and risk of death and hospitalizations in diabetic dialysis patients. *Clin J Am Soc Nephrol* 2011;6:1635–1643.

86. Murea M, Moran T, Russell GB, et al. Glycated albumin, not hemoglobin A1c, predicts cardiovascular hospitalization and length of stay in diabetic patients on dialysis. *Am J Nephrol* 2012;36:488–496.

87. Qunibi WY. Dyslipidemia in dialysis patients. *Semin Dial* 2015;28:345–353.

88. Randomised trial of cholesterol lowering in 4444 patients with coronary heart disease: the Scandinavian Simvastatin Survival Study (4S). *Lancet* 1994;344:1383–1389.

89. Long-Term Intervention with Pravastatin in Ischaemic Disease (LIPID) Study Group. Prevention of cardiovascular events and death with pravastatin in patients with coronary heart disease and a broad range of initial cholesterol levels. *N Engl J Med* 1998;339:1349–1357.

90. Heart Protection Study Collaborative Group. MRC/BHF heart protection study of cholesterol lowering with simvastatin in 20,536 high-risk individuals: a randomised placebo-controlled trial. *Lancet* 2002;360:7–22.

91. LaRosa JC, Grundy SM, Waters DD, et al. Intensive lipid lowering with atorvastatin in patients with stable coronary disease. *N Engl J Med* 2005;352:1425–1435.

92. Epstein M, Vaziri ND. Role of statins in the management of dyslipidemia of chronic kidney disease: current concepts and emerging treatment paradigms. *Nat Rev Nephrol* 2012;8(4):214–223.

93. Kassimatisa TI, Goldsmith DJA. Statins in chronic kidney disease and kidney transplantation. *Pharmacol Res* 2014;88:62–73.

94. Kasiske BL. Hyperlipidemia in patients with chronic renal disease. *Am J Kidney Dis* 1998;32(5 Suppl 3):S142–S156.

95. Vaziri ND. Dyslipidemia of chronic renal failure: the nature, mechanisms, and potential consequences. *Am J Physiol Renal Physiol* 2006;290:F262–F277.

96. Wan RK, Mark PB, Jardine AG. The cholesterol paradox is flawed; cholesterol must be lowered in dialysis patients. *Semin Dial* 2007;20:504–509.

97. Drueke T, Lacour B, Roullet JB, et al. Recent advances in factors that alter lipid metabolism in chronic renal failure. *Kidney Int* 1983;24(Suppl):S134–S138.

98. Rapoport J, Aviram M, Chaimovitz C, et al. Defective high-density lipoprotein composition in patients on chronic hemodialysis. *N Engl J Med* 1978;299:1326–1329.

99. Fuh M, Lee CM, Jeng CY, et al. Effect of chronic renal failure on high-density lipoprotein kinetics. *Kidney Int* 1990;37:1295–1300.

100. Hahn R, Oette K, Mondorf H, et al. Analysis of cardiovascular risk factors in chronic hemodialysis patients with special attention to the hyperlipoproteinemias. *Atherosclerosis* 1983;48:279–288.

101. Nestel P, Fidge NH, Tan MH. Increased lipoprotein-remnant formation in chronic renal failure. *N Engl J Med* 1982;307:329–333.

102. Weintraub M, Burstein A, Rassin T, et al. Severe defect in clearing postprandial chylomicron remnants in dialysis patients. *Kidney Int* 1992;42:1247–1252.

103. Bostom AG, Shemin D, Lapane KL, et al. Hyperhomocystinemia, hyperfibrinogenemia, and lipoprotein (a) excess in maintenance dialysis patients: a matched case-control study. *Atherosclerosis* 1996;125:91–101.

104. Lowrie EG, Lew NL. Death risk in hemodialysis patients: the predictive value of commonly measured variables and an evaluation of death rate differences between facilities. *Am J Kidney Dis* 1990;15:458–482.

105. Kilpatrick RD, McAllister CJ, Kovesdy CP, et al. Association between serum lipids and survival in hemodialysis patients and impact of race. *J Am Soc Nephrol* 2007;18:293–303.

106. Kovesdy CP, Anderson JE, Kalantar-Zadeh K. Inverse association between lipid levels and mortality in men with chronic kidney disease who are not yet on dialysis: effects of case mix and the malnutrition-inflammation-cachexia syndrome. *J Am Soc Nephrol* 2007;18:304–311.

107. Liu Y, Coresh J, Eustace JA, et al. Association between cholesterol level and mortality in dialysis patients: role of inflammation and malnutrition. *JAMA* 2004;291:451–459.

108. Glavind J, Hartmann S, Clemmesen J, et al. Studies on the role of lipoperoxides in human pathology: II. The presence of peroxidized lipids in the atherosclerotic aorta. *Acta Pathol Microbiol Scand* 1952;30:1–6.

109. Cai H, Harrison DG. Endothelial dysfunction in cardiovascular diseases: the role of oxidant stress. *Circ Res* 2000;87:840–844.

110. Vaziri ND. Effect of chronic renal failure on nitric oxide metabolism. *Am J Kidney Dis* 2001;38:S74–S79.

111. Himmelfarb J. Relevance of oxidative pathways in the pathophysiology of chronic kidney disease. *Cardiol Clin* 2005;23:319–330.

112. Himmelfarb J, Stenvinkel P, Ikizler TA, et al. The elephant of uremia: oxidative stress as a unifying concept of cardiovascular disease in uremia. *Kidney Int* 2002;62:1524–1538.

113. Vaziri ND. Oxidative stress in uremia: nature, mechanisms and potential consequences. *Semin Nephrol* 2004;24:469–473.

114. Himmerfalb J, Hakim RM. Oxidative stress in uremia. *Curr Opin Nephrol Hypertens* 2003;12:593–598

115. Lucchi L, Cappelli G, Acerbi MA, et al. Oxidative metabolism of polymorphonuclear leukocytes and serum opsonic activity in chronic renal failure. *Nephron* 1989;51:44–50.

116. Shainkin-Kestenbaum R, Caruso C, Berlyne GM. Reduced superoxide dismutase activity in erythrocytes of dialysis patients: a possible factor in the etiology of uremic anemia. *Nephron* 1990;55:251–253.

117. Toborek M, Wasik T, Drózdz M, et al. Effect of hemodialysis on lipid peroxidation and antioxidant system in patients with chronic renal failure. *Metabolism* 1992;41:1229–1232.

118. Stenvinkel P, Pecoits-Filho R, Lindholm B. Coronary artery disease in end-stage renal disease: no longer a simple plumbing problem. *J Am Soc Nephrol* 2003;14:1927–1939.

119. Himmelfarb J, Ault KA, Holbrook D, et al. Intradialytic granulocyte reactive oxygen species production: a prospective crossover trial. *J Am Soc Nephrol* 1993;4:178–186.

120. Loughrey CM, Young IS, Lightbody JH, et al. Oxidative stress in hemodialysis. *QJM* 1994;87:679–683.

121. Nagasi S, Aoyagi K, Hirayama A, et al. Favorable effect of hemodialysis on decreased serum antioxidant activity in hemodialysis patients demonstrated by electron spin resonance. *J Am Soc Nephrol* 1997;8:1157–1163.

122. Ponka A, Kuhlbäck B. Serum ascorbic acid in patients undergoing chronic hemodialysis. *Acta Med Scand* 1983;213:305–307.

123. Cohen JD, Viljoen M, Clifford D, et al. Plasma vitamin E levels in a chronically hemolyzing group of dialysis patients. *Clin Nephrol* 1986;25:42–47.

124. Gey KF, Brubacher GB, Stähelin HB. Plasma levels of antioxidant vitamins in relation to ischemic heart disease and cancer. *Clin Nutr* 1987;45:1368–1377.

125. Rimm EB, Stampfer MJ, Ascherio A, et al. Vitamin E consumption and the risk of coronary heart disease in men. *N Engl J Med* 1993;328:1450–1456.

126. Jha P, Flather M, Lonn E, et al. The antioxidant vitamins and cardiovascular disease: a critical review of epidemiologic and clinical trial data. *Ann Intern Med* 1995;123:860–872.

127. Hodis HN, Mack WJ, LaBree L, et al. Serial coronary angiographic evidence that antioxidant vitamin intake reduces progression of coronary artery atherosclerosis. *JAMA* 1995;273:1849–1854.

128. Anderson TJ, Meredith IT, Yeung AC, et al. The effect of cholesterol-lowering and antioxidant therapy on endothelium-dependent coronary vasomotion. *N Engl J Med* 1995;332:488–493.

129. Levine GN, Frei B, Koulouris SN, et al. Ascorbic acid reverses endothelial vasomotor dysfunction in patients with coronary artery disease. *Circulation* 1996;93:1107–1113.

130. Tepel M, van der Giet M, Statz M, et al. The antioxidant acetylcysteine reduces cardiovascular events in patients with end-stage renal failure: a randomized, controlled trial. *Circulation* 2003;107:992–995.

131. Boaz M, Smetana S, Weinstein T, et al. Secondary prevention with antioxidants of cardiovascular disease in end-stage renal disease (SPACE): randomised placebo-controlled trial. *Lancet* 2000;356:1213–1218.

132. Bohlender JM, Franke S, Stein G, et al. Advanced glycation end products and the kidney. *Am J Physiol Renal Physiol* 2005;289:F645–F659.

133. Peppa M, Uribarri J, Vlassara H. Glucose, advanced glycation end products, and diabetes complications: what is new and what works. *Clin Diabetes* 2003;21:186–187.

134. Lin KY, Ito A, Asagami T, et al. Impaired nitric oxide synthase pathway in diabetes mellitus: role of asymmetric dimethylarginine and dimethylarginine dimethylaminohydrolase. *Circulation* 2002;106:987–992.

135. Channon KM, Qian H, George SE. Nitric oxide synthase in atherosclerosis and vascular injury. *Arteriscl Thromb Vasc Biol* 2000;20:1873–1881.

136. Baynes JW, Thorpe SR. Glycoxidation and lipidoxidation in atherogenesis. *Free Radic Biol Med* 2000;28:1708–1716.

137. Palinski W, Koschinsky T, Butler SW, et al. Immunological evidence for the presence of advanced glycosylation end products in atherosclerotic lesions of euglycemic rabbits. *Arterioscler Thromb Biol* 1995;15:571–582.

138. Hou FF, Jiang JP, Guo JQ, et al. Receptor for advanced glycation end products on human synovial fibroblasts: role in the pathogenesis of dialysis-related amyloidosis. *J Am Soc Nephrol* 2002;13:1296–1306.

139. Nishizawa Y, Koyama H, Inaba M. AGEs and cardiovascular diseases in patients with end-stage renal diseases. *J Ren Nutr* 2012;22:128–133.

140. Meerwaldt R, Hartog JW, Graaff R, et al. Skin autofluorescence, a measure of cumulative metabolic stress and advanced glycation end products, predicts mortality in hemodialysis patients. *J Am Soc Nephrol* 2005;16:3687–3693.

141. Roberts MA, Thomas MC, Fernando D, et al. Low molecular weight advanced glycation end products predict mortality in asymptomatic patients receiving chronic haemodialysis. *Nephrol Dial Transplant* 2006;21:1611–1617.

142. Wagner Z, Molnar M, Molnar GA, et al. Serum carboxymethyllysine predicts mortality in hemodialysis patients. *Am J Kidney Dis* 2006;47:294–300.

143. Schwedler SB, Metzger T, Schinzel R, et al. Advanced glycation end products and mortality in hemodialysis patients. *Kidney Int* 2002;62:301–310.

144. Busch M, Franke S, Muller A, et al. Potential cardiovascular risk factors in chronic kidney disease: AGEs, total homocysteine and metabolites, and the C-reactive protein. *Kidney Int* 2004;66:338–347.

145. Li D, Yang B, Mehta JL. OxLDL induces apoptosis in human coronary artery endothelial cells: role of PKC, PTK, bcl-2, and Fas. *Am J Physiol* 1998;275:H568–H576.

146. Parthasarathy S, Wieland E, Steinberg D. A role for endothelial cell lipoxygenase in the oxidative modification of low density lipoprotein. *Proc Natl Acad Sci U S A* 1989;86:1046–1050.

147. Bjorkhem I, Henriksson-Freyschuss A, Breuer O, et al. The antioxidant butylated hydroxytoluene protects against atherosclerosis. *Arterioscler Thromb* 1991;11:15–22.

148. Thomas JP, Geiger PG, Girotti AW. Lethal damage to endothelial cells by oxidized low density lipoprotein: role of selenoperoxidases in cytoprotection against lipid hydroperoxide-mediated and iron-mediated reactions. *J Lipid Res* 1993;332:218–220.

149. Palinski W, Ylä-Herttuala S, Rosenfeld ME, et al. Antisera and monoclonal antibodies specific for epitopes generated during oxidative modification of low density lipoproteins. *Arteriosclerosis* 1990;10:325–335.

150. Salonen JT, Ylä-Herttuala S, Yamamoto R, et al. Autoantibody against oxidized LDL and progression of carotid atherosclerosis. *Lancet* 1992;339:883–887.

151. Horkko S, Huttunen K, Kervinen K, et al. Decreased clearance of uremic and mildly carbamylated low-density lipoprotein. *Eur J Clin Invest* 1994;24:105–113.

152. Maggi E, Bellazzi R, Falaschi F, et al. Enhanced LDL oxidation in uremic patients: an additional mechanism for accelerated atherosclerosis? *Kidney Int* 1994;45:876–883.

153. Jackson P, Loughrey CM, Lightbody JH, et al. Effect of hemodialysis on total antioxidant capacity and serum antioxidants in patients with chronic renal failure. *Clin Chem* 1995;41:1135–1138.

154. Jain SK, Abreo K, Duett J, et al. Lipofuscin products, lipid peroxides and aluminum accumulation in red blood cells of hemodialyzed patients. *Am J Nephrol* 1995;15:306–311.

155. Itabe H, Yamamoto H, Imanaka T, et al. Sensitive detection of oxidatively modified low density lipoprotein using a monoclonal antibody. *J Lipid Res* 1996;37:45–53.

156. Cressmann MD, Heyka RJ, Paganini EP, et al. Lipoprotein(a) is an independent risk factor for cardiovascular disease in hemodialysis patients. *Circulation* 1992;86:475–482.

157. Kronenberg F, Kuen E, Ritz E, et al. Lipoprotein(a) serum concentrations and apolipoprotein(a) phenotypes in mild and moderate renal failure. *J Am Soc Nephrol* 2000;11:105–115.

158. Kronenberg F, König P, Neyer U, et al. Multicenter study of lipoprotein(a) and apolipoprotein(a) phenotypes in patients with end-stage renal disease treated by hemodialysis or continuous ambulatory peritoneal dialysis. *J Am Soc Nephrol* 1995;6:110–120.

159. Stenvinkel P, Heimbürger O, Tuck CH, et al. Apo(a)-isoform size, nutritional status and inflammatory markers in chronic renal failure. *Kidney Int* 1998;53:1336–1342.

160. Grainger DJ, Kirschenlohr HL, Metcalfe JC, et al. Proliferation of human smooth muscle cells promoted by lipoprotein(a). *Science* 1993;260:1655–1658.

161. Kronenberg F, Lhotta K, König P, et al. Apolipoprotein(a) isoform-specific changes of lipoprotein(a) after kidney transplantation. *Eur J Hum Genet* 2003;11:693–699.

162. Kalantar-Zadeh K, Block G, Humphreys MH, et al. Reverse epidemiology of cardiovascular risk factors in maintenance dialysis patients. *Kidney Int* 2003;63:793–808.

163. Kaysen GA, Dubin JA, Muller HG, et al. Relationships among inflammation, nutrition and physiologic mechanisms establishing albumin levels in hemodialysis patients. *Kidney Int* 2002;61:2240–2249.

164. Kalantar-Zadeh K, Kilpatrick RD, Kuwae N, et al. Revisiting mortality predictability of serum albumin in the dialysis population: time dependency, longitudinal changes and population-attributable fraction. *Nephrol Dial Transplant* 2005;20:1880–1888.

165. Ritz E, Vallance P, Nowicki M. The effect of malnutrition on cardiovascular mortality in dialysis patients: is L-arginine the answer? *Nephrol Dial Transplant* 1994;9:129–130.

166. Koch M, Kutkuhn B, Grabensee B, et al. Apolipoprotein A, fibrinogen, age, and history of stroke are predictors of death in dialysed diabetic patients: a prospective study in 412 subjects. *Nephrol Dial Transplant* 1997;12:2603–2611.

167. Kalantar-Zadeh K, Kuwae N, Wu DY, et al. Associations of body fat and its changes over time with quality of life and prospective mortality in hemodialysis patients. *Am J Clin Nutr* 2006;83:202–210.

168. Hansson GK. Inflammation, atherosclerosis, and coronary artery disease. *N Engl J Med* 2005;352(16):1685–1695.

169. Zapolski T. Malnutrition–inflammation complex syndrome: link between end-stage renal disease, atherosclerosis and valvular calcification. *Hypertens Res* 2010;33:541–543.

170. Zimmermann J, Herrlinger S, Pruy A, et al. Inflammation enhances cardiovascular risk and mortality in hemodialysis patients. *Kidney Int* 1999;55:648–658.

171. Pecoits-Filho R, Lindholm B, Axelsson J, et al. Update on interleukin-6 and its role in chronic renal failure. *Nephrol Dial Transplant* 2003;18:1042–1045.

172. Schwarz U, Buzello M, Ritz E, et al. Morphology of coronary atherosclerotic lesions in patients with end-stage renal failure. *Nephrol Dial Transplant* 2000;15:218–223.

173. Nakano T, Ninomiya T, Sumiyoshi S, et al. Association of kidney function with coronary atherosclerosis and calcification in autopsy samples from Japanese elders: the Hisayama study. *Am J Kidney Dis* 2010;55:21–30.

174. Hayano S, Ichimiya S, Ishii H, et al. Relation between estimated glomerular filtration rate and composition of coronary arterial atherosclerotic plaques. *Am J Cardiol* 2012;109(8):1131–1136.

175. Weiner DE, Tighiouart H, Amin MG, et al. Chronic kidney disease as a risk factor for cardiovascular disease and all-cause mortality: a pooled analysis of community-based studies. *J Am Soc Nephro* 2004;115:1307–1315.

176. Kidney Disease: Improving Global Outcomes (KDIGO) CKD–MBD Work Group. KDIGO clinical practice guideline for the diagnosis, evaluation, prevention, and treatment of chronic kidney disease–mineral and bone disorder (CKD–MBD). *Kidney Int* 2009;76(Suppl 113):S1–S130.

177. Qunibi WY, Nolan CR, Ayus JC. Cardiovascular calcification in patients with end-stage renal disease: a century-old phenomenon. *Kidney Int* 2002:82(Suppl):S73–S80.

178. Qunibi WY, Abouzahr F, Mizani MR, et al. Cardiovascular calcification in Hispanic Americans (HA) with chronic kidney disease (CKD) due to type 2 diabetes. *Kidney Int* 2005;68:271–277.

179. Qunibi WY. Cardiovascular calcification in nondialyzed patients with chronic kidney disease. *Semin Dial* 2007;20(2):134–138.

180. Budoff MJ, Rader DJ, Reilly MP, et al. Relationship of estimated GFR and coronary artery calcification in the CRIC (Chronic Renal Insufficiency Cohort) study. *Am J Kidney Dis* 2011;58:519–526.

181. Toussaint ND, Lau KK, Strauss BJ, et al. Associations between vascular calcification, arterial stiffness and bone mineral density in chronic kidney disease. *Nephrol Dial Transplant* 2008;23:586–593.

182. Shroff RC, McNair R, Skepper JN, et al. Chronic mineral dysregulation promotes vascular smooth muscle cell adaptation and extracellular matrix calcification. *J Am Soc Nephrol* 2010;21:103–112.

183. Fang Y, Ginsberg C, Sugatani T, et al. Early chronic kidney disease-mineral bone disorder stimulates vascular calcification. *Kidney Int* 2014;85(1):142–150.

184. McCullough PA, Agrawal V, Danielewicz E, et al. Accelerated atherosclerotic calcification and Monckeberg's sclerosis: a continuum of advanced vascular pathology in chronic kidney disease. *Clin J Am Soc Nephrol* 2008;3:1585–1598.

185. Amann K. Media calcification and intima calcification are distinct entities in chronic kidney disease. *Clin J Am Soc Nephrol* 2008;3:1599–1605.

186. Paloian NJ, Giachelli CM. A current understanding of vascular calcification in CKD. *Am J Physiol Renal Physiol* 2014;307:F891–F900.

187. Shroff R, Long DA, Shanahan C. Mechanistic Insights into vascular calcification in CKD. *J Am Soc Nephrol* 2013;24:179–189.

188. Reynolds JL, Joannides AJ, Skepper JN, et al. Human vascular smooth muscle cells undergo vesicle-mediated calcification in response to changes in extracellular calcium and phosphate concentrations: a potential mechanism for accelerated vascular calcification in ESRD. *J Am Soc Nephrol* 2004;15:2857–2867.

189. Son BK, Kozaki K, Iijima K, et al. Statins protect human aortic smooth muscle cells from inorganic phosphate-induced calcification by restoring Gas6-Axl survival pathway. *Circ Res* 2006;98:1024–1031.

190. Kestenbaum B, Sampson JN, Rudser KD, et al. Serum phosphate levels and mortality risk among people with chronic kidney disease. *J Am Soc Nephrol* 2005;16(2):520–528.

191. Tonelli M, Sacks F, Pfeffer M, et al. Relation between serum phosphate level and cardiovascular event rate in people with coronary disease. *Circulation* 2005;112:2627–2633.

192. Neves KR, Graciolli FG, dos Reis LM, et al. Vascular calcification: contribution of parathyroid hormone in renal failure. *Kidney Int* 2007;71:1262–1270.

193. Ozkok A, Kekik C, Karahan GE, et al. FGF-23 associated with the progression of coronary artery calcification in hemodialysis patients. *BMC Nephrol* 2013;14:241–247.

194. van Venrooij NA, Pereira RC, Tintut Y, et al. FGF23 protein expression in coronary arteries is associated with impaired kidney function. *Nephrol Dial Transplant* 2014;29(8):1525–1532.

195. Scialla JJ, Lau WL, Reilly MP, et al. Fibroblast growth factor 23 is not associated with and does not induce arterial calcification. *Kidney Int* 2013;83(6):1159–1168.

196. Lim K, Lu TS, Molostvov G, et al. Vascular klotho deficiency potentiates the development of human artery calcification and mediates resistance to FGF-23. *Circulation* 2012;125:2243–2255.

197. Chertow GM, Burke SK, Raggi P. Sevelamer attenuates the progression of coronary and aortic calcification in hemodialysis patients. *Kidney Int* 2002;62:245–252.

198. Block GA, Spiegel DM, Ehrlich J, et al. Effects of sevelamer and calcium on coronary artery calcification in patients new to hemodialysis. *Kidney Int* 2005;68:1815–1824.

199. Russo D, Miranda I, Ruocco C, et al. The progression of coronary artery calcification in predialysis patients on calcium carbonate or sevelamer. *Kidney Int* 2007;72:1255–1261.

200. Suki WN. Effects of sevelamer and calcium-based phosphate binders on mortality in hemodialysis patients: results of a randomized clinical trial. *J Ren Nutr* 2008;18:91–98.

201. Block GA, Raggi P, Bellasi A, et al. Mortality effect of coronary calcification and phosphate binder choice in incident hemodialysis patients. *Kidney Int* 2007;71:438–441.

202. Jamal SA, Vandermeer B, Raggi P, et al. Effect of calcium-based versus non-calcium-based phosphate binders on mortality in patients with chronic kidney disease: an updated systematic review and meta-analysis. *Lancet* 2013;382:1268–1277.

203. Qunibi W, Moustafa M, Muenz LR, et al. A 1-year randomized trial of calcium acetate versus sevelamer on progression of coronary artery calcification in hemodialysis patients with comparable lipid control: the Calcium Acetate Renagel Evaluation-2 (CARE-2) study. *Am J Kidney Dis* 2008;51:952–965.

204. Barreto DV, Barreto FdC, de Carvalho AB, et al. Phosphate binder impact on bone remodeling and coronary calcification—results from the BRiC study. *Nephron* 2008;110:c273–c283.

205. St. Peter WL, Liu J, Weinhandl E, et al. A comparison of sevelamer and calcium-based phosphate binders on mortality, hospitalization, and morbidity in hemodialysis: a secondary analysis of the Dialysis Clinical Outcomes Revisited (DCOR) randomized trial using claims data. *Am J Kidney Dis* 2008;51:445–454.

206. Tonelli M, Wiebe N, Culleton B, et al; for the Alberta Kidney Disease Network. Systematic review of the clinical efficacy and safety of sevelamer in dialysis patients. *Nephrol Dial Transplant* 2007;22(10):2856–2866.

207. Block GA, Wheeler DC, Persky MS, et al. Effects of phosphate binders in moderate CKD. *J Am Soc Nephrol* 2012;23:1407–1415.

208. Tonelli M, Pannu N, Manns B. Oral phosphate binders in patients with kidney failure. *N Engl J Med* 2010;362:1312–1324.

209. Isakova T, Gutierrez OM, Chang Y, et al. Phosphorus binders and survival on hemodialysis. *J Am Soc Nephrol* 2009;20:388–396.

210. Cannata-Andía JB, Fernández-Martín JL, Locatelli F, et al. Use of phosphate-binding agents is associated with a lower risk of mortality. *Kidney Int* 2013;84:998–1008.

211. Winkelmayer WC, Liu J, Kestenbaum B. Comparative effectiveness of calcium-containing phosphate binders in incident US dialysis patients. *Clin J Am Soc Nephrol* 2011;6:175–183.

212. London GM, Guérin AP, Marchais SJ, et al. Arterial media calcification in end-stage renal disease: impact on all-cause and cardiovascular mortality. *Nephrol Dial Transplant* 2003;18:1731–1740.

213. Blacher J, Guerin AP, Pannier B, et al. Impact of aortic stiffness on survival in end-stage renal disease. *Circulation* 1999;99:2434–2439.

214. Braun J, Oldendorf M, Moshage W, et al. Electron beam computed tomography in the evaluation of cardiac calcification in chronic dialysis patients. *Am J Kidney Dis* 1996;27:394–401.

215. Goodman WG, Goldin J, Kuizon BD, et al. Coronary-artery calcification in young adults with end-stage renal disease who are undergoing dialysis. *N Engl J Med* 2000;342:1478–1483.

216. Detrano R, Hsiai T, Wang S, et al. Prognostic value of coronary calcification and angiographic stenoses in patients undergoing coronary angiography. *J Am Coll Cardiol* 1996;27(2):285–290.

217. Arad Y, Spadaro LA, Goodman K, et al. Prediction of coronary events with electron beam computed tomography. *J Am Coll Cardiol* 2000;36:1253–1260.

218. Rumberger JA, Brundage BH, Rader DJ, et al. Electron beam computed tomographic coronary artery calcium scanning: a review and guidelines for use in asymptomatic persons. *Mayo Clin Proc* 1999;74:243–252.

219. Raggi P, Chertow GM, Torres PU, et al. The ADVANCE study: a randomized study to evaluate the effects of cinacalcet plus low-dose vitamin D on vascular calcification in patients on hemodialysis. *Nephrol Dial Transplant* 2011;26:1327–1339.

220. Chertow GM, Block GA, Correa-Rotter R, et al. Effect of cinacalcet on cardiovascular disease in patients undergoing dialysis. *N Engl J Med* 2012;367:2482–2494.

221. Conlon P, Krucoff MW, Minda S, et al. Incidence and long-term significance of transient ST segment deviation in hemodialysis patients. *Clin Nephrol* 1998;49:236–239.

222. Gowdak LHW, de Paula FJ, César LAM, et al. Screening for significant coronary artery disease in high-risk renal transplant candidates. *Coron Artery Dis* 2007;18(7):553–558.

223. Kasiske BL, Cangro CB, Hariharan S, et al. The evaluation of renal transplantation candidates: clinical practice guidelines. *Am J Transplant* 2002;1(Suppl 2):3–95.

224. Philipson J, Carpenter BJ, Itzkoff J, et al. Evaluation of cardiovascular risk for renal transplantation in diabetic patients. *Am J Med* 1986;81:630–634.

225. Ramos E, Kasiske BL, Alexander SR, et al. The evaluation of candidates for renal transplantation. *Transplantation* 1994;57:490–497.

226. Brown K, Rimmer J, Haisch C. Noninvasive cardiac risk stratification of diabetic and nondiabetic uremic renal allograft candidates using dipyridamole-thallium-201 imaging and radionuclide ventriculography. *Am J Cardiol* 1989;64:1017–1021.

227. Dubin RF, Li Y, He J, et al. CRIC Study Investigators: predictors of high sensitivity cardiac troponin T in chronic kidney disease patients: a cross-sectional study in the chronic renal insufficiency cohort (CRIC). *BMC Nephrol* 2013;14:229–236.

228. Jain N, Hedayati SS. How should clinicians interpret cardiac troponin values in patients with ESRD? *Semin Dial* 2011;24:398–400.

229. National Kidney Foundation. K/DOQI clinical practice guidelines for cardiovascular disease in dialysis patients. *Am J Kidney Dis* 2005;45:16–153.

230. Apple FS, Murakami MM, Pearce LA, et al. Multi-biomarker risk stratification of N-terminal pro-B-type natriuretic peptide, high-sensitivity C-reactive protein, and cardiac troponin T and I in end-stage renal disease for all-cause death. *Clin Chem* 2004;50:2279–2285.

231. Khan NA, Hemmelgarn BR, Tonelli M, et al. Prognostic value of troponin T and I among asymptomatic patients with end-stage renal disease: a meta-analysis. *Circulation* 2005;112:3088–3096.

232. Giannitsis E, Katus HA. Troponin T release in hemodialysis patients. *Circulation* 2004;110:e25–e26.

233. Lauer MS. Cardiac troponins and renal failure: the evolution of a clinical test. *Circulation* 2005;112:3036–3037.

234. Zoccali C, Mallamaci F, Benedetto FA, et al. Cardiac natriuretic peptides are related to left ventricular mass and function and predict mortality in dialysis patients. *J Am Soc Nephrol* 2001;12:1508–1515.

235. Aviles RJ, Askari AT, Lindahl B, et al. Troponin T levels in patients with acute coronary syndromes, with or without renal dysfunction. *N Engl J Med* 2002;346:2047–2052.

236. Antman EM. Decision making with cardiac troponin tests. *N Engl J Med* 2002;346:2079–2082.

237. Porter GA, Norton T, Bennett WM. Long-term follow p of the utility of troponin T to assess cardiac risk in stable chronic hemodialysis patients. *Clin Lab* 2000;46:469–476.

238. Iliou MC, Fumeron C, Benoit MO, et al. Factors associated with increased serum levels of cardiac troponins T and I in chronic haemodialysis patients: Chronic Haemodialysis and New Cardiac Markers Evaluation (CHANCE) study. *Nephrol Dial Transplant* 2001;16:1452–1458.

239. Mallamaci F, Zoccali C, Parlongo S, et al. Troponin is related to left ventricular mass and predicts all-cause and cardiovascular mortality in hemodialysis patients. *Am J Kidney Dis* 2002;40:68–75.

240. Sommerer C, Beimler J, Schwenger V, et al. Cardiac biomarkers and survival in haemodialysis patients. *Eur J Clin Invest* 2007;37: 350–356.

241. Zoccali C, Tripepi G, Mallamaci F. Predictors of cardiovascular death in ESRD. *Semin Nephrol* 2005;25:358–362.

242. Chang JW, Yang WS, Min WK, et al. Effects of simvastatin on high-sensitivity C-reactive protein and serum albumin in hemodialysis patients. *Am J Kidney Dis* 2002;39:1213–1217.

243. Lacson E Jr, Levin NW. C-reactive protein and end-stage renal disease. *Semin Dial* 2004;17:438–448.

244. Rao M, Guo D, Perianayagam MC, et al. Plasma interleukin-6 predicts cardiovascular mortality in hemodialysis patients. *Am J Kidney Dis* 2005;45:324–333.

245. Panichi V, Rizza GM, Paoletti S, et al; and the RISCAVID Study Group. Chronic inflammation and mortality in haemodialysis: effect of different renal replacement therapies. Results from the RISCAVID study. *Nephrol Dial Transplant* 2008;23:2337–2343.

246. Maisel AS, Krishnaswamy P, Nowak RM, et al. Rapid measurement of B-type natriuretic peptide in the emergency diagnosis of heart failure. *N Engl J Med* 2002;347:161–167.

247. Wang TJ, Larson MG, Levy D, et al. Plasma natriuretic peptide levels and the risk of cardiovascular events and death. *N Engl J Med* 2004;350:655–663.

248. Zoccali C, Mallamaci F, Tripepi G. Novel cardiovascular risk factors in end-stage renal disease. *J Am Soc Nephrol* 2004;15:S77–S80.

249. Lentine KL, Brennan DC, Schnitzler MA. Incidence and predictors of myocardial infarction after kidney transplantation. *J Am Soc Nephrol* 2005;16:496–506.

250. Kasiske BL, Maclean JR, Snyder JJ. Acute myocardial infarction and kidney transplantation. *J Am Soc Nephrol* 2006;17:900–907.

251. Lentine KL, Schnitzler MA, Abbott KC, et al. De novo congestive heart failure after kidney transplantation: a common condition with poor prognostic implications. *Am J Kidney Dis* 2005;46:720–733.

252. Lentine KL, Schnitzler MA, Abbott KC, et al. Incidence, predictors, and associated outcomes of atrial fibrillation after kidney transplantation. *Clin J Am Soc Nephrol* 2006;1:288–296.

253. de Mattos AM, Prather J, Olyaei AJ, et al. Cardiovascular events following renal transplantation: role of traditional and transplant-specific risk factors. *Kidney Int* 2006;70:757–764.

254. Briggs JD. Causes of death after renal transplantation. *Nephrol Dial Transplant* 2001;16:1545–1549.

255. Kasiske BL. Ischemic heart disease after renal transplantation. *Kidney Int* 2002;61:356–360.

256. Wheeler DC, Steiger J. Evolution and etiology of cardiovascular disease in renal transplant recipients. *Transplantation* 2000;70(Suppl 11): SS41–SS45.

257. Barrionuevo JD, Vargas-Machuca MF, Pulido FG, et al. Prevalence of cardiovascular disease in kidney transplant candidates: outpatient cardiac evaluation. *Transplant Proc* 2010;42(8):3126–3127.

258. Jeloka TK, Ross H, Smith R, et al. Renal transplant outcome in high-cardiovascular risk recipients. *Clin Transplant* 2007;21:609–614.

259. Abbott KC, Villines TC. Cardiac stress testing in patients with end-stage renal disease. *Semin Dial* 2014;27:547–549.

260. Lentine KL, Costa SP, Weir MR, et al. Cardiac disease evaluation and management among kidney and liver transplantation candidates: a scientific statement from the American Heart Association and the American College of Cardiology Foundation: endorsed by the American Society of Transplant Surgeons, American Society of Transplantation, and National Kidney Foundation. *Circulation* 2012;126(5):617–663.

261. Choi HY, Park HC, Ha SK. How do we manage coronary artery disease in patients with CKD and ESRD? *Electrolyte Blood Press* 2014;12(2):41–54.

262. Karthikeyan V, Ananthasubramaniam K. Coronary risk assessment and management options in chronic kidney disease patients prior to kidney transplantation. *Curr Cardiol Rev* 2009;5:177–186.

263. Danovitch GM, Hariharan S, Pirsch JD, et al. Management of the waiting list for cadaveric kidney transplants: report of a survey and recommendations by the Clinical Practice Guidelines Committee of the American Society of Transplantation. *J Am Soc Nephrol* 2002;13:528–535.

264. Le A, Wilson R, Douek K, et al. Prospective risk stratification in renal transplant candidates for cardiac death. *Am J Kidney Dis* 1994;24: 65–71.

265. DeLemos JA, Hillis DL. Diagnosis and management of coronary artery disease in patients with end-stage renal disease on hemodialysis. *J Am Soc Nephrol* 1996;7:2044–2054.

266. Lewis MS, Wilson RA, Walker K, et al. Factors in cardiac risk stratification of candidates for renal transplant. *J Cardiovasc Risk* 1999;6: 251–255.

267. Siedlecki A, Foushee M, Curtis JJ, et al. The impact of left ventricular systolic dysfunction on survival after renal transplantation. *Transplantation* 2007;84(12):1610–1617.

268. Murphy SW, Parfrey PS. Screening for cardiovascular disease in dialysis patients. *Curr Opin Neph Hypert* 1996;5:532–540.

269. Harnett JD, Foley RN, Kent GM, et al. Congestive heart failure in dialysis patients: prevalence, incidence, prognosis and risk factors. *Kidney Int* 1995;47:884–890.

270. Rigatto C, Foley RN, Kent GM, et al. Long-term changes in left ventricular hypertrophy after renal transplantation. *Transplantation* 2000;70:570–575.

271. Ramanathan V, Goral S, Tanriover B, et al. Screening asymptomatic diabetic patients for coronary artery disease prior to renal transplantation. *Transplantation* 2005;79(10):1453–1458.

272. Manske C, Thomas W, Wang Y, et al. Screening diabetic transplant candidates for coronary artery disease: identification of a low risk subgroup. *Kidney Int* 1993;44:617–621.

273. Stokkel M, Duchateau CS, Jukema W, et al. Noninvasive assessment of left ventricular function prior to and 6 months after renal transplantation. *Transplant Proc* 2007;39:3159–3162.

274. Camp A, Garvin PJ, Hoff J, et al. Prognostic value of intravenous dipyridamole thallium imaging in patients with diabetes mellitus considered for renal transplantation. *Am J Cardiol* 1990;65:1459–1463.

275. Reis G, Marcovitz PA, Leichtman AB, et al. Usefulness of dobutamine stress echocardiography in detecting coronary artery disease in end-stage renal disease. *Am J Cardiol* 1995;75:707–710.

276. Morrow CE, Schwartz JS, Sutherland DE, et al. Predictive value of thallium stress testing for coronary and cardiovascular events in uremic diabetic patients before renal transplantation. *Am J Surg* 1983;146:331–335.

277. Marwick TH, Steinmuller DR, Underwood DA, et al. Ineffectiveness of dipyridamole SPECT thallium imaging as a screening technique for coronary artery disease in patients with end-stage renal failure. *Transplant* 1990;49:100–103.

278. Boudreau RJ, Strony JT, duCret RP, et al. Perfusion thallium imaging of type I diabetes patients with ESRD: comparison of oral and intravenous dipyridamole administration. *Radiology* 1990;175:103–105.

279. Derfler K, Kletter K, Balcke P, et al. Predictive value of thallium-201-dipyridamole myocardial stress scintigraphy in chronic hemodialysis patients and transplant recipients. *Clin Nephrol* 1991;36:192–202.

280. Sharma R, Pellerin D, Gaze DC, et al. Dobutamine stress echocardiography and the resting but not exercise electrocardiograph predict severe coronary artery disease in renal transplant candidates. *Nephrol Dial Transplant* 2005;20:2207–2214.

281. Rabbat CG, Treleaven DJ, Russell JD, et al. Prognostic value of myocardial perfusion studies in patients with end-stage renal disease assessed for kidney or kidney-pancreas transplantation: a meta-analysis. *J Am Soc Nephrol* 2003;14:431–439.

282. Schmidt A, Stefenelli T, Schuster E, et al. Informational contribution of noninvasive screening tests for coronary artery disease in patients on chronic renal replacement therapy. *Am J Kidney Dis* 2001;37:56–63.

283. Braun W, Marwick TH. Coronary artery disease in renal transplant recipients. *Cleve Clin J Med* 1994;61:370–385.

284. Charytan D, Kuntz RE. The exclusion of patients with chronic kidney disease from clinical trials in coronary artery disease. *Kidney Int* 2006;70:2021–2030.

285. Kidney Disease: Improving Global Outcomes (KDIGO) Anemia Work Group. KDIGO clinical practice guideline for anemia in chronic kidney disease. *Kidney Int* 2012;(Suppl 2):279–335.

286. Painter P, Moore G, Carlson L, et al. Effects of exercise training plus normalization of hematocrit on exercise capacity and health-related quality of life. *Am J Kidney Dis* 2002;39:257–265.

287. Silberberg JS, Barre PE, Prichard SS, et al. Impact of left ventricular hypertrophy on survival in end-stage renal disease. *Kidney Int* 1989;36:286–290.

288. Sargoca MA, Canziani ME, Cassiolato JL, et al. Left ventricular hypertrophy as a risk factor for arrhythmias in hemodialysis patients. *J Cardiovasc Pharmacol* 1991;17(Suppl 2):S136–S138.

289. Zoccali C, Mallamaci F, Maas R, et al. Left ventricular hypertrophy, cardiac remodeling and asymmetric dimethylarginine (ADMA) in hemodialysis patients. *Kidney Int* 2002;62:339–345.

290. Selvin E, Marinopoulos S, Berkenblit G, et al. Meta-analysis: glycosylated hemoglobin and cardiovascular disease in diabetes mellitus. *Ann Intern Med* 2004;141:421–431.

291. Shurraw S, Majumdar SR, Thadhani R, et al. Glycemic control and the risk of death in 1,484 patients receiving maintenance hemodialysis. *Am J Kidney Dis* 2010;55:875–884.

292. Gottlieb SO. Asymptomatic or silent myocardial ischemia in angina pectoris: pathophysiology and clinical implications. *Cardiol Clin* 1991;9:49–61.

293. Wright RS, Reeder GS, Herzog CA, et al. Acute myocardial infarction and renal dysfunction: a high-risk combination. *Ann Intern Med* 2002;137:563–570.

294. Jardine MJ, Ninomiya T, Perkovic V, et al. Aspirin is beneficial in hypertensive patients with chronic kidney disease: a post-hoc subgroup analysis of a randomized controlled trial. *J Am Coll Cardiol* 2010;56:956–965.

295. Antithrombotic Trialists' Collaboration. Collaborative meta-analysis of randomized trials of antiplatelet therapy for the prevention of death, myocardial infarction, and stroke in high risk patients. *BMJ* 2002;324:71–86.

296. Berger AK, Duval S, Krumholz HM. Aspirin, beta-blocker, and angiotensin-converting enzyme inhibitor therapy in patients with end-stage renal disease and an acute myocardial infarction. *J Am Coll Cardiol* 2003;42:201–208.

297. Abbott KC, Trespalacios FC, Agodoa LY, et al. Beta-blocker use in long-term dialysis patients: association with hospitalized heart failure and mortality. *Arch Intern Med* 2004;164:2465–2471.

298. McCullough PA, Sandberg KR, Borzak S et al. Benefits of aspirin and beta-blockade after myocardial infarction in patients with chronic kidney disease. *Am Heart J* 2002;144:226–232.

299. Weir MA, Dixon SN, Fleet JL, et al. β-Blocker dialyzability and mortality in older patients receiving hemodialysis. *J Am Soc Nephrol* 2015;26:987–996.

300. Wanner C, Krane V, Marz W, et al. Atorvastatin in patients with type 2 diabetes mellitus undergoing hemodialysis. *N Engl J Med* 2005;353:238–248.

301. Fellstrom BC, Jardine AG, Schmieder RE, et al. Rosuvastatin and cardiovascular events in patients undergoing hemodialysis. *N Engl J Med* 2009;360:1395–1407.

302. Baigent C, Landray MJ, Reith C; for the SHARP Investigators. The effects of lowering LDL cholesterol with simvastatin plus ezetimibe in patients with chronic kidney disease (Study of Heart and Renal Protection): a randomized placebo-controlled trial. *Lancet* 2011;377:2181–2192.

303. Kasiske BL, Wanner C, O'Neill WC. An assessment of statin safety by nephrologists. *Am J Cardiol* 2006;97:82C–85C.

304. Schech S, Graham D, Staffa J, et al. Risk factors for statin-associated rhabdomyolysis. *Pharmacoepidemiol Drug Saf* 2006;16:352–358.

305. Thompson PD, Clarkson P, Karas RH. Statin-associated myopathy. *JAMA* 2003;289:1681–1690.

306. Kidney Disease: Improving Global Outcomes (KDIGO) Lipid Work Group. KDIGO Clinical Practice Guideline for lipid management in chronic kidney disease. *Kidney Int* 2013;3(Suppl):259–305.

307. Efrati S, Zaidenstein R, Dishy V, et al. ACE inhibitors and survival of hemodialysis patients. *Am J Kidney Dis* 2002;40:1023–1029.

308. McCullough PA, Sandberg KR, Yee J, et al. Mortality benefit of angiotensin-converting enzyme inhibitors after cardiac events in patients with end-stage renal disease. *J Renin Angiotensin Aldosterone Syst* 2002;3:188–191.

309. Zannad F, Kessler M, Grunfeld JP, et al. FOSIDIAL: a randomised placebo controlled trial of the effects of fosinopril on cardiovascular morbidity and mortality in haemodialysis patients. Study design and patients' baseline characteristics. *Fundam Clin Pharmacol* 2002;16:353–360.

310. Gupta T, Harikrishnan P, Kolte D, et al. Trends in management and outcomes of ST-elevation myocardial infarction in patients with end-stage renal disease in the United States. *Am J Cardiol* 2015;115(8):1033–1041.

311. Charytan D, Mauri L, Agarwal A, et al. The use of invasive cardiac procedures after acute myocardial infarction in long-term dialysis patients. *Am Heart J* 2006;152:558–564.

312. United States Renal Data System. *USRDS 2011 Annual Data Report: Atlas of Chronic Kidney Disease and End-Stage Renal Disease in the United States.* Bethesda, MD: National Institutes of Health, National Institute of Diabetes and Digestive and Kidney Diseases, 2011.

313. Marso SP, Gimple LW, Philbrick JT, et al. Effectiveness of percutaneous coronary interventions to prevent recurrent coronary events in patients on chronic hemodialysis. *Am J Cardiol* 1998;82:378–380.

314. Schoebel FC, Gradaus F, Ivens K, et al. Restenosis after elective coronary balloon angioplasty in patients with end stage renal disease: a case-control study using quantitative coronary angiography. *Heart* 1997;78:337–342.

315. Le Feuvre C, Dambrin G, Helft G, et al. Clinical outcome following coronary angioplasty in dialysis patients: a case-control study in the era of coronary stenting. *Heart* 2001;85:556–560.

316. Kahn JK, Rutherford BD, McConahay DR, et al. Short- and long-term outcome of percutaneous transluminal coronary angioplasty in chronic dialysis patients. *Am Heart J* 1990;119:484–489.

317. Ahmed WA, Kirshenbaum JM. Outcome of coronary artery angioplasty in hemodialysis patients. *Semin Dial* 1994;7:96–99.

318. Le Feuvre C, Dambrin G, Helft G, et al. Comparison of clinical outcome following coronary stenting or balloon angioplasty in dialysis versus non-dialysis patients. *Am J Cardiol* 2000;85:1365–1368.

319. Das P, Moliterno DJ, Charnigo R, et al. Impact of drug-eluting stents on outcomes of patients with end-stage renal disease undergoing percutaneous coronary revascularization. *J Invasive Cardiol* 2006;18:405–408.

320. Aoyama T, Ishii H, Toriyama T, et al. Sirolimus-eluting stents vs bare metal stents for coronary intervention in japanese patients with renal failure on hemodialysis. *Cir J* 2008;72:56–60.

321. Nishida K, Kimura T, Kawai K, et al. Comparison of outcomes using the sirolimus-eluting stent in calcified versus non-calcified native coronary lesions in patients on- versus not on-chronic hemodialysis (from the j-Cypher registry). *Am J Cardiol* 2013;112(5):647–655.

322. Best PJM, Lennon R, Ting HH, et al. The impact of renal insufficiency on clinical outcomes in patients undergoing percutaneous coronary interventions. *J Am Coll Cardiol* 2002;39:1113–1119.

323. Rubenstein MH, Harrell LC, Sheynberg BV, et al. Are patients with renal failure good candidates for percutaneous coronary revascularization in the new device era? *Circulation* 2000;102:2966–2972.

324. Gruberg L, Weissman NJ, Waksman R, et al. Comparison of outcomes after percutaneous coronary revascularization with stents in patients with and without mild chronic renal insufficiency. *Am J Cardiol* 2002;89:54–57.

325. Narala KR, Hassan S, LaLonde TA, et al. Management of coronary atherosclerosis and acute coronary syndromes in patients with chronic kidney disease. *Curr Probl Cardiol* 2013;38(5):165–206.

326. Liu JY, Birkmeyer NJ, Sanders JH, et al. Risks of morbidity and mortality in dialysis patients undergoing coronary artery bypass surgery. Northern New England Cardiovascular Disease Study Group. *Circulation* 2000;24:2973–2977.

327. Szczech LA, Reddan DN, Owen WF, et al. Differential survival after coronary revascularization procedures among patients with renal insufficiency. *Kidney Int* 2001;60:292–299.

328. Hemmelgarn BR, Southern D, Culleton BF, et al; and the Alberta Provincial Project for Outcomes Assessment in Coronary Heart Disease (APPROACH) Investigators. Survival after coronary revascularization among patients with kidney disease. *Circulation* 2004;110(14):1890–1895.

329. Zheng H, Xue S, Lian F, et al. Meta-analysis of clinical studies comparing coronary artery bypass grafting with percutaneous coronary intervention in patients with end-stage renal disease. *Eur J Cardiothorac Surg* 2013;43(3):459–467.

330. Kannan A, Poongkunran C, Medina R, et al. Coronary revascularization in chronic and end-stage renal disease: a systematic review and meta-analysis. *Am J Ther* 2016;23:e16–e28.

331. Fellner SK, Follman D, Dasgupta DS, et al. Ischemic heart disease in patients with end-stage renal disease. *Adv Ren Replace Ther* 1996;3:240–249.

332. Hillis LD. Coronary artery bypass surgery: risks and benefits, realistic and unrealistic expectations. *J Invest Med* 1995;43:17–27.

333. Franga DL, Kratz JM, Crumbley AJ, et al. Early and long-term results of coronary artery bypass grafting in dialysis patients. *Ann Thorac Surg* 2000;70:813–819.

334. Castelli P, Condemi AM, Munari M. Immediate and long-term results of coronary revascularization in patients undergoing chronic hemodialysis. *Eur J Cardiothorac Surg* 1999;15:51–54.

335. Osake S, Osawa H, Miyazawa M, et al. Immediate and long-term results of coronary artery bypass operation in hemodialysis patients. *Artif Organs* 2001;25:252–255.

336. Okamura Y, Mochizuki Y, Iida H, et al. Coronary artery bypass in dialysis patients. *Artif Organs* 2001;25:256–259.

337. Naruse Y, Makuuchi H, Kobayashi T, et al. Coronary artery bypass grafting in patients with dialysis-dependent renal failure. *Artif Organs* 2001;25:260–262.

338. Higashiue S, Nishimura Y, Shinbo M, et al. Coronary artery bypass grafting in patients with dialysis-dependent renal failure. *Artif Organs* 2001;25:263–267.

339. Nishida H, Uchikawa S, Chikazawa G, et al. Coronary artery bypass grafting in 105 patients with hemodialysis-dependent renal failure. *Artif Organs* 2001;25:268–272.

340. Hirose H, Amano A, Takahashi A. Efficacy of off-pump coronary bypass grafting for the patients on chronic hemodialysis. *Jpn J Thorac Cardiovasc Surg* 2001;49:693–699.

341. Beckermann J, Van Camp J, Li S, et al. On-pump versus off-pump coronary surgery outcomes in patients requiring dialysis: perspectives from a single center and the United States experience. *J Thorac Cardiovasc Surg* 2006;131:1261–1266.

342. Opsahl J, Husebye DG, Helseth HK, et al. Coronary artery bypass surgery in patients on maintenance dialysis: long-term survival. *Am J Kidney Dis* 1988;12:271–274.

343. Buxton AE, Calkins H, Callans DJ, et al. ACC/AHA/HRS 2006 key data elements and definitions for electrophysiological studies and procedures: a report of the American College of Cardiology/American Heart Association Task Force on Clinical Data Standards (ACC/AHA/HRS Writing Committee to Develop Data Standards on Electrophysiology). *Circulation* 2006;114:2534–2570.

344. Green D, Roberts PR, New DI, et al. Sudden cardiac death in hemodialysis patients: an in-depth review. *Am J Kidney Dis* 2011;57(6):921–929.

345. Parekh ES. Expect the unexpected: sudden cardiac death in dialysis patients. *Clin J Am Soc Nephrol* 2012;7:8–11.

346. Zachariah D, Kalra PR, Roberts PR. Sudden cardiac death in end stage renal disease: unlocking the mystery. *J Nephrol* 2015;28(2):133–141.

347. Middleton JP. Predisposition to arrhythmias: electrolytes, uremic fibrosis, other factors. *Semin Dial* 2011;24:287–289.

348. United States Renal Data System. *USRDS 2010 Annual Data Report: Atlas of Chronic Kidney Disease and End-Stage Renal Disease in the United States.* Bethesda, MD: National Institutes of Health, National Institute of Diabetes and Digestive and Kidney Diseases, 2010.

349. Jadoul M, Thumma J, Fuller DS, et al. Modifiable practices associated with sudden death among hemodialysis patients in the dialysis outcomes and practice patterns study. *Clin J Am Soc Nephrol* 2012;7(5):765–774.

350. Takeda K, Harada A, Okuda S, et al. Sudden death in chronic dialysis patients. *Nephrol Dial Transplant* 1997;12:952–955.

351. Genovesi S, Valsecchi MG, Rossi E, et al. A sudden death and associated factors in a historical cohort of chronic haemodialysis patients. *Nephrol Dial Transplant* 2009;24:2529–2536.

352. Krane V, Heinrich F, Meesmann M, et al. Electrocardiography and outcome in patients with diabetes mellitus on maintenance hemodialysis. *Clin J Am Soc Nephrol* 2009;4:394–400.

353. Bleyer AJ, Hartman J, Brannon PC, et al. Characteristics of sudden death in hemodialysis patients. *Kidney Int* 2006;69:2268–2273.

354. Mangrum AJ, Liu D, Dimarco JP, et al. Sudden cardiac death and left ventricular function in hemodialysis patients. *Heart Rhythm* 2005;2(5):S41.

355. Paoletti E, Specchia C, Di Maio G, et al. The worsening of left ventricular hypertrophy is the strongest predictor of sudden cardiac death in haemodialysis patients: a 10 year survey. *Nephrol Dial Transplant* 2004;19(7):1829–1834.

356. Pun PH, Smarz TR, Honeycutt EF, et al. Chronic kidney disease is associated with increased risk of sudden cardiac death among patients with coronary artery disease. *Kidney Int* 2009;6:652–658.

357. Amann K, Breitbach M, Ritz E, et al. Myocyte/capillary mismatch in the heart of uremic patients. *J Am Soc Nephrol.* 1998;9(6):1018–1022.

358. Mark PB, Johnston N, Groenning BA, et al. Redefinition of uremic cardiomyopathy by contrast-enhanced cardiac magnetic resonance imaging. *Kidney Int* 2006;69(10):1839–1845.

359. Schietinger BJ, Brammer GM, Wang H, et al. Patterns of late gadolinium enhancement in chronic hemodialysis patients. *JACC Cardiovasc Imaging* 2008;1(4):450–456.

360. Amann K, Ritz E, Wiest G, et al. A role of parathyroid hormone for the activation of cardiac fibroblasts in uremia. *J Am Soc Nephrol* 1994;4(10):1814–1819.

361. Burton JO, Jefferies HJ, Selby NM, et al. Hemodialysis-induced cardiac injury: determinants and associated outcomes. *Clin J Am Soc Nephrol* 2009;4(5):914–920.

362. Kovesdy C, Regidor D, Mehrotra R, et al. Serum and dialysate potassium concentrations and survival in hemodialysis patients. *Clin J Am Soc Nephrol* 2004;2:999–1007.

363. Pun PH, Lehrich RW, Honeycutt EF, et al. Modifiable risk factors associated with sudden cardiac arrest within hemodialysis clinics. *Kidney Int* 2011;79(2):218–227.

364. Karnik JA, Young BS, Lew NL, et al. Cardiac arrest and sudden death in dialysis units. *Kidney Int* 2001;60(1):350–357.

365. Movilli E, Gaggia P, Zubani R, et al. Association between high ultrafiltration rates and mortality in uraemic patients on regular haemodialysis. A 5-year prospective observational multicentre study. *Nephrol Dial Transplant* 2007;22(12):3547–3552.

366. Saran R, Bragg-Gresham JL, Levin NW, et al. Longer treatment time and slower ultrafiltration in hemodialysis: associations with reduced mortality in the DOPPS. *Kidney Int* 2006;69(7):1222–1228.

367. Flythe JE, Brunelli SM. The risks of high ultrafiltration rate in chronic hemodialysis: implications for patient care. *Semin Dial* 2011;24(3):259–265.

368. Pande S, Raja R, Bloom E, et al. Effect of dialysate baths on serum bicarbonate levels in hemodialysis patients. *Am J Kidney Dis* 2011;57(4):A75.

369. Tentori F, Karaboyas A, Robinson BM, et al. Association of dialysate bicarbonate concentration with mortality in the Dialysis Outcomes and Practice Patterns Study (DOPPS). *Am J Kidney Dis* 2013;62(4):738–746.

370. Gill GV, Woodward A, Casson IF, et al. Cardiac arrhythmia and nocturnal hypoglycaemia in type 1 diabetes—the 'dead in bed' syndrome revisited. *Diabetologia* 2009;52:42–45.

371. Drechsler C, Krane V, Ritz E, et al. Glycemic control and cardiovascular events in diabetic hemodialysis patients. *Circulation* 2009;120:2421–2428.

372. Parekh RS, Plantinga LC, Kao WH, et al. The association of sudden cardiac death with inflammation and other traditional risk factors. *Kidney Int* 2008;74(10):1335–1342.

373. Chan KE, Newton-Cheh C, Gusella JF, et al. Heritability of risk for sudden cardiac arrest in ESRD. *J Am Soc Nephrol* 2015;26:2815–2820.

374. Wan C, Herzog CA, Zareba W, et al. Sudden cardiac arrest in hemodialysis patients with wearable cardioverter defibrillator. *Ann Noninvasive Electrocardiol* 2014;19:247–257.

375. Davis TR, Young BA, Eisenberg MS, et al. Outcome of cardiac arrests attended by emergency medical services staff at community outpatient dialysis centers. *Kidney Int* 2008;73(8):933–939.

376. Hsueh CH, Chen NX, Lin SF, et al. Pathogenesis of arrhythmias in a model of CKD. *J Am Soc Nephrol* 2014;25(12):2812–2821.

377. Pun PH. The interplay between CKD, sudden cardiac death, and ventricular arrhythmias. *Adv Chronic Kidney Dis* 2014;21(6):480–488.

378. Chan KE, Maddux FW, Tolkoff-Rubin N, et al. Early outcomes among those initiating chronic dialysis in the United States. *Clin J Am Soc Nephrol* 2011;6:2642–2649.

379. Eckardt KU, Gillespie IA, Kronenberg F, et al. High cardiovascular event rates occur within the first weeks of starting hemodialysis. *Kidney Int* 2015;88:1117–1125.

380. Herzog CA, Li S, Weinhandl ED, et al. Survival of dialysis patients after cardiac arrest and the impact of implantable cardioverter defibrillators. *Kidney Int* 2005;68:818–825.

381. Ganesh SK, Stack AG, Levin NW, et al. Association of elevated serum PO(4), Ca x PO(4) product, and parathyroid hormone with cardiac mortality risk in chronic hemodialysis patients. *J Am Soc Nephrol* 2001;12(10):2131–2138.

382. Huikuri HV, Castellanos A, Myerburg RJ. Sudden death due to cardiac arrhythmias. *N Engl J Med* 2001;345(20):1473–1482.

383. Shastri S, Tangri N, Tighiouart H, et al. Predictors of sudden cardiac death: a competing risk approach in the Hemodialysis Study. *Clin J Am Soc Nephrol* 2012;7:123–130.

384. Cice G, Ferrara L, D'Andrea A, et al. Carvedilol increases two-year survival in dialysis patients with dilated cardiomyopathy: a prospective, placebo-controlled trial. *J Am Coll Cardiol* 2003;41(9):1438–1444.

385. Pun P, Lehrich RW, Smith SR, et al. Predictors of survival following cardiac arrest in outpatient hemodialysis clinics. *Clin J Am Soc Nephrol* 2007;2:491–500.

386. Tai DJ, Lim TW, James MT, et al. Cardiovascular effects of angiotensin converting enzyme inhibition or angiotensin receptor blockade in haemodialysis: a meta-analysis. *Clin J Am Soc Nephrol* 2010;5:623–630.

387. Pun PH, Horton JR, Middleton JP. Dialysate calcium concentration and the risk of sudden cardiac arrest in hemodialysis patients. *Clin J Am Soc Nephrol* 2013;8:797–803.

388. Santoro A, Mancini E, London G, et al. Patients with complex arrhythmias during and after haemodialysis suffer from different regimens of potassium removal. *Nephrol Dial Transplant* 2008;23(4):1415–1421.

389. Mendoza JM, Bayes LY, Sun S, et al. Effect of lowering dialysate sodium concentration on interdialytic weight gain and blood pressure in patients undergoing thrice-weekly in-center nocturnal hemodialysis: a quality improvement study. *Am J Kidney Dis* 2011;58(6):956–963.

390. Jefferies HJ, Burton JO, McIntyre CW. Individualized dialysate temperature improves intradialytic haemodynamics and abrogates haemodialysis-induced myocardial stunning, without compromising tolerability. *Blood Purif* 2011;32(1):63–68.

391. Pun PH, Al-Khatib SM, Han JY, et al. Implantable cardioverter-defibrillators for primary prevention of sudden cardiac death in CKD: a meta-analysis of patient-level data from 3 randomized trials. *Am J Kidney Dis* 2014;64:32–39.

392. Sakhuja R, Keebler M, Lai T-S, et al. Meta-analysis of mortality in dialysis patients with an implantable cardioverter defibrillator. *Am J Cardiol* 2009;103:735–741.

393. Dasgupta A, Montalvo J, Medendorp S, et al. Increased complication rates of cardiac rhythm management devices in ESRD patients. *Am J Kidney Dis* 2007;49(5):656–663.

394. Wase A, Basit A, Nazir R, et al. Impact of chronic kidney disease upon survival among implantable cardioverter-defibrillator recipients. *J Interv Card Electrophysiol* 2004;11(3):199–204.

395. Drew DA, Meyer KB, Weiner DE. Transvenous cardiac device wires and vascular access in hemodialysis patients. *Am J Kidney Dis* 2011;58(3):494–496.

396. Charytan DM, Patrick AR, Liu J, et al. Trends in the use and outcomes of implantable cardioverter-defibrillators in patients undergoing dialysis in the United States. *Am J Kidney Dis* 2011;58(3):409–417.

397. de Bie MK, Lekkerkerker JC, van Dam B, et al. Prevention of sudden cardiac death: rationale and design of the Implantable Cardioverter Defibrillators in Dialysis patients (ICD2) Trial—a prospective pilot study. *Curr Med Res Opin* 2008;24(8):2151–2157.

398. Herzog C. Can we prevent sudden cardiac death in dialysis patients? The WED-HED Trial. *Cardiorenal Med* 2014;4:140–145.

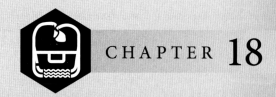

CHAPTER 18

Hemodynamic Stability and Autonomic Dysfunction in End-Stage Kidney Disease

Biff F. Palmer and William L. Henrich

The usual manifestation of hemodynamic instability during ultrafiltration dialysis (in which fluid removal is the primary goal) is hypotension. The incidence of a symptomatic reduction in blood pressure during or immediately following dialysis ranges from 15% to 50% of dialysis sessions (1). In some patients, the development of hypotension necessitates intravenous fluid replacement before the patient leaves the dialysis unit, which results in volume overload. Symptomatic hypotension may necessitate a premature discontinuation of the treatment, which if repetitive can lead to inadequate clearance. Intradialytic hypotension (IDH) and orthostatic hypotension after the procedure have been found to be independent risk factors affecting the morbidity and mortality of dialysis patients (TABLE 18.1) (2).

A second type of dialysis-related hypotension is a chronic, persistent form of hypotension that occurs in approximately 5% of dialysis patients (1). This second form of hypotension is usually observed in patients who have been on hemodialysis (HD) for at least 5 years. Such patients often come to the dialysis unit with a systolic blood pressure of less than 90 mm Hg. This form of hypotension is associated with an increased mortality and is often a manifestation of malnutrition and/or cardiovascular disease in the chronic HD patient (3–5). In one recent review of a group of such patients, chronically hypotensive patients had a lower peripheral resistance than normotensive patients (6). Of interest is that in this study, cardiac output was not significantly elevated in the hypotensive group, perhaps suggesting some decrease in cardiac reserve. This chapter focuses on the problem of episodic hypotension, which is the most frequent form of HD-related hemodynamic instability.

OVERVIEW OF THE PROBLEM

Dialysis hypotension is the result of an inadequate cardiovascular response to the reduction in blood volume that occurs when a large volume of water is removed over a short period of time. In a typical dialysis procedure, an ultrafiltrate volume that is equal to or greater that the entire plasma volume is often removed. Despite the large ultrafiltrate volume, plasma volume typically decreases by only approximately 10% to 20% (7). This ability to maintain plasma volume during ultrafiltration requires mobilization of fluid from the interstitial into the intravascular space. Adequate tone and normal compliance characteristics of the venous system is required to redistribute this fluid into the central circulation where it becomes available for cardiac refilling. Once delivered to the central circulation, normal systolic and diastolic function of the heart ensures maintenance of cardiac output. Should cardiac output begin to decline, blood pressure is stabilized by sympathetic nervous system–induced increases in peripheral vascular resistance.

Disturbances in either one or several of these steps will render the patient prone to develop hypotension in the setting of fluid removal (FIGURE 18.1). These disturbances can be the result of the chronic uremic state as well as accompanying comorbid conditions. The following sections review the various abnormalities

TABLE 18.1	Complications of Intradialytic Hypotension

Myocardial ischemia
Stroke
Mesenteric ischemia
Clotted access
Ischemic atrophy of the optic nerve with loss of vision
Inadequate clearance secondary to shortened treatment time
Persistent posttreatment volume overload

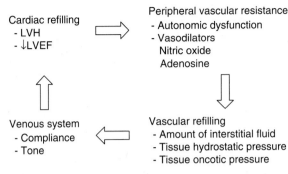

FIGURE 18.1 Overview of factors that influence vascular refilling and preservation of plasma volume in the setting of ultrafiltration. LVEF, left ventricular ejection fraction; LVH, left ventricular hypertrophy.

in the autonomic and cardiovascular systems that contribute to the development of episodic dialysis hypotension. The chapter concludes with a discussion of the prevention and management of dialysis-related hypotension.

VASCULAR REFILLING

The ability to maintain plasma volume during ultrafiltration requires mobilization of fluid from the extravascular into intravascular space. The success of vascular refilling is influenced by the stability of plasma osmolality, the rate of fluid removal, and other patient characteristics that dictate the distribution of fluid between the body fluid compartments.

Stable Plasma Osmolality

The importance of a stable plasma osmolality as a key element in preventing dialysis hypotension is discussed in detail concerning dialysate composition. The main mechanism by which a stable plasma osmolality contributes to hemodynamic stability appears to be through the maintenance of a more stable extracellular fluid volume and plasma volume (**FIGURE 18.2**) (8). The rapid fall in plasma osmolality that results from solute removal leads to the movement of water to intracellular loci. This movement of water will decrease the amount of fluid accessible for vascular refilling. The use of a higher dialysate sodium concentration (greater than 140 mEq/L) is an effective means to assure adequate vascular refilling and has proved to be

among the most effective and best-tolerated therapies for episodic hypotension. A high-dialysate sodium concentration limits the decline in plasma osmolality and therefore leads to the removal of volume during ultrafiltration from both intracellular and extracellular compartments. This effect limits the compromise in the plasma volume that normally occurs during rapid falls in plasma osmolality coupled with a very large ultrafiltration rate. Another potential mechanism by which a decline in plasma osmolality may contribute to dialysis hypotensive episodes is by impairing peripheral vasoconstriction during volume removal (9,10). A decline in plasma osmolality may also adversely affect baroreceptor function by blunting afferent sensing mechanisms, thereby contributing to autonomic dysfunction (9).

Local Starling Forces

Several patient characteristics that affect Starling forces operating at the capillary level influence the process of vascular refilling. One such characteristic is the amount of interstitial fluid present, a parameter clinically reflected by the dry weight of the patient. When the volume of interstitial fluid is small, any ultrafiltrate volume will more likely be associated with hemodynamic instability. This explains the development of hypotension when patients are dialyzed below their true dry weight. By contrast, increased amounts of interstitial fluid will expand the volume of fluid accessible for refilling of the intravascular space and, therefore, decrease the likelihood of hypotension. In most patients, a dry weight is selected that minimizes the amount of interstitial fluid present because chronic volume overload has long-term deleterious effects on the cardiovascular system. However, in patients with recurrent IDH or chronic persistent hypotension that is not amenable to other interventions, it may be necessary to purposely maintain the patient in a hypervolemic state so that the dialysis procedure can be employed with a lower likelihood of hemodynamic instability.

Determinants of the oncotic and hydrostatic pressure at the tissue level will also affect vascular refilling. For example, a well-nourished patient with a normal serum albumin concentration is more likely to have better preserved vascular refilling as compared to a patient with hypoalbuminemia. On the other hand, administration of a vasodilator has the potential to impair vascular refilling by allowing excessive transmission of arterial pressure into the capillary bed resulting in increased hydrostatic pressure.

CARDIAC REFILLING AND VENOUS DYSFUNCTION

When vascular refilling and plasma volume are normal, IDH can still occur if there is a failure to properly redistribute intravascular volume into the central circulation (11). In some patients, this failure can be traced to functional and structural abnormalities on the venous side of the circulation.

Because most plasma volume is located on the venous side of the circulation, even a small decrease in tone of the venous system can potentially limit cardiac filling because of a decrease in central blood volume. Abrupt splanchnic vasodilation can be the cause of IDH. Such vasodilation may result from ingestion of food during the dialysis procedure or withdrawal of sympathetic tone resulting from an increase in core body temperature. Increased production of vasodilators such as adenosine or nitric oxide may also play a role in this complication.

Decreased venous compliance has also been demonstrated in hypertensive HD patients (12,13). Such a disturbance in venous

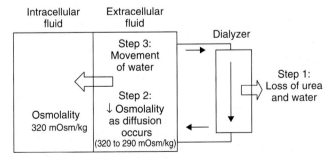

FIGURE 18.2 A decline in extracellular osmolality can contribute to hemodynamic instability. The first step is a reduction in osmolality as urea and other solutes are removed from the body across the dialyzer. This solute removal results in a decline in extracellular osmolality relative to the intracellular space. The third step is the osmotic movement of water from the extracellular to intracellular space.

compliance can lead to hemodynamic instability in at least two ways. First, decreased venous compliance leads to a steep volume-to-pressure relationship such that a major drop in cardiac filling pressure can occur with only a small decrease in plasma volume. In this regard, an inverse relationship has been observed between venous compliance and the fall in central venous pressure in dialysis patients during isolated ultrafiltration (12). Second, impaired venous compliance can lead to higher hydrostatic pressures in the upstream capillary bed resulting in reduced vascular refilling from the interstitium. Patients with evidence of decreased venous compliance exhibit a greater decrease in plasma volume during ultrafiltration as compared to those subjects with normal venous compliance characteristics (12,13). The basis for altered venous function in chronic uremia may relate to structural abnormalities of the venous wall. Morphologic studies of the iliac and inferior caval veins of hypertensive patients with end-stage kidney disease (ESKD) have shown increased thickness of the media in the venous wall (14). Such structural abnormalities may also impair the ability to mobilize erythrocytes from the splanchnic or splenic circulation into the systemic circulation during ultrafiltration (15). This mechanism may be particularly important in patients who also exhibit impaired autonomic function.

⬡ SYSTOLIC AND DIASTOLIC FUNCTION OF THE HEART

As the central circulation is filled, hemodynamic stability then becomes dependent on normal systolic and diastolic function of the heart to generate an adequate cardiac output in the face of volume removal. Myocardial dysfunction is commonly present in patients with ESKD and can be an important cofactor in dialysis-induced hypotension (16).

Diastolic Dysfunction

The frequent occurrence of hypertension and on occasion aortic stenosis contributes to pressure overload of the left ventricle and accounts for the frequent occurrence of concentric left ventricular hypertrophy (LVH). Other contributing factors include the presence of an arteriovenous fistula, anemia, and intermittent bouts of volume overload.

Left ventricular (LV) dilatation and hypertrophy lead to changes in ventricular performance that differ strikingly from that seen in the healthy heart. A high incidence of LVH and abnormal diastolic function leads to diminished diastolic distensibility, such that the volume–pressure relationship during diastolic filling is steeper and shifted to the left (**Figure 18.3**). When LV compliance is diminished, a small rise in left ventricular end-diastolic volume (LVEDV) may cause a disproportionately large increase in left ventricular end-diastolic pressure (LVEDP) with consequent pulmonary venous congestion but little or no increase in stroke volume. Even in the presence of well-preserved systolic function, the preload reserve of the left ventricle can be exceeded by abrupt or large increases in plasma volume or because decreased ventricular compliance leads to inappropriately high filling pressure and pulmonary congestion. Furthermore, decreases in plasma volume, as during ultrafiltration in the setting of a steep volume–pressure relationship, can critically decrease the filling pressure of the heart and result in hypotension. In short, many patients with ESKD operate within a narrow LV volume–pressure relationship such that changes in plasma volume are often not well tolerated.

The contribution of LVH to hemodynamic instability during dialysis is highlighted by a number of studies that have shown LVH

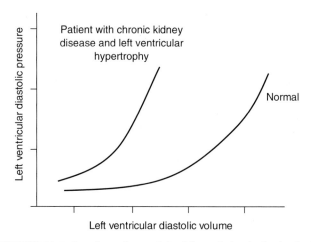

FIGURE 18.3 Compliance characteristics (left ventricular ejection fraction/left ventricular end-diastolic pressure) of the left ventricle during diastolic filling. Patients with end-stage renal disease often have the pressure–volume relationship of the left ventricle shifted to the left such that myocardial compliance is decreased.

to be more common in dialysis patients who experience episodic dialysis hypotension (17). Ritz et al. (18) observed that the LV mass-to-volume ratio was 37% greater in 27 patients with recurrent IDH than in 27 patients without this complication. Similarly, Wizemann et al. (19) noted that the incidence of dialysis hypotension was several times greater in patients with echocardiographic LVH than in those with normal ventricular mass. Another study found patients with recurrent IDH had a lower predialysis blood pressure, more severe concentric LVH, and lower LV compliance (20).

Patients with diastolic dysfunction are particularly difficult to treat. In the setting of impaired ventricular relaxation, a small amount of volume replacement can potentially trigger pulmonary edema. Therapy with inotropic agents can exacerbate the problem by further impairing ventricular relaxation. Calcium channel blockers such as verapamil or diltiazem may have some utility in this setting because these agents exert a negative inotropic effect on the heart and have the potential to improve LV relaxation. In a small series of patients, use of these drugs produced a functional improvement in cardiac performance and a reduction in the frequency of hypotension (21). However, it must be emphasized that the use of vasodilator calcium channel blockers has the potential disadvantage of lowering blood pressure. Hence, the trade-off of improving LV relaxation may not be tolerated in all patients because of the effect of the drugs to lower blood pressure.

On a more chronic basis, therapy can be instituted with the goal of reducing LV mass toward normal and presumably improve ventricular diastolic function. Partial or complete regression can be achieved by control of hypertension and by correction of anemia with erythropoietin (22). Studies in nonuremic hypertensive subjects suggest that, at equivalent blood pressure control, angiotensin-converting enzyme inhibitors, angiotensin receptor blockers, and calcium channel blockers reduce LV mass more rapidly and perhaps more effectively than most other antihypertensive drugs. It is not clear if these observations apply to the patient with renal failure. Correction of anemia with erythropoietin presumably acts by improving tissue oxygen delivery, thereby allowing the cardiac output (which is increased in anemia) and, therefore, cardiac work to fall toward normal. These changes have been associated with a 10% to 30% reduction in LV mass index (22). However, attention must also be paid to the frequent elevation in blood pressure following erythropoietin, an effect that may partially counteract the benefit associated with the elevation in hematocrit. In addition, one needs to be cautious not to increase the hemoglobin concentration to values in excess of 12 g/L because higher values have been associated with an increase in cardiovascular events (23,24).

Systolic Dysfunction

Impaired systolic function of the heart is common in dialysis patients. Depressed systolic function may be the result of a prior myocardial infarction, ischemic or hypertensive cardiomyopathy, or ischemic injury resulting from microvascular disease as in diabetes mellitus. Some patients with this disorder manifest the chronic persistent form of hypotension. More commonly impaired systolic function contributes to an increased frequency of dialysis-associated hemodynamic instability. Decreased myocardial contractility leads to poor LV performance and, importantly, a diminished cardiac reserve in the context of a hemodynamic challenge. Patients prone to hypotension during dialysis exhibit a blunted increase in cardiac index in response to a dobutamine infusion as compared to those subjects without hemodynamic instability (25). An inability to generate a sufficient cardiac output despite adequate cardiac filling can contribute to IDH and pulmonary edema.

◆ ARTERIAL DYSFUNCTION

An increase in vascular resistance on the arterial side of the circulation is an important defense against the development of hypotension when cardiac output begins to fall. Disturbances in this response can contribute to hemodynamic instability through several mechanisms. Impaired autonomic function or increases in core body temperature can lead to decreased arterial tone and result in more direct transmission of systemic pressure into the venous circulation. A sudden increase in venous pressure will increase the holding capacity of the venous compartment potentially leading to the sequestration of fluid thereby limiting cardiac refilling (7).

Disturbances in arterial function can also be the result of structural abnormalities in the arterial circulation. Vascular lesions in arteries of patients with uremia are characterized by intimal fibrosis and medial calcifications with little to no deposition of lipid droplets (26). These changes tend to be more reminiscent of accelerated aging or diabetic macroangiopathy rather than typical atherosclerosis. The causes of these pathologic changes are presumably related to age, effects of hypertension, and abnormalities of calcium and phosphorus metabolism. Such changes lead to increased wall stiffness and importantly contribute to the development of LVH.

Adenosine

Arteriolar vasoconstriction mediated by increased sympathetic nerve activity maintains blood pressure by increasing peripheral vascular resistance. In some patients, this response is inadequate due to production of vasodilators. In the setting of hypotension, no matter what the cause, tissue ischemia will result in net negative balance between the synthesis and degradation of adenosine triphosphate (ATP). As a consequence, ATP metabolites will begin to accumulate and will be released into the extracellular fluid. One such metabolite of ATP is adenosine (**FIGURE 18.4**) (27). Adenosine is an endogenous vasodilator released by endothelial cells and vascular myocytes and has been implicated in the sudden onset of decreased blood pressure during dialysis. In an attempt to demonstrate that

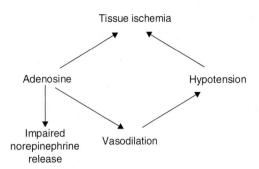

FIGURE 18.4 A cycle in which tissue ischemia can lead to intradialytic hypotension through the generation of adenosine. Adenosine can potentially exacerbate hypotension by its direct vasodilatory effects and secondarily by inhibiting norepinephrine.

accumulation of adenosine during dialysis-induced hypotension is more than just a marker of the ischemic event, Shinzato et al. (27) measured the metabolites of ATP before, during, and after dialysis-induced hypotension in a group of hypotensive-prone chronic dialysis patients. In this study, plasma levels of inosine, hypoxanthine, and xanthine rose sharply with the development of sudden IDH and quickly decreased as the blood pressure was restored. By contrast, there was no significant variation in the plasma levels of the metabolites when hypotension developed more gradually during the course of the procedure. Adenosine levels were not measured because of the short half-life of the metabolite. These patients were then treated with caffeine, a nonselective A_1 and A_2 adenosine-receptor blocker, and the frequency of hypotensive episodes was examined. A 250-mg capsule of caffeine administered 2 hours into the procedure resulted in a significant decrease in the development of hypotensive episodes.

In a prospective double-blind placebo-controlled trial in patients with frequent IDH, injection of a selective A_1 receptor blocker provided a significant but modest benefit in reducing the incidence of hypotension (28). Expression of the A_{2A} receptor is increased to a greater extent on peripheral blood mononuclear cells in dialysis patients with frequent hypotension compared to hemodynamically stable patients; suggesting A_{2A} receptors antagonism might also be of benefit (29).

Nitric Oxide

Another intriguing and as yet ill-defined contributor to the development of HD hypotension is that of nitric oxide (30). It has been proposed that blood bioincompatibility with dialysis membranes leads to the activation of monocytes in the peripheral circulation. This is thought to produce a variety of cytokines including interleukin 1 (IL-1) and tumor necrosis factor (TNF). These cytokines in turn induce the synthesis of nitric oxide by endothelial cells. The support for this hypothesis is derived from several sources. First, plasma levels of IL-1 and TNF are elevated in patients with ESKD on dialysis (31). Furthermore, IL-1 and TNF induce hypotension when administered *in vivo*, predominantly as a result of a decline in systemic vascular resistance (32). *In vitro* studies have also shown that IL-1 and TNF promote nitric oxide synthesis in endothelial cells. Nitric oxide has a direct effect as a smooth muscle vasodilator, working through intracellular cyclic guanylyl monophosphate (GMP) as a second messenger. In addition, IL-1 is also capable of inducing the synthesis of vasodilator prostaglandins (PGs), including PGE_2 and PGI_2 in human vascular smooth muscle cells and endothelial cells (33). These arachidonic acid metabolites are direct smooth muscle vasodilators as well and could thereby contribute to a decline in peripheral vascular resistance.

The concentration of the stable end products of endogenously released nitric oxide, nitrite and nitrate, is increased in chronic kidney disease patients undergoing HD as compared with healthy controls (34,35). Normally, these levels decrease significantly during a dialysis treatment in otherwise hemodynamically stable patients. By contrast, studies show these metabolites actually increase in patients who develop IDH (34,35). A higher predialysis fractional exhaled nitric oxide concentration has also been found in patients with IDH as compared with those with stable hemodynamics (35). These findings suggest that increased synthesis of nitric oxide may be contributing to hemodynamic instability in hypotensive-prone subjects. The basis for increased nitric oxide activity is unknown but may be related to the dialytic removal of the nitric oxide inhibitor, asymmetric dimethylarginine (ADMA) (36). If further studies confirm an important role for increased synthesis of nitric oxide in dialysis-associated hemodynamic instability, administration of an antagonist to nitric oxide production such as N(G)-monomethyl-arginine acetate (l-NMMA) may ultimately prove useful in the treatment of hypotensive-prone patients.

AUTONOMIC NEUROPATHY

Autonomic Dysfunction in Uremia

The importance of autonomic dysfunction as a contributing factor to dialysis hypotension has been the subject of vigorous investigation for the last 15 years. One of the first clinical associations between impaired autonomic nervous system control and hypotension was described by Bradbury and Eggelston (37) in 1925. They observed that the autonomic nervous system was essential in the orthostatic regulation of arterial pressure through baroreflex mechanisms. Subsequently, the central and peripheral neuronal pathways that control vasomotor tone, heart rate, myocardial contractility, and venous capacitance have been described in greater detail.

An autonomic reflex arc is composed of an afferent limb that consists of sensory nerve fibers originating from the vascular tree, visceral organs, and the skin. These afferent fibers travel to the central nervous system mainly through the spinal cord and vagus nerves. Arterial baroreceptors are located in the aortic arch and carotid sinus and sense changes in blood pressure; cardiopulmonary baroreceptors are located in the atrium, ventricles, great veins, and pulmonary vessels and sense changes in cardiac filling pressures. Information about these pressure changes is integrated in the central nervous system at several different levels including the brainstem, cerebellum, hypothalamus, and cerebral hemispheres. The efferent limb of the system consists of both sympathetic and parasympathetic pathways that exit the brainstem to the spinal cord and travel to the heart and circulation.

Abnormalities in autonomic function are commonly present in patients with chronic kidney disease (38,39). The presence of these abnormalities can potentially impair the patient's ability to maintain systemic blood pressure following a large degree of fluid removal by ultrafiltration. One such abnormality is an inadequate sympathetic response to volume removal in patients with recurrent IDH. The postdialysis plasma concentration of chromogranin A (a protein coreleased with catecholamines) increases to a lesser extent in patients with IDH compared to those with stable blood pressure consistent with a blunted response of sympathetic nerve activity to hypotension (40).

Under normal conditions, sympathetic neural outflow is under tonic restraint by baroreceptors in the aortic arch and carotid sinus and by baroreceptors in the cardiopulmonary region. With the volume removal that accompanies HD, reductions in central venous pressure and arterial blood pressure would be expected to unload these baroreceptors and thereby reduce their tonic restraint on the vasomotor center, resulting in reflex increases in sympathetic outflow to the heart and peripheral circulation to help maintain blood pressure. Defects in this homeostatic response may play an important role in the development of hypotension during the dialytic procedure.

Numerous tests have been employed to assess the autonomic nervous system in patients with chronic kidney disease. These tests may be used to try to localize the defect in the autonomic nervous system. For example, the Valsalva test probes the integrity of the entire autonomic nervous system: low-pressure and high-pressure baroreceptors in the cardiopulmonary circulation, the afferent and efferent limbs of these pathways, and both sympathetic and parasympathetic function. This test is, therefore, useful in detecting a defect but not in identifying the site of the abnormality. The amyl nitrite inhalation test may be used to test low-pressure baroreceptors and the resultant efferent sympathetic outflow expected when blood pressure declines. The cold pressor test (performed by placing a cold cloth on the patient's forehead or by submerging a hand in ice slush) predominantly reflects efferent sympathetic function activated by cold-induced peripheral vasoconstriction. The precise role of the autonomic nervous system in dialysis patients has been difficult to assess in part because tests of autonomic function have not been routinely included in large surveys of dialysis subjects. For this reason, the natural history of changes in the autonomic nervous system in subjects with ESKD is not presently clear.

The initial study that suggested that a defect in the autonomic nervous system could be related to HD hypotension was published in 1976 by Lilley et al. (41). These investigators performed a variety of autonomic tests and concluded that the defect in the autonomic nervous system in patients with ESKD was on the afferent side of the autonomic loop. More specifically, they concluded that the defect resided in the baroreceptors. The finding of autonomic dysfunction at the levels of the afferent branch of the baroreflex arc is consistent with numerous other studies published in the literature in which selective testing of the vasomotor center and the efferent sympathetic tract (cold pressor test, handgrip test, mental stress) showed normal function (41,42), whereas tests of the complete baroreflex arc showed a diminished response (41–44).

The precise mechanism of the autonomic dysfunction remains unclear but, because efferent sympathetic function appears to be normal, the most likely sites of primary damage are the baroreceptors or their afferent fibers or central nervous system connections. Chronic fluid overload leading to persistent overstretching has been suggested as one cause of baroreceptor dysfunction (45). In addition, there has been some sentiment that uremic "poisoning" of baroreceptors is involved in dialysis hypotension (46,47). Chronic exposure to uremic toxins has been thought to poison the baroreceptors, leading to almost complete removal of their tonic inhibitory effects on sympathetic vasomotor outflow in some patients (41,46). According to this hypothesis, uremia-induced sinoaortic baroreceptor deafferentation would cause central sympathetic outflow to be nearly maximal under basal conditions so that it could not possibly increase much further during the hypotensive stress of HD. However, the experimental support for this hypothesis is indirect, relying mainly on plasma catecholamines and semiquantitative bedside tests to assess sympathetic neural function, and a definitive relation between impaired baroreflexes and dialysis-induced hypotension has not been established. Chronic hyperkalemic depolarization of nerves has also been suggested as playing a contributory role (48).

Paradoxical Withdrawal of Sympathetic Tone in Dialysis-Induced Hypotension

To better characterize the role of autonomic dysfunction in the genesis of IDH, Converse et al. (49) examined baroreflex control of heart rate, efferent sympathetic nerve activity, and vascular resistance in 16 hypotension-resistant and 7 hypotension-prone HD patients. Hypotension-prone patients were defined as those in whom a sudden, symptomatic decrease in mean arterial pressure of greater than 30 mm Hg occurred during at least one-third of maintenance HD sessions. Patients with diabetes were excluded from the study because autonomic neuropathy is a well-known complication of diabetes mellitus. Direct measurements of sympathetic nerve activity and several quantifiable reflex maneuvers were employed to test the effects of chronic uremia on a number of specific reflexes, including arterial baroreflex control of heart rate and cardiopulmonary baroreflex control of vascular resistance. By studying the same patients both during the interdialytic period and during actual sessions of maintenance HD, these investigators were able to separate the autonomic effects of chronic uremia from the acute autonomic effects of the HD procedure.

To assess whether a chronic abnormality was present in either arterial or cardiopulmonary baroreceptors, both groups of patients were first studied during the interdialytic period. Measurement of heart rate and sympathetic nerve activity during the intravenous infusion of nitroprusside and measurement of forearm vascular resistance during the application of negative pressure to the lower body disclosed no abnormalities in either group of patients. These results suggested that there was no baseline autonomic defect chronically present to account for dialysis-induced hypotension in this select group of nondiabetic patients. It should be pointed out that in other groups of dialysis patients, such as those with diabetic autonomic neuropathy, impaired baroreflexes indeed may contribute more to hypotension during HD.

Studies were then undertaken to examine autonomic function during the dialytic procedure. In a subgroup of patients who developed severe hypotension on dialysis, baroreceptor function was again normal, that is, a small initial decrease in blood pressure was accompanied by the appropriate reflex increases in sympathetic nerve activity, heart rate, and peripheral vascular resistance. As the hypotensive episode became severe, however, normal baroreflex function was replaced by the sudden appearance of an inappropriate vasodepressor reaction. With the additional fall in blood pressure, sympathetic activity, heart rate, and vascular resistance did not increase further but rather fell paradoxically back to or below baseline levels. Shortly after the onset of the hypotension and loss of sympathetic activation, classic signs and symptoms of vasovagal syncope developed in the patients, including nausea, abdominal discomfort, diaphoresis, and giddiness.

To further examine the mechanism triggering this vasodepressor reaction, additional experiments were performed in which the normal HD procedure was separated into its component parts, ultrafiltration alone and dialysis alone. Using measurements of calf vascular resistance, it was found that ultrafiltration reproduced both the increases and decreases in vascular resistance (including vasodilation and hypotension), whereas dialysis alone had no effect on calf vascular resistance in either group of patients. These results suggested that withdrawal of volume appears to be the key stimulus triggering this vasodepressor reaction, which in turn exacerbates the volume-dependent fall in blood pressure.

An inhibitory reflex arising in the heart is the most likely mechanism causing this paradoxical bradycardia and vasodilation during hypovolemic hypotension (50–52). In addition to being a pump, the heart is also a sensory organ, being richly innervated with sensory (or afferent) nerves. Many of these sensory nerves function as mechanoreceptors and therefore signal the brain of changes in loading conditions and contractility of the ventricles. Their function is to inhibit sympathetic outflow. During euvolemia, these sensory nerves normally exert a tonic inhibitory influence on sympathetic vasomotor outflow. During mild hypovolemia, this inhibitory influence is reduced. During severe hypovolemia, however, this inhibitory influence is not reduced further but instead increases paradoxically. The theory is that the receptive fields of these endings are deformed as the adrenergically stimulated heart contracts forcefully around an almost empty ventricular chamber.

It was hypothesized that mild hypovolemia might simulate nonhypotensive HD: unloading of inhibitory ventricular afferents causing reflex sympathetic activation. In contrast, severe hypovolemia might simulate HD-induced hypotension: paradoxical activation of inhibitory ventricular afferents causing reflex inhibition of sympathetic outflow resulting in bradycardia and peripheral vasodilation. Echocardiographic measurements of LV volumes before the onset of severe hypotension showed near-obliteration of the LV cavity possibly accounting for the paradoxical activation of inhibitory LV afferents.

Therefore, in a subset of hypotensive-prone dialysis patients, a form of acute autonomic neuropathy plays an etiologic role. For this paradoxical sympathetic failure to occur, severe volume depletion must occur. To determine the prevalence of this type of hypotension (bradycardic hypotension) in the dialysis population, Zoccali et al. (53) identified 20 patients out of a total population of 106 who suffered from IDH. In 60 hypotensive episodes recorded in the 20 patients, heart rate increased in 35 episodes, remained unchanged in 19 episodes, and decreased in 6 episodes. The five patients who developed bradycardic hypotension were characterized by high ultrafiltration rates and smaller LV end-diastolic diameters as compared with those with tachycardic or fixed heart rate.

Autonomic Dysfunction and Chronic Hypotension

As mentioned previously, a small fraction of HD patients have difficulty maintaining a normal blood pressure and are chronically hypotensive between dialysis treatments. The role of autonomic dysfunction in this condition was examined in one study that compared numerous measures of autonomic function among hypotensive HD patients, normotensive HD patients, and control patients (all groups consisted of 17 individuals) (54). Chronically hypotensive individuals exhibited a significant downregulation of α- and β-adrenergic receptors, suggesting an inability to produce an adequate sympathetic response.

Autonomic Dysfunction and Arrhythmias

The development of cardiac arrhythmias in ESKD can be traced to several factors that are operative alone or in combination and include the presence of myocardial dysfunction, fluid and electrolyte shifts, and poor oxygen saturation. A previously unrecognized predisposing factor may be autonomic dysfunction. One study of 41 dialysis patients evaluated the correlation between arrhythmia (as determined by 24-hour Holter examination) and autonomic dysfunction (as determined by blood pressure and heart rate responses) (55). Compared with patients with normal autonomic function, a significantly increased incidence of atrial and/or ventricular arrhythmia was found among those with one or more autonomic abnormalities (41 abnormal rhythms in 26 patients with autonomic dysfunction vs. 1 in 15 with normal autonomic responses).

Sympathetic Nervous System and Hypertension in the Uremic State

Despite the frequent presence of autonomic dysfunction, baseline plasma catecholamine levels are often elevated in chronic kidney disease (56). Increased sympathetic tone, decreased degradation, and diminished neuronal reuptake all may contribute to this finding. The physiologic significance of this finding is uncertain, but sympathetic overactivity could contribute to the common development of hypertension in ESKD. The signal for this increased sympathetic tone may in part originate with stimulation of renal afferent nerves.

Chemosensitive renal afferent nerves have been implicated in the pathogenesis of hypertension by causing reflex activation of sympathetic outflow to the heart and peripheral circulation (57–59). Stimulation of these afferent nerves by either ischemic metabolites, such as adenosine, or by uremic toxins, such as urea, evokes reflex increases in sympathetic nerve activity and blood pressure in experimental animals (60). Reduced sympathetic activity may be one important mechanism by which bilateral nephrectomy lowers blood pressure in some HD patients (61).

In recent years, additional tests of autonomic dysfunction have been assessed. Principle among these is heart rate variability, a noninvasive measure of the autonomic system (62,63). In the most extensive of these studies, a lower heart rate variability was associated with progression to ESKD and poorer outcome. Of interest is the fact that at least one study (64) demonstrated improvement in heart rate variability after successful renal transplantation, suggesting that, to some degree, autonomic dysfunction in ESKD patients is reversible.

⬣ THERAPY FOR HEMODYNAMIC INSTABILITY DURING HEMODIALYSIS

In patients in whom dialysis hypotension has not been a problem but in whom it develops suddenly, the differential diagnoses must be expanded to include occult septicemia and unrecognized cardiac or pericardial disease. In this regard, the exclusion of a pericardial effusion and tamponade and/or a significant segmental wall motion abnormality are important in the assessment in any patient with hypotensive episodes occurring frequently. Other serious underlying conditions that can give rise to new-onset hypotension include intestinal ischemia with impending bowel infarction and occult hemorrhage. Hypotension during the early part of the procedure should make one consider exaggerated cytokine release resulting from a reaction with the dialysis membrane. After excluding these processes, there are several options available for the treatment and prevention of episodic dialysis hypotension (TABLE 18.2).

Before discussing therapies for IDH, it is important to note that there have been recent insights into the definition of IDH. Most notably, Flythe et al. (65) analyzed data from 1,409 patients in the

TABLE 18.2	**Treatment of Hemodynamic Instability**

- Exclude nondialysis related cause (cardiac ischemia, pericardial effusion, infection)
- Individualize the dialysis prescription
  - Accurate setting of the dry weight
  - Optimize dialysate composition
    - Fixed Na^+ concentration >140 mEq/L or Na^+ modeling
    - HCO_3 buffer
    - Avoid low Mg^{2+} dialysate
    - Avoid low Ca^{2+} dialysate
  - Optimize method of ultrafiltration (Uf)
    - Ultrafiltration modeling alone or with Na^+ modeling
    - Sequential Uf and isovolemic dialysis
  - Cool temperature dialysate
- Maximize cardiac performance
  - Inflatable abdominal band to enhance venous return to heart
- Avoidance of food
- Avoid antihypertensive medicines on dialysis day
- Pharmacologic interventions
  - Midodrine
  - Vasopressin
  - Adenosine antagonists
  - Others: sertraline, ephedrine, phenylephrine, carnitine

Hemodialysis (HEMO) study and concluded that a nadir-based definition of IDH was most helpful because it was associated with adverse outcomes more reliably. Thus, a systolic blood pressure <90 mm Hg was identified as a level compatible with untoward symptoms or poorer prognosis (65,66).

There are several reasons to be concerned about IDH, but among these, the recognition that IDH is associated with poor cardiovascular outcomes is particularly compelling. One longitudinal study linked IDH to major adverse cardiac events (67), while another found a greater hospitalization rate in patients with IDH (68). Perhaps even more worrisome is the association of IDH with cardiac remodeling abnormalities, a process by which a vicious cycle is established as repetitive IDH occurs (69). In any case, the recognition of the adverse consequences of IDH are recognized more frequently as new therapies to present its occurrence are evaluated (70–73).

⬣ INDIVIDUALIZING THE DIALYSIS PRESCRIPTION

Accurate Setting of the "Dry Weight"

At present, the determination of dry weight is largely assessed empirically by trial and error. The dry weight is set at the weight below which unacceptable symptoms, such as cramping, nausea and vomiting, or hypotension occur. The dry weight is highly variable in many patients and can fluctuate with intercurrent illnesses (such as diarrhea or infection) and with changes in hematocrit (as with erythropoietin). A number of methods have been proposed to more objectively define the dry weight of the patient (TABLE 18.3). Comparative studies have generally favored methods based on bioimpedance measurements, which provide an assessment of extracellular and intracellular volume and total body water (74–76). A variant of this technique in which continuous intradialytic measurements are confined to the calf shows particular promise because

TABLE 18.3	**Objective Tools to Determine Dry Weight in Hemodialysis Patients**

- Blood volume monitoring
    - Relative change during treatment
        - Blood volume with ultrafiltration pulse (to assess increment of vascular refill)
- Ultrasonographic assessment of inferior vena cava (IVC)
    - IVC diameter
    - IVC collapsibility index (fractional ↓ of diameter during breathing cycle)
- Brain natriuretic peptide (BNP), N-terminal pro-BNP, atrial natriuretic peptide levels
- Bioimpedance methodology
    - Whole body (wrist-to-ankle)
    - Segmental
    - Continuous intradialytic calf measurements
- Extravascular lung water index (invasive)

the relative volume of excess extracellular fluid is greatest in the lower extremities (77). During dialysis, plasma refilling is more dynamic from the leg in comparison to the trunk or arms suggesting the calf could be used as a window to monitor intradialytic changes in whole body extracellular fluid volume (78).

Of interest is the fact that a recent study emphasized the superiority of the absolute change in weight over a percentage weight gain in predicting IDH in dialysis patients (79). This observation was particularly true in heavier patients (79). The importance of overhydration on overall cardiovascular morbidity/mortality has also been recently emphasized (80). New insights into the complex relationship between ultrafiltration on dialysis and blood pressure suggest that in some hypertensive patients, rapid vascular refilling may inhibit an expected fall in blood pressure, thereby sustaining a higher than desired pressure (81–83). The many positive benefits of strict volume control on many cardiovascular parameters are emphasized in the literature frequently. Recently, one such paper reported an improvement in vascular function with meticulous volume management (84).

Dialysate Composition

A detailed discussion is provided elsewhere on how the composition of the dialysate can be adjusted to maximize hemodynamic stability. Summary statements regarding these components are provided in the following sections.

Dialysate Sodium Concentration and Sodium Modeling

The use of a higher dialysate Na concentration (greater than 140 mEq/L) has been among the most efficacious and best-tolerated therapies for episodic hypotension. The high Na concentration prevents a marked decline in the plasma osmolality during dialysis, thereby protecting the extracellular volume by minimizing osmotic fluid loss into the cells. Na modeling is a technique in which the dialysate Na concentration is varied during the course of the procedure. Most commonly, a high dialysate Na concentration is used initially with a progressive reduction toward isotonic or even hypotonic levels by the end of the procedure. This method of Na control allows for a diffusive Na influx early in the session to prevent the rapid decline in plasma osmolality resulting from the efflux of urea and other small molecular weight solutes. During the remainder of the procedure, when the reduction in osmolality accompanying

urea removal is less abrupt, the dialysate Na level is set at a lower level, thereby minimizing the development of hypertonicity and any resultant excessive thirst, fluid gain, and hypertension in the interdialytic period. The precise role of Na modeling has not been fully defined as yet; studies with positive and negative findings have been performed. It is a procedure associated with low morbidity and is, therefore, worthy of a trial in individual problem dialysis patients.

Dialysate Buffer

In prior years, the use of acetate as a dialysis buffer had been a potential cofactor in causing dialysis hypotension by leading to peripheral vasodilatation. The current use of high-efficiency and high-flux dialysis procedures prohibits the use of acetate as a dialysis buffer. Bicarbonate is now widely available and adaptable to all new dialysis machines. In general, blood pressure is generally better maintained with bicarbonate. The cost differential between bicarbonate dialysate and acetate dialysate has decreased sufficiently to make this issue of dialysate buffer moot.

Dialysate Magnesium Concentration

Low magnesium in the dialysate may also contribute to IDH. One study, for example, randomized 78 clinically stable patients on HD to treatment with dialysate containing low (0.38 mmol/L) or high (0.75 mmol/L) concentrations of magnesium in combination with either bicarbonate or acetate buffer (85). For both bicarbonate and acetate solutions, patients dialyzed with the low magnesium concentration solution experienced a significant increase in the number of episodes of hypotension and a lower absolute decrease in mean arterial pressure compared with those dialyzed with the higher concentration.

Dialysate Calcium Concentration

Cardiac contractility can be enhanced in many dialysis patients by increasing the dialysate calcium concentration. A limitation of this approach is the development of hypercalcemia particularly in patients being treated with calcium-containing phosphate binders and vitamin D. In patients prone to IDH who are at risk for hypercalcemia, dialysate calcium profiling can be used as a strategy to improve hemodynamic stability and yet minimize the potential for hypercalcemia (86). In one study of patients dialyzed for 4 hours, the dialysate calcium concentration was set low (1.25 mmol/L) for the first 2 hours and then increased to 1.75 mmol/L for the last 2 hours. Use of the varying dialysate calcium concentration was associated with greater hemodynamic stability as compared with a fixed dialysate calcium concentration of either 1.25 or 1.5 mmol/L. This hemodynamic benefit was accomplished by an increase in cardiac output. At the end of 3 weeks, there was no difference in the predialysis ionized calcium concentration between the three groups.

Optimized Method of Ultrafiltration
Volumetrically Controlled Ultrafiltration

Modern dialysis machines have helped in the avoidance of dialysis hypotension by allowing clinicians to program the volume removal pattern from patients during dialysis. These machines use an accurate volumetric device to evenly program ultrafiltration. Hence, a steady and even ultrafiltration rate throughout the course of dialysis is achievable. In the absence of an ultrafiltration control device, the rate of ultrafiltration can fluctuate considerably as the pressure across the membrane tends to vary. In addition, high venous pressures can lead to exaggerated rates of fluid removal. To minimize the risk for excessive fluid removal when such a device is not available, membranes with a low water permeability (K_{Uf}) should be used.

Ultrafiltration Modeling

Clinicians may desire to ultrafilter more volume at the beginning of the procedure and less toward the conclusion of the procedure. In this manner, dialysis ultrafiltration may be tailored to the individual dialysis subject. Recent studies suggest that this approach is particularly effective when combined with sodium modeling (56,87).

Sequential Ultrafiltration and Isovolemic Dialysis

A similar goal of maintenance of the plasma osmolality can be attained by initial ultrafiltration alone (without dialysis) followed by isovolemic dialysis in which little or no further fluid removal occurs because of reduced transmembrane pressures. This sequential procedure often allows a large volume of fluid to be removed without inducing hemodynamic instability. The downside to this approach is that adequacy can be impaired unless the period of dialysis is prolonged.

Blood Volume Monitoring

Devises to monitor intradialytic changes in blood volume have been advocated as a tool to minimize IDH based on the concept that the likelihood of developing hypotension will always occur at roughly the same reduction of blood volume. Unfortunately, most studies have not found a close relationship between individual changes in blood volume and occurrence of hypotension (88). In a prospective randomized trial, use of an intradialytic blood volume monitoring devise was associated with greater nonvascular and vascular access–related hospitalizations and mortality as compared to standard monitoring (89).

The lack of benefit noted with blood volume monitoring as typically employed may in part be explained by its tendency to underestimate the actual amount of volume removed. The technique is based on measuring the degree of hemoconcentration that occurs with ultrafiltration and assumes uniform mixing of plasma and red blood cells throughout the circulation. Recent observations suggest this assumption is incorrect (90). Whole body hematocrit is lower than arterial or venous blood due to a dynamic reduction in hematocrit in the capillary beds, a phenomenon known as the *Fahraeus effect*. During ultrafiltration, there is presumably a compensatory mobilization of hematocrit-poor blood from the microvasculature into the central circulation. This dilution effect minimizes the degree of hemoconcentration leading to a potential underestimation of the total ultrafiltrate volume.

Blood volume monitoring has been shown to be an effective tool when incorporated into a biofeedback system in which dialysate conductivity and ultrafiltration rate are constantly adjusted through the procedure based on input from the measured change in blood volume. The system is designed to guide the reduction in blood volume along a preset individual trajectory to avoid the acute and sudden reductions that can precipitate hypotension. This technique has been found to reduce the frequency of hypotensive episodes and provide greater stability of blood pressure both during and after the procedure (91,92). In hypertensive dialysis patients, this technique can lead to better blood pressure control through optimization of volume status and at the same time reduce the frequency of hypotensive episodes when compared to standard treatment (93).

The frequency of IDH has also been reduced using a biofeedback system in which the ultrafiltration rate is adjusted according to changes in blood pressure measured every 5 minutes during the dialysis procedure (94). This method utilizes a fuzzy logic control system that adjusts ultrafiltration according to instantaneous changes in blood pressure in the context of historical data concerning the individual's blood pressure behavior during prior treatments. One recent review of carefully conducted biofeedback dialysis technique concluded that these systems continue to hold promise in reducing IDH (81).

Cool Temperature Dialysate

In response to ultrafiltration, increased activity of the sympathetic nervous system leads to vasoconstriction of the dermal circulation. As a result, heat dissipation is impaired and core body temperature tends to increase. Indirect evidence suggests that the increase in body temperature is directly related to the amount of ultrafiltration (95). In addition to impaired heat dissipation, there is also increased central heat production that accompanies the dialysis procedure. At some point, the increase in core body temperature can overcome peripheral vasoconstriction and precipitate acute hypotension (**FIGURE 18.5**).

Recently, the simple maneuver of lowering the dialysis temperature 2°C from 37°C to 35°C has been associated with improvement in both symptoms and blood pressure. Cooling the dialysate reduces the rate of IDH by 7.1 times when compared to conventional therapy (96). Use of cooler temperature dialysate results in increased myocardial contractility in stable dialysis patients (97). In patients selected for frequent episodic hypotension or predialysis hypotension, use of the 35°C dialysate has also been shown to increase peripheral vasoconstriction (98). The peripheral vasoconstrictive response was measured directly by venous occlusion plethysmography in these studies. The increase in peripheral vasoconstriction resulted in an improvement in both supine and standing blood pressure following ultrafiltration HD in both groups of hypotensive-prone patients. No episodes of hypotension were recorded during the 35°C procedure, whereas many were noted when the patients were on the 37°C procedures. Also, the 35°C procedure was associated with an increase in plasma norepinephrine levels. In addition to increased myocardial contractility and peripheral vasoconstriction, lowering the dialysate temperature is also associated with better preservation of central blood volume through enhanced mobilization of pooled venous blood (99). Taken together, these

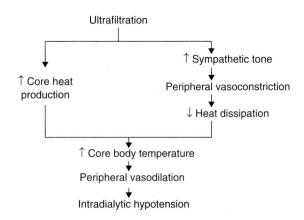

FIGURE 18.5 There is an increase in core body temperature that typically occurs during the dialysis procedure. The degree to which core body temperature rises is related to the amount of ultrafiltration. At some point, the increased body temperature overcomes peripheral vasoconstriction and leads to the sudden onset of hypotension.

findings suggest that the combination of an improvement in myocardial contractility, increased peripheral vasoconstriction, and less venous pooling add to providing improved support for blood pressure in patients undergoing ultrafiltration dialysis.

This hemodynamic protection is present even in those patients with the highest proclivity to develop dialysis hypotension. When applied to a more general dialysis population, those patients with subnormal predialysis temperatures (present in up to 23% of patients) may derive the greatest hemodynamic benefit from this procedure (100). The mechanism of the protection would appear to be an increase in efferent autonomic outflow, as deduced from the increase in plasma norepinephrine levels seen on exposure to 35°C dialysis. The improved hemodynamic stability observed with convective dialysis treatments such as hemofiltration may, in part, be related to the lower extracorporeal blood temperature typical of this procedure.

Despite the potential for cool temperature dialysis to increase the degree of urea compartmentalization as a result of peripheral vasoconstriction, the procedure has been shown to have no significant effect on dialysis efficiency (101). Although tolerated well in most patients, it should be noted that 35°C dialysis may not be tolerated in all patients. This may be particularly true of patients who are sensitive to temperature changes and in patients who develop excessive vasoconstriction and symptoms and signs of either coronary insufficiency or peripheral vascular insufficiency. The mechanism of action for vasoconstriction during cooler temperature dialysis does not appear to be a change in cytokine concentration (82).

A recent refinement in the implementation of cool temperature dialysate is the use of what has been termed *isothermic dialysis*. This technique employs a blood temperature monitor that senses temperature changes in the arterial and venous catheters of the extracorporeal circuit. This information is used to then adjust the dialysate temperature on an ongoing basis such that the body temperature remains unchanged. Use of isothermic dialysis allows for dialysate temperature to be individualized and adjusted throughout the procedure rather than subjecting every patient to the same cold stress. The procedure takes into account patient-to-patient variability in predialysis body temperature and the increase in body temperature as ultrafiltration volume varies. The effectiveness of this technique was recently verified in a large group of patients selected because of the frequent occurrence of IDH (102).

Maximize Cardiac Performance

A reduction of plasma volume will not necessarily result in symptomatic hypotension as long as the circulatory system is able to respond by compensatory vasoconstriction. Venoconstriction leads to a shift of blood into the central circulation helping to maintain cardiac output. Impaired sympathetic nerve activity or abnormalities in venous compliance can limit this response. In a study of 25 patients with intractable postdialytic orthostatic hypotension, application of an inflatable abdominal band was found to be an effective means to attenuate the fall in blood pressure immediately after the treatment (103). This device improved venous return to the heart as evidenced by an increase in ejective fraction and fall in atrial natriuretic peptide concentration.

The frequency of dialysis-associated hemodynamic instability is greatly increased in patients with a prior history of congestive heart failure, cardiomegaly, or ischemic heart disease. These conditions lead to poor LV performance and, importantly, a diminished cardiac reserve in the context of a hemodynamic challenge. As discussed

previously, cardiac contractility can be enhanced in many dialysis patients by increasing the dialysate calcium concentration, using cool temperature HD, and correcting anemia with erythropoietin.

Avoidance of Food

Food ingestion during dialysis leads to a significant decline in systemic vascular resistance that can contribute to a fall in blood pressure (104). In addition, increased splanchnic pooling of blood will impair maintenance of central blood volume and thereby limit cardiac refilling. This effect is not corrected by the concurrent intake of caffeine.

Pharmacologic Prevention of Hypotension

Erythropoietin Therapy

Correction of anemia can potentially improve hemodynamic stability in several ways. An increase in the hematocrit is associated with an exponential rise in blood viscosity that in turn is an important component of peripheral vascular resistance (105,106). Correction of the hematocrit has been shown to be beneficial in causing regression of LVH (107). An increased hematocrit may result in less tissue ischemia, thereby minimizing the release of the vasodilatory metabolite, adenosine. As mentioned previously, hemoglobin values should be maintained between 11 and 12 g/L because higher values have been associated with an increase in cardiovascular event rates (23,24).

Caffeine

Adenosine is an endogenous vasodilator that has been related to hypotensive episodes in a subset of patients on HD. This response can be blunted in some patients by the administration of caffeine, which may act as an adenosine receptor antagonist in this setting. This therapy may be limited by the fact that caffeine is rapidly removed by dialysis and chronic use may be associated with considerable tolerance to the hemodynamic effects.

Midodrine

Midodrine is a selective α_1 adrenergic pressor agent that has been used to treat patients with frequent IDH. In addition to increasing peripheral vascular resistance, midodrine has been shown to limit venous pooling and effectively restore central blood volume and maximize cardiac refilling (99). This drug may also have the additional benefit of better preserving cerebral blood flow in patients with orthostatic hypotension after HD (108).

A pilot study examining 21 patients with severe hypotension during dialysis reported a significant beneficial effect on hemodynamic stability (109). The dose was initiated at 2.5 mg given before the procedure and then titrated in 2.5-mg increments to maintain the systolic pressure above 100 mm Hg. The mean dose was 8 mg, and the drug was well tolerated. Studies examining the chronic efficacy of the drug also demonstrate a significant hemodynamic benefit in patients suffering from IDH (110). In a systematic review of the literature, 2.5 to 10 mg of the selective α_1 adrenergic agonist midodrine has proved to be an effective treatment in some patients with frequent IDH (111). It is noteworthy that many of the patients enrolled in these studies are elderly and had several comorbid conditions including diabetes mellitus, coronary artery disease, and peripheral vascular disease. Despite the high-risk nature of the patients studied, the drug is well tolerated and safe to use. The dose should be individually titrated according to blood pressure and symptoms; most patients require 10 to 20 mg administered 30 minutes before dialysis.

Sertraline

Preliminary evidence suggests that sertraline, a central nervous system serotonin reuptake inhibitor, may also be beneficial in dialysis-induced hypotension (112). A retrospective study of nine patients placed on sertraline (50 to 100 mg/d) for depression compared the blood pressure response during dialysis for the 6-week period before drug initiation to the response during an equivalent period immediately after the drug was begun. Sertraline was associated with an increase in the lowest mean blood pressure measured during dialysis (68 vs. 55 mm Hg), a lower frequency of hypotensive episodes (0.6 vs. 1.4 episodes per session), and fewer required therapeutic interventions for hypotension during the study period (1.7 vs. 11.0). This benefit may be due to an attenuation of sympathetic withdrawal. Although more data are needed, sertraline is considered a safe drug and, therefore, should be considered as a reasonable agent to administer in hypotension-prone patients.

Other Drugs

In a multicenter study of otherwise stable chronic dialysis patients, intravenous infusion of carnitine was found to significantly decrease the incidence of IDH and cramps as compared with a control group (113). Other drugs that have been used to treat patients with IDH include ephedrine (114) and phenylephrine (115). In a study of six patients with refractory HD-induced hypotension, intranasal lysine vasopressin administered 1 hour before a dialysis treatment and again 12 hours later resulted in a significant decline in the number of hypotensive episodes and in the volume of intravenous fluids used in the treatment of hypotension (116). A more recent study (117) corroborated these larger, positive results with vasopressin administration intranasally. Previous observations have found plasma vasopressin levels do not significantly increase during ultrafiltration dialysis despite an anticipated unloading of baroreceptors. In a randomized double-blind placebo-controlled trial, the continuous administration of subpressor doses of vasopressin provided for greater hemodynamic stability even in the setting where target fluid loss was set to be increased by 0.5 kg over the baseline prescription (118). Another recent study reported a similar finding: high baseline AVP levels at baseline but no increase following ultrafiltration (119).

Comparative Studies

All of the measures delineated previously provide some degree of prophylactic benefit. However, their relative efficacy in the same patient is unclear and comparative studies are limited. In one study, the efficacy and tolerability of midodrine, cool temperature dialysate, or the combination were compared in a study of 11 patients with IDH (57). All three therapies were found to be equally effective in improving hemodynamic stability. There was a trend for the combined group to have superior improvement in hemodynamic stability; however, this did not reach statistical significance.

A second study compared five different procedures in a single-blinded crossover study of 10 patients with a history of IDH (58). After 1 week of standard dialysis, all patients underwent 1 week of each of the following four strategies: high Na dialysate, Na modeling, sequential ultrafiltration and isovolemic dialysis, and cool temperature dialysis. The following results were reported: High Na dialysate, Na modeling, and cool temperature dialysis resulted in significantly fewer hypotensive events than that observed with standard dialysis. Compared with the other test strategies, sequential ultrafiltration and isovolemic dialysis had a significantly

TABLE 18.4	**Acute Treatment of Intradialytic Hypotension**

Stop or slow rate of ultrafiltration
Place patient in Trendelenburg position
Decrease blood-flow rate
Restore intravascular volume (hypertonic saline)
Assess for ischemic injury
Check patency of vascular access

---

greater number of hypotensive episodes. Postdialysis upright blood pressure was best with Na modeling and cool temperature dialysis compared with that measured with standard and isolated ultrafiltration dialysis. Weight loss was virtually identical with all protocols. In general, the best-tolerated and most effective strategy was Na modeling. High Na and cool temperature dialysis were also effective, whereas sequential ultrafiltration and isovolemic dialysis was significantly less useful.

ACUTE TREATMENT OF HYPOTENSION

Although occasionally asymptomatic, patients with hypotension may suffer from light-headedness, muscle cramps, nausea, vomiting, and dyspnea. The acute management of low blood pressure associated with HD includes stopping or slowing the rate of ultrafiltration, placing the patient in the Trendelenburg position, decreasing the blood-flow rate, and restoring intravascular volume (TABLE 18.4).

The use of hypertonic saline solutions appears to be particularly effective; it allows Na to be administered in a small volume of water, and the rapid rise in plasma osmolality may have a positive effect on cardiac inotropy (59). One study found that three different regimen safely and effectively raised the blood pressure: 10 mL of 23% saturated hypertonic saline; 30 mL of 7.5% hypertonic saline; and the latter solution with 6% dextran-70 (59). The addition of dextran appeared to prolong the duration of the blood pressure response.

Further treatment is based on the cause of the hypotension; the prompt recognition of life-threatening causes of low blood pressure is essential. Particular concerns should include occult sepsis, previously unrecognized cardiac and/or pericardial disease, and gastrointestinal bleeding.

REFERENCES

1. Palmer BF. The effect of dialysate composition on systemic hemodynamics. *Semin Dial* 1992;5:54–60.
2. Shoji T, Tsubakihara Y, Fujii M, et al. Hemodialysis-associated hypotension as an independent risk factor for two-year mortality in hemodialysis patients. *Kidney Int* 2004;66:1212–1220.
3. Zager PG, Nikolic J, Brown RH, et al. "U" curve association of blood pressure and mortality in hemodialysis patients. Medical Directors of Dialysis Clinic, Inc. *Kidney Int* 1998;54:561–569.
4. Port FK, Hulbert-Shearon TE, Wolfe RA, et al. Predialysis blood pressure and mortality risk in a national sample of maintenance hemodialysis patients. *Am J Kidney Dis* 1999;33:507–517.
5. Iseki K, Miyasato F, Tokuyama K, et al. Low diastolic blood pressure, hypoalbuminemia, and risk of death in a cohort of chronic hemodialysis patients. *Kidney Int* 1997;51:1212–1217.
6. Coll E, Larrousse M, de la Sierra A, et al. Chronic hypotension in hemodialysis patients: role of functional vascular changes and vasodilator agents. *Clin Nephrol* 2008;69:114–120.

7. Daugirdas JT. Pathophysiology of dialysis hypotension: an update. *Am J Kidney Dis* 2001;38(4 Suppl 4):S11–S17.

8. Krepel HP, Nette RW, Akçahüseyin E, et al. Variability of relative blood volume during haemodialysis. *Nephrol Dial Transplant* 2000;15:673–679.

9. Kunze DL, Brown AM. Sodium sensitivity of baroreceptors. Reflux effects on blood pressure and fluid volume in the cat. *Circ Res* 1978;42:714–720.

10. Schultze G, Maiga M, Neumayer HH, et al. Prostaglandin E2 promotes hypotension on low-sodium hemodialysis. *Nephron* 1984;37:250–256.

11. Cavalcanti S, Cavani S, Santoro A. Role of short-term regulatory mechanisms on pressure response to hemodialysis-induced hypovolemia. *Kidney Int* 2002;61:228–238.

12. Kooman JP, Gladziwa U, Böcker G, et al. Role of the venous system in hemodynamics during ultrafiltration and bicarbonate dialysis. *Kidney Int* 1992;42:718–726.

13. Kooman JP, Wijnen JA, Draaijer P, et al. Compliance and reactivity of the peripheral venous system in chronic intermittent hemodialysis. *Kidney Int* 1992;41:1041–1048.

14. Kooman JP, Daemen MJ, Wijnen R, et al. Morphological changes of the venous system in uremic patients. A histopathologic study. *Nephron* 1995;69:454–458.

15. Yu AW, Nawab ZM, Barnes WE, et al. Splanchnic erythrocyte content decreases during hemodialysis: a new compensatory mechanism for hypovolemia. *Kidney Int* 1997;51:1986–1990.

16. Parfrey PS, Foley RN. Risk factors for cardiac dysfunction in dialysis patients: implications for patient care. *Semin Dial* 1997;10:137–141.

17. Ritz E, Ruffmann K, Rambausek M, et al. Dialysis hypotension: is it related to diastolic left ventricular malfunction? *Nephrol Dial Transplant* 1987;2:293–297.

18. Ritz E, Rambausek M, Mall G, et al. Cardiac changes in uraemia and their possible relationship to cardiovascular instability on dialysis. *Nephrol Dial Transplant* 1990;5(Suppl 1):93–97.

19. Wizemann V, Timio M, Alpert MA, et al. Options in dialysis: significance of cardiovascular findings. *Kidney Int* 1993;43:S85–S91.

20. Ruffmann K, Mandelbaum A, Bommer J, et al. Doppler echocardiographic findings in dialysis patients. *Nephrol Dial Transplant* 1990;5:426–431.

21. Whelton PK, Watson AJ, Kone B, et al. Calcium channel blockade in dialysis patients with left ventricular hypertrophy and well-preserved systolic function. *J Cardiovasc Pharmacol* 1987;10(Suppl 10):S185–S186.

22. Harnett JD, Kent GM, Foley RN, et al. Cardiac function and hematocrit level. *Am J Kidney Dis* 1995;25(4 Suppl 1):S3–S7.

23. Singh A, Szczech L, Tang KL, et al. Correction of anemia with epoetin alfa in chronic kidney disease. *N Engl J Med* 2006;355:2085–2098.

24. Drüeke TB, Locatelli F, Clyne N, et al. Normalization of hemoglobin level in patients with chronic kidney disease and anemia. *N Engl J Med* 2006;355:2071–2084.

25. Poldermans D, Man in 't Veld AJ, Rambaldi R, et al. Cardiac evaluation in hypotension-prone and hypotension-resistant hemodialysis patients. *Kidney Int* 1999;56:1905–1911.

26. Ibels LS, Alfrey AC, Huffer WE, et al. Arterial calcification and pathology in uremic patients undergoing dialysis. *Am J Med* 1979;66:790–796.

27. Shinzato T, Miwa M, Nakai S, et al. Role of adenosine in dialysis-induced hypotension. *J Am Soc Nephrol* 1994;4:1987–1994.

28. Imai E, Fujii M, Kohno Y, et al. Adenosine A1 receptor antagonist improves intradialytic hypotension. *Kidney Int* 2006;69:877–883.

29. Giaime P, Carrega L, Fenouillet E, et al. Relationship between A(2A) adenosine receptor expression and intradialytic hypotension during hemodialysis. *J Investig Med* 2006;54:473–477.

30. Beasley D, Brenner BM. Role of nitric oxide in hemodialysis hypotension. *Kidney Int* 1992;42(38):S96–S100.

31. Herbelin A, Nguyen AT, Zingraff J, et al. Influence of uremia and hemodialysis on circulating interleukin-1 and tumor necrosis factor a. *Kidney Int* 1990;37:116–125.

32. Weinberg JR, Wright DJ, Guz A. Interleukin-1 and tumor necrosis factor cause hypotension in the conscious rabbit. *Clin Sci* 1988;75:251–255.

33. Rossi V, Breviaro F, Ghezzi P, et al. Prostacyclin synthesis induced in vascular cells by interleukin-1. *Science* 1985;229:174–176.

34. Yokokawa K, Mankus R, Saklayen MG, et al. Increased nitric oxide production in patients with hypotension during hemodialysis. *Ann Intern Med* 1995;123:35–37.

35. Raj DS, Vincent B, Simpson K, et al. Hemodynamic changes during hemodialysis: role of nitric oxide and endothelin. *Kidney Int* 2002;61:697–704.

36. Kang ES, Acchiardo SR, Wang YB, et al. Hypotension during hemodialysis: role for nitric oxide. *Am J Med Sci* 1997;313:138–146.

37. Bradbury S, Eggleston C. Postural hypotension: a report of three cases. *Am Heart J* 1925;1:73–86.

38. Travis M, Henrich WL. Autonomic nervous system and hemodialysis hypotension. *Semin Dial* 1989;2:158–162.

39. Henrich WL. Autonomic insufficiency. *Arch Intern Med* 1982;142:339–344.

40. Kurnatowska I, Nowicki M. Serum chromogranin A concentration and intradialytic hypotension in chronic haemodialysis patients. *Int Urol Nephrol* 2006;38:701–705.

41. Lilley JJ, Golden J, Stone RA. Adrenergic regulation of blood pressure in chronic renal failure. *J Clin Invest* 1976;57:1190–1200.

42. Ewing DJ, Winney R. Autonomic function in patients with chronic renal failure on intermittent haemodialysis. *Nephron* 1975;15:424–429.

43. Cavalcanti S, Severi S, Chiari L, et al. Autonomic nervous function during haemodialysis assessed by spectral analysis of heart-rate variability. *Clin Sci* 1997;92:351–359.

44. Enzmann G, Bianco F, Paolini F, et al. Autonomic nervous function and blood volume monitoring during hemodialysis. *Int J Artif Organs* 1995;18:504–508.

45. Heber ME, Lahiri A, Thompson D, et al. Baroreceptor, not left ventricular, dysfunction is the cause of hemodialysis hypotension. *Clin Nephrol* 1989;32:79–86.

46. Zoccali C, Ciccarelli M, Maggiore Q. Defective reflex control of heart rate in dialysis patients: evidence for an afferent autonomic lesion. *Clin Sci* 1982;63:285–292.

47. Nakashima Y, Fouad FM, Nakamoto S, et al. Localization of autonomic nervous system dysfunction in dialysis patients. *Am J Nephrol* 1987;7:375–381.

48. Krishnan AV, Kiernan MC. Uremic neuropathy: clinical features and new pathophysiological insights. *Muscle Nerve* 2007;35:273–290.

49. Converse RL Jr, Jacobsen TN, Jost CM, et al. Paradoxical withdrawal of reflex vasoconstriction as a cause of hemodialysis-induced hypotension. *J Clin Invest* 1992;90:1657–1665.

50. Henrich WL, Woodard TD, Blachley JD, et al. Role of osmolality in blood pressure stability after dialysis and ultrafiltration. *Kidney Int* 1980;18:480–488.

51. Abboud FM. Ventricular syncope: is the heart a sensory organ? *N Engl J Med* 1989;320:390–392.

52. Sander-Jensen R, Secher NH, Bie P, et al. Vagal slowing of the heart during haemorrhage: observation from 20 consecutive hypotensive patients. *Br Med J (Clin Res Ed)* 1986;292:364–366.

53. Zoccali C, Tripepi G, Mallamaci F, et al. The heart rate response pattern to dialysis hypotension in haemodialysis patients. *Nephrol Dial Transplant* 1997;12:519–523.

54. Armengol NE, Cases Amenós A, Bono Illa M, et al. Vasoactive hormones in uraemic patients with chronic hypotension. *Nephrol Dial Transplant* 1997;12:321–324.

55. Jassal SV, Coulshed SJ, Douglas JF, et al. Autonomic neuropathy predisposing to arrhythmias in hemodialysis patients. *Am J Kidney Dis* 1997;30:219–223.

56. Zhou YL, Liu HL, Duan XF, et al. Impact of sodium and ultrafiltration profiling on haemodialysis-related hypotension. *Nephrol Dial Transplant* 2006;21:3231–3237.

57. Cruz DN, Mahnensmith RL, Brickel HM, et al. Midodrine and cool dialysate are effective therapies for symptomatic intradialytic hypotension. *Am J Kidney Dis* 1999;33:920–926.

58. Dheenan S, Henrich WL. Preventing dialysis hypotension: a comparison of usual protective maneuvers. *Kidney Int* 2001;59:1175–1181.

59. Gong R, Lindberg J, Abrams J, et al. Comparison of hypertonic saline solutions and dextran in dialysis-induced hypotension. *J Am Soc Nephrol* 1993;3:1808–1812.

60. Recordati G, Moss NG, Genovesi S, et al. Renal chemoreceptors. *J Auton Nerv Syst* 1981;3:237–251.

61. Converse RL Jr, Jacobsen TN, Toto RD, et al. Sympathetic overactivity in patients with chronic renal failure. *N Engl J Med* 1992;327:1912–1918.

62. Chandra P, Sands RL, Gillespie BW, et al. Predictors of heart rate variability and its prognostic significance in chronic kidney disease. *Nephrol Dial Transplant* 2012;27:700–709.

63. Celik A, Melek M, Yuksel S, et al. Cardiac autonomic dysfunction in hemodialysis patients: the value of heart rate turbulence. *Hemodial Int* 2011;15:193–199.

64. Yang Y-W, Wu C-H, Tsai M-K, et al. Heart rate variability during hemodialysis and following renal transplantation. *Transplant Proc* 2010;42:1637–1640.

65. Flythe JE, Xue H, Lynch KE, et al. Association of mortality risk with various definitions of intradialytic hypotension. *J Am Soc Nephrol* 2014;26:724–734.

66. Daugirdas JT. Measuring intradialytic hypotension to improve quality of care. *J Am Soc Nephrol* 2015;26:512–514.

67. Stefánsson BV, Brunelli SM, Cabrera C, et al. Intradialytic hypotension and risk of cardiovascular disease. *Clin J Am Soc Nephrol* 2014;9:2014–2132.

68. Sands JJ, Usvyat LA, Sullivan T, et al. Intradialytic hypotension: frequency, sources of variation and correlation with clinical outcome. *Hemodial Int* 2014;18:415–422.

69. Chao CT, Huang J-W, Yen C-J. Intradialytic hypotension and cardiac remodeling: a vicious cycle. *Biomed Res Int* 2015;2015:724147. doi:10.1155/2015/724147.

70. Agarwal R. How can we prevent intradialytic hypotension? *Curr Opin Nephrol Hypertens* 2012;21:593–599.

71. Reilly RF. Attending rounds: a patient with intradialytic hypotension. *Clin J Am Soc Nephrol* 2014;9:798–803.

72. Schiller B, Arramreddy R, Hussein W. What are the consequences of volume expansion in chronic dialysis patients? Intra-dialytic hypotension in conventional hemodialysis: unavoidable in some, but preventable in most. *Semin Dial* 2015;28:233–235.

73. Landry DW, Oliver JA. Blood pressure instability during hemodialysis. *Kidney Int* 2006;69:1710–1711.

74. Kraemer M, Rode C, Wizemann V. Detection limit of methods to assess fluid status changes in dialysis patients. *Kidney Int* 2006;69:1609–1620.

75. Hoenich NA, Levin NW. Can technology solve the clinical problem of 'dry weight'? *Nephrol Dial Transplant* 2003;18:647–650.

76. van de Pol ACM, Frenken LA, Moret K, et al. An evaluation of blood volume changes during ultrafiltration pulses and natriuretic peptides in the assessment of dry weight in hemodialysis patients. *Hemodial Int* 2007;11:51–61.

77. Kuhlmann MK, Zhu F, Seibert E, et al. Bioimpedance, dry weight and blood pressure control: new methods and consequences. *Curr Opin Nephrol Hypertens* 2005;14:543–549.

78. Shulman T, Heidenheim AP, Kianfar C, et al. Preserving central blood volume: changes in body fluid compartments during hemodialysis. *ASAIO J* 2001;47:615–618.

79. Lai CT, Wu C-J, Chen H-H, et al. Absolute interdialytic weight gain is more important than percent weight gain for intradialytic hypotension in heavy patients. *Nephrology* 2012;17:230–236.

80. Onofriescu M, Siriopol D, Voroneanu L, et al. Overhydration, cardiac function and survival in hemodialysis patients. *PLoS One* 2015;10:e0135691. doi:10.1371/journal.pone.0135691.

81. Nesrallah GE, Suri RS, Guyatt G, et al. Biofeedback dialysis for hypotension and hypervolemia: a systematic review and meta-analysis. *Nephrol Dial Transplant* 2013;28:182–191.

82. Presta P, Mazzitello G, Fuiano L, et al. Cool temperature hemodialysis and biocompatibility in chronic hemodialysis patients: a preliminary study. *J Nephrol* 2009;22:760–765.

83. Chou K-J, Lee P-T, Chen C-L, et al. Physiological changes during hemodialysis in patients with intradialysis hypertension. *Kidney Int* 2006;69:1833–1838.

84. Günal AI, Karaca I, Ozalp G, et al. Strict volume control can improve structure and function of common carotid artery in hemodialysis patients. *J Nephrol* 2006;19:334–340.

85. Roy PN, Danziger RS. Dialysate magnesium concentration predicts the occurrence of intradialytic hypotension [abstract]. *J Am Soc Nephrol* 1996;7:1496.

86. Kyriazis J, Glotsos J, Bilirakis L, et al. Dialysate calcium profiling during hemodialysis: use and clinical implications. *Kidney Int* 2002;61:276–287.

87. Song JH, Park GH, Lee SY, et al. Effect of sodium balance and the combination of ultrafiltration profile during sodium profiling hemodialysis on the maintenance of the quality of dialysis and sodium and fluid balances. *J Am Soc Nephrol* 2005;16:237–246.

88. Dasselaar JJ, Huisman RM, de Jong PE, et al. Measurement of relative blood volume changes during haemodialysis: merits and limitations. *Nephrol Dial Transplant* 2005;20:2043–2049.

89. Reddan DN, Szczech LA, Hasselblad V, et al. Intradialytic blood volume monitoring in ambulatory hemodialysis patients: a randomized trial. *J Am Soc Nephrol* 2005;16:2162–2169.

90. Dasselaar JJ, Lub-de Hooge MN, Pruim J, et al. Relative blood volume changes underestimate total blood volume changes during hemodialysis. *Clin J Am Soc Nephrol* 2007;2:669–674.

91. Santoro A, Mancini E, Basile C, et al. Blood volume controlled hemodialysis in hypotension-prone patients: a randomized, multi-center controlled trial. *Kidney Int* 2002;62:1034–1045.

92. Franssen CFM, Dasselaar JJ, Sytsma P, et al. Automatic feedback control of relative blood volume changes during hemodialysis improves blood pressure stability during and after dialysis. *Hemodial Int* 2005;9:383–392.

93. Dasselaar JJ, Huisman RM, de Jong PE, et al. Effects of relative blood volume-controlled hemodialysis on blood pressure and volume status in hypertensive patients. *ASAIO J* 2007;53:357–364.

94. Mancini E, Mambelli E, Irpinia M, et al. Prevention of dialysis hypotension episodes using fuzzy logic control system. *Nephrol Dial Transplant* 2007;22:1420–1427.

95. Rosales LM, Schneditz D, Morris AT, et al. Isothermic hemodialysis and ultrafiltration. *Am J Kidney Dis* 2000;36:353–361.

96. Selby NM, McIntyre CW. A systematic review of the clinical effects of reducing dialysate fluid temperature. *Nephrol Dial Transplant* 2006;21:1883–1898.

97. Levy FL, Grayburn PA, Foulks CJ, et al. Improved left ventricular contractility with cool temperature hemodialysis. *Kidney Int* 1992;41:961–965.

98. Jost CM, Agarwal R, Khair-el-Din T, et al. Effects of cooler temperature dialysate on hemodynamic stability in "problem" dialysis patients. *Kidney Int* 1993;44:606–612.

99. Hoeben H, Abu-Alfa AK, Mahnensmith R, et al. Hemodynamics in patients with intradialytic hypotension treated with cool dialysate or midodrine. *Am J Kidney Dis* 2002;39:102–107.

100. Fine A, Penner B. The protective effect of cool dialysate is dependent on patients' predialysis temperature. *Am J Kidney Dis* 1996;28:262–265.

101. Yu AW, Ing TS, Zabaneh RI, et al. Effect of dialysate temperature on central hemodynamics and urea kinetics. *Kidney Int* 1995;48:237–243.

102. Maggiore Q, Pizzarelli F, Santoro A, et al; and the Study Group of Thermal Balance and Vascular Stability. The effects of control of thermal balance on vascular stability in hemodialysis patients: results of the European randomized clinical trial. *Am J Kidney Dis* 2002;40:280–290.

103. Yamamoto N, Sasaki E, Goda K, et al. Treatment of post-dialytic orthostatic hypotension with an inflatable abdominal band in hemodialysis patients. *Kidney Int* 2006;70:1793–1800.

104. Barakat MM, Nawab ZM, Yu AW, et al. Hemodynamic effects of intradialytic food ingestion and the effects of caffeine. *J Am Soc Nephrol* 1993;3:1813–1818.

105. Radermacher J, Koch KM. Treatment of renal anemia by erythropoietin substitution. The effects on the cardiovascular system. *Clin Nephrol* 1995;44(Suppl 1):S56–S60.

106. Bode-Böger SM, Böger RH, Kuhn M, et al. Recombinant human erythropoietin enhances vasoconstrictor tone via endothelin-1 and constrictor prostanoids. *Kidney Int* 1996;50:1255–1261.

107. Portolés J, Torralbo A, Martin P, et al. Cardiovascular effects of recombinant human erythropoietin in predialysis patients. *Am J Kidney Dis* 1997;29:541–548.

108. Fujisaki K, Kanai H, Hirakata H, et al. Midodrine hydrochloride and L-threo-3,4-dihydroxy-phenylserine preserve cerebral blood flow in hemodialysis patients with orthostatic hypotension. *Ther Apher Dial* 2007;11:49–55.

109. Flynn JJ III, Mitchell MC, Caruso FS, et al. Midodrine treatment for patients with hemodialysis hypotension. *Clin Nephrol* 1996;45: 261–267.

110. Cruz DN, Mahnensmith RL, Brickel HM, et al. Midodrine is effective and safe therapy for intradialytic hypotension over 8 months of follow-up. *Clin Nephrol* 1998;50:101–107.

111. Prakash S, Garg AX, Heidenheim AP, et al. Midodrine appears to be safe and effective for dialysis-induced hypotension: a systematic review. *Nephrol Dial Transplant* 2004;19:2553–2558.

112. Dheenan S, Venkatesan J, Grubb BP, et al. Effect of sertraline hydrochloride on dialysis hypotension. *Am J Kidney Dis* 1998;31:624–630.

113. Ahmad S, Robertson HT, Golper TA, et al. Multicenter trial of L-carnitine in maintenance hemodialysis patients. II. Clinical and biochemical effects. *Kidney Int* 1990;38:912–918.

114. Hirszel IP, Martin RH, Mizell MW, et al. Uremic autonomic neuropathy: evaluation of ephedrine sulphate therapy for hemodialysis-induced hypotension. *Int Urol Nephrol* 1976;8:313–321.

115. Warren SE, Olshan A, Beck CH Jr. Use of phenylephrine HCL for treatment of refractory dialysis-aggravated hypotension. *Dial Transplant* 1980;9:492–496.

116. Lindberg JS, Copley JB, Melton K, et al. Lysine vasopressin in the treatment of refractory hemodialysis-induced hypotension. *Am J Nephrol* 1990;10:269–275.

117. van der Zee S, Thompson A, Zimmerman R, et al. Vasopressin administration facilitates fluid removal during hemodialysis. *Kidney Int* 2007;71:318–324.

118. Ettema EM, Zittema D, Kuipers J, et al. Dialysis hypotension: a role for inadequate increase in arginine vasopressin levels? A systematic literature review and meta-analysis. *Am J Nephrol* 2014;29:100–109.

119. Kuhn C, Kuhn A, Rykow K, et al. Extravascular lung water index: a new method to determine dry weight in chronic hemodialysis patients. *Hemodial Int* 2006;10:68–72.

CHAPTER 19

Oxidant Stress in End-Stage Kidney Disease

Ravinder K. Wali

 DEFINITION OF OXIDANT STRESS

Oxidative stress is a pathologic state in which reactive oxygen intermediates (ROI) or reactive oxygen species (ROS) can cause oxidation of cellular and matrix macromolecules including sugars, proteins, deoxyribonucleic acid (DNA) bases, and lipids (1). ROS are generated in mitochondria from the use of molecular oxygen for the efficient cellular energy production for routine aerobic metabolic activity. ROS are the detrimental by-products resulting in oxidative damage to cellular organelles and have been associated with several disease states, including cancer, diabetes, Alzheimer's disease, Parkinson's disease, aging, inflammation, and atherosclerosis (2,3). Oxidative stress is an imbalance between the quantities of oxidants produced during normal metabolism of our cells and the quantities of antioxidant gene products [superoxide dismutase (SOD), catalases (CATs), glutathione (GSH) peroxidases, etc.], required to maintain the equipoise to prevent accumulation of oxidant molecules.

Increasing evidence suggests that oxidative stress may have a significant role in the development of complications in patients with chronic kidney disease (CKD). Understanding the role of oxidant stress in the pathogenesis of multisystem involvement in patients with CKD or dialysis-associated pathology will ultimately help to develop the strategies for the prevention and treatment of increased oxidative stress in CKD and its associated complications.

GENERATION OF REACTIVE OXYGEN SPECIES IN THE BIOLOGIC SYSTEM

In biologic systems, cells generate energy aerobically to produce adenosine triphosphate (ATP) by reducing molecular oxygen

(O_2) to water. The cytochrome-C oxidase-catalyzed reactions involve transfer of four electrons (e^-) to oxygen; the consumption of oxygen at the mitochondrial level is associated with production of oxygen intermediates. One percent to 2% of total oxygen consumption may, in fact, be converted to superoxide anion radical ($O2^-$). Formation of $O2^-$ anion radical leads to a cascade of other ROS production (4) (**FIGURE 19.1**). The biologic toxicity of superoxide is due to its capacity to inactivate iron-sulfur containing enzymes (these enzymes are critical for

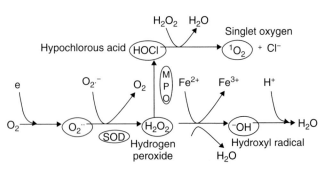

FIGURE 19.1 Generation of reactive oxygen species. The biologically active oxygen free radicals are the radical ion superoxide O_2^-, hydroxide ion OH^-, and peroxide ion O_2^{2-}. These radicals are intermediates in the respiratory process at the mitochondrial level, in which peroxide ion (O_2^{2-}) is reduced to water in a stepwise six-electron process in the presence of glutathione(s) and catalases. H_2O_2 rapidly diffuses across the lipid membranes and is converted into strong oxidants. H_2O_2 in the presence of cytoplasmic MPO produces HOCl, a free radical ion with toxic effects. MPO, myeloperoxidase; SOD, superoxide dismutase.

different metabolic pathways) and liberate free iron in the cell, which can undergo Fenton chemical reaction and generate highly reactive hydroxyl radicals (OH^-). Hydroxyl radical immediately develops into HO_2 (hydroperoxyl radical), HO_2 in combination with superoxide anion can initiate lipid peroxidation of polyunsaturated fatty acids, react with carbonyl compounds and halogenated carbons to create toxic peroxy radicals. Superoxide reacts avidly with nitric oxide (NO) to form peroxynitrite ($ONOO^-$). As such, superoxide in combination with HO_2, and $ONOO^-$ are the main causes of oxidative stress.

Superoxide dismutase (SOD) rapidly converts O_2^- to hydrogen peroxide (H_2O_2) and oxygen. Because O_2^- is more toxic than H_2O_2, its rapid removal is of paramount importance for the proper function of the microenvironment (5). H_2O_2 is a versatile ROS because it can cross plasma membranes, increase intracellular hydroxyl radicals, trigger peroxidation of cell membrane lipids (CMLs), promote protein aggregation, and damage and/or cleave DNA (5,6). H_2O_2 converts carboxylic acid (RCOOH) into peroxy acids (PRCOOH), which are used as oxidizing agents. H_2O_2 reacts with acetone to form acetone peroxide, and it interacts with ozone to form hydrogen trioxide. Its reaction with urea produces carbamide peroxide. In aqueous solution, hydrogen peroxide can oxidize or reduce a variety of inorganic ions. When H_2O_2 acts as a reducing agent, oxygen gas is also produced. In acid solution, Fe^{2+} is oxidized to Fe^{3+} (**EQUATION 19.1**).

$$2Fe^{2+}(aq) + H_2O_2 + 2H^+(aq) \rightarrow 2Fe^{3+}(aq) + 2H_2O \quad (19.1)$$

Also, through catalysis, H_2O_2 can be converted into hydroxyl radicals (.OH), the most powerful ROS in the biologic system. H_2O_2 is removed by several different pathways *in vivo*.

1. Catalase (CAT) and the reduced form (GSH) of glutathione peroxidase (GPx) catalyze H_2O_2 to $H_2O + O_2$. This is presumably a detoxification mechanism.
2. H_2O_2 is converted by the abundant myeloperoxidase (MPO) enzyme in neutrophils to hypochlorous acid (HOCl) (6). HOCl is a strong oxidant that acts as a bactericidal agent in phagocytic cells. Reaction of HOCl with H_2O_2 yields singlet oxygen ($^1O_2$) and H_2O.
3. H_2O_2 also reacts spontaneously with intracellular iron to form highly reactive hydroxy radical (OH^-) (7) by the Haber-Weiss cycle or Fenton reaction (8). The hydroxyl radical reacts instantaneously with the hydrogen moiety of other biologic molecule to produce long-lived ROS called *reactive amines* (RH) (9).
4. Superoxide (O_2^-) anion regulates the bioavailability of NO. Superoxide anion can react with NO and result in the formation of peroxynitrite ($ONOO^-$) (9). $ONOO^-$ is a strong oxidant with vasoconstrictor activities as compared with the vasodilator potential of NO (10). In addition, $ONOO^-$ reacts nonenzymatically with arachidonic acid components of phospholipids resulting in the formation of isoprostanes (8-iso-PGF2α), a potent vasoconstrictor with a long half-life.

ROS have a very short life, and excessive production and prolonged exposure of cell constituents to these evanescent radicals can result in oxidative modification of cellular macromolecules. *In vivo* measurements of ROS-modified cellular macromolecules serve as indirect markers of prevailing oxidative stress. These include products of carbohydrate and protein oxidation (11), lipid peroxidation (12), and nucleic acid oxidation with DNA fragmentation leading to DNA instability and mutation (13).

PHYSIOLOGIC ANTIOXIDANT SYSTEM

An imbalance due to increased production of ROS and the available antioxidants results in the excessive exposure of the tissue macromolecules to ROS, resulting in the production of biomarkers of oxidant stress. Under physiologic conditions, protection against oxidant stress is offered by the presence of different types of antioxidants—enzymatic and nonenzymatic antioxidants (1).

Enzymatic antioxidants include glutathione dismutase (GPx), glutathione reductase (GR) and glutathione transferase (GT), SOD, and CAT. GPx is a selenium-dependent enzyme present in the plasma and red blood cell (RBC) and is mainly produced in the kidneys. GPx exists in three different forms [GST, oxidized glutathione (GSSG), and GSH]. GR uses nicotinamide adenine dinucleotide phosphate (NADPH) to convert GSSG to its reduced form (GSH).

Recent discovery of the crystal structure of nicotinamide nucleotide transhydrogenase (TH) that facilitates the disposal of ROS and prevents the development of oxidative stress at the cellular level has further advanced the basic mechanisms of how ROS are disposed (14). The mitochondrial ROS defense system transforms reactive superoxide anions (O_2^-) formed by electrons leaking to molecular oxygen during aerobic respiration to hydrogen peroxide (H_2O_2). H_2O_2 is detoxified to water by peroxidases that use reduced GSH as a substrate. Cellular levels of GSH are maintained by reduced NADPH-dependent GR (**FIGURE 19.2** and **EQUATION 19.2**).

$$NADH = NADP^+ + H^+out \Longleftrightarrow NAD^+ + NADP^+ + H^+in \quad (19.2)$$

The resultant NADPH is used for amino acid biosynthesis and by GR and GPx to remove ROS (15).

Nonenzymatic antioxidants: Majority of nonenzymatic antioxidants have a thiol as a functional group—SH (reduced) and can be oxidized via disulphide bond formation (oxidized). Thiols have the ability to react with almost all the tissue oxidants and maintain the tissue redox (reduction/oxidation) state. The major biologic thiol/disulphide couples include GSH, thioredoxin, and other cysteine-containing proteins. GSH is particularly unique as it is able to detoxify H_2O_2, OH^-, and chlorinated oxidants. Extracellular thiols present in the plasma and interstitial fluid are important antioxidants to promote redox state. When these protective thiols are decreased as in acute as well as CKD patients, oxidized thiols lead to endothelial injury, and increased vascular morbidity (16).

Other nonenzymatic antioxidants: Important ones include α-tocopherol (vitamin E); vitamin C (ascorbic acid); albumin; and other proteins such as transferrin, ceruloplasmin, and microamounts of extracellular superoxide dismutases (ecSOD) (17). α-Tocopherol (vitamin E) is perhaps the major lipid-soluble chain-breaking antioxidant (reacting with chain-propagating radicals such as peroxyl radicals) (18). This antioxidant is particularly important because it prevents lipid peroxidation. Ascorbic acid, on the other hand, has mostly scavenging properties and other minor antioxidant properties. It scavenges the singlet oxygen ($^1O_2$), O_2^-, and H_2O_2 at a constant rate at optimal pH (7.4). It is a powerful scavenger of HOCl and also can be a substrate for the enzyme MPO to prevent the generation of HOCl (19). Vitamin C deficiency in CKD and dialysis patients is perhaps more common than thought given that such patients often avoid the consumption of fresh fruits, vegetables, and also loss of water-soluble vitamins with dialysis therapy. However, ascorbic acid in high doses can also be a pro-oxidant (20).

Acute-phase reactive proteins such as ferritin, transferrin, ceruloplasmin, haptoglobin, and others also function as effective

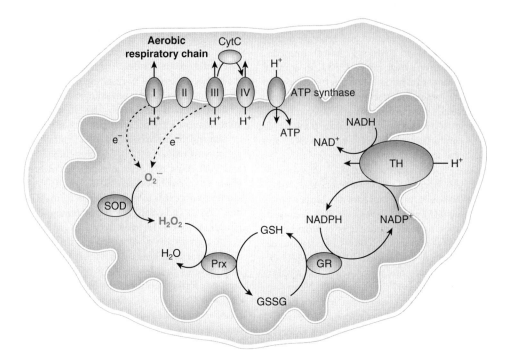

FIGURE 19.2 Mitochondrial reactive oxygen species (ROS) defense. Transhydrogenase (TH) contributes to mitochondrial ROS defense by producing NADPH. During aerobic respiration, electrons leak to molecular oxygen, primarily from complexes I and III. This results in "superoxide anions" $O_2{}^-$, which is converted to H_2O_2 by mitochondrial superoxide dismutase (SOD) and finally to water by peroxidases (Prx), using reduced glutathione (GSH). GSH levels are maintained by glutathione reductase (GR), which uses NADPH formed by TH to reduce glutathione (GSSG). CytC, cytochrome C; ATP, adenosine triphosphate. (Modified and reproduced from Krengel U, Törnroth-Horsefield S. Coping with oxidative stress. *Science* 2015;347:125–126.)

antioxidants by binding to transitional metals such as iron, copper, and bromide to prevent the formation of halides, hemes, and chloramines (21).

PATHOPHYSIOLOGY OF OXIDATIVE STRESS IN DIALYSIS PATIENTS

CKD is associated with qualitative and quantitative changes in the physiologic antioxidants. This is further complicated by the increased production or decreased removal of ROS and its related oxidation products. These sequences of events culminate in excessive tissue damage from the ROS and its end products.

Increased Generation of Oxidant Radicals (Reactive Oxygen Species) in Dialysis Patients

Advanced kidney disease is associated with increased production of ROS, and this oxidant stress is further aggravated with the initiation of dialysis therapy. There are several pathways involved in the excessive generation of ROS in CKD and dialysis population.

1. Activation of neutrophil-macrophage system

   The increased oxidative stress in CKD as well as in dialysis patients could be due to activation of monocyte-macrophage cells by the uremic milieu and further aggravated by exposure of blood to extracorporeal circulation (see Chapter 20).

   Activation of phagocytes results in respiratory burst activity with the production of ROS, necessary for host defenses, cell activation, and cell signaling (22). The respiratory burst activity is associated with activation of mitochondrial NADPH-oxidases that catalyzes the single electron transfer

and generates superoxide anion $(O_2{}^-)$ at the electron transfer chain level (23). The NADPH-oxidases are highly regulated group of homologous proteins comprising of cytoplasmic (p47, p67, p40) and membrane-bound proteins (gp91 and p22) domains (24). Deficiency or dysfunction of NADPH-oxidases is associated with increased risk of bacterial infections and results in the development of chronic granulomatous disease (CGD). Similar deficiency can lead to unbalanced effects of $O_2{}^-$.

In addition, phagocytic cells have abundant MPO in the azurophilic granules, which is released on stimulation of mononuclear cells. The MPO enzyme system in phagocytic cells catalyzes the oxidation of halides like chloride, bromide, and iodide. MPO in the presence of chloride (Cl^-) ions converts H_2O_2 to HOCl. In addition to its primary function of bactericidal killing, HOCl is a potent oxidant as it can oxidate the thiol groups of membrane proteins and intracellular enzymes, and it also inhibits the mitochondrial cytochrome system, perpetuating the production of ROS. HOCl can react with endogenous amines (R-NHI) to result in the production of long-lasting oxidants called *chloramines* (RNH-Cl) (6).

Himmelfarb et al. (25) studied phagocytic function in patients on hemodialysis (HD) and peritoneal dialysis (PD) and demonstrated an exaggerated respiratory burst activity of phagocytes after *in vitro* stimulation. This respiratory burst production of ROS coincides with the peak of complement activation during dialysis treatment (26). Furthermore, Tepel et al. (27) showed that increased ROS production from peripheral blood cells either spontaneously or after phorbol-myristate-acetate (PMA)-induced stimulation in patients on maintenance dialysis, remained unchanged before and after dialysis using biocompatible membranes.

In summary, during the last 10 years, despite the advances in dialysis therapy and introduction of high-performance dialysis membranes and improvements in the quality of dialysates and water purification methods, the rate of progression of chronic inflammation and vascular disease in dialysis-dependent patients has remained unchanged due to inability of conventional dialysis membranes to remove unconventional uremic toxins such as the products of glycation and oxidation (28,29). Therefore, the burden of proinflammatory and pro-oxidant state associated with chronic dialysis therapy has not changed (**FIGURE 19.3**). On the other hand, evidence supports that the levels of proinflammatory and pro-oxidant levels decrease significantly following kidney transplantation (30).

During maintenance dialysis, exposure of monocyte-macrophage system to the uremic solutes along with exposure to extracorporeal circulation, the two in combination, changes the phenotype of these cells to the state of proinflammatory phenotype with unbalanced production of both pro- and anti-inflammatory cytokines. These phenotypic changes result in increased production of adhesion molecules and chemotactic factors such as vascular cell adhesion molecules (VCAM), leukocyte adhesion molecules [intercellular adhesion molecule (ICAM-1) and P-selectins], monocyte chemoattractant protein-1 (MCP-1), and others (31). These changes increase leukocyte activation with migration and adhesion to subendothelial space and to atherosclerotic plaques (32), particularly in the presence of already activated platelets and endothelial cells (33). Cumulatively, these dynamic interactions at the molecular level may contribute to the pathogenesis of accelerated atherosclerosis in dialysis patients (34).

2. **Qualitative or quantitative changes in physiologic antioxidants**
The effects of increased production of ROS in dialysis patients are further aggravated by decreased levels or impaired function of both enzymatic and nonenzymatic antioxidants. Therefore, imbalance between the increased ROS production and reduced availability of antioxidants aggravates the prevailing oxidative stress.

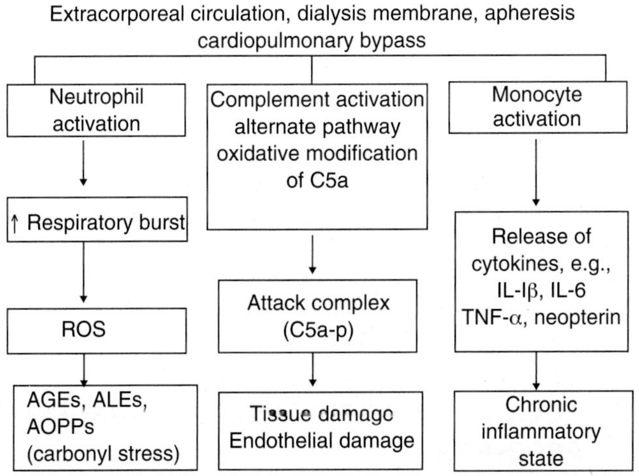

FIGURE 19.3 Different pathways of reactive oxygen species (ROS) production on exposure to extracorporeal circulation. IL, interleukin; TNF, tumor necrosis factor; AGEs, advanced glycation end products; ALEs, atomic layer epitaxies; AOPPs, advanced oxidized protein products.

GPx converts H_2O_2 to $2H_2O$. GPx is mainly produced in the kidney, and its levels in both serum and RBC decreases in proportion to the decreasing glomerular filtration rate (GFR). All three forms of glutathione (GST, GSSG, and GSH) decrease in patients with advanced kidney disease and in patients on kidney replacement therapy (HD or PD). Ross et al. (35) and Mimić-Oka et al. (36) demonstrated that whole blood and RBC glutathione and CAT levels (CATs also convert H_2O_2 to H_2O and O_2) were significantly decreased in patients with kidney disease (CKD) as well as in dialysis-dependent patients.

The levels of nonenzymatic antioxidants like vitamin C and vitamin E have been demonstrated to be low normal in dialysis patients as compared with healthy controls. The reasons for decreased levels of antioxidants in patients with kidney disease are multifactorial: increased consumption resulting from increased burden of ROS, relative deficiency of vitamin C and vitamin E (possibly related to a decreased intake and dietary restriction of fresh fruits and vegetables to avoid hyperkalemia), and the excessive losses of nutrients of different molecular weights with dialysis (37,38). It is also possible that uremic toxins that persist despite an adequate dialysis dose may cause functional deficiency of these physiologic antioxidants. Hypoalbuminemia is often present in dialysis-dependent patients and results in decreased antioxidant stores in blood (37,39).

BIOMARKERS OF OXIDATIVE STRESS

Because ROS have a very short half-life, their *in vivo* presence is extremely transient. Therefore, to understand the consequences of the presence of excessive amounts of ROS, one has to study the downstream effects of excessive ROS, called *footprints of increased oxidative stress*. Wolff and Dean (1987) introduced the concept of the Maillard reaction to describe the role of reducing sugars as catalysts in the oxidative modification and cross-linking of proteins, defined as reactive carbonyls (RCO): autoxidative glycosylation leading to production of reactive dicarbonyls such as methylglyoxal, 3-deoxyglucosone, and glyoxal. These Schiff bases undergo spontaneous rearrangements (Amadori products) resulting in the formation of advanced glycation end products (AGEs) (40).

ADVANCED GLYCATION END PRODUCTS

Aging and hyperglycemia are associated with increased production of ROS resulting in the modification of long-lived extracellular proteins such as collagen, elastin, laminin, and myelin sheath proteins. Similar phenomenon has been demonstrated in patients with CKD (41,42).

Three different carbohydrate-derived oxidation products are identified as N^ε-(carboxymethyl)lysine (CML), N^ε-(carboxymethyl) hydroxylysine (CMhL), and pentosidine (41). Intravenous administration of experimentally prepared AGE-modified albumin or enzymatically prepared AGE-peptides results in widespread vascular leakage, increased macrophage chemotactic activity, impaired NO-induced vasodilatation, and glomerulosclerosis (42).

Sell and Monnier (43) reported increased tissue levels of the AGE-specific moiety pentosidine in collagen tissues of patients with end-stage kidney disease (ESKD) and aging patients. Makita et al. (44), with the use of radioreceptor assays, demonstrated significantly higher levels of AGEs in medium-sized arteries of diabetic patients and nondiabetic subjects. Diabetic patients with ESKD had twice the levels of tissue AGEs as compared with diabetic patients without kidney disease. Dialysis-dependent diabetic patients had mean AGE levels five times higher than those diabetic patients without kidney disease. Although serum creatinine decreases by 75% with each dialysis session, AGE levels decreases by less than 25%. Successful kidney transplantation, however, is associated with a decrease in the plasma levels of AGEs commensurate with the decrease in creatinine, but levels of AGEs continue to remain higher than in healthy controls.

Different sizes of AGEs have been noted in the blood of patients with diabetes and uremia: those with AGEs less than 10 kDa versus greater than 10 kDa. Makita et al. (44) measured peptide-linked degradation products of AGEs, labeled as low molecular weight AGE-modified molecules (LMW-AGEs), with a molecular weight of 2,000 to 6,000. Serum levels of LMW-AGE remain five- to sixfold higher in patients undergoing dialysis therapy with cuprophane or high-flux membranes as well as in PD patients than in healthy controls (45).

The use of high-flux membranes was associated with at least a 50% decrease in LMW-AGE in both diabetic and nondiabetic dialysis patients. However, these levels returned to baseline values within first 4 hours after dialysis. *In vitro* experiments demonstrated that LMW-AGEs retain strong chemical activity against tissue collagen and vascular endothelium; this interaction was abrogated with the use of inhibitors of AGE-cross-linking, such as aminoguanidine (AGN). These results suggest that LMW-AGEs are refractory to removal by current modes of dialysis therapy and may be a component of the "middle molecule" uremic toxin (46).

ADVANCED LIPID PEROXIDATION PRODUCTS

Nonenzymatic oxidation of polyunsaturated fatty acids either in the plasma or cell membranes by H_2O_2, and HOCl results in the formation of lipid hydroperoxides and reactive aldehydes (47,48). These lipid hydroperoxides and reactive aldehydes are unstable and undergo spontaneous rearrangements or break down into different smaller and stable compounds such as malondialdehyde (MDA), 4-hydroxynonenal, glyoxal, and acrolein (49). Boaz et al. (50) found that patients with highest levels of post-HD MDA were almost four times more likely to have accelerated atherosclerosis.

Isoprostanes (8-iso-PGF2a) are generated by peroxidation of arachidonic acid of CMLs. The peroxidation occurs *in situ* in membrane phospholipids; these are then cleaved by endogenous phospholipases and circulate as isoprostanes. These new classes of oxidative stress by-products are strong vasoconstrictors (51). Elevated levels of urinary isoprostanes decrease with antioxidant treatment in healthy volunteers (52).

ADVANCED OXIDIZED PROTEIN PRODUCTS

ROS can alter the primary, secondary, or tertiary structure of proteins resulting initially in denaturation and fragmentation and finally cross-linking of protein moieties (11). Such cross-linked proteins are less susceptible to proteolytic digestion, resulting in long-term accumulation. Witko-Sarsat et al. (53) developed a novel spectrophotometric assay for the detection of oxidatively modified proteins called *advanced oxidized protein product* (AOPP). The plasma levels of AOPP were significantly increased in patients on dialysis (HD or PD) and in patients with advanced kidney disease but not on dialysis when compared with healthy controls.

The plasma levels of AOPP in dialysis patients correlated well with increased levels of methylguanidine (a marker of oxidant-induced

protein cross-linking and aggregation), thiobarbituric acid reactive substances (TBARS), and pentosidine as markers of advanced lipid oxidation product (ALE) and AGE, respectively. Similarly, the levels of AOPP were closely related to soluble markers of monocyte activation such as neopterin and tumor necrosis factor alpha (TNF-α) (54).

In vitro exposure of control plasma samples and human serum albumin (HSA) to HOCl (a strong oxidizing agent) results in the dose-dependent formation of AOPP. *In vitro* exposure of HSA-AOPP aggregate is capable of triggering the respiratory burst of isolated neutrophils in a dose-dependent manner. In view of these findings, it is postulated that neutrophils generate HOCl leading to the formation of AOPP, and these molecules will in turn stimulate phagocytes and release more HOCl (53). The molecular mechanisms that allow AOPP to stimulate monocytes may be dependent on ligand–receptor type interaction. These *in vitro* experiments demonstrate that AOPPs *per se* can perpetuate oxidative stress (54).

THE EUROPEAN UREMIC TOXIN WORK GROUP

Owing to recent advances in proteomics and metabolomics and a reanalysis of uremic solutes, "The European Uremic Toxin (EUTox) Work Group" defined more than 90 compounds that were classified as uremic toxins. These toxins have different molecular weights and have been distributed in three different groups based on their molecular weights; of these 96 toxins, 68 are smaller than 500 Da (*small molecules*), another 10 toxins are between 500 and 12,000 Da (*middle molecules*), and the remaining exceed 12,000 Da (*large molecules*). More than 25% of these toxins are protein-bound (46). This definition was later revised to classify uremic molecules into two categories: protein-bound solutes and middle molecules. For the latter group, the Work Group proposed that middle molecules comprise a group of proteins with a molecular weight (500 to 60,000 Da), which incorporates many toxins identified since the original middle molecule hypothesis, for which the upper molecular weight limit was approximately 2,000 Da. The low molecular weight peptides and proteins (LMWPs) comprise nearly the entire middle molecule category in the new scheme (55,56). Most of the toxins generated under the influence of increased oxidative stress fall in the category of middle molecules and are not amenable to removal by the routinely available dialysis techniques. In addition, the EUTox group demonstrated that kinetics of urea removal do not correlate with clearance of the middle and the large molecules, hence leading to the accumulation of these molecules that could potentially perpetuate the oxidative stress (46,57).

As middle molecules are modified by the ROS and reactive nitrogen species (RNS), such modifications affect their mass transfer (filterability), molecular weight, and net charge. These physiochemical changes impede their removal by the conventional dialysis methods (55–57). This concept is important to understand so that effective strategies for the removal of these factors can be developed in the future to prevent the progression in atherosclerosis and inflammation in dialysis patients.

ADVANCED NUCLEIC ACID PEROXIDATION PRODUCTS

The interaction of OH^- with nucleobases of DNA strand, such as guanine, leads to the formation of C8-hydroxyguainine or its nucleoside form named 8-hydroxy 28-deoxyguanosine (8-OH-dG). 8-OH-dG undergoes keto-reaction and results in the formation of oxidized product leading to the formation of 8-oxo-dG. Both 8-OH-dG and 8-oxo-dG are important biomarkers of free radical–induced oxidative DNA damage. Increased levels of these compounds have been demonstrated in HD as well as continuous ambulatory peritoneal dialysis (CAPD) patients (58,59). Electron spin resonance spectroscopy can be used to measure plasma oxidant activity. Roselaar et al. (60) used this technique to measure 8-OH-dG in CKD patients, and these levels did not change with dialysis therapy. Similarly, increased levels of 8-OH-dG levels in peripheral mononuclear cells have been demonstrated in dialysis patients compared to healthy controls (59).

CONSEQUENCES OF INCREASED OXIDATIVE STRESS

Increased markers of oxidant stress (especially in patients with diabetes mellitus) correlate with the severity of diabetic complications. In patients with kidney disease, oxidant stress-related processes are more diverse and intense, with an attendant alteration of a variety of cellular components irrespective of the level of blood glucose. These oxidized products play a prominent role in a variety of complications and may contribute a significant degree of morbidity and mortality in dialysis patients (**FIGURES 19.4** and **19.5**).

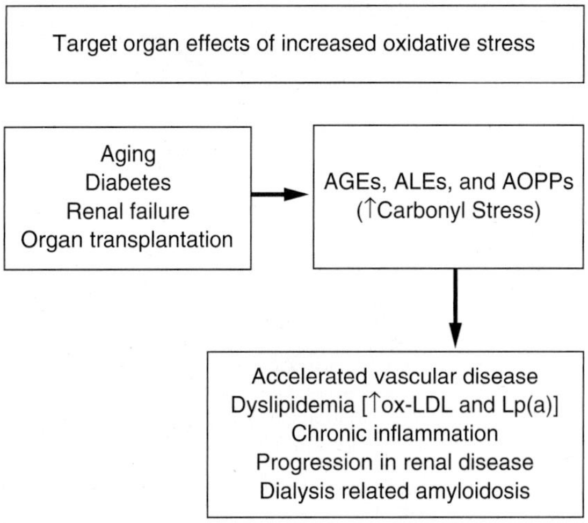

Role of Low-Density Lipoprotein Oxidation

Perhaps the most common modification is the oxidation of LDL, resulting in the formation of ox-LDL. As LDL becomes oxidized, the lipoprotein loses its ability to be recognized by the LDL receptor, and it becomes easily available to be phagocytosed by other scavenger cells such as macrophages. The macrophages become lipid loaded with decreased degradation and decreased mobility, and these changes result in the conversion of such macrophages into foam cells. The accumulation of foam cells in the intima of blood vessels is an initial step in the development of the fatty streak of the atherosclerotic lesion. Steinberg and others demonstrated the

FIGURE 19.5 Target organ effects of increased oxidative stress. AGEs, advanced glycation end products; ALEs, atomic layer epitaxies; AOPPs, advanced oxidized protein products; ox-LDL, oxidized low-density lipoprotein.

role of the early fatty streak (the precursor lesion) that subsequently leads to the development of an intermediate lesion and finally the complicated lesion of atherosclerotic plaques leading to the development of plaque rupture and acute cardiovascular event (61,62).

Increased levels of autoantibodies against the epitopes of ox-LDL and MDA-LDL have been demonstrated in the atherosclerotic plaques of coronary arteries and in the blood of dialysis patients with and without coronary artery disease. Several longitudinal studies in subjects with normal renal function have shown that the titers of circulating antibodies against ox-LDL are independent cardiovascular risk factors for progression in atherosclerosis (63). Maggi et al. (64) showed that LDL from patients with uremia and those dependent on dialysis is easily susceptible to *in vitro* oxidation.

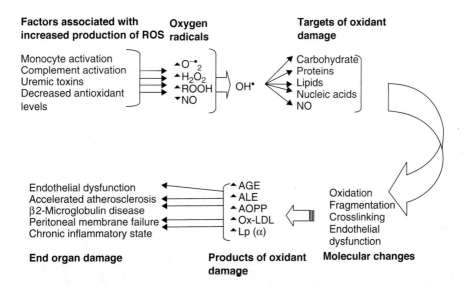

FIGURE 19.4 General pathway by which increased production of reactive oxygen species may contribute to the development of complications in patients with end-stage kidney disease. Intermediate oxygen radicals such as ($O^{-\bullet}_2$) superoxide, (H_2O_2) hydrogen peroxide, and lipid hydroperoxide (ROOH) lipid peroxides are precursors of toxic reactive species, such as (OH•) hydroxyl radicals. These radicals can cause chemical modifications of biologic molecules. These include advanced glycation end products (AGEs), advanced lipid oxidation products (ALEs), advanced oxidized protein products (AOPPs), oxidized low-density lipoprotein (ox-LDL), and increased lipoprotein (a) with decreased availability of nitric oxide.

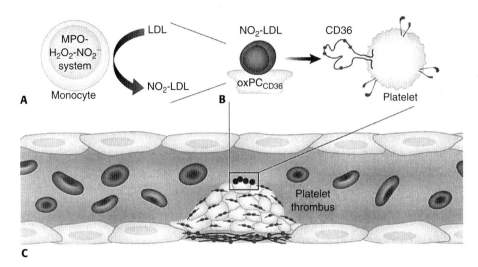

FIGURE 19.6 Role of oxidized products of low-density lipoprotein (LDL) in promoting platelet activation and thrombus formation in vivo. **A:** LDL cholesterol can be modified by monocytes through the myeloperoxidase (MPO)-H₂O₂-NO₂⁻ system to form ligands that have a high affinity for CD36 (oxPCCD36). **B,C:** oxPCCD36 interaction with platelet CD36 results in increased platelet activation **(B)** and enhanced thrombus formation **(C)** at sites of vascular injury *in vivo*. (Modified and reproduced with permission from Jackson SP, Calkin AC. The clot thickens—oxidized lipids and thrombosis. *Nat Med* 2007;13:1015–1016.)

Increased ratio of plasma antioxidized LDL antibodies to anti-native LDL was present in patients with advanced uremia and in patients on maintenance dialysis compared with healthy controls (**FIGURE 19.5**).

Ox-LDL is generated by a number of pathways, including the MPO–hydrogen peroxide–nitrite (MPO–H₂O₂–NO₂–) system (65). MPO is activated during each dialysis session due to the exposure of blood with extracorporeal circulation and other dialysis-related factors. This pathway is particularly relevant in dialysis patients (**FIGURE 19.6**). During the oxidation process of LDL, there is a concomitant generation of atherogenic oxidized choline glycerophospholipids (oxPCCD36) which reacts with its ligand called *CD36* and had been demonstrated *in vivo* at sites of increased oxidative stress (66). CD36 is expressed on macrophages and endothelial cells. It functions as a signaling molecule and stimulates macrophage foam cell formation by uptake of ox-LDL. Recent evidence has shown that CD36 is also expressed on platelets. Interaction of oxPCCD36 with platelet CD36 increases platelet reactivity and facilitates prothrombotic phenotype (66). Therefore, it establishes a strong link between oxidant stress, dyslipidemia, and prothrombotic events in the vascular system.

Role of Urea Oxidation

Carbamylation of amino acids and proteins can develop in dialysis patients due to spontaneous generation of cyanate from urea (67). The active form of cyanate (OCN⁻) is isocyanic acid that carbamylates amino acids, proteins, and other molecules. The carbamylation process changes their structure, charge, as well as function. In addition, carbamylated molecules can inhibit or potentiate other non-carbamylated proteins, producing various metabolic derangements including the production of reactive oxidant molecule, ε-N-C-lysine (homocitrulline) (67) (**FIGURE 19.7**). Using monoclonal antibodies, ε-N-C-lysine (homocitrulline) was demonstrated in neutrophils, monocytes, and more importantly, conjugated with low-density lipoprotein (called *carbamylated-LDL*); this transformation enhances the atherogenicity of LDL (68) (**FIGURE 19.8**).

Treatment with an antioxidant drug such as probucol without lipid-lowering potential has been reported to reduce the extent and the progression of atherosclerotic lesions in Watanabe heritable hyperlipidemic rabbits (WHHL) (69). On the basis of these data, it is reasonable to speculate that, in addition to the usual lipid abnormalities, enhanced *in vivo* LDL oxidation plays an important role in the process of accelerated atherosclerosis. Therefore, pharmacologic interventions that can decrease LDL oxidation should provide an important tool to ameliorate the accelerated progression in atherosclerosis in dialysis-dependent patients.

Recent introduction of vitamin E–bonded dialysis membranes may have the potential to reduce the overall oxidant stress, decrease lipid peroxidation, and LDL oxidation by providing site-specific high-dose vitamin E to prevent the release of ROS in the extracorporeal circulation (70).

◆ ROLE OF REACTIVE OXYGEN SPECIES IN THE PATHOGENESIS OF β₂-MICROGLOBULIN DISEASE

Progression in kidney disease and subsequently the need for dialysis is associated with accumulation of middle molecular weight proteins (11.8 kDa) called *β₂-microglobulin* (β₂-M) (levels in dialysis patients are usually 30-fold higher than normal healthy controls) (71,72).

Gejyo et al. (72) described increased serum levels of β₂-M in patients on maintenance HD that did not correlate with the joint or bone disease as seen in dialysis-related amyloidosis (DRA). This questioned the concept of simple deposition disease of dialysis amyloidosis. It is postulated that unknown amyloid-enhancing factors result in the qualitative or conformational changes in the β₂-molecule that plays an important role in the pathogenesis of amyloid disease. Subsequently, Miyata et al. (73,74) demonstrated that β₂-M produces tissue injury after it is modified by products of oxidant stress such as AGE, ALE, or AOPP.

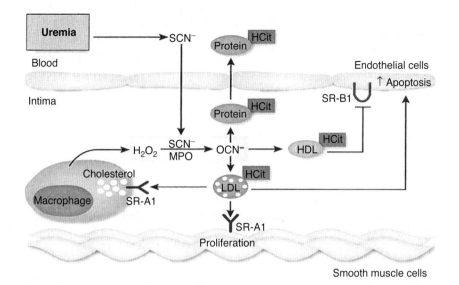

FIGURE 19.7 Role of myeloperoxidase (MPO) in the generation of cyanates in uremia. The chemical reaction catalyzed by MPO that generates cyanate (OCN⁻). The substrate for this reaction is thiocyanate (SCN⁻), which can accumulate in the body either from urea, cigarette smoking, or other dietary sources. Cyanate (OCN⁻) modifies lysine residues to form homocitrulline (HCit) on proteins and lipoproteins, in a process called *carbamylation*. The carbamylation of proatherogenic low-density lipoproteins (LDLs) promotes their binding by the scavenger receptor (SR)-A1, leading to increased macrophage LDL uptake and proliferation of smooth muscle cells, as well as increased endothelial cell apoptosis. The antiatherosclerotic high-density lipoproteins (HDLs) are also modified by this reaction, and HDL loses antiatherogenic potential. (Modified and reproduced with permission from Rader DJ, Ischiropoulos H. 'Multipurpose oxidase' in atherogenesis. *Nat Med* 2007;13:1146–1147.)

AGE-modified β₂-M stimulates monocyte-macrophage cells, releases cytokines TNF-α and IL-1β, and induces collagenase gene expression in rabbit synovial cells (73). In addition, β₂-M increases the expression of IL-8 and profibrogenic cytokine TGF-β (75) with increased recruitment of polymorphonuclear neutrophils (PMNs) (76) and increased expression of fibroblasts

in the synovial membranes of DRA-affected joints. These markers of neutrophil activation and tissue damage were absent in the presence of β₂-M deposition but without accompanying joint damage.

Further insights about the AGE and ALE modification of β₂-M were demonstrated by the use of anti-AGE monoclonal antibodies

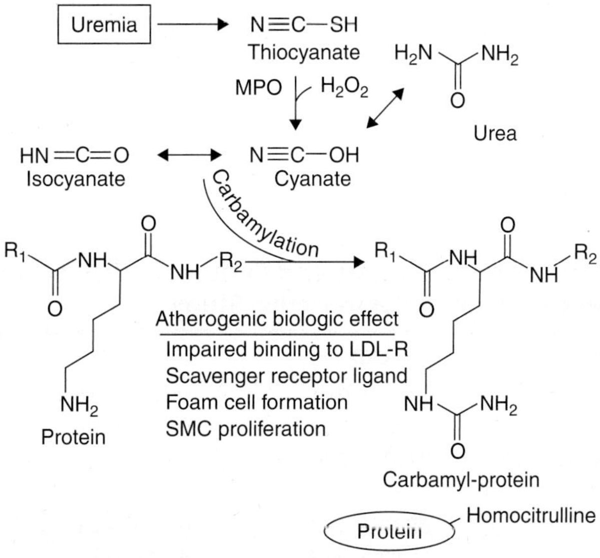

FIGURE 19.8 Schematic illustration of different pathways for protein carbamylation in uremia. Leukocyte myeloperoxidase (MPO) uses H₂O₂ and SCN⁻ as cosubstrates to generate OCN⁻ and promote protein carbamylation at sites of inflammation such as atherosclerotic plaque. Protein carbamylation is also increased in patients with chronic kidney disease as well as uremia as urea is a rich source of OCN⁻. (Modified and reproduced with permission from Wang Z, Nicholls SJ, Rodriguez ER, et al. Protein carbamylation links inflammation, smoking, uremia and atherogenesis. *Nat Med* 2007;13:1176–1184.)

for the epitopes of imidazoline and Nε-carboxymethyllysine adducts of β2-M in the synovial tissues of patients with dialysis-related arthropathy along with increased serum levels of both imidazolone and CML-modified β2-M (74).

These studies support the evidence that excessive generation of ROS in dialysis patients results in β2-M modification by AGEs, AOPPs, and ALEs; such a modification could be an important factor in the pathogenesis of tissue injury at the site of deposition of β2-M and subsequent development of DRA (73). The combined use of hemoperfusion and HD increases the rate of removal of β2-M and prevents the development of DRA (77).

REACTIVE OXYGEN SPECIES AND THEIR ROLE IN PERITONEAL MEMBRANE FAILURE IN PERITONEAL DIALYSIS PATIENTS

Progressive loss of ultrafiltration is the most common cause of PD failure. The morphologic changes associated with ultrafiltration failure include mesothelial denudation, interstitial fibrosis, and increase in extracellular matrix proteins; the end result is peritoneal membrane thickening (78). Electron microscopy reveals a characteristic replication of the basement membrane of the peritoneal capillaries and hyalinization of vascular media. These structural changes are well described in diabetic nephropathy (79). AGEs and pentosidine have been demonstrated in the peritoneal tissues and peritoneal blood vessel walls. Increased levels of AGEs and pentosidine have been correlated with the degree of peritoneal fibrosis and have been linked to the cumulative peritoneal glucose load (78,79). Whether the use of low glucose or nonglucose dialysate solutions will prevent the production of local AGEs remains to be studied and could provide new therapeutic strategies for the preservation of peritoneal function in long-term CAPD patients.

It is clear that CKD patients treated with different modes of dialysis invariably demonstrated increased levels of ROS and decreased levels of almost all the biologic antioxidants.

A recent comparative study demonstrated increased levels of different products of oxidation in three different groups (CKD, HD, and PD) of patients along with decreased levels of different antioxidants (TABLE 19.1) (80).

OXIDANT STRESS–RELATED INFLAMMATION, ACCELERATED ATHEROSCLEROSIS, AND CARDIOVASCULAR DISEASE

Patients with CKD as well as patients on long-term dialysis are characterized by a vasculopathic state as 50% patients with CKD or ESKD die of cardiovascular disease (see Chapter 17). This vasculopathic state is not completely explained by the presence of traditional risk factors known to be associated with the development of atherosclerosis (81,82).

Neutrophil–Macrophage Interactions Facilitate Inflammation and Atherosclerosis

Neutrophil extracellular traps (NETs) play a critical role to prime macrophages for inflammatory responses, these mechanisms of communication has been shown to play a critical role in the inflammation-atherosclerosis pathology (83). For example, recent study by Warnatsch et al. (84) demonstrated how NETs set the stage for inflammatory atherosclerosis. In this case, extracellular cholesterol crystals interact with neutrophils to trigger NET formation (NETosis), triggering burst of ROS, and neutrophil elastase translocation to the nucleus; an important determinant for NETosis. ROS plays a critical role in NETosis since inhibitors of reduced NADPH oxidase as well as inhibitors of neutrophil-specific proteases (NE) and proteinase 3 (PR3) were able to prevent NETosis. In-addition, NETs, which in turn primes the macrophages to produce a precursor of interleukin-1B (pro-IL-1B). Furthermore, cholesterol crystals bind to the cell surface protein CD36 on macrophages (66), which are internalized by endocytosis, activate the signaling complex called inflammasome. Activation of inflammasome results in activation of pro-IL-1b to IL-IB with its plethoric cytokine and paracrine effects on other tissue inflammatory processes (84) (**FIGURE 19.9**).

It has been demonstrated that AGEs can react with corresponding receptors called *receptors for advanced glycation end products* (RAGE) (85) and other scavenger receptors on macrophages, vascular endothelial cells, and smooth muscle cells. Such a receptor/ligand interaction leads to the activation of endothelial cells and release of VCAM-1 which further attracts monocytes to the vessel wall (86). AGE interaction with binding sites on monocytes and macrophages activates a host of intracellular signaling pathways.

TABLE 19.1	Effect of Hemodialysis and Peritoneal Dialysis on Redox Status: A Comparative Study		
Products of ROS	**CKD**	**HD**	**CAPD**
TBARS (μmol/L)	0.21 ± 0.01	0.23 ± 0.02	0.18 ± 0.01
Carbonyl (μmol/L)	0.3 ± 0.16	0.92 ± 0.15	1.90 ± 0.10
Nitric oxide (μmol/L)	22.53 ± 7.24	30.57 ± 8.7	20.52 ± 1.58
Anti-oxidant levels			
SOD (U/mL)	82.10 ± 1.53	70.08 ± 4.20	80.12 ± 0.38
GSH-Px (U/mL)	5.92 ± 0.53	4.12 ± 0.3	4.08 ± 0.06
Catalase (U/mL)	85.45 ± 4.74	80.18 ± 1.32	65.78 ± 3.45

ROS, reactive oxygen species; CKD, chronic kidney disease; HD, hemodialysis; CAPD, continuous ambulatory peritoneal dialysis; TBARS, thiobarbituric acid reactive substances; SOD, superoxide dismutase; GSH-Px, glutathione peroxidase.
Modified and reproduced from Mekki K, Taleb W, Bouzidi N, et al. Effect of hemodialysis and peritoneal dialysis on redox stats in chronic renal failure patients: a comparative study. *Lipids Health Dis* 2010;9:93.

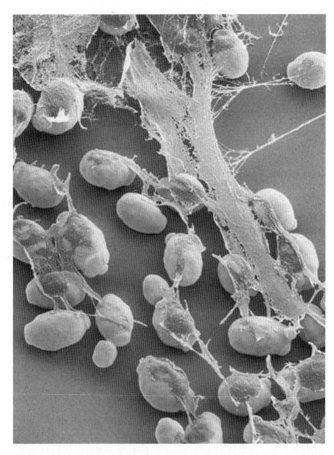

FIGURE 19.9 Deploying NETs. Colored scanning electron micrograph of neutrophil extracellular traps (NETs, brown) capturing spores from the yeast *Candida albicans* (*yellow*). [Modified and reproduced from Nahrendorf M, Swirski FK. Immunology. Neutrophil-macrophage communication in inflammation and atherosclerosis. *Science* 2015;349(6245):237–238.]

Activation of these signaling pathways results in the release of IL-1β, IL-6, TNF-α, and stimulation of NADPH oxidases with release of superoxide (O_2^-), thereby aggravates the already existent oxidative state (87).

IL-6 is one of the mediators of increased production of acute-phase proteins of acute inflammatory response. IL-6 acts directly on the hepatocytes and increases the synthesis of C-reactive protein (CRP), fibrinogen, and serum amyloid A (88). Whether AGE can act directly on the hepatocytes and increase the synthesis and/or release of CRP remains to be determined.

Increased levels of CRP and other acute-phase proteins in apparently healthy people (89) and in dialysis patients have been demonstrated to be the potential marker of predicting cardiovascular and overall mortality independent of other well-defined traditional risk factors for cardiovascular disease (3,90).

REACTIVE OXYGEN SPECIES AND ENDOTHELIAL DYSFUNCTION

CKD is associated with impaired endothelium-derived NO bioavailability and endothelial dysfunction in the absence of other associated conventional risk factors that can lead to endothelial dysfunction. Similar findings have been demonstrated even in children with CKD. The reduced NO bioavailability in kidney disease and

in dialysis patients is perhaps multifactorial such as decreased NO production (91), increased NO degradation, or both. Also, decreased NO production could be related to low levels of nitric oxide synthase (NOS) activity, as a result of decreased clearance of the endogenous NOS inhibitor such as asymmetric dimethylarginine (ADMA) in dialysis patients (92), or due to decreased bioavailability of the NOS substrate such as L-arginine, due to combination of factors such as poor intake, accompanying malnutrition, or increased losses through dialysis therapy. Another important mechanism that can deplete NO is the ability of AGEs to quench NO (92). The use of vitamin E–bonded dialyzers can reduce the level of oxidant stress and improve the endothelial function by preventing NO degradation (93).

Role of Asymmetric Dimethylarginine (ADMA) in Endothelial Nitric Oxide Synthase Uncoupling: Link between Oxidative Stress and Endothelial Dysfunction

Production of Asymmetric Dimethylarginine

ADMA is generated from posttranslational methylation of arginine residues present in a variety of specific proteins that are predominantly found in the cell nucleus (94). A number of cells elaborate ADMA, including human endothelial cells. ADMA is metabolized by the enzyme dimethylarginine dimethyl-aminohydrolase (DDAH) (95). DDAH metabolizes ADMA to L-citrulline and dimethylamine (96). ADMA and DDAH are widely distributed in tissues and may provide a mechanism for controlling NO synthesis in physiologic as well as in pathologic states. Increased ADMA levels can decrease NO synthesis by inhibiting endothelial nitric oxide synthase (eNOS) and also enhance oxidative stress by uncoupling eNOS enzyme and releasing nascent oxygen (97). However, it remains to be established whether ADMA concentrations *in vivo* in different disease states except in uremia are sufficient enough to effectively interact with eNOS activity (98).

Recently, it was demonstrated that increased levels of ADMA can further escalate the oxidative stress (97). Exposure of endothelial cells to ox-LDL and TNF-α resulted in the reduction of DDAH activity by more than 50% (99). Similarly, a high-cholesterol diet was associated with decreased DDAH activity without a change in protein expression and increased levels of ADMA. Decreased activity of DDAH may lead to local accumulation or release of intracellular ADMA and inhibition of NO synthase in disease states, including uremia. In addition, increased ADMA levels that can significantly inhibit NOS activity has been demonstrated in other disease states such as hypercholesterolemia, hypertension (HTN), hyperhomocysteinemia, tobacco exposure, and hyperglycemia (99–102) (**FIGURE 19.10**).

ADMA plasma levels (normally less than 1.060 mmol/L in healthy humans) are significantly increased in different disease states associated with increased burden of atherosclerosis, such as twofold increase in subjects with hypercholesterolemia (99), threefold increase in elderly patients with peripheral arterial occlusive disease and generalized atherosclerosis (99), and severalfold higher in dialysis patients (103). Increased levels of ADMA are independently associated with increased mortality in dialysis patients (103). Reduced clearance of ADMA in kidney disease is associated with endothelial vasodilator dysfunction, reversible by administration of L-arginine (104) or by high-flux dialysis therapy (105).

Can We Decrease the Levels of Plasma Asymmetric Dimethylarginine (Therapeutic Options)?

Plasma ADMA levels have been shown to be amenable to modification by different interventions based on the underlying etiology for such an increase in ADMA levels. Improvement of glycemic

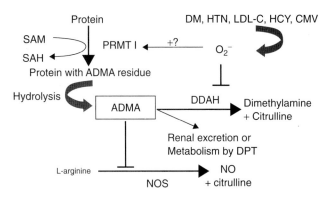

FIGURE 19.10 Biochemical pathways for generation, elimination, and degradation of asymmetric dimethylarginine (ADMA). ADMA derives from methylation of arginine residues in proteins. The reaction is catalyzed by protein arginine N-methyltransferases (PRMTs) that transfer a methyl group from S-adenosyl-L-methionine (SAM) to each guanidino nitrogen of an arginine residue. This reaction results in a methylated arginine derivative. Hydrolysis of the methylated proteins releases ADMA, a competitive inhibitor of endothelial nitric oxide synthase (NOS). All methylarginines are excreted into the urine and are in part metabolized to keto acids by dimethylarginine dimethyl-aminohydrolase (DDAH). The enzyme DDAH hydrolyzes ADMA to dimethylamine and L-citrulline. SAH, S-adenosyl homocysteine; NO, nitric oxide; DM, diabetes mellitus; HTN, hypertension; LDL-C, low-density lipoprotein cholesterol; HCY, hyperhomocysteinemia; CMV, cytomegalovirus. (Modified and reproduced with permission from Cooke JP. Asymmetrical dimethylarginine. The Über marker? *Circulation* 2004;109:1813–1818.)

control with the use of metformin resulted in decreased levels of ADMA (106). In patients with insulin resistance, rosiglitazone improved insulin resistance and lowered plasma ADMA levels (107). Use of angiotensin-converting enzyme inhibitor or angiotensin receptor antagonist in patients with HTN reduced plasma ADMA levels (108). L-Arginine is a precursor of NO and its supplements can improve the endothelial dysfunction (109). Other strategies to ameliorate the magnitude of oxidative stress could also indirectly decrease the levels of ADMA (108–111).

⬡ CAN DIALYSIS-ASSOCIATED INCREASED OXIDATIVE STRESS BE PREVENTED?

Therapeutic approaches to prevent or to decrease the oxidant stress are aimed at minimizing inflammatory cell activation, removing inflammatory cytokines or mediators, maintaining host antioxidant defenses, and using strategies to adsorb or to chelate the ROS.

Minimizing Inflammatory Cell Activation and Release of Reactive Oxygen Species

The use of biocompatible membranes (to some extent) prevents complement activation and neutrophil sequestration and activation (23), although it does not completely abrogate the production of ROS. Hence, ROS continue to have a significant effect on the generation and maintenance of oxidative stress and lipid peroxidation as measured by serum levels of MDA and ox-LDL (112).

Other investigators have demonstrated that use of ultrapure water and sterile dialysate (113) could possibly decrease the inflammatory responses. These steps (combined with use of biocompatible membranes, ultrapure water, and sterile dialysate) can decrease the production of ROS and minimize the inflammatory response.

Measures to Improve the Removal of Inflammatory Cytokines

Hemolipodialysis (HLD) improves oxidant stress by decreasing inflammatory cell activation, removing inflammatory mediators, and maintaining antioxidant levels (114). HLD uses liposomes with vitamin E added in the liposomal bilayer and vitamin C added directly in the dialysate. Liposomes have a high affinity for proteins, drugs, and cytokines. Use of liposomes can increase the removal of inflammatory mediators, whereas vitamin E in the liposomal bilayer and vitamin C in the dialysate will act synergistically to replenish the antioxidant levels ordinarily lost through diffusion during dialysis (115).

Treatment Strategies for the Removal of Products of Reactive Oxygen Species/Reactive Nitrogen Species and Other Inflammatory Biomarkers
Use of Evolving Dialysis Membranes

During the last 10 years with the introduction of high-performance dialysis membranes and improvements in the quality of dialysate and water purification methods, the rate of progression of chronic inflammation and vascular disease in dialysis-dependent patients has remained unchanged due to inability of conventional dialysis membranes to remove unconventional uremic toxins such as the products of glycation and oxidation (28,29). New dialysis membranes that provide different spectrum of diffusive-convective and adsorption properties have been developed with the aim of increasing the clearance of middle molecules including LMWPs (56). Among the high-flux membranes, modified polymethylmethacrylate (PMMA) with protein-leaking dialyzer (PLD) properties, thereby defined as ultrahigh-flux protein-leaking dialyzer (HF-PLD) compared to high-flux non–protein-leaking dialyzers (HF-NPLD), has the advantage of direct removal and adsorption of LMWPs. The use of HF-PLD is devoid of other adverse events such as hypoalbuminemia and backfiltration (115). In addition, dialysis membranes that have intrinsic adsorption properties such as PMMA and polyacrylonitrile (AN 69 membranes) increase the removal of large solutes, cytokines, and LMWPs including native and oxidized β_2-microglobulin (116,117).

By combining high-volume ultrafiltration with dialysis increases connective clearance that increases the clearance of large molecular weight solutes including LMWPs along with diffusion of small solutes; it accelerates the removal of products of oxidation. High-volume ultrafiltration with regular dialysis can be achieved by using the technique of on-line hemodiafiltration (OL-HDF) which offers the advantage of removing small to large molecular solutes. Use of this dialytic technique has been shown to reduce the burden of inflammation and endothelial dysfunction with improved patient survival (118–120).

Role of Vitamin E–Modified Hemodialysis Filters

Improved bioreactivity and biocompatibility of vitamin E–modified multilayer HD filters can reduce the production of ROS. Galli et al. (70) showed that vitamin E–modified HD filters (CL-E) as compared with cuprammonium rayon (CL-S) filters provide site-specific and time-dependent protection against ROS at the site of their generation by activated PMNs in the extracorporeal circulation. Such membranes have the potential to replenish antioxidant stores in plasma and RBCs, and inhibit the leukocyte respiratory burst and ROS production (119).

TABLE 19.2	Effect of Vitamin E–Modified Dialysis Membrane on Oxidized Low-Density Lipoprotein and Malondialdehyde Levels after 9 Months of Treatment	
	Oxidized LDL ng/µg LDL Protein	MDA nmol/mg LDL Protein
Normal range	0.257 ± 0.132	1.9 ± 0.5
Hemodialysis group	–	–
Month		
0	1.653 ± 0.76	4.329 ± 0.955
1	1.623 ± 0.966	4.091 ± 0.891
3	1.592 ± 1.064	3.997 ± 1.045
6	1.406 ± 0.568	3.656 ± 0.788
9	1.357 ± 0.852	3.459 ± 0.658[a]

Results are expressed as mean ± standard deviation (SD). Plasma oxidized-LDL and MDA levels were significantly higher in hemodialysis (HD) patients compared to controls. These values slowly decreased and were significantly lower after 9 months of treatment using vitamin E–modified dialyzer. LDL, low-density lipoprotein; MDA, malondialdehyde.
[a]$p < 0.05$ versus 0 month (before using the vitamin E–modified dialyzer).
Modified from Shimazu T, Ominato M, Toyama K, et al. Effects of a vitamin E-modified dialysis membrane on neutrophil superoxide anion radical production. Kidney Int 2001;59(Suppl 78):S137–S143, with permission.

Vitamin E–coated membrane filters have been shown to prevent dialysis-induced endothelial dysfunction by maintaining the bioreactivity of endothelium-derived NO and also decreasing the levels of ox-LDL as compared with dialysis treatment with cellulose or other synthetic membranes (93). HD using vitamin E–modified membranes increases plasma and erythrocyte vitamin E content, increases plasma levels of reduced glutathione, improves leukocyte function, and decreases mononuclear cell apoptosis and complement activation (121) (TABLE 19.2).

Taken together, these recent studies show that vitamin E–modified dialysis membranes can reduce the release of ROS and could reduce the oxidant stress. Prospective randomized studies to compare the patient outcomes with new techniques of dialysis such as HLD, high-flux polysulfones, and vitamin E–modified filters are clearly needed.

Restoring the Host Antioxidant Defenses

Role of Vitamin E and Vitamin Supplements

Several observational and epidemiologic studies in the general population have demonstrated conflicting evidence about the efficacy of various antioxidants such as vitamins A, E, and C and beta-carotene in reducing the incidence of secondary cardiovascular outcomes or death from any cause (122,123).

Vitamin E (α-tocopherol): Vitamin E (α-tocopherol) has biochemical properties to suppress generation of ROS from monocyte-macrophage cells, along with inhibition of monocyte adhesion to endothelial cells, thereby preventing endothelial damage. Vitamin E also stabilizes the atherosclerotic plaques (124).

Secondary Prevention with Anti-Oxidants of Cardiovascular Disease in ESRD (SPACE) study: Boaz et al. (125) used vitamin E 800 IU (as naturally occurring α-tocopherol) and demonstrated significantly lower primary and secondary cardiovascular events in the treatment group as compared with the placebo group, nearly 54% reduction in cardiovascular disease events in patients who are treated with vitamin E compared to placebo. However, Heart Outcomes Prevention Evaluation (HOPE) study that enrolled nearly 993 patients with mild to moderate CKD and were treated with natural source vitamin E (400 IU/d) versus placebo, did not show any benefit with vitamin E therapy (126). There were so many

differences in study designs between HOPE and SPACE study, such as HOPE enrollees received a very low dose of vitamin E, patient with mild to moderate CKD have low event rates for CVD compared to those with ESKD on dialysis as were the participants in SPACE study. Also, more than 40% of SPACE subjects used vitamin C in combination with vitamin E.

Other studies with vitamin E in other population subgroups have also yielded negative results, such as Selenium and Vitamin E Cancer Prevention Trial (SELECT) which demonstrated that use of vitamin E significantly increased the risk of prostate cancer among healthy subjects (127). A meta-analysis of several studies demonstrated that use of high-dose vitamin E (>400 IU/d) in patients with chronic disease was associated with increased risk of all-cause mortality (128).

N-Acetylcysteine: N-Acetylcysteine (NAC) is a thiol-containing antioxidant and is a potent free radical scavenger, and hence, it is considered a potent antioxidant. Tepel et al. (129) used acetylcysteine (oral dose of 600 mg twice a day) versus placebo (n = 134), and dialysis patients and demonstrated a 30% reduction in the primary end point [composite of acute myocardial infarction (AMI), cardiovascular (CV) death, percutaneous coronary intervention (PCI), coronary artery bypass grafting (CABG), cerebrovascular accident (CVA), or pulmonary vascular accident (PVD)] with the use of NAC compared to placebo. Another small study demonstrated 36% reduction in CVD events using NAC versus placebo. In the absence of power-based randomized controlled trial (RCT), it is premature to assume the efficacy of either vitamin E or acetylcysteine for prevention of atherosclerotic cardiovascular disease (ASCVD) events in patients with CKD. Hsu et al. (130) demonstrated that treatment with NAC in HD patient resulted in improvement of anemia and decreased plasma levels of 8-isoprostane and oxidized LDL. Similarly, NAC use was associated with decreased levels of 8-isoprostane and IL-6 levels in patients on PD (131). Other studies have demonstrated that NAC use is associated with decrease in homocysteine levels and improvement in endothelial function (132). Treatment with NAC in patients with nondiabetic CKD was really disappointing (133).

Treatment of hyperhomocysteinemia (Hcy) and its role in oxidative stress: Hcy is a risk factor for vascular disease, and one of the pathways is perhaps by increasing the oxidative stress (134). Increased levels of ADMA are often noted in patients with H-Hcy. Hcy is an important risk factor for atherosclerotic disease progression. However, strategies to decrease homocysteine level did not translate in decreasing the events related to vascular disease either in the general population (135) or in patients with CKD (136). Despite a marked decrease in the homocysteine levels, there was no difference in the mortality or cardiovascular outcomes among the three treatment groups. Another RCT (the Homocysteinemia in Kidney and End Stage Renal disease study) enrolled 2,056 patients with CKD, and 751 of these were on maintenance HD. The patients were assigned to receive a combination of high-dose folic acid (40 mg daily), pyridoxine (100 mg daily), and cyanocobalamin (2 mg daily) or placebo. It was not associated with any benefit (137).

Treatment with bardoxolone methyl: Use of bardoxolone methyl in mitigating increased oxidant stress in CKD population. Recently, a transcription factor named Nrf2 was found to be a positive regulator of human antioxidant response element (ARE) that drives expression of antioxidant enzymes such as NAD (P)H and quinone oxidoreductase 1 (NQO1) (138). A suppressor protein called Keap1 that is present in cytoplasm physically binds Nrf2, and preventing its translocation to the nucleus, and its access to ARE-containing promoters, such as those involved in glutathione synthesis and genes involved in limiting the inflammatory processes. Thus, Nrf2 activation modulates the expression of several different antioxidant gene products that protects the cells from the oxidative damage. Among one of the Nrf2 activators, bardoxolone methyl (methyl2-cyano-3,12-dioxooleana-1,9 dien-28-oate) interacts with cysteine residues on Keap1, allowing Nrf2 translocation to the nucleus, that results in upregulation of a multitude of cytoprotective genes. Additionally, bardoxolone methyl also produces anti-inflammatory effects by reducing the proinflammatory NF-KB pathway (139). A recent study demonstrated that use of bardoxolone methyl in patients with CKD had significant and sustained improvements in estimated GFR in a 52-week study (140).

Role of statins: Statins in general are considered to be antilipidemic agents to lower cholesterol and LDL levels. However, statins also have anti-inflammatory and antioxidant properties (141) and remain the cornerstone of treatment for primary as well as secondary prevention of acute coronary events as well as stroke in the general population. Three different RCT evaluated the efficacy of statins in dialysis patients and reported different results. Wanner et al. (142) reported (4D study: statin vs. placebo; $n = 1,255$) that despite an effective reduction in the LDL cholesterol as well as CRP, treatment with statin in dialysis patients had no effect on the primary outcome. An Assessment of Survival and Cardiovascular Events (AURORA), using rosuvastatin, again demonstrated effective reduction in the LDL cholesterol and CRP but without an impact on the primary outcome compared to the placebo group (143). Study of Heart and Renal Protection (SHARP) was an international RCT that enrolled 9,438 patients with CKD, and 3,191 were on maintenance dialysis therapy. There was a significant 17% reduction in primary outcome when all study patients were included. When primary outcome was analyzed based on patient population such as CKD versus dialysis patients, statin use resulted in 22% reduction in the primary end point in patients with CKD and only by a nonsignificant 5% reduction in primary outcome in HD-dependent patients (144). In summary, these three RCTs with different statins only resulted in less than 5% reduction

in mortality from cardiovascular disease–related events in HD patients. This rate was consistent across the spectrum of RCT (4D, AURORA, and SHARP).

Treatment with folic acid and vitamin B$_{12}$: Use of folic acid alone or in combination with vitamin B$_{12}$ is associated with reduction in homocysteine levels in ESKD patients. Although use of different doses of folic acid and vitamin B$_{12}$ supplements can lower Hcy levels, such reduction in Hcy levels have not produced positive impact on cardiovascular disease outcomes (135). However, recent meta-analysis reported that use of folic acid and vitamin B$_{12}$ may be beneficial to reduce the cardiovascular disease events in dialysis population (Heinz, 2009 #180, 137). Use of these supplements besides lowering the Hcy levels, folic acid, and vitamin B$_{12}$ use is also associated with reduction in the circulating precursors of oxidative injury such as reduction in the levels of micronuclei in peripheral blood lymphocytes (PBL); (micronuclei are chromatin rich products surrounded by a membrane that develop due to DNA damage and are formed during cell mitosis). Micronuclei are very sensitive indicators of exogenous as well as endogenous DNA damage if detected in PBL (146).

Omega-3 polyunsaturated fatty acids: These compounds are known to have anti-inflammatory and antioxidant properties. Long-chain omega-3 polyunsaturated fatty acids enhance endogenous antioxidant substrates such as gamma-glutamyl-cysteinyl ligase and GR (147). Experimental study in obstructive renal injury model in rats showed decreased rate of progression along with reduction in the molecular signatures of oxidative stress with the use of long chain omega-3 polyunsaturated fatty acids containing eicosapentaenoic acid and docosahexaenoic acid supplements (148).

Use of Angiotensin-Converting Enzyme Inhibitors

The use of angiotensin-converting enzyme inhibitors is associated with decreased incidence of cardiovascular events in high-risk populations, and this effect is remarkable even without significant changes in blood pressure as was demonstrated in the HOPE study. De Cavanagh et al. (149) demonstrated that treatment of dialysis patients with enalapril at 10 mg/d for 6 months resulted in higher levels of antioxidants and reduced levels of ROS. Therefore, enalapril treatment may have the potential of enhancing the endogenous antioxidant defenses and, hence, protect the cells from the oxidant-related injury.

Value and Efficacy of Chelators of Reactive Oxygen Species

Use of BetaSorb in Dialysis

BetaSorb HD is an accessory device for HD, placed upstream from the dialyzer in the HD circuit. Its intended use is to improve the removal of middle molecular weight uremic toxins like β_2-M, ROS, and proinflammatory cytokines such as complement factors, TNF-α, IL-1, and IL-8 (150,151). Hence, BetaSorb polymers remove size-selective toxins by adsorption. The BetaSorb device has been approved for human clinical testing by the U.S. Food and Drug Administration (FDA), and clinical trials are underway to assess the efficacy of BetaSorb devices to remove β_2-M in HD patients using the combination of high-flux dialyzer and BetaSorb as compared with the use of high-flux membrane dialyzers (Clinical trials.Gov: NCT00561093, NCT02461953).

◆ CAN OXIDATIVE STRESS BE USEFUL?

Cerebral arteries constantly regulate their tone to maintain constant blood flow to the brain regardless of variations in mean arterial pressure. ROS produce different effects on the vasomotor tone in the different arteries such as peripheral vessels compared to cerebral vessels. In the cerebral blood vessels, calcium permeable transient receptor potential ankyrin 1 (TRPA1) channels are linked to the NADPH (reduced NADPH) oxidase 2 (NOX2), a major source of ROS and is predominantly present in the cerebral vessels and has not been demonstrated in other vascular beds. Recent evidence demonstrates that ROS play an important role to maintain blood flow in the cerebral vessels. ROS produced in the endothelial cells oxidize lipids (lipid peroxidation), which triggers influx of calcium by stimulating the ion channel TRPA1. This calcium influx in turn activates calcium-dependent potassium-permeable channel, resulting in the dilatation of cerebral arteries, thus facilitating blood flow (152). However, more work needs to be done to establish the paradoxical effects of ROS in the cerebral vessels in different disease states.

SUMMARY

Patients with CKD receiving different types of dialysis are at risk for increased oxidative stress as measured by the biomarkers of oxidant stress such as ROS, AGEs, ALEs, AOPP, and ox-LDL. Increased oxidative stress may contribute directly or indirectly in the pathogenesis of accelerated atherosclerosis, the chronic inflammatory state, and the development of DRA. In light of these findings, clinical trials are needed to assess the efficacy and safety of different interventions that can abrogate the production of ROS and/or restore the function of antioxidants in the early stages of development of kidney disease and after the initiation of dialysis therapy. Similarly, dialysis modalities using high-flux polysulfones in combination with other evolving modalities of dialysis, such as the use of BetaSorb cartridges or vitamin E–modified HD filters, can be used to reduce the burden of oxidative stress and, hopefully, prevent the associated complications in patient with CKD.

REFERENCES

1. Halliwell B, Gutteridge JM, Cross CE. Free radicals, antioxidants, and human disease: where are we now? *J Lab Clin Med* 1992;119(6): 598–620.
2. Figueira TR, Barros MH, Camargo AA, et al. Mitochondria as a source of reactive oxygen and nitrogen species: from molecular mechanisms to human health. *Antioxid Redox Signal* 2013;18(16):2029–2074.
3. Nahrendorf M, Swirski FK. Immunology. Neutrophil-macrophage communication in inflammation and atherosclerosis. *Science* 2015;349 (6245):237–238.
4. Malech HL, Gallin JI. Current concepts: immunology. Neutrophils in human diseases. *N Engl J Med* 1987;317(11):687–694.
5. Weiss SJ. Tissue destruction by neutrophils. *N Engl J Med* 1989;320 (6):365–376.
6. Weiss SJ, Lampert MB, Test ST. Long-lived oxidants generated by human neutrophils: characterization and bioactivity. *Science* 1983;222(4624):625–628.
7. Nemoto S, Takeda K, Yu ZX, et al. Role for mitochondrial oxidants as regulators of cellular metabolism. *Mol Cell Biol* 2000;20(19):7311–7318.
8. Britigan BE, Cohen MS, Rosen GM. Hydroxyl radical formation in neutrophils. *N Engl J Med* 1988;318(13):858–859.
9. Radi R, Beckman JS, Bush KM, et al. Peroxynitrite-induced membrane lipid peroxidation: the cytotoxic potential of superoxide and nitric oxide. *Arch Biochem Biophys* 1991;288(2):481–487.
10. Nathan C. Nitric oxide as a secretory product of mammalian cells. *FASEB J* 1992;6(12):3051–3064.
11. Dean RT, Fu S, Stocker R, et al. Biochemistry and pathology of radical-mediated protein oxidation. *Biochem J* 1997;324(Pt 1):1–18.
12. Peuchant E, Carbonneau MA, Dubourg L, et al. Lipoperoxidation in plasma and red blood cells of patients undergoing haemodialysis: vitamins A, E, and iron status. *Free Radic Biol Med* 1994;16(3):339–346.
13. Imlay JA, Chin SM, Linn S. Toxic DNA damage by hydrogen peroxide through the Fenton reaction in vivo and in vitro. *Science* 1988;240(4852):640–642.
14. Leung JH, Schurig-Briccio LA, Yamaguchi M, et al. Structural biology. Division of labor in transhydrogenase by alternating proton translocation and hydride transfer. *Science* 2015;347(6218):178–181.
15. Arkblad EL, Tuck S, Pestov NB, et al. A *Caenorhabditis elegans* mutant lacking functional nicotinamide nucleotide transhydrogenase displays increased sensitivity to oxidative stress. *Free Radic Biol Med* 2005;38(11):1518–1525.
16. Himmelfarb J, Stenvinkel P, Ikizler TA, et al. The elephant in uremia: oxidant stress as a unifying concept of cardiovascular disease in uremia. *Kidney Int* 2002;62(5):1524–1538.
17. Fang X, Weintraub NL, Rios CD, et al. Overexpression of human superoxide dismutase inhibits oxidation of low-density lipoprotein by endothelial cells. *Circ Res* 1998;82(12):1289–1297.
18. Ingold KU, Webb AC, Witter D, et al. Vitamin E remains the major lipid-soluble, chain-breaking antioxidant in human plasma even in individuals suffering severe vitamin E deficiency. *Arch Biochem Biophys* 1987;259(1):224–225.
19. Frei B, England L, Ames BN. Ascorbate is an outstanding antioxidant in human blood plasma. *Proc Natl Acad Sci U S A* 1989;86(16):6377–6381.
20. Levine M, Daruwala RC, Park JB, et al. Does vitamin C have a pro-oxidant effect? *Nature* 1998;395(6699):231.
21. Halliwell B, Gutteridge JM. The antioxidants of human extracellular fluids. *Arch Biochem Biophys* 1990;280(1):1–8.
22. Henson PM, Johnston RB Jr. Tissue injury in inflammation. Oxidants, proteinases, and cationic proteins. *J Clin Invest* 1987;79(3):669–674.
23. Himmelfarb J, Ault KA, Holbrook D, et al. Intradialytic granulocyte reactive oxygen species production: a prospective, crossover trial. *J Am Soc Nephrol* 1993;4(2):178–186.
24. Griendling KK, Sorescu D, Ushio-Fukai M. NAD(P)H oxidase: role in cardiovascular biology and disease. *Circ Res* 2000;86(5):494–501.
25. Himmelfarb J, Lazarus JM, Hakim R. Reactive oxygen species production by monocytes and polymorphonuclear leukocytes during dialysis. *Am J Kidney Dis* 1991;17(3):271–276.
26. Descamps-Latscha B, Goldfarb B, Nguyen AT, et al. Establishing the relationship between complement activation and stimulation of phagocyte oxidative metabolism in hemodialyzed patients: a randomized prospective study. *Nephron* 1991;59(2):279–285.
27. Tepel M, Echelmeyer M, Orie NN, et al. Increased intracellular reactive oxygen species in patients with end-stage renal failure: effect of hemodialysis. *Kidney Int* 2000;58(2):867–872.
28. Bordoni V, Piroddi M, Galli F, et al. Oxidant and carbonyl stress-related apoptosis in end-stage kidney disease: impact of membrane flux. *Blood Purif* 2006;24(1):149–156.
29. Piroddi M, Depunzio I, Calabrese V, et al. Oxidatively-modified and glycated proteins as candidate pro-inflammatory toxins in uremia and dialysis patients. *Amino Acids* 2007;32(4):573–592.
30. Simmons EM, Langone A, Sezer MT, et al. Effect of renal transplantation on biomarkers of inflammation and oxidative stress in end-stage renal disease patients. *Transplantation* 2005;79(8):914–919.
31. Musial K, Zwolińska D, Polak-Jonkisz D, et al. Serum VCAM-1, ICAM-1, and L-selectin levels in children and young adults with chronic renal failure. *Pediatr Nephrol* 2005;20(1):52–55.
32. Wautier JL, Schmidt AM. Protein glycation: a firm link to endothelial cell dysfunction. *Circ Res* 2004;95(3):233–238.
33. Ballow A, Gader AM, Huraib S, et al. Platelet surface receptor activation in patients with chronic renal failure on hemodialysis, peritoneal dialysis and those with successful kidney transplantation. *Platelets* 2005;16(1):19–24.
34. Hörl WH, Cohen JJ, Harrington JT, et al. Atherosclerosis and uremic retention solutes. *Kidney Int* 2004;66(4):1719–1731.
35. Ross EA, Koo LC, Moberly JB. Low whole blood and erythrocyte levels of glutathione in hemodialysis and peritoneal dialysis patients. *Am J Kidney Dis* 1997;30(4):489–494.

36. Mimić-Oka J, Simić T, Djukanović L, et al. Alteration in plasma antioxidant capacity in various degrees of chronic renal failure. *Clin Nephrol* 1999;51(4):233–241.

37. Ikizler TA, Flakoll PJ, Parker RA, et al. Amino acid and albumin losses during hemodialysis. *Kidney Int* 1994;46(3):830–837.

38. Lim VS, Bier DM, Flanigan MJ, et al. The effect of hemodialysis on protein metabolism. A leucine kinetic study. *J Clin Invest* 1993;91(6):2429–2436.

39. Stenvinkel P, Heimbürger O, Paultre F, et al. Strong association between malnutrition, inflammation, and atherosclerosis in chronic renal failure. *Kidney Int* 1999;55(5):1899–1911.

40. Brownlee M, Cerami A, Vlassara H. Advanced glycosylation end products in tissue and the biochemical basis of diabetic complications. *N Engl J Med* 1988;318(20):1315–1321.

41. Miyata T, Fu MX, Kurokawa K, et al. Autoxidation products of both carbohydrates and lipids are increased in uremic plasma: is there oxidative stress in uremia? *Kidney Int* 1998;54(4):1290–1295.

42. Vlassara H, Fuh H, Makita Z, et al. Exogenous advanced glycosylation end products induce complex vascular dysfunction in normal animals: a model for diabetic and aging complications. *Proc Natl Acad Sci U S A* 1992;89(24):12043–12047.

43. Sell DR, Monnier VM. End-stage renal disease and diabetes catalyze the formation of a pentose-derived crosslink from aging human collagen. *J Clin Invest* 1990;85(2):380–384.

44. Makita Z, Radoff S, Rayfield EJ, et al. Advanced glycosylation end products in patients with diabetic nephropathy. *N Engl J Med* 1991;325(12):836–842.

45. Miyata T, Ueda Y, Yoshida A, et al. Clearance of pentosidine, an advanced glycation end product, by different modalities of renal replacement therapy. *Kidney Int* 1997;51(3):880–887.

46. Yavuz A, Tetta C, Ersoy FF, et al. Uremic toxins: a new focus on an old subject. *Semin Dial* 2005;18(3):203–211.

47. Miyata T, Kurokawa K, van Ypersele de Strihou C. Relevance of oxidative and carbonyl stress to long-term uremic complications. *Kidney Int* 2000;58(Suppl 76):S120–S125.

48. Ramos R, Martínez-Castelao A. Lipoperoxidation and hemodialysis. *Metabolism* 2008;57(10):1369–1374.

49. Esterbauer H, Schaur RJ, Zollner H. Chemistry and biochemistry of 4-hydroxynonenal, malonaldehyde and related aldehydes. *Free Radic Biol Med* 1991;11(1):81–128.

50. Boaz M, Matas Z, Biro A, et al. Serum malondialdehyde and prevalent cardiovascular disease in hemodialysis. *Kidney Int* 1999;56(3):1078–1083.

51. Morrow JD, Awad JA, Boss HJ, et al. Non-cyclooxygenase-derived prostanoids (F2-isoprostanes) are formed in situ on phospholipids. *Proc Natl Acad Sci U S A* 1992;89(22):10721–10725.

52. Meagher EA, Barry OP, Lawson JA, et al. Effects of vitamin E on lipid peroxidation in healthy persons. *JAMA* 2001;285(9):1178–1182.

53. Witko-Sarsat V, Friedlander M, Nguyen Khoa T, et al. Advanced oxidation protein products as novel mediators of inflammation and monocyte activation in chronic renal failure. *J Immunol* 1998;161(5):2524–2532.

54. Descamps-Latscha B, Witko-Sarsat V. Importance of oxidatively modified proteins in chronic renal failure. *Kidney Int* 2001;59(Suppl 78):S108–S113.

55. Clark WR, Winchester JF. Middle molecules and small-molecular-weight proteins in ESRD: properties and strategies for their removal. *Adv Ren Replace Ther* 2003;10(4):270–278.

56. Winchester JF, Audia PF. Extracorporeal strategies for the removal of middle molecules. *Semin Dial* 2006;19(2):110–114.

57. Vanholder R, De Smet R, Glorieux G, et al. Review on uremic toxins: classification, concentration, and interindividual variability. *Kidney Int* 2003;63(5):1934–1943.

58. Tarng DC, Huang TP, Wei YH, et al. 8-Hydroxy-2′-deoxyguanosine of leukocyte DNA as a marker of oxidative stress in chronic hemodialysis patients. *Am J Kidney Dis* 2000;36(5):934–944.

59. Tarng DC, Wen Chen T, Huang TP, et al. Increased oxidative damage to peripheral blood leukocyte DNA in chronic peritoneal dialysis patients. *J Am Soc Nephrol* 2002;13(5):1321–1330.

60. Roselaar SE, Nazhat NB, Winyard PG, et al. Detection of oxidants in uremic plasma by electron spin resonance spectroscopy. *Kidney Int* 1995;48(1):199–206.

61. Steinberg D, Parthasarathy S, Carew TE, et al. Beyond cholesterol. Modifications of low-density lipoprotein that increase its atherogenicity. *N Engl J Med* 1989;320(14):915–924.

62. Witztum JL, Steinberg D. Role of oxidized low density lipoprotein in atherogenesis. *J Clin Invest* 1991;88(6):1785–1792.

63. Salonen JT, Yla-Herttuala S, Yamamoto R, et al. Autoantibody against oxidised LDL and progression of carotid atherosclerosis. *Lancet* 1992;339(8798):883–887.

64. Maggi E, Bellazzi R, Falaschi F, et al. Enhanced LDL oxidation in uremic patients: an additional mechanism for accelerated atherosclerosis? *Kidney Int* 1994;45(3):876–883.

65. Jackson SP, Calkin AC. The clot thickens—oxidized lipids and thrombosis. *Nat Med* 2007;13(9):1015–1016.

66. Podrez EA, Byzova TV, Febbraio M, et al. Platelet CD36 links hyperlipidemia, oxidant stress and a prothrombotic phenotype. *Nat Med* 2007;13(9):1086–1095.

67. Kraus LM, Kraus AP Jr. Carbamoylation of amino acids and proteins in uremia. *Kidney Int* 2001;59(Suppl 78):S102–S107.

68. Wang Z, Nicholls SJ, Rodriguez ER, et al. Protein carbamylation links inflammation, smoking, uremia and atherogenesis. *Nat Med* 2007;13(10):1176–1184.

69. Carew TE, Schwenke DC, Steinberg D. Antiatherogenic effect of probucol unrelated to its hypocholesterolemic effect: evidence that antioxidants in vivo can selectively inhibit low density lipoprotein degradation in macrophage-rich fatty streaks and slow the progression of atherosclerosis in the Watanabe heritable hyperlipidemic rabbit. *Proc Natl Acad Sci U S A* 1987;84(21):7725–7729.

70. Galli F, Rovidati S, Chiarantini L, et al. Bioreactivity and biocompatibility of a vitamin E-modified multi-layer hemodialysis filter. *Kidney Int* 1998;54(2):580–589.

71. Capeillere-Blandin C, Delaveau T, Descamps-Latscha B. Structural modifications of human beta 2 microglobulin treated with oxygen-derived radicals. *Biochem J* 1991;277(Pt 1):175–182.

72. Gejyo F, Yamada T, Odani S, et al. A new form of amyloid protein associated with chronic hemodialysis was identified as beta 2-microglobulin. *Biochem Biophys Res Commun* 1985;129(3):701–706.

73. Miyata T, Inagi R, Iida Y, et al. Involvement of beta 2-microglobulin modified with advanced glycation end products in the pathogenesis of hemodialysis-associated amyloidosis. Induction of human monocyte chemotaxis and macrophage secretion of tumor necrosis factor-alpha and interleukin-1. *J Clin Invest* 1994;93(2):521–528.

74. Miyata T, Oda O, Inagi R, et al. beta 2-Microglobulin modified with advanced glycation end products is a major component of hemodialysis-associated amyloidosis. *J Clin Invest* 1993;92(3):1243–1252.

75. Matsuo K, Ikizler TA, Hoover RL, et al. Transforming growth factor-beta is involved in the pathogenesis of dialysis-related amyloidosis. *Kidney Int* 2000;57(2):697–708.

76. Takayama F, Miyazaki T, Aoyama I, et al. Involvement of interleukin-8 in dialysis-related arthritis. *Kidney Int* 1998;53(4):1007–1013.

77. Schwalbe S, Holzhauer M, Schaeffer J, et al. Beta 2-microglobulin associated amyloidosis: a vanishing complication of long-term hemodialysis? *Kidney Int* 1997;52(4):1077–1083.

78. Honda K, Nitta K, Horita S, et al. Accumulation of advanced glycation end products in the peritoneal vasculature of continuous ambulatory peritoneal dialysis patients with low ultra-filtration. *Nephrol Dial Transplant* 1999;14(6):1541–1549.

79. Nakayama M, Kawaguchi Y, Yamada K, et al. Immunohistochemical detection of advanced glycosylation end-products in the peritoneum and its possible pathophysiological role in CAPD. *Kidney Int* 1997;51(1):182–186.

80. Mekki K, Taleb W, Bouzidi N, et al. Effect of hemodialysis and peritoneal dialysis on redox status in chronic renal failure patients: a comparative study. *Lipids Health Dis* 2010;9:93.

81. London GM, Drueke TB. Atherosclerosis and arteriosclerosis in chronic renal failure. *Kidney Int* 1997;51(6):1678–1695.

82. Luke RG. Chronic renal failure—a vasculopathic state. *N Engl J Med* 1998;339(12):841–843.

83. Brinkmann V, Reichard U, Goosmann C, et al. Neutrophil extracellular traps kill bacteria. *Science* 2004;303(5663):1532–1535.

84. Warnatsch A, Ioannou M, Wang Q, et al. Inflammation. Neutrophil extracellular traps license macrophages for cytokine production in atherosclerosis. *Science* 2015;349(6245):316–320.

85. Neeper M, Schmidt AM, Brett J, et al. Cloning and expression of a cell surface receptor for advanced glycosylation end products of proteins. *J Biol Chem* 1992;267(21):14998–15004.

86. Schmidt AM, Hori O, Chen JX, et al. Advanced glycation endproducts interacting with their endothelial receptor induce expression of vascular cell adhesion molecule-1 (VCAM-1) in cultured human endothelial cells and in mice. A potential mechanism for the accelerated vasculopathy of diabetes. *J Clin Invest* 1995;96(3):1395–1403.

87. Abo A, Pick E, Hall A, et al. Activation of the NADPH oxidase involves the small GTP-binding protein p21rac1. *Nature* 1991;353(6345):668–670.

88. Herbelin A, Ureña P, Nguyen AT, et al. Elevated circulating levels of interleukin-6 in patients with chronic renal failure. *Kidney Int* 1991;39(5):954–960.

89. Ridker PM, Cushman M, Stampfer MJ, et al. Inflammation, aspirin, and the risk of cardiovascular disease in apparently healthy men. *N Engl J Med* 1997;336(14):973–979.

90. Zimmermann J, Herrlinger S, Pruy A, et al. Inflammation enhances cardiovascular risk and mortality in hemodialysis patients. *Kidney Int* 1999;55(2):648–658.

91. Lau T, Owen W, Yu YM, et al. Arginine, citrulline, and nitric oxide metabolism in end-stage renal disease patients. *J Clin Invest* 2000;105(9):1217–1225.

92. Bucala R, Tracey KJ, Cerami A. Advanced glycosylation products quench nitric oxide and mediate defective endothelium-dependent vasodilatation in experimental diabetes. *J Clin Invest* 1991;87(2):432–438.

93. Miyazaki H, Matsuoka H, Itabe H, et al. Hemodialysis impairs endothelial function via oxidative stress: effects of vitamin E-coated dialyzer. *Circulation* 2000;101(9):1002–1006.

94. Tran CT, Leiper JM, Vallance P. The DDAH/ADMA/NOS pathway. *Atheroscler* 2003;4(Suppl 4):33–40.

95. Kimoto M, Whitley GS, Tsuji H, et al. Detection of NG, NG-dimethylarginine dimethylaminohydrolase in human tissues using a monoclonal antibody. *J Biochem* 1995;117(2):237–238.

96. Murray-Rust J, Leiper J, McAlister M, et al. Structural insights into the hydrolysis of cellular nitric oxide synthase inhibitors by dimethylarginine dimethylaminohydrolase. *Nat Struct Biol* 2001;8(8):679–683.

97. Sydow K, Münzel T. ADMA and oxidative stress. *Atheroscler* 2003;4(Suppl 4):41–51.

98. Förstermann U, Münzel T. Endothelial nitric oxide synthase in vascular disease: from marvel to menace. *Circulation* 2006;113(13):1708–1714.

99. Böger RH, Bode-Böger SM, Szuba A, et al. Asymmetric dimethylarginine (ADMA): a novel risk factor for endothelial dysfunction: its role in hypercholesterolemia. *Circulation* 1998;98(18):1842–1847.

100. Böger RH, Sydow K, Borlak J, et al. LDL cholesterol upregulates synthesis of asymmetrical dimethylarginine in human endothelial cells: involvement of S-adenosylmethionine-dependent methyltransferases. *Circ Res* 2000;87(2):99–105.

101. Fard A, Tuck CH, Donis JA, et al. Acute elevations of plasma asymmetric dimethylarginine and impaired endothelial function in response to a high-fat meal in patients with type 2 diabetes. *Arterioscler Thromb Vasc Biol* 2000;20(9):2039–2044.

102. Stühlinger MC, Tsao PS, Her JH, et al. Homocysteine impairs the nitric oxide synthase pathway: role of asymmetric dimethylarginine. *Circulation* 2001;104(21):2569–2575.

103. Zoccali C, Bode-Böger S, Mallamaci F, et al. Plasma concentration of asymmetrical dimethylarginine and mortality in patients with end-stage renal disease: a prospective study. *Lancet* 2001;358(9299):2113–2117.

104. Vallance P, Leone A, Calver A, et al. Endogenous dimethylarginine as an inhibitor of nitric oxide synthesis. *J Cardiovasc Pharmacol* 1992;20(Suppl 12):S60–S62.

105. Kielstein JT, Böger RH, Bode-Böger SM, et al. Asymmetric dimethylarginine plasma concentrations differ in patients with end-stage renal disease: relationship to treatment method and atherosclerotic disease. *J Am Soc Nephrol* 1999;10(3):594–600.

106. Asagami T, Abbasi F, Stuelinger M, et al. Metformin treatment lowers asymmetric dimethylarginine concentrations in patients with type 2 diabetes. *Metabolism* 2002;51(7):843–846.

107. Stühlinger MC, Abbasi F, Chu JW, et al. Relationship between insulin resistance and an endogenous nitric oxide synthase inhibitor. *JAMA* 2002;287(11):1420–1426.

108. Delles C, Schneider MP, John S, et al. Angiotensin converting enzyme inhibition and angiotensin II AT1-receptor blockade reduce the levels of asymmetrical N(G), N(G)-dimethylarginine in human essential hypertension. *Am J Hypertens* 2002;15(7 Pt 1):590–593.

109. Lerman A, Burnett JC Jr, Higano ST, et al. Long-term L-arginine supplementation improves small-vessel coronary endothelial function in humans. *Circulation* 1998;97(21):2123–2128.

110. Engler MM, Engler MB, Malloy MJ, et al. Antioxidant vitamins C and E improve endothelial function in children with hyperlipidemia: Endothelial Assessment of Risk from Lipids in Youth (EARLY) Trial. *Circulation* 2003;108(9):1059–1063.

111. Saran R, Novak JE, Desai A, et al. Impact of vitamin E on plasma asymmetric dimethylarginine (ADMA) in chronic kidney disease (CKD): a pilot study. *Nephrol Dial Transplant* 2003;18(11):2415–2420.

112. Panichi V, De Pietro S, Andreini B, et al. Cytokine production in haemodiafiltration: a multicentre study. *Nephrol Dial Transplant* 1998;13(7):1737–1744.

113. Baz M, Durand C, Ragon A, et al. Using ultrapure water in hemodialysis delays carpal tunnel syndrome. *Int J Artif Organs* 1991;14(11):681–685.

114. Wratten ML, Sereni L, Tetta C. Hemolipodialysis attenuates oxidative stress and removes hydrophobic toxins. *Artif Organs* 2000;24(9):685–690.

115. Ziouzenkova O, Asatryan L, Tetta C, et al. Oxidative stress during ex vivo hemodialysis of blood is decreased by a novel hemolipodialysis procedure utilizing antioxidants. *Free Radic Biol Med* 2002;33(2):248–258.

116. Macleod AM, Campbell M, Cody JD, et al. Cellulose, modified cellulose and synthetic membranes in the haemodialysis of patients with end-stage renal disease. *Cochrane Database Syst Rev* 2005;(3):CD003234.

117. Randoux C, Gillery P, Georges N, et al. Filtration of native and glycated beta2-microglobulin by charged and neutral dialysis membranes. *Kidney Int* 2001;60(4):1571–1577.

118. Carracedo J, Merino A, Nogueras S, et al. On-line hemodiafiltration reduces the proinflammatory CD14+CD16+ monocyte-derived dendritic cells: a prospective, crossover study. *J Am Soc Nephrol* 2006;17(8):2315–2321.

119. Mydlík M, Derzsiová K, Rácz O, et al. A modified dialyzer with vitamin E and antioxidant defense parameters. *Kidney Int* 2001;59(Suppl 78):S144–S147.

120. Ramirez R, Carracedo J, Merino A, et al. Microinflammation induces endothelial damage in hemodialysis patients: the role of convective transport. *Kidney Int* 2007;72(1):108–113.

121. Shimazu T, Ominato M, Toyama K, et al. Effects of a vitamin E-modified dialysis membrane on neutrophil superoxide anion radical production. *Kidney Int* 2001;(Suppl 78):S137–S143.

122. Davey PJ, Schulz M, Gliksman M, et al. Cost-effectiveness of vitamin E therapy in the treatment of patients with angiographically proven coronary narrowing (CHAOS trial). Cambridge Heart Antioxidant Study. *Am J Cardiol* 1998;82(4):414–417.

123. Virtamo J, Rapola JM, Ripatti S, et al. Effect of vitamin E and beta carotene on the incidence of primary nonfatal myocardial infarction and fatal coronary heart disease. *Arch Intern Med* 1998;158(6):668–675.

124. Diaz MN, Frei B, Vita JA, et al. Antioxidants and atherosclerotic heart disease. *N Engl J Med* 1997;337(6):408–416.

125. Boaz M, Smetana S, Weinstein T, et al. Secondary prevention with antioxidants of cardiovascular disease in endstage renal disease (SPACE): randomised placebo-controlled trial. *Lancet* 2000;356(9237): 1213–1218.

126. Mann JF, Lonn EM, Yi Q, et al. Effects of vitamin E on cardiovascular outcomes in people with mild-to-moderate renal insufficiency: results of the HOPE study. *Kidney Int* 2004;65(4):1375–1380.

127. Klein EA, Thompson IM Jr, Tangen CM, et al. Vitamin E and the risk of prostate cancer: the Selenium and Vitamin E Cancer Prevention Trial (SELECT). *JAMA* 2011;306(14):1549–1556.

128. Miller ER III, Pastor-Barriuso R, Dalal D, et al. Meta-analysis: high-dosage vitamin E supplementation may increase all-cause mortality. *Ann Intern Med* 2005;142(1):37–46.

129. Tepel M, van der Giet M, Statz M, et al. The antioxidant acetylcysteine reduces cardiovascular events in patients with end-stage renal failure: a randomized, controlled trial. *Circulation* 2003;107(7):992–995.

130. Hsu SP, Chiang CK, Yang SY, et al. N-acetylcysteine for the management of anemia and oxidative stress in hemodialysis patients. *Nephron Clin Pract* 2010;116(3):c207–c216.

131. Nascimento MM, Suliman ME, Silva M, et al. Effect of oral N-acetylcysteine treatment on plasma inflammatory and oxidative stress markers in peritoneal dialysis patients: a placebo-controlled study. *Perit Dial Int* 2010;30(3):336–342.

132. Scholze A, Rinder C, Beige J, et al. Acetylcysteine reduces plasma homocysteine concentration and improves pulse pressure and endothelial function in patients with end-stage renal failure. *Circulation* 2004;109(3):369–374.

133. Renke M, Tylicki L, Rutkowski P, et al. The effect of N-acetylcysteine on proteinuria and markers of tubular injury in non-diabetic patients with chronic kidney disease. A placebo-controlled, randomized, open, cross-over study. *Kidney Blood Press Res* 2008;31(6):404–410.

134. Rogers EJ, Chen S, Chan A. Folate deficiency and plasma homocysteine during increased oxidative stress. *N Engl J Med* 2007;357(4):421–422.

135. Lonn E, Yusuf S, Arnold MJ, et al. Homocysteine lowering with folic acid and B vitamins in vascular disease. *N Engl J Med* 2006;354(15):1567–1577.

136. Wrone EM, Hornberger JM, Zehnder JL, et al. Randomized trial of folic acid for prevention of cardiovascular events in end-stage renal disease. *J Am Soc Nephrol* 2004;15(2):420–426.

137. Jamison RL, Hartigan P, Kaufman JS, et al. Effect of homocysteine lowering on mortality and vascular disease in advanced chronic kidney disease and end-stage renal disease: a randomized controlled trial. *JAMA* 2007;298(10):1163–1170.

138. Venugopal R, Jaiswal AK. Nrf1 and Nrf2 positively and c-Fos and Fra1 negatively regulate the human antioxidant response element-mediated expression of NAD(P)H:quinone oxidoreductase1 gene. *Proc Natl Acad Sci U S A* 1996;93(25):14960–14965.

139. Sporn MB, Liby KT, Yore MM, et al. New synthetic triterpenoids: potent agents for prevention and treatment of tissue injury caused by inflammatory and oxidative stress. *J Nat Prod* 2011;74(3):537–545.

140. Pergola PE, Raskin P, Toto RD, et al. Bardoxolone methyl and kidney function in CKD with type 2 diabetes. *N Engl J Med* 2011;365(4): 327–336.

141. Jain MK, Ridker PM. Anti-inflammatory effects of statins: clinical evidence and basic mechanisms. *Nat Rev Drug Discov* 2005;4(12): 977–987.

142. Wanner C, Krane V, März W, et al. Atorvastatin in patients with type 2 diabetes mellitus undergoing hemodialysis. *N Engl J Med* 2005;353(3):238–248.

143. Fellström BC, Jardine AG, Schmieder RE, et al. Rosuvastatin and cardiovascular events in patients undergoing hemodialysis. *N Engl J Med* 2009;360(14):1395–1407.

144. Baigent C, Landray MJ, Reith C, et al. The effects of lowering LDL cholesterol with simvastatin plus ezetimibe in patients with chronic kidney disease (Study of Heart and Renal Protection): a randomised placebo-controlled trial. *Lancet* 2011;377(9784):2181–2192.

145. Heinz J, Kropf S, Luley C, et al. Homocysteine as a risk factor for cardiovascular disease in patients treated by dialysis: a meta-analysis. *Am J Kid Dis* 2009;54(3):478–489.

146. Wang X, Fenech M. A comparison of folic acid and 5-methyltetrahydrofolate for prevention of DNA damage and cell death in human lymphocytes in vitro. *Mutagenesis* 2003;18(1): 81–86.

147. Arab K, Rossary A, Flourié F, et al. Docosahexaenoic acid enhances the antioxidant response of human fibroblasts by upregulating gamma-glutamyl-cysteinyl ligase and glutathione reductase. *Br J Nutr* 2006;95(1):18–26.

148. Fassett RG, Gobe GC, Peake JM, et al. Omega-3 polyunsaturated fatty acids in the treatment of kidney disease. *Am J Kidney Dis* 2010;56(4):728–742.

149. de Cavanagh EM, Ferder L, Carrasquedo F, et al. Higher levels of antioxidant defenses in enalapril-treated versus non-enalapril-treated hemodialysis patients. *Am J Kidney Dis* 1999;34(3):445–455.

150. Dhondt A, Vanholder R, Van Biesen W, et al. The removal of uremic toxins. *Kidney Int Suppl* 2000;58(Suppl 76):S47–S59.

151. Tetta C, Biasioli S, Schiavon R, et al. An overview of haemodialysis and oxidant stress. *Blood Purif* 1999;17(2–3):118–126.

152. Sullivan MN, Gonzales AL, Pires PW, et al. Localized TRPA1 channel Ca2+ signals stimulated by reactive oxygen species promote cerebral artery dilation. *Sci Signal* 2015;8(358):ra2.

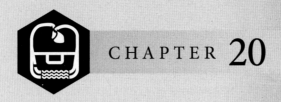

CHAPTER 20

Immune Dysfunction and Low-Grade Persistent Inflammation in Uremia

Gabriela Cobo, Juan Jesus Carrero, Bengt Lindholm, and Peter Stenvinkel

During the last two decades, the clinical phenomenon of low-grade persistent inflammation—its prevalence, root causes, implications, and possibilities for interventions—in patients with chronic kidney disease (CKD) has been a topic that has attained a great deal of attention in the nephrology community. It is now well established that systemic inflammation is a prominent, perhaps even inherent, feature of advanced CKD. Whereas inflammation is also common in other chronic diseases, such as advanced cardiovascular disease (CVD) that—like CKD—involve premature aging, accelerated vascular alterations, and muscle wasting (1), there are some unique aspects of inflammation in CKD which are mainly related to the decline of renal function that inevitably leads to retention of excess fluid and small- and medium-sized water-soluble molecules. Furthermore, a plethora of larger uremic toxins (including also proinflammatory cytokines that cannot be removed by the failing kidneys) accumulate in patients with advanced CKD and may aggravate immune dysfunction and other abnormalities in patients with CKD.

Inflammation (Latin, *inflammatio*, to set on fire) may be defined as a complex biologic response of vascular tissues to harmful stimuli, such as pathogens, damaged cells, or irritants. Although the inflammatory process should be regarded as a protective attempt by the organism to remove injurious stimuli and to initiate the healing process for the tissue, the problem faced in CKD, as well as in many other chronic debilitating disorders, is that it often leads to a state of persistent inflammation, which can last for months, or even indefinitely.

Chronic inflammation is characterized by the persistent effect of the causative stimulus, leading to destruction of cells and tissues, and provoking deleterious effects at different levels (2,3). Indeed, there is a convincing body of literature demonstrating the association between inflammation and disturbances in nutrition state, CVD and premature death in patients with CKD. The concurrence of all these disturbances has been denoted as the malnutrition-inflammation-atherosclerosis

(MIA) syndrome (4) or the malnutrition–inflammation complex syndrome (MICS) (5); however, the International Society of Renal Nutrition and Metabolism (ISRNM) recommended a few years ago that the malnutrition component in these syndromes should be termed *protein-energy wasting* (PEW) (6). Regardless of the nomenclature, inflammation is a major feature in the uremic milieu (7–12) (**FIGURE 20.1**). In a survey including 663 patients with CKD stage 5 (160 patients evaluated close to the start of dialysis and 503 patients on dialysis) from Sweden, Germany, and Italy, approximately two-thirds of the patients had C-reactive protein (CRP) levels above 3.4 mg/L (8). Similar findings are observed in patients with CKD stages 3 to 5 not yet on dialysis. According to data from the National Health and Nutrition Examination Survey III (NHANES III, $n = 15,594$), approximately 54% of the patients with glomerular filtration rate (GFR) between 15 and 60 mL/min had some degree of inflammation (CRP greater than 2.1 mg/L). In addition, the age-adjusted probability of having elevated CRP (greater than 2.1 mg/L) rose from 44% to 69% when estimated GFR was 60 and 30 mL/min, respectively (13). The close association between low-grade inflammation, comorbidities, and poor outcome highlights the importance of searching for strategies to ameliorate and avoid such conditions. This chapter describes CKD-associated immune dysregulation as it relates to clinical aspects of inflammation and susceptibility to infection, causes and consequences of inflammation in CKD, and finally, current and novel experimental strategies to avoid and treat the inflammatory burden in this patient group.

ALTERED IMMUNITY IN CHRONIC KIDNEY DISEASE

The immune system is a complex orchestration of cells, cytokines, and other molecules that act in a paracrine, autocrine, or endocrine manners to protect the human organism against disease. Uremia is

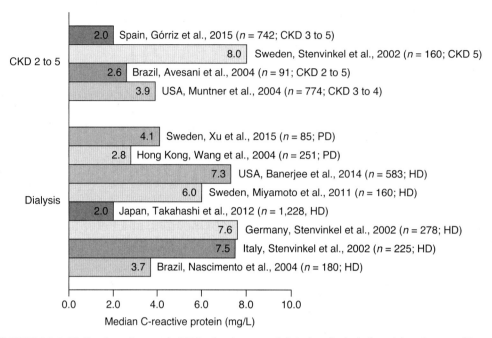

FIGURE 20.1 Median C-reactive protein (CRP) values in reported clinical studies including adult patients on different chronic kidney disease (CKD) stages. As the median CRP in the North American general population is approximately 1 mg/L, even patients with mild to moderate CKD show signs of enhanced inflammatory activity. HD, hemodialysis; PD, peritoneal dialysis.

known to be associated with a state of immune dysfunction characterized by both immune depression—that likely contributes to increased incidence and severity of microbial infections and impaired response to vaccination—and immune activation that results in a persistent inflammatory state that might contribute to PEW, atherosclerosis, CVD, and high mortality observed in this group of patients (14).

Within the complex immune system, the two major branches, innate and acquired immunity, are altered in uremic patients. The possible causes responsible for these disturbances in the uremic milieu are linked to the decline of GFR and the noxious effect of uremic toxins that accumulate due to kidney disease; however, numerous other factors such as comorbidities, other superimposed illnesses, genetic predisposition, and therapeutic interventions including the dialysis procedure, to name a few, play important roles in the pathophysiology of these immune disturbances.

With regard to the immune disorders observed in CKD, disturbances in the number and especially the function of basically all immune cells have been described. In general, the functional alterations observed include spontaneous activation, decreased phagocytic capacity, and increased apoptosis, leading to increased generation of cytokines and reactive oxygen species (ROS) and diminished defensive capacity (15). The different immune cells abnormalities observed in uremic patients are summarized in TABLE 20.1.

Among the mechanisms responsible for the compromised function of the immune cells, those concerning the pattern-recognition receptors, especially the Toll-like receptors (TLR), deserve a special mention. Pattern-recognition receptors play a role in innate immunity by recognizing pathogens through specific pathogen-associated molecular patterns (PAMPs) (16) and triggering effector cells

to perform their functions. In uremic patients, disorders in the pattern-recognition receptors system result in impaired function of cells engaged in innate immunity, leading among others, to decreased endocytosis and impaired maturation (17). In the uremic milieu, some of these receptors have been shown to be upregulated, while others are downregulated, leading to different consequences. For instance, upregulation of mannose-binding lecithin (a type of pattern-recognition receptor) is associated with worse patient and graft survival after simultaneous pancreas-kidney transplantation (18), while low levels associated with increased mortality in infected hemodialysis (HD) patients (19). Toll-like receptors belong also to the family of signaling pattern-recognition receptors that is involved in the maturation of dendritic cells, phagocytic functions, and activation of the complement pathway and production of numerous cytokines, such as interleukin 1β (IL-1β), interleukin 6 (IL-6), and TNF (20). Disorders in this group of receptors are responsible for impaired function of antigen-presenting cells (APCs), leading to more severe illness and increased mortality in case of invading pathogens diseases (14). Interestingly, a study by Kiechl et al. (21) reported that, although subjects with TLR4 polymorphism, which led to TLR4 downregulation, were found to be more susceptible to severe bacterial infections; they had a lower risk of carotid atherosclerosis and reduced intima-media thickness. These results suggest that impaired innate immunity might protect against atherosclerosis, thus resulting in lower cardiovascular mortality because of attenuated receptor signaling and diminished inflammatory response. If a similar situation is present in end-stage kidney disease (ESKD) patients, ESKD patients with impairment of immunity may have a survival advantage in the form of lower risk of CVD. But, again, this alteration may be linked to increased risk of infections and thereby inflammation.

TABLE 20.1	Alterations of Immunocompetent Cells in Chronic Kidney Disease		
		Normal Function	**Alterations in Chronic Kidney Disease**
Monocytes and macrophages		Host defense against microbial infection Tissue healing process Production of cytokines and ROS	General expansion of circulating monocytes (322) Spontaneous activation and decreased phagocyte capacity (323) Overproduction of IL-1β, IL-6, IL-12, and TNF (324)
Polymorphonuclear leukocytes (PMNL)		First line of defense against invading microbes	Spontaneous activation (103) Decreased phagocytic capacity and reduced bactericidal capabilities (325) Altered apoptosis (326)
Lymphocytes B		Production of antigen-specific antibodies	B-cell lymphopenia (327) Impaired differentiation and maturation (327) Increased apoptosis (328)
Lymphocytes T	Helper (CD4+)	Activation of cytotoxic T cells and macrophages Maturation of B-cells and antibody production from these cells Recruitment of PMNL, eosinophil, and basophils Amplification of inflammatory response	Decreased proliferation (329) Depletion of naive and central memory T cells (330) Increased apoptosis (331) Reduced ratio CD4/CD8 (330) Increased Th1/Th2 ratio (332)
	Cytotoxic (CD8+)	Destroy virally infected cells and tumor cells Participate in transplant rejection	
	Regulatory (previously known as secretory)	Central role in immunologic self-tolerance Limitation of the inflammatory response	
	Natural killer (NK)	Recognize and eliminate virally infected cells and tumor cells Can serve as helper agent by secreting cytokines	
Dendritic cells		Major antigen-presenting cells Initiation and maintenance of both innate and adaptive immunity Sensors of microbial invasion and tissue damage Regulate immune response in T, B cells, and NK	Depletion of cell (333) Decreased antigen presentation capabilities (17)

ROS, reactive oxygen species; IL-1β; interleukin 1β; IL-6, interleukin 6; IL-12, interleukin 12; TNF, tumor necrosis factor; CD4, cluster of differentiation 4; CD8, cluster of differentiation 8; Th1 and Th2, T helper cells.

Cytokine Dysregulation in Chronic Kidney Disease

As a consequence of the altered function of the immune cells, a state of hypercytokinemia is characteristic in the uremic milieu, where the delicate equilibrium between proinflammatory cytokines and their inhibitors is clearly dysregulated (22,23). Also, due to the fact that the kidneys are major sites for elimination of many of these cytokines, renal failure contributes notably to the hypercytokinemic state. Additionally, the dialysis procedure *per se* stimulates circulating nuclear cells, inducing cytokine production (24) and making them respond more vigorously after exposure to endotoxin (25).

To properly understand the state of cytokine dysregulation present in CKD patients, a number of considerations involving cytokine measurements should be made (26). First, most of the published studies focus on selected cytokines measured in plasma, culture supernatants, or in association with circulating cells. However, cytokines are "moving targets" counterbalanced by inhibitors or other cytokines with opposite effects. Second, cytokines rarely act alone because they stimulate a variety of cell types to produce and secrete other cytokines in a cascade fashion. Elevation of one cytokine immediately leads to up- or downregulation of several others. As many of the effects of cytokines are local, not systemic, these paracrine effects of cytokines are hard to detect. Third, pro- and anti-inflammatory cytokines bind to specific cytokine carriers (such as α_2-macroglobulin) and these different binding proteins may serve as extracellular cytokine reservoirs and protective shields against degradation. Therefore, it is important to take into account that established immunoassays to detect cytokines usually are not able to distinguish between active proteins and those proteins that are blocked by their specific inhibitors. To understand this complex orchestration, selected cytokines will be reviewed with regard to our current understanding of the uremic cytokine misbalance.

Interleukin 6

Different cells, including T-lymphocytes, macrophages, monocytes, endothelial cells, adipocytes, and fibroblasts, produce IL-6. IL-6 is involved in the production of neutrophils and proliferation of B-lymphocytes as well as in the stimulation of the liver to produce acute-phase proteins. IL-6 also regulates the production of adhesion molecules and induces the secretion of monocyte chemotactic protein, an important mediator for the release of other cytokines, such as TNF and IL-1β, which subsequently amplify the inflammatory response (27). Notably, IL-6 exhibits both pro- and anti-inflammatory effects and promotes inflammatory events through the activation and proliferation of lymphocytes as well as differentiation of B cells and leukocyte recruitment.

Numerous factors in the uremic *milieu* may stimulate the production of IL-6, and the kidney has been suggested to play an important role in the clearance of IL-6 (28–30). Indeed, Bolton et al. (31) found in a multiple regression analysis that serum creatinine was the sole determinant of plasma IL-6 levels in a group of predialysis and dialysis patients. Other causes responsible for the elevated IL-6 levels in CKD include comorbidities, persistent infections, such as *Chlamydia pneumoniae* (32), fluid overload, sympathetic overactivation, and oxidative stress, conditions that often appear as renal function declines (33).

Elevated concentration of circulating IL-6 is strongly associated with comorbidity and is a powerful predictor of CVD and all-cause mortality in dialysis patients (34,35). This prognostic value might be related to some independent proatherogenic properties showed by IL-6 in the early stages of atherosclerosis (36), in contrast to the putative antiatherogenic effects of CRP (37). Increased expression of IL-6 has been observed at the fibrous plaque stage of the atherosclerotic process (38), and elevated IL-6 levels have been linked to the progression of carotid atherosclerosis in patients with CKD stage 5 (32). The pathways by which IL-6 could contribute to the development of atherosclerosis include diverse metabolic, endothelial, and coagulant mechanisms (39).

Tumor Necrosis Factor

TNF is a pleiotropic inflammatory cytokine that has a pivotal role in regulating both pro- and anti-inflammatory mediators. TNF is an acute-phase protein that initiates the cytokine cascade and thereby increases vascular permeability. TNF is produced mainly by monocytes, macrophages, dendritic cells, and Th1 cells and is in charge of recruiting macrophages and neutrophils to the site of infection. This cytokine holds both growth-stimulating and growth inhibitory properties, and it appears to have self-regulatory properties as well. Deterioration of renal function may be one of the most important factors associated with a significant increase in TNF activity (28,40). TNF is highly multifunctional, affecting insulin resistance (41), coagulation cascade, lipid metabolism, and endothelial dysfunction (42). TNF is also associated with increased catabolism and may promote both atherosclerosis and PEW, and, consequently, higher levels of TNF associate with poor outcomes in patients with CKD (29).

Interleukin 10

Interleukin 10 (IL-10) is an essential anti-inflammatory cytokine produced mainly by immunoactive cells, such as monocytes and lymphocytes, and has been regarded as one of the most important anti-inflammatory immune-regulating cytokines. In fact, IL-10 not only downregulates proinflammatory cytokines, such as IL-1, IL-6, and TNF, but also reduces the production of chemotactic factors, such as IL-8 or CC chemokines, which may attract leukocytes to the location of inflammatory activity (43). Apart from the inhibition of proinflammatory cytokines, several other properties like antiatherogenic and antithrombotic effects have been related to IL-10 (26). IL-10 is capable of preventing the attachment of circulating immune cells to the endothelium (44) by inhibiting the secretion of chemotactic proteins from macrophages; signaling further recruitment of leukocytes to the subendothelial location of inflammation (43); and reducing the production of matrix metalloproteinases and superoxide anions (45). Additionally, it has been suggested that IL-10 prevent destabilization of the atherogenic plaque (46). As IL-10 is mainly cleared through the kidneys, its half-life is markedly increased and its plasma levels commonly elevated in CKD (47). Furthermore, uremic monocytes produce higher amounts of this cytokine compared to those of healthy individuals (48), probably as a consequence of chronic monocyte activation in patients with uremia. In patients with CKD, the most relevant production of IL-10 seems to occur in monocytes and macrophages, in response to endotoxins and activated complement fragments, agents known to mediate bioincompatibility reactions during renal replacement therapy (RRT). Therefore, dialysis treatment may contribute to the overall level of this long-acting cytokine. Despite the positive features assigned to IL-10, previous studies in CKD have failed to show an association between IL-10 and better outcomes. In fact, higher serum IL-10 levels have also been associated with increased risk of cardiovascular events during follow-up (49), results that can be explain as a consequence of the global proinflammatory uremic milieu that as a compensatory sequel also involves increased release of IL-10.

● ENHANCED SUSCEPTIBILITY TO BACTERIAL INFECTIONS IN UREMIA

As mentioned above, CKD is a condition associated with a state of immune dysfunction affecting both innate and acquired immunity and therefore leading to increased susceptibility to infections. Indeed, the incidence of bacterial infections is 50-fold higher in dialysis patients in comparison to the general population (32,50,51). Aside from being a consequence of altered immunity, the high infectious morbidity observed in CKD is multifactorial and the main factors involved are summarized in **TABLE 20.2**. The occurrence of bacterial infections in CKD is commonly related to the dialysis procedure and to the vascular access [especially central dialysis catheters (52)] that represents a continuous portal of entry for pathogens. Additionally, respiratory and urinary tract infections have a high prevalence in CKD patients. Likewise, comorbidity, especially diabetes and peripheral vascular pathology, have an important role in the incidence and prevalence of foot or leg ulcers infection commonly seen in this group of patient.

Among the septicemia episodes in CKD patients, around 40% to 70% of them are caused by gram-positive microorganisms (53–55), being *Staphylococcus aureus* the most commonly encountered gram-positive agent and mainly associated with vascular access infection (54). The high prevalence of *S. aureus* asymptomatic carriers in nose, throat, and skin, and the required repetitive punctures of the vascular access (55–57) represent important risk factors.

TABLE 20.2	Risk Factors and Main Pathogens for Bacterial Infections in Chronic Kidney Disease

Risk Factors
- Depressed immunity
- History of bacterial infection (at least one previous episode)
- Vascular access [central venous catheters, use of polytetrafluoroethylene (PTFE) prosthetic devices]
- Dialysis technique (bioincompatible membranes)
- Poor nutritional status
- Comorbidity (diabetes mellitus, peripheral vascular pathology)
- Iron overload (ferritin >500 μg/L)
- Immunosuppressive treatment

Main Pathogens

Gram-positive	Gram-negative
Staphylococcus aureus	Chlamydia pneumoniae
Staphylococcus epidermidis	Escherichia coli
	Pseudomonas

In peritoneal dialysis (PD) patients, formation of a bacterial biofilm on the walls of the peritoneal catheter is also a frequent cause of *S. aureus* peritonitis (58). Interestingly, aspirin treatment was recently associated with decreased rate of catheter-associated *S. aureus* bacteremia in HD patients (59). On the other hand, gram-negative bacteria infections are present in approximately 25% of the episodes of bacteremia of CKD patients, and are linked to vascular access infections (53) and gastrointestinal and genitourinary tract infections (57,60), where *Escherichia coli* is the most common gram-negative pathogen isolated (54,55). Moreover, there is a link between the intracellular gram-negative pathogen *C. pneumoniae* and atherosclerotic complications in dialysis patients (51). Although this causative link remains to be demonstrated, ongoing trials using macrolide therapy will allow assessment of whether eradication of this type of infection could result in reduced atherosclerotic morbidity (61).

Furthermore, among other infectious diseases observed in CKD patients, tuberculosis deserves to be mentioned. Due to their particular immune characteristics, patients with CKD are at increased risk of development and reactivation of latent tuberculosis and exhibit a much higher prevalence than the general population (62,63). The presentation of the disease is frequently atypical, with accelerated wasting being one possible consequence of *Mycobacterium tuberculosis* infection. Indeed, in ancient times, tuberculosis was referred to as "phthisis," which means "consumption." The diagnosis of tuberculosis infection is specially challenging in CKD due to its frequent extrapulmonary location (64,65) and the scarce sensitivity of tuberculin skin test in dialysis patients, who show anergy in more than 50% of the patients (66). In the last years, new techniques like blood tests determination using stimulation of gamma interferon have been developed with better results (67); however, sometimes, a biopsy of extrapulmonary tissue is required.

Moreover, hidden infectious process, like periodontitis (68) and bowel bacterial overgrowth (69), are prevalent conditions that are usually overlooked, although they are related to deleterious outcomes. In any case, independent of the type of infection, even asymptomatic infections contribute considerably to the persistent inflammatory state observed in CKD patients and result in increased risk of morbidity and mortality (70). Emphasis on the importance of good dialysis care and implementation of routines to avoid infection in this group of susceptible patients are of fundamental importance.

⬡ LOW-GRADE PERSISTENT INFLAMMATORY STATE

Systemic inflammation is a common feature in the uremic phenotype (7–12) and is linked to poor outcomes (71). While immune system dysfunction associated to CKD leads to a persistent inflammatory state (72,73) partially due to impaired renal elimination of proinflammatory cytokines and partially due to increased generation of cytokines (29), other factors related to dialysis technique and lifestyle are also important contributors. Moreover, it has recently become apparent that stress-induced premature senescence contributes significantly to the chronic inflammatory state of advanced CKD (74). If persistent, injurious triggers by oxidative stress, hyperphosphatemia, and uremic toxins will prevent DNA damage from being repaired, and cells will undergo senescence and secrete cytokines and growth factors (the so called senescence-associated secretory phenotype; SASP) (75).

Causes of Persistent Inflammatory State

General

A number of factors, both related and unrelated to CKD or dialysis technique, contribute to systemic inflammation in patients with uremia (FIGURE 20.2). A reduction of kidney function *per se* is associated with an increased inflammatory response due to the retention of circulating cytokines (26), advanced glycation end products (AGEs) (76), and pro-oxidants (33). Additional mechanisms include sympathetic overactivity (and/or blunted vagal nerve activity) and reduced production of specific cytokine inhibitors [suppressors of cytokine signaling (SOCS)]. As the cholinergic anti-inflammatory pathway is a neural mechanism that inhibits local cytokine release, blunted vagal activity may be a mechanism leading to increased inflammatory activity (77). Overhydration, a frequent complication in CKD, is also an indirect contributor to inflammation. Volume overload, via bacterial or endotoxin translocation in patients with severe gut edema, leads to immune activation and increased inflammatory cytokine production (78). Also, a strong relation between inflammation, residual renal function, and cardiac hypertrophy has been documented (79). Notwithstanding, other inflammatory diseases, such as systemic lupus erythematosus, rheumatoid arthritis and malignancies, are commonly observed in dialysis patients and can contribute to the inflammatory state, like intercurrent clinical events, that not surprisingly seem to be the most important predicting factor of elevation of CRP values in the context of uremia (80).

Causes Related to Dialysis Technique

In addition to the intrinsic inflammation accompanying CKD, patients undergoing RRT are subject to additional potential inflammation-activating factors. Factors associated with the dialysis technique itself include bioincompatible membranes and solutions, dialysate back flow, clotted access grafts, and catheter infections. Other factors, such as failed kidney transplants (81), endotoxemia (71,82), and fluid overload (83) may also influence the inflammatory process in this group of patients.

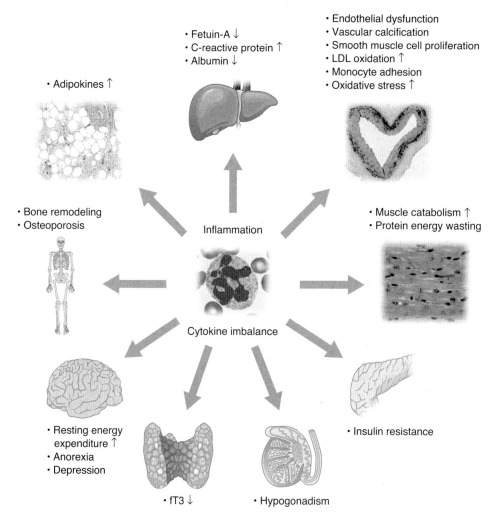

FIGURE 20.2 Putative organ effects of an altered proinflammatory cytokine balance in chronic kidney disease. fT3, free triiodothyronine; LDL, low-density lipoprotein; ↑, increase; ↓, decrease.

Additional Causes of Inflammation in Hemodialysis Patients

A number of factors related to HD procedure *per se* promote inflammation. While interestingly, dialysis-related inflammation seems to be associated with a specific genomic pattern (84); several *in vivo* studies imply that the membrane composition, the type and quality of dialysis, and the type of vascular access may contribute to inflammatory processes. In a randomized study, Schindler et al. (85) demonstrated that HD patients treated with polyamide membranes presented lower CRP levels compared to those exposed to cuprophane or polycarbonate membranes (see Chapter 1). In accordance, Memoli et al. (86) showed that a significant relation exists between membrane bioincompatibility and circulating levels of CRP, IL-6, and serum albumin. Likewise, it has been proposed that the amount of convective transport and the frequency of dialysis might influence in the level of inflammation (87). Short daily HD (six sessions per week of 3 hours each) was associated with a reduction in left ventricular hypertrophy and inflammatory mediators compared to conventional HD (three sessions per week of 4 hours each) (88) (see Chapters 8 and 10). Instead, in a multicenter, open-label, randomized controlled trial including 906 chronic HD patients and comparing the benefits

of conventional versus high-efficiency postdilution HD, a reduction in all-cause mortality was associated with the latter; however, no difference in predialysis CRP values was found between the groups (89).

As cytokine-inducing substances present in the dialysis fluid may penetrate intact dialyzer membranes, impure dialysate is yet another factor to bear in mind (90). Indeed, Schindler et al. (91) have shown that small bacterial DNA fragments in dialysis fluid can pass through dialyzer membranes. In accordance, Sitter et al. (92) showed that a switch from conventional to online-produced ultrapure dialysate resulted in lower bacterial contamination with a significant decrease in CRP and IL-6 levels. Likewise, Shiffl et al. (93) showed that changing from conventional to ultrapure dialysate reduced the levels of IL-6 and CRP and improved nutritional status. Small studies have demonstrated that ultrapure dialysate is related to a slower loss of residual renal function (94) and a lower cardiovascular morbidity (95) in HD patients. Furthermore, vascular access is fundamental in HD patients, and an appropriate manipulation of it has a major impact on the prevalence of inflammation at the dialysis unit. Both clotted access grafts (96) and catheter infections (97) are significant contributors to the inflammatory process in HD patients. Biofilm formation might be also a cause of inflammation in this patient group (98). In summary, while adequate dialysis treatment to some extent can ameliorate some uremia-related proinflammatory factors, there are many dialysis-related factors that can contribute to the inflammatory state observed in CKD.

Additional Causes of Inflammation in Patients Undergoing Peritoneal Dialysis

The PD procedure *per se* may also induce systemic inflammation. Conventional bioincompatible glucose-based PD solutions, for instance, are thought to be important contributors (99), especially due to their content of glucose degradation products (GDPs) generated during heat sterilization. GDPs have been shown to induce peritoneal inflammation and the formation of AGEs. Additionally, glucose-based solutions lead to a substantial uptake of glucose, which may induce oxidative stress, a potent cause of inflammation (100). Peritoneal transport status is another important factor to consider in PD patients. Several years ago, it was suggested that patients presenting high peritoneal transport rate have worse clinical condition characterized by worse nutritional status and inflammation (101). However, it is now thought that the worse clinical situation and the high risk of death observed in the group of high transporters may be more closely related to volume overload from inadequate drainage in the exchanges. As volume overload occurs frequently in PD patients (78), this may be another reason for immune activation in this patient group. Additionally, concomitant infections especially peritonitis and percutaneous PD catheter infections are important contributors to inflammation in PD patients.

Activation of Polymorphonuclear Leukocytes

Although polymorphonuclear leukocytes (PMNLs) under noninfectious conditions are quiescent and release little ROS, there are reports

that in the uremic milieu, PMNLs are primed long before RRT is initiated (**FIGURE 20.3**) (102). A study by Sela et al. (102) showed that PMNL priming as well as neutrophil counts were directly related to severity of kidney disease. When patients with CKD start dialysis treatment, PMNL priming seems to be further augmented (103). As PMNL priming is believed to be one important contributor to systemic oxidative stress and chronic low-grade inflammation in CKD (102), the characteristics of priming agents in the uremic milieu need to be elucidated. Although most uremic retention molecules have not yet been characterized with regard to their specific pro- and/or anti-inflammatory effects, some interesting observations have recently been reported. Glorieux et al. (104) showed that genuine AGE compounds activate the leukocyte response in the uremic condition. Moreover, the same group recently showed that *p*-cresylsulphate (the main product of the protein-bound uremic retention solute *p*-cresol) activates leukocyte free radical production (105). As *p*-cresol recently was shown to predict mortality in HD patients (106), the potential proinflammatory and proatherogenic effects of *p*-cresylsulphate need further consideration.

Causes Related to Comorbidity and Lifestyle

Comorbidities and unhealthy lifestyle issues like proinflammatory diets (107) and sedentary behavior (108) can contribute and potentiate the degree of inflammation and deserve special attention.

Oral Health and Periodontal Disease

It is appreciated that oral health is an important aspect in many chronic diseases. In CKD patients, diverse changes in the oral cavity like xerostomia and modifications in the microbial community are seen (109). These conditions together with the impaired immunity, poor oral hygiene, and malnutrition enhance the incidence of

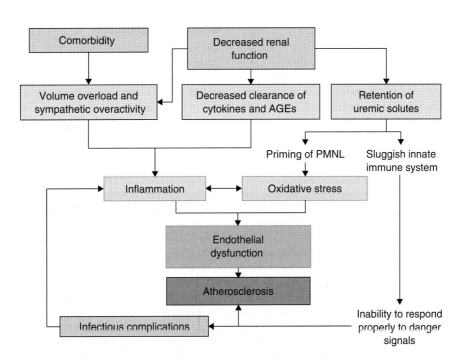

FIGURE 20.3 The interrelations by which inflammation and oxidative stress (through polymorphonuclear leukocyte activation) may lead to accelerated atherosclerosis. AGE, advanced glycation end products; PMNL, polymorphonuclear leukocyte. [Modified from Yilmaz MI, Carrero JJ, Axelsson J, et al. Low-grade inflammation in chronic kidney disease patients before the start of renal replacement therapy: sources and consequences. *Clin Nephrol* 2007;68(1):1–9].

periodontitis and other manifestations of poor oral health (110). Although oral cavity health is often overlooked, poor oral health in CKD patients has been associated with systemic consequences as infections, PEW, and atherosclerotic complications (111). Moreover, several studies have shown that patients with periodontitis have elevated levels of CRP, and periodontal disease is thought to be an important contributor to local and chronic systemic inflammation in CKD (112). Given that oral health problems could constitute a permanent source of inflammation, poor dentition and other signs of poor oral health should be an alarm clock also at early stages of CKD. However, it remains to be determined whether more successful management of poor oral health and periodontitis will reduce the risk of inflammation, infections, PEW, and atherosclerotic complications in CKD.

Bowel Bacteria Overgrowth and Altered Gut Microbiota

Uremia results in profound alterations of the gut microbial flora, also called gastrointestinal dysbiosis, and provokes impairment in the structure and function of the intestinal epithelial barrier structure (113). The causes responsible for these derangements are related not only to uremia *per se* but also to other commonly observed conditions like fluid overload, dietary fiber intake, frequent use of antibiotics, slow colonic transit, metabolic acidosis, intestinal wall edema, and oral iron intake. Alterations of the gut microbial flora in CKD are related to systemic inflammation and accumulation of gut-derived uremic toxins. Some of the uremic toxins generated by colonic bacteria include alfa-phenylacetyl-l-glutamine, 5-hydroxyindole, indoxyl glucuronide, *p*-cresol sulfate, and indoxyl sulfate (114). It is thought that they might play a role in the progression of kidney disease and in the pathogenesis of accelerated CVD and numerous other CKD-associated complications (115). In this sense, using pre/probiotics in order to attenuate the imbalance in the microbiota has been proposed as an intervention to minimize inflammation in this group of patients (116). It also has been described that beside the effect of the composition of the intestinal microbiota, uremia leads to an altered function of the intestinal barrier by provoking increased intestinal permeability (117,118). As a consequence of the disrupted intestinal epithelial junctions, an increased translocation of bacterial products across the intestinal barrier is observed, leading to an activation of innate immunity and therefore yielding to systemic inflammation (113).

Obesity and Fat Mass

Obesity, a common feature of CKD, may also contribute to an enhanced inflammatory activity (119). Adipokines and proinflammatory cytokines have a tightly link to fat and muscle tissue (120). Considering the important effect that loss of renal function has on the clearance of these substances (121), the systemic effects of adipokines in patients with CKD appear to be greater than in the general population. It has been estimated that approximately 20% of circulating IL-6 originate from fat tissue, and a significant amount of the circulating TNF comes from macrophages resident in the adipose tissue (122). As visceral fat appears to produce adipokines more actively than subcutaneous adipose tissue, visceral abdominal fat may be a main producer of IL-6. In accordance, in CKD patients evaluated shortly before the start of RRT, a significant association between serum IL-6 and truncal fat, but not between IL-6 and nontruncal fat, was documented (123). This association has also been seen in nondialyzed CKD stage 3 to 5 patients, where increased amount of visceral fat associated with higher inflammatory

parameters (124) and increased coronary artery calcification (125). Adding to the importance of fat mass distribution, rather than fat mass as such, in the same cohort, patients with more epicardial adipose tissue presented higher levels of inflammatory parameters as well as higher risk or CVD events (126).

Lifestyle Factors

Many lifestyle factors have been reported to potentiate the inflammatory status in CKD patients. Diet is a source of both anti- and proinflammatory constituents. In a study analyzing two community-based cohorts of elderly individuals, it was demonstrated that a proinflammatory diet is associated with systemic inflammation as well as with reduced kidney function (127). In this regard, dietary habits and food patterns are probably a target of major relevance in modifying systematic inflammatory levels. Moreover, both dialyzed and nondialyzed CKD patients have been reported to have a sedentary lifestyle that associate with higher values of inflammatory markers (108,128). Additionally, the implementation of programs devoted to increase physical activity in this group of patients has shown improvement in the levels of inflammatory parameters (129).

Obstructive sleep apnea syndrome is a common complication in patients with CKD (130) associated with endothelial damage, inflammation, and oxidative stress, which constitute an independent risk factor for CVD (112). Tobacco is probably the single most significant source of toxic chemical exposure to humans. Smoking is a central factor in many pathologic conditions, and its role in neoplasm, lung, and CVD has been well established for years. In recent years, cigarette smoking was shown to be able to alter both innate and immune systems and augment the production of numerous proinflammatory cytokines such as TNF, IL-1, IL-6, IL-8 GM-CSF, and a decrease in the levels of anti-inflammatory cytokines like IL-10 have been related to this (131,132).

Genetic Predisposition

Phenotypic variation is traditionally divided into a genetic and an environmental component. Undoubtedly, variations in the genome play an important role for the development of specific phenotype in CKD (133,134). Different types of genetic variants, such as insertion/deletions, mini- and microsatellites, or single nucleotide polymorphisms (SNPs), lead to a great variability in human genome, making human beings such unique individuals (134). Our understanding on the genetic predisposition to inflammation in patients with CKD has increased enormously the last decade. Because genetic variations are randomly assorted during gamete formation (independent of environmental factors), this approach, although being an association study, allows distinguishing a cause from an effect. For instance, the IL-6 gene has functional variants that affect inflammation and risk for CVD among dialysis patients, supporting a causal role for IL-6 in CVD (135). Interestingly, the IL-6 gene variants, together with those from the lymphotoxin-α gene, independently predicted risk for CVD in a rather big cohort of dialysis patients (136). Moreover, genetic variations in the IL-6 gene seem to influence inflammatory and peritoneal transport parameters, thereby contributing to the interpatient variability in small solute transport rate at the start of PD (137). Also, genetically determined interindividual differences in TNF (138), IL-10 (139), myeloperoxidase (140), and peroxisome proliferator-activated receptor (PPAR) γ (141) release have been associated with the prevalence of inflammation, CVD, and survival in CKD. Zhang et al. (142) found that although a haplotype consisting of several SNPs in the CRP gene was related to CRP levels measured over time in African American dialysis patients, there was no association between these SNPs and the presence of CVD. This finding is consistent with the growing belief that although CRP is a strong and independent risk marker of cardiovascular death, it is not a risk factor for vascular disease.

External and internal environmental stresses may also affect the phenotype via changes in the epigenome. Aberrant DNA methylation may, in relation to uremic dysmetabolism, have complex interactions for the development of premature CVD. As epigenetic mechanisms regulating the functional properties of the genome are heritable through cell divisions and may be sensitive to an abnormal environment (such as the uremic milieu), they could be potential new targets for interventions. Lastly, shortening of telomeres (nucleoprotein complexes protecting the chromosome ends that are involved in chromosome stability and repair) has been associated with an inflammatory phenotype and increased mortality in HD patients (143). In this context, it is of interest that telomere shortening to a critical length results in loss of histone and DNA methylation at mammalian telomeres, concomitant with increased histone acetylation (144). To conclude, the inflamed uremic phenotype is also the result of genetic factors. This is supported by the observation that Asian dialysis patients treated in the United States also have a markedly lower adjusted relative risk of mortality than Caucasians (145). Indeed, a substantial heritability (35% to 40%) has been found for CRP and IL-10 production (146,147), and many studies demonstrate a significant impact of genetic variations on the uremic inflammatory response (148,149).

Markers of Inflammation and Implications on Outcome

Prospective studies in patients both on HD (150–152) and PD (153–155) and after kidney transplantation (156) show that even a single measurement of an inflammatory biomarker is an independent predictor of poor outcome in patients with advanced CKD. In addition, results from the Modification of Diet in Renal Disease (MDRD) study showed that elevation of CRP (3 mg/L or more) and hypoalbuminemia predicted outcome in patients with mild to moderate CKD (157). In this regard, based on the large body of evidence available about the association of inflammation and poor outcomes in CKD population, an increased awareness of the importance of regular monitoring of inflammatory status has emerged in the nephrology community. For this purpose, a wide array of measurements are available (158), including among others, CRP, PMNL count, serum albumin, pentraxin-3 (PTX-3), IL-6, and TNF-like weak inducer of apoptosis (TWEAK) to name a few. However, there is poor agreement regarding which is the parameter that best predicts all-cause and cardiovascular mortality in patients with CKD.

In clinical practice, CRP is the most commonly used inflammatory marker. CRP is an acute-phase protein, produced by human hepatocytes in response to proinflammatory cytokines. Its measurement is cheap, reliable, easily obtained, and widely used in many centers around the world, and its interesting profile of features [stability over time (159), unaffected by circadian variation and by food intake] facilitates the use of it in dialysis patients attending different HD schedules. The use of CRP in dialysis units around the world has increased considerably in the last decade according to data from the Dialysis Outcomes and Practice Patterns Study (DOPPS) registry (160), and, interestingly, the dialysis facilities with higher percentage of patients with available CRP measurements reported lower cardiovascular-related mortality. In the uremic *milieu*, CRP

levels have shown to be associated with a number of both traditional and nontraditional cardiovascular risk factors, including dyslipidemia, oxidative stress, homocysteine levels, endothelial dysfunction, insulin resistance, and vascular calcification (26). A disadvantage faced with the use of CRP is its intra- and interindividual variability (161) and its variation over time, that in dialysis patients depend mainly on clinical events like transient infections, changes in volume status, or the intermittent stimulus of the dialysis procedure (162). Additionally, there is scarce information regarding the time-dependent predictive value of this measurement in patients with mild to moderate CKD. Moreover, whereas serial CRP measurements predict outcome better than a single CRP measurement in a group of prevalent HD patients (163), no data on serial determinations of inflammatory biomarkers are yet available in mild to moderate CKD. Therefore, prospective studies with careful serial monitoring of inflammatory biomarkers in patients with CKD are needed to evaluate if such an approach will yield more precise information to assess the disease severity.

IL-6 is considered as the key factor in the acute-phase response, and it has been suggested that this proinflammatory cytokine plays a strategic role in the pathogenesis of both PEW and atherosclerosis in the dialysis population (164). Some studies have assessed the predictive value of IL-6 over other inflammatory markers in dialysis patients, finding that IL-6 present the highest predictive value with regard to all-cause and cardiovascular mortality (34,35). Likewise, a comparative study based on ROC analysis also showed that the prediction power of the combined inflammatory burden of a number of commonly measured cytokines and adhesion molecules was identical to that provided by the sole measurement of IL-6 (165). Notwithstanding this advantage of risk prediction showed by IL-6, in a recent meta-analysis, Zhang et al. (166) found that CRP versus IL-6 had a similar predictive value for cardiovascular and all-cause mortality; CRP [hazard ratio (HR) 1.14 and 1.18, respectively] and IL-6 (HR 1.15 vs. 1.18, respectively). Thus, based on available data, it seems that the prognostic estimation provided by CRP is not much inferior to that by IL-6. Thus, the use of CRP would be sufficient to grade the inflammation status in clinical practice.

Other inflammatory markers that have attained increased interest in recent years are pentraxins. Pentraxins are a superfamily of evolutionarily conserved proteins characterized by a cyclic multimeric structure (167). On the basis of the primary structure of the subunit, the pentraxins are divided into two groups: short pentraxins (e.g., CRP and serum amyloid P) and long pentraxins. The prototype protein of the long pentraxin group is PTX-3. Whereas CRP and serum amyloid P are produced primarily in the liver in response to IL-6 (168), PTX-3 is produced by a variety of tissues and cells, particularly by innate immunity cells in response to proinflammatory signals and endothelial cells (169–171). Because of the extrahepatic synthesis and in contrast to CRP, PTX-3 levels are believed to be a true independent indicator of disease activity, produced at sites of inflammation and intimately linked to endothelial dysfunction (172). PTX-3 is elevated in HD patients as compared to healthy individuals (173) and identified as a novel mortality risk factor in CKD stage 5, independent of traditional risk factors, but most importantly independent of CRP itself (174). This suggests that this protein may have an additional role in the atherogenic process to common inflammatory mediators, perhaps reflecting endothelial damage.

Another novel inflammatory biomarker is TWEAK, (TNFSF12) is a member of the TNF superfamily of structurally related cytokines

(175) that can be expressed as a full-length membrane-bound protein or as a soluble protein (sTWEAK) that results from proteolysis of TWEAK (176,177). TWEAK gene is expressed in many tissues, including brain, kidney, heart, arterial wall, monocytes, and macrophages, and it has been found to be involved in different biologic processes, such as induction of cellular growth and proliferation (178,179), osteoclastogenesis (180), angiogenesis (181), and stimulation of apoptosis (182), favoring in that manner an inflammatory microenvironment. Moreover, TWEAK attenuates the transition from innate to adaptive immunity (183), activates nuclear factor-κB (NF-κB) signaling pathway, and induces the expression of different proinflammatory cytokines and cell adhesion molecules (184,185). In CKD, sTWEAK levels are significantly decreased compared to healthy subjects; however, high sTWEAK plasma levels have been reported to have additive effects to the high cardiovascular and all-cause mortality of HD patients with systemic inflammation (186).

⬡ CONSEQUENCES OF INFLAMMATION IN THE CLINICAL SETTING OF UREMIA

In the CKD population, persistent inflammation has been associated with several negative outcomes (71), including PEW, atherosclerosis, as well as increased cardiovascular and all-cause mortality (7,187,188). The specific pathways by which this association might be mediated are still not well known; however, it is thought that inflammation, beside its own direct effect, potentiates other known risk factors, like oxidative stress (189), insulin resistance (190), endothelial dysfunction (191), vascular calcification (192), bone mineral disorders (193), and depression (194). Additionally, inflammation may magnify the risk for poor outcomes via mechanisms related to self-enhancement of the inflammatory cascade and exacerbation of both the wasting and the vascular calcification processes (195).

Protein-Energy Wasting

The term *protein-energy wasting* describes the loss of muscle mass and fuel reserves of the body (6). PEW is observed in as many as

18% to 75% of patients with CKD (196,197), and inflammation appears to be an important contributor of this complex syndrome, both by direct and indirect mechanisms of muscle proteolysis and by impinging upon and magnifying other causes of PEW in a vicious circle. In several studies, inflammatory markers have continuously been related to markers of muscle mass (198), indicating an important role of cytokines in the development of PEW and muscle catabolism (199). Muscle mass was inversely correlated to both IL-6 and CRP in HD patients, even after adjustments for age and gender (10). Also, markers of decreasing muscle mass during a 1-year period on HD were associated with higher IL-1β concentrations (200). Besides that skeletal muscle–derived IL-6 may contribute to the production of IL-6 and oxidative stress during the HD session (201,202), IL-6 *per se* may stimulate muscle protein breakdown and promote cancer-related wasting (203,204) and wasting observed in uremic patients (198). On the other hand, while IL-6 inhibits the secretion of insulin-like growth factor 1 (IGF-1), decreased IGF-1 signaling may also be involved in the sarcopenia process (205). Some of the known related mechanisms between PEW and inflammation are described below (**FIGURE 20.4**).

Anorexia

Anorexia represents a complex and multifactorial disorder with a high prevalence among CKD patients (206). Although anorexia is a typical consequence of CKD, other metabolic abnormalities that are not fully corrected by dialysis therapy are also involved. In these derangements, given that some inflammatory markers like CRP, IL-6, and TNF have been described as related to uremic anorexia (207,208), systemic inflammation is likely to play an integrative role in the physiopathology of anorexia in CKD. Inflammatory cytokines have the capacity to regulate the appetite through disturbing specific brain areas related to appetite regulation (209). Specific cytokines access the brain and act directly on hypothalamic neurons and/or generate mediators targeting both peripheral and/or brain target sites (209,210); thus, inflammation may influence the size, duration, and frequency of meals.

A difference in the relation between inflammation and anorexia among genders needs to be pointed out. A recent study showed that

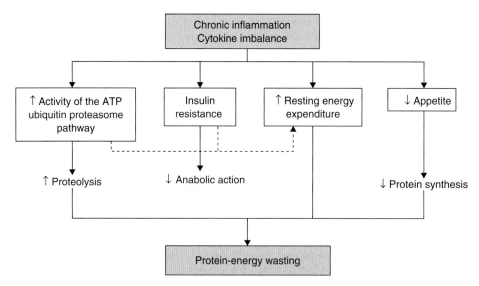

FIGURE 20.4 Potential mechanisms by which chronic inflammation may lead to protein-energy wasting. ATP, adenosine triphosphate, ↑, increase; ↓, decrease. (Modified from Avesani CM, Carrero JJ, Axelson J, et al. Inflammation and wasting in chronic kidney disease: partners in crime. *Kidney Int* 2006;70:S8–S13.)

among CKD patients, anorectic women exhibited a more favorable inflammatory and nutritional status than anorectic men (155). This difference where apparently uremic men are more prone to inflammation-induced anorexia might be explained by a possible protective role of sex hormones against the burden of inflammation. Indeed, gender is physiologically associated with feeding behavior (158) and inflammatory status (159), and men with inflammation on dialysis seem to have a worse survival as compared to women with the same conditions (5). Although the role of sex-specific regulation of feeding is unclear, increased anorectic signals and earlier satiety have been reported in men suffering from chronic illnesses (160,161), perhaps contributing to a different response pattern to anorexigenic diseases (such as heart failure and cancer) among men and women (162). An indirect support of this hypothesis is that novel anorexigenic agents, such as megestrol acetate or nandrolone decanoate, have a chemical structure similar to sex hormones.

Increased Insulin Resistance

An increased insulin resistance predisposes to a loss of muscle mass by decreasing the anabolic action of insulin. Type 2 diabetic HD patients have significantly increased skeletal muscle protein breakdown (211). Thus, dialysis patients and patients with diabetes mellitus had significantly accelerated loss of lean body mass (LBM) during the first year of RRT (212). The link between inflammation and insulin resistance occurs mainly through (a) a defect in insulin intracellular signaling pathways during inflammation, (b) induction of lipolysis by TNF, and (c) a decrease in the secretion of adiponectin caused by TNF (213). Additionally, the administration of recombinant TNF to cultured cells or to animals impairs insulin action, and obese mice lacking functional TNF or TNF receptors have improved insulin sensitivity compared with wild-type counterparts (214).

Activation of the Adenosine Triphosphate Ubiquitin-Proteolytic System

Metabolic acidosis is a common phenomenon in progressive CKD that may lead to stimulation of protein breakdown and subsequent muscle wasting through stimulation of the ATP-ubiquitin-proteolytic pathway (215). Because TNF increases ubiquitin gene expression in skeletal muscle, it is possible that it causes muscle wasting by stimulating protein catabolism through the ubiquitin proteosome pathway (215,216).

Increased Resting Energy Expenditure

The diverse metabolic abnormalities present during the inflammatory response, like fever, elevated oxygen consumption, enhanced lipolysis and fat utilization, increased concentration of catabolic hormones, and extensive protein catabolism, consume high quantities of energy that account for as much as 15% of the daily energy expenditure (217). Studies in predialysis and dialysis patients have consistently shown that inflammatory markers are associated with increased resting energy expenditure (10,218,219) and an increased mortality risk (10).

Depression

Depressive symptoms are related to poor outcomes and higher mortality in CKD and in other patient groups, and they are seen more frequently with the gradual reduction in renal function (220–222). Cytokines are thought to be important mediators of brain immune connections and may play an important role in the pathogenesis of depression due to their effect on neurotransmitters

and neurohormones (220,223). In dialysis patients, depressive symptoms seemed to worsen in the presence of increased IL-6 levels (222–226), and 8 weeks of fluoxetine treatment in depressed HD patients decreased serum IL-1β levels (227). Depression may undeniably link to fatigue (228) and unwillingness to eat (206), contributing in a vicious circle to anorexia, physical inactivity, PEW, and worse outcome, all of which have also been attributed, in part, to the effects of systemic inflammation.

Vascular Calcification

Although vascular calcification (or rather ossification) can be observed in the general population (229), CKD is a condition associated with a markedly increased prevalence of both intima and media arterial calcification (230). Indeed, several studies indicate that large artery calcification (assessed by computer tomography or chest x-ray) is present in 30% to 70% of patients with CKD (231,232), and even in approximately 15% of uremic pediatric patients (233). The presence of arterial ossification is associated with functional estimates of arterial dysfunction, such as NO-dependent vasodilation in dialysis patients (234) and pulse wave velocity (235), both of which have been associated with adverse outcome in patients with CKD (236,237). Indeed, vascular ossification is associated with increased risk of CVD (231,238,239) and mortality (238). Currently, there are a wealth of data evidencing intimate links between vascular calcification and systemic inflammation (TABLE 20.3). TNF can induce mineralization of calcifying vascular cells *in vitro* (240), and coculture of these cells with monocyte/macrophages (the source of most cytokines) can accelerate this process (241). Receptor activator of NF-κB ligand (RANKL) is a membrane-bound or soluble cytokine essential for osteoclast differentiation, whereas the decoy receptor osteoprotegerin (OPG) masks RANKL activity. Although both seem to influence the inflammatory component of atherosclerosis (242), it is of interest that OPG upregulates endothelial cell adhesion molecule in response to TNF (243). These findings suggest a mechanism by which OPG may stimulate inflammation in atheroma and thereby promote the progression and complications of atherosclerosis, which would agree with the observed detrimental effects on

TABLE 20.3	Factors Related with Vascular Calcification through Inflammation in the Uremic Milieu
Factors	**Association with Inflammation**
Inhibiting calcification	
Osteoprotegerin	+
Osteopontin	+
Bone morphogenic protein-7	+
Fetuin-A	++
HDL-cholesterol	+
Matrix gla protein	unknown
Promoting calcification	
Leptin	+
TNF	++
Genetic factors	+
Diabetes mellitus	+

HDL, high-density lipoprotein; TNF, tumor necrosis factor; +, association; ++, strong association.

survival of both increased inflammation and OPG levels in HD patients (244). On the other hand, vascular calcification, as part of the atherosclerotic process, is due to the deposition in the arterial intima of basic calcium phosphate (BCP) crystals, similar to those that mineralize bone. It was recently shown that BCP crystals could interact with human monocyte-derived macrophages, inducing a proinflammatory state through protein kinase C and mitogen-activated protein (MAP) kinase pathways (245). This implies a vicious circle of inflammation and arterial calcification that could explain the associations between inflammation and outcome in CKD.

Among the inhibitor factors of ossification, fetuin-A is the most studied. Mice lacking the gene encoding for fetuin-A rapidly develop ectopic soft tissue ossification and die at an early age (246). In CKD, low levels of circulating fetuin-A are associated with increased cardiovascular burden and mortality (247–249). Inflammation and PEW may be important causes of a decrease in serum fetuin-A level in patients with CKD, as increased proinflammatory molecules and the presence of wasting downregulate its plasma levels (250,251). Also, fetuin-A was associated with cardiac valve calcification and inflammation in PD patients (252). Taken together, these data suggest the existence of an active interplay between vascular calcification and atherosclerosis through inflammation, against a background of severe calcium-phosphorus disturbances. If the above mentioned theory is further supported by forthcoming studies, then the treatment of all three entities (atherosclerosis, calcium-phosphorus disturbances, and inflammation) have to be instituted early, concomitantly, and intensively in these patients.

Endocrine Disorders

The kidney is a key modulator of the endocrine function and an important target for hormonal action. As a direct consequence, the uremic state is associated with abnormalities in the synthesis or action of many hormones (253). Evidence suggests that this hormonal dysmetabolism may be aggravated by persistent inflammation.

Thyroid Hormones

CKD *per se* causes alterations in thyroid hormones in the absence of an underlying intrinsic thyroid disorder (254,255) characterized by a decrease in total (T_3) and free (fT_3) triiodothyronine plasma concentration, whereas thyroid-stimulating hormone (TSH) levels are usually normal. Indeed, the so-called low T_3 condition is present in approximately one-fourth of patients with CKD (256). Traditionally, decreases in plasma T_3 concentration have been interpreted as an attempt to conserve body energy stores by reducing metabolic rate. However, recent data suggest that low T_3 levels may not just be an innocent bystander and could be involved in the increased mortality risk in CKD. Low T_3 levels are independent predictors of all-cause mortality in HD (257) and PD patients (258) and even in patients with clinical and biochemical euthyroid CKD stage 5 (259). Although the reasons for this observation are as yet unknown, they may connect a state of subclinical hypothyroidism with low-grade persistent inflammation (260). Indeed, IL-6 signaling has been reported to downregulate the peripheral conversion of total thyroxine (T_4) into T_3 in both experimental (261) and clinical (262) studies. Low T_3 levels specifically predicted cardiovascular mortality (**FIGURE 20.5**) in patients with CKD stage 5 (259), whereas in a PD cohort, these levels were associated with left ventricular hypertrophy (257). This working hypothesis merits further consideration.

Sex Hormones

Testosterone deficiency or hypogonadism is common in men with CKD, with a prevalence ranging from 35% to 50% of men undergoing RRT (263,264). Although the high prevalence of hypogonadism observed in this group of patients to a large extent may be a consequence of the failing kidney *per se* (265), inflammation is thought to have an important contributory role in the physiopathology of hypogonadism. Thus, the hypothalamic–pituitary–testicular axis is suppressed by different inflammatory cytokines (266,267), and therefore, an inflammatory state may induce testosterone deficiency. In support of this, studies depict a strong inverse association between endogenous testosterone and surrogate markers of inflammation in CKD populations (268–271). However, it is also possible that testosterone has immune-modulatory actions *per se*, as suggested by the suppression of cytokine production in hypogonadal men with diabetes, coronary heart disease, and metabolic syndrome after supplementation with testosterone (272–274).

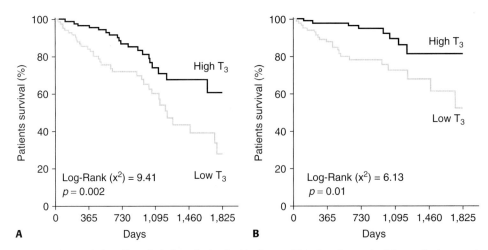

FIGURE 20.5 Association of low triiodothyronine levels with all-cause **(A)** and cardiovascular **(B)** mortality in 187 patients with clinical and biochemical euthyroid stage 5 CKD. [Modified from Carrero JJ, Qureshi AR, Axelsson J, et al. Clinical and biochemical implications of low thyroid hormone levels (total and free forms) in euthyroid patients with chronic kidney disease. *J Intern Med* 2007;262(6):690–701.]

Other Hormones

The inflammatory response inhibits growth hormone (GH) action (275), and GH forearm perfusion demonstrated that a resistance to pharmacologic doses of GH is not related to uremia *per se* but rather to an increased inflammatory state (276).

 ## PREVENTION AND TREATMENT OF INFLAMMATION

Because persistent inflammation may be a silent reflection of various pathophysiologic alterations in CKD, and as its presence is associated with many deleterious outcomes, it is essential that inflammatory markers are regularly monitored and therapeutic attempts be made to target inflammation (**FIGURE 20.6**). While a heightened attentiveness to the presence of inflammation will lead first of all to treatment of comorbidities (especially infections), other interventions are valuable in the clinical management of "uremic inflammation" (277) (**TABLE 20.4**). These include improvements in dialysis therapy (278) and fluid status (279) as well as implementation of healthy lifestyle habits, including diet modifications (280,281) and an increase in physical activity (129). As the use of central venous catheters is a common source of inflammation in HD patients (282), their use should be limited and as short as possible. Some of the possible interventions are described more in detail below.

Lifestyle and Nutritional Measures

At first, given the documented associations between proinflammatory cytokines and lifestyle factors (283), appropriate lifestyle modifications, such as weight loss or exercise training (284), may be an important component in normalizing deregulated cytokine system activity in CKD (284). Dietary interventions could also play an important role that has been, up to now, underestimated. According to *in vitro* and animal studies, different bioactive food components exert a positive effect on oxidative stress and inflammation (285); however, whether these effects can be extrapolated to humans will require further studies. HD patients who are fish eaters have been reported to have lower mortality (286), and small studies in HD patients suggest that omega-3 fatty acids have beneficial effects in different clinical conditions related to CKD (287); however, the potential

beneficial effects of fish oil or omega-3 fatty acids consumption on inflammation needs to be confirmed by further investigation. Of interest, a small randomized controlled trial with fish oil in HD patients found significant reductions in CRP concomitant with rise in blood omega-3 levels (288). Flavonoid compounds like genistein (present in soy) are also of potential interest due to their similarity with sexual hormones and protective impact on cardiovascular functions, that it is thought to be mediated by their ability to interfere with cytokine production by repression of IL-6 mRNA (289). A small interventional study using isoflavone soy in HD patients showed inverse correlations between changes in serum isoflavone levels and CRP levels (290).

Resveratrol, a phenolic compound found in various plants, including grapes, berries, and peanuts, has also anti-inflammatory properties by antagonizing the activity of NF-κB (291). Although it is conceivable that resveratrol supplementation in CKD patients could be beneficial, there are yet no studies documenting the effect on uremic inflammation. In mice, however, it has been shown that that resveratrol treatment inhibits oxidative stress and renal interstitial fibrosis (292). Other natural antioxidants like vitamin E and *N*-acetylcysteine may inhibit proinflammatory cytokine release (293,294) and improve endothelial dysfunction (295,296). They have been shown to reduce cardiovascular events in rather small cohorts of dialysis patients (297,298). Recent results from a randomized controlled trial with γ-tocopherol and docosahexaenoic acid in HD patients showed a significant reduction in selected biomarkers of inflammation (299). Increased fructose intake has recently been implicated as a potential contributor to hypertension, inflammation, and CKD, potentially via generation of uric acid. The reduction in inflammatory markers observed in 28 CKD patients on a low-fructose diet (300) indicates the need for further studies on the putative long-term anti-inflammatory effects of such a diet. Finally, a number of other nutritional interventions, such as fiber-rich food, nuts, probiotics, and diets with low content of AGEs, may have anti-inflammatory properties and should be evaluated in CKD (301,302).

Nonspecific Anti-Inflammatory Pharmacologic Interventions

The role of unspecific anti-inflammatory pharmacologic treatment strategies either alone or combined as a preventive therapy needs

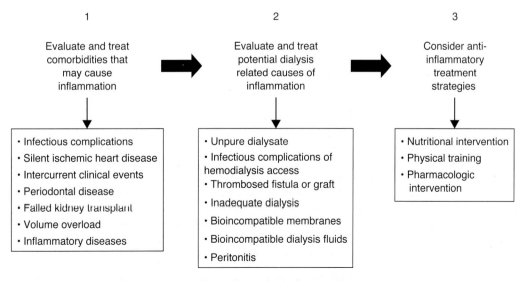

FIGURE 20.6 Suggested steps to target persistent inflammation in dialysis patients.

TABLE
20.4

Currently Available Anti-Inflammatory Treatment Strategies in Patients with Chronic Kidney Disease

I. Associated with Dialysis Treatment *Per se*

Ultrapure dialysate	Repeatedly shown to reduce CRP (90–93)
Biocompatible membranes	The inflammatory reaction is affected by choice of dialyzer (85).
Hemodiafiltration (HDF)	On-line HDF did not provoke an inflammatory response (334).
Daily dialysis	Dramatic positive effect on CRP in one study (88)
Vascular access in HD	Central venous catheters are a common source of inflammation in HD patients (282) and their use should therefore be limited and as short as possible.

II. Nutritional and Lifestyle Interventions

Physical training	Both aerobic and resistance training enhance immune function and exert anti-inflammatory effects (129,284).
Cognitive-behavioral therapy for sleep disorders	Improves sleep quality and decreases inflammatory parameters in HD and PD patients (335,336)
Smoking cessation	Active smokers present higher levels of inflammatory markers. Inflammatory markers in former smokers approach levels among nonsmokers over time, suggesting that cessation may result in a reversal of smoking-associated alterations in immunity and inflammation (337).
Salt restriction	Dietary sodium restriction is associated with the attenuation of the inflammatory state depicted by a reduction in levels of CRP, IL-6, and TNF (338).
Omega-3 fatty acids	12-week fish oil supplementation decreased CRP in HD patients (288)
Gamma-tocopherol	Small RCT in HD patients shows effect on IL-6 (299).
Pomegranate juice	One year of pomegranate juice intake yielded a significant time response reduction in PMNL priming, protein oxidation, lipid oxidation, and levels of inflammation biomarkers (339).
Probiotics	After 6 months of treatment, there was a decrease of TNF, IL-5, and IL-6 levels and an increase of IL-10 (340).
High fiber intake	High dietary total fiber intake is associated with lower risk of inflammation and mortality (341).
Low-fructose diet	Changing to a low-fructose diet decreased values of hsCRP and sICAM. hsCRP values returned to baseline with resumption of regular diet (300).
Green tea	Reduces HD-induced production of hydrogen peroxide, hypochlorous acid, atherosclerotic disease risk factors, and proinflammatory cytokines (342)
Soy	Lower prevalence of inflammation and better outcome in Asian HD patients might be due to soy intake; soy supplementation decreases CRP in HD patients (290).

III. Commonly Used Pharmacologic Interventions

Statins	Inhibit cholesterol synthesis but also showed anti-inflammatory (303,304) and anti-oxidative properties (305) in HD patients; no effect on survival in 4D (306)
ACE inhibitors	Reduction in IL-6 response to coronary artery graft surgery (308); lower inflammatory (309) and adhesion molecules (310) in CKD patients using ACE inhibitors
Sevelamer	A small RCT shows decrease in CRP and increase in fetuin-A with sevelamer treatment (314).
Antidepressant	Sertraline treatment for depression significantly decreased serum IL-6, independent of its efficacy for depression treatment (343).
Allopurinol	Decreases CRP, slows down progression of kidney disease, and reduces cardiovascular and hospitalization (344)
D-vitamin	Reduction of inflammation biomarkers in patients with congestive heart failure (312)
Cholecalciferol	Reduction of inflammatory markers and left ventricular hypertrophy (345)
Paricalcitol	Significant decrease in hsCRP, TNF, and IL-6 (346)
Linagliptin	Significant decreases of IL-6 levels after 6 months treatment (347)
Heparin	Low molecular weight heparin reduces inflammation in HD patients (348).

IV. Potential Novel Anti-Inflammatory Interventions

N-Acetylcysteine	Small show effect on outcome in HD (297).
Pentoxifylline	Significantly decreased serum concentrations of TNF, IL-6, and CRP (349)
Bardoxolone	Inhibits inflammation by activating the Nrf2 pathway (350), improving of glomerular filtration rate observed in DM-2 CKD patients (351). An RCT including CKD-4 diabetic patients observed a higher rate of cardiovascular events with bardoxolone methyl than with placebo prompted termination of the trial (352).
Anticytokine drugs	Tocilizumab (353), Canakinumab (354), Anakinra (355), and Etanercept (356) have shown promising results in chronic inflammatory diseases. Lack of data regarding the safety and concrete benefits of some of these medications in dialysis patients.

CRP, C-reactive protein; HD, hemodialysis; PD, peritoneal dialysis; IL-6, interleukin 6; TNF, tumor necrosis factor; RCT, randomized controlled trial; PMNL, polymorphonuclear leukocyte; IL-5, interleukin 5; IL-10, interleukin 10; hsCRP, high-sensitivity C-reactive protein; sICAM, soluble intercellular adhesion molecule; 4D, Die Deutsche Diabetes-Dialyse; CKD, chronic kidney disease; ACE, angiotensin-converting enzyme; DM-2, type 2 diabetes mellitus; CKD-4, stage 4 chronic kidney disease.

further evaluation. It is notable that several commonly used drugs may possess significant anti-inflammatory effects. Statins not only inhibit cholesterol synthesis but also show anti-inflammatory actions (303,304) and anti-oxidative properties (305) in HD patients. However, no effect on survival was demonstrated in the Die Deutsche Diabetes-Dialyse (4D) randomized controlled trial (306). In another study, IL-8, IL-6, and TNF levels were reduced during aspirin consumption in HD patients (307). Angiotensin-converting enzyme inhibitor (ACEI) treatment is associated with a reduction in IL-6 response to coronary artery graft surgery (308). In accordance, we have found lower plasma levels of TNF, CRP (309), and adhesion molecules (310) in patients with CKD treated with ACEI. Of interest, ACEI has also been shown to prevent wasting in patients with heart failure (311). Other interesting approaches may include D-vitamin, which effectively reduced the inflammatory milieu in a randomized controlled trial performed in patients with chronic heart failure (312). Sevelamer has also been suggested to exert favorable impact on lipids and inflammatory markers with potentially useful antiatherogenic effects in HD patients (313). In addition, short-term sevelamer intake significantly increased fetuin-A levels and improved flow-mediated dilation in patients with nondiabetic CKD stage 4 (314). N-Acetylcysteine could also be an interesting option to test considering its effect on reducing atheroma progression (probably through a decrease in oxidative stress) in an animal model of uremia-enhanced atherosclerosis (315). Finally, PPAR-γ activators, such as rosiglitazone, may be another interesting strategy to explore given their anti-inflammatory effects in PD patients (316). However, as the myocardial ischemic risk associated with rosiglitazone treatment may be increased in patients with type 2 diabetes (317), these drugs should be used with caution in dialysis patients.

Targeted Anticytokine Interventions

As targeted anticytokine treatment strategies have shown interesting results in other patient groups with inflammation, these drugs may also be of interest to study in dialysis patients. Thalidomide, a drug with immunomodulatory, anti-inflammatory, and antiangiogenic properties, exerts its therapeutic effects through the modulation of TNF. As thalidomide induces a Th2 response and has been associated with weight gain in other wasted patient groups, such as those with HIV or tuberculosis (318), it would be of interest to test the effects of this drug in dialysis patients. Pentoxifylline has been shown to reduce TNF expression by more than 50% and to improve hemoglobin levels in a small group of HD patients with erythropoietin-resistant anemia (319). Finally, as promising results in patients with type 2 diabetes (320) and in patients with acute gout (321) with IL-1-receptor antagonists have been reported, this may be another future treatment of uremic inflammation. Although specific anti-inflammatory drugs (tocilizumab, canakinumab, pentoxifylline) have been found to be of value in other inflammatory diseases (281), there is still lack of data regarding the safety and concrete benefits of these medications in dialysis patients.

◢ REFERENCES

1. Kooman JP, Kotanko P, Schols AM, et al. Chronic kidney disease and premature ageing. *Nat Rev Nephrol* 2014;10:732–742.
2. Ridker PM, Cushman M, Stampfer MJ, et al. Inflammation, aspirin, and the risk of cardiovascular disease in apparently healthy men. *N Engl J Med* 1997;336(14):973–979.
3. Llorca J, Lopez-Diaz MJ, Gonzalez-Juanatey C, et al. Persistent chronic inflammation contributes to the development of cancer in patients with rheumatoid arthritis from a defined population of Northwestern Spain. *Semin Arthritis Rheum* 2007;37(1):31–38.
4. Stenvinkel P, Heimbürger O, Paultre F, et al. Strong association between malnutrition, inflammation, and atherosclerosis in chronic renal failure. *Kidney Int* 1999;55(5):1899–1911.
5. Kalantar-Zadeh K, Ikizler TA, Block G, et al. Malnutrition-inflammation complex syndrome in dialysis patients: causes and consequences. *Am J Kidney Dis* 2003;42(5):864–881.
6. Fouque D, Kalantar-Zadeh K, Kopple J, et al. A proposed nomenclature and diagnostic criteria for protein-energy wasting in acute and chronic kidney disease. *Kidney Int* 2008;73(4):391–398.
7. Nascimento MM, Pecoits-Filho R, Qureshi AR, et al. The prognostic impact of fluctuating levels of C-reactive protein in Brazilian haemodialysis patients: a prospective study. *Nephrol Dial Transplant* 2004;19(11):2803–2809.
8. Stenvinkel P, Wanner C, Metzger T, et al. Inflammation and outcome in end-stage renal failure: does female gender constitute a survival advantage? *Kidney Int* 2002;62(5):1791–1798.
9. Kaizu Y, Ohkawa S, Odamaki M, et al. Association between inflammatory mediators and muscle mass in long-term hemodialysis patients. *Am J Kidney Dis* 2003;42(2):295–302.
10. Wang AY, Sea MM, Tang N, et al. Resting energy expenditure and subsequent mortality risk in peritoneal dialysis patients. *J Am Soc Nephrol* 2004;15(12):3134–3143.
11. Muntner P, Hamm LL, Kusek JW, et al. The prevalence of nontraditional risk factors for coronary heart disease in patients with chronic kidney disease. *Ann Intern Med* 2004;140(1):9–17.
12. Avesani CM, Draibe SA, Kamimura MA, et al. Resting energy expenditure of chronic kidney disease patients: influence of renal function and subclinical inflammation. *Am J Kidney Dis* 2004;44(6):1008–1016.
13. Eustace JA, Astor B, Muntner PM, et al. Prevalence of acidosis and inflammation and their association with low serum albumin in chronic kidney disease. *Kidney Int* 2004;65(3):1031–1040.
14. Kato S, Chmielewski M, Honda H, et al. Aspects of immune dysfunction in end-stage renal disease. *Clin J Am Soc Nephrol* 2008;3(5):1526–1533.
15. Vaziri ND, Pahl MV, Crum A, et al. Effect of uremia on structure and function of immune system. *J Ren Nutr* 2012;22(1):149–156.
16. Medzhitov R, Janeway C. Innate immunity. *N Engl J Med* 2000;343(5):338–344.
17. Verkade MA, van Druningen CJ, Vaessen LM, et al. Functional impairment of monocyte-derived dendritic cells in patients with severe chronic kidney disease. *Nephrol Dial Transplant* 2007;22(1):128–138.
18. Berger SP, Roos A, Mallat MJ, et al. Low pretransplantation mannose-binding lectin levels predict superior patient and graft survival after simultaneous pancreas-kidney transplantation. *J Am Soc Nephrol* 2007;18(8):2416–2422.
19. Satomura A, Endo M, Fujita T, et al. Serum mannose-binding lectin levels in maintenance hemodialysis patients: impact on all-cause mortality. *Nephron Clin Pract* 2006;102(3–4):c93–c99.
20. Pasare C, Medzhitov R. Toll-like receptors: linking innate and adaptive immunity. *Microbes Infect* 2004;6(15):1382–1387.
21. Kiechl S, Lorenz E, Reindl M, et al. Toll-like receptor 4 polymorphisms and atherogenesis. *N Engl J Med* 2002;347(3):185–192.
22. Descamps-Latscha B, Herbelin A, Nguyen AT, et al. Immune system dysregulation in uremia. *Semin Nephrol* 1994;14(3):253–260.
23. Descamps-Latscha B, Jungers P, Witko-Sarsat V. Immune system dysregulation in uremia: role of oxidative stress. *Blood Purif* 2002;20(5):481–484.
24. Pereira BJ, Snodgrass B, Barber G, et al. Cytokine production during in vitro hemodialysis with new and formaldehyde- or renalin-reprocessed cellulose dialyzers. *J Am Soc Nephrol* 1995;6(4):1304–1308.
25. Don BR, Kaysen GA. Assessment of inflammation and nutrition in patients with end-stage renal disease. *J Nephrol* 2000;13(4):249–259.
26. Stenvinkel P, Ketteler M, Johnson RJ, et al. IL-10, IL-6, and TNF-alpha: central factors in the altered cytokine network of uremia—the good, the bad, and the ugly. *Kidney Int* 2005;67(4):1216–1233.
27. Barton BE. The biological effects of interleukin 6. *Med Res Rev* 1996;16(1):87–109.

28. Descamps-Latscha B, Herbelin A, Nguyen AT, et al. Balance between IL-1 beta, TNF-alpha, and their specific inhibitors in chronic renal failure and maintenance dialysis. Relationships with activation markers of T cells, B cells, and monocytes. *J Immunol* 1995;154(2):882–892.

29. Pecoits-Filho R, Heimbürger O, Bárány P, et al. Associations between circulating inflammatory markers and residual renal function in CRF patients. *Am J Kidney Dis* 2003;41(6):1212–1218.

30. Poole S, Bird TA, Selkirk S, et al. Fate of injected interleukin 1 in rats: sequestration and degradation in the kidney. *Cytokine* 1990;2(6):416–422.

31. Bolton CH, Downs LG, Victory JG, et al. Endothelial dysfunction in chronic renal failure: roles of lipoprotein oxidation and pro-inflammatory cytokines. *Nephrol Dial Transplant* 2001;16(6):1189–1197.

32. Stenvinkel P, Heimbürger O, Jogestrand T. Elevated interleukin-6 predicts progressive carotid artery atherosclerosis in dialysis patients: association with *Chlamydia pneumoniae* seropositivity. *Am J Kidney Dis* 2002;39(2):274–282.

33. Dounousi E, Papavasiliou E, Makedou A, et al. Oxidative stress is progressively enhanced with advancing stages of CKD. *Am J Kidney Dis* 2006;48(5):752–760.

34. Honda H, Qureshi AR, Heimbürger O, et al. Serum albumin, C-reactive protein, interleukin 6, and fetuin a as predictors of malnutrition, cardiovascular disease, and mortality in patients with ESRD. *Am J Kidney Dis* 2006;47(1):139–148.

35. Tripepi G, Mallamaci F, Zoccali C. Inflammation markers, adhesion molecules, and all-cause and cardiovascular mortality in patients with ESRD: searching for the best risk marker by multivariate modeling. *J Am Soc Nephrol* 2005;16(Suppl 1):S83–S88.

36. Huber SA, Sakkinen P, Conze D, et al. Interleukin-6 exacerbates early atherosclerosis in mice. *Arterioscler Thromb Vasc Biol* 1999; 19(10):2364–2367.

37. Kovacs A, Tornvall P, Nilsson R, et al. Human C-reactive protein slows atherosclerosis development in a mouse model with human-like hypercholesterolemia. *Proc Natl Acad Sci U S A* 2007;104(34): 13768–13773.

38. Elhage R, Clamens S, Besnard S, et al. Involvement of interleukin-6 in atherosclerosis but not in the prevention of fatty streak formation by 17beta-estradiol in apolipoprotein E-deficient mice. *Atherosclerosis* 2001;156(2):315–320.

39. Yudkin JS, Kumari M, Humphries SE, et al. Inflammation, obesity, stress and coronary heart disease: is interleukin-6 the link? *Atherosclerosis* 2000;148(2):209–214.

40. Bemelmans MH, Gouma DJ, Buurman WA. LPS-induced sTNF-receptor release in vivo in a murine model. Investigation of the role of tumor necrosis factor, IL-1, leukemia inhibiting factor, and IFN-gamma. *J Immunol* 1993;151(10):5554–5562.

41. Hotamisligil GS, Arner P, Caro JF, et al. Increased adipose tissue expression of tumor necrosis factor-alpha in human obesity and insulin resistance. *J Clin Invest* 1995;95(5):2409–2415.

42. Bhagat K, Vallance P. Inflammatory cytokines impair endothelium-dependent dilatation in human veins in vivo. *Circulation* 1997;96(9):3042–3047.

43. Olszyna DP, Pajkrt D, Lauw FN, et al. Interleukin 10 inhibits the release of CC chemokines during human endotoxemia. *J Infect Dis* 2000;181(2):613–620.

44. Song S, Ling-Hu H, Roebuck KA, et al. Interleukin-10 inhibits interferon-gamma-induced intercellular adhesion molecule-1 gene transcription in human monocytes. *Blood* 1997;89(12):4461–4469.

45. Kuga S, Otsuka T, Niiro H, et al. Suppression of superoxide anion production by interleukin-10 is accompanied by a downregulation of the genes for subunit proteins of NADPH oxidase. *Exp Hematol* 1996;24(2):151–157.

46. Lacraz S, Nicod LP, Chicheportiche R, et al. IL-10 inhibits metalloproteinase and stimulates TIMP-1 production in human mononuclear phagocytes. *J Clin Invest* 1995;96(5):2304–2310.

47. Morita Y, Yamamura M, Kashihara N, et al. Increased production of interleukin-10 and inflammatory cytokines in blood monocytes of hemodialysis patients. *Res Commun Mol Pathol Pharmacol* 1997;98(1): 19–33.

48. Brunet P, Capo C, Dellacasagrande J, et al. IL-10 synthesis and secretion by peripheral blood mononuclear cells in haemodialysis patients. *Nephrol Dial Transplant* 1998;13(7):1745–1751.

49. Yilmaz MI, Solak Y, Saglam M, et al. The relationship between IL-10 levels and cardiovascular events in patients with CKD. *Clin J Am Soc Nephrol* 2014;9(7):1207–1216.

50. Sarnak MJ, Jaber BL. Mortality caused by sepsis in patients with end-stage renal disease compared with the general population. *Kidney Int* 2000;58(4):1758–1764.

51. Haubitz M, Brunkhorst R. C-reactive protein and chronic *Chlamydia pneumoniae* infection—long-term predictors for cardiovascular disease and survival in patients on peritoneal dialysis. *Nephrol Dial Transplant* 2001;16(4):809–815.

52. Thomson PC, Stirling CM, Geddes CC, et al. Vascular access in haemodialysis patients: a modifiable risk factor for bacteraemia and death. *QJM* 2007;100(7):415–422.

53. Dobkin JF, Miller MH, Steigbigel NH. Septicemia in patients on chronic hemodialysis. *Ann Intern Med* 1978;88(1):28–33.

54. Hoen B, Paul-Dauphin A, Hestin D, et al. EPIBACDIAL: a multicenter prospective study of risk factors for bacteremia in chronic hemodialysis patients. *J Am Soc Nephrol* 1998;9(5):869–876.

55. Abbott KC, Agodoa LY. Etiology of bacterial septicemia in chronic dialysis patients in the United States. *Clin Nephrol* 2001;56(2):124–131.

56. Kirmani N, Tuazon CU, Murray HW, et al. *Staphylococcus aureus* carriage rate of patients receiving long-term hemodialysis. *Arch Intern Med* 1978;138(11):1657–1659.

57. Khan IH, Catto GR. Long-term complications of dialysis: infection. *Kidney Int Suppl* 1993;41:S143–S148.

58. Finkelstein ES, Jekel J, Troidle L, et al. Patterns of infection in patients maintained on long-term peritoneal dialysis therapy with multiple episodes of peritonitis. *Am J Kidney Dis* 2002;39(6):1278–1286.

59. Sedlacek M, Gemery JM, Cheung AL, et al. Aspirin treatment is associated with a significantly decreased risk of *Staphylococcus aureus* bacteremia in hemodialysis patients with tunneled catheters. *Am J Kidney Dis* 2007;49(3):401–408.

60. Saitoh H, Nakamura K, Hida M, et al. Urinary tract infection in oliguric patients with chronic renal failure. *J Urol* 1985;133(6):990–993.

61. Zoccali C, Mallamaci F, Tripepi G, et al. *Chlamydia pneumoniae*, overall and cardiovascular mortality in end-stage renal disease (ESRD). *Kidney Int* 2003;64(2):579–584.

62. Shu CC, Hsu CL, Lee CY, et al. Comparison of the prevalence of latent tuberculosis infection among non-dialysis patients with severe chronic kidney disease, patients receiving dialysis, and the dialysis-unit staff: a cross-sectional study. *PLoS One* 2015;10(4):e0124104.

63. Lundin AP, Adler AJ, Berlyne GM, et al. Tuberculosis in patients undergoing maintenance hemodialysis. *Am J Med* 1979;67(4):597–602.

64. Yang WF, Han F, Zhang XH, et al. Extra-pulmonary tuberculosis infection in the dialysis patients with end stage renal diseases: case reports and literature review. *J Zhejiang Univ Sci B* 2013;14(1):76–82.

65. Ganesh G, Shankaranarayanan D, Verma A, et al. Unusual presentation of a common disease in an ESRD patient. *Kidney Int* 2013; 84(5):1055.

66. Abdelrahman M, Sinha AK, Karkar A. Tuberculosis in end-stage renal disease patients on hemodialysis. *Hemodial Int* 2006;10(4):360–364.

67. Richardson RM. The diagnosis of tuberculosis in dialysis patients. *Semin Dial* 2012;25(4):419–422.

68. Craig RG, Spittle MA, Levin NW. Importance of periodontal disease in the kidney patient. *Blood Purif* 2002;20(1):113–119.

69. Aguilera A, Gonzalez-Espinoza L, Codoceo R, et al. Bowel bacterial overgrowth as another cause of malnutrition, inflammation, and atherosclerosis syndrome in peritoneal dialysis patients. *Adv Perit Dial* 2010;26:130–136.

70. Rajagopalan S, Dellegrottaglie S, Furniss AL, et al. Peripheral arterial disease in patients with end-stage renal disease: observations from the Dialysis Outcomes and Practice Patterns Study (DOPPS). *Circulation* 2006;114(18):1914–1922.

71. Carrero JJ, Stenvinkel P. Inflammation in end-stage renal disease—what have we learned in 10 years? *Semin Dial* 2010;23(5):498–509.

72. Yilmaz MI, Stenvinkel P, Sonmez A, et al. Vascular health, systemic inflammation and progressive reduction in kidney function: clinical determinants and impact on cardiovascular outcomes. *Nephrol Dial Transplant* 2011;26(11):3537–3543.

73. Betjes MG, Meijers RW, Litjens NH. Loss of renal function causes premature aging of the immune system. *Blood Purif* 2013;36(3–4): 173–178.

74. Jimenez R, Carracedo J, Santamaría R, et al. Replicative senescence in patients with chronic kidney failure. *Kidney Int* 2005;68(Suppl 99): S11–S15.

75. Shanahan CM. Mechanisms of vascular calcification in CKD-evidence for premature ageing? *Nat Rev Nephrol* 2013;9(11):661–670.

76. Suliman ME, Heimbürger O, Bárány P, et al. Plasma pentosidine is associated with inflammation and malnutrition in end-stage renal disease patients starting on dialysis therapy. *J Am Soc Nephrol* 2003;14(6): 1614–1622.

77. Tracey KJ. Fat meets the cholinergic antiinflammatory pathway. *J Exp Med* 2005;202(8):1017–1021.

78. Enia G, Mallamaci F, Benedetto FA, et al. Long-term CAPD patients are volume expanded and display more severe left ventricular hypertrophy than haemodialysis patients. *Nephrol Dial Transplant* 2001;16: 1459–1464.

79. Wang AY, Wang M, Woo J, et al. Inflammation, residual kidney function, and cardiac hypertrophy are interrelated and combine adversely to enhance mortality and cardiovascular death risk of peritoneal dialysis patients. *J Am Soc Nephrol* 2004;15(8):2186–2194.

80. van Tellingen A, Grooteman MP, Schoorl M, et al. Intercurrent clinical events are predictive of plasma C-reactive protein levels in hemodialysis patients. *Kidney Int* 2002;62(2):632–638.

81. López-Gómez JM, Pérez-Flores I, Jofré R, et al. Presence of a failed kidney transplant in patients who are on hemodialysis is associated with chronic inflammatory state and erythropoietin resistance. *J Am Soc Nephrol* 2004;15(9):2494–2501.

82. Szeto CC, Kwan BC, Chow KM, et al. Endotoxemia is related to systemic inflammation and atherosclerosis in peritoneal dialysis patients. *Clin J Am Soc Nephrol* 2008;3(2):431–436.

83. Reyes-Bahamonde J, Raimann JG, Thijssen S, et al. Fluid overload and inflammation—a vicious cycle. *Semin Dial* 2013;26(1):31–35.

84. Zaza G, Pontrelli P, Pertosa G, et al. Dialysis-related systemic microinflammation is associated with specific genomic patterns. *Nephrol Dial Transplant* 2008;23(5):1673–1681.

85. Schindler R, Boenisch O, Fischer C, et al. Effect of the hemodialysis membrane on the inflammatory reaction in vivo. *Clin Nephrol* 2000; 53(6):452–459.

86. Memoli B, Minutolo R, Bisesti V, et al. Changes of serum albumin and C-reactive protein are related to changes of interleukin-6 release by peripheral blood mononuclear cells in hemodialysis patients treated with different membranes. *Am J Kidney Dis* 2002;39(2):266–273.

87. Schindler R. Causes and therapy of microinflammation in renal failure. *Nephrol Dial Transplant* 2004;19(Suppl 5):V34–V40.

88. Ayus JC, Mizani MR, Achinger SG, et al. Effects of short daily versus conventional hemodialysis on left ventricular hypertrophy and inflammatory markers: a prospective, controlled study. *J Am Soc Nephrol* 2005;16(9):2778–2788.

89. Maduell F, Moreso F, Pons M, et al. High-efficiency postdilution online hemodiafiltration reduces all-cause mortality in hemodialysis patients. *J Am Soc Nephrol* 2013;24(3):487–497.

90. Lonnemann G. When good water goes bad: how it happens, clinical consequences and possible solutions. *Blood Purif* 2004;22(1):124–129.

91. Schindler R, Beck W, Deppisch R, et al. Short bacterial DNA fragments: detection in dialysate and induction of cytokines. *J Am Soc Nephrol* 2004;15(12):3207–3214.

92. Sitter T, Bergner A, Schiffl H. Dialysate related cytokine induction and response to recombinant human erythropoietin in haemodialysis patients. *Nephrol Dial Transplant* 2000;15(8):1207–1211.

93. Schiffl H, Lang SM, Stratakis D, et al. Effects of ultrapure dialysis fluid on nutritional status and inflammatory parameters. *Nephrol Dial Transplant* 2001;16(9):1863–1869.

94. Schiffl H, Lang SM, Fischer R. Ultrapure dialysis fluid slows loss of residual renal function in new dialysis patients. *Nephrol Dial Transplant* 2002;17(10):1814–1818.

95. Lederer SR, Schiffl H. Ultrapure dialysis fluid lowers the cardiovascular morbidity in patients on maintenance hemodialysis by reducing continuous microinflammation. *Nephron* 2002;91(3):452–455.

96. Ayus JC, Sheikh-Hamad D. Silent infection in clotted hemodialysis access grafts. *J Am Soc Nephrol* 1998;9(7):1314–1317.

97. Allon M, Depner TA, Radeva M, et al. Impact of dialysis dose and membrane on infection-related hospitalization and death: results of the HEMO Study. *J Am Soc Nephrol* 2003;14(7):1863–1870.

98. Cappelli G, Tetta C, Canaud B. Is biofilm a cause of silent chronic inflammation in haemodialysis patients? A fascinating working hypothesis. *Nephrol Dial Transplant* 2005;20(2):266–270.

99. Schwenger V, Morath C, Salava A, et al. Damage to the peritoneal membrane by glucose degradation products is mediated by the receptor for advanced glycation end-products. *J Am Soc Nephrol* 2006;17(1):199–207.

100. Himmelfarb J, Stenvinkel P, Ikizler TA, et al. The elephant in uremia: oxidant stress as a unifying concept of cardiovascular disease in uremia. *Kidney Int* 2002;62(5):1524–1538.

101. Chung SH, Heimbürger O, Stenvinkel P, et al. Influence of peritoneal transport rate, inflammation, and fluid removal on nutritional status and clinical outcome in prevalent peritoneal dialysis patients. *Perit Dial Int* 2003;23(2):174–183.

102. Sela S, Shurtz-Swirski R, Cohen-Mazor M, et al. Primed peripheral polymorphonuclear leukocyte: a culprit underlying chronic low-grade inflammation and systemic oxidative stress in chronic kidney disease. *J Am Soc Nephrol* 2005;16(8):2431–2438.

103. Ward RA, McLeish KR. Polymorphonuclear leukocyte oxidative burst is enhanced in patients with chronic renal insufficiency. *J Am Soc Nephrol* 1995;5(9):1697–1702.

104. Glorieux GL, Dhondt AW, Jacobs P, et al. In vitro study of the potential role of guanidines in leukocyte functions related to atherogenesis and infection. *Kidney Int* 2004;65(6):2184–2192.

105. Schepers E, Meert N, Glorieux G, et al. P-cresylsulphate, the main in vivo metabolite of p-cresol, activates leucocyte free radical production. *Nephrol Dial Transplant* 2007;22(2):592–596.

106. Bammens B, Evenepoel P, Verbeke K, et al. Impairment of small intestinal protein assimilation in patients with end-stage renal disease: extending the malnutrition-inflammation-atherosclerosis concept. *Am J Clin Nutr* 2004;80(6):1536–1543.

107. Huang X, Stenvinkel P, Qureshi AR, et al. Essential polyunsaturated fatty acids, inflammation and mortality in dialysis patients. *Nephrol Dial Transplant* 2012;27(9):3615–3620.

108. Cobo G, Gallar P, Gama-Axelsson T, et al. Clinical determinants of reduced physical activity in hemodialysis and peritoneal dialysis patients. *J Nephrol* 2014;28(4):503–510.

109. Araújo MV, Hong BY, Fava PL, et al. End stage renal disease as a modifier of the periodontal microbiome. *BMC Nephrol* 2015;16:80.

110. Chambrone L, Foz AM, Guglielmetti MR, et al. Periodontitis and chronic kidney disease: a systematic review of the association of diseases and the effect of periodontal treatment on estimated glomerular filtration rate. *J Clin Periodontol* 2013;40(5):443–456.

111. Akar H, Akar GC, Carrero JJ, et al. Systemic consequences of poor oral health in chronic kidney disease patients. *Clin J Am Soc Nephrol* 2011;6(1):218–226.

112. Craig RG, Kotanko P, Kamer AR, et al. Periodontal diseases—a modifiable source of systemic inflammation for the end-stage renal disease patient on haemodialysis therapy? *Nephrol Dial Transplant* 2007;22(2):312–315.

113. Anders HJ, Andersen K, Stecher B. The intestinal microbiota, a leaky gut, and abnormal immunity in kidney disease. *Kidney Int* 2013;83(6):1010–1016.

114. Evenepoel P, Meijers BK, Bammens BR, et al. Uremic toxins originating from colonic microbial metabolism. *Kidney Int* 2009;76 (Suppl 114):S12–S19.

115. Mafra D, Lobo JC, Barros AF, et al. Role of altered intestinal microbiota in systemic inflammation and cardiovascular disease in chronic kidney disease. *Future Microbiol* 2014;9(3):399–410.

116. Ramezani A, Raj DS. The gut microbiome, kidney disease, and targeted interventions. *J Am Soc Nephrol* 2014;25(4):657–670.

117. Magnusson M, Magnusson KE, Sundqvist T, et al. Impaired intestinal barrier function measured by differently sized polyethylene glycols in patients with chronic renal failure. *Gut* 1991;32(7):754–759.

118. Magnusson M, Magnusson KE, Sundqvist T, et al. Increased intestinal permeability to differently sized polyethylene glycols in uremic rats: effects of low- and high-protein diets. *Nephron* 1990;56(3):306–311.

119. Després JP, Lemieux I. Abdominal obesity and metabolic syndrome. *Nature* 2006;444(7121):881–887.

120. Wellen KE, Hotamisligil GS. Inflammation, stress, and diabetes. *J Clin Invest* 2005;115(5):1111–1119.

121. Maruyama Y, Nordfors L, Stenvinkel P, et al. Interleukin-1 gene cluster polymorphisms are associated with nutritional status and inflammation in patients with end-stage renal disease. *Blood Purif* 2005;23(5):384–393.

122. Weisberg SP, McCann D, Desai M, et al. Obesity is associated with macrophage accumulation in adipose tissue. *J Clin Invest* 2003; 112(12):1796–1808.

123. Axelsson J, Rashid Qureshi A, Suliman ME, et al. Truncal fat mass as a contributor to inflammation in end-stage renal disease. *Am J Clin Nutr* 2004;80(5):1222–1229.

124. Cordeiro AC, Qureshi AR, Stenvinkel P, et al. Abdominal fat deposition is associated with increased inflammation, protein-energy wasting and worse outcome in patients undergoing haemodialysis. *Nephrol Dial Transplant* 2010;25(2):562–568.

125. Cordeiro AC, Qureshi AR, Lindholm B, et al. Visceral fat and coronary artery calcification in patients with chronic kidney disease. *Nephrol Dial Transplant* 2013;28(Suppl 4):iv152–iv159.

126. Cordeiro AC, Amparo FC, Oliveira MA, et al. Epicardial fat accumulation, cardiometabolic profile and cardiovascular events in patients with stages 3-5 chronic kidney disease. *J Intern Med* 2015;278(1):77–87.

127. Xu H, Sjögren P, Ärnlöv J, et al. A proinflammatory diet is associated with systemic inflammation and reduced kidney function in elderly adults. *J Nutr* 2015;145(4):729–735.

128. Akber A, Portale AA, Johansen KL. Pedometer-assessed physical activity in children and young adults with CKD. *Clin J Am Soc Nephrol* 2012;7(5):720–726.

129. Viana JL, Kosmadakis GC, Watson EL, et al. Evidence for anti-inflammatory effects of exercise in CKD. *J Am Soc Nephrol* 2014;25(9):2121–2130.

130. Zoccali C, Mallamaci F, Tripepi G. Sleep apnea in renal patients. *J Am Soc Nephrol* 2001;12(12):2854–2859.

131. Arnson Y, Shoenfeld Y, Amital H. Effects of tobacco smoke on immunity, inflammation and autoimmunity. *J Autoimmun* 2010;34(3):J258–J265.

132. Rom O, Avezov K, Aizenbud D, et al. Cigarette smoking and inflammation revisited. *Respir Physiol Neurobiol* 2013;187(1):5–10.

133. Kronenberg F, Neyer U, Lhotta K, et al. The low molecular weight apo(a) phenotype is an independent predictor for coronary artery disease in hemodialysis patients: a prospective follow-up. *J Am Soc Nephrol* 1999;10(5):1027–1036.

134. Rao M, Wong C, Kanetsky P, et al. Cytokine gene polymorphism and progression of renal and cardiovascular diseases. *Kidney Int* 2007;72(5):549–556.

135. Liu Y, Berthier-Schaad Y, Fallin MD, et al. IL-6 haplotypes, inflammation, and risk for cardiovascular disease in a multiethnic dialysis cohort. *J Am Soc Nephrol* 2006;17(3):863–870.

136. Liu Y, Berthier-Schaad Y, Plantinga L, et al. Functional variants in the lymphotoxin-alpha gene predict cardiovascular disease in dialysis patients. *J Am Soc Nephrol* 2006;17(11):3158–3166.

137. Gillerot G, Goffin E, Michel C, et al. Genetic and clinical factors influence the baseline permeability of the peritoneal membrane. *Kidney Int* 2005;67(6):2477–2487.

138. Balakrishnan VS, Guo D, Rao M, et al. Cytokine gene polymorphisms in hemodialysis patients: association with comorbidity, functionality, and serum albumin. *Kidney Int* 2004;65(4):1449–1460.

139. Girndt M, Sester U, Sester M, et al. The interleukin-10 promoter genotype determines clinical immune function in hemodialysis patients. *Kidney Int* 2001;60(6):2385–2391.

140. Pecoits-Filho R, Stenvinkel P, Marchlewska A, et al. A functional variant of the myeloperoxidase gene is associated with cardiovascular disease in end-stage renal disease patients. *Kidney Int Suppl* 2003;63(Suppl 84):S172–S176.

141. Yao Q, Nordfors L, Axelsson J, et al. Peroxisome proliferator-activated receptor gamma polymorphisms affect systemic inflammation and survival in end-stage renal disease patients starting renal replacement therapy. *Atherosclerosis* 2005;182(1):105–111.

142. Zhang L, Kao WH, Berthier-Schaad Y, et al. C-Reactive protein haplotype predicts serum C-reactive protein levels but not cardiovascular disease risk in a dialysis cohort. *Am J Kidney Dis* 2007;49(1):118–126.

143. Carrero JJ, Stenvinkel P, Fellström B, et al. Telomere attrition is associated with inflammation, low fetuin-A levels and high mortality in prevalent haemodialysis patients. *J Intern Med* 2008;263(3):302–312.

144. Benetti R, García-Cao M, Blasco MA. Telomere length regulates the epigenetic status of mammalian telomeres and subtelomeres. *Nat Genet* 2007;39(2):243–250.

145. Wong JS, Port FK, Hulbert-Shearon TE, et al. Survival advantage in Asian American end-stage renal disease patients. *Kidney Int* 1999; 55(6):2515–2523.

146. Pankow JS, Folsom AR, Cushman M, et al. Familial and genetic determinants of systemic markers of inflammation: the NHLBI family heart study. *Atherosclerosis* 2001;154(3):681–689.

147. Westendorp RG, Langermans JA, Huizinga TW, et al. Genetic influence on cytokine production in meningococcal disease. *Lancet* 1997;349(9069):1912–1913.

148. Luttropp K, Stenvinkel P, Carrero JJ, et al. Understanding the role of genetic polymorphisms in chronic kidney disease. *Pediatr Nephrol* 2008;23(11):1941–1949.

149. Luttropp K, Lindholm B, Carrero JJ, et al. Genetics/genomics in chronic kidney disease—towards personalized medicine? *Semin Dial* 2009;22(4):417–422.

150. Yeun JY, Levine RA, Mantadilok V, et al. C-Reactive protein predicts all-cause and cardiovascular mortality in hemodialysis patients. *Am J Kidney Dis* 2000;35(3):469–476.

151. Zimmermann J, Herrlinger S, Pruy A, et al. Inflammation enhances cardiovascular risk and mortality in hemodialysis patients. *Kidney Int* 1999;55(2):648–658.

152. Iseki K, Tozawa M, Yoshi S, et al. Serum C-reactive protein (CRP) and risk of death in chronic dialysis patients. *Nephrol Dial Transplant* 1999;14(8):1956–1960.

153. Noh H, Lee SW, Kang SW, et al. Serum C-reactive protein: a predictor of mortality in continuous ambulatory peritoneal dialysis patients. *Perit Dial Int* 1998;18(4):387–394.

154. Ducloux D, Bresson-Vautrin C, Kribs M, et al. C-reactive protein and cardiovascular disease in peritoneal dialysis patients. *Kidney Int* 2002;62(4):1417–1422.

155. Wang AY, Woo J, Lam CW, et al. Is a single time point C-reactive protein predictive of outcome in peritoneal dialysis patients? *J Am Soc Nephrol* 2003;14(7):1871–1879.

156. Varagunam M, Finney H, Trevitt R, et al. Pretransplantation levels of C-reactive protein predict all-cause and cardiovascular mortality, but not graft outcome, in kidney transplant recipients. *Am J Kidney Dis* 2004;43(3):502–507.

157. Menon V, Greene T, Wang X, et al. C-reactive protein and albumin as predictors of all-cause and cardiovascular mortality in chronic kidney disease. *Kidney Int* 2005;68(2):766–772.

158. Stenvinkel P, Carrero JJ, Axelsson J, et al. Emerging biomarkers for evaluating cardiovascular risk in the chronic kidney disease patient: how do new pieces fit into the uremic puzzle? *Clin J Am Soc Nephrol* 2008;3(2):505–521.

159. Meier-Ewert HK, Ridker PM, Rifai N, et al. Absence of diurnal variation of C-reactive protein concentrations in healthy human subjects. *Clin Chem* 2001;47(3):426–430.

160. Kawaguchi T, Tong L, Robinson BM, et al. C-reactive protein and mortality in hemodialysis patients: the Dialysis Outcomes and Practice Patterns Study (DOPPS). *Nephron Clin Pract* 2011;117(2):c167–c178.

161. Meuwese CL, Stenvinkel P, Dekker FW, et al. Monitoring of inflammation in patients on dialysis: forewarned is forearmed. *Nat Rev Nephrol* 2011;7(3):166–176.

162. Meuwese CL, Snaedal S, Halbesma N, et al. Trimestral variations of C-reactive protein, interleukin-6 and tumour necrosis factor-α are similarly associated with survival in haemodialysis patients. *Nephrol Dial Transplant* 2011;26(4):1313–1318.

163. Snaedal S, Heimbürger O, Qureshi AR, et al. Comorbidity and acute clinical events as determinants of C-reactive protein variation in hemodialysis patients: implications for patient survival. *Am J Kidney Dis* 2009;53(6):1024–1033.

164. Stenvinkel P, Barany P, Heimbürger O, et al. Mortality, malnutrition, and atherosclerosis in ESRD: what is the role of interleukin-6? *Kidney Int Suppl* 2002;61(Suppl 80):103–108.

165. Zoccali C, Tripepi G, Mallamaci F. Dissecting inflammation in ESRD: do cytokines and C-reactive protein have a complementary prognostic value for mortality in dialysis patients? *J Am Soc Nephrol* 2006;17(12 Suppl 3):S169–S173.

166. Zhang W, He J, Zhang F, et al. Prognostic role of C-reactive protein and interleukin-6 in dialysis patients: a systematic review and meta-analysis. *J Nephrol* 2013;26(2):243–253.

167. Gewurz H, Zhang XH, Lint TF. Structure and function of the pentraxins. *Curr Opin Immunol* 1995;7(1):54–64.

168. Steel DM, Whitehead AS. The major acute phase reactants: C-reactive protein, serum amyloid P component and serum amyloid A protein. *Immunol Today* 1994;15(2):81–88.

169. Breviario F, d'Aniello EM, Golay J, et al. Interleukin-1-inducible genes in endothelial cells. Cloning of a new gene related to C-reactive protein and serum amyloid P component. *J Biol Chem* 1992;267(31):22190–22197.

170. Alles VV, Bottazzi B, Peri G, et al. Inducible expression of PTX3, a new member of the pentraxin family, in human mononuclear phagocytes. *Blood* 1994;84(10):3483–3493.

171. Mantovani A, Garlanda C, Bottazzi B, et al. The long pentraxin PTX3 in vascular pathology. *Vascul Pharmacol* 2006;45(5):326–330.

172. Witasp A, Rydén M, Carrero JJ, et al. Elevated circulating levels and tissue expression of pentraxin 3 in uremia: a reflection of endothelial dysfunction. *PLoS One* 2013;8(5):e63493.

173. Boehme M, Kaehne F, Kuehne A, et al. Pentraxin 3 is elevated in haemodialysis patients and is associated with cardiovascular disease. *Nephrol Dial Transplant* 2007;22(8):2224–2229.

174. Tong M, Carrero JJ, Qureshi AR, et al. Plasma pentraxin 3 in patients with chronic kidney disease: associations with renal function, protein-energy wasting, cardiovascular disease, and mortality. *Clin J Am Soc Nephrol* 2007;2(5):889–897.

175. Chicheportiche Y, Bourdon PR, Xu H, et al. TWEAK, a new secreted ligand in the tumor necrosis factor family that weakly induces apoptosis. *J Biol Chem* 1997;272(51):32401–32410.

176. Winkles JA. The TWEAK-Fn14 cytokine-receptor axis: discovery, biology and therapeutic targeting. *Nat Rev Drug Discov* 2008;7(5):411–425.

177. Wiley SR, Winkles JA. TWEAK, a member of the TNF superfamily, is a multifunctional cytokine that binds the TweakR/Fn14 receptor. *Cytokine Growth Factor Rev* 2003;14(3–4):241–249.

178. Desplat-Jégo S, Varriale S, Creidy R, et al. TWEAK is expressed by glial cells, induces astrocyte proliferation and increases EAE severity. *J Neuroimmunol* 2002;133(1–2):116–123.

179. Lynch CN, Wang YC, Lund JK, et al. TWEAK induces angiogenesis and proliferation of endothelial cells. *J Biol Chem* 1999;274(13):8455–8459.

180. Polek TC, Talpaz M, Darnay BG, et al. TWEAK mediates signal transduction and differentiation of RAW264.7 cells in the absence of Fn14/TweakR. Evidence for a second TWEAK receptor. *J Biol Chem* 2003;278(34):32317–32323.

181. Ho DH, Vu H, Brown SA, et al. Soluble tumor necrosis factor-like weak inducer of apoptosis overexpression in HEK293 cells promotes tumor growth and angiogenesis in athymic nude mice. *Cancer Res* 2004;64(24):8968–8972.

182. Justo P, Sanz AB, Sanchez-Niño MD, et al. Cytokine cooperation in renal tubular cell injury: the role of TWEAK. *Kidney Int* 2006; 70(10):1750–1758.

183. Maecker H, Varfolomeev E, Kischkel F, et al. TWEAK attenuates the transition from innate to adaptive immunity. *Cell* 2005;123(5):931–944.

184. Kim SH, Kang YJ, Kim WJ, et al. TWEAK can induce pro-inflammatory cytokines and matrix metalloproteinase-9 in macrophages. *Circ J* 2004;68(4):396–399.

185. Saas P, Boucraut J, Walker PR, et al. TWEAK stimulation of astrocytes and the proinflammatory consequences. *Glia* 2000;32(1):102–107.

186. Carrero JJ, Ortiz A, Qureshi AR, et al. Additive effects of soluble TWEAK and inflammation on mortality in hemodialysis patients. *Clin J Am Soc Nephrol* 2009;4(1):110–118.

187. Stenvinkel P. Inflammation in end-stage renal disease: the hidden enemy. *Nephrology (Carlton)* 2006;11(1):36–41.

188. Carrero JJ, Stenvinkel P, Cuppari L, et al. Etiology of the protein-energy wasting syndrome in chronic kidney disease: a consensus statement from the International Society of Renal Nutrition and Metabolism (ISRNM). *J Ren Nutr* 2013;23(2):77–90.

189. Xu H, Watanabe M, Qureshi AR, et al. Oxidative DNA damage and mortality in hemodialysis and peritoneal dialysis patients. *Perit Dial Int* 2015;35(2):206–215.

190. Xu H, Huang X, Arnlöv J, et al. Clinical correlates of insulin sensitivity and its association with mortality among men with CKD stages 3 and 4. *Clin J Am Soc Nephrol* 2014;9(4):690–697.

191. Ghanavatian S, Diep LM, Bárány P, et al. Subclinical atherosclerosis, endothelial function, and serum inflammatory markers in chronic kidney disease stages 3 to 4. *Angiology* 2014;65(5):443–449.

192. Suliman ME, García-López E, Anderstam B, et al. Vascular calcification inhibitors in relation to cardiovascular disease with special emphasis on fetuin-A in chronic kidney disease. *Adv Clin Chem* 2008; 46:217–262.

193. Abe M, Okada K, Soma M. Mineral metabolic abnormalities and mortality in dialysis patients. *Nutrients* 2013;5(3):1002–1023.

194. Kalender B, Ozdemir AC, Koroglu G. Association of depression with markers of nutrition and inflammation in chronic kidney disease and end-stage renal disease. *Nephron Clin Pract* 2006;102(3–4):c115–c121.

195. Carrero JJ, Stenvinkel P. Persistent inflammation as a catalyst for other risk factors in chronic kidney disease: a hypothesis proposal. *Clin J Am Soc Nephrol* 2009;4(Suppl 1):S49–S55.

196. Stenvinkel P, Heimbürger O, Lindholm B. Wasting, but not malnutrition, predicts cardiovascular mortality in end-stage renal disease. *Nephrol Dial Transplant* 2004;19(9):2181–2183.

197. Pupim LB, Ikizler TA. Uremic malnutrition: new insights into an old problem. *Semin Dial* 2003;16(3):224–232.

198. Pecoits-Filho R, Bárány P, Lindholm B, et al. Interleukin-6 is an independent predictor of mortality in patients starting dialysis treatment. *Nephrol Dial Transplant* 2002;17(9):1684–1688.

199. Carrero JJ, Chmielewski M, Axelsson J, et al. Muscle atrophy, inflammation and clinical outcome in incident and prevalent dialysis patients. *Clin Nutr* 2008;27(4):557–564.

200. Johansen KL, Kaysen GA, Young BS, et al. Longitudinal study of nutritional status, body composition, and physical function in hemodialysis patients. *Am J Clin Nutr* 2003;77(4):842–846.

201. Raj DS, Dominic EA, Pai A, et al. Skeletal muscle, cytokines, and oxidative stress in end-stage renal disease. *Kidney Int* 2005;68(5):2338–2344.

202. Garibotto G, Sofia A, Procopio V, et al. Peripheral tissue release of interleukin-6 in patients with chronic kidney diseases: effects of end-stage renal disease and microinflammatory state. *Kidney Int* 2006; 70(2):384–390.

203. Goodman MN. Interleukin-6 induces skeletal muscle protein breakdown in rats. *Proc Soc Exp Biol Med* 1994;205(2):182–185.

204. Strassmann G, Fong M, Kenney JS, et al. Evidence for the involvement of interleukin 6 in experimental cancer cachexia. *J Clin Invest* 1992;89(5):1681–1684.

205. Barbieri M, Ferrucci L, Ragno E, et al. Chronic inflammation and the effect of IGF-I on muscle strength and power in older persons. *Am J Physiol Endocrinol Metab* 2003;284(3):E481–E487.

206. Carrero JJ. Identification of patients with eating disorders: clinical and biochemical signs of appetite loss in dialysis patients. *J Ren Nutr* 2009;19(1):10–15.

207. Carrero JJ, Qureshi AR, Axelsson J, et al. Comparison of nutritional and inflammatory markers in dialysis patients with reduced appetite. *Am J Clin Nutr* 2007;85(3):695–701.

208. Kalantar-Zadeh K, Block G, McAllister CJ, et al. Appetite and inflammation, nutrition, anemia, and clinical outcome in hemodialysis patients. *Am J Clin Nutr* 2004;80(2):299–307.

209. Plata-Salamán CR. Cytokines and feeding. *Int J Obes Relat Metab Disord* 2001;25(Suppl 5):S48–S52.

210. Carrero JJ, Aguilera A, Stenvinkel P, et al. Appetite disorders in uremia. *J Ren Nutr* 2008;18(1):107–113.

211. Pupim LB, Flakoll PJ, Majchrzak KM, et al. Increased muscle protein breakdown in chronic hemodialysis patients with type 2 diabetes mellitus. *Kidney Int* 2005;68(4):1857–1865.

212. Pupim LB, Heimbürger O, Qureshi AR, et al. Accelerated lean body mass loss in incident chronic dialysis patients with diabetes mellitus. *Kidney Int* 2005;68(5):2368–2374.

213. Haffner SM. The metabolic syndrome: inflammation, diabetes mellitus, and cardiovascular disease. *Am J Cardiol* 2006;97(2A):3A–11A.

214. Hotamisligil GS, Shargill NS, Spiegelman BM. Adipose expression of tumor necrosis factor-alpha: direct role in obesity-linked insulin resistance. *Science* 1993;259(5091):87–91.

215. Mitch WE, Du J, Bailey JL, et al. Mechanisms causing muscle proteolysis in uremia: the influence of insulin and cytokines. *Miner Electrolyte Metab* 1999;25(4–6):216–219.

216. Plata-Salamán CR. Cytokines and anorexia: a brief overview. *Semin Oncol* 1998;25(1 Suppl 1):64–72.

217. Chioléro R, Revelly JP, Tappy L. Energy metabolism in sepsis and injury. *Nutrition* 1997;13(9 Suppl):45S–51S.

218. Kamimura MA, Draibe SA, Avesani CM, et al. Resting energy expenditure and its determinants in hemodialysis patients. *Eur J Clin Nutr* 2007;61(3):362–367.

219. Utaka S, Avesani CM, Draibe SA, et al. Inflammation is associated with increased energy expenditure in patients with chronic kidney disease. *Am J Clin Nutr* 2005;82(4):801–805.

220. Kimmel PL, Peterson RA, Weihs KL, et al. Multiple measurements of depression predict mortality in a longitudinal study of chronic hemodialysis outpatients. *Kidney Int* 2000;57(5):2093–2098.

221. Riezebos RK, Nauta KJ, Honig A, et al. The association of depressive symptoms with survival in a Dutch cohort of patients with end-stage renal disease. *Nephrol Dial Transplant* 2010;25(1):231–236.

222. Chilcot J, Wellsted D, Vilar E, et al. An association between residual renal function and depression symptoms in haemodialysis patients. *Nephron Clin Pract* 2009;113(2):c117–c124.

223. Schiepers OJ, Wichers MC, Maes M. Cytokines and major depression. *Prog Neuropsychopharmacol Biol Psychiatry* 2005;29(2):201–217.

224. Sonikian M, Metaxaki P, Papavasileiou D, et al. Effects of interleukin-6 on depression risk in dialysis patients. *Am J Nephrol* 2010;31(4):303–308.

225. Montinaro V, Iaffaldano GP, Granata S, et al. Emotional symptoms, quality of life and cytokine profile in hemodialysis patients. *Clin Nephrol* 2010;73(1):36–43.

226. Preljevic VT, Østhus TB, Sandvik L, et al. Psychiatric disorders, body mass index and C-reactive protein in dialysis patients. *Gen Hosp Psychiatry* 2011;33(5):454–461.

227. Lee SK, Lee HS, Lee TB, et al. The effects of antidepressant treatment on serum cytokines and nutritional status in hemodialysis patients. *J Korean Med Sci* 2004;19(3):384–389.

228. Jhamb M, Argyropoulos C, Steel JL, et al. Correlates and outcomes of fatigue among incident dialysis patients. *Clin J Am Soc Nephrol* 2009;4(11):1779–1786.

229. Raggi P. Coronary calcium on electron beam tomography imaging as a surrogate marker of coronary artery disease. *Am J Cardiol* 2001;87(4A):27A–34A.

230. Schwarz U, Buzello M, Ritz E, et al. Morphology of coronary atherosclerotic lesions in patients with end-stage renal failure. *Nephrol Dial Transplant* 2000;15(2):218–223.

231. Sigrist M, Bungay P, Taal MW, et al. Vascular calcification and cardiovascular function in chronic kidney disease. *Nephrol Dial Transplant* 2006;21(3):707–714.

232. Fox CS, Larson MG, Vasan RS, et al. Cross-sectional association of kidney function with valvular and annular calcification: the Framingham heart study. *J Am Soc Nephrol* 2006;17(2):521–527.

233. Civilibal M, Caliskan S, Adaletli I, et al. Coronary artery calcifications in children with end-stage renal disease. *Pediatr Nephrol* 2006; 21(10):1426–1433.

234. London GM, Guérin AP, Verbeke FH, et al. Mineral metabolism and arterial functions in end-stage renal disease: potential role of 25-hydroxyvitamin D deficiency. *J Am Soc Nephrol* 2007;18(2):613–620.

235. Raggi P, Bellasi A, Ferramosca E, et al. Association of pulse wave velocity with vascular and valvular calcification in hemodialysis patients. *Kidney Int* 2007;71(8):802–807.

236. Blacher J, Guerin AP, Pannier B, et al. Impact of aortic stiffness on survival in end-stage renal disease. *Circulation* 1999;99(18):2434–2439.

237. London GM, Pannier B, Agharazii M, et al. Forearm reactive hyperemia and mortality in end-stage renal disease. *Kidney Int* 2004; 65(2):700–704.

238. Wang AY, Wang M, Woo J, et al. Cardiac valve calcification as an important predictor for all-cause mortality and cardiovascular mortality in long-term peritoneal dialysis patients: a prospective study. *J Am Soc Nephrol* 2003;14(1):159–168.

239. Blacher J, Guerin AP, Pannier B, et al. Arterial calcifications, arterial stiffness, and cardiovascular risk in end-stage renal disease. *Hypertension* 2001;38(4):938–942.

240. Tintut Y, Patel J, Parhami F, et al. Tumor necrosis factor-alpha promotes in vitro calcification of vascular cells via the cAMP pathway. *Circulation* 2000;102(21):2636–2642.

241. Tintut Y, Patel J, Territo M, et al. Monocyte/macrophage regulation of vascular calcification in vitro. *Circulation* 2002;105(5):650–655.

242. Collin-Osdoby P. Regulation of vascular calcification by osteoclast regulatory factors RANKL and osteoprotegerin. *Circ Res* 2004; 95(11):1046–1057.

243. Mangan SH, Van Campenhout A, Rush C, et al. Osteoprotegerin upregulates endothelial cell adhesion molecule response to tumor necrosis factor-alpha associated with induction of angiopoietin-2. *Cardiovasc Res* 2007;76(3):494–505.

244. Morena M, Terrier N, Jaussent I, et al. Plasma osteoprotegerin is associated with mortality in hemodialysis patients. *J Am Soc Nephrol* 2006;17(1):262–270.

245. Nadra I, Mason JC, Philippidis P, et al. Proinflammatory activation of macrophages by basic calcium phosphate crystals via protein kinase C and MAP kinase pathways: a vicious cycle of inflammation and arterial calcification? *Circ Res* 2005;96(12):1248–1256.

246. Schafer C, Heiss A, Schwarz A, et al. The serum protein alpha 2-Heremans-Schmid glycoprotein/fetuin-A is a systemically acting inhibitor of ectopic calcification. *J Clin Invest* 2003;112(3):357–366.

247. Ketteler M, Bongartz P, Westenfeld R, et al. Association of low fetuin-A (AHSG) concentrations in serum with cardiovascular mortality in patients on dialysis: a cross-sectional study. *Lancet* 2003;361(9360):827–833.

248. Stenvinkel P, Wang K, Qureshi AR, et al. Low fetuin-A levels are associated with cardiovascular death: impact of variations in the gene encoding fetuin. *Kidney Int* 2005;67(6):2383–2392.

249. Hermans MM, Brandenburg V, Ketteler M, et al. Association of serum fetuin-A levels with mortality in dialysis patients. *Kidney Int* 2007;72(2):202–207.

250. Gangneux C, Daveau M, Hiron M, et al. The inflammation-induced down-regulation of plasma Fetuin-A (alpha2HS-Glycoprotein) in liver results from the loss of interaction between long C/EBP isoforms at two neighbouring binding sites. *Nucleic Acids Res* 2003;31(20): 5957–5970.

251. Moe SM, Chen NX. Inflammation and vascular calcification. *Blood Purif* 2005;23(1):64–71.

252. Wang AY, Woo J, Lam CW, et al. Associations of serum fetuin-A with malnutrition, inflammation, atherosclerosis and valvular calcification syndrome and outcome in peritoneal dialysis patients. *Nephrol Dial Transplant* 2005;20(8):1676–1685.

253. Ros S, Carrero JJ. Endocrine alterations and cardiovascular risk in CKD: is there a link? *Nefrologia* 2013;33(2):181–187.

254. Chopra IJ. Nonthyroidal illness syndrome or euthyroid sick syndrome? *Endocr Pract* 1996;2(1):45–52.

255. Kaptein EM. Thyroid hormone metabolism and thyroid diseases in chronic renal failure. *Endocr Rev* 1996;17(1):45–63.

256. Lo JC, Chertow GM, Go AS, et al. Increased prevalence of subclinical and clinical hypothyroidism in persons with chronic kidney disease. *Kidney Int* 2005;67(3):1047–1052.

257. Zoccali C, Benedetto F, Mallamaci F, et al. Low triiodothyronine and cardiomyopathy in patients with end-stage renal disease. *J Hypertens* 2006;24(10):2039–2046.

258. Enia G, Panuccio V, Cutrupi S, et al. Subclinical hypothyroidism is linked to micro-inflammation and predicts death in continuous ambulatory peritoneal dialysis. *Nephrol Dial Transplant* 2007;22(2): 538–544.

259. Carrero JJ, Qureshi AR, Axelsson J, et al. Clinical and biochemical implications of low thyroid hormone levels (total and free forms) in euthyroid patients with chronic kidney disease. *J Intern Med* 2007; 262(6):690–701.

260. Zoccali C, Tripepi G, Cutrupi S, et al. Low triiodothyronine: a new facet of inflammation in end-stage renal disease. *J Am Soc Nephrol* 2005;16(9):2789–2795.

261. Torpy DJ, Tsigos C, Lotsikas AJ, et al. Acute and delayed effects of a single-dose injection of interleukin-6 on thyroid function in healthy humans. *Metabolism* 1998;47(10):1289–1293.

262. Bartalena L, Brogioni S, Grasso L, et al. Relationship of the increased serum interleukin-6 concentration to changes of thyroid function in nonthyroidal illness. *J Endocrinol Invest* 1994;17(4):269–274.

263. Bello AK, Stenvinkel P, Lin M, et al. Serum testosterone levels and clinical outcomes in male hemodialysis patients. *Am J Kidney Dis* 2014;63(2):268–275.

264. Carrero JJ. Testosterone deficiency at the crossroads of cardiometabolic complications in CKD. *Am J Kidney Dis* 2014;64(3):322–325.

265. Carrero JJ, Stenvinkel P. The vulnerable man: impact of testosterone deficiency on the uraemic phenotype. *Nephrol Dial Transplant* 2012;27(11):4030–4041.

266. Fukata J, Imura H, Nakao K. Cytokines as mediators in the regulation of the hypothalamic-pituitary-adrenocortical function. *J Endocrinol Invest* 1994;17(2):141–155.

267. Jones TH, Kennedy RL. Cytokines and hypothalamic-pituitary function. *Cytokine* 1993;5(6):531–538.

268. Carrero JJ, Qureshi AR, Nakashima A, et al. Prevalence and clinical implications of testosterone deficiency in men with end-stage renal disease. *Nephrol Dial Transplant* 2011;26(1):184–190.

269. Carrero JJ, Qureshi AR, Parini P, et al. Low serum testosterone increases mortality risk among male dialysis patients. *J Am Soc Nephrol* 2009;20(3):613–620.

270. Kyriazis J, Tzanakis I, Stylianou K, et al. Low serum testosterone, arterial stiffness and mortality in male haemodialysis patients. *Nephrol Dial Transplant* 2011;26(9):2971–2977.

271. Karakitsos D, Patrianakos AP, De Groot E, et al. Androgen deficiency and endothelial dysfunction in men with end-stage kidney disease receiving maintenance hemodialysis. *Am J Nephrol* 2006;26(6): 536–543.

272. Kalinchenko SY, Tishova YA, Mskhalaya GJ, et al. Effects of testosterone supplementation on markers of the metabolic syndrome and inflammation in hypogonadal men with the metabolic syndrome: the double-blinded placebo-controlled Moscow study. *Clin Endocrinol (Oxf)* 2010;73(5):602–612.

273. Malkin CJ, Pugh PJ, Jones RD, et al. The effect of testosterone replacement on endogenous inflammatory cytokines and lipid profiles in hypogonadal men. *J Clin Endocrinol Metab* 2004;89(7):3313–3318.

274. Corrales JJ, Almeida M, Burgo R, et al. Androgen-replacement therapy depresses the ex vivo production of inflammatory cytokines by circulating antigen-presenting cells in aging type-2 diabetic men with partial androgen deficiency. *J Endocrinol* 2006;189(3):595–604.

275. Cooney RN, Shumate M. The inhibitory effects of interleukin-1 on growth hormone action during catabolic illness. *Vitam Horm* 2006;74:317–340.

276. Garibotto G, Russo R, Sofia A, et al. Effects of uremia and inflammation on growth hormone resistance in patients with chronic kidney diseases. *Kidney Int* 2008;74(7):937–945.

277. Machowska A, Carrero JJ, Lindholm B, et al. Therapeutics targeting persistent inflammation in chronic kidney disease. *Transl Res* 2015; 167(1):204–213.

278. Leurs P, Lindholm B, Stenvinkel P. Effects of hemodiafiltration on uremic inflammation. *Blood Purif* 2013;35(Suppl 1):11–17.

279. Ortega O, Rodriguez I, Gracia C, et al. Strict volume control and longitudinal changes in cardiac biomarker levels in hemodialysis patients. *Nephron Clin Pract* 2009;113(2):c96–c103.

280. Xu H, Huang X, Risérus U, et al. Dietary fiber, kidney function, inflammation, and mortality risk. *Clin J Am Soc Nephrol* 2014;9(12):2104–2110.

281. Stenvinkel P. Can treating persistent inflammation limit protein energy wasting? *Semin Dial* 2013;26(1):16–19.

282. Sabry AA, Elshafey EM, Alsaran K, et al. The level of C-reactive protein in chronic hemodialysis patients: a comparative study between patients with noninfected catheters and arteriovenous fistula in two large Gulf hemodialysis centers. *Hemodial Int* 2014;18(3):674–679.

283. Gielen S, Adams V, Möbius-Winkler S, et al. Anti-inflammatory effects of exercise training in the skeletal muscle of patients with chronic heart failure. *J Am Coll Cardiol* 2003;42(5):861–868.

284. Castaneda C, Gordon PL, Parker RC, et al. Resistance training to reduce the malnutrition-inflammation complex syndrome of chronic kidney disease. *Am J Kidney Dis* 2004;43(4):607–616.

285. Cardozo LF, Pedruzzi LM, Stenvinkel P, et al. Nutritional strategies to modulate inflammation and oxidative stress pathways via activation of the master antioxidant switch Nrf2. *Biochimie* 2013;95(8):1525–1533.

286. Friedman AN, Moe SM, Perkins SM, et al. Fish consumption and omega-3 fatty acid status and determinants in long-term hemodialysis. *Am J Kidney Dis* 2006;47(6):1064–1071.

287. Friedman A, Moe S. Review of the effects of omega-3 supplementation in dialysis patients. *Clin J Am Soc Nephrol* 2006;1(2):182–192.

288. Saifullah A, Watkins BA, Saha C, et al. Oral fish oil supplementation raises blood omega-3 levels and lowers C-reactive protein in haemodialysis patients—a pilot study. *Nephrol Dial Transplant* 2007;22(12):3561–3567.

289. Ershler WB, Keller ET. Age-associated increased interleukin-6 gene expression, late-life diseases, and frailty. *Annu Rev Med* 2000;51:245–270.

290. Fanti P, Asmis R, Stephenson TJ, et al. Positive effect of dietary soy in ESRD patients with systemic inflammation—correlation between blood levels of the soy isoflavones and the acute-phase reactants. *Nephrol Dial Transplant* 2006;21(8):2239–2246.

291. Saldanha JF, Leal Vde O, Stenvinkel P, et al. Resveratrol: why is it a promising therapy for chronic kidney disease patients? *Oxid Med Cell Longev* 2013;2013:963217.

292. Liang J, Tian S, Han J, et al. Resveratrol as a therapeutic agent for renal fibrosis induced by unilateral ureteral obstruction. *Ren Fail* 2014;36(2):285–291.

293. Lappas M, Permezel M, Rice GE. N-Acetyl-cysteine inhibits phospholipid metabolism, proinflammatory cytokine release, protease activity, and nuclear factor-kappaB deoxyribonucleic acid-binding activity in human fetal membranes in vitro. *J Clin Endocrinol Metab* 2003;88(4):1723–1729.

294. Jiang Q, Elson-Schwab I, Courtemanche C, et al. γ-Tocopherol and its major metabolite, in contrast to α-tocopherol, inhibit cyclooxygenase activity in macrophages and epithelial cells. *Proc Natl Acad Sci U S A* 2000;97(21):11494–11499.

295. Scholze A, Rinder C, Beige J, et al. Acetylcysteine reduces plasma homocysteine concentration and improves pulse pressure and endothelial function in patients with end-stage renal failure. *Circulation* 2004;109(3):369–374.

296. Kinlay S, Fang JC, Hikita H, et al. Plasma α-tocopherol and coronary endothelium-dependent vasodilator function. *Circulation* 1999; 100(3):219–221.

297. Tepel M, van der Giet M, Statz M, et al. The antioxidant acetylcysteine reduces cardiovascular events in patients with end-stage renal failure: a randomized, controlled trial. *Circulation* 2003;107(7):992–995.

298. Boaz M, Smetana S, Weinstein T, et al. Secondary prevention with antioxidants of cardiovascular disease in endstage renal disease (SPACE): randomised placebo-controlled trial. *Lancet* 2000;356(9237):1213–1218.

299. Himmelfarb J, Phinney S, Ikizler TA, et al. Gamma-tocopherol and docosahexaenoic acid decrease inflammation in dialysis patients. *J Ren Nutr* 2007;17(5):296–304.

300. Brymora A, Flisiński M, Johnson RJ, et al. Low-fructose diet lowers blood pressure and inflammation in patients with chronic kidney disease. *Nephrol Dial Transplant* 2012;27(2):608–612.

301. Stenvinkel P, Lindholm B, Heimbürger O. Novel approaches in an integrated therapy of inflammatory-associated wasting in end-stage renal disease. *Semin Dial* 2004;17(6):505–515.

302. Bengmark S. Bioecologic control of inflammation and infection in critical illness. *Anesthesiol Clin* 2006;24(2):299–323, vi.

303. Vernaglione L, Cristofano C, Muscogiuri P, et al. Does atorvastatin influence serum C-reactive protein levels in patients on long-term hemodialysis? *Am J Kidney Dis* 2004;43(3):471–478.

304. Panichi V, Paoletti S, Mantuano E, et al. *In vivo* and *in vitro* effects of simvastatin on inflammatory markers in pre-dialysis patients. *Nephrol Dial Transplant* 2006;21(2):337–344.

305. Stenvinkel P, Rodríguez-Ayala E, Massy ZA, et al. Statin treatment and diabetes affect myeloperoxidase activity in maintenance hemodialysis patients. *Clin J Am Soc Nephrol* 2006;1(2):281–287.

306. Wanner C, Krane V, März W, et al. Atorvastatin in patients with type 2 diabetes mellitus undergoing hemodialysis. *N Engl J Med* 2005; 353(3):238–248.

307. Goldstein SL, Leung JC, Silverstein DM. Pro- and anti-inflammatory cytokines in chronic pediatric dialysis patients: effect of aspirin. *Clin J Am Soc Nephrol* 2006;1(5):979–986.

308. Brull DJ, Sanders J, Rumley A, et al. Impact of angiotensin converting enzyme inhibition on post-coronary artery bypass interleukin-6 release. *Heart* 2002;87(3):252–255.

309. Stenvinkel P, Andersson P, Wang T, et al. Do ACE-inhibitors suppress tumour necrosis factor-alpha production in advanced chronic renal failure? *J Intern Med* 1999;246(5):503–507.

310. Suliman ME, Qureshi AR, Heimbürger O, et al. Soluble adhesion molecules in end-stage renal disease: a predictor of outcome. *Nephrol Dial Transplant* 2006;21(6):1603–1610.

311. Anker SD, Negassa A, Coats AJ, et al. Prognostic importance of weight loss in chronic heart failure and the effect of treatment with angiotensin-converting-enzyme inhibitors: an observational study. *Lancet* 2003;361(9363):1077–1083.

312. Schleithoff SS, Zittermann A, Tenderich G, et al. Vitamin D supplementation improves cytokine profiles in patients with congestive heart failure: a double-blind, randomized, placebo-controlled trial. *Am J Clin Nutr* 2006;83(4):754–759.

313. Ferramosca E, Burke S, Chasan-Taber S, et al. Potential antiatherogenic and anti-inflammatory properties of sevelamer in maintenance hemodialysis patients. *Am Heart J* 2005;149(5):820–825.

314. Caglar K, Yilmaz MI, Saglam M, et al. Short-term treatment with sevelamer increases serum fetuin-a concentration and improves endothelial dysfunction in chronic kidney disease stage 4 patients. *Clin J Am Soc Nephrol* 2008;3(1):61–68.

315. Ivanovski O, Szumilak D, Nguyen-Khoa T, et al. The antioxidant N-acetylcysteine prevents accelerated atherosclerosis in uremic apolipoprotein E knockout mice. *Kidney Int* 2005;67(6):2288–2294.

316. Wong TY, Szeto CC, Chow KM, et al. Rosiglitazone reduces insulin requirement and C-reactive protein levels in type 2 diabetic patients receiving peritoneal dialysis. *Am J Kidney Dis* 2005;46(4): 713–719.

317. Nissen SE, Wolski K. Effect of rosiglitazone on the risk of myocardial infarction and death from cardiovascular causes. *N Engl J Med* 2007;356(24):2457–2471.

318. Haslett PA. Anticytokine approaches to the treatment of anorexia and cachexia. *Semin Oncol* 1998;25(2 Suppl 6):53–57.

319. Cooper A, Mikhail A, Lethbridge MW, et al. Pentoxifylline improves hemoglobin levels in patients with erythropoietin-resistant anemia in renal failure. *J Am Soc Nephrol* 2004;15(7):1877–1882.

320. Larsen CM, Faulenbach M, Vaag A, et al. Interleukin-1 receptor antagonist in type 2 diabetes mellitus. *N Engl J Med* 2007;356(15): 1517–1526.

321. So A, De Smedt T, Revaz S, et al. A pilot study of IL-1 inhibition by anakinra in acute gout. *Arthritis Res Ther* 2007;9(2):R28.

322. Gollapudi P, Yoon JW, Gollapudi S, et al. Leukocyte toll-like receptor expression in end-stage kidney disease. *Am J Nephrol* 2010;31(3): 247–254.

323. Alexiewicz JM, Smogorzewski M, Fadda GZ, et al. Impaired phagocytosis in dialysis patients: studies on mechanisms. *Am J Nephrol* 1991;11(2):102–111.

324. Girndt M, Köhler H, Schiedhelm-Weick E, et al. Production of interleukin-6, tumor necrosis factor alpha and interleukin-10 in vitro correlates with the clinical immune defect in chronic hemodialysis patients. *Kidney Int* 1995;47(2):559–565.

325. Anding K, Gross P, Rost JM, et al. The influence of uraemia and haemodialysis on neutrophil phagocytosis and antimicrobial killing. *Nephrol Dial Transplant* 2003;18(10):2067–2073.

326. Glorieux G, Vanholder R, Lameire N. Uraemic retention and apoptosis: what is the balance for the inflammatory status in uraemia? *Eur J Clin Invest* 2003;33(8):631–634.

327. Pahl MV, Gollapudi S, Sepassi L, et al. Effect of end-stage renal disease on B-lymphocyte subpopulations, IL-7, BAFF and BAFF receptor expression. *Nephrol Dial Transplant* 2010;25(1):205–212.

328. Fernández-Fresnedo G, Ramos MA, González-Pardo MC, et al. B lymphopenia in uremia is related to an accelerated in vitro apoptosis and dysregulation of Bcl-2. *Nephrol Dial Transplant* 2000;15(4):502–510.

329. Stachowski J, Pollok M, Burrichter H, et al. Signalling via the TCR/CD3 antigen receptor complex in uremia is limited by the receptors number. *Nephron* 1993;64(3):369–375.

330. Yoon JW, Gollapudi S, Pahl MV, et al. Naïve and central memory T-cell lymphopenia in end-stage renal disease. *Kidney Int* 2006;70(2): 371–376.

331. Meier P, Dayer E, Blanc E, et al. Early T cell activation correlates with expression of apoptosis markers in patients with end-stage renal disease. *J Am Soc Nephrol* 2002;13(1):204–212.

332. Sester U, Sester M, Hauk M, et al. T-cell activation follows Th1 rather than Th2 pattern in haemodialysis patients. *Nephrol Dial Transplant* 2000;15(8):1217–1223.

333. Agrawal S, Gollapudi P, Elahimehr R, et al. Effects of end-stage renal disease and haemodialysis on dendritic cell subsets and basal and LPS-stimulated cytokine production. *Nephrol Dial Transplant* 2010;25(3):737–746.

334. Vaslaki LR, Berta K, Major L, et al. On-line hemodiafiltration does not induce inflammatory response in end-stage renal disease patients: results from a multicenter cross-over study. *Artif Organs* 2005; 29(5):406–412.

335. Chen HY, Cheng IC, Pan YJ, et al. Cognitive-behavioral therapy for sleep disturbance decreases inflammatory cytokines and oxidative stress in hemodialysis patients. *Kidney Int* 2011;80(4):415–422.

336. Chen HY, Chiang CK, Wang HH, et al. Cognitive-behavioral therapy for sleep disturbance in patients undergoing peritoneal dialysis: a pilot randomized controlled trial. *Am J Kidney Dis* 2008;52(2):314–323.

337. Shiels MS, Katki HA, Freedman ND, et al. Cigarette smoking and variations in systemic immune and inflammation markers. *J Natl Cancer Inst* 2014;106(11).

338. Rodrigues Telini LS, de Carvalho Beduschi G, Caramori JC, et al. Effect of dietary sodium restriction on body water, blood pressure, and inflammation in hemodialysis patients: a prospective randomized controlled study. *Int Urol Nephrol* 2014;46(1):91–97.

339. Shema-Didi L, Sela S, Ore L, et al. One year of pomegranate juice intake decreases oxidative stress, inflammation, and incidence of infections in hemodialysis patients: a randomized placebo-controlled trial. *Free Radic Biol Med* 2012;53(2):297–304.

340. Wang IK, Wu YY, Yang YF, et al. The effect of probiotics on serum levels of cytokine and endotoxin in peritoneal dialysis patients: a randomised, double-blind, placebo-controlled trial. *Benef Microbes* 2015;6(4):423–430.

341. Krishnamurthy VM, Wei G, Baird BC, et al. High dietary fiber intake is associated with decreased inflammation and all-cause mortality in patients with chronic kidney disease. *Kidney Int* 2012;81(3):300–306.

342. Hsu SP, Wu MS, Yang CC, et al. Chronic green tea extract supplementation reduces hemodialysis-enhanced production of hydrogen peroxide and hypochlorous acid, atherosclerotic factors, and proinflammatory cytokines. *Am J Clin Nutr* 2007;86(5):1539–1547.

343. Taraz M, Khatami MR, Dashti-Khavidaki S, et al. Sertraline decreases serum level of interleukin-6 (IL-6) in hemodialysis patients with depression: results of a randomized double-blind, placebo-controlled clinical trial. *Int Immunopharmacol* 2013;17(3):917–923.

344. Goicoechea M, de Vinuesa SG, Verdalles U, et al. Effect of allopurinol in chronic kidney disease progression and cardiovascular risk. *Clin J Am Soc Nephrol* 2010;5(8):1388–1393.

345. Bucharles S, Barberato SH, Stinghen AE, et al. Impact of cholecalciferol treatment on biomarkers of inflammation and myocardial structure in hemodialysis patients without hyperparathyroidism. *J Ren Nutr* 2012;22(2):284–291.

346. Navarro-González JF, Donate-Correa J, Méndez ML, et al. Antiinflammatory profile of paricalcitol in hemodialysis patients: a prospective, open-label, pilot study. *J Clin Pharmacol* 2013;53(4):421–426.

347. Nakamura Y, Tsuji M, Hasegawa H, et al. Anti-inflammatory effects of linagliptin in hemodialysis patients with diabetes. *Hemodial Int* 2014;18(2):433–442.

348. Poyrazoglu OK, Dogukan A, Yalniz M, et al. Acute effect of standard heparin versus low molecular weight heparin on oxidative stress and inflammation in hemodialysis patients. *Ren Fail* 2006;28(8):723–727.

349. González-Espinoza L, Rojas-Campos E, Medina-Pérez M, et al. Pentoxifylline decreases serum levels of tumor necrosis factor alpha, interleukin 6 and C-reactive protein in hemodialysis patients: results of a randomized double-blind, controlled clinical trial. *Nephrol Dial Transplant* 2012;27(5):2023–2028.

350. Van Laecke S, Van Biesen W, Vanholder R. The paradox of bardoxolone methyl: a call for every witness on the stand? *Diabetes Obes Metab* 2015;17(1):9–14.

351. Pergola PE, Raskin P, Toto RD, et al. Bardoxolone methyl and kidney function in CKD with type 2 diabetes. *N Engl J Med* 2011;365(4):327–336.

352. de Zeeuw D, Akizawa T, Audhya P, et al. Bardoxolone methyl in type 2 diabetes and stage 4 chronic kidney disease. *N Engl J Med* 2013;369(26):2492–2503.

353. Smolen JS, Beaulieu A, Rubbert-Roth A, et al. Effect of interleukin-6 receptor inhibition with tocilizumab in patients with rheumatoid arthritis (OPTION study): a double-blind, placebo-controlled, randomised trial. *Lancet* 2008;371(9617):987–997.

354. Ridker PM, Thuren T, Zalewski A, et al. Interleukin-1β inhibition and the prevention of recurrent cardiovascular events: rationale and design of the Canakinumab Anti-inflammatory Thrombosis Outcomes Study (CANTOS). *Am Heart J* 2011;162(4):597–605.

355. Hung AM, Ellis CD, Shintani A, et al. IL-1β receptor antagonist reduces inflammation in hemodialysis patients. *J Am Soc Nephrol* 2011;22(3):437–442.

356. Don BR, Kim K, Li J, et al. The effect of etanercept on suppression of the systemic inflammatory response in chronic hemodialysis patients. *Clin Nephrol* 2010;73(6):431–438.

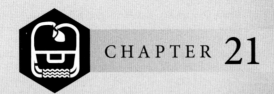

CHAPTER 21

Hepatitis and Human Immunodeficiency Virus Infections in End-Stage Kidney Disease Patients

Ruth Berggren

Despite widespread implementation of universal precautions, chronic dialysis patients remain at risk for parenterally transmitted infections including with hepatitis B virus (HBV), hepatitis C virus (HCV), or human immunodeficiency virus (HIV) from blood product transfusions or nosocomial transmission in hemodialysis units (1–4). Adverse outcomes, including increased mortality rates, are noted among dialysis patients with chronic viral hepatitis (5). Yet not all dialysis patients are appropriately screened or considered for hepatitis treatment nor are they consistently vaccinated appropriately against HBV. In this chapter, the epidemiologic significance, morbidity, and mortality of HIV, HBV, and HCV infections in the chronic hemodialysis population are examined. Methods for preventing transmission and management recommendations for dialysis patients with chronic viral hepatitis or HIV infection are reviewed. Of these three parenterally transmissible viruses, HBV is the most likely to be transmitted in the setting of hemodialysis, and infection control guidelines reflect this difference (6). As of 2008, U.S. hemodialysis facilities must follow Centers for Disease Control and Prevention (CDC) guidelines in order to receive Medicare reimbursement for outpatient hemodialysis (7). This chapter reviews guidelines for immunization of the hemodialysis population against HBV, which differ from those for the general population, and summarizes postexposure prophylaxis (PEP) guidelines for personnel and/or patients accidentally exposed to HIV. GB virus C (GBV/HGV) is not addressed because although recent evidence reveals HGV can be transmitted in hemodialysis units, this is a relatively nonpathogenic virus with no known long-term sequelae for dialysis patients (8).

EPIDEMIOLOGY OF HEPATITIS B VIRUS, HEPATITIS C VIRUS, AND HUMAN IMMUNODEFICIENCY VIRUS INFECTIONS IN HEMODIALYSIS PATIENTS

National surveillance of dialysis-associated diseases in the United States in 2002 demonstrated the prevalence of hepatitis B surface antigen (HBsAg), anti-HCV antibody, and HIV infection at 1.0%, 7.8%, and 1.5%, respectively (9). In 2002, a minority of hemodialysis centers were routinely screening for HIV, so the 1.5% HIV prevalence in dialysis centers may be an underestimate. These data are the result of surveillance questionnaires administered by the CDC to all chronic hemodialysis centers licensed by the Centers for Medicare and Medicaid Services (CMS). The 4,035 centers representing 263,820 patients and 58,043 staff were surveyed regarding hemodialysis practices, disposable dialyzer reuse, cleaning and disinfection procedures for dialysis equipment, HIV prevalence, HBV vaccination coverage, and the results of testing patients for HBsAg and anti-HCV antibody (10). The study found that the incidence of viral hepatitis did not differ substantially according to infection control practices.

In 2002, 27.3% of U.S. centers reported at least one patient with chronic HBV and 2.8% of centers reported at least one newly acquired HBV infection. Patients still acquire HBV infection in hemodialysis centers due to inadequate infection control or breaches of technique (9). The risk of seroconversion for patients with untreated percutaneous exposure to HBV is as high as 30% (11). In 2002, HBV incidence was 0.12% overall but higher in centers where injectable medications were prepared on medication carts in treatment areas compared to centers with a separate medication room. According to a cross-sectional study of 8,615 adult hemodialysis patients in Western Europe and the United States, the prevalence of HBV infection in this population ranges between 0% and 7% (4,12). In developing countries, rates of chronic HBsAg carriers range from 2% to 20% (4). Higher rates in developing countries are attributed to the higher background prevalence of HBV and difficulties following infection control strategies against HBV in the setting of lack of infrastructure and financial resources (4).

Although HCV seroprevalence among U.S. dialysis patients is 5 times higher than in the general population (7.8% vs. 1.6%), HCV incidence has been declining (13). In 2002, HCV incidence at U.S. dialysis centers was 0.34%, representing a significant decline from the previous decade (6). Centers using disposable containers for priming dialyzers demonstrated significantly lower HCV incidence (9). HCV transmission may occur in centers having opportunities for cross-contamination among dialysis patients, including failure to disinfect contaminated equipment or shared environmental surfaces. The duration of time on dialysis is the most important risk factor independently associated with HCV infection (6). Employment of nurses with at least 2 years of formal dialysis training is associated with lower seroconversion risk (14).

The proportion of U.S. hemodialysis patients with HIV increased from 0.3% to 1.4% from 1985 to 1999 (6); more recent estimates show stability with about 1.5% since 2002 (9). Patient-to-patient transmission of HIV infection has not been reported in American hemodialysis centers. In other countries, however, HIV transmission has been attributed to mixing of reused access needles and inadequate equipment disinfection procedures (15).

MORBIDITY AND MORTALITY OF HUMAN IMMUNODEFICIENCY VIRUS, HEPATITIS C VIRUS, AND HEPATITIS B VIRUS INFECTION IN HEMODIALYSIS PATIENTS

With the advent of highly active antiretroviral therapy (HAART), survival of HIV-infected patients on hemodialysis has vastly improved. A 2-year prospective French study followed all HIV-infected patients on hemodialysis in France through 2003. Survival was compared with that of 584 hemodialysis patients who did not have HIV infection in the same period. The 2-year survival rate was statistically indistinguishable from the survival of the control cohort. However, there were some significant mortality risk factors including low CD4+ T cell count (hazard ratio [HR] 1.4/100 CD4+ T cells per mm^3 lower), high viral load (HR 2.5/1 log10 per mL), absence of HAART (HR 2.7), and a history of opportunistic infection (HR 3.7) (16). Nevertheless, HIV-infected patients who are taking appropriate HAART and getting proper follow-up are comparable to non–HIV-infected end-stage kidney disease (ESKD) patients with regard to morbidity and mortality.

Among maintenance hemodialysis patients, HCV is associated with higher all-cause and cardiovascular mortality across almost all clinical and demographic groups (17,18). A database of 13,664 dialysis patients who underwent HCV testing during a 3-year interval (through June 2004) was analyzed. In logistic regression models, HCV infection was linked to younger age, male gender, black race,

Hispanic ethnicity, Medicaid insurance, longer dialysis duration, unmarried status, HIV infection, and smoking. The mortality HR associated with HCV infection was 1.25 (95% confidence interval 1.12 to 1.39; $p <0.001$) (5). A longitudinal study showed a mortality rate of 33% for HCV-infected dialysis patients, compared with 23.2% mortality for the HCV-uninfected dialysis group over a 6-year follow-up (18).

In contrast to HCV, HBV-related liver disease in the hemodialysis population has a relatively benign course (19). Although HBV infection in hemodialysis patients more often results in a chronic carrier state compared to patients without kidney disease, the risk of death from liver disease is low (11,20). No significant difference in mortality between dialysis patients according to HBsAg status has been consistently shown (4,21,22). There are contradictory data from a small study in India, which indicates that HBsAg-positive hemodialysis patients had a higher mortality rate (72.7% vs. 21.4%)` than HBsAg-negative hemodialysis patients due to fulminating hepatic failure in these individuals (4,23).

SCREENING AND PREVENTION RECOMMENDATIONS FOR HUMAN IMMUNODEFICIENCY VIRUS, HEPATITIS B VIRUS, AND HEPATITIS C VIRUS IN HEMODIALYSIS PATIENTS

In 2006, the CDC issued revised guidelines for HIV screening in the general population as follows: "HIV screening is recommended for patients in all health-care settings after the patient is notified that testing will be performed unless the patient declines (opt-out screening). Persons at high risk for HIV infection should be screened for HIV at least annually (TABLE 21.1). Separate written consent for HIV testing should not be required; general consent for medical care should be considered sufficient to encompass consent for HIV testing" (24). These guidelines apply equally to the population receiving chronic hemodialysis. Therefore, all individuals should be screened before the initiation of hemodialysis (FIGURE 21.1) and annually thereafter if they are at high risk. The definition of individuals at high risk for HIV infection includes injection drug users, men who have sex with men and persons with multiple sexual partners including those who exchange drugs or money for sex, and heterosexual partners of HIV-infected persons. There is no recommendation to segregate HIV-positive from HIV-negative dialysis patients or to dedicate dialysis machines solely to HIV-positive patients. As of 2015, there is no effective vaccine for the prevention of HIV, and prevention of infection requires education of patients and staff to minimize risk (25).

Hepatitis B Virus Screening and Immunization

Hepatitis B screening is especially critical in hemodialysis units because HBV-infected patients need to be isolated in a separate room and assigned dialysis equipment, instruments, supplies, and staff members that are not shared by HBV-susceptible patients (6). Several tests for which serologic assays are commercially available may be used to diagnose HBV infection. These include HBsAg and anti-HBs, anti-HBc, hepatitis B envelope antigen (HBeAg), and antibody to HBeAg (anti-HBe) (TABLE 21.2). One or more of these markers are detectable during phases of HBV infection (6).

HBsAg indicates ongoing HBV infection and the potential for transmission to others. Among newly infected patients

TABLE 21.1	Screening Schedule for Hemodialysis Patients: Hepatitis B (HBV), Hepatitis C (HCV), and Human Immunodeficiency Virus (HIV)			
Patient	**Admission**	**Monthly**	**Twice Yearly**	**Yearly**
All	HBsAg	–	–	–
	Total anti-HBc	–	–	–
	Anti-HBs	–	–	–
	Anti-HCV, ALT	–	–	–
	Anti-HIV	–	–	–
		–	–	–
HBV nonimmune[a]	–	HBsAg	–	–
HBV-immune[b] but HBc negative	–	–	–	Anti-HBs[c]
Anti-HBs+ and anti-HBc+[d]	–	–	–	No additional testing
Anti-HCV–	–	ALT	Anti-HCV	–
Anti-HIV–	–	–	–	Anti-HIV if high risk

[a]All nonimmune persons should be immunized against HBV.
[b]A patient is HBV-immune if anti-HBs is greater than or equal to 10 mIU/mL.
[c]Boost HBV vaccine if anti-HBs declines to less than 10 mIU/mL.
[d]A patient who is both anti-HBc+ and anti-HBs+ demonstrates immunity due to prior infection does not need annual screening.
HBsAg, hepatitis B surface antigen; ALT, alanine aminotransferase.
From Centers for Disease Control and Prevention. Recommendations for preventing transmission of infections among chronic hemodialysis patients. *MMWR Recomm Rep* 2001;50(RR-5):1–43.

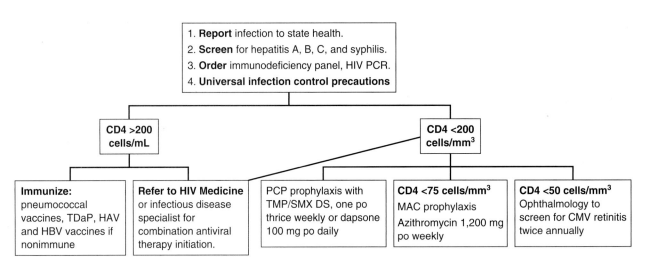

FIGURE 21.1 Incidentally discovered HIV in a dialysis patient. CD4: absolute CD4 + T lymphocyte count measured by immunodeficiency panel. All HIV infections must be reported to state health department to permit contact tracing. All newly diagnosed HIV-infected patients should have an immunodeficiency panel ordered right away to determine need for potentially life-saving prophylaxis against opportunistic infections, which can be initiated prior to seeing a specialist. Antiviral therapy is now recommended for all HIV-infected patients regardless of CD4 cell count; do not wait for CD4 cell count to drop below a certain threshold to make referral for therapy. If specialist cannot see new HIV patient right away, initiate standard vaccines noted as appropriate. HBV or HCV coinfected patients have special management considerations in selecting antiviral therapy for HIV. Unlike the case for hepatitis B infection, hemodialysis patients with HIV infection do not require segregation or use of a dedicated hemodialysis machine. HIV, human immunodeficiency virus; PCR, polymerase chain reaction; TDaP, tetanus, diphtheria, and pertussis; HAV, hepatitis A virus; HBV, hepatitis B virus; PCP, pneumocystis pneumonia; TMP/SMX, trimethoprim/sulfamethoxazole; DS, double strength; MAC, *Mycobacterium* avium complex; CMV, cytomegalovirus. (From Guidelines for the prevention and treatment of opportunistic infections in HIV-infected adults and adolescents. http://aidsinfo.nih.gov/guidelines. Accessed July 9, 2016.)

TABLE 21.2	Hepatitis B Serologic Profile Interpretation for End-Stage Kidney Disease (ESKD) Patients			
Serologic Test Profile	**Results**	**Interpretation**		**ESKD Differences**
HBsAg Total anti-HBc Anti-HBs	Negative Negative Negative	Susceptible		
HBsAg Total anti-HBc Anti HBs Anti-HBc IgM	Negative Positive Positive Negative	Immune due to natural infection		
HBsAg Total anti-HBc Anti-HBs	Negative Negative Positive	Immune due to hepatitis B vaccination		Vaccine induced transient HBsAg positivity can be seen in HD populations[a]
HBsAg Total anti-HBc IgM anti-HBc Anti-HBs	Positive Positive Positive Negative	Acutely infected		
HBsAg Anti-HBc IgM anti-HBc Anti-HBs	Positive Positive Negative Negative	Chronically infected		ESKD patients may be anti-HBc core alone positive and have +HBV DNA.
HBsAg Anti-HBc Anti-HBs	Negative Positive Negative	Four possible interpretations: 1. Resolved infection 2. False-positive anti-HBc, susceptible 3. Low-level chronic infection 4. Resolving acute infection[b]		ESKD patients with this pattern should be immunized but also have HBV DNA PCR, and if positive, evaluate for treatment criteria (see algorithm).

[a]Because of the possibility of transient vaccine-induced HBV antigenemia, defer HBsAg testing for at least 4 weeks after vaccination to avoid false positives.
[b]The pattern noted in the table, with the designation of possible "resolving acute infection" may be seen during the window period between disappearance of HBsAg and appearance of anti-HBs.
HBsAg, hepatitis B surface antigen; IgM, immunoglobulin M; HD, hemodialysis; PCR, polymerase chain reaction.
From Comprehensive immunization strategy to eliminate transmission of hepatitis B virus infection in the United States: recommendations of the advisory committee on immunization practices. Part 1: immunization of infants, children, and adolescents. *MMWR Recomm Rep* 2005;54(RR-16):1–31. http://www.cdc.gov/hepatitis. Accessed July 9, 2016; Mohan D, Railey M, Al Rukhaimi M. Vaccination and transient hepatitis B surface antigenemia. *NDT Plus* 2011;4(3):190–191; Onuigbo MA, Nesbit A, Weisenbeck J, et al. Hepatitis B surface antigenemia following recombinant Engerix B hepatitis B vaccine in an 81-year-old ESRD patient on hemodialysis. *Ren Fail* 2010;32(4):531–532; Anjum Q. False positive hepatitis B surface antigen due to recent vaccination. *Int J Health Sci (Qassim)* 2014;8(2):189–193.

(**FIGURE 21.2**), serum HBsAg is found 30 to 60 days after exposure to HBV and persists for variable periods. Anti-HBc antibody develops in all HBV infections, appearing at onset of liver enzyme elevations in acute infection and persisting for life. Acute infection can be detected by immunoglobulin M (IgM) anti-HBc antibody, which persists for up to 6 months (6).

For those who recover from HBV (>85% of adults), HBsAg is eliminated from blood in 2 to 3 months, followed by the development of anti-HBs antibody. Anti-HBs antibody indicates immunity from HBV infection. After infection, most people are positive for anti-HBs and anti-HBc antibodies. In contrast, only anti-HBs antibody develops in persons who have been vaccinated against hepatitis B. Those who do not recover from HBV become chronically infected and remain positive for HBsAg (and anti-HBc). A small number (0.3% per year) eventually clear HBsAg and develop anti-HBs antibody (2,6).

Some individuals have anti-HBc antibody as the only HBV serologic marker. Isolated anti-HBc antibody can occur after HBV infection among persons who have recovered but whose anti-HBs antibody levels have waned or among persons who failed to develop anti-HBs antibody. HBV DNA is detected in <10% of persons with isolated anti-HBc antibody, and these persons are unlikely to be infectious to others. For most people with isolated anti-HBc antibody, the result appears to be a false positive. A primary anti-HBs antibody response develops in most of these individuals after

a three-dose hepatitis B vaccine series. We have no data on response to vaccination for hemodialysis patients with this serologic pattern (2,6).

HBeAg can be detected in serum of those with acute or chronic HBV infection, usually appearing shortly after the appearance of anti-HBc. The presence of HBeAg correlates with viral replication, whereas anti-HBe correlates with the loss of replicating virus. All HBsAg-positive people should be considered infectious, regardless of HBeAg or anti-HBe status. HBV infection can also be detected using tests for HBV DNA. These tests are most commonly used for persons being treated with antivirals (2,6).

All hemodialysis patients should be screened for hepatitis B [HBsAg, anti-HBc total, anti-HBs, and alanine aminotransferase (ALT)] upon admission to the dialysis unit. It is important to note that in chronic uremia, the serum aminotransferases are spuriously low in chronic HBV infections and must not be relied upon to indicate which patients need hepatitis screening (4). Nonimmune individuals should be immunized and screening for HBsAg repeated monthly until seroconversion from vaccination has been documented. Individuals who are anti-HBs and anti-HBc positive require no additional HBV testing because they are immune. After vaccine-induced seroconversion to anti-HBs positive (≥10 mIU/mL) dialysis, patients should be screened annually for anti-HBs. A booster dose of vaccine should be given if anti-HBs declines to <10 mIU/mL, and annual testing should continue thereafter.

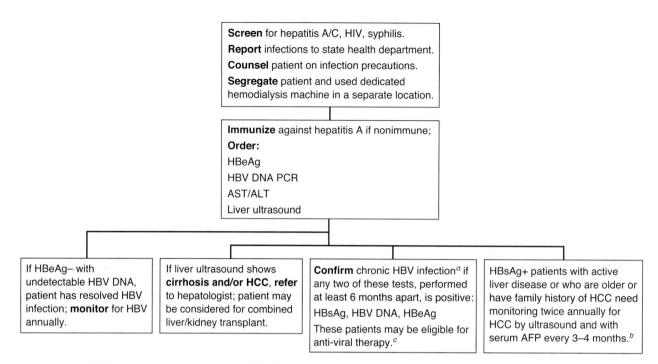

FIGURE 21.2 Incidentally discovered HBV (HBsAg+) in a dialysis patient. [a]For confirmation of chronic HBV infection, a positive result any two of these tests, performed at least 6 months apart is acceptable: HBsAg, HBV DNA, HBeAg. From Completeness of reporting of chronic hepatitis B and C virus infections–Michigan 1995–2008. *MMWR* 2013;62(06);99–102. [b]From Di Bisceglie AM. Hepatitis B and hepatocellular carcinoma. *Hepatology* 2009;49(5S)S56–S60; Chan TM. Hepatitis B virus and dialysis patients. UpToDate. Updated August 14, 2015. Accessed July 9, 2016. [c]Treat chronic HBV when abnormal ALT levels suggest liver inflammation and HBV DNA levels are greater than or equal to 4 to 5 log10 copies/mL. Optimal therapy for chronic HBV infection in dialysis patients is being studied. Clinical data support using interferon-alfa or nucleotide or nucleoside analogs for these patients (see **TABLE 21.4**). HCC, hepatocellular carcinoma; AFP, serum alpha fetoprotein, tumor marker for HCC; HBV, hepatitis B virus; PCR, polymerase chain reaction; AST, aspartate aminotransferase; ALT, alanine aminotransferase.

Since 1977, the recommendation has been that HBsAg-positive persons should be isolated in a separate room, using separate machines, equipment, instruments, and supplies. Staff members assigned to HBsAg-positive patients should not be assigned to HBV-susceptible patients during the same shift. Dialysis equipment assigned to HBsAg-positive patients must not be shared by HBV-susceptible patients, and the routine cleaning and disinfection of equipment and environmental surfaces is of paramount importance. HBV is viable for up to 7 days on environmental surfaces and has been detected in dialysis centers on clamps, scissors, dialysis machine controls, and doorknobs. Blood-contaminated surfaces are a reservoir for HBV transmission, and dialysis staff members must take great care not to transfer virus to patients from these contaminated surfaces by their hands or gloves or through contaminated supplies (6).

Hepatitis B Virus Vaccine Recommendations

HBV vaccination recommendations for susceptible hemodialysis patients and staff include documentation of baseline serologies followed by three intramuscular doses of vaccine, with the second and third doses given at 1 month and 6 months after the first dose. Because immunocompromised persons have lower vaccine response rates, both the Recombivax HB and Engerix-B vaccine formulations have separate, U.S. Food and Drug Administration (FDA)-approved, recommendations for predialysis versus dialysis-dependent persons. With Recombivax HB, dialysis-dependent

patients should receive 40 μg in 1 mL at 0, 2, and 6 months, whereas the recommended Engerix schedule for dialysis patients is for 40 μg at 0, 1, 2, and 6 months. All doses should be administered in the deltoid by the intramuscular route. Since hepatitis B vaccine became available, no HBV infections have been reported among vaccinated hemodialysis patients if they maintained protective levels of antibody to HBV. Fifty percent to 70% of nonresponders will respond to three additional doses. For nonresponders after six doses of vaccine, no data support additional doses. Among successfully immunized hemodialysis patients whose antibody titers subsequently declined below protection, data show that most respond to a booster dose. Periodic hepatitis B antibody screening of vaccine responders in the hemodialysis unit should permit identification of individuals in need of a booster dose to maintain immunity (6,11).

HEPATITIS C VIRUS SCREENING

Because morbidity and mortality rates are higher in HCV-infected hemodialysis patients, these individuals should be screened at initial entry to hemodialysis, and annually thereafter if they engage in high risk behaviors, including injection drug use, intranasal cocaine use, or are men who have sex with men. Screening should use both ALT and an enzyme immunoassay (EIA) or the supplemental recombinant immunoassay (RIBA) that detects anti-HCV antibodies. The CDC has recommended monthly ALT screening for HCV-negative persons, regardless of risk factors, as early detection of an infection

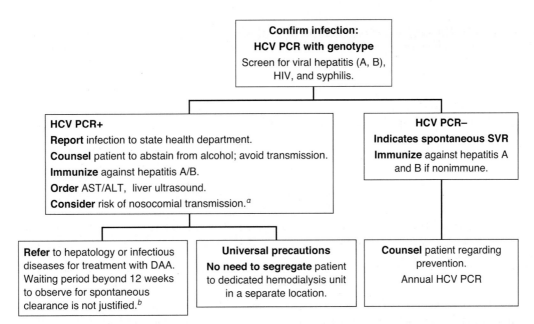

FIGURE 21.3 Incidentally discovered HCV (Aby+) in a dialysis patient. All oral regimens available depending on HCV genotype. [a]If nosocomial HCV transmission is suspected, HCV PCR should be performed and repeated in 2 to 12 weeks for each potentially exposed patient. There is a risk of false-negative PCR early after infection. [b]https://www.kidney.org/professionals /kdoqi/12-10-1601. HCV, hepatitis C virus; PCR, polymerase chain reaction; AST, aspartate aminotransferase; alanine aminotransferase; DAA, directly acting antiviral therapy; SVR, sustained virologic response.

would permit consideration of therapy (**FIGURE 21.3**) (6). The EIA is at least 97% sensitive, but it does not distinguish between acute, chronic, or resolved HCV infection, and therefore, a positive antibody test should be followed by a reverse transcriptase polymerase chain reaction (RT-PCR) assay for HCV, which is commonly used in clinical practice and commercially available. Persistent viremia with HCV defines chronicity, which is seen in some 85% of infections. After treatment, or after spontaneous viral clearance (which may occur in 15% to 45% of infected persons), a sustained virologic response (SVR) is defined by finding undetectable HCV by RT-PCR after a 12- (SVR12) or 24-week (SVR24) interval (26). Regardless of whether a hemodialysis patient with HCV is a candidate for specific HCV therapy, knowledge of this comorbidity allows the clinician to counsel the patient about prognosis and about basic health maintenance measures that may improve outcomes. HCV-infected persons should abstain from alcohol because it accelerates fibrosis progression; avoid excessive acetaminophen use; avoid behaviors such as sharing of needles, razor blades, or toothbrushes which may result in transmission of viral infection to others; and they should be immunized against both hepatitis A and B to prevent fulminant hepatitis superinfection (27). There is no vaccine available for prevention of HCV in 2015.

TREATMENT OF HEPATITIS C, HEPATITIS B, AND HUMAN IMMUNODEFICIENCY VIRUS IN HEMODIALYSIS PATIENTS

Treatment of Hepatitis C in Hemodialysis Patients

The higher mortality rate of HCV-infected hemodialysis patients creates a significant motivation to consider HCV treatment in these individuals, especially if kidney transplantation is being considered.

HCV infection results in worse survival of both patients and organ grafts after transplantation. Posttransplant diabetes mellitus is also more common in patients with HCV infection. Because organ transplant is associated with accelerated fibrosis progression (28), it is advisable to consider treating HCV before kidney transplant. Direct-acting, all oral antiviral drugs for hepatitis C have simplified therapy and improved SVR rates to over 90% for many patient populations. Still, treatment of HCV during hemodialysis requires ongoing study due to limited information about safety and efficacy of anti-HCV drugs in this setting. Current guidelines continue to recommend pegylated interferon and dose-adjusted ribavirin for patients with HCV genotype 2,3,5, or 6 infections and creatinine clearance (CrCl) below 30 mL/min (rating: class IIb level B) (**TABLE 21.3**). For genotypes 1a, 1b, and 4, patients with CrCl below 30 mL/min, who do not have cirrhosis, can be treated with daily fixed dose combination oral combination therapies (in 2015, these included paritaprevir, ritonavir, ombitasvir, and dasabuvir with or without ribavirin at reduced doses) (28). Some of these oral combinations have been used successfully during hemodialysis; however, anemia and other side effects (liver enzyme elevations) may be severe, and these patients must be managed in consultation with hepatology or infectious disease specialists.

Because studies of all oral direct-acting antiviral drugs for HCV during hemodialysis are ongoing, we continue to rely on interferon-based regimens for non-genotype 1 or 4 patients in 2015 (28). Studies of interferon α (IFN-α) monotherapy in hemodialysis patients demonstrate SVR rates of 33% to 40%, which are generally higher than for those without kidney disease. High adverse event rates are reported for these studies as well, leading to caution in making generalized recommendations for the HCV-infected dialysis patient. Pegylated interferon is still used in combination with oral antivirals in certain patients with HCV genotypes 3, 4, 5, and 6 (28). Because ribavirin is cleared by

TABLE 21.3 Dosing of Hepatitis C Medications in Dialysis			
HCV Genotype	**Drug**	**Normal Dose**	**Hemodialysis Adjustment**
	Ribavirin (RBV)[a]	1,000–1,200 mg daily (weight based)	200 mg daily or thrice weekly; after dialysis
1a or 1b	Ombitasvir/ paritaprevir/ritonavir (part of dose pack)[b]	12.5 mg/75 mg/50 mg 2 tablets po daily × 12–24 wk	Not defined; limited clinical data, no adjustment
1a or 1b	Dasabuvir (part of dose pack)[b]	250 mg 2 tablets po daily × 12–24 wk	Limited clinical data exist, no adjustment
1a or 1b	Four-drug dose pack +/− RBV	RBV added for HCV genotype 1a; not needed for genotype 1b	A recommended regimen for HCV genotype 1b
1a, 1b, 4	Elbasvir/grazoprevir	50 mg/100 mg po daily for 12–16 wk	Limited clinical data no adjustment
2,3,5, or 6	Pegylated interferon 2a	180 μg sc weekly with daily RBV	135μg sc weekly with daily RBV

[a]RBV should be discontinued if hemoglobin level declines by more than 2 g/dL despite erythropoietin.
HCV, hepatitis C virus; po, by mouth; sc, subcutaneous.
From Recommendations for Testing, managing, and treating hepatitis C. http://hcvguidelines.org/sites/default/files/HCV-Guidance_April_2016_d1.pdf. Accessed July 9, 2016.

the kidney and causes a dose-related hemolysis, HCV-infected hemodialysis patients who need this drug must be carefully monitored for hemolysis and require significant dose reduction. Treatment should be individualized, focused primarily on patients who are renal transplant candidates, and undertaken only by experienced clinicians who can inform patients about potential benefits and risks. Proactive screening for HCV in chronic kidney disease (CKD) patients should lead to HCV treatment during earlier stages of CKD, allowing better tolerability of the best antiviral regimens and avoiding some of the toxicities that cause concern during hemodialysis (13). Publication of data for specifically targeted antiviral therapy for hepatitis C will be a welcome development for the HCV infected patient on chronic hemodialysis (29).

Treatment of Hepatitis B in Hemodialysis Patients

Recommendations for the treatment of HBV infection, including for hemodialysis patients, have been published in the guidelines of the American Association for the Study of Liver Diseases (AASLD) (30). Antiviral therapy should be provided to patients with established chronic infection (HBsAg+ for more than 6 months) who have evidence of viral replication (HBV DNA >20,000 IU/mL if HBeAg positive; HBV DNA >2,000 IU/mL if HBeAg negative)

and evidence of liver disease (ALT greater than 2 times normal or moderate/severe hepatitis on biopsy) (30,31). The goal of therapy is viral suppression and prevention of viral complications such as cirrhosis or hepatocellular carcinoma. In patients with HBV-associated kidney diseases, including polyarteritis nodosa or immune complex glomerulonephropathy, HBV treatment before the patient requires dialysis is important and can facilitate remission of proteinuria and preservation of renal function (31). Treatment should be with one of six approved antiviral medications. While pegylated IFN-α adefovir or entecavir is the preferred initial antiviral for the general population with chronic HBV, interferon is poorly tolerated. Entecavir is favored in patients with kidney disease because of a high genetic barrier to resistance and favorable renal safety profile (31). Although lamivudine has the longest track record in hemodialysis, it engenders high rates of viral resistance and is considered suboptimal as a first-line treatment option (31). Prior treatment with lamivudine leads to resistance mutations for entecavir; such patients may be treated with tenofovir or adefovir in hemodialysis (30,31). Adjustments of adult dosage of nucleoside/nucleotide analogues should be in accordance with CrCl (**TABLE 21.4**). In hemodialysis patients, adefovir dose is only 10 mg weekly following dialysis;

TABLE 21.4 Dosing of Hepatitis B Medications in Dialysis		
Drug	**Normal Dose**	**Hemodialysis Adjustment**
Adefovir	10 mg po q24 h	10 mg po weekly (dose after dialysis)
Entecavir	0.5 mg po daily	0.05 mg q24 h or 0.5 mg po q7 d
Entecavir	For lamivudine refractory or decompensated liver disease	0.1 mg q24 h or 1 mg q7 d
Lamivudine	300 mg po daily	50 mg po once, and then 25 mg q24 h (dose after dialysis on dialysis day)
Telbivudine	600 mg po daily	Tablets: 600 mg po q96 h Solution: 120 mg po q24 h (after dialysis on dialysis day)
Tenofovir	300 mg po daily	300 mg po once weekly dose after dialysis; consider alternative for treatment of HBV and/or HIV

po, by mouth; HBV, hepatitis B virus; HIV, human immunodeficiency virus.
From Guidelines for the prevention and treatment of opportunistic infections in HIV-infected adults and adolescents. https://aidsinfo.nih.gov/guidelines. Accessed July 9, 2016; Table 7.

entecavir dose is .05 mg (nucleoside analogue naive) to 0.1 mg daily in lamivudine refractory patients, or 0.5 mg every 7 days (32). Telbivudine is dosed at 600 mg every 96 hours, with no supplement following dialysis. Tenofovir is given at 300 mg every 7 days after dialysis. Patients who fail to respond to IFN-α may be re-treated with nucleoside analogues. Those who fail to achieve a primary response as evidenced by <2 log10 decrease in serum HBV DNA level after 6 months of nucleic acid therapy may be switched to an alternative treatment (30). A test for HBV resistance mutations should be performed to differentiate primary nonresponse from breakthrough infection and to guide subsequent therapeutic choices. The recommended treatment duration for HBeAg-positive HBV is 48 weeks for peg IFN-α. Duration of nucleoside analogue treatment depends on HBeAg status. Most patients will require very long-term suppressive therapy. All patients with cirrhosis require life-long treatment with nucleoside/nucleotide analogues (32). However, for noncirrhotic, HBeAg-positive chronic HBV, treatment may be discontinued if the patient has achieved HBeAg seroconversion and completed at least 12 months of additional treatment after appearance of anti-HBe, with persistently normal ALT and undetectable HBV DNA. If HBV DNA testing is not available, treatment should be continued until 12 months after the patient has achieved HBsAg

clearance, regardless of prior HBeAg status (32). Patients with compensated cirrhosis should receive long-term treatment (2,4).

Treatment of Human Immunodeficiency Virus in Hemodialysis Patients

With the advent of HAART, survival of HIV-infected dialysis patients has significantly improved in the United States. Using the United States Renal Data System database, 6,166 HIV-infected patients with ESKD who received dialysis in the United States were evaluated. The majority of the patients were black (89%), 7.4% white, and 3% other. From 1990 to 1999, the annual death rates in HIV-infected dialysis patients declined from 458 to 240 deaths per 1,000 patient-years, reflecting the introduction of HAART in 1995 to 1996 (33). Detailed information exists regarding the metabolism and pharmacokinetics of HIV therapeutics in renal insufficiency (34), and quite a few of these medications (including abacavir, efavirenz, etravirine, rilpivirine, nevirapine, most protease inhibitors, enfuvirtide, dolutegravir, elvitegravir, and raltegravir) require no dosage adjustment in renal insufficiency. Thus, HIV-infected patients on chronic hemodialysis may continue with HAART, so long as their regimen has been reviewed for drugs which require dose adjustment in kidney disease (**TABLE 21.5**). Regularly updated

TABLE 21.5	Dosing of Human Immunodeficiency Virus Medications in Dialysis	
Drug	**Normal Dose**	**Hemodialysis Adjustment**
Abacavir	300 mg po bid	None
Didanosine	250 mg (<60 kg)/400 mg (>60 kg) po qd	75 mg (solution) to 125 mg po qd (weight based)
Emtricitabine	200 mg tablet po qd	200 mg tablet po q96 h or 60 mg po q24 h (solution)
Lamivudine	300 mg po qd or 150 mg po bid	1 × 50 mg, then 25 mg po q24 h
Tenofovir	300 mg po qd	300 mg po q7 d
Zidovudine	300 mg po bid	300 mg po qd
Efavirenz	600 mg po qd	None
Etravirine	200 mg po bid	None
Nevirapine	200 mg po bid	Limited data
Rilpivirine	25 mg po qd	None
Atazanavir	400 mg po qd	300 mg qd with 100 mg ritonavir qd if treatment naive
Darunavir/ritonavir	800 mg/100 mg po qd	None
Darunavir/cobicistat	1 tablet po qd	None
Fosamprenavir	1,400 mg po bid	None
Indinavir	800 mg po qd	None
Lopinavir/ritonavir	400 mg/100 mg po bid	None
Nelfinavir	1,250 mg po bid	None
Ritonavir (rtv) (booster)	100–400 mg po qd	None
Saquinavir/rtv	1,000 mg/100 mg po bid	None
Tipranavir/rtv	500 mg/200 mg po bid	None
Dolutegravir	50 mg po qd–bid	None
Elvitegravir	85–50 mg po qd	None
Raltegravir	400 mg po bid	None
Enfuvirtide (T-20)	90 mg sc bid	None
Maraviroc	Dose differs based on concomitant medications or potential drug–drug interactions.	Without CYP 3A inhibitors; 300 mg po bid; for orthostasis reduce to 150 mg po bid

Coformulated HIV drugs are to be avoided in hemodialysis.
From Panel on Antiretroviral Guidelines for Adults and Adolescents. Guidelines for the use of antiretroviral agents in HIV-1-infected adults and adolescents. Washington, DC: U.S. Department of Health and Human Services. http://aidsinfo.nih.gov/contentfiles/lvguidelines/AdultandAdolescentGL.pdf. Accessed July 9, 2016; Appendix B, Table 7.

guidelines regarding HIV therapy and dose adjustment for renal insufficiency may be found at https://aidsinfo.nih.gov/guidelines. HIV patients require no additional management considerations in the hemodialysis setting other than universal precautions and patient education regarding preventing transmission to others.

INFECTION CONTROL MEASURES IN THE DIALYSIS UNIT

In 2001, the CDC issued recommendations for preventing transmission of infections among chronic hemodialysis patients. These recommendations were updated and clarified in 2008 and also incorporated by reference into the CMS conditions for coverage for ESKD facilities. As a result, since October 2008, all ESKD facilities must follow CDC recommendations in order to receive Medicare reimbursement for outpatient dialysis (7). Knowledge of guidelines for prevention of HBV and HCV in the dialysis setting and infection control practices were assessed in a CDC national survey. In 2002, 63% of these centers reported reuse of disposable dialyzers, most of whom reprocessed them at their own facilities. Most centers reported using per acetic acid (72%), while 20% used formaldehyde, and 4% used heat or glutaraldehyde for disinfection. The practice of dialyzer reuse is considered safe if performed according to recognized protocols (10).

General infection control precautions for all patients include wearing disposable gloves during patient care, with removal of gloves and hand washing between patients. Nondisposable items that are not disinfectable (such as cloth covered blood pressure cuffs) should be dedicated for use on a single patient (6).

Multiple-dose vials containing medications or diluents taken to a patient station should be used only for the designated patient. This guideline was updated and clarified by CDC in August 2008 to specify that all single-use injectables must be dedicated for use on a single patient and be entered one time only to prevent transmission of both bacteria and blood-borne viruses. When multiple-dose medication vials are used, they should be assigned to a single patient whenever possible; patient doses should be individually prepared in a centralized area away from the dialysis stations. Multiple-dose medication vials should not be carried from station to station. Medication vials, syringes, or supplies should not be carried in pockets. All units need clean areas that are clearly designated for preparation and storage of medications and unused equipment (6). In addition, dialysis centers are required to report clusters of infections and adverse events to local public health authorities (7).

External venous and arterial pressure transducer filters/protectors should be used for each patient treatment to prevent contamination of dialyzer pressure monitors. Filters and protectors should be changed between each patient and not reused. However, internal transducer filters are not changed routinely between patients. Dialysis stations must be disinfected between patients, with special attention to cleaning control panels and frequently touched surfaces. All fluid should be properly discarded; used dialyzers and tubing must be placed in leak-proof containers during transport to disposal or reprocessing areas (6).

The HBsAg-positive patient must be dialyzed in a separate room using separate equipment, machines, and supplies. Staff taking care of HBsAg-positive patients may not care for HBV-susceptible patients during the same shift (6). Neither HIV- nor HCV-infected patients require dialysis in separate rooms.

POSTEXPOSURE PROPHYLAXIS GUIDELINES FOR PATIENTS AND STAFF

Human Immunodeficiency Virus

Recommendations from the U.S. Public Health Service were updated in 2013 and reflect better safety and tolerability of new antiviral medications (35,36). PEP with a three-drug antiviral regimen (emtricitabine, tenofovir, and raltegravir) is recommended whenever occupational exposure to HIV has occurred. It is important to document the HIV status of the source patient to determine management (36). Rapid HIV tests for source patients of unknown serostatus can expedite decisions regarding HIV PEP after occupational exposures. If PEP is offered, and the source patient is later determined to be uninfected, the PEP should be discontinued. Most HIV exposures do not result in the transmission of infection. The average risk for acquisition of HIV, after exposure to a known HIV-infected patient, is 0.3% per needle stick exposure and only .09% per mucous membrane blood splash. Therefore, the potential toxicity of antiretroviral drugs must be carefully considered before making a decision about PEP (35). After an exposure, the injured site or splashed mucous membrane should be immediately and thoroughly washed for 10 minutes with soap and water. The injury report should be made as soon as possible after the exposure to facilitate the institution of PEP within a few hours and no longer than 24 to 36 hours. Guidelines no longer recommend a two-drug regimen for lower risk exposures (i.e., those that did not involve large-bore hollow needles, deep punctures, visible blood on device, or needle used in patient artery or vein). Now, all occupational exposures require greater than or equal to three-drug PEP (e.g., emtricitabine, tenofovir, and raltegravir). If the patient is known or suspected to have drug-resistant HIV infection, expert consultation should be sought to customize the regimen; however, PEP administration should not be delayed (36). The duration of PEP for a confirmed exposure is 28 days, during which time the exposed health care worker should be counseled to abstain from unprotected sex, blood or tissue donation, or breastfeeding. PEP should be discontinued if the source patient is later determined to be HIV negative. Further details regarding risk assessment and PEP may be found at https://aidsinfo.nih.gov.

Expert Consultation Is Advised in the Following Situations

A report of an occupational exposure should be done no later than 72 hours after the incident and should include whether it is an unknown source, known or suspected pregnancy in the exposed person, breastfeeding in the exposed person, suspected resistance of the source virus to antiretroviral agents, toxicity of the initial PEP regimen, or serious medical illness in the exposed person (36). For all of these situations, local experts may be consulted and/or the National Clinician's Postexposure Prophylaxis hotline (PEP line; 1-888-448-4911) should be contacted. Whether or not expert consultation is sought, PEP should be initiated within hours of the exposure, not days later.

Serologic Follow-up after Exposure to Human Immunodeficiency Virus

Follow-up for the HIV-exposed health care worker should start with a baseline HIV antibody test by EIA and a follow-up appointment within 72 hours of exposure. HIV testing is repeated at 6 weeks, 12 weeks, and 6 months after the exposure. If a newer, fourth-generation combination HIVp24 antigen–antibody test is utilized, then HIV testing may be concluded after the 12-week test (36). In the particular circumstance where the exposure source is coinfected with HIV and HCV and the exposed person becomes HCV infected, an additional 12-month serologic follow-up to exclude HIV infection is recommended (35,36).

Hepatitis B Virus

The risk of HBV infection from a needle stick contaminated by HBV-infected blood ranges from 6% to 30% depending on the HBeAg status of the source. Patients who are both HBsAg and HBeAg positive are more likely to transmit HBV (37). In contrast, the risk of developing clinical hepatitis from a needle carrying HBsAg-positive, HBeAg-negative blood is 1% to 6%, and the risk of developing serologic evidence of HBV infection in this instance is 23% to 37% (6).

Percutaneous injuries actually account for the minority of HBV infections among health care providers. In fact, most infected health workers do not recall an overt needle stick, but up to a third of infected providers do recall caring for an HBsAg-positive patient. It is important to remember that HBV can survive at room temperature in dried blood on environmental surfaces for at least 7 days. Thus, HBV infections in health providers with no history of occupational injury come from blood or body fluid exposures that inoculated virus into scratches or abrasions, or on mucosal surfaces. HBV transmission via contact with contaminated surfaces has been repeatedly demonstrated in hemodialysis units (6).

PEP for an occupational exposure to hepatitis B in a nonimmune person should include both hepatitis B immune globulin (HBIG) and the hepatitis B vaccine series. Regimens consisting of multiple doses of HBIG alone or hepatitis B vaccine series are 70% to 75% effective in preventing HBV infection. After a percutaneous exposure to HBsAg-positive blood, multiple doses of HBIG should be initiated within 1 week. Although the efficacy of combining HBIG and the vaccine has not been formally evaluated for occupational settings, the superior efficacy of this protocol after perinatal exposure, compared with HBIG alone, is extrapolated to the occupational setting. As individuals requiring PEP at their work are continually at risk for HBV infection, they should receive the hepatitis B vaccine series.

Hepatitis C Virus

HCV is not efficiently transmitted via occupational blood exposures. The incidence of HCV seroconversion after a needle stick from an HCV-positive source is 1.8%. Transmission seldom results from mucous membrane exposures to infected blood, and no transmission in health workers has been documented from skin exposures. Unlike HBV, environmental contamination with blood containing HCV is not a meaningful risk for transmission in the health care setting (with the exception of hemodialysis units where HCV transmission has been associated with poor infection control practices). The risk of transmission from exposure to fluids other than HCV-infected blood is probably quite low (6).

After a percutaneous exposure to HCV, the exposed person should have baseline HCV antibody and RNA testing within 48 hours. If negative, follow-up HCV RNA and ALT testing every 4 to 6 weeks for 6 months is recommended to permit identification and treatment of acute infection (28). HCV clearance after acute infection is most likely to occur within 12 weeks of the onset of symptoms and is more likely in patients with symptomatic hepatitis. Safety and efficacy data for IFN-sparing oral therapy for HCV are not yet available, *but* current guidelines advise at 4 to 6 months of monitoring for spontaneous virologic clearance before initiating treatment. If the decision is made to initiate treatment after 6 months, treatment as described for chronic hepatitis C is recommended (28).

REFERENCES

1. Thornton L, Fitzpatrick F, De La Harpe D, et al. Hepatitis B reactivation in an Irish dialysis unit, 2005. *Euro Surveill* 2007;12:E7–E8.
2. Lok AS, McMahon BJ. Chronic hepatitis B. *Hepatology (Baltimore, Md.)* 2007;45:507–539.
3. Pereira BJ, Levey AS. Hepatitis C virus infection in dialysis and renal transplantation. *Kidney Int* 1997;51:981–999.
4. Fabrizi F, Messa P, Martin P. Hepatitis B virus infection and the dialysis patient. *Semin Dial* 2008;21:440–446.
5. Kalantar-Zadeh K, Kilpatrick RD, McAllister CJ, et al. Hepatitis C virus and death risk in hemodialysis patients. *J Am Soc Nephrol* 2007;18: 1584–1593.
6. Centers for Disease Control and Prevention. Recommendations for preventing transmission of infections among chronic hemodialysis patients. *MMWR Recomm Rep* 2001;50(RR-5):1–43.
7. Centers for Disease Control and Prevention. Infection control requirements for dialysis facilities and clarification regarding guidance on parenteral medication vials. *MMWR Morb Mortal Wkly Rep* 2008;57(32):875–876.
8. Fallahian F, Alavian S, Rasoulinejad M. Epidemiology and transmission of hepatitis G virus infection in dialysis patients. *Saudi J Kidney Dis Transpl* 2010;21:831–834.
9. Finelli L, Miller JT, Tokars JI, et al. National surveillance of dialysis-associated diseases in the United States, 2002. *Semin Dial* 2005;18: 52–61.
10. Tokars JI, Finelli L, Alter MJ, et al. National surveillance of dialysis-associated diseases in the United States, 2001. *Semin Dial* 2004;17:310–319.
11. Edey M, Barraclough K, Johnson D. Review article: hepatitis B and dialysis. *Nephrology* 2010;15:137–145.
12. Burdick RA, Bragg-Gresham JL, Woods JD, et al. Patterns of hepatitis B prevalence and seroconversion in hemodialysis units from three continents: the DOPPS. *Kidney Int* 2003;63:2222–2229.
13. Carrion A, Martin P. What are the management issues for hepatitis C in dialysis patients? Natural history of hepatitis C in dialysis populations. *Semin Dial* 2014;27:446–448.
14. Goodkin DA, Young EW, Kurokawa K, et al. Mortality among hemodialysis patients in Europe, Japan, and the United States: case-mix effects. *Am J Kidney Dis* 2004;44:16–21.
15. Velandia M, Fridkin SK, Cardenas V, et al. Transmission of HIV in dialysis centre. *Lancet* 1995;345:1417–1422.
16. Tourret J, Tostivint I, du Montcel ST, et al. Outcome and prognosis factors in HIV-infected hemodialysis patients. *Clin J Am Soc Nephrol* 2006;1:1241–1247.
17. Polenakovic M, Dzekova P, Sikole A. Hepatitis C in dialysis patients. *Prilozi* 2007;28:239–265.
18. Ramamurthy M, Muir AJ. Treatment of hepatitis C in special populations. *Clinics in Liver Disease* 2006;10:851–865.
19. Fabrizi F, Martin P, Lunghi G, et al. Natural history of HBV in dialysis population [in Italian]. *G Ital Nefrol* 2004;21:21–28.
20. Harnett JD, Parfrey PS, Kennedy M, et al. The long-term outcome of hepatitis B infection in hemodialysis patients. *Am J Kidney Dis* 1988;11:210–213.
21. Fabrizi F, Bunnapradist S, Lunghi G, et al. Epidemiology and clinical significance of hepatotropic infections in dialysis patients. Recent evidence. *Minerva Urol Nefrol* 2004;56:249–257.
22. Josselson J, Kyser BA, Weir MR, et al. Hepatitis B surface antigenemia in a chronic hemodialysis program: lack of influence on morbidity and mortality. *Am J Kidney Dis* 1987;9:456–461.
23. Chadha MS, Arankalle VA, Jha J, et al. Prevalence of hepatitis B and C virus infections among haemodialysis patients in Pune (western India). *Vox Sang* 1993;64:127–128.
24. Branson BM, Handsfield HH, Lampe MA, et al. Revised recommendations for HIV testing of adults, adolescents, and pregnant women in health-care settings. *MMWR Recomm Rep* 2006;55:1–17, quiz CE1–4.
25. Weiss RA. Special anniversary review: twenty-five years of human immunodeficiency virus research: successes and challenges. *Clin Exp Immunol* 2008;152:201–210.

26. European Association for the Study of the Liver. EASL Recommendations on Treatment of Hepatitis C 2015. *J Hepatol* 2015;63:199–236.

27. NIH Consensus Statement on Management of Hepatitis C: 2002. *NIH Consens State Sci Statements* 2002;19:1–46.

28. HCV Guidelines. www.hcvguidelines.org. Accessed July 9, 2016.

29. Soriano V, Madejon A, Vispo E, et al. Emerging drugs for hepatitis C. *Expert Opin Emerg Drugs* 2008;13:1–19.

30. Terrault N, Bzowej N, Chang K, et al. AASLD guidelines for treatment of chronic hepatitis B. *Hepatology* 2016;63:261–283. doi:10.1002/hep.28156.

31. Pipili C, Papatheodoridis G, Cholongitas E. Treatment of hepatitis B in patients with chronic kidney disease. *Kidney Int* 2013;84:880–885.

32. World Health Organization. *Guidelines for the Prevention, Care and Treatment of Persons with Chronic Hepatitis B Infection.* Geneva, Switzerland: World Health Organization. http://www.who.int/hiv/pub/hepatitis/hepatitis-b-guidelines/en/. Accessed July 9, 2016.

33. Ahuja TS, Kumar S, Mansoury H, et al. Hepatitis B vaccination in human immunodeficiency virus-infected adults receiving hemodialysis. *Kidney Int* 2005;67:1136–1141.

34. Dolin R, Masur H, Saag M, eds. *AIDS Therapy.* 3rd ed. Philadelphia, PA: Churchill Livingstone Elsevier, 2008.

35. Panlilio AL, Cardo DM, Grohskopf LA, et al. Updated U.S. Public Health Service guidelines for the management of occupational exposures to HIV and recommendations for postexposure prophylaxis. *MMWR Recomm Rep* 2005;54:1–17.

36. Kuhar D, Henderson D, Struble K, et al; for US Public Health Service Working Group. Updated US Public Health Service guidelines for the management of occupational exposures to human immunodeficiency virus and recommendations for postexposure prophylaxis. *Infect Control Hosp Epidemiol* 2013;34:875–892.

37. Centers for Disease and Control Prevention. Infection control. Updated October 25, 2013. http://www.cdc.gov/oralhealth/infectioncontrol/faq/bloodborne_exposures.htm. Accessed July 9, 2016.

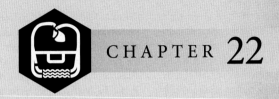

CHAPTER 22

Endocrine Disorders in Dialysis Patients

Yin Oo, Naim Maalouf, and R. Tyler Miller

Patients with renal insufficiency or who are receiving dialysis may develop the same endocrine disorders that are found in the general population including thyroid, adrenal, gonadal, and pituitary diseases, the areas addressed in this chapter. The symptoms of diseases of these hormone systems may overlap and be confused with the symptoms of kidney disease. Patients with kidney disease are also subject to endocrine disorders that arise as a consequence of their kidney disease. These disorders include infertility, impotence, growth hormone (GH) resistance, and disorders of mineral and bone metabolism. Additionally, uremia, metabolic acidosis, and chronic inflammation, which frequently accompany chronic kidney disease and end-stage kidney disease (ESKD), cause a generalized hormone insensitivity syndrome, a situation that contributes to illness in dialysis patients and complicates the diagnosis of many endocrine disorders. In this chapter, thyroid, adrenal, and pituitary diseases are discussed because they occur in patients with kidney disease, may not be suspected, and may be difficult to diagnose because many tests of endocrine function are altered, or are not possible to carry out in kidney disease. Fertility and impotence will also be considered because these are important problems for many patients. In each section, the physiology of the endocrine system, the most common diseases that affect it, and the diagnosis and therapy if they differ from diagnosis and therapy in the normal patient population are reviewed. Disorders of vitamin D, parathyroid hormone (PTH), bone metabolism, and lipids are considered elsewhere.

 THYROID DISORDERS

Introduction

An appropriate supply of thyroid hormone is essential for normal metabolism, cardiovascular function, mental status, and muscle strength. Diagnosis of thyroid disease in patients on dialysis is complicated by the fact that kidney disease can produce many of the same findings as thyroid disease and is often caused or accompanied by diseases such as diabetes, connective tissue diseases, and liver disease. These conditions can confound physical findings or alter standard tests used to evaluate thyroid function. Thyroid physiology, the effects of kidney disease, the most common thyroid disorders, and their evaluation, and management are described in this section.

Thyroid Physiology

Thyroid function is regulated at multiple levels to ensure that only minimal variation in circulating thyroid hormone levels occurs. The complexity of regulation of thyroid hormone reflects its importance as a regulator of development as well as metabolism and essential systemic functions. The synthesis and secretion of thyroid hormone are primarily controlled by the hypothalamus and pituitary. Although T_4 is the predominant circulating form of thyroid hormone, T_3 is the biologically active form and is responsible for negative feedback at the levels of the hypothalamus and pituitary that can reduce thyrotropin-releasing hormone (TRH) and thyroid-stimulating hormone (TSH) secretion, respectively. The hypothalamus produces TRH, and TRH stimulates TSH production and release by the thyrotrophic cells in the anteromedial region of the pituitary. TRH production and secretion increase in response to reduced circulating levels of T_3. TSH is the primary trophic hormone for the thyroid gland and is responsible for its size, vascularity, and the level of thyroid hormone production as well as the release of thyroid hormone.

Iodine, an essential substrate of thyroid hormone synthesis that is concentrated in the thyroid by an active transport mechanism, contributes to control of thyroid hormone synthesis and release. Excess iodine inhibits iodine uptake and thyroid hormone synthesis by the thyroid. High levels or acute high doses (such as given with Lugol's solution or with iodinated contrast dye) reduce thyroid hormone synthesis and secretion. The primary route of iodine excretion is the kidney, and as renal insufficiency progresses, one would expect iodine to be retained. Dialysis patients have increased serum inorganic iodine and thyroid iodine content as well as an increased incidence of enlarged thyroid glands, but the full physiologic implications of this situation are not understood (1).

Both T_4 and T_3 are produced in the thyroid, but T_4 is the predominant secreted form. T_3 levels in the systemic circulation primarily reflect peripheral conversion of T_4 to T_3 by a monodeiodinase, a metabolic step that is also subject to regulation. Several proteins in the blood bind and transport thyroid hormone, including thyroid-binding globulin (TBG), prealbumin, and albumin. Except in rare circumstances, the effects of the other proteins are negligible compared to that of TBG. Loss of thyroid hormone through hemo- or peritoneal dialysis is negligible under normal circumstances (1). Finally, the sensitivity of tissues to thyroid hormone can be altered through changes in thyroid hormone receptor expression (2).

Serum thyroid hormone levels vary with changes in the concentration of serum thyroid hormone–binding proteins. In states such as liver disease (acute and chronic hepatitis, primary biliary cirrhosis), HIV infection, use of estrogen, tamoxifen, or pregnancy, TBG levels are increased, which will be reflected in increased total thyroid hormone. In the nephrotic syndrome, following administration of androgens, or high-dose glucocorticoids, and in major systemic illnesses or acromegaly, TBG levels are decreased, and total serum thyroid hormone levels are reduced. In the absence of other complicating factors, serum free T_3 (fT_3) and free T_4 (fT_4) levels, the biologically important parameters, are normal.

Peripheral conversion of T_4 to T_3 is controlled by at least three enzymes, types 1 (5′), 2 (5′), and 3 (5′) deiodinases. Type 1

deiodinase is expressed in liver, kidney, thyroid, the central nervous system (CNS), and the pituitary and is responsible for conversion of T_4 to T_3 in these tissues. This enzyme is primarily responsible for systemic T_3 levels but may also produce reverse T_3 (rT_3), a metabolically inactive form of T_3. The peripheral conversion of T_4 to T_3 (presumably through inhibition of this enzyme) is reduced in a number of conditions that are important in nephrology including renal failure, malnutrition, liver disease, other systemic illnesses, and following trauma or surgery (euthyroid sick syndrome, nonthyroidal illness syndrome, or NTIS). Drugs that impair conversion of T_4 to T_3 include glucocorticoids, propranolol (>200 mg/d), amiodarone, and oral cholecystographic agents. The type 2 deiodinase is expressed in the CNS, pituitary, brown fat, and placenta. In states (see subsequent text) where peripheral conversion of T_4 to T_3 is reduced, type 2 deiodinase may maintain the CNS, pituitary, brown fat, and placenta in a relatively euthyroid state through *in situ* production of T_3. Type 3 deiodinase is expressed in the CNS, placenta, and skin and is the primary source of rT_3. rT_3 is an inactive metabolite of T_4 that increases in some conditions including burns, trauma, and uremia. The fact that local concentrations of T_3 may differ because of differential regulation of the deiodinases can make it difficult to determine if a hypothyroid state truly exists.

Measurement of Thyroid Function

The suspicion of thyroid disease is raised by the patient's history and physical findings and confirmed with laboratory measurement of thyroid hormone levels. Described below are the most commonly used assays with an emphasis on the laboratory characterization of the euthyroid-sick, NTISs because renal failure produces this pattern of laboratory values in up to 65% of dialysis patients (**FIGURE 22.1** and **TABLE 22.1**) (3–5). Sensitive assays are available for measuring fT_4, fT_3, rT_3, and TSH, and these measurements are

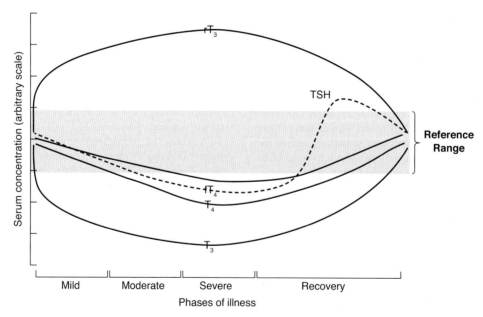

FIGURE 22.1 The varying levels of thyroid hormones, thyroid-stimulating hormone (TSH), and free T_4 (fT_4) in the "euthyroid-sick syndrome." Patients with kidney disease and receiving dialysis treatment may have thyroid function test values that correspond to any severity of illness shown on the graph when they do not have intrinsic thyroid, pituitary, or hypothalamic pathology. (Adapted from Meuwese CL, Dekkers OM, Stenvenkel P, et al. Nonthyroidal illness and the cardiorenal syndrome. *Nat Rev Nephrol* 2013;9:599–609.)

TABLE 22.1	**Changes in Thyroid Function Tests in Euthyroid/Sick, Hypothyroid, and Thyrotoxic States**			
	Normal	**Euthyroid/Sick**	**Hypothyroid**	**Thyrotoxic**
TSH	0.5–5 mIU/L	Normal to slightly decreased early; increased during recovery	Increased	Decreased
Free T_3	2.0–3.5 pg/mL	Decreased	Decreased	Increased
Free T_4	0.9–1.7 ng/dL	Decreased	Decreased	Increased
rT_3	10–24 ng/dL	Increased	Decreased to normal	Normal

Reference values for TSH (0.5 to 5 mU/L or 0.5 to 5 μU/mL), free T_3 (2.0 to 3.5 pg/mL) or free T_4 (0.9–1.7 ng/dL), and reverse T_3 (10–24 ng/dL) are given as the normal values. The direction of the change in the serum value is shown under the heading for each condition. In many situations, not all values will be abnormal but may be at the upper or lower limits of the normal range.
TSH, thyroid-stimulating hormone; rT_3, reverse T_3.
From Larsen PR, Davies TF, Hay ID. The thyroid gland. In: Wilson JD, Foster DW, Kronenberg HM, et al., eds. *Williams Textbook of Endocrinology.* 9th ed. Philadelphia, PA: WB Saunders, 1998:389–515.

the clinical tests used most commonly to establish the diagnosis of thyroid hormone excess or deficiency. Total serum T_4, T_3, and rT_3 are measured by radioimmunoassay (RIA for rT_3 is measured in special circumstances). Its level increases with alterations in peripheral deiodinase activity in systemic illnesses. T_4 is tightly bound by serum proteins (primarily TBG), and the level of total T_4 changes substantially with changes in the level of TBG. TBG may change markedly with disease or nutritional state so that a high or low total T_4 level may not be meaningful if the level of the thyroid hormone–binding protein is also high or low. Renal failure and dialysis do not directly affect TBG levels, although its levels may be reduced with persistent nephrotic range proteinuria, high rates of peritoneal protein loss, or following androgen administration for anemia in patients who might not also be receiving erythropoietin.

The biologically active form of the hormone is that which is "free" in the serum and not protein bound. In the past two decades, improved assays have allowed for more accurate measurement of true free thyroid hormone levels. Thus, in states of "pure" thyroid disease, the lack of specificity for total T_4 or T_3 is no longer a diagnostic problem because the level of fT_3 is a function of the level of fT_4. However, in conditions such as kidney disease, malnutrition, or other systemic diseases (euthyroid sick or NTISs), the activity of the peripheral deiodinases is altered, and conversion of T_4 to T_3 is not regulated normally (5,6). In these situations, serum fT_4 and fT_3 measurement are essential to fully characterize thyroid function.

Sensitive assays exist that allow direct measurement of TSH, the trophic hormone from the pituitary that participates in feedback regulation of thyroid function. TSH levels are a function of T_3 biologic activity in the hypothalamus where TRH production and release respond to T_3 levels and T_3 biologic activity in the pituitary. In primary thyroid disease, if T_3 levels are reduced, TSH levels rise. If T_3 levels are elevated, TSH levels are suppressed. However, hypothyroidism can occur as a result of a failure of the hypothalamopituitary axis resulting in low or inappropriately normal TSH levels, and thyrotoxicosis can result from increased secretion of TSH such as from a pituitary tumor. The normal range for TSH is 0.5 to 5 mU/mL. Patients who are thyrotoxic have serum TSH levels below 0.5 mU/mL, and patients who have hypothyroid have serum levels above 5 mU/mL. If pituitary failure is suspected, a TRH stimulation test can be performed.

Dialysis patients have at least one systemic illness, chronic kidney disease, and frequently others such as malnutrition and diabetes. These chronic illnesses (and others) alter the activity of peripheral deiodinases and cause an abnormal pattern of thyroid function tests, termed the *euthyroid-sick syndrome* (3,5). This patient population is also characterized by increased levels of circulating cytokines such as interleukin 6 (IL-6) that may also contribute to biochemical abnormalities including the euthyroid sick state (6). The euthyroid sick syndrome is characterized by reduced total and free serum T_3 and increased serum rT_3 as a result of increased peripheral deiodination of T_4 to rT_3. The degree of reduction of the serum T_3 level corresponds to the severity of the systemic illness (**FIGURE 22.1**). In mild to moderately severe illnesses, fT_3 is reduced, rT_3 is increased, but T_4, fT_4, and TSH levels are normal. With severe illness, the fT_4 levels may fall in the subnormal range. During recovery from a severe illness, the TSH level may rise to levels slightly above normal before normalizing. Consequently, thyroid hormone levels in dialysis patients must be interpreted using a euthyroid-sick pattern as normal.

Whether patients with the NTIS are in fact physiologically hypothyroid is not known. fT_4, fT_3, and rT_3 levels reflect systemic metabolism of T_4, while TSH levels reflect hypothalamic and pituitary levels of T_3. In the presence of illness where peripheral conversion of T_4 to T_3 is reduced, TSH levels may not reflect low T_3 levels because the conversion of T_4 to T_3 in the tissue responsible for sensing T_3 activity (hypothalamus and pituitary) is mediated by a deiodinase whose activity does not appear to change with systemic illness. In contrast, systemic measurement of thyroid hormones reflects metabolism by different deiodinases whose activity may change with systemic illness. Consequently, the CNS and pituitary may appear euthyroid, while the remainder of the body is hypothyroid. Administration of L T_4 to severely ill patients has been studied but does not alter their outcomes (7,8). Survivors could be identified by their high baseline T_3:T_4 ratios. Low serum T_3 levels in dialysis patients are associated with reduced survival (4). Preliminary studies in dialysis patients suggest that treatment of dialysis patients with low doses of T_3 results in a less favorable nitrogen balance and increased protein degradation (1).

Thyroid Diseases

Thyroid diseases can be separated into those that cause increased hormone levels (thyrotoxicosis), decreased hormone levels (hypothyroidism), those that produce nonfunctional nodules, and the inflammatory diseases of the thyroid.

Thyrotoxicosis

Thyrotoxicosis is a pathophysiologic condition that results from excess thyroid hormone. The precise manifestations of thyrotoxicosis depend on the magnitude of hormone excess, the age of the patient, and the presence of other illnesses such as cardiovascular disease and diabetes. In general, the effects of thyroid hormone excess represent an exaggeration of its normal physiologic response and are usually most prominent on metabolism and on the cardiovascular and nervous systems.

Elevated thyroid hormone levels cause an increase in metabolic rate that is reflected in increased calorie utilization, oxygen consumption, heat generation, and increased basal body temperature. Protein synthesis and breakdown are increased, but degradation exceeds synthesis, leading to weight loss and decreased body mass. Many such patients have an abnormal glucose tolerance that may simulate diabetes mellitus. Lipid metabolism is also altered with both increased synthesis and degradation of lipids, but with degradation exceeding synthesis, leading to increased serum free fatty acid levels, while triglyceride and cholesterol levels are decreased. The metabolic manifestations of thyrotoxicosis may be difficult to detect in patients with renal disease and those who are on dialysis because they overlap with those of renal failure or with chronic diseases such as diabetes mellitus that are commonly found in the dialysis population. Although kidney disease patients rarely are hyperthermic, they commonly are catabolic and glucose intolerant.

Thyroid hormone has a direct cardiostimulatory activity that leads to increased cardiac output through resting tachycardia (heart rate greater than 100 bpm), increased stroke volume, and decreased peripheral resistance. The increased cardiac output is a response to supply the increased oxygen demands and the requirement to dissipate heat. Patients with hyperthyroidism may also have increased blood pressure and a widened pulse pressure. Because of the high frequency of hypertension and alterations in total body volume in dialysis patients, these findings may not be valuable in identifying patients with thyrotoxicosis. However, arrhythmias, congestive heart failure, and a change in pattern of angina may provide excellent clues to the presence of thyrotoxicosis. Supraventricular arrhythmias, especially atrial fibrillation, are common and may be the presenting complaint in patients with thyrotoxicosis. In the absence of preexisting heart disease, congestive heart failure is an uncommon presentation of thyrotoxicosis. Patients with thyrotoxicosis and atrial fibrillation are commonly resistant to heart rate control with digitalis. The frequency, pattern, or severity of angina is frequently increased in thyrotoxic patients with coronary artery disease. Patients may complain of shortness of breath in the absence of congestive heart failure. This sensation may be due to reduced lung compliance and muscle weakness in some circumstances.

Thyrotoxicosis usually produces prominent effects in the nervous system. Patients complain of nervousness that is characterized by a short attention span, restlessness, and compulsion to move despite fatigue. These patients often have fast jerky movements and a fine rhythmic tremor of hands and tongue. They are emotionally labile and often complain of insomnia. Psychiatric disorders occur including manic-depressive, schizoid, and paranoid states.

In patients with seizure disorders, the seizure threshold is lowered resulting in an increased frequency of seizures. The hyperkinetic state described is uncommon in dialysis patients, but fatigue, restlessness, inattention, psychiatric and emotional disturbances, and changes in seizure frequency occur frequently. Consequently, the existence of any one of this constellation of findings in a patient may not be helpful in suggesting thyrotoxicosis, but their appearance in a patient who was previously stable may be of diagnostic value.

Common gastrointestinal (GI) symptoms include increased motility (faster gastric and intestinal emptying and transit times) with less well-formed stools, and increased stool frequency. Overt diarrhea is rare. Appetite is generally increased in hyperthyroid patients, although it may be decreased in severe cases or in the elderly. Patients with kidney disease usually have decreased bowel motility, so apparent normalization of bowel function may be a clue to thyrotoxicosis. Hepatic dysfunction with elevated transaminases has been reported in thyrotoxicosis, possibly due in part to increased O_2 extraction in the splanchnic bed (9).

Increased levels of thyroid hormone alter the structure and function of muscle and bone. Patients complain of proximal muscle weakness and fatigability. These symptoms are usually partly due to wasting and loss of muscle mass but are also due to primary changes in the muscles. Myopathy is more common in men than women. In patients with normal kidney function, thyrotoxicosis leads to loss of bone mass with increased bone turnover, greater urinary excretion of Ca and PO_4, and turnover markers such as deoxypyridinoline, with reduced levels of serum PTH and vitamin D. In dialysis patients, the effects of excess thyroid hormone on bone mass presumably are similar, but they have not been reported.

Causes of Thyrotoxicosis

Dialysis patients develop thyrotoxicosis for the same reasons as patients with normal kidney function. The causes include Graves' disease or toxic diffuse goiter, toxic thyroid nodule, toxic multinodular goiter, thyroiditis, and rarely due to increased secretion of TSH due to a pituitary adenoma, increased secretion of TRH, or resistance of either the hypothalamus or pituitary to T_3. Graves' disease is the most common cause of thyrotoxicosis and is an autoimmune disease that results from circulating autoantibodies (thyroid-stimulating immunoglobulins or TSIs) that appear to be directed against the TSH receptor on the thyroid cell membrane. The disease is characterized not only by thyrotoxicosis but also by an infiltrative ophthalmopathy producing exophthalmos and dermopathy. Toxic multinodular goiter usually arises in a multinodular thyroid gland. The thyrotoxicosis is usually less severe than in Graves' disease, but it occurs in an older population so cardiovascular symptoms may be more prominent (2). Thyroid nodules may be more common in patients receiving chronic dialysis (10). Thyroiditis may be triggered by a viral infection, exposure to iodinated contrast material, or medications such as amiodarone.

Diagnosis of Thyrotoxicosis

Thyrotoxicosis may not be suspected in dialysis patients because the symptoms of thyrotoxicosis may be ascribed to other underlying illnesses such as cardiovascular disease, hypertension, and volume overload. Many of the symptoms may be masked by medications such as β-blockers or other blood pressure medications. Weight loss may be masked by retained fluid or ascribed to gastroparesis. Nevertheless, new symptoms that are consistent with thyrotoxicosis, particularly cardiovascular symptoms, should suggest the possibility of thyrotoxicosis (**TABLE 22.1** and **FIGURE 22.2**).

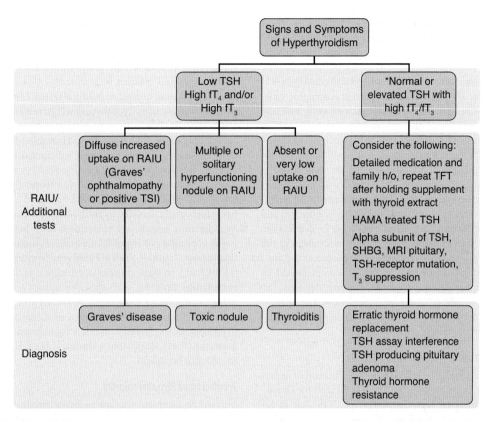

FIGURE 22.2 The detail diagnostic workup of this category is beyond the scope of this review. RAIU, radioactive iodine uptake scan; TSI, thyroid-stimulating immunoglobulin; TFT, thyroid function tests; HAMA, human anti-mouse monoclonal antibody; SHBG, sex hormone–binding globulin.

The complaint or finding of increasing neck size or a lump in the anterior neck is particularly valuable in identifying patients who may be thyrotoxic. Thyrotoxicosis is caused by elevated T_3, and a diagnosis of thyrotoxicosis requires elevated levels of fT_3 and/or fT_4, so these hormones should be measured. If thyrotoxicosis is caused by primary overproduction of thyroid hormone by the entire gland (Graves' disease) or by nodules (95% of cases), the TSH level will be suppressed. If thyrotoxicosis is caused by overproduction of TSH (pituitary tumor, hypothalamic lesion or ectopic production, <5% of cases), the TSH level will be elevated.

Treatment of Thyrotoxicosis

The immediate treatment of thyrotoxicosis in patients with kidney disease is the same as other patients and includes the use of β-blockers, dexamethasone, and agents that block thyroid hormone synthesis and release (propylthiouracil and methimazole). In patients with renal failure, propylthiouracil can cause granulocytopenia, agranulocytosis, rheumatic syndromes, and hepatitis. However, the doses of both propylthiouracil and methimazole are not changed in dialysis patients. Radioactive ^{131}iodine (^{131}I) ablation may also be used, although it is cleared by both peritoneal and hemodialysis (11). Disposal of the radioactive effluent can be a problem for which guidelines do not exist.

Hypothyroid States

Hypothyroidism occurs for three general reasons: (a) most commonly, loss of functional thyroid tissue; (b) loss of trophic activity by TSH; and (c) defective hormone synthesis (as with iodine deficiency). Loss of trophic activity in pituitary or hypothalamic lesions

represents approximately 5% of all cases of hypothyroidism. The symptoms of hypothyroidism are generally the opposite of those of thyrotoxicosis. They are even more difficult to identify in kidney disease and dialysis because like kidney disease, hypothyroidism results in generalized constitutional symptoms and gradual loss of function. Reduced glomerular filtration rate (GFR) is associated with hypothyroidism, and a GFR of <30 mL/min confers a risk of hypothyroidism that is increased approximately twofold over the normal population (GFR >90 mL/min) (12).

In hypothyroidism, the metabolic rate slows, resulting in decreased oxygen consumption; heat generation decreases; appetite decreases; and the rate of protein synthesis is reduced. The latter may be due to decreased effectiveness of GH and insulin-like growth factor 1 (also known as *somatomedin C*). The oral glucose tolerance test is flat, and the peak insulin response is delayed. The rate of degradation of insulin is decreased leading to an increased sensitivity to exogenous insulin. Patients also have increased capillary permeability which leads to peripheral edema. Cholesterol and triglyceride circulating concentration levels are elevated as a consequence of their decreased clearance, and high-density lipoprotein (HDL) levels are reduced. Superficially, none of these findings are specific for hypothyroidism and are seen frequently in dialysis patients.

Hypothyroidism reduces heart rate and myocardial contractility, diminishing pulse pressure and reducing cardiac output. The heart is enlarged, and a pericardial effusion frequently develops. Pleural effusions are also common. Electrocardiogram (ECG) abnormalities include sinus bradycardia, prolonged PR interval, reduced amplitude of the P wave and QRS complex, and nonspecific ST-segment and T-wave changes. These changes may contribute to congestive heart failure. Other than the bradycardia, these findings are commonly seen to progress slowly over months and are commonly seen on dialysis services in patients with normal thyroid function.

In hypothyroidism, GI motility is decreased and constipation is a frequent complaint. The mucosa of the GI tract is atrophic causing reduced absorption, but the decreased transit time partially compensates for the decreased absorption rate. Ascites consisting of mucopolysaccharide- and protein-rich fluid is common. Superficially, these findings are not pathognomonic for hypothyroidism and can occur for a variety of reasons in the dialysis population.

The most prominent symptoms in hypothyroidism are frequently found in the nervous system. They include reduced cognitive function, deterioration of memory, slow speech, syncope, and coma. Psychiatric symptoms may include paranoia or depression. Speech is thick and slurred as a consequence of infiltration of the larynx and tongue by mucopolysaccharides. Movements are slow and appear uncoordinated and may be further compromised by compression of peripheral nerves by myxedematous deposits. Reflexes are slow due to altered nerve responses including delayed relaxation time. Myxedematous patients complain of stiff, sore muscles, but muscle strength usually remains intact.

Causes of Hypothyroidism

Loss of functional thyroid tissue occurs following ablation of hyperactive thyroid tissue (such as following ablative therapy for Graves' disease with ^{131}I), idiopathic hypothyroidism, or in the late stages of Hashimoto's thyroiditis (autoimmune thyroiditis). Excess iodine inhibits thyroid function by inhibiting thyroid uptake of iodine and thyroid hormone synthesis and release. As the primary route of excretion of iodine is the urine, one might expect high levels of iodine to accumulate in patients with renal failure. Regulation of iodine metabolism in kidney disease and dialysis patients has not been studied systematically, but ^{131}I is removed by hemodialysis and peritoneal dialysis (11). One report of three cases exists of hypothyroidism due to iodine accumulation in dialysis patients eating a high-iodine diet (13). Iodinated contrast agents may also represent an iodine load for dialysis patients that could affect thyroid function. Another group of patients who may be at risk for hypothyroidism are patients with iron overload syndromes (14). Metabolic acidosis causes reduced T_3, and T_4, levels and increased TSH levels with an increased sensitivity of TSH secretion to TRH stimulation (15). In dialysis patients, correction of metabolic acidosis increases TSH levels so the metabolic acidosis associated with kidney disease is a treatable cause of hypothyroidism (16).

Diagnosis of Hypothyroidism

Many of the symptoms of hypothyroidism are nonspecific and overlap with those of chronic kidney disease (17). Consequently, hypothyroidism may not be suspected and may go undiagnosed. Patients who are at particular risk for hypothyroidism are those who have a history of previous ablative treatment of thyroid disease, possibly those with other autoimmune endocrine diseases, or those whose general condition deteriorates for unexplained reasons. The physical signs of hypothyroidism such as delayed reflexes may be undetectable in a diabetic patient with neuropathy, or a slow pulse may be masked in a patient taking β-blockers, and may also be difficult to identify in dialysis patients who have many comorbid conditions and take many medications. Nevertheless, if present, delayed reflexes are valuable in making the diagnosis of hypothyroidism as

long as other neurologic disorders are not present. If a patient is not taking medications that could slow the heart rate, then heart rate is also valuable in screening patients for hypothyroidism. Measurement of circulating thyroid hormone levels will usually reveal a "sick-euthyroid" pattern with a variable (low or normal) fT_4, low rT_3U, low fT_3, and normal or mildly elevated TSH. However, dialysis patients who are truly hypothyroid will have elevations of TSH with normal hypothalamopituitary function, so primary hypothyroidism can be diagnosed with a serum TSH in most situations. Whether mild elevations of TSH represent subclinical hypothyroidism, or whether this state represents a euthyroid CNS and pituitary with a hypothyroid periphery is not clear (2). Normal patients with minimal elevations of their TSH levels (<10 to 15 mU/mL) are usually not symptomatic. Isolated hypothyroidism is unusual in pituitary or hypothalamic lesions (see subsequent text), but if hypothyroidism is due to pituitary or hypothalamic failure (tumors, following radiation therapy, trauma), the TSH level may be extremely low (less than 0.5 mU/mL). In these situations, evaluation of the pituitary and hypothalamus structure with either computed tomography (CT) or magnetic resonance imaging (MRI) scans and function with TSH and TRH stimulation tests is indicated. Corroborative evidence of hypothalamic or pituitary disease with reduced follicle-stimulating hormone (FSH), luteinizing hormone (LH), GH, and cortisol levels should also be sought.

Treatment of Hypothyroidism

Thyroid replacement therapy in hypothyroid patients on chronic dialysis is the same as that in other populations. In general, patients with kidney disease are at risk for cardiovascular disease if they have not already been diagnosed with it. Consequently, their thyroid hormone should be replaced slowly to avoid precipitating angina or congestive heart failure, unless the patient is comatose or severely ill with another diagnosis. The usual replacement dose of levothyroxine (T_4) is around 1.6 μg per kilogram body weight per day. Some physicians use thyroid extract (120 mg/d) or T_3 (liothyronine or cytomel, replacement dose 50 to 100 μg/d), but levothyroxine (T_4) has the advantage that the body can regulate its conversion to T3 and the serum half-life is longer (18). A role for T_3 in euthyroid-sick patients has not been established (2). The effectiveness and dosing of thyroid replacement therapy is usually followed by measuring serum TSH because no other physiologic or symptomatic parameter is sufficiently sensitive.

⬡ ANTERIOR PITUITARY DISORDERS

Introduction

The anterior pituitary gland integrates information from the brain (hypothalamus) and feedback from peripheral hormones to control production of its trophic hormones (19,20). The hormones produced by the anterior pituitary, adrenocorticotropic hormone (ACTH), GH, prolactin, TSH, FSH, and LH, all have specific effects on different tissues in the body, and their excess production as well as loss of their production produces specific syndromes. In general, syndromes of pituitary hormone excess can be related to individual hormones because they are individually controlled and produced in distinct cell types. In contrast, deficiency syndromes involve multiple or all of the hormones secreted because they are caused by processes that destroy the hypothalamus and/or pituitary. Prolactin is the exception because its synthesis and release are under tonic inhibitory control by the hypothalamus. Chronic kidney disease alters the regulation and response to GH, prolactin, FSH, and LH. The biology of these hormones is complex and not fully understood in normal conditions, and their biology remains only partially characterized in dialysis patients. TSH is discussed earlier in the section "Thyroid Diseases."

Physiology

The anterior pituitary contains cells that produce several hormones including ACTH, GH, prolactin, TSH, FSH, and LH. Each hormone is produced by an individual cell type. Functioning tumors of the pituitary are usually clonal and produce one hormone of the anterior pituitary. The venous system that drains the hypothalamus forms a plexus in the anterior pituitary so that peptide-releasing factors descending from the hypothalamus control the activity of the pituitary cells and the release of ACTH, GH, prolactin, TSH, FSH, and LH. The six peptide-releasing factors are corticotrophin-releasing factor (CRF) that stimulates ACTH release, TRH that stimulates TSH release, gonadotropin-releasing hormone (GnRH) that simulates FSH and LH release, growth hormone–releasing hormone (GHRH) that stimulate GH release, somatostatin that inhibits secretion of all of the pituitary hormones but is most potent in inhibiting GH release, and prolactin inhibitory activity (PRIH) that tonically inhibits prolactin release. PRIH may be several factors including dopamine. These hormones are also subject to regulation at the level of the pituitary by direct feedback mechanisms.

Growth Hormone

GH has a variety of growth-promoting and metabolic effects (19,20). GH is produced in the somatotrophs of the pituitary and is secreted under the dual control of GHRH (stimulatory) and somatostatin (inhibitory), which results in a pulsatile pattern of release. GHRH secretion is increased by dopamine, serotonin, α-adrenergic agonists, hypoglycemia, exercise, protein-rich food, and emotional stress and is inhibited by β-adrenergic agonists, free fatty acids, insulin-like growth factor 1, and GH. GH is carried in the serum primarily by a binding protein, growth hormone–binding protein (GHBP), which is derived from the GH receptor. Although GH has direct differentiating effects on some cell types, most of its effects are through stimulation of production of somatomedins or insulin-like growth factors 1 and 2 (IGF-1 and IGF-2). IGF-1 appears to replicate many of the biologic effects of GH, but the function of IGF-2 is less well defined. IGF-1 is produced locally in small quantities in response to GH, but the liver appears to be the main site of production. IGF is carried in the serum by a six-member family of binding proteins (IGFBP 1–6) and is so tightly bound that only approximately 1% of the hormone is free.

The growth-promoting effects of GH are primarily to increase cell number and produce a positive nitrogen balance, with accumulation of Ca, Mg, K, Na, and PO_4. Before puberty and the closure or epiphyses, GH increases bone length and thickness and produces a proportional increase in the size of other organs and tissues except the CNS. In adulthood (after the closure of epiphyses), bones cannot grow in length and only become thicker while other organs increase in size. Like insulin, GH is an anabolic hormone, but in contrast to insulin, it leads to carbohydrate intolerance, inhibits lipogenesis, increases mobilization of fat, and promotes ketosis. In nondiabetic patients with even low amounts of insulin present, these effects of GH are anabolic, but in diabetic patients, its effects are diabetogenic. In the absence of insulin, GH does not have anabolic activity. GH levels increase with exercise, hypoglycemia, and sleep.

GH excess causes gigantism if it occurs before puberty, and acromegaly if it occurs after epiphyseal closure. The most common cause of GH excess is a microadenoma of the pituitary. GH deficiency may occur as a consequence of hypothalamic disease or as a result of loss of GH receptors (Laron dwarfism). If it occurs in infancy or childhood, growth failure results. In adults who are fully grown at the time GH deficiency develops, the consequences appear to be minimal and may involve mild loss of muscle mass and impaired nutrient utilization, but the condition has not been studied well.

Chronic kidney disease and dialysis alter the GHRH-GH-IGF-1 system such that uremic patients appear to be insensitive to GH and IGF-1 and have higher GH levels due to increased secretory bursts and an increased half-life of GH with reduced IGF-1 levels (16,21–25). This resistance to GH and IGF-1 may explain why acromegaly is so rare in dialysis patients. This field is complicated because the nutritional and metabolic status (metabolic acidosis) of the patient and chronic illnesses alter the GH/IGF axis (16). Consequently, the relative importance of malnutrition, acidosis, uremic toxins, and decreased clearance of peptides by the kidney are difficult to determine. This remains an area of intense investigation in both clinical and basic science. Most of the recent information is from the pediatric literature because of interest in the growth retardation found in pediatric renal failure and dialysis patients. In the adult population, insensitivity to GH and IGF-1 may contribute to the catabolism and wasting that commonly occur. Information on the mechanisms of resistance to GH and IGF-1 has not been completely established in humans. Some information is available from human studies and more can be inferred from animal disease models.

In kidney disease, GH levels are increased due to reduced clearance of GH by the kidney and an increased number of secretory bursts. In one study, the circulating concentrations in controls were 0.7 μg/mL versus 1.22 μg/mL in dialysis patients (21). In prepubertal patients, secretion is increased, but in pubertal patients and presumably adults, it is decreased (23,26). The level of GHBP (which reflects hepatic GH receptor expression levels) is reduced, providing a possible mechanism for GH insensitivity. Studies in humans and experimental animals indicate that metabolic acidosis is sufficient to confer resistance to GH (16,24,27,28). Dialysis patients are resistant to the short-term metabolic effects of IGF-1, IGF-1-stimulated reductions in plasma insulin, cortisol, C-peptide, and amino acid levels (29). Although the levels of IGF-1 are normal to slightly reduced, the levels of IGFBP (particularly IGFBP-2, 3, and 5) are increased (30). Because these IGFBPs bind IGF-1 tightly, the bioavailability of IGF-1 is reduced (23). The levels of the IGFBPs appear to be increased because of their reduced clearance by the kidney. In experimental systems, excess IGFBP is sufficient to inhibit the growth-promoting effects of IGF-1 (23). The half-life ($t_{1/2}$) and volume of distribution of recombinant human IGF-1 are reduced in dialysis patients (31). Low molecular weight substances in uremic serum also appear to inhibit the action of IGF-1 (23,32).

The biologic effects of GH and IGF-1 are inhibited at many levels in uremia, and tissue resistance to these hormones may contribute to morbidity and mortality in this patient population. The benefits of human growth hormone (hGH) therapy are most clear in the pediatric population, and recombinant human growth hormone (rhGH) treatment is now established therapy for children with growth failure due to ESKD and renal insufficiency once nutritional and metabolic deficiencies (including acidosis, PO_4 levels, and PTH levels) have been corrected or optimized (33).

Long-term (4 to 8 years) administration of recombinant hGH (achieving supranormal levels and increasing IGF-1 levels) to children with chronic renal insufficiency and failure can restore linear growth and result in catch-up growth so that they achieve normal height (34,35). rhGH treatment may also improve muscle mass and bone density. This therapy does not have adverse effects on Ca, PO_4, bone metabolism, glucose tolerance (although insulin levels may be elevated), the incidence of malignancy, or benign intracranial hypertension, and for patients with kidney insufficiency, the rate of progression of kidney disease was not accelerated (33–35). The dose of rhGH is higher than for patients with GH deficiency, on the order of 0.35 mg/kg/wk (28 IU/m^2/wk), and may be higher during puberty. Nutritional requirements may increase in patients treated with rhGH. Methods for following dosing of the drug (e.g., serum IGF-1 levels) have not been established. Factors that contribute to a favorable response to hGH are increased height at the initiation of therapy, young age at the start of therapy, and shorter duration of dialysis treatment (33,35).

The role for recombinant hGH in the treatment of adults on dialysis is less clear because long-term, large-scale studies have not been performed. Patients treated with rhGH for 6 months show an increase in muscle mass, hand grip strength, albumin levels, and increased bone turnover with a decrease in bone density and total body mineral content (36–40). Shorter term metabolic studies demonstrate that rhGH treatment leads to a positive nitrogen balance (40). Although these studies support an anabolic effect of rhGH in dialysis patients and do not report complications of therapy, they are of relatively short duration, so the risk of potential complications of elevated levels of GH and IGF-1 that include insulin resistance and glucose intolerance, hypertension, cardiomyopathy, abnormal bone growth, and an increased incidence of colonic polyps cannot be determined. Optimal treatment of acidosis may restore the sensitivity of patients to GH and IGF-1, so improvements in the GH-IGF-1 system may be effected without administration of rhGH (41,42). Erythropoietin may sensitize the pituitary to the effects of GHRH, so optimal therapy with this agent may also have anabolic effects (43,44). The leptin system does not appear to play a major role in the catabolic state of dialysis patients (45,46).

Prolactin

Prolactin is produced by the lactotrophs in the pituitary, and it is secreted in a pulsatile fashion. In contrast to other pituitary hormones, prolactin is under tonic negative control by inhibitory factors from the hypothalamus. Its normal function in women is to promote lactation in cooperation with estrogen and progesterone, but its function in men is not established. Increased prolactin levels are caused by dopamine antagonists, oral contraceptives, diseases of the hypothalamus or pituitary that interfere with tonic suppression of prolactin secretion, and tumors. Up to 30% of pituitary tumors secrete prolactin. Prolactin is a stress response hormone, and its blood levels may rise with stress or pain. Normal prolactin levels are 2 to 15 µg/mL, levels in dialysis patients are often in the range of 15 to 50 µg/mL, and levels greater than 250 µg/mL are suggestive of first trimester pregnancy or a prolactin-secreting tumor (20,21). In women, excess production of prolactin results in galactorrhea, suppression of menstrual cycles, and infertility, and in men, infertility (47).

In dialysis patients, prolactin levels are elevated because of increased secretion and decreased clearance (21,47). Elevated prolactin levels may be responsible for some of the gonadal abnormalities found in kidney disease. Recent reports indicate that erythropoietin reduces prolactin levels by mechanisms that may be independent of the improvement in anemia (48). Hypothyroidism, pregnancy, and medication-induced hyperprolactinemia should be excluded by careful history, physical exam, TSH, and human chorionic gonadotropin (hCG) measurements. Prolactinomas can be effectively treated with dopamine agonist that suppresses prolactin production. Sexual function in dialysis patients has improved in response to bromocriptine, a dopamine agonist that suppresses prolactin production (49). Cabergoline is more effective than bromocriptine because cabergoline is better tolerated and has higher affinity for dopamine receptor binding sites (50,51). However, about 10% to 15% of patients with prolactinomas are resistant to dopamine agonist therapy and may require additional therapy such as transsphenoidal surgery or radiotherapy (52).

Follicle-Stimulating Hormone, Luteinizing Hormone, and Gonadal Function

FSH and LH are secreted by the same pituitary cell, the gonadotrope. Their secretion is controlled by the integration of signals from luteinizing hormone–releasing hormone (LHRH) and feedback signals from estrogen, progesterone, and androgens, and gonadal peptides such as inhibin (20). Pulsatile, rather than continuously elevated, levels of LHRH are required for normal gonadal function. The frequency and amplitude of the pulses is controlled by the hypothalamus through hypothalamic function and feedback mechanisms from the periphery. LH controls production of estrogen and progesterone in the ovary and testosterone in the testis. FSH stimulates sertoli cells to produce sperm and expression of LH receptors by Leydig cell. In women, FSH stimulates follicle development. These systems are abnormal in both men and women with kidney disease or who are on dialysis. Although psychological factors may contribute to sexual dysfunction, abnormalities at the levels of the hypothalamus and gonads are probably the predominant cause.

Reproduction in Women

Female dialysis patients frequently exhibit amenorrhea, dysmenorrhea, dysfunctional uterine bleeding, and cystic ovarian disease. These disorders occur because of disruption of normal menstrual cycles at the level of the hypothalamus and ovary (47,53). LH levels are tonically elevated due to increased release, the estrogen-induced LH surge does not occur, and FSH levels are normal or slightly elevated (53). Suppression of pulsatile LHRH secretion by prolactin may contribute to this problem. Additionally, the ovaries have a subnormal steroidogenic response to LH. The frequency of menstruation has risen from 10% to 20% 20 years ago to approximately 40% at this time which may reflect improved dialysis quality or care, but these cycles are generally thought to be anovulatory (54).

Conception occurs with a frequency of approximately 0.3% to 2.2% per year in Western countries, although these numbers represent estimates because accurate records are not kept (54–58). The frequency of conception on dialysis appears to be increasing, which may reflect improved dialysis techniques, beneficial effects of erythropoietin, and in some cases the effects of frequent dialysis regimens. Of the patients who conceive and progress to the first trimester, approximately 50% deliver viable infants. In two studies of patients who were treated with dialysis when they were pregnant, those who conceived before starting dialysis delivered viable infants in 75% to 80% of the cases, and those who conceived on dialysis delivered viable infants in 40% to 50% of cases (55,58,59).

Pregnancies are complicated by intrauterine death, hypertension, intrauterine growth retardation, premature labor, premature birth of babies with low birth weights for gestational age, and an increased frequency of congenital malformations (60). Neonatal care is an important factor in the survival of these infants (55–58). Deliveries of viable infants occur at approximately 32 weeks, and the outcome improves with longer gestation. The infants weigh on the order of 1,200 to 1,550 g at birth. An increased dose of dialysis appears to be beneficial with reports of weekly Kt/V values of 6 to 8, or dialysis 5 to 6 days per week (55–57,61,62). Increased doses of erythropoietin are required to maintain hemoglobin levels in an acceptable range, and transfusions are sometimes required in addition (55,58). In many cases, patients are hospitalized around week 20 of gestation for management of blood pressure, dialysis fluid balance, nutrition, and anemia (63). Transplantation provides the best outcomes in fertility and pregnancy for patients with ESKD.

Evaluation for amenorrhea, dysmenorrhea, or dysfunctional uterine bleeding in women receiving dialysis should be carried out in consultation with a gynecologist. The evaluation should include a thorough pelvic examination, Pap smear, and may also include measurement of serum prolactin, LH and FSH levels, a pelvic ultrasound, and endometrial biopsy.

Reproduction in Men

In men, erectile dysfunction, impotence, decreased libido, and decreased sperm count are manifestations of uremia. LH is elevated due to increased secretion and decreased clearance. The increased LH production may be caused by low levels of testosterone synthesis by the testes. FSH levels are usually normal but may be high with severe testicular dysfunction. Presumably, increased prolactin levels would interfere with normal regulation of LHRH secretion. Evaluation of men for impotence should include measurement of serum prolactin, testosterone, FSH, and LH levels. Correction of anemia with erythropoietin may improve the function of the hypothalamo–pituitary–testicular axis in dialysis patients (64). Patients should also be evaluated for autonomic neuropathy and peripheral vascular disease since these two entities are relatively common in dialysis patients, especially those with hypertension and diabetes. Following kidney transplantation in young men, testicular size, sperm counts, and fertility commonly remain abnormal. These findings may reflect effects of antirejection regimens but nevertheless are a consequence of ESKD (65).

In contrast to women whose primary reproductive endocrinologic defect appears to be hypothalamic, hypogonadism is more prominent in men (66). These men, who have reduced testosterone levels, may respond to replacement testosterone. Erectile dysfunction is common in dialysis patients, affecting 70% to 80% of men (67). The incidence is higher in men with diabetes and who have been on dialysis for long periods, and these men tend to have reduced testosterone levels and reduced penile blood flow. Approximately 80% of men with erectile dysfunction respond to sildenafil (Viagra) (68). The level of penile blood flow is the most important parameter for predicting a response to sildenafil.

Adrenocorticotropic Hormone

ACTH stimulates steroidogenesis in the glomerulosa and fasciculata layers of the adrenal glands. ACTH is derived from proopiomelanocortin (POMC), a peptide that is produced by the corticotrope cells of the anterior pituitary and cleaved to ACTH and β-lipotropin (LPH). ACTH is further cleaved into α-melanocyte-stimulating hormone (α-MSH or ACTH 1-13) and ACTH-like peptide (ACTH 18-39). β-Lipotropin is processed to lipotropin (LPH) and β-endorphin. Secretion of ACTH is stimulated by corticotropin-releasing hormone (CRH) and vasopressin. Negative feedback control is provided by suppression of CRH, vasopressin, and ACTH secretion by cortisol, and inhibition of CRH secretion by ACTH. ACTH is secreted in a pulsatile fashion in a diurnal pattern that is maximal in the early morning and minimal in the evening.

In dialysis patients, ACTH levels are normal or slightly increased compared to normal controls, and its metabolism does not appear to be altered. Normal and abnormal responses to dexamethasone and metyrapone suppression tests have been reported. The circadian rhythms and levels of cortisol are normal, and the response of the adrenals to ACTH stimulation is normal. Consequently, a number of the tests of pituitary–adrenal function used in normal patients are applicable to dialysis patients.

◆ DISORDERS OF THE ADRENAL CORTEX

Introduction

The adrenal cortex produces two physiologically important steroid hormones, cortisol and aldosterone. The primary physiologic effect of aldosterone is on the kidneys, where it acts on the distal nephron to promote Na reabsorption and K and H excretion. Aldosterone also affects transport in the colon, but this appears to be a minor effect, and disorders of aldosterone metabolism in dialysis patients have not been reported. Consequently, this section deals with glucocorticoid excess or insufficiency.

Glucocorticoids are essential for life and affect glucose and lipid metabolism, the immune system, and bone and mineral metabolism. No tissue or organ system including the cardiovascular, GI, or CNS functions normally in the absence of glucocorticoids. Glucocorticoid activity is required for glycogen synthesis and maintenance of glycogen stores, gluconeogenesis, and has a permissive effect on lipolysis. The effects of glucocorticoids on the immune system under normal physiologic conditions are not fully understood, but pharmacologic concentrations decrease the number of peripheral lymphocytes, inhibit T-cell activation, macrophage proliferation, and inhibit the actions of a number of mediators of inflammation including chemokines, prostaglandins, and histamine. Glucocorticoids affect bone formation by reducing osteoblast numbers, decreasing intestinal Ca reabsorption, and increasing serum PTH levels.

Adrenal Insufficiency

In the general population, primary adrenal insufficiency usually presents as adrenal crisis following some form of stress such as surgery or an acute illness. Patients complain of anorexia, nausea, vomiting, and weakness with a history of weight loss. The findings may include volume depletion, hypotension and shock, hypoglycemia, fever, and possibly hyperpigmentation. This constellation of findings is caused by loss of both cortisol and aldosterone. The loss of aldosterone is largely responsible for the symptoms and findings related to volume depletion. Patients who are receiving renal replacement therapy but who encounter a physiologic stress can also develop adrenal crisis (25,69).

Dialysis patients have minimal renal function and therefore do not develop the salt-losing nephropathy associated with adrenal insufficiency. Presumably, if dialysis patients develop adrenal insufficiency, they present more like patients with secondary adrenal insufficiency (pituitary lesions with loss of ACTH production) or tertiary

TABLE 22.2	Tests for Primary or Secondary Adrenal Insufficiency		
	Normal	**Primary Adrenal Insufficiency**	**Pituitary/Hypothalamic Insufficiency**
ACTH (8 AM)	4.5–12 pmol/L (20–52 pg/mL)	Increased	Low or normal range
Cortisol (8 AM)	10–20 μg/dL (275–550 nmol/L)	<275 nmol/L	Low or normal range
Cosyntropin stimulation	Peak cortisol ≥18–20 μg/dL (500–550 nmol/L) after 30–60 min	<18 μg/dL (500 nmol/L) after 30–60 min	Normal or low if adrenals are atrophic
Metyrapone	8 AM ACTH ≥17 pmol/L, 11-deoxycortisol 210–660 nmol/L	8 AM ACTH ≥17 pmol/L, 11-deoxycortisol <210 nmol/L	8 AM ACTH ≤17 pmol/L, 11-deoxycortisol <210 nmol/L

Reference values or normal responses are shown for normal patients.
ACTH, adrenocorticotropic hormone.
From Melmed S, Casanueva FF, Hoofman AR, et al. Diagnosis and treatment of hyperprolactinemia: an Endocrine Society Clinical Practice Guideline. *J Clin Endocrinol Metab* 2011;96:273–288; and Fiad TM, Kirby JM, Cunningham SK, et al. The overnight single-dose metyrapone test is a simple and reliable index of the hypothalamic-pituitary-adrenal axis. *Clin Endocrinol (Oxf)* 1994;40:603–609.

(hypothalamic lesions with loss of CRF production). In these patients, adrenal crisis is rare, and they present with insidious onset of generalized symptoms of malaise and signs and symptoms of hypoglycemia.

Primary adrenal insufficiency is caused by tuberculosis, fungal diseases, metastases from tumors, and autoimmune disease. As dialysis patients are at increased risk for tuberculosis, they are also presumably at increased risk for adrenal insufficiency due to tuberculosis. Autoimmune adrenalitis is associated with polyglandular autoimmune syndromes I and II which are associated with mucocutaneous candidiasis and hypoparathyroidism, and thyroid disorders and insulin-dependent diabetes, respectively. Primary autoimmune polyglandular syndrome type II is more common than the autosomal recessive type I syndrome. Patients with HIV infections and with cytomegalovirus, mycobacterium avium intracellulare, cryptococcus, or Kaposi's sarcoma may manifest partial adrenal insufficiency. Adrenal insufficiency can be precipitated by ketoconazole because it inhibits cortisol synthesis, or rifampin because it increases cortisol metabolism (69). Secondary or tertiary

adrenal insufficiency is associated with destructive lesions of the pituitary or hypothalamus such as tumors, postradiation therapy, trauma, or use of anticoagulants. In these situations, other pituitary hormones are usually lost in addition to ACTH. Adrenal insufficiency is also caused by long-term use of glucocorticoids for immune suppression as in patients with systemic lupus erythematosus, other glomerular diseases, or following renal transplantation.

Diagnosis of Adrenal Insufficiency

Renal failure and dialysis do not alter the diurnal variation of cortisol or the adrenal response to ACTH (25). Consequently, AM and PM cortisol levels and the ACTH stimulation test can be used to demonstrate adrenal or hypothalamic–pituitary–adrenal function (**TABLE 22.2** and **FIGURE 22.3**). As serum cortisol concentrations are normally highest in the early morning hours ranging between 10 and 20 μg/dL (275 to 555 nmol/L), inappropriately low cortisol less than 3.6 μg/dL (100 nmol/L) strongly suggest adrenal insufficiency (70). Values below 10 μg/dL (275 nmol/L) make the diagnosis likely

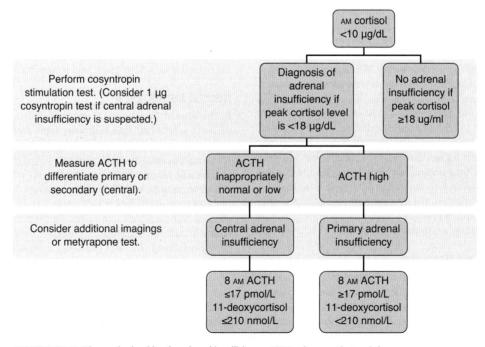

FIGURE 22.3 Diagnostic algorithm for adrenal insufficiency. ACTH, adrenocorticotropic hormone.

but require additional standard or low-dose ACTH stimulation test (cosyntropin test). In the standard ACTH stimulation test, plasma cortisol is measured before, 30 minutes after, and 60 minutes after intravenous injection of 250 μg of synthetic ACTH (ACTH 1-24). A cortisol value ≥18 to 20 μg/dL (500 to 550 nmol/L) at any of the time points in the test indicates normal adrenal function. The low-dose ACTH stimulation test is preferred and has improved sensitivity in cases of secondary adrenal insufficiency of recent onset or partial adrenal insufficiency. The prolonged ACTH stimulation test or an in-sulin-induced hypoglycemia test helps differentiate between primary and secondary or tertiary adrenal insufficiency (71–73). The over-night, single-dose metyrapone suppression test with measurement of serum cortisol, 11-deoxycortisol, and ACTH is useful for making a diagnosis of complete or partial pituitary-adrenal insufficiency and is the most sensitive test of pituitary-adrenal reserve (69). Patients may have a normal response of ACTH and cortisol to hypoglycemia but have an abnormal response to metyrapone suppression. Metyrapone blocks conversion of 11-deoxycortisol, a compound with no gluco-corticoid activity and that does not participate in feedback to corti-sol. As cortisol production decreases, ACTH rises and stimulates the production of cortisol precursors which can be measured as 11-de-oxycortisol. Metyrapone (30 mg/kg body weight) is given orally at midnight, and 8 AM cortisol, 11-deoxycortisol, and ACTH levels are measured. A normal response is a rise in 11-deoxycortisol from 210 to 660 nmol and a level of ACTH greater than 17 pmol/L. If the cor-tisol level is normal or greater than 210 nmol/L in the 8-AM sample, the dose of metyrapone was inadequate to block cortisol synthesis. A normal response to the metyrapone suppression test excludes abnor-malities of the hypothalamo–pituitary–adrenal axis. ACTH release

can also be measured in response to CRF to document intact pituitary function (69). Patients who are addisonian may become symptomatic with the metyrapone suppression test, so it should be supervised. If primary adrenal insufficiency is suspected, a CT scan of the abdomen to evaluate the size of the adrenal glands is warranted.

Adrenal Hyperfunction

The adrenal glands may overproduce aldosterone or cortisol. Over-production of aldosterone is caused by adrenal adenomas of the glomerulosa layer (either single or multiple). In patients with kidney disease who are on dialysis, it is not clear if aldosterone excess causes clinical abnormalities. Consequently, this section deals with gluco-corticoid excess or Cushing's syndrome. Cushing's syndrome may be caused by excess ACTH (usually due to a pituitary adenoma, see preceding text), adrenal hyperplasia, or exogenous glucocorticoids for inflammatory diseases or antirejection therapy. Cushing's syn-drome is characterized by centripetal obesity, glucose intolerance, weakness (due to proximal myopathy), hypertension, psychological changes (depression or mania), bruisability, striae, osteopenia, men-strual irregularities or impotence, acne or oily skin, hypertension, edema, and hirsutism. None of these findings is diagnostic of corti-sol excess, but the occurrence of several of them in the same patient is suggestive of Cushing's syndrome. In dialysis patients, hyperten-sion and edema and menstrual irregularities or impotence may not be valuable because they are so common in the dialysis population.

Diagnosis of Hypercortisolism

The diagnosis of Cushing's syndrome in dialysis patients can be based on most of the same criteria as the general population (TABLE 22.3

TABLE 22.3	**Serum Assays and Provocative Tests for Hypercortisolism**		
	Normal	**Primary Adrenal Overproduction**	**Pituitary or Hypothalamic or Ectopic Adrenocorticotropic Hormone**
ACTH	4.5–12 pmol/L (20–52 pg/mL)	Reduced (usually <2 pmol/L)	Normal or modestly increased in Cushing's disease Elevated, usually >20 pmol/L (>90 pg/mL) in ectopic ACTH syndrome
Serum cortisol	Normal diurnal variation Highest at 8 AM 220–660 nmol/L Lowest at midnight <50 nmol/L (<2 μg/dL)	Loss of diurnal variation with midnight elevation >200 nmol/L (>7.5 μg/dL)	Loss of diurnal variation with midnight elevation >200 nmol/L (>7.5 μg/dL)
Low-dose dexamethasone suppression	8 AM cortisol ≤140 nmol/L (<5 μg/dL),ᵃ 8 AM ACTH ≤4.4 pmol/L	8 AM cortisol ≥220 nmol/L, low ACTH	8 AM cortisol ≥220 nmol/L, elevated ACTH
High-dose dexamethasone suppression	8 AM cortisol ≤140 nmol/L	No suppression on AM cortisol	>50% suppression of plasma or urinary cortisol from baseline value in Cushing's disease Cortisol is not suppressible in ectopic ACTH syndrome.
Metyrapone test	8 AM ACTH ≥17 pmol/L, 11-deoxycortisol 210–660 nmol/L	8 AM ACTH no change to increased, 11-deoxycortisol no change to decreased	Cushing's disease 8 AM ACTH ≥17 pmol/L, 11-deoxycortisol 210–660 nmol/L (typically, >1,000 nmol/l) Ectopic ACTH syndrome No change or increased

Reference values and normal responses are shown in the normal column.
ᵃEndocrine society suggests cortisol cut-off point of <50 nmol/L (1.8 μg/dL) to improve the sensitivity of diagnosis of hypercortisolism.
ACTH, adrenocorticotropic hormone.
From Melmed S, Casanueva FF, Hoofman AR, et al. Diagnosis and treatment of hyperprolactinemia: an Endocrine Society Clinical Practice Guideline. *J Clin Endocrinol Metab* 2011;96:273–288; and Fiad TM, Kirby JM, Cunningham SK, et al. The overnight single-dose metyrapone test is a simple and reliable index of the hypothalamic-pituitary-adrenal axis. *Clin Endocrinol (Oxf)* 1994;40:603–609.

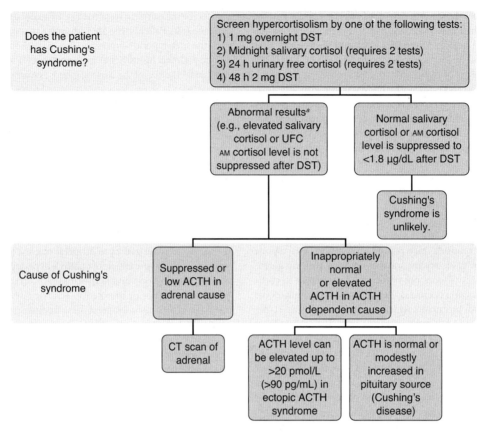

FIGURE 22.4 Diagnostic algorithm for Cushing's syndrome. DST, dexamethasone suppression test; ACTH, adrenocorticotropic hormone; UFC, urinary free cortisol; CT, computed tomography. [a]Abnormal results should be confirmed with one of other additional screening tests.

and **FIGURE 22.4**). Glucocorticoid use for inflammatory diseases of the kidney or as part of an antirejection regimen are probably the most common causes of Cushing's syndrome in the dialysis population. In the absence of such a history, glucocorticoid excess may be either primary or secondary. Renal failure and dialysis do not alter the diurnal variation of cortisol or the adrenal response to ACTH, so AM and PM cortisol levels can be used to demonstrate abnormal diurnal variation (loss of the PM fall) in cortisol.

Screening for hypercortisolism can be achieved using 8-AM cortisol measurement after a low-dose overnight dexamethasone (1 mg DST), the 2-mg/48-h dexamethasone suppression test, midnight salivary cortisol (requires two measurements on separate days), or urinary free cortisol (UFC) (requires two measurements on separate days). Biochemical excess of cortisol in an initial screening test should be confirmed by performing different provocative tests before looking for the source of the excess cortisol or cause of Cushing's syndrome (74). The sensitivity of UFC is diminished in chronic kidney disease patients when creatinine clearance falls below 60 mL/min as kidney filtration of cortisol fall linearly with more severe kidney disease (75).

Dexamethasone suppresses ACTH secretion through negative feedback at the levels of the pituitary and hypothalamus. The low-dose dexamethasone suppression test (1 mg PO between 11 PM and midnight with measurement of 8-AM cortisol and ACTH) is designed to distinguish patients with glucocorticoid excess for any reason from patients with normal hypothalamo–pituitary–adrenal function. If the patient is normal, the low dose of dexamethasone

will suppress cortisol production, and the 8-AM plasma cortisol level should be less than 140 nmol/L (5 µg/dL) and the ACTH should be less than 4.4 pmol/L (20 pg/mL). Most experts advocate usage of lower cortisol cut-off point below 50 nmol/L (1.8 µg/dL) to improve diagnostic sensitivity to over 95% (74,76). Initial screening tests for hypercortisolism are 1 mg dexamethasone suppression test, UFC, or midnight salivary cortisol. In some cases, the 2-day low-dose dexamethasone suppression test is used. The high-dose dexamethasone suppression test and metyrapone are used to identify the source of cortisol after two different screening tests confirm cortisol excess. As UFC is not reliable in chronic kidney disease, if 1 mg dexamethasone suppression test is positive, the midnight salivary cortisol level should be measured to confirm cortisol excess.

The midnight salivary cortisol value measured by RIA greater than 2.0 ng/mL (5.5 nmol/L) on two separate days has 100% sensitivity and 96% specificity for diagnosis of Cushing's syndrome (77).

The distinction between primary and secondary or tertiary hypercortisolism can be made measuring ACTH level (**FIGURE 22.4**), using high-dose dexamethasone suppression test (**FIGURE 22.5**) or the single-dose metyrapone test with measurement of serum 11-deoxycortisol and cortisol (59,62). The morning plasma ACTH measured by two-site immunoradiometric assay helps in differentiating ACTH-dependent from ACTH-independent causes. ACTH is undetectable (<1 pmol/L) in patients with adrenal tumors; normal at 2 to 11 pmol/L (9 to 52 pg/mL) or modestly elevated in Cushing's disease and elevated up to >20 pmol/L (>90 pg/mL) in ectopic ACTH syndrome (51).

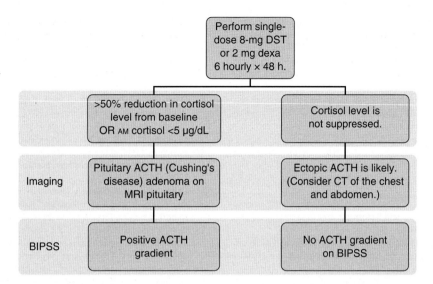

FIGURE 22.5 Further diagnostic workup for ACTH dependent Cushing's syndrome. DST, dexamethasone suppression test; ACTH, adrenocorticotropic hormone; MRI, magnetic resonance imaging; CT, computed tomography; BIPSS, bilateral inferior petrosal sinus sampling.

In patients with pituitary adenomas or increased hypothalamic activity, ACTH can be undetectable and 8-AM cortisol levels can be suppressed to less than 140 nmol/l (5 μg/dL) on high doses of dexamethasone (8 mg of dexamethasone given between 11 PM and midnight). If the hypercortisolism is due to ectopic ACTH, ACTH and cortisol will not typically suppress with either high or low dose of dexamethasone. However, there are some exceptions as approximately 50% of patients with ectopic ACTH syndrome due to indolent bronchial carcinoid tumors may show some suppression after high-dose dexamethasone. The "gold standard" test for distinguishing between Cushing's disease and an ectopic source of ACTH is bilateral inferior petrosal sinus sampling with CRH. The finding of central (inferior petrosal) to peripheral plasma ACTH gradient greater than 2:1 or 3:1 after CRH administration is consistent with Cushing's disease (51).

The metyrapone suppression test can also be used to distinguish primary adrenal overproduction of cortisol from excess ACTH secretion due to pituitary or hypothalamic disease. Metyrapone blocks conversion of 11-deoxycortisol, a compound with no glucocorticoid activity and that does not participate in feedback, to cortisol. The reduced cortisol levels stimulate ACTH production which in turn stimulate the cortisol synthetic pathway. A pituitary adenoma responds to reduced cortisol with increased ACTH production resulting in an increase in 11-deoxycortisol production. In contrast, in the presence of an adrenal adenoma, the hypothalamopituitary axis is atrophic, the increase in ACTH is minimal, and 11-deoxycortisol levels fall or do not change. Approximately half of adrenal adenomas and most adrenal carcinomas do not respond to ACTH. The uninvolved contralateral adrenal gland may be atrophic and unable to respond to ACTH (69). If a pituitary or hypothalamic lesion is suspected, structural evaluation of the pituitary and hypothalamus with CT or MRI scans is indicated (**FIGURES 22.4** and **22.5**). The metyrapone test is no longer widely used to differentiate patients with Cushing's disease from those with a primary adrenal cause as these conditions can be more reliably distinguished by measurement of plasma ACTH followed by CT scanning of the adrenals (51).

⬡ REFERENCES

1. Lim VS. Thyroid function in patients with chronic renal failure. *Am J Kidney Dis* 2001;38:S80–S84.
2. Larsen PR, Davies TF, Hay ID. The thyroid gland. In: Wilson JD, Foster DW, Kronenberg HM, et al, eds. *Williams Textbook of Endocrinology*. 9th ed. Philadelphia, PA: WB Saunders, 1998:389–515.
3. Brent GA, Hershman GM. Effects of nonthyroidal illness on thyroid function tests. In: Van Middlesworth L, ed. *The Thyroid Gland: A Practical Clinical Treatise*. Chicago, IL: Year Book Medical Publishers, 1986:83–110.
4. Zoccali C, Mallamaci F, Tripepi G, et al. Low triiodothyronine and survival in end-stage renal disease. *Kidney Int* 2006;70:523–528.
5. de Vries E, Fliers E, Boelen A. The molecular basis of the non-thyroidal illness syndrome. *J Endocrinol* 2015;225:R67–R81.
6. Bartalena L, Bogazzi F, Brogioni S, et al. Role of cytokines in the pathogenesis of euthyroid sick syndrome. *Eur J Endocrinol* 1998;138:603–614.
7. Becker RA, Vaughan GM, Zeigler MG, et al. Hypermetabolic low triiodothyronine syndrome of burn injury. *Crit Care Med* 1982;10:870–875.
8. Brent GA, Hershman JM. Thyroxine therapy in patients with severe nonthyroidal illness and low serum thyroxine concentration. *J Clin Endocrinol Metab* 1986;63:1–8.
9. Myers JD, Brannon ES, Holland BC. A correlative study of the cardiac output and the hepatic circulation in hyperthyroidism. *J Clin Invest* 1950;29:1069–1077.
10. Miki H, Oshimo K, Inoue H, et al. Thyroid nodules in female uremic patients on maintenance hemodialysis. *J Surg Oncol* 1993;54:216–218.
11. Culpepper RM, Hirsch JI, Fratkin MJ. Clearance of ^{131}I by hemodialysis. *Clin Nephrol* 1992;38:110–114.
12. Lo JC, Chertow GM, Go AS, et al. Increased prevalence of subclinical and clinical hypothyroidism in persons with chronic kidney disease. *Kidney Int* 2005;67:1047–1052.
13. Takeda S, Michigishi T, Takazukura E. Iodine-induced hypothyroidism in patients on regular dialysis treatment. *Nephron* 1993;65:51–55.
14. Shirota T, Shinoda T, Aizawa T, et al. Primary hypothyroidism and multiple endocrine failure in association with hemochromatosis in a long-term hemodialysis patient. *Clin Nephrol* 1992;38:105–109.
15. Brüngger M, Hulter HN, Krapf R. Effect of chronic metabolic acidosis on thyroid homeostasis in humans. *Am J Physiol* 1997;272:F648–F653.
16. Wiederkehr MR, Kalogiros J, Krapf R. Correction of metabolic acidosis improves thyroid and growth hormone axes in haemodialysis patients. *Nephrol Dial Transplant* 2004;19:1190–1197.

17. Lim VS, Fang VS, Katz AI, et al. Thyroid dysfunction in chronic renal failure. A study of the pituitary-thyroid axis and peripheral turnover kinetics of thyroxine and triiodothyronine. *J Clin Invest* 1974;60:522–534.

18. Haynes RC. Thyroid and antithyroid drugs. In: Gilman AG, Rall TW, Nies AS, et al, eds. *The Pharmacological Basis of Therapeutics.* 8th ed. New York, NY: Pergammon Press, 1990:1361–1383.

19. Kuret JA, Murad F. Adenohypophyseal hormones and related substances. In: Gilman AG, Rall TW, Nies AS, et al, eds. *The Pharmacological Basis of Therapeutics.* 8th ed. New York, NY: Pergammon Press, 1990:1334–1360.

20. Thorner MO, Vance ML, Horvath E, et al. The anterior pituitary. In: Wilson JD, Foster DW, Kronenberg HM, et al, eds. *Williams Textbook of Endocrinology.* 9th ed. Philadelphia, PA: WB Saunders, 1998: 249–340.

21. Veldhuis JD, Iranmanesh A, Wilkowski MJ, et al. Neuroendocrine alterations in the somatotropic and lactotropic axes in uremic men. *Eur J Endocrinol* 1994;131:489–498.

22. Haffner D, Schaefer F, Girard J, et al. Metabolic clearance of recombinant human growth hormone in health and chronic renal failure. *Clin Invest* 1994;93:1163–1171.

23. Tönshoff B, Blum WF, Mehls O. Derangements of the somatotropic hormone axis in chronic renal failure. *Kidney Int* 1997;51:S106–S113.

24. Kuemmerle N, Krieg RJ Jr, Latta K, et al. Growth hormone and insulin-like growth factor in non-uremic acidosis and uremic acidosis. *Kidney Int* 1997;51:S102–S105.

25. Emmanouel DS, Lindheimer MD, Katz AI. Endocrine abnormalities in chronic renal failure: pathogenic principles and clinical implications. *Semin Nephrol* 1981;1:151–174.

26. Tönshoff B, Veldhuis JD, Heinrich U, et al. Deconvolution analysis of spontaneous nocturnal growth hormone secretion in prepubertal children with preterminal chronic renal failure and with end-stage renal disease. *Pediatr Res* 1995;37:86–93.

27. Maniar S, Kleinknecht C, Zhou X, et al. Growth hormone action is blunted by acidosis in experimental uremia or acid load. *Clin Nephrol* 1996;46:72–76.

28. Kleinknecht C, Maniar S, Zhou X, et al. Acidosis prevents growth hormone-induced growth in experimental uremia. *Pediatr Nephrol* 1996;10:256–260.

29. Fouque D, Peng SC, Kopple JD. Impaired metabolic response to recombinant insulin-like growth factor-1 in dialysis patients. *Kidney Int* 1995;47:876–883.

30. Ulinski T, Mohan S, Kiepe D, et al. Serum insulin-like growth factor binding protein (IGFBP)-4 and serum IGFBP-5 in children with chronic renal failure: relationship to growth and glomerular filtration rate. *Pediatr Nephrol* 2000;14:589–597.

31. Fouque D, Peng SC, Kopple JD. Pharmacokinetics of recombinant human insulin-like growth factor-1 in dialysis patients. *Kidney Int* 1995;47:869–875.

32. Kreig RJ Jr, Santos F, Chan JC. Growth hormone, insulin-like growth factor and the kidney. *Kidney Int* 1995;48:321–326.

33. Mahan JD, Warady BA. Assessment and treatment of short stature in pediatric patients with chronic kidney disease: a consensus statement. *Pediatr Nephrol* 2006;21:917–930.

34. Haffner D, Schaefer F, Nissel R, et al. Effect of growth hormone treatment on the adult height of children with chronic renal failure. *N Engl J Med* 2000;343:923–930.

35. Hokken-Koelega A, Mulder P, De Jong R, et al. Long-term effects of growth hormone treatment on growth and puberty in patients with chronic renal insufficiency. *Pediatr Nephrol* 2000;14:701–706.

36. Gram J, Hansen B, Jensen PB, et al. The effect of recombinant human growth hormone treatment on bone and mineral metabolism in haemodialysis patients. *Nephrol Dial Transplant* 1998;13:1529–1534.

37. Jensen PB, Hansen TB, Frystyk J, et al. Growth hormone, insulin-like growth factors and thier binding proteins in adult hemodialysis patients treated with recombinant human growth hormone. *Clin Nephrol* 1999;52:103–109.

38. Johannsson G, Bengtsson BA, Ahlmén J. Double-blind, placebo-controlled study of growth hormone treatment in elderly patients undergoing chronic hemodialysis: anabolic effect and functional improvement. *Am J Kidney Dis* 1999;33:709–717.

39. Feldt-Rasmussen B, Lange M, Sulowicz W, et al. Growth hormone treatment during hemodialysis in a randomized trial improves nutrition, quality of life, and cardiovascular risk. *J Am Soc Nephrol* 2007;18: 2161–2171.

40. Pupim LB, Flakoll PJ, Yu C, et al. Recombinant human growth hormone improves muscle amino acid uptake and whole-body protein metabolism in chronic hemodialysis patients. *Am J Clin Nutr* 2005;82: 1235–1243.

41. Sicuro A, Mahlbacher K, Hulter HN, et al. Effect of growth hormone on renal and systemic acid-base homeostasis in humans. *Am J Physiol* 1998;274:F650–F657.

42. Ballmer PE, McNurlan MA, Hulter HN, et al. Chronic metabolic acidosis decreases albumin synthesis and induces negative nitrogen balance in humans. *J Clin Invest* 1995;95:39–45.

43. Díez JJ, Iglesias P, Sastre J, et al. Growth hormone responses to growth hormone-releasing hormone and clonidine before and after erythropoietin therapy in CAPD patients. *Nephron* 1996;74:548–554.

44. Cremagnani L, Cantalamessa L, Orsatti A, et al. Recombinant human erythropoietin (rhEPO) treatment potentiates growth hormone (GH) response to growth hormone releasing hormone (GHRH) stimulation in hemodialysis patients. *Clin Nephrol* 1993;39:282–286.

45. Garibotto G, Barreca A, Sofia A, et al. Effects of growth hormone on leptin metabolism and energy expenditure in hemodialysis patients with protein-calorie malnutrition. *J Am Soc Nephrol* 2000;11:2106–2113.

46. Rodriguez-Carmona A, Perez Fontan M, Cordido F, et al. Hyperleptinemia is not correlated with markers of protein malnutrition in chronic renal failure. A cross-sectional study in predialysis, peritoneal dialysis and hemodialysis patients. *Nephron* 2000;86:274–280.

47. Mujais SK, Sabatini S, Kurtzman NA. Pathophysiology of the uremic syndrome. In: Brenner BM, Rector FC Jr, eds. *The Kidney.* 3rd ed. Philadelphia, PA: WB Saunders, 1986:1587–1630.

48. Yeksan M, Tamer N, Cirit M, et al. Effect of recombinant human erythropoietin (r-HuEPO) therapy on plasma FT3, FT4, TSH, FSH, LH, free testosterone and prolactin levels in hemodialysis patients. *Int J Artif Organs* 1992;15:585–589.

49. Bommer J, Ritz E, del Pozo E, et al. Improved sexual function in male hemodialysis patients on bromocriptine. *Lancet* 1979;2:496–497.

50. Verhelst J, Abs R, Maiter D, et al. Cabergoline in the treatment of hyperprolactinemia: a study of 455 patients. *J Clin Endocrinol Metab* 1999; 84:2518–2522.

51. Melmed S, Casanueva FF, Hoofman AR, et al. Diagnosis and treatment of hyperprolactinemia: an Endocrine Society Clinical Practice Guideline . *J Clin Endocrinol Metab* 2011;96:273–288.

52. Molitch ME. Pharmacologic resistance in prolactinoma patients. *Pituitary* 2005;8:43–52.

53. Lim VS, Henriquez C, Sieversten G, et al. Ovarian function in chronic renal failure: evidence suggesting hypothalamic anovulation. *Ann Int Med* 1980;93:21–27.

54. Hou S. Pregnancy in chronic renal insufficiency and end-stage renal disease. *Am J Kidney Dis* 1999;33:235–252.

55. Bagon J, Vernaeve H, De Muylder X, et al. Pregnancy and dialysis. *Am J Kidney Dis* 1998;31:756–765.

56. Chao AS, Huang JY, Lein R, et al. Pregnancy in women who undergo long-term hemodialysis. *Am J Obstet Gynecol* 2002;187:152–156.

57. Toma H, Tanabe K, Tokumoto T, et al. Pregnancy in women receiving renal dialysis or transplantation in Japan: a nationwide survey. *Nephrol Dial Transplant* 1999;14:1511–1516.

58. Okundaye I, Abrinko P, Hou S. Registry of pregnancy in dialysis patients. *Am J Kidney Dis* 1998;31:766–773.

59. Imbasciati E, Gregorini G, Cabbidu G, et al. Pregnancy in CKD stages 3 to 5: fetal and maternal outcomes. *Am J Kidney Dis* 2007;49:753–762.

60. Panaye M, Jolivot A, Lemoine S, et al. Pregnancies in hemodialysis patients with end-stage renal disease: epidemiology, management and prognosis. *Nephrol Ther* 2014;10:485–491.

61. Nadeau-Fredette AC, Hladunewich M, Hui D, et al. End-stage renal disease and pregnancy. *Adv Chron Kidney Dis* 2013;20:246–252.

62. Chou C-Y, Ting I-W, Lin T-H, et al. Pregnancy in patients on chronic dialysis: a single center experience and combined analysis of reported results. *Eur J Obstet Gynecol Reprod Biol* 2008;136:165–170.

63. Haase M, Morgera S, Bamberg C, et al. A systematic approach to managing pregnant dialysis patients—the importance of an intensified haemodiafiltration protocol. *Nephrol Dial Transplant* 2005;20:2537–2542.

64. Tokgöz B, Utaş C, Dogukan A, et al. Effects of long-term erythropoietin therapy on the hypothalamo-pituitary-testicular axis in male CAPD patients. *Perit Dial Int* 2001;21:448–454.

65. Tainio J, Jahnukainen K, Nurmio M, et al. Testicular function, semen quality, and fertility in young men after renal transplantation during childhood or adolescence. *Transplantation* 2014;98:987–993.

66. Palmer BF. Sexual dysfunction in uremia. *J Am Soc Nephrol* 1999; 10:1381–1388.

67. Türk S, Karalezli G, Tonbul HZ, et al. Erectile dysfunction and the effects of sildenafil treatment in patients on haemodialysis and continuous ambulatory peritoneal dialysis. *Nephrol Dial Transplant* 2001;16:1818–1822.

68. Chen J, Mabjeesh NJ, Greenstein A, et al. Clinical efficacy of sildenafil in patients on chronic dialysis. *J Urol* 2001;165:819–821.

69. Orth DN, Kovacs WJ. The adrenal cortex. In: Wilson JD, Foster DW, Kronenberg HM, et al, eds. *Williams Textbook of Endocrinology*. 9th ed. Philadelphia, PA: WB Saunders, 1998:517–664.

70. Hägg EA, Asplund K, Lithner F. Value of basal plasma cortisol assays in the assessment of pituitary-adrenal insufficiency. *Clin Endocrinol* 1987;26:221–226.

71. Nye EJ, Grice JE, Hockings GI, et al. Comparison of adrenocorticotrophin (ACTH) stimulation tests and insulin hypoglycemia in normal humans: low dose, standard high dose, and 8-hour ACTH-(1-24) infusion tests. *J Clin Endocrinol Metab* 1999;84:3648–3655.

72. Kaslauskaite R, Evans AT, Villabona CV, et al. Corticotrophin tests for hypothalamic-pituitary-adrenal insufficiency: a metaanalysis. *J Clin Endocrinol Metab* 2008;93:4245–4253.

73. Grossman AB. The diagnosis and management of central hypoadrenalism. *J Clin Endocrinol Metab* 2010;95:4855–4863.

74. Nieman LK, Biller BM, Findling JW, et al. The diagnosis of Cushing's syndrome: an Endocrine Society Clinical Practice Guideline. *J Clin Endocrinol Metab* 2008;93:1526–1540.

75. Chan KC, Lit LC, Law EL, et al. Diminished urinary free cortisol excretion in patients with moderate and severe renal impairment. *Clin Chem* 2004;50:757–759.

76. Wood PJ, Barth JH, Freedman DB, et al. Evidence for the low-dose dexamethasone suppression test to screen for Cushing's syndrome—recommendations for a protocol for biochemistry laboratories. *Ann Clin Biochem* 1997;34:222–229.

77. Yaneva M, Mosnier-Pudar H, Dugué MA, et al. Midnight salivary cortisol for for the initial diagnosis of Cushing's syndrome of various causes. *J Clin Endocrinol Metab* 2004;89:3345–3351.

CHAPTER 23

Gastrointestinal Complications in End-Stage Kidney Disease

George T. Fantry, Seema Patil, and Donna S. Hanes

Gastrointestinal symptoms are very common in patients with end-stage kidney disease (ESKD) (1), occurring in 77% to 79% of patients undergoing hemodialysis (2,3). Before the widespread use of dialysis, gastrointestinal complications accounted for a large part of the uremic syndrome. Uremia causes pathologic and physiologic changes throughout the gastrointestinal tract, which results in gastrointestinal disturbances involving both the upper and lower gastrointestinal tract (4,5) as well as the pancreas, leading to a broad spectrum of gastrointestinal complaints (TABLE 23.1) (2). There is an increased frequency of gastroesophageal reflux disease (GERD), gastritis, gastrointestinal bleeding, pancreatitis, ascites, and constipation. These gastrointestinal complications of ESKD have a negative impact on quality of life (1), increase morbidity, and may contribute to death. This chapter reviews the pathophysiology,

diagnosis, and management of these common gastrointestinal disorders in dialysis patients.

 ESOPHAGUS

Upper gastrointestinal symptoms, including nausea, vomiting, heartburn, and epigastric pain are common in patients with chronic kidney disease. In addition to dialysis-related nausea and vomiting, potential esophageal causes of these symptoms include GERD or reflux esophagitis and esophageal motility disorders.

Multiple studies have found an increased prevalence of GERD-related symptoms in chronic kidney disease and hemodialysis patients (6–8). Additionally, the prevalence of GERD, as assessed by endoscopy and 24-hour pH monitoring in patients with GERD-related symptoms and ESKD, has been demonstrated to be very high (81%), suggesting that upper gastrointestinal symptoms in patients with chronic kidney disease are important in predicting the presence of GERD (9). Furthermore, continuous ambulatory peritoneal dialysis (CAPD) was a risk factor for the development of GERD (9,10). This association is likely due to increased intra-abdominal pressure when the abdominal cavity is filled with dialysate fluid and its effect on lower esophageal sphincter pressure.

A potential relationship between kidney disease and GERD-associated esophagitis was suggested in an autopsy series of patients with ESKD revealing a high prevalence of mild to severe esophagitis (36%) (11). However, in prospective studies of patients with chronic kidney disease on hemodialysis, the prevalence of esophagitis was much lower, ranging from 5.8% to 13% (12–14). The prevalence rate of endoscopic esophagitis in these studies is similar to or slightly greater than that in the general population. In a case-controlled study showing that the prevalence of GERD symptoms and esophagitis was increased in chronic kidney disease patients, multifactorial

TABLE 23.1	Prevalence of Gastrointestinal Symptoms in Patients on Hemodialysis	
Symptoms	**Percentage**	
Nausea	74	
Vomiting	68	
Anorexia	64	
Constipation	59	
Heartburn	52	
Abdominal distension	51	
Abdominal pain	49	
Diarrhea	25	
Dysphagia	16	

logistic regression analysis revealed a negative relationship between the presence *Helicobacter pylori* infection in the stomach and reflux esophagitis (8). This finding suggests that *H. pylori* infection may protect against the development reflux esophagitis which has been previously proposed by others (15,16).

A high prevalence of hiatal hernia has been reported in patients with ESKD (2,17,18). Hiatal hernias are known to play a role in the pathophysiology of GERD by altering the antireflux barrier and by acting as a reservoir for potential acid refluxate. Nonspecific esophageal motility disorders have been identified in chronic hemodialysis patients (19–21); however, the clinical significance of these findings is uncertain.

A presumptive diagnosis of GERD can be made when esophageal symptoms such as heartburn and regurgitation are present, and empiric therapy with acid-suppressive therapy with a proton pump inhibitor should be instituted. Symptom response to therapy confirms the diagnosis. Endoscopy should be performed in patients with persistent symptoms. Early endoscopy is indicated for unexplained nausea and vomiting or when alarm symptoms such as dysphagia are present.

STOMACH/DUODENUM

Dyspeptic symptoms are very common in patients with chronic kidney disease leading to investigation for possible gastroduodenal pathology, such as gastritis, duodenitis, and peptic ulcer disease. Many decades ago, a high prevalence of diffuse hemorrhagic gastritis and duodenitis was described in patients with fatal acute uremia (22,23). A subsequent autopsy study of chronic hemodialysis patients revealed a similar frequency of gastritis, which was less extensive and severe (11). More recent radiologic and endoscopic studies have confirmed a high prevalence of gastroduodenal lesions—such as gastritis, gastric erosions, duodenitis, and duodenal erosions—in patients with chronic kidney disease with endoscopic or histologic evidence of peptic disease found in up to 60% to 74% of the patients (12,14,24–27). There is a strong association between *H. pylori* infection and gastritis; however, poor correlation between endoscopic and histologic findings was seen (24).

Physiologic abnormalities in the presence of ESKD—such as decreases in pancreatic and duodenal bicarbonate secretion and elevated serum gastrin levels—led to speculation of an association between chronic kidney disease and peptic ulcer disease. Early clinical studies of small numbers of patients utilizing diagnostic radiology techniques suggested that chronic kidney disease was a risk factor for the development of peptic ulcers, but more recent endoscopic studies in patients on chronic hemodialysis have found a prevalence of peptic ulcers similar to that of the general population (12,14,28). Identified risk factors for the development of peptic ulcers include age, peritoneal dialysis, diabetes mellitus, congestive heart failure, and low serum albumin (29). There is a difference in the clinical presentation and endoscopic features of peptic ulcers in uremic patients compared with patients with normal kidney function. Uremic patients are more likely to be asymptomatic (13) or have low symptom scores (27) and to present with hemorrhage (30,31). In addition, uremic patients are more likely to have giant and multiple ulcers as well as *H. pylori*–negative and postbulbar duodenal ulcers (30,32).

Given the frequency of dyspepsia in patients with chronic kidney disease and the known role of *H. pylori* as a pathogen in the development of gastritis and peptic ulcer disease, a number of

studies have addressed the prevalence of *H. pylori* in ESKD. Most studies have demonstrated that the prevalence of *H. pylori* infection in patients with ESKD is similar to or possibly less than that of the general population (33–40), and there appears to be an inverse association between the duration of dialysis treatments and the presence of *H. pylori* infection (38,39). Dyspepsia is not associated with *H. pylori* infection in patients with chronic kidney disease (26,41), a finding that is similar to the lack of a clear association between *H. pylori* infection and functional dyspepsia in the general population. These findings suggest that other factors likely contribute to the development of gastritis and dyspepsia.

Multiple diagnostic tests are available to detect *H. pylori* infection including histology, rapid urease test (RUT), *H. pylori* stool-specific antigen (HpSA), and [13] C-urea breath test ([13] C-UBT). Using histology as the gold standard, the diagnostic accuracy of RUT is decreased in patients on hemodialysis compared to patients with chronic kidney disease and patients with normal kidney function (27). However, the diagnostic accuracy of the noninvasive tests, [13] C-UBT and HpSA, remains high in hemodialysis patients (27,42). Standard treatment of *H. pylori* infection with proton pump inhibitor–based triple therapy (i.e., omeprazole, amoxicillin, clarithromycin) twice daily for 2 weeks is as effective in patients with chronic kidney disease on hemodialysis or CAPD as in those individuals with normal kidney function (43,44).

Another potential cause of frequent dyspeptic symptoms— such as nausea, vomiting, abdominal bloating, early satiety, and anorexia—in dialysis patients with chronic kidney disease is abnormal or delayed gastric emptying (41,45–48). Gastroparesis is a common complication of diabetes mellitus, the most common cause of chronic kidney disease requiring dialysis, particularly in the presence of other end-organ damage such as chronic kidney disease. In addition to diabetic gastroparesis, gastric emptying can be significantly delayed in nondiabetic dialysis patients as well (48–51). Potential causes of abnormal gastric emptying in these patients include neuropathy directly related to the uremia and alterations in gastrointestinal hormones that can affect gastric emptying. The prevalence of dysmotility-like dyspepsia has been shown to be higher in CAPD patients than in hemodialysis patients (41). In CAPD patients, studies showing delayed gastric emptying when the abdominal cavity is filled with dialysate and absent when the abdominal cavity is empty suggest that increased intra-abdominal pressure may play an important role (52); however, this remains controversial (53). Delayed gastric emptying in patients with chronic kidney disease is not associated with *H. pylori* infection (41,51,54).

Upper gastrointestinal symptoms due to gastroparesis may have an adverse effect on nutritional status and may be one of the important factors that lead to malnutrition in dialysis patients. Delayed gastric emptying in chronic hemodialysis patients is associated with changes in biochemical indicators of nutritional status such as albumin and prealbumin (49). Furthermore, treatment of gastroparesis in nondiabetic dialysis patients with promotility agents such as erythromycin or metoclopramide can significantly improve gastric emptying and short-term nutritional status as measured by serum albumin (50).

There are several therapeutic options for the management of patients with dyspepsia. An empiric trial of a proton pump inhibitor can be considered. Alternatively, a serum *H. pylori* antibody can be obtained. If the *H. pylori* antibody is positive, appropriate treatment with a 2-week course of proton pump inhibitor–based triple therapy should be instituted. In patients with persistent dyspepsia, endoscopy is warranted. Early endoscopy should be pursued in older patients and in those with associated vomiting, anorexia, and unexplained weight loss. When empiric therapy fails and a diagnostic esophagogastroduodenoscopy (EGD) is unrevealing, it may be useful to obtain a gastric emptying study to assess for gastroparesis that can be treated with a promotility agent such as metoclopramide.

GASTROINTESTINAL BLEEDING

Gastrointestinal bleeding is a common complication of ESKD, accounting for up to 8% to 12% of cases of upper gastrointestinal bleeding (55,56). The frequency of bleeding in patients with chronic kidney disease with underlying gastrointestinal pathology may be partially explained by a high occurrence of clotting abnormalities in this patient population (56). These are primarily due to multifactorial platelet dysfunction, but abnormalities in clearance of anticoagulant medications in ESKD can contribute to increased risk of bleeding (57). Treatment options to restore platelet function in patients with ESKD and active bleeding include correction of anemia (58), administration of desmopressin [1-deamino-8-D-arginine vasopressin (DDAVP)] (59), and cryoprecipitate infusion (60). Most studies have found that peptic ulcer disease (gastric or duodenal ulcers) is the most common cause of upper gastrointestinal bleeding in patients with chronic kidney disease, accounting for 30% to 60% of bleeding episodes (55,56,61). Risk factors for upper gastrointestinal bleeding among patients with ESKD include cardiovascular disease, current smoking, and inability to ambulate independently (62).

The association of chronic kidney disease with bleeding upper gastrointestinal angiodysplasias is controversial. A few studies have shown that angiodysplasias of the stomach and duodenum are a significantly more common source of upper gastrointestinal bleeding in patients with chronic kidney disease (55,56,63,64), with angiodysplasias identified as the cause of bleeding in 13% to 23% of patients (55,56). However, this has not been a universal finding (61,65,66). In one study, the prevalence of angiodysplasias as a cause of upper gastrointestinal bleeding was related to the duration of kidney disease and the need for dialysis (55). The lesions are often multiple and can also be found in the small bowel and colon (56,63,67,68). Recurrent bleeding is frequent and more common in patients with chronic kidney disease (56,64). In addition to acute gastrointestinal hemorrhage, patients with bleeding angiodysplasias often present with chronic gastrointestinal blood loss manifested by chronic anemia and hemoccult-positive stool (65). Erosive esophagitis and erosive gastritis may also be more common causes of upper gastrointestinal bleeding in chronic kidney disease patients (56,61).

The diagnosis of angiodysplasias in the appropriate clinical setting is usually made by endoscopy with upper endoscopy and/or colonoscopy. The diagnosis of angiodysplasia can sometimes be difficult to make, as the lesions may be very small and hidden between or behind folds. A high index of suspicion for the possibility of angiodysplasias should be maintained in patients with recurrent acute bleeding episodes, which are undiagnosed after conventional endoscopy with upper endoscopy and colonoscopy, and in patients with unexplained chronic iron deficiency anemia and hemoccult-positive stool. In this subset of patients, small bowel angiodysplasia is the most common cause of bleeding, and further endoscopic evaluation of the small bowel with enteroscopy and/or wireless capsule endoscopy is warranted. Chronic kidney disease is a predictive factor for positive findings on enteroscopy and wireless capsule endoscopy (69,70). When identified endoscopically, the lesions can be successfully treated with thermal therapy using contact probes (71) or argon plasma coagulation (72).

Endoscopic intervention for gastrointestinal angiodysplasias is ineffective when the vascular lesions are diffuse, inaccessible, or escape identification. Additionally, rebleeding is an important clinical issue after endoscopic therapy. Estrogen and progesterone therapy has been proposed for the prevention of recurrent bleeding from angiodysplasias. Potential mechanisms for the beneficial effect of estrogen on bleeding gastrointestinal telangiectasias include improvement in coagulation status with decreased bleeding time and improvement in the integrity of the vascular endothelial lining. Studies of hormonal therapy have had mixed results with two small studies showing cessation of bleeding and decreased transfusion requirement (68,73), but a more recent larger trial finding no significant benefit with hormonal therapy (74). Other therapies for recurrent bleeding from angiodysplasias have been studied. Treatment with thalidomide, an angiogenesis inhibitor, improved outcomes in a small study as compared to iron supplementation (75). Octreotide has been shown to benefit patients in small studies, and a decrease in transfusion requirement with octreotide treatment was confirmed in a meta-analysis (76). However, a recent systematic review found low quality or insufficient evidence to support treatment of angiodysplasia with hormonal therapy, thalidomide, or octreotide (77).

PANCREAS

Abnormal glandular morphology and pancreatic exocrine function are very common in ESKD. Pancreatic endocrine function as measured by beta-cell response has been consistently shown to produce normal glucose and insulin levels which do not differ between groups of patients with ESKD regardless of dialysis modality. In contrast, C-peptide concentrations are markedly increased over controls, and the return of insulin to basal levels is delayed with ESKD (78). Several mechanisms have been postulated to explain this finding. Iron deposition from chronic administration and elevated levels of islet amyloid polypeptide may contribute to beta-cell dysfunction (79,80). Aggressive iron depletion with phlebotomy and recombinant human erythropoietin reverses some of these defects, and recently, deferoxamine therapy has shown substantial promise in reducing insulin resistance and improving B-cell function (81). L-carnitine nutritional supplements may provide additional benefit by improving some of the beta-cell responsiveness, but the clinical benefit remains to be proven (82).

Approximately 70% of patients have abnormal pancreatic exocrine function (83). Investigators have demonstrated reduced duodenal amylase, lipase, bicarbonate, and protein levels in response to secretory stimulation tests (84,85). In addition, fecal chymotrypsin levels are significantly reduced in chronic kidney disease (86). These changes in excretory pancreatic function are infrequently associated with ultrasonographic changes within the pancreas. Autopsy studies reveal a correlation between pancreatic disease and elevated intact parathyroid hormone (PTH) levels (87). Whether these abnormalities are part of the clinical spectrum of chronic pancreatitis or represent a distinct uremic pancreatopathy is unclear. Other possible causes of pancreatic disease in dialysis patients include hypercalcemia, hypertriglyceridemia, vascular insufficiency, and drug toxicity [such as long-standing diuretic use,

TABLE 23.2	Potential Causes of Pancreatic Disease in Dialysis Patients

Alcoholism

Gallstones

Hyperparathyroidism

Hypercalcemia

Hypertriglyceridemia

Vascular insufficiency

Drug toxicity

    Diuretics

    Antibiotics

    Nonsteroidal anti-inflammatory agents

    Heparin (transient)

    Dialysate

Systemic lupus erythematosus

Polycystic kidney disease

antibiotics, and nonsteroidal anti-inflammatory drugs (NSAIDs)] (**TABLE 23.2**). The clinical result of these changes may lead to steatorrhea, which may contribute to the malnutrition seen commonly in dialysis patients (88).

Patients with chronic kidney disease frequently have elevated serum amylase and lipase levels in the absence of clinical pancreatitis, probably related to diminished kidney clearance. The kidney is responsible for 20% of the clearance of these enzymes. Serum amylase, lipase, and trypsin values remain normal until the creatinine clearance is less than 50 mL/min (89). The levels then rise to approximately two to three times normal, which may correlate with the duration of chronic kidney disease (90). Total serum amylase, pancreatic amylase, and salivary amylase isoenzymes are elevated, but isoenzymes are not routinely measured in clinical practice (86,91). Serum amylase in asymptomatic patients rarely exceeds 500 IU/L and is unaffected by dialysis (89,92). The predialysis serum lipase activity is also increased in patients with ESKD and rises further after hemodialysis. This effect is related to the lipolytic effect of intradialytic heparin and dose. Patients on CAPD and with peritonitis also have mild elevations in serum and peritoneal amylase (up to 100 IU/L); however, marked elevations, as seen in patients with pancreatitis or cholecystitis, are not found (93,94).

Acute pancreatitis has been reported to be more common in ESKD than in the general population. Several series report an incidence of 2.3% to 6.4% in patients with kidney disease (95,96). Pancreatitis is significantly more common in those with alcohol abuse, systemic lupus erythematosus, and polycystic kidney disease. It is not significantly associated with biliary tract disease, hyperlipidemia, or hypercalcemia. The mortality is 20% to 50%. Acute pancreatitis is equally common in patients on CAPD and on hemodialysis (96–98). The dialysate may be clear, hemorrhagic, or cloudy. It has been suggested that metabolic abnormalities related to absorption of glucose and buffer from dialysate, hypertriglyceridemia, or absorption of a toxic substance in the dialysate, bags, or tubing may increase the risk of pancreatitis in dialysis patients (99).

Chronic pancreatitis can interfere with absorption and may result in malnutrition, vitamin deficiencies, and chronic wasting in dialysis patients (88). Histologic evidence of pancreatitis can be

seen in greater than 50% of patients with ESKD, 85% of which is chronic (100). Pathologic changes include calcifications, fibrosis, abscess formation, and deposition of hemosiderin. However, despite the frequency of chronic morphologic findings and functional abnormalities of the pancreas associated with ESKD, clinically significant chronic pancreatitis is rare. Most patients are asymptomatic; rarely, symptoms suggestive of malabsorption, such as steatorrhea, develop (101).

Diagnosing pancreatitis in dialysis patients can be very difficult. Dialysis patients frequently experience abdominal discomfort, nausea, and vomiting as a result of uremia or dialysis treatments. Nonspecific elevations of serum amylase and lipase are common. Therefore, interpretation of hyperamylasemia must be approached with caution. Clinicians should maintain a high level of suspicion if values exceed three times the normal limit. Abdominal computed tomography (CT) can be useful to confirm pancreatic inflammation and peripancreatic abnormalities suspicious for pancreatitis. Early diagnosis and therapy may reduce the progression or severity of disease. Acute pancreatitis is more likely to be severe and is associated with a worse prognosis in dialysis patients than in the general population (102). Using Ranson's criteria, the mortality for patients with three or more (including kidney insufficiency) criteria approaches 70%, compared to 11% for patients without kidney disease. Complications such as pancreatic abscesses, pseudocysts, and necrosis occur with the same frequency as in the general population. However, dialysis patients develop twice as many systemic complications, such as cardiovascular and pulmonary complications, and sepsis (103). Treatment should be similar to that for nondialysis patients, including bowel rest, volume resuscitation as needed with frequent dialysis to maintain euvolemia, and pain control. Pain management strategies should avoid the use of meperidine (Demerol), which may lower the threshold for seizures in ESKD.

NEPHROGENIC ASCITES

Nephrogenic ascites (NA) or idiopathic dialysis ascites (IDA) is an uncommon but important cause of morbidity in dialysis patients. By definition, it is a disorder that manifests as massive, refractory ascites in chronic hemodialysis patients where all other causes of ascites have been excluded (104). The incidence appears to be decreasing with improved volumetrically controlled dialysis and nutrition and is center-dependent (104,105). Most patients present with sustained volume overload, arterial hypertension, large interdialytic weight gains, minimal extremity edema, cachexia, and a history of dialysis-associated hypotension (104–107). NA is frequently associated with hyperparathyroidism, hypoalbuminemia, and uremia; has a male predominance; and is unrelated to age or race (108). It is associated with a grave prognosis, with a 1-year mortality rate of more than 30% (106) (**TABLE 23.3**).

The pathophysiology of NA is complex, probably multifactorial, and incompletely understood. Many patients have a history of previous CAPD, suggesting persisting abnormalities of the peritoneal membrane. However, the syndrome also occurs in patients even before the initiation of dialysis (106). The accumulation of ascites may occur up to 18 months preceding dialysis to as late as 5 years after initiation of dialysis. The characteristics of the ascitic fluid indicate that the underlying pathogenesis is an alteration of the balance between peritoneal membrane permeability and impaired resorption due to peritoneal lymphatic obstruction, without a significantly

TABLE 23.3	Causes and Characteristics of Nephrogenic Ascites

Possible causes

Sustained volume overload

Impaired lymphatic drainage

Elevated hepatic venous hydrostatic pressure

Increased peritoneal membrane permeability resulting from

  Dialysate solutions

  Uremic toxins

  Hyperparathyroidism

  Hypoalbuminemia

  Circulating immune complexes

  Hemosiderosis

  Activation of the renin-angiotensin system

  Celiac disease

Clinical characteristics

  Refractory ascites in the absence of hepatic, neoplastic, or infectious disease

  Arterial hypertension

  Minimal extremity edema

  Cachexia

  History of intradialytic hypotension

  Exudative ascites

Adapted from Hammond TC, Takiyyuddin MA. Nephrogenic ascites: a poorly understood syndrome. *J Am Soc Nephrol* 1994;5:1173–1177.

elevated hepatic vein hydrostatic pressure (107,109). The ascitic fluid is straw colored and exudative, with a total protein of more than 3 g/dL; ratio of serum albumin to ascites albumin of less than 0.9 g/dL; and a low ascites total protein/serum total protein of more than 0.72. Therefore, NA must be differentiated from pancreatitis, malignancy, and tuberculous peritonitis (110). Changes in membrane permeability as a result of dialysis membranes and fluid, circulating immune complexes, iron deposition, abnormal sodium transport, or activation of the renin-angiotensin system have been proposed (104,107,111–113). Celiac disease has also been described as a rare cause (114). Histologic examination of the peritoneum typically demonstrates chronic inflammation, fibrosis, and mesothelial cell proliferation (105).

The diagnosis of NA is one of exclusion. Examination of the ascitic fluid is critical to establish an exudative pattern. Diagnostic paracentesis is central to establish the protein content and rule out infectious or neoplastic causes. Ultrasonography or CT may help delineate hepatic structure, but peritoneoscopy with biopsy is generally more definitive.

The treatment of NA is multimodal and includes strict volume control, daily hemodialysis for several weeks, frequent paracentesis, and optimization of protein nutrition. Other strategies have been employed with varying and unsatisfactory success. Ascites may respond to ascitic fluid reinfusion, peritoneal venous shunts, CAPD, bilateral nephrectomy, intraperitoneal corticosteroids, and possibly angiotensin-converting enzyme (ACE) inhibitor therapy (105,109,115–119) and iron depletion (120). However, kidney transplantation remains the definitive treatment for NA and offers the best hope for cure. Patients experience complete resolution

of ascites within 6 weeks of graft functioning but may have a recurrence after graft failure (121,122). Such measures can reverse the progressive course of cachexia and malnutrition, improve the quality of life, and improve survival.

CONSTIPATION

Functional constipation consists of decreased bowel frequency with fewer than three stools per week or frequent straining, incomplete evacuation, hard or lumpy stools, and the need for manual maneuvers. In the general population, the prevalence of constipation rises with age, affecting more than 25% of patients older than 65 years (123,124). Approximately 63% of hemodialysis patients experience constipation, possibly as a result of associated comorbidities, poor nutritional status, and increased colonic transit time or medications (**TABLE 23.4**) (125). Among CAPD patients, the prevalence of constipation is 29% and is age-related (126). The lower rate of constipation in CAPD has been attributed to better metabolic and potassium control and increased dietary fiber intake. In most patients, constipation is bothersome and may interfere with the quality of life; however, in rare instances, severe obstipation can be associated with colonic perforation and death.

TABLE 23.4	Factors Commonly Associated with Constipation in Dialysis Patients

Drugs

Analgesics

  Anticholinergics

Antidepressants

  Anticholinergics

  Serotonin antagonists

Antipsychotics

Antihypertensives

  Calcium channel antagonists

Calcium-containing drugs

  Iron supplements

  Aluminum binders

  Calcium acetate binders

  Calcium carbonate

Opiates

Neurogenic disorders

  Autonomic neuropathy

  Diabetic enteropathy

  Intestinal pseudoobstruction

Metabolic problems

  Hypercalcemia

  Hypocalcemia

  Hypothyroidism

Nutritional factors

  Malnutrition

  Dehydration

  Low dietary fiber

  Hyperkalemia

Inactivity

Uremic patients having chronic constipation, abdominal pain, and distension should be evaluated for colonic pseudoobstruction. This is associated with colonic perforation in up to 50% of cases, particularly if the bowel wall diameter exceeds 12 cm (127). Neostigmine can be considered in the absence of contraindications unrelated to ESKD but may require dose adjustment. Early endoscopic or surgical decompression may result in complete recovery. Aluminum hydroxide binders have been associated with 78% of these cases as well as drugs and autonomic neuropathy (128). Plain abdominal films can be helpful to confirm the diagnosis, and CT scan or colonoscopy can rule out potential causes of mechanical obstruction. Antacid impactions should be considered in patients with ESKD, as they can ingest a large volume of antacids for dyspepsia and control of phosphorus absorption. Complications of antacid impactions such as stercoral ulceration and perforation are not uncommon (129).

The initial evaluation of a patient with constipation should include a careful history and physical examination, with emphasis on recent changes in bowel movements, and medications. If no cause is identified, imaging studies to rule out mass lesions, megacolon, and strictures may be useful. If these studies are normal, studies to assess for prolonged fecal transit time and pelvic floor dysfunction should be considered, in conjunction with consultation with a gastroenterologist.

Early and aggressive measures to reduce constipation are important, as uremic patients have a greater risk of developing diverticula and perforation than the general population (130). This is particularly true in patients with polycystic kidney disease, approximately 80% of whom have diverticuli, compared with 49% of patients with other causes of chronic kidney disease (131). Medical management of constipation in dialysis patients can begin with increasing dietary fiber and activity and avoiding volume depletion. Medications should be tailored to reduce the number of drugs associated with constipation (TABLE 23.4). Hyperosmolar, magnesium-containing compounds can cause hypermagnesemia in kidney disease and are contraindicated. Phosphate-containing enemas are also contraindicated. Stool softeners with docusate sodium may improve the ability of water to enter the stool but are not very effective. Chronic use of aluminum binders may worsen constipation, renal osteodystrophy, and encephalopathy. Chronic use of intestinal wall stimulants such as bisacodyl may induce hypokalemia and protein malnutrition; their use should be restricted to short-term management only. Lactulose, sorbitol, and polyethylene glycol are helpful in dialysis patients and can be used occasionally for refractory constipation (132). Lubiprostone and linaclotide are newer agents that can be employed for treatment of chronic constipation. For severe incapacitating constipation, surgical measures may be necessary.

REFERENCES

1. Strid H, Simrén M, Johansson AC, et al. The prevalence of gastrointestinal symptoms in patients with chronic renal failure is increased and associated with impaired psychological general well being. *Nephrol Dial Transplant* 2002;17:1434–1439.
2. Abu Farsakh NA, Roweily E, Rababaa M, et al. Brief report: evaluation of the upper gastrointestinal tract in uraemic patients undergoing haemodialysis. *Nephrol Dial Transplant* 1996;11:847–850.
3. Hammer J, Oesterreicher C, Hammer K, et al. Chronic gastrointestinal symptoms in hemodialysis patients. *Wien Klin Wochenschr* 1998;110:287–291.
4. Kahvecioglu S, Akdag I, Kiyici M, et al. High prevalence of irritable bowel syndrome and upper gastrointestinal symptoms in patients with chronic renal failure. *J Nephrol* 2005;18:61–66.
5. Cano AE, Neil AK, Kang JY, et al. Gastrointestinal symptoms in patients with end-stage renal disease undergoing treatment by hemodialysis or peritoneal dialysis. *Am J Gastroenterol* 2007;102:1990–1997.
6. Strid H, Fjell A, Simrén M, et al. Impact of dialysis on gastroesophageal reflux, dyspepsia, and proton pump inhibitor treatment in patients with chronic renal failure. *Eur J Gastroenterol Hepatol* 2009;21:137–142.
7. Kawaguchi Y, Mine T, Kawana I, et al. Gastroesophageal reflux disease in hemodialysis patients. *Tokai J Exp Clin Med* 2009;34:48–52.
8. Abdulrahman IS, Al-Quorain AA. Prevalence of gastroesophageal reflux disease and its association with *Helicobacter pylori* infection in chronic renal failure patients and in renal transplant recipients. *Saudi J Gastroenterol* 2008;14:183–186.
9. Cekin AH, Boyacioglu S, Gursoy M, et al. Gastroesophageal reflux disease in chronic renal failure patients with upper GI symptoms: multivariate analysis of pathogenic factors. *Am J Gastroenterol* 2002;97:1352–1356.
10. Kim MJ, Kwon KH, Lee SW. Gastroesophageal reflux disease in CAPD patients. *Adv Perit Dial* 1998;14:98–101.
11. Vaziri ND, Dure-Smith B, Miller R, et al. Pathology of gastrointestinal tract in chronic hemodialysis patients: an autopsy study of 78 cases. *Am J Gastroenterol* 1985;80:608–611.
12. Andriulli A, Malfi B, Recchia S, et al. Patients with chronic renal failure are not at risk of developing chronic peptic ulcers. *Clin Nephrol* 1985;23:245–248.
13. Sotoudehmanesh R, Ali Asgari A, Ansari R, et al. Endoscopic findings in end-stage renal disease. *Endoscopy* 2003;35:502–505.
14. Margolis DM, Saylor JL, Geisse G, et al. Upper gastrointestinal disease in chronic renal failure. A prospective evaluation. *Arch Intern Med* 1978;138:1214–1217.
15. El-Serag HB, Sonnenberg A, Jamal MM, et al. Corpus gastritis is protective against reflux esophagitis. *Gut* 1999;45:181–185.
16. Varanasi RV, Fantry GT, Wilson KT. Decreased prevalence of *Helicobacter pylori* infection in gastroesophageal reflux disease. *Helicobacter* 1998;3:188–194.
17. Kawaguchi Y, Mine T, Kawana I, et al. Gastroesophageal reflux disease in chronic renal failure patients: evaluation by endoscopic evaluation. *Tokai J Exp Clin Med* 2009;34:80–83.
18. Mora Fernández C, del Castillo N, Medina ML, et al. High incidence of hiatal hernia in patients with end-stage renal disease. *Clin Nephrol* 1996;46:218.
19. Francos GC, Besarab A, Joseph RE. Disorders of oesophageal motility in chronic haemodialysis patients. *Lancet* 1984;1:219.
20. Siamopoulos KC, Tsianos EV, Dardamanis M, et al. Esophageal dysfunction in chronic hemodialysis patients. *Nephron* 1990;55:389–393.
21. Doğan I, Unal S, Sindel S, et al. Esophageal motor dysfunction in chronic renal failure. *Nephron* 1996;72:346–347.
22. Jaffe RH, Laing DR. Changes of the digestive tract in uremia: a pathologic anatomic study. *Arch Intern Med* 1934;53:851–864.
23. Mason EE. Gastrointestinal lesions occurring in uremia. *Ann Intern Med* 1952;37:96–105.
24. Moustafa FE, Khalil A, Abdel Wahab M, et al. *Helicobacter pylori* and uremic gastritis: a histopathologic study and correlation with endoscopic and bacteriologic findings. *Am J Nephrol* 1997;17:165–171.
25. Fabbian F, Catalano C, Bordin V, et al. Esophagogastroduodenoscopy in chronic hemodialysis patients: 2-year clinical experience in a renal unit. *Clin Nephrol* 2002;58:54–59.
26. Al-Mueilo SH. Gastroduodenal lesions and *Helicobacter pylori* infection in hemodialysis patients. *Saudi Med J* 2004;25:1010–1014.
27. Nardone G, Rocco A, Fiorillo M, et al. Gastroduodenal lesions and *Helicobacter pylori* infection in dyspeptic patients with and without chronic renal failure. *Helicobacter* 2005;10:53–58.
28. Kang JY, Wu AY, Sutherland IH, et al. Prevalence of peptic ulcer in patients undergoing maintenance hemodialysis. *Dig Dis Sci* 1988;33:774–778.

29. Chen YT, Yang WC, Lin CC, et al. Comparison of peptic ulcer disease risk between peritoneal and hemodialysis patients. *Am J Nephrol* 2010;32:212.

30. Troskot B, Kes P, Duvnjak M, et al. Giant peptic ulcers in patients undergoing maintenance hemodialysis. *Acta Med Croatica* 1995;49:59–64.

31. Huang K, Leu HB, Luo JC, et al. Different peptic ulcer bleeding risk in chronic kidney disease and end-stage renal disease patients receiving different dialysis. *Dig Dis Sci* 2014;59:807–813.

32. Kang JY, Ho KY, Yeoh KG, et al. Peptic ulcer and gastritis in uraemia, with particular reference to the effect of *Helicobacter pylori* infection. *J Gastroenterol Hepatol* 1999;14:771–778.

33. Ozgür O, Boyacioğlu S, Ozdoğan M, et al. *Helicobacter pylori* infection in haemodialysis patients and renal transplant recipients. *Nephrol Dial Transplant* 1997;12:289–291.

34. Gladziwa U, Haase G, Handt S, et al. Prevalence of *Helicobacter pylori* in patients with chronic renal failure. *Nephrol Dial Transplant* 1993;8: 301–306.

35. Davenport A, Shallcross TM, Crabtree JE, et al. Prevalence of *Helicobacter pylori* in patients with end-stage renal failure and renal transplant recipients. *Nephron* 1991;59:597–601.

36. Jaspersen D, Fassbinder W, Heinkele P, et al. Significantly lower prevalence of *Helicobacter pylori* in uremic patients than in patients with normal renal function. *J Gastrenterol* 1995;30:585–588.

37. Krawczyk W, Górna E, Suwala J, et al. Frequency of *Helicobacter pylori* infection in uremic hemodialyzed patients with antral gastritis. *Nephron* 1996;74:621–622.

38. Ala-Kaila K, Vaajalahti P, Karvonen AL, et al. Gastric *Helicobacter* and upper gastrointestinal symptoms in chronic renal failure. *Ann Med* 1991;23:403–406.

39. Nakajima F, Sakaguchi M, Amemoto K, et al. *Helicobacter pylori* in patients receiving long term dialysis. *Am J Nephrol* 2002;22:468–472.

40. Gu M, Xiao S, Pan X, et al. *Helicobacter pylori* infection in dialysis patients: a meta-analysis. *Gastroenterol Res Pract* 2013;2013:785892.

41. Schoonjans R, Van VB, Vandamme W, et al. Dyspepsia and gastroparesis in chronic renal failure: the role of *Helicobacter pylori*. *Clin Nephrol* 2002;57:201–207.

42. Huang JJ, Huang CJ, Ruaan MK, et al. Diagnostic efficacy of (13)C-urea breath test for *Helicobacter pylori* infection in hemodialysis patients. *Am J Kidney Dis* 2000;36:124–129.

43. Mak SK, Loo CK, Wong AM, et al. Efficacy of a 1-week course of proton-pump inhibitor-based triple therapy for eradicating *Helicobacter pylori* in patients with and without chronic renal failure. *Am J Kidney Dis* 2002;40:576–581.

44. Suleymanlar I, Tuncer M, Tugrul Sezer M, et al. Response to triple treatment with omeprazole, amoxicillin, and clarithromycin for *Helicobacter pylori* infections in continuous ambulatory peritoneal dialysis patients. *Adv Perit Dial* 1999;15:79–81.

45. Van Vlem B, Schoonjans R, Vanholder R, et al. Delayed gastric emptying in dyspeptic chronic hemodialysis patients. *Am J Kidney Dis* 2000;36:962–968.

46. Hirako M, Kamiya T, Misu N, et al. Impaired gastric motility and its relationship to gastrointestinal symptoms in patients with chronic renal failure. *J Gastroenterol* 2005;40:1116–1122.

47. Guz G, Bali M, Poyraz NY, et al. Gastric emptying in patients on renal replacement therapy. *Ren Fail* 2004;26:619–624.

48. Van Vlem B, Schoonjans R, Vanholder R, et al. Dyspepsia and gastric emptying in chronic renal failure patients. *Clin Nephrol* 2001;56:302–307.

49. De Schoenmakere G, Vanholder R, Rottey S, et al. Relationship between gastric emptying and clinical and biochemical factors in chronic hemodialysis patients. *Nephrol Dial Transplant* 2001;16:1850–1855.

50. Ross EA, Koo LC. Improved nutrition after the detection and treatment of occult gastroparesis in nondiabetic dialysis patients. *Am J Kidney Dis* 1998;31:62–66.

51. Strid H, Simrén M, Stotzer PO, et al. Delay in gastric emptying in patients with chronic renal failure. *Scand J Gastroenterol* 2004;39:516–520.

52. Schoonjans R, Van Vlem B, Vandamme W, et al. Gastric emptying of solids in cirrhotic and peritoneal dialysis patients: influence of peritoneal volume load. *Eur J Gastroenterol Hepatol* 2002;14:395–398.

53. Hubalewska A, Stompór T, Płaczkiewicz E, et al. Evaluation of gastric emptying in patients with chronic renal failure on continuous ambulatory peritoneal dialysis using 99mTc-solid meal. *Nucl Med Rev Cent East Eur* 2004;7:27–30.

54. Kao CH, Hsu YH, Wang SJ. Delayed gastric emptying and *Helicobacter pylori* infection in patients with chronic renal failure. *Eur J Nucl Med* 1995;22:1282–1285.

55. Chalasani N, Cotsonis G, Wilcox CM. Upper gastrointestinal bleeding in patients with chronic renal failure: role of vascular ectasia. *Am J Gastroenterol* 1996;91:2329–2332.

56. Zuckerman GR, Cornette GL, Clouse RE, et al. Upper gastrointestinal bleeding in patients with chronic renal failure. *Ann Intern Med* 1985;102:588–592.

57. Lutz J, Menke J, Sollinger D, et al. Hemostasis in chronic kidney disease. *Nephrol Dial Transplant* 2014;29(1):29–40.

58. Livio M, Gotti E, Marchesi D, et al. Uremic bleeding: role of anemia and beneficial effects of red cell transfusion. *Lancet* 1982;2:1013–1015.

59. Mannucci PM, Remuzzi G, Pusineri F, et al. Deamino-8-D-arginine vasopressin shortens the bleeding time in uremia. *N Engl J Med* 1983; 308(1):8–12.

60. Janson PA, Jubelirer SJ, Weinstein MJ, et al. Treatment of the bleeding tendency in uremia with cryoprecipitate. *N Engl J Med* 1980;303(23):1318.

61. Tsai C, Hwang JC. Investigation of upper gastrointestinal hemorrhage in chronic renal failure. *J Clin Gastroenterol* 1996;22:2–5.

62. Wasse H, Gilen DL, Ball AM, et al. Risk factors for upper gastrointestinal bleeding among end-stage renal disease patients. *Kidney Int* 2003;64:1455–1461.

63. Clouse RE, Costigan DJ, Mills BA, et al. Angiodysplasia as a cause of upper gastrointestinal bleeding. *Arch Intern Med* 1985;145:458–461.

64. Navab F, Masters P, Subramani R, et al. Angiodysplasia in patients with renal insufficiency. *Am J Gastroenterol* 1989;84:1297–1301.

65. Cappell MS, Gupta A. Changing epidemiology of gastrointestinal angiodysplasia with increasing recognition of clinically milder cases: angiodysplasia tend to produce mild chronic gastrointestinal bleeding in a study of 47 consecutive patients admitted from 1980-1989. *Am J Gastroenterol* 1992;87:201–206.

66. Alvarez L, Puleo J, Balint JA. Investigation of gastrointestinal bleeding in patients with end stage renal disease. *Am J Gastroenterol* 1993;88:30–33.

67. Marcuard SP, Weinstock JV. Gastrointestinal angiodysplasia in renal failure. *J Clin Gastroenterol* 1988;10:482–484.

68. Bronner MH, Pate MB, Cunningham JT, et al. Estrogen-progesterone therapy for bleeding gastrointestinal telangiectasias in chronic renal failure. *Ann Intern Med* 1986;105:371–374.

69. Lepère C, Cuillerier E, Van Gossum A, et al. Predictive factors of positive findings in patients explored by push enteroscopy for unexplained GI bleeding. *Gastrointest Endosc* 2005;61:709–714.

70. Karagiannis S, Goulas S, Kosmadakis G, et al. Wireless capsule endoscopy in the investigation of patients with chronic renal failure and obscure gastrointestinal bleeding (preliminary data). *World J Gastroenterol* 2006;12:5182–5185.

71. Stefanidis I, Liakopoulos V, Kapsoritakis AN, et al. Gastric antral vascular ectasia (watermelon stomach) in patients with ESRD. *Am J Kidney Dis* 2006;47:77–82.

72. Tomori K, Nakamoto H, Kotaki S, et al. Gastric angiodysplasia in patients undergoing maintenance dialysis. *Adv Perit Dial* 2003;19:136–142.

73. van Cutsem E, Rutgeerts P, Vantrappen G. Treatment of bleeding gastrointestinal vascular malformations with oestrogen-progesterone. *Lancet* 1990;335:953–955.

74. Junquera F, Feu F, Papo M, et al. A multicenter, randomized, clinical trial of hormonal therapy in the prevention of rebleeding from gastrointestinal angiodysplasia. *Gastroenterology* 2001;121:1073–1079.

75. Ge ZZ, Chen HM, Gao YJ, et al. Efficacy of thalidomide for refractory gastrointestinal bleeding from vascular malformation. *Gastroenterology* 2011;141(5):1629.e4–1637.e4.

76. Brown C, Subramanian V, Wilcox CM, et al. Somatostatin analogues in the treatment of recurrent bleeding from gastrointestinal vascular malformations: an overview and systematic review of prospective observational studies. *Dig Dis Sci* 2010;55(8):2129–2134.

77. Swanson E, Mahgoub A, MacDonald R, et al. Medical and endoscopic therapies for angiodysplasia and gastric antral vascular ectasia: a systematic review. *Clin Gastroenterol Hepatol* 2014;12(4):571–582.

78. Smith WG, Hanning I, Johnston DG, et al. Pancreatic beta-cell function in CAPD. *Nephrol Dial Transplant* 1988;3:448–452.

79. el-Reshaid K, Seshadri MS, Hourani H, et al. Endocrine abnormalities is hemodialysis patients with iron overload: reversal with iron depletion. *Nutrition* 1995;11:521–526.

80. de Koning EJ, Fleming KA, Gray DW, et al. High prevalence of pancreatic islet amyloid in patients with end-stage renal failure on dialysis treatment. *J Pathol* 1995;175:253–258.

81. Alnahal AA, Tahan M, Fathy A, et al. Effect of deferoxamine therapy on insulin resistance in end-stage renal disease patients with iron overload. *Saudi J Kidney Dis Transpl* 2014;25:808–813.

82. Vazelov E, Borissova AM, Kirilov G, et al. L-carnitine consecutively administered to patients on dialysis improves beta-cell response. *Int J Artif Organs* 2003;26:304–307.

83. Bartos B, Melichar J, Erben J. The function of the exocrine pancreas in chronic renal disease. *Digestion* 1970;3:33–40.

84. Sachs EF, Hurwitz FJ, Bloch HM, et al. Pancreatic exocrine hypofunction in the wasting syndrome of end-stage renal disease. *Am J Gastroenterol* 1983;78:170–176.

85. Malyszko J, Sosnowski S, Mazerska M, et al. Gastric and pancreatic function in hemodialyzed patients. *Int Urol Nephrol* 1995;27:471–478.

86. Ventrucci M, Campieri C, Di Stefano M, et al. Alterations of exocrine pancreas in end-stage renal disease. Do they reflect a clinically relevant uremic pancreatopathy? *Dig Dis Sci* 1995;40:2576–2581.

87. Avram RM, Iancu M. Pancreatic disease in uremia and parathyroid hormone excess. *Nephron* 1982;32:60–62.

88. Griesche-Philippi J, Otto J, Schwörer H, et al. Exocrine pancreatic function in patients with end-stage renal disease. *Clin Nephrol* 2010;74:457–464.

89. Collen MJ, Ansher AF, Chapman AB, et al. Serum amylase in patients with renal insufficiency and renal failure. *Am J Gastroenterol* 1990;85:1377–1380.

90. Bardella MT, Bianchi ML, Molteni N, et al. Serum amylase and isoamylase in chronic renal failure. *Int J Artif Organs* 1987;10:259–262.

91. Tsianos EV, Dardamanis MA, Elisaf M, et al. The value of alpha-amylase and isoamylase determination in chronic renal failure patients. *Int J Pancreatol* 1994;15:105–111.

92. Vaziri ND, Chang D, Malekpour A, et al. Pancreatic enzymes in patients with end-stage renal disease maintained on hemodialysis. *Am J Gastroenerol* 1988;83:410–412.

93. Caruana RJ, Burkart J, Segraves D, et al. Serum and peritoneal fluid amylase levels in CAPD. Normal values and clinical usefulness. *Am J Nephrol* 1987;7:169–172.

94. Gupta A, Yuan ZY, Balaskas EV, et al. CAPD and pancreatitis: no connection. *Perit Dial Int* 1992;12:309–316.

95. Padilla B, Pollak VE, Pesce A, et al. Pancreatitis in patients with end-stage renal disease. *Medicine* 1994;73:8–20.

96. Quaraishi ER, Goel S, Gupta M, et al. Acute pancreatitis in patients on chronic peritoneal dialysis: an increased risk? *Am J Gastroenterol* 2005;100:2288–2293.

97. Pannekeet MM, Kredeit RT, Boeschoten EW, et al. Acute pancreatitis during CAPD in The Netherlands. *Nephrol Dial Transplant* 1993;8:1376–1381.

98. Bruno MJ, van Westerloo DJ, van Dorp WT, et al. Acute pancreatitis in peritoneal dialysis and haemodialysis: risk, clinical course, outcome, and possible aetiology. *Gut* 2000;46:385–389.

99. Caruana RJ, Wolfman NT, Karstaedt N, et al. Pancreatitis: an important cause of abdominal symptoms in patients on peritoneal dialysis. *Am J Kidney Dis* 1986;7:135–140.

100. Araki T, Ueda M, Ogawa K, et al. Histological pancreatitis in end-stage renal disease. *Int J Pancreatol* 1992;12:263–269.

101. Masoero G, Bruno M, Gallo L, et al. Increased serum pancreatic enzymes in uremia: relation with treatment modality and pancreatic involvement. *Pancreas* 1996;13:350–355.

102. Joglar FM, Saadé M. Outcome of pancreatitis in CAPD and HD patients. *Perit Dial Int* 1995;15:264–266.

103. Pitchumoni CS, Arguello P, Agarwal N, et al. Acute pancreatitis in chronic renal failure. *Am J Gastroenterol* 1996;91:2477–2482.

104. Glück Z, Nolph KD. Ascites associated with end-stage renal disease. *Am J Kidney Dis* 1987;10:9–18.

105. Singh S, Mitra S, Berman LB. Ascites in patients on maintenance hemodialysis. *Nephron* 1974;12:114–120.

106. Mauk PM, Schwartz JT, Lowe JE, et al. Diagnosis and course of nephrogenic ascites. *Arch Intern Med* 1988;148:1577–1579.

107. Hammond TC, Takiyyuddin MA. Nephrogenic ascites: a poorly understood syndrome. *J Am Soc Nephrol* 1994;5:1173–1177.

108. Nasr EM, Joubran NI. Is nephrogenic ascites related to secondary hyperparathyroidism? *Am J Kidney Dis* 2001;37:E16.

109. Han SH, Reynolds TB, Fong TL. Nephrogenic ascites. Analysis of 16 cases and review of the literature. *Medicine* 1998;77:233–245.

110. Tannenberg AM. Ascites in dialysis patients. In: Nissenson AR, Fine RN, eds. *Dialysis Therapy*. Philadelphia, PA: Hanley & Belfus, 1993:299–301.

111. Gotloib L, Servadio C. Ascites in patients undergoing maintenance hemodialysis. Report of six cases and physiopathologic approach. *Am J Med* 1976;61:465–470.

112. Twardowski ZJ, Alpert MA, Gupta KD, et al. Circulating immune complexes: possible toxins responsible for serositis (pericarditis, pleuritis, peritonitis) in renal failure. *Nephron* 1983;35:190–195.

113. Beşbaş N, Söylemezoğlu O, Saatçi U, et al. Peritoneal hemosiderosis in pediatric patients with nephrogenic ascites. *Nephron* 1992;62:292–295.

114. Al-bderat J, Hazza I, Haddad R. Celiac disease a rare cause of nephrogenic ascites. *Saudi J Kidney Dis Transpl* 2013;24:1262–1264.

115. Rubin J, Kiley J, Pay R, et al. Continuous ambulatory peritoneal dialysis. Treatment of dialysis-related ascites. *Arch Intern Med* 1981;14:1093–1095.

116. Roy-Chaudhury P, Edward N. ACE inhibitors in the management of hemodialysis ascites. *Nephrol Dial Transplant* 1994;9:1695–1696.

117. Gunal AI, Karaca I, Celiker H, et al. Strict volume control in the treatment of nephrogenic ascites. *Nephrol Dial Transplant* 2002;17:1248–1251.

118. Buselmeier TJ, Simmons RL, Duncan DA, et al. Local steroid treatment of intractable ascites in dialysis patients. *Proc Clin Dial Transplant Forum* 1975;5:9–11.

119. Liu J, Zhang C, Zhu X, et al. Intravenous infusion ascitic fluid during hemodialysis: a study of 108 treatments in 13 uremic patients. *Artif Cells Substit Immobil Biotechnol* 1999;27:153–162.

120. Nomura S, Osawa G, Karai M. Treatment of a patient with end-stage renal disease, severe iron overload and ascites by weekly phlebotomy combined with recombinant human erythropoietin. *Nephron* 1990;55:210–213.

121. Markov M, Van Theil DH, Nadir A. Ascites and kidney transplantation: case report and critical appraisal of the literature. *Dig Dis Sci* 2007;52(12):3383–3388.

122. Melero M, Rodriguez M, Araque A, et al. Idiopathic dialysis ascites in the nineties: resolution after renal transplantation. *Am J Kidney Dis* 1995;26:668–670.

123. Murtagh FE, Addington-Hall J, Higginson IJ. The prevalence of symptoms in end-stage renal disease: a systematic review. *Adv Chronic Kidney Dis* 2007;14:82–99.

124. Talley NJ, O'Keefe EA, Zinsmeister AR, et al. Prevalence of gastrointestinal symptoms in the elderly: a population-based study. *Gastroenterology* 1992;102:895–901.

125. Wu MJ, Chang CS, Cheng CH, et al. Colonic transit time in long-term dialysis patients. *Am J Kidney Dis* 2004;44:322–327.

126. Yasuda G, Shibata K, Takizawa T, et al. Prevalence of constipation in continuous ambulatory peritoneal dialysis patients and comparison with hemodialysis patients. *Am J Kidney Dis* 2002;39:1292–1299.

127. Nanni G, Garbini A, Luchetti P, et al. Ogilvie's syndrome (acute colonic pseudo-obstruction): review of the literature (October 1948 to

March 1980) and report of four additional cases. *Dis Colon Rectum* 1982;25(2):157–166.

128. Adams DL, Rutsky EA, Rostand SG, et al. Lower gastrointestinal tract dysfunction in patients receiving long-term hemodialysis. *Arch Intern Med* 1982;142:303–306.

129. Welch JP, Schweizer RT, Bartus SA. Management of antacid impactions in hemodialysis and renal transplant patients. *Am J Surg* 1980; 139:561–568.

130. Flynn CT, Chandran PK. Renal failure and angiodysplasia of the colon. *Ann Intern Med* 1985;103:154.

131. Scheff RJ, Zuckerman G, Harter H, et al. Diverticular disease in patients with chronic renal failure due to polycystic kidney disease. *Ann Intern Med* 1980;92(2 Pt 1):202–204.

132. Mimidis K, Mourvati E, Kaliontzidou M, et al. Efficacy of polyethylene glycol in constipated CAPD patients. *Perit Dial Int* 2005;25: 601–603.

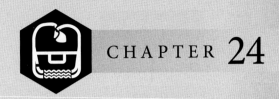

CHAPTER 24

Chronic Kidney Disease-Mineral Bone Disorder in Patients with End-Stage Kidney Disease

Wajeh Y. Qunibi

Chronic kidney disease (CKD) is a global epidemic affecting 5% to 10% of the world population (1). Historically, nephrologists have been primarily concerned about of CKD progression to end-stage kidney disease (ESKD). However, we now realize that CKD is associated with a number of other comorbidities that contribute to the high risk of death. Among these comorbidities, three interrelated disorders have recently been the subject of intense interest and debate. First, disorders of mineral metabolism including those of calcium, phosphorus, parathyroid hormone (PTH), fibroblast growth factor-23 (FGF-23), and vitamin D metabolism. These disorders are very prevalent in CKD patients (2), usually become manifest when the glomerular filtration rate (GFR) falls below 60 mL/min, and worsen with progressive loss of kidney function. Some mineral disorders, such as the increase in FGF-23 and the decrease in klotho and calcitriol, may be observed early in the course of CKD and precede the onset of clinically detectable abnormalities in serum phosphorus, calcium, and PTH. The nature and degree of the changes in mineral metabolism may be influenced by various therapeutic interventions, such as phosphate binders, vitamin D, or calcimimetic agents. Second, bone disease, previously called renal osteodystrophy, which is also common in patients with CKD and universally present in patients with ESKD. Bone disease can be a consequence and/or a cause of abnormal mineral metabolism. Third and more serious component of CKD comorbidities is the accelerated cardiovascular disease (CVD), particularly cardiovascular calcification, which is now established as the leading cause of morbidity and mortality in patients with CKD (3,4). Age, gender, and race-adjusted cardiovascular mortality rate has been found to be 30- to more than 100-fold greater in dialysis patients than that in age- and race-matched individuals from the general population (3).

Increasing evidence has shown that the aforementioned abnormalities, singly and in combination, contribute to adverse outcomes of patients with CKD. For example, disturbances in mineral metabolism are known to be associated with bone disorders, cardiovascular calcification, and arterial stiffness but more importantly associated with all-cause and cardiovascular mortality in CKD patients (2,5,6). Indeed, abnormalities in mineral metabolism are among the most important factors that contribute to the high cardiovascular mortality in these patients. Similarly, bone disease may lead to abnormalities in mineral metabolism and predispose to cardiovascular calcification and increases the risk of cardiovascular mortality. Because these disorders are deemed causally interrelated, the Work Group of the Kidney Disease: Improving Global Outcomes (KDIGO) (7) recommend using the term *chronic kidney disease-mineral and bone disorder* (CKD-MBD) to describe such a systemic disorder that occurs as a result of CKD (**FIGURE 24.1**). The new definition of CKD-MBD has now replaced the traditional term *renal osteodystrophy* since the latter does not incorporate the broad clinical spectrum described above. Indeed, the KDIGO Work Group recommends to restrict the use of the term *renal osteodystrophy* to describe the bone pathology associated with CKD, as seen on bone biopsy, using an expanded classification system based on parameters of bone turnover, mineralization, and volume (8).

BIOCHEMICAL ABNORMALITIES IN PATIENTS WITH CHRONIC KIDNEY DISEASE-MINERAL AND BONE DISORDER

The first component of CKD-MBD is abnormal mineral metabolism including that of serum calcium, phosphate, PTH, vitamin D, and FGF-23. The pathophysiology of CKD-MBD comprises a number of feedback loops involving the kidney, bone, intestine, heart, and the vasculature, with the aim of maintaining the calcium and phosphate balance, often at the expense of abnormalities in other components of the system. The kidney plays a central role in regulating mineral

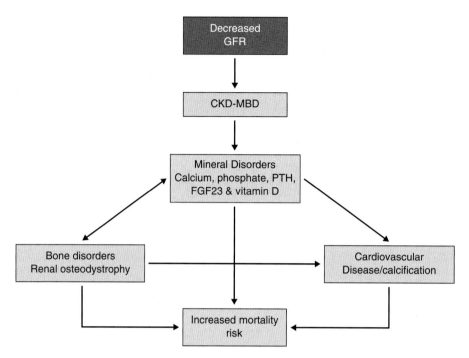

FIGURE 24.1 Chronic kidney disease-mineral bone disorder (CKD-MBD).

metabolism, and as such, disturbances in mineral metabolism may occur early in the course of CKD because of the inability of the failing kidneys to maintain the levels of serum phosphate and calcium in the normal range. Bone disease develops as early as CKD stage 2 and becomes almost universal in patients with CKD stage 5 (9,10). Vascular calcifications also develop early, and its prevalence increases as the GFR declines such that approximately 80% of incident dialysis patients have evidence of coronary artery calcification (11–13). Given that these abnormalities are interrelated, and that they worsen with progressive loss of GFR, a clear understanding of the central role of the kidney in calcium and phosphate homeostasis will certainly help in understanding the pathophysiology of CKD-MBD.

In order to document the various abnormalities relevant to CKD-MBD, laboratory evaluation of serum phosphate, calcium, PTH, alkaline phosphatase, as well as selective imaging for soft-tissue calcification should be done. In this regard, several studies have shown that serum calcium and phosphate values do not become abnormal until the GFR falls below 40 mL/min/1.73 m² and are relatively stable until GFR falls below 20 mL/min/1.73 m² (14,15). However, 12% of patients with GFR >80 mL/min/1.73 m² had a high PTH (defined as >65 pg/mL, the upper limit of normal of the assay used), and almost 60% of patients with GFR <60 mL/min/1.73 m² had elevated PTH levels (14). In incident dialysis patients, serum levels of calcium and phosphate at the start of dialysis were 9.35 mg/dL and 5.23 mg/dL, respectively, but increase over the initial 6 months of renal replacement therapy (16). High levels of serum alkaline phosphatase greater than 120 U/L were reported in almost 30% of prevalent dialysis patients and found to be associated with mortality (17). In this chapter, these abnormalities are discussed, and current therapeutic options are summarized.

The Role of Phosphorus in Chronic Kidney Disease-Mineral and Bone Disorder

Phosphate is an inorganic molecule with a central phosphorus atom and four oxygen atoms. Although the terms *phosphorus* and *phosphate* are often used interchangeably, the term *phosphate* refers to the sum of the two physiologically occurring inorganic ions, hydrogen phosphate (HPO_4^{2-}) and dihydrogen phosphate ($H_2PO_4^{-}$), but most laboratories report this measurable, inorganic component as phosphorus. Inorganic phosphorus is critically important for a number of physiologic functions including cell membrane phospholipid content and function, cell signaling, energy transfer through mitochondrial metabolism, platelet aggregation, mineral metabolism, and skeletal development. As a result, the body has developed homeostatic mechanisms to maintain serum phosphate in the range of 2.5 to 4.5 mg/dL.

Phosphorus is the sixth most abundant element in the human body. The adult human body contains between 700 and 1,000 g of phosphorus, of which 85% is in bone, 14% is in the intracellular compartment, and the remaining 1% is in the extracellular fluids (**FIGURE 24.2**) (18). Normal daily dietary intake varies from 800 to 1,500 mg. Absorption of dietary phosphate occurs along the entire length of the small intestine, but absorption occurs mainly in the small intestine (19,20). Intestinal phosphate absorption occurs through two well-defined mechanisms (21). Most of the phosphate absorption occurs by a passive, concentration-dependent diffusion process. It is still unclear whether this passive absorption takes place by a paracellular or transcellular transport pathway. Of note, this pathway for sodium-independent phosphate transport is unregulated (22). Even in patients with severe hyperphosphatemia, phosphate absorption from the diet is only slightly lower than that in normal subjects. A smaller fraction of phosphorus is absorbed through a saturable, active transport pathway through the intestinal epithelial brush border sodium phosphate cotransporter 2b (Npt2b) which is regulated by dietary phosphate and 1,25 dihydroxyvitamin D [1,25(OH)₂ D₃] (21,22). These transporters are expressed in the small intestine and are upregulated under conditions of dietary phosphate deprivation. It is this active phosphate transport mechanism that becomes important under conditions of low phosphate intake. For example, during dietary phosphate restriction, 80% to

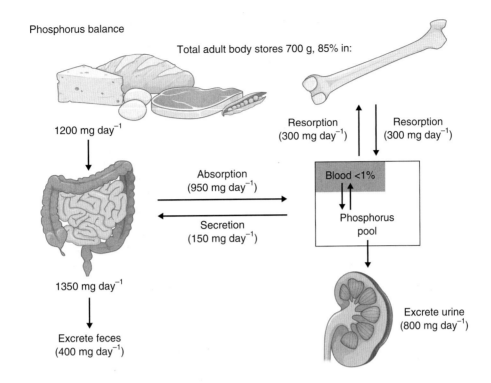

FIGURE 24.2 Normal phosphorus homeostasis. (Reprinted from Hruska KA, Mathew S, Lund R, et al. Hyperphosphatemia of chronic kidney disease. *Kidney Int* 2008;74:148–157.)

90% of phosphorus is absorbed. Approximately 150 mg of phosphorus is secreted daily into the gastrointestinal (GI) tract.

To maintain phosphate balance, the kidneys are responsible for excreting an amount of phosphorus equals to that absorbed from the intestine. The main factors that regulate proximal tubular phosphate excretion are the serum phosphate concentration itself, PTH, as well as FGF-23. These factors act on the proximal tubular epithelial brush border sodium phosphate cotransporters (Npt2a and Npt2c). Thus, serum phosphate concentration is primarily determined by the ability of the kidneys to excrete dietary phosphate. Interestingly, there is a diurnal variation in both serum phosphate levels and urinary phosphate excretion. Serum phosphate levels reach a nadir in the early hours of the morning, increasing to a plateau at 4 PM, and further increasing to a peak from 1 to 3 AM (23,24). A similar circadian pattern of serum phosphate was reported in CKD with lowest concentrations at 8 AM and highest at 4 PM and 4 AM (25). However, no diurnal variation was found in patients on dialysis when studied on a nondialysis day (26).

Phosphorus is present in most food products, particularly those with high protein content (27,28). In general, the higher the protein intake, the higher the phosphorus load, particularly in foods with a high phosphate-to-protein ratio as well as those with food additives and preservatives (27,20). In the steady state, serum phosphate concentration is primarily determined by the ability of the kidneys to excrete dietary phosphate (29). However, a tendency toward phosphate retention due to decreased phosphate filtration and excretion occurs as the GFR declines, but hyperphosphatemia is not commonly seen until the GFR drops to <25 to 40 mL/min/1.73 m². This is due to the actions of PTH, FGF-23, and klotho on the proximal tubular phosphate reabsorption. In patients with advanced kidney disease, hyperphosphatemia results

from a decrease in functioning nephrons, a decrease in the amount of filtered phosphate, and a subsequent decrease in excreted phosphate. Thus, in patients with CKD stage 4 or 5, the dietary intake of phosphate will likely exceed urinary excretion which leads to a positive phosphate balance. Hyperphosphatemia occurs almost universally in patients undergoing dialysis despite an apparent dietary phosphate restriction. Initially, excess phosphate will be buffered by bone, but once bone buffering is saturated, soft tissue phosphate deposition, usually in combination with calcium, ensues.

Consequences of Hyperphosphatemia

High serum phosphate is not a benign biochemical abnormality as it has been shown to be associated with a number of adverse clinical consequences (**FIGURE 24.3**). In this review, I will focus on the effects that hyperphosphatemia exerts in CKD-MBD. In the parathyroid gland (PTG), hyperphosphatemia directly stimulates parathyroid cells leading to increased PTH secretion. Also, it suppresses the 1-α-hydroxylase activity in the kidney which contributes to calcitriol deficiency. Finally, hyperphosphatemia stimulates the secretion of FGF-23 from osteocytes as will be discussed later.

Perhaps, the most important consequence of hyperphosphatemia is on the cardiovascular system where it stimulates osteoblastic transformation of the vascular smooth muscle cell (VSMC) in the vasculature and directly contributes to extraskeletal calcification. This was supported by finding an association of high serum phosphate with increased mortality risk was demonstrated in patients with CKD, particularly those on maintenance dialysis. Epidemiologic studies in the last two decades have consistently identified serum phosphate as an independent predictor of cardiovascular mortality in dialysis patients (2,30,31). In 25,588 patients on

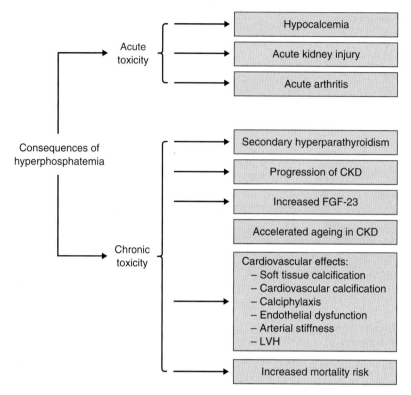

FIGURE 24.3 Clinical consequences of hyperphosphatemia.

hemodialysis from Dialysis Outcomes and Practice Patterns Study (DOPPS), serum phosphate level of 3.6 to 5 mg/dL was associated with the lowest risk of cardiovascular mortality, while serum phosphate level greater than 7 mg/dL was associated with the greatest risk of mortality (32). Serum phosphate levels are also associated with cardiovascular outcomes in non-CKD individuals. Higher serum phosphate, even within the normal range, was found to be associated with a greater risk of carotid atherosclerosis, coronary calcification, and cardiovascular mortality in patients with CKD (33,34). Moreover, in 15,732 patients from the Atherosclerosis Risk in Communities (ARIC) Study followed for 12.6 years, serum phosphate adjusted for GFR was associated with coronary events, stroke, and cardiovascular death (35). Higher serum phosphate is also associated with arterial stiffness, a marker of cardiovascular risk that may be related to vascular calcification (36). A recent meta-analysis of 47 cohort studies in 327,644 patients with CKD found an 18% increased risk of death for every 1-mg/dL increase in serum phosphate, while there was no significant association between all-cause mortality and serum PTH or calcium (6). Even in individuals with GFR >70 mL/min, higher serum phosphate levels were associated with a greater risk of cardiovascular events in a 15-year follow-up (37). However, these epidemiologic studies suffer from a number of limitations such as the level of serum phosphate above which there is increased risk of mortality in dialysis and CKD patients and the circadian variability in serum phosphate levels, which can be as high as 1 mg/dL, making interpretation of serum phosphate levels in the aforementioned studies difficult (24). Also, no clinical trial has shown that lowering serum phosphate to any specific level is associated with improvement in patients' outcomes. Nonetheless, a number of pathophysiologic mechanisms underlie the association between higher serum phosphate and CVD. These include

cardiovascular calcification, endothelial dysfunction, and left ventricular hypertrophy (LVH) (see below).

The Role of Phosphate in Secondary Hyperparathyroidism

It has been recognized for decades that persistent hyperphosphatemia plays a key role in the pathogenesis of secondary hyperparathyroidism (SHPT). The mechanism by which phosphate plays such a role are both indirect and direct. Elevations in serum PTH levels may become evident usually when the GFR falls below 60 mL/min/1.73 m² before hyperphosphatemia or hypocalcemia are detectable by routine laboratory measurements. To explain this phenomenon, it was initially proposed that reduced GFR leads to retention of phosphate, transiently increasing serum phosphate level which in turn leads to a reduction in the level of serum ionized calcium in the blood, which then triggers an increase in the secretion of PTH. The goal for the increase in PTH level is to restore the serum calcium back to normal. Thus, PTH increases renal phosphate excretion by decreasing proximal tubular resorption of phosphate, mobilizing calcium from bone, and by stimulating the production of calcitriol by the kidney, which in turn increases intestinal absorption of calcium. As a result, a new steady state is reached where serum phosphate and calcium are normal at the expense of a higher level of PTH. This "trade-off" continues as the GFR declines further until severe SHPT develops (38). In this regard, several studies have shown that high-phosphate diet results in parathyroid hyperplasia (39,40). Moreover, dietary phosphate restriction in proportion to the reduction in GFR was effective in preventing the initial rise in PTH secretion and the development of hyperparathyroidism (41,42). Beside the reciprocal decline in serum ionized calcium due to transient hyperphosphatemia, phosphate retention may also inhibit the 1-α-hydroxylase enzyme in the kidney and thus may decrease the production of calcitriol. Moreover, it is now clear that high serum phosphate may directly stimulate the production and secretion of PTH, independent of its effects on serum ionized calcium and calcitriol (42–45). This effect is posttranscriptional and suggests that the stability of PTH mRNA may be regulated by phosphate and that this effect is mediated by proteins within the PTG that bind to the 3′ untranslated region of the PTH gene transcript (46–49). Furthermore, phosphate retention seems to reduce the production of arachidonic acid by parathyroid tissue; this signaling mechanism may be due to the effect of changes in cytosolic calcium on the phospholipase A2–arachidonic acid pathway (50). On the other hand, the effect of a low-phosphate diet in preventing parathyroid growth seems to be mediated by an increase in the cell cycle regulator p21 (51). Therefore, there are both indirect and direct mechanisms by which serum phosphate initially promotes PTH secretion (**FIGURE 24.3**). However, as will be discussed later, the recent discovery of FGF-23 has changed our understanding of the pathogenesis of SHPT.

The Role of Serum Calcium in Chronic Kidney Disease-Mineral Bone Disorder

Dietary calcium is also absorbed by two different mechanisms. First is an active, transcellular pathway via the transient receptor potential vanilloid 6 (TRPV6) channel on the apical membrane of the duodenum and proximal jejunum, and second by a paracellular pathway that occurs throughout the length of the intestine (52,53). Of the average 1,000-mg calcium ingested by a normal adult per day, 800 to 900 mg of these appear in the feces. Of the ingested calcium, 400 to 500 mg may be absorbed and 300 mg is secreted via the intestinal secretions, thus leaving a net calcium absorption of only 100 to 200 mg per day (54). In healthy adults who are in calcium balance, this net amount of absorbed calcium is excreted in the urine. The adult human body contains approximately 1,200 g of calcium, 99% of which is stored in bone as calcium–phosphate complexes, primarily as hydroxyapatite. Skeletal mineralization is one of the most important functions of calcium as it provides skeletal strength and a dynamic store to maintain the intra- and extracellular calcium pools. Less than 1% of the total body calcium is present in the serum, and its concentration is tightly regulated within a narrow physiologic range that is optimal for its functions. This range is between 8.5 and 10.5 mg/dL, but serum calcium is not a good indicator of the total body calcium. Moreover, it should be realized that the ionized component, which represents 40% of the total serum calcium, is the fraction of serum calcium that is closely regulated. In persons with healthy kidneys, normal serum level of calcium is maintained through the interaction of PTH and $1,25(OH)_2 D_3$ (calcitriol), the active metabolite of vitamin D. Decreased ionized calcium level stimulates secretion of PTH which in turn acts to increase serum calcium (55).

The kidneys play a critical role in the regulation of normal serum calcium concentration which is maintained in the normal range until very late in CKD when it may decrease slightly. Although calcium balance in CKD is poorly understood, two recent balance studies in patients with CKD not yet on dialysis have shed some light on this subject. In the first study, Spiegel and Brady (56) found that subjects with late stage 3 and stage 4 CKD were in slightly negative to neutral calcium balance on a daily calcium intake of 800 mg but were in markedly positive balance on 2,000 mg calcium intake per day. In the second study, Hill et al. (57) studied eight patients with stage 3 or 4 CKD who received a controlled diet

with or without 1,500 mg/d calcium carbonate supplement during two 3-week balance periods in a randomized placebo-controlled crossover design. The study found that patients were in neutral calcium balance while consuming a diet containing 957 mg calcium per day. However, increasing calcium intake with 500 mg calcium from calcium carbonate taken three times daily with meals produced positive calcium balance. The authors attributed this positive calcium balance to increased intestinal calcium absorption and net retention in the face of the kidneys' failure to increase urine calcium excretion. As will be discussed later, the adverse consequences of positive calcium balance on mortality and cardiovascular calcification continue to be hotly debated.

Effects of Calcium on the Parathyroid Hormone

Since calcium plays a critical role in a wide range of biologic functions, its serum concentration is maintained within a very narrow range by a number of hormones including PTH, vitamin D, FGF-23, calcitonin, and estrogen. Among these, PTH is the primary regulator of serum calcium. On the other hand, ionized calcium is the primary regulator of PTH secretion (**FIGURE 24.4**). This bidirectional relationship has been described by an inverse sigmoidal curve (58). The midpoint or set point of this curve is the calcium-stimulated PTH, which is a key determinant of the serum ionized calcium concentration *in vivo*. In normal subjects, a small decrease in serum ionized calcium results in a sharp increase in serum PTH level within minutes. Also, an equally small increase in serum ionized calcium results in rapid decrease in the serum PTH level. Decreased serum ionized calcium triggers a sharp increase in PTH secretion which in turn acts to increase the plasma calcium by activating the 1-α-hydroxylase enzyme in the kidney and increasing the synthesis of calcitriol $[1,25(OH)_2 D_3]$, which in turn enhances intestinal calcium absorption. PTH also mobilizes calcium from the readily available bone calcium stores and activates bone resorption indirectly by binding to PTH receptors on osteoblasts, which in turn increase osteoclast number and activity but also directly by binding and stimulating osteoclasts which lead to bone resorption (59). Finally, PTH increases calcium reabsorption in the distal nephron by activating adenylyl cyclase, which increases cyclic AMP levels and protein kinase A. The latter then phosphorylates and activates the transient receptor potential vanilloid 5 (TRPV5) which leads to increased transcellular calcium transport. Moreover, PTH increases the expression of several calcium transport proteins such as TRPV5, calbindin-D28k, and other transport proteins in the distal nephron, which also enhance renal calcium reabsorption (60). As a result, free serum calcium concentration is maintained in the normal range.

Total serum calcium usually decreases during the course of CKD. This is due to several factors including phosphate retention, decreased calcitriol $[1,25(OH)_2 D_3]$ level, and resistance to the calcemic actions of PTH on bone. Phosphate retention may cause calcium precipitation in soft tissues, decreases calcium efflux from bone by increasing resistance of bone to PTH action, and inhibits the 1-α-hydroxylase enzyme, leading to further reduction in the already decreased level of calcitriol and decreased intestinal absorption of calcium (61). However, hypocalcemia is relatively uncommon in CKD patients and may not be critical in the development of SHPT (62). Moreover, the increase in PTH level first become evident when the GFR drops below 60 mL/min/1.73 m², despite normal serum calcium and phosphate concentrations (15). On the other hand, circulating calcitriol concentrations begin to

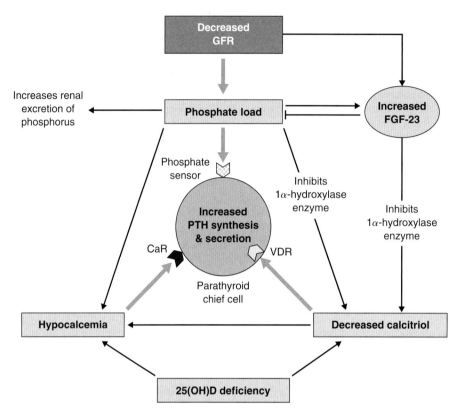

FIGURE 24.4 Pathogenesis of secondary hyperparathyroidism in chronic kidney disease (CKD).

fall much earlier when the GFR is even above 60 mL/min/1.73 m² and are markedly decreased in subjects with ESKD (63). The primary reason for the decline in calcitriol concentration is increased FGF-23 concentration, rather than the loss of functioning renal tissue (64). Hyperphosphatemia may also contribute to the decline in calcitriol synthesis late in the course of CKD by suppressing the 1-α-hydroxylase enzyme. Thus, the primary stimulus for PTH secretion in CKD is the low calcitriol level. However, when hypocalcemia is present and persistent, it directly increases PTH mRNA concentrations via posttranscriptional actions and stimulates the proliferation of parathyroid cells over days or weeks leading to the development of PTG hyperplasia (65).

Changes in serum ionized calcium are sensed by the calcium-sensing receptor (CaSR) on parathyroid cells. More than two decades ago, it was shown that the secretion of PTH is mainly regulated by the CaSR, a membrane receptor that responds to small changes in serum ionized calcium (66). This receptor, a member of the G-protein-coupled membrane receptors on the parathyroid chief cells, enables the parathyroid cells to act as calcium electrodes and thus sense and respond rapidly to very small changes in the level of extracellular calcium. Hypocalcemia stimulates PTH secretion by inactivating the CaSR while hypercalcemia activates the CaSR and inhibits the secretion of PTH. Also, CaSR inhibits PTH gene expression at the transcriptional and/or posttranscriptional level, and thus, it can inhibit parathyroid cellular proliferation. The discovery and cloning of the CaSR in the PTG has increased our awareness of the importance of calcium ion in regulating PTH secretion. Kovacs et al. (67) have shown that CaSR knockout mice develop severe parathyroid hyperplasia and hyperparathyroidism despite significantly increased 1,25(OH)₂ D₃ levels. By contrast, studies in vitamin D

receptor (VDR) knockout mice show that these VDR-deficient animals develop hyperparathyroidism that can be reversed by the administration of calcium and normalizing serum calcium levels (68). Therefore, it was not surprising that CaSR became a rational target for therapeutic intervention by agents that either mimic the actions of calcium ion on PTH secretion (type I calcimimetics) or induce changes in the structural conformation of the CaSR and thus increase the sensitivity of the receptor to extracellular ionized calcium (type II calcimimetics) and can lower PTH secretion from the PTG. In CKD, the number of CaSRs may be reduced in hypertrophied PTGs, particularly in areas of nodular hypertrophy (69–71). Decreased expression of the CaSR appears to be related to the proliferation of parathyroid tissue, and both may be related to increased serum phosphate (70,72). Such decrease in CaSR number can lead to inadequate suppression of PTH secretion by calcium, resulting in inappropriately high PTH concentrations in the setting of normal or even high calcium concentrations. However, experimental studies suggest that calcimimetic agents may even suppress PTH secretion in human parathyroid cells with pathologically reduced CaSR levels (73) and attenuate parathyroid hyperplasia (74).

Role of Vitamin D in Chronic Kidney Disease-Mineral Bone Disorder

Calcitriol [1,25(OH)₂ D₃] is a key hormone in the regulation of mineral metabolism. It acts by binding to a nuclear VDR, which is ubiquitously distributed in most tissues, leading to transcriptional regulation of target genes. Calcitriol is a critical factor in the regulation of serum calcium, phosphate, PTH, and FGF-23. It enhances the absorption of phosphate from the small intestinal cells by upregulating the apical membrane sodium-dependent phosphate cotransporter 2b (Npt2b), the rate-limiting step in intestinal phosphate absorption. It also helps to maintain the plasma calcium concentration through actions on the intestine, bone, and the kidney. In the intestine, it acts by increasing the expression of TRPV6 while in the kidney, it enhances calcium reabsorption by increasing the expression of the transporter protein TRPV5 in the distal renal tubular and connecting tubular cells (75). However, its effect on bone with regard to regulating serum calcium is not entirely clear but may involve increasing calcium release from bone by binding to osteoblasts and osteocytes and suppressing bone matrix mineralization during negative calcium balance (76).

CKD is both a state of calcitriol deficiency and resistance. Nutritional vitamin D deficiency (25-hydroxyvitamin D), which is very common in CKD, is an important contributor to calcitriol deficiency (64,77). In general, 25-hydroxyvitamin D is not biologically active, and thus, it must be metabolized in the kidney to its active form, the $1,25(OH)_2 D_3$ or calcitriol, by the enzyme 1-α-hydroxylase in the renal proximal tubular cells and several other extrarenal cells. There are a number of factors that regulate the activity of this enzyme, the most important of which is PTH, serum phosphate, serum calcium, and various hormones (**FIGURE 24.4**). More recently, FGF-23 and secreted frizzled related protein 4 (sFRP4) have been shown to inhibit the 1-α-hydroxylase enzyme activity (78,79). In fact, it has been shown that the primary cause of the low calcitriol level in patients with CKD is increased FGF-23 concentration rather than the loss of functioning renal tissue (64). Also, hyperphosphatemia may contribute to the decline in calcitriol synthesis late in the course of CKD by suppressing the 1-α-hydroxylase enzyme. Given that calcitriol exerts a potent negative feedback on the PTG, thereby decreasing PTH production and release, its low level in CKD is now believed to trigger the initial increase in PTH secretion. However, when hypocalcemia is present and persistent, it directly increases PTH mRNA concentrations via posttranscriptional actions and stimulates the proliferation of parathyroid cells over days or weeks leading to the development of PTG hyperplasia (65).

Role of Parathyroid Hormone

PTH (1-84) is a single-chain polypeptide of 84 amino acids that is cleaved from pre-pro-PTH, where it is stored along with its fragments in secretory granules in the PTG. PTH is synthesized as a pre-pro-PTH and then is proteolytically processed to pro-PTH in the endoplasmic reticulum and then to PTH in the Golgi and secretory vesicles. All intracellular pro-PTH is normally converted to PTH before secretion. Once released, PTH has a short half-life of 2 to 4 minutes as it is cleaved after secretion into N-terminal, carboxy C-terminal, and midregion fragments. These fragments are usually metabolized by the liver and in the kidney (80). In patients with reduced GFR, the renal excretion of the C-fragment is reduced, resulting in marked elevation of PTH levels. PTH 1-84 is the biologically active hormone that exerts its effects through the interaction of its first 34 amino acids with the type 1 parathyroid hormone receptor (PTHR1). Some of PTH fragments lacking residues at the extreme N-terminus such as PTH (7-84) is believed to interact with its own distinct receptors and may have antagonistic effects to the calcemic action of PTH (1-84) and PTH (1-34) (81,82).

The serum concentrations of PTH depend on its release from stores in secretory granules within the PTG and also by synthesis of new PTH. The primary stimulus for PTH secretion is reduction in serum ionized calcium concentration. Hypocalcemia, acting through the CaSR, induces a rapid release of stored PTH in secretory

granules and retards its degradation within the PTG. Moreover, it increases division of the parathyroid cells in the PTG likely through the action of the CaSR (55). In addition to calcium, high serum phosphate levels also increase PTH secretion independently of changes in serum calcium or serum levels $1,25(OH)_2 D_3$. However, it is not clear how the parathyroid cell senses changes in the serum phosphate level. Also, vitamin D alters the transcription of PTH and may indirectly inhibit its release by increasing the expression of CaSR in the PTG (**FIGURE 24.4**). Low vitamin D level removes the inhibitory effect of vitamin D on transcription and thus stimulates PTH synthesis and secretion. On the other hand, hypercalcemia, administration of the active vitamin D analogs, as well as high FGF-23 level inhibit PTH synthesis or release (55,83,84).

PTH is considered a systemic toxin that has been implicated in the pathogenesis of various uremic complications including CKD-MBD (85). It acts by binding to its receptor, the PTHR1, which is widely expressed in many tissues including bone, kidney, and the vasculature. As discussed above, PTH increases extracellular fluid calcium by mobilizing calcium from its readily available stores in bone and also by increasing osteoclastic bone resorption. Moreover, it increases calcium reabsorption in the distal nephron by upregulating the TRPV5 and TRPV6, calbindin-D28K, and other transport proteins in the distal nephron (60). Another important function of PTH is its phosphaturic effect which is mediated by rapid internalization and subsequent degradation of Npt2a and Npt2c proteins in the apical membrane of the proximal tubule. PTH also stimulates the 1-α-hydroxylase enzyme in the kidney which in turn converts 25OHD into its active form, the $1,25(OH)_2 D_3$. Lastly, PTH enhances the synthesis and secretion of FGF-23 from bone cells. Studies have shown that continuous infusion of (1-34) PTH for 24 to 46 hours increased serum FGF-23 levels in healthy volunteers and in patients with ESKD (86,87). By contrast, parathyroidectomy decreased serum FGF-23 levels (88,89). However, since PTH stimulates the production of $1,25(OH)_2 D_3$, it is difficult to determine whether its effect on FGF-23 is the result of a direct stimulatory effect on osteocytes or to an indirect effect of elevated $1,25(OH)_2 D_3$ levels (90). Finally, because of its effect on bone, both high and low PTH levels may increase the risk of vascular calcification (91). The systemic toxic effects of PTH are many and include cardiomyopathy, hyperlipidemia, carbohydrate intolerance, bone marrow fibrosis, and anemia resistant to erythropoietin, pruritus, peripheral neuropathy, and encephalopathy (85,92,93). Moreover, high PTH serum levels have been shown to be associated with higher mortality rates in dialysis patients (2,31,94). In a recent study from DOPPS, the mortality risk in dialysis patients was higher for PTH level of 301 to 450 pg/mL and >600 pg/mL compared with the group with PTH of 150 to 300 pg/mL. Also, cardiovascular mortality and the risk of hospitalization were higher for PTH >600 pg/mL. On the other hand, PTH level <50 pg/mL was also associated with mortality, particularly among patients with diabetes and those with lower body mass index (95).

Accurate measurement of the serum PTH concentration is essential for the proper evaluation and management of patients with CKD-MBD. Measurements and interpretation of PTH values in patients with CKD, particularly those on chronic dialysis, remain challenging with wide variations among various assays in current use (96). What constitutes an appropriate assay for PTH measurement remains unclear. PTH level was initially measured by radioimmunoassay (RIA) (first-generation assays) using various polyclonal antibodies directed against epitopes that are located within the mid- or C-terminal portion of the PTH molecule. However, these assays proved to be inaccurate and have been replaced by two-site immunometric assay (IMAs) (second- and third-generation assays). The second-generation assays, so-called "intact PTH" assays, not only measure the full-length PTH molecule (1-84) but also detect the PTH (7-84) fragment (97,98). On the other hand, the more recent third-generation assay measures only PTH (1-84) and is referred to as the whole, bioactive or biointact PTH assay. However, the role of this assay in the diagnosis of renal osteodystrophy remains to be established.

The difficulty in interpreting PTH values led some authors to suggest that measurements of PTH levels in CKD and dialysis patients are not even necessary because there is inadequate evidence to link PTH to skeletal and cardiovascular end points in CKD (80). However, others believe that there is sufficient evidence that links PTH with adverse outcomes, especially when levels are toward the extremes of the KDIGO recommendations, and thus, PTH measurements are helpful in evaluating CKD-MBD in such patients (99). In our opinion, a single value of PTH measured at a single time point is unlikely to precisely reflect the underlying bone disease in patients with CKD, but the trend of serial measurements of PTH, using the same PTH assay, would be more informative. Another important but difficult issue is what represents an appropriate target range for PTH level. The 2009 KDIGO clinical practice guidelines suggest a broad range of PTH values, ranging from 2 to 9 times the upper limit of normal (7). Although very high or very low PTH values can predict with some certainty the nature of the underlying bone disease, we believe that the higher end of the KDIGO recommended value for PTH is bound to increase the prevalence of osteitis fibrosa (100). Indeed, a recent study from DOPPS showed that SHPT is on the rise since the KDIGO guidelines were released (95). Moreover, data from the Control of Renal Osteodystrophy in South America study and the Analyzing Data, Recognizing Excellence, and Optimizing Outcomes study from Europe showed that PTH values as recommended by the 2003 KDOQI guidelines may be associated with the best clinical outcomes (101,102). Thus, as we previously suggested, a PTH level in the 100 to 400 range may minimize both low turnover bone disease and osteitis fibrosa (100). This range is also supported by recent data from the Japanese Society for Dialysis Therapy (JSDT) which showed that patients with PTH levels outside their recommend target range of intact PTH between 60 and 240 pg/mL have increased mortality risk (100,103). The adverse consequences of high PTH levels was recently reported from the Cardiovascular Health Study which showed that serum PTH levels >65 pg/mL were associated with greater N-terminal pro-B-type natriuretic peptide, cardiac troponin T, and left ventricular mass, particularly in patients with CKD (104).

Role of Fibroblast Growth Factor-23 in Chronic Kidney Disease-Mineral Bone Disorder

FGF-23 is a circulating peptide that plays a key role in the control of serum phosphate concentrations (105,106). FGF-23 is produced by bone osteocytes and osteoblasts in response to calcitriol, increased dietary phosphate load, PTH, and calcium (106,107). The primary function of FGF-23 is to maintain normal serum phosphate concentration by reducing renal phosphate reabsorption and by reducing intestinal phosphate absorption through decreased calcitriol production (**FIGURE 24.4**). In the renal proximal tubular cells, FGF-23 binds to the fibroblast growth factor receptor (FGFR) and its coreceptor, klotho, causing inhibition of the expression of the Npt2a

and possibly Npt2c (108). As discussed earlier, FGF-23 also inhibits expression of 1-α-hydroxylase enzyme, leading to decreased calcitriol synthesis by the kidney (109).

FGF-23 and PTH mutually regulate each other in a negative feedback loop (110). Studies have shown that PTH stimulates synthesis and secretion of FGF-23 by activation of PTH/PTHrP receptor on osteocytes and osteoblasts (88,90,111). On the other hand, other studies showed that FGF-23 suppresses PTH synthesis (112,113). However, among CKD patients, the presence of high PTH concentrations, despite high FGF-23 concentrations, suggests that the PTG is relatively resistant to the elevated concentrations of FGF-23 in uremia. This may be related to the markedly decreased expression of FGFR 1 and klotho protein in the hyperplastic PTG (114,115). Klotho is a transmembrane protein that is produced by osteocytes and is essential for FGF-23 receptor activation (116). Klotho is expressed in the kidney and the PTGs, making these organs the target for FGF-23. Unlike FGFRs which are quite ubiquitously distributed, klotho expression is restricted, and thus, its presence may control whether a cell is an FGF-23 target. Its expression in the kidney and PTGs decreases during CKD progression in mice and humans (113,114,117). Klotho itself is a target gene of calcitriol (118,119). Moreover, klotho extracellular domain does not directly bind to FGF-23 but enhances FGF-23 binding to its receptor complex with a much higher affinity than to the FGFR alone (120). Decreases in klotho induce resistance to FGF-23 in these target organs, which further increases blood FGF-23 levels (113,114,117). It has been shown that a 50% decrease in klotho expression results in approximately 300% increase in blood FGF-23 levels in mice (121).

Patients with CKD have increased FGF-23 concentrations due to increased secretion by osteocytes and decreased catabolism by the diseased kidney (122,123). Klotho expression declines early in the course of CKD and then progressively with decreasing GFR (124). The reduction in klotho temporally coincides with the rise in FGF-23, suggesting that this decline may be partially responsible for the progressive rise in FGF-23 concentration. Moreover, the decrease in klotho expression on hyperplastic PTGs may contribute to the resistance and impaired parathyroid suppression by FGF-23 (114). On the other hand, FGF-23 may be a regulator of klotho expression in the kidney (121). Klotho deficiency is bound to decrease its regulation of FGF-23 production and thus allows hyperphosphatemia to become the principal regulator of FGF-23 secretion in CKD. Moreover, the decrease in membrane-bound klotho expression curbs FGF-23 actions on FGFR/klotho complexes leading to loss of negative feedback to FGF-23 secretion and continued production of FGF-23 by the osteocyte. Interestingly, in the absence of klotho expression as in the heart, the very high levels of FGF-23 in advanced stages of CKD enable FGF receptor activation in the heart, independent of klotho, leading to direct pathologic effects such as left ventricular hypertrophy (125).

FGF-23 level increases prior to changes in calcium, phosphorus, calcitriol, or PTH levels and therefore is now recognized as one of the earliest detectable biomarkers of the CKD-MBD (**FIGURE 24.5**) (126). Patients with advanced CKD have increased FGF-23 and PTH levels but decreased calcitriol levels. This constellation of compensatory changes initially result in normal serum calcium and phosphate levels, but eventually, such mechanisms become overwhelmed in patients with ESKD resulting in the full expression of the syndrome of CKD-MBD. One component of CKD-MBD that FGF-23 and/or klotho may play a role is vascular calcification. Some studies reported an independent

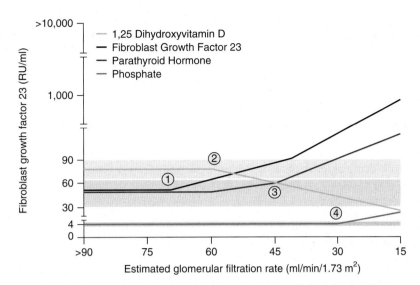

FIGURE 24.5 Biochemical phenotype of disordered mineral metabolism in CKD. The graph summarizes evolution of abnormal mineral metabolism along the spectrum of CKD. Depicted values are based on published literature. (Reproduced with permission from Isakova T, Ix JH, Sprague SM, et al. Rationale and approaches to phosphate and fibroblast growth factor 23 reduction in CKD. *J Am Soc Nephrol* 2015;26:2328–2339.). The x-axis represents glomerular filtration. The y-axis represents circulating levels of individual analytes with temporal changes in and normal ranges of fibroblast growth factor-23 (FGF-23), 1,25 dihydroxyvitamin D (1,25D), parathyroid hormone (PTH), and phosphate. Elevated FGF-23 is the earliest alteration in mineral metabolism in CKD (**1**). Elevations in FGF-23 levels cause the early decline in 1,25D levels (**2**) that leads to secondary hyperparathyroidism (**3**). All of these changes occur prior to elevations in serum phosphate levels (**4**).

association between circulating FGF-23 level with the progression of coronary calcifications (127,128), but more recent data indicate that FGF-23 is not involved in vascular calcification (129), while klotho deficiency is a recognized factor in that process (129). However, robust data are currently available to implicate the high levels of FGF-23 in dialysis and CKD patients with left ventricular mass, heart failure, and mortality but not with ischemic heart disease (125,130–132).

 CARDIOVASCULAR CALCIFICATION

The second important component of CKD-MBD is vascular calcification. This type of calcification results from abnormal deposition of calcium phosphate salts into the vascular wall as well as in other cardiac structures including the aorta, coronary arteries, cardiac valves, as well as peripheral vessels. Vessels from healthy control subjects do not calcify even after long-term exposure to supraphysiologic levels of phosphate and/or calcium *in vitro*, whereas vessels from CKD and dialysis patients calcify (133). Calcification starts as early as CKD stage 2, as shown in an animal model of CKD equivalent to human CKD stage 2 (134) but becomes accelerated with progressive loss of GFR particularly in patients with ESKD who are receiving dialysis. Several studies have documented that patients with ESKD on dialysis have a higher prevalence and severity of cardiovascular calcification than age- and gender-matched healthy subjects. Vascular calcification in patients with CKD can be either atherosclerotic affecting the intima, or medial calcification with calcium phosphate deposition in the media of the vessel wall. It has been argued that medial calcification is a manifestation of accelerated atherosclerosis in patients with CKD (135), but others

believe that atherosclerotic and medial calcification are two distinct entities, with the latter developing more commonly in patients with CKD particularly those with diabetes mellitus (136). Clearly, both forms of calcification can occur concomitantly in patients with CKD.

The cause of accelerated calcification in patients with ESKD is multifactorial and include both the traditional CVD risk factors and uremia-related risk factors (12,137). Vascular calcification in patients with CKD was initially thought to be a passive, physicochemical process in which serum phosphate and calcium are deposited in the arterial wall. However, we now know that vascular calcification is more complex and involves an active, cell-mediated, and highly regulated process similar to bone formation with VSMC playing a critical role. Just as in bone formation, vascular calcification results from either an imbalance between factors that promote calcification and those regulatory molecules that act to inhibit calcification (12,137,138). Incubation of human aortic smooth muscle (SM) cells in high phosphate medium similar to those regularly seen in dialysis patients directly enhanced extracellular calcification in these cells via a sodium-dependent phosphate cotransporter-sensitive mechanism (139). In this scenario, serum phosphate induces transformation of VSMC to an osteoblast-like cell by simultaneously downregulating the production of SM genes such as α-actin and SM22 and upregulating Runx2 (Cbfa1), osterix, osteopontin, osteocalcin, and alkaline phosphatase. Similarly, high calcium in the medium also induces transformation of VSMC to an osteoblast-like cell (133). It is likely that calcium and phosphate have synergistic procalcification effects in mediating VSMC cell apoptosis, osteochondrocytic differentiation, and matrix vesicle release (140). However, recent *in vitro* studies have found calcium to be a stronger procalcification factor than phosphate. Experimental studies utilizing human VSMC explant cultures or aortic ring cultures clearly document a role for calcium in the pathogenesis of vascular calcification in CKD and dialysis patients. In one study, when arterial rings obtained during abdominal surgery from children with normal renal function, those with impaired renal function, and from those on dialysis were exposed to high phosphate and calcium media, calcium-induced calcification more potently than phosphate, but only in rings from patients with CKD or those on dialysis (133). This suggests that VSMCs from healthy vessels have effective inhibitory mechanisms that prevent calcification, while those with CKD, particularly dialysis patients, become susceptible to calcification.

The now phenotypically transformed VSMCs lose their contractile function and behave like bone-forming cells that lay down a collagen-1 rich extracellular matrix and pinch-off matrix vesicles that are rich in calcium and phosphate. These vesicles are capable of initiating mineralization of the vascular wall just as they do so in bone (138). The key transcription factor here is Runx2 without which no such transformation of VSMCs or mineralization of the vessel wall can occur. Increased calcium levels promote calcification further by inducing apoptosis of VSMCs (133,141,142). Both matrix vesicles and apoptotic bodies serve as nucleation sites for hydroxyapatite, particularly in the presence of low calcification inhibitors such as matrix-Gla protein (MGP) and fetuin-A. Thus, unlike vessels from healthy individuals, vessels from predialysis and, to a much greater extent, dialysis patients have been primed to calcify (133). Susceptibility to calcification in CKD may be related to a decrease in matrix vesicles calcification inhibitors such as fetuin-A and MGP and to degradation of the elastin by matrix metalloproteases (MMP), such as MMP-2 and MMP-9, which are upregulated in the arterial wall in CKD (138). The degradation of elastin leads to overexpression of transforming growth factor (TGF)-β, which is thought to be involved in osteoblast differentiation and in enhancing VSMC calcification and arterial stiffness (138). From the above, it can be deduced that vascular calcification is the result of interaction between factors that promote calcification and those that normally inhibit calcification in the microenvironment of the vessel wall and not simply by spontaneous deposition of calcium phosphate.

One of the factors that was suspected of enhancing vascular calcification in dialysis and CKD patients is the calcium load provided from use of calcium-based phosphate binders (CBPBs). While a number of clinical trials (143–145), epidemiologic studies (146), and meta-analysis (147) have shown increased risk of all-cause mortality or progression of cardiovascular calcification in CKD patients treated with CBPB, other clinical trials (148,149), epidemiologic studies (150), and meta-analysis (151) did not show a difference between calcium-based and non–calcium-based phosphate binders. In fact, a recent randomized placebo-controlled pilot clinical trial by Block et al. (152) showed that therapy with both non–calcium- and calcium-based phosphate binders resulted in progression of vascular calcification, albeit to a smaller degree in noncalcium phosphate binders. Thus, the effects of calcium load from use of CBPB on progression of cardiovascular calcification, while plausible, remain controversial (153). An important issue that needs to be investigated is whether slowing vascular calcification by any means, including phosphate binders, would translate into improvements in clinical outcomes. Two epidemiologic studies have in fact reported that use of any type of phosphate binder, possibly with

the exception of aluminum-based binders, is independently associated with improved survival in dialysis patients compared with no use of binder at all (154,155). A third study in an incident United States Renal Data System (USRDS) cohort that started dialysis in 1996 to 1997, when only CBPBs were used in the United States, found no association between the use of these agents and mortality (156). As a result, the KDIGO Work Group stated that "there were inconclusive data to indicate that any one binder has beneficial effects on mortality or other patient-centered outcomes when compared with any other binder" (7). However, 16 of 17 members of the KDIGO Work Group felt that the weight of evidence is in favor of the non-CBPBs. In patients with CKD stages 3 to 5D, the Work Group recommend restricting the dose of CBPBs and/or the dose of calcitriol or vitamin D analog in the presence of persistent or recurrent hypercalcemia, arterial calcification, or adynamic bone disease (ABD).

The clinical consequences of vascular calcification in patients with CKD are serious. Cardiovascular calcification increases the risk of cardiovascular events including myocardial infarction, fatal arrhythmia, congestive heart failure, and valvular heart disease (4,157). Hyperphosphatemia may be associated with increased cardiac stroke index, increased systolic and decreased diastolic blood pressure, increased pulse pressure, and increased pulse wave velocity (4,157). Moreover, these patients had higher common carotid artery diameter and lower wall-to-lumen ratios. The authors speculated that these changes were due to medial calcification of the arterial wall, which leads to arterial stiffness. These hemodynamic disturbances may result in LVH and compromise coronary artery blood flow during diastole. It is noteworthy that in the Framingham Heart Study, abdominal aortic calcification identified by plain radiographs was independently predictive of subsequent vascular morbidity and mortality (158).

 RENAL OSTEODYSTROPHY

The third component of CKD-MBD is renal bone disease. Abnormal bone lesions are common in patients with CKD and usually start early when most biochemical measures of mineral metabolism are still normal. Most patients with early stages of CKD (stages 1 to 3) have age-related osteoporosis, while those with the more advanced stages of CKD (stages 3 to 5D), particularly those who have abnormalities of mineral metabolism, usually have renal osteodystrophy (159). Abnormal bone quality and quantity can lead to increased bone fragility, resulting in fracture. Both osteoporosis and renal osteodystrophy may coexist and can lead to increased bone fragility and fractures in all stages of CKD.

In patients with CKD, progressive bone lesions may result in bone pain, fractures, and deformities in growing children, reduced growth velocity, and abnormal height, particularly in those on maintenance dialysis. The prevalence of fractures among the dialysis population is between 10% and 40% (7). Such complication is often associated with serious consequences. As an example, hip fractures may be associated with bleeding, infection, and increased risk of mortality. Osteoporosis is traditionally diagnosed by finding low bone mineral density (BMD). By contrast, CKD-MBD can lead to an abnormal bone quality even in the setting of a normal or high bone mineral content in patients with CKD stages 3 to 5D. Thus, measurement of BMD by dual-energy x-ray absorptiometry (DXA) scan may not distinguish between the various types of renal osteodystrophy as seen with bone histology (7). A more accurate but also more expensive is the use of quantitative computed tomography (QCT), which was recently shown to prospectively identify more bone loss at the hip than DXA (160). However, bone biopsy is the gold standard as it provides information on the three variables suggested by KDIGO: bone turnover, mineralization, and volume (TMV). Turnover refers to a spectrum of bone formation rates from abnormally low to very high. Mineralization reflects the amount of unmineralized osteoid. Bone volume, which is the end result of changes in bone formation and resorption rates, contributes to bone fragility. In a recent review of studies dating from 1969 to 2007, the KDIGO group reported that bone volume/trabecular volume (BV/TV) is generally lower in dialysis patients compared with that in nondialysis CKD patients across all renal osteodystrophy categories (7).

Renal osteodystrophy encompasses four different types of bone lesions including osteitis fibrosa cystica, ABD, osteomalacia, and mixed lesions (TABLE 24.1). The prevalence of these types of bone diseases, as determined by bone biopsy carried out in adult dialysis patients between 1983 and 2006, showed that osteitis fibrosa was present in 34% of patients, ABD in 19%, osteomalacia in 10%, and mixed lesions in 32%. Only 2% of bone biopsies in dialysis patients were reported as normal (7). However, the prevalence of these bone lesions have changed over the last two to three decades, largely due to changes in patients' demographics and in therapeutic strategies. In the early dialysis era, aluminum-based phosphate binders were the predominant phosphate binders, vitamin D therapy was not routinely used, dialysis patients were younger, diabetes was not as prevalent, and multiple renal transplantations were not frequently done. Also, clinical studies of the relationship between plasma PTH levels and bone histology among dialysis patients during the 1980s and early 1990s reflected the impact of the changes in therapeutic strategies and the demographics of the dialysis population during that period. Of note, nearly all studies during this period used a first-generation RIA for PTH from Nichols Institute Diagnostics. In the present era, more than half of patients receiving dialysis are 65 years of age or older, and nearly 50% of them have diabetes, and one-third of diabetic patients are African Americans. Moreover, aluminum-based phosphate binders were replaced by CBPB and more recently with non–calcium-containing binders such as sevelamer hydrochloride and lanthanum carbonate. Also, large intermittent intravenous doses of vitamin D analogs as well as cinacalcet are being used to treat the bone lesion associated with SHPT. Consequently, aluminum-induced bone disease has decreased from 40% of biopsies carried out before 1995 to 20% in patients biopsied after 1995 (7).

| TABLE 24.1 | **Histopathologic Classification of Renal Bone Disease "Renal Osteodystrophy"** |

- High turnover bone disease
  - Mild secondary hyperparathyroidism
  - Osteitis fibrosa
  - Mixed bone lesions
- Low turnover bone disease
  - Aluminum-induced osteomalacia
  - Osteomalacia
  - Adynamic bone disease
- Others
  - Dialysis-related amyloidosis

Unfortunately, few studies have assessed the impact of these demographic and therapeutic changes on bone histology among patients with CKD. However, in a seminal paper, Sherrard et al. (161) reported the results of their bone biopsy study in 259 patients from their dialysis program. Their results showed an increased incidence of the so-called aplastic bone lesion, particularly in patients treated with peritoneal dialysis. Sixty-six percent of these patients had low turnover bone lesions, whereas 62% of those treated with hemodialysis had the high turnover bone lesion of SHPT. Aluminum-associated osteomalacia was noted less frequently than before, largely due to the substantial decline in the use of aluminum-based phosphate binders. This spectrum of bone lesions is considerably different from that previously reported. Indeed, in hemodialysis patients, the frequency of osteitis fibrosa and ABD are currently similar, but ABD is the predominant lesion in peritoneal dialysis patients. Yet, the increasing use of non–calcium-containing phosphate binders and cinacalcet may result in a change in the histologic bone lesions in the future. Moreover, the higher target for PTH level recommended by the KDIGO clinical practice guidelines may also result in resurgence of predominant lesions of osteitis fibrosa (7).

PATHOPHYSIOLOGY OF RENAL BONE DISEASE

High Bone Turnover Bone Disease

Osteitis Fibrosa and Secondary Hyperparathyroidism

Bone is the main reservoir for both calcium and phosphate, and its turnover is regulated by PTH and vitamin D. Thus, disturbances in these mineral metabolism are expected to result in bone disease. Normal bone histology is illustrated in FIGURE 24.6A. The classical histopathologic form of renal bone disease is osteitis fibrosa, an entity caused mainly by SHPT (TABLE 24.1 and FIGURE 24.6B). The disease begins quite early in the course of CKD when the GFR declines to less than 60 mL/min/1.73 m^2, in response to a series of abnormalities that initiate and maintain increased PTH secretion (162,163). The hallmark of osteitis fibrosa is marrow fibrosis and increased bone remodeling (164). There is increased bone formation rate, which is characterized by increased amount of osteoid, and increase in the number of osteoblasts. Concomitantly, there is increased resorption of bone caused by increased number and activity of osteoclasts. Many of the histologic features occur in response to the high PTH level with contributions from local cytokines and low level of calcitriol. The degree to which these features develop is generally proportional to the PTH level and the duration of exposure to such levels. In the aforementioned study, Sherrard et al. (161) noted that 45 of their 259 unselected patients had mild and 57 had severe hyperparathyroidism. Those with more severe disease had a longer duration of renal failure. As discussed above, a number of factors play a role in triggering increased synthesis and secretion of PTH by the PTGs in patients with CKD. These include decreased serum ionized calcium, phosphate retention, decreased plasma levels of 1,25(OH)$_2$D$_3$ (calcitriol), the active form of vitamin D, and skeletal resistance to the calcemic actions of PTH.

The Role of Ionized Calcium in Secondary Hyperparathyroidism

PTH level undergoes diurnal variations, primarily due to changes in serum ionized calcium which modulate the minute-to-minute secretion of PTH. Consequently, ionized calcium concentration remains maintained in the normal range in CKD, largely due to

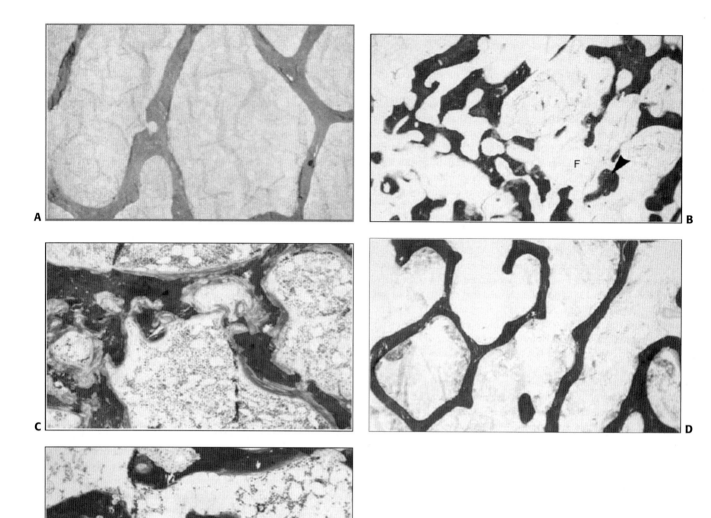

FIGURE 24.6 A: Normal bone. **B:** Osteitis fibrosa where there is prominent peritrabecular fibrosis (*F*) which is the hallmark of the disease. Increased rates of bone remodeling are demonstrated by numerous resorption lacunae, resulting in scalloped trabeculae, loss of trabecular connections, and the appearance of bone islands. At a higher magnification, more osteoblasts and osteoclasts can be seen. **C:** Osteomalacia. **D:** Adynamic bone disease. **E:** Mixed bone lesion. (Reproduced with permission from Hruska K, Teitelbaum S. Renal osteodystrophy. *N Engl J Med* 1995;333:166–174.)

mobilization of calcium from bone by PTH (165). Total serum calcium usually decreases during the course of CKD. This is due to several factors including phosphate retention, decreased $1,25(OH)_2$ D_3 level, and resistance to the calcemic actions of PTH on bone. Hypocalcemia is relatively uncommon in CKD patients and may not be critical in the development of SHPT (62). However, when present and persistent, it enhances the pre-pro-PTH gene transcription and ultimately promotes the development of PTG hyperplasia. Phosphate retention may cause calcium precipitation in soft tissues, decreases calcium efflux from bone by increasing resistance of bone to PTH action, and inhibits the 1-α-hydroxylase enzyme, leading to further reduction in the already decreased level of calcitriol and decreased intestinal absorption of calcium (61).

More than two decades ago, it was shown that the secretion of PTH is mainly regulated by CaSR, a membrane receptor that responds to small variations in serum ionized calcium (66). The CaSR

is a member of the G-protein-coupled membrane receptors that is highly expressed in multiple tissues including the surface of the chief cells of the PTG, kidneys, bone marrow, osteoclasts, osteoblasts, and others (166). It enables the parathyroid cells to sense very small changes in the level of extracellular ionized calcium and rapidly responds to bring about the required changes in PTH secretion. In turn, by increasing bone resorption, stimulating the formation of the active vitamin D (calcitriol) in the kidney and by reducing renal calcium excretion, PTH acts to raise the serum ionized calcium concentration toward normal. In the kidney, CaSR, which is expressed on the basolateral membrane on the cells of the thick ascending limb of the loop of Henle, is a major regulator of urinary calcium excretion (167,168). In addition to calcium, the CaSR can also be activated by magnesium and certain amino acids (169). In summary, CaSR orchestrates changes in the PTG and kidney functions in order to normalize serum calcium concentration.

Consequently, CaSR became a target for therapeutic intervention for SHPT and osteitis fibrosa. Calcimimetic agents are now routinely used in clinical practice for treatment of SHPT in patients with ESKD (170).

The Role of Phosphate Retention in and Secondary Hyperparathyroidism

As explained earlier, hyperphosphatemia does not become evident until stage 4 CKD, a tendency toward phosphate retention due to decreased phosphate filtration and excretion occurs as the GFR declines (15,171). Elevations in serum PTH levels may become evident when the GFR falls below 60 mL/min/1.73 m^2 before hyperphosphatemia and hypocalcemia are detectable by routine laboratory measurements. Initially, the "trade-off" hypothesis was proposed to explain this phenomenon, where progressive decline in renal function leads to a new steady state where serum phosphate and calcium are normal at the expense of a higher level of PTH. This "trade-off" continues as the GFR declines further until severe SHPT develops. In this regard, several studies have shown that high phosphate diet results in parathyroid hyperplasia (39,40). Moreover, dietary phosphate restriction in proportion to the reduction in GFR was effective in preventing the initial rise in PTH secretion and the development of hyperparathyroidism (41,42). The mechanism by which phosphate retention plays a role in the pathogenesis of SHPT includes both indirect and direct actions. Beside the reciprocal decline in serum ionized calcium due to transient hyperphosphatemia, phosphate retention may also inhibit the 1-α-hydroxylase enzyme in the kidney and thus may decrease the production of calcitriol. Moreover, it is now clear that phosphorus may directly inhibit the production and secretion of PTH, independent of its effects on serum ionized calcium and calcitriol (43–45). This effect is posttranscriptional and suggests that the stability of PTH mRNA may be regulated by phosphorus and that this effect is mediated by proteins within the PTG that bind to the 3′ untranslated region of the PTH gene transcript (46,47,49). Furthermore, phosphate retention seems to reduce the production of arachidonic acid by parathyroid tissue; this signaling mechanism may be due to the effect of changes in cytosolic calcium on the phospholipase A2–arachidonic acid pathway (50). On the other hand, the effect of a low-phosphorus diet to prevent parathyroid growth seems to be mediated by an increase in the cell cycle regulator p21 (51).

The Role of Calcitriol

Decreased production of calcitriol in CKD patients removes the inhibitory action of calcitriol on the PTG and leads to increased production of PTH. In turn, high PTH level enhances the activity of 1-α-hydroxylase enzyme in the kidney and tends to increase the plasma level of calcitriol back to the normal range. This action is counter balanced by several other factors: First and most important is the increased level of the phosphaturic hormone FGF-23 in patients with CKD which decreases the production of calcitriol by suppressing the activity of 1-α-hydroxylase enzyme (64,172). Second, phosphate retention resulting from decreased renal function contribute to suppression of 1-α-hydroxylase enzyme and decreased calcitriol production. Third, decreased level of 25(OH) D, the precursor for calcitriol is very common in CKD patients (64,173). Finally, decreased delivery of 25(OH)D that is bound to the vitamin D–binding protein into the cell. This compound is filtered through the glomerulus and is reabsorbed in the proximal tubules by the endocytic receptor megalin. Endocytosis is required

to preserve 25(OH)D and to deliver it into the cell for generation of 1,25(OH)$_2$ D$_3$. In CKD, there is decreased delivery of 25OHD to the 1-α-hydroxylase enzyme, particularly in presence of proteinuria due to loss of vitamin D–binding protein in the urine (174). These events lead to decreased intestinal absorption of calcium and hypocalcemia, which in turn stimulates PTH secretion. However, *in vitro* and *in vivo* studies have shown that calcitriol directly inhibits PTH synthesis by acting through the VDR in parathyroid cell nuclei leading to decreased pre-pro-PTH messenger RNA in a dose-dependent manner (175,176). In contrast, calcitriol deficiency may lead to increased PTH production, even in the absence of overt hypocalcemia, by removing its direct suppressive action on PTH secretion. A decrease in calcitriol concentrations also lowers the number of VDRs in the parathyroid cells in experimental animals and in uremic patients (177–180). Moreover, the role of uremic toxins in inhibiting calcitriol receptor binding to vitamin D response elements may contribute to the calcitriol resistance of renal failure (181,182).

The Role of Parathyroid Gland Structure and Function

One of the earliest changes in the PTG during the course of CKD is parathyroid hyperplasia. This structural change develops within few days following experimental CKD and increases in parallel with the progression of renal disease (183). Factors that are involved in triggering hyperplasia are still unclear but include persistent hypocalcemia, calcitriol deficiency, and hyperphosphatemia (184,185). Hypocalcemia is a potent stimulus for PTG growth, and its effect is mediated by the CaSR (184). Moreover, studies have suggested that the set point for calcium-regulated PTH secretion is abnormal in the hyperplastic PTG (186). This is likely due to decreased expression of the CaSR in the hyperplastic PTG of CKD patients (69,187). The CaSRs themselves may contribute to PTG hyperplasia because the use of calcimimetic agents have been shown to prevent PTG hyperplasia (74,170,188).

Decreased calcitriol levels may also contribute to parathyroid hyperplasia. Pertinent to this mechanism is that VDR expression is downregulated in hyperplastic PTG (178,180) and administration of calcitriol is associated with upregulation of expression of VDRs as well as the CaSRs (176,189). The severity of parathyroid hyperplasia in patients with CKD correlates directly with the reduction of PTG VDR (180). Prolonged PTG stimulation initially leads to diffuse polyclonal hyperplasia, but in patients in whom hyperplasia was allowed to continue, monoclonal expansion of the parathyroid cells develops, leading to the formation of nodules within the PTG (190–192). Studies in genetically modified mice indicate that signal transduction via the CaSR is a key determinant of parathyroid cell proliferation and PTG hyperplasia (193). It seems that parathyroid cell hyperplasia precedes the downregulation of CaSR expression in a uremic rat model (194). When nodular hyperplasia is present, there is decreased expression of both VDRs and CaSRs. This in turn leads to increased set point for the concentration of calcium that is needed to decrease PTH secretion and the response of the PTG to therapeutic maneuvers becomes more difficult leading to refractory SHPT.

The Role of Skeletal Resistance to the Actions of Parathyroid Hormone

Patients with CKD are known to have reduced calcemic response to PTH and thus require a higher PTH level to maintain normal bone turnover (195,196). Thus, in order to keep a normal bone turnover in patients with CKD, the level of PTH must be 2 to 3 times its normal level. On the other hand, excessive suppression of PTH secretion will lower the bone turnover (197). This skeletal resistance to the calcemic action of PTH was demonstrated in patients with acute kidney injury, CKD patients acutely infused with PTH, early CKD patients with high PTH level, advanced CKD, hemodialysis patients, and renal transplant recipients with decreased renal function. The pathogenesis of skeletal resistance to PTH is multifactorial and includes phosphate retention (198), downregulation of the PTH receptors (199,200), low levels of calcitriol (201–203), and inhibition of PTH binding to receptors by the 7-84 PTH fragment (81). Other factors include increased level of osteoprotegerin (OPG), which acts as a decoy receptor for osteoclastogenesis-promoting factor in patients with CKD (204,205) and decreased level of BMP-7 (206). The calcemic response to high PTH may be restored after adequate amounts of both $1,25(OH)_2 D_3$ and $24,25(OH)_2 D_3$ (207).

Low Bone Turnover Bone Disease

Adynamic Bone Disease and Osteomalacia

The low turnover lesions are categorized into osteomalacia and ABD. Osteomalacia is characterized by very low rate of bone turnover and marked accumulation of unmineralized osteoid (**FIGURE 24.6C**). Until a decade ago, the most common cause of osteomalacia in patients with ESKD was aluminum toxicity which is known to inhibit bone mineralization. However, the incidence of osteomalacia has decreased with the abandonment of aluminum-based phosphate binders and the introduction of more efficient techniques for treatment of water used in preparing the dialysate. Another possible cause of osteomalacia in CKD patients is deficiency of 25-hydroxyvitamin D.

On the other hand, ABD is being seen with increasing frequency in dialysis and CKD patients, particularly those with diabetes (161,208–210). Moreover, variations in its prevalence can be seen in different geographic regions (211,212). ABD is characterized by low bone turnover in the absence of aluminum overload. The KDIGO Work Group examined bone biopsy studies between 1983 and 2006 and found the prevalence of ABD to be 18% in CKD stages 3 to 5 not yet on dialysis, 19% in hemodialysis patients, and 50% in peritoneal dialysis patients (7). In these studies, ABD has replaced osteomalacia and exceeded that of osteitis fibrosa (213). Even in patients with advanced CKD not yet on dialysis, the prevalence of low turnover disease has reportedly increased to between 12% and 23% (10,214). Definitive diagnosis of ABD requires bone biopsy showing an overall reduction in cellular activity in bone, including both the number of osteoblasts and osteoclasts (**FIGURE 24.6D**), which leads to very low rate of bone turnover. In contrast to osteomalacia, ABD is characterized by low bone turnover without osteoid accumulation. Moreover, both the rate of collagen synthesis by osteoblasts and its subsequent mineralization are subnormal (208,213).

The pathogenesis of ABD is poorly understood but likely involves multiple factors (215,216). In some patients, bone lesions may be irreversible as seen in patients with diabetes mellitus and those associated with osteoporosis due to old age, menopause, or steroid therapy. ABD may also be caused by the malnutrition–inflammation–cachexia syndrome (MICS) (217). However, in other patients, the bone lesions are reversible and are amenable to therapeutic maneuvers. This is particularly true in patients who develop the disease due to aluminum toxicity; parathyroidectomy; and treatment with large doses of CBPBs, calcitriol, or the use of high dialysate calcium, factors suspected of oversuppressing PTH secretion.

High doses of calcitriol may also have PTH-independent inhibitory effects on osteoblastic proliferation and function and thus may induce ABD even in presence of high PTH levels. Interestingly, oxacalcitriol has been shown to control SHPT in uremic dogs without inducing low bone turnover (218). Patients undergoing peritoneal dialysis are particularly at increased risk of developing ABD due to sustained exposure to high calcium concentration in the dialysate. Use of low dialysate calcium concentration or non–calcium-containing binders have been reported to lead to reversal of ABD lesion (219,220). An additional pathogenetic mechanism for ABD was also described. Studies in animal models showed that CKD directly produces ABD by diminishing skeletal growth factors or by producing anabolic inhibitors or both (221). Interestingly, ABD developed when CKD was induced despite the presence of SHPT. Pertinent to this mechanism is the fact that ABD has been described in CKD patients before dialysis (222,223). The mechanism by which CKD causes ABD is not clear but may involve several factors such as uremic toxins, acidosis, increased concentration of OPG and N-terminally truncated PTH fragments, prior use of steroid therapy, malnutrition, and disturbances in growth factors and cytokines. The importance of growth factors in the pathogenesis of ABD was demonstrated in experimental animals in that treatment with the anabolic factor bone morphogenetic protein (BMP)-7 reversed the adynamic bone lesions (224).

Most patients with ABD are asymptomatic, although some may develop bone pain (208,216). Moreover, patients with ABD are at increased risk of fractures and hypercalcemia (225–227). Importantly, patients with ABD are at increased risk of vascular calcification. One study in hemodialysis patients (228) reported an association between low bone turnover and vascular calcification. Another study by the same authors found a significant interaction between the dose of CBPBs and bone activity such that calcium load had a significantly greater impact on aortic calcification and stiffness in patients with ABD (229).

Other Bone Lesions

Mixed bone lesions are now commonly encountered in bone biopsies of patients with CKD. This was observed in 18 of the 259 patients reported by Sherrard et al. (161). The lesion is characterized by an increase in unmineralized osteoid as seen in osteomalacia and an increase in marrow fibrosis similar to that found in the severe hyperparathyroidism (**FIGURE 24.6E**). Bone formation is increased in this group as a result of elevated PTH level. Sherrard et al. (161) speculated that the high PTH level in patients with this bone lesion was almost certainly due to inadequate calcium replacement as lack of adequate calcium may result in a large amount of unmineralized osteoid. Therefore, under these conditions, although calcium may have been deposited at a very high rate, the overstimulated osteoblasts were forming osteoid at an even higher rate giving rise to the mixed bone lesion. This entity has also been described with a normal or low bone formation. Such a picture may be seen when aluminum toxicity and hyperparathyroidism coexist and produce normal bone formation or even a low bone formation if aluminum toxicity dominates the picture.

Dialysis-related amyloidosis (DRA) is another bone lesion that results from amyloid deposits in articular and periarticular tissues in dialysis patients, particularly in those who have been receiving dialysis for over 10 years (230,231). This entity is not caused by abnormalities in mineral metabolism and has no effect on bone morphology or vascular calcification. As a result, it is not currently included in the KDIGO clinical practice guidelines for the diagnosis, evaluation, prevention, and treatment of CKD-MBD. DRA is a disabling disease characterized by accumulation and tissue deposition of amyloid fibrils consisting of β_2-microglobulin in the bone, periarticular structures, and viscera of patients with CKD (208). This is because reduced renal clearance of this protein in patients with decreased GFR leads to plasma accumulation and slow tissue deposition. β_2-Microglobulin amyloid deposits may also be found at subperiosteal locations (232). There are a number of risk factors associated with DRA including older age, dialysis vintage, use of low-flux dialysis membranes and/or bioincompatible dialysis membrane, and lack of residual renal function (233,234).

Patients with DRA usually complain of shoulder pain related to scapulohumeral periarthritis and rotator cuff infiltration by amyloid. Also, patients may develop symptoms of carpal tunnel syndrome due to amyloid deposition in the carpal tunnel which causes hand pain and numbness and dysesthesias in the distribution of the median nerve. Carpal tunnel syndrome is a recognized complication of amyloid deposits and develops frequently in patients on long-term hemodialysis therapy (235). Large cystic deposits can be seen in the long bones, clavicles, phalanges, carpal or tarsal bones, and pelvis. Fractures through these cysts or into infiltrates in the femoral head are particularly common and heal with difficulty. Of particular note, these large, often cystic deposits are commonly misdiagnosed by radiologists as the "brown tumors" of osteitis fibrosa cystica. In fact, cysts, particularly large cysts, are distinctly uncommon in SHPT. When hyperparathyroid cysts do occur, they are more likely to be found in the mandible or skull, and are usually quite small (230,232). Renal transplant is the most effective treatment modality for amyloid-induced symptoms, but the use of biocompatible dialysis membranes may also be helpful (236). Beside enhancing β_2-microglobulin clearance by dialysis or renal transplantation, treatment of DRA is otherwise palliative. Analgesics help with periarticular and bone pain, but since DRA is a progressive disease, early surgical correction of CTS is warranted.

Diagnosis of Renal Osteodystrophy

Clinical Presentation

Renal bone disease is usually asymptomatic, particularly in the earlier stages of CKD. Even in advanced stages of CKD, symptoms are often nonspecific and include bone pain, arthralgia, proximal muscle weakness, and spontaneous tendon rupture (**TABLE 24.2**). These symptoms are not helpful in differentiating between SHPT and low turnover bone diseases. However, patients with low turnover disorders, not due to aluminum, have increased incidence of asymptomatic hypercalcemia. Moreover, in one study, 34% of the patients with ABD but without significant aluminum deposition who were reevaluated after 5 years developed bone pain and fractures and had increased mortality (209).

Clinical presentation of renal osteodystrophy may also involve extraosseous manifestations that are caused by the pathophysiologic entities that contribute to the development of bone lesions. Widespread calcification of various cardiac structures including the coronary and peripheral arteries, cardiac valves, and skin—the so-called calcemic uremic arteriolopathy (CUA) may be seen particularly in patients with ESKD, even among young adults (11,12,137,148,208,237,238).

Bone Biopsy and Other Laboratory Parameters

The gold standard for precise diagnosis of renal bone lesions is bone biopsy. The procedure involves administration of tetracycline on

TABLE 24.2	**Diagnostic Approach for Renal Bone Disease "Renal Osteodystrophy"**

- Clinical presentation
  - Pruritus
  - Bone pain
  - Proximal muscle weakness
  - Arthralgia
  - Spontaneous tendon rupture
  - Fractures
  - Extraskeletal calcification, particularly calciphylaxis
- Laboratory parameters
  - Bone biopsy (gold standard)
  - Serum calcium and phosphorus
  - PTH level
  - 25-Hydroxyvitamin D level
  - Alkaline phosphatases
  - Bone specific alkaline phosphatase
  - Others: osteocalcin, procollagen, propeptides, collagen breakdown products, tartrate-resistant acid phosphatase, and collagen C-terminal telopeptide
- Radiologic diagnosis
  - Subperiosteal bone erosion
  - Rugger-jersey spine
  - Ground glass appearance of skull "pepper pot skull"
  - Brown tumors and bone cysts
  - Bone deformity
  - Chest wall deformity
  - Slipped epiphysis
  - Kyphoscoliosis
  - Growth retardation in children
- Bone mineral density (BMD)

PTH, parathyroid hormone.

two occasions separated by 2 weeks (**TABLE 24.3**). This is followed by obtaining bone biopsy, usually from the iliac crest. Quantitation of bone mineralization rate is done by measuring the distance between the two fluorescent tetracycline layers. Based on histomorphometric analysis, Sherrard et al. (161) proposed classification of renal bone disease using parameters of bone turnover, percentage of unmineralized bone (osteoid) and fibrosis. They further divided the various forms of renal osteodystrophy into three groups: high turnover disease (osteitis fibrosa cystica), low turnover bone disease (ABD or osteomalacia), and mixed uremic bone lesions. More recently, the KDIGO initiative recommended standardization of the nomenclature for reporting bone biopsy to reflect the role of

TABLE 24.3	**Procedure for Obtaining Bone Biopsy**

- Labeling schedule
  - Tetracycline 1,000 mg (15 mg/kg) PO 3 wk before biopsy
  - Demeclocycline 600 mg (9 mg/kg) PO 1 wk before biopsy
- Characteristics of biopsy (iliac crest)
  - Site: 2 cm posterior to anterior superior iliac spine
  - Size: >3 × 8 mm
  - Cancellous (trabecular) bone should predominate
- Fixation[a]
  - Place sample in 10% buffered formalin for 8–24 h
  - Transfer to 70% ethanol for shipping

[a]If osteoclast evaluation is important, specimens should be kept cold (32°F–40°F) but not frozen.

TABLE 24.4	**Clinical Indications for Bone Biopsy**

- Inconsistencies among biochemical parameters that preclude a definitive interpretation
- Unexplained skeletal fracture or bone pain
- Severe progressive vascular calcification
- Unexplained hypercalcemia
- Suspicion of overload or toxicity from aluminum and possibly other metals
- Before parathyroidectomy if there has been significant exposure to aluminum in the past or if the results of biochemical determinations are not consistent with advanced secondary or tertiary hyperparathyroidism
- Before beginning treatment with bisphosphonates

turnover and also incorporate mineralization and volume (8). However, the fact that bone biopsy is quite invasive, requires expertise in processing and interpreting the biopsy, is expensive, and may not be suitable to study progression of renal bone disease or its response to therapies makes it impractical for routine clinical use. Hence, most nephrologists resort to utilizing noninvasive means including biomarkers as well as imaging methods for the diagnosis and follow-up of renal bone disease. TABLE 24.4 lists the current indications for bone biopsy.

Laboratory Tests

Laboratory parameters that are useful in the diagnosis of renal bone disease include measurement of serum calcium, phosphate, PTH, and alkaline phosphatase since these factors are known to contribute to the pathogenesis of bone disease particularly osteitis fibrosa. These parameters should be routinely and frequently obtained, and every attempt should be made to keep their values within the goals recommended by the recent KDIGO Clinical Practice Guidelines for Bone Metabolism and Disease in Chronic Kidney Disease guidelines (7). Unfortunately, the use of various PTH assays in the management of renal bone disease is problematic. The first generation two-site immunometric PTH assay used two different affinity-purified antibodies, one directed toward the C-terminal region of PTH and the second directed toward an amino terminal epitope of PTH. This assay has high sensitivity and specificity. The current therapeutic guidelines for treatment of SHPT were based on this assay which was thought to measure intact PTH. However, Brossard et al. (239), using high-performance liquid chromatography (HPLC) to separate the molecular forms of circulating PTH, noted that the two-site IMA appeared to react with an additional molecular form of PTH, the N-terminally truncated PTH fragments such as the PTH 7-84. Consequently, newer PTH assays that specifically measure the PTH 1-84 molecule became available. However, despite initial enthusiasm for these newer assays and the introduction of the ratio between PTH 1-84 and PTH fragments such as 7-84, the intact PTH assays remain widely used in clinical practice. One issue that is troubling in all intact PTH assays is the significant variation in the results obtained with assays from different manufacturers. These variations are mainly caused by the degree of cross-reactivity of these assays with the circulating N-terminally truncated PTH fragments (240).

An even more relevant issue is the concern about the precision of intact PTH as a surrogate marker of the underlying bone lesions in ESKD patients. Although a decade ago the intact assay

was a strong predictor, with values of less than 100 suggesting low turnover bone disorders and those of more than 300 suggesting high turnover lesions (241,242), this may no longer be the case. It has been suggested that this might result from the recent change in therapy in regard to parenteral vitamin D, because these agents may have direct effects on bone, independent of their effects on PTH (243,244). To improve the usefulness of these assays, it was recently proposed to use of the "ratio" of intact PTH 1-84 to C-fragment (245). Unfortunately, this has not been supported by subsequent reports (246).

Besides calcium, phosphorus, and PTH measurements, other biologic markers of bone formation and resorption have been investigated. Of these, the most useful are serum alkaline phosphatase and bone-specific alkaline phosphatase. Circulating alkaline phosphatase is considered a marker of bone turnover in the absence of liver and biliary disease and thus was initially advocated for the diagnosis and management of renal osteodystrophy (247). Recent publications have highlighted the role of bone alkaline phosphatase as a marker of CKD-MBD. Bone alkaline phosphatase is directly related to bone turnover, reflects bone histomorphometry, and predicts outcomes in hemodialysis patients to a better degree than PTH (247,248). A recent study in 185,277 prevalent hemodialysis patients from Japan found that patients in the highest quartile of serum alkaline phosphatase had 46% and 25% higher all-cause and cardiovascular death risk, respectively, as well as a 71% higher incidence of hip fracture events, than those within the lowest quartile (249). The study also found that a higher serum alkaline phosphatase was more strongly linked to a higher mortality in the patients with lower PTH levels.

Procollagen type 1N propeptide (s-P1NP) and procollagen type 1C propeptide (s-P1CP) are markers for bone formation. On the other hand, tartrate-resistant acid phosphatase 5b (TRAP5b) is released by osteoclasts during bone resorption. A recent study in patients with CKD stages 3 to 5 showed that the highest tertile of formation (s-P1NP) and resorption (TRAP5b) markers were independently and positively associated with prevalent fracture (250). However, more studies are needed for further evaluation of these and other biomarkers in patients with renal osteodystrophy. Other biomarkers such as osteocalcins are used mainly for research purposes and do not add significantly to the information obtained from measurement of the parameters described above.

Radiologic Techniques and Bone Mineral Density

The utility of radiologic techniques in the diagnosis of renal bone disease has also changed over the years (251). In the early dialysis era, radiographic features of SHPT were common and florid. However, with adequate dialysis and treatment of abnormalities of mineral metabolism and the use of high doses of vitamin D, radiographic features of SHPT have become less common. Therefore, x-rays are not routinely performed now because they are relatively insensitive for the diagnosis of early renal bone disease. The classical radiologic features that are pathognomonic of severe SHPT include subperiosteal erosion of the radial aspect of the middle phalanges of the second and third phalanges, clavicles, and pelvis, the ground-glass or "pepper pot" appearance of the skull, and osteosclerosis of the vertebrae, the "rugger-jersey" spine (FIGURE 24.7A–D). On the other hand, brown tumors, which represent focal accumulation of giant cells, are usually seen in the long bones of patients with severe hyperparathyroidism and should be differentiated from bone metastases or amyloid bone cysts (FIGURE 24.7E).

In the general population, measurement of BMD by DXA is predictive of fractures. The value of measuring BMD in patients with CKD is not well established (252). KDIGO recommends DXA to assess fracture risk in patients with CKD stages 1 to 3, if biochemical testing does not suggest CKD-MBD (7). However, for patients with CKD stages 3B to 5, the guideline did not recommend DXA owing to the lack of definitive data demonstrating that DXA predicts fracture in CKD-MBD. Also, DXA evaluates BMD, a measure of bone mass but does not measure bone quality, and there is no correlation between DXA and bone histomorphometry. This is likely due to the multitude of

histologic bone lesions encountered in CKD patients. Moreover, the influence of age, diabetes, prior treatment with corticosteroids, extraosseous calcification, as well as vitamin D deficiency makes BMD results difficult to interpret. Despite these limitations, measuring BMD is becoming increasingly popular in the assessment of renal bone disease. In fact, data from two studies support the claim that DXA can predict fracture risk in patients with CKD. In the first study, meta-analysis of six studies totaling 683 dialysis subjects showed that those with fractures had significantly lower BMD at all sites except for the femoral neck (253). Moreover, in a recent study, Yenchek et al. (254) analyzed

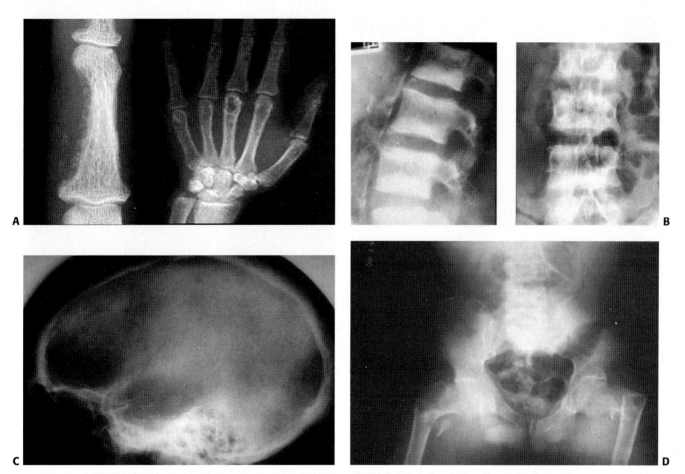

FIGURE 24.7 **A:** Subperiosteal bone erosion in secondary hyperparathyroidism. **B:** Osteosclerosis or "rugger-jersey" spine in secondary hyperparathyroidism. Osteosclerosis (related to hyperparathyroidism) in the spine that involves the end plates of the vertebrae, giving a striped ("rugger-jersey" spine) appearance. There is an erosion of the upper, anterior margin of one of the vertebra; this may be present in 25% of patients with ESKD and on hemodialysis, and may be an early feature of amyloid deposition disease. Arterial calcification is also present in the abdominal aorta. **C:** Ground glass appearance or "pepper-pot" skull in secondary hyperparathyroidism. **D:** Horizontal fracture of the left femoral neck in a patient with adynamic bone disease. Adynamic bone disease. There is reduced osteoid formation and reduced bone turnover. This results radiographically in reduced bone density and fractures that may appear rather bizarre (horizontal across the bone in this radiograph) and occur in unusual sites (second to the fourth ribs, odontoid process). This is related to aluminum toxicity related to treatment with aluminum hydroxide to reduce serum phosphate or from aluminum in the hemodialysis fluid. **E:** Bone cysts (*arrows*) in a uremic patient with amyloidosis. Amyloid deposition disease. The accumulation of β2-microglobulin (β₂-M) results in juxta-articular, well-corticated cysts in the carpal bones (*right upper panel*) (which precedes the development of carpal tunnel syndrome), and around the large joints (*right lower panel*), as seen in the acetabular margin of the left hip. **C:** Computed tomography (CT) scan showing cystic lesions in the anterior margin of the left femoral neck associated with an adjacent anterior soft tissue mass, which is the inflammatory response found in amyloid deposition disease (*left panel*). (Figures A and C courtesy of Dr. Alison Bradley, consultant radiologist, South Manchester University Hospitals, United Kingdom. The rest reproduced with permission from Adams JE. Dialysis bone disease. *Semin Dial* 2002;15:277–289.)

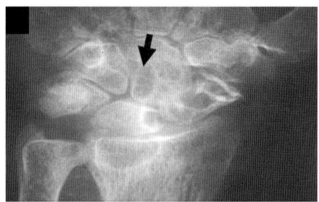

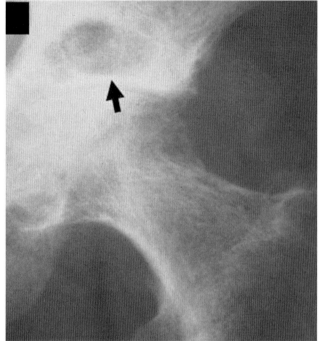

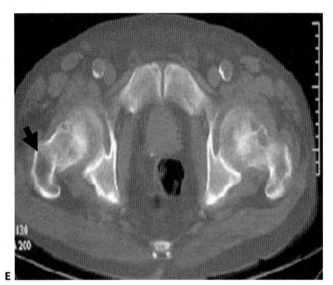

FIGURE 24.7 *(Continued)*

the effect of CKD on fracture risk prediction by DXA in 587 older adults with an eGFR <60 mL/min/1.73 m² followed for 11.3 years per participant. They found that a low femoral neck BMD was associated with greater than a twofold increased risk of fracture in patients with CKD compared with those without CKD (254).

QCT allows three-dimensional imaging of cross-sections of the central and axial skeleton to provide spatial or volumetric bone mineral density (vBMD). It also allows distinction between cortical and trabecular compartments. The technique also allows the calculation of biomechanical parameters, such as the ability of a bone to resist bending. A recent study which compared DXA with QCT in detection of osteoporosis in dialysis patients found that QCT identified prospectively more bone loss at the hip than DXA (160). However, QCT is expensive and requires high radiation exposure. By contrast, peripheral QCT avoids large dose of radiation exposure for patients by focusing on the tibia and distal radius. A small study in dialysis patients reported that a decrease in distal radial cortical vBMD, cortical area, and cortical thickness as well as decreases in torsional strength and bending strength all associated with the odds of a fracture (255).

MANAGEMENT OF CHRONIC KIDNEY DISEASE-MINERAL BONE DISORDER

In order to manage CKD-MBD, it will be necessary to treat each and every component of this syndrome to the extent possible. Thus, the goals of management should include (a) prevention of the development and control of hyperphosphatemia, hypocalcemia, hypercalcemia, or positive calcium balance; (b) correction of vitamin D deficiency; (c) prevention and treatment of abnormal PTH secretion and avoidance of the development of PTG hyperplasia; (d) decreasing the risk of bone disease and fractures; (e) prevention or reducing the risk of progressive cardiovascular calcification; (f) and finally, and most importantly, is reducing the risk of mortality in CKD patients (**TABLE 24.5**). To achieve these goals, the KDIGO guidelines suggest maintaining serum calcium in the normal range in all stages of CKD, maintaining phosphate levels in the normal range in CKD stages 3 to 5 and decreasing serum phosphate levels toward the normal range in dialysis patients, and maintaining PTH level at >2 to <9 times the upper limit of normal (7) (**TABLE 24.6**). To successfully achieve these goals, the use of combination of measures that simultaneously target most, if not all, components of CKD-MBD is required.

TABLE 24.5	Goals of Management of Chronic Kidney Disease-Mineral Bone Disorder

- Immediate goals: maintenance of calcium, phosphorus, and PTH in the range recommended by the KDIGO guidelines
  - Dietary restriction of phosphorus to 800–1,000 mg/d
  - Prevent hypocalcemia
  - Phosphate binders for hyperphosphatemia
  - Dialysate calcium between 2.0 and 2.5 mEq/L
  - Monitor mineral metabolism monthly
- Long-term goals
  - Start treatment early in the course of CKD
  - Prevent the development of parathyroid gland hyperplasia
    - Dietary restriction of phosphorus early in the course of CKD
    - Calcium supplements to prevent hypocalcemia
  - Treatment of established secondary hyperparathyroidism
    - Phosphate binders for hyperphosphatemia
    - Dialysate calcium between 2.0 and 2.5 mEq/L
    - Vitamin D sterols
    - Calcimimetic agents
    - Parathyroidectomy
    - Monitor mineral metabolism monthly
  - Prevent risk of extraosseous calcification
  - Reduce morbidity and mortality
- Avoid
  - Delaying treatment of secondary hyperparathyroidism or osteomalacia
  - Hypercalcemia
  - Hypocalcemia
  - Oversuppression of PTH

PTH, parathyroid hormone; KDIGO, Kidney Disease: Improving Global Outcomes; CKD, chronic kidney disease.

Prevention and Treatment of Hyperphosphatemia

The principles of therapy for SHPT involve correcting the reversible causes of increased PTH secretion such as hypocalcemia, hyperphosphatemia, and low vitamin D levels. In order to prevent the development of SHPT, therapy should be initiated early in the course of CKD when the GFR decreases to less than 70 mL/min. The primary goal here is to prevent the development of parathyroid hyperplasia. Hypocalcemia is a potent stimulus for PTH secretion and thus should be corrected with calcium supplement taken between meals. Given that phosphate plays a key role in CKD-MBD, potential benefits from controlling serum phosphate are many and may include amelioration of SHPT, avoidance of hypocalcemia, less inhibition

TABLE 24.6	Kidney Disease: Improving Global Outcomes Treatment Goals for Serum Calcium, Phosphate, and Parathyroid Hormone in Chronic Kidney Disease Stages 3 to 5 and Stage 5D

Mineral	CKD 3–5	CKD 5D
Serum calcium	Within normal range	Within normal range
Serum phosphate	Within normal range	Toward normal
Serum PTH	Unknown	2–9 times upper limit of normal

CKD, chronic kidney disease; PTH, parathyroid hormone.

of calcitriol production, decreased FGF-23 levels, decreased risk of cardiovascular calcification, and most importantly decreased risk of death. Although the benefits of lowering serum phosphate to a certain target level has not been proved in randomized controlled trials (RCTs), the KDIGO guidelines suggest maintaining phosphate levels in the normal range in CKD stages 3 to 5 and decreasing serum phosphate levels toward the normal range in dialysis patients (7).

Dietary phosphate restriction and use of phosphate binders are necessary for lowering PTH level and prevention of PTG hyperplasia (7). The typical American diet contains about 1,000 to 1,400 mg/d of phosphate. Dietary phosphate restriction to 800 to 1,000 mg/d should be encouraged as soon as the renal function begins to fall and phosphate intake should be decreased in proportion to the decrease in the GFR (256). This can be accomplished by restricting intake of dairy products, but protein restriction should be modest to avoid malnutrition. In addition, the protein source is also important. Phosphate in plant-based foods is bound to phytic acid or phytate and may be less bioavailable because humans lack the enzyme phytase that is required to degrade the phosphorus-phytate bond. In a crossover trial in nine patients with a mean eGFR of 32 mL/min to directly compare vegetarian and meat diets with equivalent protein and phosphorus contents, subjects had lower serum phosphate levels, a trend toward decreased urine 24-hour phosphorus excretion, and significantly decreased FGF-23 levels in the vegetarian diet compared with the meat-based diet (257). Another aspect of dietary counseling is to encourage consumption of foods with a low phosphate to protein ratio such as egg white (19,27). Finally, counseling patients to avoid processed foods with large amounts of phosphate additives such as soft drinks and cheese can be very effective in treating hyperphosphatemia. This is because processed foods contain a high amount of inorganic phosphate which is more readily absorbed. In fact, >90% of inorganic phosphate may be absorbed from the intestine, as opposed to only 40% to 60% of the organic phosphate present in natural foods (19). Food additives may contribute as much as 1,000 mg/d phosphate to the average American diet (20,258). If serum phosphate remains elevated despite careful dietary restriction, as is the case in stage 4 to 5D CKD, then phosphate binders are indicated. One retrospective study in nondialyzed CKD patients showed that phosphate binder therapy was associated with 23% decrease in mortality (259).

CBPBs such as calcium acetate and calcium carbonate are the preferred agents in patients with CKD not yet on dialysis because these agents correct hypocalcemia, a potent stimulus for PTH secretion. However, other non–calcium-based phosphate binders such as sevelamer and lanthanum carbonate can also be used. A recent randomized placebo-controlled pilot clinical trial by Block et al. (152) showed that therapy with both non–calcium- and calcium-based phosphate binders significantly lower serum and urinary phosphorus and attenuate progression of SHPT among patients with CKD who have normal or near-normal levels of serum phosphorus. However, they also resulted in progression of vascular calcification, albeit to a smaller degree in non–calcium- than in calcium-based phosphate binders.

Management of Dialysis Patients

In patients with ESKD, the use of phosphate binders and active vitamin D sterols is necessary to control SHPT. In general, the same approach as outlined earlier for predialysis patients should be continued. Foremost among the measures needed is control of hyperphosphatemia, an abnormality that is invariably present among patients with ESKD. Hyperphosphatemia remains a very common mineral disorder in patients with ESKD and is considered an important clinical entity. Unfortunately, despite concerted efforts by patients, dietitians, and nephrologists to control serum phosphate, the most recent report by DOPPS show that in the United States, at least 35% of patients had serum phosphate above 5.5 mg/dL and 65% had phosphate above normal (3.5 to 4.5 mg/dL) as recommended by KDIGO (7,260).

Dietary phosphate restriction should be encouraged in patients with ESKD. Unfortunately, although important, it is difficult to accomplish the goal serum phosphate with dietary restriction of phosphorus alone since these patients are encouraged to consume a diet that contains at least 1.2 g of protein/kg/d in order to prevent protein malnutrition. Intermittent hemodialysis can remove approximately 1,000 mg of phosphate per session. However, since patients may absorb more than 1,000 mg each day, their net phosphate balance is usually greater than 4,000 mg/wk. Intermittent hemodialysis thrice weekly alone also does not adequately control serum phosphorus in most patients (261). However, the use of more frequent dialysis such as short daily dialysis or long nocturnal hemodialysis may be effective in achieving the recommended goal serum phosphate level without the use of phosphate binders (262,263). Unfortunately, these dialysis modalities are not practical and have not yet been widely applied in clinical practice. Consequently, phosphate binders are routinely prescribed for most patients with ESKD in order to reduce intestinal absorption of dietary phosphorus and prevent hyperphosphatemia. To be effective, these medications should be taken with meals in order to bind the phosphate in the food and prevent its intestinal absorption.

Phosphate Binders

Two large observational studies have reported that phosphate binders are associated with decreased mortality among dialysis patients (154,155). The ideal phosphate binder should be effective in small number of pills in binding most dietary phosphate in the intestine without producing significant adverse effects. It should also be safe, not absorbed, and relatively inexpensive because most dialysis patients usually consume relatively large daily doses of the binder. An important but often ignored aspect of phosphate binder therapy is to divide the number of daily binder pills according to the size of the meal. The largest dose should be taken with the main meal. By contrast, no binder should be given if no food is consumed. Unfortunately, none of the currently used phosphate binders fulfill all these requirements. This is best exemplified by aluminum hydroxide which is probably the most cost-effective phosphate binder we ever had. This drug has largely been abandoned because of the risks of aluminum intoxication leading to encephalopathy, microcytic anemia, and osteomalacia (264). Calcium acetate and calcium carbonate replaced aluminum hydroxide as the most widely prescribed phosphate binders. Although cost-effective, concern about the possible role of calcium loading from these binders in progression of cardiovascular calcification has led to more frequent use of the considerably more expensive noncalcium, non-aluminum phosphate binders such as sevelamer hydrochloride and to a much lower extent lanthanum carbonate (265–267). We have shown in an earlier randomized double-blind trial that calcium acetate is significantly more effective than sevelamer in controlling serum phosphorus to the recommended goal levels (268). More recently, Daugirdas et al. (269) showed that sevelamer has the least phosphate binder equivalent dose compared with other phosphate binders. In our experience, patients frequently require higher number of sevelamer pills per meal than other binders to control serum

phosphate, and its use may be associated with significant GI adverse events; both are common triggers for patients' nonadherence. On the other hand, two published clinical trials reported that treatment of hyperphosphatemia in hemodialysis patients with sevelamer was associated with slower progression of coronary artery calcification compared with that of CBPB (143,144). However, two other studies have not confirmed these findings (148,149). In the Calcium Acetate Renagel Evaluation-2 (CARE-2) study, we found that treatment with calcium acetate plus atorvastatin for 1-year period was associated with similar degrees of progression of coronary artery calcification to sevelamer in hemodialysis patients (148). Nonetheless, an important issue that is still unclear is whether a decrease in vascular calcification by any means is associated with improved patients' outcomes. The KDIGO clinical practice guidelines suggest restricting use of CBPB in patients with hypercalcemia, those with low PTH level or ABD and in those with evidence of vascular calcification (7).

Lanthanum carbonate is a potent noncalcium phosphate binder. Its main advantages include a relatively low pill burden, favorable effects on bone turnover, and lowering of serum FGF-23 (270,271). Unfortunately, a small amount of lanthanum is absorbed from the intestine and deposited in various organs including liver and bone (272). Although there was no demonstrable toxicity from lanthanum in these tissues, long-term safety remains a great concern. However, post hoc analysis of four phase III trials with a follow-up of up to 6 years did not find evidence of hepatotoxicity or other organ damage in patients with CKD (273). Other phosphate binders include magnesium salts which bind phosphorus but are less potent than either aluminum or calcium salts (274). Experimental studies suggest that magnesium inhibits phosphate-induced calcification *in vitro* and has a protective role on vascular calcification (275,276). However, large amounts of magnesium can be absorbed and may produce hypermagnesemia unless the dialysate magnesium is reduced. More troubling is the diarrhea produced by virtually all magnesium salts when large doses are ingested. Both magnesium hydroxide and magnesium carbonate have been studied and, although neither is particularly effective, the carbonate salt is the better phosphorous-binding agent.

Finally, a new era of phosphate binders has begun (277). Two iron-based phosphate binders were recently approved by the U.S. Food and Drug Administration (FDA) for clinical use (278,279). In a large phase III RCT, treatment with ferric citrate resulted in significantly higher serum ferritin and transferrin saturation (TSAT) levels compared with active control. Also, subjects receiving ferric citrate required less IV iron than controls over 52 weeks, the percentage of subjects not requiring IV iron was significantly higher and the cumulative erythropoietin-stimulating agent (ESA) dose over 52 weeks was lower than in the control group (278,280). Similar results were also reported in nondialysis CKD patients who had iron deficiency anemia but were not allowed to receive ESA or IV iron (281). Therefore, it appears that ferric citrate not only controls serum phosphate but also simultaneously provides a source of maintenance iron that leads to reduction in IV iron and ESA use while maintaining hemoglobin (Hb) levels in dialysis and CKD patients. By contrast, sucroferric oxyhydroxide, also an iron-based phosphate binder, does not seem to significantly increase iron stores since its active moiety, polynuclear ferric-oxyhydroxide, is insoluble and does not release ferric iron for absorption. However, it has been shown to be as effective as sevelamer in controlling serum phosphate level in dialysis patients with much lower pill burden (279).

Other means of controlling serum phosphate is to inhibit the intestinal sodium-phosphate cotransporter 2b (NaPi-2b) with nicotinamide or niacin (282,283). Nicotinamide is associated with less adverse reactions than niacin. These compounds are particularly useful in nonadherent patients since intermittent phosphate restriction and/or phosphate binder treatment trigger an upregulation of intestinal NaPi-2b allowing greater phosphate absorption after phosphate binder doses are missed. Also the use of chitosan chewing gum as an adjunct to phosphate binders has been shown to help in controlling serum phosphate (284).

Vitamin D Therapy

KDIGO guidelines recommend "maintaining PTH in the normal range for the assay in patients with CKD stages 3 to 5 and of approximately 2 to 9 times the upper limit of normal in CKD stage 5D." The guidelines further recommend to first correct hypocalcemia, elevated phosphate levels, and vitamin D deficiency by reducing dietary phosphate intake and administering phosphate binders, calcium supplements, and/or native vitamin D (7). The Kidney Disease Outcomes Quality Initiative (KDOQI) guidelines recommend treating 25OHD level <5 ng/mL with ergocalciferol 50,000 IU/wk orally for 12 weeks then monthly for 6 months (285). For levels between 5 and 15 ng/mL, ergocalciferol 50,000 IU/wk orally for 4 weeks and monthly for 6 months should be given. For 25OHD levels that are 16 to 30 ng/mL, treatment with 50,000 IU monthly for 6 months should be given. In all cases, the level of 25OHD should be remeasured at the end of the treatment period. However, our own experience, and those of others, cast doubt on the efficacy of this approach in controlling SHPT (77,256,286). If serum calcium, phosphate and 25OHD levels are normal, but the PTH level remains elevated, active vitamin D preparations such as calcitriol should be added. Given the important role of decreased calcitriol level in the pathogenesis of SHPT, the use of active vitamin D sterols is considered the main treatment modality for lowering the PTH levels among patients with all stages of CKD. Minimal doses should be used first and the dose should be increased slowly, probably no more often than every 3 months. Calcitriol will increase intestinal absorption of both calcium and phosphorous, so their levels will need to be monitored closely and therapy adjusted promptly if elevations occur. Other active vitamin D analogs can also be used in patients with CKD.

For dialysis patients, a number of active vitamin D agents are available for clinical use in the United States, including calcitriol, paricalcitol, and doxercalciferol. There are potential differences between these compounds that should be considered. Calcitriol is effective whether given orally or by intravenous boluses during the hemodialysis procedure. However, it may cause hypercalcemia particularly when used in combination with CBPB (287). Moreover, it has been shown to induce vascular calcification in experimental animals (139,288). Consequently, the search for other vitamin D sterols leads to the introduction of vitamin D prohormones such as 1-α-hydroxyl vitamin D_2 (doxercalciferol) and 1-α-hydroxyvitamin D_3. These two preparations undergo 25 hydroxylation in the liver and are metabolized to the active 1,25-hydroxyvitamin D_2 and 1,25-hydroxyvitamin D_3. Furthermore, in an attempt to selectively suppress PTH production while minimizing the effects of vitamin D on calcium and phosphate metabolism, structural changes in the vitamin D molecule were made and lead to the introduction of several analogs such as 19-nor-1,25-dihydroxyvitamin D_2 (paricalcitol), 22-oxacalcitriol, and 26, 27-hexafluorocalcitriol (falecalcitriol).

Although direct head-to-head randomized studies in patients are limited, few studies that compared paricalcitol with doxercalciferol showed more episodes of hyperphosphatemia with doxercalciferol (289). Moreover, in experimental animals, calcitriol and doxercalciferol are associated with vascular calcification, while paricalcitol was not (290).

The value of vitamin D administration to CKD patients may extend beyond its effect on calcium, phosphate, and PTH levels. Teng et al. (291) reported in a historical cohort study that hemodialysis patients who were administered paricalcitol had better survival than those who received calcitriol. However, in a follow-up retrospective study on incident hemodialysis patients, they found that the administration of any vitamin D sterols to dialysis patients may confer survival advantage over that of patients who were not given any vitamin D preparation (291,292). In multivariable analyses, the association of paricalcitol treatment with survival persisted without regard to the serum concentrations of calcium or phosphate. Moreover, vitamin D administration has been shown in observational studies to be associated with improved survival in predialysis patients with CKD (293,294). The exact mechanism of the beneficial effect of vitamin D on patients' outcome may be related to its antiproliferative effects on myocardial cell hypertrophy and proliferation, its negative regulatory effect on the renin-angiotensin system, as well as its ability to inhibit inflammatory changes that have been established as key in the pathogenesis of atherosclerosis (295). It is interesting that a meta-analysis of 76 clinical trials showed that the use of vitamin D therapy in patients with CKD does not reduce the risk of death or vascular calcification (296). Moreover, administration of active vitamin D analogs has been shown to increase FGF-23 in ESKD patients (297), which has been shown in other studies to be an independent predictor of mortality in patients with ESKD (131). Finally, the Paricalcitol Capsule Benefits in Renal Failure Induced Cardiac Morbidity (PRIMO) study randomized 227 patients with stage 3 and 4 CKD, mild left ventricular hypertrophy, but normal systolic function to either paricalcitol or placebo. The study was based on the hypothesis that paricalcitol directly reduces the adverse effects of the renin-angiotensin system on cardiac remodeling by activation of the VDR in cardiac myocytes. The primary end point was a change in ventricular mass over 48 weeks as assessed by magnetic resonance imaging (MRI). The results showed no significant difference between the two groups (298). Other measures of LV function such as the end-systolic index, end-diastolic index, ejection fraction, aorta compliance, and aorta volume were also not different. However, the risk of hospitalizations was significantly decreased in the paricalcitol group (1.1 per 100 person-years vs. 8.8 per 100 person-years, $p = 0.04$) likely due to decrease in episodes of congestive heart failure and a reduction in atrial enlargement.

Calcimimetic Agents

Although the use of vitamin D has been effective in lowering markedly elevated PTH levels, a number of patients eventually become refractory to vitamin D therapy or become intolerant because of hypercalcemia which often demands cessation of vitamin D therapy. Consequently, the percentage of vitamin D–treated patients who actually achieved and maintain the recommended clinical practice targets for mineral metabolism is rather small. Given that changes in serum ionized calcium are sensed by the CaSRs on parathyroid cells, these receptors became a target for therapeutic intervention by agents that activate the CaSR and lower PTH secretion from the PTG. Cinacalcet is a calcimimetic agent that became commercially available in the United States in May 2004. It binds reversibly to the membrane-spanning portion of the CaSR and lowers the threshold for its activation by ionized calcium (299). This agent results in leftward shift of the set point and in a significant fall in PTH levels at any level of serum ionized calcium. Some authors believe that cinacalcet is the most effective agent currently available for reducing PTH levels in dialysis patients that can be used as an alternative treatment modality for the control of SHPT (300). Studies in hemodialysis patients with SHPT have shown that a single oral dose of cinacalcet resulted in a rapid drop in PTH level to a nadir after 2 to 4 hours (300,301). The degree of reduction in PTH level attributed to cinacalcet correlates with pretreatment PTH level; the higher the PTH level, the greater the reduction in PTH level (302). Of interest, cinacalcet lowers serum calcium and phosphate as well as PTH (170,303). Indeed, concomitant use of cinacalcet and vitamin D in dialysis patients with persistently elevated PTH levels resulted in significantly higher percentage of patients who achieved the KDOQI targets for mineral metabolism (303). Cinacalcet is clearly useful in patients who are receiving CBPB as well as in those who develop hypercalcemia with high doses of vitamin D. However, cinacalcet should not be prescribed to patients with serum calcium concentration <8.4 mg/dL. Cinacalcet may reduce parathyroid cell proliferation and retard the development of PTG hyperplasia, thus diminishing the need for parathyroidectomy (74,304,305). Also, calcimimetic therapy have been shown to decrease FGF-23 by decreasing PTH levels, whereas vitamin D therapy increases FGF-23 production by a direct effect on gene transcription (306). The implications for these actions of cinacalcet are not clear at the present time.

Two major recent studies that compared outcomes of treatment of SHPT with either cinacalcet or paricalcitol, a vitamin D analog, have been published. The recent Action in Diabetes and Cardiovascular Disease: Preterax and Diamicron Modified Release Controlled Evaluation (ADVANCE) trial in 360 patients showed a trend toward decreasing the progression of vascular and valvular calcification but was only significant for aortic valvular calcification (307). In the Evaluation of Cinacalcet Hydrochloride Therapy to Lower Cardiovascular Events (EVOLVE) study, cinacalcet was compared with placebo in 3,883 hemodialysis patients with SHPT for up to 64 months (308). Most patients in the study were receiving phosphate binders and vitamin D analogs. The study showed that cinacalcet is effective in the treatment of SHPT either as monotherapy or with vitamin D therapy. The unadjusted intention to treat analysis showed that cinacalcet does not significantly reduce the risk of death or major cardiovascular events in patients with moderate-to-severe SHPT who were undergoing hemodialysis (308). Also, after adjustment for differences in baseline characteristics, multiple fractures, and/or events prompting discontinuation of study drug, the trial showed that treatment with cinacalcet reduced the rate of clinical fracture by 16% to 29% (309). Therefore, cinacalcet seems to be a very useful drug for lowering the PTH level, for decreasing PTG hyperplasia, and for decreasing fracture rate in dialysis patients, but the claim that it has beneficial effects on progression of cardiovascular calcification and patient survival remain unsubstantiated.

Two other studies have evaluated the safety and efficacy of cinacalcet in patients with CKD not receiving dialysis (310,311). In both studies, cinacalcet was found to be effective in lowering PTH levels but at the expense of frequent development of hypocalcemia, increased urinary calcium excretion, hyperphosphatemia, and decreased urinary phosphate and citrate excretion. In the only randomized controlled trial in this population, patients randomized to cinacalcet required more active vitamin D analogs and more phosphate binders than the control group (311). Based on the results of these trials, KDIGO Work Group felt that more data were needed before recommending calcimimetics for patients with CKD stages 3 to 5 and SHPT (7). Similarly, the FDA has not approved cinacalcet for use in predialysis patients with CKD.

Parathyroidectomy

Approximately 10% of patients with ESKD undergo parathyroidectomy for refractory SHPT (312). However, the rate of parathyroidectomy in the dialysis population has varied substantially over the past few decades from 12.5 per 1,000 patient-years in 1992 to 5.5 per 1,000 patient-years in 2005 but increased again to 9 per 1,000 patient-years in 2007 (312). A more recent study by Tentori et al. (95) on 35,655 participants from the DOPPS phases 1 to 4 (1996 to 2011) confirmed that, despite increased PTH levels, rates of parathyroidectomy has indeed declined in all regions over the 15-year study period. This decrease is likely related to multiple factors including the new KDIGO recommended level of PTH and the use of cinacalcet which was shown in the aforementioned EVOLVE trial to reduce the rate of parathyroidectomy by more than half (313).

Currently, KDIGO recommends targeting PTH levels to within 2 to 9 times the upper limit of normal for the dialysis population (7). KDIGO also recommend parathyroidectomy for patients with CKD stages 3 to 5D with severe hyperparathyroidism who fail to respond to medical/pharmacologic therapy but did not specify threshold PTH level for parathyroidectomy (7). As a practical guideline, parathyroidectomy is indicated for patients with severe hyperparathyroidism, defined as PTH level greater than 800 pg/mL, particularly if accompanied by symptoms (**TABLE 24.7**). This is because observational studies have consistently showed a higher risk of adverse clinical outcomes in patients whose PTH levels are outside those recommended by KDIGO for dialysis patients. Parathyroidectomy is specially indicated in patients who are noncompliant with diet and phosphate binders and in whom medical therapy becomes ineffective, impractical, or even contraindicated particularly with the

TABLE 24.7	Indications for Parathyroidectomy

- Refractory secondary hyperparathyroidism
  - Persistently elevated PTH level (>800 pg/mL)
  - Persistent hypercalcemia when using vitamin D
- Severe symptomatic disease
  - Refractory pruritus
  - Fractures
  - Unexplained myopathy
  - Tendon rupture
  - Bone pain
  - Severe bone disease
  - Severe pruritus in presence of high PTH level
  - Calciphylaxis
- Should not wait too long when parathyroidectomy is indicated
- Exclude aluminum toxicity before parathyroidectomy

PTH, parathyroid hormone.

development of hypercalcemia (TABLE 24.7). A relatively urgent indication for parathyroidectomy is the presence of high PTH level in patients with CUA or calciphylaxis, although its benefits have not been convincingly shown (208).

There are presumed benefits of parathyroidectomy on both laboratory parameters and clinical outcomes including fractures. Patients who undergo parathyroidectomy usually experience improvement in various biochemical parameters. However, comparisons between medical and surgical therapy for outcomes of morbidity and mortality are difficult to evaluate. Parathyroidectomy may be associated with adverse events. Only a few studies have systematically evaluated the risks associated with parathyroidectomy. Using USRDS data (1988 to 1999), Kestenbaum et al. (314) found increased 30-day mortality for patients who underwent parathyroidectomy compared with those who did not (3.1% vs. 1.2%). The increased risk continued for 90 days and then inverted at 1 year. Also, Rudser et al. (315) reported a 32% lower risk of hip, vertebra, and distal radius-wrist fractures after parathyroidectomy in a nationwide cohort of patients who underwent parathyroidectomy compared with matched controls. More recently, Ishani et al. (316) reported that parathyroidectomy is associated with significant morbidity in the 30 days after hospital discharge and in the year after the procedure. Most pronounced were high rehospitalization rates, more intensive care unit (ICU) visits, more hospital days, and 2% mortality within 30 days of hospital discharge after the procedure.

The choice of surgical procedure depends on the experiences of the surgeon. An important factor to consider is that 5% of patients have fewer than four PTG and 10% have more than four. The most commonly performed procedure is subtotal parathyroidectomy or total parathyroidectomy with reimplantation of non-nodular parathyroid tissue in the forearm. However, another option is total parathyroidectomy for patients who are not renal transplant candidates because recurrence of hyperparathyroidism may develop in 10% of patients who have subtotal resections (317). There is no evidence that total parathyroidectomy with immediate ectopic parathyroid tissue reimplantation is superior or inferior to subtotal parathyroidectomy (7). In patients with severe hyperparathyroidism who are likely to be transplanted, total parathyroidectomy with reimplantation of a remnant into the arm may be preferred. Unfortunately, identifying and removing the parathyroid tissue from the forearm may be difficult in case of recurrent hyperparathyroidism. Moreover, malignancy in these transplanted remnant parathyroid tissue may develop (318). Persistent hyperparathyroidism after surgery indicates the presence of an extra gland that was missed during surgery. An essential point to consider before parathyroidectomy is to rule out coexisting aluminum toxicity by using deferoxamine (DFO) testing or even bone biopsy in patients who have history of use of aluminum-based phosphate binders. This is because parathyroidectomy in this situation may precipitate the development of osteomalacia.

Hungry bone syndrome usually occurs in parathyroidectomized uremic patients who had successful surgery. This syndrome is defined as development of serum calcium <6.0 mg/dL immediately after parathyroidectomy requiring intravenous calcium infusion to control such severe degree of hypocalcemia despite higher dialysate calcium concentration, calcitriol, and oral calcium carbonate supplementation. The syndrome has been reported in 27.8% to 51.2% of patients in different studies (319,320). Due to the development of an abrupt decrease in the plasma concentrations of calcium and

phosphate, these patients experience muscle cramps, tingling, tetany, seizures, and cardiac arrhythmias. The sudden decrease in PTH levels results in an almost immediate decrease in bone resorption, while bone formation continues at a very high rate. Thus, large amounts of calcium are shifted to the skeleton, but little moves out. Patients who received high-dose parenteral vitamin D for hyperparathyroidism before parathyroidectomy may not develop hungry bone syndrome. This may be due to PTH-independent actions of vitamin D on bone (205,243). Witteveen et al. (321) suggested that between 6 and 12 g/d of calcium supplementation will be required to treat the severe hypocalcemia. They also suggested that initially, calcium should be given intravenously, but treatment with oral preparations should be initiated as early as possible. Serum calcium must then be measured every 6 hours for 24 to 48 hours. Moreover, calcitriol should be administered in 2 to 4 μg daily doses or even higher along with magnesium to correct concomitant hypomagnesemia. Finally, they suggested that preoperative administration of bisphosphonates may reduce the severity and duration of hypocalcemia.

The weight of the parathyroid tissue removed may predict the degree of hypocalcemia and also provides an excellent guide to the amount of calcium required postoperatively. For every gram of tissue resected, patients will require 1 g of calcium chloride over the following 24 hours. This rule has been useful in the management of more than 50 patients with removed tissue weighing 1.5 to 17 g (161). In some patients, high doses of oral calcium (up to 10 g daily) and calcitriol (up to 4 μg daily) may be necessary for as long as 1 to 2 months after surgery.

⬡ BONE DISEASE IN RENAL TRANSPLANT RECIPIENTS

Renal transplantation is recognized as the optimal treatment for patients with ESKD. Besides improving the quality of life, transplantation is clearly associated with improved patient survival compared to dialysis. Moreover, clinical consequences of renal failure such as anemia and mineral metabolism substantially improve after transplantation. Unfortunately, CKD-MBD may worsen after renal transplantation despite restoring near-normal renal function in most patients. The fracture risk for a kidney transplant recipient is fourfold higher than in the general population (322), and the high fracture rate seen in dialysis patients increases even further after successful kidney transplantation, especially in diabetics (323–325). The pathophysiology of bone disease in renal transplant recipients is complex since it may represent a continuum of structural changes in bone from the earlier stages of CKD, throughout the dialysis period and then after renal transplantation. The prevalence of various histologic patterns of bone disease after transplantation is not well described but almost all types of renal osteodystrophy are represented, with low turnover bone disease being the most prevalent (326). Prior to transplantation, many patients have been exposed to treatments with active vitamin D analogs, steroids, other immunosuppressive drugs, or anticonvulsant medications. Moreover, some may suffer from preexisting diabetes, osteoporosis, immobilization, malnutrition, and impaired gonadal function. Thus, patients awaiting renal transplantation already have significant underlying bone pathologies.

Unfortunately, this picture does not improve but instead accelerates, particularly in the first 6 to 12 months after transplantation. Julian et al. (327) reported a 6.8% decrease in vertebral BMD

6 months after renal transplantation compared to baseline. This is because renal transplant recipients are subjected to many risk factors that contribute to the type and/or severity of posttransplant bone disease. Besides the aforementioned preexisting renal osteodystrophy, the use of immunosuppressive drugs such as steroids and calcineurin inhibitors and other transplantation-specific therapies as well as worsening graft function also contribute to the transplant bone disease (323). Persistent hyperparathyroidism, hypercalcemia, hypophosphatemia, hypomagnesemia, and loop diuretics also increase the risk for bone disease after transplantation. Other immunosuppressive agents such as azathioprine, mycophenolate mofetil, and sirolimus have not been shown to have any negative effects on bone health. It must be emphasized, however, that the bone diseases associated with transplantation are not unique to kidney transplants but may develop with other types of organ transplants (323).

Steroids play a major role in accelerating bone loss during the first 6 months after transplantation (328,329). Rojas et al. (330) performed serial bone biopsies in 20 renal transplant recipients at 22 and 160 days after transplantation and found impaired osteoblastogenesis and early osteoblast apoptosis. Steroids increase bone resorption and decrease bone formation by numerous mechanisms, including reduction of osteoblast proliferation, increased osteoblast apoptosis, downregulation of collagen I, osteocalcin, BMPs, and TGF-β. Moreover, steroids accelerate osteoclastogenesis as a result of their action in decreasing OPG and increase in receptor activator of nuclear factor κB ligand (RANKL). These detrimental effects of steroids on bone are attributed to the cumulative dose in renal transplant recipients. Steroids may also induce negative calcium balance by reducing intestinal calcium absorption and increasing urinary calcium excretion which in turn may play a role in the development of osteoporosis and hyperparathyroidism (331). On the other hand, the effects of the two calcineurin inhibitors, cyclosporine and tacrolimus, on bone are incompletely understood but their main effect includes acceleration of bone resorption (329,332). One study that examined the independent potential of cyclosporine and tacrolimus on bone formation and bone resorption using serum markers to measure bone turnover found no significant difference between these two immunosuppressive drugs (333).

Avascular Necrosis

Avascular necrosis (AVN) is a debilitating complication of renal and other organ transplantation. Previous studies suggested an incidence of approximately 15% within 3 years of the transplant (334). In an interesting prospective study of 48 patients without evidence of femoral osteonecrosis prior to renal transplantation, AVN was documented in 4% by MRI at 6 months following the procedure (334). AVN affects all weight-bearing joints, particularly the hip, and more than half of affected patients have more than one joint involved. In this disorder, the weight-bearing surface such as the femoral head undergoes necrosis. This results in additional stress on adjacent bone, which may also be damaged. AVN occurs in 5% to 30% of renal transplant patients, usually in the first year after transplant (335). It occurs more frequently in patients who receive high doses of steroid. The exact etiology is not well understood but is likely multifactorial. One theory suggests that steroids induce fat cells to proliferate in the marrow space leading to marked increase in intraosseous pressure which in turn interferes with perfusion of bone leading to ischemic necrosis. The diagnosis of AVN is usually made after the patient presents with hip pain. Routine x-rays are not sensitive and are usually negative but may eventually show a defect in the femoral head. MRI is the most sensitive and definitive diagnostic test and often reveals the lesion even before symptoms develop (**FIGURE 24.8**) (336). It is likely that the frequency of AVN will decrease with the current trend for using lower dose protocols for renal transplant recipients.

Management of Posttransplant Bone Disease

Unfortunately, the lack of RCTs in renal transplant recipients with bone disease makes it difficult to recommend bone-specific therapies, particularly during the first 12 months after kidney transplantation. However, prevention and/or treatment of pretransplant bone disease clearly have an impact on the management of posttransplant

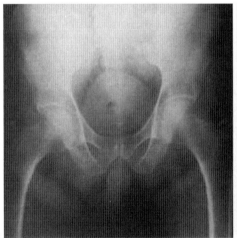
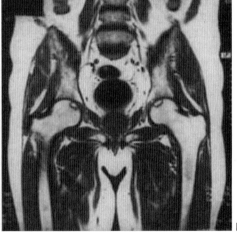

FIGURE 24.8 Magnetic resonance images from a transplant patient. **A:** Normal x-ray of the pelvis with no pathologic findings in the femoral heads 3 months after renal transplantation. **B:** Avascular necrosis of the femoral heads 3 months after transplantation. The T1-weighted image 3 months after transplantation showed small isointense necrotic areas and hypointense demarcation rims in both femoral heads. X-ray image of the pelvis 3 months after transplantation. No pathologic findings in both femoral heads. (Reproduced with permission from Fink B, Degenhardt S, Paselk C, et al. Early detection of avascular necrosis of the femoral head following renal transplantation. *Arch Orthop Trauma Surg* 1997;116:151–156.)

bone disease. Every effort should be made to avoid significant bone disease at the time of transplantation. Moreover, it is suggested that potential transplant recipients undergo assessment of their bone status before transplantation. This assessment should include parameters of mineral metabolism, PTH level, x-rays of the spine, and measurement of BMD of the hip, spine, and radius. KDIGO developed recommendations for the evaluation and treatment of bone disease in renal transplant recipients (7). These recommendations include monitoring serum calcium, phosphate, 25OHD, PTH, and alkaline phosphatase at specific intervals. Moreover, the guidelines also recommended measuring BMD in the first 3 months after kidney transplant if they receive corticosteroids or have risk factors for osteoporosis. Strategies to avoid or slow the bone loss that routinely develops in transplant recipients include: *First,* calcium supplements (800 to 1,200 mg elemental calcium per day) can be given along with nutritional vitamin D to correct vitamin D deficiency and active vitamin D analogs in order to increase positive calcium balance. *Second,* use the lowest possible dose of steroids. As cyclosporine has also been incriminated, replacing steroids with high doses of this agent is also problematic. Newer agents that permit very low doses of steroids or even steroid-free regimens offer great hope. *Third,* the use of antiresorptive agents such as bisphosphonates should be considered in patients who are at high fracture risk (337). Bisphosphonates are used to prevent bone mass loss and to treat osteoporosis. In renal transplant recipients, small doses of intravenous pamidronate, ibandronate, or zoledronate given at the time of transplantation have been reported to be associated with prevention of bone loss (338). A recent meta-analysis of RCTs concluded that bisphosphonates are effective in preventing bone loss in the early posttransplant period (339). Similar efficacy has been reported for heart transplantation, and others have found pamidronate very effective in preventing bone loss in patients treated with steroids for a variety of reasons (339). Its safety is well established in patients with renal disease (340). However, caution should be exercised with all bisphosphonates since they may induce or worsen the development of low turnover bone disease. Thus, KDIGO suggests to consider bone biopsy before the use of bisphosphonates due to the high incidence of ABD (7).

Unfortunately, once AVN develops, hip replacement will usually be required. However, for a small, asymptomatic lesion, inactivity and limited weight bearing may permit healing and recovery. Lesions greater than about 5 mm, however, usually will not respond to this conservative approach.

◈ REFERENCES

1. Eknoyan G, Lameire N, Barsoum R, et al. The burden of kidney disease: improving global outcomes. *Kidney Int* 2004;66:1310–1314.
2. Block GA, Klassen PS, Lazarus JM, et al. Mineral metabolism, mortality, and morbidity in maintenance hemodialysis. *J Am Soc Nephrol* 2004;15:2208–2218.
3. Foley RN, Parfrey PS, Sarnak MJ. Clinical epidemiology of cardiovascular disease in chronic renal disease. *Am J Kidney Dis* 1998;32(Suppl 3): S112–S119.
4. London GM, Guérin AP, Marchais SJ, et al. Arterial media calcification in end-stage renal disease. impact on all-cause and cardiovascular mortality. *Nephrol Dial Transplant* 2003;18:1731–1740.
5. Drüeke TB, Massy ZA. Atherosclerosis in CKD: differences from the general population. *Nat Rev Nephrol* 2010;6:723–735.
6. Palmer SC, Hayen A, Macaskill P, et al. Serum levels of phosphorus, parathyroid hormone, and calcium and risks of death and cardiovascular disease in individuals with chronic kidney disease: a systematic review and meta-analysis. *JAMA* 2011;305:1119–1127.

7. Kidney Disease: Improving Global Outcomes (KDIGO) CKD–MBD Work Group. KDIGO clinical practice guideline for the diagnosis, evaluation, prevention, and treatment of chronic kidney disease–mineral and bone disorder (CKD–MBD). *Kidney Int* 2009;76(Suppl 113):S1–S130.
8. Moe S, Drüeke T, Cunningham J, et al. Definition, evaluation, and classification of renal osteodystrophy: a position statement from Kidney Disease: Improving Global Outcomes (KDIGO). *Kidney Int* 2006;69:1945–1953.
9. Hamdy NA, Kanis JA, Beneton MN, et al. Effect of alfacalcidol on natural course of renal bone disease in mild to moderate renal failure. *BMJ* 1995;310:358–363.
10. Coen G, Ballanti P, Bonucci E, et al. Renal osteodystrophy in predialysis and hemodialysis patients: comparison of histologic patterns and diagnostic predictivity of intact PTH. *Nephron* 2002;91:103–111.
11. Qunibi WY, Abouzahr F, Mizani MR, et al. Cardiovascular calcification in Hispanic Americans (HA) with chronic kidney disease (CKD) due to type 2 diabetes. *Kidney Int* 2005;68:271–277.
12. Qunibi WY. Cardiovascular calcification in nondialyzed patients with chronic kidney disease. *Semin Dial* 2007;20:134–138.
13. Budoff MJ, Rader DJ, Reilly MP, et al. Relationship of estimated GFR and coronary artery calcification in the CRIC (Chronic Renal Insufficiency Cohort) study. *Am J Kidney Dis* 2011;58:519–526.
14. Levin A, Bakris GL, Molitch M, et al. Prevalence of abnormal serum vitamin D, PTH, calcium, and phosphorus in patients with chronic kidney disease: results of the study to evaluate early kidney disease. *Kidney Int* 2007;71:31–38.
15. Vassalotti JA, Uribarri J, Chen SC, et al. Trends in mineral metabolism: Kidney Early Evaluation Program (KEEP) and the National Health and Nutrition Examination Survey (NHANES) 1999–2004. *Am J Kidney Dis* 2008;51:S56–S68.
16. Melamed ML, Eustace JA, Plantinga LC, et al. Third-generation parathyroid hormone assays and all-cause mortality in incident dialysis patients: the CHOICE study. *Nephrol Dial Transplant* 2008;23: 1650–1658.
17. Regidor DL, Kovesdy CP, Mehrotra R, et al. Serum alkaline phosphatase predicts mortality among maintenance hemodialysis patients. *J Am Soc Nephrol* 2008;19:2193–2203.
18. Hruska KA, Mathew S, Lund R, et al. Hyperphosphatemia of chronic kidney disease. *Kidney Int* 2008;74(2):148–157.
19. Kalantar-Zadeh K, Gutekunst L, Mehrotra R, et al. Understanding sources of dietary phosphorus in the treatment of patients with chronic kidney disease. *Clin J Am Soc Nephrol* 2010;5:519–530.
20. Uribarri J. Phosphorus additives in food and their effect in dialysis patients. *Clin J Am Soc Nephrol* 2009;4:1290–1292.
21. Weinman EJ, Light PD, Suki WN. Gastrointestinal phosphate handling in CKD and its association with cardiovascular disease. *Am J Kidney Dis* 2013;62:1006–1011.
22. Marks J, Debnam ES, Unwin RJ. The role of the gastrointestinal tract in phosphate homeostasis in health and chronic kidney disease. *Curr Opin Nephrol Hypertens* 2013;22:481–487.
23. Portale AA, Halloran BP, Morris RC Jr. Dietary intake of phosphorus modulates the circadian rhythm in serum concentration of phosphorus. Implications for the renal production of 1,25-dihydroxyvitamin D. *J Clin Invest* 1987;80:1147–1154.
24. de Boer IH, Rue TC, Kestenbaum B. Serum phosphorus concentrations in the Third National Health and Nutrition Examination Survey (NHANES III). *Am J Kidney Dis* 2009;53:399–407.
25. Ix JH, Anderson CAM, Smits G, et al. Effect of dietary phosphate intake on the circadian rhythm of serum phosphate concentrations in chronic kidney disease: a crossover study. *Am J Clin Nutr* 2014;100:1392–1397.
26. Trivedi H, Moore H, Atalla J. Lack of significant circadian and postprandial variation in phosphate levels in subjects receiving chronic hemodialysis therapy. *J Nephrol* 2005;18:417–422.
27. Noori N, Kalantar-Zadeh K, Kovesdy CP, et al. Association of dietary phosphorus intake and phosphorus to protein ratio with mortality in hemodialysis patients. *Clin J Am Soc Nephrol* 2010;5:683–692.
28. Fouque D, Horne R, Cozzolino M, et al. Balancing nutrition and serum phosphorus in maintenance dialysis. *Am J Kidney Dis* 2014;64: 143–150.

29. Tonelli M. Serum phosphorus in people with chronic kidney disease: you are what you eat. *Kidney Int* 2013;84:871–873.

30. Lowrie EG, Lew NL. Death risk in hemodialysis patients: the predictive value of commonly measured variables and an evaluation of death rate differences between facilities. *Am J Kidney Dis* 1990;15:458–482.

31. Kalantar-Zadeh K, Kuwae N, Regidor DL, et al. Survival predictability of time-varying indicators of bone disease in maintenance hemodialysis patients. *Kidney Int* 2006;70:771–780.

32. Tentori F, Blayney MJ, Albert JM, et al. Mortality risk for dialysis patients with different levels of serum calcium, phosphorus, and PTH: the Dialysis Outcomes and Practice Patterns Study (DOPPS). *Am J Kidney Dis* 2008;52:519–530.

33. Kestenbaum B, Sampson JN, Rudser KD, et al. Serum phosphate levels and mortality risk among people with chronic kidney disease. *J Am Soc Nephrol* 2005;16:520–528.

34. Tonelli M, Sacks F, Pfeffer M, et al. Relation between serum phosphate level and cardiovascular event rate in people with coronary disease. *Circulation* 2005;112:2627–2633.

35. Foley RN, Collins AJ, Ishani A, et al. Calcium-phosphate levels and cardiovascular disease in community-dwelling adults: the Atherosclerosis Risk in Communities (ARIC) Study. *Am Heart J* 2008;156:556–563.

36. Kendrick J, Ix JH, Targher G, et al. Relation of serum phosphorus levels to ankle brachial pressure index (from the Third National Health and Nutrition Examination Survey). *Am J Cardiol* 2010;106:564–568.

37. Dhingra R, Sullivan LM, Fox CS, et al. Relations of serum phosphorus and calcium levels to the incidence of cardiovascular disease in the community. *Arch Intern Med* 2007;167:879–885.

38. Bricker NS. On the pathogenesis of the uremic state. An exposition of the "trade-off hypothesis." *N Engl J Med* 1972;286:1093–1099.

39. Laflamme GH, Jowsey J. Bone and soft tissue changes with oral phosphate supplements. *J Clin Invest* 1972;51:2834–2840.

40. Jowsey J, Reiss E, Canterbury JM. Long-term effects of high phosphate intake on parathyroid hormone levels and bone metabolism. *Acta Orthop Scand* 1974;45:801–808.

41. Rutherford WE, Bordier P, Marie P, et al. Phosphate control and 25-hydroxycholecalciferol administration in preventing experimental renal osteodystrophy in the dog. *J Clin Invest* 1977;60:332–341.

42. Slatopolsky E, Finch J, Denda M, et al. Phosphorus restriction prevents parathyroid gland growth. High phosphorus directly stimulates PTH secretion in vitro. *J Clin Invest* 1996;97:2534–2540.

43. Tanaka Y, Deluca HF. The control of 25-hydroxyvitamin D metabolism by inorganic phosphorus. *Arch Biochem Biophys* 1973;154:566–574.

44. Almaden Y, Hernandez A, Torregrosa V, et al. High phosphate level directly stimulates parathyroid hormone secretion and synthesis by human parathyroid tissue in vitro. *J Am Soc Nephrol* 1998;9:1845–1852.

45. Almaden Y, Canalejo A, Hernandez A, et al. Direct effect of phosphorus on PTH secretion from whole rat parathyroid glands in vitro. *J Bone Miner Res* 1996;11:970–976.

46. Kilav R, Silver J, Naveh-Many T. Parathyroid hormone gene expression in hypophosphatemic rats. *J Clin Invest* 1995;96:327–333.

47. Yalcindag C, Silver J, Naveh-Many T. Mechanism of increased parathyroid hormone mRNA in experimental uremia: roles of protein RNA binding and RNA degradation. *J Am Soc Nephrol* 1999;10:2562–2568.

48. Sela-Brown A, Naveh-Many T, Silver J. Transcriptional and posttranscriptional regulation of PTH gene expression by vitamin D, calcium and phosphate. *Miner Electrolyte Metab* 1999;25:342–344.

49. Sela-Brown A, Silver J, Brewer G, et al. Identification of AUF1 as a parathyroid hormone mRNA 3′-untranslated region-binding protein that determines parathyroid hormone mRNA stability. *J Biol Chem* 2000;275:7424–7429.

50. Almadén Y, Canalejo A, Ballesteros E, et al. Effect of high extracellular phosphate concentration on arachidonic acid production by parathyroid tissue in vitro. *J Am Soc Nephrol* 2000;11:1712–1718.

51. Dusso AS, Pavlopoulos T, Naumovich L, et al. p21(WAF1) and transforming growth factor-alpha mediate dietary phosphate regulation of parathyroid cell growth. *Kidney Int* 2001;59:855–865.

52. Hoenderop JG, Nilius B, Bindels RJ. Calcium absorption across epithelia. *Physiol Rev* 2005;85:373.

53. Bronner F, Pansu D, Stein WD. An analysis of intestinal calcium transport across the rat intestine. *Am J Physiol* 1986;250:G561.

54. Kumar R. Vitamin D and calcium transport. *Kidney Int* 1991;40:1177.

55. Kumar R, Thompson JR. The regulation of parathyroid hormone secretion and synthesis. *J Am Soc Nephrol* 2011;22:216–224.

56. Spiegel DM, Brady K. Calcium balance in normal individuals and in patients with chronic kidney disease on low- and high-calcium diets. *Kidney Int* 2012;81:1116–1122.

57. Hill KM, Martin BR, Wastney ME, et al. Oral calcium carbonate affects calcium but not phosphorus balance in stage 3-4 chronic kidney disease. *Kidney Int* 2013;83:959–966.

58. Brown EM. Four-parameter model of the sigmoidal relationship between parathyroid hormone release and extracellular calcium concentration in normal and abnormal parathyroid tissue. *J Clin Endocrinol Metab* 1983;56:572.

59. Talmage RV, Mobley HT. Calcium homeostasis: reassessment of the actions of parathyroid hormone. *Gen Comp Endocrinol* 2008;156:1–8.

60. de Groot T, Lee K, Langeslag M, et al. Parathyroid hormone activates TRPV5 via PKA-dependent phosphorylation. *J Am Soc Nephrol* 2009;20:1693.

61. Slatopolsky E, Brown A, Dusso A. Role of phosphorus in the pathogenesis of secondary hyperparathyroidism. *Am J Kidney Dis* 2001;37(Suppl 2):S54–S57.

62. Lopez-Hilker S, Galceran T, Chan YL, et al. Hypocalcemia may not be essential for the development of secondary hyperparathyroidism in chronic renal failure. *J Clin Invest* 1986;78:1097–1102.

63. Pitts TO, Piraino BH, Mitro R, et al. Hyperparathyroidism and 1,25-dihydroxyvitamin D deficiency in mild, moderate, and severe renal failure. *J Clin Endocrinol Metab* 1988;67:876.

64. Gutierrez O, Isakova T, Rhee E, et al. Fibroblast growth factor-23 mitigates hyperphosphatemia but accentuates calcitriol deficiency in chronic kidney disease. *J Am Soc Nephrol* 2005;16:2205.

65. Silver J, Levi R. Cellular and molecular mechanisms of secondary hyperparathyroidism. *Clin Nephrol* 2005;63:119.

66. Brown EM, Gamba G, Riccardi D, et al. Cloning and characterization of an extracellular Ca(2+)-sensing receptor from bovine parathyroid. *Nature* 1993;366:575–580.

67. Kovacs CS, Ho-Pao CL, Hunzelman JL, et al. Regulation of murine fetal-placental calcium metabolism by the calcium-sensing receptor. *J Clin Invest* 1998;101:2812–2820.

68. Li YC, Amling M, Pirro AE, et al. Normalization of mineral ion homeostasis by dietary means prevents hyperparathyroidism, rickets, and osteomalacia, but not alopecia in vitamin D receptor-ablated mice. *Endocrinology* 1998;139:4391–4396.

69. Gogusev J, Duchambon P, Hory B, et al. Depressed expression of calcium receptor in parathyroid gland tissue of patients with hyperparathyroidism. *Kidney Int* 1997;51:328–336.

70. Yano S, Sugimoto T, Tsukamoto T, et al. Association of decreased calcium-sensing receptor expression with proliferation of parathyroid cells in secondary hyperparathyroidism. *Kidney Int* 2000;58:1980–1986.

71. Cañadillas S, Canalejo A, Santamaría R, et al. Calcium-sensing receptor expression and parathyroid hormone secretion in hyperplastic parathyroid glands from humans. *J Am Soc Nephrol* 2005;16:2190–2197.

72. Brown AJ, Ritter CS, Finch JL, et al. Decreased calcium-sensing receptor expression in hyperplastic parathyroid glands of uremic rats: role of dietary phosphate. *Kidney Int* 1999;55:1284–1292.

73. Kawata T, Imanishi Y, Kobayashi K, et al. Direct in vitro evidence of the suppressive effect of cinacalcet HCl on parathyroid hormone secretion in human parathyroid cells with pathologically reduced calcium-sensing receptor levels. *J Bone Miner Metab* 2006;24:300–306.

74. Colloton M, Shatzen E, Miller G, et al. Cinacalcet HCl attenuates parathyroid hyperplasia in a rat model of secondary hyperparathyroidism. *Kidney Int* 2005;67:467–476.

75. Gkika D, Hsu YJ, van der Kemp AW, et al. Critical role of the epithelial Ca2+ channel TRPV5 in active Ca2+ reabsorption as revealed by TRPV5/calbindin-D28K knockout mice. *J Am Soc Nephrol* 2006;17:3020–3027.

76. Lieben L, Carmeliet G. Vitamin D signaling in osteocytes: effects on bone and mineral homeostasis. *Bone* 2013;54:237–243.

77. Qunibi W, Abdellatif A, Sankar S, et al. Treatment of vitamin D deficiency in CKD patients with ergocalciferol: are current KDOQI treatment guidelines adequate? *Clin Nephrol* 2010;73:276–285.

78. Shimada T, Hasegawa H, Yamazaki Y, et al. FGF-23 is a potent regulator of vitamin D metabolism and phosphate homeostasis. *J Bone Miner Res* 2004;19:429–435.

79. Taal MW, Thurston V, McIntyre NJ, et al. The impact of vitamin D status on the relative increase in fibroblast growth factor 23 and parathyroid hormone in chronic kidney disease. *Kidney Int* 2014;86:407–413.

80. Garrett G, Sardiwal S, Lamb EJ, et al. PTH—a particularly tricky hormone: why measure it at all in kidney patients? *Clin J Am Soc Nephrol* 2013;8:299–312.

81. Slatopolsky E, Finch J, Clay P, et al. A novel mechanism for skeletal resistance in uremia. *Kidney Int* 2000;58:753–761.

82. Murray TM, Rao LG, Divieti P, et al. Parathyroid hormone secretion and action: evidence for discrete receptors for the carboxyl-terminal region and related biological actions of carboxyl-terminal ligands. *Endocr Rev* 2005;26:78–113.

83. Habener JF, Rosenblatt M, Potts JT Jr. Parathyroid hormone: biochemical aspects of biosynthesis, secretion, action, and metabolism. *Physiol Rev* 1984;64:985–1053.

84. Kumar R. Metabolism of 1,25-dihydroxyvitamin D3. *Physiol Rev* 1984;64:478–504.

85. Klahr S, Slatopolsky E. Toxicity of parathyroid hormone in uremia. *Annu Rev Med.* 1986;37:71–78.

86. Burnett-Bowie SM, Henao MP, Dere ME, et al. Effects of hPTH(1-34) infusion on circulating serum phosphate, 1,25-dihydroxyvitamin D, and FGF23 levels in healthy men. *J Bone Miner Res* 2009;24:1681–1685.

87. Wesseling-Perry K, Harkins GC, Wang HJ, et al. The calcemic response to continuous parathyroid hormone (PTH)(1-34) infusion in end-stage kidney disease varies according to bone turnover: a potential role for PTH(7-84). *J Clin Endocrinol Metab* 2010;95:2772–2780.

88. Lavi-Moshayoff V, Wasserman G, Meir T, et al. PTH increases FGF23 gene expression and mediates the high-FGF23 levels of experimental kidney failure: a bone parathyroid feedback loop. *Am J Physiol Renal Physiol* 2010;299:F882–F889.

89. Kawata T, Imanishi Y, Kobayashi K, et al. Parathyroid hormone regulates fibroblast growth factor-23 in a mouse model of primary hyperparathyroidism. *J Am Soc Nephrol* 2007;18:2683–2688.

90. Lopez I, Rodriguez-Ortiz ME, Almaden Y, et al. Direct and indirect effects of parathyroid hormone on circulating levels of fibroblast growth factor 23 in vivo. *Kidney Int* 2011;80:475–482.

91. Neves KR, Graciolli FG, dos Reis LM, et al. Vascular calcification: contribution of parathyroid hormone in renal failure. *Kidney Int* 2007;71:1262–1270.

92. Feinfeld D. The role of parathyroid hormone as a uremic toxin: current concepts. *Semin Dial* 1992;5:48–53.

93. Rodriguez M, Lorenzo V. Parathyroid hormone, a uremic toxin. *Semin Dial* 2009;22:363–368.

94. Young EW, Albert JM, Satayathum S, et al. Predictors and consequences of altered mineral metabolism: the Dialysis Outcomes And Practice Patterns Study. *Kidney Int* 2005;67:1179–1187.

95. Tentori F, Wang M, Bieber BA, et al. Recent changes in therapeutic approaches and association with outcomes among patients with secondary hyperparathyroidism on chronic hemodialysis: the DOPPS study. *Clin J Am Soc Nephrol* 2015;710:98–109.

96. Souberbielle JC, Roth H, Fouque DP. Parathyroid hormone measurement in CKD. *Kidney Int* 2010;77:93–100.

97. Hecking M, Kainz A, Bielesz B, et al. Clinical evaluation of two novel biointact PTH(1-84) assays in hemodialysis patients. *Clin Biochem* 2012;45:1645–1651.

98. Tan K, Ong L, Sethi SK, et al. Comparison of the Elecsys PTH(1-84) assay with four contemporary second generation intact PTH assays and association with other biomarkers in chronic kidney disease patients. *Clin Biochem* 2013;46:781–786.

99. Sprague SM, Moe SM. The case for routine parathyroid hormone monitoring. *Clin J Am Soc Nephrol* 2013;8:313–318.

100. Qunibi W, Kalantar-Zadeh K. Target levels for serum phosphorus and parathyroid hormone. *Semin Dial* 2011;24:29–33.

101. Floege J, Kim J, Ireland E, et al. Serum iPTH, calcium and phosphate, and the risk of mortality in a European haemodialysis population. *Nephrol Dial Transplant* 2011;26:1948–1955.

102. Naves-Díaz M, Passlick-Deetjen J, Guinsburg A, et al. Calcium, phosphorus, PTH and death rates in a large sample of dialysis patients from Latin America. The CORES Study. *Nephrol Dial Transplant* 2011;26:1938–1947.

103. Fukagawa M, Yokogama K, Koiiwa F, et al. Clinical practice guideline for the management of chronic kidney disease-mineral and bone disorder. *Ther Apher Dial* 2013;17:247–288.

104. van Ballegooijen AJ, Visser M, Kestenbaum B, et al. Relation of vitamin D and parathyroid hormone to cardiac biomarkers and to left ventricular mass (from the Cardiovascular Health Study). *Am J Cardiol* 2013;111:418–424.

105. Liu S, Gupta A, Quarles LD. Emerging role of fibroblast growth factor 23 in a bone-kidney axis regulating systemic phosphate homeostasis and extracellular matrix mineralization. *Curr Opin Nephrol Hypertens* 2007;16:329–335.

106. Liu S, Quarles LD. How fibroblast growth factor 23 works. *J Am Soc Nephrol* 2007;18:1637–1647.

107. Quinn SJ, Thomsen AR, Pang JL, et al. Interactions between calcium and phosphorus in the regulation of the production of fibroblast growth factor 23 in vivo. *Am J Physiol Endocrinol Metab* 2013;304:E310–E20.

108. Miyamoto K, Ito M, Tatsumi S, et al. New aspect of renal phosphate reabsorption: the type IIc sodium-dependent phosphate transporter. *Am J Nephrol* 2007;27:503–515.

109. Saito H, Kusano K, Kinosaki M, et al. Human fibroblast growth factor-23 mutants suppress Na+-dependent phosphate co-transport activity and 1alpha,25-dihydroxyvitamin D3 production. *J Biol Chem* 2003;278:2206–2211.

110. Hu MC, Shiizaki K, Kuro-o M, et al. Fibroblast growth factor 23 and Klotho: physiology and pathophysiology of an endocrine network of mineral metabolism. *Annu Rev Physiol* 2013;75:503–533.

111. Rhee Y, Bivi N, Farrow E, et al. Parathyroid hormone receptor signaling in osteocytes increases the expression of fibroblast growth factor-23 in vitro and in vivo. *Bone* 2011;49:636–643.

112. Ben-Dov IZ, Galitzer H, Lavi-Moshayoff V, et al. The parathyroid is a target organ for FGF23 in rats. *J Clin Invest* 2007;117:4003–4008.

113. Krajisnik T, Bjorklund P, Marsell R, et al. Fibroblast growth factor-23 regulates parathyroid hormone and 1alpha-hydroxylase expression in cultured bovine parathyroid cells. *J Endocrinol* 2007;195:125–131.

114. Komaba H, Goto S, Fujii H, et al. Depressed expression of Klotho and FGF receptor 1 in hyperplastic parathyroid glands from uremic patients. *Kidney Int* 2010;77:232–238.

115. Canalejo R, Canalejo A, Martinez-Moreno JM, et al. FGF23 fails to inhibit uremic parathyroid glands. *J Am Soc Nephrol* 2010;21:1125–1135.

116. Urakawa I, Yamazaki Y, Shimada T, et al. Klotho converts canonical FGF receptor into a specific receptor for FGF23. *Nature* 2006;444:770–774.

117. Galitzer H, Ben-Dov IZ, Silver J, et al. Parathyroid cell resistance to fibroblast growth factor 23 in secondary hyperparathyroidism of chronic kidney disease. *Kidney Int* 2010;77:211–218.

118. Forster RE, Jurutka PW, Hsieh JC, et al. Vitamin D receptor controls expression of the anti-aging klotho gene in mouse and human renal cells. *Biochem Biophys Res Commun* 2011;414:557–562.

119. Tsujikawa H, Kurotaki Y, Fujimori T, et al. Klotho, a gene related to a syndrome resembling human premature aging, functions in a negative regulatory circuit of vitamin D endocrine system. *Mol Endocrinol* 2003;17:2393–2403.

120. Kuro-o M. Klotho as a regulator of fibroblast growth factor signaling and phosphate/calcium metabolism. *Curr Opin Nephrol Hypertens* 2006;15:437–441.

121. Kuro-o M. Klotho in health and disease. *Curr Opin Nephrol Hypertens* 2012;21:362–368.

122. Larsson T, Nisbeth U, Ljunggren O, et al. Circulating concentration of FGF-23 increases as renal function declines in patients with chronic kidney disease, but does not change in response to variation in phosphate intake in healthy volunteers. *Kidney Int* 2003;64:2272–2279.

123. Imanishi Y, Inaba M, Nakatsuka K, et al. FGF-23 in patients with end-stage renal disease on hemodialysis. *Kidney Int* 2004;65:1943–1946.

124. Asai O, Nakatani K, Tanaka T, et al. Decreased renal α-Klotho expression in early diabetic nephropathy in humans and mice and its possible role in urinary calcium excretion. *Kidney Int* 2012;81:539–547.

125. Faul C, Amaral AP, Oskouei B, et al. FGF23 induces left ventricular hypertrophy. *J Clin Invest* 2011;121:4393–4408.

126. Isakova T, Ix JH, Sprague SM, et al. Rationale and approaches to phosphate and fibroblast growth factor 23 reduction in CKD. *J Am Soc Nephrol* 2015;26(10):2328–2339.

127. Hu MC, Shi M, Zhang J, et al. Klotho deficiency causes vascular calcification in chronic kidney disease. *J Am Soc Nephrol* 2011;22:124–136.

128. Ozkok A, Kekik C, Karahan GE, et al. FGF-23 associated with the progression of coronary artery calcification in hemodialysis patients. *BMC Nephrol* 2013;14:241–247.

129. Scialla JJ, Lau WL, Reilly MP, et al. Fibroblast growth factor 23 is not associated with and does not induce arterial calcification. *Kidney Int* 2013;83:1159–1168.

130. Lim K, Lu TS, Molostvov G, et al. Vascular Klotho deficiency potentiates the development of human artery calcification and mediates resistance to fibroblast growth factor 23. *Circulation* 2012;125:2243–2255.

131. Gutiérrez OM, Mannstadt M, Isakova T, et al. Fibroblast growth factor 23 and mortality among patients undergoing hemodialysis. *N Engl J Med* 2008;359:584–592.

132. Isakova T, Xie H, Yang W, et al. Fibroblast growth factor 23 and risks of mortality and end-stage renal disease in patients with chronic kidney disease. *JAMA* 2011;305:2432–2439.

133. Shroff RC, McNair R, Skepper JN, et al. Chronic mineral dysregulation promotes vascular smooth muscle cell adaptation and extracellular matrix calcification. *J Am Soc Nephrol* 2010;21:103–112.

134. Fang Y, Ginsberg C, Sugatani T, et al. Early chronic kidney disease-mineral bone disorder stimulates vascular calcification. *Kidney Int* 2014;85:142–150.

135. McCullough PA, Agrawal V, Danielewicz E, et al. Accelerated atherosclerotic calcification and Monckeberg's sclerosis: a continuum of advanced vascular pathology in chronic kidney disease. *Clin J Am Soc Nephrol* 2008;3:1585–1598.

136. Amann K. Media calcification and intima calcification are distinct entities in chronic kidney disease. *Clin J Am Soc Nephrol* 2008;3:1599–1605.

137. Qunibi WY, Nolan CR, Ayus JC. Cardiovascular calcification in patients with end-stage renal disease: a century-old phenomenon. *Kidney Int* 2002;(82):S73–S80.

138. Paloian NJ, Giachelli CM. A current understanding of vascular calcification in CKD. *Am J Physiol Renal Physiol* 2014;307:F891–F900.

139. Jono S, McKee MD, Murry CE, et al. Phosphate regulation of vascular smooth muscle cell calcification. *Circ Res* 2000;87:e10–e17.

140. Shroff R, Long DA, Shanahan C. Mechanistic insights into vascular calcification in CKD. *J Am Soc Nephrol* 2013;24:179–189.

141. Reynolds JL, Joannides AJ, Skepper JN, et al. Human vascular smooth muscle cells undergo vesicle-mediated calcification in response to changes in extracellular calcium and phosphate concentrations: a potential mechanism for accelerated vascular calcification in ESRD. *J Am Soc Nephrol* 2004;15:2857–2867.

142. Son BK, Kozaki K, Iijima K, et al. Statins protect human aortic smooth muscle cells from inorganic phosphate-induced calcification by restoring Gas6-Axl survival pathway. *Circ Res* 2006;98:1024–1031.

143. Chertow GM, Burke SK, Raggi P. Sevelamer attenuates the progression of coronary and aortic calcification in hemodialysis patients. *Kidney Int* 2002;62:245–252.

144. Block GA, Spiegel DM, Ehrlich J, et al. Effects of sevelamer and calcium on coronary artery calcification in patients new to hemodialysis. *Kidney Int* 2005;68:1815–1824.

145. Russo D, Miranda I, Ruocco C, et al. The progression of coronary artery calcification in predialysis patients on calcium carbonate or sevelamer. *Kidney Int* 2007;72:1255–1261.

146. Suki WN; for the Dialysis Clinical Outcomes Revisited Investigators. Effects of sevelamer and calcium-based phosphate binders on mortality in hemodialysis patients: results of a randomized clinical trial. *J Ren Nutr* 2008;18:91–98.

147. Jamal SA, Vandermeer B, Raggi P, et al. Effect of calcium-based versus non-calcium-based phosphate binders on mortality in patients with chronic kidney disease: an updated systematic review and meta-analysis. *Lancet* 2013;382:1268–1277.

148. Qunibi W, Moustafa M, Muenz LR, et al. A 1-year randomized trial of calcium acetate versus sevelamer on progression of coronary artery calcification in hemodialysis patients with comparable lipid control: the Calcium Acetate Renagel Evaluation-2 (CARE-2) study. *Am J Kidney Dis* 2008;51:952–965.

149. Barreto DV, Barreto Fde C, de Carvalho AB, et al. Phosphate binder impact on bone remodeling and coronary calcification—results from the BRiC study. *Nephron* 2008;110:c273–c283.

150. St. Peter WL, Liu J, Weinhandl E, et al. A comparison of sevelamer and calcium-based phosphate binders on mortality, hospitalization, and morbidity in hemodialysis: a secondary analysis of the Dialysis Clinical Outcomes Revisited (DCOR) randomized trial using claims data. *Am J Kidney Dis* 2008;51:445–454.

151. Tonelli M, Wiebe N, Culleton B, et al. Systematic review of the clinical efficacy and safety of sevelamer in dialysis patients. *Nephrol Dial Transplant* 2007;22:2856–2866.

152. Block GA, Wheeler DC, Persky MS, et al. Effects of phosphate binders in moderate CKD. *J Am Soc Nephrol* 2012;23:1407–1415.

153. Tonelli M, Pannu N, Manns B. Oral phosphate binders in patients with kidney failure. *N Engl J Med* 2010;362:1312–1324.

154. Isakova T, Gutierrez OM, Chang Y, et al. Phosphorus binders and survival on hemodialysis. *J Am Soc Nephrol* 2009;20:388–396.

155. Cannata-Andía JB, Fernández-Martín JL, Locatelli F, et al. Use of phosphate-binding agents is associated with a lower risk of mortality. *Kidney Int* 2013;84:998–1008.

156. Winkelmayer WC, Liu J, Kestenbaum B. Comparative effectiveness of calcium-containing phosphate binders in incident U.S. dialysis patients. *Clin J Am Soc Nephrol* 2011;6:175–183.

157. Blacher J, Guerin AP, Pannier B, et al. Impact of aortic stiffness on survival in end-stage renal disease. *Circulation* 1999;99:2434–2439.

158. Wilson PW, Kauppila LI, O'Donnell CJ, et al. Abdominal aortic calcific deposits are an important predictor of vascular morbidity and mortality. *Circulation* 2001;103:1529–1534.

159. Miller PD. Bone disease in CKD: a focus on osteoporosis diagnosis and management. *Am J Kidney Dis* 2014;64:290–304.

160. Malluche HH, Davenport DL, Cantor T, et al. Bone mineral density and serum biochemical predictors of bone loss in patients with CKD on dialysis. *Clin J Am Soc Nephrol* 2014;9:1254–1262.

161. Sherrard DJ, Hercz G, Pei Y, et al. The spectrum of bone disease in end-stage renal failure: an evolving disorder. *Kidney Int* 1993; 43:436–442.

162. Malluche H, Ritz E, Lange H. Bone histology in incipient and advanced renal failure. *Kidney Int* 1976;9:355–362.

163. Cunningham J, Locatelli F, Rodriguez M. Secondary hyperparathyroidism: pathogenesis, disease progression, and therapeutic options. *Clin J Am Soc Nephrol* 2011;6:913–921.

164. Hruska K, Teitelbaum S. Renal osteodystrophy. *N Engl J of Med* 1995;333:166–174.

165. Martinez I, Saracho R, Montenegro J, et al. The importance of dietary calcium and phosphorous in the secondary hyperparathyroidism of patients with early renal failure. *Am J of Kidney Dis* 1997;29:496–502.

166. Riccardi D, Brown EM. Physiology and pathophysiology of the calcium-sensing receptor in the kidney. *Am J Physiol Renal Physiol* 2010;298:F485–F499.

167. Tu Q, Pi M, Karsenty G, et al. Rescue of the skeletal phenotype in CasR-deficient mice by transfer onto the Gcm2 null background. *J Clin Invest* 2003;111:1029.

168. Houillier P, Paillard M. Calcium-sensing receptor and renal cation handling. *Nephrol Dial Transplant* 2003;18:2467–2470.

169. Tfelt-Hansen J, Brown EM. The calcium-sensing receptor in normal physiology and pathophysiology: a review. *Crit Rev Clin Lab Sci* 2005;42:35–70.

170. Block GA, Martin KJ, de Francisco AL, et al. Cinacalcet for secondary hyperparathyroidism in patients receiving hemodialysis. *N Engl J Med* 2004;350:1516–1525.

171. Craver L, Marco MP, Martínez I, et al. Mineral metabolism parameters throughout chronic kidney disease stages 1-5—achievement of K/DOQI target ranges. *Nephrol Dial Transplant* 2007;22:1171–1176.

172. Fukagawa M, Kazama JJ. With or without the kidney: the role of FGF23 in CKD. *Nephrol Dial Transplant* 2005;20:1295–1298.

173. Gonzalez EA, Sachdeva A, Oliver DA, et al. Vitamin D insufficiency and deficiency in chronic kidney disease. A single center observational study. *Am J Nephrol* 2004;24:503–510.

174. Nykjaer A, Dragun D, Walther D, et al. An endocytic pathway essential for renal uptake and activation of the steroid 25-(OH) vitamin D3. *Cell* 1999;96:507–515.

175. Silver J, Russell J, Sherwood LM. Regulation by vitamin D metabolites of messenger ribonucleic acid for preproparathyroid hormone in isolated bovine parathyroid cells. *Proc Natl Acad Sci U S A* 1985;82:4270–4273.

176. Naveh-Many T, Silver J. Regulation of parathyroid hormone gene expression by hypocalcemia, hypercalcemia, and vitamin D in the rat. *J Clin Invest* 1990;86:1313–1319.

177. Merke J, Hügel U, Zlotkowski A, et al. Diminished parathyroid $1,25(OH)_2D_3$ receptors in experimental uremia. *Kidney Int* 1987;32:350–353.

178. Korkor AB. Reduced binding of [3H]1,25-dihydroxyvitamin D3 in the parathyroid glands of patients with renal failure. *N Engl J Med* 1987;316:1573–1577.

179. Brown AJ, Dusso A, Lopez-Hilker S, et al. 1,25-(OH)2D receptors are decreased in parathyroid glands from chronically uremic dogs. *Kidney Int* 1989;35:19–23.

180. Fukuda N, Tanaka H, Tominaga Y, et al. Decreased 1,25-dihydroxyvitamin D3 receptor density is associated with a more severe form of parathyroid hyperplasia in chronic uremic patients. *J Clin Invest* 1993;92:1436–1443.

181. Patel SR, Ke HQ, Vanholder R, et al. Inhibition of calcitriol receptor binding to vitamin D response elements by uremic toxins. *J Clin Invest* 1995;96:50–59.

182. Sawaya BP, Koszewski NJ, Qi Q, et al. Secondary hyperparathyroidism and vitamin D receptor binding to vitamin D response elements in rats with incipient renal failure. *J Am Soc Nephrol* 1997;8:271–278.

183. Dusso AS, Sato T, Arcidiacono MV, et al. Pathogenic mechanisms for parathyroid hyperplasia. *Kidney Int* 2006;70:S8–S11.

184. Naveh-Many T, Rahamimov R, Livni N, et al. Parathyroid cell proliferation in normal and chronic renal failure rats. The effects of calcium, phosphate, and vitamin D. *J Clin Invest* 1995;96:1786–1793.

185. Denda M, Finch J, Slatopolsky E. Phosphorus accelerates the development of parathyroid hyperplasia and secondary hyperparathyroidism in rats with renal failure. *Am J Kidney Dis* 1996;28:596–602.

186. Goodman WG, Belin T, Gales B, et al. Calcium-regulated parathyroid hormone release in patients with mild or advanced secondary hyperparathyroidism. *Kidney Int* 1995;48:1553–1558.

187. Kifor O, Moore FD Jr, Wang P, et al. Reduced immunostaining for the extracellular Ca2+-sensing receptor in primary and uremic secondary hyperparathyroidism. *J Clin Endocrinol Metab* 1996;81:1598–1606.

188. Mizobuchi M, Hatamura I, Ogata H, et al. Calcimimetic compound upregulates decreased calcium-sensing receptor expression level in parathyroid glands of rats with chronic renal insufficiency. *J Am Soc Nephrol* 2004;15:2579–2587.

189. Brown AJ, Zhong M, Finch J, et al. Rat calcium-sensing receptor is regulated by vitamin D but not by calcium. *Am J Physiol* 1996;270:F454–F460.

190. Drueke T, Martin D, Rodriguez M. Can calcimimetics inhibit parathyroid hyperplasia? Evidence from preclinical studies. *Nephrol Dial Transplant* 2007;22:1828–1839.

191. Tominaga Y, Takagi H. Molecular genetics of hyperparathyroid disease. *Curr Opin Nephrol Hypertens* 1996;5:336–341.

192. Drüeke TB. Cell biology of parathyroid gland hyperplasia in chronic renal failure. *J Am Soc Nephrol* 2000;11:1141–1152.

193. Goodman WG, Quarles LD. Development and progression of secondary hyperparathyroidism in chronic kidney disease: lessons from molecular genetics. *Kidney Int* 2008;74:276–288.

194. Ritter CS, Finch JL, Slatopolsky EA, et al. Parathyroid hyperplasia in uremic rats precedes down-regulation of the calcium receptor. *Kidney Int* 2001;60:1737–1744.

195. Evanson JM. The response to the infusion of parathyroid extract in hypocalcaemic states. *Clin Sci* 1966;31;63–75.

196. Massry SG, Coburn JW, Lee DB, et al. Skeletal resistance to parathyroid hormone in renal failure. Studies in 105 human subjects. *Ann Intern Med* 1973;78:357–364.

197. Fukagawa M, Iwasaki Y, Kazama JJ. Skeletal resistance to parathyroid hormone as a background abnormality in uremia. *Nephrology (Carlton)* 2003;(8 Suppl):S50–S52.

198. Somerville PJ, Kaye M. Evidence that resistance to the calcemic action of parathyroid hormone in rats with acute uremia is caused by phosphate retention. *Kidney Int* 1979;16:552–560.

199. Olgaard K, Arbelaez M, Schwartz J, et al. Abnormal skeletal response to parathyroid hormone in dogs with chronic uremia. *Calcif Tissue Int* 1982;34:403–407.

200. Picton ML, Moore PR, Mawer EB, et al. Down-regulation of human osteoblast PTH/PTHrP receptor mRNA in end-stage renal failure. *Kidney Int* 2000;58:1440–1449.

201. Somerville PJ, Kaye M. Resistance to parathyroid hormone in renal failure: role of vitamin D metabolites. *Kidney Int* 1978;14:245–254.

202. Massry SG, Stein R, Garty J, et al. Skeletal resistance to the calcemic action of parathyroid hormone in uremia: role of 1,25 (OH)2 D3. *Kidney Int* 1976;9:467–474.

203. Galceran T, Martin KJ, Morrissey JJ, et al. Role of 1,25-dihydroxyvitamin D on the skeletal resistance to parathyroid hormone. *Kidney Int* 1987;32:801–807.

204. Kazama JJ, Shigematsu T, Yano K, et al. Increased circulating levels of osteoclastogenesis inhibitory factor (osteoprotegerin) in patients with chronic renal failure. *Am J Kidney Dis* 2002;39:525–532.

205. Coen G, Ballanti P, Balucci A, et al. Serum osteoprotegerin and renal osteodystrophy. *Nephrol Dial Transplant* 2002;17:233–238.

206. Hruska K. New concepts in renal osteodystrophy. *Nephrol Dial Transplant* 1998;13:2755–2760.

207. Massry SG, Tuma S, Dua S, et al. Reversal of skeletal resistance to parathyroid hormone in uremia by vitamin D metabolites: evidence for the requirement of $1,25(OH)_2D_3$ and 24,25(OH)2D3. *J Lab Clin Med* 1979;94:152–157.

208. Morrow B, Qunibi W. Specific bone and mineral disorders in patients with chronic kidney disease. *Clin Rev Bone Miner Metab* 2012;10:184–209.

209. Hercz G, Pei Y, Greenwood C, et al. Aplastic osteodystrophy without aluminum: the role of "suppressed" parathyroid function. *Kidney Int* 1993;44:860–866.

210. Ferreira A, Frazão JM, Monier-Faugere MC, et al. Effects of sevelamer hydrochloride and calcium carbonate on renal osteodystrophy in hemodialysis patients. *J Am Soc Nephrol* 2008;19:405–412.

211. Martin KJ, Olgaard K, Coburn JW, et al. Diagnosis, assessment, and treatment of bone turnover abnormalities in renal osteodystrophy. *Am J Kidney Dis* 2004;43:558–565.

212. Changsirikulchai S, Domrongkitchaiporn S, Sirikulchayanonta V, et al. Renal osteodystrophy in Ramathibodi Hospital: histomorphometry and clinical correlation. *J Med Assoc Thai* 2000;83:1223–1232.

213. Brandenburg VM, Floege J. Adynamic bone disease—bone and beyond. *NDT Plus* 2008;1.135–147.

214. Spasovski GB, Bervoets AR, Behets GJ, et al. Spectrum of renal bone disease in end-stage renal failure patients not yet on dialysis. *Nephrol Dial Transplant* 2003;18:1159–1166.

215. Couttenye MM, D'Haese PC, Verschoren WJ, et al. Low bone turnover in patients with renal failure. *Kidney Int Suppl* 1999;73:S70–S76.

216. Andress DL. Adynamic bone in patients with chronic kidney disease. *Kidney Int* 2008;73:1345–1354.

217. Heaf J. Adynamic bone disease and malnutrition-inflammation-cachexia syndrome. *Kidney Int* 2007;71:1326.
218. Monier-Faugere MC, Geng Z, Friedler RM, et al. 22-oxacalcitriol suppresses secondary hyperparathyroidism without inducing low bone turnover in dogs with renal failure. *Kidney Int* 1999;55:821–832.
219. Spasovski G, Gelev S, Masin-Spasovska J, et al. Improvement of bone and mineral parameters related to adynamic bone disease by diminishing dialysate calcium. *Bone* 2007;41:698–703.
220. Mathew S, Lund RJ, Strebeck F, et al. Reversal of the adynamic bone disorder and decreased vascular calcification in chronic kidney disease by sevelamer carbonate therapy. *J Am Soc Nephrol* 2007;18:122–130.
221. Davies MR, Lund RJ, Mathew S, et al. Low turnover osteodystrophy and vascular calcification are amenable to skeletal anabolism in an animal model of chronic kidney disease and the metabolic syndrome. *J Am Soc Nephrol* 2005;16:917–928.
222. Hernandez D, Concepcion MT, Lorenzo V, et al. Adynamic bone disease with negative aluminium staining in predialysis patients: prevalence and evolution after maintenance dialysis. *Nephrol Dial Transplant* 1994;9:517–523.
223. Torres A, Lorenzo V, Hernandez D, et al. Bone disease in predialysis, hemodialysis, and CAPD patients: evidence of a better bone response to PTH. *Kidney Int* 1995;47:1434–1442.
224. Lund RJ, Davies MR, Brown AJ, et al. Successful treatment of an adynamic bone disorder with bone morphogenetic protein-7 in a renal ablation model. *J Am Soc Nephrol* 2004;15:359–369.
225. Piraino B, Chen T, Cooperstein L, et al. Fractures and vertebral bone mineral density in patients with renal osteodystrophy. *Clin Nephrol* 1988;30:57.
226. Coco M, Rush H. Increased incidence of hip fractures in dialysis patients with low serum parathyroid hormone. *Am J Kidney Dis* 2000;36:1115–1121.
227. Kurz P, Monier-Faugere MC, Bognar B, et al. Evidence for abnormal calcium homeostasis in patients with adynamic bone disease. *Kidney Int* 1994;46:855–861.
228. London GM, Marty C, Marchais SJ, et al. Arterial calcifications and bone histomorphometry in end-stage renal disease. *J Am Soc Nephrol* 2004;15:1943–1951.
229. London GM, Marchais SJ, Guérin AP, et al. Association of bone activity, calcium load, aortic stiffness, and calcifications in ESRD. *J Am Soc Nephrol* 2008;19:1827–1835.
230. Kleinman KS, Coburn JW. Amyloid syndromes associated with hemodialysis. *Kidney Int* 1989;35:567–575.
231. Kessler M, Netter P, Azoulay E, et al. Dialysis-associated arthropathy: a multicenter survey of 171 patients receiving hemodialysis for over 10 years. The Co-operative Group on Dialysis-associated Arthropathy. *Br J Rheumatol* 1992;31:157–162.
232. Onishi S, Andress DL, Maloney NA, et al. Beta 2-microglobulin deposition in bone in chronic renal failure. *Kidney Int* 1991;39:990–995.
233. Cianciolo G, Colí L, La Manna G, et al. Is beta2-microglobulin-related amyloidosis of hemodialysis patients a multifactorial disease? A new pathogenetic approach. *Int J Artif Organs* 2007;30:864–878.
234. Fry AC, Singh DK, Chandna SM, et al. Relative importance of residual renal function and convection in determining beta-2-microglobulin levels in high-flux haemodialysis and on-line haemodiafiltration. *Blood Purif* 2007;25:295–302.
235. Chanard J, Bindi P, Lavaud S, et al. Carpal tunnel syndrome and type of dialysis membrane. *BMJ* 1989;298:867–868.
236. Saito A, Gejyo F. Current clinical aspects of dialysis-related amyloidosis in chronic dialysis patients. *Ther Apher Dial* 2006;10:316–320.
237. Goodman WG, Goldin J, Kuizon BD, et al. Coronary-artery calcification in young adults with end-stage renal disease who are undergoing dialysis. *N Engl J Med* 2000;342:1478–1483.
238. Nigwekar SU, Kroshinsky D, Nazarian RM, et al. Calciphylaxis: risk factors, diagnosis, and treatment. *Am J Kidney Dis* 2015;66(1):133–146.
239. Brossard JH, Cloutier M, Roy L, et al. Accumulation of a non-(1-84) molecular form of parathyroid hormone (PTH) detected by intact PTH assay in renal failure: importance in the interpretation of PTH values. *J Clin Endocrinol Metab* 1996;81:3923–3929.
240. Souberbielle JC, Boutten A, Carlier MC, et al. Inter-method variability in PTH measurement: implication for the care of CKD patients. *Kidney Int* 2006;70:345–350.
241. Quarles LD, Lobaugh B, Murphy G. Intact parathyroid hormone overestimates the presence and severity of parathyroid-mediated osseous abnormalities in uremia. *J Clin Endocrinol Metab* 1992;75:145–150.
242. Wang W, Hercz G, Sherrard DJ, et al. Relationship between intact I-84 parathyroid hormone and bone histomorphometric parameters in dialysis patients without aluminum toxicity. *Am J Kidney Dis* 1995;26:836–844.
243. Andress DL, Norris KC, Coburn JW, et al. Intravenous calcitriol in the treatment of refractory osteitis fibrosa of chronic renal failure. *N Engl J Med* 1989;321:274–279.
244. Coen G, Bonucci E, Ballanti P, et al. PTH 1-84 and PTH "7-84" in the non-invasive diagnosis of renal bone disease. *Am J Kid Dis* 2002;40:348–354.
245. Monier-Faugere MC, Geng Z, Mawad H, et al. Improved assessment of bone turnover by the PTH-(1-84)/large C-PTH fragments in ESRD patients. *Kidney Int* 2001;60:1460–1468.
246. Goodman WG. Comments on plasma parathyroid hormone levels and their relationship to bone histopathology among patients undergoing dialysis. *Semin Dial* 2007;20:1–4.
247. Lau WL, Kalantar-Zadeh K. Towards the revival of alkaline phosphatase for the management of bone disease, mortality and hip fractures. *Nephrol Dial Transplant* 2014;29:1450–1452.
248. Sardiwal S, Magnusson P, Goldsmith DJ, et al. Bone alkaline phosphatase in CKD–mineral bone disorder. *Am J Kidney Dis* 2013;62:810–822.
249. Maruyama Y, Taniguchi M, Kazama JJ, et al. A higher serum alkaline phosphatase is associated with the incidence of hip fracture and mortality among patients receiving hemodialysis in Japan. *Nephrol Dial Transplant* 2014;29:1532–1538.
250. Nickolas TL, Cremers S, Zhang A, et al. Discriminants of prevalent fractures in chronic kidney disease. *J Am Soc Nephrol* 2011;22:1560–1572.
251. Adams JE. Dialysis bone disease. *Semin Dial* 2002;15:277–289.
252. Moorthi RN, Moe SM. Recent advances in the noninvasive diagnosis of renal osteodystrophy. *Kidney Int* 2013;84:886–894.
253. Jamal SA, Hayden JA, Beyene J. Low bone mineral density and fractures in long-term hemodialysis patients: a meta-analysis. *Am J Kidney Dis* 2007;49:674–681.
254. Yenchek RH, Ix JH, Shlipak MG, et al. Bone mineral density and fracture risk in older individuals with CKD. *Clin J Am Soc Nephrol* 2012;7:1130–1136.
255. Jamal SA, Gilbert J, Gordon C, et al. Cortical pQCT measures are associated with fractures in dialysis patients. *J Bone Miner Res* 2006;21:543–548.
256. Moorthi RN, Moe SM. CKD—mineral and bone disorder: core curriculum 2011. *Am J Kidney Dis* 2011;58:1022–1036.
257. Moe SM, Zidehsarai MP, Chambers MA, et al. Vegetarian compared with meat dietary protein source and phosphorus homeostasis in chronic kidney disease. *Clin J Am Soc Nephrol* 2011;6:257–264.
258. Sullivan C, Sayre SS, Leon JB, et al. Effect of food additives on hyperphosphatemia among patients with end-stage renal disease: a randomized controlled trial. *JAMA* 2009;301:629–635.
259. Kovesdy CP, Kuchmak O, Lu JL, et al. Outcomes associated with phosphorus binders in men with non-dialysis-dependent CKD. *Am J Kidney Dis* 2010;56:842–851.
260. United States Dialysis Outcomes and Practice Patterns Study. DOPPS Practice Monitor. http//www.dopps.org/DPM. Accessed April 2016.
261. Hou SH, Zhao J, Ellman CF, et al. Calcium and phosphorus fluxes during hemodialysis with low calcium dialysate. *Am J Kidney Dis* 1991;18:217–224.
262. Musci I, Hercz G, Uldall R, et al. Control of serum phosphate without any phosphate binders in patients treated with nocturnal hemodialysis. *Kidney Int* 1998;53:1399–1404.
263. Chertow GM, Levin NW, Beck GJ, et al. In-center hemodialysis six times per week versus three times per week. *N Engl J Med* 2010;363:2287–2300.

264. K/DOQI clinical practice guidelines and clinical practice recommendations for anemia in chronic kidney disease in adults. *Am J Kidney Dis* 2006;47(5 Suppl 3):S11–S145.

265. Slatopolsky EA, Burke SK, Dillon MA, et al. RenaGel, a nonabsorbed calcium- and aluminum-free phosphate binder, lowers serum phosphorus and parathyroid hormone. *Kidney Int* 1999;55:299–307.

266. Hutchison AJ. Lanthanum carbonate: a novel non-calcemic phosphate binder in dialysis patients. *Nephrol Dial Transplant* 2000;15:113.

267. Joy MS, Finn WF; for the LAM-302 Study Group. Randomized, double-blind, placebo-controlled, dose-titration, phase III study assessing the efficacy and tolerability of lanthanum carbonate: a new phosphate binder for the treatment of hyperphosphatemia. *Am J Kidney Dis* 2003;42:96–107.

268. Qunibi WY, Hootkins RE, McDowell LL, et al. Treatment of hyperphosphatemia in hemodialysis patients: the Calcium Acetate Renagel Evaluation (CARE Study). *Kidney Int* 2004;65:1914–1926.

269. Daugirdas JT, Finn WF, Emmett M, et al. The phosphate binder equivalent dose. *Semin Dial* 2011;24:41–49.

270. D'Haese PC, Spasovski GB, Sikole A, et al. A multicenter study on the effects of lanthanum carbonate (Fosrenol™) and calcium carbonate on renal bone disease in dialysis patients. *Kidney Int* 2003;63(Suppl 85): S73–S78.

271. Gonzalez-Parra E, Gonzalez-Casaus ML, Galan A, et al. Lanthanum carbonate reduces FGF23 in chronic kidney disease stage 3 patients. *Nephrol Dial Transplant* 2011;26:2567–2571.

272. Lacour B, Lucas A, Auchère D, et al. Chronic renal failure is associated with increased tissue deposition of lanthanum after 28-day oral administration. *Kidney Int* 2005;67:1062–1069.

273. Hutchison AJ, Barnett ME, Krause R, et al. Lanthanum carbonate treatment, for up to 6 years, is not associated with adverse effects on the liver in patients with chronic kidney disease stage 5 receiving hemodialysis. *Clin Nephrol* 2009;71:286–295.

274. Spiegel DM. The role of magnesium binders in chronic kidney disease. *Semin Dial* 2007;20:333–336.

275. De Schutter TM, Behets GJ, Geryl H, et al. Effect of a magnesium-based phosphate binder on medial calcification in a rat model of uremia. *Kidney Int* 2013;83:1109–1117.

276. Louvet L, Büchel J, Steppan S, et al. Magnesium prevents phosphate-induced calcification in human aortic vascular smooth muscle cells. *Nephrol Dial Transplant* 2013;28(4):869–878.

277. Qunibi WY. Is it too much of a good thing? A new era in phosphate binder therapy in ESRD. *J Am Soc Nephrol* 2015;26(10):2311–2313.

278. Lewis JB, Sika M, Koury MJ, et al; for the Collaborative Study Group. Ferric citrate controls phosphorus and delivers iron in patients on dialysis. *J Am Soc Nephrol* 2015;26:493–503.

279. Floege J, Covic AC, Ketteler M, et al. A phase III study of the efficacy and safety of a novel iron-based phosphate binder in dialysis patients. *Kidney Int* 2014;86:638–647.

280. Umanath K, Jalal DI, Greco BA, et al. Ferric citrate reduces intravenous iron and erythropoiesis-stimulating agent use in ESRD. *J Am Soc Nephrol* 2015;26:2578–2587.

281. Block GA, Fishbane S, Rodriguez M, et al. A 12-week, double-blind, placebo-controlled trial of ferric citrate for the treatment of iron deficiency anemia and reduction of serum phosphate in patients with CKD stages 3-5. *Am J Kidney Dis* 2014;65:728–736.

282. Maccubbin D, Tipping D, Kuznetsova O, et al. Hypophosphatemic effect of niacin in patients without renal failure: a randomized trial. *Clin J Am Soc Nephrol* 2010;5:582–589.

283. Cheng SC, Young DO, Huang Y, et al. A randomized, double-blind, placebo-controlled trial of niacinamide for reduction of phosphorus in hemodialysis patients. *Clin J Am Soc Nephrol* 2008;3:1131–1138.

284. Savica V, Calò LA, Monardo P, et al. Salivary phosphate binding chewing gum reduces hyperphosphatemia in dialysis patients. *J Am Soc Nephrol* 2009;20:639–644.

285. K/DOQI clinical practice guidelines for bone metabolism and disease in chronic kidney disease. *Am J Kidney Dis* 2003;42:S1–S201.

286. Kooienga L, Fried L, Scragg R, et al. The effect of combined calcium and vitamin D3 supplementation on serum intact parathyroid hormone in moderate CKD. *Am J Kidney Dis* 2009;53:408–416.

287. Milliner DS, Zinsmeister AR, Leiberman E, et al. Soft tissue calcification in pediatric patients with end-stage renal disease. *Kidney Int* 1990;38:931–936.

288. Merke J, Hofmann W, Goldschmidt D, et al. Demonstration of 1,25(OH)₂ vitamin D3 receptors and actions in vascular smooth muscle cells in vitro. *Calcif Tissue Int* 1987;41:112–114.

289. Joist HE, Ahya SN, Giles K, et al. Differential effects of very high doses of doxercalciferol and paricalcitol on serum phosphorus in hemodialysis patients. *Clin Nephrol* 2006;65(5):335–341.

290. Mizobuchi M, Finch JL, Martin DR, et al. Differential effects of vitamin D receptor activators on vascular calcification in uremic rats. *Kidney Int* 2007;72(6):709–715.

291. Teng M, Wolf M, Lowrie E, et al. Survival of patients undergoing hemodialysis with paricalcitol or calcitriol therapy. *N Engl J Med* 2003;349:446.

292. Teng M, Wolf M, Ofsthun MN, et al. Activated injectable vitamin D and hemodialysis survival: a historical cohort study. *J Am Soc Nephrol* 2005;16:1115.

293. Kovesdy CP, Ahmadzadeh S, Anderson JE, et al. Association of activated vitamin D treatment and mortality in chronic kidney disease. *Arch Intern Med* 2008;168:397–403.

294. Shoben AB, Rudser KD, de Boer IH, et al. Association of oral calcitriol with improved survival in nondialyzed CKD. *J Am Soc Nephrol* 2008;19:1613–1619.

295. Levin A, Li YC. Vitamin D and its analogues: do they protect against cardiovascular disease in patients with kidney disease? *Kidney Int* 2005;68:1973–1981.

296. Palmer SC, McGregor DO, Macaskill P, et al. Meta-analysis: vitamin D compounds in chronic kidney disease. *Ann Intern Med* 2007;147:840–853.

297. Nishi H, Nii-Kono T, Nakanishi S, et al. Intravenous calcitriol therapy increases serum concentrations of fibroblast growth factor-23 in dialysis patients with secondary hyperparathyroidism. *Nephron Clin Pract* 2005;101:C94–C99.

298. Thadhani R, Appelbaum E, Pritchett Y, et al. Vitamin D therapy and cardiac structure and function in patients with chronic kidney disease: the PRIMO randomized controlled trial. *JAMA* 2012;307:674–684.

299. Nemeth EF, Shoback D. Calcimimetic and calcilytic drugs for treating bone and mineral-related disorders. *Best Pract Res Clin Endocrinol Metab* 2013;27(3):373–384.

300. Quarles LD. Cinacalcet HCl: a novel treatment for secondary hyperparathyroidism in stage 5 chronic kidney disease. *Kidney Int* 2005;96:S24–S28.

301. Goodman WG, Hladik GA, Turne SA, et al. The calcimimetic agent AMG 073 lowers plasma parathyroid hormone levels in hemodialysis patients with secondary hyperparathyroidism. *J Am Soc Nephrol* 2002;13:1017–1024.

302. Harris RZ, Padhi D, Marbury TC, et al. Pharmacokinetics, pharmacodynamics, and safety of cinacalcet hydrochloride in hemodialysis patients at doses up to 200 mg once daily. *Am J Kidney Dis* 2004;44:1070–1076.

303. Moe SM, Cunningham J, Bommer J, et al. Long-term treatment of secondary hyperparathyroidism with the calcimimetic cinacalcet HCl. *Nephrol Dial Transplant* 2005;20:2186–2193.

304. Cunningham J, Danese M, Olson K, et al. Effects of the calcimimetic cinacalcet HCl on cardiovascular disease, fracture, and health-related quality of life in secondary hyperparathyroidism. *Kidney Int* 2005;68: 1793–1800.

305. Wada M, Furuya Y, Sakiyama J, et al. The calcimimetic compound NPS R-568 suppresses parathyroid cell proliferation in rats with renal insufficiency. Control of parathyroid cell growth via a calcium receptor. *J Clin Invest* 1997;100:2977–2983.

306. Finch JL, Tokumoto M, Nakamura H, et al. Effect of paricalcitol and cinacalcet on serum phosphate, FGF-23, and bone in rats with chronic kidney disease. *Am J Physiol Renal Physiol* 2010;298:F1315–F1322.

307. Raggi P, Chertow GM, Torres PU, et al. The ADVANCE study: a randomized study to evaluate the effects of cinacalcet plus low-dose vitamin D on vascular calcification in patients on hemodialysis. *Nephrol Dial Transplant* 2011;26:1327–1339.

308. Chertow GM, Block GA, Correa-Rotter R, et al. Effect of cinacalcet on cardiovascular disease in patients undergoing dialysis. *N Engl J Med* 2012;367:2482–2494.

309. Moe SM, Abdalla S, Chertow GM, et al. Effects of cinacalcet on fracture events in patients receiving hemodialysis: the EVOLVE Trial. *J Am Soc Nephrol* 2015;26:1466–1475.

310. Charytan C, Coburn JW, Chonchol M, et al. Cinacalcet hydrochloride is an effective treatment for secondary hyperparathyroidism in patients with CKD not receiving dialysis. *Am J Kidney Dis* 2005;46: 58–67.

311. Chonchol M, Locatelli F, Abboud HE, et al. A randomized, double-blind, placebo-controlled study to assess the efficacy and safety of cinacalcet HCl in participants with CKD not receiving dialysis. *Am J Kidney Dis* 2009;53:197–207.

312. Foley RN, Li S, Liu J, et al. The fall and rise of parathyroidectomy in U.S. hemodialysis patients, 1992 to 2002. *J Am Soc Nephrol* 2005;16: 210–218.

313. Parfrey PS, Chertow GM, Block GA, et al. The clinical course of treated hyperparathyroidism among patients receiving hemodialysis and the effect of cinacalcet: the EVOLVE Trial. *J Clin Endocrinol Metab* 2013;98:4834–4844.

314. Kestenbaum B, Andress DL, Schwartz SM, et al. Survival following parathyroidectomy among United States dialysis patients. *Kidney Int* 2004;66:2010–2016.

315. Rudser KD, de Boer IH, Dooley A, et al. Fracture risk after parathyroidectomy among chronic hemodialysis patients. *J Am Soc Nephrol* 2007;18:2401–2407.

316. Ishani A, Liu J, Wetmore JB, et al. Clinical outcomes after parathyroidectomy in a nationwide cohort of patients on hemodialysis. *Clin J Am Soc Nephrol* 2015;10:90–97.

317. Kaye M, D'Amour P, Henderson J. Elective total parathyroidectomy without autotransplant in end-stage renal disease. *Kidney Int* 1989;35:1390–1399.

318. Hampl H, Steinmüller T, Stabell U, et al. Recurrent hyperparathyroidism after total parathyroidectomy and autotransplantation in patients with long-term hemodialysis. *Miner Electrolyte Metab* 1991;17: 256–260.

319. Goldfarb M, Gondek SS, Lim SM, et al. Postoperative hungry bone syndrome in patients with secondary hyperparathyroidism of renal origin. *World J Surg* 2012;36:1314–1319.

320. Latus J, Roesel M, Fritz P, et al. Incidence of and risk factors for hungry bone syndrome in 84 patients with secondary hyperparathyroidism. *Int J Nephrol Renovasc Dis* 2013;6:131–137.

321. Witteveen JE, van Thiel S, Romijn JA, et al. Hungry bone syndrome: still a challenge in the post-operative management of primary hyperparathyroidism: a systematic review of the literature. *Eur J Endocrinol* 2013;168: R45–R53.

322. Palmer S, McGregor D, Strippoli G. Interventions for preventing bone disease in kidney transplant recipients. *Cochrane Database Syst Rev* 2007;(3):CD005015.

323. Cunningham J. Posttransplantation bone disease. *Transplantation* 2005;79:629–634.

324. Ball AM, Gillen DL, Sherrard D, et al. Risk of hip fracture among dialysis and renal transplant recipients. *JAMA* 2002;288:3014–3018.

325. Abbott KC, Oglesby RJ, Hypolite IO, et al. Hospitalizations for fractures after renal transplantation in the United States. *Ann Epidemiol* 2001;11:450–457.

326. Molnar MZ, Naser MS, Rhee CM, et al. Bone and mineral disorders after kidney transplantation: therapeutic strategies. *Transplant Rev (Orlando)* 2014;28(2):56–62.

327. Julian BA, Quarles LD, Niemann KM. Musculoskeletal complications after renal transplantation: pathogenesis and treatment. *Am J Kidney Dis* 1992;19:99–120.

328. Lukert BP, Raisz LG. Glucocorticoid-induced osteoporosis: pathogenesis and management. *Ann Intern Med* 1990;112:352–364.

329. Rich GM, Mudge GH, Laffel GL, et al. Cyclosporin A and prednisone-associated osteoporosis in heart transplant recipients. *J Heart Lung Transplant* 1992;11:950–958.

330. Rojas E, Carlini RG, Clesca P, et al. The pathogenesis of osteodystrophy after renal transplantation as detected by early alterations in bone remodeling. *Kidney Int* 2003;63:1915–1923.

331. Canalis E, Mazziotti G, Giustina A, et al. Glucocorticoid-induced osteoporosis: pathophysiology and therapy. *Osteoporos Int* 2007;18: 1319–1328.

332. Dumoulin G, Hory B, Nguyen NU, et al. Lack of evidence that cyclosporine treatment impairs calcium-phosphorus homeostasis and bone remodeling in normocalcemic long-term renal transplant recipients. *Transplantation* 1995;59:1690–1694.

333. Bozkaya G, Nart A, Uslu A, et al. Impact of calcineurin inhibitors on bone metabolism in primary kidney transplant patients. *Transplant Proc* 2008;40:151–155.

334. Lopez-Ben R, Mikuls TR, Moore DS, et al. Incidence of hip osteonecrosis among renal transplantation recipients: a prospective study. *Clin Radiol* 2004;59:431–438.

335. Braun WE, Richmond BJ, Protiva DA, et al. The incidence and management of osteoporosis, gout, and avascular necrosis in recipients of renal allografts functioning more than 20 years (level 5A) treated with prednisone and azathioprine. *Transplant Proc* 1999;31(1–2): 1366–1369.

336. Fink B, Degenhardt S, Paselk C, et al. Early detection of avascular necrosis of the femoral head following renal transplantation. *Arch Orthop Trauma Surg* 1997;116:151–156.

337. Brandenburg VM, Floege J. Transplantation: an end to bone disease after renal transplantation? *Nat Rev Nephrol* 2013;9:5–6.

338. Coco M, Glicklich D, Faugere MC, et al. Prevention of bone loss in renal transplant recipients: a prospective, randomized trial of intravenous pamidronate. *J Am Soc Nephrol* 2003;14:2669–2676.

339. Mitterbauer C, Schwarz C, Haas M, et al. Effects of bisphosphonates on bone loss in the first year after renal transplantation—a meta-analysis of randomized controlled trials. *Nephrol Dial Transplant* 2006;21: 2275–2281.

340. Boutsen Y, Jamart J, Esselinckx W, et al. Primary prevention of glucocorticoid induced osteoporosis with intravenous pamidronate and calcium. *J Bone Min Res* 2001;16:104–112.

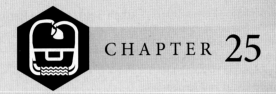

CHAPTER 25

Acid–Base Considerations in End-Stage Kidney Disease

F. John Gennari and Dana Negoi

Maintenance of normal body pH and P_{CO_2} depends on daily replenishment of body alkali stores that are either consumed, neutralizing strong acids produced by normal body metabolism, or lost in the stool (1–4). This task is normally accomplished by the kidneys through an incompletely defined system of sensors and effectors that regulate H^+ and NH_4^+ excretion (4). The result is acid balance, achieved by reabsorption of all the filtered HCO_3^- and, in addition, excretion of just enough acid (primarily as NH_4^+) to replenish the HCO_3^- lost from the body (**FIGURE 25.1**). This balance is flexible, responding rapidly to changes in acid production, and precise, maintaining blood $[HCO_3^-]$ remarkably constant from day to day.

As kidney disease progresses, renal regulation of acid balance is lost and metabolic acidosis ensues, due primarily to impaired acid excretion. Initiation of renal replacement therapy addresses this problem not by removing H^+ but by adding HCO_3^- to the body on a regular basis. Net addition of HCO_3^- during dialysis therapy is regulated not by any physiologic feedback mechanism but by the physical principles of diffusion and convection (5–7). This switch has major implications for acid–base homeostasis, changing the way one thinks about both normal and disordered acid balance.

Throughout this chapter, the term $[HCO_3^-]$ is used both for serum and bath concentrations. In most instances, however, serum $[HCO_3^-]$ is actually measured as serum [total CO_2]. Keep in mind that serum [total CO_2] includes dissolved CO_2 as well as HCO_3^- and is on average about 1 mmol/L higher than serum $[HCO_3^-]$.

⬡ GENERAL PRINCIPLES

Regardless of the alkali source added to the dialysis bath or infused during renal replacement therapy, a new equilibrium is achieved that is driven primarily by variations in endogenous acid production, just as in individuals with normal kidney function (5–7). The fundamental reason for this linkage is that the net gain of HCO_3^- is directly related to its transmembrane concentration gradient. Therefore, the lower the concentration of HCO_3^- in the body fluids at the onset of treatment, the greater will be the net entry of alkali. In patients receiving renal replacement therapy, the prevailing serum $[HCO_3^-]$ is determined jointly by the dialysis

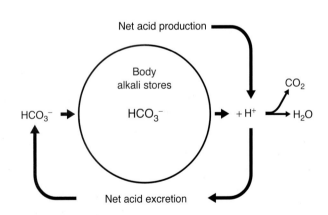

In steady state: net acid excretion = net acid production

FIGURE 25.1 Normal acid–base balance. Net acid production, comprising endogenous acid production and the difference between the alkali added by the diet and the alkali lost in the stool, adds new H^+ to the body fluids. These ions react with HCO_3^-, yielding CO_2 and H_2O. In the steady state, through a complex signal pathway that is incompletely understood, the kidney adjusts net acid excretion (NH_4^+ plus titratable acid excretion minus any HCO_3^- lost in the urine) to match net acid production, thereby adding back an equivalent amount of HCO_3^-.

treatment itself and by endogenous acid production. Because the dialysis prescription is fixed, the variable component is endogenous acid production, which likely accounts for most of the variability in serum $[HCO_3^-]$ in patients with end-stage kidney disease (ESKD) (5–7). Although less flexible than functioning kidneys, this property of dialysis therapy allows for variations in endogenous acid production to be matched by variable amounts of net HCO_3^- addition during treatment. The details of how this equilibrium is achieved are discussed first for peritoneal dialysis (PD) and then for hemodialysis (HD).

ACID–BASE HOMEOSTASIS IN PERITONEAL DIALYSIS

In recent years, there has been a resurgence of PD as a treatment for ESKD. The number of incident PD patients increased from 7,588 in 2000 to 9,451 in 2012 (8). Monthly prevalent counts increased by 24% between January 2010 and October 2012, compared to only 9.6% increase in HD (9). This resurgence is likely due to the finding that PD is as beneficial as HD but less expensive and also to new financial incentives for initiation of PD (9).

Automated peritoneal dialysis (APD) is now more commonly used than continuous ambulatory peritoneal dialysis (CAPD) as a result of improvement in technology and better perceived quality of life (10); patients have more freedom during the day as the therapy is delivered primarily at night with the help of a machine that is easy to use. With this resurgence, attention has been directed at trying to identify the best solution to restore body alkali stores and at the same time minimize damage to the peritoneal membrane. In general, it is recommended that plasma bicarbonate be maintained in the high normal range: Protein catabolism is reduced at bicarbonate levels around 30 mmol/L and nutritional status seems to be improved (11). On the other hand, there is a concern that higher bicarbonate levels may be associated with soft tissue calcifications and adynamic bone disease, but these complications have not been shown to occur in PD so far (11).

Alkali Source in the Peritoneal Dialysis Solutions

As in the case of HD, the first PD solutions contained bicarbonate (12). At that time, commercially prepared dialysis solutions were not available for clinical use, and fresh solutions were prepared in the hospital at the time PD was performed. In order to avoid precipitation of calcium carbonate if bicarbonate solutions were to be stored for longer periods of time, calcium was added shortly before inflow into the abdomen (12). As commercial solutions were developed in the 1950s, another problem became apparent. The high pH in bicarbonate-based PD solutions facilitated caramelization of glucose during the sterilization process and generation of glucose degradation products that were thought to contribute to peritoneal membrane damage after prolonged exposure. In short order, bicarbonate was removed from most PD solutions and replaced with acetate or lactate, organic anions that are absorbed and metabolized to bicarbonate in the body. Acetate-containing solutions were abandoned quickly because of the untoward effects on the peritoneal membrane from local vasodilation. These effects included increased membrane permeability with loss of ultrafiltration, and encapsulating peritoneal sclerosis (13). Lactate quickly became the standard alkali source because it is rapidly metabolized to HCO_3^- while serum lactate concentration remains low. Initially, solutions contained sodium lactate at a concentration 35 mmol/L, but almost all standard solutions now contain at a concentration of 40 mmol/L because serum $[HCO_3^-]$ is higher using the latter concentration (14–16) (**TABLE 25.1**). Lactate-based solutions have been well tolerated, but concerns remain about damage to the peritoneal membrane after long-term exposure to the low pH of the solution when first introduced into the abdomen. Within 15 minutes, of course, pH rises in the peritoneal space due to rapid entry of HCO_3^- across the peritoneal membrane (**FIGURE 25.2**) (13).

The search for biocompatible PD solutions has brought bicarbonate-based solutions back into the forefront (13,20–22). Packaging the PD solution in a two-compartment bag system allows for separation of HCO_3^- from glucose, calcium, and magnesium salts. The two bags are mixed just prior to infusion into the abdomen, and rapid equilibration of the mixed solution with body

TABLE 25.1	**Steady-State Acid–Base Values in Patients Treated with Peritoneal Dialysis**				
Type	**Bath [Lactate] mmol/L**	**N**	**Venous [Total CO₂] mmol/L**	**Year**	**Reference**
CAPD[a]	35	31	23.9 ± 4.0	1983	(16)
CAPD	35	33	21.5 ± 2.4	2003	(13)
CAPD	40	25	27.4 ± 3.3	1983	(16)
		20	26.3 ± 2.5	1990	(17)
		8	28.8 ± 3.0	1983	(15)
		175	25.3 ± 3.2	2003	(18)
		11	27.5 ± 3.3	1995	(19)
APD[b]	40	75	25.7 ± 3.2	2003	(18)
CAPD[c]	0	13	27.1 ± 2.1	2004	(20)
CAPD[d]	15	70	27.7 ± 2.7	2000	(21)

All values, mean ± 1 SD
[a]Continuous ambulatory peritoneal dialysis, four exchanges per day.
[b]APD, automated overnight cycling peritoneal dialysis.
[c]Bath contains HCO_3^-, 34 mmol/L, arterial $[HCO_3^-]$ calculated from pH and P_{CO_2}.
[d]Bath contains HCO_3^-, 25 mmol/L in addition to 15 mmol/L lactate.

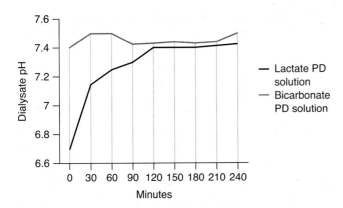

FIGURE 25.2 Changes in dialysate pH over time during equilibrium in abdomen. The *black line* indicates a dialysis solution containing 40 mmol/L of lactate and no bicarbonate. The *gray line* indicates a solution containing 25 mmol/L of bicarbonate and 15 mmol/L of lactate. [Redrawn using data in Heimburger O, Mujais S. Buffer transport in peritoneal dialysis. *Kidney Int* 2003;64(Suppl 88):S37–S42.]

TABLE 25.2	Composition of Standard 40 mmol/L Lactate Peritoneal Dialysis Solution
Sodium (mmol/L)	134
Potassium (mmol/L)	2
Calcium (mmol/L)	0–1.75
Magnesium (mmol/L)	0.25–0.75
Chloride (mmol/L)	95
Lactate (mmol/L)	40
Glucose (g/dl)	1.5–4.25
pH	5.2–5.5
Osmolality (mOsm/kg H$_2$O)	358–511

P_{CO_2} keeps the pH in a range at which calcium and magnesium salts do not precipitate. This solution can be used in both APD and CAPD. Another advantage of the bicarbonate-based solutions is the lower incidence of in-flow pain due to the physiologic pH of the solution as compared to low initial pH in lactate-based solutions (22).

Buffer Transport in Peritoneal Dialysis Using a Lactate-Containing Solution

During PD, the peritoneal cavity is filled with fresh dialysis solution, which is allowed to dwell for a variable amount of time. The standard lactate-based PD fluid composition is shown in **TABLE 25.2**. During the dwell, HCO_3^- and lactate cross the peritoneal membrane down their respective concentration gradients causing a gradual decline in dialysate [lactate] and increase in dialysate [HCO_3^-]. The rate of HCO_3^- movement into the bath diminishes as the concentration rises in the dialysate, but even after a 6-hour dwell, equilibrium is not achieved (**FIGURE 25.3**) (19). At the end of the dwell, the spent dialysate is drained, and fresh PD fluid is infused into the peritoneal

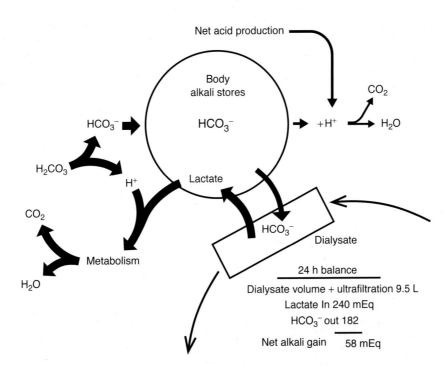

FIGURE 25.3 Acid balance in peritoneal dialysis. To replenish HCO_3^- stores that have been consumed in buffering endogenous acid production, lactate is added from the dialysis fluid and metabolized to produce new HCO_3^-. A large portion of the newly generated HCO_3^- is lost by diffusing back into the peritoneal dialysis fluid. The rate of HCO_3^- loss (and therefore the net gain of alkali) depends on its transmembrane concentration gradient. As shown in the example, the serum [HCO_3^-] is maintained at a level at which the difference between lactate added and HCO_3^- lost each day is equal to daily net acid production.

cavity. PD is in most instances a continuous procedure; PD fluid is present in the peritoneal space 24 hours a day, 7 days a week. As a result, serum [HCO$_3^-$] is stable and does not fluctuate as it does with intermittent HD (see later).

Because blood lactate concentration is approximately 1 mmol/L, lactate diffuses from the peritoneal cavity into the systemic circulation across the peritoneal membrane. The absorbed lactate is metabolized primarily in the liver to generate an equivalent amount of new HCO$_3^-$. As a result of rapid metabolism, serum [lactate] does not increase notably during PD, allowing for a favorable concentration gradient to be maintained during the dwell. When the PD fluid is left in the peritoneal cavity for 6 hours, approximately 75% of the lactate is absorbed and metabolized, yielding an equivalent amount of new bicarbonate (19). A portion of the newly generated HCO$_3^-$ is consumed in buffering endogenous acids produced by body metabolism on a daily basis. Because the PD solution contains no HCO$_3^-$, a large portion of the newly generated HCO$_3^-$ also diffuses from the patient into the peritoneal cavity down its concentration gradient (5,7,23). Its rate of diffusion is determined by the same principles that govern lactate transport, and its concentration in the peritoneal cavity increases during the dwell. After 6 hours, PD fluid [HCO$_3^-$] is about 80% of the serum level (**FIGURE 25.3**) (19). The net alkali gained for any given period is equal to the difference between the systemically added lactate and the loss of HCO$_3^-$ into the PD fluid. (5,7,19).

Based on the relative diffusion rates of HCO$_3^-$ and lactate, one can estimate the net alkali gain for a standard CAPD prescription (23). In the model shown in **FIGURE 25.3**, serum [HCO$_3^-$] is 24 mmol/L and the patient is receiving four 2-L exchanges, each with a dialysate lactate concentration of 40 mmol/L each day. For this prescription, total lactate content in the PD fluid each day will be 8 × 40 = 320 mmol/d, and total lactate added to the body fluids is 320 × 0.75 = 240 mmol/d. If dialysate [HCO$_3^-$] is 80% of the serum concentration at the end of the dwell period, dialysate [HCO$_3^-$] will be 24 × 0.8 = 19 mmol/L. Assuming the additional removal of 1.5 L of fluid during a 24-hour period of dialysis, the total spent dialysate volume will be 8 + 1.5 = 9.5 L. Total HCO$_3^-$ content in the spent dialysate will be 9.5 × 19 = 182 mmol/d. Total systemic alkali gain is therefore 240 − 182 = 58 mmol/d. If this net alkali gain exceeds the rate of endogenous acid production, serum [HCO$_3^-$] will rise, increasing the amount of HCO$_3^-$ lost, until net alkali gain matches endogenous acid production. At this point, an equilibrium will be achieved in which net alkali gained will equal net acid production. These theoretical considerations are supported

by direct measurements, showing that patients treated with PD are in acid balance, with serum [HCO$_3^-$] related inversely to endogenous acid production (19).

Bicarbonate-Based Solutions

Bicarbonate-based PD solutions are now commercially available in Europe and Canada, using a two-bag system to prevent precipitation of calcium and magnesium salts during storage. When this system is used, acid–base status is improved in patients with low serum [HCO$_3^-$] when bath [HCO$_3^-$] is increased from 34 to 39 mmol/L (14,20). Newer solutions are now available containing a mixture of bicarbonate and lactate (B/L) (11,13,21). The B/L solutions are also packed in a two-bag system. The B/L dialysis solutions made by Baxter contain [HCO$_3^-$] at 25 mmol/L and [lactate] at either 10 or 15 mmol/L. Unfortunately, neither bicarbonate nor B/L solutions are available for use in the United States.

The proposed advantage of the B/L solutions is a physiologic pH and Pco$_2$, thereby reducing glucose-degradation products (11). Clinical experience with B/L solutions showed efficient acid–base control and reduction in infusion pain due to physiologic pH of the solution (pH of 7.4) compared to 5.5 in lactate-only solutions (10,13,21,22). A modest but significant increase in ultrafiltration was observed in patients using a B/L solution compared to lactate (21).

Effect of Automated Peritoneal Dialysis on Serum [HCO$_3^-$]

As APD is the predominant form of PD, it is important to consider its effect on the patient's acid–base status. In APD, patients are exposed to higher total volume of dialysis solutions, but most of the dwells are shorter in duration. Current experience shows that good control of acid–base balance can be obtained regardless of whether CAPD or APD is used (**FIGURE 25.4**). As seen in the figure, most patients achieve a plasma bicarbonate concentration of 22 to 30 mmol/L, irrespective of modality status, and there is no notable difference in average serum [HCO$_3^-$] (10,18).

Lactate and bicarbonate are transported faster across the peritoneal membrane in high transporters compared to low transporters. For this reason in CAPD, serum bicarbonate concentration might be slightly higher in high transporters compared to low transporters, but the difference has no physiologic consequence (18). In APD, there is no difference in serum [HCO$_3^-$] among different type of transporters due to higher volume of dialysate used (10).

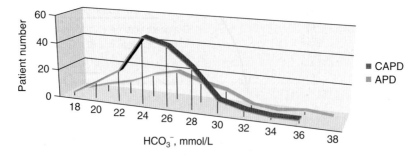

FIGURE 25.4 Ranges of steady-state serum [HCO$_3^-$] in 175 patients treated with continuous ambulatory peritoneal dialysis (CAPD) and in 77 patients treated with automated peritoneal dialysis (APD). Bicarbonate concentration is plotted against the number of patients for each value. [Redrawn from data in Mujais S. Acid-base profile in patients on PD. *Kidney Int* 2003;64(Suppl 88):S26–S36.]

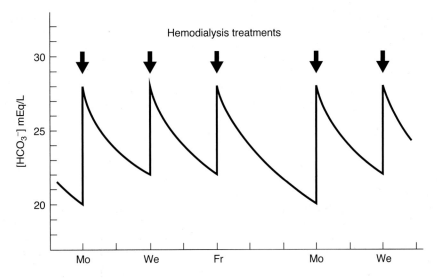

FIGURE 25.5 Schematic representation of the pattern of serum [HCO₃⁻] in a patient receiving hemodialysis treatments thrice weekly [Monday (Mo), Wednesday (We), and Friday (Fr)]. Serum [HCO₃⁻] rises with each dialysis and then falls during the interval between treatments, reaching a nadir once a week at the end of the long interval between treatments.

⬡ ACID–BASE HOMEOSTASIS IN HEMODIALYSIS

Conventional HD is an intermittent treatment, in contrast to the continuous nature of PD. As a result, there is no day-to-day steady state with regard to alkali stores and serum [HCO₃⁻]. As shown in **FIGURE 25.5**, alkali is added rapidly during a 3- to 4-hour treatment three times a week. This added alkali then gradually dissipates during the period between treatments, as HCO₃⁻ is consumed by endogenous acid production and diluted by fluid retention (7). Thus, from an acid–base perspective, HD patients undergo a continuous back-and-forth fluctuation from a postdialysis serum [HCO₃⁻] in the high normal or slightly alkaline range to a predialysis serum [HCO₃⁻] in a range that is usually slightly below normal. Given that serum [HCO₃⁻] falls by as much as 7 to 8 mmol/L from the end of one dialysis to the beginning of the next, it is important to note when acid–base status is assessed. By convention, one usually reports the predialysis value and, ideally, the nadir value obtained after the longest interval between treatments (**TABLE 25.3**).

Alkali Source

When HD was first developed, the bath solution contained HCO₃⁻ in a concentration of 26 mmol/L (32), but the concentration was empirically increased to 35 mmol/L over the next decade to improve

TABLE 25.3	**Steady-State Predialysis Acid–Base Values in Stable Patients Treated with Conventional Hemodialysis[a]**			
Year	**N**	**[Total CO₂] mmol/L**		**Reference**
1990[b]	22	21.4 ± 2.4		(17)
1993	38	19.0 ± 3.1		(24)
1999	995	21.6 ± 3.4		(25)
2000[c]	7,123	22.8 ± 3.5		(26)
2006	56,385	21.8 ± 2.8		(27)
2010	196	24.5 ± 2.8		(28)
2015[b]	175	23.9 ± 2.1		Gennari[d]
		Arterial Blood Values		
		[HCO⁻][e] mmol/L	**Pco₂ mm Hg**	**pH**
1982	10	18.9 ± 2.5	33 ± 2.5	7.37 ± 0.09	(29)
1985	16	19.0 ± 1.2	36 ± 1.9	7.37 ± 0.02	(30)
2015	30	21.6 ± 2.4	37 ± 4.5	7.39 ± 0.04	(31)

[a]Thrice weekly with a bicarbonate bath (final concentration 32 to 36 mmol/L).
[b]Values obtained after longest interval between treatments.
[c]Midweek predialysis value.
[d]Unpublished observations.
[e]Recall that serum [HCO₃⁻] is lower than serum [total CO₂] by approximately 1 mmol/L because the latter measurement includes dissolved CO₂.

alkali transfer (33). To prevent precipitation of $CaCO_3$, bath pH had to be adjusted to 7.4 by aeration with a carbon dioxide/oxygen gas mixture. Acetate was first introduced as an alkali precursor in 1964 (34). This organic anion was chosen because it was metabolized readily by most tissues in the body (35), allowing for rapid HCO_3^- production during treatment. Because acetate obviated the need for aerating the bath with CO_2, it allowed for a central bath solution preparation system that could be used for multiple patients, and it quickly replaced HCO_3^- as an alkali source.

This change created a bidirectional dynamic similar to that for PD with lactate, although much more rapid and impressive in magnitude. Almost as quickly as the acetate added from the bath to the patient was metabolized to HCO_3^- during HD, the new HCO_3^- diffuses back into the bath (6). As a result, the only way to add substantial amounts of HCO_3^- to the body stores was to add sufficient acetate to overcome its rate of metabolic conversion and raise its concentration in the blood by the end of the treatment. After the dialysis session, this unmetabolized acetate (as high as 3 to 4 mmol/L) is converted to HCO_3^- and the new HCO_3^- is now retained by the patient. By trial and error, a bath acetate concentration of 37 mmol/L was settled on to achieve this goal. This concentration represented a compromise between providing sufficient substrate for HCO_3^- generation during each treatment and limiting the rate of acetate delivery to an amount that could be metabolized without producing toxic levels (36–38).

Despite the ease of bath preparation, alkali repletion using acetate is a remarkably inefficient process. During a 4-hour HD treatment, for example, more than 700 mmol of HCO_3^- is lost into the bath (6,37). This loss limits alkali replenishment, so that patients receiving this form of dialysis have predialysis serum [HCO_3^-] values of less than 18 mmol/L, on average (6,17,37,39). As blood-flow rates and dialyzer membrane permeability increased, the amount of acetate delivered also increased and serum acetate concentration often reached toxic levels, causing hypotension and other symptoms (30,36,38,40–42). An additional problem with using acetate-based dialysis solutions was CO_2 loss from the patient to the bath, an effect that decreased ventilatory drive and contributed to dialysis-induced hypoxemia (42,43).

Because of these problems, HCO_3^- was again introduced as the source for alkali replenishment in the early 1980s (29,43,44). Reintroduction of HCO_3^- into the bath solution was made possible by a new technology, the use of a proportioning system that allowed continuous production of dialysate from concentrated salt solutions either in a central delivery system or individually for each patient. In such a system, $NaHCO_3$ is added to the rest of the bath solution just before delivery to the dialysis membrane. At the moment of HCO_3^- addition, the pH of the bath is prevented from rising too high by the presence of a small amount of acetic acid. The acetic acid reacts rapidly with the added HCO_3^-, yielding carbonic acid and acetate anions. The final bath solution after $NaHCO_3$ addition has a pH of approximately 7.05 and contains HCO_3^- (most commonly at a concentration of 35 mmol/L), acetate (4 mmol/L in most systems), and dissolved CO_2 (4 mmol/L, equivalent to a Pco_2 of 133 mm Hg). The Pco_2 in the bath falls rapidly as it diffuses across the dialysis membrane, raising the Pco_2 in the postfilter blood to only approximately 50 mm Hg (37). The inward diffusion of CO_2 reverses the loss from the patient that occurred with acetate dialysis (see earlier) but has no notable impact on systemic Pco_2 or ventilation (43,44). The acetate produced by this reaction also diffuses across the dialysis membrane into the blood, providing a small additional source of new HCO_3^- as it is metabolized.

Reintroduction of HCO_3^- into the HD bath solution increased predialysis serum [HCO_3^-] by 3 to 4 mmol/L (29,30,42,45–47) and decreased patient symptoms dramatically (29,30,45,48). By 1990, this technology essentially completely replaced acetate HD. Bath solutions currently used for conventional HD most commonly combine a 39-mmol/L HCO_3^- solution with a solution containing 4 mmol/L of acetic acid, yielding a final bath [HCO_3^-] of 35 mmol/L and [acetate] of 4 mmol/L when mixed. One formulation uses sodium diacetate, which yields an [acetate] of 8 mmol/L. The acetate anions cross the dialysis membrane into the blood and are rapidly metabolized, producing 4 or 8 mmol/L of new HCO_3^-. This additional HCO_3^-, however, has no impact on end-dialysis [HCO_3^-] because, to the extent the new HCO_3^- is not consumed by buffering or organic acid production and is retained in the blood, it simply reduces the transmembrane HCO_3^- gradient and slows the rate of HCO_3^- entry from the bath. The end-dialysis [HCO_3^-] is determined by the bath [HCO_3^-] and by the magnitude of the increase in organic acid production during the treatment engendered by the abrupt alkalinization of the body fluids (see later). Because of continued concerns about the effects of acetate on body metabolism even at low concentrations, citric acid has replaced acetic acid in many dialysis units as the organic acid used to control bath pH before HCO_3^- addition. This trivalent acid is effective at lower concentrations, and the citrate anions produced are rapidly metabolized to generate bicarbonate. In a standard citrate-based dialysis bath solution, metabolism of citrate yields 2.7 mmol/L of HCO_3^-.

Acid–Base Balance

Although the transient events are more complex than in PD, a similar equilibrium is established between net acid production and alkali addition in patients receiving intermittent HD. The amount of HCO_3^- added from the bath to the patient during an HD session is primarily dependent on the dialysance of this anion (a function of dialysis membrane surface area and permeability) and the transmembrane concentration gradient (**FIGURE 25.6**). Because the bath [HCO_3^-] is fixed, as are the surface area and permeability of the membrane, the variable factor in this relationship is serum [HCO_3^-]. The serum [HCO_3^-] at the beginning of each treatment is determined primarily by the rate of acid production in the interdialytic period and to a lesser extent by fluid retention (see later). The lower the initial value, the greater the initial rate of HCO_3^- addition, and vice versa.

The total amount of HCO_3^- added during each HD treatment is determined not only by the initial transmembrane concentration gradient but also by the rate of change in the gradient as the treatment progresses. To the extent that newly added HCO_3^- is retained in the extracellular fluid (ECF) compartment, its concentration in the blood will rise, diminishing the gradient across the dialysis membrane. The minute-to-minute change in this gradient is determined by the extent to which the added HCO_3^- is consumed by the production of new H^+ in the body (**FIGURE 25.6**). The response to rapid alkalinization of the body fluids includes not only the release of H^+ from nonbicarbonate buffers but also the stimulation of cellular organic acid production (4,7,47,48).

Increases in the production of organic acids that dissociate at the pH of the body fluid can produce almost unlimited amounts of new H^+ to titrate and remove added HCO_3^- from the extracellular compartment. If the organic anions produced by this titration were retained, they would eventually be metabolized and thereby regenerate the HCO_3^- titrated by their formation. Organic anions, however, readily cross the dialysis membrane and are lost into the

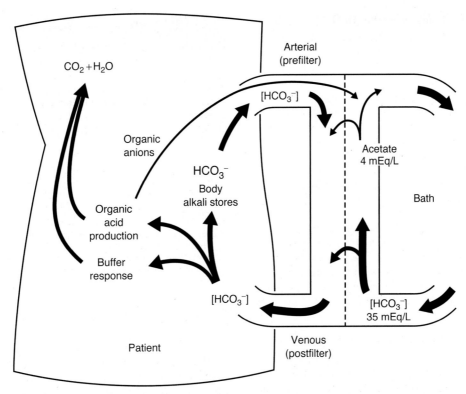

$$HCO_3^- \text{ added} = D_{HCO3} \times o\!\int^t (\text{Bath } [HCO_3^-] - \text{Blood} [HCO_3^-])$$
In steady state: alkali gained = net acid production

FIGURE 25.6 Alkali addition and disposition during hemodialysis. During each treatment, body HCO_3^- stores are replenished by the addition of HCO_3^- and acetate from the bath (the latter anion metabolized to form HCO_3^-). Added and newly generated HCO_3^- is partially consumed by titration with body buffers and by organic acid production. The remaining HCO_3^- is added to the pool and raises $[HCO_3^-]$ in the blood returning to the hemodialysis membrane, reducing the transmembrane concentration gradient, and limiting further HCO_3^- addition. The total HCO_3^- added is determined by its dialysance (D_{HCO3}) and by the integrated transmembrane HCO_3^- concentration gradient over the time of treatment, $o\!\int^t$ (Bath $[HCO_3^-]$ − Blood $[HCO_3^-]$). Because the variable component of this gradient is blood $[HCO_3^-]$, equilibrium is achieved at a predialysis blood $[HCO_3^-]$ at which the alkali added with each treatment is equivalent to endogenous acid production over the interval between treatments.

dialysate (**FIGURE 25.6**) (46,47). At blood-flow rates much lower than are now customarily used, losses of 30 to 50 mmol of organic anions have been measured during a standard HD treatment (46,47). Because many more organic acids are produced than were measured in these studies, and because blood-flow and therefore clearance rates have increased, it seems likely that organic anion losses are now even higher (7). The magnitude of this response to added HCO_3^- remains undefined, but it is clear that organic acid production and loss of the organic anions formed can have a major influence on net alkali addition during HD.

The transmembrane HCO_3^- concentration gradient could also be influenced if the blood returning to the dialyzer contained an admixture of slowly mixing pools with differing HCO_3^- concentrations, but whether this occurs to any measurable degree is unknown. In addition, there may be ionic constraints on HCO_3^- diffusion, despite the presence of a favorable chemical concentration gradient, as it competes with Cl^- and negatively charged proteins (Gibbs-Donnan effect) for charge balance with the cations in the blood, particularly during the latter half of the treatment. These factors probably influence net alkali addition to a much smaller extent than the buffer and organic acid responses, but their contribution remains undefined.

Assuming the factors controlling alkali addition during HD are constant from treatment to treatment, the amount of HCO_3^- added with each treatment is determined primarily by the predialysis serum $[HCO_3^-]$. This value, in turn, is determined by the rate of endogenous acid production in the period between treatments and to a lesser degree by the amount of fluid retained. Eventually, a new equilibrium is achieved in which the interplay between intradialytic and interdialytic events serves to maintain predialysis serum $[HCO_3^-]$ relatively constant. One should emphasize, of course, that the predialysis value for serum $[HCO_3^-]$ is the nadir in a descending trend, with the peak value occurring immediately after dialysis and falling gradually until the next session (**FIGURE 25.5**). Because of the complex nature of the response to alkali addition during HD and its variability from patient to patient, as well as differences in net acid production and fluid retention between treatments, predialysis serum $[HCO_3^-]$ varies more widely in patients receiving intermittent HD than in individuals with normal kidney function (25,26).

Determinants of Postdialysis Serum [HCO₃⁻]

FIGURE 25.7 shows the pattern and magnitude of the increase in serum [HCO₃⁻] during a single HD treatment in seven stable patients. This figure shows the increase in serum [HCO₃⁻] induced by 4 hours of HD (7). The striking feature shown in this figure is that serum [HCO₃⁻] changes little, if at all, during the last 2 hours of dialysis, despite a 4- to 6-mmol/L concentration gradient (after Gibbs-Donnan adjustment) for HCO₃⁻ entry across the dialysis membrane. This pattern has been confirmed by other investigators (44,49). While the observations shown in FIGURE 25.7 are characteristic, serum [HCO₃⁻] actually falls during dialysis in a small subset of patients (7). The fall in these patients most likely is due to a surge in lactic acid production, resulting from tissue hypoxia and hypotension.

Although the factors responsible for determining end-dialysis serum [HCO₃⁻] remain to be completely elucidated, this value is of critical importance because it sets the platform from which [HCO₃⁻] slowly falls in the period between treatments. Assuming no intervening events, the postdialysis serum [HCO₃⁻] is normally determined primarily by the specific dialysis [HCO₃⁻] prescribed for any given patient.

Determinants of Predialysis Serum [HCO₃⁻]

In the interval between HD sessions, the two major determinants of the rate of fall in serum [HCO₃⁻] are the rate of endogenous acid production and the rate of fluid retention. Endogenous acid production between treatments is determined primarily by diet; patients ingesting a diet low in sulfur-containing proteins will have low rates of endogenous acid production and *vice versa* (1,2). Although there is no information on the effect of specific diets on predialysis serum [HCO₃⁻], a clear inverse correlation between normalized protein catabolic rate (an indirect measure of dietary protein intake) and predialysis serum [HCO₃⁻] is evident in patients receiving HD (25–27,50).

TABLE 25.4	Effect of Endogenous Acid Production and Fluid Retention on Predialysis Serum [HCO₃⁻] in Patients Treated with Conventional Hemodialysis

Acid Production mmol/d	Fluid Retention[a] L per Interval	Predialysis [HCO₃⁻][b] mmol/L
40	2	23.4
80	2	20.4
120	2	17.3
60	0	23.1
60	3	21.3
60	6	19.8

Assumptions: weight = 70 kg, postdialysis serum [HCO₃⁻] = 28 mmol/L, and HCO₃⁻ buffer space = 0.5 × body weight (kg).
[a]Liters retained during longest interval between treatments.
[b]After longest interval between treatments (68 hours).

On the basis of these observations and a few assumptions, one can estimate the magnitude of the effect of variations in endogenous acid production on predialysis serum [HCO₃⁻]. If one assumes that all the acid produced is retained and that the buffer space for the retained H⁺ is 50% of body weight [an assumption supported by measurements in HD patients (50)], such an analysis predicts that variations in acid production will alter predialysis serum [HCO₃⁻] by as much as 6 mmol/L (TABLE 25.4). Given these assumptions, variations in daily acid production can mean the difference between a low normal and frankly acidotic predialysis serum [HCO₃⁻] in patients receiving exactly the same dialysis prescription. Although the major determinant of endogenous acid production is dietary protein intake, the catabolic state of the patient will also influence acid production.

For the analysis shown in the first half of TABLE 25.4, it is assumed that 2 L of fluid is retained between each treatment, highlighting the importance of the second factor, fluid retention between runs. For any given rate of endogenous acid production, fluid retained without proportionate alkali between treatments will also decrease predialysis serum [HCO₃⁻]. This is a true "dilution acidosis" caused by an increase in the fluid compartment in which the existing HCO₃⁻ stores are distributed. Using a fixed value for endogenous acid production of 60 mmol/d, keeping the same assumptions for buffering, and assuming that changes in ECF volume do not have any special effects on the buffer response, one can also predict the effect of variations in fluid retention on predialysis serum [HCO₃⁻]. As shown in the lower portion of TABLE 25.4, this effect is almost as profound as changes in acid production. This theoretic analysis also has experimental support. A difference of only 1 L in fluid retention between dialysis treatments has been shown to affect predialysis serum [HCO₃⁻] by more than 1 mmol/L (51). The implications of these effects for the management of acid–base equilibrium in patients receiving HD are discussed further later.

Normal Values for Predialysis Serum [HCO₃⁻]

The average predialysis serum [HCO₃⁻] (measured in most instances as [total CO₂]) for stable patients receiving three HD treatments a week ranges from 20 to 24 mmol/L (TABLE 25.3) (7,24–28). These values are generally lower than those in individuals with normal renal function and in patients receiving PD therapy, and they

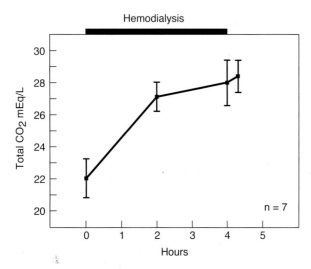

FIGURE 25.7 Pattern of change in serum [total CO₂] during 4 hours of hemodialysis treatment based on measurements in seven stable, nondiabetic patients (7). In these patients, [total CO₂] was measured before dialysis, after 2 hours, at the end of dialysis, and 15 minutes after completion of dialysis. The brackets around the data points are equal to ± standard error. Note that virtually the entire increase in [total CO₂] occurs during the first 2 hours of treatment.

show a much wider range. For reasons that are unclear, average predialysis serum [HCO$_3^-$] has risen by approximately 2 mmol/L over the last 10 to 15 years without any major change in dialysis technique or bath composition (**TABLE 25.3**). This increase may reflect the aging of our dialysis population and the likely associated decrease in dietary intake. The respiratory response to hypobicarbonatemia is normal in ESKD (6,30,38,39,47,52), and therefore, PCO_2 is appropriately reduced when serum [HCO$_3^-$] is low. As a result, average blood pH is either within the normal range or only slightly reduced (**TABLE 25.3**) (29–31,46).

EFFECTS OF METABOLIC ACIDOSIS ON BONE AND MUSCLE METABOLISM

In two studies, a steady-state predialysis serum [HCO$_3^-$] of less than 19 mmol/L was associated with impaired parathyroid hormone responsiveness to changes in serum calcium concentration and with more severe bone disease (53,54). In one of these studies, predialysis serum [HCO$_3^-$] was increased from 15.6 to 24 mmol/L by increasing bath [HCO$_3^-$] (Table 23.5). This change arrested the progression of both high- and low-turnover bone disease, despite otherwise equivalent management (53). In the second study, predialysis serum [HCO$_3^-$] was increased from 18.6 to 25.3 mmol/L using the same approach (**TABLE 25.5**), and this maneuver improved the sensitivity of parathyroid hormone to changes in serum calcium concentration (53).

A low predialysis serum [HCO$_3^-$] also appears to have adverse effects on protein metabolism. In one study, a low predialysis serum [HCO$_3^-$] (18.5 mmol/L) was associated with abnormally high muscle protein turnover, a measure of muscle catabolism (55). When predialysis serum [HCO$_3^-$] was increased to 24.8 mmol/L by raising bath [HCO$_3^-$] (**TABLE 25.5**), muscle protein turnover was reduced. Additional studies have shown a beneficial effect on increasing predialysis serum [HCO$_3^-$] on muscle metabolism (57,58). A similar reduction in protein turnover in patients receiving PD was seen when steady-state serum [HCO$_3^-$] was increased from 19 to 26 mmol/L by giving oral NaHCO$_3$ supplements (59).

EFFECT OF PREDIALYSIS SERUM [HCO$_3^-$] ON MORTALITY

The relative risk of death in HD patients dialyzed with the same bath [HCO$_3^-$] is increased in patients who either have very low or very high values for predialysis serum [HCO$_3^-$] (as compared with a reference group with values between 19 and 23 mmol/L) (27,28,60,61). In two large cohort studies (7,000 and 20,000 patients, respectively), the relative risk of mortality increased by 10% to 15% for predialysis [total CO$_2$] values less than 19 mmol/L, as compared to patients with values of 19 to 22 mmol/L, and 19 to 24 mmol/L, respectively (60,61). In a third cohort study, with an even larger number of patients, mortality risk increased by 10% for patients with serum [total CO$_2$] values less than 19 mmol/L (27). All three studies also showed a higher mortality risk when serum [total CO$_2$] was high, but this effect largely disappeared when the cases were adjusted for indicators of malnutrition and inflammation (27). As discussed earlier, a high predialysis serum [HCO$_3^-$] occurring without an upward adjustment in bath [HCO$_3^-$] likely reflects low dietary protein intake, which may be a marker of other comorbidities that increase mortality risk. A low predialysis serum [HCO$_3^-$] appears to have a more direct effect on mortality. It should be emphasized that none of these studies assessed pH and PCO_2, and it is likely the effect of changes in pH on cell function and is more important than the prevailing serum [HCO$_3^-$] with regard to mortality. In one study in which pH was measured predialysis, mortality risk was increased only when the value was ≥7.40, underscoring concerns about excess alkalinity (62).

MANAGEMENT OF PATIENTS WITH LOW SERUM [HCO$_3^-$]

Based on the evidence cited above for patients with low predialysis serum [HCO$_3^-$], the 2000 Kidney Disease Outcome Quality Initiative (KDOQI) guidelines recommended increasing the value to 22 mmol/L or higher in all patients by increasing bath [HCO$_3^-$] if necessary (63). Many dialysis units have worked to meet this guideline, but it is unclear whether such an effort is justified. A recent large cohort study has found an increase in mortality risk of 8% for every 4 mmol/L increase in bath [HCO$_3^-$] (64). This risk is independent of the predialysis serum [HCO$_3^-$]. Although this is a single study, one should probably not raise bath [HCO$_3^-$] more than 1 to 3 mmol/L, and such an intervention should be limited to patients with predialysis values of <19 mmol/L.

Before considering any increase in bath [HCO$_3^-$], one should try to determine the cause of the low predialysis serum value. This assessment should include an analysis of both the events between treatments and during dialysis. The rate of fall in serum [HCO$_3^-$] between treatments can be assessed by comparing the postdialysis

		[HCO$_3^-$] mmol/L			
N	**Duration (mo)**	**Baseline**	**Treatment**	**Technique**	**Reference**
11	18	15.6	24.0	↑ Bath [HCO$_3^-$] to 40–48 mmol/L	(54)
38	3	19.0	24.8	↑ Bath [HCO$_3^-$] to 39 mmol/L	(24)
8	1	18.6	25.3	↑ Bath [HCO$_3^-$] to 40 mmol/L	(53)
21	6	20.4	23.3	↑ Bath [HCO$_3^-$] to 40 mmol/L	(55)
25	6	22.5	26.7	↑ Bath [HCO$_3^-$] to 40 mmol/L	(55)
6	1	18.5	24.8	↑ Bath [HCO$_3^-$] to 40 + oral NaHCO$_3$	(56)
9	1	20.0	25.0	↑ Bath [HCO$_3^-$] to 40 + oral NaHCO$_3$	(49)
12	6	18.8	23.1	↑ Bath [HCO$_3^-$] to 36 + oral NaHCO$_3$	(57)

TABLE 25.5 Studies in which Predialysis Serum [HCO$_3^-$] Was Increased in Conventional Hemodialysis: Techniques and Results

value with the next predialysis value. As discussed earlier, the key factors influencing the rate of decline are nutrition (specifically, protein intake) and fluid retention. If dietary adjustments are called for, one must be careful to ensure that overall nutrition remains adequate, as protein malnutrition will certainly not be beneficial for the patient (26,60). If fluid retention is excessive, a reduction in intake between treatments should be encouraged, recognizing that this is a difficult undertaking. For completeness, one should also determine whether patients are losing large amounts of HCO_3^- in their urine (if they still have significant urine output) or in their stool (diarrhea states, see later). To assess net alkali gain during dialysis, serum $[HCO_3^-]$ can be measured before and immediately after the treatment. This measurement can answer the question of whether the alkali added from the bath has been retained or consumed by excessive organic acid production. Normally, serum $[HCO_3^-]$ should increase by 6 to 10 mmol/L during each treatment (**FIGURE 25.7**).

Regardless of the cause, predialysis serum $[HCO_3^-]$ can easily be increased by increasing bath $[HCO_3^-]$ (23,47,53–57,59). **TABLE 25.5** summarizes the results of studies in which bath $[HCO_3^-]$ was increased to improve predialysis serum $[HCO_3^-]$. These studies demonstrate that postdialysis $[HCO_3^-]$ is directly related to bath $[HCO_3^-]$, and this value in turn exerts a parallel effect on the nadir serum $[HCO_3^-]$ before the next treatment. In these studies, postdialysis serum $[HCO_3^-]$ increased to between 30 and 34 mmol/L, and this relative (and transient) alkalemia was not associated with any adverse events. However, given the possible long-term risk to the patient of increasing bath $[HCO_3^-]$ (see above) (64), this maneuver is no longer recommended, unless predialysis serum $[HCO_3^-]$ is persistently less than 19 mmol/L and cannot be corrected by any other means. An alternative (or supplemental) approach is to administer oral sodium bicarbonate on a daily basis. This supplement will effectively increase predialysis serum $[HCO_3^-]$ but may also increase fluid retention (49,56,57).

MANAGEMENT OF PATIENTS WITH HIGH SERUM $[HCO_3^-]$

A new concern is in patients with very high predialysis serum $[HCO_3^-]$ who clearly have an increased mortality risk (65). As many as 15% of patients now receiving dialysis have values >26 mmol/L. The available evidence suggests that, unlike low predialysis serum $[HCO_3^-]$, high values are a marker for nutritional deficiency or inflammatory events, rather than an independent risk factor, and thus reducing bath $[HCO_3^-]$ is unlikely to be beneficial (27). In these patients, attention should be focused on addressing nutrition and modifiable inflammatory factors, rather than making any adjustments in the HD prescription. These patients represent a quandary, however, and the best approach to treatment remains to be determined.

DAILY HEMODIALYSIS

The use of daily HD treatments, either in critically ill inpatients or in stable outpatients, quickly normalizes serum $[HCO_3^-]$ and pH (see Chapter 8) (66–69). In stable outpatients receiving daily nocturnal HD treatments, the difference between predialysis and postdialysis serum $[HCO_3^-]$ is reduced to less than 1 mmol/L, and bath $[HCO_3^-]$ has been reduced to 28 to 32 mmol/L to avoid metabolic alkalosis. Similar outcomes have been observed with daily short HD treatments. These results are not surprising, given the dynamic changes in serum $[HCO_3^-]$ described earlier for intermittent HD.

One form of daily HD differs from the others: It uses a lactate-containing bath in an enclosed cartridge (70). In this form of HD, the dynamics of alkali addition are similar to PD—loss of HCO_3^- into the bath and gain of lactate into the blood, and serum $[HCO_3^-]$ levels are maintained in the normal range by adjusting bath lactate concentration.

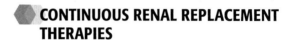

CONTINUOUS RENAL REPLACEMENT THERAPIES

Continuous hemofiltration, hemofiltration plus dialysis, and slow low-efficiency HD are all currently used for the treatment of kidney failure in critically ill patients (see Chapter 10) (66,71–74). With these techniques, the same principles hold with regard to acid–base homeostasis as discussed earlier for conventional HD. With continuous hemofiltration, HCO_3^- loss is related to the serum concentration and the ultrafiltration rate as well as to the ongoing rate of endogenous acid production. Replacement is achieved with a continuous infusion of either an HCO_3^- or lactate-containing solution (74,75), and serum $[HCO_3^-]$ is readily maintained within the range of normal (66). With continuous slow, low-efficiency dialysis, serum $[HCO_3^-]$ becomes essentially equal to the concentration in the dialysis bath solution and the latter must be reduced to 24 to 28 mmol/L to prevent the development of metabolic alkalosis.

Hemofiltration and Hemodiafiltration

Hemofiltration uses the principle of convection rather than diffusion for toxin removal and can be used as an intermittent therapy. To achieve adequate toxin removal, high-volume ultrafiltration occurs during the procedure necessitating the rapid infusion of replacement fluids (at ~100 mL/min) (76). Although acetate-containing solutions were originally used for this procedure, replacement solutions containing HCO_3^- are necessary for adequate acid–base homeostasis (76). The high-volume ultrafiltration and rapid infusion of replacement solutions make the technique more complex and subject to risk than conventional HD, and it is rarely used.

Hemodiafiltration combines the high convective characteristics of intermittent hemofiltration with a bath solution containing either acetate or HCO_3^- (77,78). For this treatment, replacement solutions containing HCO_3^- are necessary to achieve positive net alkali addition, and the procedure has the same complexity as hemofiltration and little advantage over conventional HD from an acid–base perspective.

Acetate-free biofiltration is a hemodiafiltration technique in which the dialysate contains no HCO_3^- or acetate but does contain other key solutes (79). High-volume ultrafiltration is carried out, and isotonic $NaHCO_3$ is continually infused into the postfilter blood. One proposed advantage for this procedure is the removal of all acetate from the bath, but there is no evidence that the small amount of acetate currently used in bath solutions has any clinically important toxicity. As opposed to regular hemodiafiltration where the replacement solution contains all electrolytes, only $NaHCO_3$ is reinfused with this procedure, allowing for high concentrations of HCO_3^- to be used. Using this technique, one can predictably increase serum $[HCO_3^-]$ to the level desired in each patient (79). As discussed earlier, the same goal can be achieved with conventional HD by simply adjusting the bath $[HCO_3^-]$, and acetate-free biofiltration is only rarely used for the treatment of ESKD. Despite the lack of evidence for acetate toxicity at low levels, conventional HD bath solutions are also now commonly using citric acid rather than acetic acid to stabilize pH for HCO_3^- addition (see earlier), eliminating the rationale for this complex dialysis technique.

ACID–BASE DISORDERS IN PATIENTS WITH END-STAGE KIDNEY DISEASE

Thus far, we have considered the factors determining the "normal" values for serum $[HCO_3^-]$ in patients receiving renal replacement therapy. This section is directed at identifying and managing acute or chronic superimposed acid–base disorders in this population of patients. Such disorders are heralded by deviations from the expected normal values for serum $[HCO_3^-]$ and Pco_2 (**TABLES 25.1** and **25.3**). In general, an abrupt change in serum $[HCO_3^-]$ of 3 mmol/L or greater from the usual value should signal the presence of a new metabolic acid–base disorder. Respiratory acid–base disorders, by contrast, are not associated with any change in serum $[HCO_3^-]$ and must be suspected by the clinical presentation and history (80,81).

Given the wide variation in predialysis serum $[HCO_3^-]$ in this unique group of patients, identification of superimposed disorders seems a formidable task. Fortunately, an ongoing log of monthly values for serum $[HCO_3^-]$ is available to use for comparison with a suspected abnormal value. Identifying an abnormality in Pco_2 is a more difficult undertaking because no laboratory trail exists for this parameter. The ventilatory response to variations in serum $[HCO_3^-]$ is normal in patients with kidney failure (6,30,38,39,46,47), and so one can use the following formulas to estimate the expected Pco_2 for any given serum $[HCO_3^-]$ if one has a clinical suspicion that a ventilatory problem is present:

For serum $[HCO_3^-]$ values 24 mmol/L or less:

$$Pco_2 \text{ (mm Hg)} = 40 - 1.2 \times (24 - [HCO_3^-]) \quad (25.1)$$

For serum $[HCO_3^-]$ values greater than 24 mmol/L:

$$Pco_2 \text{ (mm Hg)} = 40 + 0.7 \times ([HCO_3^-] - 24) \quad (25.2)$$

These equations should be considered only as approximations, but they can be used to determine whether a measured Pco_2 deviates notably from the expected value. Given the normal variability in the ventilatory response to a given serum $[HCO_3^-]$, one should consider the measured Pco_2 to be abnormal only if it is 5 mm Hg or more different from the expected value.

Once an abnormal Pco_2 or serum $[HCO_3^-]$ has been identified, the approach to characterizing the abnormality is the same as that in patients with normal kidney function:

1. Identify the primary disorder (e.g., metabolic acidosis or alkalosis, respiratory acidosis or alkalosis).
2. Determine whether the secondary response is appropriate.
3. Determine the cause of the disorder.

Although the general approach is the same, the diagnostic process is actually simpler than in patients with kidney function (**FIGURE 25.8**). In patients with ESKD, for example, there is no kidney adaptive response to respiratory acid–base disorders. In addition, one need not consider kidney causes for either metabolic acidosis or alkalosis. The approach to each of the four cardinal acid–base disorders is discussed in following sections.

Metabolic Acidosis

A new metabolic acidosis can be diagnosed in a patient with ESKD when serum $[HCO_3^-]$ falls by 3 mmol/L or more from the usual value (80,81). Unlike patients with kidney function, one does not have to consider the possibility that chronic respiratory alkalosis is responsible because the secondary reduction in $[HCO_3^-]$ induced by hypocapnia requires kidney function. Although a primary respiratory alkalosis cannot be the cause of the low serum $[HCO_3^-]$ in patients with ESKD, blood pH and Pco_2 should be measured to

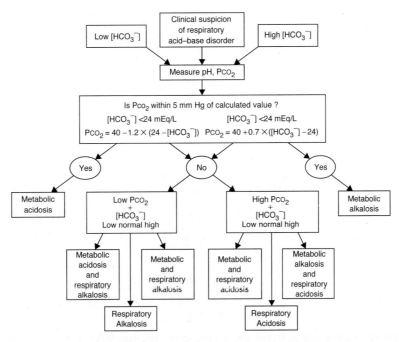

FIGURE 25.8 Approach to the evaluation of acid–base disorders in patients with end-stage kidney disease (ESKD). The terms *low [HCO₃⁻]* and *high [HCO₃⁻]* in the diagram refer to values that are 3 mmol/L or more either lower or higher than the average values found in patients receiving renal replacement therapy (**TABLES 25.1** and **25.2**).

determine whether the ventilatory response to metabolic acidosis is appropriate. In patients with functioning fistulas, this information can be easily obtained without a separate arterial puncture (82). The expected ventilatory response to metabolic acidosis decreases Pco_2 by approximately 1.2 mm Hg for each 1 mmol/L fall in serum $[HCO_3^-]$ (**EQUATION 25.1**) (52). If the measured Pco_2 deviates from the expected value by 5 or more mm Hg, then the patient likely has a mixed disorder (see later). If the fall in Pco_2 is within the expected range, then the patient most likely has an uncomplicated metabolic acidosis (**FIGURE 25.8**), and attention should be directed at diagnosing its cause. In all instances, the history and physical examination findings should be used in conjunction with these equations to determine whether a simple or mixed disorder is present.

Causes

Metabolic acidosis can be produced either by the sudden addition of a new acid to the body fluids or by the loss of HCO_3^- (**TABLE 25.6**). The most common cause is acid generation as a result of abnormalities in body metabolism or through toxin-induced stimulation of acid production. The only site for abnormal HCO_3^- losses in patients without kidney function is from the gastrointestinal tract.

Separation of the causes of metabolic acidosis by assessment of whether the anion gap is increased or not is less useful in patients with ESKD than in patients with functioning kidneys. The anion gap must be corrected for the serum albumin concentration and is often already increased in these patients (80,81). In addition, most causes of metabolic acidosis in HD patients are associated with a further increase. The most useful tool is a baseline anion gap to allow assessment of any change. In the absence of baseline data, an anion gap of more than 20 mmol/L should be considered abnormally high.

Organic Acidosis

The most common cause of a new metabolic acidosis in patients with ESKD is a pathologic process that leads to overproduction of one or more organic acids. Diabetic ketoacidosis is the most common culprit, but one also should consider other causes such

TABLE 25.6	Causes of Metabolic Acidosis in End-Stage Kidney Disease	
Increased Anion Gap[a]	**No Increase in Anion Gap**
Diabetic ketoacidosis	Gastrointestinal alkali loss
Lactic acidosis	Diarrhea
Alcoholic ketoacidosis	Pancreatic drainage
Toxin ingestions	Hemofiltration with NaCl replacement
Methyl alcohol	Ammonium chloride ingestion
Ethylene glycol	
Salicylates	
Paraldehyde	
Catabolic state	
High protein intake	
High salt and water intake	

[a]Increase from the usual level in the patient by greater than 3 mmol/L.

as alcoholic ketoacidosis, lactic acidosis, and toxin ingestions (**TABLE 25.6**). The organic acids produced by these disorders titrate and replace HCO_3^- in the body fluids, causing the anion gap to increase as the anions of these acids accumulate in the serum. In contrast to patients with functioning kidneys, patients with ESKD cannot excrete these newly formed anions, and they remain available to be metabolized unless they are removed by dialysis. Thus, once the pathologic process leading to their generation is reversed, they are able to regenerate all the HCO_3^- that was consumed. This sequence of events is illustrated in **FIGURE 25.9** in a patient with ESKD with diabetes mellitus who developed diabetic ketoacidosis (83). In this patient, the ketoacidosis rapidly lowered serum $[HCO_3^-]$ and increased the anion gap. Insulin therapy alone decreased the anion gap and increased serum $[HCO_3^-]$ from 14 to 25 mmol/L over 10 hours. Note that this recovery occurred without

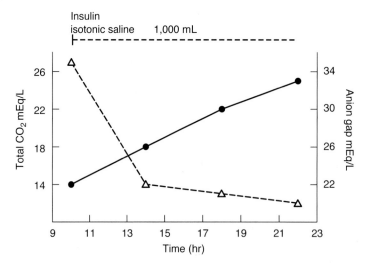

FIGURE 25.9 Correction of diabetic ketoacidosis in a patient with end-stage kidney disease (ESKD) without HCO_3^- administration or dialysis treatment. Serum [total CO_2] and serum anion gap were restored to preacidosis levels by the administration of insulin and 1 L of isotonic saline. (Reprinted with permission from Gennari FJ. Acid–base disorders in end-stage renal disease. Part I. *Semin Dial* 1990;3:81–85.)

an intervening dialysis treatment and required only minimal fluid replacement and no exogenous alkali; these patients lose neither fluid nor organic anions when they develop ketoacidosis.

Although diabetic ketoacidosis is rapidly reversed by insulin therapy, production of other organic acids cannot be so easily halted. Therefore, dialysis is often required both to remove the organic anions and to rapidly replace them with HCO_3^-. HD therapy is particularly useful when toxin ingestions lead to metabolic acidosis in anephric individuals, as this mode of therapy is the most effective in removing the offending toxins. In some types of lactic acidosis, production of lactic acid cannot be halted (84,85), and HD in this setting offers a means to replace HCO_3^- rapidly without causing fluid overload. Although rapid alkalinization using HD accelerates lactic acid production (84), continuous HD can overcome this increase and can produce a sustained increase in serum $[HCO_3^-]$ until lactic acid production can be halted (86). As with all organic acidosis, reversal of the cause of the increase in acid production is key to sustained correction of the metabolic acidosis.

Other Causes

As discussed earlier, an increase in dietary protein intake or an increase in body protein catabolism will reduce predialysis serum $[HCO_3^-]$ (TABLE 25.6). Because the increase in endogenous acid production engendered is associated with anions other than chloride, this type of acidosis also increases the anion gap. An increase in fluid retention, due to high NaCl and water intake between HD treatments, will also lower predialysis serum $[HCO_3^-]$ by diluting body alkali stores (TABLE 25.4). The dilution occurs without a change in the concentration of other electrolytes, and therefore, the anion gap increases, although the change in this instance is likely to be minimal. Neither an increase in ECF volume nor an increase in protein catabolism is likely to produce a severe metabolic acidosis. If serum $[HCO_3^-]$ falls by more than 6 to 8 mmol/L acutely, one can be virtually certain that an organic acidosis is responsible.

Induction of metabolic acidosis from gastrointestinal HCO_3^- losses requires the development of severe diarrhea or could occur from surgical drainage of fluid rich in pancreatic secretion. This form of metabolic acidosis does not increase the anion gap above the usual level, as the acidosis is associated with the disproportionate loss of HCO_3^- and therefore an increase in serum $[Cl^-]$. Inadvertent replacement of alkali in the bath with a chloride-containing solution is a technique error that will induce a severe metabolic acidosis without increasing the anion gap (87). An extremely rare cause of metabolic acidosis without a further increase in the anion gap is the deliberate or accidental ingestion of ammonium chloride. In patients with no kidney function, renal tubule acidosis need not be considered as a cause of metabolic acidosis.

In patients treated with continuous hemofiltration, metabolic acidosis can be induced if an inappropriate replacement solution is used. If Ringer's lactate is used in a patient who is unable to metabolize this organic anion, the resulting metabolic acidosis will be associated with an increase in the anion gap, although the acidosis is induced by HCO_3^- loss through hemofiltration. If sodium chloride is used as the replacement solution, then the acidosis will be associated with hyperchloremia and no increase in anion gap.

Metabolic Alkalosis

Metabolic alkalosis is diagnosed by the finding of an increase in serum $[HCO_3^-]$. In patients with ESKD, chronic respiratory acidosis is not a consideration because the increase in serum $[HCO_3^-]$

engendered by sustained respiratory acidosis requires kidney function. Metabolic alkalosis is generated by the selective loss of chloride from the body fluids (e.g., from vomiting or nasogastric drainage) or by the addition of new alkali. Unlike patients with functioning kidneys, the disorder is sustained once initiated, regardless of dietary intake (88,89). In addition, because the hypokalemia associated with metabolic alkalosis is primarily caused by renal K^+ losses, serum $[K^+]$ is unchanged from its usual value when metabolic alkalosis occurs in patients with ESKD (88,89). In these patients, vomiting or nasogastric drainage can cause very severe metabolic alkalosis because they cannot excrete any of the newly generated HCO_3^- (89). Kidney causes of metabolic alkalosis (e.g., Bartter syndrome, primary hyperaldosteronism) need not be considered, nor is it necessary to partition the causes into chloride-sensitive and chloride-resistant groups.

An increase in serum $[HCO_3^-]$ of 3 mmol/L or more from the usual value in a patient with ESKD is the working rule for diagnosing a new metabolic alkalosis, but because serum $[HCO_3^-]$ is lower than that of individuals with normal renal function, the diagnosis is often not recognized unless a much larger increase is present—some 8 to 10 mmol/L (90). Although one does not have to consider chronic respiratory acidosis as a cause of the increase in serum $[HCO_3^-]$, one should measure blood pH and Pco_2 to ensure that the respiratory response to the metabolic alkalosis is in the expected range. The normal response to an increase in serum $[HCO_3^-]$ is hypoventilation: for each 1 mmol/L increase in $[HCO_3^-]$, Pco_2 increases by 0.7 mm Hg (EQUATION 25.2). If the measured Pco_2 is within 5 mm Hg of the expected value, the patient has an uncomplicated metabolic alkalosis (FIGURE 25.8). If the value deviates from this range, the patient likely has a mixed disorder (see later).

Causes

TABLE 25.7 presents the causes of metabolic alkalosis in patients with ESKD. There are only two categories to consider: loss of acid or the addition of new alkali. The former occurs only with vomiting or nasogastric drainage, and the diagnosis is almost always immediately apparent. However, bulimic patients may deny vomiting (90). The potential sources of alkali range from $NaHCO_3$ to certain anionic amino acids (TABLE 25.7). Administration of $NaHCO_3$ in a dose of 2 mmol/kg body weight will increase serum $[HCO_3^-]$ by 4 to 5 mmol/L (91). Calcium salts containing carbonate, acetate,

TABLE 25.7	Causes of Metabolic Alkalosis in End-Stage Kidney Disease
Vomiting	
Nasogastric drainage	
Exogenous alkali/alkali precursor	
Sodium bicarbonate	
Potassium bicarbonate	
Calcium carbonate	
Lactate	
Acetate	
Citrate	
Glutamate	
Proprionate	
Aluminum hydroxide + Kayexalate	

or citrate only add alkali to the body to the extent that calcium is ionized and absorbed. Therefore, they rarely cause significant metabolic alkalosis.

A rare cause of metabolic alkalosis in patients with ESKD is the combined use of sodium polystyrene sulfonate (Kayexalate) and aluminum hydroxide (92). Aluminum hydroxide is usually converted to aluminum phosphate or chloride by gastric acid, and a portion of these salts dissociate in the duodenum, allowing aluminum ions to bind to HCO_3^- secreted by the pancreas. When Kayexalate is present, however, aluminum ions bind to it instead forming a compound that does not dissociate. As a result, HCO_3^- is neither neutralized nor bound, and this alkali is reabsorbed by the small intestine and retained in the body fluids.

Management

Management of metabolic alkalosis in patients with ESKD should be directed at removing the cause. Treatment of the cause of vomiting and removal of any sources of exogenous alkali in most instances will lead to eventual correction of the disorder. If these interventions fail to correct the disorder and if the high serum $[HCO_3^-]$ is causing symptoms or interfering with management (e.g., ventilator dependence), serum $[HCO_3^-]$ can be reduced by decreasing bath $[HCO_3^-]$, an option easily managed with the dialysis machines now available (89). Metabolic alkalosis in the anephric patient in the intensive care unit can also be corrected by using continuous hemofiltration and replacing losses with only sodium chloride (88) or by using slow, low-efficiency HD with a bath $[HCO_3^-]$ of 25 mmol/L.

Respiratory Acidosis

Respiratory acidosis is caused by alveolar hypoventilation and is manifested by an increase in arterial P_{CO_2}. The normal secondary response to this disorder has two components (93). The first is an acute buffer response that produces a very small increase in serum $[HCO_3^-]$; the second and major component is produced by renal HCO_3^- generation. In patients with ESKD, this latter response cannot occur; therefore, no notable increase in serum $[HCO_3^-]$ occurs to signal the presence of hypercapnia. One must have a clinical suspicion for the disorder and measure blood pH and P_{CO_2} to confirm it (**FIGURE 25.8**). A P_{CO_2} value of 5 mm Hg or higher than the expected value for the prevailing serum $[HCO_3^-]$ establishes the diagnosis (**EQUATIONS 25.1** and **25.2**). One need not evaluate whether the serum $[HCO_3^-]$ is appropriate; serum $[HCO_3^-]$ is determined by the dialysis treatment rather than by P_{CO_2} in patients with ESKD.

Because there is no renal secondary response, hypercapnia leads to a sustained and severe acidemia in patients with ESKD. In a patient with kidney function, a sustained P_{CO_2} level of 55 mm Hg will result in only a minor reduction in blood pH because this increment in P_{CO_2} will induce a secondary increase in serum $[HCO_3^-]$ to 30 to 33 mmol/L. By contrast, a patient with ESKD with the same P_{CO_2} level may have a predialysis serum $[HCO_3^-]$ of 20 to 22 mmol/L with a resultant blood pH of 7.18 to 7.22.

Management

Management of respiratory acidosis should be directed at reversing the hypercapnia if at all possible. If the P_{CO_2} cannot be reduced to a safe level, one can increase bath $[HCO_3^-]$ to try to raise the serum level. Other approaches include daily or continuous HD or PD. Bicarbonate supplementation is also an option, but this therapy may lead to fluid overload, further embarrassing pulmonary gas exchange.

Respiratory Alkalosis

Respiratory alkalosis is caused by alveolar hyperventilation and is manifested by a decrease in arterial blood P_{CO_2}. The normal secondary response to this disorder has two components: an acute buffer response that lowers serum $[HCO_3^-]$ within minutes and a chronic kidney response that lowers serum $[HCO_3^-]$ further (94). Both responses are obliterated in patients receiving dialysis therapy. The chronic response requires kidney function and the acute response is overwhelmed by the effect of dialysis on serum $[HCO_3^-]$. Therefore, severe alkalemia is to be expected in patients with ESKD. Because serum $[HCO_3^-]$ does not change notably, one must have a clinical suspicion that the disorder is present and measure blood pH and P_{CO_2} to establish the diagnosis. The presence of a P_{CO_2} level that is 5 mm Hg or more lower than expected for the prevailing serum $[HCO_3^-]$ indicates the presence of respiratory alkalosis (**EQUATIONS 25.1** and **25.2** and **FIGURE 25.8**).

Causes and Management

Many pathologic events can cause respiratory alkalosis (**TABLE 25.8**). In contrast to patients with normal kidney function who can tolerate hypocapnia without serious complications, patients with renal failure can develop severe and sustained life-threatening alkalemia. Blood pH levels greater than 7.70 have been reported in patients with sustained respiratory alkalosis receiving PD therapy (83,95). In one patient with sustained respiratory alkalosis receiving conventional HD, an arterial pH greater than 7.90 was observed. If hypocapnia cannot be corrected, one can attempt to reduce serum $[HCO_3^-]$ by continuous hemofiltration without alkali replacement (using only saline) in an intensive care unit setting, but mortality is high if the problem persists.

TABLE 25.8	**Causes of Respiratory Alkalosis**
Hypoxemia (PO_2 <60 mm Hg)	
Anxiety hyperventilation syndrome	
Central nervous system disorders	
Stroke	
Infection	
Trauma	
Tumors	
Pulmonary disease[a]	
Pneumonia	
Pulmonary edema	
Pulmonary embolus	
Interstitial fibrosis	
Sepsis (most commonly gram negative)	
Hepatic failure	
Pregnancy	
Drugs	
Salicylates	
Nicotine	
Progesterone	

[a]Independent of hypoxemia.

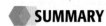 TABLE 25.9	Mixed Acid–Base Disorders in End-Stage Kidney Disease

Mixed Metabolic and Respiratory Disorders

↓[HCO₃⁻]

Pco₂ > expected = metabolic + respiratory acidosis

Pco₂ < expected = metabolic acidosis + respiratory alkalosis

↑[HCO₃⁻]

Pco₂ > expected = metabolic alkalosis + respiratory acidosis

Pco₂ < expected = metabolic + respiratory alkalosis

Metabolic alkalosis + metabolic alkalosis

Serum [HCO₃⁻] + Δ anion gap[a] >30 mmol/L

Triple disorders

Metabolic acidosis + metabolic alkalosis +:

Pco₂ > expected = respiratory acidosis

Pco₂ < expected = respiratory alkalosis

[a]Δ anion gap = anion gap at time of presentation–usual anion gap in that patient.

Mixed Acid–Base Disorders

Mixed acid–base disorders occur when two or more primary acid–base abnormalities are present at the same time. In patients with ESKD, the spectrum of possible mixed disorders is narrower than in patients with kidney function because of the absence of any secondary response to hypo- and hypercapnia (**TABLE 25.9**). The most common mixed disorders are a combination of metabolic and respiratory disturbances. These are diagnosed by measuring Pco₂ and using **EQUATIONS 25.1** and **25.2** to determine if the value is appropriate for the concomitantly measured serum [HCO₃⁻]. If the serum [HCO₃⁻] is low (metabolic acidosis), the ventilatory response can be inadequate (superimposed respiratory acidosis) or greater than expected (respiratory alkalosis). The former is more common and can be associated with severe acidemia. Urgent intubation and assisted ventilation is needed for such patients in addition to management of the metabolic acidosis. If the serum [HCO₃⁻] is high (metabolic alkalosis), this disorder can also be associated with an inadequate or greater than normal ventilatory response. When primary hyperventilation (respiratory alkalosis) complicates metabolic alkalosis, life-threatening increases in pH can occur. Attention should be directed at increasing Pco₂ if possible, or urgently reducing serum [HCO₃⁻].

More rarely, a mixed metabolic alkalosis and acidosis can occur. The sequence that might cause such a disorder in a dialysis patient would be the administration of exogenous alkali, increasing serum [HCO₃⁻], followed by the development of a lactic acidosis or diabetic ketoacidosis. Such a sequence might fortuitously result in a serum [HCO₃⁻] at or near normal levels, but the disorder is uncovered by finding an increase in the anion gap. Because of the variability in anion gap, such a diagnosis should only be made if the value is increased by 6 or more mmol/L. If the respiratory response to the final serum [HCO₃⁻] in such a patient is abnormal, then a triple disorder is diagnosed.

SUMMARY

From an acid–base perspective, two issues should be addressed in the management of patients with ESKD. First, one must understand the forces determining the steady-state serum [HCO₃⁻], so that modifications in treatment can be instituted as necessary to maintain this value in an optimal range. Second, one must recognize and treat superimposed acid–base disorders in these patients. The approach to diagnosing these disorders is less complex in patients with no kidney function. One need not consider metabolic acid–base disorders caused by changes in kidney alkali or acid excretion, nor need one consider secondary kidney responses to respiratory acidosis or alkalosis. The laboratory data normally accumulated in these patients facilitate the quick identification of changes in serum [HCO₃⁻] caused by either metabolic acidosis or alkalosis, but respiratory acid–base disorders must be suspected on clinical grounds. Diagnosis and management of uncomplicated acid–base disorders are straightforward. Although relatively uncommon, mixed disturbances can occur in patients with renal failure, and their recognition and management can be lifesaving.

REFERENCES

1. Kurtz I, Maher T, Hulter HN, et al. Effect of diet on plasma acid-base composition in normal humans. *Kidney Int* 1983;24:670–680.
2. Lennon EJ, Lemann J Jr, Litzow JR. The effects of diet and stool composition on the net external acid balance of normal subjects. *J Clin Invest* 1966;45:1601–1607.
3. Relman AS, Lennon EJ, Lemann J Jr. Endogenous production of fixed acid and the measurement of the net balance of acid in normal subjects. *J Clin Invest* 1961;40:1621–1630.
4. Gennari FJ. Regulation of acid-base balance: overview. In: Gennari FJ, Adrogue HJ, Galla JH, et al, eds. *Acid–Base Disorders and Their Treatment*. Boca Raton, FL: Taylor & Francis, 2005:177–208.
5. Gennari FJ. Effect of renal replacement therapy on acid-base homeostasis. In: Gennari FJ, Adrogue HJ, Galla JH, et al, eds. *Acid–Base Disorders and Their Treatment*. Boca Raton, FL: Taylor & Francis, 2005:697–716.
6. Gennari FJ. Acid-base balance in dialysis patients. *Kidney Int* 1985; 28:678–688.
7. Gennari FJ. Acid-base homeostasis in end-stage renal disease. *Semin Dial* 1996;9:404–411.
8. United States Renal Data System. Incidence, prevalence, patient characteristics, and treatment modalities. In: *2014 USRDS Annual Data Report: Vol. 2, End-Stage Renal Disease in the United States*. Bethesda, MD: National Institutes of Health, National Institute of Diabetes and Digestive and Kidney Diseases, 2014.
9. Watnick S. The state of peritoneal dialysis in the United States: from inertia to resurgence. *NephSAP* 2014;13(5):311–315.
10. Mujais S, Childers RW. Profiles of automated peritoneal dialysis prescriptions in the US 1997–2003. *Kidney Int* 2006;70(Suppl):S84–S90.
11. Pecoits-Filho R, Tranaeus A, Lindholm B. Clinical trial experience with Physioneal™. *Kidney Int* 2003;64(Suppl 88):S100–S104.
12. Boen ST. Kinetics of peritoneal dialysis. a comparison with the artificial kidney. *Medicine* 1961;40(3):243–288.
13. Heimburger O, Mujais S. Buffer transport in peritoneal dialysis. *Kidney Int* 2003;64(Suppl 88):S37–S42.
14. Feriani M. Use of different buffers in peritoneal dialysis. *Semin Dial* 2000;13:256–260.
15. Mandelbaum JM, Heistand ML, Schardin KE. Six months' experience with PD-2 solution. *Dial Transplant* 1983;12:259–260.
16. Nolph KD, Prowant B, Serkes KD, et al. Multicenter evaluation of a new peritoneal dialysis solution with a high lactate and a low magnesium concentration. *Perit Dial Bull* 1983;3:63–65.
17. Gennari FJ, Rimmer JM. Acid-base disorders in end stage renal disease. *Semin Dial* 1990;3:81–85.
18. Mujais S. Acid-base profile in patients on PD. *Kidney Int* 2003;64(Suppl 88): S26–S36.
19. Uribarri J, Buquing J, Oh MS. Acid-base balance in chronic peritoneal dialysis patients. *Kidney Int* 1995;47:269–273.
20. Feriani M, Passlick-Deetjen J, Jaeckle-Meyer I, et al. Individualized bicarbonate concentrations in the peritoneal dialysis fluid to optimize

acid-base status in CAPD patients. *Nephrol Dial Transplant* 2004;19: 195–202.

21. Tranaeus A. A long-term study of a bicarbonate/lactate-based peritoneal dialysis solution—clinical benefits. *Perit Dial Int* 2000;20:516–523.
22. Mactier RA, Sprosen TS, Gokal R, et al. Bicarbonate and bicarbonate/lactate peritoneal dialysis solutions for the treatment of infusion pain. *Kidney Int* 1998;53:1061–1067.
23. Gennari FJ. Acid-base balance in dialysis patients. *Semin Dial* 2000; 13:235–239.
24. Oettinger CW, Oliver JC. Normalization of uremic acidosis in hemodialysis patients with a high bicarbonate dialysate. *J Am Soc Nephrol* 1993; 3:1804–1807.
25. Uribarri J, Levin NW, Delmez J, et al. Association of acidosis and nutritional parameters in hemodialysis patients. *Am J Kidney Dis* 1999; 34:493–499.
26. Chauveau P, Fouque D, Combe C, et al. Acid-base in renal failure: acidosis and nutritional status in hemodialyzed patients. *Semin Dial* 2000;13:241–246.
27. Wu DY, Shinaberger CS, Regidor DL, et al. Association between serum bicarbonate and death in hemodialysis patients: is it better to be acidotic or alkalotic? *Clin J Am Soc Nephrol* 2006;1:70–78.
28. Gennari FJ. Very low and high predialysis serum bicarbonate levels are risk factors in mortality: What are the appropriate interventions? *Semin Dial* 2010;23(3):253–257.
29. Man NK, Fournier G, Thireau P, et al. Effect of bicarbonate-containing dialysate on chronic hemodialysis patients: a comparative study. *Artif Organs* 1982;6:421–428.
30. Hakim RM, Pontzer MA, Tilton D, et al. Effects of acetate and bicarbonate dialysate in stable chronic dialysis patients. *Kidney Int* 1985;28: 535–540.
31. Marano M, D'Amato A, Marano S. A very simple formula to compute pCO2 in hemodialysis patients. *Int Urol Nephrol* 2015;47(4):691–694.
32. Murphy WP Jr, Swan RC Jr, Walter CW, et al. Use of an artificial kidney. III. Current procedures in clinical hemodialysis. *J Lab Clin Med* 1952;40:436–444.
33. Brandon JM, Nakamoto S, Rosenbaum JL, et al. Prolongation of survival by periodic prolonged hemodialysis in patients with chronic renal failure. *Am J Med* 1962;33:538–544.
34. Mion CM, Hegstrom RM, Boen ST, et al. Substitution of sodium acetate for sodium bicarbonate in the bath fluid for hemodialysis. *Trans Am Soc Artif Intern Organs* 1964;10:110–113.
35. Mudge GH, Manning JA, Gilman A. Sodium acetate as a source of fixed base. *Proc Soc Exp Biol Med* 1949;71:136–138.
36. Kveim M, Nesbakken R. Utilization of exogenous acetate during hemodialysis. *Trans Am Soc Artif Intern Organs* 1975;21:138–143.
37. Tolchin N, Roberts JL, Hayashi J, et al. Metabolic consequences of high mass-transfer hemodialysis. *Kidney Int* 1977;11:366–378.
38. Vreman HJ, Assomull VM, Kaiser BA, et al. Acetate metabolism and acid-base homeostasis during hemodialysis: influence of dialyzer efficiency and rate of acetate metabolism. *Kidney Int* 1980;10(Suppl): S62–S74.
39. Cohen E, Liu K, Batlle DC. Patterns of metabolic acidosis in patients with chronic renal failure: impact of hemodialysis. *Int J Artif Organs* 1988; 11:440–448.
40. Vinay P, Prud'Homme M, Vinet B, et al. Acetate metabolism and bicarbonate generation during hemodialysis: 10 years of observation. *Kidney Int* 1987;31:1194–1204.
41. Kveim MH, Nesbakken R. Acetate metabolizing capacity in man. *J Oslo City Hosp* 1980;30:101–104.
42. Graefe U, Milutinovich J, Follette WC, et al. Less dialysis-induced morbidity and vascular instability with bicarbonate in dialysate. *Ann Intern Med* 1978;88:332–336.
43. Hunt JM, Chappell TR, Henrich WL, et al. Gas exchange during dialysis. Contrasting mechanisms contributing to comparable alterations with acetate and bicarbonate buffers. *Am J Med* 1984;77:255–260.
44. Symreng T, Flanigan MJ, Lim VS. Ventilatory and metabolic changes during high efficiency hemodialysis. *Kidney Int* 1992;41:1064–1069.

45. Ward RA, Wathen RL, Williams TE. Effects of long-term bicarbonate hemodialysis (BHD) on acid-base status. *Trans Am Soc Artif Intern Organs* 1982;28:295–298.
46. Ward RA, Wathen RL, Williams TE, et al. Hemodialysate composition and intradialytic metabolic, acid-base and potassium changes. *Kidney Int* 1987;32:129–135.
47. Gotch FA, Sargent JA, Keen ML. Hydrogen ion balance in dialysis therapy. *Artif Organs* 1982;6:388–395.
48. Diamond SM, Henrich WL. Acetate dialysate versus bicarbonate dialysate: a continuing controversy. *Am J Kidney Dis* 1987;9:3–11.
49. Harris DC, Yuill E, Chesher DW. Correcting acidosis in hemodialysis: effect on phosphate clearance and calcification risk. *J Am Soc Nephrol* 1995;6:1607–1612.
50. Uribarri J, Zia M, Mahmood J, et al. Acid production in chronic hemodialysis patients. *J Am Soc Nephrol* 1998;9:114–120.
51. Fabris A, LaGreca G, Chiaramonte S, et al. The importance of ultrafiltration on acid-base status in a dialysis population. *ASAIO Trans* 1988; 34:200–201.
52. Bushinsky DA, Coe FL, Katzenberg C, et al. Arterial PCO2 in chronic metabolic acidosis. *Kidney Int* 1982;22:311–314.
53. Graham KA, Hoenich NA, Tarbit M, et al. Correction of acidosis in hemodialysis patients increases the sensitivity of the parathyroid glands to calcium. *J Am Soc Nephrol* 1997;8:627–631.
54. Lefebvre A, de Vernejoul MC, Gueris J, et al. Optimal correction of acidosis changes progression of dialysis osteodystrophy. *Kidney Int* 1989;36:1112–1118.
55. Williams AJ, Dittmer ID, McArley A, et al. High bicarbonate dialysate in haemodialysis patients: effects on acidosis and nutritional status. *Nephrol Dial Transplant* 1997;12:2633–2637.
56. Graham KA, Reaich D, Channon SM, et al. Correction of acidosis in hemodialysis decreases whole-body protein degradation. *J Am Soc Nephrol* 1997;8:632–637.
57. Kooman JP, Deutz NE, Zijlmans P, et al. The influence of bicarbonate supplementation on plasma levels of branched-chain amino acids in haemodialysis patients with metabolic acidosis. *Nephrol Dial Transplant* 1997;12:2397–2401.
58. Bergström J, Alvestrand A, Fürst P. Plasma and muscle free amino acids in maintenance hemodialysis patients without protein malnutrition. *Kidney Int* 1990;38:108–114.
59. Graham KA, Reaich D, Channon SM, et al. Correction of acidosis in CAPD decreases whole body protein degradation. *Kidney Int* 1996; 49:1396–1400.
60. Lowrie EG, Lew NL. Death risk in hemodialysis patients: the predictive value of commonly measured variables and an evaluation of death rate differences between facilities. *Am J Kidney Dis* 1990;15:458–482.
61. Bommer J, Locatelli F, Satayathum S, et al. Association of predialysis serum bicarbonate levels with risk of mortality and hospitalization in the Dialysis Outcomes and Practice Patterns Study (DOPPS). *Am J Kidney Dis* 2004;44:661–671.
62. Yamamoto T, Shoji S, Yamakawa T, et al. Predialysis and postdialysis pH and bicarbonate and risk of all-cause and cardiovascular mortality in long-term hemodialysis patients. *Am J Kidney Dis* 2015;66(3): 469–478.
63. National Kidney Foundation. K/DOQI clinical practice guidelines for nutrition in chronic renal failure. *Am J Kidney Dis* 2000;35:S1–S140.
64. Tentori F, Karaboyas A, Robinson BM, et al. Association of dialysate concentration with mortality in the Dialysis Outcomes and Practice Patterns Study (DOPPS). *Am J Kidney Dis* 2013:62(4):738–746.
65. Lisawat P, Gennari FJ. Approach to the hemodialysis patient with an abnormal serum bicarbonate concentration. *Am J Kidney Dis* 2014; 64(1):151–155.
66. Zimmerman D, Cotman P, Ting R, et al. Continuous veno-venous haemodialysis with a novel bicarbonate dialysis solution: prospective cross-over comparison with a lactate buffered solution. *Nephrol Dial Transplant* 1999;14:2387–2391.
67. Buoncristiani U. Fifteen years of clinical experience with daily haemodialysis. *Nephrol Dial Transplant* 1998;13(Suppl 6):148–151.

68. Buoncristiani U, Quintaliani G, Cozzari M, et al. Daily dialysis: long-term clinical metabolic results. *Kidney Int* 1988; 24(Suppl):S137–S140.

69. Pierratos A, Ouwendyk M, Francoeur R, et al. Nocturnal hemodialysis: three-year experience. *J Am Soc Nephrol* 1998;9:859–868.

70. Kraus M, Burkart J, Hegeman R, et al. A comparison of center-based vs. home-based daily hemodialysis for patients with end-stage renal disease. *Hemodial Int* 2007;11:468–477.

71. Marshall MR, Ma T, Galler D, et al. Sustained low-efficiency daily diafiltration (SLEDD-f) for critically ill patients requiring renal replacement therapy: towards an adequate therapy. *Nephrol Dial Transplant* 2004; 19:877–884.

72. Marshall MR, Golper TA, Shaver MJ, et al. Sustained low-efficiency dialysis for critically ill patients requiring renal replacement therapy. *Kidney Int* 2001;60:777–785.

73. Forni LG, Hilton PJ. Continuous hemofiltration in the treatment of acute renal failure. *N Engl J Med* 1997;336:1303–1309.

74. Manns M, Sigler MH, Teehan BP. Continuous renal replacement therapies: an update. *Am J Kidney Dis* 1998;32:185–207.

75. McLean AG, Davenport A, Cox D, et al. Effects of lactate-buffered and lactate-free dialysate in CAVHD patients with and without liver dysfunction. *Kidney Int* 2000;58:1765–1772.

76. Santoro A, Ferrari G, Bolzani R, et al. Regulation of base balance in bicarbonate hemofiltration. *Int J Artif Organs* 1994;17:27–36.

77. Feriani M, Ronco C, Biasioli S, et al. Effect of dialysate and substitution fluid buffer on buffer flux in hemodiafiltration. *Kidney Int* 1991;39:711–717.

78. Biasioli S, Feriani M, Chiaramonte S, et al. Different buffers for hemodiafiltration: a controlled study. *Int J Artif Organs* 1989;12:25–30.

79. Santoro A, Spongano M, Ferrari G, et al. Analysis of the factors influencing bicarbonate balance during acetate-free biofiltration. *Kidney Int* 1993;41(Suppl):S184–S187.

80. Gennari FJ. Acid-base disorders in end-stage renal disease. Part I. *Semin Dial* 1990;3:81–85.

81. Gennari FJ. Acid-base disorders in dialysis patients. In: Gennari FJ, Adrogue HJ, Galla JH, et al, eds. *Acid–Base Disorders and Their Treatment*. Boca Raton, FL: Taylor & Francis, 2005:717–730.

82. Santiago-Delpin EA, Buselmeier TJ, Simmons RL, et al. Blood gases and pH in patients with artificial arteriovenous fistulas. *Kidney Int* 1972;1:131–133.

83. Gennari FJ. Acid-base disorders in end-stage renal disease: part II. *Semin Dial* 1990;3:161–165.

84. Fraley DS, Adler S, Bruns FJ, et al. Stimulation of lactate production by administration of bicarbonate in a patient with a solid neoplasm and lactic acidosis. *N Engl J Med* 1980;303:1100–1102.

85. Fields AL, Wolman SL, Halperin ML. Chronic lactic acidosis in a patient with cancer: therapy and metabolic consequences. *Cancer* 1981;47(8):2026–2029.

86. Prikis M, Bhasin V, Young MP, et al. Sustained low-efficiency dialysis as a treatment modality in a patient with lymphoma-associated lactic acidosis. *Nephrol Dial Transplant* 2007;22:2383–2385.

87. Brueggemeyer CD, Ramirez G. Dialysate concentrate: a potential source for lethal complications. *Nephron* 1987;46:397–398.

88. Rimmer JM, Gennari FJ. Metabolic alkalosis. *J Intensive Care Med* 1987; 2:137–150.

89. Huber L, Gennari FJ. Severe metabolic alkalosis in a hemodialysis patient. *Am J Kidney Dis* 2011;58(1):144–149.

90. Gennari FJ. A normal serum bicarbonate in a woman receiving chronic hemodialysis. *Semin Dial* 1991;4:59–61.

91. Van Stone JC. Oral base replacement in patients on hemodialysis. *Ann Intern Med* 1984;101:199–201.

92. Madias NE, Levey AS. Metabolic alkalosis due to absorption of "nonabsorbable" antacids. *Am J Med* 1983;74:155–158.

93. Adrogue HJ, Madias NE. Respiratory acidosis. In: Gennari FJ, Adrogue HJ, Galla JH, et al, eds. *Acid–Base Disorders and Their Treatment*. Boca Raton, FL: Taylor & Francis, 2005:597–640.

94. Krapf R, Hulter HN. Respiratory alkalosis. In: Gennari FJ, Adrogue HJ, Galla JH, et al, eds. *Acid–Base Disorders and Their Treatment*. Boca Raton, FL: Taylor & Francis, 2005:641–680.

95. Kenamond TG, Graves JW, Lempert KD, et al. Severe recurrent alkalemia in a patient undergoing continuous cyclic peritoneal dialysis. *Am J Med* 1986;81:548–550.

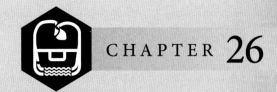

CHAPTER 26

Respiratory Disorders in End-Stage Kidney Disease

Vibhu Sharma and Michael Achilles Markos

The kidneys and the lungs are responsible for acid–base homeostasis. Pulmonary kidney cross talk is intimate and denotes, on a macroscopic and microscopic level, interactions between the pulmonary and kidney circulation and physiology. This chapter reviews basic physiology as it relates to pulmonary kidney interactions, and offer practical narratives on the most common conditions that a nephrologist might encounter that have a direct bearing on the pulmonary system.

 PHYSIOLOGY

The lungs and the kidneys interact closely to maintain an acid–base balance. HL Mencken, a noted American satirist, wrote in the *Baltimore Sun*, "Life is a battle against hydrogen ions." Any perturbation in the hydrogen ion balance whether by addition of mineral (nonvolatile) acid such as lactic acid, formic acid, or hydrochloric/sulfuric acid; by a reduction in serum HCO_3; or by an increase in carbon dioxide (volatile acid: carbonic acid) in an organism stimulates a compensatory response that attempts to revert the organism closer to a steady state. In the first two scenarios (metabolic acidosis, as defined by a reduction in serum HCO_3) (1), an immediate respiratory compensation develops that can drive the $Paco_2$ to ≤ 10 mm Hg in an attempt to maintain a life-conserving pH. This extreme compensation is illustrated dramatically in presentations of diabetic ketoacidosis (DKA). An increased secretion of hydrogen ions eventually occurs in the kidneys with an attempt to further normalize pH if the metabolic acidosis persists.

In the third scenario above (respiratory acidosis, defined by an increase in $Paco_2$) (2), the kidneys retain HCO_3 to allow for a more normal pH. Respiratory acidosis is typically seen in patients with chronic obstructive pulmonary disease (COPD) and obesity hypoventilation syndrome (OHS) in addition to respiratory failure

due to neuromuscular disease (e.g., myasthenia gravis and acute inflammatory demyelinating polyneuropathy).

Conversely, the emergence of a primary metabolic alkalotic state (defined by an increase in serum HCO_3) (3) produces a drop in alveolar ventilation mediated by medullary chemoreceptors to allow carbon dioxide levels (and thus hydrogen ion concentration borne of carbonic acid) to rise to allow reversion closer to steady state. Compensatory hypercapnia in this setting is usually modest (expected $Paco_2$ 48 to 50 mm Hg with arterial pH not infrequently in excess of 7.60). Primary metabolic alkalosis is most frequently seen in the setting of vomiting and diuretic use.

A reduction in carbon dioxide tension in the organism due to primary respiratory alkalosis triggers an "alkaliuresis," again with the goal to revert pH to a more normal state. Primary respiratory alkalosis may be seen in patients presenting with stroke, head injury, or salicylate intoxication, in addition to asthma and pulmonary embolism (PE), for example.

Respiratory responses to primary acid–base perturbations occur almost instantly (minutes), while kidney compensation is slower, taking days to reach a peak response, and therefore, the ability of an organism to respond to a major insult to the acid–base balance is limited by the intensity of response that may be required and coexistent morbidities affecting either organ system. For example, a limitation in ventilation due to airway disease may prevent an adequate response to a severe metabolic acidosis in the setting of sepsis or poisoning, similarly, presence of end-stage kidney disease (ESKD) and a concomitant new respiratory acidosis may result in a lower pH than if the kidneys were functional. Given the rapidity of respiratory perturbations in acid–base disturbances, more extreme changes in arterial pH can be expected compared to the relatively slower (and weaker) perturbations in metabolic alterations.

There are three major methods by which physiologic interactions between the lung and kidney may be described: using HCO_3 to quantify the metabolic component, the strong ion difference (SID), and the standard base excess (SBE). All three are essentially clinically indistinguishable (4,5) with regard to predicting secondary directional changes in metabolic parameters.

Pulmonary kidney interactions are defined mathematically by the Henderson-Hasselbalch equation (5) encapsulating the essential and intimate relationship between the lungs and the kidney to maintain life (**Equation 26.1**):

$$pH = 6.1 + \log$$
$$(\text{serum } HCO_3 \text{ concentration} / 0.03 \times Paco_2) \quad (26.1)$$

Detailed acid–base disturbance reviews have recently been published and are out of the scope of this basic review (6).

The kidneys also play a major role in the regulation of volume status; major perturbations in kidney function will necessarily impact pulmonary function due to changes in total lung water. This is discussed further below.

Key Points

- Respiratory perturbations in acid–base disturbances result in more extreme changes in arterial pH compared to the relatively slower (and weaker) perturbations in metabolic alterations.
- There are three major methods to describe secondary directional changes in acid–base disturbances: using HCO_3 to quantify the metabolic component, the strong ion difference (SID), and the standard base excess (SBE). All three are essentially clinically indistinguishable and may be used interchangeably.

⬢ CHRONIC KIDNEY DISEASE AND LUNG FUNCTION

A major consideration in patients with chronic kidney disease (CKD) is volume status; this may be especially important not only in patients in the intensive care unit (ICU) but also in the ambulatory patient assessed for dyspnea. Volume homeostasis is typically preserved until the estimated glomerular filtration rate (eGFR) falls to 10 to 15 mL/min/1.73m². These patients may however be at risk for volume overload with small perturbations in sodium and/or water intake.

For the physician caring for a dyspneic patient with ESKD on hemodialysis (HD), it is important to assess interdialytic weight gain

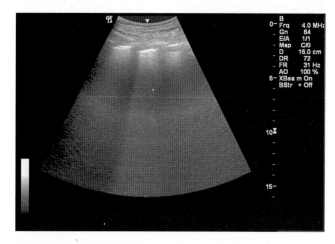

FIGURE 26.2 B-line count 2.

which may be a marker for hypervolemia (7). Pulmonary edema is a recognized complication of fluid overload in patients with CKD stage 5 whether or not dialysis is ongoing and substantial pulmonary congestion in patients with ESKD may be present without symptoms or signs or with subtle signs (8). Lung ultrasound is a useful noninvasive technique to determine lung congestion in the setting of HD.

B-lines (also called "comet tails," "ultrasound comets," or "lung comets") (**Figures 26.1–26.4**) are reverberation artifacts that occur due to reflection of the ultrasound beam off thickened interlobular septae in the setting of pulmonary congestion (9). The absence of

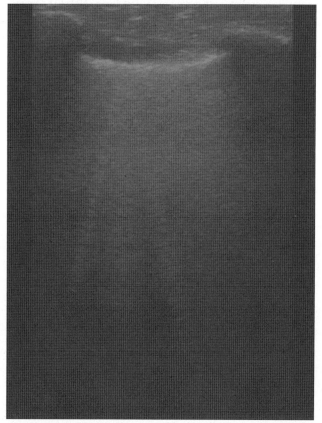

FIGURE 26.3 B-line count 3.

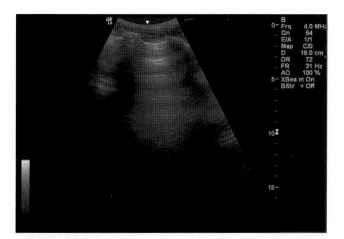

FIGURE 26.1 Normal lung.

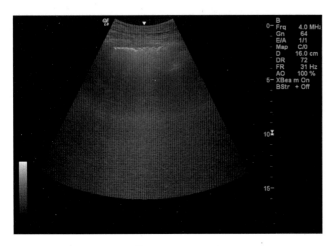

FIGURE 26.4 Numerous B-lines.

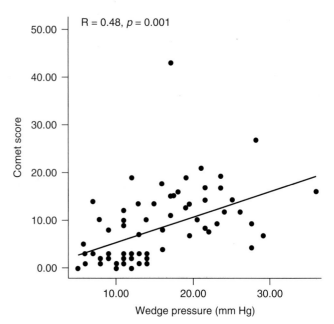

FIGURE 26.6 Positive linear correlation between comet score and wedge pressure determined using the pulmonary artery catheter.

B-lines is a good predictor of a low-wedge pressure (9), and positive correlations have been found between extravascular lung water (EVLW) determined by the PiCCO system, wedge pressure, and the number of B-lines counted across the chest ("comet-score") (10) (**Figures 26.5** and **26.6**).

Pulmonary congestion as determined by B-line scores on lung ultrasound is highly prevalent in both symptomatic and asymptomatic patients on HD (11). These scores increase as New York Heart Association (NYHA) functional class worsens. B-line scores have been shown to decrease as fluid is removed during the course of dialysis in linear fashion and can be followed in real time (12); these scores also correlate with weight reduction during HD (13). Quantification of B-lines (a surrogate for lung congestion) has been shown to predict mortality in asymptomatic outpatients on HD (8). Lung ultrasound is easy to learn and is thus an attractive noninvasive test to assess pulmonary congestion in patients with CKD whether

or not they are being dialyzed. Automated counting of B-lines is a promising technique described recently (14) that may standardize B-line scoring allowing for wider use in the setting of ESKD.

A hyperinflation pattern on pulmonary function testing (increased total lung capacity and residual volume), diminished inspiratory respiratory muscle strength (**Table 26.1**) (15), and a reduced diffusion capacity for carbon monoxide (DLCO or KCO) (**Table 26.1** and **Figure 26.7**) (16) may be seen among patients with CKD. Other studies (17) have shown a restrictive pattern, reduced DLCO, and diminished inspiratory respiratory muscle strength in patients on HD. These abnormalities seem to remit slowly with transplantation (**Table 26.2**) (17).

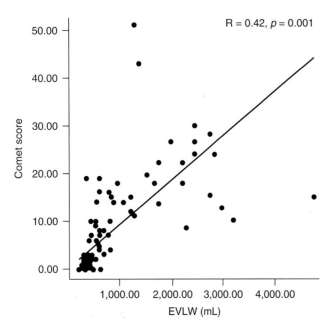

FIGURE 26.5 Correlation of ultrasound determined comet score and extravascular lung water determined by thermodilution. EVLW, extravascular lung water.

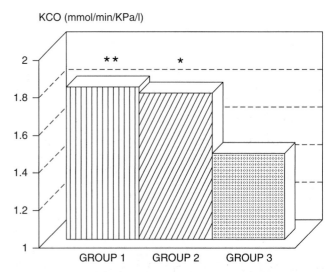

FIGURE 26.7 Absolute values of KCO in the three groups of patients (*$p < 0.05$ and **$p < 0.01$ vs group 3). Group 1: CKD EGFR <25 mL not on HD. Group 2: HD <12 months. Group 3: HD × >5 years. CKD, chronic kidney disease; EGFR, estimated glomerular filtration rate; HD, hemodialysis.

TABLE 26.1	**The Pulmonary Function Test Results for the Study Groups (All Values Expressed as Percentage of Predicted Value)**			
	CAPD (n = 22)	**HD (n = 27)**	**RT (n = 24)**	**p**
FVC (%)	83.0 ± 19.3	82.6 ± 13.5	84.7 ± 11.5	NS
FEV_1 (%)	88.95 ± 15.2	85.0 ± 16.1	90.1 ± 14.7	NS
FEF_{25-75} (%)	86.9 ± 29.4	80.6 ± 26.4	91.7 ± 29.1	NS
TLC (%)	104.7 ± 18.5	105.5 ± 17.0	84.5 ± 18.2	<0.001
VC (%)	89.0 ± 21.7	84.8 ± 14.7	86.1 ± 11.9	NS
RV (%)	139.6 ± 43.5	148.8 ± 44.5	79.0 ± 38.0	<0.001
DLCO (%)	94.8 ± 20.8	112.4 ± 28.0	96.2 ± 19.7	<0.05
PI_{max} (%)	49.9 ± 19.9	66.5 ± 23.4	54.7 ± 19.5	<0.05
PE_{max} (%)	31.1 ± 12.1	34.7 ± 13.3	31.5 ± 11.9	NS

CAPD, continuous ambulatory peritoneal dialysis; HD, hemodialysis; RT, renal transplantation; FVC, forced vital capacity; FEV_1; forced expiratory volume in 1 second; FEF_{25-75}, forced expiratory flow between 25% and 75% of vital capacity; TLC, total lung capacity; VC, vital capacity; RV, residual volume; DLCO, diffusion capacity of the lung for carbon monoxide; PI_{max}, inspiratory muscle strength; PE_{max}, expiratory muscle strength; NS, not significant.
From Karacan O, Tutal E, Colak T, et al. Pulmonary function in renal transplant recipients and end-stage renal disease patients undergoing maintenance dialysis. *Transplant Proc* 2006;38:396–400.

For the patient in the ICU presenting with dyspnea due to pulmonary congestion, supportive measures include noninvasive ventilation, oxygen, and fluid removal with dialysis as soon as feasible. Nondialytic measures to treat pulmonary edema in the setting of hypertensive urgencies or emergencies include intravenous nicardipine (slow onset of action and long half-life) (18), intravenous labetalol, or intravenous fenoldopam (19). Intravenous nitroglycerine may also be indicated in the right clinical setting (e.g., coronary ischemia). Studies of the effect of loop diuretics on central hemodynamics in this setting are conflicting, some showing favorable improvement (20) and others no change (21). Patient characteristics may account for some of the differences in the outcomes of these studies.

TABLE 26.2	**The Effect of Kidney Transplantation on Pulmonary Function and Respiratory Muscle Strength in Patients with End-Stage Kidney Disease**			
Parameter	**Predicted (SD)**	**Preop (SD)**	**Postop 2 (SD)**	**Postop 3 (SD)**
Chest expansion (cm)		3.24 (±1.13)	4.27 (±1.39)	4.31 (±1.23)
OCD (mm)		69.82 (±20.29)	86.17 (±16.91)	86.17 (±18.36)
MIP (cm H_2O)	113.115	101.8 (±37.53)	140.48 (±43.30)	134.2 (±41.99)
MEP (cm H_2O)		98.55 (±30.03)	122.27 (±34.05)	122.55 (±37.37)
SNIP (cm H_2O)		7.8 (±24.6)	84.59 (±19.7)	95.18 (±28.53)
Inspiratory capacity (IC in L)	2.73 (±0.30002)	2.15 (±0.611)	2.25 (±0.664)	2.36 (±0.5151)
Tidal volume (VT in L)	0.453 (±0.796)	1.16 (±0.794)	0.965 (±0.7)	0.815 (±0.401)
Forced vital capacity (FVC in L)	4.064 (±0.558)	3.18 (±0.818)	3.327 (±0.811)	3.365 (±0.745)
Forced expiratory volume (FEV1 in L)	3.463 (±0.494)	2.675 (±0.682)	2.83 (±0.783)	2.93 (±0.678)
Maximum midexpiratory flow rate (MMEFR in L/s)	3.703 (±0.557)	3.081 (±1.079)	3.249 (±1.199)	3.621 (±1.277)
Peak expiratory flow rate (PEFR in L/s)	8.428 (±0.973)	6.552 (±2.218)	6.862 (±2.098)	7.813 (±2.131)
Diffusion capacity of carbon monoxide (DLCO in mL/min/mm Hg)	19.8 (±2.29)	9.71 (±2.58)	11.1 (±3.69)	12.45 (±3.732)
Arterial blood gas analysis				
pH		7.392 (±0.067)	7.383 (±0.040)	7.34 (±0.059)
pO_2 (mm Hg)		94.34 (±26.29)	93.82 (±28.9)	92.95 (±25.01)
pco_2 (mm Hg)		32.61 (±5.11)	33.72 (±5.06)	34.06 (±6.05)
HCO_3 (mmol/L)		19.48 (±4.08)	19.76 (±3.46)	18.51 (±3.88)
SpO_2 (%)		95.61 (±3.52)	95.12 (±7.92)	95.49 (±6.05)
$AaDO_2$ (mm Hg)		15.85 (±25.34)	13.14 (±22.87)	11 (±17.1)

Predicted, predicted values; Preop, mean of preop values recorded; Postop 2, mean of postop day 30 values; Postop 3, mean of postop day 90 values; SD, standard deviation; OCD oxygen cost diagram; MIP, maximal inspiratory pressure; MEP, maximal expiratory pressure; SNIP, sniff nasal inspiratory pressure; pO_2, partial pressure of oxygen; Pco_2, partial pressure of carbon dioxide; HCO_3, bicarbonate; SpO_2, estimate of arterial oxygen saturation; $AaDO_2$, alveolar–arterial oxygen difference.
From Guleria S, Agarwal RK, Guleria R, et al. The effect of renal transplantation on pulmonary function and respiratory muscle strength in patients with end-stage renal disease. *Transplant Proc* 2005;37:664–665.

Key Points

- Interdialytic weight gain may be a marker for hypervolemia in apparently stable outpatients with ESKD.
- Assessment of B-lines using ultrasound is a useful and validated technique to assess congestion in relatively stable outpatients with ESKD. Pulmonary congestion assessed by ultrasound correlates with mortality among patients with ESKD.
- Restrictive and obstructive pulmonary function abnormalities remit with dialysis.

CHRONIC KIDNEY DISEASE AND PULMONARY HYPERTENSION

The Fifth World Symposium on Pulmonary Hypertension (PH) classifies PH-associated with ESKD as Group 5 ("of unknown or multifactorial origin") (22). Dyspnea in a patient with CKD that remains unexplained ought to trigger a workup for PH. The diagnosis of PH requires right heart catheterization (RHC), performed after HD in the dialysis-dependent patient.

PH, defined as a mean pulmonary artery pressure ≥25 mm Hg determined by RHC (23), is common among patients with both dialysis-dependent and non–dialysis-dependent CKD stage 5. The prevalence of PH in non–dialysis-dependent CKD stage 5 ranges from 9% to 39% (24) and is higher in patients on HD (25). While connective tissue disorders and systemic illnesses may contribute, it is increasingly being recognized that abnormal kidney function *per se* is a trigger for the development of PH. Endothelial dysfunction is universal in patients with CKD and may contribute with other kidney-specific factors thought to be important including the presence of arteriovenous fistulas, exposure to dialysis membranes, secondary hyperparathyroidism, and anemia (24).

Most cases of PH in the setting of CKD, however, are Group 2 (secondary to left heart dysfunction) (26). It is important to ensure that reversible and treatable causes of PH are systematically investigated, the two major ones being venous thromboembolism and sleep apnea. PE is more frequent in patients with ESKD on HD than those with CKD. ESKD and CKD independently confer an increased risk of PE compared with patients with normal kidney function (27).

Sleep apnea (discussed later in this chapter) is intimately linked with volume overload both of which lead to nocturnal hypoxemia that may drive the development or progression of PH (28,29).

Assessment of pulmonary congestion with ultrasound as described previously in this chapter may assist in identifying some of these patients. The treatment of PH in the setting of CKD centers on the treatment of modifiable risk factors, aggressive control of blood pressure, and pulmonary congestion. In the absence of trials of specific vasodilator agents in this setting, a recommendation for vasodilator therapy cannot be made, although PH-specific therapies can be considered on a case-by-case basis for those with defined class I disease.

It is important to note that kidney transplantation results in substantial improvements in left ventricular (LV) dysfunction and PH (30,31). Established PH, while not a contraindication to kidney transplantation, was associated with an increased risk of mortality in kidney transplant recipients especially if it was severe [defined as pulmonary artery systolic pressure (PASP) >50 mm Hg] (32). Severe PH despite aggressive treatment is typically considered a contraindication to kidney transplantation.

Key Points

- The prevalence of PH in non–dialysis-dependent CKD stage 5 is higher than in the general population and is even higher in patients on HD.
- Most cases of PH in the setting of CKD are Group 2 (secondary to left heart dysfunction).
- PE is more frequent in patients with ESKD on HD than those with CKD.
- ESKD and CKD independently confer an increased risk of PE compared with patients with normal kidney function.
- Kidney transplantation results in substantial improvements in LV dysfunction and PH.
- Severe PH despite aggressive treatment is typically considered a contraindication to kidney transplantation.

PULMONARY KIDNEY INTERACTIONS IN SEPSIS

There is increasing appreciation for pulmonary kidney cross talk in the setting of acute kidney injury (AKI). Preexisting AKI increases the susceptibility of the lungs to an endotoxin insult (33). Additionally, in animal studies, absent obvious fluid overload, ischemic AKI has been demonstrated to increase lung water via altered Na-K aquaporin channels and pulmonary endothelial cell death (34). Increased lung endothelial cell apoptosis and increased lung inflammation as demonstrated by increased bronchoalveolar lavage fluid (BALF) protein, myeloperoxidase activity, and neutrophil cell counts has been demonstrated with primary ischemic AKI (35,36). This response is distinct from the response to experimental nephrectomy (37). AKI also induces cardiac cell apoptosis, which in turn may worsen EVLW (38). These cardiopulmonary effects are mediated by host activation of the tumor necrosis factor receptor 1 (TNFR1) gene superfamily and other proapoptotic pathways that activate programmed cell death and vascular leak (38). An upregulation of complement, proinflammatory cytokines, and Toll-like receptors has been shown after AKI has occurred (39).

Sepsis is a multisystem disorder; AKI independently predicts mortality in the setting of sepsis. AKI is defined as an absolute increase of ≥0.3 mg/dL in serum creatinine from baseline within 48 hours from the presumed insult (40). Fluid management is a key intervention in the management of sepsis and affects both kidney outcomes and pulmonary outcomes. The Fluid and Catheter Treatment Trial (FACTT) (41) assessed the outcomes of patients with sepsis assigned to two arms, a fluid conservative management arm whereby fluid balance was net zero at 7 days, or usual therapy where fluid balance was substantially positive at day 7. Patients with positive fluid balance had prolonged lengths of stay in the ICU and prolonged mechanical ventilation.

Fluid administration itself may influence serum creatinine by causing dilution. There is an important relationship between fluid balance and the newer definitions of AKI, and it has been suggested that creatinine be adjusted for fluid balance to better quantify changes in creatinine and account for the dilutional effect of fluid expansion. In one retrospective analysis of the FACTT (42), once serum creatinine had been adjusted for fluid balance, the incidence of mild AKI (AKIN1) increased in patients managed with a liberal fluid strategy. In a second retrospective analysis of the FACTT (43), 306 patients developed AKI in the first 2 days after randomization. In this group of patients, a net positive fluid balance was associated with increased mortality; diuretic therapy to reduce net positive fluid balance was associated with reduced mortality.

Both these retrospective analyses of the FACTT from a kidney perspective suggest that early AKI and AKI adjusted for creatinine are associated with a positive fluid balance. Low tidal volume ventilation is the cornerstone of management of the acute respiratory distress syndrome (ARDS); this intervention attenuates the risk of AKI resulting in a reduction in the need for kidney replacement therapy. Application of positive end expiratory pressure (PEEP) is a key intervention in the management of ARDS as well and may result in a reduction in cardiac output and kidney perfusion, and those patients with severe ARDS requiring PEEP greater than 10 cm H_2O are also at greater risk for alterations in kidney hemodynamics, especially if not adequately fluid resuscitated (44). High levels of PEEP lead to an increase in the levels of renin and aldosterone, further impairing kidney microcirculation (45).

For reasons delineated above, close attention to fluid management is imperative to improve not just lung-specific outcomes but kidney outcomes as well. Not infrequently, fluid management requirements will need to be balanced to keep the lungs "dry" and the kidney well perfused.

Early in sepsis while diuresis is preserved, the kidney removes cytokines from the systemic circulation (46). Some studies (47) have assessed the efficacy of dialytic removal of inflammatory cytokines and endotoxin in the setting of sepsis and AKI, and a few have shown improvement in survival among ICU patients (48). While this is an exciting development, the larger scale impact of these technologies remains to be proven.

Patients with ESKD frequently have multiple comorbidities and may need care in critical care settings. A recent systematic review (49) of ICU-specific outcomes among patients with ESKD addressed frequency of admission to the ICU (more frequent than patients without ESKD), reasons for admission of these patients to the critical care unit (most frequently for pulmonary edema), outcomes in the setting of sepsis (noting an increased incidence of sepsis and risk of death from sepsis in ESKD compared to those without), and outcomes by type of ICU (higher mortality if admitted for a medical compared to a surgical reason). When compared to AKI requiring renal replacement therapy (RRT), however, patients with ESKD admitted to the ICU have a more favorable short- and long-term prognosis (49).

Key Points

- AKI is defined as an absolute increase of ≥0.3 mg/dL in serum creatinine from baseline within 48 hours from a presumed insult.
- AKI independently predicts mortality in the setting of sepsis.
- Antecedent AKI increases the susceptibility of the lungs to an endotoxin insult.
- Ischemic AKI increases lung water via altered Na-K aquaporin channels and pulmonary endothelial cell death.
- Serum creatinine adjusted for fluid balance in the setting of "resuscitated sepsis" increases the incidence of mild AKI (AKIN1) in patients managed with a liberal fluid strategy.
- Diuretic therapy to reduce net positive fluid balance in resuscitated sepsis is associated with reduced mortality.
- High levels of applied PEEP (≥10 cm H_2O) in mechanically ventilated patients with ARDS can impair kidney microcirculation.
- Patients with ESKD have better outcomes in ICU settings compared to those with AKI requiring RRT.

THE PLEURA AND PERICARDIUM IN CHRONIC KIDNEY DISEASE

Uremic pericarditis and pleuritis are common complications of CKD that remain undiagnosed until late in the course. Both are intensely inflammatory and for the most part reverse with HD.

Cardiac tamponade is not infrequently the first presentation of ESKD. A classic study published in 1968 (50) described the epidemiology of this condition noting that while pleuritic symptoms accompanied most presentations, pleural effusions were unusual. A friction rub was usual but may be intermittent. All had an abnormal chest x-ray, but only the minority had an abnormal diagnostic electrocardiogram (ECG) with nonspecific ST-T changes being most common. The pericarditis is fibrinous, maybe hemorrhagic, and may be associated with adhesions and loculations.

Pleural effusions related to uremia are uncommon (~3%) but may be large, are usually unilateral and are usually exudative, and may be hemorrhagic (51). All acute and chronic complications associated with intensely inflammatory effusions can occur in this setting (fever, severe pleuritic chest pain, and fibrothorax) (52).

Hydrothorax associated with peritoneal dialysis (PD) ("sweet hydrothorax") (53) has been described and occurs due to translocation of fluid across defects in the diaphragm. Large collections can lead to dyspnea and pose diagnostic dilemmas. These usually remit with surgical closure of diaphragmatic defects, and PD can usually resume (54).

It is important to remember that patients with CKD are immunocompromised, and therefore, pleural effusions or pericardial effusions due to tuberculosis ought to be kept in mind (55).

Key Points

- Cardiac tamponade is not infrequently the first presentation of ESKD.
- A minority of patients with uremic pericarditis have an abnormal diagnostic ECG with nonspecific ST-T changes being most common.
- Pleural effusions related to uremia are uncommon.
- Hydrothorax associated with PD (sweet hydrothorax) is due to anatomical defects in the diaphragm and usually remit with surgical closure of these defects.
- Tuberculosis should be considered a major differential in pleuro-pericardial disease associated with CKD.

CHRONIC KIDNEY DISEASE AND SLEEP-RELATED DISORDERS

Sleep disorders are categorized broadly as sleep apnea (obstructive or central), insomnia, excessive daytime sleepiness, restless legs syndrome (RLS), and periodic limb movement disorder (PLMD). Obstructive sleep apnea (OSA) is more common in the patient population with ESKD than in the general population (50% to 70% vs. 3% to 4%) (56,57). Patients with ESKD may lack classic risk factors (e.g., obesity) for OSA (58), thus necessitating a high index of suspicion for sleep apnea.

While it is apparent that preexisting upper airway (UAW) abnormalities are important prerequisites for development of OSA, nocturnal changes in neck circumference correlate with the amount of fluid displaced from the legs (59), and thus, volume shifts to the oropharynx are thought to play an important role in the pathogenesis of OSA in patients with ESKD. The coexistence of congestive heart failure in many of these patients adds another dimension to sleep-disordered breathing. It is important to pay special attention to the volume status of these patients given that apparently euvolemic patients on conventional HD (CHD) or PD may have significant congestion (60).

Pulmonary congestion is easily assessed with lung ultrasound as has been discussed elsewhere in this chapter. Pulmonary congestion also causes restrictive abnormalities in the lung and also allows for development of airway obstruction (61), both of which contribute to hypoxia and ventilatory instability during sleep. Experimental volume expansion seems to worsen OSA (62) rounding out the importance of volume status contributing to OSA. In a recent study (63), ultrafiltration alone ameliorated sleep apnea severity as assessed by the apnea hypopnea index without changes in metabolic parameters. Patients converted from CHD to nocturnal hemodialysis (NHD) seem to have improvement in OSA severity as measured by the apnea–hypopnea index (AHI) (64). The mechanism goes beyond improvement in UAW diameter, perhaps relating to enhanced chemoreceptor sensitivity and ventilation stability. Patients on PD have similar risk profiles as it relates to OSA when compared to patients on HD. Nocturnal PD seems to ameliorate OSA better than continuous ambulatory PD (65).

A few cases of resolution of sleep apnea syndromes with kidney transplantation have been reported (66).

Excessive daytime sleepiness, RLS, and PLMD occur with increased frequency in patients with ESKD (67). While the true pathophysiology of RLS and PLMD are unknown, the major driving factors are thought to be uremia and/or iron deficiency (67). The diagnosis of RLS is based on a characteristic history of an incessant sensation of needing to move the legs with associated paresthesias. PLMD is diagnosed during an overnight polysomnogram and is characterized by a sudden repetitive movement of the legs that have a characteristic appearance and is thought to be rare in the general population (68). The true prevalence of both disorders among patients with ESKD has been difficult to discern given the small sample size in studies assessing prevalence and the small number of studies. Gabapentin (69), intravenous iron (70), and ropinirole (71) are useful in treating sleep-related RLS. RLS may occur while patients are on dialysis, and in this setting, aerobic exercise during dialysis (72) and pramipexole (73) as well as cooling the dialysate (74) have been shown in small trials to improve symptoms. RLS has been reported to improve (75) and in one case report (76) resolve after kidney transplantation. The etiology of excessive daytime sleepiness among patients with ESKD is thought to be due to day/night sleep reversal attributed to uremia (67,77) but also hypothesized to be associated with abnormal melatonin dynamics (78), tyrosine deficiency leading to neurotransmitter deficiency (79), and possibly up titration of inflammatory and sleep-inducing cytokines during dialysis (80,81), making the treatment of excessive daytime sleepiness in this population difficult.

Key Points

- Patients with ESKD may lack classic risk factors (obesity or large neck circumference) for OSA.
- Nocturnal fluid shifts to the oropharynx play an important role in the pathogenesis of OSA in patients with ESKD.
- Ultrafiltration alone ameliorates OSA in patients with OSA.
- Nocturnal HD and PD ameliorate OSA better than diurnal HD and PD perhaps relating to enhanced chemoreceptor sensitivity.

- Excessive daytime sleepiness, RLS, and PLMD occur with high frequency in patients with ESKD.
- Sleep-related disorders improve after kidney transplantation; case reports have informed the possibility of almost complete resolution of all categories of sleep disorders after kidney transplantation.

◆ SUMMARY

The lungs and the kidneys work in tandem to maintain life. HD is a lifesaving and life-preserving modality with an immeasurable impact on kidney disease. Respiratory failure remains a difficult problem and a prominent cause of mortality in patients with severe multiorgan failure where the kidneys have been artificially replaced. Respiratory dialysis (RD) with extracorporeal removal of CO_2 (82–85) promises to revolutionize the management of these patients closing a large gap in the treatment of severely ill patients and hopefully making RD as commonplace as HD.

◆ REFERENCES

1. Swenson ER. Metabolic acidosis. *Respir Care* 2001;46:342–353.
2. Epstein SK, Singh N. Respiratory acidosis. *Respir Care* 2001;46:366–383.
3. Khanna A, Kurtzman NA. Metabolic alkalosis. *Respir Care* 2001;46: 354–365.
4. Schlichtig R, Grogono AW, Severinghaus JW. Human PaCO2 and standard base excess compensation for acid-base imbalance. *Crit Care Med* 1998;26:1173–1179.
5. Kellum JA. Determinants of blood pH in health and disease. *Crit Care* 2000;4:6–14.
6. Berend K, de Vries AP, Gans RO. Physiological approach to assessment of acid-base disturbances. *N Engl J Med* 2014;371:1434–1445.
7. Kalantar-Zadeh K, Regidor DL, Kovesdy CP, et al. Fluid retention is associated with cardiovascular mortality in patients undergoing long-term hemodialysis. *Circulation* 2009;119:671–679.
8. Zoccali C, Torino C, Tripepi R, et al. Pulmonary congestion predicts cardiac events and mortality in ESRD. *J Am Soc Nephrol* 2013;24: 639–646.
9. Lichtenstein DA, Meziere GA, Lagoueyte JF, et al. A-lines and B-lines: lung ultrasound as a bedside tool for predicting pulmonary artery occlusion pressure in the critically ill. *Chest* 2009;136:1014–1020.
10. Agricola E, Bove T, Oppizzi M, et al. "Ultrasound comet-tail images": a marker of pulmonary edema: a comparative study with wedge pressure and extravascular lung water. *Chest* 2005;127:1690–1695.
11. Mallamaci F, Benedetto FA, Tripepi R, et al. Detection of pulmonary congestion by chest ultrasound in dialysis patients. *JACC Cardiovasc Imaging* 2010;3:586–594.
12. Noble VE, Murray AF, Capp R, et al. Ultrasound assessment for extravascular lung water in patients undergoing hemodialysis. Time course for resolution. *Chest* 2009;135:1433–1439.
13. Vitturi N, Dugo M, Soattin M, et al. Lung ultrasound during hemodialysis: the role in the assessment of volume status. *Int Urol Nephrol* 2014;46:169–174.
14. Brattain LJ, Telfer BA, Liteplo AS, et al. Automated B-line scoring on thoracic sonography. *J Ultrasound Med* 2013;32:2185–2190.
15. Karacan O, Tutal E, Colak T, et al. Pulmonary function in renal transplant recipients and end-stage renal disease patients undergoing maintenance dialysis. *Transplant Proc* 2006;38:396–400.
16. Herrero JA, Alvarez-Sala JL, Coronel F, et al. Pulmonary diffusing capacity in chronic dialysis patients. *Respir Med* 2002;96:487–492.
17. Guleria S, Agarwal RK, Guleria R, et al. The effect of renal transplantation on pulmonary function and respiratory muscle strength in patients with end-stage renal disease. *Transplant Proc* 2005;37:664–665.
18. Neutel JM, Smith DH, Wallin D, et al. A comparison of intravenous nicardipine and sodium nitroprusside in the immediate treatment of severe hypertension. *Am J Hypertens* 1994;7:623–628.

19. Murphy MB, Murray C, Shorten GD. Fenoldopam: a selective periph-eral dopamine-receptor agonist for the treatment of severe hyperten-sion. *N Engl J Med* 2001;345:1548–1557.

20. Dikshit K, Vyden JK, Forrester JS, et al. Renal and extrarenal hemody-namic effects of furosemide in congestive heart failure after acute myo-cardial infarction. *N Engl J Med* 1973;288:1087–1090.

21. Hayashi SY, Seeberger A, Lind B, et al. Acute effects of low and high intravenous doses of furosemide on myocardial function in anuric haemodialysis patients: a tissue Doppler study. *Nephrol Dial Transplant* 2008;23:1355–1361.

22. Simonneau G, Gatzoulis MA, Adatia I, et al. Updated clinical classifica-tion of pulmonary hypertension. *J Am Coll Cardiol* 2013;62:D34–D41.

23. Hoeper MM, Bogaard HJ, Condliffe R, et al. Definitions and diagnosis of pulmonary hypertension. *J Am Coll Cardiol* 2013;62:D42–D50.

24. Bolignano D, Rastelli S, Agarwal R, et al. Pulmonary hypertension in CKD. *Am J Kidney Dis* 2013;61:612–622.

25. Agarwal R. Prevalence, determinants and prognosis of pulmonary hypertension among hemodialysis patients. *Nephrol Dial Transplant* 2012;27:3908–3914.

26. Pabst S, Hammerstingl C, Hundt F, et al. Pulmonary hypertension in patients with chronic kidney disease on dialysis and without dialysis: results of the PEPPER-study. *PLoS One* 2012;7:e35310.

27. Kumar G, Sakhuja A, Taneja A, et al. Pulmonary embolism in patients with CKD and ESRD. *Clin J Am Soc Nephrol* 2012;7:1584–1590.

28. Sakaguchi Y, Shoji T, Kawabata H, et al. High prevalence of obstructive sleep apnea and its association with renal function among nondialysis chronic kidney disease patients in japan: a cross-sectional study. *Clin J Am Soc Nephrol* 2011;6:995–1000.

29. Zoccali C, Mallamaci F, Tripepi G. Nocturnal hypoxemia predicts inci-dent cardiovascular complications in dialysis patients. *J Am Soc Nephrol* 2002;13:729–733.

30. Casas-Aparicio G, Castillo-Martinez L, Orea-Tejeda A, et al. The effect of successful kidney transplantation on ventricular dysfunction and pulmonary hypertension. *Transplant Proc* 2010;42:3524–3528.

31. Bozbas SS, Kanyilmaz S, Akcay S, et al. Renal transplant improves pul-monary hypertension in patients with end stage renal disease. *Multidis-cip Respir Med* 2011;6:155–160.

32. Issa N, Krowka MJ, Griffin MD, et al. Pulmonary hypertension is asso-ciated with reduced patient survival after kidney transplantation. *Trans-plantation* 2008;86:1384–1388.

33. Basu RK, Donaworth E, Wheeler DS, et al. Antecedent acute kidney injury worsens subsequent endotoxin-induced lung inflammation in a two-hit mouse model. *Am J Physiol Renal Physiol* 2011;301:F597–F604.

34. White LE, Cui Y, Shelak CM, et al. Lung endothelial cell apoptosis during ischemic acute kidney injury. *Shock* 2012;38:320–327.

35. Campanholle G, Landgraf RG, Goncalves GM, et al. Lung inflamma-tion is induced by renal ischemia and reperfusion injury as part of the systemic inflammatory syndrome. *Inflamm Res* 2010;59:861–869.

36. Hoke TS, Douglas IS, Klein CL, et al. Acute renal failure after bilateral nephrectomy is associated with cytokine-mediated pulmonary injury. *J Am Soc Nephrol* 2007;18:155–164.

37. Hassoun HT, Grigoryev DN, Lie ML, et al. Ischemic acute kidney injury induces a distant organ functional and genomic response distinguishable from bilateral nephrectomy. *Am J Physiol Renal Physiol* 2007;293:F30–F40.

38. Kelly KJ. Distant effects of experimental renal ischemia/reperfusion in-jury. *J Am Soc Nephrol* 2003;14:1549–1558.

39. Grigoryev DN, Liu M, Hassoun HT, et al. The local and systemic in-flammatory transcriptome after acute kidney injury. *J Am Soc Nephrol* 2008;19:547–558.

40. Mehta RL, Kellum JA, Shah SV, et al. Acute kidney injury network: re-port of an initiative to improve outcomes in acute kidney injury. *Crit Care* 2007;11:R31.

41. Wiedemann HP, Wheeler AP, Bernard GR, et al. Comparison of two fluid-management strategies in acute lung injury. *N Engl J Med* 2006;354:2564–2575.

42. Macedo E, Bouchard J, Soroko SH, et al. Fluid accumulation, recog-nition and staging of acute kidney injury in critically-ill patients. *Crit Care* 2010;14:R82.

43. Grams ME, Estrella MM, Coresh J, et al. Fluid balance, diuretic use, and mortality in acute kidney injury. *Clin J Am Soc Nephrol* 2011;6:966–973.

44. Seeley EJ. Updates in the management of acute lung injury: a focus on the overlap between AKI and ARDS. *Adv Chronic Kidney Dis* 2013;20:14–20.

45. Annat G, Viale JP, Bui Xuan B, et al. Effect of PEEP ventilation on renal function, plasma renin, aldosterone, neurophysins and urinary ADH, and prostaglandins. *Anesthesiology* 1983;58:136–141.

46. Graziani G, Bordone G, Bellato V, et al. Role of the kidney in plasma cyto-kine removal in sepsis syndrome: a pilot study. *J Nephrol* 2006;19:176–182.

47. Haase M, Bellomo R, Baldwin I, et al. Hemodialysis membrane with a high-molecular-weight cutoff and cytokine levels in sepsis compli-cated by acute renal failure: a phase 1 randomized trial. *Am J Kidney Dis* 2007;50:296–304.

48. Matsumura Y, Oda S, Sadahiro T, et al. Treatment of septic shock with continuous HDF using 2 PMMA hemofilters for enhanced intensity. *Int J Artif Organs* 2012;35:3–14.

49. Arulkumaran N, Annear NM, Singer M. Patients with end-stage renal disease admitted to the intensive care unit: systematic review. *Br J An-aesth* 2013;110:13–20.

50. Bailey GL, Hampers CL, Hager EB, et al. Uremic pericarditis. clinical features and management. *Circulation* 1968;38:582–591.

51. Nidus BD, Matalon R, Cantacuzino D, et al. Uremic pleuritis—a clini-copathological entity. *N Engl J Med* 1969;281:255–256.

52. Berger HW, Rammohan G, Neff MS, et al. Uremic pleural effusion. A study in 14 patients on chronic dialysis. *Ann Intern Med* 1975;82:362–364.

53. Yang PJ, Liu TH. Massive "sweet" hydrothorax. *CMAJ* 2010;182:1883.

54. Lang CL, Kao TW, Lee CM, et al. Video-assisted thoracoscopic surgery in continuous ambulatory peritoneal dialysis-related hydrothorax. *Kid-ney Int* 2008;74:136.

55. Hussein MM, Mooij JM, Roujouleh H. Tuberculosis and chronic renal disease. *Semin Dial* 2003;16:38–44.

56. Unruh ML, Sanders MH, Redline S, et al. Sleep apnea in patients on con-ventional thrice-weekly hemodialysis: comparison with matched controls from the sleep heart health study. *J Am Soc Nephrol* 2006;17:3503–3509.

57. Kuhlmann U, Becker HF, Birkhahn M, et al. Sleep-apnea in patients with end-stage renal disease and objective results. *Clin Nephrol* 2000;53:460–466.

58. Sim JJ, Rasgon SA, Derose SF. Review article: Managing sleep apnoea in kidney diseases. *Nephrology (Carlton)* 2010;15:146–152.

59. Beecroft JM, Hoffstein V, Pierratos A, et al. Pharyngeal narrowing in end-stage renal disease: implications for obstructive sleep apnoea. *Eur Respir J* 2007;30:965–971.

60. Panuccio V, Enia G, Tripepi R, et al. Chest ultrasound and hidden lung congestion in peritoneal dialysis patients. *Nephrol Dial Transplant* 2012;27:3601–3605.

61. Pierson DJ. Respiratory considerations in the patient with renal failure. *Respir Care* 2006;51:413–422.

62. Yadollahi A, Gabriel JM, White LH, et al. A randomized, double cross-over study to investigate the influence of saline infusion on sleep apnea severity in men. *Sleep* 2014;37:1699–1705.

63. Lyons OD, Chan CT, Yadollahi A, et al. Effect of ultrafiltration on sleep apnea and sleep structure in patients with end-stage renal disease. *Am J Respir Crit Care Med* 2015;191:1287–1294.

64. Hanly PJ, Pierratos A. Improvement of sleep apnea in patients with chronic renal failure who undergo nocturnal hemodialysis. *N Engl J Med* 2001;344:102–107.

65. Tang SC, Lam B, Ku PP, et al. Alleviation of sleep apnea in patients with chronic renal failure by nocturnal cycler-assisted peritoneal dialysis compared with conventional continuous ambulatory peritoneal dialy-sis. *J Am Soc Nephrol* 2006;17:2607–2616.

66. Langevin B, Fouque D, Leger P, et al. Sleep apnea syndrome and end-stage renal disease: cure after renal transplantation. *Chest* 1993;103:1330–1335.

67. Perl J, Unruh ML, Chan CT. Sleep disorders in end-stage renal disease: "markers of inadequate dialysis"? *Kidney Int* 2006;70:1687–1693.

68. Aurora RN, Kristo DA, Bista SR, et al. The treatment of restless legs syndrome and periodic limb movement disorder in adults—an update for 2012: practice parameters with an evidence-based systematic review and meta-analyses: an American Academy of Sleep Medicine Clinical Practice Guideline. *Sleep* 2012;35:1039–1062.

69. Thorp ML, Morris CD, Bagby SP. A crossover study of gabapentin in treatment of restless legs syndrome among hemodialysis patients. *Am J Kidney Dis* 2001;38:104–108.

70. Sloand JA, Shelly MA, Feigin A, et al. A double-blind, placebo-controlled trial of intravenous iron dextran therapy in patients with ESRD and restless legs syndrome. *Am J Kidney Dis* 2004;43:663–670.

71. Pellecchia MT, Vitale C, Sabatini M, et al. Ropinirole as a treatment of restless legs syndrome in patients on chronic hemodialysis: an open randomized crossover trial versus levodopa sustained release. *Clin Neuropharmacol* 2004;27:178–181.

72. Sakkas GK, Hadjigeorgiou GM, Karatzaferi C, et al. Intradialytic aerobic exercise training ameliorates symptoms of restless legs syndrome and improves functional capacity in patients on hemodialysis: a pilot study. *ASAIO J* 2008;54:185–190.

73. Miranda M, Kagi M, Fabres L, et al. Pramipexole for the treatment of uremic restless legs in patients undergoing hemodialysis. *Neurology* 2004;62:831–832.

74. Kerr PG, van Bakel C, Dawborn JK. Assessment of the symptomatic benefit of cool dialysate. *Nephron* 1989;52:166–169.

75. Kahvecioglu S, Yildiz D, Buyukkoyuncu N, et al. Effect of renal transplantation in restless legs syndrome. *Exp Clin Transplant* 2016; 14:45–49.

76. Yasuda T, Nishimura A, Katsuki Y, et al. Restless legs syndrome treated successfully by kidney transplantation—a case report. *Clin Transpl* 1986;138.

77. Hanly P. Sleep apnea and daytime sleepiness in end-stage renal disease. *Semin Dial* 2004;17:109–114.

78. Vaziri ND, Oveisi F, Wierszbiezki M, et al. Serum melatonin and 6-sulfatoxymelatonin in end-stage renal disease: effect of hemodialysis. *Artif Organs* 1993;17:764–769.

79. Furst P. Amino acid metabolism in uremia. *J Am Coll Nutr* 1989;8:310–323.

80. Entzian P, Linnemann K, Schlaak M, et al. Obstructive sleep apnea syndrome and circadian rhythms of hormones and cytokines. *Am J Respir Crit Care Med* 1996;153:1080–1086.

81. Vgontzas AN, Papanicolaou DA, Bixler EO, et al. Sleep apnea and daytime sleepiness and fatigue: relation to visceral obesity, insulin resistance, and hypercytokinemia. *J Clin Endocrinol Metab* 2000;85:1151–1158.

82. Zanella A, Castagna L, Salerno D, et al. Respiratory electrodialysis: a novel, highly efficient extracorporeal CO removal technique. *Am J Respir Crit Care Med* 2015;19(6):719–726.

83. Hermann A, Riss K, Schellongowski P, et al. A novel pump-driven veno-venous gas exchange system during extracorporeal CO2-removal. *Intensive Care Med* 2015;41(10):1773–1780.

84. Batchinsky AI, Jordan BS, Regn D, et al. Respiratory dialysis: reduction in dependence on mechanical ventilation by venovenous extracorporeal CO2 removal. *Crit Care Med* 2011;39:1382–1387.

85. Kaushik M, Wojewodzka-Zelezniakowicz M, Cruz DN, et al. Extracorporeal carbon dioxide removal: the future of lung support lies in the history. *Blood Purif* 2012;34:94–106.

CHAPTER 27

Malnutrition and Intradialytic Parenteral Nutrition in End-Stage Kidney Disease Patients

Joel D. Kopple, Anuja Shah, and Kamyar Kalantar-Zadeh

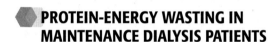
PROTEIN-ENERGY WASTING IN MAINTENANCE DIALYSIS PATIENTS

Causes and Treatment of Protein-Energy Wasting

Protein-energy wasting (PEW) refers to the loss or reduced amounts of protein, fat, and/or carbohydrates in the body to an unhealthy degree. The term PEW rather than protein-energy malnutrition (PEM) is used because there are many causes of PEW which are not related to suboptimal nutrient intake. The many causes for PEW in maintenance dialysis (MD) patients are listed in TABLE 27.1 (1).

Reduced nutrient intake and nutrient losses into dialysate are important causes of PEW. Many studies indicate that dietary protein and energy intake are frequently low in MD patients (1,2). Dietary protein and energy intake often average 20% and 30%, respectively, below recommended intakes for maintenance hemodialysis (MHD) and chronic peritoneal dialysis (CPD) patients (1,2). Reports from uncontrolled studies of patients undergoing MHD at more frequent intervals (e.g., daily hemodialysis) and/or for more hours than the usual 3 to 4 hours of hemodialysis three times weekly indicate that their appetite and nutritional status improve (3). These findings suggest that MHD patients treated with standard dialysis therapy tend to remain somewhat anorexic, possibly because their uremia is less adequately treated. Hemodialysis with high-flux membranes removes about 8.0 ± 2.8 (SD) g and 9.3 ± 2.7 g of amino acids from postabsorptive and postprandial patients, respectively (4,5). Approximately 2 to 3.5 g/d of free amino acids are removed during continuous ambulatory peritoneal dialysis (CAPD) (6). Normally, little protein, perhaps 1 or 2 g of protein, is lost during hemodialysis. About 8.8 ± 0.5 standard error of the mean (SEM) g/d of total protein and 5.7 ± 0.4 g/d of albumin are lost into the dialysate with

CAPD (7). With mild peritonitis, the quantity of protein removed increases to an average of 15.1 ± 3.6 g/d (7); protein losses can rise markedly with severe peritonitis. Such losses fall rapidly with antibiotic therapy but may remain elevated for many days to weeks, particularly if the peritoneal infection becomes well established before it is eradicated (7).

In normoglycemic individuals, approximately 15 to 25 g of glucose may be removed during hemodialysis when glucose-free dialysate is used (8). When the hemodialysate contains 200 mg/dL of glucose (180 mg/dL of anhydrous glucose), there is net absorption of approximately 10 to 12 g of glucose with each dialysis. Water-soluble vitamins and other bioactive compounds are removed by both hemodialysis and peritoneal dialysis (PD) (4–6,9). These vitamin losses can be easily replaced from the diet, but in patients with poor nutrient intake, such losses may enhance vitamin malnutrition. Patients with kidney disease often lose substantial quantities of blood secondary to occult gastrointestinal bleeding, frequent blood sampling for laboratory testing, and the sequestration of blood in the hemodialyzer (10). Since blood is rich in protein, these blood losses may contribute to protein wasting. The problem of maintaining adequate protein nutrition is potentially more difficult for CPD patients because the combined losses of proteins, peptides, and amino acids are greater than they are in patients undergoing hemodialysis, particularly since the losses with CPD occur every day, whereas hemodialysis is usually performed only three times weekly. Although the nutritional disorders most commonly associated with chronic kidney disease (CKD) are PEM and iron and vitamin D (e.g., 25-hydroxycholecalciferol and 1,25-dihydroxycholecalciferol) deficiencies (1,2,10–12), other deficiencies, particularly for vitamins B₆ and C, folic acid, and possibly carnitine and zinc, occur frequently if the patient does not receive supplemental nutrients (9,13,14).

It is apparent from **TABLE 27.1** that some of the causes of PEW in MD patients are not nutrition related. Other etiologic factors engendering PEW include inflammatory processes, the altered hormonal milieu of the patient with kidney disease, and both oxidant and carbonyl stress (15). Acidemia and physical deconditioning, which may be profound, may contribute to PEW. Because of the multifactorial nature of the wasting syndrome in patients with CKD, the term PEW (1) has been proposed as a more appropriate appellation for the wasting syndrome that occurs in CKD (16).

The multiple causes of PEW in MD patients require that therapeutic strategies to prevent and treat this condition should be directed into several areas. Some of these are indicated in **TABLE 27.2**.

Therapeutic strategies should be directed toward inaugurating MD in a timely manner, before patients with end-stage kidney failure develop frank PEW. PEW tends to occur as patients approach end-stage kidney failure (17,18) and inauguration of chronic dialysis treatment is associated with an improvement in PEW (19). In this regard, chronic dialysis patients are frequently anorectic (20). Therapeutic strategies for reduced nutritional intake include dietary counseling, food supplementation, intradialytic parenteral nutrition (IDPN), gastric or intestinal tube feeding, nutritional PD, or nutritional hemodialysis. In exceptional cases, total parenteral nutrition, given on a continuing basis, may be necessary (15).

Since MD patients frequently sustain intercurrent catabolic illnesses, it is important to treat such comorbid conditions aggressively and to ensure that there is adequate nutritional support during such treatment. MD patients are often in an inflammatory state and may have oxidant and/or carbonyl stress—even when there are no apparent superimposed complicating illnesses. It is

TABLE 27.2	**Therapeutic Strategies to Prevent and Treat Protein-Energy Wasting in Maintenance Dialysis Patients**

1. Start maintenance dialysis in a timely manner before clinically apparent anorexia, reduced nutrient intake, and protein-energy wasting occur.
2. Ensure optimal frequency/duration/dose of dialysis.
3. Appropriate dietary energy and protein intake with periodic dietary counseling and monitoring of nutrient intake and protein-energy status, as needed
4. Maintain or increase protein/amino acid and energy intake.
5. Food supplements, intradialytic nutrition, tube feeding, and possibly nutritional peritoneal dialysis, nutritional hemodialysis, and total parenteral nutrition as needed
6. Treat acute and chronic superimposed illnesses aggressively.
7. Prevent or treat acidemia.
   - Optimal arterial blood pH 7.40 to 7.45?
8. Less well-proven methods to maintain healthy protein-energy status
   a. Hormones and other compounds with anabolic effects[a]
      - Pentoxifylline
      - Insulin
      - Growth hormone
      - Insulin-like growth factor-I (IGF-I)
      - Testosterone
      - Carnitine
   b. Anti-inflammatory agents, antioxidants, anticarbonyl compounds. Several clinical trials are in progress.
   c. Exercise training
   d. Ketoacid supplements

[a]Except when the patient is deficient in a hormone, there is currently no strong evidence for the effectiveness of these compounds as anabolic or anticatabolic agents when given chronically to advanced chronic kidney disease patients.

believed that that elevated levels of inflammatory, oxidant, and carbonyl reactive compounds are important causes of morbidity and PEW in MD patients. CKD patients often have low circulating levels of certain anabolic hormones, increased levels of some catabolic hormones, and resistance to other anabolic hormones (15), and a number of studies have examined whether anabolic hormones may improve the protein-energy state of MD patients with PEW. Short-term studies in MHD or CPD patients given repetitive doses of growth hormone, insulin-like growth factor-1, or carnitine have shown anabolic effects of each of these agents (21–23).

Since acidemia can promote protein degradation (24), it is important to prevent and treat acidemia in these patients. In patients undergoing MHD thrice weekly, acidemia is particularly likely to occur immediately prior to a hemodialysis treatment, and it may be necessary to give such individuals alkali supplements during the end of their interdialytic period. MD patients with substantial residual renal function also may develop hyperchloremic acidosis due to excessive urinary bicarbonate losses. The optimal arterial blood pH for such patients has been reexamined in clinically stable patients undergoing CAPD. Metabolic balance studies in these patients indicate that arterial blood pH in the range of 7.43 to 7.45 is often associated with more positive protein balance than when their arterial blood pH is 7.36 to 7.38 (25).

Exercise training can improve both cardiopulmonary exercise capacity and strength in MD patients (26). Whether this treatment may be associated with protein accrual or increased muscle mass is not clear. We have found that exercise training in such patients is associated in skeletal muscle with increases in the gene transcripts for a number of growth factors and a reduction in the gene transcripts for myostatin, an antihypertrophic protein (27). However, these changes were not associated with an increase in skeletal muscle mass possibly because patients did not exercise sufficiently vigorously or that kidney failure is an antianabolic state. The increased gene transcripts may have induced protein remodeling that resulted in the increased exercise capacity that occurs in MD patients who exercise train (26). It should be emphasized that there are no randomized, prospective, controlled clinical trials that have examined whether improving the protein-energy state of wasted MD patients will reduce morbidity or mortality or improve quality of life. However, retrospective analyses of patients receiving intradialytic nutrition suggest that nutritional support in these patients is associated with reduced mortality (28–30), and exercise training, at least in the short term, may improved quality of life scores.

Effects of Protein-Energy Wasting on the Clinical Course of Maintenance Dialysis Patients

Many epidemiologic studies indicate that the PEW status of MHD and CPD patients is strongly associated with increased morbidity and mortality. MD patients who either have PEW or who have worsening protein-energy status have substantially higher mortality rates; the increase in mortality is largely due to cardiovascular events (20,31). MD patients who ingest inadequate quantities of protein and energy are more likely to develop PEW and to have higher mortality (20,32). Serum albumin is one of the strongest predictors of mortality in MHD patients (31,33,34). There is a direct relationship morbidity or mortality rates in MHD patients and poor appetite; spontaneous low dietary protein intake; decreased body-weight-for-height [i.e., body mass index (BMI)]; anthropometric measures of skeletal muscle mass and total body fat; and low serum albumin, urea, creatinine, cholesterol, and potassium (20,31–34). Similar relationships with morbidity and mortality, based on smaller sample sizes, usually (33,35), but not always (36), have been shown for CPD patients. The relative contributions of PEM and inflammation to the high morbidity and mortality of CKD patients are unclear, particularly because the syndrome of PEM shares many clinical manifestations with inflammation. Because inflammatory processes may cause endothelial injury and/or predispose to atherosclerosis and vascular thrombosis, it is easy to perceive why there could be a causal connection between inflammation and morbidity and mortality from vascular disease.

⬡ DIETARY THERAPY FOR MAINTENANCE DIALYSIS PATIENTS

General Approach to Dietary Management

The widespread nutritional and metabolic alterations and high incidence of malnutrition in CKD patients indicate that nutritional therapy is a critical aspect of their management. The three main goals for dietary treatment are to maintain good nutritional status; to prevent or ameliorate uremic toxicity and the metabolic disorders of kidney disease; and to reduce the risks of cardiovascular, cerebrovascular, and peripheral vascular disease. Adherence to specialized diets is often a difficult and frustrating endeavor for patients and their families. Patients following low-protein diet usually must make fundamental changes in their behavior patterns and forsake some of their traditional sources of daily pleasure. Often, the patients must procure special foods, prepare special recipes, forego or severely limit their intake of favorite foods, or eat foods that they

may not desire. To ensure successful dietary therapy, patients with kidney disease must undergo extensive training concerning the principles of nutritional therapy and the design and preparation of diets, and they need to be repetitively encouraged to adhere to the prescribed diet. They usually require repeated training regarding their nutritional therapy. Without careful monitoring of nutritional intake, retraining, encouragement, and sensitivity to their cultural background, psychosocial condition, and lifestyle, patients will be more likely to adhere poorly to their dietary prescription. They may eat too little rather than too much of some essential nutrients.

Monitoring Compliance

In general, to maintain good dietary adherence and to maintain a healthy clinical, fluid and electrolyte, and nutritional status, the physician must review the patient's nutritional status and dietary compliance at frequent intervals. Since nutritional status may begin to deteriorate in patients with chronic progressive kidney disease when the glomerular filtration rate (GFR) falls below 35 to 50 mL/min/l.73m^2 (17,18), careful attention to nutritional status should begin at this time or earlier. This is particularly important because CKD patients appear to be at greatest risk for malnutrition from the time that the GFR falls below 10 mL/min until the patient is established on MD therapy (18,37). Also, although nutritional status often improves after commencing hemodialysis (19), nutritional status of patients at the onset of chronic dialysis treatment is a good predictor of their nutritional status 2 to 3 years later (37,38). Moreover, measures indicating PEW at the onset of MD therapy predict increased morbidity and mortality (33,39). Hence, particular effort should be given to prevent malnutrition as the patient approaches dialysis therapy and during the first few weeks of MD treatment. These efforts should be directed toward maintaining good nutritional intake during this period, rapidly instituting therapy for superimposed illnesses, and maintaining good nutritional support during such illnesses.

Monitoring Nutritional-Inflammatory Status

Since diets prescribed for renal insufficiency are often marginally low in some nutrients (e.g., protein) and high in others (e.g., calcium) and PEW is not infrequent, it is important to periodically evaluate the adequacy of the patient's diet and protein-energy status. The National Kidney Foundation Kidney Disease Outcomes Quality Initiative (NKF K/DOQI) Clinical Practice Guidelines for Nutrition in Chronic Renal Failure (40) recommends that panels of nutritional measures should be used to assess protein-energy nutritional status in MD patients. The recommended panel of measurements of PEW status for MHD and CPD patients is indicated in TABLE 27.3. A predialysis serum specimen for these measurements is obtained from an individual immediately before the initiation of a chronic hemodialysis or intermittent peritoneal dialysis (IPD) treatment. A stabilized serum measurement is obtained after the patient has stabilized on a given dose of CAPD or IPD. There are other nutrition-related parameters that often will require monitoring, for example, serum albumin, potassium, phosphorus, calcium, parathyroid hormone, iron, ferritin, transferrin, total low-density lipoprotein (LDL) and high-density lipoprotein (HDL) cholesterol and triglycerides, interdialytic weight gain, and, if relevant, bone densitometry or radiography (15). Measures of inflammation or oxidant or carbonyl stress are often very helpful. Such measures usually include serum quantitative high sensitivity C-reactive protein (CRP) and serum interleukin-6 (15). Dietitians are often best qualified to perform anthropometric measurements of nutritional status because of training and experience.

TABLE 27.3	**Recommended Methods for Assessing Protein-Energy Status**[a]	
Category	**Measure**	**Minimum Frequency of Measurement**
I. Measurements that should be performed routinely in all patients	• Body weight predialysis or post peritoneal dialysis drain	• Monthly
	• BMI	• Monthly
	• Predialysis or stabilized serum albumin	• Every 1–2 mo
	• Appetite	• Monthly
	• Percentage of usual postdialysis (MHD) or postdrain (CPD) body weight or percentage of standard (NHANES II) body weight	• Every 6 mo
	• Subjective global assessment (SGA)	• Every 6 mo
	• Dietary history with or without a diary	• Monthly for MHD; every 2–3 mo for CPD
	• nPNA	• Monthly for MHD; every 2–3 mo for CPD
	Simple screening studies	
	• Predialysis or stabilized serum	
	- Creatinine	• Every 1–2 mo
	- Urea nitrogen	• Every 1–2 mo
	- Cholesterol	• Every 1–2 mo
II. Measures that can be useful for a more rigorous assessment of protein-energy status but that may be more costly or labor intensive	• Predialysis or stabilized serum prealbumin (<30 mg/dL)	• All as needed
	• Serum CRP	
	• Serum IL-6	
	• Skinfold thickness	
	• Mid arm muscle area, circumference, or diameter	
	• Dual energy x-ray absorptiometry	
	• Bioelectric impedance assessment	

BMI, body mass index; MHD, maintenance hemodialysis; CPD, chronic peritoneal dialysis; NHANES II, Second National Health and Nutrition Evaluation Survey; nPNA, normalized protein equivalent of total nitrogen appearance [determined from the urea nitrogen appearance (38,40)]; CRP, C-reactive protein; IL, interleukin.
Adapted from K/DOQI Nutrition Workgroup. National Kidney Foundation Kidney Disease Outcomes Quality Initiative. Clinical practice guidelines for nutrition in chronic renal failure. *Am J Kid Dis* 2000;35(Suppl 2):S19–S56.

RECOMMENDED DIETARY INTAKES

The nutritional needs of patients treated with more frequent hemodialysis have not been systematically investigated. Uncontrolled reports indicate that patients treated with more frequent hemodialysis have greater appetites and food intake (3). It is anticipated that such individuals will probably have increased daily needs for certain nutrients than are discussed in this chapter and listed in TABLE 27.4. Such patients may also have greater tolerance for some nutrients than is indicated here. The benefits of more frequent hemodialysis have not yet been established in randomized, prospective clinical trials, although less well controlled data are very encouraging (41,42).

Protein

Maintenance Hemodialysis

Protein requirements are increased in MHD patients because of the removal of amino acids and peptides by the dialysis procedure (4,5) and because the hemodialysis treatment appears to stimulate protein catabolism by engendering an inflammatory, catabolic response (43). Nitrogen balance studies suggest that many MHD patients may require at least 1.0 g protein/kg/d to maintain both protein balance and normal total body protein mass (44). However, for a safe protein intake that will maintain protein balance in almost all clinically stable MHD patients, the NKF K/DOQI Clinical Practice Guidelines on Nutrition in CKD

recommend 1.2 g protein per kilogram body weight per day (40) and the European Best Practice Guidelines (EBPG) recommend at least 1.1 g protein per kilogram ideal body weight (IBW) per day (45). To ensure adequate intake of essential amino acids, it is recommended that at least half of the dietary protein should be of high biologic value, although experimental evidence to prove this contention is lacking. For most individuals undergoing more frequent MHD, 1.2 g protein/kg/d probably will also provide an adequate protein intake.

Chronic Peritoneal Dialysis

A diet providing 1.2 to 1.3 g protein/kg/d appears to be a safe protein intake for CAPD patients and is consistent with the recommendations of the NKF K/DOQI Clinical Practice Guidelines on Nutrition in CKD (40) and with complete nitrogen balance studies on CAPD patients (46). Daily losses of amino acids and protein into dialysate of patients undergoing automated daily peritoneal dialysis (APD) are similar to the losses with CAPD (6,7,47). Thus, although there are no complete nitrogen balance studies of dietary protein requirements in APD patients, one would expect that the dietary protein requirements would be similar to those of patients undergoing CAPD. Again, it is recommended that at least 50% of the dietary protein should be of high biologic value (40). It is possible that CAPD and APD patients who are protein depleted or hypercatabolic may become more anabolic when they ingest up to 1.5 g protein/kg/d, although this has not been clinically investigated.

TABLE 27.4	**Recommended Dietary Protein, Energy, and Fiber Intake for Patients Undergoing Maintenance Hemodialysis or Chronic Peritoneal Dialysis**	
	Maintenance Hemodialysis	**Continuous Ambulatory Peritoneal Dialysis or Automated Peritoneal Dialysis**
Protein	1.1–1.2 g/kg/d 50% high biologic value[a]	1.2–1.3 g/kg/d 50% high biologic value protein[a]
Energy (kcal/kg/d)	35 kcal/kg/d for individuals younger than 60 years old and 30–35 kcal/kg/d for patients 60 years old or older. Patients with relative body weight >120% or patients who are afraid of gaining unwanted weight may be prescribed lower energy intakes. Energy intake includes energy obtained from diet and, if applicable, from hemodialysate or peritoneal dialysate.	
Fat (percentage of total energy intake)[b,c]	25–35	25–35
Polyunsaturated fatty acids[b,c]	Up to 10% of total calories	Up to 10% of total calories
Monounsaturated fatty acids[b,c]	Up to 20% of total calories	Up to 20% of total calories
Saturated fatty acids[b,c]	<7% of total calories	<7% of total calories
Cholesterol[c]	250 mg/d or lower	250 mg/d or lower
Carbohydrate[b,c,d]	50%–65% of total calories	50%–65% of total calories
Total fiber intake (g/d)[b,c]	20–30	20–30

[a]When recommended intake is expressed per kilogram body weight, this refers to the adjusted edema-free body weight. Some studies, not widely confirmed, recommend for CPD patients an 0.8 g protein/kg/d diet supplemented with about 0.1–0.12 g/kg of a mixture of four ketoacid analogs of essential amino acids, one hydroxy acid analog of methionine, and the other four essential amino acids, sometimes with one urea cycle amino acid added (56).

[b]Refers to percentage of total energy intake (diet plus dialysate); if triglyceride levels are very high, the percentage of fat in the diet may be increased to about 40% (to decrease the amount of carbohydrate consumed). Otherwise, 35% or less of total calories from fat is preferable. The recommendations regarding fat, carbohydrate, and fiber intake follow the NCEP TLC (National Cholesterol Education Program Therapeutic Lifestyle Changes) diet.

[c]These dietary recommendations are considered less crucial than the others. They are only emphasized if the patient has a specific disorder that may benefit from this modification or is complying well to the other, more important aspects of the dietary treatment (see text).

[d]Should be primarily complex carbohydrates.

Patients classified as high peritoneal transporters by the peritoneal equilibration test lose more protein and amino acids into peritoneal dialysate than those classified as low transporters (e.g., typical 24-hour losses in high vs. low transporters: albumin, 4.9 ± 2 (SD) vs. 3.2 ± 1 g/d, $p < 0.03$, total free amino acids, 15.4 ± 4 vs. 10 ± 4 mmol/d, $p = 0.002$) (48,49). This trend is shown in all studies of high versus low transporters. The high transporters also have, on average, lower serum albumin levels (48,49). However, the difference in protein and amino acid losses with high versus low transporters is not great, and dietary protein intakes of 1.2 to 1.3 g/kg/d should provide sufficient amounts of protein and amino acids to compensate for these increased peritoneal losses if the ability to synthesize these serum proteins is normal.

Some nephrologists report MHD or CPD patients who habitually ingest somewhat lesser amounts of protein or calories than are recommended and yet do not show evidence of PEW and lead physically active, rehabilitated lives. These observations raise questions as to whether the foregoing recommended dietary protein and energy intakes for chronic dialysis patients may be excessive. Several comments may be pertinent in this regard. First, some MD patients who appear to be doing well will, on close inspection, turn out to have evidence for malnutrition. Epidemiologic studies have associated protein depletion, even in mild forms, with increased mortality (31–35,50). Second, subtle forms of malnutrition are particularly difficult to detect, and the recommended intakes may provide some protection against mild forms of PEM. Third, the concept of dietary allowances presupposes that in order to ensure a sufficient nutrient intake for virtually all individuals (i.e., about 97%) in a given

population, the recommended allowance must be greater than the actual requirement for a large proportion of that population (51). This reasoning is similar to that used by the World Health Organization and the Food and Nutrition Board of the National Academy of Sciences to determine the recommended dietary protein intakes for normal adults (52). Thus, it is expected that some individuals will ingest less protein or calories than is recommended without developing protein malnutrition. At present, there is no method that will identify in advance, under the conditions of clinical practice, which patients can safely ingest lower protein or energy intakes. Hence, to be safe, unless the patient can be shown to maintain a healthy nutritional status on a lower nutrient intake, he or she should be prescribed the dietary allowances described here.

Recently, a number of studies have reported that patients with far advanced or end-stage CKD may be treated with low-protein or very low-protein diets (e.g., 0.60 g protein/kg/d or 0.3 to 0.4 g protein/kg/d) supplemented with ketoacid or hydroxyacid analogs of usually five essential amino acids plus the other four essential amino acids. These studies indicate that for many patients, this treatment may safely delay the need for chronic dialysis therapy (53), may safely allow time for a PD access or a hemodialysis vascular access to mature without, for example, resorting to tunnel catheters (54), or may allow for a lower dose of dialysis treatment, at least as long as some residual kidney function is preserved (55). Some data suggest that these low-protein or supplemented very low-protein diets may delay the loss of residual kidney function (55,56). These diets appear to attain these results without inducing protein or energy wasting, serious metabolic abnormalities, or uremic toxicity. Some data suggest that the ketoacid and essential amino acid preparations may induce an anti-inflammatory effect (57). For the low-protein diets or a combination of low-protein diets and dialysis treatments to be safe and effective for patients with advanced CKD or end-stage kidney disease (ESKD), it would seem that the patient must be very motivated to adhere to the protein-restricted diets.

Energy

In most studies, energy expenditure in patients undergoing MHD or CAPD, measured by indirect calorimetry, appears to be normal during resting and sitting, following ingestion of a standard meal, and with defined exercise (58). What is most impressive about these foregoing studies is that there is no report of decreased energy expenditure in CKD, MHD, or CPD patients. Dietary energy intake in MHD and CPD patients is commonly reported to be lower than their recommended intakes (1,2). Many CPD patients tend to gain body fat and weight, probably due to the glucose uptake from peritoneal dialysate. The surges in plasma insulin that accompany the glucose absorbed from peritoneal dialysate may contribute to the increase in body fat that is not uncommonly observed in CPD patients.

The NKF K/DOQI Clinical Practice Guidelines for Nutrition in CKD recommend an energy intake of 35 kcal/kg/d for MHD and CPD patients who are younger than 60 years of age and 30 to 35 kcal/kg/d for those who are 60 years of age or older (**Table 27.4**) (40). This intake includes energy derived from the diet as well as from any fuels taken up from dialysate. Because individuals older than 60 years old tend to be more sedentary and their muscles often constitute a smaller proportion of their body mass, their recommended energy intake is somewhat lower. These recommendations are similar to the EBPG of 30 to 40 kcal/kg IBW/d adjusted for age, gender, and estimated physical activity (45). These intakes are also rather similar to those for normal individuals engaged in light to moderate activity as put forth in the RDA by the Food and Nutrition Board, National Academy of Sciences (51). Patients who are obese with an edema-free body weight greater than 120% of desirable body weight may be treated with lower calorie intakes. Some patients, particularly young or middle-aged women, may become obese on this energy intake or may refuse to ingest the recommended calories out of fear of obesity. These individuals may require a lower energy prescription. There are many readily prepared or commercially available high-calorie foodstuffs that are low in protein, sodium, and potassium which can be recommended by the renal dietitian.

⬡ TREATMENT OF RISK FACTORS FOR VASCULAR DISEASE

Lipids

There are a number of reviews of the causes for the abnormal serum lipids and lipoproteins in MHD and CPD patients, and space constraints do not allow a full discussion of these abnormalities or their causes (59). In brief, MHD and CPD patients often have increased serum triglyceride levels, intermediate density lipoprotein (IDL), and very low-density lipoprotein (VLDL), and serum lipoprotein(a) [Lp(a)]; serum HDL cholesterol is often low. CPD patients often have higher serum total cholesterol, triglycerides, LDL cholesterol, and apolipoprotein B levels than do MHD patients. Qualitative changes in the apolipoprotein concentrations also occur; among these is an increase in small dense low-density lipoprotein (sd LDL) (60). Since alterations in lipid metabolism and

serum lipids may contribute to the high incidence of atherosclerosis and cardiovascular cerebrovascular and peripheral vascular disease in CKD patients, attention has been directed toward reducing serum triglycerides and LDL cholesterol and increasing HDL cholesterol.

Treatment of altered lipid levels and the risk of cardiac and vascular disease normally involves three components: nutrient intake, medicines, and exercise. In MHD patients, clinical trials do not indicate that cholesterol-lowering agents reduce adverse cardiovascular events (59), and there are no clinical trials examining whether any dietary lipid therapy reduces cardiovascular risk. On the other hand, *epidemiologic studies* indicate that serum levels that are low in phosphorus and a lower serum calcium–phosphorus product are associated with less cardiovascular disease (61,62).

Until more evidence is available, based on data from the general population, we encourage MD patients to follow a dietary plan that is based upon the National Cholesterol Education Program (NCEP) Therapeutic Lifestyle Changes (TLC) diet for all MHD and CPD patients, especially if their serum LDL levels are over 100 mg/dL (63). Since these patients are at high risk for cardiovascular, cerebrovascular, and peripheral vascular disease, we prefer to set a target LDL cholesterol of 70 mg/dL. The TLC diet provides the following (63): no more than 25% to 35% of total calories from fat, polyunsaturated fatty acids providing up to 10% of total calories, monounsaturated fatty acids providing up to 20% of total calories, saturated fatty acids providing less than 7% of total calories, and a cholesterol content of 200 mg/d or lower. Carbohydrate intake should be 50% to 60% of total calories and derived predominantly from foods rich in complex carbohydrates. Fiber intake should be 20 to 30 g/d (63). Since the TLC diet may be less palatable to many patients, their energy intake should be monitored to ensure that it remains adequate (see the subsequent text). Patients are encouraged to control calorie intake to avoid becoming substantially overweight or frankly obese. (i.e., avoid a BMI greater than about 28 kg/m^2). It is recognized that most individuals will not be able to adhere exactly to the TLC diet. However, there is reason to believe that even some modifications of dietary intake in the direction of lowering serum cholesterol may reduce the risk of adverse vascular events (64). Moreover, if MD patients are not counseled on the characteristics and rationale underlying this diet, they may eat even a less healthy diet as they grow older.

Omega-3 fatty acids (e.g., eicosapentaenoic acid and docosahexaenoic acid, which are found in fish oil) lower serum triglycerides and have more variable effects on serum LDL cholesterol and HDL cholesterol (65). Fish oil also decreases platelet aggregation and appears to exert anti-inflammatory effects, and omega-3 fatty acids may enhance immune function. 3-Hydroxy-3-methylglutaryl coenzyme A reductase inhibitors (statins) lower LDL-cholesterol; may slightly increase serum HDL-cholesterol; appear to be anti-inflammatory, antithrombotic, and fibrinolytic; improve impaired endothelial function; and, in animals, protect against progressive renal injury (66). It is emphasized that evidence that manipulation of lipid intake may reduce cardiovascular risk in MHD and CPD patients is currently lacking.

Other Potential Nonnutritional Techniques for Reducing Cardiovascular Risk

Evidence for the protective nature of other methods for reducing cardiovascular risk is largely obtained from clinical trials in the general population. Antiplatelet therapy, such as aspirin, has been shown to reduce the risk of myocardial infarction in adult high-risk CKD patients (67,68). In CKD patients, impaired hemostasis caused by aspirin may increase the risk of bleeding. However, 100 mg aspirin per day taken by MD patients increased the risk of minor bleeding (e.g., epistaxis, ecchymoses, or bruising) by three-fold ($p = 0.001$) but not the risk of major bleeding episodes (e.g., leading to hospitalization or fatality) (69).

Multifactorial intervention may reduce the risk of adverse cardiovascular events in patients with type 2 diabetes mellitus without advanced kidney failure (70). The intervention consisted of dietary treatment (fat intake less than 30% of daily energy intake, saturated fatty acids less than 10% of daily intake), 30 minutes of light to moderate exercise three to five times per week, smoking cessation classes for smokers, daily intake of angiotensin-converting enzyme (ACE) inhibitors or angiotensin receptor blockers (ARBs) irrespective of blood pressure, daily vitamin-mineral supplements providing vitamin C 250 mg, D-α-tocopherol 100 mg, folic acid 400 μg, chromium picolinate 100 μg, aspirin (unless there were contraindicators), and aggressive control of blood glucose, blood pressure, and hypercholesterolemia and hypertriglyceridemia. The patients receiving this intensive therapy had a significantly lower risk of adverse cardiovascular events, kidney disease (albuminuria greater than 300 mg/24 h in two of three consecutive urine specimens), retinopathy, and autonomic neuropathy. We treat hypertriglyceridemia by dietary modification or medicines only when fasting serum triglycerides are very high (i.e., 500 mg/dL or more), because in the general population, these triglyceride levels increase the risk of adverse cardiovascular events and pancreatitis. In this situation, dietary fat intake may be increased but not above 40% of total calories. A high proportion of dietary carbohydrates should be complex. These modifications often lower the palatability of the diet; therefore, the patient's total energy intake must be monitored closely to ensure that it does not fall to levels that are inadequate to maintain desirable body and protein mass. With high serum triglyceride levels that are unresponsive to dietary therapy, a fibrate (e.g., fenofibrate) may be tried cautiously while monitoring the patient for myopathy.

Oxidant and Carbonyl Stress

As indicated earlier, end-stage kidney disease is associated with increased levels of compounds that promote oxidant and carbonyl stress and chronic inflammation, all of which may promote atherosclerotic and proliferative vascular disease (71,72). Although there are few interventional trials evaluating the effects of reduction of these risk factors on morbidity or mortality of MD patients, the following treatments may be considered for MHD patients, particularly given their high risk of cardiovascular disease: (a) larger flux dialyzers that remove greater amounts of advanced glycation end products and other reactive carbonyl compounds; (b) antioxidants or antioxidant precursors, such as vitamins E or C (see the section "Vitamins" in the subsequent text) or selenium; supplemental selenium must be taken with caution because selenium is primarily excreted in the urine and may accumulate in kidney disease (73); (c) one glass per day of an alcoholic drink, perhaps particularly red wine; (d) statins, notwithstanding the lack of evidence for their effectiveness in MHD patients; and (e) regular exercise.

Carnitine

Carnitine, which is essential for life (74), is both ingested and synthesized *in vivo*. Carnitine facilitates the transfer of long-chain (greater than 10 carbon) fatty acids into muscle mitochondria. Since fatty acids are the major fuel source for skeletal and myocardial muscle

at rest and during mild to moderate exercise, carnitine is considered necessary for normal skeletal and cardiac muscle function. MD patients and particularly MHD patients display low serum-free carnitine and, in some but not all studies, low skeletal muscle-free and total carnitine levels (74). Also, in MHD patients, serum and sometimes muscle acylcarnitines (fatty acid-carnitine compounds) and serum total carnitines are increased (75). The low serum and skeletal muscle-free carnitine levels led some investigators to postulate that many MD patients are carnitine deficient. Clinical trials of oral or intravenous carnitine administration to MD patients have led to conflicting results. Most students of this problem believe that evidence for beneficial effects of carnitine supplements to MD patients is unconvincing.

Carbohydrates

Patients should be encouraged to eat complex rather than purified carbohydrates to reduce triglyceride synthesis and to improve glucose tolerance if it is abnormal.

Minerals and Vitamins

Sodium

Hypertension in MD patients generally is more easily controlled when they are sodium restricted, and hypertension may be accentuated by an increased sodium intake, probably because of expanded extracellular fluid volume (76) and possibly due to altered intracellular electrolyte composition within arteriolar smooth muscle cells that increase contractility. Cross-sectional studies indicate that the blood pressure that is associated with lowest mortality are increased in MHD patients. The range of prehemodialysis systolic and diastolic blood pressures associated with the lowest mortality in MHD patients is approximately 160 to 189 mm Hg and 70 to 99 mm Hg, respectively (77). However, longitudinal studies of MHD patients indicates blood pressures closer to healthy levels for the general population are associated with improved survival.

It is recommended that blood pressures for CPD patients and for MHD patients, obtained prehemodialysis, should be no higher than 140/90 mm Hg (78). If sodium and water balance are tightly controlled in MHD patients, most such individuals will require little or no antihypertensive medications to maintain a desirable blood pressure. However, this level of sodium control is difficult to attain with hemodialysis performed only thrice weekly for ≤4 hours per hemodialysis treatment. Usually, when sodium balance is well controlled, the thirst mechanism will adequately regulate water balance. In patients with diabetes mellitus, hyperglycemia may also increase thirst and enhance positive water balance. Some MD patients are at risk for overhydration from excessive water intake independent of sodium intake, and their water intake should be controlled independently of sodium. In patients undergoing MD who are not anuric and who gain excessive sodium or water despite attempts at dietary restriction, a potent loop diuretic, such as furosemide or bumetanide, may be tried to increase urinary sodium and water excretion.

Patients undergoing MHD or CPD frequently are oliguric or anuric. For MHD patients, sodium and total fluid intake generally should be restricted to 1,000 to 2,000 mg/d and 1,000 to 1,500 mL/d, respectively. Because sodium and water can be removed easily with CAPD or other forms of daily PD, a more liberal salt and water intake is usually allowed. Indeed, by maintaining a larger dietary sodium and water intake, the quantity of fluid removed from the CPD patient and hence the daily dialysate outflow volume can be increased. This may be advantageous, since with CPD, the daily clearance of small- and middle-sized molecules is directly related to the volume of dialysate outflow. Therefore, for some CPD patients, a higher sodium and water intake (e.g., 6 to 8 g/d of sodium and 3 L/d of water) may enable the patient to use more hypertonic or hyperoncotic dialysate to increase the dialysate outflow volume, thereby increasing dialysate clearances and energy uptake from dialysate, if hypertonic glucose is used. This treatment may be undesirable for obese or severely hypertriglyceridemic patients because the greater use of hypertonic glucose exchanges will increase their glucose load. Also, there is the potential disadvantage that some patients may become habituated to high salt and water intakes; if they change to hemodialysis therapy, they may have difficulty curtailing their sodium and water intake.

Potassium

MD patients exhibit increased fecal potassium (46), which slightly increases the tolerance to dietary potassium. Loss of renal function, acidemia, catabolic stress, hypoinsulinism or insulin resistance, and catecholamine antagonists may each be associated with increased risk of hyperkalemia in MD patients (79). Hyperkalemia can usually be prevented in MD patients if they ingest no more than 70 mEq of potassium per day. Refractory hyperkalemia may require treatment with lower dialysate potassium, oral intake of potassium binders, or more frequent hemodialysis.

Magnesium

The optimal dietary magnesium allowance for MD patients has not been well defined. Experience suggests that when the magnesium content is about 1.0 mEq/L in hemodialysate or 0.50 to 0.75 mEq/L in peritoneal dialysate, a dietary magnesium intake of 200 to 300 mg/d will maintain the serum magnesium at normal or only slightly elevated levels.

Phosphorus and Phosphate Binders

The rationale for controlling dietary phosphorus and methods to prevent and treat hyperphosphatemia, a high serum calcium–phosphorus product, calcium phosphate deposition in soft tissue, hyperparathyroidism, and altered bone mineral metabolism are discussed in Chapter 24. This section considers the prescription of dietary phosphorus intake and phosphate binders. In MD patients, a large dietary phosphorus intake can lead to a high plasma calcium–phosphorus product with increased risk of calcium and phosphate deposition in soft tissues including arteries. Moreover, hyperphosphatemia, by lowering serum calcium, provides a strong stimulus to the development of hyperparathyroidism and increased serum FGF-23 levels. Hyperphosphatemia, hyperparathyroidism, and increased FGF-23 are independently associated with increased mortality in MHD patients (33,80). The NKF KDOQI Clinical Practice Guidelines recommend for MHD and CPD patients that serum phosphorus be maintained between 3.5 and 5.5 mg/dL (11). This often requires a low phosphorus intake not to exceed 1,000 to 1,200 mg/d, (i.e., about 12 to 15 mg phosphorus/kg/d), particularly when MD patients have moderate or severe hyperparathyroidism (see the subsequent text). This higher upper limit was chosen because with their greater protein intakes, dialysis patients cannot readily ingest less phosphorus without making the diet too restrictive and unattractive. Without phosphate binders, there is a net intestinal phosphate absorption (diet minus fecal phosphorus) of roughly 60% of the phosphorus intake (46). Therefore, even with this level of dietary phosphorus restriction, MHD and CPD patients almost always require phosphate binders to prevent hyperphosphatemia, unless MHD patients undergo hemodialysis more than thrice weekly. Serum phosphorus levels should be monitored monthly after starting MD, and dietary phosphorus restriction should be employed with use of phosphate binders as necessary to ensure that serum phosphorus remains within the normal range.

The phosphate binders, aluminum carbonate and aluminum hydroxide, are uncommonly used now because of aluminum toxicity (81). Phosphate binders in current use include calcium carbonate, calcium acetate, sevelamer hydrochloride (82), sevelamer carbonate, lanthanum carbonate (83), and several iron preparations (84,85). These phosphate binders are discussed in greater detail in Chapter 24. Phosphate binders vary somewhat as to the effectiveness at binding phosphate in the intestinal tract and not uncommonly cause such mild gastrointestinal distress as anorexia, nausea, diarrhea, or constipation which may reduce compliance (86). Often, with more time taking the same binder, these symptoms will abate. Calcium binder doses should not provide more than about 600 to 1,500 mg of elemental calcium per day [total calcium intake (from diet plus binders) should not exceed 1,000 to 2,000 mg/d] to prevent excessive accumulation of calcium in soft tissues and especially arteries (11,13). Treatment with 1,25-dihydroxycholecalciferol (calcitriol) or its analogs may decrease tolerance to calcium binders by enhancing intestinal calcium absorption. Calcium binders should be taken in divided doses with meals and should not be prescribed if the serum phosphorus level is very high in order to avoid precipitation of calcium and phosphate in soft tissues. Therefore, hyperphosphatemic patients may be treated with other binders of phosphate until serum phosphorus falls to normal or near normal. At that time, the regimen may be changed to a calcium binder. Calcium comprises 40% of calcium carbonate and 25% of calcium acetate.

Noncalcium binders have the advantage that they should pose no increased risk of calcium deposition in soft tissues including arteries. Sevelamer HCl is often given in doses of two to six 800 mg capsules three or four times per day with meals. Sevelamer HCl also has the benefit of lowering serum LDL-cholesterol and increasing serum HDL-cholesterol (87). Some individuals taking this drug can become acidemic because of the large hydrochloride content of this preparation. Sevelamer carbonate, which should not induce acidemia, can be prescribed instead (88). Lanthanum carbonate appears to be one of the more effective phosphate binders and is generally well tolerated. Small quantities of lanthanum accumulate in tissues of MD patients with daily doses (89); at present, there is no evidence that this is harmful to patients. Lanthanum carbonate is often given in doses of 0.5 to 1.5 g three times daily with meals. Ferric citrate and sucroferric oxyhydroxide are currently available iron-based phosphate binders (85,90). These compounds may also provide an iron supplement and may decrease the amount of intravenous iron and the dosage of erythropoiesis-stimulating agents that MD patients may require (84,91). Bixalomer, a phosphate-binding polymer, may also be tried (92). If MD patients are intolerant to recommended doses of any of these binders or if they remain hyperphosphatemic despite maximal or maximally tolerated doses of a binder (serum phosphorus greater than greater than 5.5 mg/dL), two or more phosphate binders may be given simultaneously. Phosphate binders, in general, bind only up to 300 to 500 mg phosphorus per day, even when given in maximum doses. Since people absorb roughly 60% of ingested phosphorus, the use of phosphate binders does not substitute for the need to restrict dietary phosphorus unless patients are receiving quotidian dialysis (93).

Some studies indicate that compounds that impair phosphate transport in the intestinal tract may also decrease serum phosphorus and the body phosphate burden. This has been shown for niacin and tenapanor (94,95).

Calcium, Vitamin D, and Parathyroid Hormone

The NKF DOQI guidelines recommend the serum calcium–phosphorus product should be maintained below 55 mg^2/dL^2 (11). This product should be attained primarily by controlling serum levels of phosphorus within the target range as indicated earlier. Frequent monitoring of serum calcium is important because hypercalcemia may develop, particularly if serum phosphorus should fall to low-normal or low levels. This is especially likely to occur if the patient also has hyperparathyroidism, a common complication of CKF, or is receiving larger doses of calcitriol. The NKF DOQI guidelines recommend that serum calcium levels, corrected for any alteration in serum albumin (see the subsequent text), should be maintained within the normal range for the laboratory used but preferably toward the lower end of normal (8.4 to 9.5 mg/dL) (11). As indicated earlier, it is the authors' policy that total calcium intake from the diet and calcium-based phosphate binders combined should not exceed 1,000 to 2,000 mg/d. If the serum total corrected calcium is below the lower limit for the laboratory used (less than 8.4 mg/dL), the patient may receive a higher dose of calcitriol or other vitamin D analog, a lower intake of the calcium receptor agonist, cinacalcet, or a greater intake of calcium to increase serum calcium levels. Serum calcium corrected for serum albumin may be calculated as follows (**EQUATION 27.1**) (11):

$$\text{Corrected serum calcium (mg/dL)} = \text{Total serum} \quad (27.1)$$
$$\text{calcium (mg/dL)} + 0.0704 \times$$
$$[34 - \text{serum albumin (g/L)}]$$

A simpler equation, which is about as accurate, is as follows (**EQUATION 27.2**):

$$\text{Corrected serum calcium (mg/dL)} = \text{Total serum} \quad (27.2)$$
$$\text{calcium (mg/dL)} + 0.8 \times [4 - \text{serum albumin (g/dL)}]$$

MD patients have an increased dietary requirement for calcium because they have vitamin D deficiency and resistance to the actions of vitamin D which may impair the intestinal absorption of calcium. The risk of calcium deficiency in these patients is enhanced because the diets prescribed for MHD patients are almost always low in calcium, because foods high in calcium are usually high in phosphorus (e.g., dairy products) and are therefore restricted for uremic patients.

On the other hand, MHD and CPD patients often have extensive calcification of their arteries including the coronary arteries (96). In the general population, the extent of coronary artery calcification is directly related to the risk of myocardial infarction (97). Therefore, for MHD or CPD patients, it may be preferable to maintain total calcium intake closer to 1,000 mg/d or even lower if serum calcium is greater than 9.4 mg/dL. It is emphasized that when patients take l,25-dihdroxycholecalciferol (calcitriol) or other vitamin D analogs that increase intestinal calcium absorption, lower calcium intake may be indicated. Serum calcium should be monitored frequently because hypercalcemia may develop with these treatments.

To reduce the total daily calcium load to the dialysis patient who is taking calcium binders of phosphate, the calcium content of dialysate is often reduced. This is a somewhat more effective method

for controlling calcium balance with daily CPD than with thrice-weekly MHD. The usual dialysate calcium concentration for MHD or CPD patients is 2.5 mEq/L. Secondary hyperparathyroidism can be treated in patients with CKD with vitamin D analogs. In general, serum intact parathyroid hormone in MD patients should be maintained within a target range of 150 to 300 pg/mL. If the serum level of 25-hydroxyvitamin D is less than 30 ng/mL, supplementation with vitamin D$_2$ (ergocalciferol) or vitamin D$_3$ (cholecalciferol) should be initiated. For MD patients, therapy with an active vitamin D sterol (1,25-dihdroxycholecalciferol, alphacalcidol, paricalcitol, or doxercalciferol) should be provided if the plasma levels of intact parathyroid hormone are greater than 300 pg/mL (11). Retrospective studies indicate that MHD patients treated with calcitriol or paricalcitol had lower mortality than patients not receiving these medicines ($p < 0.001$) (98,99). Vitamin D has many other actions in addition to its effects on calcium absorption, parathyroid hormone secretion, and bone metabolism. These effects include regulation of immune function, antiproliferative, differentiating effects (100), promotion of muscle strength, and possibly hypertrophy (101). Thus, it is not surprising if vitamin D and its congeners may affect survival rates. Moreover, another retrospective study indicates that MHD patients treated with the vitamin D analog paricalcitol had a lower mortality rate than MHD patients who received calcitriol (98). Cinacalcet increases the sensitivity of the calcium receptor in the parathyroid gland to calcium so that parathyroid hormone secretion can be suppressed or inhibited at lower serum calcium levels (102). This medicine is effective at suppressing hyperparathyroidism in MD patients.

The syndrome of aplastic or hypoplastic bone disease in MD patients is characterized by relatively low serum parathyroid hormone concentrations, decreased bone osteoblasts, and marked reduction in bone turnover. The syndrome can be caused by aluminum toxicity and probably excess iron (11,103). Large doses of calcium binders of phosphate or vitamin D with consequent suppression of parathyroid hormone also appear to cause this disorder (11,103).

Trace Elements

Many trace elements are excreted primarily in urine and may accumulate with kidney failure. Excessive uptake from dialysate or losses of trace elements into dialysate may occur during dialysis therapy depending on the relative concentrations in plasma and dialysate of the trace element and the degree of its binding to protein or red cells (104). Hemodialysance of copper, strontium, zinc, and lead, for example, which are largely bound to plasma proteins or red cells, should be minimal (105). Hemodialysis or hemodiafiltration may remove some trace elements if the dialysate concentrations are sufficiently low (e.g., bromide, iodine, lithium, rubidium, cesium, and zinc) (105,106). Zinc may be taken up and copper lost from peritoneal dialysate. Because many trace elements are avidly bound to serum proteins, they may be taken up by blood against a concentration gradient when present in even small quantities in dialysate (105,107). These observations provide part of the justification for intensive purification of dialysate. Inhalation may result in increased intake of certain trace elements. This may occur in people exposed to certain industrial processes, fertilizers, insecticides, herbicides, or burning of fossil fuels.

PEW, which can be associated with lowered serum concentrations of proteins that bind trace elements, may decrease the serum levels of a number of these elements including zinc, manganese, and nickel (108). Occupational exposure or pica may increase the burden of some trace elements. Therapeutic doses of trace elements may be administered through dialysis, as has been done for zinc (109). Reduced dietary intake of many nutrients by the uremic patient might lower body pools of trace elements, but there is little scientific evidence that bears on this hypothesis (108).

Assessment of trace element burden in kidney disease patients is difficult because the binding protein concentrations may be decreased, thereby lowering serum trace element levels, and the binding characteristics of these proteins may be altered in kidney disease as well. Also, red cell concentrations of trace elements may not reflect levels in other tissues. Trace element supplementation should be undertaken with caution because impaired urinary excretion and poor dialysance of most trace elements, due to protein binding, increase the risk of overdosage.

Dietary requirements for trace elements have not been well defined in MD patients. Iron deficiency is common, particularly in MHD patients because intestinal iron absorption is sometimes impaired, there are often substantial blood losses; iron may bind to the dialyzer membrane, and the erythropoietin-induced rise in hemoglobin concentrations may deplete the body's iron supply (110). Not only do iron requirements increase during the time when erythropoietin therapy is initiated and hemoglobin concentrations rise, but higher serum iron levels and body iron burden are associated with a greater response to erythropoietin (111). Some researchers recommend that, in general, MHD or CPD patients should maintain serum transferrin saturation (TSAT) at 30% to 50% and serum ferritin at about 400 to 800 ng/mL (111). Although some MD patients may maintain these iron values with oral iron supplements, many such individuals will not be able to do so unless they receive parenteral iron therapy (12,111). Oral ferrous sulfate, 300 mg three times per day one-half hour after meals, may be tried. Some patients develop anorexia, nausea, constipation, or abdominal pain with ferrous sulfate; these individuals sometimes will tolerate other iron compounds better, such as ferrous fumarate, gluconate, or lactate. Patients may satisfy some of their iron requirement by taking such iron salts as ferric citrate and sucroferric oxyhydroxide that are also phosphate binders (see above). Patients who are intolerant to oral iron supplements and the preponderance of MHD or CPD patients who will not maintain TSAT at 30% to 50% and serum ferritin levels of 400 to 800 ng/mL with oral iron may be treated with intravenous iron (12,111).

As indicated earlier, MHD patients may have an increased body burden of aluminum, often from ingesting aluminum salts used as phosphate binders or from contaminated dialysate. Increased serum aluminum has been implicated as a cause of a progressive dementia syndrome, osteomalacia, weakness of the muscles of the proximal limbs, impaired immune function, and anemia (81,103). Current methods of water treatment have removed virtually all aluminum from dialysate. Increased body burden and toxicity of iron or aluminum in MHD or CPD patients may be reduced by reduction of intake or by infusion of deferoxamine, which is dialyzable (112). Care must be taken because deferoxamine may promote infection, particularly mucormycosis (113). Injections of erythropoietin with repeated phlebotomy are another method for removing excess body iron (114).

Although the zinc content of most tissues is normal in kidney disease patients, usually serum and hair zinc are reported to be low and red cell zinc increased (13,108,115). Fecal zinc is increased (115), and the dietary requirement for zinc may be increased. Further studies are needed to confirm this possibility. Some reports

indicate that dysgeusia, poor food intake, and impaired sexual function, which are common problems of MD patients, may be improved by giving patients zinc supplements (13,115). Other studies, however, have not confirmed these findings (116). The finding that serum selenium is low in dialysis patients has raised the question of whether selenium supplements are indicated (117). This question is of particular importance because selenium participates in the defense against oxidative damage of tissues, which may be increased in kidney disease (118).

Vitamins

Among MD patients who do not take vitamin supplements, vitamin deficiencies are not uncommon because of reduced intake, dialysis losses and altered absorption, metabolism, or activity of some vitamins (119). The low potassium and phosphorus diets prescribed for MD patients often lead to low intake of some vitamins. Some medicines interfere with the actions of certain vitamins. Vitamin deficiencies are particularly frequent for 25 hydroxycholecalciferol and 1,25-dihydroxycholecalciferol (calcitriol) (discussed above), folic acid, vitamin B_6 (pyridoxine), vitamin C, and, to a lesser extent, other water-soluble vitamins (119,120). Vitamin B_{12} deficiency is uncommon in MD patients, even in patients undergoing hemodiafiltration (121) because it is protein bound in plasma and therefore poorly dialyzable and because body vitamin B_{12} stores are quite large.

There is a high prevalence of vitamin C deficiency in MHD and CPD patients who do not take vitamin supplements, which is probably due to reduced vitamin C in their diets and losses into dialysate. Zhang et al. (122) reported that in 64% of 284 MHD and CPD patients who were not receiving supplements, plasma vitamin C levels were insufficient or deficient. The amount of vitamin C lost in hemodialysate is reported to range from 92 to 334 mg per treatment (123). Plasma ascorbic acid fell by 50% during an individual MHD treatment (123). Morena et al. (124) reported that with hemodiafiltration, two-thirds of dialysate vitamin C losses are due to diffusion and one-third to convection, and the convection volume in this study was substantially lower than what is currently recommended. Scurvy is seldom reported in MD patients (125), but it is not unlikely that less severe vitamin C deficiency may be unrecognized. Raimann et al. (126) found that in comparison with MD patients who had plasma vitamin C levels above the normal range, those with plasma vitamin C below the normal range had more severe periodontal disease and teeth losses, signs consistent with scurvy. Only a supplement providing the RDA for vitamin C is recommended because larger doses can increase plasma oxalate levels (127).

Vitamin B_6 is composed of three compounds: pyridoxine, pyridoxal, and pyridoxamine. Pyridoxal-5-phosphate (PLP), a key phosphorylated metabolic product of vitamin B_6, is a coenzyme for almost 100 enzymatic reactions, particularly for enzymes involved in the metabolism of amino acids and lipids. Corken and Porter (128) reported a 33% to 56% prevalence of vitamin B_6 deficiency when low plasma PLP was used as the criterion for deficiency. Removal of PLP in high-flux dialysis is significantly increased even though it is bound to albumin; PLP is often low in serum of PD patients. The dietary requirement for vitamin B_6 is increased to 10 mg/d, given as a pyridoxine HCl supplement (8.2 mg/d of free pyridoxine, **TABLE 27.5**). Some but not all studies suggest that treatment with large doses of pyridoxine HCl can decrease elevated plasma oxalate levels in MHD patients, although not to normal values (129).

Low plasma niacin concentrations are reported in some patients receiving MD therapy (119,120). Nicotinamide has been

| TABLE 27.5 | Recommended Mineral and Vitamin Intake for Patients Undergoing Maintenance Hemodialysis or Chronic Peritoneal Dialysis[a] | |

	Maintenance Hemodialysis	Continuous Ambulatory Peritoneal Dialysis or Automated Peritoneal Dialysis
Minerals and water (range of intake)		
Sodium (mg/d)	1,000–2,000[b]	1,000–3,000[b]
Potassium (mEq/d)	40–70[c]	40–70[c]
Phosphorus (mg/kg/d)	12–15[c] (not to exceed 1,000–1,200 mg/d)	12–15[c] (not to exceed 1,000–1,200 mg/d)
Calcium (mg/d)	500–2,000[d]	500–2,000[d]
Magnesium (mg/d)	200–300	200–300
Iron (mg/d)	See text[e]	See text[e]
Zinc (mg/d)	15[b]	15[b]
Water (mL/d)	≤1,500[f]	≤1,500[f]
Vitamins	Diets to be supplemented with these quantities	
Thiamin (mg/d)	1.5	1.5
Riboflavin (mg/d)	1.8	1.8
Pantothenic acid (mg/d)	5	5
Niacin (mg/d)	20	20
Pyridoxine HCl (mg/d)	10	10
Vitamin B_{12} (mg/d)	3	3
Vitamin C (mg/d)	75–90	75–90
Folic acid (mg/d)	0.8–1[g]	0.8–1[g]
Vitamin A	No addition	No addition
Vitamin D	See text	See text
Vitamin E (IU/d)	15	15
Vitamin K	None[h]	None[h]

[a]When recommended intake is expressed per kilogram of body weight, this refers to the adjusted edema-free body weight (see text).
[b]Can be higher in continuous ambulatory peritoneal dialysis (CAPD) patients or in hemodialysis patients who have greater urinary losses.
[c]Phosphate binders, calcium carbonate, acetate, or citrate, sevelamer carbonate or hydrochloride, lanthanum carbonate, ferric citrate, or other iron binders of phosphate are generally needed to maintain normal serum phosphorus levels. Inhibitors of intestinal phosphate transport may also reduce body phosphate burden.
[d]Prescribed dietary calcium intake will depend on the dialysate calcium concentration, the dose and type of vitamin D compound administered and the intake of any calcium-based binders of phosphate. The indicated Ca intake in this table includes any calcium-based binders of phosphate ingested.
[e]Iron needs may be increased because of the rapid rise in hemoglobin after commencing erythropoietin therapy, blood losses, possibly because of impaired intestinal absorption, and adherence of iron to dialyzer membranes. Since oral iron supplements may not maintain adequate iron stores and may cause gastrointestinal symptoms, iron is not uncommonly given intravenously. Iron-based binders of phosphate may increase serum iron and reduce the needed doses of erythropoiesis-stimulating agents.
[f]Water intake may be greater in patients with substantial daily urine volumes.
[g]Folic acid, 0.8–1 mg/d, is adequate for maintenance hemodialysis (MHD) and chronic peritoneal hemodialysis (CPD) patients (see text).
[h]Vitamin K supplements may be needed for patients who are not eating and who receive antibiotics.

shown to inhibit the Na/Pi type IIb cotransporter (Na Pi-2b) in the intestinal brush border and the type IIa cotransporter (NaPi-2a) in the proximal renal tubular epithelial cells of the kidneys (130). Large doses of nicotinamide, 500 to 1,500 mg/d taken twice daily, can reduce serum phosphorus concentrations in hemodialysis patients by inhibiting intestinal phosphate absorption and increasing fecal phosphate excretion.

Low plasma folate levels are not uncommon in advanced CKD patients who do not take vitamin supplements. Folates losses into dialysate may be substantial because it is water soluble, not very large, and not protein bound. Because many patients eat poorly, some patients present with low serum folate levels, and some medications may interfere with folate metabolism, a daily supplement of about 0.8 to 1 mg of folic acid is recommended for MHD and CPD patients (**TABLE 27.5**). Possible mild side effects of folate, such as

nausea, headache, or vivid dreams, have been reported with folate supplements, usually with a dose of 5 mg/d or greater (131).

Despite the water solubility of riboflavin, thiamin, pantothenic acid, and biotin, plasma concentrations of these vitamins are usually not decreased in patients undergoing MHD. Nonetheless, because of their water solubility, a daily supplement equal to the RDA or average intake (for biotin) is recommended. Functional thiamin deficiency has been reported both in MHD and CPD patients even when the plasma thiamin levels are normal (132). The hemodialysis procedure induces a greater decrease in plasma thiamin levels with high-flux versus low-flux membranes (133). Plasma thiamin levels are reported to be lower but not outside the normal range in patients treated with longer MHD treatment times (134). Beriberi, a disease associated with thiamin deficiency, is rarely described in dialysis patients. Hung et al. (135) found thiamin deficiency in

10 out of 30 MHD and CPD patients presenting with mental disturbances. Half of these patients were taking vitamin supplements containing vitamin B_1. In 9 out of these 10 patients, their mental disorder improved with intravenous thiamin supplements (135). Infection, surgery, and large glucose loads may increase the nutritional needs for thiamin and may precipitate clinical manifestations of thiamin deficiency in people who have marginal thiamin levels.

Vitamin K, available as phylloquinone (vitamin K_1) and menaquinone (vitamin K_2), is a coenzyme involved in the posttranslational carboxylation of glutamate residues in several proteins. This produces gamma-carboxyglutamate (Gla) residues on proteins which can bind to calcium. Gla-proteins are found in the coagulation cascade. Several inhibitors of coagulation are also vitamin K-dependent, including proteins C, S, and Z. The anticoagulation effect of coumarin-like compounds is related to blockade of the vitamin K participation in the formation of the Gla residues. Two Gla-proteins are present in bone, osteocalcin and matrix Gla protein (MGP). Osteocalcin is the most abundant noncollagenous protein of bone and is a specific marker for osteoblast activity. *In vitro*, osteocalcin binds to hydroxyapatite in bone and regulates its formation. MGP is also expressed in smooth muscle cells of the arterial wall and regulates calcium deposition in bone and in vascular tissue. Knock-out mice for MGP develop extensive lethal vascular calcifications (136).

Vitamin K is bound to lipoproteins; hence, no losses should occur during dialysis. Reports indicate that there is an increased serum uncarboxylated fraction in vitamin K–dependent proteins in many dialysis patients (137). These proteins include prothrombin, MGP, and osteocalcin and indicate a functional deficiency of vitamin K in some patients with kidney failure. Patients with elevated plasma dephosphorylated-uncarboxylated MGP may have increased vascular calcification (137). The need for vitamin K to maintain normal levels of certain anticoagulant factors and to maintain normal levels of MGP and osteocalcin may explain why coumarin-derivatives are risk factors for calciphylaxis stimulated by bone mineral metabolism imbalance in kidney failure patients (138). It has been proposed that measuring the uncarboxylated fractions of vitamin K–dependent proteins can indicate vitamin K deficiency. In support of this, vitamin K_2 supplements were able to reduce dephosphorylated-uncarboxylated MGP (139). This raises the possibility of a therapy to prevent vascular calcification. Several trials are currently being conducted to evaluate the effectiveness of vitamin K supplements for reducing vascular calcification. Patients who do not eat (and hence do not ingest foods containing vitamin K) and who are receiving antibiotics that suppress intestinal bacteria for extended periods of time may be at particular risk for vitamin K deficiency (140).

Serum total vitamin A, retinol binding protein (RBP), RBP-bound vitamin A, and free vitamin A are increased in CKD patients (141). Moreover, even relatively small supplements of vitamin A, that is, 7,500 to 15,000 IU/d [about 2,250 to 4,500 μg retinal equivalents (RE) per day], appear to cause bone toxicity and hypercalcemia in some CKD patients (142). On the other hand, Espe et al. (143) found that the lower quartiles of plasma retinol and RBP4 were associated with increased risk of sudden death, infection-related mortality, and overall mortality. It is noteworthy that the lower quartile of plasma retinol remained above the normal range for plasma retinol. One possible interpretation is that the lower retinol level is a marker of inflammation. In dialysis patients, plasma vitamin A levels are elevated, and vitamin A deficiency is rarely observed.

Moreover, even small vitamin A supplements (7,500 to 15,000 IU; i.e., 2,250 to 4,500 μg of RE) may cause vitamin A toxicity. Hence, there is a consensus that supplemental doses of vitamin A larger than the RDA for vitamin A in normal healthy adults (i.e., 700 to 900 μg of RE) should not be given (**TABLE 27.5**).

Normal, low, and increased plasma or red cell vitamin E (α-tocopherol) levels have been described in nondialyzed MHD and CPD patients (119,120). Several studies indicate that administration of 1,200 IU of vitamin E (all-racemic α-tocopherol acetate) to MHD patients may decrease oxidative stress induced by 100 mg of iron sucrose, and this antioxidant effect may be enhanced with the use of a combination of vitamins E and C (144). In the Secondary Prevention with Antioxidants of Cardiovascular Disease (SPACE) study of MHD patients with preexisting cardiovascular disease, treatment with vitamin E (α-tocopherol), 800 IU/d, is reported to significantly reduce [relative risk (RR) = 0.46] the primary composite end point (fatal and nonfatal myocardial infarction, ischemic stroke, peripheral vascular disease, and unstable angina) (145). This trial has never been confirmed. The Heart Outcomes Prevention Evaluation (HOPE) trial did not find a reduction in cancer and cardiovascular events with vitamin E supplements in patients with diabetes mellitus or a history of adverse cardiovascular events (146). When the duration of this trial was extended (HOPE-TOO trial), these initial results were confirmed; unexpectedly in the HOPE-TOO trial, an increased risk of heart failure was observed in the patients receiving vitamin E supplements. It has been suggested that vitamin E–coated dialyzer membranes might reduce oxidative stress during MHD treatment. Most clinical trials with these membranes reported an increase in plasma or red blood cell (RBC) vitamin E levels. However, currently, no trial has clearly shown improvement in important clinical outcomes with the use of these membranes (147). More research will be necessary before the routine use of daily vitamin E supplements or vitamin E–coated dialyzer membranes can be recommended for MD patients (**TABLE 27.3**).

Since a low intake of several vitamins from foods is common in patients with kidney disease, many reports continue to show that substantial numbers of patients with kidney disease not taking supplements show evidence for vitamin deficiencies. Because water-soluble vitamin supplements are generally safe, it would seem wise to use these supplements routinely (119,120). The Dialysis Outcomes and Practice Study (DOPPS) report showed a survival advantage in MD patients who were vitamin-supplemented. Analysis of the composition of the supplements, which was available only for the U.S. patients, indicated that vitamins C, B_6 and B_{12}, and folate were present in all of the multivitamin preparations used. However, it was not possible to determine the contribution of each of these vitamins to the greater survival of these patients. Recommended nutritional intakes for vitamins are shown in **TABLE 27.5**. Recommendations for vitamin D intake are given in Chapter 24.

Homocysteine

Increased plasma homocysteine is a risk factor for adverse cardiovascular events in the general population (148), and plasma homocysteine is increased in about 90% to 95% of MHD and CPD patients (15,148). Epidemiologic studies in large numbers of MHD patients indicate that a high plasma homocysteine may indicate a better prognosis, because malnutrition and/or inflammation may lower plasma homocysteine levels (149). Homocysteine is an intermediary product of sulfur amino acid metabolism. Plasma homocysteine levels are not affected by membrane flux, and dialysis treatment is not sufficiently effective to normalize plasma homocysteine levels. Three vitamins, vitamins B_6, B_{12}, and folate, are directly involved in its synthesis and metabolism. The Homocysteinemia in Kidney and End Stage Renal Disease (HOST) study indicated that megavitamin therapy that lowers hyperhomocysteinemia in advanced CKD and MHD patients is not associated with reduced cardiovascular events (150). Heinz et al. (151) reported similar findings in another randomized controlled study of vitamin therapy in ESKD patients.

Alkalinization

A high serum anion gap is associated with greater survival in MHD patients (152). This relation is considered to be due to greater appetite and protein intake, which are signs of health in patients but also lead to higher anion gaps (20,152,153). After adjustment for measures indicating protein intake, PEM, or inflammation, it turns out that individuals with lower serum anion gaps (i.e., who are less acidotic) have greater survival (20,153–155). Since the level of acidemia at which amino acid or protein loss or bone reabsorption is stimulated is not well defined, it would seem prudent to prevent any degree of chronic acidemia. Indeed, evidence indicates that CPD patients are more anabolic or less catabolic when their arterial blood pH is 7.42 to 7.45 as compared to 7.35 to 7.38 (25). Also, in nondialyzed CKD patients, both observational studies and randomized controlled clinical trials indicate that when serum bicarbonate is about ≤24 mmol/L, the rate of loss of GFR appears to be more rapid (156–159). Two National Kidney Foundation K/DOQI Practice Guidelines recommend that the serum bicarbonate should be measured once monthly in MHD and CPD patients and that the predialysis or stabilized serum bicarbonate should be maintained at or greater than 22 mmol/L in these individuals (40,160). Because of the above-mentioned potential advantages of completely eradicating acidemia and the safety of giving bicarbonate, the authors believe that these KDOQI guidelines are no longer acceptable. A normal serum bicarbonate (i.e., about 25 mEq/L) is now recommended. In nondialyzed CKD patients, urine also should be continuously maintained alkaline (urine pH >7.0) to slow progression of kidney failure. Alkali therapy probably should be initiated if the arterial blood pH is less than approximately 7.38 regardless of the serum bicarbonate level. Sodium bicarbonate tablets, Shohl's solution, or Bicitra (citric acid and sodium citrate, 1.0 mEq of alkali per milliliter of solution) may be given. For most nondialyzed CKD patients, a dose of about 1 mEq alkali/kg/d, split into at least two doses per day, will usually ensure that there is no acidemia and an alkaline urine. MD patients with large protein intakes or who have a large residual GFR and excrete substantial urinary bicarbonate may also need alkali supplements. MHD patients are often alkalemic immediately postdialysis; if they become acidemic before their next dialysis, they may need to take alkali starting 1 or 2 days postdialysis but excluding the hemodialysis day.

Fiber

In normal individuals, a high dietary fiber intake may lower the incidence of constipation, irritable bowel syndrome, diverticulitis, and neoplasia of the colon and possibly, improve glucose tolerance (161,162). It seems reasonable that the benefits of a high dietary fiber intake in normal people would also occur in MD patients. A high dietary fiber intake of 20 to 30 g/d is therefore recommended.

PRIORITIZING DIETARY GOALS

Since the number and magnitude of the changes in the dietary intake for MD patients are rather numerous, some patients could become discouraged if these recommendations were all presented to the patient at once; the patient could become demoralized and lose his motivation to comply with the diet. We therefore prioritize goals for dietary treatment. Usually, we emphasize the importance of controlling the protein, phosphorus, sodium, potassium, water, energy, and magnesium intake and the need to take vitamin supplements. Statins or fibric acid derivatives are usually better tolerated than dietary modifications, and prescription of these medicines, if lipid disorders are apparent, may enable patients to initially focus on other pressing aspects of dietary modification. If the patient has complied well with the more critical elements of dietary therapy, has a specific lipid disorder that may benefit from dietary therapy, or has expressed an interest in modifying fat, carbohydrate, or fiber intake, then the modifications of the dietary intake of these latter nutrients are explored more intensively with the patient.

ADJUSTED EDEMA-FREE BODY WEIGHT

Many recommended nutrient intakes are given in terms of the patient's body weight. Since MD patients often are underweight, obese, and/or overhydrated or frankly edematous, the NKF practice guidelines issued the following statement (40): "The body weight to be used for assessing or prescribing protein or energy intake is the aBW_{ef} [sic, adjusted edema-free body weight]. For MHD patients, this should be obtained postdialysis. For CPD patients, this should be obtained after drainage of dialysate." The adjusted edema-free body weight (aBW_{ef}) should be used for MD patients, who have an edema-free body weight that is less than 95% or greater than 115% of the median standard weight, as determined from the National Health and Nutrition Evaluation Survey II (NHANES II) data. For individuals with an edema-free body weight between 95% and 115% of the median standard weight, the actual edema-free body weight may be used. The guideline goes on to state, "For DXA measurements of total body fat and fat-free mass, the actual edema-free body weight obtained at the time of the DXA measurement should be used. For anthropometric calculations, the postdialysis (for MHD) or postdrain (for CPD) actual edema-free body weight should be used." Clinical judgment and, if desired, body composition measurements can be used to estimate the magnitude of the edema, if any. The aBW_{ef} may be calculated as follows (**Equation 27.3**) (40):

$$aBW_{ef} = BW_{ef} + [(SBW - BW_{ef}) \times 0.25] \qquad (27.3)$$

where aBW_{ef} is the actual edema-free body weight and SBW is the standard body weight as determined from the NHANES II data (163). If possible, the BW_{ef} should be measured after the patient has fasted for at least 8 hours. The NHANES II weights are used for SBW because Americans as a group were less fat at the time that the NHANES II data were collected than they are today.

ORAL AND ENTERAL NUTRITION

Provision of increased nutrients to chronic dialysis patients with PEW who are not eating well is best accomplished by nutritional counseling, oral nutritional supplements, or, if these maneuvers fail, enteral nutrition. In general, feeding by the gastrointestinal tract is safer, maintains the gastrointestinal tract in a healthier state, and is less expensive than parenteral nutrition (164). Intensive nutritional counseling may improve nutritional status in some chronic dialysis patients (165). When nutritional counseling is not sufficient, supplements may be tried. A number of clinical trials, usually rather small in sample size and often without randomized prospective controls, indicate that oral or enteral nutrition often improves nutritional or protein-energy status in CKD or MD patients with PEW (166,167). Some studies have examined oral nutritional supplements during the dialysis procedure. Giving nutritional supplements in this manner may increase adherence to the nutritional prescription and mitigate the marked disruption in extracellular and intracellular amino acid pools that occurs when patients undergo hemodialysis in the fasting state. Protein anabolism also increases acutely when patients receive oral nutrition containing protein during hemodialysis (168). A longer term randomized, prospective controlled clinical trial of routine feeding of a nutritional supplement during the hemodialysis procedure describes improvement in nutritional status (169). This nutritional supplement also contained compounds considered to be anti-inflammatory and antioxidant and measures of inflammation and oxidant stress also decreased in the patients who received this supplement. A retrospective analysis of a large cohort of MHD patients indicated that intradialytic provision of oral nutritional supplements in MHD patients with PEW is associated with increased survival (30). Some nephrologists are reluctant to allow feeding during hemodialysis because feeding may cause changes in hemodynamics that may promote hypotension during hemodialysis (170). Our experience indicates that intradialytic hypotension or nausea and vomiting are not common complications associated with intradialytic feeding. Possibly, feeding during hemodialysis should not be offered to patients with a history of intradialytic hemodynamic instability. Many patients tire of taking nutritional supplements, and after about 3 to 4 months, adherence rates to such supplements often decrease. One possible solution to this dilemma is to prescribe the nutritional supplements to be given in the hemodialysis unit by the nurses, like a medicinal prescription (171). Another possibility is to use enteral tube feeding, which in the opinion of the authors is an underused therapy. Finally, there is the option of IDPN, nutrition through dialysate, or, in extreme cases, total parenteral nutrition.

◆ INTRADIALYTIC PARENTERAL NUTRITION

For patients who have marginally adequate intakes and who will not ingest more nutrients through foods or food supplements or take enteral tube feedings (166), supplemental amino acids, glucose, and lipids may be infused intravenously during hemodialysis treatment (i.e., IDPN) (28,29,172,173). The preparation is infused into the blood leaving the dialyzer to reduce dialysate losses of amino acids and glucose.

Evidence does not clearly show that IDPN is beneficial or that patients may not receive similar advantages from oral supplements or tube feeding (28,29,172,173). Large-scale prospective, randomized controlled appropriately performed clinical trials that test the clinical value or indications for use of IDPN have not been performed. Studies describe acute increases in total body and muscle protein synthesis and positive-energy balance during IDPN (174). However, protein anabolism also increased acutely if patients received oral nutrition during hemodialysis (175). Improved serum albumin and edema-free body mass have been described in a number of studies, which often involved small numbers of patients, no randomized control group, or no strict control or monitoring of oral nutrient intake (172,176,177). Exercise on a stationary bicycle during hemodialysis in patients receiving IDPN promotes more positive protein balance (178). Reference is made to a recently published detailed review of IDPN (173).

A case control retrospective study (28) and a nonrandomized retrospective report (29) provide suggestive data that IDPN increases survival in malnourished MHD patients. In the case control study, those patients with a serum albumin of 3.3 g/dL or lower who were given IDPN had greater survival than those who were not (28). In the retrospective comparison of nonrandomized MHD patients, those individuals who received IDPN had a reduced mortality rate (29). The French Intradialytic Nutrition Evaluation (FINE) Study involved 186 MHD patients with PEW who received an oral nutritional supplement for 1 year that provided approximately 5.8 kcal/kg/d and 0.38 g protein/kg/d. During this same time, patients were randomized to receive IDPN or no IDPN with each hemodialysis (179). The recommended IDPN was designed to bring the total intake (oral plus intravenous) 30 to 35 kcal/kg/d and 1.2 g/protein/kg/d. The patients randomized to receive IDPN, in comparison to those not receiving IDPN, did not show, over 2 years, improved mortality or hospitalization rates, or reduced evidence for PEW. This lack of beneficial nutritional effect from IDPN may have been due to the fact that almost all IDPN-treated and control patients received an oral nutritional supplement as well (179).

TABLE 27.6 summarizes the potential advantages and limitations of IDPN. Some reports concerning indications for IDPN emphasize that IDPN is only indicated for malnourished MHD patients who ingest inadequate nutrients and for whom counseling, food supplements, and enteral tube feeding are not helpful or are contraindicated (173,180). IDPN is probably of value only for clinically stable or only modestly inflamed MHD patients who have a slightly or moderately suboptimal intake of nutrients (i.e., perhaps 60% to 80% or greater of the patient's recommended daily intake). This technique is probably inadequate for severely ill MHD patients because their oral or enteral intake is usually very low, their nutrient needs are high, and the nutritional supplements can be given only intermittently, when the patient undergoes hemodialysis. Of course, if the patient is hospitalized and receiving continuous venovenous hemodialysis or daily hemodialysis—particularly if the daily hemodialysis extends for more than 4 hours each day, then intravenous nutrition can provide all of the patient's nutritional needs and can be completely substituted for oral or enteral feeding.

Since most patients who need IDPN do ingest energy sources and protein/amino acids, but in suboptimal amounts, we generally give about 40 to 42 g of essential and nonessential amino acids and 200 g of D-glucose (150 g of D-glucose if the dialysate contains glucose) and usually 250 mL of a 10% or 20% lipid solution (i.e., 25 to 50 g of fat). The nutrients are administered at a constant rate throughout the dialysis procedure to minimize the decrease in plasma glucose that occurs with the use of glucose-free hemodialysate and the fall in amino acid pools in the body that normally occur with a hemodialysis treatment. In the authors' experience, about 85% to 90% of the amino acids and a large proportion of the glucose infused during hemodialysis are retained; the amino acid losses in dialysate rise by an average of only 4 to 5 g (181). The nutrients may be utilized more efficiently because they are given continuously rather than as a bolus.

Patients who have low serum concentrations of potassium or phosphorus at the start of the dialysis treatment may need supplements of these minerals during the amino acid and glucose infusions to prevent worsening of hypokalemia or hypophosphatemia due to both intracellular movement as well as dialysis losses of these minerals. If the dialysate is glucose-free, the infusion is not stopped until the end of the hemodialysis session to prevent hypoglycemia.

TABLE 27.6	Advantages and Disadvantages of Intradialytic Parenteral Nutrition

Advantages

1. IDPN can be provided with each dialysis session (usually thrice weekly) through the blood tubing without the need for additional venipuncture or placement of a central catheter.

2. It provides nutritional support to patients independent of anorexia, appetite, willingness or ability to cooperate, gastrointestinal function or disease states.

3. All needed nutrients can be provided through IDPN in contrast to nutrition provided through the dialysate.

4. The quantity and nutrient composition of the nutritional intake can be regulated.

5. Excess fluid and minerals and metabolic products can be removed during the course of dialysis; therefore, undesirable positive fluid or mineral balance and probably increased accrual of potentially toxic metabolites can be prevented.

6. It is a convenient way to provide supplemental nutrition with little or no effort by the patient and does not interfere with the patient's daily activities.

Disadvantages

1. The nutritional intake is given only during hemodialysis, which typically is provided for 3–4 h thrice weekly or ~12 h/wk; therefore, IDPN is not very effective as the sole source of nutrition.

2. Nutrients given intravenously are cleared very rapidly from blood.

3. The short intense duration of intravenous feeding by IDPN is unphysiologic because normal nutrient-gut interactions are lacking and also because adult humans eating three or four meals daily spend most of their lives in the postprandial state, in contrast to the short intense duration of intravenous nourishment by IDPN.

4. It often is expensive, although theoretically it does not have to be.

5. It requires time and effort from the nursing staff.

6. Microbial contamination with ensuing infection in the patient can occur.

7. There is a risk of reactive hypoglycemia, particularly if patients are infused with large quantities of D-glucose over a short period of time.

8. Oral nutritional supplements, if tolerated, appear to be just as effective as a nutritional source (179).

IDPN, intradialytic parenteral nutrition.
This table is reproduced, with modifications. (Dukkipati R, Kalantar-Zadeh K, Kopple JD. Is there a role for intradialytic parenteral nutrition? A review of the evidence. *Am J Kidney Dis* 2010;55(2):352–364. Courtesy of the editor.)

Also, the patient may eat a source of carbohydrates 20 to 30 minutes before the end of the IDPN infusion if there is any concern that the patient may develop reactive hypoglycemia. The infusion may be tapered or a peripheral infusion of glucose started to avoid hypoglycemia. Since lipids have been added to the IDPN solutions and the glucose dose from IDPN has been correspondingly reduced, the risk of developing postinfusion hypoglycemia appears to be reduced.

Nutritional Hemodialysis and Nutritional Peritoneal Dialysis

Amino acids may be added to the dialysate of patients undergoing CPD or MHD (182,183). With hemodialysis, additional glucose also may be added. The nutrients diffuse into the body during dialysis. These techniques have the potential advantages of consolidating nutritional and dialysis treatment into one procedure, reducing the risk of fluid and electrolyte disturbances from intravenous nutrition, and decreasing the considerable costs of intravenous feeding. When the nutrients are added to the hemodialysate, some investigators have reduced the dialysis flow rate to increase the fractional extraction of amino acids and glucose from dialysate. This has the benefit of reducing the cost of the nutrients given to the patient, but it also decreases the efficiency of dialysis; hence, these patients may require more hours of dialysis therapy, which raises nursing costs. Also, nutritional hemodialysis would have to be performed daily if it were the only or the main source of nutrition for a patient. Daily nutritional hemodialysis is probably only of benefit only for hospitalized patients, and it would have to be designed so that it was performed by intensive care unit personnel rather than by hemodialysis nurses in order to save costs. Under these conditions, it would be a variant of continuous venovenous hemodialysis (CVVHD).

Chazot et al. (5) added amino acids to hemodialysate during a standard hemodialysis using a cellulose triacetate hemodialyzer. When about 46 g of a mixture of 20 amino acids were added to the concentrate to provide a final dialysate amino acid concentration similar to fasting plasma levels, the amino acid losses into hemodialysate were prevented. When 139 g of these amino acids were added to the hemodialysate concentrate, there was a net transfer of about 39 g of amino acids from the dialysate to the patient during the hemodialysis.

Amino acids maybe added to peritoneal dialysate for protein-wasted CPD patients (182,183). By adding amino acids, the glucose load from the dialysate can be reduced. Also, for malnourished patients who are ingesting low-protein diets, the supplemental amino acids appear to increase protein synthesis, nitrogen balance, and serum levels of several proteins (182,183). In general, a mixture of both essential and nonessential amino acids are provided in about a 1.1% solution of standard peritoneal dialysate with the glucose contented deleted. One or two peritoneal dialysate exchanges of this solution are substituted each day for the patient's usual exchanges. Dwell times should last about 4 to 6 hours to ensure an uptake of about 80% of the total dialysate amino acid content and to prevent excessive reabsorption of other compounds in dialysate by an excessively long dwell time. It is to be emphasized that the calorie load from these solutions is very small. Hence, it is preferable that these exchanges are given during the major meals of the day. Again, it should be emphasized that dietary counseling and food supplements should be attempted and tube feeding should be considered before turning to these more expensive and incomplete nutritional supplements.

[*Note*: When the recommended nutrient intake is given in terms of body weight, the latter refers to standard body weight as determined from the NHANES data from 1976 to 1980 (40,163)].

REFERENCES

1. Mehrotra R, Kopple JD. Causes of protein-energy malnutrition in chronic renal failure. In: Kopple JD, Massry SG, eds. *Nutritional Management of Renal Disease*. Philadelphia, PA: Lippincott Williams & Wilkins, 2004:167–182.

2. Rocco MV, Paranandi L, Burrowes JD, et al. Nutritional status in the HEMO study cohort at baseline. *Am J Kidney Dis* 2002;39(2):245–256. doi:10.1053/ajkd.2002.30543.

3. Schulman G. Nutrition in daily hemodialysis. *Am J Kidney Dis* 2003;41(3 Suppl 1):S112–S115. doi:10.1053/ajkd.2003.50098.

4. Alp Ikizler T, Flakoll PJ, Parker RA, et al. Amino acid and albumin losses during hemodialysis. *Kidney Int* 1994;46(3):830–837. doi:10.1038/ki.1994.339.

5. Chazot C, Shahmir E, Matias B, et al. Dialytic nutrition: provision of amino acids in dialysate during hemodialysis. *Kidney Int* 1997;52(6):1663–1670. doi:10.1038/ki.1997.500.

6. Kopple JD, Blumenkrantz MJ, Jones MR, et al. Plasma amino acid levels and amino acid losses during continuous ambulatory peritoneal dialysis. *Am J Clin Nutr* 1982;36(3):395–402.

7. Blumenkrantz MJ, Gahl GM, Kopple JD, et al. Protein losses during peritoneal dialysis. *Kidney Int* 1981;19(4):593–602.

8. Wathen RL, Keshaviah P, Hommeyer P, et al. The metabolic effects of hemodialysis with and without glucose in the dialysate. *Am J Clin Nutr* 1978;31(10):1870–1875.

9. Gilmour ER, Hartley GH, Goodship THJ. Trace elements and vitamins in renal disease. In: Mitch WE, Klahr S, eds. *Nutrition and the Kidney.* Boston, MA: Little, Brown and Company, 1993:114–131.

10. Linton AL, Clark WF, Driedger AA, et al. Correctable factors contributing to the anemia of dialysis patients. *Nephron* 1977;19(2):95–98. doi:10.1159/000180871.

11. National Kidney Foundation. K/DOQI clinical practice guidelines for bone metabolism and disease in chronic kidney disease. *Clinic Rev Bone Miner Metab* 2007;5(1):53–67. doi:10.1007/bf02736671.

12. NKF-DOQI clinical practice guidelines for the treatment of anemia of chronic renal failure. National Kidney Foundation-Dialysis Outcomes Quality Initiative. *Am J Kidney Dis* 1997;30(4 Suppl 3):S192–S240.

13. Mahajan SK, Prasad AS, Lambujon J, et al. Improvement of uremic hypogeusia by zinc: a double-blind study. *Am J Clin Nutr* 1980;33: 1517–1521. doi:10.1097/00002480-197902500-00085.

14. Bellinghieri G, Savica V, Mallamace A, et al. Correlation between increased serum and tissue L-carnitine levels and improved muscle symptoms in hemodialyzed patients. *Am J Clin Nutr* 1983;38(4):523–531.

15. Kopple JD. Dietary considerations in patients with chronic renal failure, acute renal failure, and transplantation. In: Shrier RW, ed. *Diseases of the Kidney and Urinary Tract.* 8th ed. Philadelphia, PA: Lippincott Williams & Wilkins, 2006;2709–2764.

16. Fouque D, Kalantar-Zadeh K, Kopple J, et al. A proposed nomenclature and diagnostic criteria for protein–energy wasting in acute and chronic kidney disease. *Kidney Int* 2007;73(4):391–398. doi:10.1038/sj.ki.5002585.

17. Ikizler TA, Greene JH, Wingard RL, et al. Spontaneous dietary protein intake during progression of chronic renal failure. *J Am Soc Nephrol* 1995;6(5):1386–1391.

18. Kopple JD, Greene T, Chumlea WC, et al. Relationship between nutritional status and GFR: results from the MDRD Study. *Kidney Int* 2000;57(4):1688–1703. doi:10.1046/j.1523-1755.2000.00014.x.

19. Mehrotra R, Berman N, Alistwani A, et al. Improvement of nutritional status after initiation of maintenance hemodialysis. *Am J Kidney Dis* 2002;40(1):133–142. doi:10.1053/ajkd.2002.33922.

20. Kalantar-Zadeh K, Block G, McAllister CJ, et al. Appetite and inflammation, nutrition, anemia, and clinical outcome in hemodialysis patients. *Am J Clin Nutr* 2004;80(2):299–307.

21. Fouque D, Peng SC, Shamir E, et al. Recombinant human insulin-like growth factor-1 induces an anabolic response in malnourished CAPD patients. *Kidney Int* 2000;57(2):646–654. doi:10.1046/j.1523-1755.2000.057002646.x.

22. Kopple JD, Brunori G, Leiserowitz M, et al. Growth hormone induces anabolism in malnourished maintenance hemodialysis patients. *Nephrol Dial Transplant* 2005;20(5):952–958. doi:10.1093/ndt/gfh731.

23. Kopple J, Qing DP. Effect of L-carnitine on nitrogen balance in CAPD patients. *Journal J Am Soc Nephrol* 1999;10:264A.

24. Mitch WE, Medina R, Grieber S, et al. Metabolic acidosis stimulates muscle protein degradation by activating the adenosine triphosphate-dependent pathway involving ubiquitin and proteasomes. *J Clin Invest* 1994;93(5):2127–2133. doi:10.1172/jci117208.

25. Mehrotra R, Bross R, Wang H, et al. Effect of high-normal compared with low-normal arterial pH on protein balances in automated peritoneal dialysis patients. *Am J Clin Nutr* 2009;90(6):1532–1540. doi:10.3945/ajcn.2009.28285.

26. Chan M, Singh B, Cheema B, et al. Progressive resistance training and nutrition in renal failure. *J Ren Nutr* 2007;17(1):84–87. doi:10.1053/j.jrn.2006.10.014.

27. Kopple JD, Wang H, Casaburi R, et al. Exercise in maintenance hemodialysis patients induces transcriptional changes in genes favoring anabolic muscle. *J Am Soc Nephrol* 2007;18(11):2975–2986. doi:10.1681/ASN.2006070794.

28. Chertow GM, Ling J, Lew NL, et al. The association of intradialytic parenteral nutrition administration with survival in hemodialysis patients. *Am J Kidney Dis* 1994;24(6):912–920. doi:10.1016/s0272-6386(12)81060-2.

29. Capelli JP, Kushner H, Camiscioli TC, et al. Effect of intradialytic parenteral nutrition on mortality rates in end-stage renal disease care. *Am J Kidney Dis* 1994;23(6):808–816.

30. Lacson E Jr, Wang W, Zebrowski B, et al. Outcomes associated with intradialytic oral nutritional supplements in patients undergoing maintenance hemodialysis: a quality improvement report. *Am J Kidney Dis* 2012;60(4):591–600. doi:10.1053/j.ajkd.2012.04.019.

31. Kalantar-Zadeh K, Kopple JD, Humphreys MH, et al. Comparing outcome predictability of markers of malnutrition-inflammation complex syndrome in haemodialysis patients. *Nephrol Dial Transplant* 2004;19(6):1507–1519. doi:10.1093/ndt/gfh143.

32. Shinaberger CS, Kilpatrick RD, Regidor DL, et al. Longitudinal associations between dietary protein intake and survival in hemodialysis patients. *Am J Kidney Dis* 2006;48(1):37–49. doi:10.1053/j.ajkd.2006.03.049.

33. Avram MM, Mittman N, Bonomini L, et al. Markers for survival in dialysis: a seven year prospective study. *Am J Kidney Dis* 1995;26(1): 209–219. doi:10.1016/0272-6386(95)90176-0.

34. Iseki K, Uehara H, Nishime K, et al. Impact of the initial levels of laboratory variables on survival in chronic dialysis patients. *Am J Kidney Dis* 1996;28(4):541–548. doi:10.1016/s0272-6386(96)90465-5.

35. Churchill DN, Taylor DW, Cook RJ, et al. Canadian Hemodialysis Morbidity Study. *Am J Kidney Dis* 1992;19(3):214–234. doi:10.1016/s0272-6386(13)80002-9.

36. Blake PG, Sombolos K, Abraham G, et al. Lack of correlation between urea kinetic indices and clinical outcomes in CAPD patients. *Kidney Int* 1991;39(4):700–706. doi:10.1038/ki.1991.84.

37. Kopple JD. McCollum Award Lecture, 1996: protein-energy malnutrition in maintenance dialysis patients. *Am J Clin Nutr* 1997;65(5): 1544–1557.

38. Kopple JD. Nutritional status as a predictor of morbidity and mortality in maintenance dialysis patients. *ASAIO J* 1997;43(3):246–250. doi:10.1097/00002480-199743030-00026.

39. Chung SH, Lindholm B, Lee HB. Influence of initial nutritional status on continuous ambulatory peritoneal dialysis patient survival. *Perit Dial Int* 2000;20(1):19–26.

40. National Kidney Foundation K/DOQI clinical practice guidelines for nutrition in chronic renal failure. *Am J Kidney Dis* 2001;37(1 Suppl 2):S66–S70. doi:10.1053/ajkd.2001.20748.

41. Galland R, Traeger J. Short daily hemodialysis and nutritional status in patients with chronic renal failure. *Semin Dial* 2004;17(2):104–108. doi:10.1111/j.0894-0959.2004.17205.x.

42. Spanner E, Suri R, Heidenheim AP, et al. The impact of quotidian hemodialysis on nutrition. *Am J Kidney Dis* 2003;42(1 Suppl): 30–35.

43. Lindsay RM, Bergstrom J. Membrane biocompatibility and nutrition in maintenance haemodialysis patients. *Nephrol Dial Transplant* 1994; (9 Suppl 2):150–155.

44. Kopple JD, Wang H, Bross R, et al. Dietary protein requirements in maintenance hemodialysis patients. *J Am Soc Nephrol* 2006;17:725A.

45. Fouque D, Vennegoor M, Ter Wee P, et al. EBPG guideline on nutrition. *Nephrol Dial Transplant* 2007;22(Suppl 2):ii45–ii87. doi:10.1093/ndt/gfm020.

46. Blumenkrantz MJ, Kopple JD, Moran JK, et al. Metabolic balance studies and dietary protein requirements in patients undergoing continuous ambulatory peritoneal dialysis. *Kidney Int* 1982;21(6):849–861. doi:10.1038/ki.1982.109.

47. Westra WM, Kopple JD, Krediet RT, et al. Dietary protein requirements and dialysate protein losses in chronic peritoneal dialysis patients. *Perit Dial Int* 2007;27(2):192–195.

48. Nolph KD, Moore HL, Prowant B, et al. Continuous ambulatory peritoneal dialysis with a high flux membrane. *ASAIO J* 1993;39(4):904–909. doi:10.1097/00002480-199310000-00015.

49. Ahmed KR, Scognamillo B, Kopple JD. Relationship of peritoneal transport kinetics and nutritional status in chronic peritoneal dialysis patients. *Perit Dial Int* 1995;15:S5.

50. Lowrie EG, Lew NL. Death risk in hemodialysis patients: the predictive value of commonly measured variables and an evaluation of death rate differences between facilities. *Am J Kidney Dis* 1990;15(5):458–482. doi:10.1016/s0272-6386(12)70364-5.

51. Trumbo P, Schlicker S, Yates AA, et al. Dietary reference intakes for energy, carbohydrate, fiber, fat, fatty acids, cholesterol, protein and amino acids. *J Am Diet Assoc* 2002;102(11):1621–1630. doi:10.1016/s0002-8223(02)90346-9.

52. Livesey G. Energy and protein requirements the 1985 report of the 1981 Joint FAO/WHO/UNU Expert Consultation. *Nutr Bulletin* 1987;12(3):138–149. doi:10.1111/j.1467-3010.1987.tb00040.x.

53. Brunori G, Viola BF, Parrinello G, et al. Efficacy and safety of a very-low-protein diet when postponing dialysis in the elderly: a prospective randomized multicenter controlled study. *Am J Kidney Dis* 2007;49(5):569–580. doi:10.1053/j.ajkd.2007.02.278.

54. Duenhas M, Goncalves E, Dias M, et al. Reduction of morbidity related to emergency access to dialysis with very low protein diet supplemented with ketoacids (VLPD+KA). *Clin Neprol* 2013;79(5):387–393. doi:10.5414/CN107460.

55. Caria S, Cupisti A, Sau G, et al. The incremental treatment of ESRD: a low-protein diet combined with weekly hemodialysis may be beneficial for selected patients. *BMC Nephrol* 2014;15:172. doi:10.1186/1471-2369-15-172.

56. Jiang N, Qian J, Sun W, et al. Better preservation of residual renal function in peritoneal dialysis patients treated with a low-protein diet supplemented with keto acids: a prospective, randomized trial. *Nephrol Dial Transplant* 2009;24(8):2551–2558.

57. Dong J, Li YJ, Xu R, et al. Ketoacid supplementation partially improves metabolic parameters in patients on peritoneal dialysis. *Perit Dial Int* 2015;35(7):736–742. doi:10.3747/pdi.2014.00151.

58. Olevitch LR, Bowers BM, DeOreo PB. Measurement of resting energy expenditure via indirect calorimetry during adult hemodialysis treatment. *J Ren Nutr* 1994;4:192.

59. Wanner C. Altered lipid metabolism and serum lipids in renal disease and renal failure. In: Kopple JD, Massry SG, eds. *Nutritional Management of Renal Disease*. 2nd ed. Philadelphia, PA: Lippincott Williams & Wilkins, 2004:41.

60. Deighan CJ, Caslake MJ, McConnell M, et al. Atherogenic lipoprotein phenotype in end-stage renal failure: origin and extent of small dense low-density lipoprotein formation. *Am J Kidney Dis* 2000;35(5):852–862. doi:10.1016/s0272-6386(00)70255-1.

61. Slinin Y, Foley RN, Collins AJ. Calcium, phosphorus, parathyroid hormone, and cardiovascular disease in hemodialysis patients: the USRDS waves 1, 3, and 4 study. *J Am Soc Nephrol* 2005;16(6):1788–1793. doi:10.1681/ASN.2004040275.

62. Tentori F, Blayney MJ, Albert JM, et al. Mortality risk for dialysis patients with different levels of serum calcium, phosphorus, and PTH: the Dialysis Outcomes and Practice Patterns Study (DOPPS). *Am J Kidney Dis* 2008;52(3):519–530. doi:10.1053/j.ajkd.2008.03.020.

63. National Cholesterol Education Program. Executive summary of the third report of the National Cholesterol Education Program (NCEP) Expert Panel on Detection, Evaluation, and Treatment of High Blood Cholesterol in Adults (Adult Treatment Panel III). *JAMA* 2001;285(19):2486–2497. doi:10.1001/jama.285.19.2486.

64. LaRosa JC, Grundy SM, Waters DD, et al. Intensive lipid lowering with atorvastatin in patients with stable coronary disease. *N Engl J Med* 2005;352(14):1425–1435. doi:10.1056/nejmoa050461.

65. Bradberry JC, Hilleman DE. Overview of omega-3 fatty acid therapies. *P T* 2013;38(11):681–691.

66. Kidney Disease Outcomes Quality Initiative (K/DOQI) Group. K/DOQI clinical practice guidelines for management of dyslipidemias in patients with kidney disease. *Am J Kid Dis* 2003;41(4 Suppl 3):I–IV, S1–S91.

67. McCullough PA, Sandberg KR, Borzak S, et al. Benefits of aspirin and beta-blockade after myocardial infarction in patients with chronic kidney disease. *Am Heart J* 2002;144(2):226–232. doi:10.1067/mhj.2002.125513.

68. Berger AK, Duval S, Krumholz HM. Aspirin, beta-blocker and angiotensin-converting enzyme inhibitor therapy in patients with end-stage renal disease and an acute myocardial infarction. *J Am Coll Cardiol* 2003;42:201. doi:10.1016/j.accreview.2003.08.055.

69. Baigent C, Landray M, Leaper C, et al. First United Kingdom Heart and Renal Protection (UK-HARP-I) study: biochemical efficacy and safety of simvastatin and safety of low-dose aspirin in chronic kidney disease. *Am J Kidney Dis* 2005;45(3):473–484.

70. Gæde P, Vedel P, Larsen N, et al. Multifactorial intervention and cardiovascular disease in patients with type 2 diabetes. *N Engl J Med* 2003;348(5):383–393.

71. Loughrey CM, Young IS, Lightbody JH, et al. Oxidative stress in haemodialysis. *QJM* 1994;87(11):679–683.

72. Miyata T, Horie K, Ueda Y, et al. Advanced glycation and lipoxidation of the peritoneal membrane in peritoneal dialysis: respective roles of serum and peritoneal dialysis fluid reactive carbonyl compounds. *Kidney Int* 2000;58(1):425–435. doi:10.1046/j.1523-1755.2000.00182.x.

73. Burk RF, Brown DG, Seely RJ, et al. Influence of dietary and injected selenium on whole-body retention, route of excretion, and tissue retention of 75SeO32-in the rat. *J Nutr* 1972;102(8):1049–1055.

74. Guarnieri G, Toigo G, Crapesi L, et al. Carnitine metabolism in chronic renal failure. *Kidney Int Suppl* 1987;22:S116–S127.

75. Wanner C, Forstner-Wanner S, Schaeffer G, et al. Serum free carnitine, carnitine esters and lipids in patients on peritoneal dialysis and hemodialysis. *Am J Nephrol* 1986;6(3):206–211. doi:10.1159/000167119.

76. Shaldon S, Vienken J. The long forgotten salt factor and the benefits of using a 5-g-salt-restricted diet in all ESRD patients. *Nephrol Dial Transplant* 2008;23(7):2118–2120. doi:10.1093/ndt/gfn175.

77. Kalantar-Zadeh K, Kilpatrick RD, McAllister CJ, et al. Reverse epidemiology of hypertension and cardiovascular death in the hemodialysis population: the 58th Annual Fall Conference and Scientific Sessions. *Hypertension* 2005;45(4):811–817.

78. K/DOQI Workgroup. K/DOQI clinical practice guidelines for cardiovascular disease in dialysis patients. *Am J Kidney Dis* 2005;45(4 Suppl 3):S1–S153.

79. DeFronzo RA, Smith JD. Clinical disorders of hyperkalemia. In: Narins RG, ed. *Maxwell & Kleeman's Clinical Disorders of Fluid and Electrolyte Metabolism*. New York, NY: McGraw-Hill, 1994:697.

80. Kalantar-Zadeh K, Kuwae N, Regidor DL, et al. Survival predictability of time-varying indicators of bone disease in maintenance hemodialysis patients. *Kidney Int* 2006;70(4):771–780. doi:10.1038/sj.ki.5001514.

81. Cannata JB, Briggs JD, Junor BJR. Aluminium hydroxide intake: real risk of aluminium toxicity. *Br Med J* 1983;286(6382):1937–1938.

82. Slatopolsky EA, Burke SK, Dillon MA. RenaGel, a nonabsorbed calcium- and aluminum-free phosphate binder, lowers serum phosphorus and parathyroid hormone. *Kidney Int* 1999;55(1):299–307. doi:10.1046/j.1523-1755.1999.00240.x.

83. Al-Baaj F, Speake M, Hutchison AJ. Control of serum phosphate by oral lanthanum carbonate in patients undergoing haemodialysis and continuous ambulatory peritoneal dialysis in a short-term, placebo-controlled study. *Nephrol Dial Transplant* 2005;20(4):775–782. doi:10.1093/ndt/gfh693.

84. Floege J, Covic AC, Ketteler M, et al. Long-term effects of the iron-based phosphate binder, sucroferric oxyhydroxide, in dialysis patients. *Nephrol Dial Transplant* 2015;30(6):1037–1046. doi:10.1093/ndt/gfv006.

85. Van Buren PN, Lewis JB, Dwyer JP, et al. The phosphate binder ferric citrate and mineral metabolism and inflammatory markers in maintenance dialysis patients: results from prespecified analyses of a randomized clinical trial. *Am J Kidney Dis* 2015;66(3):479–488.

86. Pflanz S, Henderson IS, McElduff N, et al. Calcium acetate versus calcium carbonate as phosphate-binding agents in chronic haemodialysis. *Nephrol Dial Transplant* 1994;9(8):1121–1124.

87. Chertow GM, Burke SK, Dillon MA, et al. Long-term effects of sevelamer hydrochloride on the calcium x phosphate product and lipid profile of haemodialysis patients. *Nephrol Dial Transplant* 2000;15(4):2907–2914. doi:10.1093/oxfordjournals.ndt.a027950.

88. Perry CM, Plosker GL. Sevelamer carbonate: a review in hyperphosphataemia in adults with chronic kidney disease. *Drugs* 2014;74(7):771–792. doi:10.1007/s40265-014-0215-7.

89. Lacour B, Lucas A, Auchere D, et al. Chronic renal failure is associated with increased tissue deposition of lanthanum after 28-day oral administration. *Kidney Int* 2005;6 7(3):1062–1069. doi:10.1111/j.1523-1755.2005.00171.x.

90. Negri AL, Ureña Torres PA. Iron-based phosphate binders: do they offer advantages over currently available phosphate binders? *Clin Kidney J* 2015;8(2):161–167. doi:10.1093/ckj/sfu139.

91. Umanath K, Jalal DI, Greco BA, et al. Ferric citrate reduces intravenous iron and erythropoiesis-stimulating agent use in ESRD. *J Am Soc Nephrol* 2015;26(10):2578–2587. doi:10.1681/ASN.2014080842.

92. Akizawa T, Origasa H, Kameoka C, et al. Dose-finding study of bixalomer in patients with chronic kidney disease on hemodialysis with hyperphosphatemia: a double-blind, randomized, placebo-controlled and sevelamer hydrochloride-controlled open-label, parallel group study. *Ther Apher Dial* 2014;18(Suppl 2):24–32. doi:10.1111/1744-9987.12202.

93. Achinger SG, Ayus JC. The role of daily dialysis in the control of hyperphosphatemia. *Kidney Int Suppl* 2005;(95):S28–S32. doi:10.1111/j.1523-1755.2005.09504.x.

94. Cheng SC, Young DO, Huang Y, et al. A randomized, double-blind, placebo-controlled trial of niacinamide for reduction of phosphorus in hemodialysis patients. *Clin J Am Soc Nephrol* 2008;3(4):1131–1138. doi:10.2215/CJN.04211007.

95. Labonte ED, Carreras CW, Leadbetter MR, et al. Gastrointestinal inhibition of sodium-hydrogen exchanger 3 reduces phosphorus absorption and protects against vascular calcification in CKD. *J Am Soc Nephrol* 2015;26(5):1138–1149.

96. Goodman WG, Goldin J, Kuizon BD, et al. Coronary-artery calcification in young adults with end-stage renal disease who are undergoing dialysis. *N Engl J Med* 2000;342(20):1478–1483. doi:10.1056/nejm200005183422003.

97. Budoff MJ, Achenbach S, Berman DS, et al. Task force 13: training in advanced cardiovascular imaging (computed tomography) endorsed by the American Society of Nuclear Cardiology, Society of Atherosclerosis Imaging and Prevention, Society for Cardiovascular Angiography and Interventions, and Society of Cardiovascular Computed Tomography. *J Am Coll Cardiol* 2008;51(3):409–414.

98. Teng M, Wolf M, Lowrie E, et al. Survival of patients undergoing hemodialysis with paricalcitol or calcitriol therapy. *N Engl J Med* 2003;349(5):446–456.

99. Teng M. Activated injectable vitamin D and hemodialysis survival: a historical cohort study. *J Am Soc Nephrol* 2005;16(4):1115–1125.

100. Holick MF. Noncalcemic actions of 1,25-dihydroxyvitamin D3 and clinical applications. *Bone* 1995;17(2 Suppl):107S–111S. doi:10.1016/8756-3282(95)00195-j.

101. Owens DJ, Sharples AP, Polydorou I, et al. A systems based investigation into vitamin D and skeletal muscle repair, regeneration and hypertrophy. *Am J Physiol Endocrinol Metab* 2015;309(12):E1019–E1031. doi:10.1152/ajpendo 00375.2015.

102. Block GA, Martin KJ, de Francisco ALM, et al. Cinacalcet for secondary hyperparathyroidism in patients receiving hemodialysis. *N Engl J Med* 2004;350(15):1516–1525.

103. Sherrard DJ, Hercz G, Pei Y, et al. The spectrum of bone disease in end-stage renal failure—an evolving disorder. *Kidney Int* 1993;43(2):436–442.

104. Padovese P, Gallieni M, Brancaccio D, et al. Trace elements in dialysis fluids and assessment of the exposure of patients on regular hemodialysis, hemofiltration and continuous ambulatory peritoneal dialysis. *Nephron* 1992;61(4):442–448.

105. Van Renterghem D, Cornelis R, Vanholder R. Behaviour of 12 trace elements in serum of uremic patients on hemodiafiltration. *J Trace Elem Electrolytes Health Dis* 1992;6(3):169–174.

106. Krachler M, Scharfetter H, Wirnsberger GH. Exchange of alkali trace elements in hemodialysis patients: a comparison with Na(+) and K(+). *Nephron* 1999;83(3):226–236. doi:10.1159/000045515.

107. Manzler AD, Schreiner AW. Copper-induced acute hemolytic anemia. *Ann Intern Med* 1970;73(3):409. doi:10.7326/0003-4819-73-3-409.

108. Hosokawa S, Oyamaguchi A, Yoshida O. Trace elements and complications in patients undergoing chronic hemodialysis. *Nephron* 1990;55(4):375–379. doi:10.1159/000186003.

109. Sprenger KBG, Bundschu D, Lewis K, et al. Improvement of uremic neuropathy and hypogeusia by dialysate zinc supplementation: a double-blind study. *Kidney Int Supplement* 1983;16:S315–S318.

110. Lawson DH, Boddy K, King PC, et al. Iron metabolism in patients with chronic renal failure on regular dialysis treatment. *Clin Sci* 1971;41(4):345–351. doi:10.1042/cs0410345.

111. Macdougall IC. Strategies for iron supplementation: oral versus intravenous. *Kidney Int* 1999;69:S61–S66. doi:10.1046/j.1523-1755.1999.055suppl.69061.x.

112. von Bonsdorff M, Sipila R, Pitkanen E. Correction of haemodialysis-associated anaemia by deferoxamine. Effects on serum aluminum and iron overload. *Scand J Urol Nephrol Suppl* 1990;131:49–54.

113. Boelaert JR, de Locht M, Van Cutsem J, et al. Mucormycosis during deferoxamine therapy is a siderophore-mediated infection—*in vitro* and *in vivo* animal studies. *J Clin Invest* 1993;91(5):1979–1986. doi:10.1172/jci116419.

114. Nomura S, Osawa G, Karai M. Treatment of a patient with end-stage renal disease, severe iron overload and ascites by weekly phlebotomy combined with recombinant human erythropoietin. *Nephron* 1990;55(2):210–213. doi:10.1159/000185954.

115. Rudolph H, Alfrey AC, Smythe WR. Muscle and serum trace element profile in uremia. *Trans Am Soc Artif Intern Organs* 1973;19(1):456–461.

116. Rodger RS, Sheldon WL, Watson MJ, et al. Zinc deficiency and hyperprolactinemia are not reversible causes of sexual dysfunction in uremia. *Nephrol Dial Transplant* 1989;4(10):888–892.

117. Richard MJ, Arnaud J, Jurkovitz C, et al. Trace elements and lipid peroxidation abnormalities in patients with chronic renal failure. *Nephron* 1991;57(1):10–15. doi:10.1159/000186208.

118. Taccone-Gallucci M, Lubrano R, Del Principe D, et al. Platelet lipid peroxidation in haemodialysis patients: effects of vitamin E supplementation. *Nephrol Dial Transplant* 1989;4(11):975–978.

119. Chazot C, Kopple JD. Vitamin metabolism and requirements in renal disease and renal failure. In: Kopple JD, Massry SG, eds. *Nutritional Management of Renal Disease*. 2nd ed. Philadelphia, PA: Lippincott Williams & Wilkins, 2004:315.

120. Kalantar-Zadeh K, Kopple JD. Trace elements and vitamins in maintenance dialysis patients. *Adv Ren Replace Ther* 2003;10(3):170–182. doi:10.1053/j.arrt.2003.09.002.

121. Fehrman-Ekholm I, Lotsander A, Logan K, et al. Concentrations of vitamin C, vitamin B12 and folic acid in patients treated with hemodialysis and on-line hemodiafiltration or hemofiltration. *Scand J Urol Nephrol* 2008;42(1):74–80.

122. Zhang K, Liu L, Cheng X, et al. Low levels of vitamin C in dialysis patients is associated with decreased prealbumin and increased C-reactive protein. *BMC Nephrol* 2011;12:18.

123. Böhm V, Tiroke K, Schneider S, et al. Vitamin C status of patients with chronic renal failure, dialysis patients and patients after renal transplantation. *Int J Vitam Nutr Res* 1997;67(4):262–266.

124. Morena M, Cristol J-P, Bosc J-Y, et al. Convective and diffusive losses of vitamin C during haemodiafiltration session: a contributive factor to oxidative stress in haemodialysis patients. *Nephrol Dial Transplant* 2002;17:422–427.

125. Ihle BU, Gillies M. Scurvy and thrombocytopathy in a chronic hemodialysis patient. *Aust N Z J Med* 1983;13(5):523.

126. Raimann JG, Levin NW, Craig RG, et al. Is vitamin C intake too low in dialysis patients? *Semin Dial* 2013;26(1):1–5.

127. Canavese C, Petrarulo M, Massarenti P, et al. Long-term, low-dose, intravenous vitamin C leads to plasma calcium oxalate supersaturation in hemodialysis patients. *Am J Kidney Dis* 2005;45(3):540–549.

128. Corken M, Porter J. Is vitamin B(6) deficiency an under-recognized risk in patients receiving haemodialysis? A systematic review: 2000–2010. *Nephrology (Carlton)* 2011;16(7):619–625.

129. Tomson CRV, Channon SM, Parkinson IS, et al. Effect of pyridoxine supplementation on plasma oxalate concentrations in patients receiving dialysis. *Eur J Clin Invest* 1989;19(2):201–205.

130. Berns JS. Niacin and related compounds for treating hyperphosphatemia in dialysis patients. *Semin Dial* 2008;21(3):203–205.

131. Zazgornik J, Druml W, Balcke P, et al. Diminished serum folic acid levels in renal transplant recipients. *Clinical Nephrol* 1982;18(6):306–310.

132. Descombes E, Hanck AB, Fellay G. Water soluble vitamins in chronic hemodialysis patients and need for supplementation. *Kidney Int* 1993;43(6):1319–1328.

133. Heinz J, Domröse U, Westphal S, et al. Washout of water-soluble vitamins and of homocysteine during haemodialysis: effect of high-flux and low-flux dialyser membranes. *Nephrology (Carlton)* 2008;13(5):384–389.

134. Coveney N, Polkinghorne KR, Linehan L, et al. Water-soluble vitamin levels in extended hours hemodialysis. *Hemodial Int* 2011;15(1):30–38.

135. Hung SC, Hung SH, Tarng DC, et al. Thiamine deficiency and unexplained encephalopathy in hemodialysis and peritoneal dialysis patients. *Am J Kidney Dis* 2001;38(5):941–947.

136. Shanahan CM, Proudfoot D, Tyson KL, et al. Expression of mineralisation-regulating proteins in association with human vascular calcification. *Z Kardiol* 2000;89(Suppl 2):63–68.

137. Delanaye P, Krzesinski JM, Warling X, et al. Dephosphorylated -uncarboxylated Matrix Gla protein concentration is predictive of vitamin K status and is correlated with vascular calcification in a cohort of hemodialysis patients. *BMC Nephrol* 2014;15:145.

138. Mehta RL, Scott G, Sloand JA, et al. Skin necrosis associated with acquired protein C deficiency in patients with renal failure and calciphylaxis. *Am J Med* 1990;88(3):252–257.

139. Westenfeld R, Krueger T, Schlieper G, et al. Effect of vitamin K_2 supplementation on functional vitamin K deficiency in hemodialysis patients: a randomized trial. *Am J Kidney Dis* 2012;59(2):186–195.

140. Udall JA. Human sources and absorption of vitamin K in relation to anticoagulation stability. *JAMA* 1965;194(2):127–129.

141. Stein G, Schöne S, Geinitz D, et al. No tissue level abnormality of vitamin A of uremic patients. *Clin Nephrol* 1986;25(2):87–93.

142. Farrington K, Miller P, Varghese Z, et al. Vitamin A toxicity and hypercalcaemia in chronic renal failure. *Br Med J* 1981;282(6281):1999–2002. doi:10.1136/bmj.282.6281.1999.

143. Espe KM, Raila J, Henze A, et al. Impact of vitamin A on clinical outcomes in haemodialysis patients. *Nephrol Dial Transplant* 2011;26(12):4054–4061.

144. Winklhofer-Roob BM, Rock E, Ribalta J, et al. Effects of vitamin E and carotenoid status on oxidative stress in health and disease. Evidence obtained from human intervention studies. *Mol Aspects Med* 2003;24(6):391–402.

145. Boaz M, Smetana S, Weinstein T, et al. Secondary prevention with antioxidants of cardiovascular disease in endstage renal disease (SPACE): randomised placebo-controlled trial. *Lancet* 2000;356(9237):1213–1218.

146. Yusuf S, Dagenais G, Pogue J, et al. Vitamin E supplementation and cardiovascular events in high-risk patients. The Heart Outcomes Prevention Evaluation Study Investigators. *N Engl J Med* 2000;342(3):154–160. doi:10.1056/NEJM200001203420302.

147. Huang J, Yi B, Li AM, et al. Effects of vitamin E-coated dialysis membranes on anemia, nutrition and dyslipidemia status in hemodialysis patients: a meta-analysis. *Ren Fail* 2015;37(3):398–407.

148. Klusmann A, Ivens K, Schadewaldt P, et al. Is homocysteine a risk factor for coronary heart disease in patients with terminal renal failure? *Med Klin (Munich)* 2000;95(4):189–194.

149. Kalantar-Zadeh K, Block G, Humphreys MH, et al. A low, rather than a high, total plasma homocysteine is an indicator of poor outcome in hemodialysis patients. *J Am Soc Nephrol* 2004;52:S386–S7.

150. Jamison RL, Hartigan P, Kaufman JS, et al. Effect of homocysteine lowering on mortality and vascular disease in advanced chronic kidney disease and end-stage renal disease: a randomized controlled trial. *JAMA* 2007;298(10):1163–1170.

151. Heinz J, Kropf S, Domröse U, et al. B vitamins and the risk of total mortality and cardiovascular disease in end-stage renal disease: results of a randomized controlled trial. *Circulation* 2010;121(12):1432–1438. doi:10.1161/CIRCULATIONAHA.109.904672.

152. Lowrie EG, Zhu X, Lew NL. Primary associates of mortality among dialysis patients: trends and reassessment of Kt/V and urea reduction ratio as outcome-based measures of dialysis dose. *Am J Kidney Dis* 1998;32(6 Suppl 4):S16–S31.

153. Ravel VA, Molnar MZ, Streja E, et al. Low protein nitrogen appearance as a surrogate of low dietary protein intake is associated with higher all-cause mortality in maintenance hemodialysis patients. *J Nutr* 2013;143(7):1084–1092.

154. Wu DYJ, Kilpatrick RD, Dadres S, et al. Association between serum bicarbonate and death in hemodialysis patients: is it better to be acidotic or alkalotic? *Hemodial Int* 2005;9(1):87.

155. Kopple JD, Kalantar-Zadeh K, Mehrotra R. Risks of chronic metabolic acidosis in patients with chronic kidney disease. *Kidney Int* 2005;67:S21–S27.

156. Shah SN, Abramowitz M, Hostetter TH, et al. Serum bicarbonate levels and the progression of kidney disease: a cohort study. *Am J Kidney Dis* 2009;54(2):270–277.

157. de Brito-Ashurst I, Varagunam M, Raftery MJ, et al. Bicarbonate supplementation slows progression of CKD and improves nutritional status. *J Am Soc Nephrol* 2009;20(9):2075–2084.

158. Goraya N, Simoni J, Jo CH, et al. Treatment of metabolic acidosis in patients with stage 3 chronic kidney disease with fruits and vegetables or oral bicarbonate reduces urine angiotensinogen and preserves glomerular filtration rate. *Kidney Int* 2014;86(5):1031–1038.

159. Kraut JA. Effect of metabolic acidosis on progression of chronic kidney disease. *Am J Physiol Renal Physiol* 2011;300(4):F828–F829.

160. KDIGO 2012 clinical practice guideline for the evaluation and management of chronic kidney disease. *Kidney Int Suppl* 2013;3(1):1–150.

161. Chutkan R, Fahey G, Wright WL, et al. Viscous versus nonviscous soluble fiber supplements: mechanisms and evidence for fiber-specific health benefits. *J Am Acad Nurse Pract* 2012;24(8):476–487.

162. Otles S, Ozgoz S. Health effects of dietary fiber. *Acta Sci Pol Technol Aliment* 2014;13(2):191–202.

163. Frisancho AR. New standards of weight and body composition by frame size and height for assessment of nutritional status of adults and the elderly. *Am J Clin Nutr* 1984;40(4):808–819.

164. Kalantar-Zadeh K, Cano NJ, Budde K, et al. Diets and enteral supplements for improving outcomes in chronic kidney disease. *Nat Rev Nephrol* 2011;7(7):369–84.

165. Garagarza CA, Valente AT, Oliveira TS, et al. Effect of personalized nutritional counseling in maintenance hemodialysis patients. *Hemodial Int* 2015;19(3):412–418.

166. Stratton RJ, Bircher G, Fouque D, et al. Multinutrient oral supplements and tube feeding in maintenance dialysis: a systematic review and meta-analysis. *Am J Kidney Dis* 2005;46(3):387–405.

167. Ikizler TA, Cano NJ, Franch H, et al. Prevention and treatment of protein energy wasting in chronic kidney disease patients: a consensus statement by the International Society of Renal Nutrition and Metabolism. *Kidney Int* 2013;84(6):1096–1107.

168. Sundell MB, Cavanaugh KL, Wu P, et al. Oral protein supplementation alone improves anabolism in a dose-dependent manner in chronic hemodialysis patients. *J Ren Nutr* 2009;19(5):412–421.

169. Rattanasompattikul M, Molnar MZ, Lee ML, et al. Anti-Inflammatory and Anti-Oxidative Nutrition in Hypoalbuminemic Dialysis Patients (AIONID) study: results of the pilot-feasibility, double-blind, randomized, placebo-controlled trial. *J Cachexia Sarcopenia Muscle* 2013;4(4):247–257.

170. Barakat MM, Nawab ZM, Yu AW, et al. Hemodynamic effects of intradialytic food ingestion and the effects of caffeine. *J Am Soc Nephrol* 1993;3(11):1813–1818.

171. Kalantar-Zadeh K, Ikizler TA. Let them eat during dialysis: an overlooked opportunity to improve outcomes in maintenance hemodialysis patients. *J Ren Nutr* 2013;23(3):157–163.

172. Foulks CJ. An evidence-based evaluation of intradialytic parenteral nutrition. *Am J Kidney Dis* 1999;33(1):186–192.

173. Dukkipati R, Kalantar-Zadeh K, Kopple JD. Is there a role for intradialytic parenteral nutrition? A review of the evidence. *Am J Kidney Dis* 2010;55(2):352–364.

174. Pupim LB, Flakoll PJ, Brouillette JR, et al. Intradialytic parenteral nutrition improves protein and energy homeostasis in chronic hemodialysis patients. *J Clin Invest* 2002;110(4):483–492.

175. Caglar K, Fedje L, Dimmitt R, et al. Therapeutic effects of oral nutritional supplementation during hemodialysis. *Kidney Int* 2002;62(3):1054–1059.

176. Cherry N, Shalansky K. Efficacy of intradialytic parenteral nutrition in malnourished hemodialysis patients. *Am J Health Syst Pharm* 2002;59(18):1736–1741.

177. Blondin J, Ryan C. Nutritional status: a continuous quality improvement approach. *Am J Kidney Dis* 1999;33(1):198–202.

178. Pupim LB, Flakoll PJ, Levenhagen DK, et al. Exercise augments the acute anabolic effects of intradialytic parenteral nutrition in chronic hemodialysis patients. *Am J Physiol Endocrinol Metab* 2004;286(4):E589–E597.

179. Cano NJM, Fouque D, Roth H, et al. Intradialytic parenteral nutrition does not improve survival in malnourished hemodialysis patients: a 2-year multicenter, prospective, randomized study. *J Am Soc Nephrol* 2007;18(9):2583–2591.

180. Kopple JD, Foulks CJ, Piraino B, et al. Proposed health care financing administration guidelines for reimbursement of enteral and parenteral nutrition. *Am J Kidney Dis* 1995;26(6):995–997.

181. Wolfson M, Jones MR, Kopple JD. Amino acid losses during hemodialysis with infusion of amino acids and glucose. *Kidney Int* 1982;21(3):500–506.

182. Kopple JD, Bernard D, Messana J, et al. Treatment of malnourished CAPD patients with an amino acid based dialysate. *Kidney Int* 1995;47(4):1148–1157.

183. Jones MR, Gehr TW, Burkart JM, et al. Replacement of amino acid and protein losses with 1.1% amino acid peritoneal dialysis solution. *Perit Dial Int* 1998;18(2):210–216.

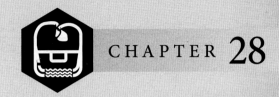

CHAPTER 28

Disorders of Hemostasis in Dialysis Patients

Federica Mescia, Miriam Galbusera, Paola Boccardo, and Giuseppe Remuzzi

The association between bleeding and kidney disease was first described by Morgagni (1) in 1794. The advent of modern dialysis techniques and the use of erythropoietin to correct anemia definitively reduced the incidence of severe hemorrhages, but bleeding diathesis still represents a relevant problem for uremic patients. For instance, among the control group of a clinical trial, 24% of hemodialysis patients experienced clinically significant bleeding over less than 1 year (2). Compared to the general population, patients with end-stage kidney disease (ESKD) have around a 10-fold greater risk of cerebral hemorrhage (3), subdural hematoma (4), and gastrointestinal bleeding (5). Surgery and invasive procedures, such as biopsies, pose additional hemorrhagic risks.

On the other hand, abnormalities in blood coagulation and fibrinolysis may predispose uremic patients to a hypercoagulable state rather than hemorrhage, and patients undergoing hemodialysis are exposed to thrombotic complications of vascular access.

PATHOGENESIS OF UREMIC BLEEDING

The causes of uremic bleeding have been the subject of a major debate since the 1970s. Most landmark studies in the field were indeed conducted in the 1970s to 1980s, when, in the early days of dialysis, hemorrhagic issues often posed major clinical challenges. In the following decades, widespread adoption of erythropoiesis-stimulating agents substantially reduced the clinical relevance of uremic bleeding. Nonetheless, a deep understanding of the hemostatic derangements in ESKD remains pivotal to provide optimal patient care. The pathogenesis of uremic bleeding is multifactorial, and the major defects involve primary hemostasis (**FIGURE 28.1**), that is, platelet–vessel wall and platelet–platelet interactions.

Platelet Abnormalities and Uremic Toxins

Moderate thrombocytopenia is commonly found in uremic patients, suggesting inadequate production or platelet overconsumption (6). Nonetheless, thrombocytopenia rarely is severe enough to cause bleeding. Numerous biochemical changes have been reported in platelets from ESKD patients. Dense granule content is altered in uremic platelets, with reduced levels of the aggregation agonists serotonin and adenosine diphosphate (ADP) (7). Granule secretion is defective too: Release of adenosine triphosphate (ATP) from dense granules (8) and of α-granule proteins, including β-thromboglobulin (9), are impaired. Calcium content is increased in platelets from uremic patients (10), and its mobilization in response to stimulation is abnormal (11), leading to functional defects. Anomalies in the platelet cytoskeleton contribute to defective hemostasis in chronic kidney disease (CKD): Cytoskeletal proteins are quantitatively reduced, and their assembly upon stimulation is qualitatively abnormal (12), hindering cellular contraction and motility. Platelets from uremic patients also display defects in two adhesion receptors, glycoprotein (Gp) Ib and the Gp IIb–IIIa complex. Gp Ib is fundamental for platelet adhesion to the subendothelium at high shear rates, like those found in the capillary circulation. Availability of Gp Ib on the platelet surface is decreased in CKD, likely because of enhanced proteolysis of the receptor (13). Platelet adhesion to subendothelial surfaces leads to activation of the Gp IIb–IIIa receptor complex, that in turn binds von Willebrand factor (vWF) and fibrinogen. The number of Gp IIb–IIIa receptors expressed on the platelet membrane of uremic patients is normal, but their function is impaired (14,15). This has been ascribed to competitive binding of the receptor by fibrinogen fragments and, possibly, other dialyzable toxic substances that accumulate in uremic plasma.

465

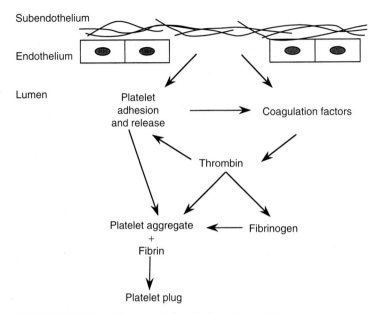

FIGURE 28.1 Schematic representation of primary hemostasis.

Arachidonic acid and prostaglandin metabolism is deregulated in uremia: A relative deficiency of the platelet agonist thromboxane A_2 and an excess of the potent platelet inhibitor and vasodilator prostacyclin are found, tipping the balance toward defective platelet function. Production of thromboxane A_2 by platelets in response to endogenous and exogenous stimuli is impaired (16,17). On the other hand, formation of prostacyclin is increased in uremic patients (18), and their plasma contains higher than normal amounts of a factor that stimulates vascular production of prostacyclin (19). Elevation in prostacyclin and pathologic hyperactivity of platelet adenylate cyclase (20) cooperate in increasing intracellular levels of cyclic adenosine monophosphate (cAMP) (21), which in turn contributes to impaired platelet function.

Nitric oxide (NO) is another key player in uremic bleeding (22,23) that interferes with hemostasis by inhibiting platelet aggregation and by preventing the vasoconstriction that normally follows vessel injury. Rats made uremic by extensive surgical ablation of kidney mass display bleeding time prolongation and elevated plasma levels of the stable NO metabolites nitrites and nitrates (24). In this animal model, increased expression of both inducible nitric oxide synthase (iNOS) and endothelial nitric oxide synthase (eNOS) is found in the aorta (24), consistently with enhanced vascular release of NO. Higher plasma levels of ʟ-arginine, the substrate for NO synthesis, have been documented in uremic patients, compared with healthy volunteers. Platelets taken from CKD patients generate more NO than control platelets (25), and uremic plasma, unlike plasma from controls, potently induces *in vitro* NO production in cultured human umbilical vein or microvascular endothelial cells (26). Increased NO synthesis is likely the main mechanism by which the uremic toxins guanidinosuccinic acid and methylguanidine interfere with platelet function (26). Cytokines such as tumor necrosis factor-α (TNF-α) and interleukin-1β (IL-1β), which rise in ESKD, are also potent inducers of iNOS (27).

After mixing with plasma from healthy subjects, uremic platelets show improvement of many functional parameters, while mixing of uremic plasma with normal platelets leads to platelet dysfunction. These findings highlight the key role of soluble plasma factors in determining platelet defects. The already cited elevation in prostacyclin, fibrinogen fragments, and inducers of NO synthesis, together with reduced thromboxane A_2 in uremia, partially account for these effects. The metabolites phenol, phenolic acid (28), and guanidinosuccinic acid (29) rise in CKD and impair platelet aggregation to ADP *in vitro*. Also, parathyroid hormone (PTH) has been consistently shown to inhibit platelets *in vitro* (30). Nonetheless, a clear correlation between skin bleeding time and the serum concentrations of these substances has not been demonstrated in ESKD patients (31,32). Other uremic retention solutes, like urea, creatinine, and guanidinoacetic acid, do not significantly interfere with platelet function when added to normal plasma (33).

Chronic volume overload in dialysis patients has been proposed to be an additional factor that increases bleeding risk, in particular of spontaneous subdural hematomas. The putative pathogenic mechanism entails venous hypertension, predisposing to small venous tears of dural bridging veins (4).

Anemia

Anemia is a common finding in ESKD patients and has a multifactorial origin, encompassing shortened survival of red blood cells in the uremic milieu, reduced responsiveness of the erythroid marrow induced by uremic toxins (34), repeated blood loss during dialysis, and, most importantly, defective secretion of erythropoietin. Anemia plays a key role in uremic bleeding, mainly through rheologic factors. At a low hematocrit, platelets tend to be dispersed along the blood vessels, which impairs their interaction with the vascular walls (35). At a hematocrit above 30% instead, erythrocytes mainly localize at the center of the vessels and platelets are displaced more peripherally, closer to the endothelial surface where their efficiency in forming a plug, in case of exposure of the subendothelium, is optimized. Erythrocytes also directly enhance platelet function by releasing platelet aggregation agonists ADP and thromboxane A_2, by inactivating prostacyclin, and by scavenging NO through hemoglobin (35).

Skin bleeding time is inversely correlated with hematocrit and significantly shortened after red blood cell transfusion (36,37).

Treatment with recombinant human erythropoietin also reduces bleeding time and increases hemostatic efficiency (38). In a randomized study, erythropoietin normalized the bleeding time in all uremic patients as hematocrits rose from 27% to 32% (39).

Effects of Dialysis

Dialysis has opposing effects on hemostasis. On the one hand, it allows removal of some of the uremic toxins that induce platelet dysfunction and hemostatic derangements. As a proof of concept, for example, skin bleeding time is significantly shortened, albeit rarely normalized, in uremic patients after the first dialysis sessions (40). However, dialysis cannot effectively remove all uremic retention solutes, especially those with high molecular weight or protein-bound, and only partially corrects uremia and the associated bleeding tendency (31).

Importantly, dialysis itself can increase bleeding risk, especially in the case of hemodialysis, where blood gets in contact with the extracorporeal circuit and systemic anticoagulation is usually required (41). In patients on chronic hemodialysis, skin bleeding time is often longer right after the dialysis session than before, an effect not attributable to heparin use (42). In spite of significant advances in biocompatibility with current hemodialysis technology, exposure of blood to the dialyzer membrane, to circuit tubing, to microbubbles in the circuit, and to shear stress, particularly in the roller pump segment, inevitably leads to a certain degree of activation of platelets, inflammatory cells, coagulation, and complement system. As well documented also in the setting of cardiopulmonary bypass, continual platelet activation can bring about mild thrombocytopenia and transient functional platelet exhaustion due to reiterated degranulation and loss of Gp receptors (41).

In the course of the hemodialysis session, hemostasis is modulated also by oscillations in the plasma levels of NO, which are the result of two opposing processes. Hemodialysis removes uremic toxins that stimulate NO synthesis and, at the same time, activates inflammation pathways in the extracorporeal circuit, raising the levels of potent NO inducers like the cytokines TNF-α and IL-lβ (25,43). In particular, NO induction has been attributed to complement-activating dialyzer membranes, acetate-containing dialysate, and dialysate contamination by intact endotoxin, endotoxin fragments, and other bacterial components that may cross the dialysis membranes. The current use of synthetic, more biocompatible, membranes, the widespread availability of bicarbonate dialysis, and the adoption of more and more stringent standards of dialysate purity could hopefully tip the balance toward a net reduction in NO during hemodialysis, thus improving hemostasis.

Administration of anticoagulants to avoid circuit clotting during hemodialysis is an additional factor that can increase bleeding risk. In particular, heparin, the drug most widely used for this purpose, is known to promote platelet self-aggregation and activation through nonimmunogenic mechanisms, which can exacerbate the functional alterations generated by the extracorporeal circulation.

From the standpoint of bleeding risk, peritoneal dialysis presents clear theoretical advantages over hemodialysis by avoiding the need of intradialytic anticoagulation and the exposure of blood to the extracorporeal circuit. Along the same line, epidemiologic studies have documented a lower incidence of gastrointestinal and intracranial bleeding in peritoneal dialysis, compared to hemodialysis patients (5,44).

Medications

Dialysis patients are often prescribed anticoagulant and antiplatelet agents due to their cardiovascular conditions or to preserve vascular access. Compared to the general population, these drugs put uremic patients at higher bleeding risk (45,46), exacerbating their hemorrhagic diathesis. Particular caution must be exercised prescribing drugs like low molecular weight heparins, which rely on a primarily kidney metabolism and tend to accumulate in ESKD (47). Bleeding risk due to bioaccumulation is significantly raised also with the new oral anticoagulants, targeting either thrombin (e.g., dabigatran) or factor Xa (e.g., apixaban), which are contraindicated in dialysis (48). The effects of aspirin on hemostasis are potentiated in the uremic milieu: In addition to the well-known irreversible blocking of platelet cyclooxygenase, aspirin also causes a cyclooxygenase-independent marked prolongation of the bleeding time in uremic patients but not in normal subjects (49). In addition, aspirin and the other nonsteroidal anti-inflammatory drugs directly hamper integrity of the gastrointestinal mucosa through inhibition of prostaglandin synthesis (50). This effect may be of particular relevance in dialysis patients, that are especially prone to gastrointestinal bleeding.

Other drugs that can contribute to uremic bleeding are β-lactam antibiotics. They accumulate in advanced kidney disease and may perturb platelet membrane, interfering with the ADP receptor and therefore inhibiting platelet aggregation (51). These effects are dose- and duration-dependent and resolve after drug discontinuation. Among the β-lactam antibiotics, third-generation cephalosporins may affect hemostasis the most, due to concomitant interference with intrahepatic vitamin K metabolism, in addition to platelet inhibition (52).

CLINICAL FINDINGS

The most common bleeding complications in uremia are petechial hemorrhages, blood blisters, and ecchymoses at the site of fistula puncture or temporary venous access insertion. Less frequent but more serious bleeding problems are discussed below.

Gastrointestinal Bleeding

The gastrointestinal tract is the most frequent site of major bleeding in ESKD patients (53). The sources of gastrointestinal hemorrhage are similar to those in patients with normal kidney function and include gastric and duodenal ulcers/erosions, vascular ectasias, esophagitis, gastritis, Mallory-Weiss tears, gastric cancer (54), hemorrhoids, colonic diverticular disease, and polyps (55).

Angiodysplasias (telangiectasias, arteriovenous malformations) are small vascular lesions of the gastrointestinal mucosa and submucosa that have been observed all along the digestive tract and may cause acute or subacute hemorrhage. They have been reported as a cause of bleeding more frequently in dialysis patients than in the general population (56). It is not clear whether this finding reflects a higher incidence of angiodysplasias in the setting of CKD and/or an increased risk for these lesions to bleed and thus to be diagnosed in uremic patients.

Ischemic colitis is another important differential diagnosis in dialysis patients with lower gastrointestinal bleeding, especially in those with widespread vascular disease and prone to intradialytic hypotension (57).

Alternative rare causes of digestive hemorrhage, like Kaposi's sarcoma, cytomegalovirus colitis, and non–Hodgkin's lymphoma, need to be considered in patients with concomitant severe immunodepression, such as those with HIV nephropathy or a history of long-term exposure to immunosuppressant drugs for kidney transplantation or immune-mediated systemic diseases (55).

Intracranial Hemorrhage

ESKD patients are more prone than the general population to intracranial bleedings, including subdural hematomas, intracerebral hemorrhages, and subarachnoid hemorrhages (4,58,59). Such events are often spontaneous, without recallable trauma, and are associated with higher mortality in dialysis patients. For instance, data from a large U.S. database showed that the incidence rate of subarachnoid hemorrhages was more than sixfold higher in patients on dialysis, who had a mortality of 38.4% versus 21.9% in the general population (59).

Brain magnetic resonance imaging (MRI) studies have also shown that small hemosiderin deposits, indicative of prior microscopic cerebral hemorrhage, are highly prevalent among hemodialysis patients. These alterations, known as cerebral microbleeds, are closely associated with other cerebral small-vessel diseases and likely contribute to cognitive dysfunction; age and high blood pressure are significant risk factors (60,61).

Hemorrhagic Pericarditis and Pleuritis

Limited, fibrinous pericardial and pleural effusions are common findings in patients with advanced kidney disease. Without adequate dialysis, serous effusion can undergo hemorrhagic transformation, leading to life-threatening uremic pericarditis, with possible tamponade (62), or pleuritis (63). These presentations used to be frequent in the predialysis era and are now rarely encountered. Nonetheless, they remain medical emergencies that require prompt recognition and treatment, the core of management being intensive, anticoagulant-free dialysis.

Other Hemorrhagic Presentations

Women on dialysis frequently present abnormal uterine bleedings, with a high prevalence of uncontrolled menorrhagia, contributing to symptomatic anemia (64). Kidney cysts are a common finding in dialysis-associated cystic kidney disease and occasionally give rise to unprovoked bleeding. Presentations range from asymptomatic, trivial intracystic hemorrhage to massive retroperitoneal hematomas (65).

Subcapsular liver hematoma is another serious hemorrhagic complication that has been rarely observed in uremic patients (66).

Notably, patients with CKD from autosomal dominant polycystic kidney disease may be at higher than average bleeding risk, due to predisposing anatomic abnormalities like kidney and liver cysts, an elevated frequency of colon diverticulosis and susceptibility to develop intracranial aneurysms (67).

Finally, in spite of the current improvements in standards of care, major surgery and invasive procedures still entail perioperative hemorrhagic risks that are more elevated in dialysis patients than in the general population, with subsequent higher morbidity and mortality rates (68).

⬡ LABORATORY ASSESSMENT OF THE BLEEDING RISK

The single assay that best correlates with uremic bleeding is skin bleeding time, an *in vivo* test that gives an overall assessment of primary hemostasis (69). Among the factors that influence skin bleeding time, there are platelet number and functionality, hematocrit,

vascular integrity, and activity of vWF. The skin bleeding time is most commonly determined using the Ivy method. A blood pressure cuff is applied above the cubital fossa and inflated at 40 mm Hg to elevate venous pressure and increase test sensitivity. A small cut is made on the ventral side of the subject's forearm, in an area where there are no hairs or visible veins. The cut is done quickly by an automatic device, which provides a standardized width and depth. The blood is blot away every 30 seconds by filter paper, until the platelet plug forms and the bleeding terminates. The time it takes for the bleeding to stop is measured and represents the skin bleeding time. Normal values are below 7 minutes; prolongation above 10 minutes correlates with a significantly increased risk of bleeding in uremic patients. The skin bleeding time was established as a predictor of hemorrhagic events in CKD patients in the 1970s and suffers from poor reproducibility and accuracy; nonetheless, it remains the best available test at present.

Several *in vitro* assays of platelet function have been developed, such as closure time test (also known as platelet function analyzer or PFA-100, that measures platelet aggregation in response to ADP and epinephrine), whole blood platelet aggregation (WBPA), thromboelastography (TEG), and cone platelet analyzer (CPA) (70). However, none of these tests has been validated in clinical practice in the setting of uremic bleeding, and their use remains investigational.

⬡ PREVENTION AND TREATMENT

We will focus on the following key points that should be systematically addressed in all dialysis patients in order to prevent bleeding and optimize treatment of active hemorrhage (TABLE 28.1): the dialysis prescription, correction of anemia, appropriateness of

TABLE 28.1	**Guidelines for the Prevention and Management of Hemorrhagic Complications of Uremia**

- For all patients with hemorrhagic complications or undergoing major surgery, the dialysis prescription should be carefully reviewed, ensuring adequacy and personalizing intradialytic anticoagulation.
- Correction of anemia by red blood cell transfusion and/or erythropoiesis-stimulating agents is the first key step in the prevention and treatment of uremic bleeding. The hematocrit should be kept above 30% in order to improve hemostasis.
- Indications for prescription of antiplatelet/anticoagulant agents in dialysis patients should be regularly reassessed, focusing on risk/benefit profile.
- Desmopressin acetate can be useful to improve hemostasis during acute bleeding episodes. It can be administered intravenously (0.3 μg/kg added to 50 mL of saline over 30 min), subcutaneously (0.3 μg/kg) or intranasally (3 μg/kg). The effect of desmopressin acetate has a fast onset but lasts only a few hours and loses efficacy after repeated administrations.
- Tranexamic acid can be used as a second-line agent in acute bleeding, paying attention to the risk of bioaccumulation in dialysis patients.
- Conjugated estrogens, given by intravenous infusion in a cumulative dose of 3 mg/kg as a daily divided dose (i.e., 0.6 mg/kg for 5 consecutive days), can help to achieve long-lasting hemostasis in case of persistent chronic bleeding.
- Because the favorable effect of cryoprecipitate on bleeding time has not been uniformly observed, we do not recommend its use.

concomitant antiplatelet/anticoagulant therapies, and use of specific agents to improve hemostasis.

In case of ongoing hemorrhage, first-line management is not specific for dialysis patients and includes hemodynamic support; identification of the hemorrhagic source and, possibly, subsequent treatment by surgical, endovascular, or endoscopic techniques. ESKD should be accounted for in the risk assessment of bleeding patients and in the subsequent planning of therapeutic interventions. For example, markedly higher rebleeding rates from endoscopically treated peptic ulcers have been documented in dialysis patients, even when these patients had low-risk ulcer stigmata on endoscopy (71). While awaiting more comprehensive data, it could thus be reasonable to manage all dialysis patients with peptic ulcer bleeding, and maybe other hemorrhagic disorders as well, as high-risk patients.

Dialysis Prescription

Adequate dialysis is a mainstay in the prevention of uremic bleeding. However, as already discussed, current dialysis technologies allow only partial correction of the bleeding diathesis associated with uremia, and hemodialysis in particular interferes with hemostasis. For these reasons, in the absence of other contraindications, peritoneal dialysis is a reasonable choice for patients at particularly high hemorrhagic risk.

In the hemodialysis prescription, intradialytic anticoagulation needs to be personalized, balancing individual thrombotic and hemorrhagic risks. The minimum dose of heparin effective in preventing circuit clotting should be determined for each patient. Reduced-intensity intradialytic anticoagulation is a sensible option in patients treated with oral anticoagulants: In many of such cases, even complete avoidance of intradialytic anticoagulation is feasible, provided that the international normalized ratio (INR) is within the target range, there is minimal inflammation, a native vascular access with adequate blood-flow rate is available, and synthetic high-flux membranes are used (72). As detailed elsewhere in this book, use of minimum-dose heparin or no-heparin hemodialysis is possible in patients at high bleeding risk or with ongoing hemorrhage, at the cost of increasing the possibilities of circuit clotting. Regional citrate anticoagulation is a valid alternative. In case of life-threatening bleeding, like intracranial hemorrhages, complete avoidance of anticoagulants is advised, usually for a period of at least 2 weeks.

Dialytic adequacy must be carefully considered, especially in patients presenting with uremic or dialysis-associated pericarditis. In this setting, it is mandatory to make a trial of intensive dialysis, usually defined, in the case of hemodialysis, as daily sessions for 10 to 15 days, preferably without heparin to minimize the risk of hemopericardium and cardiac tamponade (62).

In case central venous catheters are used as hemodialysis access, heparin lock is an often under recognized factor possibly concurring to bleeding risk. In fact, a certain degree of spillage of lock solution in the systemic circulation is practically inevitable, and if high-concentration heparin (5,000 to 10,000 U/mL) is employed, this can occasionally contribute to clinical bleeding. Use of 4% citrate or low-dose heparin (1,000 U/mL) is safe and effective alternative as lock solution (73,74).

Correction of Anemia

Management of anemia is pivotal in the prevention and treatment of uremic bleeding. Use of recombinant human erythropoietin has largely replaced transfusions and significantly lowered hemorrhagic risk. A randomized study established that a threshold hematocrit

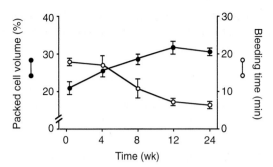

FIGURE 28.2 Effect of recombinant human erythropoietin therapy on packed cell volume and bleeding time in uremic patients.

between 27% and 32% effectively normalized bleeding time in uremic patients on erythropoietin (**FIGURE 28.2**) (39). Treatment of anemia likely improves hemostasis by displacing platelets from a midstream position toward the vessel wall, thus encouraging platelet–endothelium interactions. In addition, recombinant human erythropoietin affects hemostasis also independently of amelioration of anemia. For instance, it increases the number of reticulated platelets, which are more metabolically active (75), improves platelet calcium signaling (76), and enhances thrombin-induced phosphorylation of platelet proteins (77).

In case of ongoing hemorrhage, correction of anemia should be prompt, applying a lower transfusion trigger than in nonuremic patients, in order to steadily keep the hematocrit above 30%. Erythropoiesis-stimulating agents need a long time—at least 7 days—to significantly increase the red blood cell mass; nonetheless, it is reasonable to start their administration or increase dosing also in the acute setting, due to the direct effects on platelet activation and to limit the need for future transfusions.

Appropriateness of Concomitant Antiplatelet/ Anticoagulant Therapies

Dialysis patients frequently take antiplatelet and anticoagulant medications for primary or secondary cardiovascular prevention. These drugs often result in a relatively higher increase in bleeding risk in ESKD patients than in those with preserved kidney function. For instance, absolute risk of major bleeding in dialysis patients on warfarin ranged from 0.10 to 0.54 events per patient-year, which was 10 times higher than rates in the general population (46). Antiplatelet agents, especially when taken in combination, also significantly raise hemorrhagic risk in patients on hemodialysis. For example, major hemorrhage was noted in 7.6% of hemodialysis patients on a trial of aspirin and clopidogrel (2), compared with 3.7% of nonuremic patients enrolled in the Clopidogrel in Unstable Angina to Prevent Recurrent Events (CURE) trial, despite the use of the same two drugs (78).

To further complicate decision making, we must consider that the indications for antiplatelet and anticoagulant medications derive from clinical trials that excluded patients with advanced CKD. It is therefore unknown whether the risk/benefit profile demonstrated for these therapies in the general population can be reliably extrapolated to dialysis patients. For instance, based on retrospective case series, efficacy of warfarin to prevent stroke in dialysis patients with atrial fibrillation has not been consistently demonstrated, while increased hemorrhagic risk clearly emerged (79).

Anticoagulant/antiplatelet agents are frequently prescribed also for preservation of hemodialysis access patency, despite the lack of clinical studies demonstrating clear-cut evidence of benefit for this indication (46). Prescription appropriateness needs to be carefully evaluated on a case-by-case basis.

Ongoing bleeding should prompt assessment of the opportunity to discontinue any medication that interferes with hemostasis. Treatments to quickly reverse the effects of anticoagulant medications are available too, such as protamine for heparin and vitamin K, alone or in association with prothrombin complex concentrates, for warfarin.

Use of Specific Agents to Improve Hemostasis

In selected cases, it is possible to use medications that directly affect the hemostatic system and ameliorate uremic bleeding, like desmopressin acetate, cryoprecipitate, estrogens, or tranexamic acid.

Desmopressin and Cryoprecipitate

Even if quantitative or qualitative defects in vWF have not been consistently demonstrated in uremia, therapies that increase vWF plasma levels, such as desmopressin acetate and cryoprecipitate, improve platelet–vWF interaction and significantly shorten bleeding time in patients with advanced CKD.

Desmopressin acetate [1-deamino-8-D-arginine vasopressin (DDAVP)] is a synthetic derivative of the antidiuretic hormone with fewer vasopressor effects. It induces the release of autologous vWF from storage sites and may also increase platelet membrane Gp expression. In two randomized, double-blind, crossover trials in uremic patients, DDAVP was effective in shortening bleeding time at the dose of 0.3 μg/kg, administered either intravenously (added to 50 mL of saline over 30 minutes) or subcutaneously (80,81). Peak responses are achieved 1 hour after intravenous administration or 1.5 to 2 hours after subcutaneous dosing. The effect lasts 6 to 8 hours, and bleeding time subsequently returns to basal values. Desmopressin can also be given by the intranasal route, which is well tolerated and safe, at 10 to 20 times the intravenous dose (3 to 6 μg/kg) (82). Desmopressin loses its efficacy when repeatedly administered, probably due to a progressive depletion of vWF stores in endothelial cells (83). Adverse effects include mild to moderate decreases in platelet count, facial flushing, transient headache, nausea, abdominal cramps, and tachycardia. Thrombotic events following DDAVP administration have been rarely reported, particularly in patients with underlying advanced cardiovascular disease. Contraction of urinary volume and hyponatremia may also seldom occur if residual diuresis is present. Thanks to its rapid onset of action, DDAVP is commonly used as the first-line hemostatic agent in patients with active severe bleeding or those who are about to undergo surgery (84).

Cryoprecipitate is a transfusional product obtained when plasma is frozen and thawed, enriched with factor VIII/vWF multimers and fibrinogen. It shortens bleeding time, enhances resolution of hemorrhages in uremic patients, and reduces blood losses in ESKD patients undergoing major surgery (85). The effect of cryoprecipitate on bleeding time is detectable by 1 hour after infusion, maximal after 4 to 12 hours (on average 8 hours) and vanishes by 24 to 36 hours. The usual dose is 10 units given intravenously over 30 minutes. Cryoprecipitate has important drawbacks: As many as 50% of patients fail to respond to it, and being a blood product, it carries a minimum, yet not negligible, risk of transmission of infectious agents. Rare but severe reactions are possible, including anaphylaxis, pulmonary edema, and intravascular hemolysis. For these reasons, the use of cryoprecipitate for uremic bleeding has been largely abandoned.

Conjugated Estrogens

The anecdotal observation of reduced gastrointestinal bleeding in uremic patients treated with conjugated estrogens and of improved hemostasis in von Willebrand disease during pregnancy led to investigations of the effect of estrogens on the bleeding tendency in uremia (86,87). Estrogens mainly ameliorate uremic bleeding by decreasing the production of L-arginine, which is a precursor of NO. Although none of the studies in this specific setting have looked into the effects of estrogens on coagulation, it is plausible that the well-documented capacity of these hormones to decrease the levels of antithrombin III and protein S and to increase factor VII concentrations play a role as well.

The minimum dose of conjugated estrogens to reduce bleeding time is 0.6 mg/kg, administered intravenously over 30 to 40 minutes. Dosing is the same in women and men. Four or five daily infusions are needed to shorten bleeding time by at least 50% (88). The effect manifests only after several hours, becomes maximum over 5 to 7 days, and lasts up to 14 to 21 days. More data exist to support the use of intravenous estrogens, but the oral and transdermal routes have been shown to be effective as well. One oral dose of 25 mg of conjugated estrogens (Premarin) normalizes bleeding time for 3 to 10 days (88). Courses of 25 to 50 mg/day, for an average of 5 to 7 days, have been used with success in clinical studies (89). Low-dose transdermal estrogens (estradiol 50 to 100 μg/24 h), applied as a patch twice a week, effectively reduced bleeding time and lowered the risk of recurrent gastrointestinal bleeding (90). In all the clinical trials on estrogens in uremic bleeding, the hormones were administered only for a few days. With such short courses of treatment, no significant adverse effects were reported, other than hot flashes. The clinical use of estrogens in uremic bleeding is mainly reserved for selected cases where long-lasting effects are needed, for example, in the preparation of elective surgery at high hemorrhagic risk.

Tranexamic Acid

Tranexamic acid (TXA) is a potent inhibitor of the fibrinolytic system that stabilizes clots by preventing the binding of plasminogen to fibrin and the activation of plasminogen to plasmin. TXA rapidly decreases bleeding time in uremia (91). Case reports showed that TXA was effective in controlling chronic bleeding from colonic angiodysplasias (92) and spontaneous subdural and cerebral hematomas in dialysis patients (93). In a pilot study, adjunctive therapy with TXA effectively reduced rates of rebleeding in dialysis patients with major upper gastrointestinal hemorrhage. The dosage used was 20 mg intravenously, followed by 10 mg/kg/48 h orally for the next 4 weeks (94). TXA may accumulate in kidney insufficiency, and there is no evidence that it is more effective than desmopressin. Severe side effects, such as seizures (95) and visual impairment (96), have been linked to TXA overdose in dialysis patients. Intravenous TXA should therefore be considered only in the acute setting and as a second-line agent.

ABNORMALITIES OF COAGULATION AND FIBRINOLYSIS

Paradoxically, despite the hemorrhagic diathesis, uremic patients also run an increased risk of thrombosis, in particular thrombosis of the hemodialysis access and cardiovascular events.

PATHOGENESIS

Several prothrombotic alterations have been reported in uremia. Plasma levels of coagulation cascade proteins, like fibrinogen, factor VII, factor VIII (97), and tissue factor (98), rise in the setting of CKD. On the other hand, uremic patients display a downregulation in anticoagulant pathways, such as protein C activity (99) and antithrombin III activity (100). Contrasting results have been obtained regarding fibrinolysis. Seminal studies documented a decrease in fibrinolytic activity in uremia, concurring to the hypercoagulable state (101,102). Instead, later reports found evidence of enhanced activation of fibrinolysis in uremia, consistent with increases in plasmin–antiplasmin complexes and fibrinogen\fibrin degradation products, together with reduced plasminogen activator inhibitor activity (103). These findings probably reflect fibrinolytic responses secondary to fibrin deposition, taking place even if the overall fibrinolytic activity is depressed.

Chronic endothelial injury and activation (104), with subsequent loss of thromboresistance, contribute to the prothrombotic environment. CKD patients display increased plasma levels of markers of thrombosis, like thrombin–antithrombin III complex, D-dimer (105), activated factor XII, and activated factor VII (106). Activation of coagulation parallels the low-grade inflammation of uremia that is reflected, for instance, by the rise in C-reactive protein and interleukin-6 and the decrease in albumin levels (97,107). Inflammation in turn has been increasingly recognized as a key player in the pathogenesis of atherosclerosis and cardiovascular diseases, also independently of kidney insufficiency (108). Hyperhomocysteinemia, a common finding in dialysis patients, has also been associated with endothelial dysfunction and cardiovascular events (109,110).

In the case of vascular access thrombosis, local factors, such as surgical trauma, hemodynamic shear stress, and vessel wall injury, play a prominent pathogenetic role too (111).

Additional conditions that may further increase thrombotic risk in specific subsets of dialysis patients include nephrotic syndrome, heparin-induced thrombocytopenia type 2 (HIT-II), and antiphospholipid antibodies.

Nephrotic syndrome significantly raises the risk of deep venous thrombosis and renal vein thrombosis. The latter has been reported in as many as 37% of adult patients with membranous nephropathy, who are—for unknown reasons—the group of nephrotic subjects at highest risk of thrombotic complications. Some of the best defined pathophysiologic mechanisms of thrombophilia in nephrotic syndrome include urinary loss of antithrombin III and increased synthesis of fibrinogen and coagulation factors V and VIII by the liver (112).

HIT-II is an acquired prothrombotic state due to the formation of platelet-activating antibodies following exposure to heparin. Typical manifestations include thrombocytopenia, venous or arterial thrombosis, skin necrosis at heparin injection sites, and acute systemic reactions after an intravenous bolus of heparin. In spite of frequent exposure of hemodialysis patients to heparin, full-blown HIT-II syndrome is rare. On the other hand, HIT antibodies are frequently detected in ESKD patients; for example, they were documented in 8.1% of 1,450 patients exposed to unfractionated heparin and in 1.8% of 218 patients dialyzed with low molecular weight heparin (113). The clinical significance of these findings is unclear. Several studies have reported absence of clinical sequelae despite positive antibody tests (114–116). Other authors instead have proposed that isolated thrombocytopenia, frequent clotting of the extracorporeal circuit, and higher risk of vascular access thrombosis are putative manifestations of HIT-II peculiar to dialysis patients (117,118).

Like HIT-II antibodies, antiphospholipid antibodies can be frequently detected in hemodialysis patients but in most cases are not associated with the typical syndrome of recurrent arterial/venous thrombosis and pregnancy-related adverse events. Their clinical significance in the dialysis setting has not been clearly established. An increased risk of vascular access thrombosis has been reported (119) but has not been confirmed in all settings (120).

 CLINICAL FINDINGS AND TREATMENT

The most frequent thrombotic complications in dialysis patients are related to the vascular access and include thrombosis of native arteriovenous fistulae, arteriovenous grafts, and central venous catheters. Vascular access–related thromboses account for a substantial percentage of hospital admission of dialysis patients and have a multifactorial pathogenesis. Local hemodynamic factors play a prominent role and are probably more relevant than hemostatic alterations in most cases. In particular, stenosis in the anastomosis region or the draining veins of arteriovenous fistulae and grafts, due to neointimal hyperplasia, are the usual harbinger of thrombosis (121). In the case of central venous catheters, thrombosis stems from a variable combination of the Virchow triad, including endothelial damage (initial insertion of the catheter leading to disruption in vessel walls), coagulability, and stasis (intraluminal stasis of blood in the interdialytic period) (122). Central vein thrombosis and right atrial thrombus can be serious complications.

No intervention, including administration of anticoagulant and antiplatelet agents, has been demonstrated to consistently improve vascular access patency with a favorable risk/benefit profile. Management is based on clinical monitoring of the vascular access and multidisciplinary approach in case of thrombosis, including personalized prescription of antithrombotic therapy and surgical/interventional radiology maneuvers.

Cardiovascular events are the predominant cause of morbidity and mortality in uremic patients and include acute coronary syndromes, heart failure, cerebrovascular events, and peripheral artery diseases. Even after adjustment for other risk factors, cardiovascular mortality is 10 to 20 times higher in dialysis patients than in the general population (123). Pathogenesis is complex, and hemostatic alterations alone likely play only a marginal role. An intricate, only partially understood interaction between traditional cardiovascular risk factors and elements peculiar to the uremic milieu, like uremic toxins and derangements in mineral metabolism, probably takes place.

There have not been major clinical trials directly addressing the management of cardiovascular events in dialysis patients. The therapeutic approach is therefore not significantly different from that adopted in the general population and includes a combination of pharmacologic, endovascular, and surgical treatments.

 REFERENCES

1. Morgagni GB. *Opera Omnia.* Venece, Italy: Ex Typographia Remondiniana, 1764.
2. Kaufman JS, O'Connor TZ, Zhang JH, et al. Randomized controlled trial of clopidogrel plus aspirin to prevent hemodialysis access graft thrombosis. *J Am Soc Nephrol* 2003;14(9):2313–2321.

3. Iseki K, Kinjo K, Kimura Y, et al. Evidence for high risk of cerebral hemorrhage in chronic dialysis patients. *Kidney Int* 1993;44(5):1086–1090.

4. Sood P, Sinson GP, Cohen EP. Subdural hematomas in chronic dialysis patients: significant and increasing. *Clin J Am Soc Nephrol* 2007;2(5):956–959.

5. Huang KW, Leu HB, Luo JC, et al. Different peptic ulcer bleeding risk in chronic kidney disease and end-stage renal disease patients receiving different dialysis. *Dig Dis Sci* 2014;59(4):807–813.

6. Eknoyan G, Wacksman SJ, Glueck HI, et al. Platelet function in renal failure. *N Engl J Med* 1969;280(13):677–681.

7. Eknoyan G, Brown CH III. Biochemical abnormalities of platelets in renal failure. Evidence for decreased platelet serotonin, adenosine diphosphate and Mg-dependent adenosine triphosphatase. *Am J Nephrol* 1981;1(1):17–23.

8. Di Minno G, Martinez J, McKean ML, et al. Platelet dysfunction in uremia. Multifaceted defect partially corrected by dialysis. *Am J Med* 1985;79(5):552–559.

9. Kyrle PA, Stockenhuber F, Brenner B, et al. Evidence for an increased generation of prostacyclin in the microvasculature and an impairment of the platelet alpha-granule release in chronic renal failure. *Thromb Haemost* 1988;60(2):205–208.

10. Gura VD, Creter D, Levi J. Elevated thrombocyte calcium content in uremia and its correction by 1 alpha (OH) vitamin D treatment. *Nephron* 1982;30(3):237–239.

11. Ware JA, Clark BA, Smith M, et al. Abnormalities of cytoplasmic Ca2+ in platelets from patients with uremia. *Blood* 1989;73(1):172–176.

12. Escolar G, Díaz-Ricart M, Cases A, et al. Abnormal cytoskeletal assembly in platelets from patients with uremia. *Am J Pathol* 1993;143(3):823–831.

13. Sloand EM, Sloand JA, Prodouz K, et al. Reduction of platelet glycoprotein Ib in uraemia. *Br J Haematol* 1991;77(3):375–381.

14. Benigni A, Boccardo P, Galbusera M, et al. Reversible activation defect of the platelet glycoprotein IIb-IIIa complex in patients with uremia. *Am J Kidney Dis* 1993;22(5):668–676.

15. Escolar G, Cases A, Bastida E, et al. Uremic platelets have a functional defect affecting the interaction of von Willebrand factor with glycoprotein IIb-IIIa. *Blood* 1990;76(7):1336–1340.

16. Smith MC, Dunn MJ. Impaired platelet thromboxane production in renal failure. *Nephron* 1981;29(3–4):133–137.

17. Remuzzi G, Benigni A, Dodesini P, et al. Reduced platelet thromboxane formation in uremia. Evidence for a functional cyclooxygenase defect. *J Clin Invest* 1983;71(3):762–768.

18. Remuzzi G, Cavenaghi AE, Mecca G, et al. Prostacyclin-like activity and bleeding in renal failure. *Lancet* 1977;2(8050):1195–1197.

19. Defreyn G, Dauden MV, Machin SJ, et al. A plasma factor in uraemia which stimulates prostacyclin release from cultured endothelial cells. *Thromb Res* 1980;19(4–5):695–659.

20. Jacobsson B, Ransnäs L, Nyberg G, et al. Abnormality of adenylate cyclase regulation in human platelet membranes in renal insufficiency. *Eur J Clin Invest* 1985;15(2):75–81.

21. Vlachoyannis J, Schoeppe W. Adenylate cyclase activity and cAMP content of human platelets in uraemia. *Eur J Clin Invest* 1982;12(5):379–381.

22. Remuzzi G, Perico N, Zoja C, et al. Role of endothelium-derived nitric oxide in the bleeding tendency of uremia. *J Clin Invest* 1990;86(5):1768–1771.

23. Radomski MW, Palmer RM, Moncada S. The role of nitric oxide and cGMP in platelet adhesion to vascular endothelium. *Biochem Biophys Res Commun* 1987;148(3):1482–1489.

24. Aiello S, Noris M, Todeschini M, et al. Renal and systemic nitric oxide synthesis in rats with renal mass reduction. *Kidney Int* 1997;52(1):171–181.

25. Noris M, Benigni A, Boccardo P, et al. Enhanced nitric oxide synthesis in uremia: implications for platelet dysfunction and dialysis hypotension. *Kidney Int* 1993;44(2):445–450.

26. Noris M, Remuzzi G. Uremic bleeding: closing the circle after 30 years of controversies? *Blood* 1999;94(8):2569–2574.

27. Hörl WH. Hemodialysis membranes: interleukins, biocompatibility, and middle molecules. *J Am Soc Nephrol* 2002;13(Suppl 1):S62–S71.

28. Rabiner SF, Molinas F. The role of phenol and phenolic acids on the thrombocytopathy and defective platelet aggregation of patients with renal failure. *Am J Med* 1970;49(3):346–351.

29. Horwitz HI, Stein IM, Cohen BD, et al. Further studies on the platelet-inhibitory effect of guanidinosuccinic acid and its role in uremic bleeding. *Am J Med* 1970;49(3):336–345.

30. Remuzzi G, Benigni A, Dodesini P, et al. Parathyroid hormone inhibits human platelet function. *Lancet* 1981;2(8259):1321–1323.

31. Remuzzi G, Livio M, Marchiaro G, et al. Bleeding in renal failure: altered platelet function in chronic uraemia only partially corrected by haemodialysis. *Nephron* 1978;22(4–6):347–353.

32. Viganò G, Gotti E, Combeti E, et al. Hyperparathyroidism does not influence the abnormal primary haemostasis in patients with chronic renal failure. *Nephrol Dial Transplant* 1989;4(11):971–974.

33. Maejima M, Takahashi S, Hatano M. Platelet aggregation in chronic renal failure—whole blood aggregation and effect of guanidino compounds. *Nihon Jinzo Gakkai Shi* 1991;33(2):201–212.

34. Macdougall IC. Role of uremic toxins in exacerbating anemia in renal failure. *Kidney Int Suppl* 2001;78:S67–S72.

35. Turitto VT, Weiss HJ. Red blood cells: their dual role in thrombus formation. *Science* 1980;207(4430):541–543.

36. Livio M, Gotti E, Marchesi D, et al. Uraemic bleeding: role of anaemia and beneficial effect of red cell transfusions. *Lancet* 1982;2(8306):1013–1015.

37. Fernandez F, Goudable C, Sie P, et al. Low haematocrit and prolonged bleeding time in uraemic patients: effect of red cell transfusions. *Br J Haematol* 1985;59(1):139–148.

38. Moia M, Mannucci PM, Vizzotto L, et al. Improvement in the haemostatic defect of uraemia after treatment with recombinant human erythropoietin. *Lancet* 1987;2(8570):1227–1229.

39. Viganò G, Benigni A, Mendogni D, et al. Recombinant human erythropoietin to correct uremic bleeding. *Am J Kidney Dis* 1991;18(1):44–49.

40. Soroyal YU, Demir C, Begenik H, et al. Skin bleeding time for the evaluation of uremic platelet dysfunction and effect of dialysis. *Clin Appl Thromb Hemost* 2012;18(2):185–188.

41. Daugirdas JT, Bernardo AA. Hemodialysis effect on platelet count and function and hemodialysis-associated thrombocytopenia. *Kidney Int* 2012;82(2):147–157.

42. Sloand JA, Sloand EM. Studies on platelet membrane glycoproteins and platelet function during hemodialysis. *J Am Soc Nephrol* 1997;8(5):799–803.

43. Herbelin A, Nguyen AT, Zingraff J, et al. Influence of uremia and hemodialysis on circulating interleukin-1 and tumor necrosis factor alpha. *Kidney Int* 1990;37(1):116–125.

44. Wang IK, Cheng YK, Lin CL, et al. Comparison of subdural hematoma risk between hemodialysis and peritoneal dialysis patients with ESRD. *Clin J Am Soc Nephrol* 2015;10(6):994–1001.

45. Hiremath S, Holden RM, Fergusson D, et al. Antiplatelet medications in hemodialysis patients: a systematic review of bleeding rates. *Clin J Am Soc Nephrol* 2009;4(8):1347–1355.

46. Harmon JP, Zimmerman DL, Zimmerman DL. Anticoagulant and antiplatelet therapy in patients with chronic kidney disease: risks versus benefits review. *Curr Opin Nephrol Hypertens* 2013;22(6):624–628.

47. Symes J. Low molecular weight heparins in patients with renal insufficiency. *CANNT J* 2008;18(2):55–61.

48. Savelieva I, Camm AJ. Practical considerations for using novel oral anticoagulants in patients with atrial fibrillation. *Clin Cardiol* 2014;37(1):32–47.

49. Gaspari F, Viganò G, Orisio S, et al. Aspirin prolongs bleeding time in uremia by a mechanism distinct from platelet cyclooxygenase inhibition. *J Clin Invest* 1987;79(6):1788–1797.

50. Wallace JL. Prostaglandins, NSAIDs, and gastric mucosal protection: why doesn't the stomach digest itself? *Physiol Rev* 2008;88(4):1547–1565.

51. Shattil SJ, Bennett JS, McDonough M, et al. Carbenicillin and penicillin G inhibit platelet function in vitro by impairing the interaction of agonists with the platelet surface. *J Clin Invest* 1980;65(2):329–337.

52. Andrassy K, Ritz E. Antimicrobial therapy in dialysis patients. I. Penicillins and cephalosporins. *Blood Purif* 1985;3(1–3):94–103.

53. Holden RM, Harman GJ, Wang M, et al. Major bleeding in hemodialysis patients. *Clin J Am Soc Nephrol* 2008;3(1):105–110.

54. Margolis DM, Saylor JL, Geisse G, et al. Upper gastrointestinal disease in chronic renal failure. A prospective evaluation. *Arch Intern Med* 1978;138(8):1214–1217.

55. Doherty CC. Gastrointestinal bleeding in dialysis patients. *Nephron* 1993;63(2):132–139.

56. Dave PB, Romeu J, Antonelli A, et al. Gastrointestinal telangiectasias. A source of bleeding in patients receiving hemodialysis. *Arch Intern Med* 1984;144(9):1781–1783.

57. Gutiérrez-Sánchez MJ, Petkov-Stoyanov V, Martín-Navarro JA, et al. Ischaemic colitis in haemodialysis. *Nefrologia* 2013;33(5):736–737.

58. Ovbiagele B, Schwamm LH, Smith EE, et al. Hospitalized hemorrhagic stroke patients with renal insufficiency: clinical characteristics, care patterns, and outcomes. *J Stroke Cerebrovasc Dis* 2014;23(9):2265–2273.

59. Sakhuja A, Schold JD, Kumar G, et al. Nontraumatic subarachnoid hemorrhage in maintenance dialysis hospitalizations: trends and outcomes. *Stroke* 2014;45(1):71–76.

60. Li L, Fisher M, Lau WL, et al. Cerebral microbleeds and cognitive decline in a hemodialysis patient: case report and review of literature. *Hemodial Int* 2015;19(3):E1–E7.

61. Naganuma T, Takemoto Y, Yamasaki T, et al. Factors associated with silent cerebral microbleeds in hemodialysis patients. *Clin Nephrol* 2011; 75(4):346–355.

62. Alpert MA, Ravenscraft MD. Pericardial involvement in end-stage renal disease. *Am J Med Sci* 2003;325(4):228–236.

63. Maher JF. Uremic pleuritis. *Am J Kidney Dis* 1987;10(1):19–22.

64. Cochrane R, Regan L. Undetected gynaecological disorders in women with renal disease. *Hum Reprod* 1997;12(4):667–670.

65. Stein J, Brewster UC, Perazella MA. Retroperitoneal bleed from acquired renal cysts. *Semin Dial* 2006;19(3):256.

66. Borra S, Kleinfeld M. Subcapsular liver hematomas in a patient on chronic hemodialysis. *Ann Intern Med* 1980;93(4):574–575.

67. Srivastava A, Patel N. Autosomal dominant polycystic kidney disease. *Am Fam Physician* 2014;90(5):303–307.

68. Cherng YG, Liao CC, Chen TH, et al. Are non-cardiac surgeries safe for dialysis patients?—a population-based retrospective cohort study. *PLoS One* 2013;8(3):e58942.

69. Mattix H, Singh AK. Is the bleeding time predictive of bleeding prior to a percutaneous renal biopsy? *Curr Opin Nephrol Hypertens* 1999;8(6):715–718.

70. Ho SJ, Gemmell R, Brighton TA. Platelet function testing in uraemic patients. *Hematology* 2008;13(1):49–58.

71. Cheung J, Yu A, LaBossiere J, et al. Peptic ulcer bleeding outcomes adversely affected by end-stage renal disease. *Gastrointest Endosc* 2010; 71(1):44–49.

72. Krummel T, Scheidt E, Borni-Duval C, et al. Haemodialysis in patients treated with oral anticoagulant: should we heparinize? *Nephrol Dial Transplant* 2014;29(4):906–913.

73. Zhao Y, Li Z, Zhang L, et al. Citrate versus heparin lock for hemodialysis catheters: a systematic review and meta-analysis of randomized controlled trials. *Am J Kidney Dis* 2014;63(3):479–490.

74. Thomson PC, Morris ST, Mactier RA. The effect of heparinized catheter lock solutions on systemic anticoagulation in hemodialysis patients. *Clin Nephrol* 2011;75(3):212–217.

75. Tàssies D, Reverter JC, Cases A, et al. Effect of recombinant human erythropoietin treatment on circulating reticulated platelets in uremic patients: association with early improvement in platelet function. *Am J Hematol* 1998;59(2):105–109.

76. Zhou XJ, Vaziri ND. Defective calcium signalling in uraemic platelets and its amelioration with long-term erythropoietin therapy. *Nephrol Dial Transplant* 2002;17(6):992–997.

77. Diaz-Ricart M, Etebanell E, Cases A, et al. Erythropoietin improves signaling through tyrosine phosphorylation in platelets from uremic patients. *Thromb Haemost* 1999;82(4):1312–1317.

78. Fox KA, Mehta SR, Peters R, et al. Benefits and risks of the combination of clopidogrel and aspirin in patients undergoing surgical revascularization for non-ST-elevation acute coronary syndrome: the Clopidogrel in Unstable Angina to Prevent Recurrent Ischemic Events (CURE) Trial. *Circulation* 2004;110(10):1202–1208.

79. Zimmerman D, Sood MM, Rigatto C, et al. Systematic review and meta-analysis of incidence, prevalence and outcomes of atrial fibrillation in patients on dialysis. *Nephrol Dial Transplant* 2012;27(10):3816–3822.

80. Mannucci PM, Remuzzi G, Pusineri F, et al. Deamino-8-D-arginine vasopressin shortens the bleeding time in uremia. *N Engl J Med* 1983;308(1):8–12.

81. Viganò GL, Mannucci PM, Lattuada A, et al. Subcutaneous desmopressin (DDAVP) shortens the bleeding time in uremia. *Am J Hematol* 1989;31(1):32–35.

82. Shapiro MD, Kelleher SP. Intranasal deamino-8-D-arginine vasopressin shortens the bleeding time in uremia. *Am J Nephrol* 1984;4(4):260–261.

83. Canavese C, Salomone M, Pacitti A, et al. Reduced response of uraemic bleeding time to repeated doses of desmopressin. *Lancet* 1985; 1(8433):867–868.

84. Mannucci PM. Desmopressin (DDAVP) in the treatment of bleeding disorders: the first 20 years. *Blood* 1997;90(7):2515–2521.

85. Janson PA, Jubelirer SJ, Weinstein MJ, et al. Treatment of the bleeding tendency in uremia with cryoprecipitate. *N Engl J Med* 1980;303(23): 1318–1322.

86. Livio M, Mannucci PM, Viganò G, et al. Conjugated estrogens for the management of bleeding associated with renal failure. *N Engl J Med* 1986;315(12):731–735.

87. Liu YK, Kosfeld RE, Marcum SG. Treatment of uraemic bleeding with conjugated oestrogen. *Lancet* 1984;2(8408):887–890.

88. Viganò G, Gaspari F, Locatelli M, et al. Dose-effect and pharmacokinetics of estrogens given to correct bleeding time in uremia. *Kidney Int* 1988;34(6):853–858.

89. Hedges SJ, Dehoney SB, Hooper JS, et al. Evidence-based treatment recommendations for uremic bleeding. *Nat Clin Pract Nephrol* 2007; 3(3):138–153.

90. Sloand JA, Schiff MJ. Beneficial effect of low-dose transdermal estrogen on bleeding time and clinical bleeding in uremia. *Am J Kidney Dis* 1995;26(1):22–26.

91. Mezzano D, Muñoz B, Pais E, et al. Fast decrease of bleeding time by tranexamic acid in uremia. *Thromb Haemost* 2000;83(5):785.

92. Vujkovac B, Lavre J, Sabovic M. Successful treatment of bleeding from colonic angiodysplasias with tranexamic acid in a hemodialysis patient. *Am J Kidney Dis* 1998;31(3):536–538.

93. Vujkovac B, Sabovic M. Treatment of subdural and intracerebral haematomas in a haemodialysis patient with tranexamic acid. *Nephrol Dial Transplant* 2000;15(1):107–109.

94. Sabovic M, Lavre J, Vujkovac B. Tranexamic acid is beneficial as adjunctive therapy in treating major upper gastrointestinal bleeding in dialysis patients. *Nephrol Dial Transplant* 2003;18(7):1388–1391.

95. Bhat A, Bhowmik DM, Vibha D, et al. Tranexamic acid overdosage-induced generalized seizure in renal failure. *Saudi J Kidney Dis Transpl* 2014;25(1):130–132.

96. Kitamura H, Matsui I, Itoh N, et al. Tranexamic acid-induced visual impairment in a hemodialysis patient. *Clin Exp Nephrol* 2003;7(4):311–314.

97. Shlipak MG, Fried LF, Crump C, et al. Elevations of inflammatory and procoagulant biomarkers in elderly persons with renal insufficiency. *Circulation* 2003;107(1):87–92.

98. Pawlak K, Tankiewicz J, Mysliwiec M, et al. Tissue factor/its pathway inhibitor system and kynurenines in chronic kidney disease patients on conservative treatment. *Blood Coagul Fibrinolysis* 2009;20(7):590–594.

99. Faioni EM, Franchi F, Krachmalnicoff A, et al. Low levels of the anticoagulant activity of protein C in patients with chronic renal insufficiency: an inhibitor of protein C is present in uremic plasma. *Thromb Haemost* 1991;66(4):420–425.

100. Tomura S, Nakamura Y, Deguchi F, et al. Coagulation and fibrinolysis in patients with chronic renal failure undergoing conservative treatment. *Thromb Res* 1991;64(1):81–90.

101. Opatrný K Jr, Vít L, Opatrná S, et al. Hypofibrinolysis after venous occlusion in patients treated with long-term hemodialysis. *Cas Lek Cesk* 1994;133(11):346–349.

102. Opatrný K Jr, Zemanová P, Opatrná S, et al. Fibrinolysis in chronic renal failure, dialysis and renal transplantation. *Ann Transplant* 2002;7(1):34–43.

103. Mezzano D, Tagle R, Panes O, et al. Hemostatic disorder of uremia: the platelet defect, main determinant of the prolonged bleeding time, is correlated with indices of activation of coagulation and fibrinolysis. *Thromb Haemost* 1996;76(3):312–321.

104. Gris JC, Branger B, Vécina F, et al. Increased cardiovascular risk factors and features of endothelial activation and dysfunction in dialyzed uremic patients. *Kidney Int* 1994;46(3):807–813.

105. Sagripanti A, Cupisti A, Baicchi U, et al. Plasma parameters of the prothrombotic state in chronic uremia. *Nephron* 1993;63(3):273–278.

106. Matsuo T, Koide M, Kario K, et al. Extrinsic coagulation factors and tissue factor pathway inhibitor in end-stage chronic renal failure. *Haemostasis* 1997;27(4):163–167.

107. Adams MJ, Irish AB, Watts GF, et al. Hypercoagulability in chronic kidney disease is associated with coagulation activation but not endothelial function. *Thromb Res* 2008;123(2):374–380.

108. Libby P. Inflammation in atherosclerosis. *Arterioscler Thromb Vasc Biol* 2012;32(9):2045–2051.

109. Mallamaci F, Zoccali C, Tripepi G, et al. Hyperhomocysteinemia predicts cardiovascular outcomes in hemodialysis patients. *Kidney Int* 2002;61(2):609–614.

110. Bostom AG, Shemin D, Verhoef P, et al. Elevated fasting total plasma homocysteine levels and cardiovascular disease outcomes in maintenance dialysis patients. A prospective study. *Arterioscler Thromb Vasc Biol* 1997;17(11):2554–2558.

111. Remuzzi A, Ene-Iordache B. Novel paradigms for dialysis vascular access: upstream hemodynamics and vascular remodeling in dialysis access stenosis. *Clin J Am Soc Nephrol* 2013;8(12):2186–2193.

112. Kerlin BA, Ayoob R, Smoyer WE. Epidemiology and pathophysiology of nephrotic syndrome-associated thromboembolic disease. *Clin J Am Soc Nephrol* 2012;7(3):513–520.

113. Syed S, Reilly RF. Heparin-induced thrombocytopenia: a renal perspective. *Nat Rev Nephrol* 2009;5(9):501–511.

114. Sitter T, Spannagl M, Banas B, et al. Prevalence of heparin-induced PF4-heparin antibodies in hemodialysis patients. *Nephron* 1998;79(2):245–246.

115. Zhao D, Sun X, Yao L, et al. The clinical significance and risk factors of anti-platelet factor 4/heparin antibody on maintenance hemodialysis patients: a two-year prospective follow-up. *PLoS One* 2013;8(4):e62239.

116. de Sancho M, Lema MG, Amiral J, et al. Frequency of antibodies directed against heparin-platelet factor 4 in patients exposed to heparin through chronic hemodialysis. *Thromb Haemost* 1996;75(4):695–696.

117. Yu A, Jacobson SH, Bygdé A, et al. The presence of heparin-platelet factor 4 antibodies as a marker of hypercoagulability during hemodialysis. *Clin Chem Lab Med* 2002;40(1):21–26.

118. Matsuo T, Kobayashi H, Matsuo M, et al. Frequency of anti-heparin-PF4 complex antibodies (HIT antibodies) in uremic patients on chronic intermittent hemodialysis. *Pathophysiol Haemost Thromb* 2006;35(6):445–450.

119. Prakash R, Miller CC III, Suki WN. Anticardiolipin antibody in patients on maintenance hemodialysis and its association with recurrent arteriovenous graft thrombosis. *Am J Kidney Dis* 1995;26(2):347–352.

120. Chew SL, Lins RL, Daelemans R, et al. Are antiphospholipid antibodies clinically relevant in dialysis patients? *Nephrol Dial Transplant* 1992;7(12):1194–1198.

121. Riella MC, Roy-Chaudhury P. Vascular access in haemodialysis: strengthening the Achilles' heel. *Nat Rev Nephrol* 2013;9(6):348–357.

122. Niyyar VD, Chan MR. Interventional nephrology: catheter dysfunction—prevention and troubleshooting. *Clin J Am Soc Nephrol* 2013;8(7):1234–1243.

123. Foley RN, Parfrey PS, Samak MJ. Epidemiology of cardiovascular disease in chronic renal disease. *J Am Soc Nephrol* 1998;9(12 Suppl):S16–S23.

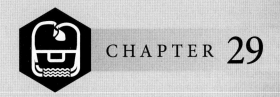

CHAPTER 29

Treatment of Anemia in Patients with End-Stage Kidney Disease

Yaakov Liss and Jeffrey S. Berns

 ANEMIA AND END-STAGE KIDNEY DISEASE: THE MAGNITUDE OF THE PROBLEM

Anemia, or reduced erythrocyte mass, is one of the most clinically significant complications of chronic kidney disease (CKD) and is associated with increased mortality and decreased quality of life. Although there is no universal definition of anemia, recent guidelines recommend diagnosing anemia in adult men with a hemoglobin (Hb) <13.0 g/dL and in adult females with an Hb <12.0 g/dL (1). Anemia is highly prevalent among patients with CKD and endstage kidney disease (ESKD), with an increase in the rate and severity of anemia associated with a decrease in glomerular filtration rate (GFR) and the near universal prevalence of anemia in patients on chronic dialysis (2,3). Recent data from the National Health and Nutrition Examination Survey (NHANES) demonstrated a prevalence of anemia in predialysis patients with CKD stage 5 of 53.4%. The prevalence of anemia increases as patients initiate chronic dialysis therapy, with 85% of patients on chronic dialysis reported to have an Hb <12.0 g/dL by the 2014 United States Renal Data System (USRDS) annual report (4).

Numerous observational studies have shown that the presence and severity of anemia correlate with numerous adverse outcomes including increased mortality (5–7), left ventricular hypertrophy (LVH) (8,9), and decreased health-related quality of life (10,11). However, randomized control trials have not demonstrated a mortality benefit for the treatment of anemia with the use of erythropoiesis-stimulating agents (ESAs) in patients with CKD or ESKD, and some studies even suggest harm.

Despite the overwhelming prevalence of anemia in patients with ESKD and the clear association of anemia with significant morbidity and mortality, the degree to which anemia should be corrected and the optimal strategy for doing so is controversial.

This chapter focuses on the treatment of anemia in patients with ESKD. We first review normal erythrocyte production and the normal response to anemia followed by a discussion of the various pathophysiological processes which lead to anemia in patients with ESKD before discussing treatment directly, as an understanding of the former topics are vital to successfully employing the latter.

 NORMAL ERYTHROCYTE PRODUCTION

Under normal conditions, approximately 1% of circulating erythrocytes are replaced daily. Erythrocyte production occurs in the bone marrow and depends on erythropoietin (EPO), a hormone which is mainly produced in the kidneys, and regulates erythropoiesis via binding to EPO receptors on erythroid precursor cells located in the bone marrow. The proper functioning of this process requires additional cofactors including iron, vitamin B_{12}, and folic acid.

EPO is the major regulatory hormone of erythropoiesis and is produced primarily in peritubular interstitial cells of the kidney with lesser production in the liver postnatally (12,13). EPO production is modulated by the delivery of oxygen from circulating erythrocytes; in the presence of tissue hypoxia, EPO production is increased. On a cellular level, this process occurs due to the presence of hypoxia-inducible factors (HIFs) in EPO-producing cells, specifically HIFα and HIFβ (14). Under normoxic conditions, HIFα is constitutively produced and subsequently degraded by the ubiquitin-proteasome system. This degradation is dependent on the hydroxylation of HIFα via specific hydroxylase enzymes, which allow for the binding of HIFα to the tumor suppressor protein von Hippel-Lindau (VHL). This leads to the HIFα molecule being tagged for proteasomal degradation. Under hypoxic conditions, HIFα degradation is inhibited, allowing for the successful production of EPO. EPO is then secreted into the systemic circulation where it binds with EPO receptors on erythroid precursor cells in the bone marrow, leading to increased production of erythrocytes by preventing erythroid cell apoptosis (15).

In order for successful erythropoiesis to occur, an adequate supply of iron, B_{12}, and folate are necessary. Iron balance is a highly regulated process, and iron deficiency, either absolute or functional, significantly contributes to anemia of CKD. The successful production of erythrocytes depends on both adequate nutritional iron stores and the mobilization of these stores for use by the bone marrow. The master regulator of this process is hepcidin (16,17). Elevated hepcidin levels inhibit duodenal iron absorption and iron release from macrophages, whereas decreased hepcidin levels promote gastrointestinal (GI) absorption and mobilization from macrophages. Hepcidin production is stimulated by total body iron overload and infection (18).

⬡ UNDERLYING ETIOLOGIES OF ANEMIA OF CHRONIC KIDNEY DISEASE

Anemia in patients with CKD is, as a rule, a multifactorial process. While EPO deficiency is usually the primary pathophysiological process (19), iron deficiency anemia related to chronic blood loss and anemia of chronic disease related to comorbidity burden and the malnutrition–inflammation complex syndrome (20) both play significant contributory roles. Other causes for anemia found in the general population can also be superimposed on the above processes and should be considered when evaluating a patient with CKD and anemia.

In healthy patients, EPO levels increase in response to anemia. In patients with CKD, there is an inadequate response, and EPO levels are inappropriately low relative to the degree of anemia (21,22). While patients with CKD and ESKD (including anephric patients) continue to produce EPO and have been shown to increase EPO production (23), the response in EPO production is blunted and inadequate to sufficiently correct the anemia. The explanation for inadequate EPO production has historically implicated reduced nephron mass and loss of EPO-producing peritubular interstitial cells. However, recent evidence including clinical trials that have demonstrated that EPO production can be increased in patients with ESKD via pharmacological stabilization of HIF using prolyl hydroxylase inhibitors (24) raises the possibility that a disturbed oxygen-sensing mechanism rather than a lack of capacity for EPO production may be the primary cause of anemia.

ESKD and chronic hemodialysis (HD) inevitably lead to negative iron balance, primarily as a result of chronic blood loss through several different mechanisms. Patients with ESKD are more likely to have both overt and occult GI bleeding (25,26). Additionally, significant blood loss occurs both due to frequent phlebotomy as well as due to the HD procedure itself (27). In addition to absolute iron deficiency, patients with ESKD have a frequently impaired ability to absorb iron or utilize their existent iron stores due to ongoing inflammation (20).

There are several other processes that may contribute to anemia in patients with CKD that are worth mentioning. It has been known for some time that patients with CKD have a shortened erythrocyte survival time (28). Neither the precise pathophysiological cause of this phenomenon nor the degree to which this shortened survival contributes to anemia is entirely clear. However, it is unlikely that dialysis modality plays a significant role, as studies have shown no significant difference in the decrease in erythrocyte survival time

between peritoneal dialysis, conventional thrice-weekly HD, nocturnal HD, or short daily HD (29,30). Furthermore, while the toxic uremic milieu is frequently cited as the probable cause for shortened erythrocyte survival, more frequent HD has shown no benefit in improving anemia (31).

Folate and vitamin B_{12} deficiency, while not common, are both readily reversible causes of anemia. These diagnoses should be tested for, particularly in the setting of macrocytosis. While there is loss of folate with dialysis, normal dietary intake should exceed such losses (32).

Historically, aluminum toxicity was a significant cause of anemia in patients with ESKD on dialysis, both due to the use of aluminum-containing phosphate binders and due to the presence of aluminum in water used for dialysis (33). Its incidence has waned significantly due to the now routine removal of aluminum from dialysis water and due to the wide availability of non–aluminum-containing phosphate binders. Aluminum toxicity–related anemia presents as a microcytic anemia in the presence of adequate iron stores (34).

Given the universal polypharmacy of patients with ESKD, it is important to consider medications and their potentially contributory role to anemia. The myelosuppressive effects of immunosuppressants, commonly used in the setting of solid organ transplants or systemic autoimmune conditions, are well known and well described. Angiotensin-converting enzyme (ACE) inhibitors and angiotensin receptor blockers (ARBs) have also been causally implicated in CKD-related anemia, although the evidence is primarily composed of case reports and small case series (35–37). Experimental data in rats demonstrates that angiotensin plays a role in EPO production (38), and it is therefore plausible that angiotensin blockade would impair EPO production and lead to anemia. While observational studies in patients on chronic dialysis have shown mixed results regarding the relationship between ACE inhibitor and ARB use with ESA dose (39,40), several uncontrolled studies did show the need for increased ESA dosing in patients receiving ACE inhibitors or ARBs (41,42).

⬡ TREATMENT OF ANEMIA OF CHRONIC KIDNEY DISEASE

The initial step in the treatment of anemia in patients with ESKD involves a basic diagnostic workup to identify the numerous processes that may be contributing to the anemia. Recent Kidney Disease Improving Global Outcomes (KDIGO) guidelines recommend that initial testing for patients with CKD and anemia includes complete blood count (CBC), absolute reticulocyte count, serum ferritin level, serum transferrin saturation (TSAT), and serum vitamin B_{12} and folate levels (1).

While tests for serum EPO levels are commercially available, these tests are not recommended since they are unlikely to affect clinical care given the lack of correlation between absolute EPO levels and the degree of anemia in patients with a creatinine clearance of less than 40 mL/min (43). As such, it can be assumed that all patients with advanced CKD and ESKD have EPO deficiency; however, it is recommended to first treat any correctable causes of anemia prior to initiating treatment with ESAs (1). This recommendation is predicated upon the fact that ESA responsiveness is unlikely in patients with additional causes of hypoproliferative anemia such as iron, vitamin B_{12}, or folate deficiency. Furthermore, correction of these underlying issues can significantly reduce the dose of or need for ESA use. In particular, iron deficiency is exceedingly common in patients with CKD and ESKD, and numerous randomized studies have demonstrated that iron supplementation reduces ESA requirements (44–48).

 ## DETERMINATION OF IRON STATUS

In healthy patients with an isolated finding of anemia, the diagnosis of iron deficiency anemia is generally clinically obvious and determined by the presence of numerous consonant factors including a low-reticulocyte index, low mean corpuscular volume (MCV), decreased iron stores based on decreased serum ferritin levels, and decreased iron availability based on decreased serum TSAT. In patients with anemia of CKD, straightforward determination of iron status is generally the exception rather than the rule. Iron stores may be present but not available for erythropoiesis, and serum ferritin levels are frequently normal or even increased without a concomitant increase in serum TSAT or even a decreased TSAT. Despite this laboratory discrepancy in iron status, studies have demonstrated that the administration of supplemental iron to patients with elevated ferritin levels can still improve the anemia (48,49), rendering serum ferritin a rather poor marker of ESA response. Given the complexity with accurately determining the iron status of patients with CKD, numerous additional serologic tests have been explored, including erythrocyte zinc protoporphyrin (50), percentage of hypochromic red blood cells (51), reticulocyte Hb content (52), and serum hepcidin (53). Thus far, none of these tests have been incorporated into routine clinical practice due to a lack of consistent results over numerous studies, lack of commercial availability, or lack of utility in meaningfully impacting current clinical practice. For now, guidelines recommend determining iron status by serum ferritin and TSAT alone; ultimately, when uncertainty still remains, iron status is determined by the administration of supplemental iron and the presence or absence of an erythropoietic response.

 ## TREATMENT OF IRON DEFICIENCY

Therapeutic Targets

The treatment of anemia in patients with ESKD almost always involves both the use of intravenous (IV) iron and the use of ESAs, and an increased dose in the first of these agents generally allows for a reduced dose in the last. Safety concerns related to ESA use, shifting market pressures, and small studies demonstrating the ability to decrease ESA use by targeting higher levels of ferritin and TSAT have led to changing serum iron marker targets over time. The 2006 Kidney Disease Outcomes Quality Initiative (KDOQI) guidelines recommended administering IV iron to achieve a serum ferritin greater than 200 ng/mL and a TSAT greater 20% (54). The 2012 KDIGO guidelines recommend the administration of IV iron if serum ferritin is less than 500 ng/mL or TSAT is less than 30% and an increase in Hb or decrease in ESA dose is desired (1). Routine administration of iron to patients with serum ferritin levels greater than 500 ng/mL or TSAT greater than 30% is recommended against due to a lack of data demonstrating the safety of this approach, but this may be considered on an individual patient basis, particularly when a reduction in ESA dose is desired.

Two randomized control studies specifically evaluated the use of IV iron to achieve different iron targets and its effect on anemia parameters. A study by Besarab et al. (48) randomized 43 patients to receive maintenance IV iron dextran to maintain TSAT 20% to

30% versus increased doses of IV iron dextran to achieve TSAT 30% to 50% over 6 months and demonstrated comparable Hb levels in both groups with increased ferritin levels and a 40% decrease in ESA dosing in the increased IV iron group. The Dialysis Patients' Response to IV Iron with Elevated Ferritin (DRIVE) study by Coyne et al. (49) randomized 134 patients with a serum ferritin of 500 to 1,200 ng/mL, and a TSAT <25% over a 6-week period to 1 g of IV ferric gluconate administered with HD over eight doses versus placebo while receiving EPO at a 25% increased dose from baseline with further titration prohibited over the duration of the study. Results demonstrated a 0.5 g/dL increase in Hb in the IV ferric gluconate group versus the placebo group.

While the above studies demonstrate that iron supplementation can improve anemia parameters even in patients with significantly elevated iron stores, there are no studies adequately powered with long enough follow-up to demonstrate long-term benefit or harm related to employing a strategy that favors the administration of iron over the use of ESAs (55).

Route of Administration

There is general agreement that IV iron is the preferred route of iron administration to patients with ESKD and that oral iron is inadequate to replete deficient iron stores. A recent meta-analysis of 28 studies involving 2,098 subjects demonstrated increased ferritin, increased TSAT, increased Hb, and decreased ESA dose with the use of IV versus oral iron (56). The accepted explanation for reduced effectiveness of oral iron has implicated elevated hepcidin levels from chronic inflammation leading to poor GI absorption. Interestingly, recent trials involving ferric citrate, an oral iron-containing phosphate binder, have demonstrated a decreased need for IV iron and ESA doses (57). It remains to be seen how the use of oral iron-containing phosphate binders will impact the overall management of anemia in patients with CKD.

Parenteral Iron Preparations

Sixty-two percent of patients with ESKD on HD regularly received IV iron in 2012 according to data from the USRDS (4). There are currently several parenteral iron preparations available for use in the United States: iron dextran, iron sucrose, ferric gluconate, ferric carboxymaltose, and ferumoxytol. Iron isomaltoside is available for use in Europe but is not currently U.S. Food and Drug Administration (FDA) approved. Data from Dialysis Outcomes and Practice Pattern Study (DOPPS) demonstrate that approximately 90% of IV iron administered in the United States in 2015 was an iron sucrose formulation, with the remainder consisting almost entirely of ferric gluconate (58).

Most IV iron preparations consist of iron associated with a carbohydrate shell. The infusion of IV iron and the release of free iron can lead to a range of anaphylactoid and other reactions including myalgias, arthralgias, facial flushing, and hypotension, although there is a relatively low risk for the occurrence of serious adverse events (59), with a predicted absolute risk of life-threatening events ranging from 0.6 to 11.3 events per million depending on the IV iron preparation used (60). Details of the various IV iron preparations are discussed below (**TABLE 29.1**).

Iron Dextran

Iron dextran is available in the United States in both a high molecular weight formulation (Dexferrum) and a low molecular weight formulation (INFeD). While KDIGO guidelines strongly recommend close monitoring of all patients during their initial dose of iron

TABLE 29.1	**Intravenous Iron Preparations**				
Generic Drug	**Trade Name**	**Commonly Used Single Dose**	**Elemental Iron Concentration (mg/mL)**	**Test Dose?**
Iron dextran (high molecular weight)	Dexferrum	100 mg	50	Yes
Iron dextran (low molecular weight)	INFeD	100 mg	50	Yes
Iron sucrose	Venofer	200–300 mg	20	No
Ferric gluconate	Ferrlecit	125 mg	12.5	No
Ferumoxytol	Feraheme	510 mg	30	No
Ferric carboxymaltose	Ferinject	20 mg/kg (maximum 1,000 mg)	50	No
Iron isomaltoside	Monofer (not available in United States)	20 mg/kg	100	No

dextran (1) due to an increased risk of severe anaphylactic reactions, several studies suggest that the increased risk of severe anaphylactic reactions is limited largely to the use of high molecular weight formulations (61,62). The use of low molecular weight iron dextran appears to have an equivalent risk of adverse reactions to other commonly used IV iron preparations (63). Iron dextran is available in 1- or 2-mL solutions of 50 mg/mL. The package insert recommends administration of a test dose of 25 mg prior to the administration of a full dose. Furthermore, KDIGO guidelines recommend that patients be monitored for 60 minutes after their initial infusion of iron dextran and that resuscitative personnel be available at the time of infusion. While the package insert recommends a maximum dose of 100 mg daily, the administration of 1,000 mg of iron dextran over 1 hour has been shown to be safe and effective (64).

Iron Sucrose

Iron sucrose (Venofer) is widely used in the United States and worldwide for the treatment of CKD-associated anemia. It appears to have a superior safety profile to iron dextran and an equivalent safety and efficacy profile to other IV iron preparations (65,66). It is available in 2.5-, 5-, or 10-mL solutions of 20 mg/mL. The package insert states that there is no need for a test dose in product-naive patients. KDIGO guidelines suggest monitoring patients for 60 minutes after the initial infusion of iron sucrose but mention that the data to support this suggestion is not strong. The package insert states that a dose of up to 200 mg can be given over a 2- to 5-minute IV infusion. Doses of 300 mg should be given over 1.5 hours. It is not recommended to administer doses above 300 mg, as this has been associated with a significant rate of adverse reactions including dizziness, nausea, and hypotension (67).

Ferric Gluconate

Ferric gluconate (Ferrlecit) was available for use in Europe for many decades before being FDA approved in 1999. It is safer than iron dextran with comparable safety and efficacy to other IV iron preparations (68,69). It is available in 5-mL solutions of 12.5 mg/mL. The package insert states that prior labeling recommended a test dose of 2 mL, but a test dose is no longer recommended. KDIGO guidelines suggest monitoring patients for 60 minutes after the initial infusion of ferric gluconate but mention that the data to support this suggestion is not strong. The package insert recommends a maximum dose of 125 mg which can be infused over 1 hour, although the infusion of 250 mg over 1 hour appears to be safe (70). There is little data available to support the safety of administering larger one-time doses.

Ferumoxytol

Ferumoxytol (Feraheme) was FDA approved for the treatment of anemia in patients with CKD in 2009. It possess supermagnetic properties and can affect magnetic resonance imaging (MRI) for days to months after its administration (71). Randomized trials have demonstrated ferumoxytol to have comparable efficacy and safety to other IV iron preparations (65,72). It is available in 17-mL solutions of 510 mg/17 mL. The package insert does not indicate the need for a test dose but recommends patient monitoring for at least 30 minutes after infusion in a setting where proper personnel and therapies are immediately available. While ferumoxytol was initially recommended to be administered as a rapid injection of 510 mg over 17 to 60 seconds, this was suggested to lead to an increased rate of anaphylactic reactions (73); subsequent recommendations suggest administering ferumoxytol in a diluted form over a slow infusion of at least 15 minutes. Although the maximum recommended dose is 510 mg, administering 1,020 mg as a one-time dose has been shown to be safe and efficacious (74).

Ferric Carboxymaltose

Ferric carboxymaltose (Injectafer) was FDA approved for anemia in non–dialysis-dependent CKD in 2013. Several randomized trials demonstrated superior efficacy with comparable safety of ferric carboxymaltose versus oral iron in patients with anemia not related to CKD (75–77). Additionally, one randomized trial demonstrated superior efficacy with comparable safety of ferric carboxymaltose versus oral iron in patients with non–dialysis-dependent CKD (78), and one randomized trial demonstrated comparable efficacy and safety between two injections of 750 mg of ferric carboxymaltose given over 1 week versus five injections of 200 mg of iron sucrose given over 2 weeks in patients with non–dialysis-dependent CKD (79). There is very little published data available at this time evaluating the safety and efficacy of ferric carboxymaltose in patients with ESKD. Ferric carboxymaltose is available in 15-mL solutions of 750 mg/15 mL. There is no mention of requiring a test dose in the package insert, and there is no specific recommendation by the FDA to monitor patients after their initial infusion. Of note, ferric carboxymaltose infusion was associated with transient hypertensive episodes (79).

Iron Isomaltoside

Iron isomaltoside (Monofer) is currently not FDA approved and is only in use outside of the United States. It can be administered as a 15-minute infusion with doses of >1,000 mg given at one time.

Iron Loading and Maintenance Therapy

There are generally two phases in the treatment of iron deficiency in anemic patients with ESKD: iron loading and maintenance therapy. Iron loading is the use of IV iron to correct iron deficiency. Maintenance therapy is the ongoing administration of IV iron in iron-replete patients who are usually receiving concurrent ESA therapy. As discussed earlier, current guidelines (1) recommend administering IV iron to patients with a TSAT <30% and a ferritin <500 ng/dL when an increase in Hb is desired. Most iron loading regimens recommend the intensive administration of approximately 1,000 mg of IV iron over a relatively short time period. This can be done over relatively few treatments with the use of iron dextran, ferumoxytol, or ferric carboxymaltose but would require more treatments with the use of iron sucrose and ferric gluconate. During the iron loading phase, it is recommended to check the CBC, TSAT, and ferritin frequently to ensure that the treatment is achieving its goals. It is recommended to ensure that iron stores are replete prior to initiating ESA therapy, as the administration of an ESA to an iron deficient patient has a high probability of failure. Once iron stores are replete and Hb and iron indices are stable, laboratory test results can be checked every 3 months (1).

Once iron stores are replete, there are two possible strategies regarding maintenance therapy: intermittent dosing of IV iron when iron indices fall below target or continuous dosing of IV iron to maintain iron indices above target. Theoretically, continuous dosing of IV iron is more likely to ensure that iron stores remain adequate, allowing for the possibility of continued, effective erythropoiesis (80). Several randomized trials evaluated the use of continuous IV iron versus intermittent administration in iron-replete patients and demonstrated superiority of a continuous dosing regimen with either a higher Hb achieved or an equivalent Hb with a reduced ESA dose (81,82).

Maintenance Therapy via Iron-Containing Dialysate

A newly tested method of maintenance administration of IV iron to patients with ESKD who are iron replete involves the addition of ferric pyrophosphate citrate (FPC) (Triferic), a water-soluble iron salt, to the dialysis solution, allowing for routine administration of low doses of IV iron with each dialysis treatment. Two identical randomized trials, Continuous Replacement Using Iron Soluble Equivalents (CRUISE) 1 and 2 (83), evaluated the effects of the use of dialysate containing 2 μmol/L of FPC iron versus standard dialysate in 599 patients on a fixed dose of ESA with prohibited supplemental iron use and demonstrated that FPC-containing dialysate maintained steady Hb levels with less of a decrease in ferritin levels versus the placebo group. An additional randomized trial, Physiological Replenishment Iron Maintenance Equivalency (PRIME) (84), evaluated the use of dialysate containing 2 μmol/L FPC iron versus standard dialysate in 103 patients on adjustable doses of ESAs and IV iron to be administered when serum ferritin levels decreased below 200 μg/L and demonstrated a decrease in ESA dose and decrease in IV iron need versus placebo. FPC (Triferic) was FDA approved as an iron replacement product to maintain Hb in adult patients with HD-dependent CKD in January 2015.

Adverse Effects of Intravenous Iron

As discussed earlier, all IV iron preparations are associated with anaphylactic-type reactions which at times can be life threatening. Excluding high molecular weight iron dextran which carries an increased risk, the absolute risk of a life-threatening serious adverse event has been estimated to be approximately 1 in 200,000 with commonly used IV iron preparations (60).

Theoretically, an iron-rich environment can promote bacterial growth, and the administration of IV iron to patients with active infection is contraindicated (1). Despite this recommendation, the evidence linking the administration of IV iron to an increased infection risk is mixed and of low quality. A retrospective study of 32,566 patients (85) showed no association between IV iron dose and infection-related mortality; a prospective, observational study of 985 patients (86) showed no association between IV iron use and infection risk; a retrospective study of 117,050 patients (87) demonstrated an increased risk of infection-related hospitalization in patients receiving higher dose intermittent versus lower dose maintenance IV iron therapy; a meta-analysis of 72 randomized controlled trials involving 10,605 patients (88) demonstrated an increased risk of infection with the use of IV versus oral or no iron; a retrospective study of 14,078 patients (89) showed no significant increased risk of infection-related mortality with IV iron dose but did demonstrate a nonsignificant trend of increased infection-related mortality in patients receiving >1,050 mg of IV iron over 3 months or >2,100 mg IV iron over 6 months; and a retrospective study of 22,820 patients on chronic HD (90) demonstrated that IV iron administration in the setting of hospitalization for infection was not associated with an increased risk of readmission for infection, increased length of stay, or mortality. A recent trial by Agarwal et al. (91) randomized 136 patients with CKD stage 3 or CKD stage 4 to IV versus oral iron and·demonstrated no significant difference in serious adverse events between the two groups. However, there was incomplete randomization, and adjustment after randomization did demonstrate a significant increase in the adjusted risk of serious adverse events including infection-related adverse events in patients receiving IV iron versus oral iron. Given the incomplete randomization, the findings of this study are difficult to interpret.

The relationship between IV iron use and overall mortality is not entirely clear at this time. A retrospective study of 32,566 patients (85) showed no association between IV iron dose and overall mortality; a retrospective study of 32,435 patients (92) demonstrated an increased risk of mortality in those receiving >300 mg/mo of IV iron; a prospective study of 58,058 patients (93) demonstrated a decreased risk of overall mortality with the use of up to 400 mg/mo of IV iron versus no iron but an increased risk of mortality with a dose of >400 mg/mo of IV iron; and a retrospective study of 14,078 patients (89) showed a decreased risk of overall mortality with the use of 150 to 350 mg/mo or >350 mg/mo of IV iron compared to 0 to150 mg/mo.

A paucity of adequately powered randomized trials of sufficient duration makes it difficult to evaluate the long-term risks and benefits of IV iron use at this time.

⬡ ERYTHROPOIESIS-STIMULATING AGENTS

Historically, anemia was an inevitable consequence of ESKD and was only treatable by regular blood transfusions, presenting a significant source of morbidity in patients with ESKD. With the advent of recombinant human erythropoietin (rHuEPO) in the 1980s, anemia became a treatable problem, with the potential of improving Hb to normal levels. Over time, additional drugs have been developed which are either derivatives of the EPO molecule or are different molecules which can directly or indirectly stimulate the EPO receptor. These medications are all grouped under the class of drugs commonly referred to as ESAs.

Epoetin

Epoetin is a term generally applied to rHuEPO preparations produced using recombinant technology via the overexpression of the human EPO gene in mammalian cell lines. Epoetin-α and epoetin-β were the first two of these compounds developed, and both are produced in Chinese hamster ovary cells. Epoetin-α is the only epoetin currently available in the United States. Several nonrandomized trials in the late 1980s demonstrated the ability of rHuEPO to increase Hb levels in patients with ESKD (94–97), leading to FDA approval of epoetin-α (Epogen; Procrit).

A number of additional epoetin preparations have been developed and are available for use outside of the United States. In particular, epoetin biosimilars, which are drugs designed as copies of either epoetin-α or epoetin-β, have been available in Europe since 2007 (98). Due to the high molecular complexity of biological medications, small changes can have a significant impact on clinical outcomes. Therefore, the FDA and other international drug-related authorities have a rigorous approval process for biosimilar medications. The potential effects of changing the formulation process of epoetins was demonstrated by the global increase in cases of pure red cell aplasia (PRCA) that occurred after subcutaneous (SC) Eprex, an epoetin-α product, was changed to an albumin-free formulation (99). There are currently no biosimilar epoetins available for use in the United States, but these drugs are expected to become available within the next few years. Details of the various epoetins are discussed below (TABLE 29.2).

Epoetin Route of Administration

Several routes of epoetin administration have been studied including IV, SC, and intraperitoneal. Intraperitoneal epoetin was found to have a bioavailability of only 3% to 8% (100) with a requirement for significantly higher doses compared to the SC route (101); it is therefore not commonly used in clinical practice. IV epoetin has a half-life of approximately 4 to 12 hours, and levels return to baseline after 2 to 3 days (100). SC epoetin has 20% to 30% bioavailability with a peak concentration at 18 hours, which is only 5% to 10% of the level that would be detected with an equivalent dose of IV epoetin; however, the levels decay much more slowly with SC administration and are still detectable 4 days later. The pharmacokinetic profile of SC epoetin appears to possess advantages over the IV route, and it has been shown that SC epoetin can maintain the same levels of Hb as IV epoetin with a 30% decrease in dose (102). Additionally, given the slower rate of decay, weekly administration of SC epoetin appears to be as effective as IV epoetin (103), whereas IV epoetin is recommended to be given thrice weekly.

The 2012 KDIGO guidelines (1) suggest that for patients with ESKD on HD, either the IV or SC route is acceptable for ESA administration, and data from DOPPS demonstrates that over 90% of patients on HD in the United States receive ESA therapy intravenously (58). A retrospective study of 62,710 patients on HD (104) demonstrated a small but significant increase in a composite outcome of death and/or cardiovascular hospitalizations among patients receiving IV versus SC epoetin-α. The study authors attributed this increased risk to the 25% increased dose of ESA used in the IV group, although they acknowledge that any conclusion from this study must be further qualified given its retrospective nature.

Darbepoetin-α

Darbepoetin-α is an EPO derivative with additional glycosylation sites which allows for an increased plasma half-life. The half-life for IV use is 25.3 hours versus 8.5 hours for epoetin (105), and SC administration has a bioavailability of 37% with a half-life of 48.8 hours. Darbepoetin appears to have comparable safety and efficacy to epoetin at a reduced dosing interval of weekly or every other week (106,107). As opposed to epoetin, there appears to be similar efficacy between IV and SC dosing (108). The conversion factor of epoetin to darbepoetin is approximately 200 U of epoetin to 1 μg of darbepoetin-α.

Methoxypolyethylene Glycol Epoetin-β

Methoxypolyethylene glycol-epoetin β, also called continuous EPO receptor activator (CERA), is a pegylated epoetin-β derivative with a half-life of approximately 130 hours when administered intravenously or subcutaneously (109). Numerous studies have shown that CERA has comparable safety and efficacy to EPO when given either once every 2 weeks or every 4 weeks (110). CERA is currently FDA approved for use in the United States under the brand name Mircera but is not commonly available for use at this time.

A meta-analysis comparing the safety and efficacy of epoetin-α, epoetin-β, darbepoetin-α, methoxypolyethylene glycol-epoetin β, and biosimilar ESAs concluded that there is insufficient evidence to suggest the superiority of any ESA formulation over another and suggested that consideration of drug cost, availability, and dosing frequency should be used to determine choice of specific ESA therapy (111).

Peginesatide

Peginesatide is an EPO-mimetic peptide that binds to the EPO receptor and increases Hb by stimulating EPO production (112). It has an amino acid sequence unrelated to that of rHuEPO

TABLE 29.2	Epoetins			
Generic Drug	**Trade Name**	**Recommended Single Dose**	**Recommended Dosing Frequency**	**Route of Administration**
Epoetin-α	Epogen; Procrit	50–100 U/kg	Three times per week	IV or SC
Epoetin-β	NeoRecormon (not available in United States)	40–100 U/kg	Three times per week	IV or SC
Darbepoetin-α	Aranesp	0.45 μg/kg weekly or 0.75 μg/kg every 2 weeks	Weekly or every 2 weeks	IV or SC
Methoxy polyethylene glycol-epoetin β	Mircera (limited United States availability)	0.6 μg/kg	Once every 2 weeks	IV or SC

IV, intravenous; SC, subcutaneous.

and was specifically recommended for use in patients with antibody-mediated red cell aplasia (1). Peginesatide was FDA approved for use in 2012, but the product was subsequently removed from the market due to a high rate of hypersensitivity reactions occurring in 0.2% of patients and fatal reactions occurring in 0.02% of patients. Peginesatide is no longer available for use.

Hypoxia-Inducible Factor Stabilizers

The HIF stabilizers are a class of oral medications that are currently undergoing clinical trials to assess their efficacy and safety in the treatment of anemia in patients with CKD and ESKD. They increase endogenous EPO production by inhibiting prolyl hydroxylase, which subsequently prevents degradation of HIFα, leading to increased endogenous EPO production by renal peritubular cells and hepatocytes (14). In addition to stimulating endogenous EPO production, HIF also plays a role in iron metabolism, and HIF stabilizers may also improve anemia by enhancing iron absorption and iron mobilization. A randomized trial of 4 weeks of oral roxadustat (FG-4592), a first-in-class prolyl hydroxylase inhibitor, versus placebo in patients with non–dialysis-dependent CKD demonstrated an average of a 1.7-g/dL increase in Hb with a concurrent decrease in serum hepcidin levels with roxadustat use (113). There are currently six different drugs in the HIF stabilizer class undergoing phase I to III clinical trials testing their overall safety and efficacy, with numerous trials comparing various HIF stabilizers to epoetin-α or darbepoetin-α. Given their success thus far in early trials, there is a strong possibility that in the next several years, HIF stabilizers will provide an additional option to the nephrologist managing anemia in patients with CKD and ESKD.

CLINICAL TRIALS: RISKS, BENEFITS, AND TARGET HEMOGLOBIN

With the advent of rHuEPO, the management of anemia in patients with ESKD dramatically improved, with a significant decrease in transfusion requirements, a decrease in iron overload caused by frequent transfusions, and the ability to achieve an almost normal Hb value in the overwhelming majority of patients with ESKD with relative ease. However, despite these apparent benefits, initial studies that first lead to FDA approval of rHuEPO in 1989 were generally nonrandomized studies involving relatively small numbers of patients being monitored for a relatively short duration. As such, the long-term safety and overall benefit of ESAs were never established initially. Since that time, several large-scale randomized controlled trials have been done in several different patient populations including patients with malignancy-associated anemia, patients with CKD not on dialysis, and patients with ESKD on dialysis. As will be discussed in greater detail, in each of these populations, these trials have raised concerns with the overall safety of ESAs.

Erythropoiesis-Stimulating Agent Use in Patients with Malignancy-Associated Anemia

Epoetin-α and darbepoetin-α are both FDA approved for the treatment of malignancy-associated anemia. While studies have consistently shown that ESAs are effective in raising Hb levels, decreasing transfusion requirements, and improving quality of life, several meta-analyses have raised concerns with the long-term safety of ESAs in this patient population. A meta-analysis from 2012 of 91 trials involving 20,102 patients being treated with ESAs for malignancy-associated anemia demonstrated a decrease

in transfusions and an improvement in quality of life but an increase in mortality during the active study period and an increase in thromboembolic events (114). A randomized trial of epoetin-β versus placebo in 351 patients with head and neck cancer demonstrated increased tumor progression with ESA use (115), but an adverse relationship of ESA use and tumor growth has not been consistently shown, with no relationship between ESA use and tumor growth seen in the aforementioned meta-analysis and several other randomized trials (116,117). Given the safety concerns of ESA use in patients with malignancy, with a possible increase in tumor growth, thromboembolic events, and death, current guidelines recommend against the use of ESAs in patients receiving myelosuppressive chemotherapy when the anticipated outcome is cure and recommend a target Hb level of 10 to 12 g/dL when using ESAs for malignancy-associated anemia.

Erythropoiesis-Stimulating Agents Use in Patients with End-Stage Kidney Disease

Several large randomized trials have been done comparing various Hb targets in patients with ESKD which have raised concerns with the overall safety of ESAs. The largest trial done in patients with ESKD was the U.S. Normal Hematocrit (HCT) Trial (118) which randomized 1,233 patients with ESKD on HD and evidence of congestive heart failure (CHF) or ischemic heart disease to receive increasing doses of epoetin to achieve a hematocrit target of 42% versus a hematocrit target of 30%. The trial was halted early due to an increase in both deaths and nonfatal myocardial infarctions in the normal hematocrit group, although this result did not achieve statistical significance since the trial was stopped prior to the possibility of this occurring. The normal hematocrit group required significantly fewer transfusions and had a significant improvement in their physical function score but also had a significant increase in the incidence of thrombosis of the vascular access site. While numerous past studies have demonstrated that ESA use increases blood pressure and the rate of hypertension (95,119), there was no significant difference in blood pressure between the two groups in the Normal HCT Trial. Given that the Normal HCT Trial included only ESKD patients with underlying cardiac disease, an additional trial was conducted in patients with ESKD on HD with an absence of symptomatic cardiac disease and a lack of left ventricular dilatation on cardiac imaging to determine if normalization of the Hb in this subpopulation of patients with ESKD had a beneficial effect on cardiac remodeling and ultimately cardiovascular events. The trial done by Parfrey et al. (120) randomized 596 patients with ESKD who had recently initiated HD to increasing doses of epoetin to achieve a target Hb of 13.5 to 14.5 g/dL versus a target of Hb of 9.5 to 11.5 g/dL and assessed left ventricular volume index (LVVI) as a primary outcome measure. The results demonstrated that despite an achieved Hb of 13.3 g/dL versus 10.9 g/dL in the higher versus lower Hb groups, there was no difference in LVVI or left ventricular mass index (LVMI). The higher Hb group had improved quality of life as demonstrated by an improved SF-36 vitality score. There was no overall difference in adverse events including death, cardiac events, and vascular access thrombosis, but there was a small but statistically significant increase in stroke in the higher Hb group.

Erythropoiesis-Stimulating Agent Use in Patients with Chronic Kidney Disease Not on Dialysis

Although initial trials in patients with ESKD demonstrated no long-term benefit to achieving a normal Hb value and even raised concerns for possible harm, given that patients with CKD are a distinct patient population with improved prognosis and decreased comorbidity burden, several randomized trials were done to evaluate the risks and benefits of targeting a normal Hb in this patient population.

The Cardiovascular Reduction Early Anemia Treatment Epoetin β (CREATE) trial (121) randomized 603 patients with an estimated glomerular filtration rate (eGFR) of 15.0 to 35.0 mL/min to SC epoetin-β treatment to an Hb target of 13.0 to 15.0 g/dL versus an Hb target of 10.5 to 11.5 g/dL. Results demonstrated no significant difference between the groups in the incidence of cardiovascular events, death, or LVMI. The higher Hb group had improved quality of life scores. There was no change in overall eGFR or eGFR decline between the two groups, although the higher Hb group had a significant increase in number of patients initiating dialysis, a finding that the study investigators found difficult to interpret. There was a higher rate of hypertension in the higher Hb group, but no change in overall adverse events and no change in AV fistula thromboses.

The Correction of Hemoglobin and Outcomes in Renal Insufficiency (CHOIR) trial (122) randomized 1,432 patients with an eGFR of 15 to 50 mL/min to SC epoetin-α to a target Hb of 13.5 g/dL versus a target Hb of 11.3 g/dL. The trial was stopped early due to a statistically significant increase in the primary end point of a composite of death, myocardial infarction, hospitalization for CHF, and stroke in the higher Hb group. None of the composite end points individually achieved statistical significance, but a near-significant increase in both deaths and CHF hospitalizations led to a statistically significant increase in the overall primary end point. Additionally, there was no improvement in quality of life scores in the higher Hb group, nor was there a significant difference in progression to ESKD. There was also an increase in serious adverse events in the higher Hb group.

The Time to Reconsider Evidence for Anaemia Treatment (TREAT) trial (123) is the largest trial to date of an ESA and randomized 4,038 patients with diabetes and an eGFR of 20 to 60 mL/min to SC darbepoetin-α to a target Hb of 13 g/dL versus placebo with the availability of darbepoetin-α rescue therapy only when the Hb decreased below 9.0 g/dL. There was no significant difference between the two groups in the incidence of death or cardiovascular events, although there was a significant increase in stroke, arterial thromboembolic events, and venous thromboembolic events in the higher Hb group. The higher Hb group also had a significant decrease in transfusions and a modest improvement in patient-reported fatigue scores. There was no difference in the incidence of progression to ESKD between the two groups, but the higher Hb group did have a significant decrease in cardiac revascularization procedures. Although not a prespecified outcome, among patients with a baseline history of cancer, there was a nonsignificant increase in deaths and a significant increase in cancer-related deaths in the higher Hb group.

Summarizing the Data

The aforementioned randomized trials of ESA use in patients with CKD and ESKD (**Table 29.3**) have demonstrated that achieving normal Hb values provides modest benefits including decreased transfusion requirements and improved physical functioning and quality of life, but there are consistently no significant long-term benefits such as a decrease in mortality or cardiac events. Furthermore, all of the studies showed increased risks, although the

precise risks were inconsistent from study to study. For example, the Parfrey et al. study (120) and the TREAT trial (123) showed a significant increase in stroke, but this finding was absent in the CREATE (121) and CHOIR (122) trials. The Normal HCT trial (118) and the CHOIR trial (122) both demonstrated an increase in mortality, but this finding was absent in CREATE (121) and TREAT (123) trials. The CREATE trial showed a significant increase in the rate of progression to ESKD, and the Normal HCT Trial demonstrated an increased rate of vascular access thrombosis, but neither of those findings were consistently seen throughout the other trials.

The results of the aforementioned trials which have demonstrated very modest benefits with a concern for significant harm has led to recommendations for judicious use of ESAs in patients with CKD and ESKD, with current guidelines recommending great caution when considering ESA use in patients with active malignancy, a history of malignancy, or a history of stroke (1). Furthermore, the epoetin-α package insert recommends using the lowest dose sufficient to reduce the need for blood transfusions.

Target Hemoglobin

All of the aforementioned trials randomized patients to a normal Hb target versus an Hb target of 9 to 11.3 g/dL depending on the trial. While it is generally accepted that the risks of achieving a normal Hb level outweigh the benefits, there is little data to determine what the ideal Hb target should be. As such, the most optimal approach at this time is an individualized one which takes into account the patient's particular risks as related to his comorbidities and his particular benefits as related to his transfusion needs and anemia symptom burden. KDIGO guidelines recommend initiating the use of ESAs in patients with ESKD when the Hb level decreases below 10 g/dL with a goal of maintaining the Hb up to 11.5 g/dL (1); however, the guidelines state that one can consider initiating ESA use when the Hb is above 10.0 g/dL and maintaining an Hb level greater than 11.5 g/dL for individual patients who may have an improvement in quality of life with higher Hb levels and are prepared to accept the added risks of treatment. Intentionally maintaining an Hb level above 13.0 g/dL is recommended against under all circumstances. In addition to maintaining higher Hb levels for specific individual patients, there are specific patient populations for whom a lower Hb target may be indicated such as patients with sickle cell anemia or cirrhosis, as studies in these patient populations have demonstrated increased risk even with Hb levels above 10 g/dL (124,125).

Erythropoiesis-Stimulating Agent Dosing

The initial dose of ESA used should be individualized based on the patient's initial Hb, body weight, and clinical circumstances (1). Generally speaking, it is recommended to start with a lower dose of ESA to minimize ESA-related cardiovascular risks, and it is recommended to avoid raising the Hb by more than 2.0 g/dL per month. If the Hb level is increasing by more than 2.0 g/dL per month, the dose should be held or reduced by 50%. While initiating ESA therapy, Hb levels should be checked at least monthly and up to weekly, and a time period of 2 to 4 weeks should generally be allowed to assess the full effect of the ESA dose prior to making dose adjustments. If the Hb value increases above the target, the ESA dose can be held or continued at a reduced dose, the latter being recommended by KDIGO (1). Once a stable Hb level is achieved on a steady dose of ESA, Hb levels need not be monitored more frequently than monthly.

TABLE 29.3	Summary of Randomized Controlled Trials of Erythropoiesis-Stimulating Agent Use in Patients with Chronic Kidney Disease and End-Stage Kidney Disease					
Randomized Controlled Trials	Number of Patients	Intervention	Inclusion Criteria	Exclusion Criteria	Primary Outcome	Results	Adverse Events
U.S. Normal HCT Trial (118)	1,233	Epoetin-α administration to target HCT of 42% versus 30%	Patients with CHF or ischemic heart disease on chronic hemodialysis	DBP >100 mm Hg; severe cardiac disability; MI, PTCA, CABG in prior 3 mo	Time to death or nonfatal MI	Nonsignificant increase in primary outcome (CI 0.9–1.9)	Significant increase in vascular access thrombosis; nonsignificant increase in deaths
Canadian Normal HCT Trial (12C)	596	Epoetin-α administration to target Hb range of 13.5–14.5 g/dL versus 9.5–11.5 g/dL	Patients who initiated hemodialysis during the prior 3–18 months with an LVVI <100 mL/m²	Symptomatic ischemic heart disease or heart failure; angiographic critical CAD	Difference in change in LVVI	No difference between groups in LVVI or LVMI change	Significant increase in strokes
CREATE (121)	603	Epoetin-β administration to a target Hb of 13.0–15.0 g/dL versus 10.5–11.5 g/dL	Patients with an eGFR 15–35 mL/min, Hb 11.0–12.5 g/dL, and a BP less than 170/95 mm Hg	Anticipated need for RRT in the next 6 mo; advanced cardiovascular disease; nonrenal cause of anemia	Time to first cardiovascular event	No significant difference between groups in cardiovascular events, death, or LVMI	Significant increase in progression to ESKD
CHOIR (122)	1,432	Epoetin-α administration to a target Hb of 13.5 g/dL versus 11.3 g/dL	Patients with an eGFR 15–50 mL/min, Hb <11.0 g/dL	Uncontrolled HTN; active GI bleeding; iron overload state; active cancer; prior ESA use	Time to composite of death, MI, hospitalization for CHF, or stroke	Significant increase in the composite outcome, primarily driven by a near significant increase in both deaths and hospitalization for CHF	Increased risk of serious adverse events overall, including a significant increase in CHF episodes
TREAT (123)	4,038	Darbepoetin-α administration to a target Hb of 13 g/dL versus placebo with darbepoetin-α rescue therapy available only when the Hb decreased below 9.0 g/dL	Patients with type 2 DM, eGFR 20–60 mL/min, Hb <11.0 g/dL, and TSAT >15%	Uncontrolled HTN; prior receipt of or planning for upcoming kidney transplant; current use of IV antibiotics, chemotherapy, or radiation therapy; cancer; HIV; active bleeding; hematologic disease	Time to composite of death or cardiovascular event; time to composite of death or ESKD	No significant difference between groups in both composite outcomes of death and cardiovascular events or death and ESKD; significant increase in fatal and nonfatal strokes	Significant increase in fatal and nonfatal strokes; significant increase in venous and arterial thromboembolic events; significant decrease in cardiac revascularization procedures

HCT, hematocrit; CHF, congestive heart failure; DBP, diastolic blood pressure; MI, myocardial infarction; PTCA, percutaneous transluminal coronary angioplasty; CABG, coronary artery bypass grafting; CI, confidence interval; Hb, hemoglobin; LVVI, left ventricular volume index; CAD, coronary artery disease; LVMI, left ventricular mass index; CREATE, Cardiovascular Reduction Early Anemia Treatment Epoetin β; eGFR, estimated glomerular filtration rate; BF, blood pressure; RRT, renal replacement therapy; ESKD, end-stage kidney disease; CHOIR, Correction of Hemoglobin and Outcomes in Renal Insufficiency; HTN, hypertension; GI, gastrointestinal; ESA, erythropoiesis-stimulating agent; TREAT, Time to Reconsider Evidence for Anaemia Treatment; DM, diabetes mellitus; TSAT, transferrin saturation; IV, intravenous.

Erythropoiesis-Stimulating Agent Hyporesponsiveness

Lack of an appropriate response in erythropoiesis despite appropriate weight-based ESA dosing is a commonly encountered problem while managing anemia in patients with ESKD and has been shown to correlate to poor outcomes including increased cardiovascular events and death (126). Poor response to ESA therapy may portend a poor prognosis as a result of representing a significant disease marker or by leading to escalating doses of ESA therapy which itself may lead to an increased risk of cardiovascular events and death. For this reason, ESA hyporesponsiveness should be managed by initiating a search for reversible causes of ESA hyporesponsiveness and, if no reversible cause can be identified, the acceptance of a lower Hb target with a limited increase in ESA dose and the possible need for regular blood transfusions; it should not be managed through ever escalating doses of ESA therapy.

KDIGO defines initial ESA hyporesponsiveness as a lack of increase in Hb level after 1 month of treatment with appropriate weight-based dosing and acquired ESA hyporesponsiveness as the need to increase the ESA dose twice up to an increase of 50% of the prior dose to maintain a stable Hb value from prior. In the setting of initial or acquired ESA hyporesponsiveness, the ESA dose should not be increased by more than two times the initial weight-based dose or the prior dose on which the patient had achieved a target Hb level (1).

Workup for ESA hyporesponsiveness should include evaluation for iron, vitamin B_{12}, and folate deficiency. Medications should be carefully reviewed, and discontinuation of ACE inhibitors and ARBs should be considered. Secondary hyperparathyroidism has been associated with ESA hyporesponsiveness (127), and parathyroid hormone levels should be optimized. Underlying causes of ongoing inflammation such as infection, chronic rejection of a prior failed transplant, or malnutrition should be considered. Additional causes of ESA hyporesponsiveness include primary marrow disorders such hemoglobinopathies, aluminum toxicity, occult malignancy, and antibody-mediated PRCA and should be evaluated for when appropriate. PRCA should be suspected in the setting of a decreasing Hb level or new transfusion requirements on a steady dose of ESA and an absolute reticulocyte count of less than 10,000/μL.

Often, despite an exhaustive search, no reversible cause of ESA hyporesponsiveness is identified, and management needs to be adjusted toward a lower Hb target with the possible need for regular blood transfusions.

CONCLUSION

Anemia is a nearly universal complication of ESKD and contributes significantly to the morbidity of patients with ESKD. It is usually multifactorial due to relative EPO deficiency, negative iron balance, and chronic inflammation leading to poor iron absorption and utilization, and its treatment consists of ESA administration, iron supplementation, and ongoing surveillance for underlying causes of chronic inflammation. Despite significant advances in the treatment of anemia in patients with ESKD over the last several decades, the long-term benefits of Hb correction have never been rigorously demonstrated, concerns abound related to the safety of ESA use, and the ideal balance of iron supplementation and ESA use have not been rigorously tested. Several new medications are either now FDA approved or in the process of being tested for the management of anemia in patients with ESKD including iron-containing oral phosphate binders and HIF stabilizers, and only time will tell how these new options will affect the treatment of anemia in patients with ESKD.

REFERENCES

1. Kidney Disease: Improving Global Outcomes. KDIGO Clinical Practice Guideline for anemia in chronic kidney disease. *Kidney Int* 2012;2: 279–335.
2. Stauffer ME, Fan T. Prevalence of anemia in chronic kidney disease in the United States. *Plos One* 2014;9(1):e84943.
3. Astor BC, Muntner P, Levin A, et al. Association of Kidney Function with Anemia: the Third National Health and Nutrition Examination Survey (1988-1994). *Arch Intern Med* 2002;162(12):1401–1408.
4. Saran RN, Li Y, Robinson B, et al. US Renal Data System 2014 annual data report: epidemiology of kidney disease in the United States. *Am J Kidney Dis* 2015;66(1 Suppl 1):S1–S305.
5. Regidor DL, Kopple JD, Kovesdy CP, et al. Associations between changes in hemoglobin and administered erythropoiesis-stimulating agent and survival in hemodialysis patients. *J Am Soc Nephrol* 2006;17(4): 1181–1191.
6. Servilla KS, Singh AK, Hunt WC, et al. Anemia management and association of race with mortality and hospitalization in a large not-for-profit dialysis organization. *Am J Kidney Dis* 2009;54(3):498–510.
7. Fort J, Cuevas X, García F, et al. Mortality in incident haemodialysis patients: time-dependent haemoglobin levels and erythropoiesis-stimulating agent dose are independent predictive factors in the ANSWER study. *Nephrol Dial Transplant* 2010;25(8):2702–2710.
8. Eckardt KU. Pathophysiology of renal anemia. *Clin Nephrol* 2000;53 (1 Suppl):S2–S8.
9. Metivier F, Marchais SJ, Guerin AP, et al. Pathophysiology of anaemia: focus on the heart and blood vessels. *Nephrol Dial Transplant* 2000;15(Suppl 3):14–18.
10. Mujais SK, Story K, Brouillette J, et al. Health-related quality of life in CKD patients: correlates and evolution over time. *Clin J Am Soc Nephrol* 2009;4(8):1293–1301.
11. Finkelstein FO, Story K, Firanek C, et al. Health-related quality of life and hemoglobin levels in chronic kidney disease patients. *Clin J Am Soc Nephrol* 2009;4(1):33–38.
12. Suzuki N, Obara N, Yamamoto M. Use of gene-manipulated mice in the study of erythropoietin gene expression. *Methods Enzymol* 2007;435:157–177.
13. Obara N, Suzuki N, Kim K, et al. Repression via the GATA box is essential for tissue-specific erythropoietin gene expression. *Blood* 2008;111(10):5223–5232.
14. Koury MJ, Haase VH. Anaemia in kidney disease: harnessing hypoxia responses for therapy. *Nat Rev Nephrol* 2015;11(7):394–410.
15. Silva M, Grillot D, Benito A, et al. Erythropoietin can promote erythroid progenitor survival by repressing apoptosis through Bcl-XL and Bcl-2. *Blood* 1996;88(5):1576–1582.
16. Hamada Y, Fukagawa M. Is hepcidin the star player in iron metabolism in chronic kidney disease? *Kidney Int* 2009;75(9):873–874.
17. Young B, Zaritsky J. Hepcidin for clinicians. *Clin J Am Soc Nephrol* 2009;4(8):1384–1387.
18. Nemeth E, Valore EV, Territo M, et al. Hepcidin, a putative mediator of anemia of inflammation, is a type II acute-phase protein. *Blood* 2003;101(7):2461–2463.
19. Erslev AJ, Besarab A. Erythropoietin in the pathogenesis and treatment of the anemia of chronic renal failure. *Kidney Int* 1997;51(3): 622–630.
20. Kalantar-Zadeh K, Ikizler TA, Block G, et al. Malnutrition-inflammation complex syndrome in dialysis patients: causes and consequences. *Am J Kidney Dis* 2003;42(5):864–881.
21. Eschbach JW. Erythropoietin 1991—an overview. *Am J Kidney Dis* 1991;18(4 Suppl 1):3–9.
22. Erslev AJ. Erythropoietin. *N Engl J Med* 1991;324(19):1339–1344.
23. Radtke HW, Claussner A, Erbes PM, et al. Serum erythropoietin concentration in chronic renal failure: relationship to degree of anemia and excretory renal function. *Blood* 1979;54(4):877–884.
24. Bernhardt WM, Wiesener MS, Scigalla P, et al. Inhibition of prolyl hydroxylases increases erythropoietin production in ESRD. *J Am Soc Nephrol* 2010;21(12):2151–2156.

25. Wasse H, Gillen DL, Ball AM, et al. Risk factors for upper gastrointestinal bleeding among end-stage renal disease patients. *Kidney Int* 2003;64(4):1455–1461.

26. Bini EJ, Kinkhabwala A, Goldfarb DS. Predictive value of a positive fecal occult blood test increases as the severity of CKD worsens. *Am J Kidney Dis* 2006;48(4):580–586.

27. Otti T, Khajehdehi P, Fawzy A, et al. Comparison of blood loss with different high-flux and high-efficiency hemodialysis membranes. *Am J Nephrol* 2001;21(1):16–19.

28. Eschbach JW Jr, Funk D, Adamson J, et al. Erythropoiesis in patients with renal failure undergoing chronic dialysis. *N Engl J Med* 1967;276(12):653–658.

29. Ly J, Marticorena R, Donnelly S. Red blood cell survival in chronic renal failure. *Am J Kidney Dis* 2004;44(4):715–719.

30. Vos FE, Schollum JB, Coulter CV, et al. Red blood cell survival in long-term dialysis patients. *Am J Kidney Dis* 2011;58(4):591–598.

31. Chertow GM, Levin NW, Beck GJ, et al. In-center hemodialysis six times per week versus three times per week. *N Engl J Med* 2010;363(24):2287–2300.

32. Teschner M, Kosch M, Schaefer RM. Folate metabolism in renal failure. *Nephrol Dial Transplant* 2002;17(Suppl 5):24–27.

33. Jaffe JA, Liftman C, Glickman JD. Frequency of elevated serum aluminum levels in adult dialysis patients. *Am J Kidney Dis* 2005;46(2):316–319.

34. Touam M, Martinez F, Lacour B, et al. Aluminium-induced, reversible microcytic anemia in chronic renal failure: clinical and experimental studies. *Clin Nephrol* 1983;19(6):295–298.

35. Gossmann J, Thürmann P, Bachmann T, et al. Mechanism of angiotensin converting enzyme inhibitor-related anemia in renal transplant recipients. *Kidney Int* 1996;50(3):973–978.

36. Korzets A, Zevin D, Chagnac A, et al. Angiotensin-converting enzyme inhibition and anaemia in renal patients. *Acta Haematol* 1993;90(4):202–205.

37. Graafland AD, Doorenbos CJ, van Saase JC. Enalapril-induced anemia in two kidney transplant recipients. *Transpl Int* 1992;5(1):51–53.

38. Cole J, Ertoy D, Lin H, et al. Lack of angiotensin II-facilitated erythropoiesis causes anemia in angiotensin-converting enzyme-deficient mice. *J Clin Invest* 2000;106(11):1391–1398.

39. Saudan P, Halabi G, Perneger T, et al. ACE inhibitors or angiotensin II receptor blockers in dialysed patients and erythropoietin resistance. *J Nephrol* 2006;19(1):91–96.

40. Grzegorzewska AE. Erythropoietin dose and angiotensin-converting enzyme inhibitors. *Perit Dial Int* 2007;27(1):102–103.

41. Albitar S, Genin R, Fen-Chong M, et al. High dose enalapril impairs the response to erythropoietin treatment in haemodialysis patients. *Nephrol Dial Transplant* 1998;13(5):1206–1210.

42. Ertük S, Nergizoğlu G, Ateş K, et al. The impact of withdrawing ACE inhibitors on erythropoietin responsiveness and left ventricular hypertrophy in haemodialysis patients. *Nephrol Dial Transplant* 1999;14(8):1912–1916.

43. Fehr T, Ammann P, Garzoni D, et al. Interpretation of erythropoietin levels in patients with various degrees of renal insufficiency and anemia. *Kidney Int* 2004;66(3):1206–1211.

44. Nyvad O, Danielsen H, Madsen S. Intravenous iron-sucrose complex to reduce epoetin demand in dialysis patients. *Lancet* 1994;344(8932):1305–1306.

45. Fishbane S, Frei GL, Maesaka J. Reduction in recombinant human erythropoietin doses by the use of chronic intravenous iron supplementation. *Am J Kidney Dis* 1995;26(1):41–46.

46. Taylor JE, Peat N, Porter C, et al. Regular low-dose intravenous iron therapy improves response to erythropoietin in haemodialysis patients. *Nephrol Dial Transplant* 1996;11(6):1079–1083.

47. Macdougall IC, Tucker B, Thompson J, et al. A randomized controlled study of iron supplementation in patients treated with erythropoietin. *Kidney Int* 1996;50(5):1694–1699.

48. Besarab A, Amin N, Ahsan M, et al. Optimization of epoetin therapy with intravenous iron therapy in hemodialysis patients. *J Am Soc Nephrol* 2000;11(3):530–538.

49. Coyne DW, Kapoian T, Suki W, et al. Ferric gluconate is highly efficacious in anemic hemodialysis patients with high serum ferritin and low transferrin saturation: results of the Dialysis Patients' Response to IV Iron with Elevated Ferritin (DRIVE) Study. *J Am Soc Nephrol* 2007;18(3):975–984.

50. Braun J, Hammerschmidt M, Schreiber M, et al. Is zinc protoporphyrin an indicator of iron-deficient erythropoiesis in maintenance haemodialysis patients? *Nephrol Dial Transplant* 1996;11(3):492–497.

51. Braun J, Lindner K, Schreiber M, et al. Percentage of hypochromic red blood cells as predictor of erythropoietic and iron response after i.v. iron supplementation in maintenance haemodialysis patients. *Nephrol Dial Transplant* 1997;12(6):1173–1181.

52. Brugnara C, Zelmanovic D, Sorette M, et al. Reticulocyte hemoglobin: an integrated parameter for evaluation of erythropoietic activity. *Am J Clin Pathol* 1997;108(2):133–142.

53. Tessitore N, Girelli D, Campostrini N, et al. Hepcidin is not useful as a biomarker for iron needs in haemodialysis patients on maintenance erythropoiesis-stimulating agents. *Nephrol Dial Transplant* 2010;25(12):3996–4002.

54. National Kidney Foundation. II. Clinical practice guidelines and clinical practice recommendations for anemia in chronic kidney disease in adults. *Am J Kidney Dis* 2006;47(5 Suppl 3):S16–S85.

55. Spiegel DM, Chertow GM. Lost without directions: lessons from the anemia debate and the drive study. *Clin J Am Soc Nephrol* 2009;4(5):1009–1010.

56. Albaramki J, Hodson EM, Craig JC, et al. Parenteral versus oral iron therapy for adults and children with chronic kidney disease. *Cochrane Database Syst Rev* 2012;(1):CD007857.

57. Nakanishi T, Hasuike Y, Nanami M, et al. Novel iron-containing phosphate binders and anemia treatment in CKD: oral iron intake revisited [published online ahead of print July 3, 2015]. *Nephrol Dial Transplant*.

58. Arbor Research Collaborative for Health. DOPPS practice monitor. http://www.dopps.org/dpm/DPMSlideBrowser.aspx. Accessed October 26, 2015.

59. Auerbach M, Macdougall IC. Safety of intravenous iron formulations: facts and folklore. *Blood Transfus* 2014;12(3):296–300.

60. Chertow GM, Mason PD, Vaage-Nilsen O, et al. Update on adverse drug events associated with parenteral iron. *Nephrol Dial Transplant* 2006;21(2):378–382.

61. Chertow GM, Mason PD, Vaage-Nilsen O, et al. On the relative safety of parenteral iron formulations. *Nephrol Dial Transplant* 2004;19(6):1571–1575.

62. Fletes R, Lazarus JM, Gage J, et al. Suspected iron dextran-related adverse drug events in hemodialysis patients. *Am J Kidney Dis* 2001;37(4):743–749.

63. Auerbach M, Al Talib K. Low-molecular weight iron dextran and iron sucrose have similar comparative safety profiles in chronic kidney disease. *Kidney Int* 2008;73(5):528–530.

64. Auerbach M, Pappadakis JA, Bahrain H, et al. Safety and efficacy of rapidly administered (one hour) one gram of low molecular weight iron dextran (INFeD) for the treatment of iron deficient anemia. *Am J Hematol* 2011;86(10):860–862.

65. Macdougall IC, Strauss WE, McLaughlin J, et al. A randomized comparison of ferumoxytol and iron sucrose for treating iron deficiency anemia in patients with CKD. *Clin J Am Soc Nephrol* 2014;9(4):705–712.

66. Sheashaa H, El-Husseini A, Sabry A, et al. Parenteral iron therapy in treatment of anemia in end-stage renal disease patients: a comparative study between iron saccharate and gluconate. *Nephron Clin Pract* 2005;99(4):c97–c101.

67. Chandler G, Harchowal J, Macdougall IC. Intravenous iron sucrose: establishing a safe dose. *Am J Kidney Dis* 2001;38(5):988–991.

68. Okam MM, Mandell E, Hevelone N, et al. Comparative rates of adverse events with different formulations of intravenous iron. *Am J Hematol* 2012;87(11):E123–E124.

69. Bailie GR, Clark JA, Lane CE, et al. Hypersensitivity reactions and deaths associated with intravenous iron preparations. *Nephrol Dial Transplant* 2005;20(7):1443–1449.

70. Folkert VW, Michael B, Agarwal R, et al. Chronic use of sodium ferric gluconate complex in hemodialysis patients: safety of higher-dose (≥250 mg) administration. *Am J Kidney Dis* 2003;41(3):651–657.

71. McCullough BJ, Kolokythas O, Maki JH, et al. Ferumoxytol in clinical practice: implications for MRI. *J Magn Reson Imaging* 2013;37(6):1476–1479.

72. Hetzel D, Strauss W, Bernard K, et al. A phase III, randomized, open-label trial of ferumoxytol compared with iron sucrose for the treatment of iron deficiency anemia in patients with a history of unsatisfactory oral iron therapy. *Am J Hematol* 2014;89(6):646–650.

73. Rosner MH, Auerbach M. Ferumoxytol for the treatment of iron deficiency. *Expert Rev Hematol* 2011;4(4):399–406.

74. Auerbach M, Strauss W, Auerbach S, et al. Safety and efficacy of total dose infusion of 1,020 mg of ferumoxytol administered over 15 min. *Am J Hematol* 2013;88(11):944–947.

75. Onken JE, Bregman DB, Harrington RA, et al. A multicenter, randomized, active-controlled study to investigate the efficacy and safety of intravenous ferric carboxymaltose in patients with iron deficiency anemia. *Transfusion* 2014;54(2):306–315.

76. Van Wyck DB, Mangione A, Morrison J, et al. Large-dose intravenous ferric carboxymaltose injection for iron deficiency anemia in heavy uterine bleeding: a randomized, controlled trial. *Transfusion* 2009;49(12):2719–2728.

77. Anker SD, Comin Colet J, Filippatos G, et al. Ferric carboxymaltose in patients with heart failure and iron deficiency. *N Engl J Med* 2009;361(25):2436–2448.

78. Macdougall IC, Bock AH, Carrera F, et al. FIND-CKD: a randomized trial of intravenous ferric carboxymaltose versus oral iron in patients with chronic kidney disease and iron deficiency anaemia. *Nephrol Dial Transplant* 2014;29(11):2075–2084.

79. Onken JE, Bregman DB, Harrington RA, et al. Ferric carboxymaltose in patients with iron-deficiency anemia and impaired renal function: the REPAIR-IDA trial. *Nephrol Dial Transplant* 2014;29(4):833–842.

80. Besarab A. Resolving the paradigm crisis in intravenous iron and erythropoietin management. *Kidney Int Suppl* 2006;(101):S13–S18.

81. Besarab A, Kaiser JW, Frinak S. A study of parenteral iron regimens in hemodialysis patients. *Am J Kidney Dis* 1999;34(1):21–28.

82. Bolaños L, Castro P, Falcón TG, et al. Continuous intravenous sodium ferric gluconate improves efficacy in the maintenance phase of EPOrHu administration in hemodialysis patients. *Am J Nephrol* 2002;22(1):67–72.

83. Fishbane SN, Singh AK, Cournoyer SH, et al. Ferric pyrophosphate citrate (Triferic™) administration via the dialysate maintains hemoglobin and iron balance in chronic hemodialysis patients. *Nephrol Dial Transplant* 2015;30(12):2019–2026.

84. Gupta A, Lin V, Guss C, et al. Ferric pyrophosphate citrate administered via dialysate reduces erythropoiesis-stimulating agent use and maintains hemoglobin in hemodialysis patients. *Kidney Int* 2015;88(5):1187–1194.

85. Feldman HI, Joffe M, Robinson B, et al. Administration of parenteral iron and mortality among hemodialysis patients. *J Am Soc Nephrol* 2004;15(6):1623–1632.

86. Hoen B, Paul-Dauphin A, Kessler M. Intravenous iron administration does not significantly increase the risk of bacteremia in chronic hemodialysis patients. *Clin Nephrol* 2002;57(6):457–461.

87. Brookhart MA, Freburger JK, Ellis AR, et al. Infection risk with bolus versus maintenance iron supplementation in hemodialysis patients. *J Am Soc Nephrol* 2013;24(7):1151–1158.

88. Litton E, Xiao J, Ho KM. Safety and efficacy of intravenous iron therapy in reducing requirement for allogeneic blood transfusion: systematic review and meta-analysis of randomised clinical trials. *BMJ* 2013;347:f4822.

89. Miskulin DC, Tangri N, Bandeen-Roche K, et al. Intravenous iron exposure and mortality in patients on hemodialysis. *Clin J Am Soc Nephrol* 2014;9(11):1930–1939.

90. Ishida JH, Marafino BJ, McCulloch CE, et al. Receipt of intravenous iron and clinical outcomes among hemodialysis patients hospitalized for infection. *Clin J Am Soc Nephrol* 2015;10(10):1799–1805.

91. Agarwal R, Kusek JW, Pappas MK. A randomized trial of intravenous and oral iron in chronic kidney disease. *Kidney Int* 2015;88(4):905–914.

92. Bailie GR, Larkina M, Goodkin DA, et al. Data from the Dialysis Outcomes and Practice Patterns Study validate an association between high intravenous iron doses and mortality. *Kidney Int* 2015;87(1):162–168.

93. Kalantar-Zadeh K, Regidor DL, McAllister CJ, et al. Time-dependent associations between iron and mortality in hemodialysis patients. *J Am Soc Nephrol* 2005;16(10):3070–3080.

94. Eschbach JW, Egrie JC, Downing MR, et al. Correction of the anemia of end-stage renal disease with recombinant human erythropoietin. Results of a combined phase I and II clinical trial. *N Engl J Med* 1987;316(2):73–78.

95. Eschbach JW, Abdulhadi MH, Browne JK, et al. Recombinant human erythropoietin in anemic patients with end-stage renal disease. Results of a phase III multicenter clinical trial. *Ann Intern Med* 1989;111(12):992–1000.

96. Eschbach JW, Kelly MR, Haley NR, et al. Treatment of the anemia of progressive renal failure with recombinant human erythropoietin. *N Engl J Med* 1989;321(3):158–163.

97. Winearls CG, Oliver DO, Pippard MJ, et al. Effect of human erythropoietin derived from recombinant DNA on the anaemia of patients maintained by chronic haemodialysis. *Lancet* 1986;2(8517):1175–1178.

98. Mikhail A, Farouk M. Epoetin biosimilars in Europe: five years on. *Adv Ther* 2013;30(1):28–40.

99. Eckardt KU, Casadevall N. Pure red-cell aplasia due to anti-erythropoietin antibodies. *Nephrol Dial Transplant* 2003;18(5):865–869.

100. Macdougall IC, Roberts DE, Coles GA, et al. Clinical pharmacokinetics of epoetin (recombinant human erythropoietin). *Clin Pharmacokinet* 1991;20(2):99–113.

101. Johnson CA, Wakeen M, Taylor CA III, et al. Comparison of intraperitoneal and subcutaneous epoetin alfa in peritoneal dialysis patients. *Perit Dial Int* 1999;19(6):578–582.

102. Kaufman JS, Reda DJ, Fye CL, et al. Subcutaneous compared with intravenous epoetin in patients receiving hemodialysis. Department of Veterans Affairs Cooperative Study Group on Erythropoietin in Hemodialysis Patients. *N Engl J Med* 1998;339(9):578–583.

103. Macdougall IC. Once-weekly erythropoietic therapy: is there a difference between the available preparations? *Nephrol Dial Transplant* 2002;17(12):2047–2051.

104. Wright DG, Wright EC, Narva AS, et al. Association of erythropoietin dose and route of administration with clinical outcomes for patients on hemodialysis in the United States. *Clin J Am Soc Nephrol* 2015;10(10):1822–1830.

105. Macdougall IC, Gray SJ, Elston O, et al. Pharmacokinetics of novel erythropoiesis stimulating protein compared with epoetin alfa in dialysis patients. *J Am Soc Nephrol* 1999;10(11):2392–2395.

106. Locatelli F, Olivares J, Wlaker R, et al. Novel erythropoiesis stimulating protein for treatment of anemia in chronic renal insufficiency. *Kidney Int* 2001;60(2):741–747.

107. Vanrenterghem Y, Bárány P, Mann JF, et al. Randomized trial of darbepoetin alfa for treatment of renal anemia at a reduced dose frequency compared with rHuEPO in dialysis patients. *Kidney Int* 2002;62(6):2167–2175.

108. Aarup M, Bryndum J, Dieperink H, et al. Clinical implications of converting stable haemodialysis patients from subcutaneous to intravenous administration of darbepoetin alfa. *Nephrol Dial Transplant* 2006;21(5):1312–1316.

109. Macdougall IC. CERA (Continuous Erythropoietin Receptor Activator): a new erythropoiesis-stimulating agent for the treatment of anemia. *Curr Hematol Rep* 2005;4(6):436–440.

110. Ohashi N, Sakao Y, Yasuda H, et al. Methoxy polyethylene glycol-epoetin beta for anemia with chronic kidney disease. *Int J Nephrol Renovasc Dis* 2012;5:53–60.

111. Palmer SC, Saglimbene V, Mavridis D, et al. Erythropoiesis-stimulating agents for anaemia in adults with chronic kidney disease: a network meta-analysis. *Cochrane Database Syst Rev* 2014;(12):CD010590.

112. Macdougall IC. Hematide, a novel peptide-based erythropoiesis-stimulating agent for the treatment of anemia. *Curr Opin Investig Drugs* 2008;9(9):1034–1047.

113. Besarab A, Provenzano R, Hertel J, et al. Randomized placebo-controlled dose-ranging and pharmacodynamics study of roxadustat (FG-4592) to treat anemia in nondialysis-dependent chronic kidney disease (NDD-CKD) patients. *Nephrol Dial Transplant* 2015;30(10): 1665–1673.

114. Tonia T, Mettler A, Robert N, et al. Erythropoietin or darbepoetin for patients with cancer. *Cochrane Database Syst Rev* 2012;(12):CD003407.

115. Henke M, Laszig R, Rübe C, et al. Erythropoietin to treat head and neck cancer patients with anaemia undergoing radiotherapy: randomised, double-blind, placebo-controlled trial. *Lancet* 2003;362(9392): 1255–1260.

116. Aapro M, Leonard RC, Barnadas A, et al. Effect of once-weekly epoetin beta on survival in patients with metastatic breast cancer receiving anthracycline- and/or taxane-based chemotherapy: results of the Breast Cancer-Anemia and the Value of Erythropoietin (BRAVE) study. *J Clin Oncol* 2008;26(4):592–598.

117. Fujisaka Y, Sugiyama T, Saito H, et al. Randomised, phase III trial of epoetin-β to treat chemotherapy-induced anaemia according to the EU regulation. *Br J Cancer* 2011;105(9):1267–1272.

118. Besarab A, Bolton WK, Browne JK, et al. The effects of normal as compared with low hematocrit values in patients with cardiac disease who are receiving hemodialysis and epoetin. *N Engl J Med* 1998;339(9):584–590.

119. Krapf R, Hulter HN. Arterial hypertension induced by erythropoietin and erythropoiesis-stimulating agents (ESA). *Clin J Am Soc Nephrol* 2009;4(2):470–480.

120. Parfrey PS, Foley RN, Wittreich BH, et al. Double-blind comparison of full and partial anemia correction in incident hemodialysis patients without symptomatic heart disease. *J Am Soc Nephrol* 2005;16(7):2180–2189.

121. Drüeke TB, Locatelli F, Clyne N, et al. Normalization of hemoglobin level in patients with chronic kidney disease and anemia. *N Engl J Med* 2006;355(20):2071–2084.

122. Singh AK, Szczech L, Tang KL, et al. Correction of anemia with epoetin alfa in chronic kidney disease. *N Engl J Med* 2006;355(20): 2085–2098.

123. Pfeffer MA, Burdmann EA, Chen CY, et al. A trial of darbepoetin alfa in type 2 diabetes and chronic kidney disease. *N Engl J Med* 2009;361(21):2019–2032.

124. Boyle SM, Jacobs B, Sayani FA, et al. Management of the dialysis patient with sickle cell disease. *Semin Dial* 2015;29(1):62–70.

125. Villanueva C, Colomo A, Bosch A, et al. Transfusion strategies for acute upper gastrointestinal bleeding. *N Engl J Med* 2013;368(1):11–21.

126. Solomon SD, Uno H, Lewis EF, et al. Erythropoietic response and outcomes in kidney disease and type 2 diabetes. *N Engl J Med* 2010;363(12):1146–1155.

127. Gaweda AE, Goldsmith LJ, Brier ME, et al. Iron, inflammation, dialysis adequacy, nutritional status, and hyperparathyroidism modify erythropoietic response. *Clin J Am Soc Nephrol* 2010;5(4):576–581.

CHAPTER 30

Neurologic Complications Associated with Dialysis and Chronic Kidney Disease

Imran I. Ali and Noor A. Pirzada

Chronic kidney disease (CKD) is associated with neurologic derangements that involve both the central and the peripheral nervous system (1–4). Several of these neurologic syndromes are well defined, and their clinical characteristics are protean and nonspecific (2,3). The diagnosis of these disorders is sometimes straightforward, although a high index of suspicion is required to exclude other potentially serious and possibly reversible causes. Moreover, it is important to remember that some systemic disorders that result in kidney disease may also cause neurologic symptoms. For example, polyarteritis nodosa may present with kidney disease and mononeuritis multiplex or central nervous system involvement requiring a more detailed evaluation for prompt diagnosis.

The clinician must distinguish the neurologic symptoms and signs associated with the primary disease from those associated with uremia. This requires familiarity not only with the neurologic features of renal insufficiency but also with those of disorders that may present with neurologic and renal involvement (TABLE 30.1). A comprehensive neurologic evaluation is necessary for precise diagnosis and subsequent management of these disorders. The spectrum of neurologic disorders seen in association with CKD is listed in TABLE 30.2.

This chapter is divided into two sections. The first discusses central nervous system disorders in patients with CKD and dialysis patients, and the second addresses the peripheral nervous system in patients with CKD and in dialysis patients.

◆ CENTRAL NERVOUS SYSTEM ABNORMALITIES

Uremic Encephalopathy

CKD may result in cognitive impairment associated with clouding of consciousness, especially when the glomerular filtration rate (GFR) falls below 10 mL/min (4). The clinical features of uremic

TABLE 30.1	Systemic Disorders with Renal and Nervous System Involvement	
Disease	**Clinical Presentation**
Polyarteritis nodosa	Mononeuritis multiplex, CNS vasculitis
Systemic lupus erythematosus	Neuropsychiatric disease, cerebral infarction, myelitis, neuropathy
Wegener's granulomatosis	Midline granulomatous inflammation, peripheral neuropathy
Thrombotic thrombocytopenic purpura	Cerebral edema, seizures, fluctuating focal deficits
Rheumatoid arthritis	CNS vasculitis, cervical myelopathy, neuropathy
Hypertensive encephalopathy	Headaches, seizures, altered sensorium, coma
Autosomal dominant polycystic kidney disease	Intracranial aneurysms

CNS, central nervous system.

encephalopathy are nonspecific and include confusion, psychomotor agitation, alteration of sleep–wake cycle, disorientation, impaired memory, inattention, paranoid ideation, impaired abstraction, visual hallucinations, myoclonus, and seizures (4–8). The clinical course is usually insidious in onset with waxing and waning of intellectual function, a typical feature of most metabolic encephalopathies.

Progression of renal insufficiency may subsequently result in gradual obtundation followed by coma unless dialysis is performed. Dialysis initiation usually results in gradual clinical improvement (4).

TABLE 30.2	Neurologic Disorders Associated with Kidney Disease and Dialysis

Central nervous system disorders
  Uremic encephalopathy
    Dialysis dysequilibrium syndrome
    Dialysis dementia
    Cerebrovascular disease
  Peripheral nervous system disorders
    Uremic neuropathy
    Autonomic and cranial neuropathy
  Mononeuropathies
    Carpal tunnel syndrome
    Ischemic monomelic neuropathy
    Compressive neuropathies

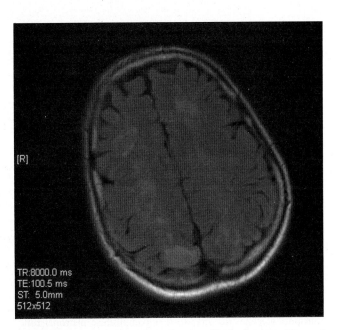

FIGURE 30.1 Magnetic resonance imaging of brain showing evidence of T2 white matter hyperintensities in a patient with posterior reversible leukoencephalopathy. These resolved completely on a repeat scan a month later.

There is no absolute correlation between neurologic impairment and the blood urea nitrogen level, although it has been suggested that the rate of rise of urea and creatinine may be related to the development of neurologic symptoms (6,8). Neurologic examination is usually nonlateralizing; impaired higher cortical functions, hyperreflexia, and asterixis may be present.

Asterixis, a sudden loss of muscle tone that results in a "flapping" tremor, is best assessed by having the patient hyperextend at the elbow and wrist with the fingers spread apart; the asterixis is then best seen at the metacarpophalangeal joints and the wrist. This phenomenon is also seen in hepatic and other metabolic encephalopathies, and, although a nonspecific finding, it may be useful in assessment of a patient with declining renal function (2).

Patients with uremic encephalopathy characteristically may also manifest multifocal myoclonus. Myoclonus is a sudden rhythmic movement of muscle groups; it is asymmetric and usually not related to seizures. In addition, focal neurologic findings such as extensor plantar response and grasp or snout reflexes have been described. Myoclonus may also occur in kidney disease patients associated with medications such as but not limited to serotonin reuptake inhibitors and narcotic analgesics.

The presence of focal neurologic findings should be fully investigated to look for other causes of altered mentation. Neuroimaging studies such as computed tomography (CT) or magnetic resonance imaging (MRI) typically show cortical atrophy (9,10). Rarely, changes suggestive of edema are seen involving the basal ganglia, cerebral cortex, and centrum semiovale (10). Interestingly, these changes are similar to those seen in hypertensive encephalopathy. The cause and significance of these changes are unknown in the absence of marked hypertension, but they are thought to be related to transient ischemia or cerebral edema. The possibility that these changes are related to uremic toxins or other metabolic derangement cannot be excluded because these changes usually resolve after dialysis (10).

Posterior reversible leukoencephalopathy syndrome (PRLS) is a well-defined syndrome seen in associated with severe hypertension and acute renal insufficiency (11). Clinical features include headaches, altered mentation, visual changes, and even cortical blindness related to the predilection for involvement of the occipital lobes (12). These findings have also been described in patients with organ transplantation and with use of certain immunosuppressant

medications such as cyclosporine and tacrolimus (13,14). Typically, this condition is reversible with complete resolution of symptoms, clinical and radiologic changes with control of blood pressure and/or discontinuation of offending agents (**FIGURE 30.1**).

Cerebrospinal fluid (CSF) examination usually is normal, although mildly elevated protein is seen in more than half of the patients with uremia and lymphocytic pleocytosis may be seen in up to 10% of patients (2,15). It is of critical importance that encephalitis, meningitis, and other causes of CSF abnormalities be excluded before attributing the CSF changes to uremia alone.

One of the most interesting questions in uremia relates to the pathogenesis of uremic encephalopathy. The substance responsible for the encephalopathy is not known. There is no direct relationship between urea or creatinine levels and the level of encephalopathy (5–7). Most likely, uremic encephalopathy is a result of a combination of factors, including accumulation of various organic acids and substances such as urea guanidine (16–17), myoinositol, purines, organic phosphates, oxalate, ascorbic acid, amino acid peptides, parathyroid hormone (PTH), β_2-microglobulin, methylguanidine, guanidinosuccinic acid, hippuric acid, polyamines, phenols, and indoles, in addition to urea and creatinine (6,7,18–20). In animal models, a number of these compounds of different molecular weights produce toxicity similar to that seen in uremic syndrome.

Urea and creatinine are considered low molecular weight compounds (less than 300 Da), whereas myoglobulin is considered high molecular weight (greater than 12,000 Da). Similarly, compounds with molecular weight between 300 and 12,000 Da such as β_2-microglobulins are considered "middle molecules." Because the middle molecules are removed less efficiently than urea and creatinine during hemodialysis, these are considered likely candidates that contribute to uremic encephalopathy. These compounds include PTH, peptides, glucuronated conjugates, and β_2-microglobulin. Compounds such as methylguanidine, hippuric acid, polyamines, phenols, and indoles have lower molecular weight, but their kinetics of removal during dialysis are similar to the "classic" middle molecules (19).

As stated previously, PTH has been implicated in the pathogenesis of uremic encephalopathy (20–22) because of secondary hyperparathyroidism and effect of PTH on neuronal function (21). Even in the absence of renal insufficiency, elevated levels of PTH can result in confusion and altered mental status. In animal models of uremia, there is a marked increase in intracellular calcium (7,20), suggesting a possible link between PTH and neuronal dysfunction. In these animals, blockade of PTH function reverses the symptoms associated with uremic encephalopathy. Increased intracellular calcium results in impairment of energy metabolism with reduced adenosine triphosphate (ATP) levels because of abnormal mitochondrial function. There is also evidence to suggest abnormal phospholipid metabolism related to the previously mentioned events causes membrane instability and further neuronal injury (3,15–20).

Accumulation of various organic acids and the middle molecules described previously (6,7,18,19), either from increased permeability of the blood–brain barrier or from impaired cellular transport mechanisms, may further compromise neuronal function. Biasioli et al. (8) describe an alteration in amino acid profile in serum and CSF of uremic patients, which indicates an increase in glycine, dopamine, and serotonin and a decrease in γ aminobutyric acid (GABA). Increased dopamine, serotonin, and glycine accumulation may result in increased irritability, sensorial clouding, tremors, and unsteadiness. Low GABA levels may lead to seizures and myoclonus and may exacerbate other uremic symptoms (8,20). However, no single abnormality fulfills all the criteria for being the putative neurotoxin, and uremic encephalopathy is most likely the result of derangements of neuronal function at multiple levels. Positron emission tomography (PET) scans in patients with CKD show reduced brain metabolism that correlates well with cognitive dysfunction and may be explained by the molecular events discussed previously (23). Additional metabolic derangements such as hyponatremia and hypernatremia have been associated with CKD and dialysis, these may result in altered mental status, encephalopathy, and seizures and addressed elsewhere in this text.

Seizures

Seizures may occur during the course of uremic encephalopathy in as many as 10% to 20% of patients and are usually generalized tonic clonic, although simple or complex partial seizures may also be seen (2,6). It is important to exclude drug toxicity as a reversible cause of seizures, because a number of commonly used drugs are associated with seizures in kidney disease. Drugs such as quinolones, penicillins, cephalosporins, acyclovir, and erythropoietin lower the seizure threshold and can lead to clinical seizure activity (24,25). The diagnosis is one of exclusion, and withdrawal of the presumed offending agent is enough to control the seizure activity.

Electroencephalography (EEG) in patients with seizures usually shows marked slowing of the background with increased θ (4 to 7 Hz) and δ (1 to 3 Hz) activity, as well as bilateral frontal paroxysmal slowing and occasional frontal epileptiform activity in the form of spikes and sharp waves (**FIGURE 30.2**) (6–8,26). It is important to note that these epileptiform abnormalities may be seen in patients with uremia and without a history of seizures as well. This finding in patients without seizures most likely represents evidence of cortical irritability and by themselves do not require any treatment. A characteristic EEG finding in patients with uremic encephalopathy is triphasic waves, which are seen with advanced stages (**FIGURE 30.3**). However, this pattern may also be seen in other metabolic disorders such as hepatic encephalopathy, severe hyponatremia, and certain drug intoxications (e.g., lithium) (26).

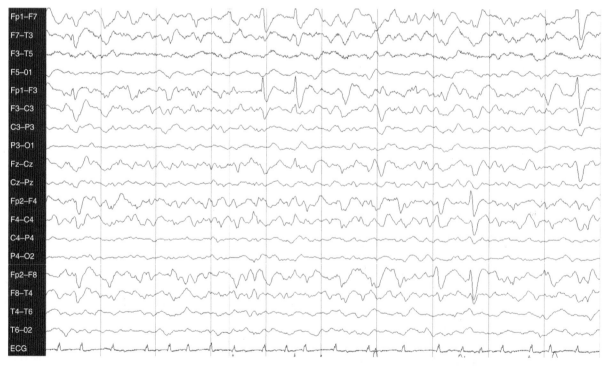

FIGURE 30.2 An electroencephalography showing bilateral frontal epileptiform discharges in a patient with uremic encephalopathy. ECG, electrocardiogram.

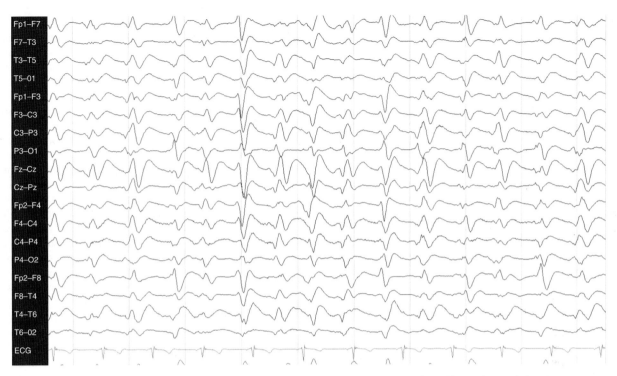

FIGURE 30.3 An electroencephalography showing classical triphasic waves in a patient with uremic encephalopathy. ECG, electrocardiogram.

The seizures should be treated the same as in other patients with metabolic encephalopathies. Long-term antiepileptic drug (AED) therapy is only required in patients with a high risk of recurrence, such as those with multiple seizures, history of recent status epilepticus, focal neurologic deficits, focal abnormality involving the cerebral cortex on imaging, and seizures in the absence of any specific metabolic derangement. If long-term antiepileptic medication is indicated, the impact of renal insufficiency and dialysis on drug metabolism should be taken into account (**TABLE 30.3**) (27–30). Phenytoin, carbamazepine, and valproic acid are all reasonable first-line agents for the treatment of seizures, although the newer agents have less systemic toxicity associated with them and are preferred by most neurologists. Phenytoin, levetiracetam, lacosamide, and valproate have the advantage of being available in intravenous (IV)

TABLE 30.3	Selected Antiepileptic Drug Therapy in Kidney Disease					
AED	**Typical Daily Dose Range with Normal Renal Function (mg/d)**	**Plasma Concentration in CRF**	**Plasma Half-Life**	**Dose Adjustment**	**Removal by Dialysis**	**Post-HD Supplementation**
Phenytoin	300–600	Total ↓, free ↑	Decreased	Based on free levels	Negligible	No
Carbamazepine	600–1,600	No change	No change	None	None	No
Oxcarbazepine	600–2,400	Increased	Increased	Yes	Insignificant	No
Phenobarbital	60–200	No change	Increased or no change	Slight reduction: avoid in most cases	Significant	Possibly
Lacosamide	200–400	Increased	Increased	Yes	Significant	Yes
Gabapentin	1,200–3,600	Increased	Increased	Yes	Significant	Yes
Pregabalin	150–600	Increased	Increased	Yes	Significant	Yes
Lamotrigine	100–600	Increased	Increased	Yes	Significant	Yes
Valproic acid	1000–3,000	Decreased	No change	No	Negligible	No
Topiramate	100–400	Increased	Increased	Yes: avoid if possible	Significant	Yes
Zonisamide	100–400	Increased	Increased	Yes: unknown	Unknown	Unknown

AED, antiepileptic drug; CRF, chronic renal failure; HD, hemodialysis.
Data related to other less commonly prescribed AEDs such as clobazam, perampanel, eslicarbazepine, rufinamide, ezogabine, and felbamate can be found elsewhere (79).

form and can be given rapidly in an emergency. Because phenytoin is one of the most commonly used antiepileptic medications and its metabolism is affected by uremia (2,31,32) the pharmacokinetics in kidney disease must be well understood before using them in these medically complex patients. Because of expanded volume of distribution there is a reduction in total level, although this is offset by a marked increase of the free fraction of the drug from 10% to 25% (31,32). This may result in clinical toxicity, even though the total level may be low; therefore, free phenytoin levels, which are easily available in most centers, should be used as a guide to dosing. The half-life of phenytoin is also reduced from 13 hours to approximately 8 hours; therefore, three times a day dosing is recommended.

Valproic acid is now also available in IV formulation as is levetiracetam and lacosamide, although there is very little confirmatory data regarding its use in management of status epilepticus. We prefer to use these agents for seizures initially, and it requires careful monitoring for toxicity due to the impact of renal insufficiency on their respective serum levels (as noted in **TABLE 30.3**). Drugs that are metabolized by the cytochrome P-450 such as phenytoin, carbamazepine, oxcarbazepine, and phenobarbital are enzyme inducers and may interfere with metabolism of a number of other drugs including tacrolimus, a commonly used antirejection drug; therefore, caution is advised when using these antiepileptic agents in medically complex patients. We typically tend to avoid use of phenobarbital in most patients due to numerous other options available and its significant toxicity. A number of new antiepileptic agents have been approved by the U.S. Food and Drug Administration (FDA) over the last few years and may be a reasonable alternative for these patients (**TABLE 30.3**). The choice of AED is based on the need for rapid dosing (phenytoin, valproic acid, levetiracetam, lacosamide), side effect profile (potential renal toxicity with topiramate and zonisamide), and significant dosing adjustment of the drug (gabapentin, levetiracetam, lacosamide, oxcarbazepine). Phenytoin is still preferentially used for rapid IV dosing in a patient with acute repetitive seizures or status epilepticus. However, in a patient with focal seizures who does not have status epilepticus one may choose a drug like carbamazepine as dosing adjustments are not necessary in patients with renal insufficiency. AEDs such as lamotrigine and levetiracetam are additional exceedingly effective and safe options for add-on therapy if a single drug is ineffective at its maximally tolerable dose. However, these drugs are renally excreted and substantial dose adjustments are required especially with hemodialysis. A neurologic consultation may also be helpful in choosing the most appropriate AED.

Cerebrovascular Disease in Chronic Kidney Disease

Patients on chronic hemodialysis have a fivefold higher risk of cerebrovascular disease compared with the normal population (33–36). This may be related to the high prevalence of hypertension (33), underlying diabetes, hyperhomocysteinemia, dyslipidemia, and atherosclerosis in hemodialysis patients (34). There are considerable data that suggest hyperhomocysteinemia is an important risk factor in patients with ischemic cerebrovascular disease and chronic renal insufficiency (34). It is important to identify the cause of hyperhomocysteinemia, which may be related to folate, cobalamin, or pyridoxine deficiency or because of a mutation of methylene tetrahydrofolate reductase (MTHFR) enzyme. Folic acid at 1 to 5 mg is recommended for most patients with MTHFR mutation, for folate deficiency, or when no other cause of hyperhomocysteinemia is identified.

The stroke risk is increased in patients with CKD and those undergoing dialysis. In a paper published recently (35), stroke occurred at a rate of 49.2/1,000 patient-years with a greater risk of ischemic stroke in patients undergoing hemodialysis compared to peritoneal dialysis. However, the risk of hemorrhagic stroke did not appear to show such an association. The management of ischemic cerebrovascular disease is the same as in patients without kidney disease. Addressing associated risk factors such as hypertension, hypercholesterolemia, and other modifiable risk factors is critically important. Antiplatelet agents such as aspirin and clopidogrel are recommended for atherothrombotic disease, whereas patients with embolic infarction may need to be anticoagulated with warfarin. The decision to anticoagulate is based on the size of the infarct, the risk of recurrence, and the risk of systemic or intracranial bleeding in a particular patient.

In another older study intracerebral hemorrhage was seen more commonly than cerebral infarct as the cause of stroke and most likely is related to hypertension (36). The actual incidence of intracerebral hemorrhage was noted to be *12.3 per 1,000 patient-years, and that of cerebral infarct is 3.9 per 1,000 patient-years* (32). This was also associated with an overall 30-day stroke mortality that is 74.4%, compared with 12.3% in the general population. This high mortality could be partly related to the disproportionately high incidence of intracerebral hemorrhage and associated systemic disease that was noted in this particular study. However, a more recent study has shown a higher incidence of ischemic infarction compared to intracerebral hemorrhage in patients with CKD who are receiving hemodialysis (35).

Patients with autosomal dominant polycystic kidney disease (ADPKD) have a higher prevalence of intracranial aneurysms (35). These aneurysms are usually small, involve the anterior circulation, and are frequently multiple. The prevalence of these aneurysms is approximately 5% to 12%, depending on the screening method used. Cerebral angiography is the gold standard diagnostic method for locating these aneurysms (**FIGURE 30.4**) (11);

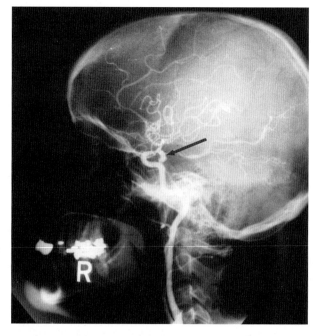

FIGURE 30.4 A cerebral angiogram showing a posterior communicating artery aneurysm (*arrow*). (Courtesy Brinker RA, MD, Department of Radiology, formerly Medical College of Ohio, Toledo, Ohio.)

however, magnetic resonance angiography (MRA) is sometimes a useful screening tool. It is safe in patients with kidney disease when no contrast is needed.

Screening is recommended for patients above the age of 20 as aneurysms are typically not noted in individuals younger than that. Risk factors for aneurysms include a family history of aneurysms, a previous history of aneurysm or subarachnoid hemorrhage, polycystic kidney disease, as well as certain connective tissue disorders such as Marfan or Ehler-Danlos syndrome type IV (35).

Clinical features may be related to mass effect in the case of a large aneurysm or because of a sudden rupture. Patients with subarachnoid hemorrhage usually present with sudden explosive headache that is frequently described as the "worst headache of their life." Nuchal rigidity and third cranial nerve (CN) palsy may also be present but are not seen in all patients. The initial evaluation must be rapid in patients with suspected subarachnoid hemorrhage, and urgent admission to an intensive care unit is warranted. The overall mortality of a ruptured aneurysm is approximately 30% to 50% in patients with or without ADPKD. Timely intervention can be life-saving, and most of interventions are now planned and done before development of vasospasm, which usually occurs 3 to 4 days after rupture. In addition to open craniotomy, endovascular procedures are being more commonly utilized in these medically challenging patients (37).

Management of asymptomatic aneurysms guidelines have previously been published (38). Patients with ADPKD should undergo screening every 5 years due to a high prevalence of intracranial aneurysms (39). There is a strong correlation between size of the aneurysm, location (posterior circulation > anterior circulation), family history, and risk of rupture. Aneurysm location does also affect management because those located in the posterior circulation such as the basilar artery or posterior communicating arteries are more likely to rupture irrespective of size. Other factors that may have an impact on management of unruptured aneurysms include previous subarachnoid hemorrhage; age; family history; coexisting medical conditions; aneurysm characteristics such as size, location, and morphology; and neurosurgical expertise. In the authors' opinion, surgical decisions in an asymptomatic patient with intracranial aneurysms should be individualized after an informed discussion between the neurosurgeon, endovascular neurologist, nephrologist (in case of associated renal disease), and the patient.

Approach to a Patient with Confusion and Kidney Disease

In a patient who develops confusion associated with renal insufficiency, it is imperative to exclude other causes that may mimic uremic encephalopathy. A complete history and physical including a careful neurologic examination is mandatory. A systematic approach should be adopted to evaluate these patients. In these medically complex patients, systemic infections may result in profound confusion and should be looked for in addition to a complete neurologic evaluation. The differential diagnosis and the diagnostic workup for some of the neurologic diseases are listed in TABLE 30.4. It is important to exclude nonconvulsive status epilepticus as a cause of confusion in a patient with uremia. It is a potentially life-threatening disorder that can be easily diagnosed by EEG and responds to antiepileptic therapy. If unrecognized and untreated, nonconvulsive status epilepticus can lead to irreversible neurologic injury.

Dialysis Disequilibrium Syndrome

The dialysis disequilibrium syndrome is an unusual complication in current dialysis practice. It presents with a variety of constitutional and neurologic symptoms that include headache, fatigue, nausea, vomiting, hypertension, tremors, seizures, agitation, delirium, and subsequent coma (1–3,5,40–43). These symptoms usually appear within 24 hours of dialysis completion and last for a few hours (1). The syndrome is usually seen in patients who are severely uremic and are dialyzed aggressively. The EEG may show generalized and paroxysmal slowing during this period (3,26).

With regard to cause, some patients develop elevated intracranial pressure (ICP) during dialysis (19,43). This increase may be explained on the basis of reverse urea effect (40). Reverse urea effect results from more efficient removal of urea from plasma, as compared with the brain, with development of a reverse osmotic gradient. This intracellular accumulation of solutes such as urea favors movement of water to the intracellular space, leading to cerebral edema and the increase in ICP. The finding of more efficient removal of urea from the plasma compared with the brain during hemodialysis is disputed by some, but it is a plausible explanation for much of the clinical symptomatology seen.

Urea is, however, not the only compound responsible for the osmotic gradient, and other compounds such as idiogenic osmoles

TABLE 30.4	Approach to a Patient with Confusion in Kidney Disease		
Clinical Features	**Diagnosis**	**Diagnostic Tests**
Head trauma, headaches, falls	Subdural hematoma	CT or MRI
Focal neurologic findings (hemiparesis, homonymous hemianopsia, aphasia, etc.)	Infarct or intracerebral hemorrhage	CT or MRI
Fever, headaches, nuchal rigidity, seizures	Meningitis (bacterial, fungal, or mycobacterial)	CSF examination
Worst-ever headache, nuchal rigidity, subhyaloid hemorrhage on funduscopy	Subarachnoid hemorrhage	CT, cerebral angiography, neurosurgical evaluation
Altered sensorium, nonlateralizing examination	Hepatic encephalopathy, hyponatremia, hypoxia, hypercarbia gases	Liver function chemistries, arterial blood
Intermittent confusion, stereotypical behavior, automatisms	Nonconvulsive status epilepticus	EEG
Seizures with or without any other symptoms	Drug toxicity (penicillins, cephalosporins, carbapenems acyclovir, erythropoietin)	History, drug withdrawal

CT, computed tomography; MRI, magnetic resonance imaging; CSF, cerebrospinal fluid; EEG, electroencephalogram.

may also be involved (1,40). Idiogenic osmoles are thought to be organic acids that are formed intracellularly in the brain and also contribute to the increased brain osmolality. Support for this comes from studies that show that the urea concentration in the brain can only account for 50% to 60% of the increase in brain osmolality; the rest is presumably related to these idiogenic osmoles (8).

Another somewhat controversial explanation for the development of cerebral edema is paradoxical intracellular acidosis (7,20), which may also be related to accumulation of organic acids. A fall in CSF pH is noted during dialysis in patients and in experimental animal models. This increase in the intracellular H^+ ion concentration in the brain results in increased osmolar content with a secondary increase in brain water. This would then result in cerebral edema and the symptoms of dialysis disequilibrium syndrome. This finding has, however, been refuted by other studies (8), which have not been able to demonstrate acidosis within the central nervous system. Similarly, the possible association of hemodynamic alterations and electrolyte shifts to the genesis of this syndrome is also unclear.

Dialysis Dementia or Dialysis Encephalopathy

Patients with CKD on hemodialysis undergoing neuropsychologic testing show impaired performance on tests of short-term memory, attention, concentration span, and sequential information processing (4,44). This cognitive decline may or may not improve with therapy and is associated with diffuse cerebral atrophy, which may be seen on routine studies such as CT or MRI (9). Pathologically, there is neuronal cell loss and other nonspecific changes. The pathophysiology of these changes are unknown but are thought to be related to a combination of chronic aluminum toxicity, impaired cerebrovascular autoregulation, and breakdown of blood–brain barrier (9). Interestingly, patients undergoing peritoneal dialysis perform better on cognitive testing than those patients receiving hemodialysis (44).

Unlike the benign course described previously, some patients on hemodialysis for a period of greater than 2 years may develop a progressive dementia that is irreversible and invariably fatal (45–51). This form of dementia is exceedingly rare now; because of *the reduction in the use of aluminum-containing phosphate binders* and improved screening for aluminum in dialysate water (see also Chapter 25) (20). However, rare cases have been described in association with contamination of the dialysate water supply, such as when well water high in aluminum was used for home dialysis. The clinical features include aphasia, apraxia, myoclonus, seizures, progressive intellectual decline, confusion, auditory or visual hallucinations, and dysarthria (1–4). The symptoms are initially intermittent and may worsen immediately after dialysis (47).

As the disease progresses, there is persistent cognitive impairment, and an increase in seizures may also occur. These seizures are poorly responsive to AED therapy but may initially respond to benzodiazepines. EEG may initially show paroxysmal slowing with predominant frontal spikes and sharp waves intermixed with normal background. As the disease progresses, the EEG may also show more severe background abnormalities (7,26,52). There is evidence that EEG changes may precede the clinical picture by months (4). Neuroimaging is usually unremarkable but may be useful in excluding tumors, subdural hematoma, or chronic infections.

The occurrence of dialysis dementia has been linked by a number of epidemiologic studies to aluminum intoxication (45–52). These patients have a high serum aluminum level and may also show increased brain levels, especially in the gray matter (1,51). Removing aluminum from the dialysate and reducing intake of

phosphate-binding gels that have a high aluminum content have resulted in a dramatic decline in the incidence of this disease (2–4). However, there are patients who develop this disease with no evidence of exposure or evidence of aluminum intoxication (49). Children with CKD may develop this syndrome without ever undergoing dialysis or being exposed to aluminum. In such cases, it is hypothesized that uremia may result in development of this syndrome through its effect on the developing brain (7).

Aluminum is normally absorbed in the gastrointestinal tract and is excreted through the kidneys. Increased absorption is probably the effect of PTH (21) on the gastrointestinal tract; in combination with reduced excretion, patients on dialysis have plasma levels that are six to eight times higher than normal (normal, 0 to 20 mg/L). At levels above 200 mg/L, chelating agents such as deferoxamine are recommended (2). To prevent the development of this complication, dialysate aluminum is kept below 20 mg/L by deionization (4,7). This process also removes other compounds such as cadmium, mercury, lead, manganese, copper, nickel, thallium, boron, and tin. The relationship of other substances including trace elements to dialysis dementia is not known (see Chapter 3) (7).

⬡ PERIPHERAL NERVOUS SYSTEM INVOLVEMENT IN UREMIA

Involvement of the peripheral nervous system in CKD was described initially in the 19th century. Kussmaul (1864), Charcot (1870), and Osler (1892) wrote on various aspects of this condition. However, in the first half of the 20th century descriptions of peripheral neuropathy in CKD were uncommon in the medical literature, which was instead dominated by central nervous system manifestations such as coma and seizures. After hemodialysis was introduced and patients began to live longer, peripheral neuropathy was reported more frequently and now is considered an integral part of the uremic syndrome.

Uremic Polyneuropathy

Uremic polyneuropathy is the most common type of peripheral nerve involvement, and typically occurs when the creatinine clearance is less than 10 mL/min. As determined by electrophysiologic studies and careful clinical examination, evidence of peripheral neuropathy is seen in 50% to 60% of patients with ESKD who require hemodialysis (53). It is more common in men than in women.

Usually the neuropathy has an insidious onset. Muscle cramps have been thought to herald peripheral nerve involvement, but many patients with similar complaints have no other manifestation of neuropathy. In such cases, the cramps probably are a nonspecific manifestation of uremia. Patients experience distal dysesthesias which are described as painful tingling, aberrant sensation of swelling of fingers and toes, and a constrictive feeling around the feet and ankles. These prominent sensory manifestations may be accompanied by slowly progressive distal weakness and atrophy. Restless legs syndrome is seen in 20% of patients with CKD (54). Contributing factors in such patients include peripheral neuropathy and iron deficiency anemia. The syndrome of restless legs consists of creeping, crawling, prickling, and pruritic sensations deep within the legs that worsen during periods of inactivity and become particularly bothersome before the onset of sleep. The sensations disappear temporarily when the legs are moved, only to recur within a few seconds. The symptoms last from minutes to hours; they can significantly delay sleep onset and result in sleep deprivation.

The earliest signs on examination are impaired vibration sense in the lower extremities associated with loss of deep tendon reflexes—first the Achilles reflex, then the patellar responses. Advanced cases display distal decrease in touch and position sense and may also show weakness and atrophy of distal muscles.

When fully developed, uremic polyneuropathy is a distal symmetric mixed motor and sensory polyneuropathy involving the legs more than the arms. The major factors correlating with the appearance of neuropathy are the degree and duration of CKD. No correlation has been demonstrated with other factors such as age, race, levels of specific uremic metabolites, or type of underlying renal disease. Although most commonly uremic polyneuropathy evolves over many months, there have been reports of severe fulminant motor neuropathies, sometimes associated with sepsis (55).

CSF protein levels are usually normal but may be elevated up to 100 to 200 mg/dL (normal 15 to 45 mg/dL) in patients with severe uremic polyneuropathy.

The most significant abnormality on electrophysiologic study is a reduction in the amplitude of the compound muscle and sensory action potential, a finding typical of axonal neuropathy. Both motor and sensory conduction velocities are mildly reduced and the late reflexes (H reflex and F wave) become abnormally prolonged, more commonly in the lower extremities. There is a high correlation between declining creatinine clearance and reduction in conduction velocities (56). Specific predictors that herald the appearance of clinical symptoms and signs have not been identified. Quantitative sensory testing, especially the vibratory threshold, is a sensitive indicator of peripheral neuropathy in CKD and correlates well with severity (57). An early and unusual sign is the perception of heat in response to low temperature stimuli. This paradoxical heat sensation to cold can precede other signs of neuropathy (58).

Pathologically, uremic polyneuropathy represents a primary axonal disease with secondary segmental demyelination. All fiber sizes, both myelinated and unmyelinated, are affected, although the largest and the most distal are especially vulnerable. The pathologic findings are not specific for uremia and cannot be distinguished from other causes of axonal degeneration such as alcoholic neuropathy.

The fact that the appearance of peripheral neuropathy correlates with reduction in GFR and the neuropathy improves after dialysis or transplantation implies that a uremic toxin impairs peripheral nerve function. However, in spite of intensive research no specific substance has been shown to correlate with the development or severity of peripheral neuropathy in CKD. Initially attention centered on the so-called middle molecules, substances of molecular weight between 500 and 5,000 as the cause. However, this has not been substantiated. Many other agents including PTH, myoinositol, calcium, magnesium, and methylguanidine have been investigated and discarded as possible culprits in the development of neuropathy in CKD. Some studies indicate that hyperkalemia may contribute to the development of neuropathy in CKD (59).

In most patients on long-term dialysis, the neuropathy will stabilize, but improvement is less consistent (60,61). Progressive neuropathy is an indication for starting dialysis therapy and is also an indicator of insufficient dialysis. Earlier reports indicated that patients on peritoneal dialysis do not develop uremic polyneuropathy with the same frequency as patients on hemodialysis, but these observations have not been substantiated (62).

Successful renal transplantation has a more predictable and clear-cut beneficial effect on uremic polyneuropathy and remains the only cure. Provided that the transplant is successful, progressive improvement has been the rule, with substantial clinical recovery. Recovery often occurs in two phases, initial rapid improvement over days to weeks and then more protracted improvement over a period of months (63,64). Even in severe cases, walking is possible within 2 to 3 months, although some residual clinical signs such as absent ankle reflexes may persist. Serial electrophysiologic studies following transplantation have demonstrated rapid improvement in nerve conduction velocities (65). Patients with neuropathic pain can benefit from treatment with tricyclic antidepressants like amitriptyline or anticonvulsants medications such as gabapentin. Neuropathic symptoms may also improve after supplementation with biotin, pyridoxine, thiamine, and cobalamin (66). The restless legs syndrome responds poorly to dialysis. Symptomatic relief can be provided by a number of medications, including dopamine agonists, levodopa, gabapentin, and opioids. Treatment of the iron deficiency anemia can reduce symptom severity. Substantial improvement of restless legs symptoms can occur after kidney transplantation (67).

Autonomic and Cranial Neuropathies

Uremic neuropathy is not confined to motor and sensory nerves. Autonomic dysfunction is a well-known complication (see Chapter 19) (68,69). Patients with CKD demonstrate abnormal responses to the Valsalva maneuver, abnormal heart rate responses to atropine, and reduced baroreceptor sensitivity. Symptoms that indicate disordered autonomic function include orthostatic hypotension, impotence, diarrhea, and excessive perspiration. Reduced baroreceptor activity may be an important factor in producing hemodialysis-induced hypotension (see Chapter 19) (70). However, overt signs of autonomic dysfunction may be uncommon during the course of CKD. Renal transplantation can lead to considerable improvement of autonomic function while dialysis is not associated with any significant change.

Increased incidence of eighth cranial nerve (CN VIII) dysfunction, both auditory and vestibular, has been noted (71). The pathogenesis is obscure and is most likely multifactorial, potentially related to uremic toxins and prior exposure to ototoxic drugs such as aminoglycosides. There have been reports of esophageal dysfunction in patients with CRF, and uremic neuropathy of the vagus nerve (CN X) has been postulated (72).

Diabetes mellitus can also involve peripheral, cranial, and autonomic nerves. Because 40% to 45% of all patients with ESKD have diabetes, it is important to distinguish diabetic from uremic neuropathy. The clinical picture in diabetic and uremic neuropathy can be similar, but there are some differences. In diabetic neuropathy overt autonomic dysfunction, cranial nerve involvement, and compressive neuropathies are more common. Diabetic neuropathy can be asymmetric and could present with a distinctive clinical picture, as in diabetic amyotrophy that manifests with painful proximal leg weakness. Electrophysiologic studies and nerve biopsy are not helpful in making this distinction, with both disorders showing evidence of axonal disease. Importantly, diabetic polyneuropathy will not respond to hemodialysis or transplantation.

Mononeuropathies

Carpal Tunnel Syndrome

Carpal tunnel syndrome is the most common mononeuropathy in patients with CKD, just as it is in patients without renal insufficiency. However, in certain situations, kidney disease patients are especially liable to develop median nerve entrapment. In patients with CKD, carpal tunnel syndrome has been associated with arteriovenous fistulas between the radial artery and the cephalic vein in the forearm (73). The symptoms of tingling dysesthesias in the median nerve distribution with nocturnal exacerbation are similar to those reported by nonuremic patients, although in uremic patients, these symptoms may get worse during dialysis. This exacerbation is most likely related to a combination of compression and median nerve ischemia within the carpal tunnel because of venous congestion and edema. In refractory cases, treatment may ultimately require closure of the fistula.

Amyloidosis will develop in some patients on chronic hemodialysis because of β_2-microglobulin deposition and may produce carpal tunnel syndrome (this is discussed in detail in Chapter 23).

Ischemic Monomelic Neuropathy

Rarely, an arteriovenous fistula placed in the proximal upper arm can induce severe ischemia involving the median, ulnar, or radial nerve (see Chapter 4) (74,75). Pathologically, the shunting of blood in the arm and transient loss of blood flow produces acute multiple mononeuropathies, with axon loss that is most marked distally. Clinical manifestations consist of acute onset of limb pain associated with distal weakness and sensory loss. Nerve conduction studies demonstrate abnormalities in multiple distal nerves in the affected limb, and electromyography (EMG) also shows distal greater than proximal abnormalities in muscles consistent with the clinical picture. Ischemic monomelic neuropathy is considered a medical emergency and requires prompt surgical closure of the fistula or shunt. Severe or permanent neurologic sequelae may occur even after the fistula or shunt has been closed.

Compressive Neuropathies

Compressive neuropathies involving the ulnar nerve at the elbow and the peroneal nerve at the fibular head occasionally occur during ESKD, particularly if the patient is malnourished and bedridden for any length of time. Uremic toxins make the nerves more susceptible to damage from focal compression. Successful renal transplantation restores the function of these nerves.

Myopathy

Myopathy can occur in CKD and usually appears when the GFR falls under 25 mL/min and can affect up to 50% of patients on dialysis. The clinical features include proximal muscle weakness, muscle wasting, bone pain, increased fatigability, and reduced exercise tolerance. EMG and creatine kinase levels are often normal while muscle biopsy may show type 2 muscle fiber atrophy. Possible etiologic factors for myopathy include accumulation of uremic toxins, abnormalities of vitamin D metabolism, insulin resistance, malnutrition, and carnitine deficiency (76). The myopathy of CKD may respond to high doses of vitamin D while supplementation with L-carnitine has produced mixed results. Successful renal transplantation can cause significant improvement of symptoms but may not fully restore muscle function to normal (77). Rarely CKD may be associated with widespread arterial calcification in small subcutaneous and intramuscular arteries with skin necrosis, painful myopathy, and myoglobinuria. The incidence of this complication has been greatly reduced by improvement in dialysis techniques (78). The differential diagnosis of chronic myopathy also includes the nonspecific cachexia associated with CKD. Acute myopathy can be caused by abnormalities of potassium metabolism, and muscle weakness resulting from defective transmission

at the neuromuscular junction occurs as a complication of aminoglycoside antibiotics.

 REFERENCES

1. De Deyn PP, Saxena VK, Abts H, et al. Clinical and pathophysiological aspects of neurological complications in kidney disease. *Acta Neurol Belg* 1992;92:191–206.
2. Raskin NH. Neurological aspects of kidney disease. In: Aminoff MJ, ed. *Neurology and General Medicine*. New York, NY: Churchill Livingston, 1989:231–246.
3. Lockwood AH. Neurological complications of renal disease. *Neurol Clin* 1989;7:617–627.
4. Fraser CL, Arieff AI. Nervous system complications in uremia. *Ann Intern Med* 1988;109:143–153.
5. Burn DJ, Bates D. Neurology and the kidney. *J Neurol Neurosurg Psychiatry* 1998;65:810–821.
6. Moe SM, Sprague SM. Uremic encephalopathy. *Clin Nephrol* 1994;42:251–256.
7. Mahoney CA, Arieff AI. Uremic encephalopathies: clinical, biochemical and experimental features. *Am J Kidney Dis* 1982;2:324–336.
8. Biasioli S, D'Andrea G, Feriani M, et al. Uremic encephalopathy: an updating. *Clin Nephrol* 1986;25(2):57–63.
9. Savazzi GM. Pathogenesis of cerebral atrophy in uremia. *Nephron* 1988;49:94–103.
10. Okada J, Yoshikawa K, Matsuo H, et al. Reversible MRI and CT findings in uremic encephalopathy. *Neuroradiology* 1991;33:524–526.
11. Hinchey J, Chaves C, Appignani B, et al. A reversible posterior leukoencephalopathy syndrome. *N Eng J Med* 1996;334:494–500.
12. Bansal VK, Bansal S. Nervous system disorders in dialysis patients. *Handb Clin Neurol* 2014;119:395–404.
13. Singh N, Bonham A, Fukui M. Immunosuppressive-associated leukoencephalopathy in organ transplant recipients. *Transplantation* 2000;69:467–472.
14. Vaughn BV, Ali II, Olivier KN, et al. Seizures in lung transplant recipients. *Epilepsia* 1996;37(12):1175–1179.
15. Freeman RB, Sheff MF, Maher JF, et al. The blood-cerebrospinal fluid barrier in uremia. *Ann Intern Med* 1962;56:233–240.
16. Meyer TW, Hostetter TH. Uremia. *N Engl J Med* 2007;357:1316–1325.
17. Baumgaertel M, Kraemer M, Berlit P. Neurologic complications of acute and chronic renal disease. *Handb Clin Neurol* 2014;119:383–393.
18. Costigan MG, Callaghan CA, Lindup WE. Hypothesis: is accumulation of a furan dicarboxylic acid (3-carboxy-4-methyl-5-propyl-2-furanpropanoic acid) related to neurologic abnormalities in patients with kidney disease? *Nephron* 1996;73:169–173.
19. Vanholder R, De Smet R, Hsu C, et al. Uremic toxicity: the middle molecule hypothesis revisited. *Semin Nephrol* 1994;14:205–218.
20. Smogorzewski MJ. Central nervous dysfunction in uremia. *Am J Kidney Dis* 2001;38:S122–S128.
21. Parfitt AM. The hyperparathyroidism of chronic kidney disease: a disorder of growth. *Kidney Int* 1997;52:3–9.
22. Cooper JD, Lazarowitz VC, Arieff AI, et al. Neurodiagnostic abnormalities in patients with acute kidney injury (AKI): evidence for neurotoxicity of parathyroid hormone. *J Clin Invest* 1978;61:1448–1455.
23. Kanai H, Hirakata H, Nakane H, et al. Depressed cerebral oxygen metabolism in patients with chronic kidney disease: a positron emission tomography study. *Am J Kidney Dis* 2001;38:S129–S133.
24. Norrby SR. Neurotoxicity of carbapenem antibacterials. *Drug Safety* 1996;15(2):87–90.
25. Massetani R, Galli R, Calabrese R, et al. Status epilepticus in chronically dialyzed patients treated with erythropoietin. *Riv Neurol* 1991;61(6):215–218.
26. Vas GA, Cracco JB. Diffuse encephalopathies. In: Daly DD, Pedley TA, eds. *Current Practice of Clinical Electroencephalography*. 2nd ed. New York, NY: Raven Press, 1990:371–399.
27. Brewster D, Muir NC. Valproate plasma protein binding in the uremic condition. *Clin Pharmacol Ther* 1980;27:76–82.

28. Boggs JG. Seizures in medically complex patients. *Epilepsia* 1997;38(Suppl 4):S55–S59.

29. Matzke GR, Frye RF. Drug administration in patients with renal insufficiency: minimizing renal and extrarenal toxicity. *Drug Saf* 1997;16(3):205–231.

30. Bansal AD, Hill CE, Berns JS. Use of antiepileptic drugs in patients with chronic kidney disease and end stage renal disease. *Semin Dial* 2015;28:404–412.

31. Letteri JM, Mellk H, Louis S, et al. Diphenylhydantoin metabolism in uremia. *N Engl J Med* 1971;285:648–652.

32. Burgess ED, Friel PN, Blair AD Jr, et al. Serum phenytoin concentrations in uremia. *Ann Intern Med* 1981;94:59–60.

33. Iseki K, Fukiyama K. Predictors of stroke in patients receiving chronic hemodialysis. *Kidney Int* 1996;50:1672–1675.

34. Bostom A, Lathrop L. Hyperhomocysteinemia in end-stage renal disease: prevalence, etiology, and potential relationship to arteriosclerotic outcomes. *Kidney Int* 1997;52:10–20.

35. Fu J, Huang J, Lei M, et al. Prevalence and impact on stroke in patients receiving maintenance hemodialysis versus peritoneal dialysis: a prospective observational study. *PLoS One* 2015;10(10):e0140887.

36. Iseki K, Kinjo K, Kimura Y, et al. Evidence for high risk of cerebral hemorrhage in chronic dialysis patients. *Kidney Int* 1993;44:1086–1090.

37. Brinjikji W, Rabinstein AA, Nasr DM, et al. Better outcomes with treatment by coiling relative to clipping of unruptured intracranial aneurysms in the United States, 2001-2008. *AJNR Am J Neuroradiol* 2011;32(6):1071–1075.

38. Bederson JB, Awad IA, Weibers DO, et al. Recommendations for management of patients with unruptured intracranial aneurysms: a statement of healthcare professionals from the Stroke Council of the American Heart Association. *Circulation* 2000;102(18):2300–2308.

39. Xu HW, Yu SQ, Mei CL, et al. Screening for intracranial aneurysms in 355 patients with autosomal-dominant polycystic kidney disease. *Stroke* 2011;42(1):204–206.

40. Silver SM, Sterns RH, Halperin ML. Brain swelling after dialysis: old urea or new osmoles? *Am J Kidney Dis* 1996;28:1–13.

41. Schilling L, Wahl M. Brain edema: pathogenesis and therapy. *Kidney Int* 1997;59:S69–S75.

42. Yoshida S, Tajika T, Yamasaki N, et al. Dialysis dysequilibrium syndrome in neurosurgical patients. *Neurosurgery* 1987;20:716–721.

43. Wolcott DL, Wellisch DK, Marsh JT, et al. Relationship of dialysis modality and other factors to cognitive function in chronic dialysis patients. *Am J Kidney Dis* 1988;12:275–284.

44. Arieff AI, Cooper JD, Armstrong D, et al. Dementia, renal failure, and brain aluminum. *Ann Intern Med* 1979;90:741–747.

45. Alfrey A. Dialysis encephalopathy. *Kidney Int* 1986;29(18):S53–S57.

46. Mayor G, Burnatowska-Hledin M. The metabolism of aluminum and aluminum related encephalopathy. *Semin Nephrol* 1986;6(4):1–4.

47. Platts MM, Anastassiades E. Dialysis encephalopathy: precipitating factors and improvement in prognosis. *Clin Nephrol* 1981;15:223–228.

48. Russo LS, Beale G, Sandroni S, et al. Aluminum intoxication in undialyzed adults with chronic kidney disease. *J Neurol Neurosurg Psychiatry* 1992;55:697–700.

49. Bates D, Parkinson IM, Ward MK, et al. Aluminum encephalopathy. *Contrib Nephrol* 1985;45:29–41.

50. Reusche E, Koch V, Friedrich HJ, et al. Correlation of drug-related aluminum intake and dialysis treatment with deposition of argyrophilic aluminum-containing inclusions in CNS and in organ systems of patients with dialysis-associated encephalopathy. *Clin Neuropathol* 1996;15:342–347.

51. La Greca G, Biasioli S, Borin D, et al. Dialytic encephalopathy. *Contrib Nephrol* 1985;45:9–28.

52. Nortega-Sanchez A, Martinez-Maldonado M, Haiffe RM. Clinical and electroencephalographic changes in progressive uremic encephalopathy. *Neurology* 1978;28:667–669.

53. Asbury AK. Uremic polyneuropathy. In: Dyck PJ, Thomas PK, Lambert EH, et al, eds. *Peripheral Neuropathy*. 2nd ed. Philadelphia, PA: WB Saunders, 1994:1811–1825.

54. Musci I, Molnar MZ, Ambrus C, et al. Restless legs syndrome, insomnia and quality of life in patients on maintenance dialysis. *Nephrol Dial Transplant* 2005;20(3):571–577.

55. McGonigle RJS, Bewick M, Weston MJ, et al. Progressive, predominantly motor, uremic neuropathy. *Acta Neurol Scand* 1985;71:379–384.

56. Nielsen VK. The peripheral nerve function in chronic kidney disease. VI. The relationship between sensory and motor nerve conduction and kidney function, azotemia, age, sex, and clinical neuropathy. *Acta Med Scand* 1973;194:455–462.

57. Tegnér R, Lindholm B. Vibratory perception threshold compared with nerve conduction velocity in the evaluation of uremic neuropathy. *Acta Neurol Scand* 1985;71:285–289.

58. Yosipovitch G, Yarnitsky D, Mermelstein V, et al. Paradoxical heat sensation in uremic polyneuropathy. *Muscle Nerve* 1995;18:768–771.

59. Krishnan AV, Phoon RK, Pussell BA, et al. Sensory nerve excitability and neuropathy in end-stage kidney disease. *J Neurol Neurosurg Psychiatry* 2006;77:548–551.

60. Nielsen VK. The peripheral nerve function in chronic renal failure. VII. Longitudinal course during terminal kidney disease and regular hemodialysis. *Acta Med Scand* 1974;195:155–162.

61. Cadilhac J, Mion C, Duday H, et al. Motor nerve conduction velocities as an index of maintenance dialysis in patients with end-stage kidney disease. In: Canal N, Pozza G, eds. *Peripheral Neuropathies*. New York, NY: Elsevier, 1978:372–380.

62. Tegnér R, Lindholm B. Uremic polyneuropathy: different effects of hemodialysis and continuous ambulatory peritoneal dialysis. *Acta Med Scand* 1985;218:409–416.

63. Bolton CF, Baltzan MA, Baltzan RB. Effects of renal transplantation on uremic neuropathy. *N Engl J Med* 1971;284:1170–1174.

64. Nielsen VK. The peripheral nerve function in chronic renal failure. VIII. Recovery after renal transplantation. *Acta Med Scand* 1974;195:163–170.

65. Funck-Brentano JL, Chaumont P, Vantelon J, et al. Polyneuritis during the course of chronic kidney disease: follow up after renal transplantation (10 personal cases). *Nephron* 1968;5:31–42.

66. Kuwabara S, Nakazawa R, Azuma N, et al. Intravenous methylcobalamin treatment for uremic and diabetic neuropathy in chronic hemodialysis patients. *Intern Med* 1999;38(6):472–475.

67. Winkelmann J, Stautner A, Samtleben W, et al. Long-term course of restless legs syndrome in dialysis patients after kidney transplantation. *Mov Disord* 2002;17(5):1072–1076.

68. Zucchelli P, Sturani A, Zuccalà A, et al. Dysfunction of the autonomic nervous system in patients with end-stage renal failure. *Contrib Nephrol* 1985;45:69–81.

69. Solders G, Persson A, Gutierrez A. Autonomic dysfunction in non-diabetic terminal uremia. *Acta Neurol Scand* 1985;71:321–327.

70. Kersh E, Kronfield SJ, Unger A, et al. Autonomic insufficiency as a cause of hemodialysis-induced hypotension. *N Engl J Med* 1974;290:650–653.

71. Kusakari J, Kobayashi T, Rokugo M, et al. The inner ear dysfunction in hemodialysis patients. *Tohoku J Exp Med* 1981;135:359–369.

72. Siamopolous KC, Tsianos EV, Dardamanis M, et al. Esophageal dysfunction in chronic hemodialysis patients. *Nephron* 1990;55:389–393.

73. Harding AE, Le Fanu J. Carpal tunnel syndrome related to antebrachial Cimino-Brescia fistula. *J Neurol Neurosurg Psychiatry* 1977;40:511–513.

74. Wilbourn AJ, Furlan AJ, Hulley W, et al. Ischemic monomelic neuropathy. *Neurology* 1983;33:447–451.

75. Bolton CF, Driedger AA, Lindsay RM. Ischemic neuropathy in uremic patients caused by bovine arteriovenous shunt. *J Neurol Neurosurg Psychiatry* 1979;42:810–814.

76. Kunis CL, Markowitz GS, Liu-Jarin X, et al. Painful myopathy and end-stage renal disease. *Am J Kidney Dis* 2001;37(5):1098–1104.

77. Campistol JM. Uremic myopathy. *Kidney Int* 2002;62(5):1901–1913.

78. Goodhue WW, Davis JN, Porro RS. Ischemic myopathy in uremic hyperparathyroidism. *JAMA* 1972;221:911–912.

79. Diaz D, Deliz B, Benbadis S. The use of newer antiepileptical drugs in patients with kidney disease. *Expert Rev Neurother* 2014;12(1):99–105.

CHAPTER 31

Diabetes Management in a Patient with End-Stage Kidney Disease

Andrew Kowalski, Ruchita Patel, Armand Krikorian, and Edgar V. Lerma

 EPIDEMIOLOGY

For some time, diabetes mellitus (DM) has been known to be the leading cause of chronic kidney disease (CKD) in the world. Diabetic kidney disease (DKD) is a well-known complication hastened by uncontrolled diabetes, and unfortunately, it is a condition that affects millions around the world. Estimations in the United States demonstrate that diabetes is responsible for approximately 50% of all end-stage kidney disease (ESKD) in the developed world (1). Although the number of ESKD patients due to diabetes continues to rise, with nearly 50,000 new cases in 2011, the incidence has seemed to have plateaued over the last decade (2). This plateau may be attributed, in part, to an increase in education and awareness, easy accessibility to supportive medications, and due diligence in screening on the part of primary care providers. Despite this trend, the prevalence of DKD is increasing in the United States with an increase from 7.4% to 9.6% in adults over the age of 20 years from 1998 to 2006 (3). Differences remain among socioeconomic classes and ethnic subgroups such as African Americans, Hispanics, and Native Americans having a higher rate of ESKD (4). This is likely in response to the increase in incidence of type 2 diabetes and obesity that is plaguing younger generations allowing the expansion of diabetes at younger ages (4).

Current advances in renal replacement therapy, especially dialytic modalities, have slowly decreased mortality rates over the past years. According the United States Renal Data System, mortality rates have declined 26% since 1985 and 21% since 2000 in patients receiving hemodialysis (1). Additionally, 52% and 61% of patients receiving hemodialysis and peritoneal dialysis, respectively, are still alive after 3 years of therapy. Despite these advances, the all-cause mortality rate still remains high in patients receiving dialysis, 6.5 to 7.9 times greater than in the general population (1). Moreover, diabetic dialysis patients have a worse survival than those with

other ESKD etiologies with a survival of 34% at 5 years (2). It can be inferred that if this trend continues, then two probable paths will emerge, either the incidence will continue to increase proportionally with an increase in DKD and progression to ESKD or there will be a maintained plateau or even fall in ESKD prevalence with continued focus of prevention of DKD (3). That is why it is imperative that continued education, perseverance of screening, and appropriate pharmacotherapy be implemented.

 IMPACT ON PATIENTS AND RESOURCES

DKD continues to have a large impact on patient morbidity and financial institutions. Kidney disease, notably albuminuria, and declining glomerular filtration rates are independent risk factors for cardiovascular disease and noncardiovascular mortality (4). These consequences are related to the micro- and macrovascular sequelae that arise from repeated insults of oxidative stresses and inflammatory mediators as a result of chronic diabetes. Furthermore, ESKD confers a risk of cardiovascular disease about 40 to 50 times greater than the general population (5).

The financial burden of ESKD is high and has been steadily increasing. In 2012, Medicare's expenses for ESKD had risen 3.2% from the previous year, the highest in the last 20 years, accounting for a total of $28.6 billion and 5.6% of the total Medicare expenditure (1). These expenses cover 5,525,481 ESKD patients in the prevalent Medicare population, along with 111,418 non-Medicare patients, with the latter adding an additional estimated $14.93 billion (1). The total fee-for-service in the hemodialysis population in per person per year (PPPY) were $87,945 in 2011 and for peritoneal dialysis patients $71,630 PPPY (1). These costs have led to significant economic strain on the U.S. health care system especially in light of budget cuts in recent years.

MORTALITY IN PATIENTS WITH DIABETES AND END-STAGE KIDNEY DISEASE

Although there is an increased risk of mortality related to end-stage microvascular events such as progressive nephropathy and retinopathy, cardiovascular events have escalated rates of morbidity and mortality in patients with DM (6). Multiple studies have been conducted to evaluate cardiovascular and all-cause mortality in diabetic patients with comparison between intensive versus conventional/ standard glycemic control therapy.

In patients with type 1 DM, Diabetes Control and Complications Trial (DCCT) demonstrated that intensive glycemic control [targeting a glycated hemoglobin (Hb$_{A1c}$) level of less than 7% vs. 9%] delayed the onset of microvascular complications and nephropathy with a 34% and 56% reduction in microalbuminuria and macroalbuminuria over a mean follow-up period of 6.5 years (7). In Epidemiology of Diabetes Interventions and Complications (EDIC), a follow-up study was completed to evaluate cardiovascular outcomes in this population. DCCT could not assess such results because of the younger population demography (ages 13 to 39 years). EDIC monitored patients for an 11-year period and found that intensive glycemic control lowered the risk of a cardiovascular event by 42% and by 57% for a severe cardiovascular event. It was extrapolated that those patients with cardiovascular events also had some level of retinopathy or nephropathy concurrently. Thus, EDIC demonstrated that intensive glycemic control contributed to a decrease in end organ damage, including nephropathy (7).

There are four significant trials that examined cardiovascular events in patients with type 2 DM, in comparing intensive versus conventional glucose control. In the United Kingdom Prospective Diabetes Study (UKPDS), intensive glycemic control (fasting glucose <108 mg/dL, median Hb$_{A1c}$ 7.0%) led to a 25% reduction in microvascular complications (mainly retinopathy requiring photocoagulation) in patients with newly diagnosed with type 2 DM. There was also a reduction in myocardial infarctions and all-cause mortality that was ascertained during a 10-year follow-up period (8). This amount of extended follow-up could not be replicated in the other studies analyzing similar variables (8).

Afterward, in the Action to Control Cardiovascular Risk in Diabetes (ACCORD) trial, the initial goal aimed to see if the results from DCCT crossed over to patients with type 2 DM. In ACCORD trial, the intensive glycemic control group had an average Hb$_{A1c}$ <6%, while the standard glycemic control group had an average Hb$_{A1c}$ of 7% to 7.9%. Diverging from similar studies, ACCORD trial found that patients in the intensive therapy group had increased mortality, with no improvement in cardiovascular risk reduction. The original study was prematurely halted due to this statistically significant and surprising finding. A follow-up of the study illustrated a reduction in nonfatal cardiovascular events (9).

Concurrently, in the Action in Diabetes and Vascular Disease: Preterax and Diamicron Modified Release Controlled Evaluation (ADVANCE) trial, patients with onset of DM after age 30 years were examined. There was a 23% reduction of microvascular events such as nephropathy in the intensive glycemic control (Hb$_{A1c}$ less than or equal to 6.5%) study group compared to the standard one at a mean 5-year follow-up period. In contrast to the ACCORD trial, there was not an increased risk of mortality in the intensive glycemic control study group. An additional 5-year follow-up demonstrated similar findings as well (9).

In Glucose Control and Vascular Complications in Veterans with Type 2 Diabetes [Veterans Affairs Diabetes Trial (VADT)],

a similar group of patients was found to have no significant improvement in cardiovascular event rate after randomization to intensive versus standard glycemic control study groups. After a 5.6-year follow-up, the constricted group (average Hb$_{A1c}$ 6.5%) had a decreased occurrence of microvascular events, in mainly the incidence of nephropathy. However, the number of deaths did not significantly differ between the two study groups (10).

In review of these trials, it is concluded that long-term intensive glucose control (Hb$_{A1c}$ around 7%) corresponds to the delay in developing kidney disease secondary to DM. The question of whether CKD itself presents a risk factor for cardiovascular mortality is not addressed in these studies, as most of the selected patients did not have preexisting CKD from another known etiology. Unfortunately, there have been no randomized controlled trials assessing mortality in patients with diabetes and ESKD. Therefore, the clinician's goal is to aim for optimal glycemic control in patients, with the hope to prevent DKD or delay the progression.

GLUCOSE HOMEOSTASIS IN RENAL DYSFUNCTION

Insulin utilization in muscle and adipose tissue is the rate-limiting step that sets into action specific transporter proteins to translocate glucose into cells (11). These actions are precipitated by the phosphorylation of the insulin receptor substrate 1 (IRS-1), thereby leading to the activation of other downstream proteins, namely, protein kinase C, glycogen synthase, and endothelial nitric oxide synthase, and ultimately leading to the uptake of glucose (11).

In light of renal dysfunction, glucose homeostasis experiences altered functions, with episodes of sustained or periodic hyper- or hypoglycemia (12). Abnormal glucose control has been a known manifestation of renal dysfunction, notably ESKD, for many decades (13). Although diabetes plays a key role, patients with ESKD from other etiologies have also been noted to experience altered glucose metabolism leading to a mild fasting hyperglycemia and episodes of spontaneous hypoglycemia (14).

Insulin Clearance

One of the key abnormal factors that surround glucose homeostasis in ESKD is the clearance of insulin by the kidneys. Insulin clearance is mediated by its uptake and degradation in the peritubular and endothelial cells of the kidney (13). Glomerular filtration has little effect on insulin clearance until the filtration rate drops below 40 mL/min. The uptake and degradation of insulin is increased as the filtration rate decreased, until the filtration rate reaches 15 to 20 mL/min, and then the rate of insulin clearance declines proportionally (13). The rate of insulin uptake and degradation is also affected by other factors that lead to a prolonged half-life of the compound. As kidney function begins to decline, other toxins begin to accumulate and sites of nonrenal insulin degradation such as muscle and liver begin to experience impaired function contributing to a longer circulating time (13).

Hyperglycemia

In the advanced stages of CKD, hyperglycemia and glucose intolerance continue to progress until a decline in insulin secretion and insulin resistance is observed (13). Hyperglycemia, as a manifestation of insulin resistance and glucose intolerance, has also been observed in nondiabetic patients. This suggests that one of the presenting features of ESKD is insulin dysregulation and that it possibly plays a role in the alteration of glucose regulation (13). Studies have looked at insulin receptor sites in uremic patients and through the investigation of muscle biopsies rendered normal insulin binding and activation of downstream proteins (15). This suggests that in uremic patients, the mechanisms are not related to alterations in the protein complexes themselves but may be related to an outside influence. One suggestion is the possibility of oxidative and nonoxidative pathways augmenting insulin resistance (16). Although the exact pathogenesis is not known, it is speculated that accumulation of uremic toxins, such as pseudouridine and asymmetric dimethyl arginine (ADMA), may play a role in insulin resistance, as improvements in sensitivity has been observed when patients began dialysis (17). Additionally, urea, which was never given weight in terms of toxicity, has been shown in animal models to induce reactive oxygen species and lead to insulin resistance (18). Long-standing metabolic acidosis may also play a role in insulin resistance as it has been associated with progressive inflammation and protein-energy malnutrition due to its influence on catabolic effects at the cellular level (19). Administration of bicarbonate has been shown to mitigate its effects with improved insulin sensitivity and insulin secretion in uremic patients (20).

Chronic inflammation, as in ESKD, also leads to impaired glucose uptake due to the release of inflammatory mediators such as interleukin 6 (IL-6), C-reactive protein (CRP), interleukin 1 beta (IL-1-β), and tumor necrosis factor alpha (TNF-α) (21). TNF-α appears to play a major role in insulin resistance through multiple mechanisms. Downstream effects of TNF-α mediation have been shown to induce the phosphorylation of muscle cell IRS-1 that is linked to two main pathways: phosphatidylinositol 3-kinase and protein kinase B (18). These two pathways are metabolically responsible for the majority of glucose transport. With the phosphorylation of IRS-1, downstream effects are activated in the insulin receptor that ultimately leads to a failure of the signaling pathway and disrupts glucose transporter type 4 (GLUT4) translocation, thereby interfering with glucose uptake (22). This was observed after the infusion of TNF-α in healthy humans, where downstream effects lead to the dysfunction in the GLUT4 transporter (23). TNF-α is also responsible for the induction of lipolysis and accumulation of free fatty acids that contribute to insulin resistance through the induction of additional inflammatory markers in the hepatic system (24). IL-6 contributes to insulin resistance by the induction of suppressors of cytokine signaling (SOCS) proteins responsible for feedback regulation (25). These proteins directly affect the insulin receptor and IRS-1 resulting in an inhibition of glucose translocation into muscle and adipose tissue (25).

Other factors have also emerged that lead to the suggestion that alterations in metabolism, primarily adipose tissue, have played a role in insulin resistance. Adipose tissue, accounting for less than 2% of glucose load usage, is now acknowledged as an active organ that secretes numerous enzymes, hormones, and cytokines (26). The tissue is rich in macrophages and adipocytes, and it is speculated that these cells release TNF-α and IL-6 among other cytokines, commonly referred to as adipokines (26). Data suggests that in uremic patient's adipose tissue, primarily visceral fat, is an important source of these inflammatory molecules (27). The progressive reduction in renal function contributes to the imbalance of these adipokines, along with decreased clearance of proinflammatory cytokines leading to a state of chronic inflammation (26).

Many adipokines play a role in the augmentation of insulin sensitivity. Leptin is a small peptide responsible for energy expenditure and the feeling of satiety that is commonly filtered by the kidney and degraded in the renal tubules (28). This peptide appears to have a correlation with CRP and has been suggested that elevation in its plasma concentration may be a major contributor in uremic cachexia (29). Interestingly, additional studies in animal models have proposed that hyperleptinemia may lead to increased expression of TGF-β and therefore contribute to the development of tubulointerstitial fibrosis and nephron destruction further decreasing renal clearance (30). Although chronic plasma elevations of leptin may contribute to worsening kidney disease, its association with insulin resistance is not quite understood. It has been observed that elevated plasma concentrations of leptin appear to be associated with elevated insulin levels leading to the speculation that resistance is present (31).

Adiponectin is another small adipokine peptide that is predominantly secreted by adipocytes. Unlike other cytokines, adiponectin has many protective biologic roles as it appears to have anti-inflammatory and antiatherogenic properties along with an insulin sensitizing effect by inducing GLUT4 (32). Its actions are primarily responsible for assisting in the production on nitric oxide in the endothelial cells, fatty acid oxidation, and inhibition of hepatic gluconeogenesis (33). Although adiponectin is a desirable peptide, lower levels are a result of chronic inflammation and have been implicated in increasing the risk for cardiovascular disease and the development of insulin resistance (34). Although lower concentrations are associated with resistance, patients undergoing hemodialysis were found to have exceptionally high levels of adiponectin (35). The elevation is likely related to the decrease in renal function; however, there is some minor evidence that there might be an upregulation in adiponectin synthesis in response to the uremic inflammatory state (36). Despite ESKD patients having elevations in adiponectin, it is currently unknown as to how this relates to insulin resistance.

Recent evidence has pointed to the role of vitamin D deficiency and secondary hyperparathyroidism in insulin resistance, suggesting that there is an inverse relationship between serum 25-hydroxyvitamin D and insulin resistance (13). One of the nonclassical effects of vitamin D is the effect on the islet cells in the pancreas and the stimulation of insulin secretion (37). Vitamin D repletion has been shown to increase insulin secretion and improve glucose tolerance in hemodialysis patients without changes in parathyroid hormone concentration (37).

Finally, a major contribution to hyperglycemia in patients undergoing dialysis is the use of larger glucose concentrations in peritoneal dialysis. Glucose concentrations in dialysate can range from 1,360 to 3,860 mg/dL and can contribute to as much as 10% to 30% of a patient's total caloric intake (38).

Hypoglycemia

Alterations in renal physiology compounded with dialytic therapy have been observed to change the natural course of diabetes, leaving the patient with variability in glucose homeostasis (39). The uremic milieu has been thought to contribute to poor glucose tolerance and a decrease in insulin sensitivity leaving the patient with episodes of hyperglycemia (2). Despite these observations, spontaneous resolution of hyperglycemia, along with an impressive normalization of Hb$_{A1c}$, has been seen in patients undergoing dialysis, regardless of other treatment modalities (39). This phenomenon has been described as "burnt-out" diabetes, where in many diabetic patients undergoing dialysis, the occurrence of glucose normalization with spontaneous hypoglycemia results in the cessation of antidiabetic therapy in hopes of mitigating the potentially fatal episodes (40).

This condition appears to be multifactorial, with numerous factors contributing to glucose normalization. As progression to ESKD occurs, there is an observed reduction in the nephron mass (41). This reduction, likely related to nephron scarring and an attenuation of function, may lead to the reduced renal gluconeogenesis (42). Additionally, the uremic milieu asserts its deleterious effect on hepatic functions by disrupting the mechanisms of insulin clearance, thus contributing to an increase in the half-life of circulating insulin (13). The process of insulin clearance and degradation is affected once the filtration rate declines to below 15 to 20 m/min (39).

Along this thought, the decline in filtration rate leads to the accumulation of multiple uremic toxins (39). Guanidine solutes contribute to a large variety of compounds that make up the uremic milieu (43). Several have been implicated in vascular disease acceleration and have been identified as players in neuronal, cardiovascular, leukocyte, erythrocyte, and platelet dysfunction (43). Biguanides are frequently used to treat type 2 diabetes, and interestingly, their structure is composed of a simple marriage between two guanidine with the loss of an ammonia group (2). It has been suggested that the accumulation of these guanidine groups may contribute to the stabilization of blood glucose and the normalization of Hb_{A1c} (2).

These metabolic instabilities have been observed to extend beyond the context of glucose homeostasis. Physical fitness has long been advised a method of glucose control (13). Observations have been made with dialysis patients who participate in a long-term fitness program resulting in improved glucose tolerance, normalizations of glycemic, and exercise capacity (44).

Existing evidence has shown that uremia contributes to muscle protein catabolism and likely other metabolic defects (12). Nondiabetic and nonobese patients undergoing dialysis have also been observed to undergo similar muscle protein catabolism (12). This breakdown has been implicated through the ubiquitin–proteasome pathway due to the suppression of phosphatidylinositol-3 kinase (39).

Glucose utilization may also be improved by the influence of diabetes in the mechanics of gut motility. Diabetic gastroparesis leads to slowing of gut motility leading to early satiety and contributes to poor oral intake and malnutrition (13). Along that thought, distention of the abdominal cavity caused by peritoneal dialysate may also contribute to the delayed gastric emptying and interfere with food intake and utilizations (45). Additionally, there is evidence that suggests that hemodialysis may also lead to dysfunction of myenteric activity, thereby contributing to the gastric dysfunction in ESKD patients (46). Long durations of poor glycemic control has been associated with a higher incidence of gastroparesis; fortunately, prokinetic agents have been shown to ameliorate the effects and lead to improved absorption in this population (47).

 MONITORING

Management of diabetic patients undergoing dialysis has numerous challenges as previously stated. The question arises as to how to monitor such a patient to mitigate the complications associated with attempting to achieve glucose homeostasis. Guidelines have proposed the use of Hb_{A1c} as a tool with a goal of <7% and a slightly less stringent goal for the elderly (48). Dialysis patients pose a challenge as their comorbidities and metabolic derangements often lead to inaccuracies in laboratory methods. These inaccuracies have led to the investigation of other laboratory modalities, namely, fructosamine and glycated albumin (2).

Fructosamine

Fructosamine is a measurement of nonenzymatically glycated serum proteins that have stable ketoamines (49). This measurement has become increasingly popular as a metric for short-term glucose monitoring in ESKD patients, with an assessment period of about 7 to 14 days (12). Fructosamine has been of interest because of its ability to more accurately predict glycemic control in states of chronic anemia regardless of the use of erythrocyte-stimulating agents (40). Despite these accuracies in altered hemoglobin levels, fructosamine has been observed to underestimate glucose control in states of dysproteinemias, such as malnutrition, protein-energy wasting, hepatic disease, steroid use, and in peritoneal dialysis (50). Although fructosamine's accuracy offers diminishing returns in states of hypoproteinemia, studies have shown that its use may be beneficial as a predictor of increased hospitalization and infection (51). Additionally, fructosamine has been observed as a marker of cardiovascular mortality, with evidence supporting a doubling of fructosamine correlating with a twofold increase in cardiovascular disease (52).

Glycated Albumin

Similar to the formation of fructosamine, glycated albumin is a nonenzymatic reaction of glucose with albumin that is able to measure glucose control within a similar time frame of 7 to 14 days (53). Studies have proposed that glycated albumin is a better measure of glycemic control in patients with diabetes and CKD, although few studies have looked into its impact on ESKD (12). As with fructosamine, glycated albumin is not influenced by erythrocyte lifespan, anemia, or erythropoietin stimulants but is influenced by abnormal protein turnover, peritoneal dialysis, infections, malnutrition, and steroids (2). Although fructosamine and glycated albumin have many similarities, improved assays have allowed glycated albumin greater accuracy in settings of hypoalbuminemia (54). Glycated albumin has also been noted to be superior to Hb_{A1c} as large studies discovered lower values of Hb_{A1c} when compared to direct glucose measurements and glycated albumin suggesting a better representation of overall glucose control (54). Additionally, increasing concentrations of glycated hemoglobin were believed to be a strong predictor of hospitalization and overall mortality as compared to glucose levels and Hb_{A1c} (55). Despite the limitations of fructosamine and glycated albumin, further research and deeper investigation is warranted into these novel metrics as interest has shown a specific niche and predictive value in patients with ESKD.

Hemoglobin A1c

Hb_{A1c} is typically described as a nonenzymatic reaction between hemoglobin β chains and glucose and is typically illustrated as a percentage of the total hemoglobin exposed to glucose over time (39). This measurement offers a rough 120-day timeline of a patient's average blood glucose concentration. The value is influenced by numerous factors: glucose concentration, anemia, length of glucose exposure, serum pH, and temperature; therefore, it is not unreasonable to expect alterations in Hb_{A1c} in dialysis patients with their prevalence of metabolic derangements (50). Exposures to elevated urea concentrations have been shown to lead to the formation of carbamylated hemoglobin, which is indistinguishable from Hb_{A1c} in certain assays (2). Furthermore, Hb_{A1c} appears to normalize in the dialysis population, and this can be attributed to a number of factors. With progression to ESKD, erythropoietin production diminishes leading to a state of chronic anemia. The uremic milieu also contributes to a decreased erythrocyte lifespan by leading to hemoglobinopathies and an increase in erythrocyte fragility (12). Erythropoietin has thus been frequently utilized as a stimulating agent to increase the production of erythrocytes (56). All of these factors have led to the phenomena of Hb$_{A1c}$ normalization. Additionally, chronic anemia and a decreased erythrocyte lifespan have led to an underestimation of Hb$_{A1c}$, compounded by the utilization of erythrocyte-stimulating agents, which lead to the production of new, nonglycated erythrocytes and thus leading to a further decrease in Hb$_{A1c}$ (56).

Despite the evidence of uremia and anemia affecting the value of Hb$_{A1c}$, guidelines from the Kidney Disease Improving Global Outcomes (KDIGO) and the Kidney Disease Outcomes Quality Initiative (KDOQI) recommend long-term and routine Hb$_{A1c}$ measurements along with home blood glucose monitoring as a staple in the management of diabetes in patients with ESKD (57).

OPTIMUM GLUCOSE CONTROL

Appropriate glucose control in ESKD patients has long been a concern and struggle for health care professionals. Large trials have demonstrated that uncontrolled blood glucose predisposes patients to micro- and macrovascular disease and have stressed the importance of targeting Hb$_{A1c}$ to <7% (39). More recent landmark trials such as ADVANCE trial, the VADT, and ACCORD trial pointed out that intensive glycemic control may have no benefit on cardiovascular outcomes and in patients with preexisting cardiovascular disease may even increase the risk of mortality (58). This has led to some concerns as normalization of blood glucose in patients with underlying cardiovascular disease may potentially lead to an increase in mortality (59).

As previously mentioned, ESKD patients are at risk for hypoglycemia and have been observed to normalize their Hb$_{A1c}$ over time, with one study suggesting that about 33% of diabetic dialysis patients have an Hb$_{A1c}$ of <6% (60). This leads to the uncertainty of an optimal glycemic target in dialysis patients (2). In an attempt to answer this question, there was a small study that showed no correlation between Hb$_{A1c}$ and mortality. It was quickly criticized due to the lack of repeated Hb$_{A1c}$ measurements and multiple confounders (61). A subsequent study with a longer duration of follow-up initially suggested an increase in mortality with lower Hb$_{A1c}$ levels. This study was also criticized when adjusted for other confounders such as malnutrition and inflammation: Higher Hb$_{A1c}$ levels correlated with mortality (60). Building on these two studies, subsequent research has pointed out that Hb$_{A1c}$ exhibits a J-shaped curve with mortality being prevalent at <6.5% and >11% (62). More recent work has suggested that Hb$_{A1c}$ values of <6% and >8% were associated with an increase in mortality (63). Additionally, analysis has also suggested that a lower Hb$_{A1c}$ may be a marker for malnutrition and worsening illness (2). Currently, KDIGO and KDOQI recommend that Hb$_{A1c}$ in dialysis patients be maintained >7% in those with comorbidities and decreased life expectancy to minimize the risk of hypoglycemia and death (57).

Although no studies have looked at a comparison of hemodialysis to peritoneal dialysis, observational data supports that both modalities might be equally efficacious (12). When diving deeper into recent literature, suggestions have arisen that hemodialysis might have a slightly better advantage in survival, but this appears to be short lived with disadvantages emerging after 2 years of use (64). Further differences appear between the two modalities in regard to diabetic patients with abnormal glucose homeostasis. Patients undergoing peritoneal dialysis, especially diabetic patients, are at risk of developing

peritoneal fibrosis at a faster rate and ultimately compromising ultrafiltration (12). Additional challenges in glucose management stem from the high glucose concentration in the peritoneal dialysate. This large glucose load often contributes to the patient's morbidity and offers additional challenges in achieving glucose control (12). Glucose control may be achieved with the substitution of dextrose with icodextrin. This polymer is advantageous in that it is minimally absorbed across the peritoneal membrane, although lymphatic absorption does occur (65). While safe, its use may lead to confusion and difficulty with glucose management by the development of spurious hyperglycemia. After being absorbed by the lymphatic system, icodextrin is metabolized to maltose metabolites, which some on glucometers will register as significant hyperglycemia and if not educated properly may lead the patient to receive a larger insulin load (65).

THERAPEUTIC MANAGEMENT OF DIABETICS IN END-STAGE KIDNEY DISEASE POPULATION

There is a continuing challenge in treating patients with progressive diabetic nephropathy and specifically ESKD. Not only is mortality linked to medication side effects, namely, hypoglycemia, but cardiovascular risk of death is heightened in this population as well (57). Insulin therapy is mainstay therapy in diabetic patients with ESKD, largely due to contraindication of most oral hypoglycemic agents in severe renal impairment. In general, oral medications are not indicated in this group because of increased drug accumulation with decreased renal clearance leads to adverse drug effects such has hypoglycemia. Dose adjustments are required in CKD and ESKD in those medications that can be used in diabetic patients in ESKD (**TABLE 31.1**) (66).

Biguanides

Metformin has been the most widely studied oral antidiabetic agent. By decreasing hepatic gluconeogenesis, its prevalent use stems from the mostly tolerable side effects. Most commonly, gastrointestinal disturbance is experienced with initial therapy that is titrated up in a stepwise manner. A benefit of the medication is the lack of weight gain observed (8). In addition, monitoring of vitamin B$_{12}$ and folate levels is required with long-term therapy. Historically, metformin has been contraindicated in patients with renal impairment [plasma creatinine >1.5 mg/dL for men and >1.4 mg/dL in women, estimated glomerular filtration rate (eGFR) <40 mL/min/1.73 m^2]. Lactic acidosis is the rare complication most concerning with metformin use and occurs at a rate of less than 0.01 to 0.08 cases per 1,000 patient-years. Renal impairment is the greatest risk factor for the development of lactic acidosis (67). However, through review of observational and retrospective studies, metformin will not likely increase the risk of lactic acidosis in patients with CKD stage 3 (eGFR 30 to 60 mL/min/1.73 m^2), but no randomized controlled trials exist as of yet (68). About 90% of metformin is excreted through the kidneys, and thus, there is decreased elimination of the drug in patients with reduced kidney function. It is recommended the dose be halved in patients with eGFR <60 mL/min/1.73 m^2 and completely avoided in patients on dialysis (69).

Sulfonylureas

Sulfonylureas stimulate insulin secretion by binding to sulfonylurea receptors, leading to closure of adenosine triphosphate (ATP)-sensitive potassium channels on pancreatic β cells and then

TABLE 31.1	Summary of Antidiabetic Medications and Their Use in End-Stage Kidney Disease						
Drug Class	Drug	Mechanism of Action/Pharmacokinetics	Adverse Side Effects	Use in HD	Use in PD	Dose Adjustment (if Used in PD/HD)	Dialyzable?
Sulfonylureas: First generation	Acetohexamide Chlorpropamide Tolazamide Tolbutamide	Closes potassium channel on pancreatic β cell membrane, promoting insulin secretion; longer half-lives than second generation — Excreted in urine	Hypoglycemia, nausea, affects liver enzymes, hypersensitivity in patients with sulfa allergies, weight gain	No No No No	No No No No		
Sulfonylureas: Second generation	Glipizide Gliclazide Glyburide Glimepiride	Closes potassium channel on pancreatic β cell membrane, promoting insulin secretion — Excreted in urine; 20% excreted in urine; 50% excreted in urine; Excreted in urine	Hypoglycemia, nausea, affects liver enzymes, hypersensitivity in patients with sulfa allergies, weight gain	Yes Yes No No	Yes Yes No No	None None	
Meglitinides (can be used as monotherapy in some ESKD patients)	Repaglinide	Insulin secretagogue; act at ATP-dependent potassium channels on pancreatic β cells (different site than sulfonylureas) — Excreted in feces	Hypoglycemia	Yes, with caution	Yes, with caution	Initiate 0.5 mg before each meal (not done in United States)	
	Nateglinide Mitiglinide (only approved in Japan)	Decreases postprandial glucose levels — Excreted in urine		Yes, with caution	Yes, with caution	Initiate dose of 120 mg daily	
Biguanides	Metformin	Inhibits hepatic gluconeogenesis, increases peripheral sensitivity to insulin — Excreted in urine	Nausea, diarrhea, metallic taste, lactic acidosis (0.03 cases per 1,000 patient-years), weight loss	No	No		Yes
Thiazolidinediones	Rosiglitazone	Decreases hepatic gluconeogenesis; increases peripheral sensitivity to insulin by acting on PPAR-γ receptor — Primarily excreted in urine	Increase LDL-C, increased cardiovascular related mortality, volume expansion	Avoid	Avoid		
	Pioglitazone	Excreted in urine and feces	Bladder cancer, volume expansion	Avoid	Avoid		
Incretin-based: dipeptidyl peptidase 4 (DPP4) inhibitors	Sitagliptin	Increase GLP-1 activity by blocking DPP4 — Excreted in urine	Hepatotoxicity, acute pancreatitis (both rare)	Yes	Yes	Initiate 25 mg/d	<15% dialyzable
	Saxagliptin	Excreted in feces		Yes	Yes	Initiate 2.5 mg/d	25% dialyzable
	Vildagliptin			Yes	Yes	Initiate low dose	
	Alogliptin			Yes	Yes	Initiate 6.25 mg/d	
	Linagliptin			Yes	Yes	None	

(Continued)

TABLE 31.1 Continued

Drug Class	Drug	Mechanism of Action/Pharmacokinetics	Adverse Side Effects	Use in HD	Use in PD	Dose Adjustment (if Used in PD/HD)	Dialyzable?
Incretin-based: glucagon-like peptide-1 (GLP-1) agonists	Exenatide	Resistant to metabolism by DPP4; increase insulin secretion and suppress glucagon secretion in a glucose-dependent manner	Nausea, vomiting, weight loss, pancreatitis, thyroid C-cell hyperplasia, and tumors (liraglutide and weekly exenatide)	No	No		
	Liraglutide	Excreted in urine and feces		Avoid	Avoid		
	Albiglutide			No	No		
α-Glucosidase inhibitors	Acarbose	Inhibits gastrointestinal α-glucosidases and pancreatic α-amylases, affecting gastrointestinal glucose absorption	Flatulence, diarrhea, abdominal pain	No	No		
	Miglitol	Excreted in urine		No	No		
	Voglibose			No	No		
Sodium-glucose cotransporter 2 (SGLT2) inhibitors	Canagliflozin	Inhibits glucose absorption at the SGLT2 receptor in the renal proximal tubule, promoting glucosuria	Genitourinary tract infections, hypotension, diabetic ketoacidosis, dehydration	No	No		
	Dapagliflozin			No	No		
	Empagliflozin			No	No		
Amylin analogs	Pramlintide	Stimulates glucose dependent insulin release from pancreatic β cells, inhibits glucagon release, decreases appetite, delays gastric emptying	Nausea, hypoglycemia	Avoid	Avoid		
Dopamine 2 agonists	Bromocriptine	Unknown mechanism, may reset hypothalamic circadian activities which have been altered by obesity	Dizziness, headache, fatigue, constipation, low efficacy	No data	No data		
Bile acid sequestrant	Colesevelam	Binds with bile acids in intestine to form insoluble complex, eliminated in feces	Constipation, lowers LDL	No data	No data		
Insulin	Aspart, lispro, glulisine Regular Neutral protamine hagedorn (NPH) Detemir Glargine	Supplements endogenous insulin	Hypoglycemia, weight gain	Yes	Yes (can use intraperitoneal vs. subcutaneous)	Initiate 50% dose reduction; those on PD may require increase in dosage due to absorption of glucose from the dialysate through the peritoneal cavity	No

HD, hemodialysis; PD, peritoneal dialysis; ESKD, end-stage kidney disease; ATP, adenosine triphosphate; PPAR, peroxisome proliferator-activated receptor; LDL-C, low-density lipoprotein cholesterol; LDL, low-density lipoprotein.
Avoid = limited data on use in patients with estimated glomerular filtration rate less than 30 mL/min/1.73 m².

insulin release (69). Because of their mechanism, the most common side effects are hypoglycemia and weight gain, and its effectiveness decreases with prolonged history of DM and reduction in β cell function. The United Kingdom Prospective Diabetes Study and ADVANCE trial demonstrated sulfonylureas' success in achieving tight glycemic control (8). They are excreted mainly in the urine. First-generation sulfonylureas (acetohexamide, chlorpropamide, tolazamide, and tolbutamide) were known to have longer duration of action and so, contraindicated in dialysis patients (66). They have since fallen out of clinical practice. The second-generation medications (glipizide, gliclazide, glyburide, glimepiride) are shorter acting and subsequently have a safer side effect profile. In patients on dialysis, the only available medications are glipizide and gliclazide (not available in United States) (69). The major metabolites of glipizide, through aromatic hydroxylation, have no hypoglycemic activity. These two agents do not require dose adjustments in dialysis patients; however, initial doses are low with titration every 1 to 4 weeks (69).

Meglitinides

Similar to sulfonylureas, meglitinides are also insulin secretagogues. Their mechanism of action relies upon closure of ATP-dependent potassium channels on pancreatic β cells at a different site than sulfonylureas. Their role is utilized in lowering postprandial blood glucose levels. With its recommended use to be taken before meals, basal insulin levels are achieved 2 hours after ingestion of the drug (70). The meglitinides (repaglinide, nateglinide, and mitiglinide) are approved for use in dialysis patients. Mitiglinide is only available in Japan. Repaglinide is preferred in dialysis patients because 80% of the drug is metabolized by the liver and about 8% is excreted unchanged in the urine, so there is a lower risk of hypoglycemia (71). Initial dose is 0.5 mg taken prior to meals in dialysis patients (69). Nateglinide has renally excreted metabolites that cause a higher risk of hypoglycemia (72). In ESKD patients, meglitinides can be used as monotherapy agents (73).

Thiazolidinediones

The thiazolidinediones (TZDs), rosiglitazone and pioglitazone, are medications that activate peroxisome proliferator-activated receptors (PPARs). They lower blood glucose levels by increasing peripheral sensitivity to insulin, in addition to decreasing hepatic gluconeogenesis (70). The side effect profiles of both of these medications have led to its infrequent use in recent years. Rosiglitazone was initially thought to lead to increased myocardial infarctions, but a large randomized controlled trial did not show similar results (74). That same randomized controlled trial did show increased risk of heart failure and fractures with rosiglitazone, compared with standard glucose-lowering agents such as metformin and sulfonylureas. However, there was no increased risk of overall cardiovascular morbidity and mortality with its use compared with standard therapy (74). Rosiglitazone can be administered in dialysis patients because less than 1% of its active metabolites are excreted unchanged in the urine. There is no dose adjustment required. Pioglitazone has been linked to increased bladder cancer risk in a large randomized controlled trial (75). Both medications are shown to cause weight gain, along with fluid retention, and thus are generally avoided in ESKD patients (66).

Incretin-Based Therapies

Among the newer antidiabetic agents, the incretin-based therapies have provided an addition to the list of possible medications appropriate for use in dialysis patients. Glucagon-like peptide-1

(GLP-1) is an intestinal hormone that is secreted in response to food, triggering insulin secretion, along with a decrease in glucagon secretion, gut motility, and increase in satiety (70). Dipeptidyl peptidase 4 (DPP4) is an enzyme that breaks down GLP-1.

Glucagon-Like Peptide-1 Agonists

GLP-1 agonists include exenatide, liraglutide, and albiglutide. In contrast to previously mentioned antidiabetic agents, GLP-1 agonists are administered subcutaneously and, in addition, only recommended for adjunct therapy (70). Exenatide is not recommended for use in dialysis patients, and ingestion leads to intolerable nausea, diarrhea, and headache (57). In studies with rats, liraglutide use has led to C-cell hyperplasia, raising concerns for risks of medullary thyroid carcinoma. A randomized controlled trial with 24 patients with type 2 DM and ESKD and 23 control subjects with just type 2 DM demonstrated statistically significant increased plasma through levels of liraglutide in ESKD patients compared to the control group, with increased temporary nausea and vomiting as well (76). Therefore, liraglutide use is not advised in ESKD patients. There is limited data with albiglutide use in severe renal impairment, and thus, its use is not advised.

Dipeptidyl Peptidase 4 Inhibitors

DPP4 inhibitors include sitagliptin, saxagliptin, linagliptin, alogliptin, and vildagliptin (not approved for use in the United States). By increasing GLP-1 activity, these agents work by decreasing postprandial hyperglycemia. Aside from linagliptin, all other members of this class are excreted by the kidneys and require dose adjustments in ESKD patients. The main side effects include weight neutrality and possible hepatotoxicity (70). Sitagliptin dosing is initiated at 25 mg daily in ESKD patients (77). Saxagliptin had similar results in an open-label study with severe renal impairment patients, and recommended initial dose is 2.5 mg daily (78). In addition, about 23% of the drug will be removed with a 4-hour hemodialysis session, so an additional dose may need to be given after it is completed (79,80). Alogliptin dose is adjusted to 6.25 mg daily in ESKD patients, but caution is advised (69). Vildagliptin use in patients with moderate or severe CKD had similar adverse event profiles in the placebo and vildagliptin groups and also labeled with the same warnings as the alogliptin (81). Linagliptin is not renally excreted and therefore does not require dose adjustment; however, its safety has not been extensively studied in the dialysis population (66).

α-Glucosidase Inhibitors

The α-glucosidase inhibitors include acarbose, miglitol, and voglibose (not available in the United States). This class of medications inhibits the enzyme α-glucosidase from metabolizing polysaccharides to monosaccharides (70). Glycemic control is achieved through maintaining homeostatic glucose levels postprandially. The side effect profile limits its use, mainly gastrointestinal: abdominal discomfort, diarrhea, flatulence (2). These medications are not advised in ESKD because of the accumulation of metabolites in severe renal impairment, along with lack of clinical trials, on its use in diabetic patients with ESKD (69).

Sodium-Glucose Cotransporter 2 Inhibitors

The sodium-glucose cotransporter 2 (SGLT2) receptor is found in the proximal renal tubule and responsible for about 90% of glucose reabsorption. Currently, there are three medications in this class: canagliflozin, dapagliflozin, and empagliflozin. The main side effects of these medications include glucosuria, dehydration, and natriuresis. As being the only antidiabetic agent to exhibit its effects on the kidney itself, this class of medications is contraindicated in ESKD patients (82). Canagliflozin is the only SGLT2 inhibitor that can be used in patients with eGFR of 45 mL/min/1.73 m² and greater (83). Recent data from four randomized placebo controlled phase 3 studies indicated that canagliflozin dosed at 100 mg daily will lead to a 0.47% reduction in Hb_{A1c} with a greater number of patients reaching target Hb_{A1c} of <7.0%, compared to placebo. This effect was largely seen in patients with stage 3a CKD (eGFR 45 to <60 mL/min/1.73 m²), as opposed to stage 3b CKD (83). Even though there was a slight decrease in eGFR (10% to 15%) after initiation of therapy, kidney function trended toward baseline after 6 weeks of therapy. This transient decline in kidney function is secondary to intravascular hemodynamic changes after initial therapy and does not suggest progression of CKD (83).

Amylin Analogs

Another medication available to assist in lowering postprandial hyperglycemia is pramlintide, an amylin analog. This medication is appropriate for use in both type 1 and 2 DM. It is an endogenous hormone secreted by pancreatic β cells in response to postprandial hyperglycemia. As an adjunct therapy to mealtime insulin, its use enhances satiety, delays gastric emptying, increases hepatic glycogen synthesis, and subdues postprandial glucagon secretion. Pramlintide has not been studied well in dialysis patients, and therefore, its use in this population is not advised (84).

Bile Acid Sequestrants and Dopamine-2 Agonists

Colesevelam is an antihyperglycemic agent used in type 2 DM with a poorly understood mechanism of action. Its use has been beneficial in diabetic patients with elevated low-density lipoprotein cholesterol levels (85). For dopamine agonists, the antihyperglycemic effect is theorized around the proposed reset of the circadian rhythm in the hypothalamus, leading to less insulin resistance (86). No clinical studies have been conducted for either class on diabetic patients with CKD and ESKD.

Insulin

Insulin therapy is recommended for most patients with ESKD. However, even though it is the most commonly used medication in diabetics with ESKD, it carries a significant risk of hypoglycemia. Insulin's half-life is prolonged since the diseased kidney cannot metabolize it effectively. In addition, there is decreased first-pass hepatic metabolism in ESKD with exogenous use. The improved insulin sensitivity that occurs with the start of hemodialysis contributes to an increased risk of hypoglycemia as well (17). In general, there is basal (glargine, detemir, neutral protamine hagedorn) and mealtime or correction (aspart, regular, lispro, glulisine) insulin therapies. It is recommended to decrease the insulin dose by 50% in patients with ESKD (87). The approach for insulin dosing in ESKD patients is individualized because of variable meal schedules, and thus, no superior treatment, basal, or mealtime has demonstrated a reduction in Hb_{A1c} or other clinical outcomes (88). There are no studies conducted regarding insulin pump use in patients with CKD (12).

In peritoneal dialysis, insulin can be administered subcutaneously or intraperitoneally. In a meta-analysis performed on intraperitoneal insulin use in diabetic patients on peritoneal dialysis, three studies showed that optimal glycemic control was achieved with intraperitoneal insulin versus standard subcutaneous insulin

use. However, insulin use was twofold higher in the intraperitoneal group and showed worsening lipid profiles (89,90). Also, there is an increased risk of bacterial contamination with injection into the dialysate bag, possible peritoneal fibroblastic proliferation, and can cause hepatic subcapsular steatonecrosis (91–93).

 REFERENCES

1. Collins AJ, Foley RN, Chavers B, et al. US Renal Data System 2013 annual data report. *Am J Kidney Dis* 2014;63:A7.
2. Rhee CM, Leung AM, Kovesdy CP, et al. Updates on the management of diabetes in dialysis patients. *Semin Dial* 2014;27:135–145.
3. Cowie CC, Rust KF, Byrd-Holt DD, et al. Prevalence of diabetes and high risk for diabetes using A1C criteria in the U.S. population in 1988-2006. *Diabetes Care* 2010;33:562–568.
4. Tuttle KR, Bakris GL, Bilous RW, et al. Diabetic kidney disease: a report from an ADA Consensus Conference. *Am J Kidney Dis* 2014;64:510–533.
5. Palmer SC, Craig JC, Navaneethan SD, et al. Benefits and harms of statin therapy for persons with chronic kidney disease: a systematic review and meta-analysis. *Ann Intern Med* 2012;157:263–275.
6. Haffner SM, Lehto S, Rönnemaa T, et al. Mortality from coronary heart disease in subjects with type 2 diabetes and in nondiabetic subjects with and without prior myocardial infarction. *N Engl J Med* 1998;339:229–234.
7. The effect of intensive treatment of diabetes on the development and progression of long-term complications in insulin-dependent diabetes mellitus. The Diabetes Control and Complications Trial Research Group. *N Engl J Med* 1993;329:977–986.
8. King P, Peacock I, Donnelly R. The UK prospective diabetes study (UKPDS): clinical and therapeutic implications for type 2 diabetes. *Br J Clin Pharmacol* 1999;48:643–648.
9. Gerstein HC, Miller ME, Byington RP, et al. Effects of intensive glucose lowering in type 2 diabetes. *N Engl J Med* 2008;358:2545–2559.
10. Duckworth W, Abraira C, Moritz T, et al. Glucose control and vascular complications in veterans with type 2 diabetes. *N Engl J Med* 2009;360:129–139.
11. Goldstein BJ, Mahadev K, Wu X. Redox paradox: insulin action is facilitated by insulin-stimulated reactive oxygen species with multiple potential signaling targets. *Diabetes* 2005;54:311–321.
12. Williams ME, Garg R. Glycemic management in ESRD and earlier stages of CKD. *Am J Kidney Dis* 2014;63:S22–S38.
13. Mak RH. Impact of end-stage renal disease and dialysis on glycemic control. *Semin Dial* 2000;13:4–8.
14. Comenzo RL. LECT2 makes the amyloid list. *Blood* 2014;123:1436–1467.
15. Friedman JE, Dohm GL, Elton CW, et al. Muscle insulin resistance in uremic humans: glucose transport, glucose transporters, and insulin receptors. *Am J Physiol* 1991;261:E87–E94.
16. Alvestrand A. Carbohydrate and insulin metabolism in renal failure. *Kidney Int Suppl* 1997;62:S48–S52.
17. DeFronzo RA, Tobin JD, Rowe JW, et al. Glucose intolerance in uremia. Quantification of pancreatic beta cell sensitivity to glucose and tissue sensitivity to insulin. *J Clin Invest* 1978;62:425–435.
18. Liao MT, Sung CC, Hung KC, et al. Insulin resistance in patients with chronic kidney disease. *J Biomed Biotechnol* 2012;2012:691369.
19. Chiu YW, Kopple JD, Mehrotra R. Correction of metabolic acidosis to ameliorate wasting in chronic kidney disease: goals and strategies. *Semin Nephrol* 2009;29:67–74.
20. Kalantar-Zadeh K, Mehrotra R, Fouque D, et al. Metabolic acidosis and malnutrition-inflammation complex syndrome in chronic renal failure. *Semin Dial* 2004;17:455–465.
21. Ikizler TA. Nutrition, inflammation and chronic kidney disease. *Current Opin Nephrol Hypertens* 2008;17:162–167.
22. de Alvaro C, Teruel T, Hernandez R, et al. Tumor necrosis factor alpha produces insulin resistance in skeletal muscle by activation of inhibitor kappaB kinase in a p38 MAPK-dependent manner. *J Biol Chem* 2004;279:17070–17078.

23. Plomgaard P, Bouzakri K, Krogh-Madsen R, et al. Tumor necrosis factor-alpha induces skeletal muscle insulin resistance in healthy human subjects via inhibition of Akt substrate 160 phosphorylation. *Diabetes* 2005;54:2939–2945.

24. Plomgaard P, Fischer CP, Ibfelt T, et al. Tumor necrosis factor-alpha modulates human *in vivo* lipolysis. *J Clin Endocrinol Metab* 2008;93:543–549.

25. Ueki K, Kondo T, Kahn CR. Suppressor of cytokine signaling 1 (SOCS-1) and SOCS-3 cause insulin resistance through inhibition of tyrosine phosphorylation of insulin receptor substrate proteins by discrete mechanisms. *Mol Cell Biol* 2004;24:5434–446.

26. Manolescu B, Stoian I, Atanasiu V, et al. Review article: the role of adipose tissue in uraemia-related insulin resistance. *Nephrology (Carlton)* 2008;13:622–628.

27. Axelsson J, Rashid Qureshi A, Suliman ME, et al. Truncal fat mass as a contributor to inflammation in end-stage renal disease. *Am J Clin Nutr* 2004;80:1222–1229.

28. Meyer C, Robson D, Rackovsky N, et al. Role of the kidney in human leptin metabolism. *Am J Physiol* 1997;273:E903–E907.

29. Cumin F, Baum HP, Levens N. Mechanism of leptin removal from the circulation by the kidney. *J Endocrinol* 1997;155:577–585.

30. Kumpers P, Gueler F, Rong S, et al. Leptin is a coactivator of TGF-beta in unilateral ureteral obstructive kidney disease. *Am J Physiol Renal Physiol* 2007;293:F1355–F1362.

31. Stenvinkel P, Heimbürger O, Lönnqvist F. Serum leptin concentrations correlate to plasma insulin concentrations independent of body fat content in chronic renal failure. *Nephrol Dial Transplant* 1997;12: 1321–1325.

32. Wiecek A, Adamczak M, Chudek J. Adiponectin—an adipokine with unique metabolic properties. *Nephrol Dial Transplant* 2007;22:981–988.

33. Chen H, Montagnani M, Funahashi T, et al. Adiponectin stimulates production of nitric oxide in vascular endothelial cells. *J Biol Chem* 2003;278:45021–45026.

34. Spranger J, Kroke A, Möhlig M, et al. Adiponectin and protection against type 2 diabetes mellitus. *Lancet* 2003;361:226–228.

35. Abdallah E, Waked E, Nabil M, et al. Adiponectin and cardiovascular outcomes among hemodialysis patients. *Kidney Blood Press Res* 2012;35:247–253.

36. Shen YY, Charlesworth JA, Kelly JJ, et al. Up-regulation of adiponectin, its isoforms and receptors in end-stage kidney disease. *Nephrol Dial Transplant* 2007;22:171–178.

37. Mak RH. 1,25-Dihydroxyvitamin D3 corrects insulin and lipid abnormalities in uremia. *Kidney Int* 1998;53:1353–1357.

38. Grodstein GP, Blumenkrantz MJ, Kopple JD, et al. Glucose absorption during continuous ambulatory peritoneal dialysis. *Kidney Int* 1981;19:564–567.

39. Park J, Lertdumrongluk P, Molnar MZ, et al. Glycemic control in diabetic dialysis patients and the burnt-out diabetes phenomenon. *Curr Diab Rep* 2012;12:432–439.

40. Kovesdy CP, Park JC, Kalantar-Zadeh K. Glycemic control and burnt-out diabetes in ESRD. *Semin Dial* 2010;23:148–156.

41. Cano N. Bench-to-bedside review: glucose production from the kidney. *Crit Care* 2002;6:317–321.

42. Arem R. Hypoglycemia associated with renal failure. *Endocrinol Metab Clin North Am* 1989;18:103–121.

43. Eloot S, van Biesen W, Dhondt A, et al. Impact of increasing haemodialysis frequency versus haemodialysis duration on removal of urea and guanidino compounds: a kinetic analysis. *Nephrol Dial Transplant* 2009;24:2225–2232.

44. Rhee CM, Kalantar-Zadeh K. Resistance exercise: an effective strategy to reverse muscle wasting in hemodialysis patients? *J Cachexia Sarcopenia Muscle* 2014;5:177–180.

45. Sutton D, Higgins B, Stevens JM. Continuous ambulatory peritoneal dialysis patients are unable to increase dietary intake to recommended levels. *J Ren Nutr* 2007;17:329–335.

46. Ko CW, Chang CS, Wu MJ, et al. Transient impact of hemodialysis on gastric myoelectrical activity of uremic patients. *Dig Dis Sci* 1998;43:1159–1164.

47. Eisenberg B, Murata GH, Tzamaloukas AH, et al. Gastroparesis in diabetics on chronic dialysis: clinical and laboratory associations and predictive features. *Nephron* 1995;70:296–300.

48. National Kidney Foundation. KDOQI clinical practice guideline for diabetes and CKD: 2012 update. *Am J Kidney Dis* 2012;60:850–886.

49. Armbruster DA. Fructosamine: structure, analysis, and clinical usefulness. *Clin Chem* 1987;33:2153–2163.

50. Kalantar-Zadeh K, Derose SF, Nicholas S, et al. Burnt-out diabetes: impact of chronic kidney disease progression on the natural course of diabetes mellitus. *J Ren Nutr* 2009;19:33–37.

51. Mittman N, Desiraju B, Fazil I, et al. Serum fructosamine versus glycosylated hemoglobin as an index of glycemic control, hospitalization, and infection in diabetic hemodialysis patients. *Kidney Int* 2010;78(Suppl 117):S41–S45.

52. Shafi T, Sozio SM, Plantinga LC, et al. Serum fructosamine and glycated albumin and risk of mortality and clinical outcomes in hemodialysis patients. *Diabetes Care* 2013;36:1522–1533.

53. Alskär O, Korell J, Duffull SB. A pharmacokinetic model for the glycation of albumin. *J Pharmacokinet Pharmacodyn* 2012;39:273–282.

54. Inaba M, Okuno S, Kumeda Y, et al. Glycated albumin is a better glycemic indicator than glycated hemoglobin values in hemodialysis patients with diabetes: effect of anemia and erythropoietin injection. *J Am Soc Nephrol* 2007;18:896–903.

55. Freedman BI, Andries L, Shihabi ZK, et al. Glycated albumin and risk of death and hospitalizations in diabetic dialysis patients. *Clin J Am Soc Nephrol* 2011;6:1635–1643.

56. Nakao T, Matsumoto H, Okada T, et al. Influence of erythropoietin treatment on hemoglobin A1c levels in patients with chronic renal failure on hemodialysis. *Intern Med* 1998;37:826–830.

57. KDIGO 2012 clinical practice guideline for the evaluation and management of chronic kidney disease. *Kidney Int* 2013;3(1):1–150.

58. Patel A, MacMahon S, Chalmers J, et al. Intensive blood glucose control and vascular outcomes in patients with type 2 diabetes. *New Engl J Med* 2008;358:2560–2572.

59. Cushman WC, Evans GW, Byington RP, et al. Effects of intensive blood-pressure control in type 2 diabetes mellitus. *N Engl J Med* 2010;362:1575–1585.

60. Kalantar-Zadeh K, Kopple JD, Regidor DL, et al. A1C and survival in maintenance hemodialysis patients. *Diabetes Care* 2007;30:1049–1055.

61. Williams ME, Lacson E Jr, Teng M, et al. Hemodialyzed type I and type II diabetic patients in the US: characteristics, glycemic control, and survival. *Kidney Int* 2006;70:1503–1509.

62. Williams ME, Lacson E Jr, Wang W, et al. Glycemic control and extended hemodialysis survival in patients with diabetes mellitus: comparative results of traditional and time-dependent Cox model analyses. *Clinn J Am Soc Nephrol* 2010;5:1595–1601.

63. Ricks J, Molnar MZ, Kovesdy CP, et al. Glycemic control and cardiovascular mortality in hemodialysis patients with diabetes: a 6-year cohort study. *Diabetes* 2012;61:708–715.

64. Mehrotra R, Chiu YW, Kalantar-Zadeh K, et al. Similar outcomes with hemodialysis and peritoneal dialysis in patients with end-stage renal disease. *Arch Intern Med* 2011;171:110–118.

65. Riley SG, Chess J, Donovan KL, et al. Spurious hyperglycaemia and icodextrin in peritoneal dialysis fluid. *BMJ* 2003;327:608–609.

66. Flynn C, Bakris GL. Noninsulin glucose-lowering agents for the treatment of patients on dialysis. *Nat Rev Nephrol* 2013;9:147–153.

67. Bailey CJ, Turner RC. Metformin. *N Engl J Med* 1996;334:574–579.

68. Inzucchi SE, Lipska KJ, Mayo H, et al. Metformin in patients with type 2 diabetes and kidney disease: a systematic review. *JAMA* 2014;312:2668–2675.

69. Abe M, Okada K, Soma M. Antidiabetic agents in patients with chronic kidney disease and end-stage renal disease on dialysis: metabolism and clinical practice. *Curr Drug Metab* 2011;12:57–69.

70. Boyle SM, Simon B, Kobrin SM. Antidiabetic therapy in end stage renal disease. *Semin Dial* 2015;28:337–344.

71. Reilly JB, Berns JS. Selection and dosing of medications for management of diabetes in patients with advanced kidney disease. *Semin Dial* 2010;23:163–168.

72. Devineni D, Walter YH, Smith HT, et al. Pharmacokinetics of nateglinide in renally impaired diabetic patients. *J Clin Pharmacol* 2003;43:163–170.

73. Phillippe HM, Wargo KA. Mitiglinide for type 2 diabetes treatment. *Expert Opin Pharmacother* 2013;14:2133–2144.

74. Home PD, Pocock SJ, Beck-Nielsen H, et al. Rosiglitazone evaluated for cardiovascular outcomes in oral agent combination therapy for type 2 diabetes (RECORD): a multicentre, randomised, open-label trial. *Lancet* 2009;373:2125–2135.

75. Dormandy JA, Charbonnel B, Eckland DJ, et al. Secondary prevention of macrovascular events in patients with type 2 diabetes in the PROactive Study (PROspective pioglitAzone Clinical Trial In macroVascular Events): a randomised controlled trial. *Lancet* 2005;366:1279–1289.

76. Idorn T, Knop FK, Jorgensen MB, et al. Safety and efficacy of liraglutide in patients with type 2 diabetes and end-stage renal disease: an investigator-initiated, placebo-controlled, double-blinded, parallel group, randomized trial. *Diabetes Care* 2016;39:206–213.

77. Chan JC, Scott R, Arjona Ferreira JC, et al. Safety and efficacy of sitagliptin in patients with type 2 diabetes and chronic renal insufficiency. *Diabetes Obes Metab* 2008;10:545–555.

78. Nowicki M, Rychlik I, Haller H, et al. Saxagliptin improves glycaemic control and is well tolerated in patients with type 2 diabetes mellitus and renal impairment. *Diabetes Obes Metab* 2011;13:523–532.

79. Boulton DW, Li L, Frevert EU, et al. Influence of renal or hepatic impairment on the pharmacokinetics of saxagliptin. *Clin Pharmacokinet* 2011;50:253–265.

80. Scheen AJ. Pharmacokinetics of dipeptidylpeptidase-4 inhibitors. *Diabetes Obes Metab* 2010;12:648–658.

81. Lukashevich V, Schweizer A, Shao Q, et al. Safety and efficacy of vildagliptin versus placebo in patients with type 2 diabetes and moderate or severe renal impairment: a prospective 24-week randomized placebo-controlled trial. *Diabetes Obes Metab* 2011;13:947–954.

82. Kaushal S, Singh H, Thangaraju P, et al. Canagliflozin: a novel sglt2 inhibitor for type 2 diabetes mellitus. *N Am J Med Sci* 2014;6:107–113.

83. Yamout H, Perkovic V, Davies M, et al. Efficacy and safety of canagliflozin in patients with type 2 diabetes and stage 3 nephropathy. *Am J Nephrol* 2014;40:64–74.

84. Younk LM, Mikeladze M, Davis SN. Pramlintide and the treatment of diabetes: a review of the data since its introduction. *Expert Opin Pharmacother* 2011;12:1439–1451.

85. Zieve FJ, Kalin MF, Schwartz SL, et al. Results of the glucose-lowering effect of WelChol study (GLOWS): a randomized, double-blind, placebo-controlled pilot study evaluating the effect of colesevelam hydrochloride on glycemic control in subjects with type 2 diabetes. *Clinical Ther* 2007;29:74–83.

86. Gaziano JM, Cincotta AH, O'Connor CM, et al. Randomized clinical trial of quick-release bromocriptine among patients with type 2 diabetes on overall safety and cardiovascular outcomes. *Diabetes Care* 2010;33:1503–1508.

87. Charpentier G, Riveline JP, Varroud-Vial M. Management of drugs affecting blood glucose in diabetic patients with renal failure. *Diabetes Metab* 2000;26(Suppl 4):73–85.

88. Raz I, Wilson PW, Strojek K, et al. Effects of prandial versus fasting glycemia on cardiovascular outcomes in type 2 diabetes: the HEART2D trial. *Diabetes Care* 2009;32:381–386.

89. Almalki MH, Altuwaijri MA, Almehthel MS, et al. Subcutaneous versus intraperitoneal insulin for patients with diabetes mellitus on continuous ambulatory peritoneal dialysis: meta-analysis of non-randomized clinical trials. *Clin Invest Med* 2012;35:E132–E143.

90. Quellhorst E. Insulin therapy during peritoneal dialysis: pros and cons of various forms of administration. *J Am Soc Nephrol* 2002;13(Suppl 1): S92–S96.

91. Selgas R, Diez JJ, Munoz J, et al. Comparative study of two different routes for insulin administration in CAPD diabetic patients. A multicenter study. *Adv Perit Dial* 1989;5:181–184.

92. Selgas R, Lopez-Rivas A, Alvaro F, et al. Insulin influence (used as an additive to dialysate) on the mitogenic-induced effect of the peritoneal effluent in CAPD patients. *Adv Perit Dial* 1989;5:161–164.

93. Wanless IR, Bargman JM, Oreopoulos DG, et al. Subcapsular steatonecrosis in response to peritoneal insulin delivery: a clue to the pathogenesis of steatonecrosis in obesity. *Mod Pathol* 1989;2:69–74.

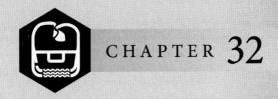

CHAPTER 32

Pregnancy in the Chronic Dialysis Patient

Lakshmi Kannan and Janani Rangaswami

Confortini et al. (1) reported the first successful pregnancy in a dialysis patient in 1971. Despite improving results with pregnancy outcomes, 44 years after this initial success, pregnancy in a long-term dialysis patient is still a challenging situation (2). In 1980, the European Dialysis and Transplant Association reported that only 23% of 115 pregnancies in dialysis ended with surviving infants (3). Since then, fetal survival rate in pregnant dialysis patients has increased by approximately 25% per decade, and recent estimate of live birth rates in pregnant dialysis patients touched an all-time high of 86.4%, as reported from the Toronto Pregnancy and Kidney Disease Clinic Registry (4). With prolonged waiting times for transplantation, the need to optimize maternal and fetal outcomes with pregnancy and dialysis is more relevant than ever. This chapter discusses the diagnosis and management of pregnancy in the setting of maintenance dialysis and summarizes maternal and fetal outcomes.

INCIDENCE AND DIAGNOSIS

Infertility is common in dialysis patients, with the incidence of pregnancy in end-stage kidney disease (ESKD) being approximately 2.2% per year in the United States (5).The luteal hormone surge and the estradiol peak that occurs mid to late menstruation with ovulation are absent in uremia, possibly due to the hyperprolactinemic state found in ESKD (6,7). While transplantation is the most effective way to restore fertility in these patients, intensification of the dialysis prescription by switching from intermittent dialysis to nocturnal hemodialysis increased the conception rate to 16.5% in a small series (8). The preponderance of anovulatory cycles with dialysis makes amenorrhea difficult to interpret in women with suspected pregnancy. While this should be investigated with β-human chorionic gonadotropin (β-hCG) serum testing, caution should be exercised when interpreting hCG test results in ESKD

owing to high number of false-positive results (7). The half-life of circulating hCG is increased in these patients, making the test unreliable for calculation of gestational age as well. Obstetric ultrasound is favored for estimation of gestational age in pregnant women with ESKD, with the mean gestational age at which the diagnosis of pregnancy is made being 16.5 weeks (9).

DIALYSIS PRESCRIPTION IN THE PREGNANT PATIENT

Poor outcomes for pregnancy in ESKD have been attributed to uremia-induced disturbances in hormonal homeostasis and the ensuing effects on placentation and fetal growth. The increasing success with fetal and maternal outcomes with dialysis over the last decade are largely due to intensification of the dialysis prescription, with the best results coming from long, nocturnal dialysis–based regimens (8,10,11). Nocturnal dialysis with a mean dialysis duration of 36 hours preconception and 48 hours during pregnancy in a cohort of seven pregnancies resulted in a mean gestational age of 36.2 weeks and a mean birth weight of 2,417.5 ± 657 g (8). In a study by Hladunewich et al. (4) that compared outcomes between a Canadian and American cohort of pregnant dialysis women, the live birth rates were 86.4% and 61.4%, respectively ($p = 0.03$), and the mean gestational ages was 36.2 weeks and 27 weeks, respectively ($p = 0.002$) (4). Notably, the Canadian cohort received a mean of 43 hours of dialysis compared to the 17 hours provided in the United States (4). Intense dialysis regimens of five to seven times a week, with each session lasting 8 to 10 hours, are associated with improved outcomes leading to improved live birth rates, decrease in prematurity, and improved blood pressure (BP) control. Intensive dialysis improves urea clearance, lowers peripheral vascular resistance, and ameliorates fluctuations in volume status (12,13).

TABLE 32.1	Commonly Used Drugs in Hemodialysis and Their Use in Pregnancy	
Drug	**Safety Data**	**Dosing and Pharmacology**
Erythropoietin	FDA category C	Dosing similar to nonpregnant state, typical pregnancy requirement is double the baseline dose, placental kinetics unknown
Paricalcitol	FDA category C	Similar to nonpregnant state
Calcitriol	FDA category B	Similar to nonpregnant state
Calcium acetate	FDA category C	Similar to nonpregnant state
Sevelamer/lanthanum	FDA category C	No safety data/guidelines available
Intravenous iron	FDA category B	Similar to nonpregnant state
Heparin	FDA category C	Similar to nonpregnant state, does not cross the placental barrier

FDA, U.S. Food and Drug Administration.

Daily dialysis offers the advantage of decreased risk of hypotension owing to decreased fluid removal per session and allows for high protein intake to meet caloric needs of the fetus and mother. It is also hypothesized that increased solute clearance with daily dialysis reduces placental urea and thus reduces fetal osmotic diuresis and resulting complications such as polyhydramnios (12).

While maternal and fetal outcomes do not significantly differ between hemodialysis and peritoneal dialysis (9), intensification of the dialysis prescription is easier on hemodialysis. As with hemodialysis, a patient's treatment requirements will increase with peritoneal dialysis especially during the latter half of gestation (14). A switch to continuous cyclical peritoneal dialysis (CCPD) with an increased frequency of small volume exchanges, with supplemental manual exchanges, is often required in late pregnancy to achieve adequate clearance (14). Using tidal peritoneal dialysis to successfully optimize solute clearance in pregnancy with restricted abdominal volumes has been reported (15). There are no changes in peritoneal dialysis efficacy in pregnancy as measured by a standard peritoneal equilibration test (PET) of glucose and creatinine and ultrafiltration efficacy (14). Rarely, complications such as lacerations of the gravid uterine veins from trauma to the peritoneal dialysis catheter and preterm delivery from peritonitis during pregnancy have been reported (14).

Dialyzers used during pregnancy range from standard high-flux dialyzers to nonreusable biocompatible dialyzers with blood flows ranging from 200 to 400 mL/min (4). There is little data reported on vascular access for maintenance hemodialysis in pregnancy influencing the outcome. In patients dialyzing with arteriovenous fistulae, the risk of aneurysmal dilation of the fistula due to histologic changes in the vessel wall associated with the hormonal changes in pregnancy and altered pregnancy-related hemodynamics must be factored into the routine examination of the pregnant dialysis patient (16). Heparin does not cross the placental barrier and can be used safely with hemodialysis in pregnancy, without necessitating a dose reduction.

The physiologic weight gain associated with pregnancy, which is recommended to be 1 to 1.5 kg within the first trimester and thereafter 0.3 to 0.5 kg/wk (9), should be factored into dry weight assessment. With daily dialysis, fluid gains should be minimal, and BP goals of <140/90 mm Hg should be achievable with minimal antihypertensives (9). Persistent elevations in BP despite optimal fluid removal should raise the suspicion of preeclampsia.

Target values of the main laboratory parameters suggested for pregnant women on dialysis are similar to those advised in nonpregnant dialysis patients. The pregnant patient is predisposed to respiratory alkalosis as a result of progesterone-induced hyperventilation. Hence, a bicarbonate solution concentration as low as 25 mM is preferred to standard higher concentrations to avoid superimposed metabolic alkalosis (9). With a standard 2.5 mEq/L calcium dialysate solution, the mother will need 2 g of oral calcium per day to keep a positive calcium balance and ensure the fetal calcium requirement of 25 to 30 g during pregnancy (17). The placenta secretes calcitriol which also aids in positive calcium balance.

Intensive dialysis regimens during pregnancy can result in hypophosphatemia. Most patients often do not require any phosphate binders, and at times, addition of phosphorus to the dialysate may be necessary (18). In patients with hyperphosphatemia, calcium-containing binders are preferred due to their safety profile (9). There is no experience with sevelamer or lanthanum in pregnancy (9). There is limited data currently on the effects of pregnancy on dialysis-associated metabolic bone disease profiles. Activated vitamin D analogs such as paricalcitol (pregnancy category C) and calcitriol (pregnancy category B) are dosed based on the individual nephrologist's discretion (**TABLE 32.1**).

MANAGEMENT OF ANEMIA

Anemia is common in pregnancy due to volume expansion. Daily iron losses are also frequent in pregnancy. In pregnant patients with ESKD, this physiologic anemia is exaggerated, and most patients will require erythropoietin and iron supplementation. Accentuated anemia and increased erythropoiesis-stimulating agent (ESA) requirements are attributed to cytokine-induced erythropoietin resistance and the effect of plasma volume expansion leading to hemodilution (19). ESA is not associated with fetal congenital anomalies at usual doses, and if patients are on ESA when they become pregnant, the dose is typically doubled for the length of the pregnancy (9). Intravenous iron supplementation can be given in pregnant dialysis patients, given the expected physiologic need for an extra 700 to 1,150 mg of elemental iron during pregnancy. The U.S. Food and Drug Administration has labeled intravenous iron as category B for pregnancy.

NUTRITION

Protein intake should be increased to meet the metabolic needs of the mother and the growing fetus. For this, a daily protein intake of 1.8 g/kg is recommended (9). Folate supplementation at higher than usual doses (around 4 mg/d) is recommended for the pregnant mother on dialysis to compensate for losses from intensification of dialysis and prevention of neural tube defects (9).

PREGNANCY OUTCOMES

Fetal Outcomes

With intensification of dialysis dose, the rate of live births has escalated from 23% in the 1970s (3) to a high of 87% (20). In the Canadian cohort (4) and in the nocturnal hemodialysis cohort reported by Barua et al. (8), the mean duration of the pregnancy was 36 weeks compared to 32 weeks on previous reports (20). Enhanced solute clearance with these regimens appears directly related to fetal outcomes with a significant negative correlation noted between blood urea nitrogen (BUN) and birth weight/gestational age (21). In a large registry performed in the United States (5), there was a nonsignificant trend toward better survival and decreased prematurity in patients who received >20 hours of dialysis per week. The ability to maintain maternal BP throughout pregnancy with minimal to no antihypertensives also offers improved fetal perfusion, in regimens such as described by Barua et al. (8).

The Australian and New Zealand Dialysis and Transplantation (ANZDATA) registry compiled all pregnancy data in dialysis patients between 1996 and 2008 (22). This registry noted superior live birth rates among women who conceived prior to dialysis initiation compared with those on dialysis at the time of conception (91% vs. 63%, $p = 0.03$). This study further noted that this significant difference in live birth rate was secondary to early pregnancy losses (<20 weeks of gestation) in established dialysis patients. However, beyond 20 weeks, these pregnancies were similar with no significant difference in gestational age or birth weight.

 MATERNAL COMPLICATIONS

Hypertension is the major clinical concern with regard to the pregnant mother on dialysis. This could manifest as gestational hypertension, preeclampsia, or eclampsia. High placental urea leads to increased fetal solute diuresis resulting in complications such as polyhydramnios (23). Other frequently reported complications include gestational diabetes mellitus, premature rupture of membranes, chorioamnionitis, placental abruption, and hemorrhage postpartum (8).

 MANAGEMENT OF HYPERTENSION IN PREGNANCY

Hypertension is notable for earlier onset (<24 weeks) in pregnant dialysis patients compared to pregnant women without ESKD. About 80% of all pregnant women on dialysis have a BP of 140/90 mm Hg or above, and 40% have severe hypertension as defined by systolic BP >200 mm Hg and/or diastolic BP >110 mm Hg (9). Improved surveillance measures that include weekly weight change assessments and daily BP measurements at home are therefore recommended. Fluid status is first determined when the mother is found to be hypertensive. Once euvolemia is established, persistent elevations in BP are managed with medications. Safe options include methyldopa (class B), labetalol (class C; selective β-blockers are associated with intrauterine growth restriction), and calcium channel blockers (class C). Hypertensive crises are treated with intravenous labetalol or hydralazine (class C), and magnesium loading for seizure prophylaxis should be cautious with careful monitoring of serum levels (9). Recently, endothelial dysfunction and cardiovascular outcomes in chronic kidney disease (CKD) and ESKD patients have been linked to an increase in soluble fms-related tyrosine kinase 1 (sFlt1), an inhibitor of the vascular endothelial growth factor (VEGF) (24). The "antiangiogenic" milieu created by a relative VEGF deficiency with preeclampsia is reflected with persistent elevations of sFlt1 in this population at baseline (25), making it a possible nontraditional cardiovascular risk marker in these women, in addition to serving as a marker for superimposed preeclampsia.

 LABOR AND DELIVERY

Pregnant women on dialysis are considered high-risk pregnancies and need close coordination care between the nephrologist and obstetrician. Biweekly antenatal monitoring to screen for fetal well-being, biometry, amniotic fluid index, cervical length, and umbilical artery pulsatility should begin at 26 weeks of gestation and increased to weekly profiles near term (4). Combinations of calcium channel blockers and magnesium should be avoided due to profound maternal hypotension. Cesarean sections are performed for obstetric indications and can be performed in patients on peritoneal dialysis if indicated (9). Newborns should be monitored in high-risk neonatal care units. The baby's BUN and creatinine will initially be elevated. This leads to solute diuresis necessitating careful monitoring of volume status and electrolytes. A snapshot of key concepts during and after the course of the pregnancy is summarized in **Table 32.2**.

 SUMMARY AND RECOMMENDATIONS

In summary, while the management of pregnancy in a patient on dialysis remains complex and challenging, huge strides have been made over the last decade in terms of gestational age, live birth rate, and minimizing maternal complications with intensification of the dialysis prescription. Having an international registry for pregnancy outcomes in dialysis patients will help pool experience

TABLE 32.2	**Highlights of Hemodialysis Management during Pregnancy**	
Prepregnancy	**During Pregnancy**	**After Delivery**
• High risk for fetal loss (<20 weeks) • Stop ACEI and ARB before or right after conception. • Confirm pregnancy with obstetric ultrasound in addition to β-hCG results. • Preconception counseling about higher risks of early pregnancy losses, stillbirth, fetal prematurity, and preeclampsia	• Best results with intense dialysis regimens of 5–7 times/wk of 8–10 h/session • Expected weight gain 1–1.5 kg in first trimester and 0.3–0.5 kg/wk thereafter • Oral calcium and phosphate supplements may be needed. • ESA dose is typically doubled for the length of pregnancy. • Intravenous iron to supplement the extra 700–1,100 mg of elemental iron needed • Protein intake of 1.8 g/kg/d and folate dose of 4–5 mg/d • Close surveillance for preeclampsia	• Readjust dry weight and antihypertensives. • Watch for postpartum preeclampsia.

ACEI, angiotensin-converting enzyme inhibitor; ARB, angiotensin receptor blocker; β-hCG, β-human chorionic gonadotropin; ESA, erythropoiesis-stimulating agent.

with the complex interface of pregnancy-related physiologic needs and the absence of the optimal renal adaptive response to this state. Close multispecialty monitoring and communication is the key to successful maternal and fetal outcomes, which will hopefully be the standard of care with pregnancy in this population.

REFERENCES

1. Confortini P, Galanti G, Ancona G, et al. Full term pregnancy and successful delivery in a patient on chronic hemodialysis. *Proc Eur Dial Transplant Assoc* 1971;8:74–80.
2. Hou S. Pregnancy in dialysis patients: where do we go from here? *Semin Dial* 2003;16:376–378.
3. Successful pregnancies in women treated by dialysis and kidney transplantation. Report from the Registration Committee of the European Dialysis and Transplant Association. *Br J Obstet Gynaecol* 1980;87:839–845.
4. Hladunewich MA, Hou S, Odutayo A, et al. Intensive hemodialysis associates with improved pregnancy outcomes: a Canadian and United States cohort comparison. *J Am Soc Nephrol* 2014;25:1103–1109.
5. Okundaye IB, Abrinko P, Hou S. Registry for pregnancy in dialysis patients. *Am J Kidney Dis* 1998;31:766–773.
6. Palmer BF. Sexual dysfunction in uremia. *J Am Soc Nephrol* 2003;10:1381–1388.
7. Schwarz A, Post KG, Keller F, et al. Value of human chorionic gonadotropin measurements in blood as a pregnancy test in women on maintenance hemodialysis. *Nephron* 1985;39(4):341–343.
8. Barua M, Hladunewich M, Keunen J, et al. Successful pregnancies on nocturnal home hemodialysis. *Clin J Am Soc Nephrol* 2008;3:392–396.
9. Hou S, Grossman S. Obstetric and gynecologic issues. In: Daugirdas J, Blake P, Ing T, eds. *Handbook of Dialysis*. 4th ed. Philadelphia, PA: Lippincott Williams & Wilkins, 2007:672–684.
10. Bamberg C, Diekmann F, Haase M, et al. Pregnancy on intensified hemodialysis: fetal surveillance and perinatal outcome. *Fetal Diagn Ther* 2007;22:289–293.
11. Haase M, Morgera S, Bamberg C, et al. A systematic approach to managing pregnant dialysis patients—the importance of an intensified haemodiafiltration protocol. *Nephrol Dial Transplant* 2006;21:1443–1457.
12. Chan CT. Cardiovascular effects of frequent intensive hemodialysis. *Semin Dial* 2004;17:99–103.
13. Chan CT, Harvey PJ, Picton P, et al. Short term blood pressure, nor adrenergic and vascular effects of nocturnal hemodialysis. *Hypertension* 2003;42:925–931.
14. Deering S, Seiken G. Dialysis. In: Belfort M, Saade G, Foley M, et al, eds. *Critical Care Obstetrics*. 5th ed. Chichester, United Kingdom: Wiley-Blackwell, 2010:188–195.
15. Chang H, Miller MA, Bruns FJ, et al. Tidal peritoneal dialysis during pregnancy improves clearance and abdominal symptoms. *Perit Dial Int* 2002;22:272–274.
16. Stephenson MA, Neate EC, Mistry H, et al. A large aneurysm in an arteriovenous fistula for renal access in a pregnancy young woman. *J Vasc Access* 2013;14(1):94–95.
17. Hou S. Pregnancy in chronic renal insufficiency and end stage renal disease. *Am J Kidney Dis* 1999;33(2):235–252.
18. Hussain S, Savin V, Piercing W, et al. Phosphorus enriched dialysis during pregnancy: two case reports. *Hemodial Int* 2005;9(2):147–152.
19. Bagon JA, Vernaeve H, De Muylder X, et al. Pregnancy and dialysis. *Am J Kidney Dis* 1998;31:756–765.
20. Luders C, Castro MC, Titan SM, et al. Obstetric outcomes in pregnant women on long-term dialysis: a case series. *Am J Kidney Dis* 2010;56:77–85.
21. Asamiya Y, Otsubo S, Matsuda Y, et al. The importance of low blood urea nitrogen levels in pregnant patients undergoing hemodialysis to optimize birth weight and gestational age. *Kidney Int* 2009;75:1217–1222.
22. Shahir AK, Briggs N, Katsoulis J, et al. An observational outcomes study from 1996-2008, examining pregnancy and neonatal outcomes from dialysed women using data from the ANZDATA registry. *Nephrology* 2013;18:276–284.
23. Reddy SS, Holly JL. Management of the pregnancy chronic dialysis patient. *Adv Chronic Kidney Dis* 2007;14:146–155.
24. Hladenuwich M, Karumanchi SA, Lafayette R, et al. Pathophysiology of the clinical manifestations of pre eclampsia. *Clin J Am Soc Nephrol* 2007;2:543–549.
25. DiMarco GS, Reuter S, Hillebrand U, et al. The soluble VEGF receptor sFlt1 contributes to endothelial dysfunction in CKD. *J Am Soc Nephrol* 2009;20:2235–2245.

CHAPTER 33

Acquired Cystic Kidney Diseases in Dialysis Patients

Judy K. Tan, Jonathan Silverman, and Edgar V. Lerma

In 1977, Dunnill et al. (1) first described the presence of acquired cystic kidney disease (ACKD) in patients with end-stage kidney disease (ESKD) on hemodialysis examined on autopsy. Since then, there have been a number of reports that have been published on the association of ACKD and kidney disease.

ACKD is characterized by the development of multiple fluid-filled cysts in the kidneys of patients who do not have a hereditary cause of cystic kidney disease. A diagnosis requires the involvement of both kidneys, four or more cysts being present, and that the cysts are confined in the kidney. ESKD is frequently associated with ACKD. It occurs in patients on long-term renal replacement therapy either in the form of hemodialysis or peritoneal dialysis. During the past years, ACKD has become more prevalent with the widespread use of dialysis and as patients with ESKD tend to live longer and undergo more diagnostic imaging studies.

 ## EPIDEMIOLOGY

The incidence of acquired cystic disease increases progressively with the duration of renal replacement therapy—hemodialysis or peritoneal dialysis. However, ACKD can occur in some patients even before dialysis is initiated. In one study of 130 patients with advanced kidney disease or ESKD, the incidence of multiple cysts was noted to be 7% in those with chronic kidney disease (CKD) and 22% in those on maintenance dialysis (2). The duration of dialysis was 15 months in patients with no cysts, 28 months in those with one to three cysts, and 49 months in those with acquired cystic disease (2). Fifty percent to 80% of patients are affected after 10 or more years on dialysis (3–5). In a similar study of 48 patients with ESKD on continuous ambulatory peritoneal dialysis (CAPD), the incidence of both solitary and multiple renal cysts was noted to be 52% in patients on CAPD for 23 ± 16 months (6). The frequency however

may be underestimated on the basis of imaging studies alone. In a single-center study in which most renal transplant patients undergo ipsilateral native nephrectomy at the time of transplant surgery, the prevalence of ACKD was reported to be at 33% based on strict pathologic criteria, which may still be lower than the true incidence given that only one kidney was removed (7) (**FIGURE 33.1**).

 ## RISK FACTORS

Researchers have shown that time spent on hemodialysis was the most important risk factor for the development of ACKD (8). Men and African Americans have been reported to be at much higher risk than women or Caucasians (8,9).

 ## PATHOGENESIS

The exact pathogenesis of ACKD in humans is not known, but its understanding has been aided by available *in vivo* and *in vitro* animal models. The slow progressive loss of functioning renal tissue in ESKD promotes initial compensatory hypertrophy and later hyperplasia of the residual nephrons (3,9). The cysts being confined to the kidneys suggest that local intrarenal events are of primary importance (9). Analysis of the cyst fluid, which is thought to derive from ultrafiltrate secreted into the cyst, typically has a composition similar to that in the plasma; this finding plus the presence of a brush border on the luminal membrane on microdissection studies suggests that the cysts arise primarily from proliferation of proximal tubular epithelial cells (3,9).

Compensatory renal hypertrophy is influenced by many factors, the most important of which is activation of oncogenes and release of growth factors, which, over a prolonged period of time, promote progressive tubular hyperplasia and cyst formation (10,11).

513

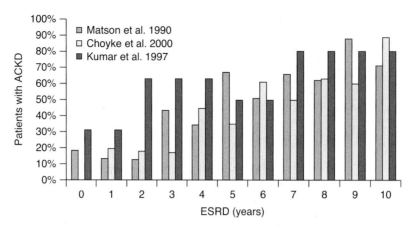

FIGURE 33.1 Prevalence of acquired cystic kidney disease (ACKD) in hemodialysis patients in relation to their duration of hemodialysis treatment.

Alternatively, other provoking factors might emerge, such as environmental chemicals, transforming viruses, or male sex hormones, that lead to the transition of the proliferative process into malignant growth.

CLINICAL MANIFESTATIONS

ACKD is usually asymptomatic and discovered incidentally during imaging studies. In one review, for example, only 14% of patients developed symptoms, with hematuria being most common, followed by pain and urinary tract infection. Some may manifest with potential complications of ACKD such as cystic hemorrhage that may present with or without hematuria, cyst rupture with consequent perinephric or retroperitoneal hemorrhage, and cyst infection or abscess formation or erythrocytosis.

COMPLICATIONS

Renal Cell Carcinoma

As with ACKD, the incidence of renal cell carcinoma (RCC) as a complication of ACKD varies in different reports (8,12,13). Two prospective studies found an incidence of 4% (2 of 57) and 7% (2 of 30) over a 7- to 10-year period. A review of published reports estimated an incidence of 0.18% per year, compared with 0.008% in the general population in the United States.

Most reports, however, may misrepresent the true prevalence of RCC because they primarily rely upon screening radiography for detection. A single-center study in which most renal transplant patients underwent ipsilateral native nephrectomy at the time of transplant surgery showed that RCC was found in 4.2% of 260 nephrectomies, which may still be lower than the true incidence given that only one kidney was removed (7).

There are important differences between the renal cell cancer development in the setting of ACKD and in the general population. ACKD patients with renal cancer are younger, predominantly male compared with the general population. The carcinomas as a complication of ACKD are usually limited to the kidney and, in approximately 25% to 50% of cases, are multiple and bilateral (3,9,12). Whereas sporadic tumors are mostly composed of clear cell or granular carcinomas (90%), papillary cell types represent approximately 5% to 7%, in ACKD the proportion of clear-cell carcinomas to papillary carcinoma is approximately 1:1 (14). The reason for the

difference is uncertain. There seems to be a lower metastatic rate in the ACKD group compared with that in the general population, but mortality rate was similar in both groups. The similar mortality rate may partly explained by the higher prevalence of comorbid conditions associated in the ACKD group.

Men (male-to-female ratio 7:1) and patients with large cysts and an increased kidney size are at increased risk for malignant transformation (12,15).

Cystic Hemorrhage

Bleeding is usually confined within the cyst but occasionally extend into the renal collecting system causing gross or microscopic hematuria or into the perinephric or retroperitoneal space causing flank pain. Rarely, bleeding may evolve into cyst rupture severe enough to require surgical intervention or transcatheter embolization.

Other Complications

Other important complications of ACKD include cyst infection, abscess formation, erythrocytosis, and calcification in or around the cyst.

DIAGNOSIS AND SCREENING

By itself, acquired renal cysts are of limited clinical significance. However, some cysts transform into malignant lesions. In an attempt at early detection of these premalignant or malignant lesions, some investigators have suggested that periodic imaging of the native kidneys be performed in patients on long-term dialysis (3,9). However, the basis for these recommendations nor their potential consequences have been elaborated. Moreover, the relatively low incidence of RCC in addition to the high mortality of patients with ESKD from other causes and the need for computed tomography (CT) or magnetic resonance imaging for effective screening in this population has prompted others to suggest that routine imaging is not cost-effective (16). A decision analysis model performed to more precisely determine the cause of screening showed that screening could lead to a 1.6 year in life expectancy over a 25-year period provided that only young (20-year-old) patients with a long life span were screened (17). When the screening tests are applied to the young ESKD patients, the benefit ACKD screening programs appears to be comparable to the benefit of established interventions such as breast cancer screening, colon cancer screening, and cervical cancer screening. However, the benefit of screening critically on life expectancy. For middle-aged patients beginning dialysis treatments with a life expectancy of 5 years, screening by CT or ultrasound prolong average life expectancy by 4 or 5 days. For yet older patients, the gains are even smaller. Since the median age of patients beginning dialysis in the United States is about 62 years old, this analysis implies that more than half of the incident ESKD population screening of asymptomatic individuals for ACKD is unlikely to be of benefit.

Given the aforementioned data, some investigators have suggested that radiologic studies be performed only in patients with concerning symptoms such as new hematuria or flank pain, or in young patients with risk factors such as long duration of dialysis and large kidneys due to acquired cystic disease (16,18). An individualized approach to cancer screening is also recommended based on the patient's cancer expected survival and transplant status.

The optimal imaging modality for screening is uncertain. Contrast-enhanced CT scanning is more sensitive than ultrasonography in detecting and characterizing cysts but may not be superior in detecting solid tumors (2,4,19). Moreover, CT scanning has the added benefit of defining the extent of disease.

Magnetic resonance imaging (MRI) with injection of gadolinium is the best modality to explore complex renal cysts, but there is a concern of the development of nephrogenic systemic fibrosis (NSF) in patients with CKD stages 4 and 5 and in patients on dialysis.

Some experts recommend initiating screening by ultrasonography in at-risk patients. Once the ultrasonogram becomes positive for cysts, the more sensitive contrast-enhanced CT scan or MRI is performed at recommended intervals to screen for the possible occurrence of carcinoma. A classification of renal cysts, based on their appearance in CT scans, introduced by Bosniak, is now widely accepted and is also applied to ultrasound and MRI.

TREATMENT

The treatment for ACKD is supportive unless complications arise.

The treatment for renal cancer is a radical nephrectomy. The challenge is to determine if this surgical procedure is indicated in any patient with a renal mass as in some cases, it is difficult to definitively differentiate benign from malignant lesions on the basis of an imaging study. It is generally agreed that a tumor larger than 3 cm in diameter, a rapidly growing mass, or one that is associated with suspicious symptoms such as hematuria warrants a nephrectomy.

PROGNOSIS

The cysts may stabilize or regress following successful renal transplantation, a setting in which the level of growth factors is reduced due to the restoration of normal renal function. In one prospective study of patients with ESKD and patients with renal transplant, the incidence of cystic disease was lower and the native kidneys were smaller and had lower cyst grades in transplant recipients when compared with patients treated with maintenance hemodialysis (20). This benefit was limited to patients not receiving cyclosporine. Those treated with cyclosporine had an incidence of cystic disease similar to the dialyzed patients.

 REFERENCES

1. Dunnill MS, Millard PR, Oliver D. Acquired cystic disease of the kidneys: a hazard of long-term intermittent maintenance haemodialysis. *J Clin Pathol* 1977;30:868–877.
2. Narasimhan N, Golper TA, Wolfson M, et al. Clinical characteristics and diagnostic considerations in acquired renal cystic disease. *Kidney Int* 1986;30:748–752.
3. Ishikawa I. Acquired cystic disease: mechanisms and manifestations. *Semin Nephrol* 1991;11:671–684.
4. Matson MA, Cohen EP. Acquired cystic kidney disease: occurrence, prevalence, and renal cancers. *Medicine* 1990;69:217–226.
5. Kumar R, Mishra HK. Acquired cystic renal disease in patients receiving long-term hemodialysis. *Saudi J Kidney Dis Transpl* 1997;8:8–10.
6. Rodriguez-Perez JC, Vega N, Camantilde T, et al. Acquired cystic disease of the kidney in continuous ambulatory peritoneal dialysis (CAPD) patients. *Perit Dial Int* 1988;8:273–275.
7. Denton MD, Magee CC, Ovuworie C, et al. Prevalence of renal cell carcinoma in patients with ESRD pre-transplantation: a pathologic analysis. *Kidney Int* 2002;61:2201–2209.
8. Ishikawa I, Saito Y, Shikura N, et al. Ten-year prospective study on the development of renal cell carcinoma in dialysis patients. *Am J Kidney Dis* 1990;16:452–458.
9. Grantham JJ. Acquired cystic kidney disease. *Kidney Int* 1991;40: 143–152.
10. Herrera GA. C-erb B-2 amplification in cystic renal disease. *Kidney Int* 1991;40:509–513.
11. Konda R, Sato H, Hatafuku F, et al. Expression of hepatocyte growth factor and its receptor C-met in acquired renal cystic disease associated with renal cell carcinoma. *J Urol* 2004;171:2166–2170.
12. Truong LD, Krishnan B, Cao JT, et al. Renal neoplasm in acquired cystic kidney disease. *Am J Kidney Dis* 1995;26:1–12.
13. Levine E, Slusher SL, Grantham JJ, et al. Natural history of acquired renal cystic disease in dialysis patients: a prospective longitudinal CT study. *AJR Am J Roentgenol* 1991;156:501–506.
14. Ishikawa I, Kovacs G. High incidence of papillary renal cell tumours in patients on chronic haemodialysis. *Histopathology* 1993;22:135–139.
15. MacDougall ML, Welling LW, Wiegmann TB. Prediction of carcinoma in acquired cystic disease as a function of kidney weight. *J Am Soc Nephrol* 1990;1:828–831.
16. Fick GM, Gabow PA. Hereditary and acquired cystic disease of the kidney. *Kidney Int* 1994;46:951–964.
17. Sarasin FP, Wong JB, Levey AS, et al. Screening for acquired cystic kidney disease: a decision analytic perspective. *Kidney Int* 1995;48:207–219.
18. Chandhoke PS, Torrence RJ, Clayman RV, et al. Acquired cystic disease of the kidney: a management dilemma. *J Urol* 1992;147:969–974.
19. Taylor AJ, Cohen EP, Erickson SJ, et al. Renal imaging in long-term dialysis patients: a comparison of CT and sonography. *AJR Am J Roentgenol* 1989;153:765–767.
20. Lien YH, Hunt KR, Siskind MS, et al. Association of cyclosporin A with acquired cystic kidney disease of the native kidneys in renal transplant recipients. *Kidney Int* 1993;44:613–616.

CHAPTER 34

Quality of Life and Rehabilitation in Dialysis Patients

Daniel Jay Salzberg and Fathima Konari

 ## DEFINITION OF QUALITY OF LIFE

The *American Heritage Dictionary* defines life as the physical, mental, and spiritual experiences that constitute existence (1). This chapter explores how we have come to define quality of life (QOL) and various methods by which QOL is assessed in patients with chronic kidney disease (CKD) stage 5 requiring dialysis [previously called *end-stage kidney disease* (ESKD), now abbreviated CKD stage 5D]. The World Health Organization defines QOL as "an individual's perception of their position in life in the context of the culture and value system where they live, and in relation to their goals, expectations, standards, and concerns" (2). The measurement of QOL should incorporate the many factors that effect a subject's existence and satisfaction. It should include not just the physical aspect but also the emotional, intellectual, social, cultural, and ethnic components that comprise daily life.

Terms that are sometimes equated with QOL include functional status, sense of well-being, life satisfaction, and health status. Although health status is not synonymous with QOL, the two are interrelated with health affecting QOL and QOL affecting health. Illustrative of this point is that survival appears to be greater in subjects with a higher measured QOL (3–5).

Given this foundation, one can define an aspect of QOL as being health related. This health-related quality of life (HRQOL) represents the "physical, psychological, and social domains of health that are influenced by a person's experience, beliefs, expectations, and perceptions" (6). Within this context, health is defined as not only the absence of disease and infirmity but also the presence of physical, mental, and social well-being (2). HRQOL includes both an objective assessment of functional status and a subjective perception of one's health (6).

When dealing with a chronic illness like CKD, it is essential to take a multidisciplinary approach. Given the number and complexity of stressors faced by patients with CKD stage 5D, it would be naive to draw conclusions about their global health based solely on a single metric such as Kt/V or normalized protein catabolic rate (nPCR). Similarly, methodologic studies that evaluate only one primary endpoint, such as blood pressure control, may miss other significant aspects that effect health. It is with this global concept of health that HRQOL tools have been developed. The use of HRQOL instruments is even more important in subjects with CKD stage 5D, as compared with other chronic disease states, because of the associated high prevalence and severity of their comorbid conditions.

An important concept that underscores the study of QOL is that a new procedure or drug may decrease mortality but may not necessarily improve QOL and, therefore, may not be of overall benefit to the patient. To further illustrate this paradigm, take the example of two patients with virtually identical medical conditions. Despite similar care and objective disease states, they may have vastly different perceived QOL based on their social support systems, psychological outlook, and coping mechanisms. HRQOL measurements allow for the assessment of these factors contributing to QOL.

Some of the practical applications of measuring HRQOL include assessment of therapeutic interventions and their impact on QOL, effect of different modalities of renal replacement therapy and effect on QOL, determination of change in QOL within the same population over the course of the disease, and assessment of the impact of interventions on cost and/or morbidity with relation to QOL.

MEASUREMENT OF QUALITY OF LIFE

Optimal HRQOL measurement instruments capture all the nuances that disease and its treatment have on the physical, emotional, social, and mental dimensions of an individual (7). Ideally, instruments should be comprehensive, valid, have test–retest reliability, and be responsive to change and yet be brief enough to allow for quick administration. They should allow for comparisons between groups of subjects with different illnesses and be sensitive enough to pick up subtle differences within a specific group. Lastly, for an HRQOL measure to be of value, subjects' life experiences must be converted into a quantitative, numerical value.

Unfortunately, there is no one ideal tool that measures HRQOL, and therefore, multiple different instruments have been developed (**TABLE 34.1**). Most of these instruments use a psychometric approach, which is based on the item measure theory (8). This theory postulates that true QOL cannot be directly measured but can be assessed indirectly through a series of questions. These questions are defined as "items" (9). Each item is then given a numerical value based on a predetermined scale. For example, in the RAND 36-Item Health Survey 1.0 Questionnaire (10), a subject is asked to rate his or her health on a scale from 1 (excellent) to 5 (poor).

When items are rated in this way, they are often referred to as *Likert-type items*. This rating presumes the existence of an underlying continuous variable whose value characterizes the respondents'

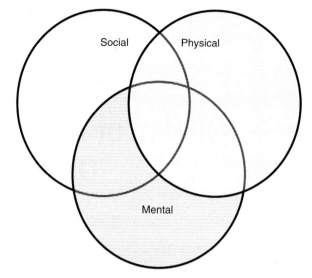

FIGURE 34.1 Domains of health-related quality of life.

TABLE 34.1	**Health-Related Quality of Life Instruments Used in Assessment of Dialysis Patients**

Generic instruments
  Global assessment instruments
    Sickness Impact Profile (SIP)
    Medical Outcomes Study 36-Item Short Form Health Survey (MOS SF-36)
    Time trade-off approach (TTO)
  Domain-specific tools
    Physical health
      Karnofsky Performance Status (KPS) Scale or the Karnofsky Index (KI)
      Symptoms and comorbidity checklist
      Sexual functioning scale
    Mental health
      Index of General Affect, Index of Life Satisfaction, and Index of Well-Being
      Affect Balance Score
      Beck Depression Inventory
      9-Question Patient Health Questionnaire (PHQ-9)
      Rosenberg's Self-Esteem Inventory
      Locus of control scales
    Social health
      Illness intrusiveness
      Employment status measures
End-stage kidney disease (ESKD) targeted instruments
  Parfrey et al. health questionnaire specific for ESKD
  Kidney Disease Questionnaire (KDQ)
  Kidney Disease Quality-of-Life Instrument (KDQOL)
  Kidney Disease Quality-of-Life Instrument Short Form (KDQOL-SF)
  CHOICE Health Experience Questionnaire (CHEQ)
  Dialysis-Quality of Life Questionnaire (DIAQOL)
  Dialysis Discontinuation Quality of Dying (DDQOD)
  Dialysis Quality of Dying Apgar (DQODA)

Adapted from Edgell ET, Coons SJ, Carter WB, et al. A review of health-related quality-of-life measures used in end-stage renal disease. *Clin Ther* 1996;18: 887–938, with permission.

attitudes and opinions. Each Likert-type item provides a discrete approximation of the variable being assessed (11). The advantage of this ordinal scale is its ability to rank order subjective responses that are otherwise difficult to quantify. When using these Likert-type items, there is no assumption that the difference between the possible responses is of the same magnitude. Said another way, the difference between responses 2 and 4 may not have the same meaning as the difference between responses 3 and 5.

The numerical score of each Likert-type item is then added together to obtain a sum score that represents the overall global HRQOL score. It is the ability of these instruments to quantify QOL and produce a meaningful numerical score that allows for intragroup and intergroup comparisons.

HRQOL instruments can be subdivided into categories based on whether the tool is global or domain specific. Three major domains comprise global HRQOL: the physical domain, the social domain, and the psychosocial or mental domain (**FIGURE 34.1**) (12). Certain HRQOL instruments examine only one domain of HRQOL such as the Karnofsky Performance Status (KPS) scale, which primarily assesses the dimension of physical health. Other instruments, such as the Sickness Impact Profile (SIP), not only examine the physical domain but also give a global, overall measurement of HRQOL.

The types of HRQOL instruments can be further grouped into disease-targeted versus generic disease nonspecific tools (**TABLE 34.1**). The major advantage of disease-targeted tools is their ability to focus on the unique aspects and treatments of the disease being studied. However, extrapolation to other disease populations is severely limited. On the other hand, generic tools allow for comparisons of HRQOL across different populations and disease states but may not be specific or sensitive for subtle changes within a specific disease.

Generic Instruments

Generic instruments are designed to be applicable to a wide variety of populations. The major advantage of using a generic measure of HRQOL is that one can compare groups of subjects across different health and disease states. A number of these HRQOL instruments, however, have not been validated in the CKD stage 5D population, and these include Spitzer QL-index, Nottingham Health Profiles, Campbell Index of Well-Being (IWB), Cantril's Self-Anchoring Scale, and the Life Satisfaction Scale (12,13). Others have been demonstrated to be valid and will, therefore, be examined further.

Generic measures of HRQOL can be further subdivided into those that give a global assessment of HRQOL and those that focus on a specific domain, that is, physical health, mental health, or social health.

Generic, global assessment instruments are designed to provide a comprehensive overview of the three domains included in HRQOL. The potential advantages of using a global assessment tool include the ability to use a single instrument instead of many domain-specific ones and the ability to combine the global tool with either a disease-specific tool or a domain-specific tool.

A classic example of these generic, global assessment tools is the SIP, which was developed by Bergner et al. (14,15). As its name implies, the SIP was designed to assess the impact of sickness on QOL. The SIP contains 136 behavior-based items that are either interviewer- or self-administered questionnaires. These 136 items are divided into 12 health-related categories, including ambulation, mobility, body care and movement (these three categories comprise the physical dimension of the SIP), social interaction, alertness, emotional behavior, communication (these four categories comprise the psychosocial dimension), sleep and rest, eating, work, home management, and recreation and pastimes. Combining the score of all the items gives a global QOL score that ranges from 0 to 100 points. A lower score indicates better QOL. The SIP has been proved to be reliable and valid in the CKD stage 5D population (7,12).

The Medical Outcomes Study Short Form 36-Item Health Survey (MOS SF-36, also abbreviated as SF-36) (16) is another widely used generic HRQOL measurement instrument. It was designed specifically to be a more time-efficient questionnaire allowing comparisons of HRQOL across different groups. As with the SIP, the SF-36 Health Survey can be either interviewer- or self-administered. Unlike the SIP, which contains 136 items, the SF-36 only contains 36 items, through which it evaluates eight health concepts of HRQOL. The eight health concepts are physical functioning (10 items), role limitations resulting from physical problems (4 items), role limitations caused by emotional or personal problems (3 items), social functioning (2 items), bodily pain (2 items), energy/fatigue (4 items), emotional well-being (5 items), and general health perceptions (5 items). In addition, there is one single item that provides an indication of perceived change, now versus 1 year ago. For example, the questions that are used to assess social functioning are "During the last 4 weeks, to what extent has your physical health or emotional problems interfered with your normal social activities with family, friends, neighbors, or groups?" ranked from 1 (not at all) to 5 (extremely) and "During the last 4 weeks, how much of the time has your physical health or emotional problems interfered with your social activities (such as visiting with friends, relatives, etc.)?" ranked from 1 (all of the time) to 5 (none of the time) (10). Two additional components can be calculated from the SF-36, and they are the Physical Component Summary (PCS) and the Mental Component Summary (MCS). There are different methods for determining an overall score within each health concept, but the overall concept is that a higher score represents a more favorable health state. The SF-36 Health Survey has been proved to be both reliable and valid in the CKD stage 5D population (7,12).

Unlike the SIP and the SF-36, the Time Trade-Off (TTO) technique of assessing HRQOL employs a preference-based approach rather than using a psychometric item-based instrument. The TTO technique employs modern utility theory, which postulates that, if presented with two alternatives with full disclosure of the risks and benefits involved, a person will choose the option that serves them best (17). In this model of decision making, subjects are first given a fixed amount of time that they will live in their current chronic disease state, defined as time (t). Next, they are presented with the theoretical question: "How many years of life would you be willing to give up in order to live the remaining years of your life in perfect health?" The utility theory postulates that everyone would choose to live in perfect health. By subtracting the subject's answer from the predefined t, this technique establishes the amount of time that the subject would live in perfect health, defined as variable x. The subject is then asked, "If the amount of time you were to live in perfect health (x) was decreased, would you still choose perfect health?" In this technique, t is a fixed number and x is varied to achieve a point of indifference. This indifference point (hi) is defined as the point at which there is no preference between shorter life with perfect health and longer life with chronic disease. Mathematically, this is expressed as hi = x / t, with a resultant single value, ranging between 0.0 and 1.0. For example, a subject who is willing to trade no more than 2 years of his or her life to achieve perfect health, when given 10 years to live with CKD stage 5D, has a hi score of 0.8. In this example, t equals 10 years and x equals 8 years. The higher the hi score, the better the estimated HRQOL (7). Although the TTO approach appears to be reliable in the setting of CKD stage 5D (18), its validity has been questioned (19–22).

Generic domain-specific instruments are less comprehensive for measuring overall HRQOL when compared with generic global tools. However, the domain-specific instruments may have the advantage of being more sensitive to changes within the assessed particular domain (**FIGURE 34.1**).

The physical health domain encompasses the concept of performance status, which can be defined as the functional capacity of an individual. These instruments were originally tested in patients with cancer and demonstrated a significant positive correlation with survival (23,24). The prototypical example of a measure of performance status is the KPS scale, also known as the *Karnofsky Index* (*KI*). The KPS scale has been used extensively in CKD stage 5D studies (7). Unlike the SIP and SF-36, it is clinician assessed, and it cannot be self-administered. There are 11 descriptive statements that rank performance status on an ordinate scale from normal (score of 100) to death (score of 0) (**TABLE 34.2**). In the CKD stage 5D population, as with cancer patients, the KPS appears to be a predictor of mortality (12).

The checklist of symptoms and sexual functioning scales are two other techniques used to assess physical health. These HRQOL instruments are exemplified by a list of physical symptoms that are rated on a numerical scale. Examples of these surveys include the Index of Comorbidity (25), the Sexual Dysfunction Scale (26), the Index of Sexual Function (27), and the checklist created by Parfrey et al. (28). Unfortunately, most of these measures have not been established to be reliable and/or valid in the CKD stage 5D population (7).

HRQOL tools that measure the mental health domain primarily assess for depression, anxiety, and psychological well-being. In CKD stage 5D, the most frequently used measures include Campbell's Indices of General Affect, Well-Being, and Life Satisfaction; the Affect Balance Scale (ABS); the Beck Depression Inventory (BDI); the Self-Esteem Inventory; and locus of control scales (7).

TABLE 34.2	The Karnofsky Performance Status Scale

Description	Scale (%)
Normal, no complaints	100
Able to carry on normal activities; minor signs or symptoms of disease	90
Normal activity with effort	80
Cares for self; able to carry on normal activity or do active work	70
Requires occasional assistance but able to care for most needs	60
Requires considerable assistance and frequent medical care	50
Disabled; requires special care and assistance	40
Severely disabled; hospitalization indicated although death not imminent	30
Very sick: hospitalization necessary; active supportive treatment necessary	20
Moribund	10
Dead	0

TABLE 34.3	The Affect Balance Scale

During the past few weeks, did you ever feel . . .
  Positive feelings: yes/no
    Pleased about having accomplished something?
    That things were going your way?
    Proud because someone complimented you on something you had done?
    Particularly excited or interested in something?
    On top of the world?
  Negative feelings: yes/no
    So restless that you could not sit long in a chair?
    Bored?
    Depressed or very unhappy?
    Very lonely or remote from other people?
    Upset because someone criticized you?

Adapted from Bradburn N. *The Structure of Psychological Well-Being. Two Dimensions of Psychological Well-Being: Positive and Negative Affect.* Chicago, IL: Aldine, 1967, with permission.

Campbell's indices combine the Index of Life Satisfaction (ILS) and the Index of General Affect (IGA) to determine the IWB (29,30). The ILS, as the name implies, explores the concept of life satisfaction. It consists of one global item, "How satisfied are you with your life as a whole these days?" rated on a 7-point scale from completely dissatisfied to completely satisfied (29). The IGA consists of eight pairs of diametrically opposed items. These items are presented at either end of a 7-point scale. For example, in the pair of adjectives "discouraging to hopeful," discouraging would be 1 and hopeful would be 7. Respondents are asked to rank how they feel about their present life for each item. This technique is called a *semantic differential scale* and was developed by Osgood. The items that comprise the IGA are "boring versus interesting," "miserable versus enjoyable," "useless versus worthwhile," "lonely versus friendly," "empty versus full," "discouraging versus hopeful," "disappointing versus rewarding," and "does not give me much chance versus brings out the best in me" (29). The IGA score is obtained by averaging all eight items and ranges from 1 to 7. The IWB is then calculated from the ILS and the IGA. Mathematically, IWB = (ILS × 1.1) + IGA, with a resultant range of scores between 2.1 and 14.7, and a higher score indicating a better level of well-being. Campbell's indices are reliable and valid in the CKD stage 5D population (7) and can be either interviewer- or self-administered.

Like Campbell's indices, the ABS is also a composite of two scales, the Positive Feeling Scale (PFS) and the Negative Feeling Scale (NFS), each consisting of five items (**TABLE 34.3**) (31). The questions are presented in a yes or no format, where yes = 1 and no = 0. A composite score is calculated using the following formula: ABS = (PFS + 5) − NFS. Scores range from 0 to 10, with 10 representing a better affect. It can be either interviewer- or self-administered. The ABS is both reliable and valid in subjects with CKD stage 5D (7).

Unlike the ABS and Campbell's indices, the BDI is used to measure the presence and intensity of depression (32,33). It consists of 21 items that deal with a specific behavioral manifestation of depression, ranked from 0 to 3. Overall scores range from 0 to 63, with higher scores correlating with more severe depression. When compared with the *Diagnostic and Statistical Manual of Mental Disorders (DSM-III)* criteria for depression, the BDI was found to be valid in the CKD stage 5D population (31). Of note, there is a new edition of the BDI, the BDI-II, which revised the BDI to match the revamped criteria for depression in the DSM-IV. Both the BDI and the BDI-II take less than 10 minutes to complete and can be either interviewer or self-administered.

An additional tool validated in patients on dialysis is the nine-question Patient Health Questionnaire (PHQ-9) (34). Scores of 5, 10, 15, and 20, on the PHQ-9, represent mild, moderate, moderately severe, and severe depression, respectively (35). Importantly, a number of electronic health records have the PHQ-9 already built into the system.

Other HRQOL instruments relating to mental health attempt to quantify one's self-esteem. Self-esteem, in this setting, is defined as an overall evaluation of one's worth or value (36). The most widely used tool for measuring self-esteem is the Rosenberg Self Esteem Inventory (SEI) scale. The SEI scale uses 10 Likert-like items, such as "On whole, I am satisfied with myself" and "At times I think I am no good at all," that are answered on a scale from strongly agree to strongly disagree. A higher score indicates a higher self-esteem (32). With regard to the CKD stage 5D population, the Rosenberg SEI scale has not been established as valid and reliable (7). These instruments are often used as a component of a battery of tests used to assess the mental domain of HRQOL.

Another type of mental health HRQOL instrument that has been used in patients with CKD stage 5D is the locus of control scales. These tools attempt to measure the extent to which a subject believes that health is or is not determined by his or her own behavior; that is, the outcomes are the result of his or her own actions (internal) or the result of external forces (external). Examples of locus of control scales include the Health Locus of Control (HLC) scale developed by Wallston et al. (37), the Internal External Locus of Control (IELC) scale developed by Rotter (38,39), and the Locus of Control of Behaviour (LCB) scale developed by Craig et al. (40). The LCB consists of 17 items, rated in a Likert-type response scale from 0 (strongly agree) to 5 (strongly disagree). One example from Craig's scale is "People are victims of circumstance beyond their control." A higher score corresponds to a stronger external locus of control. Both of the IELC and the LCB have not been established as reliable or valid in the CKD stage 5D population (7). As with the tools to assess one's self-esteem, these tools are often used as a component of a battery of tests used to assess the mental domain of HRQOL. However, it seems the field is moving away from using locus of control scales.

The social health domain of HRQOL is the least well characterized, and tools used to measure this domain focus mainly on illness intrusiveness and employment status. HRQOL tools that measure illness intrusiveness attempt to quantify the degree to which a chronic illness or treatment disrupts a patient's life. The Illness Intrusiveness Rating Scale (IIRS) was developed by Devins et al. (41) to assess perceived intrusiveness of CKD stage 5D on HRQOL. The IIRS is a self-administered scale that rates perceived intrusiveness on 11 to 13 life domains, including work, recreation, family and marital relations, sex, and diet. Each item is rated in a Likert-type response scale ranging from not very much (1) to very much (7). The IIRS is valid and reliable in the CKD stage 5D population (42–44).

Various approaches have been attempted to quantify vocational rehabilitation ranging from objective measure of working status (yes and no), to subjective determination of ability to work, to detailed self-reports such as the Psychosocial Adjustment to Illness Scale (PAIS) (45). Despite the apparent ease of determining this variable, it appears that this measure may not be a valid measure of the social domain of HRQOL (46).

The other major category of HRQOL instruments is the disease-targeted instruments, which are applicable to a defined population of subjects. Examples of these tools include Parfrey's Health Questionnaire Specific for CKD stage 5D (28), Laupacis's Kidney Disease Questionnaire (KDQ) (47), Hays's Kidney Disease QOL Instrument (48), and Wu's Choice for Health Outcomes in Caring for End-Stage Renal Disease (CHOICE) Health Experience Questionnaire (49).

Parfrey et al. (28) developed the first published ESKD-targeted HRQOL instrument in 1989. The "Health Questionnaire Specific for ESRD" goal was to measure the effect of specific ESKD therapy on QOL. They constructed two unique scales for the CKD stage 5D population exploring physical symptoms (the symptom scale) and emotional symptoms (the affect scale). The symptom scale consists of 12 items (tiredness, headache, sleep disturbance, joint pain, cramps, pruritus, dyspnea, angina, nausea/vomiting, abdominal pain, muscle weakness, and other) rated from 1 (very severe) to 5 (absent). Like the symptom scale, the affect scale also consists of 12 items (determination*, faith*, confused, different, angry, scared, helpless, alone, fed up, sad, desperate, and other) [*faith and determination are actually rated from 1 (absent) to 5 (very strong)] again rated from 1 to 5. They then combined these two indices with two subjective measures of HRQOL (Campbell's Indices of General Affect, Well-Being, and Life Satisfaction and the Spitzer Subjective QOL Index) and two objective measures of HRQOL (KPS scale and the Spitzer Concise QL-Index). Overall, this questionnaire has good reproducibility (except for the Spitzer Subjective QOL Index), is responsive to change, has construct validity, and allows for comparisons between CKD stage 5D and other disease states. The questionnaire takes between 15 and 20 minutes to complete but does require a trained interviewer to administer it.

In 1992, Laupacis et al. (47) developed the KDQ, a disease-specific HRQOL tool particularly for patients on chronic hemodialysis (HD) therapy. The KDQ contains 26 items in the following five dimensions: physical symptoms (6 items), fatigue (6 items), depression (5 items), relationships (6 items), and frustration (3 items) (47). Unlike other HRQOL questionnaires, the physical symptoms dimension of the KDQ is patient specific. The six physical symptoms that are most important to each subject are identified and used to assess that dimension. Items are ranked from 1 (all of the time) to 7 (none of the time). The KDQ has construct validity and reliability (47) and is more responsive to change than the SIP or TTO (47,50). The two major limitations of the KDQ are that it is designed for use only in subjects with CKD stage 5D undergoing HD and that there is no single overall health rating.

Like the KDQ, Hays's Kidney Disease Quality of Life (KDQOL) instrument was also developed for use in subjects with CKD stage 5D on HD. Unlike the KDQ, the KDQOL uses the SF-36 as its core and supplements this with 19 additional multi-item scales (48). The incorporation of the SF-36, a global generic assessment tool, allows for comparisons of HRQOL across disease states. Major advantages of the KDQOL are its comprehensive scope and the inclusion of a single-item overall health rating. The major limitation of the KDQOL is its length, 134 items, which takes approximately 30 minutes to complete. Rao et al. (51) have subsequently developed an 11 multi-item subscale from the KDQOL's Symptoms/Problems and Effects of Kidney Disease scales, which correlates with the SF-36 Health Survey and number of disability days.

Because of the length of the KDQOL, the KDQOL short form (KDQOL-SF) was created. It includes the core SF-36 scale, 43 kidney disease-targeted items from the original KDQOL, and a single overall health-rating item, thereby containing only 80 items. Both the KDQOL and its short form are self-administered, but the KDQOL-SF takes about half as long to complete. The KDQOL-SF can be used to determine the three components of HRQOL: PCS, MCS, and the Kidney Disease Component Summary (KDCS). Both the short and long forms appear to be reliable and have construct validity (48,52). In addition to the KDQOL-SF, there is the KDQOL-36 that only contains 36 items.

Like the KDQOL, the CHOICE Health Experience Questionnaire (CHEQ) also incorporates the SF-36 as its core (49). It consists of 83 items divided into 21 domains. It can be used for subjects on either peritoneal dialysis (PD) or HD and appears to be reliable and have construct validity (49).

We recommend the 80-item KDQOL-SF for routine clinical practice for the following reasons: It allows comparisons across diseases (by incorporation of the SF-36 Health Survey), it has proven kidney disease-targeted items, it takes a relatively short amount of time to administer, and it has a single overall health-rating item. The KDQOL-SF version 1.3 instrument and scoring programs can be downloaded at the following website: http://www.rand.org /health/surveys_tools/kdqol.html.

Although not a direct measure of QOL, there have been a number of studies looking at the quality of dying in dialysis patients. CKD stage 5D offers a unique opportunity to quantify this process because dialysis is the only life-support therapy that is frequently discontinued. An estimated 17.8% of dialysis patients between 1990 and 1995 withdrew from dialysis before death (53). To better understand this aspect of QOL, Cohen et al. (54) developed a prototype tool to assess the quality of dying, the Dialysis Discontinuation Quality of Dying (DDQOD) instrument. The DDQOD is composed of three domains: duration (of dying), pain and suffering, and psychosocial. Each domain is scored on a scale from 1 to 5. A summed score can range from 3 to 15 and is divided into three types of death: a very good death defined as a score greater than 12, a good death greater than 8 to 12, and a bad death less than or equal to 8. Using the DDQOD instrument in 131 adults discontinuing dialysis, 38% of the subjects were judged as having had very good deaths, 47% good deaths, and 15% bad deaths (54). The major drawback of this tool is that it is not applicable to death in subjects with CKD stage 5D that are not preceded termination of dialysis therapy (54,55).

The Dialysis Quality of Dying Apgar (QODA) is another tool that attempts to quantify quality of dying. It is modeled after the original pediatric Apgar assessment and consists of five domains (pain, nonpain symptoms, advanced care planning, peace, and time). Each domain is scored from 0 to 2, with a range of scores between 0 and 10. It is currently being field tested in six New England dialysis clinics, but it still requires testing for reliability and validity [see reference (56)]. At this time, QODA scores correlating to the three types of deaths (as in the DDQOD) have not been established (55).

QUALITY OF LIFE IN END-STAGE KIDNEY DISEASE

As more and more people develop advanced CKD requiring renal replacement therapy, the understanding of HRQOL becomes more pertinent, as mortality and outcome measures alone do not provide a comprehensive understanding of patient dynamics. However, there is consistent data that subjects with CKD and CKD stage 5D have impaired HRQOL. In a landmark study by Evans et al. (25), the National Kidney Dialysis and Transplant Study rigorously examined the HRQOL of 859 subjects undergoing dialysis or transplantation to determine major variables that affect patient outcomes. Using Campbell's indices (IGA, ILS, and IWB), Evans reported that 79% of the transplant recipients were able to function at nearly normal levels compared with only 59%, 44.7%, and 47.5% of subjects on home HD, in-center HD, and PD, respectively.

Overall, subjects receiving renal replacement therapy had significantly lower functional scores than the general population. Nonetheless, the study suggested that patients with CKD stage 5D are able to adapt to very adverse life circumstances.

Other studies have also demonstrated improved QOL with transplantation when compared with dialysis. In a meta-analysis of 61 published articles, kidney transplantation was associated with greater well-being and lower distress when compared with other forms of renal replacement therapy (57). Bremer et al. (58) found similar results using Campbell's Indices of General Affect, Well-Being, and Life Satisfaction. In this trial, 489 of 903 eligible subjects returned valid questionnaires (54% response rate). Regarding QOL, subjects with functioning allografts fared the best, consistent with the National Kidney Dialysis and Transplant Study. Unlike Evans's study, however, that group of subjects whose allograft failed and required reinitiation of dialysis had the greatest measured loss of HRQOL. Using the SF-36 Health Survey, DeOreo (3) demonstrated that the PCS was a significant predictor of mortality, which is equal to measured Kt/V. In the Italian "Dialysis-Quality of Life" (DIAQOL) project, 246 of 304 subjects on center dialysis completed the SF-36 questionnaire (59). Factors that effected HRQOL included the presence of diabetes and the subjects' age, whereas there was no association with Kt/V, hemoglobin (Hb) concentration, body mass index, or parathyroid level. There was, however, a strong association between the serum albumin level and the SF-36 Health Survey measurement of physical functioning.

In the Spanish Cooperative Renal Patients QOL study, HRQOL was assessed using the KI and SIP in more than 1,000 subjects, the majority on HD (60). All study participants reported a reduced HRQOL, with the most severely affected dimensions being work, activities, and sleep. There was no significant effect predicted by mode of dialysis, dialysis membrane, delivered Kt/V, or PCR. Higher Hb concentration and greater education and socioeconomic levels predicted positive measures of HRQOL. Subjects with diabetes, peripheral vascular disease (PVD), multiple comorbidities, and female gender scored lower. Unfortunately, there were variations in QOL between the different centers, thereby increasing the complexity and applicability of these results (61).

There may also be perceptual differences between a subject's HRQOL and that of health care providers. Molzahn et al. (62) explored this issue in a cross-sectional, descriptive comparative study of 215 subjects with CKD stage 5D who were administered measures of HRQOL: the Self-Anchoring Striving Scale, the IWB, and TTO. Of note, when compared to the subjects' own rated HRQOL, nurses tended to have a lower, and physicians a higher, perception of the subjects' HRQOL.

IMPACT OF QUALITY OF LIFE

The importance of assessing the HRQOL cannot be overemphasized because it not only reflects patients' satisfaction but also has been independently correlated with morbidity, hospital utilization, and survival (63). The PCS score on the SF-36 Health Survey appears to be as significant a predictor of mortality as PCR and delivered Kt/V (3). Specifically, for each 5-point increment in the PCS score the survival rate increased by 10%. In a prospective, international, observational study, the Dialysis Outcomes and Practice Patterns Study (DOPPS) used the KDQOL-SF (version 1.3) to measure HRQOL in 9,526 subjects on dialysis (64). Lower PCS and lower MCS scores were associated with significant increased risk of death (relative risk of 1.29 and 1.13, respectively, $p < 0.001$) and hospitalization (relative risk of 1.15 and 1.05, respectively, $p < 0.01$) (63).

In a longitudinal observational study by Parkerson and Gutman (65), 103 subjects on dialysis were given five questionnaires, which included the KDQOL-SF. HRQOL was measured at baseline and then after 6 months and 1 year. After adjusting for hypertension and demographic factors, a higher physical functioning dimension on the KDQOL-SF correlated with 1-year survival (odds ratio 1.050, $p = 0.008$).

A multicenter, prospective study using the SF-36 Health Survey in 226 subjects with new CKD stage 5D starting dialysis demonstrated that HRQOL was substantially impaired compared to the general population (66). Physical and mental scores greater than two standard deviations lower than the general population were predictors of poor outcomes (malnutrition, prolonged hospitalization, and death), as were baseline comorbidities and low serum albumin.

EARLY REFERRAL

Because of the substantial effect that kidney disease can have on a subject's functional status, social functioning, and overall well-being, it is important to consider HRQOL measures early in the course of kidney disease. Numerous studies have demonstrated the importance of early referral to a nephrologist (TABLE 34.4) (67,68). The National Institutes of Health recommends that patients with CKD be referred to a multidisciplinary predialysis team to

TABLE 34.4	**Prognostic Factors Associated with the Quality of Life (QOL) in Dialysis Patients**	
Improved QOL	**Reduced QOL**	
Early referral to nephrologist	Younger age	
Higher hematocrit	Diabetes	
Black race	Intermittent claudication	
Socioeconomic level	Female sex	
Educational level	Depression	
Adequate dialysis	Multiple comorbidities	
Exercise	Malnutrition	
Social support	Sleep disorders	

Adapted from Valderrábano F, Jofre R, López-Gómez JM. Quality of life in end-stage renal disease patients. *Am J Kidney Dis* 2001;38:443–464, with permission.

minimize morbidity and ease the transition to renal replacement therapy (69). Early referral affords (a) the benefit of improved patient involvement and compliance; (b) greater participation in the selection and initiation of a dialysis modality; (c) better patient education; (d) time for access maturation and avoidance of unnecessary central catheters; (e) broader employment opportunities; (f) improved ability to delay the progression of CKD stage 5D; (g) delayed development of associated comorbidities such as anemia and malnourishment; (h) improved QOL with less frustration, dissatisfaction, and depression; and (i) improved mortality rate (TABLE 34.5) (67,70–75). Patients with established predialysis care also require fewer emergency starts and in-hospital days compared with standard care (76). Although Dialysis Outcomes Quality Initiative (DOQI) guidelines advocate an early start of dialysis, the evidence is not convincing (see Chapter 6 for discussion) (77). To further assess the DOQI guidelines, the multicenter, prospective Netherlands Cooperative Study on the Adequacy of Dialysis (NECOSAD) (78) used the KDQOL-SF in 237 subjects with new CKD stage 5D starting dialysis. In this cohort, 90 subjects (38%) were classified as starting "too late," according to the DOQI guidelines. This study demonstrated that subjects starting HD "too late" uniformly had

TABLE 34.5	**Potential Benefits of Early Nephrology Referral**
Better patient involvement	
Improved compliance	
Greater participation in one's care	
Time for access maturation	
Avoidance of unnecessary catheters	
Better patient education	
Improved employment opportunities	
Delayed progression to ESKD	
Delayed development of anemia	
Delayed development of malnutrition	
Improved quality of life	
Improved mortality	

ESKD, end-stage kidney disease (chronic kidney disease stage 5D).

lower perceived HRQOL versus those that were not late starters. However, this effect was not significant after 12 months. Additionally, all subjects treated with HD demonstrated marked improvement in HRQOL when reassessed at 3 and 6 months.

A retrospective study by White et al. (67) used the SF-36 Health Survey to compare 71 incident dialysis subjects who had attended predialysis clinics with 46 who had not. Adjusting for age, sex, residual kidney function, and other comorbidities, predialysis clinic attendance was an independent predictor of higher HRQOL scores for physical function, emotional role limitation, social function, and general health. Such patients generally show improved compliance and less depression and difficulties with interpersonal relationships. These findings are exaggerated in the elderly population who may require more intensive medical education and support in the setting of already compromised physical function. The finding that subjects initiated on continuous ambulatory PD therapy have a greater HRQOL as compared with HD may be related to the fact that they often receive more intensive, individualized predialysis training (79).

Insofar as early initiation of dialysis is accompanied by increased monetary costs and earlier personal restrictions, the advantage of early initiation must be individualized. A multidisciplinary approach coupled with predialysis care should help to optimize this decision and improve overall HRQOL.

SLEEP DISTURBANCES

Sleep disturbances are one of the most common problems encountered by subjects on dialysis. The prevalence of primary dyssomnias, defined as disturbances in the amount, quality, or timing of sleep, is estimated to exceed 60% in subjects on dialysis compared to between 15% and 25% in the general population (80). In one study, subjects with diabetes on maintenance HD had a prevalence of sleep disturbances of 68% (81). Many individuals experience significant distress or impairment resulting in a compromised HRQOL as measured by physical and emotional problems, reduced general health and vitality, increased pain and social isolation, and possibly increased mortality (81).

The most commonly encountered sleep disorders in subjects on dialysis include insomnia, sleep apnea and related breathing disorders, and the restless legs syndrome. In the Kidney Outcomes Prediction and Evaluation (KOPE) study, significant number of patients report waking during the night (57%), waking too early (55%), difficulty falling asleep (41%), and excessive daytime sleepiness (31%) (82). Risk factors for sleep disturbances in subjects with diabetes on HD include advanced age, depression, and compromised nutritional status (81). Increased perception of pain and greater depressive symptoms are more likely to be related to difficulty falling asleep and excessive daytime sleepiness. Patients with reduced functional status are more likely to wake during the night or too early. Women are more than twice as likely to wake too early and experience restless sleep. Patients encounter more frequent sleep disturbances if they have bone pain, pruritus, or inadequate dialysis; if they smoke; or if they have been on dialysis for a long time (80,83–85). Interestingly, nutritional status and the dose of dialysis as measured by Kt/V do not correlate with sleep disturbances; the effect of increasing Hb concentration is controversial (82,84,86–88).

Measures to improve successful sleep habits include limitation of smoking and alcohol, relaxation and biofeedback techniques, avoiding daytime and intradialytic naps, and changes in the sleep environment. Pharmacotherapy should be avoided, and first-line therapy should include cognitive behavioral therapy (89). In a randomized control trial of cognitive behavioral therapy versus sleep hygiene education in subjects on HD, cognitive behavioral therapy significantly improved all measures (Pittsburgh Sleep Quality Index, Fatigue Severity Scale, BDI, and Beck Anxiety Inventory) when compared to controls (90). When absolutely necessary, benzodiazepines that are converted into inactive metabolites, such as clonazepam, lorazepam, oxazepam, and temazepam, or the hypnotic agent, zolpidem, can be used for sedation with appropriate dose adjustments for kidney disease (91). Initial doses should be reduced by 25% to 50%.

Sleep-related breathing disorders and pathologic breathing patterns affect up to 70% of subjects on dialysis and frequently present as excessive sleepiness (92). In addition to impairing normal cognitive function, subjects with sleep-related breathing disorders are at greater risk for cardiovascular morbidity and mortality (93). Sanner et al. (94) reported clinically significant increases in the number of apnea and hypopnea episodes that exceeded 13 per hour in most subjects on dialysis, with normal defined as less than 10 per hour. These abnormalities were associated with a median oxygen saturation of 92.5%. The severity of the breathing disorder correlated with impairments in physical functioning, social functioning, role limitation, and general health and vitality, as measured on the SF-36 Health Survey. It was also correlated with pain, sleep, social isolation, and emotional reactions. The etiology of sleep apnea remains unclear but may be related to alterations in acid–base balance, thereby favoring periodic hyperventilation/hypoventilation cycles (95,96). Because of the high prevalence of sleep apnea, clinicians should maintain a high clinical suspicion and have a low threshold to obtain polysomnography in subjects on dialysis who are hypersomnolent.

Another common cause of sleep disturbances in subjects on dialysis is the periodic limb movement/restless legs syndrome. Twenty percent to 30% of subjects with CKD stage 5D report lower extremity symptoms of ascending and migratory paresthesias or cramps so severe as to interfere with sleep (83,97). Patients typically experience prolonged muscle contractions preceded by sensory discomfort (98). These are associated with sudden jerking movements that occur two to three times per minute and can lead to sudden waking. Although fluid and electrolyte imbalances may contribute to the pathophysiology, many subjects have hyperactivity of the motor neurons (99). Anecdotal reports of improvement in cramping symptoms have been reported with quinine sulfate, which appears to interfere with the excitability of the motor end plate and subsequent contractility of the muscles. However, the U.S. Food and Drug Administration has withdrawn its use for cramps because of hypersensitivity and adverse reactions. Other agents, including levodopa (100 to 200 mg/d), gabapentin (300 mg thrice weekly), or moderate doses of carbamazepine, have been used with widely variable efficacy (100–102).

SOCIAL SUPPORT AND THE QUALITY OF LIFE FOR CAREGIVERS

The interplay between patients and their social support is multidimensional. In subjects on dialysis, social support scores correlate with depression, psychosocial measures, and compliance (103,104). Their perceptions of increased social support correlate with lower

depression scores, lower perceptions of illness burden, and higher marital and life satisfaction scores independent of age and severity of illness. Higher socioeconomic, education, and employment levels generally are associated with a greater QOL, except perhaps in African Americans (60,105). Perception of social support and living with family in CKD stage 5D are predictors of survival (65,103,106,107).

Loss of employment also affects HRQOL. Unemployed subjects with CKD stage 5D score significantly lower in the SF-36 Health Survey as compared with those employed (in physical function, role physical, bodily pain, general health, vitality, and emotional scales) (108). Multiple comorbidities, a physical occupation before the onset of significant CKD, and poor physical function are independent predictors of unemployment in CKD stage 5D. Subjects who are employed or do housework tend to be more compliant with their medical regimen (109). Stack (110) attempted to better define determinants of modality selection (HD vs. PD) among incident dialysis patients in the United States. Subjects were more likely to choose PD if they were employed, married, educationally accomplished, more autonomous, and/or living with someone, as compared to HD. In addition, the selection of PD significantly associated with younger age, white race, fewer comorbid conditions, and lower serum albumin.

An important but frequently overlooked component of a subject's well-being is the QOL of their caregivers. Healthy, well-balanced relationships can provide the support many subjects on dialysis need to maintain compliance with medications, diet, and treatments; reduce the severity or occurrence of depression; and improve the overall care that they receive. Social support from family members improves compliance with interdialytic fluid restrictions (111). It is well documented that families who live with chronically ill members have a greater frequency of physical and mental disturbances (112,113). The burden and QOL of the caregivers for subjects on HD can be substantial. In a study in Brazil by Belasco and Sesso (114), most caregivers were female (84%), married (66%), and had a low socioeconomic level. The health and vitality of the caregivers, as measured by the SF-36 Health Survey, were the most frequently effected variables and inversely correlated with the burden of the caregiver, the illness of the patient, and perceived pain of the caregiver. Other studies support this finding. In a study in Sweden, Lindqvist et al. (115) demonstrated that optimistic and palliative coping strategies and less confrontational and emotional behaviors resulted in improved HRQOL of the caregivers. Spouses who were female more frequently used these skills (115). In a study from the United States, caregiver ethnicity and mode of dialysis did not significantly affect dialysis subjects perceived QOL (116). Highly functioning patients and families report the least burden and best coping strategies. To circumvent the stress associated with the ubiquitous uncertainty about the patient's health and life expectancy, frequent dialytic treatments, and potential for transplantation, families and caregivers rely heavily on their support groups and religious beliefs, living one day at a time (117). Such family and interpersonal dynamics should be explored for all subjects with CKD to help optimize their overall well-being.

ANEMIA

The impact of anemia on the HRQOL is well described and spans the continuum from early stage CKD through ESKD (see Chapter 29). Symptoms associated with uncorrected anemia in subjects with

CKD include fatigue, sexual function, cognitive dysfunction, cold intolerance, angina, dyspnea, and an impaired HRQOL. The introduction of human recombinant erythropoietin (rHuEPO) therapy into clinical practice to increase the Hb has had a dramatic effect on these parameters, particularly HRQOL measures. In subjects on HD or PD, correction of anemia consistently results in improvement in functional status, exercise ability, cognitive function, sexual function, and somatic complaints (50,118–122). In the Spanish Cooperative Study, Hb concentrations correlated significantly with physical and global scores on the SIP (60). Other large clinical studies confirm improvements in fatigue, perceived strength, and global scores on the SIP, KI, and SF-36 Health Survey, even with only modest increases in hematocrit (Hct) to 30.1% (123,124). In these trials, subjects on HD who were not receiving rHuEPO had significantly lower scores on the SF-36 than those who were receiving rHuEPO. The gap in the scores progressively diminished as the patients were initiated on rHuEPO therapy. In a similar trial, Moreno et al. (125) observed significant improvement in all three dimensions of the SIP when subjects on dialysis were started on rHuEPO. HRQOL had a positive correlation with Hct between the levels of 29% and 35%, as assessed using the KI and SIP. Using the KI and objective measures of employment status, Evans (118) demonstrated that the perceived HRQOL of subjects on dialysis treated with rHuEPO for 10 months actually exceeded that of untreated subjects with kidney transplantation.

Anemic predialysis subjects also gain substantial improvements in HRQOL when started on rHuEPO (126,127). In a randomized prospective trial, Revicki et al. (72) compared pre-ESKD subjects treated with rHuEPO to achieve an Hct of 35% with comparable untreated cohort whose mean Hct was 26.8%. HRQOL was measured using components of the SIP (three scales), SF-36 (four scales), and Campbell's ILS. Treated subjects reported improvements in physical function, energy, health distress, sexual dysfunction, depression, and satisfaction; results correlated with the improvement in Hct (72). It has also been suggested that early correction of anemia may prevent some of the complications of CKD. Correction of anemia may lead to regression of left ventricular hypertrophy, improve myocardial contractility, and increase left ventricular ejection fraction. Early treatment of anemia, instituted when the Hct falls below 35%, may prevent cardiovascular deterioration, reduce overall morbidity and mortality, and is essential in maintaining HRQOL (128–131).

Unfortunately, the target Hg/Hct that optimizes HRQOL remains controversial. Initial National Kidney Foundation (NKF)-DOQI guidelines for the management of anemia recommended targeting Hb concentrations between 11 and 12 g/dL (132). Whether HRQOL measures are improved by further increasing the Hg remains uncertain. In the Canadian Erythropoietin Study, the increase in HRQOL effects plateaued at an Hb concentration of 11.7 g/dL (21,50). The KI and SIP scores obtained by Moreno et al. (133) showed a positive correlation with Hct between 29% and 35%; the benefits are most evident at higher Hct concentrations. Eschbach et al. (134) demonstrated continued improvement in HRQOL with increasing Hct up to 42%. In another trial by Moreno et al. (135), the Hct of subjects on dialysis was increased 5 points above their baseline Hct. Baseline Hct ranged between 28% and 35%. The increase in Hct was associated with a significant improvement in HRQOL as assessed by both the KI and SIP. Although this trial was not associated with other problems, it should be noted that the cohort tested did not have significant comorbidities.

In contrast, in subjects on HD with ischemic heart disease or congestive heart failure, normalization of the Hct may be detrimental. In the North American Multicenter Study, Besarab et al. (136) prospectively randomized 1,233 subjects with known heart disease to target Hct levels of either 42% or 30%. Given concerns regarding increased risk of morbidity and mortality in normalized Hct group, an independent data monitoring committee terminated the study early. After 29 months, there were 183 deaths and 19 nonfatal myocardial infarctions (MIs) in the normal Hct group as compared with 150 deaths and 14 MIs in the low Hct group. Of note, the mortality of both groups decreased with increasing Hct, and HRQOL, as measured by the SF-36, increased 0.6 points for each percentage increase in the Hct. Other studies have demonstrated that patients with higher Hct experience less morbidity (135). The Correction of Hemoglobin and Outcomes in Renal Insufficiency (CHOIR) study was a randomized trial in subjects with CKD not on dialysis randomized to either high-Hb group (target Hg 13.5 g/dL) or low-Hb group (target Hg 11.3 g/dL) (137). HRQOL was assessed using the following three metrics: the KDQ, SF-36 Health Survey, and the Linear Analogue Self-Assessment (LASA). The CHOIR study was terminated early due to concerns that the conditional power for demonstrating benefit for the high-Hb group was going to be less than 5%. Data from the 1,432 subjects demonstrated that both groups demonstrated improvement in HRQOL scores when anemia was treated. When comparing improvement from baseline HRQOL using the LASA and KDQ, there was no significant difference between the two groups. However, the lower Hb group had more improvement in role limitations caused by emotional or personal problems as determined by the SF-36 (137). Issues with the CHOIR study include target Hb of the high-Hb group was not achieved (median Hb 12.8 g/dL), unclear time frame when the QOL tools administered, and use of high doses of rHuEPO, which have been hypothesized as having vascular effects.

The 2006 Kidney DOQI guidelines recommend that Hb levels be maintained at or above 11 g/dL in all subjects with CKD and that Hb levels not be routinely maintained above 13 g/dL (138). However, because the HRQOL may improve more the closer the Hb is to 13 g/dL, emphasis must be placed on at least achieving currently recommended levels of Hb. The KDIGO's 2012 guidelines stated that individualization of anemia therapy will be necessary, as some patients may have improvements in QOL at Hb concentration above 11.5 g/dL, although this recommendation was not graded (139).

◆ DEPRESSION

Depression appears to be the most common psychological problem experienced by subjects on HD, effecting anywhere from 20% to 70% of patients (12,140,141). Estimates of the prevalence of depression vary widely based on the instruments used to detect it and differing diagnostic criteria. In subjects on dialysis, depression clearly correlates with a compromised HRQOL (142), is more common in women, is unrelated to satisfaction with the dialysis staff or the nephrologist, and is most common in HD as compared with PD and transplantation (143,144). The etiology of depression in dialysis patients is multifactorial. Impaired physical status; complex medical regimens; and the loss of time, finances, sexual function, and control contribute to depressive symptoms. As in other chronic illnesses, the extent of depression over time in subjects with CKD stage 5D predicts mortality (141,143,145). Kovac et al. (143) investigated whether the risk of mortality and rate of hospitalization can be predicted from physician-diagnosed depression and patients' self-reports of depressive symptoms. In their cohort of more than 5,000 HD patients, the prevalence of depression was 20%. The relative risk of mortality and hospitalization among depressed patients, as measured by medical records and the KDQOL-SF, was 23% higher than in nondepressed patients. Consequently, subjects should be evaluated periodically for depression, using sensitive tools such as the BDI, BDI-II, or PHQ9, and if found, treated accordingly (33). In a few small studies in subjects on HD, cognitive behavioral therapy has been associated with improvement in BDI-II (self-reported, $p = 0.03$) and Hamilton Depression Rating Scale (clinician-reported, $p < 0.001$) scores after intervention (146–148).

 DEMOGRAPHIC VARIABLES

Age

As the age of the dialysis and transplant population increases, it is critical to explore the impact of age on the HRQOL. Early studies indicated that advanced age has a negative impact on the HRQOL (25,66,149). These studies compared the HRQOL of subjects with CKD younger than 65 years with those older than 65 years and found that HRQOL was worse in the older cohort. In the Spanish QOL study, deterioration in the physical dimension of the SIP was strongly correlated to increased age (12,60,133). However, using the SIP and SF-36, Rebollo et al. (150) studied 485 subjects who were either on HD or posttransplant; the scores of the elderly subjects were significantly higher than those of the younger subset. Elderly renal transplant subjects had even higher scores than the reference general population. This data suggest that CKD stage 5D has less of an impact in the elderly and that transplantation in this group offers a reasonable alternative to dialysis.

A study done on nursing home residents who were initiated on HD compared functional status prior to and 3 months after initiation on HD. Functional status was measured by assessing the degree of dependence using the Minimum Data Set–Activities of Daily Living scale. After 3 months of HD, functional status was maintained in only 39% of the subjects, and after 12 months, only 13% had maintenance of their functional status, 58% of the subjects had died by 12 months (151). Using a random-effects model, the initiation of dialysis was associated with a marked decline in functional status; this decline was independent of age, sex, race, and functional-status trajectory before the initiation of dialysis.

In contrast to elderly patients living in nursing homes, as assessed by the SF-36 Health Survey, elderly subjects on dialysis living in London had better physical functioning, lower levels of pain, and better general health perceptions than their younger counterparts. Interestingly, these elderly subjects were also less likely to be hospitalized and, when they were, had shorter lengths of stay. Higher economic level, educational level, KI score, and lower number of comorbid conditions were associated with higher HRQOL (152). Elderly subjects tend to be more satisfied with their life while on dialysis and appear to accept their limitations better than younger subjects. This may be due, in part, to the fact that older individuals expect some degree of deterioration in their HRQOL and are more grateful for the extension of life provided by renal replacement therapy (4,153,154). In DOPPS, older age was not significantly associated with reduced scores in MCS, social function scales, or general health but was associated with lower scores in the PCS (64).

Among elderly subjects on PD, despite having worse appetites and moods than their younger counterparts, there is no significant difference in their overall HRQOL (155). In addition, clinical outcomes and HRQOL, as measured by the SF-36 and KDQOL, do not differ significantly among elderly subjects treated with PD or HD (156). Therefore, based on HRQOL alone, subjects should not be excluded from a treatment modality simply on the basis of age.

Gender

Studies consistently demonstrate that women have a lower HRQOL than men, regardless of the type of renal replacement modality, and this exists even among CKD subjects predialysis (60,152,157,158). It has been suggested that much of the measured decrement in HRQOL may be related more to social factors and depression, particularly the change in women's social role, rather than because of physical factors (12). However, in a study done in Sweden, women appeared to be less effective at coping with the physical aspects of CKD stage 5D as compared with their male counterparts (159). Additionally, women treated with PD had lower scores on the Swedish Health-Related Quality of Life (SWED-QUAL) questionnaire (developed from the SF-36 Health Survey) as compared with woman on HD (159). DOPPS also demonstrated that women had significantly lower scores in physical functioning, bodily pain, and vitality compared to men (64).

Ethnicity

Despite the overrepresentation of racial and ethnic minorities among subjects on dialysis and underrepresentation among transplant patients, the adjusted mortality and HRQOL for minority participants in the CKD stage 5D program are better than for the majority population (160). Using the Wisconsin QOL Index, Welch and Austin (161) evaluated the HRQOL in 79 black subjects on dialysis at two urban dialysis units. Their HRQOL was fairly high and similar to that of a non–African American cohort. In the black cohort, psychological and spiritual health ranked higher than physical functioning. Worse HRQOL was associated with more education and younger age. In a prospective, observational trial in the state of Georgia, elderly black subjects on dialysis had better perceived HRQOL than elderly white subjects (105). In this study, the elderly white subjects more frequently complained of nausea, fatigue, and postdialysis inertia. They were also more likely to perceive dialysis as an intrusion to their health and diets and to be dissatisfied with their health and life, despite a lower incidence of diabetes (105). The largest data set examining differences in HRQOL comes from the DOPPS, whose cohort was broken down into: white ($n = 3,143$), African American ($n = 2,102$), Asian ($n = 183$), Native American ($n = 50$), Hispanic ($n = 587$), and Other ($n = 86$). Compared with the non-Hispanic white group, the African American group had significantly higher mean adjusted HRQOL scores for all three components of the KDQOL-SF (162). Specifically, their mean difference was $+1.3$, $+1.1$, and $+1.8$ (PCS, MCS, and KDCS, respectively). However, the African American group had significantly lower score (mean difference, -3.2) in the item "patient satisfaction" (162).

When compared with whites, Asian subjects in England reported significantly lower HRQOL both while on dialysis and after successful transplantation, using the KDQOL-SF survey (163). Asian subjects, in particular, were noted to perceive kidney disease as a social burden. In DOPPS, the Asian group had a significantly higher score than whites for the PCS (mean difference, $+2.4$), but no significant difference was observed for the MCS and KDCS (162).

When compared with the white group, the Hispanic group from DOPPS had significantly higher adjusted scores for the PCS (mean difference, +1.6) but lower scores for the MCS and KDCS (mean difference, −1.4 and −1.7, respectively) (164).

Of concern, minorities in the United States typically have longer waiting times for transplantation, limited referral for home dialysis, fewer native fistulas placed, and higher rate of inadequate dialysis prescriptions. Correction of these inequities may have a positive effect on HRQOL.

 ## HEALTH-RELATED QUALITY OF LIFE

Comorbid Conditions

As renal function declines, many subjects experience fatigue, lethargy, muscle cramps, loss of appetite, and a sense of loss of control. This physical deterioration is accompanied by a decline in the HRQOL. In the Modification of Diet in Renal Disease (MDRD) study, the severity of physical symptoms correlated with a decline in HRQOL that paralleled the loss of kidney function (157). Some subjects experience an improvement in HRQOL after the initiation of dialysis, but the improvement was variable and depended on coexisting medical problems. In subjects both before and after initiation of dialysis, the number of comorbid conditions strongly correlates with lower physical function and worse scores on the SIP (12,60). Specifically, the presence of intermittent claudication (as a manifestation of PVD), uncontrolled hypertension, and physical symptoms has been shown to be important determinants of a poor HRQOL (59,164). Not surprisingly, diabetes is also strongly associated with a worse HRQOL (149). Subjects with diabetes mellitus (DM) consistently score lower in all variables of HRQOL measures, independent of age. This may be related to the multisystem involvement of DM and in particular, the associated neuropathy (165). Importantly, intensive education seems to improve the HRQOL in these subjects. McMurray et al. (166) randomized 83 subjects with DM on dialysis to either standard or intensive education. The control group's risk of foot disease and amputation increased over the course of a year but was unchanged in the intensive education group. The treatment group reported significant improvement in HRQOL indices when compared with the controls, highlighting the important benefits of intensive education and support. In the Hemodialysis (HEMO) study, factors that were associated with more fatigue included the presence of diabetes, a lower serum albumin, a higher index of coexistent diseases (ICED) score, non–African American race, use of medications for sleep, and poor sleep quality (167). In this study, older subjects and dialysis vintage was also associated with a higher rate of worsening fatigue, whereas a high serum albumin was associated with improvement in fatigue.

 ## DIALYSIS-RELATED FACTORS

Dialysis Modality

The effect of dialysis modality on HRQOL remains controversial. Some studies demonstrated better satisfaction in subjects on HD as compared with PD (25,57,58). In a prospective, observational study, the PCS and MCS components of the SF-36 Health Survey were used to compare HRQOL in 177 subjects over 15 months (168). Subjects on PD had a significantly lower PCS score than subjects on HD, despite having similar MCS scores and prevalence of depression. However, when corrected for the serum albumin level, this difference was eliminated. Other investigators have found that although patients on PD have a greater degree of independence, they appear to be more anxious and insecure than patients on HD (12,169).

Using the KDQOL-SF, the NECOSAD study demonstrated that subjects on PD had a greater decrease in the physical dimension of HRQOL compared with subjects on HD (170). Bakewell et al. (171) found similar results in subjects on PD using the KDQOL-SF.

Other studies have yielded the opposite results. In a meta-analysis of 61 studies comparing differences in HRQOL across renal replacement therapies demonstrated that subjects on PD enjoyed a greater sense of well-being and were less distressed than subjects on HD (57).

To determine if increased frequency of dialysis would improve HRQOL, the Frequent Hemodialysis Network randomized trials compared the effects of six versus three times per week HD on physical health (172). Subjects randomized to frequent HD had a significant increase in their physical health composite scores but no significant change in their short physical performance battery, when compared with the convention thrice-weekly dialysis group. Frequent HD was associated with favorable results with respect to the composite outcomes of death or change in left ventricular mass and the composite outcome of death or change in a physical health composite score.

Adequacy of Dialysis Clearance

Other studies have evaluated the impact of Kt/V and innovative approaches to dialysis on the HRQOL. Using the KDQOL-SF, SF-36, and EuroQol EQ-5D, Manns et al. (173) found that subjects on HD with an average Kt/V greater than or equal to 1.3 had better HRQOL. In the HEMO study, the IWB and the KDQOL (long-form) questionnaires were used to assess HRQOL. The high dose of delivered dialysis (eKt/V of 1.45) was associated with higher PCS scores and significantly less pain when compared with standard dose of delivered dialysis (eKt/V of 1.05) (174). Using the SF-36 Health Survey, Chen et al. (175) demonstrated that subjects on PD with adequate total urea clearance had a better HRQOL than those with inadequate clearance, as determined by Kt/V urea. Support of the notion that improved clearance improves HRQOL comes from a study which demonstrated that uremic subjects on PD showed increased HRQOL with the addition of once-weekly HD (176).

No long-term studies have demonstrated the effect of dialysate buffer on an individual's HRQOL. Other methods to improve the dose of delivered dialysis have been studied. The use of high-flux membranes was not associated with improved HRQOL in the HEMO study compared to low-flux membranes (174). However, both daily dialysis and nightly home HD have been reported to positively impact HRQOL, as they show promise in reducing dialysis-related symptoms and hospitalizations and in improving well-being (177–179). Because of substantial cost and the technical support needed for these interventions, further cost-benefit analysis is needed.

 ## NUTRITION AND PHYSICAL ACTIVITY

The importance of maintaining adequate nutrition in CKD stage 5D has been well established (see Chapter 27 for discussion). Multiple studies, although not examining nutrition directly, report an association between low albumin levels and a low HRQOL. In general, there is a significant inverse relationship between SF-36 scores and serum albumin and anemia, and a negative correlation with obesity (180,181). Low albumin levels are independently associated with decreased physical function, social function, and burden of kidney disease as assessed by the SF-36. Low PCR is associated with decreased physical function scores and disability, as measured by the KPS (182).

Many authors describe advantages of physical exercise in improving the HRQOL. This appears to be true both at the initiation of dialysis, when muscle deterioration begins, and throughout the course of dialytic therapy (183,184). Exercise activity independently predicts performance measures of gait speed and chair rising and perceived physical functioning (185). Interventions to improve exercise may include in-center cycling, home regimens, and rehabilitation (186,187) and should be explored for all patients.

CONCLUSION

Recognition that HRQOL is an important predictor of morbidity and mortality has been an important advancement in caring for subjects with CKD. Measurement of HRQOL is helpful in assessing the impact of interventions, increasing patients' participation in their own care, and increasing patient satisfaction (188). Improvement of anemia, malnutrition, inactivity, predialysis care, and social support systems enhance the HRQOL and are associated with improved survival. Strategies aimed at these components and in controlling blood pressure, preserving residual kidney function, and assuring adequacy of dialysis should further reduce the risk of poor outcomes. In the future, telemedicine and other technologic advances may provide additional mechanisms to improve the HRQOL (189). Presently, health care providers should focus on HRQOL issues and measure their patients' perceptions at periodic intervals using a validated tool like the KDQOL-SF.

REFERENCES

1. *The American Heritage Dictionary of the English Language*. 3rd ed. Boston, MA: Houghton Mifflin, 1992.
2. World Health Organization. *World Health Organization Handbook of Basic Documents*. 5th ed. Geneva, Switzerland: Palais des Nations, 1952: 3–20. http://www.who.int/healthinfo/survey/whoqol-qualityoflife/en/. Accessed June 22, 2016.
3. DeOreo PB. Hemodialysis patient-assessed functional health status predicts continued survival, hospitalization, and dialysis-attendance compliance. *Am J Kidney Dis* 1997;30:204–212.
4. Ifudu O, Paul HR, Homel P, et al. Predictive value of functional status for mortality in patients on maintenance hemodialysis. *Am J Nephrol* 1998;18:109–116.
5. McClellan WM, Anson C, Birkeli K, et al. Functional status and quality of life: predictors of early mortality among patients entering treatment for end stage renal disease. *J Clin Epidemiol* 1991;44:83–89.
6. Testa MA, Simonson DC. Assessment of quality-of-life outcomes. *N Engl J Med* 1996;334:835–840.
7. Edgell ET, Coons SJ, Carter WB, et al. A review of health-related quality-of-life measures used in end-stage renal disease. *Clin Ther* 1996;18:887–938.
8. Lord FM. *Applications of Item Response Theory to Practical Testing Problems*. Hillsdale, MI: Lawrence Erlbaum Associates, 1980.
9. Kimmel PL. Just whose quality of life is it anyway? Controversies and consistencies in measurement of quality of life. *Kidney Int* 2000;57:S113–S120.
10. RAND Health. *36-Item Short Form Survey from the RAND Medical Outcomes Study*. Santa Monica, CA: RAND Health, 1986. http://www.rand.org/health/surveys_tools/mos/mos_core_36item.html. Accessed June 22, 2016.
11. Clason D, Dormody T. Analyzing data measured by individual Likert-type items. *J Agric Tradit Bot Appl* 1994;35(4):31–35.
12. Valderrábano F, Jofre R, López-Gómez JM. Quality of life in end-stage renal disease patients. *Am J Kidney Dis* 2001;38:443–464.
13. Cagney KA, Wu AW, Fink NE, et al. Formal literature review of quality-of-life instruments used in end-stage renal disease. *Am J Kidney Dis* 2000;36:327–336.
14. Bergner M, Bobbitt RA, Kressel S, et al. The sickness impact profile: conceptual formulation and methodology for the development of a health status measure. *Int J Health Serv* 1976;6:393–415.
15. Bergner M, Bobbitt RA, Carter WB, et al. The sickness impact profile: development and final revision of a health status measure. *Med Care* 1981;19:787–805.
16. Ware JE Jr, Sherbourne CD. The MOS 36-item short-form health survey (SF-36). I. Conceptual framework and item selection. *Med Care* 1992;30:473–483.
17. Torrance GW. Utility approach to measuring health-related quality of life. *J Chronic Dis* 1987;40:593–603.
18. Churchill DN, Torrance GW, Taylor DW, et al. Measurement of quality of life in end-stage renal disease: the time trade-off approach. *Clin Invest Med* 1987;10:14–20.
19. Maor Y, King M, Olmer L, et al. A comparison of three measures: the time trade-off technique, global health-related quality of life and the SF-36 in dialysis patients. *J Clin Epidemiol* 2001;54:565–570.
20. Churchill DN, Wallace JE, Ludwin D, et al. A comparison of evaluative indices of quality of life and cognitive function in hemodialysis patients. *Control Clin Trials* 1991;12(Suppl 4):159S–167S.
21. Keown PA. The Canadian Erythropoietin Study Group. Quality of life in end-stage renal disease patients during recombinant human erythropoietin therapy. *Contrib Nephrol* 1991;88:81–89.
22. Laupacis A, Wong C, Churchill D, et al. The Canadian Erythropoietin Study Group. The use of generic and specific quality-of-life measures in hemodialysis patients treated with erythropoietin. *Control Clin Trials* 1991;12(Suppl 4):168S–179S.
23. Maltoni M, Pirovano M, Scarpi E, et al. Prediction of survival of patients terminally ill with cancer: results of an Italian prospective multicentric study. *Cancer* 1995;75:2613–2622.
24. Llobera J, Esteva M, Rifà J, et al. Terminal cancer: duration and prediction of survival time. *Eur J Cancer* 2000;36:2036–2043.
25. Evans RW, Manninen DL, Garrison LP Jr, et al. The quality of life of patients with end-stage renal disease. *N Engl J Med* 1985;312:553–559.
26. Revicki DA. Relationship between health utility and psychometric health status measures. *Med Care* 1992;30(Suppl 5):MS274–MS282.
27. Berkman AH, Katz LA, Weissman R. Sexuality and the life-style of home dialysis patients. *Arch Phys Med Rehabil* 1982;63:272–275.
28. Parfrey PS, Vavasour H, Bullock M, et al. Development of a health questionnaire specific for end-stage renal disease. *Nephron* 1989;52:20–28.
29. Campbell A, Converse P, Rodgers W. *The Quality of American Life: Perceptions, Evaluations, and Satisfactions*. New York, NY: Russell Sage Foundation, 1976:32–60.
30. Campbell A. Subjective measures of well-being. *Am Psychol* 1976;31: 117–124.
31. Bradburn N. *The Structure of Psychological Well-Being. Two Dimensions of Psychological Well-Being: Positive and Negative Affect*. Chicago, IL: Aldine, 1969.
32. Beck AT, Ward CH, Mendelson M, et al. An inventory for measuring depression. *Arch Gen Psychiatry* 1961;4:561–571.
33. Craven JL, Rodin GM, Littlefield C. The Beck Depression Inventory as a screening device for major depression in renal dialysis patients. *Int J Psychiatry Med* 1988;18:365–374.
34. Watnick S, Wang PL, Demadura T, et al. Validation of 2 depression screening tools in dialysis patients. *Am J Kidney Dis* 2005;46(5):919–924.
35. Kroenke K, Spitzer RL, Williams JB. The PHQ-9: validity of a brief depression severity measure. *J Gen Intern Med* 2001;16(9):606–613.
36. Silber E, Tippett J. Self-esteem: clinical assessment and measurement validation. *Psychol Rep* 1965;16:1017–1071.
37. Wallston BS, Wallston KA, Kaplan GD, et al. Development and validation of the Health Locus of Control (Hlc) Scale. *J Consult Clin Psychol* 1976;44:580–585.
38. Rotter JB. Generalized expectancies for internal versus external control of reinforcement. *Psychol Monogr* 1966;80:1–28.
39. Rotter JB. *The Development and Applications of Social Learning Theory*. New York, NY: Praeger, 1982.
40. Craig AR, Franklin JA, Andrews G, et al. A scale to measure locus of control of behaviour. *Br J Med Psychol* 1984;57(Pt 2):173–180.

41. Devins GM, Binik YM, Hutchinson TA, et al. The emotional impact of end-stage renal disease: importance of patients' perception of intrusiveness and control. *Int J Psychiatry Med* 1983–1984;13: 327–343.

42. Devins GM, Beanlands H, Mandin H, et al. Psychosocial impact of illness intrusiveness moderated by self-concept and age in end-stage renal disease. *Health Psychol* 1997;16:529–538.

43. Devins GM, Dion R, Pelletier LG, et al. Structure of lifestyle disruptions in chronic disease: a confirmatory factor analysis of the Illness Intrusiveness Ratings Scale. *Med Care* 2001;39:1097–1104.

44. Devins GM, Mandin H, Hons RB, et al. Illness intrusiveness and quality of life in end-stage renal disease: comparison and stability across treatment modalities. *Health Psychol* 1990;9:117–142.

45. Kaplan De-Nour A. Psychosocial Adjustment to Illness Scale (PAIS): a study of chronic hemodialysis patients. *J Psychosom Res* 1982;26: 11–22.

46. Kaplan De-Nour A. Renal replacement therapies. In: Spilker B, ed. *Quality of Life Assessments in Clinical Trials*. New York, NY: Raven Press, 1990:381–389.

47. Laupacis A, Muirhead N, Keown P, et al. A disease-specific questionnaire for assessing quality of life in patients on hemodialysis. *Nephron* 1992;60:302–306.

48. Hays RD, Kallich RD, Mapes DL, et al. Development of the Kidney Disease Quality of Life (KDQOL) instrument. *Qual Life Res* 1994;3: 329–338.

49. Wu AW, Fink NE, Cagney KA, et al. Developing a health-related quality-of-life measure for end-stage renal disease: the CHOICE Health Experience Questionnaire. *Am J Kidney Dis* 2001;37:11–21.

50. Association between recombinant human erythropoietin and quality of life and exercise capacity of patients receiving haemodialysis. Canadian Erythropoietin Study Group. *BMJ* 1990;300:573–578.

51. Rao S, Carter WB, Mapes DL, et al. Development of subscales from the symptoms/problems and effects of kidney disease scales of the kidney disease quality of life instrument. *Clin Ther* 2000;22:1099–1111.

52. Korevaar JC, Merkus MP, Jansen MA, et al. Validation of the KDQOL-SF: a dialysis-targeted health measure. *Qual Life Res* 2002;11: 437–447.

53. Neff MS. To be or not to be: the decision to withdraw or be withdrawn from dialysis. *Am J Kidney Dis* 1999;33:601–606.

54. Cohen LM, Germain MJ, Poppel DM, et al. Dying well after discontinuing the life-support treatment of dialysis. *Arch Intern Med* 2000;160:2513–2518.

55. Cohen LM, Poppel DM, Cohn GM, et al. A very good death: measuring quality of dying in end-stage renal disease. *J Palliat Med* 2001;4: 167–172.

56. Cohen LM, Germain MJ. Measuring quality of dying in end-stage renal disease. *Semin Dial* 2004;17(5):376–379.

57. Cameron JI, Whiteside C, Katz J, et al. Differences in quality of life across renal replacement therapies: a meta-analytic comparison. *Am J Kidney Dis* 2000;35:629–637.

58. Bremer BA, McCauley C, Wrona RM, et al. Quality of life in end-stage renal disease: a reexamination. *Am J Kidney Dis* 1989;13:200–209.

59. Mingardi G, Cornalba L, Cortinovis E, et al. Health-related quality of life in dialysis patients: a report from an Italian study using the SF-36 Health Survey. DIA-QOL group. *Nephrol Dial Transplant* 1999;14: 1503–1510.

60. Moreno F, López Gomez JM, Sanz-Guajardo D, et al. Quality of life in dialysis patients: a Spanish multi-centre study. *Nephrol Dial Transplant* 1996;11(Suppl 2):S125–S129.

61. Mozes B, Shabtai E, Zucker D. Differences in quality of life among patients receiving dialysis replacement therapy at seven medical centers. *J Clin Epidemiol* 1997;50:1035–1043.

62. Molzahn AE, Northcott HC, Dossetor JB. Quality of life of individuals with end-stage renal disease: perceptions of patients, nurses, and physicians. *ANNA J* 1997;24:325–335.

63. Mingardi G. DIA-QOL Group. Quality of life and end-stage renal disease therapeutic programs. Dialysis quality of life. *Int J Artif Organs* 1998;21:741–747.

64. Lopes AA, Bragg-Gresham JL, Goodkin DA, et al. Factors associated with health-related quality of life among hemodialysis patients in the DOPPS. *Qual Life Res* 2007;16(4):545–557.

65. Parkerson GR Jr, Gutman RA. Health-related quality of life predictors of survival and hospital utilization. *Health Care Financ Rev* 2000;21(3):171–184.

66. Merkus MP, Jager KJ, Dekker FW, et al. Quality of life in patients on dialysis: self-assessment 3 months after the start of treatment. *Am J Kidney Dis* 1997;29:584–592.

67. White CA, Pilkey RM, Lam M, et al. Pre-dialysis clinic attendance improves quality of life among hemodialysis patients. *BMC Nephrol* 2002;3:3.

68. Binik YM, Devins GM, Barre PE, et al. Live and learn: patient education delays the need to initiate renal replacement therapy in end-stage renal disease. *J Nerv Ment Dis* 1993;181:371–376.

69. NIH Consensus Statement. Morbidity and mortality of dialysis. *Ann Intern Med* 1994;121:62–70.

70. Klang B, Björvell H, Clyne N. Predialysis education helps patients choose dialysis modality and increases disease-specific knowledge. *J Adv Nurs* 1999;29:869–876.

71. Ahlmén J, Carlsson L, Schönborg C. Well-informed patients with end-stage renal disease prefer peritoneal dialysis to hemodialysis. *Perit Dial Int* 1993;12(Suppl 2):S196–S198.

72. Revicki DA, Brown RE, Feeny DH, et al. Health-related quality of life associated with recombinant human erythropoietin therapy for pre-dialysis chronic renal disease patients. *Am J Kidney Dis* 1995;25:548–554.

73. Sesso R, Yoshihiro MM. Time of diagnosis of chronic renal failure and assessment of quality of life in haemodialysis patients. *Nephrol Dial Transplant* 1997;12:2111–2115.

74. Arora P, Obrador GT, Ruthazer R, et al. Prevalence, predictors and consequences of late nephrology referral at a tertiary care center. *J Am Soc Nephrol* 1999;10:1281–1286.

75. Obrador GT, Pereira BJ. Early referral to the nephrologist and timely initiation on renal replacement therapy: a paradigm shift in the management of patients with chronic renal failure. *Am J Kidney Dis* 1998;31:398–417.

76. Holland DC, Lam M. Sub-optimal dialysis initiation in a retrospective cohort of predialysis patients. *Scand J Urol Nephrol* 2000;34:341–347.

77. Eknoyan G, Levin N. *Clinical Practice Guidelines: Final Guideline Summaries from the Work Groups of the National Kidney Foundation–Dialysis Outcomes Quality Initiative*. New York, NY: National Kidney Foundation, 1997.

78. Korevaar JC, Jansen MA, Dekker FW. National Kidney Foundation-Dialysis Outcomes Quality Initiative. Evaluation of DOQI guidelines: early start of dialysis treatment is not associated with better health-related quality of life. *Am J Kidney Dis* 2002;39:108–115.

79. Korevaar JC, Jansen MA, Merkus MP, et al. The NECOSAD Study Group. Quality of life in pre-dialysis end-stage renal disease patients at the initiation of dialysis therapy. *Perit Dial Int* 2000;20:69–75.

80. American Psychiatric Association. *Diagnostic and Statistical Manual of Mental Disorders*. 4th ed. Washington, DC: American Psychiatric Association, 2000.

81. Han SY, Yoon JW, Jo SK, et al. Insomnia in diabetic hemodialysis patients: prevalence and risk factors by a multicenter study. *Nephron* 2002;92:127–132.

82. Williams SW, Tell GS, Zheng B, et al. Correlates of sleep behavior among hemodialysis patients: the kidney outcomes prediction and evaluation (KOPE) study. *Am J Nephrol* 2002;22:18–28.

83. Walker S, Fine A, Kryger MH. Sleep complaints are common in a dialysis unit. *Am J Kidney Dis* 1995;26:751–756.

84. Holley JL, Nespor S, Rault R. A comparison of reported sleep disturbances in patients on chronic hemodialysis and continuous peritoneal dialysis. *Am J Kidney Dis* 1992;19:156–161.

85. Soldatos C, Kales JD, Scharf MD, et al. Cigarette smoking associated with sleep difficulty. *Science* 1980;207:551–553.

86. Evans RW, Rader B, Manninen DL. The quality of life of hemodialysis recipients treated with recombinant human erythropoietin. Cooperative Multicenter EPO Clinical Trial Group *JAMA* 1990;263:825–830.

87. Levin NW. Quality of life and hematocrit level. *Am J Kidney Dis* 1992;20(Suppl 1):16–20.

88. Benz RL, Pressman M, Hovick E, et al. The SLEEPO Study. A preliminary study of the effects of correction of anemia with recombinant human erythropoietin therapy on sleep, sleep disorders, and daytime sleepiness in hemodialysis patients. *Am J Kidney Dis* 1999;34:1089–1095.

89. Wilson SJ, Nutt DJ, Alford C, et al. British Association for Psychopharmacology consensus statement on evidence-based treatment of insomnia, parasomnias and circadian rhythm disorders. *J Psychopharmacol* 2010;24(11):1577–1601.

90. Chen HY, Cheng IC, Pan YJ, et al. Cognitive-behavioral therapy for sleep disturbance decreases inflammatory cytokines and oxidative stress in hemodialysis patients. *Kidney Int* 2011;80(4):415–422.

91. Salvà P, Costa J. Clinical pharmacokinetics and pharmacodynamics of zolpidem: therapeutic implications. *Clin Pharmacokinet* 1995;29:142–153.

92. Kimmel PL, Miller G, Mendelson WB. Sleep apnea syndrome in chronic renal dialysis. *Am J Med* 1989;86:308–314.

93. Partinen M, Jamieson A, Guilleminault C. Long-term outcome for obstructive sleep apnea syndrome patients. *Chest* 1988;94:1200–1204.

94. Sanner BM, Tepel M, Esser M, et al. Sleep-related breathing disorders impair quality of life in haemodialysis recipients. *Nephrol Dial Transplant* 2002;17:1260–1265.

95. Fletcher EC. Obstructive sleep apnea and the kidney. *J Am Soc Nephrol* 1993;4:1111–1121.

96. Hallett MD, Burden S, Stewart D, et al. Sleep apnea in end-stage renal disease patients on hemodialysis and continuous ambulatory peritoneal dialysis. *ASAIO J* 1995;41:M435–M441.

97. Winkelman JW, Chertow GM, Lazarus JM. Restless legs syndrome in end-stage renal disease. *Am J Kidney Dis* 1996;28:372–378.

98. Trenkwalder C, Bucher SF, Oertel WH. Electrophysiologic pattern of involuntary limb movements in the restless leg syndrome. *Muscle Nerve* 1996;19:155–162.

99. McGee SR. Muscle cramps. *Arch Intern Med* 1990;150:511–518.

100. Trenkwalder C, Stiasny K, Pollmächer T, et al. L-dopa therapy of uremic and idiopathic restless legs syndrome: a double blind, cross over trial. *Sleep* 1995;18:681–688.

101. Serrao M, Rossi P, Cardinali P, et al. Gabapentin treatment for muscle cramps: an open-label trial. *Clin Neuropharmacol* 2000;23:45–49.

102. Thorp ML, Morris CD, Bagby SP. A crossover study of gabapentin in the treatment of restless legs syndrome among hemodialysis patients. *Am J Kidney Dis* 2001;38:104–108.

103. Kimmel PL. Psychosocial factors in adult end-stage renal disease patients treated with hemodialysis: correlates and outcomes. *Am J Kidney Dis* 2000;35(4 Suppl 1):S132–S140.

104. Boyer CB, Friend R, Chlouverakis G, et al. Social support and demographic factors influencing compliance of hemodialysis patients. *J Appl Soc Psychol* 1990;20:1902–1918.

105. Kutner NG, Devins GM. A comparison of the quality of life reported by elderly whites and elderly blacks on dialysis. *Geriatr Nephrol Urol* 1998;8:77–83.

106. Christensen AJ, Wiebe JS, Smith TW, et al. Predictors of survival among hemodialysis patients: effect of perceived family support. *Health Psychol* 1994;13:521–525.

107. McClellan WM, Stanwyck DJ, Anson CA. Social support and subsequent mortality among patients with end-stage renal disease. *J Am Soc Nephrol* 1993;4:1028–1034.

108. Blake C, Codd MB, Cassidy A, et al. Physical function, employment and quality of life in end-stage renal disease. *J Nephrol* 2000;13:142–149.

109. Lamping DL, Campbell KA. Hemodialysis compliance: assessment, prediction and intervention: part II. *Semin Dial* 1990;3:105–111.

110. Stack AG. Determinants of modality selection among incident US dialysis patients: results from a national study. *J Am Soc Nephrol* 2002;13(5):1279–1287.

111. Brown J, Fitzpatrick R. Factors influencing compliance with dietary restrictions in dialysis patients. *J Psychosom Res* 1988;32:191–196.

112. Cantor MH. Strain among caregivers: a study of the experiences in the United States. *Gerontologist* 1983;23:597–604.

113. Schultz R, O'Brien AT, Bookwala J, et al. Psychiatric and physical morbidity effects of dementia caregiving: prevalence, correlates, and causes. *Gerontologist* 1995;35:771–791.

114. Belasco AG, Sesso R. Burden and quality of life of caregivers for hemodialysis patients. *Am J Kidney Dis* 2002;39:805–812.

115. Lindqvist R, Carlsson M, Sjödén PO. Coping strategies and health-related quality of life among spouses of continuous ambulatory peritoneal dialysis, haemodialysis, and transplant patients. *J Adv Nurs* 2000;31:1398–1408.

116. Wicks MN, Milstead EJ, Hathaway DK, et al. Subjective burden and quality of life in family caregivers of patients with end-stage renal disease. *ANNA J* 1997;24:531–538.

117. Pelletier-Hibbert M, Sohi P. Sources of uncertainty and coping strategies used by family members of individuals living with end-stage renal disease. *Nephrol Nurs J* 2001;28:411–419.

118. Evans RW. Recombinant human erythropoietin and the quality of life of end-stage renal disease patients: a comparative analysis. *Am J Kidney Dis* 1991;18(4 Suppl 1):62–70.

119. Delano BG. Improvements in quality of life following treatment with rHuEPO in anemic hemodialysis patients. *Am J Kidney Dis* 1989;14:14–18.

120. Auer J, Simon G, Stevens J, et al. Quality of life improvements in CAPD patients treated with subcutaneously administered erythropoietin for anemia. *Perit Dial Int* 1992;12:40–42.

121. Guthrie M, Cardenas D, Eschbach JW, et al. Effects of erythropoietin on strength and functional status of patients on hemodialysis. *Clin Nephrol* 1993;39:97–102.

122. Mayer G, Thum J, Cada EM, et al. Working capacity is increased following recombinant human erythropoietin treatment. *Kidney Int* 1988;34:525–528.

123. Bennet WM. A multicenter clinical trial of epoetin beta for anemia of end-stage renal failure. *J Am Soc Nephrol* 1991;1(7):990–998.

124. Beusterein LM, Nissenson AR, Port FK, et al. The effects of recombinant human erythropoietin on functional health and well-being in chronic dialysis patients. *J Am Soc Nephrol* 1996;7:763–773.

125. Moreno F, Valderabano F, Aracil FJ, et al. Influence of hematocrit on the quality of life of hemodialysis patients. *Nephrol Dial Transplant* 1994;9(7):1034.

126. Lim VS. Recombinant human erythropoietin in predialysis patients. *Am J Kidney Dis* 1991;18(Suppl):34–37.

127. Double-blind, placebo-controlled study of the therapeutic use of recombinant human erythropoietin for anemia associated with chronic renal failure in predialysis patients. The US Recombinant Human Erythropoietin Predialysis Study Group. *Am J Kidney Dis* 1991;18(1):50–59.

128. Drüeke TB, Eckardt KU, Frei U, et al. Does early anemia correction prevent complications of chronic renal failure? *Clin Nephrol* 1999;51:1–11.

129. Bedani PL, Verzola A, Bergami M, et al. Erythropoietin and cardiocirculatory condition in aged patients with chronic renal failure. *Nephron* 2001;89:350–353.

130. McMahon LP, Mason K, Skinner SL, et al. Effects of haemoglobin normalization on quality of life and cardiovascular parameters in end-stage renal failure. *Nephrol Dial Transplant* 2000;15:1425–1430.

131. Valderrabano F. Quality of life benefits of early anaemia treatment. *Nephrol Dial Transplant* 2000;15(Suppl 3):23–28.

132. National Kidney Foundation-Dialysis Outcomes Quality Initiative. NKF-DOQI clinical practice guidelines for the treatment of anemia of chronic renal failure. *Am J Kidney Dis* 1997;30(4 Suppl 3):S192–S240.

133. Moreno F, Aracil FJ, Pérez R, et al. Controlled study on the improvement of quality of life in elderly hemodialysis patients after correcting end-stage related anemia with erythropoietin. *Am J Kidney Dis* 1996;27:548–556.

134. Eschbach JW, Glenny R, Robertson T. Normalizing the hematocrit in hemodialysis patients improves quality of life and is safe [abstract]. *J Am Soc Nephrol* 1993;4:445.

135. Moreno F, Sanz-Guajardo D, López-Gómez JM, et al. Spanish Cooperative Renal Patients Quality of Life Study Group of the Spanish Society of Nephrology. Increasing the hematocrit has a beneficial effect on quality of life and is safe in selected hemodialysis patients. *J Am Soc Nephrol* 2000;11:335–342.

136. Besarab A, Bolton WK, Browne JK, et al. The effects of normal as compared with low hematocrit values in patients with cardiac disease who are receiving hemodialysis and epoetin. *N Engl J Med* 1998;339:584–590.

137. Singh AK, Szczech L, Tang KL, et al. CHOIR Investigators. Correction of anemia with epoetin alfa in chronic kidney disease. *N Engl J Med* 2006;355(20):2085–2098.

138. National Kidney Foundation. KDOQI Clinical practice guidelines and clinical practice recommendations for anemia in chronic kidney disease. *Am J Kidney Dis* 2006;47(5 Suppl 3):S11–S145.

139. Drüeke TB, Parfrey PS. Summary of the KDIGO guideline on anemia and comment: reading between the (guide)line(s). *Kidney Int* 2012;82(9):952–960.

140. Finkelstein FO, Finkelstein SH. Depression in chronic dialysis patients: assessment and treatment. *Nephrol Dial Transplant* 2000;15:1911–1913.

141. Kimmel PL, Peterson RA, Weihs KL, et al. Multiple measurements of depression predict mortality in a longitudinal study of urban hemodialysis patients. *Kidney Int* 2000;57:2093–2098.

142. Tsay SL, Healstead M. Self-care-efficacy, depression, and the quality of life among patients receiving hemodialysis in Taiwan. *Int J Nurs Stud* 2002;39:245–251.

143. Kovac JA, Patel SS, Peterson RA, et al. Patient satisfaction with care and behavioral compliance in end-stage renal disease patients treated with hemodialysis. *Am J Kidney Dis* 2002;39:1236–1244.

144. Zimmermann PR, Poli de Figueiredo CE, Fonseca NA. Depression, anxiety and adjustment in renal replacement therapy: a quality of life assessment. *Clin Nephrol* 2001;56:387–390.

145. Kimmel PL. Psychosocial factors in dialysis patients. *Kidney Int* 2001;59:1599–1613.

146. Cukor D. Use of CBT to treat depression among patients on hemodialysis. *Psychiatr Serv* 2007;58(5):711–712.

147. Duarte PS, Miyazaki MC, Blay SL, et al. Cognitive-behavioral group therapy is an effective treatment for major depression in hemodialysis patients. *Kidney Int* 2009;76(4):414–421.

148. Cukor D, Ver Halen N, Asher DR, et al. Psychosocial intervention improves depression, quality of life, and fluid adherence in hemodialysis. *J Am Soc Nephrol* 2014;25(1):196–206.

149. Baiardi F, Degli Esposti E, Cocchi R, et al. Effects of clinical and individual variables on quality of life in chronic renal failure patients. *J Nephrol* 2002;15:61–67.

150. Rebollo P, Ortega F, Baltar JM, et al. Is the loss of health-related quality of life during renal replacement therapy lower in elderly patients than in younger patients? *Nephrol Dial Transplant* 2001;16:1675–1680.

151. Kurella Tamura M, Covinsky KE, Chertow GM, et al. Functional status of elderly adults before and after initiation of dialysis. *N Engl J Med* 2009;361(16):1539–1547.

152. Rebollo P, Ortega F, Baltar JM, et al. Health-related quality of life (HRQOL) in end-stage renal disease (ESRD) patients over 65 years. *Geriatr Nephrol Urol* 1998;8:85–94.

153. Lamping DL, Constantinovici N, Roderick P, et al. Clinical outcomes, quality of life, and costs in the North Thames Dialysis Study of elderly people on dialysis: a prospective cohort study. *Lancet* 2000;356:1543–1550.

154. Kutner NG, Jassal SV. Quality of life and rehabilitation of elderly dialysis patients. *Semin Dial* 2002;15:107–112.

155. Trbojevic JB, Nesic VB, Stojimiovic BB, et al. Quality of life of elderly patients undergoing continuous ambulatory peritoneal dialysis. *Perit Dial Int* 2001;21(Suppl 3):S300–S303.

156. Harris SA, Lamping DL, Brown EA, et al. Clinical outcomes and quality of life in elderly patients on peritoneal dialysis versus hemodialysis. *Perit Dial Int* 2002;22:463–470.

157. Rocco MV, Gassman JJ, Wang SR, et al. The Modification of Diet in Renal Disease Study. Cross-sectional study of quality of life and symptoms in chronic renal disease patients. *Am J Kidney Dis* 1997;32:557–566.

158. Simmons RG, Abress L. Quality of life issues for end-stage renal disease patients. *Am J Kidney Dis* 1990;15:201–208.

159. Lindqvist R, Carlsson M, Sjödén PO. Coping strategies and quality of life among patients on hemodialysis and continuous ambulatory peritoneal dialysis. *Scand J Caring Sci* 1998;12:223–230.

160. Redden DN, Szczech LA, Klassen PS, et al. Racial inequities in America's ESRD program. *Semin Dial* 2000;13:399–403.

161. Welch JL, Austin JK. Quality of life in black hemodialysis patients. *Adv Ren Replace Ther* 1999;6:351–357.

162. Lopes AA, Bragg-Gresham JL, Satayathum S, et al. Health-related quality of life and associated outcomes among hemodialysis patients of different ethnicities in the United States: the Dialysis Outcomes and Practice Patterns Study (DOPPS). *Am J Kidney Dis* 2003;41(3):605–615.

163. Bakewell AB, Higgins RM, Edmunds ME. Does ethnicity influence perceived quality of life of patients on dialysis and following renal transplant? *Nephrol Dial Transplant* 2001;16:1395–1401.

164. Merkus MP, Jager KJ, Dekker FW, et al. Physical symptoms and quality of life in patients on chronic dialysis: results of the Netherlands Cooperative Study on Adequacy of Dialysis (NECOSAD). *Nephrol Dial Transplant* 1999;14:1163–1170.

165. Apostolou T, Gokal R. Neuropathy and quality of life in diabetic continuous ambulatory peritoneal dialysis patients. *Perit Dial Int* 1999;19:S242–S247.

166. McMurray SD, Johnson G, Davis S, et al. Diabetes education and care management significantly improve patient outcomes in the dialysis unit. *Am J Kidney Dis* 2002;40:566–575.

167. Jhamb M, Pike F, Ramer S, et al. Impact of fatigue on outcomes in the hemodialysis (HEMO) study. *Am J Nephrol* 2011;33(6):515–523.

168. Mittal SK, Ahern L, Flaster E, et al. Self-assessed quality of life in peritoneal dialysis patients. *Am J Nephrol* 2001;21:215–220.

169. Maiorca R, Ruggieri G, Vaccaro CM, et al. Psychological and social problems of dialysis. *Nephrol Dial Transplant* 1998;13:S89–S95.

170. Merkus MP, Jager KJ, Dekker FW, et al. NECOSAD study. Quality of life over time in dialysis: The Netherlands Cooperative Study on the Adequacy of Dialysis. *Kidney Int* 1999;56:720–728.

171. Bakewell AB, Higgins RM, Edmunds ME. Quality of life in peritoneal dialysis patients: decline over time and association with clinical outcomes. *Kidney Int* 2002;61:239–248.

172. Hall YN, Larive B, Painter P, et al. Effects of six versus three times per week hemodialysis on physical performance, health, and functioning: Frequent Hemodialysis Network (FHN) randomized trials. *Clin J Am Soc Nephrol* 2012;7(5):782–794.

173. Manns BJ, Johnson JA, Taub K, et al. Dialysis adequacy and health related quality of life in hemodialysis patients. *ASAIO J* 2002;48:565–569.

174. Unruh M, Benz R, Greene T, et al. HEMO study group. Effects of hemodialysis dose and membrane flux on health-related quality of life in the HEMO Study. *Kidney Int* 2004;66(1):355–366.

175. Chen YC, Hung KY, Kao TW, et al. Relationship between dialysis adequacy and quality of life in long-term peritoneal dialysis patients. *Perit Dial Int* 2000;20:534–540.

176. Hashimoto Y, Matsubara T. Combined peritoneal dialysis and hemodialysis therapy improves quality of life in end-stage renal disease patients. *Adv Perit Dial* 2000;16:108–112.

177. Mohr PE, Neumann PJ, Franco SJ, et al. The case for daily dialysis: its impact on costs and quality of life. *Am J Kidney Dis* 2001;37:777–789.

178. McPhatter LL, Lockridge RS Jr, Albert J, et al. Nightly home hemodialysis: improvement in nutrition and quality of life. *Adv Ren Replace Ther* 1999;6:358–365.

179. Kooistra MP, Vos J, Koomans HA, et al. Daily home hemodialysis in The Netherlands: effects on metabolic control, hemodynamics and quality of life. *Nephrol Dial Transplant* 1998;13:2853–2860.

180. Kalantar-Zadeh K, Kopple JD, Block G, et al. Association among SF36 quality of life measures and nutrition, hospitalization, and mortality in hemodialysis. *J Am Soc Nephrol* 2001;12:2979–2806.

181. Shield CH. The impact of nutrition and fitness on quality of life. *Nephrol News Issues* 2002;16:52–55.

182. Ohri-Vachaspati P, Sehgal AR. Quality of life implications of inadequate protein nutrition among hemodialysis patients. *J Ren Nutr* 1999; 9:9–13.

183. Iborra Moltó C, Picó Vicent L, Montiel Castillo A, et al. Quality of life and exercise in renal disease. *EDTNA ERCA J* 2000;26:38–40.

184. Brodin E, Ljungman S, Hedberg M, et al. Physical activity, muscle performance and quality of life in patients treated with chronic peritoneal dialysis. *Scand J Urol Nephrol* 2001;35:71–78.

185. Kutner NG, Zhang R, McClellan WM. Patient-reported quality of life early in dialysis treatment: effects associated with usual exercise activity. *Nephrol Nurs J* 2000;27:357–367.

186. Painter P, Carlson L, Carey S, et al. Physical functioning and health related quality of life changes with exercise training in hemodialysis patients. *Am J Kidney Dis* 2000;35:482–492.

187. Curtin RB, Klag MJ, Bultman DC, et al. Renal rehabilitation and improved patient outcomes in Texas dialysis facilities. *Am J Kidney Dis* 2002;40:331–338.

188. Callahan MB. Using quality of life measurement to enhance interdisciplinary collaboration. *Adv Ren Replace Ther* 2001;8:148–151.

189. Stroetmann KA, Gruetzmacher P, Stroetmann VN. Improving quality of life for dialysis patients through telecare. *J Telemed Telecare* 2000; 6:S80–S83.

CHAPTER 35

Prescribing Drugs for Dialysis Patients

Ali J. Olyaei and William M. Bennett

Acute and chronic kidney disease affects the pharmacokinetic and pharmacodynamics of most pharmacologic agents (1–3). The effect of uremia and kidney disease on individual agents varies. Clearly, uremia affects every organ system in the body. Therefore, alteration of drug absorption, distribution, metabolism, and excretion and their active or toxic metabolites must be considered when prescribing pharmacologic agents for patients with kidney disease, in particular for patients on renal replacement therapy (hemodialysis or peritoneal dialysis). In addition, most patients with kidney disease have many comorbid conditions, which often compound the complexity of drug management in this setting (4).

Health care providers who prescribe drug therapy for patients with chronic kidney disease must be familiar with basic pharmacokinetic and pharmacologic principles. Dosage adjustment is required for the drug excreted renally in patients with chronic kidney disease to ensure long-term efficacy and prevent short- and long-term toxicity. Often, a drug with a narrow therapeutic concentration or critical dosage schedule is necessary to treat a serious disease. For drugs with a narrow therapeutic window, therapeutic drug monitoring (TDM) is required to prevent both drug accumulation and subtherapeutic dosing. Many pharmacologic agents also have active metabolites that undergo renal excretion. The metabolism and elimination of these agents depend on normal renal function. Pharmacologic agents that do not undergo renal elimination may be altered and, therefore, cause adverse effects in this patient population.

The kidney plays an important role in the regulation of extracellular and intracellular fluid homeostasis. Renal dysfunction has profound effects on the volume distribution and pharmacology of many drugs. Improvements in the clinical management of patients with kidney disease, coupled with the development of new and more efficient methods of renal replacement therapy, have created a large patient population with a special need for drug management. One study indicated that 40% of patients with chronic kidney disease received excessive dose of medications. Another study observed a positive association with the number of medications administered and the mortality rate in patients with chronic kidney disease (5). These data highlight the importance of identifying patients with chronic kidney disease, estimating renal function, and adjusting the drug dosage appropriately according to renal function (6).

This chapter covers information about drug disposition in patients with chronic kidney disease and how to effectively approach pharmacotherapy in patients undergoing dialytic therapies to optimize drug efficacy while minimizing toxicity.

INITIAL PATIENT ASSESSMENT

Patient assessment begins with a complete past medical history and physical examination. Taking a thorough past medication history, drug allergy, adverse drug reactions, and concurrent medicines are vital in the initial evaluation of patients with chronic kidney disease. Patients with kidney disease receive on average 11 different medications for the treatment of cardiovascular diseases, metabolic disorders, infectious complications, and other comorbid conditions. In addition, patients with kidney disease experience a threefold higher incidence of adverse drug reactions compared to the general population with normal renal function (7–9). Pharmacotherapy should be individualized and minimized to reduce the risk of adverse drug reactions and potential drug–drug interactions.

Principles of Altered Pharmacokinetics in Kidney Disease

Several pharmacokinetic factors are altered when renal function is impaired. These factors include bioavailability, volume of distribution, protein binding, and biotransformation. Pharmacologic agents

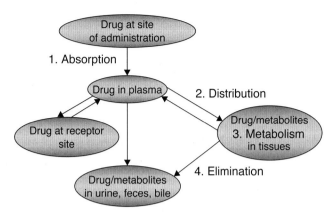

FIGURE 35.1 Pharmacologic agents may pass through several body compartments before reaching receptor site or being eliminated from body.

may pass through several body compartments before reaching receptor site or being eliminated from the body (**FIGURE 35.1**).

Bioavailability

The bioavailability of a drug refers to the fraction (expressed as a percentage) of a given dose that reaches the systemic circulation. The rate and route of administration are the primary factors which determine bioavailability. An agent that is not completely absorbed or is eliminated by the liver in its first pass has low bioavailability. Drugs administered intravenously are generally 100% bioavailable because the entire dosage reaches the systemic circulation. When given orally, subcutaneously, or intramuscularly, bioavailability decreases. For example, given intravenously, furosemide is 100% bioavailable but only approximately 50% bioavailable when given orally. In patients with right-sided heart failure or liver disease, the absorption rate may drop to 10%. For this reason, many clinicians double or triple the furosemide dose when switching a patient from IV to oral furosemide (10).

Drug absorption determines bioavailability and may be altered in patients with renal insufficiency. Many factors may account for this phenomenon. Neuropathic changes resulting from diabetes mellitus and/or aging may cause gastroparesis or uremia-induced vomiting. Patients with cirrhosis, nephrosis, or congestive heart failure (CHF) commonly have edematous gastrointestinal mucosa, causing a reduction in drug absorption. Drugs which increase gastric pH such as phosphate binders and H_2 receptor blockers may impair absorption of concomitantly administered drugs. Concomitant administration of some drugs (such as aluminum- or calcium-containing phosphate binders) with antibiotics or iron-containing supplements may result in the formation of insoluble complexes which can both decrease absorption and slow gut motility.

Volume of Distribution

The volume of distribution (Vd) of a pharmacologic agent is derived by dividing the total amount of drug in the body by the concentration of the drug in the blood. The Vd does not refer to a specific anatomic compartment, but it is useful for calculating the dose required to achieve a desired systemic drug level. An inverse correlation exists between the serum concentration and the Vd (11,12).

After a drug reaches the systemic circulation or is completely absorbed, it is distributed throughout the body. Initially, drugs are distributed to high-flow organs such as the heart, liver, kidney, and brain. In the next phase, drugs are distributed to areas with a lower extraction ratio such as fat, bone, and skin. The rate and extent of distribution of a drug throughout the body determine how much of the drug will be available to exert the pharmacologic actions and how rapidly the drug will be eliminated. Kidney disease affects both drug distribution and protein binding. Edema and ascites increase the distribution volume of many drugs, whereas volume depletion contracts this space. Fluid-volume status of patients should be assessed before administering drugs that require dose adjustment for body weight. For most drugs, ideal body weight (IBW) should be calculated. For men, IBW is 50 kg plus 2.3 kg for each inches more than 5 ft. For women, IBW is 45.5 kg plus 2.3 kg for each inches more than 5 ft.

Therefore, alterations in the extracellular fluid volume can affect the Vd. Volume contraction decreases the Vd while serum drug concentration rises. This is particularly true for hydrophilic compounds such as aminoglycosides or drugs with low Vd (less than 0.7 mL/kg). A rise in extracellular fluid volume due to edema or ascites increases the Vd, resulting in a lower serum drug concentration.

Protein Binding

Plasma contains many proteins which bind drugs. Plasma protein binding is often altered in kidney disease (**TABLE 35.1**). Most drug molecules are circulating in both bound and unbound (free) forms. It is the unbound drug which is distributed and is biologically active (13). The concentration of a given agent which is bound to plasma proteins may be considered a storage pool for that agent. The effects of diseases on drug–protein binding are complex; however, kidney disease tends to decrease protein binding for most agents and increases the free fraction. This is, in part, true because circulating organic wastes bind to carrier proteins, thereby displacing the pharmacologic agent. As a result, a larger concentration of the agent circulates in its free, active form. Most drug assays measure total drug concentration that contains both bound and free drug levels. In some cases (such as in a patient receiving phenytoin), it may be prudent to specifically monitor unbound drug when a narrow therapeutic window exists.

Biotransformation

Metabolism or biotransformation refers to the biochemical conversion of a drug from one chemical form to another (10,14). Most biotransformation occurs in the liver through hepatic metabolic pathways including oxidation, reduction, acetylation, or hydrolysis. The result is a more polar, hydrophilic metabolite which is more

TABLE 35.1	Compounds with Decreased Protein Binding in Uremic Patients
Cephalosporins	Phenytoin
Clofibrate	Primidone
Diazepam	Salicylate
Diazoxide	Sulfonamide
Furosemide	Theophylline
Morphine	Valproic acid
Penicillins	Warfarin
Phenobarbital	

TABLE 35.2	Drugs with Active or Toxic Metabolites Excreted by the Kidney
Acebutolol	Imipramine
Allopurinol	Meperidine
Cephalosporins	Methyldopa
Chlorpropamide	Nitrofurantoin
Clofibrate	Prednisone
Daunorubicin	Procainamide
Diazepam	Propoxyphene
Digoxin	Rifampin
Doxorubicin	Sodium nitroprusside
Enalapril	Succinylcholine
Flurazepam	Sulfonamides

readily excreted. Many drug metabolites are pharmacologically active and depend on renal excretion for elimination from the body. Kidney disease affects both renal and nonrenal pathways. There is some clinical evidence of slow hydrolysis and faster oxidation rates in patients with kidney disease. Toxic metabolites dependent upon renal excretion may also form (**TABLE 35.2**).

Elimination

The glomerular filtration rate (GFR) is closely correlated with renal drug elimination and is useful in determining dosage adjustments. If the total renal clearance of a drug or active metabolite is greater than 30%, a dosage adjustment is needed.

To obtain metabolic balance in patients with reduced renal function, several agents should be avoided. Some drugs increase the metabolic load by increasing creatinine production and/or urea production (glucocorticoids and androgens). Other drugs may overwhelm the kidney's capacity by increasing the metabolic load of excess acid, alkali magnesium, potassium, or sodium. Nonsteroidal anti-inflammatory agents may impair the kidney's ability to excrete free water.

Various pharmacologic agents can interfere with laboratory markers of renal function (**TABLE 35.3**). Elevated serum creatinine (Scr) from direct drug interference with the chromogen assay or by inhibition of renal tubular creatinine secretion can cause confusion to the inexperienced clinician. Similarly, a number of agents can also cause a rise in the blood urea nitrogen (BUN) through interference with the assay utilized. Temporary discontinuation of the offending medication may be necessary when the Scr or BUN rises unexpectedly. The Cockcroft-Gault (CG) formula is widely used to calculate the creatinine clearance (Clcr) and has traditionally been used to approximate the GFR (15). BUN and Scr are, at best, crude markers of kidney function. The CG formula includes the variables of age (years), IBW (kg), and Scr (mg/dL) and calculates the Scr (mL/min) (**EQUATION 35.1**):

$$*\text{Clcr} = \frac{(140 - \text{age}) \times \text{IBW}}{72 \times \text{Scr}} \quad (35.1)$$

*Multiply result by 0.85 in women

Patients with acute kidney injury should have an assumed Clcr of less than 10 mL/min, and it should be remembered that CG Clcr overestimates the GFR in these setting and should be avoided for assessment of kidney function in acute kidney injury. There are a number of new method to estimate renal function in chronic

TABLE 35.3	Drug Interference with Kidney Function Testing	
	Drug	**Test and Mechanisms of Interference**
Increased serum creatinine	Ascorbic acid	Elevates total chromogen
	Levodopa	Interferes with autoanalyzer method
	Methyldopa	—
	Aspirin	—
	Cimetidine	Blocks tubular secretion of creatinine
	Trimethoprim	—
	Cefotetan	Interferes with Jaffé reaction
	Cefoxitin	—
Increased BUN	Acetaminophen	—
	Aminophylline	Interferes with nonenzymatic method
	Ascorbic acid	—
	Salicylates	—
	Methyldopa	Interferes with phosphotungstate method
	Levodopa	Interferes with autoanalyzer method

BUN, blood urea nitrogen.

kidney disease: Modification of Diet in Renal Disease (MDRD) and Chronic Kidney Disease Epidemiology Collaboration (CKD-EPI). These new markers of GFR are currently being utilized in both the research and clinical setting to more accurately measure renal function without exposing the patient to radiolabeled material. It is important to mention that these formulas approximate GFR rather than Clcr and, therefore, may be a more accurate estimate of renal function. It has been shown to be more accurate than other formulas for predicting GFR. The formula uses a creatinine assay (the kinetic alkaline picrate reaction), which is the least subject to artifact interference. GFR was predicted over a wide range of values including variables for ethnicity and serum albumin concentration and did not rely on timed urine collections. The MDRD study equation (16) is as follows (**EQUATION 35.2**):

$$\text{GFR} = 170_{[ml]} \times [\text{Scr}]^{-0.999} \times [\text{Age}]^{-0.176} \times [0.762 \text{ if female}] \times [1.180 \text{ if patient is black}] \times [\text{BUN}]^{-0.170} \times [\text{Albumin}]^{-0.318} \quad (35.2)$$

Appropriate application of the MDRD equation requires calibration of the measured Scr. In addition, this equation has not been rigorously validated in some patient populations, such as those with a GFR greater than 60 mL/min, renal transplant recipients, some ethnic groups, and patients with extreme body weights.

The CG, MDRD, and CKD-EPI equations (**TABLE 35.4**) have been shown to have statistically significant differences in estimating GFR in various populations. It has been further improved with the MDRD, and CKD-EPI equations included more specific variable of race in addition to age, gender, and Scr. Although accuracy in GFR assessment has improved, one equation has yet to be developed to be the most accurate in all populations. Therefore, drug dosing adjustments based on the various equations may differ. However, without clinical outcome data, it is yet to be determined whether these differences are clinically significant.

TABLE 35.4	**Commonly Used Method for Estimation of Glomerular Filtration Rate (GFR) Using Serum Creatinine**

Cockroft-Gault

Clcr (mL/min) = ([140 − age] × weight) / (Scr × 72) (× 0.85 in women)

MDRD

GFR (mL/min/1.73 m²) = 186 × Scr$^{-1.154}$ × Age$^{-0.203}$ (× 0.742 if female) (× 1.212 if black)

MDRD using standard creatinine value

GFR (mL/min/1.73 m²) = 175 × Scr$^{-1.154}$ × Age$^{-0.203}$ (× 0.742 if female) (× 1.212 if black)

CKD-EPI

Women:

GFR (mL/min/1.73 m²) = 144 × (Scr/0.7)$^{-0.329}$ × 0.993^{age} (× 1.15 if black) if Scr ≤0.7 mg/dL

GFR (mL/min/1.73 m²) = 144 × (Scr/0.7)$^{-1.209}$ × 0.993^{age} (× 1.15 if black) if Scr >0.7 mg/dL

Men:

GFR (mL/min/1.73 m²) = 141 × (Scr/0.9)$^{-0.411}$ × 0.993^{age} (× 1.16 if black) if Scr ≤0.9 mg/dL

GFR (mL/min/1.73 m²) = 141 × (Scr/0.9)$^{-1.209}$ × 0.993^{age} (× 1.16 if black) if Scr >0.9 mg/dL

Clcr, creatinine clearance; Scr, serum creatinine in mg/dL; MDRD, Modification of Diet in Renal Disease; CKD-EPI, Chronic Kidney Disease Epidemiology Collaboration.

Loading Dose Determination

The half-life of many drugs may be significantly prolonged in patients with kidney disease. In patients with normal renal function, steady-state drug concentrations are achieved after approximately 3.3 half-lives. In patients with kidney disease, achievement of steady-state drug levels, which ensures therapeutic efficacy, may be greatly delayed if a loading dose (LD) is not given. Patients with renal insufficiency should, in general, receive the same LD as patients with normal renal function in order to achieve a rapid therapeutic dose. Patients with kidney disease receiving digoxin, however, should receive only 50% to 75% of the usual LD as its Vd is greatly reduced in kidney disease.

The following formula can be used to calculate the LD with Vd in L/kg, IBW in kg, Cp being the desired plasma concentration in mg/L (**EQUATION 35.3**):

$$LD = Vd \times IBW \times [Cp] \qquad (35.3)$$

Maintenance Dose Determination

Before adjusting the maintenance dose, the route of excretion should be established. The maintenance dose should be adjusted only for drugs with greater than 50% renal excretion, low rate of protein binding, and small Vd. The maintenance dosage in patients with renal insufficiency can be adjusted in three ways: dosing interval prolongation, dosage reduction, or both. Increasing the dosage interval to correspond to the degree of renal dysfunction can be calculated from the following formula (**EQUATION 35.4**):

$$\text{Dosing interval} = \frac{\text{normal Clcr} \times \text{normal interval}}{\text{patients Clcr}} \qquad (35.4)$$

Dosage reduction without changing the dosing interval can be calculated from the following formula (**EQUATION 35.5**):

$$\text{Maintenance dose} = \frac{\text{patients Clcr} \times \text{normal dose}}{\text{normal Clcr}} \qquad (35.5)$$

Dosage interval extension allows for adequate peak concentrations but may risk subtherapeutic trough levels. Dosing reduction may provide for more constant drug levels but increases the risk of toxicity from higher plasma trough concentrations. Appendix A summarizes recommendations for most drugs in patients with renal dysfunction.

Drug Level Monitoring

Dosage and interval modifications do not necessarily protect against drug toxicity in particular for drugs with a narrow therapeutic window. For such pharmacologic agents, plasma drug monitoring is important in the patient with kidney disease to avoid drug toxicity. To correctly interpret drug concentrations, it is important to know the exact dose given, the route of administration, time since the last dose, and the particular drug's half-life. Peak drug levels represent the highest drug concentration achieved after initial rapid distribution and predict drug efficacy. Trough drug levels are obtained immediately before the next dose, represent the lowest serum concentration, and predict drug toxicity. Drug level monitoring can be expensive, is not always available, and does not always reduce the incidence of toxicity. Aminoglycoside antibiotics, for instance, can concentrate in tissues such as the inner ear and renal cortex, and toxicity is not always correlated with high blood levels. Ongoing clinical assessment is important even when drug levels are within the established therapeutic range. In the presence of metabolic acidosis or hypokalemia, digoxin toxicity may occur despite therapeutic levels. Most assays do not distinguish between free and protein-bound drug in the plasma. An increase in unbound drug is common in patients with kidney disease. **TABLE 35.5** summarizes recommendations for TDM in patients with renal dysfunction (3,4,17).

Drug Removal by Dialysis

Intermittent hemodialysis necessitates high blood and dialysate flow rates, which enhances drug removal primarily by the process of diffusion down a concentration gradient from blood to dialysate, across the dialysis membrane (18). Small molecular weight drugs (less than 500 Da) cross the dialysis membrane readily and are removed from the plasma with most dialysis membranes. With the advent of high-flux membranes, drugs with higher molecular weights are also removed very effectively. For instance, vancomycin (molecular weight approximately 1,400 Da) can be significantly removed during high-flux dialysis, especially with continuous renal replacement therapy (CRRT) (19). Drugs with large volumes of distribution are less likely to be removed by dialysis than those with a small Vd (Vd less than 0.7 mL/kg). Pharmacologic agents with

TABLE 35.5	Drugs with Narrow Therapeutic Index Which Require Routine Monitoring		
Drug Name	**Therapeutic Range**	**When to Draw Sample**	**How Often to Draw Levels**
Aminoglycosides (Conventional dosing) Gentamicin, tobramycin, and amikacin	Gentamicin and tobramycin: Trough: 0.5–2 mg/L Peak: 5–8 mg/L Amikacin: Peak: 20–30 mg/L Trough: <10 mg/L 0.5–3 mg/L	Trough: immediately prior to dose Peak: 30 min after a 30- to 45-min infusion	Check peak and trough with third dose For therapy less than 72 h, levels not necessary; repeat drug levels weekly or if renal function changes
Aminoglycosides (24-h dosing) Gentamicin, tobramycin, and amikacin		Obtain random drug level 12 h after dose	After initial dose; repeat drug level in 1 wk or if renal function changes
Carbamazepine	4–12 μg/mL	Trough: immediately prior to dosing	Check 2–4 d after first dose or change in dose
Cyclosporin	150–400 ng/mL	Trough: immediately prior to dosing	Daily for first week and then weekly
Digoxin	0.8–2.0 ng/mL	12 h after maintenance dose	5–7 d after first dose for patients with normal renal and hepatic function; 15–20 d in anephric patients
Lidocaine	1–5 μg/mL	8 h after IV infusion started or changed	
Lithium	Acute: 0.8–1.2 mmol/L Chronic: 0.6–0.8 mmol/L	Trough: before morning dose at least 12 h since last dose	
Phenobarbital	15–40 μg/mL	Trough: immediately prior to dosing	Check 2 wk after first dose or change in dose; follow-up level in 1–2 mo
Phenytoin	10–20 μg/mL	Trough: immediately prior to dosing	5–7 d after first dose or after change in dose
Free phenytoin	1–2 μg/mL		
Procainamide	4–10 μg/mL	Trough: immediately prior to next dose or 12–18 h after starting or changing an infusion	
NAPA (N-acetyl procainamide) a procainamide metabolite	Trough: 4 μg/mL Peak: 8 μg/mL 10–30 μg/mL	Draw with procainamide sample	
Quinidine	1–5 μg/mL	Trough: immediately prior to next dose	
Sirolimus	10–20 ng/dL	Trough: immediately prior to next dose	
Tacrolimus (FK-506)	10–15 ng/mL	Trough: immediately prior to next dose	Daily for first week, and then weekly
Theophylline PO or aminophylline IV	15–20 μg/mL	Trough: immediately prior to next dose	
Valproic acid (divalproex sodium)	40–100 μg/mL	Trough: immediately prior to next dose	Check 2–4 d after first dose or change in dose
Vancomycin	Trough: 5–15 mg/L Peak: 25–40 mg/L	Trough: immediately prior to dose Peak: 60 min after a 60-min infusion	With third dose (when initially starting therapy, or after each dosage adjustment); for therapy less than 72 h, levels not necessary; repeat drug levels if renal function changes

IV, intravenous; PO, by mouth.

large Vd are disseminated into adipose tissue or have extensive tissue binding. In conventional hemodialysis, drug removal by diffusion is based on concentration gradients, and drug removal more closely relates to the blood and dialysate flow rates (20). High-flux dialyzers are impermeable to drugs with molecular weight up to 20,000 Da and allow most drugs to be removed during the dialysis.

In this setting, drug removal is more dependent on Vd and percentage of protein binding.

In peritoneal dialysis, the peritoneal membrane functions as the dialyzing membrane. It is much less effective than hemodialysis membranes with regard to drug clearance. In peritoneal dialysis, drug removal occurs as a result of diffusion and is dependent on the blood to dialysate concentration gradient. A smaller molecular weight, a lower protein binding, and a smaller Vd facilitate drug removal, similar to low-flux hemodialysis. Some high molecular weight drugs can be removed because of secretion into peritoneal lymphatic fluid. The most important factor in determining the percentage of drug removal during peritoneal dialysis is the rate of dialysate flow. Increasing the number of peritoneal exchanges facilitates removal of low molecular weight drugs, whereas extending the duration of the peritoneal dwell time enhances large molecular weight drug clearance (20–22).

CRRTs most often are used for the management of critically ill patients who are not able to tolerate conventional intermittent hemodialysis (23–25). There is very limited information about how CRRT affects the clearance of individual pharmacologic agents. During CRRT, most drugs can be safely dosed for a GFR of 10 to 30 mL/min. However, for some drugs, the diffusion process significantly increases drug clearance during CRRT due to high-flux dialysis. Similar to high-flux hemodialysis, molecular weight and blood and dialysate flow rates determine the rate and extent of drug removal during CRRT. However, because most drugs have a smaller molecular weight than 1,500 Da, the molecular weight *per se* does not significantly affect the extent of drug removal during CRRT. Like peritoneal dialysis, the Vd and duration of therapy are the most critical factors in influencing drug removal during CRRT (26,27).

There are number of alternative, hybrid method of renal replacement therapies that might alter drug dosing in patient with chronic kidney disease. A short 2 hours or slow over 6 to 8 hours of nocturnal dialysis have been become popular to improve the quality of life and avoid some of the complications of hemodialysis. In addition, patient residual renal function should be considered in dosage recommendations. Unfortunately, there is very limited information about drug dosing in either of these modalities. Due to lack of data in this area, for each drug, health care providers should assess risk versus benefits of each treatment closely to avoid toxicity while enhance efficacy. The limited data from number of antibiotics indicate that a more aggressive dosing schedule is needed compared to conventional hemodialysis. It is reasonable to consider dosing for Clcr 30 to 50 mL/min for patients on 6 to 8 hours nocturnal hemodialysis.

◆ CONCLUSION

Due to epidemic of obesity and diabetes, the number of patients with chronic kidney disease has increased significantly in the last 10 years. Most of these patients have number of comorbid conditions that require pharmacotherapeutic agents. Health care must be aware of changes in basic pharmacokinetic and pharmacologic principles in patients with chronic kidney disease. For most drugs that excreted renally in patients with chronic kidney disease, a dosage adjustment is required to ensure long-term efficacy and prevent short- and long-term toxicity.

◆ REFERENCES

1. Susla GM. Antibiotic dosing in critically ill patients undergoing renal replacement therapy. *AACN Adv Crit Care* 2015;26(3):244–251.
2. Udy AA, Jarrett P, Stuart J, et al. Determining the mechanisms underlying augmented renal drug clearance in the critically ill: use of exogenous marker compounds. *Crit Care* 2014;18(6):657.
3. Hudson JQ, Nyman HA. Use of estimated glomerular filtration rate for drug dosing in the chronic kidney disease patient. *Curr Opin Nephrol Hypertens* 2011;20(5):482–491.
4. Nolin TD. A synopsis of clinical pharmacokinetic alterations in advanced CKD. *Semin Dial* 2015;28(4):325–329.
5. MacCallum L. Optimal medication dosing in patients with diabetes mellitus and chronic kidney disease. *Can J Diabetes* 2014;38(5):334–343.
6. Philips BJ, Lane K, Dixon J, et al. The effects of acute renal failure on drug metabolism. *Expert Opin Drug Metab Toxicol* 2014;10(1):11–23.
7. Levey AS, Bosch JP, Lewis JB, et al; for the Modification of Diet in Renal Disease Study Group. A more accurate method to estimate glomerular filtration rate from serum creatinine: a new prediction equation. *Ann Intern Med* 1999;130:461.
8. Olyaei A, deMattos AM, Bennett WM. Drug usage in dialysis patients. In: Nissenson AR, Fine RN, eds. *Clinical Dialysis*. New York, NY: McGraw-Hill, 2005:1192.
9. Hudson JQ. Estimated glomerular filtration rate leads to higher drug dose recommendations in the elderly compared with creatinine clearance. *Int J Clin Pract* 2015;69(3):313–320.
10. Dowling TC. Glomerular filtration rate equations overestimate creatinine clearance in older individuals enrolled in the Baltimore Longitudinal Study on Aging: impact on renal drug dosing. *Pharmacotherapy* 2013;33(9):912–921.
11. Teruel Briones JL, Gomis Couto A, Sabater J, et al. Validation of the Chronic Kidney Disease Epidemiology Collaboration (CKD-EPI) equation in advanced chronic renal failure. *Nefrologia* 2011;31(6):677–682.
12. Akbari A, Clase CM, Acott P, et al. Canadian Society of Nephrology commentary on the KDIGO clinical practice guideline for CKD evaluation and management. *Am J Kidney Dis* 2015;65(2):177–205.
13. Tansley G, Hall R. Pharmacokinetic considerations for drugs administered in the critically ill. *Br J Hosp Med* 2015;76(2):89–94.
14. Twardowski ZJ. Short, thrice-weekly hemodialysis is inadequate regardless of small molecule clearance. *Int J Artif Organs* 2004;27:452–466.
15. Boffito M, Back DJ, Blaschke TF, et al. Protein binding in antiretroviral therapies. *AIDS Res Hum Retroviruses* 2003;19:825–835.
16. Nolin TD, Frye RF, Matzke GR. Hepatic drug metabolism and transport in patients with kidney disease. *Am J Kidney Dis* 2003;42:906–925.
17. Cockcroft DW, Gault MH. Prediction of creatinine clearance from serum creatinine. *Nephron* 1976;16:31–41.
18. Levey AS, Bosch JP, Lewis JB, et al. A more accurate method to estimate glomerular filtration rate from serum creatinine: a new prediction equation. Modification of Diet in Renal Disease Study Group. *Ann Intern Med* 1999;130:461–470.
19. Olyaei AJ, de Mattos AM, Bennett WM. Drug dosage in renal failure. In: DeBroe ME, Porter GA, Bennett WM, et al, eds. *Clinical Nephrotoxins: Renal Injury from Drugs and Chemicals*. 2nd ed. Dordrecht, The Netherlands: Kluwer Academic Publishers, 2003:667–679.
20. Van BW, Vanholder R, Lameire N. Dialysis strategies in critically ill acute renal failure patients. *Curr Opin Crit Care* 2003;9:491–495.
21. Kielstein JT, Czock D, Schopke T, et al. Pharmacokinetics and total elimination of meropenem and vancomycin in intensive care unit patients undergoing extended daily dialysis. *Crit Care Med* 2006;34:51–56.
22. Nolin TD, Frye RF. Stereoselective determination of the CYP2C19 probe drug mephenytoin in human urine by gas chromatography-mass spectrometry. *J Chromatogr B Analyt Technol Biomed Life Sci* 2003;783:265–271.
23. Kuang D, Verbine A, Ronco C. Pharmacokinetics and antimicrobial dosing adjustment in critically ill patients during continuous renal replacement therapy. *Clin Nephrol* 2007;67:267–284.
24. Schetz M. Drug dosing in continuous renal replacement therapy: general rules. *Curr Opin Crit Care* 2007;13:645–651.
25. Subach RA, Marx MA. Drug dosing in acute renal failure: the role of renal replacement therapy in altering drug pharmacokinetics. *Adv Ren Replace Ther* 1998;5:141–147.
26. Bohler J, Donauer J, Keller F. Pharmacokinetic principles during continuous renal replacement therapy: drugs and dosage. *Kidney Int Suppl* 1999;72:S24–S28.
27. Bugge JF. Pharmacokinetics and drug dosing adjustments during continuous venovenous hemofiltration or hemodiafiltration in critically ill patients. *Acta Anaesthesiol Scand* 2001;45:929–934.

◆ APPENDIX A

Antimicrobial Dosing in Kidney Disease

Drugs	Normal Dosage	% of Renal Excretion	Dosage Adjustment in Kidney Disease			Dosage Adjustment in CRRT	Comments
			GFR >50	GFR 10–50	GFR <10		
Aminoglycoside antibiotics							Nephrotoxic; ototoxic; toxicity worse when hyperbilirubinemic; measure serum levels for efficacy and toxicity; peritoneal absorption increases with presence of inflammation; Vd increases with edema, obesity, and ascites
Streptomycin	7.5 mg/kg q12h (1.0 g q24h for TB)	60	q24h	q24–72h	q72–96h	Unknown	For the treatment of TB; may be less nephrotoxic than other members of class
Kanamycin	7.5 mg/kg q8h	50–90	60%–90% q12h or 100% q12–24h	30%–70% q12h or 100% q24–48h	20%–30% q24–48h or 100% q48–72h	Unknown	Nephrotoxic; ototoxic; toxicity worse when hyperbilirubinemic; Vd increases with edema, obesity, and ascites; do not use once-daily dosing in patients with creatinine clearance <30–40 mL/min or in patients with acute kidney injury or uncertain level of kidney function
Gentamicin	1.7 mg/kg q8h	95	60%–90% q8–12h or 100% q12–24h	30%–70% q12h or 100% q24–48h	20%–30% q24–48h or 100% q48–72h	**Monitor levels very closely,** 1 mg/kg/d	Concurrent penicillins may result in subtherapeutic aminoglycoside levels; peak 6–8, trough <2
Tobramycin	1.7 mg/kg q8h	95	60%–90% q8–12h or 100% q12–24h	30%–70% q12h or 100% q24–48h	20%–30% q24–48h or 100% q48–72h	**Monitor levels very closely,** 1 mg/kg/d	Concurrent penicillins may result in subtherapeutic aminoglycoside levels; peak 6–8, trough <2
Netilmicin	2 mg/kg q8h	95	50%–90% q8–12h or 100% q12–24h	20%–60% q12h or 100% q24–48h	10%–20% q24–48h or 100% q48–72h		May be less ototoxic than other members of class; peak 6–8, trough <2
Amikacin	7.5 mg/kg q12h	95	60%–90% q12h or 100% q12–24h	30%–70% q12h or 100% q24–48h	20%–30% q24–48h or 100% q48–72h	7.5 mg/kg	Monitor levels; peak 20–30, trough <5
Cephalosporin							Coagulation abnormalities, transitory elevation of BUN, rash, and serum sickness-like syndrome
Oral cephalosporin							
Cefaclor	250–500 mg tid	70	100%	100%	50%	50%	
Cefadroxil	500–1,000 mg bid	80	100%	100%	50%	50%	
Cefixime	200–400 mg q12h	85	100%	100%	50%	50%	

(continued)

Continued

Drugs	Normal Dosage	% of Renal Excretion	Dosage Adjustment in Kidney Disease			Dosage Adjustment in CRRT	Comments
			GFR >50	GFR 10–50	GFR <10		
Ceftibuten	400 mg q24h	70	100%	100%	50%	50%	Malabsorbed in presence of H₂-blockers; absorbed better with food
Cefuroxime axetil	250–500 mg tid	90	100%	100%	50%	50%	
Cephalexin	250–500 mg tid	95	100%	100%	50%	50%	Rare allergic interstitial nephritis; absorbed well when given intra-peritoneally; may cause bleeding from impaired prothrombin biosynthesis
Cephradine	250–500 mg tid	100	100%	100%	50%	50%	Rare allergic interstitial nephritis; absorbed well when given intra-peritoneally; may cause bleeding from impaired prothrombin biosynthesis
IV cephalosporin						100%	
Cefamandole	1–2 g IV q6–8h	100	q6h	q8h	q12h	50%	
Cefazolin	1–2 g IV q8h	80	q8h	q12h	q12–24h	50%	
Cefepime	1–2 g IV q8h	85	q8–12h	q12h	q24h	50%	
Cefmetazole	1–2 g IV q8h	85	q8h	q12h	q24h	50%	
Cefoperazone	1–2 g IV q12h	20	No renal adjustment is required			50%	Displaced from protein by bilirubin; reduce dose by 50% for jaundice; may prolong prothrombin time
Cefotaxime	1–2 g IV q6–8h	60	q8h	50%	q12–24h	50%	Active metabolite in ESKD; reduce dose further for combined hepatic and kidney disease
Cefotetan	1–2 g IV q12h	75	q12h	50%	q24h	50%	
Cefoxitin	1–2 g IV q6h	80	q6h	100%	q12h	50%	May produce false increase in serum creatinine by interference with assay
Ceftazidime	1–2 g IV q8h	70	q8h	50%	q24h	50%	
Ceftriaxone	1–2 g IV q24h	50	No renal adjustment is required				
Cefuroxime sodium	0.75–1.5 g IV q8h	90	q8h	q8–12h	q12–24h	50%	Rare allergic interstitial nephritis; absorbed well when given intra-peritoneally; may cause bleeding from impaired prothrombin biosynthesis
Penicillin							Bleeding abnormalities, hypersensitivity; seizures

Oral penicillin							
Amoxicillin	500 mg po tid	60	100%	100%	50%–75%	70%	
Ampicillin	500 mg po q6h	60	100%	100%	50%–75%	50%	
Dicloxacillin	250–500 mg po q6h	50	100%	100%	50%–75%	50%	
Penicillin V	250–500 mg po q6h	70	100%	100%	50%–75%	50%	
IV penicillin							
Ampicillin	1–2 g IV q6h	60	q6h	q8h	q12h	50%	
Nafcillin	1–2 g IV q4h	35	No renal adjustment is required			100%	
Penicillin G	2–3 million U IV q4h	70	q4–6h	q6h	q8h	50%	Seizures; false-positive urine protein reactions; 6 million U/D upper limit dose in ESKD
Piperacillin	3–4 g IV q4–6h		No renal adjustment is required			100%	Specific toxicity: sodium, 1.9 mEq/g
Ticarcillin/clavulanate	3.1 g IV q4–6h	85	1–2 g q4h	1–2 g q8h	1–2 g q12h	50%	Specific toxicity: sodium, 5.2 mEq/g
Piperacillin/tazobactam	3.375 g IV q6–8h	75–90	q4–6h	q6–8h	q8h		Specific toxicity: sodium, 1.9 mEq/g
Quinolones							Photosensitivity, food, dairy products, tube feeding and Al (OH)$_3$ may decrease the absorption of quinolones
Cinoxacin	500 mg q12h	55	100%	50%	Avoid	Avoid	
Fleroxacin	400 mg q12h	70	100%	50%–75%	50%	50%	
Ciprofloxacin	200–400 mg IV q24h	60	q12h	q12–24h	q24h	q24h	Poorly absorbed with antacids, sucralfate, and phosphate binders; IV dose 1/3 of oral dose; decreases phenytoin levels
Lomefloxacin	400 mg q24h	76	100%	200–400 mg q48h	50%	50%	Agents in this group are malabsorbed in the presence of magnesium, calcium, aluminum, and iron; theophylline metabolism is impaired; higher oral doses may be needed to treat CAPD peritonitis.
Levofloxacin	500 mg po qd	70	q12h	250 q12h	250 q12h	250 q12h	L-Isomer of ofloxacin: appears to have similar pharmacokinetics and toxicities
Moxifloxacin	400 mg qd	20	No renal adjustment is required				
Nalidixic acid	1.0 g q6h	High	100%	Avoid	Avoid	Avoid	Agents in this group are malabsorbed in the presence of magnesium, calcium, aluminum, and iron; theophylline metabolism is impaired; higher oral doses may be needed to treat CAPD peritonitis.

(continued)

Continued

Drugs	Normal Dosage	% of Renal Excretion	Dosage Adjustment in Kidney Disease			Dosage Adjustment in CRRT	Comments
			GFR >50	GFR 10–50	GFR <10		
Norfloxacin	400 mg po q12h	30	q12h	q12–24h	q24h	q24h	Agents in this group are malabsorbed in the presence of magnesium, calcium, aluminum, and iron
Ofloxacin	200–400 mg po q12h	70	q12h	q12–24h	q24h	q24h	Agents in this group are malabsorbed in the presence of magnesium, calcium, aluminum, and iron
Pefloxacin	400 mg q24h	11	100%	100%	100%	100%	Excellent bidirectional transperitoneal movement
Sparfloxacin	400 mg q24h	10	100%	50%–75%	50% q48h	50% q48h	
Miscellaneous agents							
Azithromycin	250–500 mg po qd	6	No renal adjustment is required				No drug–drug interaction with CsA/FK
Clarithromycin	500 mg po bid		No renal adjustment is required				
Clindamycin	150–450 mg po tid	10	No renal adjustment is required				Increase CsA/FK level
Dirithromycin	500 mg po qd		No renal adjustment is required				Nonenzymatically hydrolyzed to active compound erythromycylamine
Erythromycin	250–500 mg po qid	15	No renal adjustment is required				Increase CsA/FK level; avoid in transplant patients.
Imipenem/ cilastatin	250–500 mg IV q6h	50	500 mg q8h	250–500 q8–12h	250 mg q12h	50%	Seizures in ESKD; nonrenal clearance in acute kidney injury is less than in chronic kidney disease; administered with cilastin to prevent nephrotoxicity of renal metabolite
Meropenem	1 g IV q8h	65	1 g q8h	0.5–1g q12h	0.5–1 g q24h	50%	
Metronidazole	500 mg IV q6h	20	No renal adjustment is required			50%	Peripheral neuropathy, increase LFTs, disulfiram reaction with alcoholic beverages
Pentamidine	4 mg/kg/d	5	q24h	q24h	q48h	50%	Inhalation may cause bronchospasm; IV administration may cause hypotension, hypoglycemia, and nephrotoxicity.
Trimethoprim/ sulfamethoxazole	800/160 mg po bid	70	q12h	q18h	q24h	25%	Increase serum creatinine; can cause hyperkalemia
Vancomycin	1 g IV q12h	90	q12h	q24–36h	q48–72h	Monitor levels, redoes at level <20	Nephrotoxic, ototoxic, may prolong the neuromuscular blockade effect of muscle relaxants; peak 30, trough 5–10
Vancomycin	125–250 mg po qid	0	100%	100%	100%	100%	Oral vancomycin is indicated only for the treatment of *Clostridium difficile.*

Antituberculosis antibiotics

Drug	Dose	%	GFR >50	GFR 10–50	GFR <10	Supplement	Comments
Rifampin	300–600 mg po qd	20	No renal adjustment is required				Decrease CSA/FK level; many drug interactions

Antifungal agents

Drug	Dose	%	GFR >50	GFR 10–50	GFR <10	Supplement	Comments
Amphotericin B	0.5 mg–1.5 mg/kg/d	<1	No renal adjustment is required				Nephrotoxic, infusion-related reactions, give 250 mL NS before each dose
Amphotec	4–6 mg/kg/d	<1	No renal adjustment is required				
Abelcet	5 mg/kg/d	<1	No renal adjustment is required				
AmBisome	3–5 mg/kg/d	<1	No renal adjustment is required				

Azoles and other antifungals

Drug	Dose	%	GFR >50	GFR 10–50	GFR <10	Supplement	Comments
Fluconazole	200–800 mg IV qd/bid	70	100%	100%	50%	100%	Increase CsA/FK level
Flucytosine	37.5 mg/kg	90	q12h	q16h	q24h	50%	Hepatic dysfunction; marrow suppression more common in azotemic patients
Griseofulvin	125–250 mg q6h	1	100%	100%	100%	100%	
Itraconazole	200 mg q12h	35	100%	100%	50%	50%	Poor oral absorption
Ketoconazole	200–400 mg po qd	15	100%	100%	100%	100%	Hepatotoxic
Miconazole	1,200–3,600 mg/d	1	100%	100%	100%	100%	
Terbinafine	250 mg po qd	>1	100%	100%	100%	100%	
Voriconazole	4 mg/kg q12h	>1	100%	100%	100%	100%	IV use should be limited for only few doses in patients with Clcr less than 30 mL/min.

Antiviral agents

Drug	Dose	%	GFR >50	GFR 10–50	GFR <10	Supplement	Comments
Acyclovir	200–800 mg po 5×/d	50	100%	100%	50%	25%	Poor absorption; neurotoxicity in ESKD; IV preparation can cause kidney disease injected rapidly.
Adefovir	10 mg	45	100%	10 mg q48h	10 mg q72h	10 mg q72h	Nephrotoxic
Amantadine	100–200 mg q12h	90	100%	50%	25%	25%	
Cidofovir	5 mg/kg weekly × 2 (induction) –5 mg/kg every 2 wk	90	No data: avoid	No data: avoid	No data: avoid	No data	Dose-limiting nephrotoxicity with proteinuria, glycosuria, renal insufficiency; nephrotoxicity and renal clearance reduced with coadministration of probenecid
Delavirdine	400 mg q8h	5	No data: 100%	No data: 100%	No data: 100%	No data	
Didanosine	200 mg q12h (125 mg if <60 kg)	40–69	q12h	q24h	50% q24h	50% q24h	Pancreatitis
Famciclovir	250–500 mg po bid to tid	60	q8h	q12h	q24h	q24h	VZV: 500 mg po tid HSV: 250 po bid; metabolized to active compound penciclovir

(continued)

Continued

Drugs	Normal Dosage	% of Renal Excretion	Dosage Adjustment in Kidney Disease			Dosage Adjustment in CRRT	Comments
			GFR >50	GFR 10–50	GFR <10		
Foscarnet	40–80 mg IV q8h	85	20–40 mg q8–24h according to Clcr			No data	Nephrotoxic, neurotoxic, hypocalcemia, hypophosphatemia, hypomagnesemia, and hypokalemia
Ganciclovir IV	5 mg/kg q12h	95	q12h	q24h	2.5 mg/kg qd	2.5 mg/kg qd	Granulocytopenia and thrombocytopenia
Ganciclovir po	1,000 mg po tid	95	1,000 mg tid	1,000 mg bid	1,000 mg qd	1,000 mg qd	Oral ganciclovir should be used *only* for prevention of CMV infection; always use IV ganciclovir for the treatment of CMV infection.
Indinavir	800 mg q8h	10	No data: 100%	**No data:** 100%	No data: 100%	No data: 100%	Nephrolithiasis; acute kidney injury due to crystalluria, tubulointerstitial nephritis
Lamivudine	150 mg po bid	80	q12h	q24h	50 mg q24h	50 mg q24h	For hepatitis B
Nelfinavir	750 mg q8h	No data	No data	No data	No data	No data	
Nevirapine	200 mg q24h × 14 d	<3	No data: 100%	No data: 100%	No data: 100%	No data: 100%	May be partially cleared by hemodialysis and peritoneal dialysis
Ribavirin	500–600 mg q12h	30	100%	100%	50%	25%	Hemolytic uremic syndrome
Rifabutin	300 mg q24h	5–10	100%	100%	100%	100%	
Rimantadine	100 mg po bid	25	100%	100%	50%	50%	
Ritonavir	600 mg q12h	3.50	No data: 100%	No data: 100%	No data: 100%	No data: 100%	Many drug interactions
Saquinavir	600 mg q8h	<4	No data: 100%	No data: 100%	No data: 100%	No data: 100%	
Stavudine	30–40 mg q12h	35–40	100%	50% q12–24h	50% q24h	50% q24h	
Valacyclovir	500–1,000 mg q8h	50	100%	50%	25%	25%	Thrombotic thrombocytopenic purpura/hemolytic uremic syndrome
Vidarabine	15 mg/kg infusion q24h	50	100%	100%	75%	75%	
Zanamivir	2 puffs bid × 5 d	1	100%	100%	100%	100%	Bioavailability from inhalation and systemic exposure to drug is low.
Zalcitabine	0.75 mg q8h	75	100%	q12h	q24h	q24h	
Zidovudine	200 mg q8h, 300 mg q12h	8–25	100%	100%	100 mg q8h	100 mg q8h	Enormous interpatient variation; metabolite renally excreted

GFR, glomerular filtration rate; CRRT, continuous renal replacement therapy; Vd, volume of distribution; TB, tuberculosis; BUN, blood urea nitrogen; ESKD, end-stage kidney disease; CAPD, continuous ambulatory peritoneal disease; CsA, Cyclosporine; FK, tacrolimus; LFT, liver function test; NS, normal saline; Clcr, creatinine clearance; VZV, varicella zoster virus; HSV, herpes simplex virus; CMV, cytomegalovirus.

Analgesic Drug Dosing in Kidney Disease

Analgesics	Normal Dosage	% of Renal Excretion	Dosage Adjustment in Kidney Disease				Comments
			GFR >50	GFR 10–50	GFR <10	CRRT	
Narcotics and narcotic antagonists							
Alfentanil	Anesthetic induction 8–40 μg/kg	Hepatic	100%	100%	100%	100%	Titrate the dose regimen
Butorphanol	2 mg q3–4h	Hepatic	100%	75%	50%	50%	
Codeine	30–60 mg q4–6h	Hepatic	100%	75%	50%	50%	
Fentanyl	Anesthetic induction (individualized)	Hepatic	100%	75%	50%	50%	CRRT–titrate
Meperidine	50–100 mg q3–4h	Hepatic	100%	Avoid	Avoid	Avoid	Normeperidine, an active metabolite, accumulates in ESKD and may cause seizures; protein binding is reduced in ESKD; 20%–25% excreted unchanged in acidic urine
Methadone	2.5–5 mg q6–8h	Hepatic	100%	100%	50%–75%	50%–75%	Should not be used for acute pain
Morphine	20–25 mg q4h	Hepatic	100%	75%	50%	50%	Increased sensitivity to drug effect in ESKD; active metabolites
Naloxone	2 mg IV	Hepatic	100%	100%	100%	100%	
Pentazocine	50 mg q4h	Hepatic	100%	75%	75%	75%	
Propoxyphene	65 mg po q6–8h	Hepatic	100%	100%	Avoid	Avoid	Active metabolite norpropoxyphene accumulates in ESKD; cardiotoxic
Sufentanil	Anesthetic induction	Hepatic	100%	100%	100%	100%	CRRT–titrate
Nonnarcotics							
Acetaminophen	650 mg q4h	Hepatic	q4h	q6h	q8h	q8h	Overdose may be nephrotoxic; drug is major metabolite of phenacetin.
Acetylsalicylic acid	650 mg q4h	Hepatic (renal)	q4h	q4–6h	Avoid	Avoid	Nephrotoxic in high doses; may decrease GFR when renal blood flow is prostaglandin dependent; may add to uremic GI and hematologic symptoms; protein binding reduced in ESKD

GFR, glomerular filtration rate; CRRT, continuous renal replacement therapy; ESKD, end-stage kidney disease; GI, gastrointestinal.

Antihypertensive and Cardiovascular Agent Dosing in Kidney Disease

Antihypertensive and Cardiovascular Agents	Normal Dosage	% of Renal Excretion	Dosage Adjustment in Kidney Disease				Dosage in CRRT	Comments
			GFR >50	GFR 10–50	GFR <10			
ACE inhibitors								Hyperkalemia, acute kidney injury, angioedema, rash, cough, anemia, and liver toxicity
Benazepril	80 mg qd	20	100%	75%	25%–50%	25%–50%	
Captopril	6.25–25 mg po tid	35	100%	75%	50%	50%	Rare proteinuria, nephrotic syndrome, dysgeusia, granulocytopenia; increases serum digoxin levels
Enalapril	5 mg qd	45	100%	75%	50%	50%	Enalaprilat, the active moiety formed in liver
Fosinopril	10 mg po qd	20	100%	100%	75%	75%	Fosinoprilat, the active moiety formed in liver; drug less likely than other ACE inhibitors to accumulate in kidney disease
Lisinopril	2.5 mg qd	80	100%	50%–75%	25%–50%	25%–50%	Lysine analog of a pharmacologically active enalapril metabolite
Pentopril	125 mg q24h	80–90	100%	50%–75%	50%	50%	50%
Perindopril	2 mg q24h	<10	100%	75%	50%	50%	50%
Quinapril	10 mg qd	30	100%	75%–100%	75%		Active metabolite is quinaprilat; 96% of quinaprilat is excreted renally.
Ramipril	2.5 mg qd	15	100%	50%–75%	25%–50%		Active metabolite is ramiprilat; data are for ramiprilat.
Trandolapril	1–2 mg qd	33	100%	50%–100%	50%	50%	
Angiotensin-II receptor antagonists								Hyperkalemia, angioedema (less common than ACE inhibitors
Candesartan	16 mg qd	33	100%	100%	50%	50%	Candesartan cilexetil is rapidly and completely bioactivated by ester hydrolysis during absorption from the gastrointestinal tract to candesartan.
Eprosartan	400–800 mg qd	25	100%	100%	100%	100%	Eprosartan pharmacokinetics more variable ESKD; decreased protein binding in uremia
Irbesartan	150 mg qd	20	100%	100%	100%	100%	

Drug	Dose							Comments
Losartan	50 mg qd	100 mg qd	13	100%	100%	100%	100%	
Valsartan	80 mg qd	160 mg bid	7	100%	100%	100%	100%	
Telmisartan	20–80 mg qd		<5	100%	100%	100%	100%	
β-Blockers								Decrease HDL, mask symptoms of hypoglycemia, bronchospasm, fatigue, insomnia, depression, and sexual dysfunction
Acebutolol	400 mg q24h or bid	600 mg q24h or bid	55	100%	50%	30%–50%	30%–50%	Active metabolites with long half-life
Atenolol	25 mg qd	100 mg qd	90	100%	75%	50%	50%	Accumulates in ESKD
Betaxolol	20 mg q24h	80%–90%	100	100%	50%	50%	50%	
Bopindolol	1 mg q24h	4 mg q24h	<10	100%	100%	100%	100%	
Carteolol	0.5 mg q24h	10 mg q24h	<50	100%	50%	25%	25%	
Carvedilol	3.125 mg po tid	25 mg tid	2	100%	100%	100%	100%	Kinetics are dose dependent; plasma concentrations of carvedilol have been reported to be increased in patients with renal impairment.
Celiprolol	200 mg q24h		10	100%	100%	75%	75%	
Dilevalol	200 mg bid	400 mg bid	<5	100%	100%	100%	100%	
Esmolol (IV only)	50 µg/kg/min	300 µg/kg/min	10	100%	100%	100%	100%	Active metabolite retained in kidney disease
Labetalol	50 mg po bid	400 mg bid	5	100%	100%	100%	100%	For IV use: 20 mg slow IV injection over a 2-min period; additional injections of 40 mg or 80 mg can be given at 10-min intervals until a total of 300 mg or continuous infusion of 2 mg/min.
Metoprolol	50 mg bid		100 mg bid	<5%	100%	100%	100%	
Nadolol	80 mg qd	160 mg bid	90	100%	50%	25%	25%	Start with prolonged interval and titrate.
Penbutolol	10 mg q24h	40 mg q24h	<10	100%	100%	100%	100%	
Pindolol	10 mg bid	40 mg bid	40	100%	100%	100%	100%	
Propranolol	40–160 mg po tid	320 mg/d	<5	100%	100%	100%	100%	Bioavailability may increase in ESKD; metabolites may cause increased bilirubin by assay interference in ESKD; hypoglycemia reported in ESKD

(continued)

Continued

Antihypertensive and Cardiovascular Agents	Normal Dosage	% of Renal Excretion	Dosage Adjustment in Kidney Disease			Dosage in CRRT	Comments
			GFR >50	GFR 10–50	GFR <10		
Sotalol	80 mg bid / 160 mg bid	70	100%	50%	25%–50%	25%–50%	Extreme caution should be exercised in the use of sotalol in patients with kidney disease undergoing hemodialysis; to minimize the risk of induced arrhythmia, patients initiated or reinitiated on Betapace should be placed for a minimum of 3 days (on their maintenance dose) in a facility that can provide cardiac resuscitation and continuous electrocardiographic monitoring.
Timolol	10 mg bid / 20 mg bid	15	100%	100%	100%	100%	
Calcium channel blockers							Dihydropyridine: headache, ankle edema, gingival hyperplasia, and flushing. Nondihydropyridine: bradycardia, constipation, gingival hyperplasia, and AV block
Amlodipine	2.5 po qd / 10 mg qd	10	100%	100%	100%	100%	May increase digoxin and cyclosporine levels
Bepridil	No data	<1%	No data	No data	Weak vasodilator and antihypertensive		
Diltiazem	30 mg tid / 90 mg tid	10	100%	100%	100%	100%	Acute renal dysfunction; may exacerbate hyperkalemia; may increase digoxin and cyclosporine levels
Felodipine	5 mg po bid / 20 mg qd	1	100%	100%	100%	100%	May increase digoxin levels
Isradipine	5 mg po bid / 10 mg bid	<5	100%	100%	100%	100%	May increase digoxin levels
Nicardipine	20 mg po tid / 30 mg po tid	<1%	100%	100%	100%	100%	
Nifedipine XL	30 qd / 90 mg bid	10	100%	100%	100%	100%	Avoid short-acting nifedipine formulation
Nimodipine	30 mg q8h	10	100%	100%	100%	100%	
Nisoldipine	20 mg qd / 30 mg bid	10	100%	100%	100%	100%	May increase digoxin levels
Verapamil	40 mg tid / 240 mg/d	10	100%	100%	100%	100%	Acute renal dysfunction; active metabolites accumulate particularly with sustained-release forms

Diuretics	Dose		% excreted	GFR >50	GFR 10–50	GFR <10	Comments
							Hypokalemia/hyperkalemia (potassium-sparing agents), hyperuricemia, hyperglycemia, hypomagnesemia, increase serum cholesterol
Acetazolamide	125 mg po tid	500 mg po tid	90	100%	50%	Avoid	May potentiate acidosis; ineffective as diuretic in ESKD; may cause neurologic side effects in dialysis patients
Amiloride	5 mg po qd	10 mg po qd	50	100%	100%	Avoid	Hyperkalemia with GFR <30 mL/min, especially in diabetics; hyperchloremic metabolic acidosis
Bumetanide	1–2 mg po qd	2–4 mg po qd	35	100%	100%	100%	Ototoxicity increased in ESKD in combination with aminoglycosides; high doses effective in ESKD; muscle pain, gynecomastia
Chlorthalidone	25 mg q24h		50%	q24h	q24h	50%	Avoid	Ineffective with low GFR
Ethacrynic acid	50 mg po bid	100 mg po bid	20	100%	100%	100%	Ototoxicity increased in ESKD in combination with aminoglycosides
Furosemide	40–80 mg po qd	120 mg po tid	70	100%	100%	100%	Ototoxicity increased in ESKD, especially in combination with aminoglycosides; high doses effective in ESKD
Indapamide	2.5 mg q24h		<5%	100	100%	Avoid	Ineffective in ESKD
Metolazone	2.5 mg po qd	10 mg po bid	70%	100%	100%	100%	High doses effective in ESKD; gynecomastia, impotence
Piretanide	6 mg q24h	12 mg q24h	40–60	100%	100%	100%	High doses effective in ESKD; ototoxicity
Spironolactone	100 mg po qd	300 mg po qd	25	100%	Avoid	Avoid	Active metabolites with long half-life; hyperkalemia common when GFR <30, especially in diabetics; gynecomastia, hyperchloremic acidosis; increases serum by immunoassay interference
Thiazides	25 mg bid	50 mg bid	>95%	100%	100%	Avoid	Avoid
Torasemide	5 mg po bid	20 mg qd	25	100%	100%	100%	High doses effective in ESKD; ototoxicity

(continued)

Continued

Antihypertensive and Cardiovascular Agents	Normal Dosage	% of Renal Excretion	Dosage Adjustment in Kidney Disease				Comments
			GFR >50	GFR 10–50	GFR <10	Dosage in CRRT	
Triamterene	25 mg bid / 50 mg bid	5–10	q12h	q12h	Avoid	Avoid	Hyperkalemia common when GFR <30, especially in diabetics; active metabolite with long half-life in ESKD; folic acid antagonist; urolithiasis; crystalluria in acid urine; may cause acute kidney injury
Miscellaneous agents							
Amrinone	5 mg/kg/min daily dose <10 mg/kg / 10 mg/kg/min daily dose <10 mg/kg	10–40	100%	100%	100%	100%	Thrombocytopenia; nausea, vomiting in ESKD
Clonidine	0.1 po bid/tid / 1.2 mg/d	45	100%	100%	100%	100%	Sexual dysfunction, dizziness, postal hypotension
Digoxin	0.125 mg qod/qd / 0.25 mg po qd	25	100%	100%	100%	100%	Decrease loading dose by 50% in ESKD; radioimmunoassay may overestimate serum levels in uremia; clearance decreased by amiodarone, spironolactone, quinidine, verapamil; hypokalemia, hypomagnesemia enhance toxicity; Vd and total body clearance decreased in ESKD; serum level 12 h after dose is best guide in ESKD; digoxin-immune antibodies can treat severe toxicity in ESKD.
Hydralazine	10 mg po qid / 100 mg po qid	25	100%	100%	100%	100%	Lupus-like reaction
Midodrine	No data	75–80	5–10 mg q8h	5–10 mg q8h	No data	No data	Increased blood pressure
Minoxidil	2.5 mg po bid / 10 mg po bid	20	100%	100%	100%	100%	Pericardial effusion, fluid retention, hypertrichosis, and tachycardia
Nitroprusside	1 μg/kg/min / 10 μg/kg/min	<10	100%	100%	100%	100%	Cyanide toxicity
Amrinone	5 μg/kg/min / 10 μg/kg/min	25	100%	100%	100%	100%	Thrombocytopenia; nausea, vomiting in ESKD
Dobutamine	2.5 μg/kg/min / 15 μg/kg/min	10	100%	100%	100%	100%	
Milrinone	0.375 μg/kg/min / 0.75 μg/kg/min		100%	100%	100%	100%	

GFR, glomerular filtration rate; CRRT, continuous renal replacement therapy; ACE, angiotensin-converting enzyme; ESKD, end-stage kidney disease; HDL, high-density lipoprotein; AV, arteriovenous; Vd, volume distribution.

Endocrine and Metabolic Agent Dosing in Kidney Disease

	Normal Dosage	% of Renal Excretion	Dosage Adjustment in Kidney Disease			Dosage in CRRT	Comments
			GFR >50	GFR 10–50	GFR <10		
Hypoglycemic agents							Avoid all oral hypoglycemic agents on CRRT
Acarbose	25 mg tid / 100 mg tid	35	100%	50%	Avoid	Avoid	Abdominal pain, N/V, and flatulence
Acetohexamide	250 mg q24h / 1,500 mg q24h	None	Avoid	Avoid	Avoid	Avoid	Diuretic effect; may falsely elevate serum creatinine; active metabolite has T$_{1/2}$ of 5–8 h in healthy subjects and is eliminated by the kidney; prolonged hypoglycemia in azotemic patients
Chlorpropamide	100 mg q24h	47	50%	Avoid	Avoid	Avoid	Impairs water excretion; prolonged hypoglycemia in azotemic patients
Glibornuride	12.5 mg q24h / 100 mg q14h	No data	No data	No data	No data	No data	
Gliclazide	80 mg q24h / 320 mg q24h	<20	50%–100%	Avoid	Avoid	Avoid	
Glipizide	5 mg qd / 20 mg bid	5	100%	50%	50%	Avoid	
Glyburide	2.5 mg qd / 10 mg bid	50	100%	50%	Avoid	Avoid	
Metformin	500 mg bid / 2,550 mg/d (bid or tid)	95	100%	Avoid	Avoid	Avoid	Lactic acidosis
Repaglinide	0.5–1 mg / 4 mg tid						
Tolazamide	100 mg q24h / 250 mg q24h	7	100%	100%	Avoid	Avoid	Diuretic effects
Tolbutamide	1 g q24h / 2 g q24h	None	100%	100%	Avoid	Avoid	May impair water excretion
Troglitazone	200 mg qd / 600 mg qd	3	100%	Avoid	Avoid	Avoid	Decrease CsA level; hepatotoxic
Parenteral agents							Dosage guided by blood glucose levels
Insulin	Variable	None	100%	75%	50%	50%	Renal metabolism of insulin decreases with azotemia.
Lispro insulin	Variable	No data	100%	75%	50%	50%	
Hyperlipidemic agents							Avoid all oral hypoglycemic agents on CRRT
Atorvastatin	10 mg/d / 80 mg/d	<2	100%	100%	100%	100%	Liver dysfunction, myalgia, and rhabdomyolysis with CsA/FK
Bezafibrate	200 mg bid–qid / 400 mg SR q24h	50	50%–100%	25%–50%	Avoid	Avoid	Avoid
Cholestyramine	4 g bid / 24 g/d	None	100%	100%	100%	100%	
Clofibrate	500 mg bid / 1,000 mg bid	40–70	q6–12h	q12–18h	Avoid	Avoid	Avoid

(continued)

Continued

	Normal Dosage	% of Renal Excretion	Dosage Adjustment in Kidney Disease			Dosage in CRRT	Comments
			GFR >50	GFR 10–50	GFR <10		
Colestipol	30 g/d	None	100%	100%	100%	100%	
Fluvastatin	80 mg/d	<1	100%	100%	100%	100%	
Gemfibrozil	600 bid	None	100%	100%	100%	100%	
Lovastatin	20 mg/d	None	100%	100%	100%	100%	
Nicotinic acid	2 g tid	None	100%	50%	25%	25%	
Pravastatin	10–40 mg/d	<10	100%	100%	100%	100%	
Probucol	500 mg bid	<2	100%	100%	100%	Avoid	
Rosuvastatin	5–20 mg/d		100%	100%	100%	50%	
Simvastatin	5–20 mg/d	13	100%	100%	50%	50%	
Antithyroid Dosing in Kidney Disease							
Antithyroid drugs							
Methimazole	5–20 mg tid	7	100%	100%	100%	100%	
Propylthiouracil	100 mg tid	<10	100%	100%	100%	100%	

GFR, glomerular filtration rate; CRRT, continuous renal replacement therapy; N/V, nausea, vomiting; CsA, Cyclosporine; FK, tacrolimus; SR, sustained release.

Gastrointestinal Dosing in Kidney Disease

Gastrointestinal Agents	Normal Doses		% of Renal Excretion	Dosage Adjustment in Kidney Disease			Dosage in CRRT	Comments
	Starting Dose	Maximum Dose		GFR >50	GFR 10–50	GFR <10		
Cimetidine	300 mg po tid	800 mg po bid	60	100%	75%	25%	25%	Multiple drug–drug interactions; β-blockers, sulfonylurea, theophylline, warfarin, and so forth
Famotidine	20 mg po bid	40 mg po bid	70	100%	75%	25%	25%	Headache, fatigue, thrombocytopenia, alopecia
Lansoprazole	15 mg po qd	30 mg bid	None	100%	100%	100%	100%	Headache, diarrhea
Nizatidine	150 mg po bid	300 mg po bid	20	100%	75%	25%	25%	Headache, fatigue, thrombocytopenia, alopecia
Omeprazole	20 mg po qd	40 mg po bid	None	100%	100%	100%	100%	Headache, diarrhea
Rabeprazole	20 mg po qd	40 mg po bid	None	100%	100%	100%	100%	Headache, diarrhea
Pantoprazole	40 mg po qd	80 mg po bid	None	100%	100%	100%	100%	Headache, diarrhea
Ranitidine	150 mg po bid	300 mg po bid	80	100%	75%	25%	25%	Headache, fatigue, thrombocytopenia, alopecia
Cisapride	10 mg po tid	20 mg qid	5	100%	100%	50%–75%	50%–75%	Avoid with azole antifungal, macrolide antibiotics, and other P450 IIIA-4 inhibitors.
Metoclopramide	10 mg po tid	30 mg po qid	15	100%	100%	50%–75%	50%–75%	Increase cyclosporine/tacrolimus level; neurotoxic
Misoprostol	100 μg po bid	200 μg po qid	None	100%	100%	100%	100%	Diarrhea, N/V, abortifacient agent
Sucralfate	1 g po qid	1 g po qid	None	100%	100%	100%	100%	Constipation, decrease absorption of MMF

GFR, glomerular filtration rate; CRRT, continuous renal replacement therapy; N/V, nausea, vomiting; MMF, mycophenolate mofetil.

Neurologic/Anticonvulsant Dosing in Kidney Disease

Anticonvulsants	Normal Dosage	% of Renal Excretion	Dosage Adjustment in Kidney Disease				Dosage in CRRT	Comments
			GFR >50	GFR 10–50	GFR <10			
Carbamazepine	2–8 mg/kg/d; adjust for side effect and TDM	2	100%	100%	100%	100%	Plasma concentration: 4–12, double vision, fluid retention, myelosuppression
Clonazepam	0.5 mg tid	2 mg tid	1	100%	100%	100%	100%	Although no dose reduction is recommended, the drug has not been studied in patients with renal impairment. Recommendations are based on known drug characteristics, not clinical trials data.
Ethosuximide	5 mg/kg/d; adjust for side effect and TDM	20	100%	100%	100%	100%	Plasma concentration: 40–100, headache
Felbamate	400 mg/tid	1,200 mg/tid	90	100%	50%	25%	25%	Anorexia, vomiting, insomnia, nausea
Gabapentin	150 mg tid	900 mg tid	77	100%	50%	25%	25%	Less CNS side effects compared to other agents
Lamotrigine	25–50 mg/d	150 mg/d	1	100%	100%	100%	100%	Auto-induction, major drug–drug interaction with valproate
Levetiracetam	500 mg bid	1,500 mg bid	66	100%	50%	50%	25%	Less effect on P450 compared to carbamazepine
Oxcarbazepine	300 mg bid	600 mg bid	1	100%	100%	100%	100%	Plasma concentration: 15–40, insomnia
Phenobarbital	20 mg/kg/d; adjust for side effect and TDM	1	100%	100%	100%	100%	
Phenytoin	20 mg/kg/d; adjust for side effect and TDM	1	Adjust for kidney disease and low albumin		100%	Plasma concentration: 10–20, nystagmus, check free phenytoin level
Primidone	50 mg	100 mg	1	100%	100%	100%	100%	Plasma concentration: 5–20
Sodium valproate	7.5 to 15 mg/kg/d; adjust for side effect and TDM	1	100%	100%	100%	100%	Plasma concentration: 50–150, weight gain, hepatitis, check free valproate level
Tiagabine	4 mg qd, increase 4mg/d, titrate weekly	2	100%	100%	100%	100%	Total daily dose may be increased by 4–8 mg at weekly intervals until clinical response is achieved or up to 32 mg/d. The total daily dose should be given in divided doses two to four times daily.
Topiramate	50 mg/d	70	100%	50%	50%	Avoid	Kidney stone
Trimethadione	300 mg tid–qid	600 mg tid–qid	None	q8h	q8–12h	q12–24h	Avoid	Active metabolites with long half-life in ESKD; nephrotic syndrome
Vigabatrin	1 g bid	2 g bid	70	100%	50%	25%	25%	Encephalopathy with drug accumulation
Zonisamide	100 mg qd	100–300 mg qd–bid	30	100%	75%	50%	50%	Manufacturer recommends that zonisamide should not be used in patients with kidney disease (estimated GFR <50 mL/min) as there has been insufficient experience concerning drug dosing and toxicity. Zonisamide doses of 100–600 mg/d are effective for normal renal function. Dose recommendations for renal impairment based on clearance ratios.

GFR, glomerular filtration rate; CRRT, continuous renal replacement therapy; TDM, therapeutic drug monitoring; CNS, central nervous system; ESKD, end-stage kidney disease.

Rheumatologic Dosing in Kidney Disease

Arthritis and Gout Agents	Normal Dosage	% of Renal Excretion	Dosage Adjustment in Kidney Disease				Dosage in CRRT	Comments
			GFR >50	GFR 10–50	GFR <10			
Allopurinol	300 mg q24h	30	75%	50%	25%	25%	Interstitial nephritis; rare xanthine stones; renal excretion of active metabolite with $T_{1/2}$ of 25 h in normal renal function; $T_{1/2}$ 1 wk in patients with ESKD; exfoliative dermatitis
Auranofin	6 mg q24h	50	50%	Avoid	Avoid	Avoid	Proteinuria and nephritic syndrome
Colchicine	Acute: 2 mg then 0.5 mg q6h Chronic: 0.5–1.0 mg q24h	5–17	100%	50%–100%	25%	25%	Avoid prolonged use if GFR <50 mL/min.
Gold sodium	25–50 mg	60–90	50%	Avoid	Avoid	Avoid	Thiomalate proteinuria; nephritic syndrome; membranous nephritis
Penicillamine	250–1,000 mg q24h	40	100%	Avoid	Avoid	Avoid	Nephrotic syndrome
Probenecid	500 mg bid	<2	100%	Avoid	Avoid	Avoid	Ineffective at decreased GFR
Nonsteroidal anti-inflammatory drugs							May decrease renal function; decrease platelet aggregation; nephrotic syndrome; interstitial nephritis; hyperkalemia; sodium retention
Diclofenac	25–75 mg bid	<1	50%–100%	Avoid	Avoid	Avoid	
Diflunisal	250–500 mg bid	<3	100%	50%	Avoid	Avoid	
Etodolac	200 mg bid	Negligible	50%–100%	Avoid	Avoid	Avoid	
Fenoprofen	300–600 mg qid	30	50%–100%	Avoid	Avoid	Avoid	
Flurbiprofen	100 mg bid–tid	20	50%–100%	Avoid	Avoid	Avoid	
Ibuprofen	800 mg tid	1	50%–100%	Avoid	Avoid	Avoid	
Indomethacin	25–50 mg tid	30	50%–100%	Avoid	Avoid	Avoid	
Ketoprofen	25–75 mg tid	<1	50%–100%	Avoid	Avoid	Avoid	
Ketorolac	15 mg q6h	30–60	50%–100%	Avoid	Avoid	Avoid	Acute hearing loss in ESKD
Meclofenamic acid	50–100 tid–qid	2–4	50%–100%	Avoid	Avoid	Avoid	
Mefenamic acid	250 mg qid	<6	50%–100%	Avoid	Avoid	Avoid	
Nabumetone	1.0–2.0 g q24h	<1	50%–100%	Avoid	Avoid	Avoid	
Naproxen	500 mg bid	<1	50%–100%	Avoid	Avoid	Avoid	
Oxaprozin	1,200 mg q24h	<1	50%–100%	Avoid	Avoid	Avoid	
Phenylbutazone	100 mg tid–qid	1	50%–100%	Avoid	Avoid	Avoid	
Piroxicam	20 mg q24h	10	50%–100%	Avoid	Avoid	Avoid	
Sulindac	200 mg bid	7	50%–100%	Avoid	Avoid	Avoid	Active sulfide metabolite in ESKD
Tolmetin	400 mg tid	15	100%	100%	100%	100%	

GFR, glomerular filtration rate; CRRT, continuous renal replacement therapy; ESKD, end-stage kidney disease.

Sedative Dosing in Kidney Disease

Sedatives	Normal Dosage	% of Renal Excretion	Dosage Adjustment in Kidney Disease			Dosage in CRRT	Comments
			GFR >50	GFR 10–50	GFR <10		
Barbiturates							May cause excessive sedation, increase osteomalacia in ESKD; charcoal hemoperfusion and hemodialysis more effective than peritoneal dialysis for poisoning
Pentobarbital	30 mg q6–8h	Hepatic	100%	100%	100%	100%	
Phenobarbital	50–100 mg q8–12h	Hepatic (renal)	q8–12h	q8–12h	q12–16h	q12–16h	Up to 50% unchanged drug excreted with urine with alkaline diuresis
Secobarbital	30–50 mg q6–8h	Hepatic	100%	100%	100%	100%	
Thiopental	Anesthesia induction (individualized)	Hepatic	100%	100%	100%	100%	
Benzodiazepines							May cause excessive sedation and encephalopathy in ESKD
Alprazolam	0.25–5.0 mg q8h	Hepatic	100%	100%	100%	100%	
Clorazepate	15–60 mg q24h	Hepatic (renal)	100%	100%	100%	100%	
Chlordiazepoxide	15–100 mg q24h	Hepatic	100%	100%	50%	50%	
Clonazepam	1.5 q24h	Hepatic	100%	100%	100%	100%	Although no dose reduction is recommended, the drug has not been studied in patients with renal impairment; recommendations are based on known drug characteristics not clinical trials data.
Diazepam	5–40 mg q24h	Hepatic	100%	100%	100%	100%	Active metabolites, desmethyldiazepam, and oxazepam may accumulate in kidney disease; dose should be reduced if given longer than a few days; protein binding decreases in uremia.
Estazolam	1 mg qhs	Hepatic	100%	100%	100%	100%	
Flurazepam	15–30 mg qhs	Hepatic	100%	100%	100%	100%	
Lorazepam	1–2 mg q8–12h	Hepatic	100%	100%	100%	100%	
Midazolam	Individualized	Hepatic	100%	100%	50%	50%	
Oxazepam	30–120 mg q24h	Hepatic	100%	100%	100%	100%	
Quazepam	15 mg qhs	Hepatic	No data	No data	No data	No data	

Temazepam	30 mg qhs	Hepatic	100%	100%	100%	100%	
Triazolam	0.25–0.50 mg qhs	Hepatic	100%	100%	100%	100%	Protein binding correlates with α-1 acid glycoprotein concentration.
Benzodiazepines: Benzodiazepine antagonist						100%	May cause excessive sedation and encephalopathy in ESKD
Flumazenil	0.2 mg IV over 15 s	Hepatic	100%	100%	100%	100%	
Miscellaneous sedative agents						100%	
Buspirone	5 mg q8h	Hepatic	100%	100%	100%	100%	
Ethchlorvynol	500 mg qhs	Hepatic	100%	Avoid	Avoid	100%	Removed by hemoperfusion; excessive sedation
Haloperidol	1–2 mg q8–12h	Hepatic	100%	100%	100%	100%	Hypertension, excessive sedation
Lithium carbonate	0.9–1.2 g q24h	Renal	100%	50%–75%	25%–50%	100%	Nephrotoxic; nephrogenic diabetes insipidus; nephrotic syndrome; renal tubular acidosis; interstitial fibrosis; acute toxicity when serum levels >1.2 mEq/L; serum levels should be measured periodically 12 h after dose; $T_{1/2}$ does not reflect extensive tissue accumulation; plasma levels rebound after dialysis; toxicity enhanced by volume depletion, NSAIDs, and diuretics
Meprobamate	1.2–1.6 g q24h	Hepatic (renal)	q6h	q9–12h	q12–18h	25%	Excessive sedation; excretion enhanced by forced diuresis

GFR, glomerular filtration rate; CRRT, continuous renal replacement therapy; ESKD, end-stage kidney disease; NSAIDs, nonsteroidal anti-inflammatory drugs.

Anti-Parkinson Dosing in Kidney Disease

Anti-Parkinson Agents	Normal Dosage	% of Renal Excretion	Dosage Adjustment in Renal Failure			Dosage in CRRT	Comments
			GFR >50	GFR 10–50	GFR <10		
Carbidopa	1 tablet tid to 6 tablets daily	30	100%	100%	100%	100%	Require careful titration of dose according to clinical response
Levodopa	25–500 mg bid to 8 g q24h	None	100%	50%–100%	50%–100%	100%	Active and inactive metabolites excreted in urine; active metabolites with long $T_{1/2}$ in ESKD

GFR, glomerular filtration rate; CRRT, continuous renal replacement therapy; ESKD, end-stage kidney disease.

Antipsychotic Dosing in Kidney Disease

Antipsychotics	Normal Dosage	% of Renal Excretion	Dosage Adjustment in Kidney Disease			Dosage in CRRT	Comments
			GFR >50	GFR 10–50	GFR <10		
Phenothiazines							Orthostatic hypotension, extrapyramidal symptoms, and confusion can occur.
Chlorpromazine	300–800 mg q24h	Hepatic	100%	100%	100%	100%	No comments
Promethazine	20–100 mg q24h	Hepatic	100%	100%	100%	100%	Excessive sedation may occur in ESKD.
Thioridazine	50–100 mg po tid; increase gradually; maximum of 800 mg/d	Hepatic	100%	100%	100%	100%	
Trifluoperazine	1–2 mg bid; increase to no more than 6 mg	Hepatic	100%	100%	100%	100%	
Perphenazine	8–16 mg po bid, tid, or qid; increase to 64 mg daily	Hepatic	100%	100%	100%	100%	
Thiothixene	2 mg po tid; increase gradually to 15 mg daily	Hepatic	100%	100%	100%	100%	
Haloperidol	1–2 mg q8–12h	Hepatic	100%	100%	100%	100%	Hypotension, excessive sedation
Loxapine	12.5–50 mg IM q4–6h	Hepatic	100%	100%	100%	100%	Do not administer drug IV.
Clozapine	12.5 mg po; 25–50 daily to 300–450 by end of 2 wk; maximum: 900 mg daily	Metabolism nearly complete	100%	100%	100%	100%	
Risperidone	1 mg po bid; increase to 3 mg bid		100%	100%	100%	100%	
Olanzapine	5–10 mg	Hepatic	100%	100%	100%	100%	Potential hypotensive effects
Quetiapine	25 mg po bid; increase in increments of 25–50 bid or tid; 300–400 mg daily by day 4	Hepatic	100%	100%	100%	100%	
Ziprasidone	20–100 mg q12h	Hepatic	100%	100%	100%	100%	

GFR, glomerular filtration rate; CRRT, continuous renal replacement therapy; ESKD, end-stage kidney disease.

Miscellaneous Dosing in Kidney Disease

Corticosteroids	Normal Dosage	% of Renal Excretion	Dosage Adjustment in Renal Failure			Dosage in CRRT	Comments
			GFR >50	GFR 10–50	GFR <10		
Betamethasone	0.5–9.0 mg q24h	5	100%	100%	100%	100%	May aggravate azotemia, Na$^+$ retention, glucose intolerance, and hypertension
Budesonide	No data	None	100%	100%	100%	100%	
Cortisone	25–500 mg q24h	None	100%	100%	100%	100%	
Dexamethasone	0.75–9.0 mg q24h	8	100%	100%	100%	100%	
Hydrocortisone	20–500 mg q24h	None	100%	100%	100%	100%	
Methylprednisolone	4–48 mg q24h	<10	100%	100%	100%	100%	
Prednisolone	5–60 mg q24h	34	100%	100%	100%	100%	
Prednisone	5–60 mg q24h	34	100%	100%	100%	100%	
Triamcinolone	4–48 mg q24h	No data	100%	100%	100%	100%	

GFR, glomerular filtration rate; CRRT, continuous renal replacement therapy.

Anticoagulant Dosing in Kidney Disease

Anticoagulants	Normal Dosage		% of Renal Excretion	Dosage Adjustment in Renal Failure			Dosage in CRRT	Comments
				GFR >50	GFR 10–50	GFR <10		
Alteplase	60 mg over 1 h then 20 mg/h for 2 h		No data	100%	100%	100%	100%	Tissue-type plasminogen activator
Aspirin	81 mg/d	325 mg/d	10	100%	100%	100%	100%	GI irritation and bleeding tendency
Clopidogrel	75 mg/d	75 mg/d	50	100%	100%	100%	100%	GI irritation and bleeding tendency
Dalteparin	2,500 U sc/d	5,000 U sc/d	Unknown	100%	100%	50%	Avoid	
Dipyridamole	50 mg tid		No data	100%	100%	100%	100%	
Enoxaparin	20 mg/d	30 mg bid	8	100%	50%–75%	50%	25%–50%	1 mg/kg q12h for treatment of DVT; check anti-factor Xa activity 4 h after second dose in patients with renal dysfunction; some evidence of drug accumulation in kidney disease
Heparin	75 U/kg load then 15 U/kg/h		None	100%	100%	100%	100%	Half-life increases with dose
Iloprost	0.5–2.0 ng/kg/min for 5–12 h		No data	100%	100%	50%	50%	
Indobufen	100 mg bid	200 mg bid	<15	100%	50%	25%	25%	
Streptokinase	250,000 U load then 100,000 U/h		None	100%	100%	100%	100%	
Sulfinpyrazone	200 mg bid		25–50	100%	100%	Avoid	Avoid	Acute kidney injury; uricosuric effect at low GFR
Ticlopidine	250 mg bid	250 mg bid	2	100%	100%	100%	100%	Decrease CsA level; may cause severe neutropenia and thrombocytopenia
Tranexamic acid	25 mg/kg tid–qid		90	50%	25%	10%	Avoid	
Urokinase	4,400 U/kg load then 4400 U/kg qh		No data	100%	100%	100%	100%	
Warfarin	2.5–5 mg/d	Adjust per INR	<1	100%	100%	100%	100%	Monitor INR very closely; start at 5 mg/d; 1 mg vitamin K IV over 30 min or 2.5–5 mg po can be used to normalize INR.

GFR, glomerular filtration rate; CRRT, continuous renal replacement therapy; GI, gastrointestinal; DVT, deep venous thrombosis; CsA, Cyclosporine; INR, international normalized ratio.

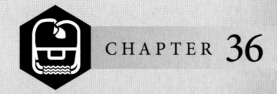

CHAPTER 36

Extracorporeal Treatment of Poisoning and Drug Overdose

Wajeh Y. Qunibi

 EPIDEMIOLOGY OF POISONING

Although poisoning has been reported to health care institutions for a long time, its incidence is clearly underestimated. The incidence of poisoning continues to increase largely due to abuse of over-the-counter medications as well as illicit drugs. Poisoning became the leading cause of accidental death in the United States in 2008, exceeding motor vehicle accident deaths for the first time since 1980 (1). In 2014, the Toxic Exposure Surveillance System (TESS) data compiled by the American Association of Poison Control Centers (AAPCC) revealed that there were almost 2.3 million reported human poison exposure cases. Over 600,000 exposures led to a visit in a health care facility (HCF), 27% of them required hospital admission resulting in 1,261 deaths in the United States (2). The majority (80%) of these cases were unintentional, but suicidal intent was suspected in 10.5% of cases. Poisoning may also result from malicious intent, drug–drug interaction (12.5%), or from occupational or environmental exposure. The top five substance classes most frequently involved in all human exposures are analgesics (11.6%), cosmetics/personal care products (7.9%), household cleaning substances (7.2%), sedatives/hypnotics/antipsychotics (6.0%), and antidepressants (4.1%) (2). Analgesics and sedative/hypnotics/antipsychotics exposures as a class increased most rapidly over the last 13 years for cases showing more serious outcomes. The National Poison Data System (NPDS) documented 2,477 human exposures resulting in death of which 2,113 human fatalities judged related. Again, analgesics were the most common cause of death, and acetaminophen is the analgesic most often implicated in fatal poisoning. Children younger than 3 years were involved in 35.5% of exposures and children younger than 6 years accounted for approximately half of all human exposures (48.0%). Male predominance was found among cases involving children younger than 13 years, but this gender distribution was

reversed in teenagers and adults, with females comprising the majority of reported exposures. Most human exposures (87.9%) were acute cases (single, repeated, or continuous exposure occurring over 8 hours or less). The route of exposure to the poison was ingestion in 83.4% of cases followed in frequency by dermal (7.0%), inhalation/nasal (6.1%), and ocular routes (4.3%). Of the 2,188,013 human exposures reported, 71.8% of calls originated from a residence (own or other), but 93.5% actually occurred at a residence. Another 20.3% of calls were made from an HCF. Beyond residences, exposures occurred in the workplace in 1.6% of cases, schools (1.3%), health care facilities (0.3%), and restaurants or food services (0.2%) (2).

Most cases reported to poison centers were managed in a non-HCF (68.7%), usually at the site of exposure, primarily the patient's own residence. Treatment in an HCF was rendered in 27.5% of cases. Of these, 16.5% were admitted for critical care, and 11.2% were admitted to a noncritical unit. Older age-groups exhibit a greater number of severe medical outcomes. Overall, the mortality rate was 0.11% of all exposures but much higher in hospitalized patients with suicidal overdose, who account for 32% of all deaths. In most of the fatal cases in adolescents and adults, poisoning was intentional. Because most poisoning fatalities occur before the patients reach an HCF, it is probable that the total number of fatalities resulting from poisoning is higher than that gathered by the AAPCC report. Extracorporeal treatments were used in 2,385 cases of poisoning; 97.5% of these were hemodialysis and 2.6 % were hemoperfusion (2).

The approach to diagnosis and treatment of poisoned individuals is usually divided into six stages. These include stabilization, laboratory assessment, decontamination of the gastrointestinal tract, administration of specific antidote if available, enhancing the elimination of the offending agent, and disposition. In this chapter, I will focus on the appropriate use of extracorporeal methods of elimination of common types of poisons.

PRINCIPLES OF MANAGEMENT OF POISONING

Diagnosis of Poisoning

In order to establish the correct diagnosis of poisoning, a systematic approach to the management of poisoned individuals must be followed. This should include careful history, physical examination, routine, and toxicologic laboratory evaluations (**FIGURE 36.1**). Moreover, particular attention should be paid to the clinical course of the patient's condition. The history is clearly of critical importance and should include the time, route of administration, duration, and intent of exposure. The exact name and amount of the drug, chemical, or ingredient involved; the time of onset, nature, and severity of symptoms; and the medical and psychiatric history should also be obtained. Unfortunately, it may not be possible to obtain this information from the victim who may be confused, comatose, unable, or unwilling to admit to self-poisoning. Under these circumstances, relevant history may be obtained from family or friends, paramedics, police, or other physicians. Sometimes, a search of the patients' belongings and residence may reveal a suicidal note or a container of drugs or chemical. Of critical importance is to establish, if possible, the timing of the exposure since this may have implications on the onset of symptoms and the patient's clinical course. It is also important to establish the reason behind the exposure and whether the exposure was a suicide attempt (3). Physical *examination* should focus initially on the vital signs, cardiopulmonary system, rate and depth of breathing, and neurologic status. Moreover, examination of the eyes for nystagmus, pupil size, and reaction; abdomen for bowel activity; and skin for color, dryness, temperature, and presence of medication patches may reveal findings of diagnostic value. It is also crucial to perform frequent reexamination since the physical findings may change rapidly and patients may abruptly deteriorate. Routine laboratory tests should include complete blood count, chemistries, and arterial blood gases. Other blood tests should be obtained for suspected drugs or toxins in which blood concentration will not only help to confirm exposure but also help to predict toxicity and guide the approach for definitive therapy (**FIGURE 36.1**).

General Treatment Measures

Administration of appropriate treatment for the patient with poisoning should be done without delay (**TABLE 36.1**). In fact, diagnosis and treatment may have to be done sequentially or simultaneously, depending on the patient's clinical course. Aggressive supportive care is of utmost importance and should follow the ABCs of emergency care; airway, breathing, and circulation for all poisoned victims in order to ensure adequate respiration; stable hemodynamics; and maintenance of fluid, electrolyte, and acid–base balance. These supportive measures have been shown to reduce mortality and morbidity to very low levels (3–6). The recognition of the critical role of supportive care in the treatment of poisoning has led to important changes in our approach to managing poisoning. *First*, abandonment of the use of stimulants (when the offending agent is a sedative). *Second*, reduced emphasis on the use of antidotes, except in a few special types of intoxications for which specific antidotes are available (**TABLE 36.2**). *Third*, decontamination which refers to preventing or reducing absorption of the suspected substance has also evolved over time. Gastric lavage, ipecac or cathartics, once mainstay of therapy of poisoning, have been questioned and deemed inappropriate since they may increase rather than reduce absorption and may even be harmful (7–12). However, administration of activated charcoal in an awake patient with intact airways may be used to enhance the elimination of ingested toxins (13). This adsorbent can be administered by mouth or by nasogastric intubation, preferably within 1 hour of ingestion and even before the identity of the toxic agent is known because of its capacity to bind a wide variety of toxins. However, activated charcoal does not bind lithium, heavy metals, or toxic alcohols. Multiple-dose activated charcoal (MDAC) can be administered over several hours in

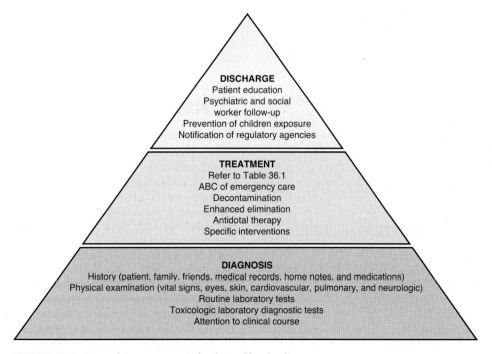

FIGURE 36.1 Approach to management of patients with poisoning.

TABLE 36.1	Management Strategies for Patients with Poisoning

1. Stabilization (supportive care)
- Admission to intensive care unit
- Secure airways:
  - Oxygenation and/or ventilation
  - Prevention of aspiration
- Treatment of cardiac arrhythmias
- Hemodynamic support
- Control of seizures
- Correction of temperature abnormalities

2. Laboratory assessment
- Complete blood count
- Serum electrolytes, calcium, and phosphorus
- Renal function including urinalysis
- Liver function tests
- Coagulation tests
- Arterial blood gases
- Calculation of anion and osmolar gaps
- Measurement of serum drug level
- Chest x-ray
- ECG

3. Decontamination
- Gastrointestinal decontamination
  - Gastric evacuation by lavage
  - Absorbents such as activated charcoal
  - Catharsis or whole bowel irrigation
- Decontamination of the eyes and skin

4. Administration of antidotes
- Neutralizing antibodies
- Chemical binding of toxins
- Antagonism of the physiologic or metabolic effects

5. Enhancement of elimination of the toxin
- Multiple-dose activated charcoal
- Forced diuresis
- Alkalinization of the urine
- Chelation
- Extracorporeal techniques
  - Peritoneal dialysis
  - Hemodialysis
  - Hemoperfusion
  - Hemofiltration
  - Plasmapheresis
  - Exchange transfusion
- Hyperbaric oxygen for carbon monoxide poisoning

6. Disposition
- Patient education
- Prevention of children exposure
- Notification of regulatory agencies
- Psychiatric evaluation
- Social worker counseling

ECG, electrocardiogram.

an attempt to enhance the elimination of a substance, such as carbamazepine and theophylline (3,14). By virtue of interrupting these toxin's enterohepatic circulation, activated charcoal is effective even when the toxin is no longer present in the stomach or, as in the case of theophylline, when the toxin has already been systemically absorbed. *Fourth*, use of "forced diuresis" which entails administration of large fluid volume coupled with a diuretic agent to ensure a urine flow rate of 3 to 6 mL/kg/h has been largely abandoned. This approach was previously popular because of the belief that it would accelerate the elimination of most intoxicants through the kidney. However, given the lack of evidence for the efficacy of forced diuresis in treatment of poisoning on the one hand, and its association with significant risk of volume overload, pulmonary edema, and electrolyte abnormalities on the other, forced diuresis is no longer recommended in the management of patients with suspected poisoning. *Finally*, alkalinization of the urine is employed to promote the elimination of toxins that are weak acids in patients who have adequate urine output and normal renal function. The basis for this approach is that renal tubular cell membranes are more readily permeated by the lipid-soluble nonionized form of the drug in question. Thus, increasing the urine pH will lead to increasing the ionized fraction of the substance which is lipid insoluble and thus cannot be reabsorbed and will be trapped in the renal tubular lumen and be excreted in the urine. Urine alkalinization is achieved by the administration of one ampule of sodium bicarbonate as a bolus followed by dextrose 5% in water (D5W) to which 100 to 150 mEq of sodium bicarbonate is added to each liter and infused at 150 to 250 mL/h. The goal is to have a urine pH >7.5 (15,16). This degree of urinary alkalinization was thought to be helpful in patients with exposure to drugs that are known to be excreted unchanged by the kidney, have low degree of protein binding, exist in a weakly acidic form, and are primarily distributed in the extracellular fluid compartment such as salicylate, phenobarbital, chlorpropamide, 2,4-dichlorophenoxyacetic acid, diflunisal, fluoride, mecoprop, and methotrexate (15,16). Urinary acidification for weak bases, such as phencyclidine or amphetamines, should not be done due to risk of rhabdomyolysis and acute kidney injury (AKI) (17). Hemodialysis and other extracorporeal methods are commonly used for removal of toxins, particularly in patients with severe acid–base or electrolyte disorders, even when the nature of the toxic agent is not known.

EXTRACORPOREAL TREATMENT OF POISONING

Available Extracorporeal Methods

Extracorporeal treatments (ECTRs) were required in 0.1% of all intoxications in the United States (1). Although the number may represent a small fraction of all toxic exposures, nephrologists are routinely consulted to help in the management of poisoned victims. The basis for their role in this clinical setting is fourfold. First, drugs and toxins may affect the renal function directly or through their effects on renal hemodynamics leading to AKI. Second, poisons may lead to serious clinical consequences such as acid–base and electrolyte abnormalities for which nephrologists are asked to manage. Third, the realization that poisons can be cleared from the body either by the kidney or by the use of extracorporeal techniques. Finally, their expertise in the dialysis procedure and presumed knowledge in the use of extracorporeal methods for enhancing toxins elimination.

The rationale for the application of extracorporeal techniques in the treatment of acute intoxication lies in their ability to increase the

TABLE 36.2	**Common Emergency Antidotes**		
Poison	**Antidote**	**Adult Dosage**	**Mechanism/Comment**
Acetaminophen	N-acetylcysteine	140 mg/kg initial oral dose, followed by 70 mg/kg q4h for 17 doses or IV as 150 mg/kg × 1 h then 50 mg/kg over 4 h then 100mg/kg over 16 h	Most effective within 16 h; may be useful after 24 h
Atropine, anticholinergics	Physostigmine	Initial dose: 0.5–2 mg (IV); children: 0.02 mg/kg	Cholinesterase inhibitor that antagonizes central and peripheral nervous system effects. May cause convulsions, bradycardia, and a systole
Benzodiazepines	Flumazenil	0.2 mg (2 mL) (IV) over 15 s; repeat 0.2 mg (IV) as necessary; initial dose not to exceed 1 mg	Recommended only for reversal of pure benzodiazepine sedation
β-Blockers	Glucagon	1 mg/mL ampoule; 5–10 (IV) initially	Stimulates cyclic adenosine monophosphate synthesis; increases myocardial contractility
Calcium channel blockers	Calcium chloride 10%	1 g (10 mL) (IV) over 5 min as initial dose; repeat as necessary to restore blood pressure	Each syringe contains 1 g or 10 mL of 10% calcium chloride; each milliliter contains 100 mg of calcium chloride or 1.4 mEq of calcium; used for hypotension, bradyarrhythmias
Carbon monoxide	Oxygen	1–3 atm	Hyperbaric oxygen in critical patients
Cyanide	Amyl nitrate Sodium nitrite	Administer pearls every 2 min. Adult: 10 mL of 3% solution over 3 min (IV). Child: 0.33 mL (10 mL 3% solution)/kg over 10 min	Methemoglobin-cyanide complex cause hypotension; dosage assume normal hemoglobin.
	Sodium thiosulphate	Adult: 25% solution 50 mL (IV) over 10 min. Child: 1.65 mL/kg	Forms harmless sodium thiocyanates
Digitalis	Digibind-FAB antibodies (antigen-binding fragments)	IV dose of Digibind in critical patient with unknown ingestion; 800 mg (20 vials); dosage if serum digoxin and patient's weight (in kg) are known: the number of vials to administer = [concentration (in ng/mL) × 5.6 × kg]/600	IV dose of Digibind should be equimolar to total body load of digoxin; one vial of Digibind contains 40 mg of FAB fragments, which neutralize 0.6 mg of digoxin; the number of milligram of digoxin ingested divided by 0.6 is the number of vials required; indicated for life–threatening cardiac arrhythmias, hyperkalemia, serum digoxin level >10 ng/mL in adults or 4 ng/mL in children
Hydrofluoric acid	Calcium	Topical exposure: Apply calcium gluconate gel or calcium carbonate paste; 10% calcium gluconate 10 mL in 40 mL D5W via intraarterial infusion over 4 h may be indicated for significant digital hydrofluoric acid burns. Ingestion: 10% calcium gluconate (IV)	An intraarterial infusion of 10 mL 10% calcium gluconate (1 syringe) provides 4.65 mEq (84 mg) of elemental calcium to bind fluoride ion, preventing cellular injury and tissue necrosis. Monitor for hypokalemia and treat electrolytes.
Iron	Deferoxamine mesylate	Initial dose: 40–90 mg/kg (IV or IM), not to exceed 1 g. Infusion: 15 mg/kg/h (IV)	Deferoxamine mesylate forms renally excretable ferrioxamine complex; IV route to be used in patients with shock
Lead	Dimercapto-succinic acid (succimer)	10 mg/kg/dose, bid × 28 days 35–50 mg/kg/dose (maximum 1.0–1.5 g), bid or as a continuous infusion	Monitor liver function tests; add BAL if lead level >70 μg/dL in children, and >100 μg/dL in adults.
Mercury, arsenic, gold	BAL (Dimercaprol)	4–6 mg/kg (IM), every 4–8 h	Each milliliter of BAL has dimercaprol, 100 mg, in 210 mg (21%) benzyl benzoate and 680 mg peanut oil; forms stable, nontoxic, excretable cyclic compound; contraindicated if patient has peanut allergy
Methyl alcohol, ethylene glycol	Ethyl alcohol	500 mg/kg of 10% ethanol, then continuous infusion of 100 mg/kg/h	Watch for hypomagnesemia, hypothermia, and lethargy in children. Maintain serum ethanol concentration at 100 mg/dL.
	Fomepizole	15 mg/kg loading dose, 10 mg/kg every 12 h IV	

(continued)

TABLE
36.2   *(Continued)*

Poison	Antidote	Adult Dosage	Mechanism/Comment
Nitrites	Methylene blue	1–2 mg/kg of 1% solution (IV) over 5 min	Accelerates methemoglobin reductase system; often, exchange transfusion is needed for severe methemoglobinemia; can produce hemolysis in high dose Maximum dose: 7 mg/kg/d in adults; 4 mg/kg/d in children
Opiates, propoxyphene, diphenoxylate	Naloxone Nalmefene	Adults: 0.4–2.0 mg (IV or IM) Children: 0.01–0.1 mg/kg (IV or IM) Adults: 1 mg IV Child: 0.25 µg/kg IV	Larger doses may be necessary after sever overdose or overdose of propoxyphene. Antagonizes opiates via its higher for some receptors; naloxone has no respiratory depression.
Organophosphates, nerve carbamates exposure	Atropine Pralidoxime [2-PAM]	Adult: 0.50–2.0 mg IV Child: 0.05 mg/kg Adult: 1g IV then 500–1000 mg/h as needed Child: 15–40mg/kg then 15–40 mg/kg/h	Very large doses of atropine may be needed in sever agents, cases. Must be added to atropine if nicotinic or central symptoms are present
Tricyclic antidepressants	Sodium bicarbonate	1–2 ampules (IV) bolus or infusion	Administer if QRS interval is ≥100 msec; maintain serum pH at 7.45–7.55; avoid severe alkalosis. One ampule of 50 mL sodium bicarbonate contains 50 mEq $NaHCO_3$; IV bolus for life threatening cardiac arrhythmia

D5W, 5% dextrose in water; BAL, British anti-Lewisite; PAM, pyridine aldoxime methyl chloride.
Modified and adapted from Shannon MW. A general approach to poisoning. In: Shannon MW, Borron SW, Burns JM, eds. *Haddad and Winchester's Clinical Management of Poisoning and Drug Overdose.* 4th ed. Philadelphia, PA: WB Saunders, 2007:13–30.

clearance of the offending toxin. Thus, active removal of toxins from blood would markedly reduce the duration of exposure to toxins and reduce the morbidity and mortality associated with poisoning and overdose. An array of methods has been proposed and studied, both singly and in combination. These include intermittent hemodialysis (IHD), sustained low-efficiency dialysis (SLED), intermittent hemofiltration (IHF) and intermittent hemodiafiltration (IHDF), continuous renal replacement therapy (CRRT), hemoperfusion (HP), therapeutic plasma exchange (TPE), exchange transfusion, peritoneal dialysis (PD), albumin dialysis, cerebrospinal fluid (CSF) exchange, extracorporeal membrane oxygenation (ECMO), and emergency cardiopulmonary bypass (**Table 36.3**) (18). The use of an optimal method of extracorporeal removal of toxins is often based on clinical judgment and anecdotal reports rather than on evidence-based controlled trials

(18,19). A large body of work has emerged in this area and consists of theoretical considerations, *in vitro* and *in vivo* laboratory studies, and clinical observations ranging from large case series to anecdotal reports. However, in the selection of one method over the others, one must consider a number of factors that influence the removal of the toxin by these techniques (**Tables 36.4** and **36.5**). The following is a brief description of the methods used for removal of toxins.

Hemodialysis

HD is the most commonly used technique for extracorporeal removal of toxins. The principles governing toxin removal by HD are

TABLE
36.3   **Extracorporeal Treatments for Toxin Removal**

- Intermittent hemodialysis (IHD)
- Sustained low-efficiency dialysis (SLED)
- Intermittent hemofiltration (IHF) and intermittent hemodiafiltration (IHDF)
- Continuous renal replacement therapy (CRRT)
- Hemoperfusion (HP)
- Therapeutic plasma exchange (TPE)
- Exchange transfusion
- Peritoneal dialysis (PD)
- Albumin dialysis
- Cerebrospinal fluid exchange
- Extracorporeal membrane oxygenation (ECMO)
- Emergency cardiopulmonary bypass

TABLE
36.4   **Factors Affecting the Removal of Toxins by Extracorporeal Techniques**

Toxin-Related Factors	Extracorporeal Therapy–Related Factors
• Water soluble • Distributed in extracellular fluids • Low volume of distribution • Molecular weight (toxins <500 Da are better removed) • Low protein binding • Lipid solubility • Rebound (diffusibility from the intracellular compartment to extracellular compartment)	• High-efficiency dialyzer membrane • High-flux membrane • Large surface area of the dialyzer • High blood and dialysate flow rates • Time on extracorporeal treatment

From Shannon MW. A general approach to poisoning. In: Shannon MW, Borron SW, Burns JM, eds. *Haddad and Winchester's Clinical Management of Poisoning and Drug Overdose.* 4th ed. Philadelphia, PA: WB Saunders, 2007:13–30.

TABLE 36.5	Factors to Be Considered When Choosing between Urinary Alkalinization, Hemodialysis, Hemoperfusion, and Continuous Renal Replacement Therapy (CRRT)			
Urine Alkalinization	**Hemodialysis**	**Hemoperfusion**	**CRRT**
Toxin characteristics • Excreted unchanged by the kidney • Low degree of protein binding • Exist in a weakly acidic form • Have extracellular distribution	Toxin characteristics • Low molecular weight • Water solubility • Low protein binding	Toxin characteristics • High molecular weight • Lipid solubility • High protein binding • Low volume of distribution	Toxin characteristics • Slow release from tissues • Large volume of distribution
Patient characteristics • Normal renal function • Adequate urine output	Patient characteristics • Presence of kidney disease • Acid–base, electrolyte • Volume problems • Low platelet count	Patient characteristics • Hemodynamic instability	Patient characteristics • Critically ill • Hemodynamic instability
Examples • Tricyclic antidepressants • Phenobarbital • Salicylates	Examples • Lithium • Salicylate • Valproate • Theophylline • Methanol • Ethylene glycol	Examples • Theophylline • Phenobarbital • Glutethimide	Examples • Lithium • Salicylate • Valproate • Metformin • Acetaminophen • Ethylene glycol

essentially similar to those for treatment of uremia (19–23). HD is based mainly on the principle of diffusion. Because small solutes exhibit random molecular motion to a greater extent than larger solutes, the former solutes can diffuse through the semipermeable membrane more readily than the latter. Hence, the efficiency of dialysis in drug removal is inversely related, other things being equal, to the molecular size of the drug involved. The availability of the more permeable high-flux dialysis membranes will facilitate removal of toxins with larger molecular weights (MWs).

Drugs present in the circulation can be removed to a variable degree by HD depending on a number of factors (TABLE 36.4). These include the blood and dialysate flow rates; the physical and biologic characteristics of the offending agent such as a molecular size below the cutoff of the dialysis membrane, the volume of distribution (Vd) in the body, degree and affinity of protein binding, water or lipid solubility, state of ionization, and the physical characteristics of the dialyzer membrane [such as surface area, mass transfer area coefficient (KoA), porosity, electric charge, ability to adsorb the offending substance]; rate of ultrafiltration; and concentration gradient between blood and dialysate. For a solute that has a low MW, is not ionized, is water-soluble, and is not protein-bound, plasma dialyzer clearance can even exceed plasma flow rate and approximate blood-flow rate if that particular solute is readily equilibrated across the red cell membrane. Methanol is a drug that best exemplifies this model. Therefore, HD should be considered for poisoning resulting from toxins that have these favorable physical characteristics (TABLES 36.5 and 36.6). By contrast, HD may not be effective for removal of toxins that are lipid-soluble, protein-bound, or possess high MWs. However, the newer dialysis membranes have the capacity for removal of larger molecules and highly protein-bound poisons such as carbamazepine and phenytoin (24–27). TABLE 36.6 lists the various drugs that can be removed by HD.

There are a number of advantages for intermittent HD use in treatment of poisoning. HD services are now widely available, even in poorer countries, are relatively easy to use and of low cost, and are associated with lower complication rate when compared to other methods of extracorporeal techniques. HD also corrects concomitant electrolyte and acid–base abnormalities and removes excess fluid with ultrafiltration. Clearly, HD should be employed whenever the intoxicated patient suffers concurrently from kidney disease or has developed acid–base, electrolyte, or volume abnormalities that can be readily rectified by HD. Finally, given that it can be quickly prepared and that outcome may be dependent on prompt removal of the poison from the body, intermittent HD remains the treatment of choice for most poisonings worldwide. However, HD treatment should be adjusted to each patient's individual needs. Therefore, in hemodynamically unstable intoxicated patients, administration of physiologic saline, the use of bicarbonate-based dialysate, cool (e.g., 35°C) dialysate, and the use of vasoconstrictors such as midodrine are helpful. The composition of the dialysate should also be individualized. Therefore, a dialysate potassium concentration of 3 to 4 mEq/L is appropriate in the absence of hyperkalemia or hypokalemia. Similarly, the bicarbonate concentration in the dialysate should be adjusted according to the patient's acid–base balance. Therefore, dialysate bicarbonate level should be lowered in patients' with metabolic alkalosis but maintained at a high value in the presence of severe metabolic acidosis.

Hemoperfusion

This method is based on the adsorption of a poison to a sorbent-containing cartridge that is perfused by blood from a poisoned patient (28–30). The column is most commonly made from activated charcoal, but resins have also been used (28). As mentioned earlier, activated charcoal is an effective and commonly used oral agent for preventing gastrointestinal absorption of poisons. On the other hand, charcoal columns were used since the 1960s in HP to enhance elimination of poisons. Most commonly used HP cartridges are packed with 100 to 300 g of activated charcoal or an exchange resin and coated with a thin (0.05 mm), relatively porous semipermeable membrane. Adsorption occurs because of the hydrophobic properties of charcoal. HP can also be performed using commercially available resins which are made from heat-stable polymeric material in the form of cross-linked insoluble beads which can either be charged (e.g., Amberlite IRA-900) or uncharged, (e.g., Amberlite XAD-4) (24,30–32). The total amount of drug removed by HP is usually small and is not of great clinical consequence. However, although the extraction of highly protein-bound poisons is less than that for unbound poisons (33), studies using an adsorbent cartridge showed extraction ratios >80% when the proportion of protein-bound poison is <90% (30,34).

TABLE 36.6	**Representative Drugs Removed by Hemodialysis**

Alcohols
- Ethanol
- Ethylene glycol
- Isopropanol
- Methanol
- Analgesics
- Acetaminophen
- Colchicine
- Salicylates

Antibiotics and chemotherapeutic agents
- Amoxicillin
- Clavulanic acid
- Penicillin
- Ticarcillin
- Cefixime
- Cefuroxime
- Cephalexin
- Amikacin
- Gentamicin
- Kanamycin
- Neomycin
- Streptomycin
- Tobramycin
- Metronidazole
- Nitrofurantoin
- Sulfisoxazole
- Sulfonamides
- Tetracycline
- Imipenem
- Ciprofloxacin
- Acyclovir
- Isoniazid
- Ethambutol
- Didanosine
- Zidovudine
- Foscarnet
- Ganciclovir
- Cyclophosphamide
- 5-Flurouracil

Sedatives-anticonvulsants
- Butabarbital
- Pentobarbital
- Phenobarbital
- Carbamazepine
- Chloral hydrate
- Ethchlorvynol
- Glutethimide
- Meprobamate
- Primidone
- (Valproic acid)

Cardiovascular drugs
- Atenolol
- Captopril
- Enalapril
- Metoprolol
- Methyldopa
- Nadolol
- Procainamide
- Propranolol
- Sotalol
- Tocainide
- Solvents
- Acetone
- Camphor
- Thiols
- Toluene
- Trichloroethylene

Miscellaneous
- Lithium
- Theophylline
- Paraquat
- Aniline
- Boric acid
- Chromic acid
- Chlorates
- Diquat
- Thiocyanate

( ), not well removed.
Reprinted from Winchester JF. Active methods for detoxification. In: Shannon MW, Borron SW, Burns MJ, eds. *Haddad and Winchester's Clinical Management of Poisoning and Drug Overdose.* 3rd ed. Philadelphia, PA: WB Saunders, 1998:175–188, with permission.

Removal of many toxins is influenced by the affinity of the charcoal for the toxin and by how avid the toxin binds to plasma proteins (28,30,32,35). In HP cartridges, the semipermeable membrane is not designed to withstand pressure but rather to impede the release of the particulate matter from the sorbent into the circulation and to prevent or reduce the adherence of platelets and other formed elements of blood onto the sorbents. Consequently, this membrane is extremely thin and does not significantly restrict solute diffusion. The process of activation of the charcoal sorbent has lead to enormous increase in the total available surface area of the sorbent. However, despite the large adsorbent area, HP cartridges may become saturated after 4 to 8

hours and lose their efficiency over time, so that they may need to be replaced. Moreover, HP can be associated with several other potential complications including a 20% to 30% decrease in the blood platelet count, leukopenia, hypocalcemia, hypoglycemia, charcoal embolism, and hypothermia. However, the frequency of these complications was reduced with the use of albumin cellulose nitrate to coat charcoal. TABLE 36.7 lists the various drugs that can be removed by HP.

A frequently asked question is whether HD or HP is superior for treatment of poisoning. Early clinical experience with HP suggested that it was more effective than HD or PD for poison removal. However, recent studies have shown comparable results with the

TABLE 36.7	Representative Drugs and Chemicals Removed by Hemoperfusion

Barbiturates
- Amobarbital
- Butabarbital
- Hexobarbital
- Pentobarbital
- Quinalbital
- Secobarbital
- Thiopental
- Vinalbital

Nonbarbiturate hypnotics, sedatives and tranquilizers
- Carbromal
- Chloral hydrate
- Chlorpromazine
- (Diazepam)
- Diphenhydramine
- Ethchlorvynol
- Glutethimide
- Meprobamate
- Methaqualone
- Methsuximide
- Methyprylon
- Promazine
- Promethazine
- (Valproic acid)

Analgesics, antirheumatic
- Acetaminophen
- Acetylsalicylic acid
- Colchicine
- d-Propoxyphene
- Methylsalicylate
- Phenylbutazone
- Salicylic acid

Antimicrobials/anticancer
- (Adriamycin)
- Ampicillin
- Carmustine
- Chloramphenicol
- Chloroquine
- Clindamycin
- Dapsone
- Doxorubicin
- Gentamicin
- Isoniazid
- (Methotrexate)
- Thiabendazole
- (5-Fluorouracil)

Antidepressants
- (Amitriptyline)
- (Imipramine)
- (Tricyclics)

Plant and animal toxins, herbicides, insecticides
- Amanitin
- Chlordane
- Demeton sulfoxide
- Dimethoate
- Diquat
- Methylparathion
- Nitrostigmine
- (Organophosphate)
- Phalloidin
- Polychlorinated biphenyls
- Paraquat
- Parathion

Cardiovascular
- Digoxin
- Diltiazem
- (Disopyramide)
- Flecainide
- Metoprolol
- *N*-acetylprocainamide
- Procainamide
- Quinidine

Miscellaneous
- Aminophylline
- Cimetidine
- (Fluoroacetamide)
- (Phencyclidine)
- Phenols
- (Podophyllin)
- Theophylline
- Solvents, gases
- Carbon tetrachloride
- Ethylene oxide
- Trichloroethane
- Xylene
- Metals
- (Aluminium)*
- (Iron)*

( ), not well removed; ( )*, removed with chelation.

Reprinted from Winchester JF. Active methods for detoxification. In: Shannon MW, Borron SW, Burns MJ, eds. *Haddad and Winchester's Clinical Management of Poisoning and Drug Overdose*. 3rd ed. Philadelphia, PA: WB Saunders, 1998:175–188, with permission.

newer high-flux, high-efficiency dialyzers (36,37). **Tables 36.4** and **36.5** list the factors that should be considered when choosing between HD and HP as a treatment modality for poisoning. HP is preferred when the toxin is lipid-soluble or significantly protein-bound (36). Activated charcoal is capable of adsorbing and, thereby, extracting lipid-soluble substances much more efficiently than HD. On the other hand, HP does not contribute to the overall treatment of the patients with kidney disease and/or with acid–base, electrolyte, and fluid problems. Also, poisons with a large Vd are not likely to be efficiently removed by HP. Moreover, HP is associated with more frequent complications and higher cost, particularly since the cartridges need to be replaced regularly because of saturation. As a result, the number of HP reports has steadily declined during the last two decades (**Figure 36.2**). It should be noted that both HD and HP require the establishment of a vascular access and the administration of anticoagulants. However, anticoagulant-free HD can be performed by infusing 100 mL of physiologic saline into the dialyzer blood inlet every 30 minutes for short-duration HD.

The earlier discussion may not be applicable to those systems that employ sorbent cartridges that regenerate dialysate. These systems employ small volumes of dialysate, and the cartridges used do not effectively bind alcohols. Consequently, such systems are not indicated in the treatment of ethylene glycol, methanol, or isopropyl alcohol poisoning. Although the cartridge may adsorb salicylate or lithium, there are, to our knowledge, no published studies documenting the effectiveness of sorbent systems in these intoxications. Finally, sorbent-based systems are said to be efficacious in the treatment of theophylline intoxication, but, again, there are no published reports available on this subject.

Sustained Low-Efficiency Dialysis

This technique allows the use of conventional HD machines to perform slow, low-efficiency HD using both reduced dialysate and blood-flow rate (32,35,38,39). Conventional hemodialyzers are used with a reduced dialyzer blood-flow rate of 200 to 300 mL/min and a slower dialysate flow rate of 300 mL/min. Each treatment can last up to 6 to 12 hours daily (35,40). The relatively long treatment duration compensates for the low efficiency of the procedure. Because of the slow blood and dialysate flow rates, the procedure is better tolerated by critically ill patients with hemodynamic instability (35,39). It is conceivable that this method may serve as an adjunctive approach to conventional extracorporeal measures in the treatment of poisoning. Although SLED uses a higher dialysate flow rate than CRRT, small solute clearance is reportedly similar (39,41). However, one study showed that the daily clearance of lithium was higher with SLED than with CRRT (42). Unfortunately, there are only a limited number of reports in the literature that describe the use of SLED in poisoning.

Continuous Renal Replacement Therapy

CRRT includes several techniques that utilize convective transport alone or in combination with diffusive transport. These techniques include (a) continuous venovenous hemodialysis (CVVHD), (b) continuous venovenous hemofiltration (CVVH), and (c) continuous venovenous hemodiafiltration (CVVHDF). The continuous venovenous techniques have largely replaced continuous arteriovenous therapies. Hemofiltration involves the removal of an ultrafiltrate from the blood through the semipermeable membrane of a filter. This is usually accompanied by the simultaneous, appropriate replacement with a physiologic solution that resembles plasma. The efficiency of the procedure is related to the total volume exchanged. Ultrafiltration is based on the principle of convection, and ultrafiltration is obtained by the application of a transmembrane pressure gradient. For all solutes that can pass through the pores of a semipermeable membrane, the relatively larger solutes and their smaller counterparts all pass through the membrane at the same rate (43,44). On the other hand, hemodiafiltration involves

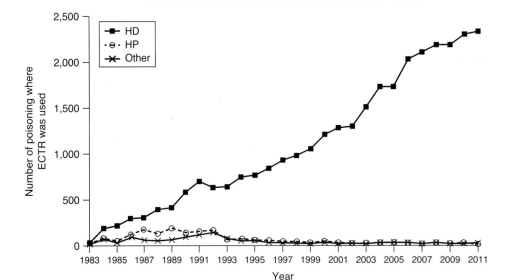

FIGURE 36.2 Temporal changes in the number of cases where hemoperfusion (HP) and hemodialysis (HD) were utilized in the treatment of poisoned patients in the United States. Data obtained from the annual reports of the American Association of Poison Control Centers' National Poison Data System (NPDS). (Reproduced with permission from Ghannoum M, Bouchard J, Nolin TD, et al. Hemoperfusion for the treatment of poisoning: technology, determinants of poison clearance, and application in clinical practice. *Semin Dial* 2014;27:350–361.)

simultaneous HD and hemofiltration using the same dialyzer/filter. The procedure is more efficient than either HD or hemofiltration alone in the removal of poisons that are small enough to pass through a semipermeable membrane (36,37,44).

These CRRT techniques were initially promoted as superior to HD in the treatment of poisoning, particularly those associated with lithium, valproic acid, and theophylline (22). However, there is no clear evidence for this assertion (20). CRRT has been proposed as effective in the removal of tissue-bound substances, such as paraquat, in which the offending agent is released slowly from its reservoir and associated with the occurrence of a "rebound phenomenon" (45). However, in most circumstances, the amount of drug removed is hampered by the slow rate of CRRT therapies. Moreover, since most toxins have a relatively small MW, they can be removed easily by HD. In most cases, the need for poison removal is urgent, and therefore, SLED and CRRT should not be used as first-line treatment. In CRRT, the blood and effluent flow rates are lower than during intermittent HD, and thus, clearance will be lower over a similar period of time (46). This has been shown to be true in methanol poisoning where the clearance is limited to <50 mL/min with CRRT compared with >200 mL/min with HD (47). Also, carbamazepine clearance is 3 times lower with CRRT compared with HD (48). However, CRRT can be used following conventional HD for treatment of poisoning with known tendency for rebound as in lithium intoxication, or they can be started as primary therapeutic modalities when hemodynamic instability militates against the use of conventional HD, hemofiltration, or hemodiafiltration (44). However, there is no clear evidence for a beneficial effect of CRRT or SLED in such circumstances (46).

Peritoneal Dialysis

PD allows the diffusion of toxins from mesenteric capillaries across the peritoneal membrane into the dialysate within the peritoneal cavity. In PD, clearance of solutes including poisons depends on the volume and number of exchanges, the peritoneal surface area, as well as the MW of the solute to be removed. In general, the clearance of solutes is quiet low in the range of 10 to 15 mL/min, and therefore, PD is not considered an effective technique for treatment of poisoning (19,49). In order to enhance clearance by PD, continuous flow peritoneal dialysis (CFPD) was developed. This technique requires the insertion of a dual-lumen PD catheter or two single-lumen catheters at opposite positions. A large volume of dialysate, up to 300 mL/min, is continuously exchanged in and out of the peritoneal cavity (50). Again, there is very limited data using this technique for removal of poisons. Therefore, PD is seldom used as a primary modality in the treatment of poisoning except in circumstances where the more efficient ECTRs are not available or cannot be performed.

Plasmapheresis or Exchange Blood Transfusion

TPE (plasmapheresis) is a process in which separation of plasma from the blood cellular components is archived by centrifugation or filtration. The volume of plasma removed during a single procedure is between 30 and 60 mL/min (51,52), and each treatment lasts 2 to 4 hours (53). The patient's plasma is replaced by other solutions such as fresh-frozen plasma, albumin, or crystalloid solution. On the other hand, exchange blood transfusion involves removal of the patient's own blood and replacing it with fresh blood. These procedures are not usually effective in the treatment of poisoning because of the limitations on the amount of plasma or of blood that

can be exchanged, especially in the case of toxins with large volumes of distribution (51,54,55). However, plasma exchange may be useful for removal of toxins that are highly protein-bound or have very low Vd. The American Society for Apheresis (ASFA) guidelines recommend an exchange volume of one to two total plasma volumes per day until clinical symptoms of poisoning have decreased and release of toxin from tissues is no longer significant (55). As of now, there are no clinical indications for the use of plasmapheresis in the treatment of poisoning and thus should be reserved for circumstances where alternative therapies are unavailable.

Albumin Dialysis

Albumin dialysis or extracorporeal liver assist devices (ELAD) includes the Molecular Adsorbent Recirculating System (MARS), the Prometheus system, and single pass albumin dialysis (SPAD) (56). With MARS, selective removal of albumin-bound substances can be achieved in a high-flux dialysis setting by the enrichment of dialysate with human albumin that functions as a molecular adsorbent. The albumin-enriched dialysate is then recirculated over sorbents. This novel dialytic approach has the theoretical advantage of enhancing elimination of protein-bound poisons in addition to excess water and water-soluble substances (57–59). With that in mind, this technique has been used successfully in anecdotal reports for the treatment of poisoning resulting from acetaminophen and cytotoxic mushrooms in the presence or absence of concomitant renal insufficiency (59,60). However, the role of albumin dialysis in poisonings remains unclear (61).

Clearance versus Drug Removal and Clinical Efficacy

A number of mathematical methods for describing the kinetics of drug removal during various extracorporeal techniques have been proposed in order to assess the efficacy of these techniques in achieving drug removal. During HD, the dialyzer clearance of a substance is defined as the volume of blood from which the substance is completely removed per unit time. If the drug concentrations in the blood entering and exiting the dialyzer and the rate of dialyzer blood flow rate are known, the dialyzer clearance of the drug can be calculated as follows (**EQUATION 36.1**):

$$C = QB (A - V) / A \qquad (36.1)$$

where

C = dialyzer clearance
QB = blood-flow rate through the dialyzer
A = the blood concentration of the drug at the blood inlet of the dialyzer
V = the blood concentration of the drug at the blood outlet of the dialyzer.

Alternatively, dialyzer clearance can be calculated by timed collection of spent dialysate from the dialysate outlet of a dialyzer and simultaneously obtaining arterial blood (or plasma) at the blood inlet at 30 seconds (62). Then the dialyzer clearance of a substance (in mL of blood or plasma/minute) will equal the amount of substance in mg collected in dialysate/arterial blood (or plasma) concentration of the substance in milligrams per milliliter.

Using either of these two methods, it can be shown that, given the proper drug characteristics and the use of appropriate dialyzers/ultrafilters or HP apparatus, drugs can be extracted from circulating blood with startling efficiency. In this example, the clearance of many toxins may approximate the blood-flow rate, and the extraction ratio may approach 100%; that is, drug concentration at the dialyzer/ultrafilter outlet may be close to zero.

Although these mathematical calculations imply that drugs are eliminated efficiently, thereby supporting the use of extracorporeal techniques for treatment of various intoxications, such an interpretation is not always accurate. An efficient extracorporeal procedure does not necessarily indicate that a clinically significant amount of intoxicant is being removed from the patient. This is because the total amount of drug removed depends, among several factors, on the apparent Vd of the toxin. A drug with a large Vd indicates that the substance is sequestered somewhere other than the vascular compartment such as the interstitial or intracellular fluid or bound to cellular proteins, cellular lipids, or cellular membranes. Under these circumstances, the extravascular distribution volume of the toxin results in slow release of the toxin into the vascular compartment. Such a scenario means that only a small fraction of the total amount of the toxin present in the body is accessible for removal by extracorporeal techniques during a given period of time. This is often the case with digoxin or tricyclic antidepressants poisoning. With these drugs, the largest amount of the ingested drug is not circulating but rather is bound to intracellular components; therefore, the total quantity of drug available for extraction from the blood is minimal. Even if one is successful in completely extracting the drug from the circulation in one treatment session by extracorporeal device, only a small fraction of the total body toxin load is removed. Therefore, efforts to remove the drug by extracorporeal techniques may be futile and may even be harmful putting in mind potential complications of the procedure and its cost. Moreover, the use of these techniques for removal of drugs with these characteristics may distract from implementing the full range of supportive measures the value of which vastly outweigh the possible minimal gain derived from the procedure (63–68).

⬡ CRITERIA FOR EXTRACORPOREAL TREATMENT OF POISONING

From the preceding discussion, it is clear that not every patient with poisoning is a candidate for ECTR. Therefore, in order to consider extracorporeal means of detoxification, one should determine that this modality will significantly augment toxin removal above that achieved by spontaneous elimination either by metabolism or by the native kidneys. Unfortunately, the indications for ECTR of poisoning are not well delineated since no randomized controlled trials have been conducted in patients with poisoning. However, the EXtracorporeal TReatments In Poisoning (EXTRIP) workgroup is developing recommendations on the use of ECTR for at least 16 poisons (69,70). In clinical practice, the following clinical and

toxicologic characteristics must be present before one can justify the use of extracorporeal techniques for toxin removal (**TABLE 36.8** and **FIGURE 36.3**) (69,71):

1. Progressive deterioration of the patient's condition thought to be related to the offending drug
   - Depression of the midbrain functions leading to hypoventilation, hypothermia, and hypotension
   - Development of coma, sepsis, or pneumonia
2. Blood levels indicating that the quantity (dose) of the drug ingested can lead to severe morbidity or mortality
3. Impairment of drug excretion by the concomitant presence of
   - Kidney disease or liver failure for drugs eliminated by the kidney or the liver, respectively
   - Ingestion or administration of "slow-release" drugs
   - Nausea or vomiting that prevents the administration of charcoal to effect drug removal from the gastrointestinal tract, especially in theophylline intoxication
4. The drug has been shown to be removed efficiently by the currently available extracorporeal techniques. This implies that the drug is not significantly bound to plasma proteins or lipids and that its molecular size, shape, and charge permit removal through dialyzer/ultrafilter membranes or by adsorption to sorbents.
5. The Vd of the drug is relatively small, implying that a large fraction of the drug is present in body water, from which it can be readily removed.
6. No effective and specific antidotes are available to reverse the effects of the toxin [e.g., in digoxin poisoning, the digoxin-specific antibody Fab fragment (Digibind) can be used].

With these criteria in mind, it becomes apparent that only few toxins can be effectively removed by extracorporeal techniques. Unfortunately, many of the toxins that account for a high percentage of total morbidity and mortality are not amenable to removal by extracorporeal techniques despite the high clearance rate achieved by extracorporeal techniques. Examples of such drugs and/or toxins include the following:

Tricyclic antidepressants. The tricyclic antidepressant (TCA) class of drugs is typified by a high Vd because of high lipid solubility. The fraction of drug available for extraction from the circulation is minuscule. The EXTRIP workgroup concluded that TCAs are not dialyzable and stated that ECTR is not recommended in severe TCA poisoning because poisoned patients with TCAs are not likely to have a clinical benefit from extracorporeal removal (72).

Barbiturates. The short-acting barbiturates are highly lipid-bound and poorly dialyzable. On the other hand, longer acting barbiturates,

TABLE 36.8	Clinical and Toxicologic Characteristics That Must Be Present Before Considering the Use of Extracorporeal Techniques for Toxin Removal

1. Progressive deterioration of the patient's condition that is thought to be related to the offending drug such as hypoventilation, hypothermia, and hypotension
2. Development of coma, sepsis, or pneumonia
3. Blood levels that indicate that the quantity of the drug ingested can lead to severe morbidity or mortality
4. Impairment of drug excretion by the concomitant presence of
   - Kidney disease or liver failure for drugs eliminated by the kidney or the liver, respectively
   - Ingestion or administration of "slow-release" drugs
   - Nausea or vomiting that prevents the administration of charcoal to effect drug removal from the gastrointestinal tract
5. The drug has been shown to be removed efficiently by the currently available extracorporeal techniques
6. The volume of distribution of the drug (Vd) is relatively small
7. No effective and specific antidotes are available to reverse the effects of the toxin

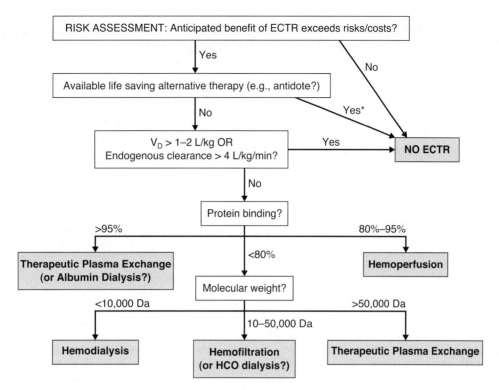

FIGURE 36.3 Stepwise approach for the initiation of extracorporeal techniques for enhanced elimination in a poisoned patients. ECTR, extracorporeal treatment. [Reproduced with permission from Ghannoum M, Roberts DM, Hoffman RS, et al. A stepwise approach for the management of poisoning with extracorporeal treatments. *Semin Dial* 2014;27(4):362–370.]

especially phenobarbital, are more water-soluble and therefore are efficiently removed by renal excretion and by HD. Alkalinization of the urine has been used to increase their rate of excretion. HP, although effective in removing circulating long-acting barbiturates, has not been proven to provide clinical benefits. HD is indicated in the patient intoxicated with long-acting barbiturates and who have poor renal function. The EXTRIP workgroup made four key recommendations. (a) The use of ECTR should be restricted to cases of severe long-acting barbiturate poisoning. (b) The indications for ECTR in this setting are the presence of prolonged coma, respiratory depression necessitating mechanical ventilation, shock, persistent toxicity, or increasing or persistently elevated serum barbiturate concentrations despite treatment with MDAC. (c) Intermittent HD is the preferred mode of ECTR, and MDAC treatment should be continued during ECTR. (d) Cessation of ECTR is indicated when clinical improvement is apparent (73).

Acetaminophen. Acetaminophen overdose is one of the most common agents leading to patients' death. Unfortunately, it is not efficiently extracted by extracorporeal procedures. Early and prolonged use of *N*-acetylcysteine (NAC) remains the therapy of choice (74). The EXTRIP workgroup agreed that acetaminophen is dialyzable but recommended ECTR only in patients with excessively large overdoses who display features of mitochondrial dysfunction manifested by early development of altered mental status and severe metabolic acidosis prior to the onset of hepatic failure. They suggested that IHD is the preferred ECTR modality in acetaminophen poisoning (75).

Narcotics and "street" drugs. A common cause of overdose and death, narcotics and other street drugs are not amenable to extraction by extracorporeal techniques. Opium antagonists and supportive therapy are the mainstays of treatment.

Nonbarbiturate hypnotics, sedatives, and tranquilizers. Many of these drugs cause little morbidity and mortality, even in apparently severely intoxicated patients. Furthermore, they all display a high apparent Vd and lipid solubility and therefore are not removed well by extracorporeal means.

Other miscellaneous toxins. This group includes paraquat, amanita mushroom toxin, and methotrexate. Contrary to some opinions and anecdotal reports, there is little evidence that extracorporeal techniques are clinically effective for the treatment of poisonings resulting from these toxins. However, because paraquat and *N*-acetyl procainamide (NAPA) are tightly tissue bound and released slowly, it has been proposed that CRRT may be efficacious (16,67). Although clinical case reports have suggested that patients suffering from life-threatening NAPA intoxication could be helped with the various extracorporeal measures, their effectiveness remains debatable (67). **TABLE 36.9** lists some agents for which various extracorporeal methods should be used for treatment of acute intoxications.

POISONING FROM TOXIC ALCOHOLS

The term *alcohol* usually implies ethyl alcohol, the predominant alcohol in alcoholic beverages. However, alcohol also includes any hydroxyl derivative of a hydrocarbon. Methanol is the simplest primary alcohol that can be produced by distillation of wood. It is used in paints, windshield washer fluid, solvents and thinners, plastics, synthetic textiles, as antifreeze, and as a fuel. Ethylene glycol is an organic compound primarily used as a raw material in polyester fibers and fabric industry, and polyethylene terephthalate resins in bottling, and is also used in other applications such as antifreeze.

TABLE 36.9	Toxic Agents for which Extracorporeal Methods Have Been Shown to Have Clinical Effectiveness and Their Main Pharmacologic Characteristics[a]			
Toxic Agent	**Molecular Weight**	**Protein Binding (%)**	**Vd**	**Toxic Levels[b]**
Ethylene glycol	62	—	0.6	unknown
Methanol	32	—	0.6	50 mg/dL
Isopropanol	60	—	0.6	400 mg/dL
Ethanol	46	—	0.6	450 mg/dL
Salicylate	138	60–90[c]	0.2	800–1,500 mg/dL
Lithium	7	—	0.8	2.5 mEq/L
Theophylline	180	40–60[c]	0.5	60 mg/mL

Vd, volume of distribution.

Modified from Garella S. Extracorporeal techniques in the treatment of exogenous intoxications. *Kidney Int* 1988;33:735–740, with permission.

[a]Please note that comments on the effectiveness of hemodialysis are not necessarily applicable to sorbent-based dialysate regeneration systems; these systems are not effective and not recommended for the treatment of ethylene glycol, methanol, or isopropyl alcohol poisonings. Furthermore, whereas the characteristics of the cartridges and/or some anecdotal reports suggest that they may be effective in the treatment of salicylate, lithium, and theophylline intoxication, no specific definitive studies documenting their effectiveness are available.

[b]Commonly accepted potentially lethal concentrations. These should be considered only as approximate guidelines, because toxicity is determined by a variety of clinical characteristics in combination with the serum concentration.

[c]Salicylate protein binding is highest at low (therapeutic) values and progressively lower with increasing (toxic) levels.

Both methanol and ethylene glycol are low MW, clear, and colorless alcohols. Methanol has an alcoholic taste, but ethylene glycol is sweet. Methanol and ethylene glycol are toxic alcohols that can result in serious morbidity and mortality. Accidental or intentional ingestion of these alcohols may result in blindness, renal dysfunction, chronic brain injury, or death (76). Factors associated with increased mortality include large osmolal gap, anion gap, and low pH <7.22. However, pH <7.22 has the highest predictive value for mortality (77). Methanol and ethylene glycol constitute medical emergencies for which early diagnosis and treatment may be lifesaving. Most of the toxicity related to methanol and ethylene glycol are related to their metabolites such as formate for methanol and oxalate and glycolate for ethylene glycol. The introduction of fomepizole as a competitive inhibitor of alcohol dehydrogenase has revolutionized treatment of toxic alcohol poisonings.

Ethylene glycol and methanol poisoning are common, but ethylene glycol poisoning is very rare in mid- and low-income countries compared to high-income countries. In 2009, there were 8,139 poisoning due to toxic alcohols in the United States. In general, poisoning with these alcohols in industrialized countries tends to be intentional in adults and accidental in children, while in developing world, it is often accidental. The minimum lethal dose for ethylene glycol is commonly cited as 100 mL or 1 to 1.5 mL/kg but also with considerable variability (76).

METHANOL POISONING

Methanol, also known as wood alcohol, is a clear, colorless, low MW alcohol commonly found in a variety of products including industrial solvents, windshield wiper fluid, windshield deicer, antifreeze, stains, dyes, varnish, shellac, canned fuel (Sterno), as well as an alternate fuel (76). Methanol poisonings most often occur from the ingestion of "moonshine" liquor (78) as well as from ingestion of windshield washer fluid but can also arise from its dermal application or inhalation. Because methanol (MW = 32 Da) possesses inebriating qualities similar to those of ethanol, is inexpensive, and widely available, it has been responsible for large outbreaks of poisoning (79–81). In the United States, during the years 2000 to 2013, there were 30,395 methanol exposures, 85,891 ethylene glycol exposures, and 3,235 combined exposures (82). Most of the exposures that have been recorded were acute and were primarily due to unintentional exposures to windshield wiper fluid and other automotive products with 25% of these occurring among children younger than 12 years old (2).

Methanol is rapidly and completely absorbed from the gastrointestinal tract with peak plasma levels attained in 30 minutes to 1 hour. It can penetrate skin, and thus, there have been reported cases of poisoning by extensive dermal contact or inhalation (83,84). Methanol does not bind to protein and has an apparent Vd of approximately 0.6 to 0.7 L/kg. Only about 5% of ingested methanol is excreted unchanged in the urine; the rest is oxidized in the liver. Some methanol is also eliminated by the lungs. If untreated, the elimination half-life of methanol is 1 to 3 hours at low concentrations and approximately 24 hours at high concentration.

Methanol is initially metabolized by alcohol dehydrogenase to formaldehyde (**FIGURES 36.4** and **36.5**). This process occurs slowly and constitutes the rate-limiting step of this reaction. Formaldehyde is cytotoxic as it may be involved in causing blindness (85,86). However, it does not accumulate because it has a very short half-life of only 1 to 2 minutes and undergoes rapid conversion to formic acid (formate). Formic acid molecule dissociates into a hydrogen ion and a formate anion, which in turn is broken down via a folic acid–dependent pathway to carbon dioxide and water. The body has limited capacity to transform formic acid; thus, accumulation of this toxin may occur increasing the susceptibility to its toxicity. The released hydrogen ion from formic acid lowers the pH of body fluids causing acidosis. In addition to formic acid, lactic acid also contributes to the severe metabolic acidosis (76,85,87). Because the first step of methanol metabolism depends on the action of alcohol dehydrogenase, which has a 10-fold greater affinity for ethanol or fomepizole than for methanol, these compounds are currently used as antidotes in the therapy of methanol poisoning (see section "Treatment"). The same mechanism explains the prolongation of the half-life of methanol to more than 30 hours (compared with the normal of 12 to 20 hours) in patients who had ingested both methanol and ethanol at the same time (88). Oxidation of methanol, like that of ethanol, proceeds independently of the serum concentration but at a rate of only 15% of that of ethanol. Thus, complete oxidation and excretion

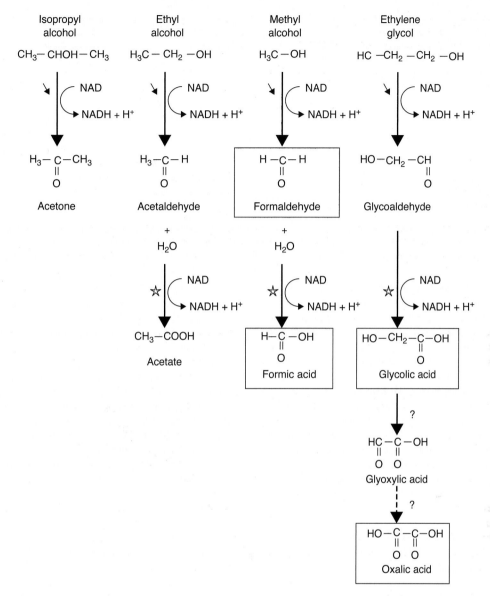

FIGURE 36.4 Pathways of metabolism of the four alcohols that most commonly cause intoxication. Alcohol dehydrogenase (*bold arrow*) is the cytosolic enzyme responsible for the first oxidative step in all four alcohols. Aldehyde dehydrogenase (*star*) is the mitochondrial enzyme responsible for catalyzing the second oxidative step in ethanol, methanol, and ethylene glycol. The main products of metabolism responsible for toxicity are enclosed in boxes. Question marks denote metabolic steps where there is uncertainty on the specific enzymes involved and on the generation of $NADH+H^+$. Note that oxalic acid represents only a small fraction of the metabolites of ethylene glycol and that other metabolites are not shown in the figure. (From Garella S. Extracorporeal techniques in the treatment of exogenous intoxications. *Kidney Int* 1988;33:735–740, with permission.)

of methanol usually requires several days which also explains the delay in the onset of toxic manifestations (84).

Clinical Picture and Laboratory Data

The clinical manifestations of methanol poisoning depend on the amount ingested, the elapsed time since ingestion, and whether there was coingestion of ethanol or other toxic substances (76). The clinical course of methanol toxicity is characterized by three distinctive stages and involves the central nervous system (CNS), the eyes, and the gastrointestinal system (**TABLE 36.10**) (88–90). An initial and fairly brief stage is characterized by CNS depression

in which the patient appears intoxicated; manifestations largely due to the effects of the parent compound. This is followed by a latent stage of 6 to 30 hours during which the patient may be asymptomatic except for blurred vision. This asymptomatic stage is followed by a third stage in which formic acid accumulates and more serious toxicity develops. Formic acid is directly toxic to the retina, and therefore, visual manifestations of methanol poisoning tend to develop rapidly (91). These manifestations include central scotoma, blurred vision, decreased visual acuity, photophobia, and progression to complete blindness. Examination reveals decreased papillary response to light and visual field defects. Later on, the

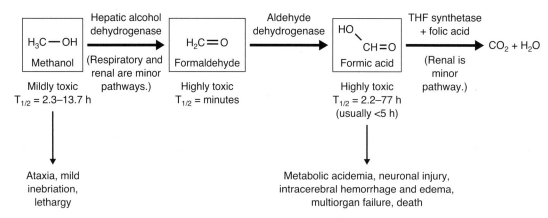

FIGURE 36.5 Metabolic biotransformation and clinical manifestations of methanol. (Modified and reproduced with permission from Roberts DM, Yates C, Megarbane B, et al. Recommendations for the role of extracorporeal treatments in the management of acute methanol poisoning: a systematic review and consensus statement. *Crit Care Med* 2015;43:461–472.)

patient develops fixed dilated pupils, hyperemia of the optic disc, papilledema, and optic atrophy (91,92). The CNS manifestations include headache, vertigo, delirium, restlessness, and confusion. These may progress to seizures, coma, and death in severe methanol intoxication. The minimal lethal doses of methanol are not well established, but it is commonly estimated at 15 mL (76,93). In 10% to 20% of cases, hemorrhagic and nonhemorrhagic necrosis of the putamen can occur (94,95). Permanent blindness and parkinsonism are common sequelae among survivors (96). Indeed, acute Parkinson's syndrome was reported in several patients with severe methanol poisoning and was thought to result from acute hemorrhagic necrosis of the basal ganglia (96–98). Lastly, methanol poisoning commonly result in significant gastrointestinal manifestations such as nausea, vomiting, diarrhea, and abdominal pain (probably as a result of gastritis and/or pancreatitis).

TABLE 36.10	Clinical and Laboratory Manifestations of Methanol Intoxication

Symptoms	Physical Findings	Laboratory Findings
First stage, <6 h • Mild and transient • Inebriation and drowsiness	Nonspecific	• May have high methanol level • Osmolal gap (31 mOsm/ 100 mg/dL)
Second stage • Asymptomatic • Blurred vision	Nonspecific	• May have high methanol level • Osmolal gap (31 mOsm/ 100 mg/dL)
Third stage, 6–30 h • Vertigo • Abdominal pain • Vomiting • Restlessness • Dyspnea • Blurred vision, blindness • Seizures, opisthotonus • Coma, death	• ± Kussmaul respiration • Papilledema, hyperemia of discs	• Metabolic acidosis • High anion gap • High formate levels • High lactate levels • Increased serum amylase • Increased mean corpuscular volume

Laboratory findings include increased serum amylase value, high anion gap metabolic acidosis, and elevated serum formate and lactate levels. The increased lactate values are, as in the case of ethylene glycol intoxication, most likely the result of both an increased nicotinamide adenine dinucleotide (NADH/NAD) ratio and a reduction in tissue perfusion. A high osmolal gap may be also apparent. Methanol contributes 31 mOsm/kg for each 100 mg/dL; therefore, a sizable osmolal gap is more likely to be present in the initial stages of the intoxication before the alcohol is metabolized. Other abnormal laboratory tests include an increased erythrocyte mean corpuscular volume attributed to a toxic effect of formaldehyde on cellular ion transport.

The quantity of ingested methanol that is required to cause serious morbidity and mortality is highly variable. While some patients may develop severe complications following the ingestion of a few milliliters of methanol, others survive the ingestion of several hundred milliliters. In addition, the serum concentration of methanol does not correlate well with the severity of the clinical picture or with prognosis (88,89). However, there are a number of findings that indicate poor prognosis (76,99). These include dyspnea and Kussmaul's respiration, which result from severe metabolic acidosis. Moreover, blindness, seizures, coma, elevated formic acid level, bradycardia, and hypotension also indicate poor prognosis (97,98). Respiratory failure is the most common cause of death in methanol poisoning. Untreated methanol poisoning is associated with death in 28% and visual deficits or blindness in 30% in survivors (78).

Laboratory Diagnosis of Methanol Intoxication

Measurements of plasma or serum methanol concentration using colorimetric or enzymatic assays can provide confirmation of toxic exposure to methanol. Unfortunately, these quantitative assays for methanol are not available in most hospitals. Even when these are available, results must be interpreted with caution. Plasma osmolality increases in proportion to the concentration of methanol or ethylene glycol, and its measurement provides a clue to ingestion of these agents if the result is abnormally high. The serum osmole gap provides a simple screening method of checking for increased osmolality that is not explained by other factors. An increased serum osmole gap in conjunction with a normal serum anion gap and absence of metabolic acidosis is frequently seen early after ingestion of methanol or ethylene glycol, before significant metabolism of methanol to formate or ethylene glycol to glycolate.

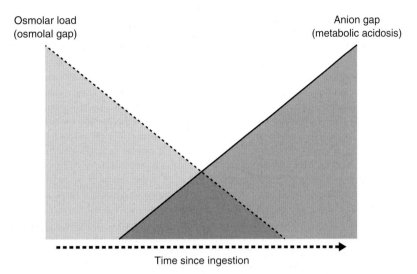

FIGURE 36.6 Schematic demonstrating the relationship between osmolal gap and anion gap in toxic alcohol poisoning. [Reproduced with permission from Mycyk MB, Aks SE. A visual schematic for clarifying the temporal relationship between the anion and osmol gaps in toxic alcohol poisoning. *Am J Emerg Med* 2003;21(4):333–335.]

However, as methanol and ethylene glycol are metabolized, their plasma concentrations decrease, and thus, their contribution to plasma osmolality and the osmolar gap also decrease (100,101). Consequently, if the patient presents after most of these alcohols have been metabolized, the serum osmolar gap may well have returned to normal despite the presence of lethal concentrations of their toxic metabolites (**Figure 36.6**). Nonetheless, metabolic acidosis develops, and the anion gap progressively increases, signifying accumulation of the toxic metabolites. The metabolic acidosis of methanol and ethylene glycol poisoning is often very severe with dangerously low blood pH as well as extremely high serum anion gap. Blood lactate levels are occasionally increased in both methanol and ethylene glycol poisoning. This may be due to use of $NAD+$ and excess accumulation of $NADH$ from the metabolism of methanol or ethylene glycol which raises the $NADH$ to $NAD+$ ratio, leading to increased transformation of pyruvate to lactate in order to replenish $NAD+$ (102). Other factors may also contribute to lactic acidosis including shock, hypoxia, and seizures. In methanol intoxication, plasma formate levels correlate with blood pH and serum anion gap (89,100,102). Other laboratory abnormalities that can be seen include hypocalcemia, increased serum amylase, and thrombocytopenia.

Treatment

Supportive care should be directed at stabilizing the airways and correcting ventilatory and circulatory disorders. Concomitantly, other interventions should be instituted with the aim to, first, correct metabolic acidosis; second, prevent other serious complications by limiting the accumulation of the toxic metabolites of methanol; and third, removal of methanol and its byproducts such as formic acid. Metabolic acidosis should be treated with intravenous (IV) infusion of sodium bicarbonate. Seizures are managed primarily with parenteral benzodiazepines. Gastrointestinal drainage can be attempted but is usually ineffective because of the rapid absorption of methanol (88,90,103,104). Folic acid administered as 50 mg IV every 4 hours for five doses then once daily may be helpful as it has been shown to increase the metabolism of formic acid to carbon dioxide and water (87,105). As with chronic ethanol use, routine

administration of thiamine to patients with known or suspected toxic alcohol ingestion may be justified (76).

In addition to the aforementioned supportive therapy, aggressive treatment must be started promptly when there is a reasonable suspicion of significant methanol intoxication. The prompt administration of inhibitors of alcohol dehydrogenase enzyme such as ethanol or fomepizole is very effective in preventing the development of metabolic acidosis by markedly decreasing the oxidative metabolism of methanol (87,90,106). Fomepizole was approved in the United States for the treatment of ethylene glycol poisoning in 1997 and in 2000 for methanol toxicity. Indications for starting IV ethanol or fomepizole administration include (a) documented recent history of ingestion of more than 0.4 mL/kg body weight of methanol; (b) a serum methanol level greater than 6 mmol/L (20 mg/dL); (c) osmolar gap greater than 10 mOsm/kg H_2O; and (d) history or strong clinical suspicion of methanol poisoning and at least two of the following findings: arterial pH <7.3, a serum bicarbonate level <20 mEq/L, or an osmolar gap >10 mOsm/kg H_2O (88,90,97) (**Table 36.11**). Ethanol administration, both oral and IV, has been used for years as an antidote for both methanol and ethylene

TABLE 36.11	Indications for Use of Fomepizole or Ethanol in Methanol Poisoning

1. Documented recent history of ingestion of toxic amounts of methanol and an osmolar gap of >10 mOsm/L
2. Strong clinical suspicion of methanol poisoning and at least two of the following criteria:
   A. Arterial pH <7.3
   B. Serum bicarbonate <20 mEq/L
   C. Osmolal gap >10 mOsm/kg
3. Plasma methanol concentration ≥6.2 mmol/L (20 mg/dL)

Modified from Barceloux DG, Bond GR, Krenzelok EP, et al. American Academy of Clinical Toxicology practice guidelines on the treatment of methanol poisoning. *J Toxicol Clin Toxicol* 2002;40:415–446; and Barceloux DG, Krenzelok EP, Olson K, et al. American Academy of Clinical Toxicology practice guidelines in the treatment of the ethylene glycol poisoning. *Clin Toxicol* 1999;37:537–560.

glycol poisoning. The basis for ethanol therapy is that both alcohol dehydrogenase and aldehyde dehydrogenase, along with nicotinamide cofactors are involved in the metabolism of both ethanol and methanol. In this reaction, ethanol is converted to acetaldehyde then to acetic acid, while methanol is converted to formaldehyde then to formic acid. Acetaldehyde is less toxic than formaldehyde, and acetic acid is essentially nontoxic, while formic acid has substantial toxicity (76). The two alcohols compete for the active sites on these two enzymes. However, the affinity of alcohol dehydrogenase for ethanol is far greater than for methanol or ethylene glycol. Thus, in presence of ethanol plus either methanol or ethylene glycol, there preferentially metabolizes ethanol and impedes that of methanol of ethylene glycol allowing time for these alcohols to be slowly excreted by the lungs and kidneys or to be slowly metabolized (107). For ethanol, a serum or blood alcohol concentration in the range of 100 to 150 mg/dL (22 to 33 mmol/L) is recommended in order to fully inhibit alcohol dehydrogenase (76). However, fomepizole, which is also a competitive inhibitor of alcohol dehydrogenase, has several advantages over ethanol and is now the preferred antidote for methanol poisoning (76,106). The doses of ethanol or of fomepizole used are similar to those recommended for ethylene glycol poisoning (90). TABLE 36.12 outlines the various dosing regimens for fomepizole before, during, and after the initiation of HD in patients with both methanol and ethylene glycol poisoning (90,104,108).

Unfortunately, ethanol or fomepizole does not completely prevent the formation of the methanol or ethylene glycol toxic metabolites. However, since these alcohols and their toxic metabolites are small molecules, they are readily dialyzable. Intermittent HD is the most effective means of removal of both methanol and formate with clearance rates of 125 to 215 and 203 mL/min, respectively (90,97,98). However, continuous modalities can be used as alternative therapeutic measures when conventional HD cannot be performed (87). HP using activated charcoal is ineffective.

HD can be critically important in patients with a significant delay between the time of ingestion and the time of administration of either ethanol or fomepizole, since significant amounts of formate or glycolate have already accumulated. The EXTRIP workgroup developed evidence-based consensus recommendations for ECTR indications in the management of methanol poisoning (TABLE 36.13) (87). HD should be performed with a bicarbonate bath because the alkali requirement may be massive due to the presence of severe metabolic acidosis associated with the intoxication (67). Methanol redistributes after discontinuation of the HD procedure and thus may result in rebound increase in

---

| TABLE 36.12 | **Fomepizole Administration for Treatment of Methanol or Ethylene Glycol Poisoning**[a] |

- Initiating dosing if patient is not on hemodialysis:
  - Give a loading dose of 15 mg/kg IV over 30 min
  - Give 10 mg/kg IV over 30 min every 12 h for four doses and then
  - Give 15 mg/kg IV over 30 min every 12 h until (a) the plasma toxin level is undetectable or (b) the plasma toxin level is <20 mg/dL, the arterial blood pH is within normal limits, and the patient is asymptomatic.

- On initiation of hemodialysis:
  - If <6 h have elapsed since the last dose, skip the next scheduled dose.
  - If >6 h have elapsed since the last dose, give the next scheduled dose (15 mg/kg) immediately.

- During ongoing hemodialysis:
  - Give 15 mg/kg IV over 30 min every 4 h.

- At time of stopping hemodialysis:
  - If <1 h has elapsed since the last dose, do not give a dose at the end of hemodialysis.
  - If 1–3 h have elapsed since the last dose, give a half-dose (7.5 mg/kg) at the end of hemodialysis.
  - If >3 h have elapsed since the last dose, give the next scheduled dose (15 mg/kg).

- Postdialysis dosing:
  - Beginning 12 h after the last dose, give 15 mg/kg IV over 30 min every 12 h until plasma toxin level is <20 mg/dL.

[a]Toxin level refers to methanol or ethylene glycol plasma concentration.
Reproduced with permission from Barceloux DG, Bond GR, Krenzelok EP, et al. American Academy of Clinical Toxicology practice guidelines on the treatment of methanol poisoning. *J Toxicol Clin Toxicol* 2002;40:415–446; Barceloux DG, Krenzelok EP, Olson K, et al. The American Academy of Clinical Toxicology practice guidelines in the treatment of ethylene glycol poisoning. *Clin Toxicol* 1999;37:537–560; and Jazz Pharmaceuticals. *Antizol-fomepizole injection, solution [package insert]*. Palo Alto, CA: Jazz Pharmaceuticals, 2006.

| TABLE 36.13 | **Role of Extracorporeal Treatment in the Treatment of a Patient with Methanol Poisoning** |

We recommend ECTR is initiated in the following circumstances:
1. Severe methanol poisoning (grade 1D), including any of:
   a. Coma (grade 1D)
   b. Seizures (grade 1D)
   c. New vision deficits (grade 1D)
   d. Metabolic acidosis from methanol poisoning
      i. Blood pH ≤7.15 (grade 1D)
      ii. Persistent metabolic acidosis despite adequate supportive measures and antidotes (grade 1D)
   e. Serum anion gap >24 mmol/L (grade 1D); calculated by serum [Na+] − [Cl−] − [HCO$_3^-$]
2. Serum methanol concentration
   a. >700 mg/L or 21.8 mmol/L in the context of fomepizole therapy (grade 1D)
   b. >600 mg/L or 18.7 mmol/L in the context of ethanol treatment (grade 1D)
   c. >500 mg/L or 15.6 mmol/L in the absence of an ADH blocker (grade 1D)
   d. In the absence of a methanol concentration, the osmolal/osmolar gap may be informative (grade 1D)
3. In context of impaired kidney function (grade 1D)

To optimize the outcomes from ECTR, we recommend:
4. Intermittent hemodialysis is the modality of choice in methanol poisoning (grade 1D). Continuous modalities are acceptable alternatives if intermittent hemodialysis is not available (grade 1D).
5. ADH inhibitors are to be continued during ECTR for methanol poisoning (grade 1D) as well as folic acid.
6. ECTR can be terminated when the methanol concentration is <200 mg/L or 6.2 mmol/L and a clinical improvement is observed (grade 1D).

ECTR, extracorporeal treatment; ADH, alcohol dehydrogenase.
Reproduced with permission from Roberts DM, Yates C, Megarbane B, et al. Recommendations for the role of extracorporeal treatments in the management of acute methanol poisoning: a systematic review and consensus statement. *Crit Care Med* 2015;43:461–472.

methanol levels which usually occurs within the 12- to 36-hour period after stopping HD. The same is true for formate necessitating prolonged HD as a therapeutic measure (109). Also, after HD, close monitoring of acid–base balance, osmolar gap, and electrolytes should be done every 2 to 4 hours for 12 to 36 hours during which fomepizole or ethanol therapy should be continued because rebound is unpredictable. Hypophosphatemia may occur in those patients who require prolonged and intensive dialysis sessions, especially in individuals who are normophosphatemic to begin with. As previously discussed, the addition of sodium phosphate salts to the dialysate (1.3 mmol/L of phosphorus in the dialysate) has been used successfully to prevent hypophosphatemia in such patients. HD must be continued until the serum methanol level is either undetectable or less than 25 mg/dL, there is no significant metabolic acidosis, and the osmolal gap becomes normal (76,88,90,97). The addition of ethanol to the dialysate has been advocated in patients with methanol poisoning in an attempt to maintain stable levels of ethanol during dialysis (110–112). Because of the possibility of intracerebral hemorrhage in methanol poisoning, dialysis should be performed with little or no anticoagulation (113).

⬡ ETHYLENE GLYCOL POISONING

Ethylene glycol (EG) poisoning may occur either as isolated single cases or as epidemics (114). The majority of clusters of EG poisoning resulted from preparing illicit beverages using EG to fortify or in place of ethanol. Cases of EG intoxication have also occurred because of contaminated water systems (115). The TESS data for the year 2005 indicate a total of 5,469 reported toxic exposures to EG resulting in 16 deaths and 176 life-threatening poisonings (116). In 2007, poison centers in the United States received reports of 5,731 possible EG exposures (117). However, because of underreporting, these data likely underestimate the total number of cases. Most (84%) of the poisonings were unintentional. More recently, a study reported that during the years 2000 to 2013, there were more than 85,000 EG exposures (82). Most of the exposures were acute and again were primarily due to unintentional exposures to windshield wiper fluid and other automotive products with 25% of these

occurring among children younger than 12 years old (2). Adults are typically exposed when they ingest EG as a cheap substitute for ethanol or in suicidal attempts. EG, also referred to as *sweet killer*, is an organic solvent commonly found in antifreeze preparations, deicers, coolants, brake and hydraulic fluids, and household cleaners. It is a sweet-tasting, viscous, colorless liquid with a molecular formula of $C_2H_6O_2$ and an MW of 62 Da (88,118). EG ingestion, like methanol, can also result in life-threatening poisoning. While ingestion is by far the most common route of poisoning, a recent case of transcutaneous diethylene glycol poisoning with severe AKI was reported (119).

Pharmacokinetics

EG is an alcohol that is rapidly absorbed from the gastrointestinal tract with peak serum concentrations 1 to 4 hours after ingestion. Being highly water-soluble and nonprotein-bound, it diffuses promptly through the total body water; its Vd is approximately 0.5 to 0.8 L/kg (120). The metabolism of EG is more complex than methanol. The liver metabolizes 80% of the absorbed EG in a stepwise NAD-dependent fashion (108,121,122). Alcohol dehydrogenase, the first enzyme in the pathway, oxidizes EG to glycoaldehyde and is competitively inhibited by both ethanol and fomepizole (**FIGURES 36.4** and **36.7**). Glycoaldehyde is then rapidly converted to glycolic acid. The next step involves the conversion of glycolic acid to glyoxylic acid. The rate-limiting step in the metabolism of EG is the conversion of glycolic acid to glyoxylic acid, which results in the accumulation of glycolic acid in massive poisonings. Glycolic acid, with contribution from lactic acid, causes severe metabolic acidosis (121,122). Finally, glyoxylic acid is converted further to oxalic acid which combines with ionized calcium in plasma to form calcium oxalate and precipitate as calcium oxalate crystals in various tissues including the kidney, brain, meninges, blood vessel walls, liver, spleen, pericardium, and cardiac conduction system. These crystals may also appear in the urine (123). Glycolic, glyoxylic, and oxalic acid all dissociate under physiologic conditions, releasing hydrogen ions from their carboxylic acid moieties (76). Minor pathways involving thiamine and pyridoxine as cofactors can also bring about the conversion of glyoxylic acid to glycine and benzoic acid. However,

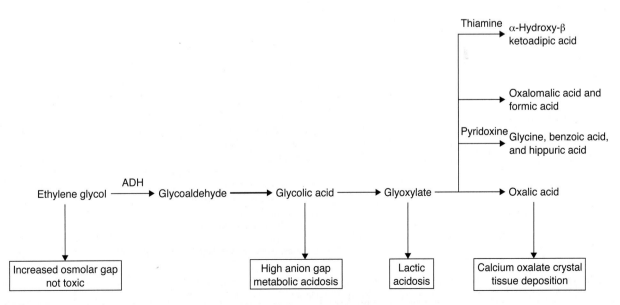

FIGURE 36.7 The oxidative pathway of ethylene glycol metabolism and its clinical effects.

these pathways are clinically insignificant, and there are no data to support the use of these cofactors in the treatment of EG intoxication (108). The average elimination half-life of EG is approximately 3 hours. Ethanol, at serum concentrations of 22 to 44 mmol/L (100 to 200 mg/dL), can effectively inhibit alcohol dehydrogenase and prolong the half-life of EG to almost 18 hours (124). Fomepizole, at serum concentrations greater than 9.8 mmol/L (0.08 mg/dL), can also prolong the half-life of EG to 20 hours (125,126).

Clinical and Pathologic Effects of Ethylene Glycol

Ingestion of EG leads to a metabolic acidosis and severe damage to the CNS, heart, lungs, and kidneys. EG itself is relatively harmless and eliminated by the kidney. The mechanism of toxicity of EG poisoning is primarily due to its conversion to four toxic metabolites (**FIGURE 36.7**). These metabolites are cell toxins that cause CNS depression and cardiopulmonary and kidney disease. The clinical course of EG develops in three different stages, but overlap is frequently seen (**TABLE 36.14**) (67,127). The stage and its severity depend on the amount of EG ingested, the possible coingestion of ethanol or other chemicals, and the timing of medical interventions (88,97,126). The presence of severe acidosis, hyperkalemia, seizures, and coma on admission indicates severe intoxication (128).

Stage 1 is predominantly neurologic and develops as a result of CNS involvement. The symptoms occur shortly after ingestion and may last for 12 hours. Initially, the patient appears intoxicated, sometimes with sustained nausea and vomiting, but without the odor of ethanol (if no ethanol has been ingested concomitantly). These symptoms are probably related to the direct effects of EG on the CNS. This is followed by hyporeflexia, coma, and focal or generalized seizures, often accompanied by ophthalmoplegia, nystagmus, and papilledema. These manifestations are most likely to reach their peak between 6 and 12 hours after ingestion and have been attributed to the toxic effects of the glycoaldehyde metabolites. Cerebral edema and diffuse petechiae are found in patients who die during this stage; focal deposition of calcium oxalate crystals is also seen. A lesser recognized devastating complication of EG is acute Parkinson's syndrome. In one such case, it was thought to result from

acute hemorrhagic necrosis of the basal ganglia (98). Moreover, EG intoxication during pregnancy may mimic eclampsia (129).

During stage 2, cardiopulmonary manifestations develop usually 12 to 24 hours after ingestion. These consist of tachycardia and mild hypertension but usually progress to pulmonary edema and cardiovascular collapse in massive poisoning. These manifestations result from deposition of calcium oxalate crystals in the vessels, myocardium, and lung parenchyma. In severe cases, multiorgan failure develops, and the patient succumbs to the poisoning. It is important to note that most lethal cases occur during this stage.

Stage 3 is predominantly renal and develops in patients who survive for more than 24 hours after ingestion of EG. These patients develop AKI, with oliguria, flank pain, and the presence of calcium oxalate crystals in the urine. Calcium oxalate precipitates in the renal tubules is thought to be the cause of EG-induced AKI, but other studies suggested involvement of other metabolites in causing acute tubular necrosis (130). The mechanisms responsible for the cardiopulmonary and renal manifestations are not entirely clear but are likely due to the toxic effects of the metabolites of EG. Prompt intervention designed at removal of EG and its more toxic metabolites may lead to complete recovery of CNS, cardiopulmonary, and renal manifestations.

Diagnosis

The diagnosis of EG poisoning should be considered in every intoxicated patient without the odor of ethanol. Moreover, the presence of severe metabolic acidosis, large anion gap and a large osmolal gap (greater than 10 mOsm/kg), hypocalcemia, neurologic manifestations, and calcium oxalate crystals in the urine are virtually diagnostic of EG poisoning. Metabolic acidosis develops as a result of the production of glycolic acid and other acidic metabolites secondary to EG breakdown. The plasma anion gap, representing unmeasured anions, is elevated as a result of the accumulation of the anions of the acid metabolites. In addition, because EG, like other alcohols, is an osmotically active compound, it contributes to the high osmolar gap. Therefore, the presence of an osmolal gap is supportive of the diagnosis of EG poisoning. Osmolal gap is the difference between the measured serum osmolality as determined by freezing

TABLE 36.14	**Stages of Ethylene Glycol Poisoning**		
Stage	**Main Manifestations**	**Signs, Symptoms, and Outcome**	**Treatment**
Stage 1: (1–12 h after ingestion)	CNS	• CNS depression, inebriation, ataxia, slurred speech, convulsions, coma, cerebral edema • Anion gap metabolic acidosis • Tachypnea • Hypocalcemia, calcium oxaluria, hematuria, proteinuria, leukocytosis	• Supportive • Fomepizole • Ethanol
Stage 2: (12–24 h after ingestion)	Cardiopulmonary	• Tachycardia, hypotension • Cardiomegaly • Tachypnea, cyanosis, pulmonary edema • Death most common in this phase • High anion metabolic acidosis • High osmolar gap • Hypocalcemia, hematuria, proteinuria, leukocytosis • Calcium oxalate crystals in urinary sediment	• Supportive • Fomepizole • Ethanol • Hemodialysis
Stage 3: (>24 h after ingestion)	Renal	• Flank pain • Acute kidney injury, anuria • Death	• Hemodialysis

CNS, central nervous system.

point depression and the osmolality calculated from the serum levels of sodium, glucose, and urea nitrogen (**Equation 36.2**).

$$\text{Calculated serum osmolality (mOsm/kg)} = 2 \times \text{Na} \text{ (mEq/L)} + \text{Glucose (mg/dL)}/18 + \text{BUN (mg/dL)}/2.8 \quad (36.2)$$

The normal osmolal gap should be between 10 and 12 mOsm/kg. Each 100 mg/dL of EG will produce an osmolal gap of 16 mOsm/kg. An elevated osmolar gap is helpful in several ways. First, it suggests the presence of EG and/or other alcohols in the serum. Second, it helps in estimating the serum concentration of any of these alcohols. Finally, serial measurement is useful in monitoring changes in EG level during removal by HD. However, a normal osmolal gap does not exclude EG intoxication as mentioned earlier. This is because only the parent compound is osmotically active, but its half-life is about 3 hours; therefore, delayed assessment after ingestion may fail to detect an osmolal gap despite the presence of toxic levels of metabolites. However, under these circumstances, the presence of the acid metabolites will still engender metabolic acidosis and an elevated anion gap (**Figure 36.6**).

Three types of crystals can be seen in the urine of patients with EG poisoning. Calcium oxalate crystals are commonly detected in the urine of these patients and are highly suggestive of EG poisoning, particularly in the presence of hypocalcemia. This is seen in nearly 50% of the patients with EG intoxication. Urinary calcium oxalate crystals usually appear after a latent period of 4 to 8 hours; consequently, repeat urinalysis should be carried out after this period (131). These crystals can have the classic appearance of "envelopes" if they consist of calcium oxalate dihydrate or more commonly the appearance of needles or prisms if they consist of calcium oxalate monohydrate (**Figure 36.8**) (132). Hippuric acid crystals have also been reported in patients with EG poisoning (133,134). The absence of calcium oxalate crystals in the urine does not exclude EG poisoning. In the rare situation where a kidney biopsy is done, calcium oxalate crystal deposition within the renal tubules and interstitial tissue can be seen even in the absence of crystalluria. Occasionally, urine of patients with EG poisoning fluoresces under Wood's lamp and was thought to be helpful in the diagnosis. This is because antifreeze, one of the most common sources for EG poisoning, contains

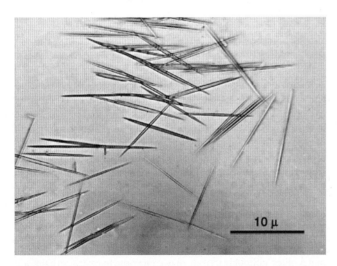

FIGURE 36.8 Urine sediment from a patient with ethylene glycol poisoning showing needle-shaped calcium oxalate monohydrate crystals. (From Marino PL. *Marino's the ICU Book*. 4th ed. Philadelphia, PA: Wolters Kluwer Health, 2014.)

sodium fluorescein, a marker geared for the detection of radiator leaks in motor vehicles (135). However, more careful studies have shown that determination of urine fluorescence is not a reliable screening tool for suspected antifreeze ingestion (136,137). Finally, the most conclusive method of diagnosis is direct measurement of serum or urine EG concentrations by gas chromatography. Unfortunately, this method is not available in most hospital laboratories, and measurement by referral laboratories may delay the diagnosis.

Treatment

Much of what has been discussed previously under treatment of methanol poisoning is applicable to EG poisoning. Again, treatment depends on the severity of the poisoning, depending on the dose ingested, time from ingestion to presentation, as well as on whether there was concomitant ethanol ingestion. Supportive measures such as securing the airway, breathing, and circulation are critically important. Due to the rapid absorption of EG from the gastrointestinal tract, gastric lavage may be beneficial but only within the first hour after ingestion, before toxic symptoms develop. Moreover, correction of severe metabolic acidosis with IV sodium bicarbonate therapy should be attempted. Aggressive treatment of acidosis and induction of an alkaline diuresis increase the renal elimination of glycolate and decrease the likelihood of AKI (138). Seizures, if present, can be treated with benzodiazepines and by correction of the severe hypocalcemia with 10 to 20 mL of 10% calcium gluconate given by slow IV infusion.

In addition to supportive care in all cases, administration of one of the two specific antidotes to delay further production of EG toxic metabolites is of paramount importance. Either ethanol or fomepizole can be used for inhibition of hepatic conversion of the parent compound by alcohol and aldehyde dehydrogenases, but they should not be used together. The indications for their use are listed in **Table 36.15**. Fomepizole, a competitive inhibitor of alcohol dehydrogenase, was approved for the treatment of EG poisoning by the U.S. Food and Drug Administration (FDA) in 1997. The Methylpyrazole For Toxic Alcohols (META) study group documented that fomepizole, if administered early in the course of intoxication, can prevent kidney injury (126). Brent et al. (126) conducted the only prospective clinical trial of fomepizole use in the treatment of EG poisoning. The drug was given intravenously at a loading dose of 15 mg/kg, followed by 10 mg/kg every 12 hours for four doses. Subsequently, it was given at as 15 mg/kg every 12 hours until the

TABLE 36.15	Indications for Use of Fomepizole or Ethanol in Ethylene

Glycol Poisoning
1. Documented recent history of ethylene glycol ingestion
2. Strong clinical suspicion of ethylene glycol poisoning and at least two of the following criteria:
   A. Arterial pH <7.3
   B. Serum bicarbonate <20 mEq/L
   C. Anion gap >16 mmol/L
   D. Osmolal gap >10 mOsm/kg
3. Plasma ethylene glycol concentration >3.2 mmol/L (20 mg/dL)
4. Presence of urinary calcium oxalate crystals
5. Unexplained metabolic acidosis with anion gap >16 mmol/L and osmolal gap >10 mOsm/kg

Data from Barceloux DG, Krenzelok EP, Olson K, et al. The American Academy of Clinical Toxicology practice guidelines in the treatment of ethylene glycol poisoning. *Clin Toxicol* 1999;37:537–560.

plasma EG concentration was less than 3.2 mmol/L (20 mg/dL). The mean time from ingestion to treatment was 11.4 hours. Seventeen of the 19 patients underwent HD, and 18 patients survived; 1 died of cardiogenic shock. Nine patients had normal renal function on presentation. The criteria for administration of fomepizole therapy are identical to those of methanol therapy (**TABLE 36.12**). As can be seen, because fomepizole is dialyzable, it is recommended to increase the frequency of its administration to every 4 hours during HD. Moreover, fomepizole should be given every 12 hours after the completion of dialysis until the EG level is less than 3.2 mmol/L (20 mg/dL) (108). Adverse effects are minimal and include bradycardia, seizure, dizziness, headache, and nausea (139).

Ethanol is also an effective antidote because it is a substrate for alcohol dehydrogenase and blocks the conversion of EG to its toxic metabolites. Serum ethanol concentration of 100 to 200 mg/dL (22 to 44 mmol/L) can saturate receptor sites of alcohol dehydrogenase enzyme and thus inhibit the metabolism of EG (124). Ethanol can be administered by any of three different routes: (a) orally or through a nasogastric tube at a loading dose of 0.8 to 1.0 mL/kg of 95% ethanol solution, followed by a maintenance of 0.15 mL/kg hourly, diluted to a 20% solution; (b) intravenously as a 10% solution with a loading dose of 7.6 to 10 mg/kg, followed by maintenance infusion of 1 to 2 mg/kg/h, titrated to achieve the desired serum concentrations; and (c) ethanol may be added to the dialysate at a concentration of 100 mg/dL using 95% ethanol (140). Because the pharmacokinetics of ethanol depend on a multitude of factors such as age, sex, chronic use of alcohol, and conditions that prolong gastric emptying, serum levels of ethanol need to be monitored frequently and the dose should be modified to achieve and maintain serum levels of 100 to 150 mg/dL (22 to 44 mmol/L). Ethanol is commonly administered until EG can no longer be detected in the serum or until the patient is asymptomatic with a normal arterial pH and a serum EG concentration of less than 20 mg/dL (3.2 mmol/L).

Ethanol is readily available and inexpensive compared with the availability and cost of fomepizole. However, ethanol therapy can be associated with intoxication with CNS depression especially in patients who have ingested other CNS depressants. Moreover, it may cause acute pancreatitis and also hypoglycemia has been noted when used in pediatric and malnourished patients (106). Consequently, patients should be monitored closely and, if necessary, treated appropriately. The lack of serious adverse effects appears to favor fomepizole over ethanol in the treatment of EG poisoning (106). Moreover, fomepizole has a longer half-life which negates the need for continuous infusion as with ethanol. Finally, it should be noted that fomepizole and ethanol can only inhibit the breakdown of EG. The elimination of EG from the body, however, still requires either adequate renal function or effective extracorporeal measures. Dialysis is also effective in rapid treatment of metabolic acidosis.

EG and its metabolites are effectively removed by HD but not by HP (85,122,141). Thus, HD has been routinely used to remove both the ingested parent compound as well as any toxic metabolites. Moreover, it should be used whenever patients with EG poisoning have deteriorating vital signs despite intensive supportive care, significant metabolic acidosis (arterial pH <7.3), and kidney disease or electrolyte abnormalities refractory to conventional therapy (67,108). It should also be used without delay in patients whom there has been significant delay between the time of ingestion and the initiation of either ethanol or fomepizole treatment, since during such time significant concentrations of glycolate have accumulated (76). A serum EG concentration greater than 50 mg/dL

(11 mmol/L) was previously used as an indication for HD. However, this approach is no longer necessary as patients with such blood levels, and normal renal function, who are asymptomatic and with no metabolic acidosis have been adequately managed with fomepizole or ethanol alone (90,108,142–147). Fomepizole and ethanol, given before or during dialysis, are removed by HD and should be replaced appropriately. In patients who have received an IV loading dose of ethanol, the maintenance dose can be discontinued during dialysis if ethanol is added to the dialysate as previously described (140).

HD should be continued until serum EG is undetectable or until it is less than 20 mg/dL (3.2 mmol/L), the disappearance of acid–base and electrolyte abnormalities, and until signs of systemic toxicity disappear. In patients with severe intoxication, it cannot be overemphasized that prolonged and intensive dialysis is often needed. In normophosphatemic patients, such aggressive dialysis may engender hypophosphatemia. Phosphate-enriched dialysates containing 1.3 mmol/L phosphorus, prepared by the addition of sodium phosphate salts to sodium bicarbonate–containing "dialysate base concentrate," have been used successfully to prevent such dialysis-induced hypophosphatemia (148,149). Hirsch et al. (150) have proposed a simple formula to estimate the required dialysis time, in hours, to reach a serum EG concentration of 5 mmol/L. Required dialysis time (hours) = $[-V \ln (5/A)]/0.06K$, where V (liter) is the Watson's estimate of total body water, A is the initial EG concentration in mmol/L, and K is 80% of the manufacturer's specified dialyzer urea clearance (mL/min) at the properly observed blood-flow rate (150).

Being slower, PD remains a less effective treatment option when HD is unavailable (97). CRRT such as hemofiltration has been used for treatment of EG poisoning and should be considered as an alternative modality in patients with circulatory instability (151).

ISOPROPANOL (ISOPROPYL ALCOHOL)

Isopropanol (MW = 60 Da), a clear, colorless liquid with a bitter taste and characteristic fruity odor, is used in the manufacture of several compounds including rubbing alcohol, acetone, and glycerin. It is present in high concentration in deicing products, solvents, cements, antifreezes, cosmetics, inks, and cleaning products. Isopropanol is readily absorbed from the gastrointestinal tract with a peak plasma concentration occurring within 30 minutes. It may also be absorbed by inhalation causing intoxication especially in small children (97,152). Isopropanol is metabolized by alcohol dehydrogenase to acetone, acetol and methylglyoxal, propylene glycol, acetate, and formate with conversion of these metabolites to glucose and other products of intermediary metabolism. The elimination of isopropanol is predominantly by the kidney and in part by the lung (152). It is, however, metabolized more slowly than ethanol, displaying an elimination half-life of 2.5 to 8 hours and a much more protracted half-life when coingested with ethanol (152). Approximately 80% of isopropanol is oxidized by alcohol dehydrogenase to acetone (**FIGURE 36.4**) (153).

Clinical Picture and Laboratory Data

In contrast to methanol and EG, the toxic effects of isopropanol appear to be mostly caused by the parent compound rather than by its metabolites, although acetone may contribute to toxicity. Therefore, no therapeutic attempts to slow its metabolism are needed (88,154). Because isopropanol is quickly absorbed, clinical signs of toxicity usually appear within 1 to 2 hours of exposure (154,155). Initially, the symptoms and signs of isopropanol intoxication may resemble those of ethanol intoxication: dizziness, incoordination, and confusion. However, these manifestations are more protracted, severe, and often progress to ataxia, coma, and death due to respiratory arrest. CNS depression is generally considered to be 2 to 2.5 times more severe compared to that produced by an equal amount of ethanol (97). Some patients may have a "fruity" odor due to the presence of acetone in the breath. The gastrointestinal manifestations, which include nausea, vomiting, abdominal pain, and hematemesis resulting from hemorrhagic gastritis, are frequent. Tachyarrhythmias and, in severe cases, shock and circulatory collapse may occur. Evidence of hepatocellular damage as well as of AKI, myoglobinuria, hypothermia, and hemolytic anemia has been reported (97,153).

Metabolic acidosis is rare because neither the parent compound nor its metabolites are organic acids (156). However, some degree of high anion gap metabolic acidosis may be seen in severe cases due to hypotension, tissue hypoperfusion, and lactic acidosis. Other laboratory tests reveal the presence of an elevated osmolal gap and a normal anion gap. The high osmolal gap results from the combination of two components: (a) isopropanol itself which contributes 17 mOsm/kg per 100 mg/dL and (b) acetone which contributes 18 mOsm/kg per 100 mg/dL. A high serum and urine acetone level in the absence of metabolic acidosis, hyperglycemia, and glycosuria is strongly suggestive of the diagnosis (97,153). Diagnosis can be made by history, the characteristic smell, clinical presentation, high osmolar gap, ketonemia, and/or ketonuria. Direct measurement of isopropanol serum concentrations can be obtained, although this may not be readily available.

Treatment

Lethal doses of isopropanol have ranged from 150 to 240 mL (157). Hypotension is the strongest predictor of mortality (153). Death has been reported to take place in 45% of patients who suffered from both coma and hypotension. Coma by itself in the absence of hypotension was not associated with a high mortality (153). Severe intoxication along with a higher mortality is seen in patients with a serum isopropanol level in excess of 400 mg/dL (67 mmol/L).

Supportive therapy is essential as previously discussed with other alcohols with emphasis on respiratory and cardiovascular systems. Inhibition of alcohol dehydrogenase with ethanol is not indicated since acetone, the major isopropanol metabolite, is less toxic than the parent compound. Moreover, it may slow the metabolism of isopropanol and lead to continued toxicity. HD is indicated in patients with an isopropanol concentration of 400 mg/dL (67 mmol/L) or higher. It is also indicated in the presence of coma, hypotension, or kidney disease (97,153). However, it is prudent to perform HD in poorly arousable or comatose patients when isopropanol ingestion is highly suspected. Studies on the kinetics of isopropanol elimination by HD have shown that the procedure is highly efficient, given its low MW, the absence of protein binding, and the low Vd (97,154,155,158,159).

◆ SALICYLATE POISONING

In 2014, the TESS data compiled by the AAPCC showed that analgesics were the most common cause of reported human poison exposures (2). Of the 2,142 fatalities due to pharmacologic agents, 946 were due to analgesics. Salicylate-containing compounds were responsible for 49 fatalities. Of these, aspirin (acetylsalicylic acid, MW = 180 Da) is the most commonly prescribed and available

preparation. Salicylates can be found in several over-the-counter and prescribed products, which are available in several formulations including liquids, powder, capsules, enteric coated tablets, and suppositories. Poisoning may occur after ingestion of salicylate-containing single agent such as aspirin or when salicylates are present in combination with other toxic compounds (97,160).

The term *salicylates* refers to all forms of salicylate including acetylsalicylic acid (aspirin) and methyl salicylate. However, the most commonly encountered form in clinical practice is acetylsalicylic acid. All salicylates are almost completely absorbed from the gastrointestinal tract. Measurable levels can be obtained within 30 minutes of ingestion of therapeutic doses. However, absorption may be considerably delayed by the dose ingested, enteric coated formulation, variability in the rate of dissolution of different pharmaceutical preparations, and the presence of food in the stomach. Therefore, the onset of symptoms or the attainment of peak serum levels may be delayed for 12 hours or more after ingestion. Methyl salicylate (oil of wintergreen) can also cause intoxication through skin absorption, but this intoxicant is seldom used at the present time. Salicylate poisoning has been reported after accidental ingestion of traditional massage oil (161) and from teething gel (162).

After intestinal absorption, aspirin is initially hydrolyzed rapidly by plasma esterase to its active metabolite salicylic acid that has a half-life of 15 to 20 minutes. Salicylic acid is then glycinated in the liver to salicyluric acid, a less toxic compound that is excreted by the kidneys. At therapeutic doses, salicylates are 90% protein-bound and only 10% of the parent compound is excreted unchanged (as salicylate) in the urine. However, in salicylate poisoning, several events occur which tend to aggravate the likelihood of toxicity. *First*, the protein-binding sites become saturated, and thereby, the ratio between the "free" to total serum salicylate levels increases. At concentrations of 80 mg/dL (5.8 mmol/L), up to 50% of salicylate is free (163,164). *Second*, the biotransformation of salicylic acid to salicyluric acid is retarded, that is, a fixed amount of salicylic acid is metabolized per unit of time regardless of the dose. This is largely due to glycine depletion as well as to the saturation of the hepatic metabolic pathways (165). This phenomenon results in a relatively higher proportion of the drug being present as salicylate, which is less efficiently excreted by the kidney than salicyluric acid. The combination of these two events engenders a greater and more prolonged toxicity. *Finally*, entry of unbound salicylate into the intracellular compartment and the CSF expands the apparent Vd from 20% at therapeutic serum levels to approximately 50% of the body weight leading to greater toxicity (163,164).

The ability of the kidneys to excrete salicylate and its metabolites is augmented by several factors including preserved glomerular filtration rate (GFR), high urine flow rates, and by an alkaline urine pH. Because this compound has an acidic pK_a, a urine pH higher than 7.0 can greatly enhance its renal excretion. In alkaline urine, salicylate and its metabolites cannot be reabsorbed by the renal tubules in their ionized forms. Entry of these compounds into cells is facilitated by acidosis and hindered by alkalosis, an observation highlighting the deleterious effect of salicylate-induced acidosis and emphasizing the need for prompt alkalinization (166).

Clinical Picture

Acute salicylate poisoning usually presents with tachypnea, hyperpnea, nausea, vomiting, abdominal pain, hyperpyrexia, diaphoresis, and tachycardia. Moreover, it may cause severe CNS symptoms including dizziness, ataxia, tinnitus, deafness, confusion, psychosis, stupor, seizures, and coma (160,167,168). These manifestations are more common in children since they predominantly have metabolic acidosis (169,170). On the other hand, chronic intoxication usually manifests as salicylism in the form of headaches, tinnitus, impaired auditory acuity, dizziness, and weakness progressing to nausea, vomiting, confusion, and hyperventilation. Severe seizures, deepening coma, and cardiovascular collapse are terminal events. Pulmonary edema, while uncommon, may also develop, particularly in patients older than 30 years of age and is considered to be the most common cause of morbidity in salicylate poisoning (171). Studies have confirmed that pulmonary edema in salicylate poisoning is noncardiogenic since the pulmonary wedge pressure in these patients is usually normal (172,173). This form of pulmonary edema is thought to result from increased pulmonary capillary permeability which results from the action of salicylate on inhibiting prostacyclin, platelet–vessel interaction as well as from cerebral edema (172–175).

Salicylates display a variety of toxic effects as a result of their interference with a number of metabolic processes (163). Prominent among these processes is uncoupling of oxidative phosphorylation, which accelerates oxygen utilization, heat generation, and CO_2 production (176). Salicylates in the CSF as well as acidemia directly stimulate the central respiratory center increasing the minute ventilation (177). The uncoupling, along with direct stimulation of the respiratory center, accounts for the characteristic hyperventilation and, at least in part, for the metabolic acidosis observed, particularly among children (178). Other mechanisms include the inhibition of the tricarboxylic acid (TCA) cycle, inhibition of amino acid metabolism leading to aminoaciduria, and a negative nitrogen balance and catabolism of proteins and fats. Also, salicylates stimulate glucocorticoids and the release of epinephrine leading to glycolysis and gluconeogenesis. Finally, in therapeutic doses, salicylates reduce urate excretion but may increase uric acid excretion at toxic doses (163).

Diagnosis

Despite the frequency of salicylate intoxication, a relatively high percentage of affected patients remain undiagnosed. Even in acute poisoning, the history may be difficult to ascertain, and therefore, physicians often depend on high degree of suspicion and laboratory investigations. In this regard, salicylate poisoning should be suspected in individuals who present with hyperventilation, diaphoresis, tinnitus, and acid–base abnormalities. In addition, routine chemistries and arterial blood gases are usually helpful and should be obtained along with blood salicylate level.

Acid–base disturbances are very common manifestation of salicylate poisoning. The generation of these acid–base abnormalities usually occurs in two phases: an initial phase of acute respiratory alkalosis followed by a high anion gap metabolic acidosis phase. The metabolic acidosis is seen primarily in children less than 4 years old, while the acute respiratory alkalosis tends to predominate in adults, at least initially. However, mixed respiratory alkalosis and metabolic acidosis are frequently encountered in adults. The pathophysiologic basis for the acid–base disturbances is not fully understood. Salicylate directly stimulates the respiratory center leading to hyperventilation. Salicylate-induced metabolic acidosis is clearly multifactorial. The low P_{CO_2} increases intracellular pH which in turn activates phosphofructokinase-1 and accelerates glycolysis. The end result is production of lactic acid. Moreover, the inhibition of TCA cycle enzymes leads to further increase in

lactic acid production. Finally, it is also possible that the ability of the liver to metabolize lactate is decreased in salicylate poisoning (179). Thus, metabolic acidosis in salicylate poisoning is primarily due to lactic acid production. Other organic acids that contribute to metabolic acidosis include ketoacids, which result from increased lipid and protein metabolism. It must be emphasized that salicylic acid contributes only a small portion to the increased anion gap metabolic acidosis (167,168,170,180). Therefore, the high anion gap in salicylate poisoning is due to many factors including lactic acid, ketoacids, salicylates, and other organic acids (180). The degree of acidosis is a major determinant of the severity of neurotoxicity and patient survival. Given that salicylic acid is a weak acid, >99% will be ionized under physiologic pH and only a minute amount will exist in the unionized form. This unionized molecule can easily move across cellular barriers, including the blood–brain barrier and the epithelium of the renal tubule while the ionized form penetrates poorly. The concentration of the unionized form increases as the blood pH falls; thus, severe academia increases the penetration of unionized fraction into the brain cells. This causes an increase in the salicylate concentration in the CNS and an increase in the amount of salicylate reabsorbed from the renal collecting system. Thus, it is the unionized fraction that is responsible for the increased mortality in patients with salicylate poisoning. In rare cases, high serum salicylate levels have been reportedly associated with false increase in serum chloride level which in turn falsely lowers the anion gap. In one such report, two cases of moderate to severe salicylate poisoning had a normal anion gap and apparent hyperchloremia (181). Other reports also reported an even negative anion gap in salicylate poisoning (182,183). This may occur with some ion-selective electrodes but not others and may be due to loss of selectivity over the operational life of the chloride electrode as well as competition between salicylate and chloride ions to bind to albumin (184).

Apart from metabolic acidosis, a number of other abnormalities can be observed in patients with salicylate poisoning. Severe hypouricemia may develop as a result of inhibition of renal tubular urate reabsorption by the high salicylate levels. Also, hypokalemia may be seen and is usually due to vomiting and potassium losses in the urine, which can be aggravated by distal tubular alkalization from respiratory alkalosis. Hypoglycemia is rare, but hyperglycemia may develop in almost 20% of cases (185). Finally, prolongation of prothrombin time, a positive ferric chloride test, and a positive Phenistix test may also be seen (186,187). The Phenistix reagent strips are impregnated with ferric and magnesium salts which produce a purple color in the presence of salicylate concentration greater than 70 mg/dL (5 mmol/L). A positive test essentially confirms the presence of salicylate in patients suspected of having salicylate intoxication (186,188).

Management of Salicylate Poisoning

The severity of salicylate poisoning can be determined by one or more of the following parameters. *First*, acute ingestion of less than 150 mg/kg is not usually associated with serious consequences. On the other hand, with ingestion of more than 150 mg/kg, toxicity is likely to occur. Clinical toxicity is usually mild with ingestion of 150 to 300 mg/kg, moderate with 300 to 500 mg/kg, and severe if the amount ingested exceeds 500 mg/kg (189). Doses of 10 to 30 g of aspirin or of sodium salicylate may result in death, although patients who ingested much larger doses have also recovered. *Second*, severe clinical symptoms and signs such as severe CNS manifestations, pulmonary edema, or AKI also indicate severe toxicity.

Lastly, it has been suggested that serum salicylate level exceeding 750 mg/L indicates severe poisoning, while levels between 500 and 700 mg/L are seen in moderate toxicity. However, symptoms of salicylism are usually present at much lower serum levels of 30 mg/dL (2.2 mmol/L). It is now believed that the serum salicylate levels may not correlate well with the severity of intoxication (190). This is particularly true in patients with chronic salicylate ingestion, those with AKI, those with acidosis, the presence of confounding factors, and the lack of knowledge of the precise time of ingestion. Moreover, one should not rely on a single blood salicylate level because of a possible delayed absorption. Therefore, the widely available nomogram that estimates the severity of intoxication from plots of salicylate levels at different times has not been predictably useful when sustained-release or enteric coated preparations have been consumed (191–193).

Supportive Care

Salicylate poisoning is a medical emergency. There is no specific antidote to treat salicylate intoxication. However, as discussed for all poisoned patients, the mainstay of therapy is supportive measures with particular attention to establishing an adequate airway. Intubation may be necessary in patients with severe tachypnea, but manual ventilation may be needed to maintain the blood pH at 7.5 to 7.55 to minimize the entry of salicylate into the CSF. Other important measures include gastric emptying should only be done for patients presenting within 1 hour of ingesting a large dose of salicylate. Moreover, administration of IV fluids that contain glucose and electrolytes is critically important in order to correct volume, electrolyte, and acid–base abnormalities as well as hypoglycemia if present.

Elimination

The above maneuvers may be adequate for patients with moderate salicylate poisoning and serum levels less than 50 mg/dL (3.6 mmol/L). However, for patients with higher serum levels of salicylate, and those with more severe clinical presentation, especially when metabolic acidosis is present, measures designed to eliminate salicylates are indicated. These maneuvers include repeated administration of activated charcoal (97,194) and alkalinization of urine. Activated charcoal is effective in decreasing the gastrointestinal absorption of salicylates, although other studies cast doubt on its effectiveness (195–197). Administration of activated charcoal is recommended especially in patients who present within 1 hour following ingestion. Dargan et al. (198) suggested an initial oral bolus of 50 g in adults or 1 g/kg for children preferably within 1 hour of ingestion followed by additional doses at 2 to 6 hours if necessary.

Alkalinization of the urine is also effective in enhancing the excretion of salicylates. This is based on the notion that the unbound fraction of salicylate undergoes glomerular filtration, tubular secretion, and absorption. In an acid medium, salicylate is maximally nonionized and can be reabsorbed across the renal tubular cell membranes. Excretion, however, is greatly accelerated in presence of high urine flow rate and alkaline urine (pH greater than 7.5) (166). Forced alkaline diuresis has been shown to be more effective than forced diuresis in augmenting salicylate excretion in the urine. Indeed, a recent position paper from the American Academy of Clinical Toxicology and the European Association of Poison Control Centers and Clinical Toxicologists recommended that urine alkalinization should be considered as first-line treatment for patients with moderately severe salicylate poisoning who do not

meet the criteria for HD (15). Forced diuresis may not only correct the commonly found dehydration of these patients but may also be deleterious as it may exacerbate the tendency of salicylates to induce pulmonary edema in overhydrated patients. Consequently, the administration of isotonic sodium bicarbonate at a rate sufficient to correct the metabolic acidosis and induce alkaline urine is now preferred (193,196). The volume of isotonic sodium bicarbonate necessary to achieve these goals may be substantial. A suggested protocol would involve administration of 225 mL of an 8.4% sodium bicarbonate intravenously in the first hour followed by additional boluses to maintain urine pH of 7.5 to 8.5. An alternative approach includes a continuous infusion of D5W mixed with 150 mmol of sodium bicarbonate. Loop diuretics should be avoided because they may decrease salicylate excretion (196).

Salicylates are readily removed by various extracorporeal techniques due to their relatively low MW, low apparent Vd, and the small degree of protein binding (97,165,199). HD is currently the preferred technique for ECTR of salicylate poisoning. PD is less efficient and should be reserved for children in whom HD may be more difficult to perform (97). Various forms of CRRT can also be used for treatment of salicylate poisoning particularly in patients who are hemodynamically unstable (200). Although HP provides a higher clearance of salicylate, HD remains the preferred technique (21,97,201,202). The indications for ECTR in patients with salicylate poisoning have been poorly defined but generally include the presence of severe clinical presentation such as seizures or coma, cerebral edema, kidney disease, severe metabolic acidosis, and clinical deterioration despite adequate therapy. Moreover, patients at risk of developing noncardiogenic pulmonary edema such as older patients, those with history of smoking, and those with inability to establish diuresis should be considered for HD (97,165,172–175,199). HD was also recommended to patients with acute salicylate poisoning and blood salicylate levels greater than 100 mg/dL or at least 60 mg/dL in those with chronic salicylate toxicity regardless of their clinical state (165). However, data from the AAPCC in 2004 showed that approximately half of the fatal acute cases reported had salicylate levels less than 100 mg/100 mL (203). Similar data were also reported from Ontario, Canada (160). Unfortunately, HD continues to be underutilized in cases of salicylate poisoning because physicians, including nephrologists, prefer to try alkalinization of urine before HD, a perceived aggressive therapy. Although urine alkalinization should be attempted as soon as the patient presents to the emergency department, it should be done in addition to, and not instead of, HD particularly in clinically severe cases of salicylate poisoning (204). The EXTRIP workgroup has recently conducted a systematic literature review and derived consensus-based recommendations for ECTR in salicylate poisoning. The workgroup concluded that ECTR is the only intervention that convincingly and rapidly reduces the burden of circulating salicylate (201). It does so efficiently (ECTR clearance can surpass 100 mL/min) and also allows correction of acidemia, which will lessen the delivery of salicylate to the brain (201).The workgroup thus recommended ECTR in patients with severe salicylate poisoning, including any patient with altered mental status, with acute respiratory distress syndrome requiring supplemental oxygen, and for those in whom standard therapy is deemed to be failing regardless of the salicylate concentration (201) (**TABLE 36.16**). High salicylate concentrations warrant ECTR regardless of signs and symptoms, with lower thresholds applied for patients with impaired kidney function. ECTR is also suggested for patients with severe academia (pH <7.20 in the absence of other

TABLE 36.16	Indications for Extracorporeal Treatment of Salicylate Poisoning

General Recommendation
ECTR is recommended in severe salicylate poisoning (1D).

Indications for ECTR
ECTR is recommended if any of the following are met:
- If [salicylate] >7.2 mmol/L (100 mg/dL) (1D)
- If [salicylate] >6.5 mmol/L (90 mg/dL) in the presence of impaired kidney function (1D)
- In the presence of altered mental status (1D)
- In the presence of new hypoxemia requiring supplemental oxygen (1D)

If standard therapy (supportive measures, bicarbonate, etc.) fails (1D), ECTR is suggested if any of the following are met:
- If [salicylate] >6.5 mmol/L (90 mg/dL) (2D)
- If [salicylate] >5.8 mmol/L (80 gm/dL) in the presence of impaired kidney function (2D)
- If the systemic pH is ≤7.20 (2D)

ECTR Cessation
ECTR cessation is indicated if
- Clinical improvement is apparent (1D) *and*
- [salicylate] <1.4 mmol/L (19 mg/dL) (1D) *or* ECTR has been performed for a period of at least 4–6 h when salicylate concentrations are not readily available (2D)

Choice of ECTR Modality
- Intermittent HD is the preferred modality in patients with salicylate poisoning (1D)
- The following are acceptable alternatives if HD is not available:
  - Intermittent HP (1D)
  - CRRT (3D)
  - Exchange transfusion in neonates (1D)
- **Miscellaneous: It is recommended to continue intravenous bicarbonate therapy between ECTR sessions (1D)**

ECTR, extracorporeal treatment; HP, hemoperfusion; CRRT, continuous renal replacement therapy.
Reproduced with permission from Juurlink DN, Gosselin S, Kielstein JT, et al. Extracorporeal treatment for salicylate poisoning: systematic review and recommendations from the EXTRIP Workgroup. *Ann Emerg Med* 2015;66(2):165–181.

indications). Intermittent HD is the preferred modality, although HP and CRRT are acceptable alternatives if HD is unavailable, as is exchange transfusion in neonates.

LITHIUM

Lithium, from the Greek word *stone*, was discovered in 1818 and used for treatment of various ailments including gout and renal stone disease. Almost a century later, lithium was used as a salt substitute in patients with hypertension or congestive heart failure and was even added to the soft drink 7 Up (205–208). However, because of its toxicity, its use was abandoned until 1950s when it was used for treatment of bipolar syndrome and remains in use for that indication until the present time (209). In addition, lithium has been successfully used in modern medicine as a mood stabilizer and for the treatment of severe depression and acute mania (210,211).

Unfortunately, lithium has a narrow therapeutic index and most patients experience some toxicity from long-term use. In the 2013 Annual Report of the AAPCC NPDS, there were 6,815 cases of toxic lithium exposures in 2012 including 11 deaths in the United States (2). Most commonly, lithium intoxication occurs in patients who have been receiving chronic lithium therapy. Acute toxicity may be superimposed on those of chronic toxicity but may also occur as a result of accidental or suicidal ingestions (97,212–214).

Lithium is dispensed in various formulations including carbonate salt in tablets, capsules, and slow-release formulations or as citrate salt in liquid preparations. It is rapidly absorbed by the gastrointestinal tract within 8 hours of ingestion. Peak serum levels are seen 1 to 3 hours after ingestion of regular formulation and 4 to 12 hours in sustained-release preparations. Lithium is a small molecule (74 Da) that is neither bound to proteins nor is it metabolized, distributes promptly in the extracellular fluid, and has a distribution volume of 0.4 L/kg. However, it slowly enters the intracellular compartment, and as a result, its Vd increases to 0.6 to 0.9 L/kg (215). Lithium is actively transported out of cells by a Na^+/Li^+ exchanger. However, because of the negative intracellular potential in certain cells, intracellular lithium concentrations may become twice as high as those of the plasma (216). Given that the rate of equilibration of

lithium across cellular membranes is slow, and that its effects occur intracellularly, it is no surprise that, at comparable serum lithium levels, chronic intoxication is more likely to be accompanied by toxic effects than acute poisoning (217,218). Lithium has a predilection to certain tissues such as the white matter of the brain, the thyroid, liver, muscle, skeleton, and the distal tubular cells of the kidney (97,212–214); its highest concentrations, however, are found in the brain and the kidney (215). Within cells, lithium is capable of inhibiting adenyl cyclase and inositol-1-phosphate, both being important intracellular messengers (97,212–214). Whether this mechanism is the one through which lithium exerts its therapeutic or toxic effects is unclear.

Lithium is almost entirely (95%) eliminated through the kidney where it is handled in a way similar to that of sodium. Therefore, it is freely filtered by the glomerulus and approximately 80% of the filtered amount is reabsorbed by the proximal tubule and a small amount is reabsorbed in the distal tubule (217). Moreover, dietary salt restriction and volume depletion profoundly increase its renal tubular reabsorption. This phenomenon accounts for the frequent occurrence of toxicity in patients receiving stable doses of lithium when they develop volume depletion from any cause such as vomiting, diarrhea, or diuretic therapy (219,220). Moreover, concomitant administration of drugs that reduce GFR such as the angiotensin-converting enzyme inhibitors and nonsteroidal anti-inflammatory drugs decrease lithium clearance and raise its serum levels (220–222). By contrast, factors that augment sodium excretion enhance lithium excretion only to a minor extent (97,212–214).

Clinical Picture

Lithium toxicity may be seen under three different patterns. Acute toxicity occurs in patients who have not previously taken the drug but overdose on lithium. Acute on chronic toxicity occurs in patients on chronic therapy but overdose on the drug. Chronic toxicity occurs in patients on maintenance lithium therapy in the clinical context of a recently increased lithium dose, a decline in kidney function, or a drug–drug interaction that impairs elimination (223,224). The last category is usually associated with the more severe toxicity. Gastrointestinal symptoms may help to distinguish between acute lithium poisoning, where they are usually present, from chronic toxicity, where they are almost invariably absent. The clinical relationship between lithium levels and toxicity is complex as clinical features are both highly variable and largely dependent on the pattern of poisoning (218,225,226). The therapeutic steady-state lithium level is 0.6 to 1.2 mEq/L (223,227), but mild lithium toxicity may be observed at lithium levels of 1.5 to 2.5 mEq/L. Moderate toxicity may develop at levels between 2.5 and 3.5 mEq/L. On the other hand, severe toxicity is usually seen when the levels exceed 3.5 mEq/L (227,228). In the elderly, toxic manifestations may appear at serum levels of 1.5 mEq/L or at even lower. Therefore, serum lithium levels should only be used as a guide to the risk of toxicity but always taken in the context of other patients' characteristics including history, clinical presentation, as well as the level of renal function.

Although lithium toxicity may lead to multiorgan dysfunction, its clinical manifestations are primarily due to CNS and renal impairment. The CNS findings may start with nervousness and agitation then followed by coarse tremors, dysarthria, confusion, delirium, ataxia, hyperpyrexia, slurred speech, stupor, seizures, and coma (212). Several case reports document the syndrome of irreversible lithium-effectuated neurotoxicity (SILENT) as a neurologic complication of lithium toxicity (229–231). Patients with this syndrome usually have chronic cerebellar sequelae, even after lithium has been discontinued and concentrations have fallen to therapeutic or undetectable levels. The clinical features of SILENT may include tremor, extrapyramidal symptoms, gait difficulties, nystagmus, dysarthria, and cognitive deficits (219–231). Unfortunately, there are no definitive treatments for SILENT at the present time (223).

Renal toxicity includes polyuria, nephrogenic diabetes insipidus, sodium-losing nephropathy, and proteinuria, which can be in the nephrotic range (232). Polyuria, which is more common with chronic therapy, occurs in up to 37% of patients with therapeutic doses of lithium before full-blown nephrogenic diabetes insipidus develop (233). Lithium is the most common cause of drug-induced nephrogenic diabetes mellitus (234). Moreover, renal acidification defects, evidence of chronic interstitial nephritis, and nephrotic syndrome are also seen (97,212–214,216). Renal biopsies in patients with lithium nephrotoxicity have documented high prevalence of focal and segmental glomerulosclerosis (232). Long-term lithium intake has also been reportedly associated with increased risk of renal tumors and renal cysts. Over a 16-year period, a recent retrospective study reported that 14 of 170 lithium-treated patients had renal tumors, including 7 malignant and 7 benign tumors. The percentage of renal tumors, particularly cancers and oncocytomas, was significantly higher in lithium-treated patients compared with 340 gender-, age-, and estimated glomerular filtration rate (eGFR)-matched lithium-free patients (235). Prolonged lithium treatment may cause hyperchloremic metabolic acidosis, which is believed to be caused by diminished net proton secretion in the collecting duct or excessive back diffusion of acid equivalents, or both (236). Interestingly, the anion gap may be low or absent in presence of exceedingly high serum level of lithium (237,238).

Other toxic effects of lithium include leukocytosis, enlargement of the thyroid gland, and evidence of hypothyroidism (97,211–214,216,224,239). Gastrointestinal symptoms are commonly encountered in acute intoxication and include nausea, vomiting, diarrhea, anorexia, and bloating (218,224,225,239,240). Lastly, cardiovascular manifestations are usually mild and include hypertension, bradycardia or tachycardia, and ST-segment depression and T-wave flattening on electrocardiogram (ECG). More serious findings include QT prolongation, QRS widening, intraventricular conduction defects due to sinus node dysfunction, ventricular arrhythmia, and myocardial infarction (241,242). Lithium toxicity is thought to correlate primarily with intracellular lithium concentrations. Therefore, at comparable serum levels, the clinical picture of the chronically intoxicated patient (with higher intracellular levels) may be more severe than that of the acutely intoxicated counterpart (224,225).

Treatment

Lithium intoxication is always a serious problem even when manifestations of toxicity appear relatively minor as seizures and other CNS complications may occur unexpectedly. There is no known antidote for lithium. Thus, supportive care including discontinuation of lithium, securing the airways and other hemodynamic parameters, as well as volume repletion with isotonic saline, must be instituted without delay. In patients with mild clinical manifestations and serum lithium level less than 2.5 mEq/L, aggressive supportive treatment may suffice. However, in patients with accidental or suicidal ingestion, gastric lavage should be employed. Administration of activated charcoal is not useful because this agent does not bind lithium ions (243). Whole bowel irrigation with polyethylene glycol electrolyte lavage solution (GoLYTELY) at 2 L/h for 5 hours after ingestion can reduce lithium absorption by 67% and reduce peak lithium levels by >50% (244). This approach may enhance the elimination of sustained-release preparations of lithium (244). Sodium polystyrene sulfonate has previously been suggested to enhance elimination of lithium but is not currently recommended.

A serum level of 2.5 mEq/L or greater typically is associated with significant morbidity and mortality and must be treated aggressively (97,212–214,218). An important goal of therapy is to maintain the GFR and urine output. This entails administration of appropriate volume of 0.9% saline IV to maintain urine output but forced diuresis is not recommended. Volume depletion can occur because of a defect in renal concentrating ability, diuretic therapy, vomiting or diarrhea. Consequently, vigorously replacing preexisting volume losses is of paramount importance in reestablishing a desirable level of renal lithium excretion (97,212–214,216–218).

HD is highly effective and currently considered the most efficient method of removing lithium from a patient with lithium poisoning (227,245). This is because its low atomic weight and minimal protein binding makes it readily diffusible across dialyzer membranes. The extraction ratio for lithium is in the range of 0.7 for plasma and 0.5 for whole blood, the discrepancy resulting from the low extraction of lithium from red blood cells (246). In view of these characteristics and of the relatively low Vd, dialysis can produce a rapid fall in total body lithium burden. In this regard, HD can reduce the half-life of lithium from 12 to 27 hours to 3.6 to 5.7 hours and can raise its clearance rate from 10 to 40 mL/min (via the patient's own kidneys) to 70 to 170 mL/min and minimize the length of time that the brain is exposed to toxic lithium levels. (97,219,228). Despite its efficacy, there is no consensus on precise indications for HD (247). This is because removal of lithium from the extracellular fluid has little effect on intracellular lithium concentration. Moreover, serum levels correlate poorly with clinical picture of toxicity. Differences in opinion in the management of lithium poisoning was highlighted at a workshop at the 2013 Annual Scientific Meeting of European Association of Poison Control

TABLE 36.17	Indications for Extracorporeal Treatment of Lithium Poisoning

- ECTR is recommended if any of the following conditions are present:
  1. If kidney function is impaired and the lithium level is >4.0 mEq/L
  2. In presence of a decreased level of consciousness, seizures, or life-threatening dysrhythmias, irrespective of the lithium level
- ECTR is suggested if any of the following conditions are present:
  3. If lithium level is >5.0 mEq/L
  4. If significant confusion is present
  5. If the expected time to reduce lithium level to <1.0 mEq/L with optimal management is >36 h
- Cessation of ECTR is recommended:
  1. If either the lithium level is <1.0 mEq/L or clinical improvement is apparent
  2. After a minimum of 6 h of ECTR if the lithium level is not readily measurable
- Choice of ECTR
  1. Intermittent hemodialysis (HD) is the preferred ECTR modality in lithium poisoning (1D).
  2. CRRT is an acceptable alternative if intermittent HD is not available (1D).
  3. After an initial treatment with intermittent HD, both CRRT and intermittent HD are equally acceptable modalities for additional lithium removal (1D).

ECTR, extracorporeal treatment.
Modified from Decker BS, Goldfarb DS, Dargan PI, et al. Extracorporeal treatment for lithium poisoning: systematic review and recommendations from the EXTRIP Workgroup. *Clin J Am Soc Nephrol* 2015;10(5):875–887.

Centers and Clinical Toxicologists in Copenhagen, Denmark (248). Nonetheless, recent recommendations from the EXTRIP workgroup on treatment of lithium poisoning were published and include the following (**TABLE 36.17**): (a) The workgroup concluded that lithium is dialyzable. (b) ECTR is recommended in severe lithium poisoning. (c) ECTR is recommended if kidney function is impaired and the lithium level is >4.0 mEq/L, or in the presence of a decreased level of consciousness, seizures, or life-threatening dysrhythmias irrespective of the lithium level. (d) ECTR is suggested if the lithium level is >5.0 mEq/L, significant confusion is present, or the expected time to reduce the lithium level to <1.0 mEq/L is >36 hours. (e) ECTR should be continued until clinical improvement is apparent or lithium level is <1.0 mEq/L. (f) ECTRs should be continued for a minimum of 6 hours if the lithium level is not readily measurable. (g) HD is the preferred ECTR, but CRRT is an acceptable alternative. Finally, the workgroup suggested that clinical decisions on when to use ECTR should take into account the lithium level, kidney function, pattern of lithium toxicity, patient's clinical status, and availability of ECTRs (223).

The relatively slow equilibration of lithium across cellular membranes may complicate response to HD treatment. This is because following dialysis and a rapid fall in extracellular lithium concentration, the patient may not improve. Indeed, the slow exit of lithium from cells often results in rebound increase in serum lithium values after dialysis cessation. Rebound may also occur in cases of poisoning resulting from the ingestion of sustained-release preparations as a result of continued gastrointestinal absorption.

Thus, rebound may result either from a redistribution of lithium from deeper compartments/red blood cells to the plasma or from ongoing absorption from the gastrointestinal tract. While the former is not usually associated with worsening symptoms, the latter, which develops from ongoing absorption from extended-release formulations or patients with decreased gastrointestinal motility, is usually associated with clinical deterioration. Consequently, HD must be repeated or continued until the serum level 6 to 8 hours after dialysis is less than 1 mEq/L (223). Prompt determination of serum lithium levels may not be readily available in many health care institutions. Under such circumstances, it would seem prudent to offer patients conventional dialysis treatment for 4 to 6 hours followed by SLED for several hours. The use of a bicarbonate bath is preferred to that of an acetate bath since acetate may reduce lithium clearance. Acetate bath, in contrast to bicarbonate bath, is thought to activate the sodium-hydrogen antiporter on the cell membrane, driving lithium (substituting for sodium) into the cells (248).

Besides HD, various CRRTs modalities [continuous arteriovenous hemodiafiltration (CAVHDF) and CVVHDF] have also been used successfully in lithium intoxication, achieving lithium clearance rates of 60 to 85 L/d (Leblanc). Because of their continuous nature, these therapies create a persistent concentration gradient between the intracellular and extracellular compartments over longer periods, allowing a gradual and more complete elimination of lithium from intracellular compartments, thereby avoiding significant rebound (249). In addition, these procedures may be especially helpful in patients with hemodynamic instability who are unable to tolerate IHD (250). Unfortunately, there are no controlled trials comparing the safety, efficacy, and cost of these CRRT techniques with those of conventional HD.

THEOPHYLLINE

Theophylline is 1,3-dimethylxanthine (MW = 180 Da) that is closely related to caffeine and is a member of the methylxanthine family of pharmacologic agents. Theophylline was popular for treatment of asthma for several decades, but its use has dramatically declined in the United States in recent years due to the introduction of newer and safer pharmacologic agents and because of concern about its toxicity. Nonetheless, it is still used as a bronchodilator in other countries in the treatment of asthma, chronic obstructive pulmonary disease, and acute mountain sickness but also used for treatment of apnea and bradycardia of premature infants (251). Theophylline intoxication is most commonly unintentional as an inadvertent consequence of chronic theophylline therapy for asthma and other chronic obstructive pulmonary diseases (252). Intoxication can also occur in toddlers or because of suicidal overdose in adults (97,251,253,254).

When taken orally, theophylline is promptly and efficiently absorbed, with peak serum levels occurring at approximately 2 hours. However, the sustained-release capsule is not completely absorbed until 6 to 8 hours after ingestion, and the peak serum levels may be delayed to 12 to 17 hours after ingestion of these agents (255). Once absorbed, theophylline is distributed predominantly in the extracellular water, with an apparent Vd of about 0.45 L/kg body weight. Infants and elderly patients tend to have larger Vds. In the circulation, theophylline is loosely bound to albumin: The fraction bound is highest (approximately 60%) at relatively low therapeutic serum concentrations but is lower at toxic serum levels as well as in adults with liver disease and in infants (256,257). The therapeutic serum concentration of theophylline is 10 to 20 μg/mL (56 to 111 μmol/L) when used for treatment of asthma. Theophylline has a narrow therapeutic index (ratio of 50% toxic dose to 50% effective dose) of 1 to 1.5.

In adults, only 10% to 15% of theophylline is excreted unchanged in the urine, the remainder is metabolized in the liver by the cytochrome P450 pathway. The rate of endogenous hepatic clearance of theophylline is relatively slow in the order of 0.7 mL/min/kg in adult nonsmokers in whom the half-life is approximately 8 hours. The metabolic clearance of theophylline is relatively slow and is influenced by many factors including age. Neonates and the elderly eliminate the drug more slowly. In infants, hepatic metabolism is also slower leading to longer half-life and higher renal excretion (50% excreted via this route). Theophylline clearance becomes maximal between the ages of 1 and 9 years but subsequently decreases by almost 50% in adults (254). Moreover, metabolism can be profoundly modified by genetic factors, environmental agents, and other drugs that alter the activity of the liver isoenzymes. Fever, severe chronic liver disease, and congestive heart failure prolong theophylline half-life, whereas smoking and hyperthyroidism reduce the half-life of the drug. The metabolism of theophylline is highly influenced by concomitant drug use. Antibiotic therapy with macrolides and quinolones prolong theophylline half-life, whereas administration of barbiturates, phenytoin, rifampin, carbamazepine, and oral contraceptives reduce the half-life of the drug (254). Theophylline exhibits Michaelis-Menten (saturable) kinetics. Consequently, increments in dose are associated with parallel increases in serum theophylline levels. With severe theophylline intoxication, drug elimination rates are very low and follow zero-order (dose-dependent) kinetics. In the latter situation, metabolic pathways may become saturated, with reduction in endogenous clearance and a consequent increment in half-life (251,253,254,257). It is usually this kinetics in addition to the drug–drug and drug–disease interactions that are often responsible for inadvertent theophylline intoxications (253,254).

Four major potential mechanisms have been proposed to explain theophylline's mode of action. First, theophylline has been thought to act as an inhibitor of cyclic nucleotide phosphodiesterase, the enzyme that breaks down intracellular cyclic adenosine monophosphate (AMP) (251,254,258). Second, recent evidence indicates that both the therapeutic and toxic effects of theophylline may be mediated by its action as a competitive antagonist at adenosine receptor sites (259,260). Third, theophylline results in a release of catecholamines and has positive inotropic and chronotropic effects on the heart (261). Lastly, its effects may result directly from changes in intracellular calcium transport.

Clinical Picture

Because theophylline has a narrow therapeutic index, it is often associated with a high rate of adverse events. Some therapeutic effects of theophylline are observed at serum levels as low as 5 mg/L (27.5 mmol/L), but response to therapy is achieved at serum concentrations in the range of 10 mg/L (55 mmol/L). On the other hand, toxic manifestations may develop in some patients at concentrations as low as 15 mg/L (82.5 mmol/L), but most patients manifest toxicity at levels greater than 25 mg/L (138 mmol/L) (262). Clinically, symptoms and signs of toxicity usually reflect the effects of theophylline on five organ systems. First, gastrointestinal symptoms are common and may include nausea, vomiting, diarrhea, heart burn, hematemesis, and abdominal pain. Second, neurologic symptoms appear at relatively low serum levels of theophylline. These include

tachypnea, anxiety, restlessness, agitation, and tremors progressing to confusion and eventually to seizures. However, the most serious of these manifestations is repeated seizures, which can be associated with hyperthermia. Third, cardiovascular effects, which can be life-threatening, include sinus tachycardia, supraventricular tachycardia (atrial flutter and fibrillation), multifocal atrial tachycardia, ventricular premature beats, ventricular tachycardia, and vasodilatation with hypotension (263). The cardiac toxicity of theophylline may be due to inhibition of the cardiac adenosine receptors or increased catecholamine release. Fourth, generalized muscle aches with occasional myoclonus and elevation of creatine phosphokinase. Fifth, metabolic consequences of theophylline intoxication such as hypokalemia and hyperglycemia are commonly observed and develop as a result of catecholamine-induced β_2-adrenergic stimulation (264). Hypokalemia is the most important metabolic abnormality and is likely due to increased shift of potassium ions to the intracellular compartment as a result of increased activity of Na-K-ATPase. Moreover, hypercalcemia, hypomagnesemia, and hypophosphatemia have also been reported. In severe and advanced cases, lactic acidosis (most likely secondary to hypotension) and rhabdomyolysis (the consequence of muscular hyperactivity, hyperthermia, and hypokalemia) are observed (252,262–265).

The development of seizures is considered the most serious of all neurologic manifestations of theophylline poisoning. The presence of seizures portends a high mortality or may result in permanent neurologic damage (266,267). Once seizures develop, they may be very difficult to control. Seizures may occur at serum theophylline concentrations less than 20 μg/mL (268). They also tend to occur at lower serum concentrations in patients receiving chronic theophylline therapy than in those with acute intoxication. The probability of seizures in patients on chronic theophylline therapy with theophylline concentration of 220 mmol/L (40 mg/L) is 50%, whereas the same probability was not reached in patients with acute intoxication until a theophylline concentration of 660 mmol/L (120 mg/L) (258,263). This observation may well be related to the fact that patients receiving chronic theophylline therapy often suffer from other concomitant diseases or receive concurrent medications that lower the seizure threshold (254,262–265). A prior history of neurologic abnormalities does appear to increase the likelihood of seizures (269,270). The exact mechanism of seizures in theophylline toxicity is unclear. However, it has been suggested that it may be related to dysfunction of the γ-aminobutyric acid-ergic (GABAergic) inhibitory neurons and depressed serum pyridoxal levels (271). Also, theophylline may reduce cerebral hyperemia and enhances brain damage induced by seizures; actions related to inhibition of brain adenosine activity (272).

Management of Theophylline Poisoning
Supportive Care

Supportive care is clearly important in theophylline poisoning. Patients should be closely monitored, preferably in the intensive care unit, where special attention can be paid for cardiac arrhythmia, hypotension, respiratory distress, and seizures. If respiratory failure or seizure develops, the patient should have immediate endotracheal intubation. Moreover, serious cardiac arrhythmias should be treated without delay. In this regard, the use of adenosine as a first-line therapy for tachyarrhythmia is recommended given the notion that these arrhythmias are due to theophylline-induced cardiac adenosine receptor antagonism. However, the use of β-blocking agents for control of cardiac arrhythmias should also be considered. Although noncardioselective agents such as propranolol may offer some advantage because of their capacity to counteract theophylline-induced vaso-dilatation and hypokalemia (273), cardioselective β-blockers are usually required in patients with bronchial asthma (274). Moreover, seizures should be anticipated and managed appropriately. Some advocate the use of prophylactic anticonvulsant therapy in patients with theophylline poisoning (275). Once they appear, seizure should be treated aggressively (253,254). The drug of choice is either benzodiazepine or a phenobarbital. If these patients do not respond to anticonvulsant therapy, general anesthesia and neuromuscular paralysis may become necessary (276). Phenytoin is relatively contra-indicated as animal studies have suggested that it may increase the risk of theophylline-induced seizures (277). It should be noted that seizures may occur hours after peak theophylline levels have been reached. Moreover, seizures may occur with slow-release preparations of the drug, and in patients with chronic overdose who may have different severities of intoxication at the same serum levels as acute overdose (258,262–267). In addition to the usual supportive measures, treatment of theophylline intoxication should include close monitoring of serum potassium and phosphorus concentrations with aggressive replacement of any deficits.

Elimination

Theophylline toxicity can be clearly life-threatening, and thus, it should be removed from the gastrointestinal tract and blood immediately if possible. The oral administration of repeated doses of activated charcoal has been proven to markedly shorten theophylline half-life, even in patients who have received theophylline by the IV route. Charcoal binds the fraction of ingested theophylline that has not yet been absorbed as well as that which diffuses into the intestine from the circulation. The latter phenomenon is referred to as *entero-capillary exsorption* (278,279). Activated charcoal is administered in the form of slurry in a dose of 1 g/kg every 4 hours or 15 to 20 g every 2 hours in adults and 2.5 to 10 g hourly in children. Alternatively, it can be given by a continuous nasogastric infusion. Activated charcoal administration should continue until serum concentrations of theophylline decrease to less than 20 mg/L (110 mmol/L), and clinical improvement can be documented (278–280). Such maneuvers should be employed routinely in all theophylline-intoxicated patients except for those with minimal signs and symptoms of toxicity. Unfortunately, the concomitant nausea and vomiting may make the use of MDAC difficult in many afflicted patients. Under such circumstances, antiemetic therapy with metoclopramide or ondansetron may be necessary. Because prochlorperazine may lower seizure threshold, its use is contraindicated (281). Use of cathartics with activated charcoal may hasten the evacuation of charcoal-theophylline complex (282). However, forced diuresis is not recommended.

Theophylline can be removed more rapidly by HP or HD. HP with either resin cartridges (such as Amberlite XAD-4) or activated charcoal cartridges is the most effective extracorporeal technique for elimination of theophylline with an extraction ratios of close to 0.75 (283–286). Indeed, because of the ease of transmembrane movement of theophylline, the drug is efficiently removed not only from the plasma but also from the erythrocytes. More than 65% of theophylline dose can be removed in 3 hours of HP; the amount can be calculated by using blood rather than plasma flow rates through the HP cartridge (287). Unfortunately, the capacity of HP cartridges to extract theophylline is not without limits, and the efficiency of theophylline elimination falls with time as the cartridge becomes saturated. Consequently, the cartridge must be replaced every 2 hours (283,285,286,288).

HD is also effective in removing theophylline but was thought to be less effective than HP (289,290). However, recent studies indicate that HD is just as effective in treating theophylline poisoning as HP (18,291–296). Substantial amounts of the drug may be removed in a relatively short period of time. This is particularly true with the use of high-efficiency hemodialyzers with a high KoA as well as high blood and dialysate flow rates. These hemodialyzers can increase the extraction ratio of theophylline to 0.5 to 0.6 (254). Prolonged HD sessions may be required to obtain results equivalent to those achieved by HP. Finally, HD may be comparable to HP in reducing the morbidity and mortality from theophylline poisoning and may be associated with fewer procedural complications (293). The simultaneous use of HD and charcoal HP (HD/HP) "in series" can increase the amount of theophylline removed. This combined procedure, if available, may also retard the saturation of the charcoal cartridge and thus represents a favorable treatment option for patients with heavy theophylline intoxication (288,289).

The indications for use of HP and/or HD are controversial. However, the EXTRIP workgroup (ECTR) recently published their recommendations for treatment of theophylline poisoning. The workgroup made the following recommendations: ECTR is recommended in severe theophylline poisoning with a theophylline concentration >100 mg/L (555 μmol/L) in acute exposure, the presence of seizures, life-threatening dysrhythmias or shock, a rising theophylline concentration despite optimal therapy, and clinical deterioration despite optimal care. In chronic poisoning, ECTR is suggested if theophylline concentration >60 mg/L (333 μmol/L) or if the theophylline concentration is >50 mg/L (278 μmol/L) and the patient is either less than 6 months of age or older than 60 years of age. ECTR is also suggested if gastrointestinal decontamination cannot be administered. ECTR should be continued until clinical improvement is apparent or the theophylline concentration is <15 mg/L (83 μmol/L). Following the cessation of ECTR, patients should be closely monitored. Intermittent HD is the preferred method of ECTR. If intermittent HD is unavailable, HP or CRRTs may be considered (292). These include sorbent-based dialysate regeneration systems such as the REDY machine (297,298), CVVH (299,300), and plasmapheresis (301). Some studies have shown no significant difference in the elimination rate of theophylline between charcoal HP and plasmapheresis (299,300). By contrast, PD is clearly not effective in the treatment of theophylline poisoning (302). Exchange transfusion is an adequate alternative to HD in neonates. MDAC should be continued during ECTR (292). In those who appear clinically stable, the administration of charcoal may suffice until serum theophylline levels become available. However, serial measurement of theophylline levels should then be obtained every 2 to 4 hours until peak levels are reached. If the level is greater than 100 μg/mL, even in the absence of major toxic manifestations, HP or HD should be started as soon as possible particularly in the presence of concomitant kidney disease, hepatic failure, cardiac failure, or advanced age (254,289).

⬡ ETHANOL

Ethanol (MW = 46 Da) is one of the most frequently encountered toxins in the emergency departments in the United States (303). Chronic alcohol-related health problems are common. Detailed description of these problems as well as ethanol pharmacokinetics and management of withdrawal syndromes are beyond the scope of this chapter. Ethanol has low MW, is highly soluble in water and lipid, and has Vd similar to water. It is rapidly absorbed from the stomach and small intestine, with a peak level at approximately 20 to 60 minutes after ingestion. Once absorbed, ethanol is initially metabolized to acetaldehyde then to acetone. Women attain higher blood ethanol levels after ingestion of equal amounts than men due to their smaller size, higher body fat content, and lower alcohol dehydrogenase enzyme in their stomach.

When ethanol is consumed in low doses, it is perceived as a stimulant owing to the suppression of central inhibitory systems. However, as the plasma levels of ethanol increase, sedation, motor incoordination, ataxia, and impaired psychomotor performance appear (304). At very high blood levels, ethanol may lead to coma and death. Acute alcoholic intoxication is responsible for a high number of deaths in the United States annually, most notably among young college students with binge drinking habits (305). Most of the deaths are caused by respiratory depression, aspiration-induced asphyxia, or traumatic injuries in severely inebriated subjects. Acute intoxication can also lead to severe hypotension and cardiac arrhythmias. Lethal level is at the realm of 450 mg/dL (98 mM) for half of the non–ethanol-dependent population, although individuals with serum concentrations as high as 1,500 mg/dL (326 mM) have survived (306,307). Most patients can be treated adequately with proper supportive care consisting of administration of fluids, electrolytes, thiamine, folate, and other vitamins in addition to the prevention of hypoglycemia and hypoxia. Gastric emptying is ineffective in decreasing the blood ethanol level due to the rapid absorption of ethanol. Charcoal may be administered if circumstances suggest the coingestion of other toxins (303). The vast majority of inebriated individuals recover on their own with supportive care (303,308). However, in severely intoxicated patients with lethal serum ethanol levels, and in those at risk of respiratory depression and circulatory failure, extracorporeal techniques such as HD, hemofiltration, and hemodiafiltration can be employed (308–310). Because of its small MW and the absence of protein-binding, ethanol is readily removed by these techniques. HD increases the plasma elimination rate of alcohol from 15 mg/dL/h to nearly 100 mg/dL/h (308).

⬡ ACETAMINOPHEN POISONING

Acetaminophen (*N*-acetyl-p-aminophenol; APAP; paracetamol) has been the most frequently used analgesic and antipyretic medication used worldwide since the advent of Tylenol in the United States in 1955 and Panadol in the United Kingdom in 1956. In therapeutic doses, APAP is usually safe. However, it has long been recognized that if APAP is taken in excessive amounts or as an overdose, it can cause fatal and nonfatal liver failure (311). Even in smaller doses, particularly in combination products, APAP can cause serious liver damage. Severe liver injury has been reported in patients who took higher than the prescribed dose of an acetaminophen-containing product in a 24-hour period, took two or more acetaminophen-containing products simultaneously, or combined alcohol with acetaminophen products (312,313). In fact, the FDA issued a statement in January 2014 stating that "combination prescription pain relievers that contain more than 325 mg of acetaminophen per tablet, capsule, or other dosage unit should no longer be prescribed because of a risk of liver damage" (313). Data from the U.S. Acute Liver Failure Study Group registry of >700 patients with acute liver failure implicates APAP poisoning in nearly 50% of all acute liver failure in the United States (314). Currently, APAP is the leading cause of acute liver failure in both United States and United Kingdom.

Acetaminophen is one of the most frequent poisoning reported to the poison centers in the United States (311). In the 2013 Annual Report of the APPCC NPDS, there were 311,347 exposures to analgesics in 2012 in the United States. There were 946 deaths involving an analgesic agent. Of these, APAP is responsible for almost one-third of poisoning-related deaths as it was recorded in 103 of acetaminophen poisoning as a single agent, 133 from acetaminophen/hydrocodone, and 24 from acetaminophen/oxycodone combinations (2). APAP toxicity is the most frequent cause of hepatic failure. Ingestion of a single dose of more than 10 to 15 g can cause severe or fatal liver injury secondary to massive hepatic necrosis (315). Moreover, ingestion of daily doses of less than 10 g on consecutive days carries a risk for liver injury in some individuals (316). It has also been suggested that APAP hepatotoxicity may even occur in those ingesting therapeutic doses under certain conditions, such as fasting or alcohol use (317,318).

APAP is rapidly and almost completely absorbed primarily in the small bowel with a peak serum level within 2 hours of ingestion, but absorption can be delayed if taken with other medications. Its Vd is 0.95 L/kg, and its half-life is 1.5 to 2 hours. Only 2% of APAP is excreted in the urine unchanged. The drug is metabolized in the liver into two major metabolites: two-thirds as glucuronide and one-third as sulfate conjugate (**FIGURE 36.9**) (319). These nontoxic inactive conjugates are largely excreted in the urine and bile. However, 5%

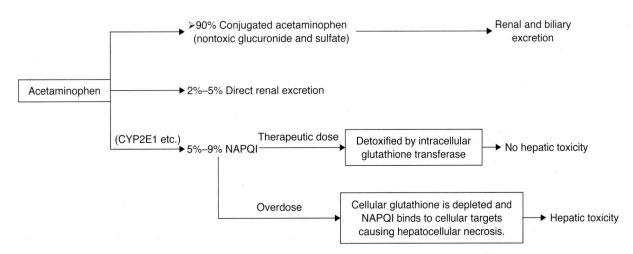

FIGURE 36.9 Acetaminophen metabolism with therapeutic doses and with overdose.

of the APAP dose ingested undergoes oxidative conversion by the cytochrome P450 (CYP2E1) enzyme system to the toxic metabolite *N*-acetyl-p-benzoquinoneimine (NAPQI). This metabolite is usually detoxified in the liver via irreversible glutathione, conjugation which helps to reduce NAPQI to cysteine, and mercapturic acid conjugates, which are safe renally excretable metabolites. Unfortunately, in overdose, large amounts of NAPQI are produced leading to overuse of this metabolic pathway and depletion of intracellular glutathione stores; thereby limiting the nontoxic metabolism of APAP, leaving NAPQI free in the liver, resulting in direct liver injury from NAPQI (**Figure 36.9**) (320). Since the glucuronide and sulfate metabolites are actively secreted by the renal tubules, it is no surprise that patients with kidney disease accumulate these metabolites which are implicated in the toxic manifestations of APAP.

Clinical Picture

Early recognition of APAP toxicity is critically important in preventing morbidity and mortality. The clinical presentation of acute APAP toxicity has been categorized into four phases (321): (a) In the first 24 hours, the patient may be totally asymptomatic or may have nonspecific symptoms such as nausea, vomiting, anorexia, diaphoresis, and lethargy. The liver function tests may initially be normal but start to increase after 16 hours of overdose. (b) The next 24 to 72 hours represent the second phase of APAP poisoning during which the patient begins to develop clinical and laboratory evidence of hepatotoxicity. The patient may develop right upper quadrant pain along with increases in transaminases, bilirubin, and prothrombin time. The kidney function may start to deteriorate. (c) In the third phase, 72 to 96 hours after overdose, the patient usually progresses to fulminant liver failure as well as kidney disease. With progression to fulminant hepatic failure, patients may develop hepatic encephalopathy, jaundice, coagulopathy, and multiorgan failure. AKI occurs in more than 50% of patients and is generally attributable to acetaminophen-induced acute tubular necrosis, which results from NAPQI production in the kidney. Patients may rarely develop severe metabolic acidosis and coma. Death usually occurs in this phase from multiorgan failure unless urgent liver transplant is done. Poor prognostic indicators include a pH less than 7.3, evidence of AKI with serum creatinine greater than 3.3 mg/dL, liver failure with international normalized ratio (INR) greater than 2 at 24 hours, 4 at 48 hours, or 6 at 72 hours, and blood lactate level greater than 3.5 mmol/L. The later criterion is often used as an indication for liver transplantation (322). Patients who present with hepatic failure have a mortality rate of 20% to 40% (323,324). (d) Patients who survive the initial insult enter into phase 4, usually 4 to 14 days after ingestion, during which resolution of liver and renal functional abnormalities and complete recovery occurs. In massive ingestions (doses >500 mg/kg), patients may present with altered level of consciousness and lactic acidosis, usually within 12 hours postingestion and often prior to biochemical or clinical evidence of hepatotoxicity. In these cases, APAP concentrations are extremely high (>750 mg/L or 5,000 µmol/L). This clinical scenario represents mitochondrial failure and early cell death from overwhelming reactive oxygen species and exhausted glutathione reserves (325,326).

Diagnosis

History, when available, often leads to the correct diagnosis. However, other causes of fulminant liver failure such as hepatotoxic mushrooms, carbon tetrachloride, halothane, viral hepatitis, Reye syndrome, acute fatty liver of pregnancy, and ischemic hepatitis must

also be considered. A characteristic finding in APAP hepatotoxicity is the marked elevations in the aminotransferases, usually greater than 3,000 IU/L, and levels as high as 48,000 have been reported (327,328). Unfortunately, history of APAP ingestion may not be readily available particularly in patients with intentional overdose. Because of the potentially disastrous consequences of unrecognized APAP ingestion, it is recommended that all intentional overdoses should be screened for APAP toxicity (329,330). The rate of potentially hepatotoxic APAP levels in patients without history of ingestion is approximately 0.3%. It should be noted, however, that false positive APAP levels have been reported in presence of high bilirubin level (331). In addition to serum APAP level and bilirubin, other laboratory data should include baseline serum transaminases, prothrombin time, arterial blood gases, and renal function tests as well as blood lactate level. Hepatotoxicity in patients with APAP overdose is defined as any increase in aspartate aminotransferase (AST) concentrations, while severe hepatotoxicity as an AST greater than 1,000 IU/L. Hepatic failure is defined as hepatotoxicity with hepatic encephalopathy.

Treatment

After attempting to establish an accurate time of ingestion, the first step in the management of APAP toxicity is aggressive supportive care. Also, activated charcoal should be given to all patients who present within 6 hours of ingestion. Subsequently, NAC should be administered since it is considered an effective antidote for APAP toxicity. NAC has been shown to limit hepatotoxicity in APAP-poisoned patients by several mechanisms (332). First, after administration, NAC is hydrolyzed in the body to cysteine, which replenishes glutathione, where glutathione covalently binds NAPQI in a 1:1 ratio preventing hepatocellular damage (333,334). Second, NAC can serve as a sulphate precursor to help maintain APAP metabolism through the sulfonation pathway. Third, NAC has been shown to blunt the hepatocellular toxicity of NAPQI (335). Finally, NAC improves hemodynamics and oxygen use and may decrease brain edema (336). NAC dramatically reduces the incidence of APAP-induced hepatotoxicity and progression to fulminant liver failure when administered within the first 8 to 10 hours following an acute overdose. Studies have shown that in patients who receive NAC within the first 8 hours after an acute overdose, the risk of hepatotoxicity is <5%, but those who receive NAC after 10 hours are at increased risk of hepatic injury (337,338).

Current treatment of APAP poisoning involves initiating a three-phase NAC infusion after comparing a plasma concentration, taken >4 hours postoverdose, to a nomogram. In this second step, the risk of hepatotoxicity after a single acute APAP ingestion should be determined by plotting the serum APAP concentration in the patient, taken between 4 hours and 24 hours postingestion on the Rumack-Matthews nomogram (339,340). The result will help to indicate whether or not a patient is at *no* risk, *possible* risk, or *probable* risk of developing APAP hepatotoxicity. Thus, patients have a 60% risk of developing fulminant liver failure if the plasma level of APAP was above the line drawn from the 200 µg/mL level at 4 hours or the 50 µg/mL level at 12 hours (339) (**Figure 36.10**). However, given that NAC is an effective antidote in patients with APAP poisoning and is relatively benign, it is my belief that it should be given to anyone with suspected or confirmed APAP overdose, regardless of the serum APAP concentration, particularly if the time of ingestion is unknown and in those with repeated supratherapeutic ingestion. However, many poison control centers in the United States and other countries still recommend NAC administration only for

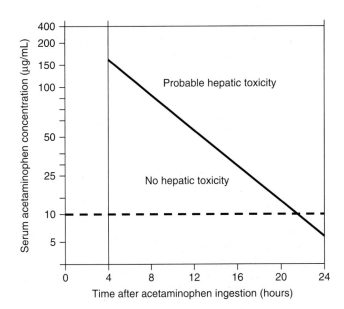

FIGURE 36.10 Acetaminophen metabolism. Relationship between plasma acetaminophen concentration, the time after ingestion, and the risk of hepatic toxicity. The *solid diagonal line* represents a 25% likelihood of hepatic injury. The *horizontal dotted line* compares the low risk at plasma concentration of 10 μg/mL soon after the ingestion versus the high risk at 24 hours since it reflects a high initial load, which has now distributed into tissues. (Reproduced with permission from Rumack BH. Acetaminophen hepatotoxicity: the first 35 years. *J Toxicol Clin Toxicol* 2002;40:3–20.)

patients who have a serum concentration that is above the "probable toxicity" line, which starts at 200 μg/mL 4 hours after ingestion (333). It should be stated here that NAC administration does affect subsequent APAP levels (333).

NAC can be administered to patients with known or suspected APAP toxicity by oral or IV routes (333,338,341). There are no clinical trials comparing the oral versus IV routes of administration. Thus, the choice of oral or IV administration will have to be determined based on the prevailing clinical circumstances. In the United States, NAC therapy is usually given orally, but since it is sterile, it can be given in identical doses by IV route in patients who cannot tolerate oral administration (342,343). An IV preparation was approved by the FDA for use in the United States. The dose of oral NAC does not have to change when activated charcoal is given concomitantly (335). Orally administered NAC has minimal adverse effect profile, consisting mostly of nausea and emesis, and increased tolerance can be achieved by coadministration of an antiemetic. On the other hand, adverse effects of IV administration include pruritus, flushing, skin rash, and anaphylactoid reactions. These adverse effects can be treated by administration of antihistamines and temporarily discontinuing the IV infusion and restarting the infusion at a lower rate (335). The FDA-approved NAC treatment protocol for the treatment of acute APAP poisoning involves a loading dose of 140 mg/kg followed by 17 maintenance doses of 70 mg/kg every 4 hours. The IV loading dose is 150 mg/kg over 1 hour, followed by an infusion of 50 mg/kg over 4 hours, and then 100 mg/kg over 16 hour period. The dose does not require adjustment for renal or hepatic impairment or for dialysis (327,333,337,344). Shorter courses as given in Canada, Europe, and Australia proved to be just as effective (345,346). Fortunately, NAC therapy is effective at any point after poisoning. Thus, it should be administered to all patients with history of APAP overdose

even if they present after 24 hours of ingestion if their APAP level is elevated (336,347). Likewise, it should be administered if there is hepatic toxicity even in the absence of measurable APAP levels. Moreover, its administration should not be restricted to the 18 doses if there is evidence of liver toxicity. In these circumstances, therapy should continue until evidence of liver injury has resolved and transaminases values have declined to near-normal levels (327).

Dialysis is not as effective as NAC therapy in APAP poisoning. The EXTRIP workgroup suggested that NAC is the mainstay of treatment of APAP poisoning and that ECTR is not warranted in most cases. However, given that APAP is dialyzable, the workgroup agreed that ECTR is suggested in patients with excessively large overdoses who display features of mitochondrial dysfunction. This is reflected by early development of altered mental status and severe metabolic acidosis prior to the onset of hepatic failure. Specific recommendations for ECTR include (a) an APAP concentration over 1,000 mg/L if NAC is not administered, (b) signs of mitochondrial dysfunction and an APAP concentration over 700 mg/L (4,630 mmol/L) if NAC is not administered, (c) signs of mitochondrial dysfunction and an APAP concentration over 900 mg/L (5,960 mmol/L) if NAC is administered, and (d) IHD is the preferred ECTR modality in APAP poisoning (**TABLE 36.18**) (348). Other forms of extracorporeal techniques have not been studied in APAP poisoning except liver dialysis, which was tried in only 4 patients (349).

TABLE 36.18	**Extracorporeal Treatment of Acetaminophen (APAP) Poisoning**

- ECTR is recommended:
  - If the [APAP] more than 1,000 mg/L (6,620 μmol/L) and NAC is NOT administered
  - If the patient presents with altered mental status, metabolic acidosis, with an elevated lactate, and an [APAP] is more than 700 mg/L (4,630 μmol/L) and NAC is NOT administered
  - If the patient presents with an altered mental status, metabolic acidosis, an elevated lactate, and an [APAP] is more than 900 mg/L (5,960 μmol/L) even if NAC is administered

- ECTR is not recommended on the basis of the reported ingested dose if NAC is administered.

- ECTR is not suggested:
  - On the basis of reported ingested dose alone even if NAC is NOT administered
  - Solely on the basis of the [APAP] if NAC is administered

- ECTR is continued until sustained clinical improvement is apparent.

- Choice of ECTR
  - Intermittent hemodialysis is the preferred ECTR in patients with APAP poisoning.
  - The following are acceptable alternatives if HD is not available:
    - Intermittent HP
    - CRRT
    - Exchange transfusion in neonates

- Miscellaneous
  - NAC therapy should be continued during ECTR at an increased rate

NAC, N-acetylcysteine; HD, hemodialysis.
Modified from Gosselin S, Juurlink DN, Kielstein JT, et al. Extracorporeal treatment for acetaminophen poisoning: recommendations from the EXTRIP workgroup. *Clin Toxicol (Phila)* 2014;52(8):856–867.

Finally, patients with repeated supratherapeutic ingestions have a worse prognosis than patients admitted after acute overdose (343,350). Approximately 30% of patients admitted for APAP overdose had repeated supratherapeutic ingestions (323). A recent systematic review with consensus recommendations stated that repeated supratherapeutic ingestions need to be referred to an emergency department only if at least 10 g or 200 mg/kg (whichever is less) during a single 24-hour period, or at least 6 g or 150 mg/kg (whichever is less) per 24-hour period for the preceding 48 hours or longer, is ingested (351). Other patients may be considered for outpatient therapy, particularly those with a supratherapeutic serum APAP concentration <70 µg/mL and less than 3 times the upper limit of alanine aminotransferase concentration (333).

⬡ REFERENCES

1. Warner M, Chen LH, Makuc DM, et al. Drug poisoning deaths in the United States, 1980–2008. *NCHS Data Brief* 2011;81:1–8.
2. Mowry JB, Spyker DA, Cantilena LR Jr, et al. 2013 annual report of the American Association of Poison Control Centers' National Poison Data System (NPDS): 31st annual report. *Clin Toxicol (Phila)* 2014;52:1032–1283.
3. Shannon MW. A general approach to poisoning. In: Shannon MW, Borron SW, Burns JM, eds. *Haddad and Winchester's Clinical Management of Poisoning and Drug Overdose.* 4th ed. Philadelphia, PA: WB Saunders, 2007:13–30.
4. Clemmesen C, Nilsson E. Therapeutic trends in the treatment of barbiturate poisoning: the Scandinavian method. *Clin Pharmacol Ther* 1961;2:220–229.
5. Lorch JA, Garella S. Hemoperfusion to treat intoxications. *Ann Intern Med* 1979;91:301–304.
6. Kirk M, Pace S. Pearls, pitfalls, and updates in toxicology. *Emerg Med Clin North Am* 1997;15:427–449.
7. Vale JA, Kulig K. Position paper: gastric lavage. *Clin Toxicol* 2004;42:933–943.
8. Position paper: ipecac syrup. *Clin Toxicol* 2004;42:133–143.
9. Position paper: cathartics. *Clin Toxicol* 2004;42:243–253.
10. Shrestha M, George J, Chiu MJ, et al. A comparison of three gastric lavage methods using the radionuclide gastric emptying study. *J Emerg Med* 1996;14:413–418.
11. Pond SM, Lewis-Driver DJ, Williams GM, et al. Gastric emptying in acute overdose: a prospective randomised controlled trial. *Med J Aust* 1995;163:345–349.
12. Smilkstein MJ. Techniques used to prevent gastrointestinal absorption of toxic compounds. In: Goldfrank LR, Floenbaum NE, Lewin NA, et al, eds. *Goldfrank's Toxicologic Emergencies.* 6th ed. Stamford, CT: Appleton & Lange, 1998:35–51.
13. McFarland AK III, Chyka PA. Selection of activated charcoal products for the treatment of poisonings. *Ann Pharmacother* 1993;27:358–361.
14. Maslov OG, Brusin KM, Kochmashev VF, et al. Comparative evaluation of methods of extracorporeal detoxification in acute carbamazepine poisoning. *Klinicheskaia Toksikologiia (Russia)* 2011;12:1169–1179.
15. Proudfoot AT, Krenzelok EP, Vale JA. Position paper on urine alkalinization. *J Toxicol Clin Toxicol* 2004;42:1–26.
16. Murphy NG, Benowitz NL, Goldschlager N. Cardiovascular toxicology. In: Shannon MW, Borron SW, Burns MJ, eds. *Haddad and Winchester's Clinical Management of Poisoning and Drug Overdose.* 3rd ed. Philadelphia, PA: WB Saunders, 2007:133–166.
17. Patel R, Connor G. A review of thirty cases of rhabdomyolysis-associated acute renal failure among phencyclidine users. *J Toxicol Clin Toxicol* 1985;23:547–556.
18. Ouellet G, Bouchard J, Ghannoum M, et al. Available extracorporeal treatments for poisoning: overview and limitations. *Semin Dial* 2014;27:342–349.
19. Holubek WJ, Hoffman RS, Goldfarb DS, et al. Use of hemodialysis and hemoperfusion in poisoned patients. *Kidney Int* 2008;74:1327–1334.
20. Feinfeld DA, Rosenberg JW, Winchester JF. Three controversial issues in extracorporeal toxin removal. *Semin Dial* 2006;19:358–362.
21. Winchester JF. Dialysis and hemoperfusion in poisoning. *Adv Ren Replace Ther* 2002;9:26–30.
22. Maher JF. Principles of dialysis and dialysis of drugs. *Am J Med* 1977;62:475–481.
23. Winchester JF. Active methods for detoxification. In: Shannon MW, Borron SW, Burns MJ, eds. *Haddad and Winchester's Clinical Management of Poisoning and Drug Overdose.* 3rd ed. Philadelphia, PA: WB Saunders, 1998:175–188.
24. Bouchard J, Roberts DM, Roy L, et al. Principles and operational parameters to optimize poison removal with extracorporeal treatments. *Semin Dial* 2014;27:371–380.
25. Ghannoum M, Troyanov S, Ayoub P, et al. Successful hemodialysis in a phenytoin overdose: case report and review of the literature. *Clin Nephrol* 2010;74:59–64.
26. Ozhasenekler A, Gokhan S, Guloglu C, et al. Benefit of hemodialysis in carbamazepine intoxications with neurological complications. *Eur Rev Med Pharmacol Sci* 2012;16(Suppl 1):43–47.
27. Tapolyai M, Campbell M, Dailey K, et al. Hemodialysis is as effective as hemoperfusion for drug removal in carbamazepine poisoning. *Nephron* 2002;90:213–215.
28. Ghannoum M, Bouchard J, Nolin TD, et al. Hemoperfusion for the treatment of poisoning: technology, determinants of poison clearance, and application in clinical practice. *Semin Dial* 2014;27:350–361.
29. Shalkham AS, Kirrane BM, Hoffman RS, et al. The availability and use of charcoal hemoperfusion in the treatment of poisoned patients. *Am J Kidney Dis* 2006;48:239–242.
30. Kawasaki CI, Nishi R, Uekihara S, et al. How tightly can a drug be bound to a protein and still be removable by charcoal hemoperfusion in overdose cases? *Clin Toxicol (Phila)* 2005;43:95–99.
31. Rosenbaum JL, Winsten S, Kramuer MS, et al. Resin hemoperfusion in the treatment of drug intoxication. *ASAIO Trans* 1970;16:134–140.
32. Marshall MR, Golper TA, Shaver MJ, et al. Sustained low-efficiency dialysis for critically ill patients requiring renal replacement therapy. *Kidney Int* 2001;60:777–785.
33. Okonek S, Reininghaus I, Setyadharma H, et al. An economical hemoperfusion system to determine *in vitro* clearances of various poisons with different adsorbents. *Arch Toxicol* 1980;46:215–220.
34. Okonek S. Intoxication with pyrazolones. *Br J Clin Pharmacol* 1980;10(Suppl 2):385S–390S.
35. Marshall MR, Golper TA, Shaver MJ, et al. Urea kinetics during sustained low-efficiency dialysis in critically ill patients requiring renal replacement therapy. *Am J Kidney Dis* 2002;39:556–570.
36. Ledebo I. Principles and practice of hemofiltration and hemodiafiltration. *Artif Organs* 1998;22:20–25.
37. Wizemann V, Külz M, Techert F, et al. Efficacy of haemodiafiltration. *Nephrol Dial Transplant* 2001;16(Suppl 4):27–30.
38. Fiaccadori E, Maggiore U, Parenti E, et al. Sustained low-efficiency dialysis (SLED) for acute lithium intoxication. *Nephrol Dial Transplant* 2008;24:329–332.
39. Berbece AN, Richardson RM. Sustained low-efficiency dialysis in the ICU: cost, anticoagulation, and solute removal. *Kidney Int* 2006;70:963–968.
40. Marshall MR. Dialytic management of acute kidney injury and intensive care unit nephrology. In: Floege JJR, Feehally J, eds. *Comprehensive Clinical Nephrology.* 4th ed. St. Louis, MO: Elsevier Saunders, 2010:843–852.
41. Liao Z, Zhang W, Hardy PA, et al. Kinetic comparison of different acute dialysis therapies. *Artif Organs* 2003;27:802–807.
42. Bailey AR, Sathianathan VJ, Chiew AL, et al. Comparison of intermittent haemodialysis, prolonged intermittent renal replacement therapy and continuous renal replacement haemofiltration for lithium toxicity: a case report. *Crit Care Resusc* 2011;13:120–122.
43. Riegel W. Use of continuous renal replacement therapy for detoxification. *Int J Artif Organs* 1996;19:111–112.
44. Ronco C, Bellomo R. Continuous renal replacement therapy: evolution in technology and current nomenclature. *Kidney Int* 1998;(Suppl 66):S160–S164.

45. Bohler J, Riegel W, Keller E, et al. Continuous arteriovenous haemoperfusion (CAVHP) for the treatment of paraquat poisoning. *Nephrol Dial Transplant* 1992;7:875–878.

46. Kim Z, Goldfarb DS. Continuous renal replacement therapy does not have a clear role in the treatment of poisoning. *Nephron Clin Pract* 2010;115:c1–c6.

47. Kan G, Jenkins I, Rangan G, et al. Continuous haemodiafiltration compared with intermittent haemodialysis in the treatment of methanol poisoning. *Nephrol Dial Transplant* 2003;18:2665–2667.

48. Harder JL, Heung M, Vilay AM, et al. Carbamazepine and the active epoxide metabolite are effectively cleared by hemodialysis followed by continuous venovenous hemodialysis in an acute overdose. *Hemodial Int* 2011;15:412–415.

49. Fertel BS, Nelson LS, Goldfarb DS. Extracorporeal removal techniques for the poisoned patient: a review for the intensivist. *J Intensive Care Med* 2010;25:139–148.

50. Amerling R, Glezerman I, Savransky E, et al. Continuous flow peritoneal dialysis: principles and applications. *Semin Dial* 2003;16:335–340.

51. Ibrahim RB, Liu C, Cronin SM, et al. Drug removal by plasmapheresis: an evidence-based review. *Pharmacotherapy* 2007;27:1529–1549.

52. Lambert C, Gericke M, Smith R, et al. Plasma extraction rate and collection efficiency during therapeutic plasma exchange with Spectra Optia in comparison with Haemonetics MCS+. *J Clin Apher* 2011;26:17–22.

53. Madore F. Plasmapheresis technical aspects and indications. *Crit Care Clin* 2002;18:375–392.

54. Jones JS, Dougherty J. Current status of plasmapheresis in toxicology. *Ann Emerg Med* 1986;15:474–482.

55. Szczepiorkowski ZM, Winters JL, Bandarenko N, et al. Guidelines on the use of therapeutic apheresis in clinical practice—evidence-based approach from the Apheresis Applications Committee of the American Society for Apheresis. *J Clin Apher* 2010;25:83–177.

56. Krisper P, Stadlbauer V, Stauber RE. Clearing of toxic substances: are there differences between the available liver support devices? *Liver Int* 2011;31(Suppl 3):5–8.

57. Wittebole X, Hantson P. Use of the molecular adsorbent recirculating system (MARS?) for the management of acute poisoning with or without liver failure. *Clin Toxicol (Phila)* 2011;49:782–793.

58. Mitzner SR, Stange J, Klammt S, et al. Albumin dialysis using the molecular adsorbent recirculating system. *Curr Opin Nephrol Hypertens* 2001;10:777–783.

59. McIntyre CW, Fluck RJ, Freeman JG, et al. Use of albumin dialysis in the treatment of hepatic and renal dysfunction due to paracetamol intoxication. *Nephrol Dial Transplant* 2002;17:316–317.

60. Shi Y, He J, Chen S, et al. MARS: optimistic therapy method in fulminant hepatic failure secondary to cytotoxic mushroom poisoning—a case report. *Liver* 2002;22(Suppl 2):78–80.

61. Karvellas CJ, Gibney N, Kutsogiannis D, et al. Bench-to-bedside review: current evidence for extracorporeal albumin dialysis systems in liver failure. *Crit Care* 2007;11:215.

62. Sam R, Patel SB, Popli A, et al. Removal of Foscarnet by hemodialysis using dialysate-side values. *Int J Artif Organs* 2000;23:165–167.

63. Gibson TP, Atkinson AJ Jr. Effect of changes in intercompartment rate constants on drug removal during hemoperfusion. *J Pharm Sci* 1978;67:1178–1179.

64. Haapanen EJ. Hemoperfusion in acute intoxication: clinical experience with 48 cases. *Acta Med Scand Suppl* 1982;668:76–81.

65. Blye E, Lorch J, Cortell S. Extracorporeal therapy in the treatment of intoxication. *Am J Kidney Dis* 1984;3:321–338.

66. Peterson RG, Peterson LN. Cleansing the blood: hemodialysis, peritoneal dialysis, exchange transfusion, charcoal hemoperfusion, forced diuresis. *Ped Clin North Am* 1986;33:675–689.

67. Garella S. Extracorporeal techniques in the treatment of exogenous intoxications. *Kidney Int* 1988;33:735–740.

68. Pentel PR. Tricyclic and newer antidepressants. In: Haddad LM, Winchester FJ, eds. *Clinical Management of Poisoning and Drug Overdose*. 3rd ed. Philadelphia, PA: WB Saunders, 1998:636–655.

69. Ghannoum M, Nolin TD, Lavergne V, et al. Blood purification in toxicology: nephrology's ugly duckling. *Adv Chronic Kidney Dis* 2011;18:160–166.

70. Lavergne V, Nolin TD, Hoffman RS, et al. The EXTRIP (Extracorporeal Treatments in Poisoning) workgroup: guideline methodology. *Clin Toxicol* 2012;50:403–413.

71. Ghannoum M, Roberts DM, Hoffman RS, et al. A stepwise approach for the management of poisoning with extracorporeal treatments. *Semin Dial* 2014;27(4):362–370.

72. Yates C, Galvao T, Sowinski KM, et al. Extracorporeal treatment for tricyclic antidepressant poisoning: recommendations from the EXTRIP Workgroup. *Semin Dial* 2014;27(4):381–389.

73. Mactier R, Laliberté M, Mardini J, et al. Extracorporeal treatment for barbiturate poisoning: recommendations from the EXTRIP Workgroup. *Am J Kidney Dis* 2014;64(3):347–358.

74. McBride PV, Rumack BH. Acetaminophen intoxication. *Semin Dial* 1992;5:292–298.

75. Gosselin S, Juurlink DN, Kielstein JT, et al. Extracorporeal treatment for acetaminophen poisoning: recommendations from the EXTRIP workgroup. *Clin Toxicol (Phila)* 2014;52(8):856–867.

76. Kruse JA. Methanol and ethylene glycol intoxication. *Crit Care Clin* 2012;28:661–711.

77. Coulter CV, Farquhar SE, McSherry CM, et al. Methanol and ethylene glycol acute poisonings—predictors of mortality. *Clin Toxicol* 2011;49:900–906.

78. Bennett IL Jr, Cary FH, Mitchell GL Jr, et al. Acute methyl alcohol poisoning: a review based on experiences in an outbreak of 323 cases. *Medicine (Baltimore)* 1953;32:431–463.

79. Zakharov S, Pelclova D, Urban P, et al. Czech mass methanol outbreak 2012: epidemiology, challenges and clinical features. *Clin Toxicol (Phila)* 2014;52:1013–1024.

80. Paasma R, Hovda KE, Tikkerberi A, et al. Methanol mass poisoning in Estonia: outbreak in 154 patients. *Clin Toxicol (Phila)* 2007;45:152–157.

81. Hovda KE, Hunderi OH, Tafjord AB, et al. Methanol outbreak in Norway 2002-2004: epidemiology, clinical features and prognostic signs. *J Intern Med* 2005;258:181–190.

82. Ghannoum M, Hoffman RS, Mowry JB, et al. Trends in toxic alcohol exposures in the United States from 2000 to 2013: a focus on the use of antidotes and extracorporeal treatments. *Semin Dial* 2014;27:395–401.

83. Bebarta VS, Heard K, Dart RC. Inhalational abuse of methanol products: elevated methanol and formate levels without vision loss. *Am J Emerg Med* 2006;24:725–728.

84. Kleiman R, Nickle R, Schwartz M. Inhalational methanol toxicity. *J Med Toxicol* 2009;5:158–164.

85. Jacobsen D, McMartin KE. Methanol and ethylene glycol poisonings. Mechanism of toxicity, clinical course, diagnosis and treatment. *Med Toxicol* 1986;1(5):309–334.

86. Martin-Amat G, McMartin KE, Hayreh SS, et al. Methanol poisoning: ocular toxicity produced by formate. *Toxicol Appl Pharmacol* 1978;45:201–208.

87. Roberts DM, Yates C, Megarbane B, et al. Recommendations for the role of extracorporeal treatments in the management of acute methanol poisoning: a systematic review and consensus statement. *Crit Care Med* 2015;43:461–472.

88. Winchester JF. Methanol, isopropyl alcohol, higher alcohols, ethylene glycol, cellosolves, acetone, and oxalate. In: Shannon MW, Borron SW, Burns MJ, eds. *Haddad and Winchester's Clinical Management of Poisoning and Drug Overdose*. 3rd ed. Philadelphia, PA: WB Saunders, 1998:491–504.

89. McMartin KE, Ambre JJ, Tephly TR. Methanol poisoning in human subjects: role for formic acid accumulation in the metabolic acidosis. *Am J Med* 1980;68:414–418.

90. Barceloux DG, Bond GR, Krenzelok EP, et al. American Academy of Clinical Toxicology practice guidelines on the treatment of methanol poisoning. *J Toxicol Clin Toxicol* 2002;40:415–446.

91. Eells JT, Salzman MM, Lewandowski MF, et al. Formate-induced alterations in retinal function in methanol-intoxicated rats. *Toxicol Appl Pharmacol* 1996;140:58–69.

92. Benton CD Jr, Calhoun FP Jr. The ocular effects of methyl alcohol poisoning: report of a catastrophe involving 320 persons. *Am J Ophthalmol* 1953;36:1677–1685.

93. Paasma R, Hovda KE, Jacobsen D. Methanol poisoning and long term sequelae—a six years follow-up after a large methanol outbreak. *BMC Clin Pharmacol* 2009;9:1–5.

94. Singh P, Paliwal VK, Neyaz Z, et al. Methanol toxicity presenting as haemorrhagic putaminal necrosis and optic atrophy. *Pract Neurol* 2013;13:204–205.

95. Phang PT, Passerini L, Mielke B, et al. Brain hemorrhage associated with methanol poisoning. *Crit Care Med* 1988;16:137–140.

96. Reddy NJ, Lewis LD, Gardner TB, et al. Two cases of rapid onset Parkinson's syndrome following toxic ingestion of ethylene glycol and methanol. *Clin Pharmacol Ther* 2007;81:114–121.

97. Seyffart G. Methyl alcohol. In: Seyffart G, ed. *Poison Index—The Treatment of Acute Intoxication.* Lengerich, Germany: Pabst Science, 1997:457–464.

98. Agency for toxic substances and disease registry. Methanol toxicity. *Am Fam Physician* 1993;47:163–171.

99. Liu JL, Daya MR, Carrasquillo O, et al. Prognostic factors in patients with methanol poisoning. *Clin Toxicol* 1998;36:175–181.

100. Hovda KE, Hunderi OH, Rudberg N, et al. Anion and osmolal gaps in the diagnosis of methanol poisoning: clinical study in 28 patients. *Intensive Care Med* 2004;30(9):1842–1846.

101. Mycyk MB, Aks SE. A visual schematic for clarifying the temporal relationship between the anion and osmol gaps in toxic alcohol poisoning. *Am J Emerg Med* 2003;21:333–335.

102. Kruse JA. Lactic acidosis. In: Carlson RW, Geheb MA, eds. *Principles and Practice of Medical Intensive Care.* Philadelphia, PA: WB Saunders, 1993:1231–1245.

103. Burns MJ, Graudins A, Aaron CK, et al. Treatment of methanol poisoning with intravenous 4-methylpyrazole. *Ann Emerg Med* 1997;30: 829–832.

104. Jazz Pharmaceuticals. Antizol-fomepizole injection, solution [package insert]. Palo Alto, CA: Jazz Pharmaceuticals, 2006.

105. Noker PE, Eells JT, Tephly TR. Methanol toxicity: treatment with folic acid and 5-formyl-tetrahydrofolic acid. *Alcohol Clin Exp Res* 1980;4:378–383.

106. Brent J. Fomepizole for ethylene glycol and methanol poisoning. *N Engl J Med* 2009;360:2216–2223.

107. Wagner FW, Burger AR, Vallee BL. Kinetic properties of human liver alcohol dehydrogenase: oxidation of alcohols by class I isoenzymes. *Biochemistry* 1983;22:1857–1863.

108. Barceloux DG, Krenzelok EP, Olson K, et al. American Academy of Clinical Toxicology practice guidelines in the treatment of the ethylene glycol poisoning. *Clin Toxicol* 1999;37:537–560.

109. Burgess E. Prolonged hemodialysis in methanol intoxication. *Pharmacotherapy* 1992;12:238–239.

110. Dorval M, Pichette V, Cardinal J, et al. The use of an ethanol and phosphate enriched dialysate to maintain stable serum ethanol levels during hemodialysis for methanol intoxication. *Nephrol Dial Transplant* 1999;14:1774–1777.

111. Chow MT, Di Silvestro VA, Yung CY, et al. Treatment of acute methanol intoxication with hemodialysis using an ethanol-enriched, bicarbonate-based dialysate. *Am J Kidney Dis* 1997;30:568–570.

112. Wadgymar A, Wu GG. Treatment of acute methanol intoxication with hemodialysis. *Am J Kidney Dis* 1998;5:897.

113. Carauna RJ, Raja RM, Bush JV, et al. Heparin-free dialysis: comparative data and results in high-risk patients. *Kidney Int* 1987;6:1351–1355.

114. Karlson-Stiber C, Persson H. Ethylene glycol poisoning: experiences from an epidemic in Sweden. *Clin Toxicol* 1992;30:565–574.

115. Schultz S, Kinde M, Johnson D, et al. Ethylene glycol intoxication due to contamination of water systems. *MMWR Morb Mortal Wkly Rep* 1987;36(36):611–614.

116. Lai MW, Klein-Schwartz W, Rodgers GC, et al. 2005 annual report of American Association of Poison Control Centers' National Poisoning and Exposure database. *Clin Toxicol* 2006;44:803–932.

117. Bronstein AC, Spyker DA, Cantilena LR Jr, et al. 2007 annual report of the American Association of Poison Control Centers' National Poison Data System (NPDS): 25th annual report. *Clin Toxicol* 2008;46: 927–1057.

118. Seyffart G. Ethylene glycol. In: Seyffart G, ed. *Poison Index—The Treatment of Acute Intoxication.* Lengerich, Germany: Pabst Science, 1997:318–328.

119. Devoti E, Marta E, Belotti E, et al. Diethylene glycol poisoning from transcutaneous absorption. *Am J Kidney Dis* 2015;65:603–606.

120. Eder AF, McGrath CM, Dowdy YG, et al. Ethylene glycol poisoning: toxicokinetic and analytical factors affecting laboratory diagnosis. *Clin Chem* 1998;44:168–177.

121. Gabow PA, Clay K, Sullivan JB, et al. Organic acids in ethylene glycol intoxication. *Ann Intern Med* 1986;105:16–20.

122. Jacobsen D, Ovrebø S, Ostborg J, et al. Glycolate causes the acidosis in ethylene glycol poisoning and is effectively removed by hemodialysis. *Acta Med Scand* 1984;216:409–416.

123. Cooper SM, Baron JM. Case records of the Massachusetts General Hospital. *N Engl J Med* 2015;372:465–473.

124. Peterson CD, Collins AJ, Himes JM, et al. Ethylene glycol poisoning: pharmacokinetics during therapy with ethanol and hemodialysis. *N Engl J Med* 1981;304:21–23.

125. McMartin KE, Hedström KG, Tolf BR, et al. Studies on the metabolic interactions between 4-methylpyrazole and methanol using the monkey as an animal model. *Arch Biochem Biophys* 1980;199:606–614.

126. Brent J, McMartin K, Phillips S, et al. Fomepizole for the treatment of ethylene glycol poisoning. *N Engl J Med* 1999;340:832–838.

127. Kahn HS, Brotchner RJ. A recovery from ethylene glycol (antifreeze) intoxication: a case of survival and two fatalities from ethylene glycol including autopsy findings. *Ann Intern Med* 1950;32:284–294.

128. Hylander B, Kjellstrand CM. Prognostic factors and treatment of severe ethylene glycol intoxication. *Intensive Care Med* 1996;22:546–552.

129. Kralova I, Stepanek Z, Dusek J. Ethylene glycol intoxication misdiagnosed as eclampsia. *Acta Anaesthesiol Scand* 2006;50:385–387.

130. Poldelski V, Johnson A, Wright S. Ethylene glycol-mediated tubular injury: identification of critical metabolites and injury pathways. *Am J Kidney Dis* 2001;38:339–348.

131. Jacobsen D, Akesson I, Shefter E. Urinary calcium monohydrate crystals in ethylene glycol poisoning. *Scand J Clin Lab Invest* 1982;42: 231–234.

132. Terlinsky AS, Grochowski J, Geoly KL, et al. Identification of atypical calcium oxalate crystalluria following ethylene glycol ingestion. *Am J Clin Pathol* 1981;76:223–226.

133. Godolphin W, Meagher EP, Sanders HD, et al. Unusual calcium oxalate crystals in ethylene glycol poisoning. *Clin Toxicol* 1980;16(4):479–486.

134. Wendland E, Yamase H, Adams N, et al. Hippuric acid not calcium oxalate crystals in the urine of a patient with ethylene glycol ingestion. *Am J Kidney Dis* 2011;57(4):A104.

135. Winter ML, Ellis MD, Snodgrass WR. Urine fluorescence using a Wood's lamp to detect the antifreeze additive sodium fluorescein: a qualitative adjunctive test in suspected ethylene glycol ingestions. *Ann Emerg Med* 1990;19:663–667.

136. Wallace KL, Suchard JR, Curry SC, et al. Diagnostic use of physicians' detection of urine fluorescence in a simulated ingestion of sodium fluorescein-containing antifreeze. *Ann Emerg Med* 2001;38: 49–54.

137. Casavant MJ, Shah MN, Battels R. Does fluorescent urine indicate antifreeze ingestion by children? *Pediatrics* 2001;109:113–114.

138. Underwood F, Bennett WN. Ethylene glycol intoxication: prevention of renal failure by aggressive management. *JAMA* 1973;226:1453–1454.

139. Jacobsen D, Sebastian CS, Barron SK, et al. Effects of 4-methylpyrazole, methanol/ethylene glycol antidote, in healthy humans. *J Emerg Med* 1990;8:455–461.

140. Noghnogh AA, Reid RW, Nawab ZM, et al. Preparation of ethanol-enriched, bicarbonate-based hemodialysis. *Artif Organs* 1999;23:208–216.

141. Cheng JT, Beysolow TD, Kaul B, et al. Clearance of ethylene glycol by kidneys and hemodialysis. *Clin Toxicol* 1987;27:95–108.

142. Watson W. Ethylene glycol toxicity: closing in a rational evidence-based treatment. *Ann Emerg Med* 2000;36:139–141.

143. Borron SW, Mégarbane B, Baud FJ. Fomepizole in treatment of uncomplicated ethylene glycol poisoning. *Lancet* 1999;354(4):831.

144. Boyer EW, Mejia M, Woolf A, et al. Severe ethylene glycol ingestion treated without hemodialysis. *Pediatrics* 2001;107(1):172–173.

145. Buchanan JA, Alhelail M, Cetaruk EW, et al. Massive ethylene glycol ingestion treated with fomepizole alone a viable therapeutic option. *J Med Toxicol* 2010;6(2):131–134.

146. Buller GK, Moskowitz CB. When is it appropriate to treat ethylene glycol intoxication with fomepizole alone without hemodialysis? *Semin Dial* 2011;24(4):441–442.

147. Levine M, Curry SC, Ruha AM, et al. Ethylene glycol elimination kinetics and outcomes in patients managed without hemodialysis. *Ann Emerg Med* 2012;59(6):527–531.

148. Chow MT, Chen J, Patel JS, et al. Use of a phosphorus-enriched dialysate to hemodialyze patients with ethylene glycol intoxication. *Int J Artif Organs* 1997;20:101–104.

149. Chow MT, Lin HJ, Mitra EA, et al. Hemodialysis-induced hypophosphatemia in a normophosphatemic patient dialyzed for ethylene glycol poisoning: treatment with phosphorus-enriched hemodialysis. *Artif Organs* 1998;22:905–913.

150. Hirsch DJ, Jindal KK, Wong P, et al. A simple method to estimate the required dialysis time for cases of alcohol poisoning. *Kidney Int* 2001;60:2021–2024.

151. Christiansson LK, Kaspersson KE, Kulling PE, et al. Treatment of severe ethylene glycol intoxication with continuous arterio-venous hemofiltration dialysis. *Clin Toxicol* 1995;33:267–270.

152. Slaughter RJ, Mason RW, Beasley DM, et al. Isopropanol poisoning. *Clin Toxicol (Phila)* 2014;52(5):470–478.

153. Lacouture PG, Wason S, Abrams A, et al. Acute isopropyl alcohol intoxication: diagnosis and management. *Am J Med* 1983;75:680–686.

154. Abramson S, Singh AK. Treatment of the alcohol intoxications: ethylene glycol, methanol and isopropanol. *Curr Opin Nephrol Hypertens* 2000;9:695–701.

155. Zaman F, Pervez A, Abreo K. Isopropyl alcohol intoxication: a diagnostic challenge. *Am J Kidney Dis* 2002;40:E12.

156. Meng X, Paul S, Federman DJ. Metabolic acidosis in a patient with isopropyl alcohol intoxication: a case report. *Ann Intern Med* 2015;162(4):322–323.

157. Lehman AJ, Chase HF. The acute and chronic toxicity of isopropyl alcohol. *J Lab Clin Med* 1944;29:561–567.

158. Rosansky SJ. Isopropyl alcohol poisoning treated with hemodialysis: kinetics of isopropyl alcohol and acetone removal. *J Toxicol Clin Toxicol* 1982;19:265–271.

159. Pappas AA, Ackerman BH, Olsen KM, et al. Isopropanol ingestion: a report of six episodes with isopropanol and acetone serum concentration time data. *J Toxicol Clin Toxicol* 1991;29:11–21.

160. Chyka PA, Erdman AR, Christianson G, et al. Salicylate poisoning: an evidence-based consensus guideline for out-of-hospital management. *Clin Toxicol (Phila)* 2007;45:95–131.

161. Muniandy RK, Sinnathamby V. Salicylate toxicity from ingestion of traditional massage oil. *BMJ Case Rep* 2012;2012:bcr2012006562.

162. Williams GD, Kirk EP, Wilson CJ, et al. Salicylate intoxication from teething gel in infancy. *Med J Aust* 2011;194(3):146–148.

163. Roberts LJ. Analgesic-antipyretics and anti-inflammatory agents and drugs employed in the treatment of gout. In: Hardman JG, Limbird LE, Gilman AG, eds. *Goodman and Gilman's the Pharmacological Basis of Therapeutics.* 10th ed. New York, NY: McGraw-Hill, 2001:687–731.

164. Wosilait WD. Theoretical analysis of the binding of salicylate by human serum albumin: the relationship between free and bound drug and therapeutic levels. *Eur J Clin Pharmacol* 1976;9:285–290.

165. Kerr F, Krenzelok EP. Salicylates. In: Shannon MW, Borron SW, Burns MJ, eds. *Haddad and Winchester's Clinical Management of Poisoning and Drug Overdose,* 4th ed. Philadelphia, PA: WB Saunders, 2007:835–848.

166. Rubin GM, Tozer TN, Fie S. Concentration-dependence of salicylate distribution. *J Pharm Pharmacol* 1983;35:115–117.

167. Hill JB. Salicylate intoxication. *N Engl J Med* 1973;288:1110–1113.

168. Proudfoot AT. Toxicity of salicylates. *Am J Med* 1983;75:88–103.

169. Gaudreault P, Temple AR, Lovejoy FH. The relative severity of acute versus chronic salicylate poisoning in children: a clinical comparison. *Pediatrics* 1982;70:566–569.

170. Winters RW, White J, Hughes MC, et al. Disturbances of acid-base equilibrium in salicylate intoxication. *Pediatrics* 1959;23:260–285.

171. Anderson RJ, Potts DE, Gabow PA, et al. Unrecognized adult salicylate intoxication. *Ann Intern Med* 1976;85:745–748.

172. Bowers RE, Brigham KL, Owen PJ. Salicylate pulmonary edema: the mechanism in sheep and review of the literature. *Am Rev Resp Dis* 1977;115:261–268.

173. Walters JS, Woodring JH, Stelling CB, et al. Salicylate-induced pulmonary edema. *Radiology* 1983;146:289–293.

174. Hormaechea E, Carlson RW, Rogove H, et al. Hypovolemia, pulmonary edema, and protein changes in severe salicylate poisoning. *Am J Med* 1979;66:1046–1050.

175. Heffner JE, Sahn SA. Salicylate-induced pulmonary edema. *Ann Intern Med* 1981;95:405–409.

176. Millhorn DE, Eldridge FL, Waldrop TG. Effects of salicylate and 2,4-dinitrophenol on respiration and metabolism. *Am J Physiol* 1982;53:925–929.

177. Ring T, Anderson PT, Knutsen F, et al. Salicylate-induced hyperventilation. *Lancet* 1985;1:1450.

178. Harrington JT. Metabolic acidosis. In: Cohen JJ, Kassirer JP, eds. *Acid-Base.* Boston, MA: Little, Brown and Company, 1982:121–225.

179. Bartels PD, Lund-Jacobsen H. Blood lactate and ketone body concentration in salicylate intoxication. *Hum Toxicol* 1986;5:363–366.

180. Gabow PA, Anderson RJ, Potts DE, et al. Acid-base disturbances in the salicylate-intoxicated adult. *Arch Intern Med* 1978;138:1481–1484.

181. Jacob J, Lavonas EJ. Falsely normal anion gap in severe salicylate poisoning caused by laboratory interference. *Ann Emerg Med* 2011;58(3):280–281.

182. Srivali N, Ungprasert P, Edmonds LC. Negative anion gap metabolic acidosis and low level of salicylate cannot ignore salicylate toxicity! *Am J Emerg Med* 2014;32(3):279–280.

183. Kaul V, Imam SH, Gambhir HS, et al. Negative anion gap metabolic acidosis in salicylate overdose—a zebra! *Am J Emerg Med* 2013;31(10):1536.e3–1536.e4.

184. Mori L, Waldhuber S. Salicylate interference with the Roche Cobas Integra chloride electrode. *Clin Chem* 1997;43:1249–1250.

185. Lim CS, Marcelo CB, Bryant SM. Those salicylate cases—how sweet are they? [published online ahead of print September 17, 2014]. *Am J Ther.*

186. Clarkson AR. Phenistix in screening. *Aust Fam Physician* 1978;7:1324–1328.

187. Brenner BE, Simon RR. Management of salicylate intoxication. *Drugs* 1982;24:335–340.

188. Johnston PK, Free HM, Free AH. A simplified urine and serum screening test for salicylate intoxication. *J Pediatr* 1963;63:949–953.

189. Temple AR. Acute and chronic effects of aspirin toxicity and their treatment. *Arch Intern Med* 1981;141:346–349.

190. Chapman J, Proudfoot AT. Adult salicylate poisoning: deaths and outcome in patients with high plasma salicylate concentration. *Q J Med* 1989;268:699–707.

191. Done AK. Aspirin overdosage: incidence, diagnosis, and management. *Pediatrics* 1978;62(5 Pt 2 Suppl):890–897.

192. Kwong TC, Laczin J, Baum J. Self-poisoning with enteric-coated aspirin. *Am J Clin Path* 1983;80:888–890.

193. Notarianni L. A reassessment of the treatment of salicylate poisoning. *Drug Saf* 1992;7:292–303.

194. Krenzelok EP. Salicylate toxicity. In: Haddad LM, Shannon MW, Winchester JF, eds. *Clinical Management of Poisoning and Drug Overdose.* 3rd ed. Philadelphia, PA: WB Saunders, 1998:675–687.

195. Mayer AL, Sitar DS, Tenenbein M. Multiple-dose charcoal and whole-bowel irrigation do not increase clearance of absorbed salicylate. *Arch Intern Med* 1992;152:393–396.

196. Prescott LF, Balali-Mood M, Critchley JA, et al. Diuresis or alkalinisation for salicylate poisoning? *BMJ* 1982;285:1383–1386.

197. Gordon IJ, Bowler CS, Coakley J, et al. Algorithm for modified alkaline diuresis in salicylate poisoning. *BMJ* 1984;289:1039–1040.

198. Dargan PI, Wallace CI, Jones AL. An evidence based flowchart to guide the management of acute salicylate (aspirin) overdose. *Emerg Med J* 2002;19:206–209.

199. Richlie DG, Anderson RJ. Contemporary management of salicylate poisoning: when should hemodialysis and hemoperfusion be used? *Semin Dial* 1996;9:257–264.

200. Wrathall G, Sinclair R, Moore A, et al. Three case reports of the use of haemodiafiltration in the treatment of salicylate overdose. *Hum Exp Toxicol* 2001;20:491–495.

201. Juurlink DN, Gosselin S, Kielstein JT, et al. Extracorporeal treatment for salicylate poisoning: systematic review and recommendations from the EXTRIP Workgroup. *Ann Emerg Med* 2015;66(2):165–181.

202. Jacobsen D, Wiik-Larsen E, Bredesen JE. Hemodialysis or hemoperfusion in severe salicylate poisoning. *Hum Toxicol* 1988;7:161–163.

203. Watson WA, Litovitz TL, Rodgers GC, et al. 2004 annual report of the American Association of Poison Control Centers Toxic Exposure Surveillance System. *Am J Emerg Med* 2005;23:589–666.

204. Fertel BS, Nelson LS, Goldfarb DS. The underutilization of hemodialysis in patients with salicylate poisoning. *Kidney Int* 2009;75: 1349–1353.

205. Aita JF, Aita JA, Aita VA. 7-Up anti-acid lithiated lemon soda or early medicinal use of lithium. *Nebr Med J* 1990;75:277–279.

206. Strobusch AD, Jefferson JW. The checkered history of lithium in medicine. *Pharm Hist* 1980;22:72.

207. Corcoran AC, Taylor RD, Page IH. Lithium poisoning from the use of salt substitutes. *J Am Med Assoc* 1949;139:685.

208. Pauzé DK, Brooks DE. Lithium toxicity from an Internet dietary supplement. *J Med Toxicol* 2007;3:61.

209. Belmaker RH. Bipolar disorder. *N Engl J Med* 2004;351:476–486.

210. Cade JF. Lithium salts in the treatment of psychotic excitement. *Med J Aust* 1949;2:349.

211. Baldessarini RJ. Drugs and the treatment of psychiatric disorders: psychosis and mania. In: Hardman JG, Limbird LE, Gilman AG, eds. *Goodman and Gilman's the Pharmacological Basis of Therapeutics.* 10th ed. New York, NY: McGraw-Hill, 2001:485–520.

212. Thundiyil JG, Olson KR. Lithium. In: Shannon MW, Borron SW, Burns MJ, eds. *Haddad and Winchester's Clinical Management of Poisoning and Drug Overdose.* 4th ed. Philadelphia, PA: WB Saunders, 2007: 579–588.

213. Winchester JF. Lithium. In: Shannon MW, Borron SW, Burns MJ, eds. *Haddad and Winchester's Clinical Management of Poisoning and Drug Overdose.* 3rd ed. Philadelphia, PA: WB Saunders, 1998:467–474.

214. Goddard J, Bloom SR, Frackowiak RS. Lithium intoxication. *BMJ* 1991;302:1267–1269.

215. Singer I, Rotenberg D. Mechanism of lithium action. *N Engl J Med* 1973;289:254–260.

216. Holstein-Rathlou NH. Lithium transport across biological membranes. *Kidney Int* 1990;37(Suppl 28):S4–S9.

217. Godinich MJ, Battle DC. Renal tubular effects of lithium. *Kidney Int* 1990;37(Suppl 28):S52–S57.

218. Hansen HE, Amdisen A. Lithium intoxication. (Report of 23 cases and review of 100 cases from the literature). *Q J Med* 1978;47:123–144.

219. Bennet WM. Drug interactions and consequences of sodium restriction. *Am J Clin Nutr* 1997;65:678–681.

220. Freeman MP, Freeman SA. Lithium: clinical considerations in internal medicine. *Am J Med* 2006;119:478–481.

221. Finley PR, Warner MD, Peabody CA. Clinical relevance of drug interactions with lithium. *Clin Pharmacokinet* 1995;29:172–191.

222. Finley PR, O'Brien JG, Coleman RW. Lithium and angiotensin-converting enzyme inhibitors: evaluation of a potential interaction. *J Clin Psychopharmacol* 1996;16:68–71.

223. Decker BS, Goldfarb DS, Dargan PI, et al. Extracorporeal treatment for lithium poisoning: systematic review and recommendations from the EXTRIP Workgroup. *Clin J Am Soc Nephrol* 2015;10(5):875–887.

224. Timmer RT, Sands JM. Lithium intoxication. *J Am Soc Nephrol* 1999;10:666–674.

225. Gadallah MF, Feinstein EI, Massry SG. Lithium intoxication: clinical course and therapeutic considerations. *Miner Electrolyte Metab* 1988;14:146–149.

226. Colak Oray N, Arici A, Yanturali S, et al. Lithium poisoning: is the lithium level a guide? *Anadolu Psikiyatri Derg* 2011;12:198–203.

227. Khasraw M, Ashley D, Wheeler G, et al. Using lithium as a neuroprotective agent in patients with cancer. *BMC Med* 2012;10:131–132.

228. Jaeger A, Sauder P, Kopferschmitt J, et al. When should dialysis be performed in lithium poisoning? A kinetic study in 14 cases of lithium poisoning. *Clin Toxicol* 1993;31:429–447.

229. Porto FH, Leite MA, Fontenelle LF, et al. The Syndrome of Irreversible Lithium-Effectuated Neurotoxicity (SILENT): one-year follow-up of a single case. *J Neurol Sci* 2009;277:172–173.

230. Adityanjee, Munshi KR, Thampy A. The syndrome of irreversible lithium-effectuated neurotoxicity. *Clin Neuropharmacol* 2005;28:38–49.

231. Zallo Atxutegi E, Pacheco MT, Izaguirre NB, et al. Syndrome of irreversible lithium-effectuated neurotoxicity. A propos of a case. *Psiquiatria Biologica* 2008;15:56–58.

232. Markowitz GS, Radhakrishnan J, Kambham N, et al. Lithium nephrotoxicity: a progressive combined glomerular and tubulointerstitial nephropathy. *Am Soc Nephrol* 2000;11:1439–1448.

233. Movig KL, Baumgarten R, Leufkens HG, et al. Risk factors for the development of lithium-induced polyuria. *Br J Psychiatry* 2003;182: 319–323.

234. Bendz H, Aurell M. Drug-induced diabetes insipidus: incidence, prevention and management. *Drug Saf* 1999;21:449–456.

235. Zaidan M, Stucker F, Stengel B, et al. Increased risk of solid renal tumors in lithium-treated patients. *Kidney Int* 2014;86(1):184–190.

236. Grünfeld JP, Rossier BC. Lithium nephrotoxicity revisited. *Nat Rev Nephrol* 2009;5(5):270–276.

237. Jurado RL, del Rio C, Nassar G, et al. Low anion gap. *South Med J* 1998; 91:624–629.

238. Kelleher SP, Raciti A, Arbeit LA. Reduced or absent serum anion gap as a marker of severe lithium intoxication. *Arch Intern Med* 1986; 146:1839–1840.

239. Oakley PW, Dawson AH, Whyte IM, et al. Lithium: thyroid effects and altered renal handling. *J Toxicol Clin Toxicol* 2000;38:333–337.

240. Sheehan GL. Lithium neurotoxicity. *Clin Exp Neurol* 1991;28:112–127.

241. Brady HR, Horgan JH. Lithium and the heart: unanswered questions. *Chest* 1988;93:166–168.

242. Perrier A, Martin PY, Favre H, et al. Very severe self-poisoning lithium carbonate intoxication causing a myocardial infarction. *Chest* 1991;100:863–865.

243. Favin F, Klein-Schwartz W, Oderda GM, et al. In-vitro study of lithium carbonate adsorption by activated charcoal. *J Toxicol Clin Toxicol* 1988;26:443–450.

244. Smith SW, Ling LJ, Halstenson CE. Whole-bowel irrigation as a treatment for acute lithium overdose. *Ann Emerg Med* 1991;20:536–539.

245. Waring WS. Management of lithium toxicity. *Toxicol Rev* 2006;25: 221–230.

246. Clendeninn NJ, Pond SM, Kaysen G, et al. Potential pitfalls in the evaluation of the usefulness of hemodialysis for the removal of lithium. *J Toxicol Clin Toxicol* 1982;19:341–352.

247. Roberts DM, Gosselin S. Variability in the management of lithium poisoning. *Semin Dial* 2014;27(4):390–394.

248. Szerlip HM, Heeger P, Feldman GM. Comparison between acetate and bicarbonate dialysis for the treatment of lithium intoxication. *Am J Nephrol* 1992;12:116–120.

249. Leblanc M, Raymond M, Bonnardeaux A, et al. Lithium poisoning treated by high-performance continuous arteriovenous and venovenous hemodiafiltration. *Am J Kidney Dis* 1996;27:365–372.

250. Beckman U, Oakley PW, Dawson AH, et al. Efficacy of continuous venovenous hemodialysis in the treatment of severe lithium toxicity. *Clin Toxicol* 2001;39:393–397.

251. Undem BJ. Drugs used in the treatment of asthma. In: Hardman JG, Limbird LE, Gilman AG, eds. *Goodman and Gilman's the Pharmacological Basis of Therapeutics.* 10th ed. New York, NY: Pergamon Press, 1990:733–754.

252. Sessler CN. Theophylline toxicity: clinical features of 116 consecutive cases. *Am J Med* 1990;88:567.

253. Seyffart G. Theophylline. In: Seyffart G, ed. *Poison Index—The Treatment of Acute Intoxication.* Lengerich, Germany: Pabst Science, 1997:638–646.

254. Shannon MW. Theophylline. In: Shannon MW, Borron SW, Burns MJ, eds. *Haddad and Winchester's Clinical Management of Poisoning and Drug Overdose.* 4th ed. Philadelphia, PA: WB Saunders, 2007:1035–1050.

255. Clayton D, Bochner F. Delayed toxicity with slow-release theophylline. *Med J Aust* 1986;144:386–387.

256. Bukowskyj M, Nakatsu K, Munt PW. Theophylline reassessed. *Ann Intern Med* 1984;101:63–73.

257. Hendeles L. Theophylline. In: Evans WE, Schentag JJ, Jusko WJ, eds. *Applied Pharmacokinetics: Principles of Therapeutic Drug Monitoring.* 2nd ed. Philadelphia, PA: Lippincott, 1986:1105–1188.

258. Shannon MW. Predictors of major toxicity after theophylline overdose. *Ann Intern Med* 1993;119:1161–1167.

259. Feoktistov I, Polosa R, Holgate ST, et al. Adenosine A2B receptors: a novel therapeutic target in asthma? *Trends Pharmacol Sci* 1998;19: 148–153.

260. Fredholm BB, Persson CGA. Xanthine derivatives as adenosine receptor antagonists. *Eur J Pharmacol* 1982;81:673–676.

261. Manns JS, Holgate ST. Specific antagonism of adenosine-induced bronchoconstriction in asthma by oral theophylline. *Br J Clin Pharmacol* 19:685–692.

262. Jacobs MH, Senior RM, Kessler G. Clinical experience with theophylline—relationships between dosage, serum concentration, and toxicity. *JAMA* 1976;235:1983–1986.

263. Olson KR, Benowitz NL, Woo OF, et al. Theophylline overdose: acute single ingestion versus chronic repeated overmedication. *Am J Emerg Med* 1985;3:386–394.

264. Kearney TE, Manoguerra AS, Curtis GP, et al. Theophylline toxicity and the beta-adrenergic system. *Ann Intern Med* 1985;102:766–769.

265. Cooling DS. Theophylline toxicity. *J Emerg Med* 1993;11:415–425.

266. Zwillich CW, Sutton FD, Neff TA, et al. Theophylline-induced seizures in adults: correlation with serum concentration. *Ann Intern Med* 1975;82:784–787.

267. Aitken ML, Martin TR. Life-threatening theophylline toxicity is not predictable by serum levels. *Chest* 1987;91:10–14.

268. American Academy of Pediatrics Committee on Drugs: precautions concerning the use of theophylline. *Pediatrics* 1992;89:781–782.

269. Covelli HD, Knodel AR, Heppner BT. Predisposing factors to apparent theophylline-induced seizures. *Ann Allerg* 1985;54:411–415.

270. Singer EP, Kolischenko A. Seizures due to theophylline overdose. *Chest* 1985;87:755–757.

271. Seto T, Inada H, Kobayashi N, et al. Depression of serum pyridoxal levels in theophylline-induced seizures. *Brain Dev* 2000;32:295–300.

272. Pinard E, Riche D, Puiroud S, et al. Theophylline reduces cerebral hyperemia and enhances brain damage induced by seizures. *Brain Res* 1990;511:303–309.

273. Biberstein MP, Ziegler MG, Ward DM. Use of beta-blockade and hemoperfusion for acute theophylline poisoning. *West J Med* 1984;141: 485–490.

274. Seneff M, Scott J, Friedman B, et al. Acute theophylline toxicity and the use of esmolol to reverse cardiovascular instability. *Ann Emerg Med* 1990;19:671–673.

275. Huber W, Ilgmann K, Page M, et al. Effect of theophylline on contrast-material nephropathy in patients with chronic renal insufficiency: controlled, randomized, double-blinded study. *Radiology* 2002;223:772–779.

276. Gaudreault P, Guay J. Theophylline poisoning—pharmacological considerations and clinical management. *Med Toxicol* 1986;1:161–191.

277. Blake KV, Massey KL, Hendeles L, et al. Relative efficacy of phenytoin and phenobarbital for the prevention of theophylline-induced seizures in mice. *Ann Emerg Med* 1988;17:1024–1028.

278. Amitai Y, Yeung AC, Moye J, et al. Repetitive oral activated charcoal and control of emesis in severe theophylline toxicity. *Ann Intern Med* 1986;105:386–387.

279. Park GD, Radomski L, Goldberg MJ, et al. Effects of size and frequency of oral doses of charcoal on theophylline clearance. *Clin Pharmacol Ther* 1983;34:663–666.

280. Goldberg MJ, Park GD, Berlinger WG. Treatment of theophylline toxicity. *J Allergy Clin Immunol* 1986;78:811–817.

281. Byrd RP, Lopez P, Mercer P, et al. Clinical theophylline toxicity: acute and chronic. *J Ky Med Assoc* 1993;91:198–202.

282. Goldberg MJ, Spector R, Park GD, et al. The effect of sorbitol and activated charcoal on serum theophyline concentrations after slow-release theophylline. *Clin Pharmacol Ther* 1987;41:108–111.

283. Russo ME. Management of theophylline intoxication with charcoal-column hemoperfusion. *N Engl J Med* 1979;300:24–26.

284. Lawyer C, Aitchison J, Sutton J, et al. Treatment of theophylline neurotoxicity with resin hemoperfusion. *Ann Intern Med* 1978;88:515–516.

285. Ehlers SM, Zaske DE, Sawchuk RJ. Massive theophylline overdose: rapid elimination by charcoal hemoperfusion. *JAMA* 1978;240:474–475.

286. Park GD, Spector R, Roberts RJ, et al. Use of hemoperfusion for treatment of theophylline intoxication. *Am J Med* 1983;74:961–966.

287. Van Kesteren RG, van Dijk A, Klein SW, et al. Massive theophylline intoxication: effects of charcoal haemoperfusion on plasma and erythrocyte theophylline concentrations. *Hum Toxicol* 1985;4:127–134.

288. Hootkins R, Lerman MJ, Thompson JR. Sequential and simultaneous "in series" hemodialysis and hemoperfusion in the management of theophylline intoxication. *J Am Soc Nephrol* 1990;1:923–926.

289. Benowitz NL, Toffelmire EB. The use of hemodialysis and hemoperfusion in the treatment of theophylline intoxication. *Semin Dial* 1993; 6:243–252.

290. Lee CS, Marbury TC, Perrin JH, Fuller TJ. Hemodialysis of theophylline in uremic patients. *J Clin Pharmacol* 1979;19:219–226.

291. Heath A, Knudsen K. Role of extracorporeal drug removal in acute theophylline poisoning: a review. *Med Toxicol* 1987;2:294–308.

292. Ghannoum M, Wiegand TJ, Liu KD, et al. Extracorporeal treatment for theophylline poisoning: systematic review and recommendations from the EXTRIP workgroup. *Clin Toxicol (Phila)* 2015;53(4):215–229.

293. Shannon MW. Comparative efficacy of hemodialysis and hemoperfusion in severe theophylline intoxication. *Acad Emerg Med* 1997;4:674–678.

294. Laurent D, Guenzet J, Bourin M. Theophylline: a haemoperfusion modelisation. *Methods Find Exp Clin Pharmacol* 1985;7:253–258.

295. Higgins RM, Hearing S, Goldsmith DJ, et al. Severe theophylline poisoning: charcoal haemoperfusion or haemodialysis? *Postgrad Med J* 1995;71:224–226.

296. Davis E, Perez A, McKay C. A novel self-contained hemoperfusion device for the treatment of theophylline overdose in a swine model [abstract]. *Clin Toxicol (Phila)* 2003;41:695–696.

297. *Guide to Custom Dialysis.* Lakewood, CO: COBE Renal Care, 1992.

298. Brezis M, Brown RS. An unsuspected cause for metabolic acidosis in chronic renal failure: sorbent system hemodialysis. *Am J Kidney Dis* 1985;6:425–427.

299. Henderson JH, McKenzie CA, Hilton PJ, et al. Continuous venovenous haemofiltration for the treatment of theophylline toxicity. *Thorax* 2001;56:242–243.

300. Urquhart R, Edwards C. Increased theophylline clearance during hemofiltration. *Ann Pharmacother* 1995;29:787–788.

301. Jacobi J, Mowry JB. Use of plasmapheresis in acute theophylline toxicity. *Crit Care Med* 1992;20:151.

302. Miceli JN, Bidani A, Aronow R. Peritoneal dialysis of theophylline. *Clin Toxicol* 1979;14:539–544.

303. Kleinschmidt KC. Ethanol. In: Shannon MW, Borron SW, Burns MJ, eds. *Haddad and Winchester's Clinical Management of Poisoning and Drug Overdose.* 4th ed. Philadelphia, PA: WB Saunders, 2007:589–604.

304. Cami J, Farre M. Drug addiction. *N Engl J Med* 2003;349:975–986.

305. Hingson R, Heeren T, Zakocs RC, et al. Magnitude of alcohol-related mortality and morbidity among U.S. college students ages 18–24. *J Stud Alcohol* 2002;63:136–144.

306. Adinoff B, Bone GH, Linnoila M. Acute ethanol poisoning and the ethanol withdrawal syndrome. *Med Toxicol Adverse Drug Exp* 1988;3:172–196.

307. O'Neill S, Tipton KF, Prichard JS, et al. Survival after high blood alcohol levels. *Arch Intern Med* 1984;144:641–642.

308. Seyffart G. Ethyl alcohol. In: Seyffart G, ed. *Poison Index—The Treatment of Acute Intoxication.* Lengerich, Germany: Pabst Science, 1997:311–317.

309. Elliot RW, Hunter PR. Acute ethanol poisoning treated by haemodialysis. *Postgrad Med J* 1974;50:515–517.

310. Atassi WA, Noghnogh AA, Hariman R, et al. Hemodialysis as a treatment of severe ethanol poisoning. *Int J Artif Organs* 1999;22:18–20.

311. Chun LJ, Tong MJ, Busuttil RW, et al. Acetaminophen hepatotoxicity and acute liver failure. *J Clin Gastroenterol* 2009;43:342.

312. Wolf MS, King J, Jacobson K, et al. Risk of unintentional overdose with non-prescription acetaminophen products. *J Gen Intern Med* 2012;27:1587.

313. U.S. Food and Drug Administration. Acetaminophen prescription combination drug products with more than 325 mg: FDA statement—recommendation to discontinue prescribing and dispensing. Silver Spring, MD: U.S. Food and Drug Administration. http://www.fda.gov/Safety/MedWatch/SafetyInformation/SafetyAlertsforHumanMedicalProducts/ucm381650.htm?source=govdelivery&utm_medium=email&utm_source=govdelivery. Accessed January 23, 2014.

314. Lee WM. Acetaminophen and the U.S. Acute Liver Failure Study Group: lowering the risks of hepatic failure. *Hepatology* 2004;40:6.

315. McJunkin B, Barwick KW, Little WC, et al. Fatal massive hepatic necrosis following acetaminophen overdose. *JAMA* 1976;236(16):1874–1875.

316. Nonprescription Drugs Advisory Committee. Safety issues related to acetaminophen. http://www.fda.gov/ohrms/dockets/ac/02/transcripts/3882T1.htm. Accessed June 26, 2007.

317. Whitcomb DC, Block GD. Association of acetaminophen hepatotoxicity with fasting and ethanol use. *JAMA* 1994;272(23):1845–1850.

318. Slattery JT, Nelson SD, Thummel KE. The complex interaction between ethanol and acetaminophen. *Clin Pharmacol Ther* 1996;60(3):241–246.

319. Josephy PD. The molecular toxicology of acetaminophen. *Drug Metab Rev* 2005;37:581–594.

320. Kaplowitz N. Acetaminophen hepatotoxicity. What do we know, what don't we know, and what do we do next. *Hepatology* 2004;40:23–26.

321. Rowden AK, Norvell J, Eldridge DL, et al. Updates on acetaminophen toxicity. *Med Clin N Am* 2005;89:1145–1159.

322. Bernal W, Donaldson N, Wyncoll D, et al. Blood lactate as an early predictor of outcome in paracetamol-induced acute liver failure: a cohort study. *Lancet* 2002;359:558–563.

323. Schiodt FV, Rochling FA, Casey DL, et al. Paracetamol toxicity in an urban county hospital. *N Engl J Med* 1997;337:1112–1117.

324. Makin AJ, Wendon J, Williams R. A 7-year experience of severe acetaminophen-induced hepatotoxicity (1987-1993). *Gastroenterology* 1995;109:1907–1916.

325. Jaeschke H, Bajt ML. Mechanisms of acetaminophen hepatotoxicity. In: McQueen CA, ed. *Comprehensive Toxicology*. 2nd ed. Philadelphia, PA: Elsevier Science, 2010;457–473.

326. Yarema MC, Johnson DW, Berlin RJ, et al. Comparison of the 20-hour intravenous and 72-hour oral acetylcysteine protocols for the treatment of acute acetaminophen poisoning. *Ann Emerg Med* 2009;54:606–614.

327. Salhanick SD, Shannon MW. Acetaminophen. In: Shannon MW, Borron SW, Burns MJ, eds. *Haddad and Winchester's Clinical Management of Poisoning and Drug Overdose*. 4th ed. Philadelphia, PA: WB Saunders, 2007;825–834.

328. Larson AM. Acetaminophen hepatotoxicity. *Clin Liver Dis* 2007;11:525–548.

329. Ashbourne JF, Olson KR, Khayam-Bashi H. Value of rapid screening for acetaminophen in all patients with intentional drug overdose. *Ann Emerg Med* 1989;18:1035–1038.

330. Sporer KA, Khayam-Bashi H. Acetaminophen and salicylate serum levels in patients with suicidal ingestion or altered mental status. *Am J Emerg Med* 1996;14:443–446.

331. Bertholf RL, Johannsen LM, Bazooband A, et al. False-positive acetaminophen results in a hyperbilirubinemic patient. *Clin Chem* 2003;49:695–698.

332. Hendrickson R. Acetaminophen. In: Nelson LS, Lewin NA, Howland MA, et al, eds. *Goldfrank's Toxicologic Emergencies*. 9th ed. New York, NY: McGraw-Hill, 2013:483–499.

333. Heard KJ. Acetylcysteine for acetaminophen poisoning. *N Engl J Med* 2008;359:285–292.

334. Shen F, Coulter CV, Isbister GK, et al. A dosing regimen for immediate N-acetylcysteine treatment for acute paracetamol overdose. *Clin Toxicol (Phila)* 2011;49(7):643–647.

335. Wolf SJ, Heard K, Sloan EP, et al. Clinical policy: critical issues in the management of patients presenting to the emergency department with acetaminophen overdose. *Ann Emerg Med* 2007;50:292–313.

336. Keays R, Harrison PM, Wendon JA, et al. Intravenous acetylcysteine in paracetamol induced fulminant hepatic failure: a prospective controlled trial. *BMJ* 1991;303:1026–1029.

337. Smilkstein MJ, Knapp GL, Kulig KW, et al. Efficacy of oral N-acetylcysteine in the treatment of acetaminophen overdose. Analysis of the national multicenter study (1976 to 1985). *N Engl J Med* 1988;319(24):1557–1562.

338. Buckley NA, Whyte IM, O'Connell DL, et al. Oral or intravenous N-acetylcysteine: which is the treatment of choice for acetaminophen (paracetamol) poisoning? *J Toxicol Clin Toxicol* 1999;37:759–767.

339. Smilkstein MJ, Bronstein AC, Linden C, et al. Acetaminophen overdose: a 48-hour intravenous N-acetylcysteine treatment protocol. *Ann Emerg Med* 1991;20:1058–1063.

340. Rumack BH. Acetaminophen hepatotoxicity: the first 35 years. *J Toxicol Clin Toxicol* 2002;40:3–20.

341. Perry HE, Shannon MW. Efficacy of oral versus intravenous N-acetylcysteine in acetaminophen overdose: results of an open-label clinical trial. *J Pediatr* 1998;132:149–152.

342. Amirzadeh A, McCotter C. The intravenous use of oral acetylcysteine (mucomyst) for the treatment of acetaminophen overdose. *Arch Intern Med* 2002;162:96–97.

343. Kanter MZ. Comparison of oral and i.v. acetylcysteine in the treatment of acetaminophen poisoning. *Am J Health Syst Pharm* 2006;63:1821–1827.

344. Prescott LF, Park J, Ballantyne A, et al. Treatment of paracetamol (acetaminophen) poisoning with N-acetylcysteine. *Lancet* 1977;2:432–434.

345. Woo OF, Mueller PD, Olson KR, et al. Shorter duration of oral N-acetylcysteine therapy for acute acetaminophen overdose. *Ann Emerg Med* 2000;35:363–368.

346. Yip L, Dart RC. A 20-hour treatment for acute acetaminophen overdose. *N Engl J Med* 2003;348:2471–2472.

347. Harrison PM, Keays R, Bray GP, et al. Improved outcome of paracetamol-induced fulminant hepatic failure by late administration of acetylcysteine. *Lancet* 1990;335:1572–1573.

348. Gosselin S, Hoffman RS, Juurlink DN, et al. Treating acetaminophen overdose: thresholds, costs and uncertainties. *Clin Toxicol (Phila)* 2013;51:130.

349. Akdoğan M, El-Sahwi K, Ahmad U, et al. Experience with liver dialysis in acetaminophen induced fulminant hepatic failure: a preliminary report. *Turk J Gastroenterol* 2003;14:164–167.

350. Daly FFS, O'Malley GF, Heard K, et al. Prospective evaluation of repeated supratherapeutic acetaminophen (paracetamol) ingestion. *Ann Emerg Med* 2004;44:393–398.

351. Dart RC, Erdman AR, Olson KR, et al. Acetaminophen poisoning: an evidence-based consensus guideline for out-of-hospital management. *Clin Toxicol (Phila)* 2006;44:1–18.

CHAPTER *37*

Chronic Dialysis in Children

Bradley A. Warady, Kathy L. Jabs, and Amy L. Skversky

This chapter reviews current approaches to the clinical application of hemodialysis (HD) and peritoneal dialysis (PD) in children. Much of the information contained in this chapter reflect current practice in the authors' pediatric dialysis centers and incorporates advancements in the provision of renal replacement therapy (RRT) to children introduced subsequent to the publication of the prior edition of this text. We have tried to focus on those areas of care in which the pediatric patient differs most from the adult patient, and we have also tried to keep the nephrologist who does not routinely care for pediatric patients in mind. Although we do not encourage those who rarely treat children to embrace this difficult patient group when referral to a pediatric dialysis center is an option, we recognize that referral is not always possible.

This chapter addresses maintenance HD and PD in children; acute dialysis in children is covered in Chapter 38.

 ## EPIDEMIOLOGIC ISSUES

Incidence and Prevalence of End-Stage Kidney Disease in Children

End-stage kidney disease (ESKD) is not a common pediatric disorder. In the United States, there are about 13 new pediatric ESKD cases per million children of similar age reported each year. A higher incidence of ESKD with older age is found within both the pediatric and adult cohorts when adjusting for differences in gender and race. In 2012, the incidence rate for children 15 to 19 years of age (23 per million) was twice the rate of children 0 to 4 years (11 per million) (1). Of note, the incidence of children treated with RRT (dialysis or transplantation) varies across the world from <4 per million (Russia) to 18 per million (New Zealand) (2). The majority of children treated with RRT live in Europe, Japan, or

North America, where there is access to this level of care for all children (2). The incidence of ESKD in children contrasts sharply with the incidence of other chronic childhood disorders such as congenital heart disease (8,000 per million) and leukemia (57 per million) (3,4). The incidence of ESKD in children is also substantially lower than the incidence among adults, as is shown by data from the United States Renal Data System (USRDS) (**TABLE 37.1**) (1). The incidence of ESKD in young children (<5 years of age) has increased over the last three decades, while there has been little change in the incidence of ESKD in older children (1). The apparent increase in the incidence in the youngest pediatric patients in the 1970s and 1980s was likely due to improvements in RRT for smaller patients, notably the availability of automated peritoneal dialysis (APD). These improvements allowed for successful treatment of the youngest pediatric patients who previously had been considered too small to survive (5).

Children account for only a small fraction of the total dialysis patient population. On December 31, 2012, the USRDS counted a total of 449,342 dialysis patients in the United States (1). Of these, only 2,060 (0.5%) were younger than 20 years (1,134 treated with HD and 898 PD) (1). Absolute pediatric dialysis patient counts increased from 1,857 to 2,060 between 1992 and 2012, compared with an adult dialysis patient count increase from 159,060 to 448,542 during the same period (1). The small number of children treated with dialysis reflects both the relatively low incidence of ESKD in children and the extensive use of renal transplantation among pediatric ESKD patients. It remains widely accepted that renal transplantation is the optimal treatment for children with irreversible, severe chronic kidney disease (CKD). Recent USRDS data show that 73% of children with ESKD in the United States are maintained by a functioning renal transplant, compared with 29% of adults (1).

TABLE 37.1	End-Stage Kidney Disease Incidence in the United States in 1982, 1992, 2002, and 2012 at the Start of End-Stage Kidney Disease Therapy (per Million Population, Adjusted for Age, Gender, and Race)			
Age Group (y)	1982	1992	2002	2012
0–4	5	7	8	11
5–9	7	6	9	7
10–14	12	13	15	12
15–19	22	29	26	23
0–19	12	14	14	13
20–44	75	119	119	122
45–64	226	500	612	570
65–74	328	1,030	1,451	1,270
75+	194	896	1,731	1,618

From United States Renal Data System. *USRDS 2014 Annual Data Report: Epidemiology of Kidney Disease in the United States*. Bethesda, MD: National Institutes of Health, National Institute of Diabetes and Digestive and Kidney Diseases, 2014.

Causes of End-Stage Kidney Disease in Children

Approximately one-half of pediatric patients with ESKD have a congenital or hereditary disorder, and one-half have an acquired renal lesion (6). This is in contrast to the adult ESKD population in whom more than 80% of patients have acquired renal disease (1). TABLE 37.2 lists the primary renal disorders of 7,039 pediatric dialysis patients reported between 1992 and 2011 to the dialysis patient database of the North American Pediatric Renal Trials and Collaborative Studies (NAPRTCS) (6). The most frequent disorders were congenital anomalies of the kidneys and urinary tract (CAKUT: aplastic/hypoplastic/dysplastic kidneys, urinary obstruction or reflux; 34.3%), focal and segmental glomerulosclerosis (14.4%), and chronic glomerulonephritis (14.5%). This is contrasted with adult patients with ESKD in whom more than 79% of prevalent cases are accounted for by only three primary renal diseases: diabetic nephropathy, hypertensive nephropathy, and chronic glomerulonephritis (1).

TABLE 37.2	Primary Renal Disease Diagnosis in Pediatric Dialysis Patients	
Diagnosis		**% of Patients**
Congenital anomalies of kidney and urinary tract		34.3
Hereditary nephropathies		6.3
Focal segmental glomerulosclerosis		14.4
Chronic glomerulonephritis		14.5
Cystic kidney disease		4.8
Hemolytic uremic syndrome		3.1
Renal infarct		1.3
Diabetic nephropathy		0.1
Miscellaneous or unknown		21.2

From North American Pediatric Renal Trials and Collaborative Studies. *Annual Dialysis Report*. Rockville, MD: EMMES Corp, 2011.

PRINCIPLES OF DIALYSIS IN CHILDREN: PERITONEAL DIALYSIS

Peritoneal Membrane Function in Children: Physiologic Concepts

It has long been held that the peritoneal membrane of the child is functionally different from that of the adult and that peritoneal transport kinetics change as a consequence of normal growth and development (7). This concept can be traced to comparative measurements of the peritoneal surface area performed more than 100 years ago. In 1884, in a paper read before the Siberian Branch of the Russian Geographic Society, Putiloff (8) presented comparative data on the peritoneal membrane surface areas of infants and adults. Using direct oiled paper tracings of peritoneal contents, Putiloff (8) found that the peritoneal surface area of an infant weighing 2.9 kg was 0.15 m², compared with 2.08 m² for an adult of unspecified weight. If a weight of 70 kg is assumed for Putiloff's adult subjects, the infant's peritoneal surface area was found to be almost twice that of the adult when scaled for body weight (522 cm²/kg vs. 285 cm²/kg). Earlier studies by Wegner (9) had suggested that the peritoneal surface area closely approximated the body surface area (BSA) of an adult.

The clinical implications of these anatomic relationships were explored in 1966 by Esperanca and Collins (10). Direct measurements of peritoneal surface areas were made during autopsies performed on six neonates and six adults. The mean peritoneal surface area to body weight ratio in the infants was found to be roughly twice that of the adults, confirming Putiloff's (8) measurements made 80 years earlier. Esperanca and Collins (10) assumed that the peritoneal surface area and peritoneal membrane function were directly correlated, postulating that "peritoneal dialysis should be twice as efficient in the infant." Peritoneal urea clearance studies in puppies and adult dogs performed by these same investigators seemed to support their hypothesis (10). When scaled for body weight, peritoneal urea clearance measured in puppies was 2 to 3 times greater than clearances measured in adult animals. However, these clearance studies were seriously flawed. Widely different dialysate delivery rates were used in the puppies and adult animals (128 vs. 42 mL/kg/h, respectively). In this range, urea clearance is directly proportional to the dialysate flow rate, providing ample explanation for the observed differences in urea clearances between the two study groups.

The report by Esperanca and Collins (10) provides an early example of the pitfalls associated with the use of variable dialysis mechanics when studying peritoneal membrane function. These pitfalls can be avoided if peritoneal transport studies are performed in accordance with the following principles, as defined by Gruskin et al. (11) in 1987:

1. Constant inflow, dwell, and outflow times must be used for all study exchanges.
2. Identical dialysate composition must be used in all study subjects.
3. Exchange volumes must be identically scaled per unit body size. Gruskin et al. (11) allow the use of body weight, height, or surface area as the scaling factor, but other work has shown BSA to be the most reliable scaling factor in pediatric patients (12).
4. Results must be reported according to the body size scaling factor used to determine the exchange volume.

Subsequent peritoneal kinetic studies performed in accordance with these principles have more clearly defined the relative performance characteristics of the peritoneal membrane in children of different ages and in adults (see subsequent text). It is also now evident that the total membrane size is likely less relevant than the total membrane pore area involved in the exchanges (see subsequent text) (13,14).

Principles of Peritoneal Membrane Solute and Fluid Transfer

The peritoneal transfer of solutes reflects two simultaneous and interrelated transport mechanisms: diffusion and convection (15). Diffusion refers to the movement of solute across a semipermeable membrane in response to differing concentrations of that solute on either side of the membrane. The solute moves from the side with higher concentration to the side with lower concentration, down an electrochemical gradient, and in accordance with basic thermodynamic principles. Convection refers to the movement of solutes swept across the membrane within the flux of fluid that arises as a consequence of ultrafiltration. Convective transport is determined by the ultrafiltration rate. Studies of peritoneal membrane function have classically characterized membrane transport properties in terms of effective membrane surface area and solute permeability, fluid transfer (ultrafiltration), and peritoneal lymphatic absorption (16,17). Characterization of the three-pore model has helped to better explain the movement of solute and water across the peritoneal membrane. This model postulates three types of pores: (a) ultrasmall transcellular water pores (aquaporin-1 channels), which account for 1% to 2% of total pore area and 40% of water flow; (b) small pores, accounting for 90% of total pore area and subject to both concentration gradients (diffusive forces) and osmotic gradients (convective forces); and (c) large pores, accounting for 5% to 7% of total pore area and allowing for movement of large molecules such as albumin. The three-pore model has been applied to studies of PD in infants and children (13,14,18).

Effective Membrane Surface Area and Solute Permeability: Diffusive Transport

In the absence of an osmotic gradient between blood and dialysate, the rate of diffusive transfer of a solute is directly related to the product of the mass transfer area coefficient (MTAC) and the concentration gradient of the solute across the peritoneal membrane. The MTAC is a single parameter that is essentially independent of dialysis mechanics (e.g., exchange volume or dialysate dextrose concentration) and represents the functional peritoneal surface area and the diffusive permeability of the membrane. The MTAC also reflects the rate of solute removal that would be achieved in the absence of ultrafiltration or solute accumulation in the dialysate. The MTAC, as applied to the current three-pore model of transperitoneal solute and water flux, is in turn equal to the product of the free diffusion coefficient for the solute, the fractional area available for diffusion, and the term A_0/D_x, the diffusion distance (19).

In an early study, Morgenstern et al. (20) found that the MTACs for urea, creatinine, uric acid, and glucose in eight children aged 1.5 to 18 years were similar to adult reference values. In contrast, Geary et al. (21) determined MTACs in 28 children and suggested that solute transport capacity varies with age and does not approach adult values until late childhood. Warady et al. (22) determined MTACs for various solutes in 83 children younger than 1 to 18 years. This study had the advantage of standardized dialysis mechanics, including a consistent test exchange volume scaled to BSA at 1,100 mL/m². Mean MTACs (normalized to BSA) for creatinine, glucose, and potassium significantly decreased with age, in support of the notion that peritoneal permeability and/or effective membrane surface area relative to BSA is greater in children than in adults. Later, MTAC studies by Bouts et al. (23) based on the three-pore model, found that the values for children, when scaled to BSA, are similar to those of adults.

Diffusive transfer, as noted earlier, is dependent on the MTAC and the transmembrane concentration gradient, which dissipates during exchanges. The amount of "wetted peritoneal membrane," or that portion of the membrane in contact with dialysate, is also of importance since this factor influences the recruitment of small pores for diffusion (24). Recognition that dissipation of the transmembrane concentration gradient is in part related to the dialysate exchange volume (e.g., geometry of diffusion) and of the importance of using a consistent test exchange volume scaled to BSA represents important advances in methodology that are essential to the proper performance of another measure of peritoneal membrane function in children, the peritoneal equilibration test (PET) (see subsequent text) (25).

Scaling the test exchange volume by BSA allows for an equivalent relationship between dialysate volume and peritoneal membrane surface area for children of all ages and sizes so that any detectable differences in solute equilibration rates in this setting are the result of true differences in diffusive transport (24). The use of BSA as the most appropriate "scaling factor" has been validated in studies conducted by Kohaut et al. (26), Warady et al. (22), de Boer et al. (27), and Schaefer et al. (13). Studying their patients in accordance with the three-pore model of peritoneal transport developed by Rippe et al. (28,29), Schaefer et al. (13) demonstrated that the functional peritoneal exchange surface is a linear function of BSA and independent of patient age.

It is also noteworthy that posture may influence the diffusion process. The proportion of the peritoneal surface area that is recruited for an exchange can be 30% higher in the supine position compared to the upright position (14).

Ultrafiltration

Ultrafiltration, the movement of fluid from blood to dialysate, is a complex process that is incompletely understood and reflects the interaction of a number of factors including the hydraulic permeability of the peritoneal membrane, the permeability of the peritoneum to the osmotically active solutes on either side of the membrane, the absorption of fluid into peritoneal tissue, and lymphatic absorption. Most important is the fact that osmotic conductance drives the transport of free water across the aquaporin-1 channels and is counteracted by the absorption of glucose via the small pores with a subsequent time-dependent loss of the crystalloid osmotic gradient (30). Convective mass transfer occurs as a consequence of ultrafiltration. When considered in the context of total solute removal during PD, convective mass transfer contributes little to the movement of small solutes but is responsible for most large solute removal (15). For example, during a 4-hour continuous ambulatory peritoneal dialysis (CAPD) exchange with 4.25% dextrose solution, the contributions of convection to total transport have been estimated by Pyle (31) to be 12% for urea, 45% for inulin, and 86% for total protein.

Early studies and much clinical experience suggested that adequate ultrafiltration could be difficult to achieve in infants and younger children. Initial studies found a more rapid decline in dialysate dextrose concentration and osmolality in younger children (32,33). Subsequent work by Kohaut et al. (26) suggested that apparent age-related differences in ultrafiltration capacity disappear when the test exchange volume is scaled to BSA rather than body weight. As mentioned earlier, proper scaling of the exchange volume is an important determinant of the rate of dissipation of the osmotic gradient that determines ultrafiltration. Finally, some data actually suggest that even the body size-normalized fluid reabsorption rate may be slightly increased in young infants compared with older children and adults and have an impact on net ultrafiltration (13). Whereas this finding may be a manifestation of a greater lymphatic absorption rate in the youngest children, it is more likely the result of a reversed movement of fluid with hydrostatic and oncotic pressure gradients as a result of greater intraperitoneal (IP) pressures being generated in the smallest patients (34,35).

Peritoneal Lymphatic Absorption

To some extent, studies of ultrafiltration in children have been hindered by the absence of information on the contribution of lymphatic absorption to net ultrafiltration. Mactier et al. (36) studied lymphatic absorption in six children aged 2 to 13 years. Peritoneal lymphatic drainage was reported to reduce mean ultrafiltration by 27%. When lymphatic absorption rates were scaled to body weight, higher values were obtained for pediatric patients when compared with adult reference values. When scaled to BSA, these differences were no longer seen. More recently, fluid absorption has been felt to primarily be related to movement directly into the tissues surrounding the peritoneal cavity. Lymphatic absorption is only thought to account for 20% of fluid absorption. The limited data on lymphatic absorption in children makes this a potential area for future investigations (34,36,37).

◆ PRINCIPLES OF DIALYSIS IN CHILDREN: HEMODIALYSIS

The principles of HD, extracorporeal perfusion, solute clearance, ultrafiltration, and mass balance, are very similar when applied in children and adult patients. Certain pediatric-specific issues with respect to patient size, however, do require comment.

Characteristics of Dialyzers

The ideal pediatric hemodialyzer would have a very small blood volume, a safe ultrafiltration coefficient, a low resistance blood circuit, a high degree of biocompatibility, and a predictable relationship between clearance and blood-flow rates (BFRs). Hollow-fiber dialyzers have now supplanted previously used flat-plate dialyzers in virtually all pediatric centers. Improvements in the manufacturing process of hollow-fiber dialyzers have led to decreased dialyzer volumes, rendering them more useful for the treatment of infants and small children in whom a small extracorporeal volume is desirable. Hollow-fiber dialyzers also have more predictable clearance characteristics and can be easily cleaned and reprocessed. There are several characteristics of dialyzers that should be considered before their clinical use: clearance, ultrafiltration, and biocompatibility.

Clearance

In the clinical setting, the clearance achieved by a dialyzer is a function of its mass transfer area coefficient (K_oA) and the blood- and dialysate flow rates (Q_B, Q_D). K_oA, expressed in mL/min, is a property of the dialyzer that describes the maximum ability of a dialyzer to clear a given solute at infinitely high blood- and dialysis flow rates (38). The relationship between BFRs and clearance for two different dialyzers is shown in **FIGURE 37.1**. In that representation, dialyzer 2 has a larger K_oA (urea) than does dialyzer 1. Several important conclusions can be drawn from the shape of the curves. First, at low BFRs, the small solute clearance is equivalent to the BFR and is the same for both dialyzers 1 and 2, and for virtually all dialyzers. Second, for each dialyzer, a maximum clearance will be achieved at a certain BFR, above which increasing the blood flow will not increase clearance. Therefore, the difference between larger and smaller dialyzers is principally the BFR at which the maximum urea clearance is achieved. Thus, when choosing a dialyzer for a pediatric patient, one must consider not only the target clearance but also the maximum achievable BFR. For example, for a large child in whom BFRs of 350 to 400 mL/min are possible, a large dialyzer would be preferable because a higher clearance could be achieved. In contrast, for a small child who achieves BFRs of 70 to 85 mL/min, the difference in clearance rates at low BFRs would be negligible, and other considerations

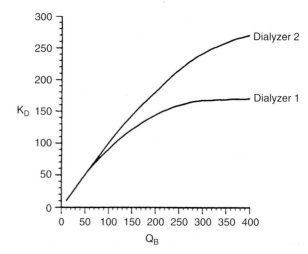

FIGURE 37.1 Relationship between blood flow (Q_B) and dialyzer clearance (K_D) for two different dialyzers. Dialyzer 2 has a K_oA for this solute that is twice that of dialyzer 1.

would be more appropriate when selecting a dialyzer, such as dialyzer volume. This will be addressed in more detail later in the chapter.

A dialyzer has different clearances for different solutes, which are generally inversely related to molecular weight. Although typically not considered in the dialysis prescription for young infants, the relatively low BFRs at which clearance of high molecular weight solutes reach their maximum levels means infants and young children usually receive high-efficiency dialysis (39). Although infants and young children receive an equivalent overall clearance of these solutes compared with adults because their volumes of distribution are significantly less, the overall mass transfer is much greater. A practical example in which this may have clinical relevance is the clearance of vancomycin as dosing intervals for vancomycin in infants receiving HD are much shorter than in adults (40).

Ultrafiltration

The ultrafiltration coefficient of the dialyzer should be sufficient to allow the desired ultrafiltration during the planned duration of a dialysis session. Concern has been raised in the past about the ultrafiltration coefficient of dialyzers used for pediatric patients because excessive ultrafiltration could lead to hypotension and shock. Theoretically, this could be a particular problem with the now standard high-efficiency dialysis. However, the routine use of dialysis machines with volumetric ultrafiltration control and noninvasive blood volume monitoring has greatly reduced these concerns.

Biocompatibility

Although there is debate concerning the preferred use of specific membranes for the chronic treatment of adults with respect to biocompatibility, there is indeed evidence that certain membranes can affect long-term leukocyte function, inflammatory markers, protein catabolism, and perhaps overall mass transfer of β_2-microglobulin, which may have long-term adverse clinical consequences (41–44). Newer generation dialysis membranes constructed from materials such as polysulfone and polymethyl methacrylate (PMMA) cause less proinflammatory cytokine activation compared with older generation membranes from cellulose or cuprophane (45). Whereas there are no data available on changes in patient outcomes with polysulfone or PMMA membranes, the incidence of anaphylactoid, complement-mediated, immediate membrane reactions are far less common with the newer biocompatible membranes that are commonly used. Although there have not been any long-term studies on this issue in pediatrics, a study from Egypt has examined the expression of adhesions molecules, particularly intercellular adhesion molecule one (ICAM-1), as a marker of biocompatibility of dialysis membranes in 80 pediatric HD patients. In this study, which compared the use of polysulfone low-flux filters and polysulfone high-flux filters, the high-flux group showed a significant decline in predialysis serum levels of ICAM-1 with decreased neutrophil activation as compared to those patients using the low-flux filters (46). At present, however, there are no clear-cut advantages associated with the use of any specific type of membrane for pediatric patients.

◆ DIALYSIS FOR END-STAGE KIDNEY DISEASE IN CHILDREN

Choice of Hemodialysis or Peritoneal Dialysis as a Chronic Renal Replacement Therapy in Children

HD, PD, and renal transplantation are all successful long-term treatments for ESKD in children. Renal transplantation has been widely recognized as the treatment of choice for children with ESKD because it can relieve the burden of continuous and repetitive treatments while restoring the child to a virtually normal metabolic homeostasis and permitting near-normal growth and development (47,48). Unfortunately, because tolerance has not yet been achieved in humans after organ transplantation, and nonadherence with medications remains a substantial issue, virtually all grafts are eventually lost and pediatric patients are on a continuous cycle of alternating between dialysis and transplantation over the course of their lifetime. Renal transplantation should, therefore, be considered a treatment rather than a cure for kidney disease. Despite the preference for renal transplantation and the fact that up to 24% of children may receive a preemptive transplant without prior dialysis, large-scale registry data indicate that a large portion of children with ESKD require a prolonged period of treatment with chronic dialysis either before or between renal transplants, making chronic dialysis a significant component of the treatment for all children with ESKD (26,49,50).

Few studies have directly compared the efficacy of chronic HD and PD in pediatric patients. The proposed advantages of HD include minimal technical assistance required for the patient and family and decreased treatment times. The proposed advantages of PD, especially APD, include decreased dependence on the treatment center, increased flexibility of the treatment schedule with improved school attendance, somewhat decreased dietary restrictions, and a decreased need for repeated venipunctures. A very early comparison of the two chronic dialysis modalities in children from a single center showed that PD appeared to be associated with lower transfusion rates, improved rehabilitation, and better metabolic control (51). However, advancements over the last two decades with respect to erythropoiesis-stimulating agent (ESA) therapy, and the availability of smaller extracorporeal circuits and volumetrically controlled HD machines, have minimized many of the previous negative aspects of HD. A 2011 review of 6,573 adult dialysis patients in Ontario, Canada, who received ≥4 months of predialysis care and who started dialysis electively demonstrated no difference in survival between PD and HD (52). The advent of nightly home HD and frequent daytime HD has made available additional effective alternative RRT options for adults that are now being used in some pediatric centers as well (see below).

There are many patient factors that play a role in the selection of a dialysis modality including patient age, lifestyle choice, parental preference, assessment of whether individual patients and families can be adherent with the dialysis regimen, and the ability of a center to provide HD or support a home-based dialysis program (53,54). Factors related to the overall success of the dialysis patients may also be involved in the selection of a dialysis modality for an individual child (e.g., children with greater social support are more likely to be treated with PD and more likely to attend school full-time). Comparison of the children in NAPRTCS has demonstrated higher full-time school attendance rates in those treated with chronic peritoneal dialysis (CPD) versus those receiving HD (e.g., 78% vs. 53% for children aged 6 to 18 years) (6). Recent reports of successful home-based HD therapies now extend the advantages of home-based programs to pediatric patients who cannot perform CPD for medical reasons (55–57).

At present, it is virtually impossible to find convincing evidence that either form of dialysis is clearly preferable for most children with ESKD, although clear preferences exist in individual cases. As noted above, the choice of dialysis treatment may be influenced by the preference of the center or by its technical capabilities. In these circumstances, it is important that patient and family choice be preserved whenever possible and not be subverted by the overt or subtle influence of the unit's personnel.

Characteristics of a Pediatric Dialysis Center

The provision of optimal chronic pediatric dialysis requires a program philosophy that is geared to the particular needs of infants, children, adolescents, and young adults. Although the equipment used for delivering pediatric dialysis is similar to that found in adult dialysis units, specialized personnel in addition to physicians and nurses with expertise in pediatric care, are necessary to ensure that children receiving dialysis can receive developmentally appropriate care in the setting of a never ending cycle of dialysis and renal transplantation (58). Child life specialists and pediatric-trained ESKD social workers are essential team members of any pediatric dialysis program (53). Child life specialists lend critical expertise to provide developmentally appropriate evaluations and assistance to children and their families during procedures and can serve as liaisons to help educate school personnel with respect to the particular medical and psychosocial needs of children with ESKD; this is especially important if a dialysis-based teacher is not available. Pediatric-trained ESKD social work personnel are essential to evaluate the psychosocial development of children with ESKD. Regular assessment of the pediatric patient's health-related quality of life (HRQOL) is mandatory, and there are a number of validated assessment tools, including the Pediatric Quality of Life Inventory generic (PedsQL4.0) and ESKD-specific (PedsQL3.0) modules. This assessment helps identify important psychosocial issues that ideally should prompt the implementation of interventions designed to address and potentially minimize the psychological stresses that negatively impact quality of life (QOL) in patients with ESKD (59,60). Assistance provided to families to help navigate complex socioeconomic challenges and barriers associated with ESKD is also crucial. Dietitians who are expert in the nutritional requirements and restrictions imposed by ESKD are vital to the development of palatable menus for children with ESKD; they also work with school lunch programs and closely monitor a multitude of nutrition status markers (see below) (61).

◆ CHRONIC PERITONEAL DIALYSIS FOR CHILDREN

Although successful as treatment for acute kidney injury (AKI), PD historically appeared to have much less to offer to the child with ESKD. Initial CPD techniques required reinsertion of the dialysis catheter for each treatment, making prolonged use in small patients difficult. The development of a permanent peritoneal catheter, first proposed by Palmer et al. (62,63) and later refined by Tenckhoff and Schechter (64), made long-term PD an accessible form of RRT for pediatric patients. When Boen et al. (65) and then Tenckhoff et al. (66) devised an automated dialysate delivery system that could be used in the home, chronic intermittent peritoneal dialysis (IPD) became a practical alternative to chronic HD for children. Largely, as a result of the pioneering efforts of the pediatric ESKD treatment team in Seattle (67,68), pediatric chronic IPD programs were established in a few prominent pediatric dialysis centers (69–72). However, enthusiasm for chronic IPD among pediatric nephrologists during this period was limited, perhaps because chronic IPD for children included many of the least desirable features of chronic

HD (e.g., substantial dietary restrictions, fluid intake limits, immobility during treatments, and complex machinery), without providing the one great advantage of HD: efficiency.

A new era in the history of PD as an RRT modality for children with ESKD was heralded by the description of CAPD in 1976 by Popovich et al. (73). CAPD appeared particularly well suited for use in children. Potential advantages of CAPD over HD of special importance to children included near steady-state biochemical control, reduced dietary restrictions and fluid limits, and freedom from repeated dialysis needle punctures. CAPD also allowed children of all ages to receive dialysis in the home, offering them the opportunity to experience a more normal childhood. Finally, CAPD made possible the routine treatment of very young infants, thereby extending the option of RRT to an entire population of patients previously considered too young for chronic dialysis.

CAPD was first used in a child in 1978 in Toronto (74,75). Subsequent experience was soon reported from growing pediatric CAPD programs in North America and Western Europe (76–78). Continuous cycling peritoneal dialysis (CCPD) was first used in a child by Price and Suki (79) in 1981. APD or cycler dialysis has since grown in popularity among many pediatric PD programs throughout North America and the world (80). In those centers where APD is freely available, this PD modality is usually preferred over CAPD. Pediatric PD registries in North America and Italy have reported that an average of 70% of children who are prescribed PD perform APD, with a substantial increase in APD usage over time (81,82). Although personal preference and lifestyle are the factors that most frequently influence the choice of CPD modality in children, individual variation in peritoneal transport characteristics may determine a patient's suitability for a particular therapy (22,83,84).

Permanent Peritoneal Dialysis Catheters for Children

A reliable peritoneal catheter is the cornerstone of successful CPD, well worth the attention and effort required to "perfect" the procedure in each center that proposes to treat children with long-term PD. There are multiple types of PD catheters presently available with a variety of configurations. In general, most long-term PD catheters are constructed of a soft material such as silicone rubber or polyurethane. The catheters can be thought of as having two separate regions, the IP portion and the extraperitoneal portion. The IP portion contains holes or slots to allow passage of peritoneal fluid. The shape of the IP portion typically is straight or curled; the latter configuration is often associated with less patient pain with dialysate inflow and a decreased predisposition to omental wrapping of the catheter. The most common catheters with these characteristics used by pediatric patients have been the straight and curled Tenckhoff catheters. The extraperitoneal portion of each of these catheters has one or two Dacron cuffs to prevent fluid leaks and bacterial migration and most importantly, to fix the catheter's position. The shape of this portion of the catheter is variable and may be straight or have a preformed angle (e.g., swan neck) to help create a downward directed catheter exit site (85).

The variability in the choice of catheter characteristics is reflected in the data from NAPRTCS, collected between 1992 and 2010 (6). Of the 4,391 catheters, 62.1% were of the Tenckhoff curled variety, and 15 different combinations of characteristics each represented at least 2.0% of the catheters placed (**TABLE 37.3**).

The two most common approaches to PD catheter placement are the open and laparoscopic techniques, as was recently reviewed in guidelines published by the Society of American Gastrointestinal and Endoscopic Surgeons (SAGES) (86). Currently, there is no data

TABLE 37.3	**Peritoneal Dialysis Access Characteristics**					
Catheter	**Cuffs**	**Tunnel**	**Exit Site**	**N (4,391)**	**% (100.0)**	
Curled	One	Straight	Lateral	619	14.1	
Curled	Two	Swan-necked/curved	Down	458	10.4	
Curled	Two	Straight	Lateral	315	7.2	
Straight	One	Straight	Lateral	313	7.1	
Curled	Two	Straight	Down	277	6.3	
Curled	One	Straight	Down	267	6.1	
Curled	One	Straight	Up	209	4.8	
Curled	Two	Swan-necked/curved	Unknown	145	3.3	
Straight	One	Straight	Up	136	3.1	
Curled	Two	Swan-necked/curved	Lateral	132	3.0	
Presternal	Two	Swan-necked/curved	Down	129	2.9	
Straight	One	Straight·	Unknown	123	2.8	
Straight	One	Swan-necked/curved	Lateral	105	2.4	
Straight	One	Straight	Down	102	2.3	
Straight	Two	Straight	Lateral	100	2.3	
Curled	One	Swan-necked/curved	Lateral	78	1.8	
Curled	One	Swan necked/curved	Down	78	1.8	
Curled	One	Straight	Unknown	76	1.7	
Curled	Two	Straight	Unknown	57	1.3	
Straight	Two	Straight	Up	54	1.2	

From North American Pediatric Renal Trials and Collaborative Studies. *Annual Dialysis Report*. Rockville, MD: EMMES Corp, 2011.

that shows the superiority of one technique over the other, and two recent meta-analyses have yielded differing results (87,88). Whichever insertion approach is used, lateral placement through the body of the rectus muscle should be encouraged as a means of decreasing the likelihood of catheter leakage (89–91). Daschner et al. (92) have reported on the laparoscopic placement of 25 two-cuff Tenckhoff catheters in 22 pediatric patients. Postoperative leakage occurred in only two patients, and the procedure facilitated the removal of adhesions and inguinal hernia repair at the time of catheter placement. Catheter placement should always be accompanied by prophylactic antibiotic therapy, a practice that has resulted in a significantly reduced risk of early peritonitis (89,93–95). Additional commentary regarding recommendations pertaining to the laparoscopic placement of PD catheters has recently been published (96).

In general, it is believed that infants and young children with vesicostomies, ureterostomies, or colostomies require placement of the PD catheter exit site as far from the stoma as possible to prevent contamination and infection. Placement of the exit site on the chest wall has successfully limited the number of infections in such high-risk situations in a small number of children and adults (97–102). The primary reason for catheter revision is catheter malfunction, often caused by omental wrapping of the catheter (103,104). In a single study of 101 pediatric PD patients who underwent reoperation for infection or malfunction of their PD catheter, lack of an omentectomy was the only independent risk factor to be associated with the need for catheter revision (105). With this in mind, an omentectomy was performed with the insertion of 82.4% of catheters in the Italian pediatric PD registry and is performed by at least 59% of North American surgeons placing chronic PD catheters (91). However, the decision to perform an omentectomy in conjunction with catheter placement is not universal (106–108).

Finally, in the most recent report of the NAPRTCS and as has been shown in previous reports, the annualized peritonitis rate decreased with increasing age and was best in association with Tenckhoff catheters with double cuffs, swan-neck tunnels, and downward-pointed exit sites (6,109). In addition, time to first peritonitis episode was longer for catheters with two cuffs compared with one, with swan-neck tunnels compared with straight tunnels, and with downward exit sites compared with lateral exit sites or exit sites directed upward. These results confirm findings from the adult PD population and prompted recommendations for use of a two-cuff Tenckhoff catheter in the *Consensus Guidelines for the Prevention and Treatment of Catheter-Related Infections and Peritonitis in Pediatric Patients Receiving Peritoneal Dialysis: 2012 Update* (95).

Role of Peritoneal Equilibration Test in Prescribing Peritoneal Dialysis for Children

The PET was developed by Twardowski et al. (83) as a simple means of characterizing solute transport rates across the peritoneum that could have direct clinical applications. The construction of reference curves based on the kinetics of solute equilibration between dialysate and plasma (D to P ratio) after a 2-L exchange volume made possible the categorization of adult patients into those with high, high-average, low-average, and low peritoneal membrane solute transport rates and served as the basis for the dialysis prescription process (see subsequent text).

However, Twardowski et al.'s (83) adult PET reference curves should not be applied to the pediatric PD population primarily because a uniform 2-L test exchange volume was provided to all study patients, regardless of their size, in the Twardowski scheme. Obviously, this approach does not allow for modification of the exchange volume to reflect differences in body size (e.g., pediatric patient, small adult, large adult) and has contributed to the limited usefulness of this approach in children.

Application of a standardized PET procedure for children has, on the other hand, resulted from an appreciation of the previously mentioned age-independent relationship between BSA and peritoneal membrane surface area and the recommended use of an exchange volume scaled to BSA whenever one conducts studies of peritoneal transport kinetics (22,26,27,110). In the largest pediatric study to date, the Pediatric Peritoneal Dialysis Study Consortium (PPDSC) evaluated 95 children for their membrane solute transport capacity (22). Similar reference data has been generated from pediatric studies in Europe with a test exchange volume of 1,000 mL/m² BSA (111). Although the standard PET is conducted over 4 hours, use of a 2-hour PET has proven reliable and less labor intensive in pediatric patients new to PD (112,113).

Because the transport capacity of a patient's peritoneal membrane is such an important factor to consider when determining the dialysis prescription, a PET evaluation should be conducted soon after the initiation of dialysis (114–116). There is, however, evidence that a PET performed within the first week after the initiation of PD may yield higher transport results than a PET performed several weeks later (117–119). Accordingly, whereas it may be most convenient to perform the initial PET at the conclusion of PD training, the Kidney Disease Outcomes Quality Initiative (KDOQI) has recommended that the PET be conducted 4 to 8 weeks following the initiation of CPD (116–118). The PET evaluation should be repeated when knowledge of the patient's current membrane transport capacity is necessary for determination of the patient's PD prescription, especially when adverse clinical events have occurred (e.g., repeated peritonitis) and are followed by clinical evidence of altered transport characteristics (e.g., worsening hypertension as a result of unexplained fluid overload, increasing need for hypertonic dialysate, ESA-resistant anemia secondary to hypervolemia) (120). In addition, knowledge of a patient's transport capacity may have a profound impact on the overall care because of the important relationships that exist between transport status and patient outcome in children and adults (121–123).

Chronic Peritoneal Dialysis Prescription

In general, the CPD prescription for children has evolved empirically from guidelines that adapted adult CAPD to the pediatric patient. A CAPD regimen of four to five exchanges per day with a fill volume of 900 to 1,100 mL/m² BSA (35 to 45 mL/kg) of 2.5% dextrose dialysis solution has routinely yielded net ultrafiltration volumes of up to 1,100 mL/m²/d. The KDOQI Clinical Practice Recommendations for Peritoneal Dialysis Adequacy that pertain to children, most of whom receive APD, target an individual fill volume of 1,000 to 1,200 mL/m² for patients older than 2 years and a lower initial volume (600 to 800 mL/m²) for younger infants (116,124,125). The greatest percentage of children receiving APD utilize a regimen consisting of 5 to 10 exchanges over 9 to 12 hours per night with a daytime dwell consisting of approximately 50% of the nocturnal fill volume, the latter to enhance solute and fluid removal particularly in anuric patients (18,126). More recently, the concept of adapted PD, with initial cycles using a relatively small fill volume and short duration to maximize ultrafiltration, followed by a larger fill volume with a longer dwell time to promote solute clearance, has been suggested as a means to improve dialysis efficiency (24).

The current goal of achieving dialysis adequacy in the most cost-effective manner has highlighted the need to be cognizant of a patient's BSA, peritoneal membrane solute transport capacity, and residual kidney function (RKF) when designing the dialysis prescription (22,84,115,116,127). The prescribed PD schedule should also be compatible with the psychosocial needs of the patient and family. In most patients (except for the rapid transporter), the most effective way to increase solute clearance is to initially increase the fill volume followed by an increase in dialysis duration by prolonging the dwell time. Measurement of the IP pressure generated by escalating fill volumes can be useful in determining the maximal tolerated IP volume because, as noted previously, an exceedingly high IP pressure (>14 cm H₂O) may result in back-filtration and compromise ultrafiltration capacity and be poorly tolerated by the patient (24,128–133). In the case of the rapid transporter, an increase in the number of exchanges and a reduction of the dwell time per cycle can result in improved solute clearance.

As mentioned earlier, the categorization of a patient's peritoneal membrane transport capacity can best be determined by the performance of a PET and comparison of the individual patient data to reference values (22,111). In turn, this information makes it possible to optimize the dialysis prescription in terms of the exchange dwell time. Recognizing that it is often impractical to consider the provision of a dialysis prescription based solely on kinetic data without reference to social constraints (e.g., school attendance, working parent), the use of the results of a PET can be particularly helpful in PD modality selection (e.g., high transporter: cycling PD; high- to low-average transporter: CAPD or APD with the option of an additional daytime exchange). Often, this selection process can be most easily achieved with the use of one of several computer modeling programs that have been validated in pediatric patients and that can provide accurate estimates of solute clearance (13,134,135). It must be emphasized that in pediatric patients, as well as in adults, predicted values are only estimates and do not substitute for actual measurements of solute clearance (see subsequent text).

The RKF, a characteristic that appears to be better preserved by PD versus HD, is calculated as the average of urea and creatinine clearance and assumes greatest importance in the patient who does not attain target clearances with dialysis alone (116,136–139). Whereas the contribution of RKF toward a target goal may be significant early in the course of dialysis, a progressive loss of RKF usually occurs and mandates an associated enhancement of the dialysis prescription if target clearances are to be maintained. Efforts to preserve RKF include the prevention of nephrotoxic insults such as exposure to radiocontrast dye and possibly the use of an angiotensin-converting enzyme inhibitor (ACEI) or angiotensin receptor blocker (116,140–142). Diuretic therapy has also recently been shown to help preserve RKF in pediatric patients receiving CPD (143).

Peritoneal Dialysis Adequacy

The goal of achieving dialysis adequacy in children emphasizes the clinical status of the patient as an important qualitative target (116). Clinical manifestations of inadequate dialysis may include congestive heart failure, hyperphosphatemia/excessive calcium–phosphorus product, overt uremia manifested as pericarditis/pleuritis or clinical, and/or biochemical signs of malnutrition or wasting. All of these outcomes may be the result of one or more of the following factors:

- Loss of RKF
- Prescription inadequate for peritoneal membrane transport characteristics

- Reduced peritoneal membrane surface area caused by extensive intra-abdominal adhesions
- Loss of peritoneal membrane solute transport/ultrafiltration capacity
- Noncompliance with PD prescription
- Poorly functioning PD catheter

Despite the emphasis on clinical parameters, PD adequacy and solute clearance have been used almost interchangeably since the performance of the National Cooperative Dialysis Study in the adult HD population. The Adequacy of Peritoneal Dialysis in Mexico (ADEMEX) study and a randomized trial of different solute clearance targets in adult CAPD patients conducted by Lo et al. have provided data that supports the current recommendation for a target total (peritoneal and kidney) Kt/V_{urea} of at least 1.7 per week in adults (116,144,145). It has also been suggested that the determination of peritoneal creatinine clearance has little added value to the prediction of outcome in adults on CAPD such that adequacy targets should be based on urea kinetics only. In contrast, due to a more variable relationship between urea and creatinine with APD, an additional target of 45 L/wk/1.73 m^2 for creatinine clearance has been recommended (146). Because there are no data that correlate solute removal with outcome in pediatrics, making it impossible to define PD adequacy in children with confidence, it has been recommended that the pediatric population should use clearance goals that meet or exceed current KDOQI adult standards. Specifically, the minimal delivered dose of total (peritoneal and kidney) small solute clearance should be a Kt/V_{urea} of at least 1.8 per week (116). Reports by Holtta et al. (147), McCauley et al. (148), Champoux (149), and Chadha et al. (150) have all presented data suggestive of a correlation between patient outcome and solute clearance. The experience of Chadha et al. (150) was also significant for demonstrating the influence that RKF has on patient outcome and the apparent contradiction of the presumed equivalence of PD and native solute clearance.

Can the solute clearance targets be achieved by children on CPD without introducing a prescription that has a significant negative impact on their QOL? Whereas data by van der Voort et al. (151) suggests otherwise, the clinical experiences of Holtta et al. (147) and Chadha et al. (150) provide good evidence that if the dialysis fill volume is maximized and if the frequency of the exchanges is individualized and adjusted according to the peritoneal membrane transport characteristics, it should be possible to achieve the current KDOQI clearance targets in most children receiving PD. In fact, data from the Clinical Performance Measures project has revealed median Kt/V_{urea} values of 2.43 and 2.45 for pediatric patients receiving CCPD and nightly intermittent peritoneal dialysis (NIPD), respectively (152).

As mentioned earlier, Kt/V_{urea} has found widespread acceptance as a marker of small-solute clearance and is calculated as the urea clearance normalized for the volume of urea distribution or total body water (TBW). Therefore, the ability to accurately estimate a patient's TBW (or V) is integral to the determination of this adequacy measure. Whereas some investigators have recommended the use of bioelectrical impedance as a means of determining V, this procedure is not regularly conducted in most pediatric dialysis centers (153). Previously published anthropometric equations and formulas derived from the study of healthy individuals also do not provide reliable information for the pediatric dialysis population (154–157). Fortunately, the publication by Morgenstern et al. (158) of data derived from studies of children on CPD conducted with

heavy water (H2 O18 or D2 O) also permitted the development of equations, which permits one to predict TBW with acceptable accuracy and precision. The gender-specific equations are as follows (**EQUATIONS 37.1** and **37.2**):

$$\text{Boys: TBW} = 0.010 \times (\text{height} \times \text{weight})^{0.68} - 0.37 \times \text{weight} \quad (37.1)$$

$$\text{Girls: TBW} = 0.14 \times (\text{height} \times \text{weight})^{0.64} - 0.35 \times \text{weight} \quad (37.2)$$

Because the height × weight parameter predicts BSA, the prediction equations can be simplified (with somewhat less precision) in the following manner (**EQUATIONS 37.3** and **37.4**):

$$\text{Boys: TBW} = 20.88 \times \text{BSA} - 4.29 \quad (37.3)$$

$$\text{Girls: TBW} = 16.92 \times \text{BSA} - 1.81 \quad (37.4)$$

In all cases, the Gehan and George (159) equation should be used to determine BSA.

Implicit in the approach to achieve and maintain dialysis adequacy is the need to repeatedly measure total solute clearance. Ideally, 24-hour collections of urine and dialysate fluid should be obtained a minimum of two times per year or when there have been significant changes in the patient's clinical status that may influence dialysis performance (e.g., severe or repeated episodes of peritonitis). For infants incontinent day and night, we currently attempt to achieve total clearance targets using dialysis clearances alone, rather than using indwelling urinary catheters for these patients to facilitate determination of RKF.

Finally, ultrafiltration capacity and overall fluid status should also be considered a component of adequate PD, and a patient's membrane transport capacity may be particularly important in this context. Adult studies have demonstrated that the relative risks of technique failure and patient mortality are significantly increased in patients categorized as high transporters by the PET (123). It is postulated that the rapid glucose absorption that characterizes the high transport state may predispose patients to chronic fluid overload and cardiovascular morbidity (160). Noteworthy is data from the NAPRTCS, which demonstrated that 57% of 4,000 pediatric PD patients had hypertension, in addition to the results of another study, which revealed that 68% of pediatric patients on CPD were found to have left ventricular hypertrophy (161,162). Additional pediatric experience with dialysis solutions characterized by improved peritoneal membrane biocompatibility, as well as with solutions using alternatives to glucose as the osmotic agent, should be a priority in view of the high incidence of hypertension and cardiovascular morbidity in children on dialysis (18,163–165). In patients experiencing decreased ultrafiltration capacity and resultant hypervolemia, therapeutic interventions may include use of a long daytime exchange with icodextrin, an increase in the number of exchanges or an increased overall treatment time, and/or an increase in the dialysate glucose concentration (18). Diuretic therapy may also be beneficial in those patients with maintained RKF (143). In some patients, however, a change in dialysis modality to HD is necessary to best control fluid status.

Nutritional Management of Children on Peritoneal Dialysis

A normal nutritional status is uncommon among children treated with CPD, despite access to a diet primarily restricted only in terms of phosphorus, and possibly sodium intake (166,167). Compared with healthy children, those on CPD have a significantly lower energy intake and diminished height, weight, triceps skinfold thickness, and mid arm muscle circumference (166). Hypoalbuminemia and hyperlipidemia are commonly seen (167,168). Anorexia and dysgeusia are often accompanied by gastroesophageal reflux and other feeding disorders (169). As part of the KDOQI process, pediatric nutritional guidelines were updated in 2009 and provide recommendations for the assessment of a patient's nutritional status and for the provision of optimal nutrition (61). In the opinion of the working group, parameters of nutritional status and growth to be followed include dietary intake, length or height, height velocity, estimated dry weight, body mass index (BMI), and head circumference (for children <3 years) (61). BMI (weight^2 / height) should be normalized to height age to account for the age dependency of the value and the growth-retarded nature of the dialysis population. Growth and nutritional parameters should be measured at the initiation of dialysis and at regular intervals as recommended in the guidelines.

Children should receive 100% of the recommended dietary reference intake (DRI) for energy, referenced to height, age, and gender (170). Whereas it is estimated that total energy intake will be augmented by an additional 8 to 20 kcal/kg/d derived from dialysate dextrose absorption, little information on this topic is available from the pediatric APD population (171).

The members of the KDOQI working group were unable to recommend with evidence the optimal protein intake for each child receiving CPD, and therefore, an initial dietary protein intake equal to 100% of the DRI for ideal body weight plus anticipated protein losses across the peritoneum is recommended (61). The efficacy of the prescribed intake must be assessed regularly to ensure that it is adequate (172). Dialysate protein losses are proportionately greater in children than in adults (173–175), and children often begin CPD with evidence of protein wasting (167,176). At the same time, excessive dietary protein intake can result in hyperphosphatemia and an increased risk for cardiovascular disease (CVD) (177–180). Therefore, current recommendations are for daily protein intakes of 1.8 g/kg for patients 0 to 6 months, 1.5 g/kg for children aged 7 to 12 months, 1.3 g/kg for children aged 1 to 3 years, 1.1 g/kg for patients 4 to 13 years, and 1.0 g/kg for the adolescent population. Supplementation of dietary protein intake with amino acids administered by the IP route has been performed on occasion, but the use of these solutions has failed to result in a significant improvement of nutritional parameters (181,182).

As suggested earlier, dietary phosphate intake must be monitored closely because of the potential adverse impact hyperphosphatemia has on bone and cardiovascular health. The guidelines recommend limiting dietary phosphorus intake to 100% of the DRI in normophosphatemic patients if the serum parathyroid hormone (PTH) concentration exceeds the target range and to 80% of the DRI when the serum phosphorus exceeds the target range and hyperparathyroidism is established (TABLE 37.4) (61). Age-appropriate serum phosphorus levels should be targeted (183).

Although there are no data on the levels of water-soluble vitamins that occur in children undergoing dialysis without vitamin supplementation, supplements of water-soluble vitamins are generally recommended for all children receiving CPD since these patients are at risk for alterations in vitamin levels as a result of decreased intake secondary to anorexia or dietary restrictions, loss per dialysis, or interference with absorption, excretion or metabolism (61,184–186). Supplements of the fat-soluble vitamin A should be avoided, and total vitamin A intake should be limited to the DRI. In the absence of the renal clearance of vitamin A metabolites, children with ESKD are at risk for hypervitaminosis A (187). Carnitine, zinc, and copper supplementation have been reported on occasion, as treatment for clinical evidence of deficiency (188–192). Because acidemia has a negative effect on growth and nutritional status, serum bicarbonate levels below 22 mmol/L should be corrected with alkali supplementation (61).

Infants receiving CPD require aggressive nutritional support. *Ad lib* food intake frequently falls below recommended levels, requiring forced feeding through nasogastric or gastrostomy tubes/buttons (61,176,193–198). Regular oral stimulation should continue irrespective of the quantity of voluntary intake to preclude problems with feeding following transplantation (199). Infants also frequently require aggressive supplementation with sodium, potassium, and phosphorus. Sodium losses into the dialysate are compounded in polyuric infants by urinary sodium losses and can result in poor growth as well as systemic hypotension and vascular events such as anterior ischemic optic neuropathy (200–203). Standard infant formulas do not contain sufficient sodium to replace these losses. Both hypophosphatemia and hypokalemia can also occur and require supplementation in the vigorously growing infant who is maintained on a low-phosphorus, low-potassium formula (204).

TABLE 37.4	Recommended Maximum Oral and/or Enteral Phosphorus Intake for Children with Chronic Kidney Disease		
		Recommended Phosphorus Intake (mg/d)	
Age	**DRI (mg/d)**	**High PTH and Normal Phosphorus**[a]	**High PTH and High Phosphorus**[b]
0–6 mo	100	<100	<80
7–12 mo	275	<275	<220
1–3 y	460	<460	<370
4–8 y	500	<500	<400
9–18 y	1,250	<1,250	<1,000

DRI, dietary reference intake; PTH, parathyroid hormone.
[a]<100% of the DRI.
[b]<80% of the DRI.
From Kidney Disease Outcomes Quality Initiative Work Group. KDOQI clinical practice guideline for nutrition in children with CKD. *Am J Kidney Dis* 2009;53(Suppl 2):S1.

The complexity of the nutritional management of pediatric CPD patients is magnified by the critical importance of proper nutrition to the growing and developing child. The crucial role of the pediatric renal dietitian in the care of these fragile patients has previously been emphasized (58,205).

COMPLICATIONS OF CHRONIC PERITONEAL DIALYSIS IN CHILDREN

Peritonitis

The single most common complication that occurs in children maintained on CPD is peritonitis (109,206–211). Data from the USRDS reveal that infection is the most common cause for hospitalization among children receiving CPD, and infection is the most common reason for modality change (212). Unfortunately, present data make it clear that children experience a significantly greater rate of peritonitis than adults, with a substantial percentage of children experiencing an episode of peritonitis during their first year of PD treatment. Reductions in observed peritonitis rates have been reported in children in association with treatment of *Staphylococcus aureus* nasal carriage or application of topical antibiotics (e.g., mupirocin or gentamicin) at the dialysis catheter exit site, use of a two-cuff catheter with a downward-oriented exit site, as well as with technical developments such as disconnect systems and the flush-before-fill technique (89,206,213–216). The important contribution of prolonged dialysis training with an emphasis on hand hygiene has also been demonstrated in children (217,218).

Evaluation of the most recent data from the NAPRTCS database has revealed a total of 4,248 reported episodes of peritonitis in 6,658 years of follow-up, resulting in an annualized peritonitis rate of 0.64 or 1 infection every 18.8 patient-months (6). The rate of peritonitis was highest in the youngest patients (0 to 1 year) who had an annualized peritonitis rate of 0.79 or 1 infection every 15.3 patient-months versus an annualized rate of 0.57 or 1 episode every 21.2 patient-months in children older than 12 years. Noteworthy is a significant improvement in the overall annualized infection rate from 0.79 in 1992 to 1996 to 0.44 in recent years, likely related to the prophylactic measures noted above, in addition to recommendations pertaining to prophylactic antibiotic usage at the time of PD catheter placement and prior to invasive procedures (e.g., gastrostomy placement) (95,219,220).

When peritonitis is suspected, empiric antibiotic therapy should be administered by the IP route and should provide coverage for gram-positive and gram-negative organisms, commonly by a combination of a first-generation cephalosporin or a glycopeptide (e.g., vancomycin), with a third-generation cephalosporin or an aminoglycoside (215). The recently published pediatric peritonitis treatment guidelines also allow for empiric monotherapy with the fourth-generation cephalosporin cefepime where available and in the absence of a history of methicillin-resistant *S. aureus* (95,215). Most important is recognition of the marked regional variation of antibiotic resistance patterns and the accompanying need to prescribe the empiric therapy based on the local antibiotic resistance profile (53,215,221,222). To minimize the risk for glycopeptide- or aminoglycoside-related toxicity, maintenance antibiotic therapy should be instituted as soon as the antibiotic susceptibilities are made known.

Finally, encapsulating peritoneal sclerosis (EPS) is a rare but extremely serious clinical entity characterized by the presence of continuous, intermittent, or recurrent bowel obstruction associated with gross thickening of the peritoneum (223–226). Although primarily diagnosed in adults, it may also occur in children, typically those who have received CPD for more than 5 years. The presence of peritoneal calcifications on abdominal computed tomographic (CT) scan in association with a long duration of dialysis and ultrafiltration failure is highly suggestive of the diagnosis and may be an indication for prompt conversion to HD (223,227). Additional management options include immunosuppressive and antifibrotic medications and surgical intervention accompanied by aggressive nutritional support.

CHRONIC HEMODIALYSIS FOR CHILDREN

The clinical use of an "artificial kidney" was pioneered in 1944 in adult patients suffering from AKI by Willem J. Kolff, a Dutch physician during World War II (228). The purification of heparin from an extract of liver tissue in 1916 by a second year medical student at Johns Hopkins was another key development in the evolution of HD. Finally, when cellophane tubes became widely used as sausage casings in the 1920s, subsequent studies in animals revealed that the casings made excellent diffusion membranes, critical to the development of Kolff's invention of the rotating drum kidney in 1944 (229).

The initial application of the drum kidney in pediatrics took place in 1950. Soon thereafter, the Children's Hospital of Pittsburgh used a coil kidney design, turning Kolff's rotating drum on its end and submerging the coils of cellophane tubing in the dialysate bath, to treat five severely uremic children on an acute basis with clinical improvement in all (230).

The development of a reusable vascular access was yet another critical requirement and was first addressed by Dr. Belding Scribner and his team in Seattle (231). Use of the Scribner shunt and a pumpless system developed by Robert Hickman and Scribner for pediatrics in the early 1960s prompted the establishment of several pediatric chronic HD programs in the United States and Europe (232).

Challenges for these initial programs included the selection of patients by the so-called "Life and Death Committees," the use of flat-plate dialyzers, the need for regular transfusions, and repeated shunt clotting and infection. However, developments that led to successful pediatric HD programs as we know them today, included (a) improved vascular access with the introduction of arteriovenous fistulas and permanent double-lumen catheters, (b) the introduction of smaller more efficient dialyzers and lower volume dialysis circuits, and (c) the development of dialysis equipment with more precise ultrafiltration monitoring and control capability (233).

Vascular Access

Adequate HD delivery depends on a functional vascular access without compromising future potential access sites. Current HD access options are divided into two categories: permanent access in the form of an arteriovenous fistula (AVF) or arteriovenous graft (AVG) and a semipermanent access in the form of catheters with a subcutaneous (SC) cuff.

The risk of death in dialysis patients 18 years of age and older is lowest in patients with AVFs, followed by AVGs and then HD catheters (234). In turn, the KDOQI Pediatric Vascular Access guidelines recommend using an AVF or AVG for HD access in children and adolescents more than 20 kg who are expected to receive HD for more than 1 year (116). The weight cutoff takes into account the fact that relatively small vessels in the youngest patients may not be able to support AVF placement and maturation. Although certain centers have reported successful AVF placement in small children, maturation can take up to 6 months, which may not be practical in many situations (235,236).

AVFs are composed of a connection between a patient's native artery and vein. The most common sites for AVFs are the wrist (radiocephalic or Brescia-Cimino) and the antecubital fossa (brachial artery to cephalic vein). AVFs require at least 4 to 12 weeks for enough venous segment dilatation or maturation to allow for successful needle placement (116,235). The most common complications of AVFs include aneurysm formation from repeated puncture at the same site, arterial inflow stenosis with resultant poststenotic vessel dilatation, and collateral vessel development.

If native blood vessels are inadequate for an AVF, artificial materials can be used to create an AVG. Currently, the most commonly used material is polytetrafluoroethylene (PTFE)/Teflon, although some vascular surgeons are now using bovine carotid artery grafts in adults with equally as good if not superior outcomes in patency rates (237). The advantages of AVGs over AVFs include an expanded variety of anatomic placement sites (distal arm, upper arm, and thigh) and configurations (loop or straight). The major disadvantage associated with an AVG is the development of intimal hyperplasia and venous outflow stenosis, which can lead to decreased intra-access flow and thrombosis. Proactive noninvasive monitoring (NIVM) of AVG blood flow coupled with rapid referral for balloon angioplasty for a low AVG blood-flow reading has led to a significant decrease in thrombosis rates (238,239).

In 2002, Sheth et al. (240) demonstrated 1-, 3-, and 5-year patency rates for AVFs (74%, 59%, 59%) and AVGs (96%, 69%, 40%), excluding primary failure, that were not statistically different. Somewhat lower but again not statistically different 1-, 2-, and 3-year survival rates were reported from Argentina, where it was also noted that access stenosis, thrombosis, and infections were more frequent in AVGs than AVFs ($p = 0.02$) (241). Finally, a recent retrospective study was conducted at the Children's Hospital of Los Angeles on 101 AVFs that were created in 93 patients at that institution between 1999 and 2012. The patients were a mean age of 14 years (range, 3 to 19 years) and had a mean weight of 51 kg (range, 12 to 131 kg). The average 2-year and 4-year primary and secondary patency rates were 83% and 92%, and 65% and 83%, respectively. During the 2.5 years of follow-up, 68 patients (75%) received a transplant, with a mean time to transplant of 556 days, arguing for concerted efforts to improve the use of AVFs in pediatric patients not likely to receive a transplant within 1 year of dialysis initiation (242).

Cuffed indwelling catheters serve as the most common form of vascular access for children receiving chronic HD in the United States (243), which is unfortunate given the higher complication rate and shorter survival time of catheters compared with AVFs and AVGs (244). Prior to 1998, dual-lumen configurations were the only options for pediatric HD catheters (245,246). Alternative catheter configurations now include dual-lumen catheters with split distal venous and arterial lumens to allow for free tip movement within the vein (Ash Split catheter) and twin separate single-lumen catheter systems inserted into the same vein with different exit sites or in different veins altogether (Tesio catheter system). Although single-center pediatric data demonstrate that Tesio catheters enjoy a longer survival and provide superior clearance more consistently than dual-lumen catheters of similar size, the use of this catheter in adults was noted to be associated with a longer insertion time (41.5 min) compared to the Ash Split (29.4 min), with increased complications and with no significant difference in BFRs at 30 and 90 days postinsertion (247,248). There are currently sufficient catheters of various designs,

TABLE 37.5	Cuffed Hemodialysis Catheter and Patient Size Guideline
Patient Size (kg)	**Catheter Options**
<20	8-Fr dual lumen
20–25	7-Fr twin Tesio
	10-Fr dual lumen
25–40	10-Fr Ash Split
	10-Fr twin Tesio
>40	12- or 14-Fr Ash Split
	10-Fr twin Tesio
	11.5- or 12.5-Fr dual lumen

diameters, and lengths to permit chronic HD in infants and children of all sizes (TABLE 37.5). The optimal site is the right internal jugular vein or femoral vein. The subclavian vein should be avoided for risk of the subsequent development of subclavian stenosis and loss of further potential access sites in that arm (249).

Equipment for Pediatric Hemodialysis

Hemodialysis Circuit

The HD circuit is composed of the patient's vascular access, blood tubing connecting the access to the hemodialyzer, and the hemodialyzer itself. Blood tubing is produced in a variety of sizes and should be matched to the patient's size to allow for optimal blood flow while minimizing the volume of the extracorporeal circuit, which is the sum of the blood tubing volume and the hollow-fiber dialyzer volume (TABLE 37.6). To prevent excessive repeated blood loss in the circuit and hemodynamic instability, the extracorporeal circuit should not exceed 10% of the patient's calculated blood volume. Neonatal lines with a volume of 40 mL are available for use in children less than 15 kg. A wide variety of dialyzers with different blood volumes are available from various manufacturers that can be matched to pediatric patient sizes. In some infants, for whom even the smallest blood tubing and dialyzer volumes exceed 10% of patient blood volume, the circuit should be primed with colloid [5% albumin or packed red blood cells (PRBCs) diluted with albumin to a measured hematocrit of 35%] instead of crystalloid.

Hemodialysis Machine

Provision of safe pediatric HD requires machines that have accurate blood pump flow rates and volumetric control of ultrafiltration. Volumetric ultrafiltration controllers are critical to prevent rapid and excessive ultrafiltration rates in infants and young children

TABLE 37.6	Hemodialysis Circuit	
	Blood Volume in Tubing (mL)[a]	**Inner Diameter of Pump Segment (mm)**[b]
Infant	29	2.6
Pediatric	52	4.8
Intermediate pediatrics	110	6.4
Adult	149	8

[a]Varies based on manufacturer. Does not include volume of dialyzer.
[b]Numbers reflective of Medisystems Combiset.

receiving HD and are now required by Centers for Medicare & Medicaid Services (CMS) in children less than 35 kg (250).

Frequent home HD (see below) is a newer modality offered to pediatric patients. Pediatric results are similar to adult data with respect to improved biochemical control and HRQOL (251,252). These studies all used conventional HD machines that rely on a treated municipal water supply, potentially repeatedly exposing patients to proinflammatory components. Goldstein et al. (253) have reported on the use of the NxStage system for frequent home HD, which uses sterile dialysis fluid to provide dialysis in the home. They found similar biochemical improvements with variable changes in proinflammatory cytokine levels.

Noninvasive Monitoring of Hematocrit

Since red blood cell volume remains constant during dialysis, changes in hematocrit will be inversely proportional to changes in intravascular volume. Continuous optical methods of NIVM of the hematocrit take advantage of this relationship to demonstrate a real-time association between fluctuating hematocrit and intravascular volume during the HD treatment, which serves as an adjunct to patient monitoring designed to decrease the frequency of adverse events (254,255). In pediatric patients, the use of NIVM has been associated with lower rates of ultrafiltration-associated event rates (defined as hypotension, headache, or cramping that required a nursing intervention such as saline bolus, Trendelenburg position, slow/stop ultrafiltration), especially for patients less than 35 kg (256,257). Analysis of the timing of events associated with different blood volume changes using NIVM has led to NIVM-guided ultrafiltration modeling algorithms that optimize fluid removal during dialysis, lessen the need for antihypertensive medications, minimize intradialytic and interdialytic patient symptoms, and decrease the need for additional HD treatments or hospitalization for treatment of fluid overload and hypertension (239,258).

Chronic Hemodialysis Prescription

Patients initiating HD may suffer from any combination of fluid overload, hypertension, malnutrition, and a variety of electrolyte abnormalities. The transition from CKD to maintenance HD must be safe and calculated with the first month goals of establishing an estimated dry weight, normalization of blood pressure (BP) and electrolyte abnormalities, as well as achieving adequate urea reduction. Rapid osmolar changes of large magnitude can be associated with cerebral edema, disequilibrium syndrome, and seizures, especially during the first few HD treatments (259). The intravenous (IV) infusion of mannitol at a dose of 0.25 to 0.50 g/kg has been proposed as a method by which these symptoms can be avoided or ameliorated in children by maintaining a relatively high extracellular fluid osmolality as urea is removed from the patient, although the clinical utility of this procedure has never been clearly established (260,261). Furthermore, accumulation of mannitol after repeated infusions may be harmful (261). An alternative method to prevent large osmolar shifts during the initial HD treatments is to limit the amount of urea clearance delivered at each treatment. Practically, this can be achieved by limiting the decrease in the blood urea nitrogen (BUN) to only 30 to 40 mg/dL at each of the first few dialysis treatments. The proportional fall in urea can be estimated by calculations using the following mass transfer equation (**Equation 37.5**):

$$C_t/C_o = e^{-Kt/V} \qquad 37.5$$

where C_t is the concentration of BUN after t minutes of dialysis, C_o is the initial concentration, K is the urea clearance (mL/min),

t is the duration of dialysis (minutes), and V is the urea volume of distribution (mL).

As noted earlier, the urea volume of distribution is equivalent to the TBW, which is approximately 60% of the patient's weight. For example, if a 10-kg child is to begin HD and has a BUN of 100 mg/dL, the following calculations could be used: At a BFR of 25 mL/min, a dialyzer will achieve a urea clearance of 25 mL/min. If the desired fall in BUN is 30 mg/dL, then C_t = 70 mg/dL at the conclusion of the dialysis treatment. Assuming an average body composition, the TBW is approximately 6,000 mL. Therefore,

$$C_t/C_o = 70/100 = 0.7 \text{ and } 0.7 = e^{-25\,mL/min \times t\,minutes/6{,}000\,mL}$$
$$Ln\,(0.7) = -25\,mL/min \times t\,minutes/6{,}000\,mL$$
$$t = 0.36 \times 6{,}000/25$$
$$t = 86\,minutes$$

The time of dialysis could be further shortened if a higher BFR and therefore a higher clearance can be tolerated. Conversely, when lower BFRs are required, proportionally longer dialysis times are necessary to achieve the same outcome. The standard BFR is 5 to 7 mL/kg/min up to 300 to 400 mL/min with a dialysis flow rate of at least 1.5 times the BFR to prevent dialysate saturation from limiting solute clearance.

While there is no standard dialysis bath, the serum targets are a normal serum sodium and potassium, bicarbonate of 22 mEq/L, and a serum calcium level which varies by age from 8.7 to 11.3 mg/dL (61). In general, the calcium target is the lower side of normal per age group in order to decrease the risk for vascular calcifications. Some centers continue to implement sodium modeling programs to create a hyperosmolar dialysate sodium concentration at the beginning of the dialysis treatment in an attempt to limit the development of hypotension during dialysis. The increased sodium concentration early in the dialysis treatment leads to an increase in serum osmolality and thereby offsets a decline of serum osmolality caused by urea clearance. A decrease of the dialysate sodium concentration subsequently occurs throughout the treatment and can be configured in an exponential, linear, or stepwise pattern. Sodium modeling has been shown to reduce dialysis morbidity in both adolescent and adult HD patients (262).

Anticoagulation

As mentioned previously, the vascular access is of utmost importance when administering HD. With that said, maintenance of access patency and prevention of clots within the extracorporeal circuit is imperative. When using a catheter for access, the vast majority of centers lock the catheter with unfractionated heparin in concentrations that vary from 1,000 to 5,000 U/mL in each lumen (263). This inactivates thrombin and inhibits fibrin formation and thrombin-induced platelet activation (264). There is some systemic infiltration of the anticoagulant, and accidental flushing of a heparin-locked catheter can result in serious bleeding and needs to be prevented by appropriate labeling of the catheter. A less common practice is to lock the HD catheter with recombinant tissue plasminogen activator (rTPA) or sodium citrate, which if accidently flushed can result in severe hypocalcemia and cardiac events. Bolus and maintenance heparin infusion are typically prescribed during the dialysis treatment to prevent clotting and blood loss in the extracorporeal circuit, with standard dosing of 10 to 20 U/kg bolus and 10 to 20 U/kg/h maintenance. Lower molecular weight heparin has also been used for maintenance anticoagulation; however, there is limited data on its efficacy and safety in pediatric HD.

Hemodialysis Adequacy

Adequate HD is usually defined as a minimum level of toxic substance clearance (usually using urea clearance as a surrogate), below which a clinically unacceptable rate of poor outcome occurs. A more complete definition of HD adequacy recognizes both HD treatment urea clearance and the patient's metabolic state as manifested by urea generation in between HD treatments. Significant research over the last 20 years has also focused on the refinement of complex mathematical models to more accurately quantify the total urea mass removed during a dialysis treatment (265–268).

The ideal parameter to use when prescribing an individual dialysis treatment should recognize the individual patient's size and metabolic state. It should be simultaneously informative of the overall production and removal of toxic substances. The conceptual basis of urea kinetic modeling (UKM) is based on the analysis of the rates of accumulation and removal of urea. Urea is generated at a constant rate that is proportional to the patient's protein catabolic rate (PCR). At the beginning of dialysis, urea is distributed in a single body pool that is equivalent to the TBW, so the distribution of urea can be described by a single-pool mathematical model. The rate of removal of urea is depicted by the term Kt/V [dialyzer urea clearance at a particular BFR (K; mL/min), HD treatment duration (t; minutes), and the patient's pretreatment and posttreatment weight (kg)]. The interdialytic accumulation of urea reflects the amount of protein catabolized during the time between dialysis treatments (269). In a steady state, this PCR (g/d) reflects the amount of protein ingested by the patient and, hence, is a marker of nutritional status (270,271).

The validity of the urea kinetic model was demonstrated in the National Cooperative Dialysis Study, which demonstrated a higher probability of "patient failure" (i.e., patient death or hospitalization) in adult patients who received lower doses of HD and/or who were in a poor state of nutrition (267). In adults, the individual dialysis treatment should be such that the single-pool Kt/V (spKt/V) is greater than 1.2 (116). Corresponding target Kt/V values for children have not been defined, although it is presumed and recommended that pediatric patients should receive dialysis that is at least equivalent to that provided for adults (116). Some initial pediatric outcome data have shown the utility of Kt/V in controlling for HD and normalized protein catabolic rate (nPCR) in the assessment of the nutrition status in malnourished patients receiving HD (272–274).

Pediatric data have demonstrated that simplified algebraic equations reliably approximate Kt/V and nPCR (275,276). Some formulas further refine urea clearance measurement to account for the double-pool distribution of urea during dialysis and the resultant BUN rebound seen in the first hour after HD ends as urea re-equilibrates between the intracellular and extracellular compartments (277–280). HD outcome study validity requires a control for HD dose, so the application of simpler and more accessible HD adequacy measurement methods should lead to an increase in pediatric HD outcome study research. Initial single-center and multicenter pediatric studies are starting to assess the impact of dialysis dose on outcome (272,281). However, a pediatric study from the CMS's Clinical Performance Measures Project demonstrated that little difference in HD prescription management would result when comparing spKt/V versus equilibrated Kt/V values from the same treatment (282). As a result, KDOQI states that spKt/V assessment is appropriate for patient management, whereas equilibrated Kt/V values should be used when an outcome study is conducted (116).

Frequent Hemodialysis

Nightly home HD has been reported by some to be associated with better survival in adults than thrice-weekly in-center HD (283). In those centers using nightly home HD, patients have experienced improved BP control, anemia management and phosphorus control, and a better HRQOL (284). In the Frequent Hemodialysis (FH) Trial Group, in which patients were randomized to either three or six weekly dialysis sessions, the latter regimen exhibited statistically significant benefits with respect to both co-primary composite end points of death or 12-month change in left ventricular mass and death or 12-month change in self-reported physical health; however, patients in the FH group experienced an increased rate of vascular access interventions (285). More recently, the Frequent Nocturnal Hemodialysis (FNH) Trial Group surprisingly reported a statistically significant increased overall mortality HR of 3.88 in the six-times weekly home nocturnal HD group compared to those patients receiving three-times weekly HD. The authors cautioned that there was a surprisingly low mortality rate for individuals randomly assigned to conventional HD (286).

In contrast to the growing experience in adults, there is limited data pertaining to home or frequent HD in children (251). Two small studies, each of four adolescents undergoing slow nocturnal HD with a follow-up of 6 to 20 months, found that the treated patients had a rapid decrease in their predialysis phosphate and PTH levels without the need for phosphate binders or diet restriction, as well as a decreased need for fluid restriction and an improved HRQOL (55,287). Fischbach et al. (288) reported improved growth of patients, with and without the need for growth hormone (GH) therapy, in association with a hemodiafiltration regimen of six times weekly, 3 hours per treatment as compared to growth with conventional dialysis plus GH therapy. In an additional experience, Goldstein et al. (253) described four patients who received home HD six times weekly over 16 weeks. The patients exhibited a decreased BP load by ambulatory BP monitoring, improved phosphorus control, and an improved nPCR. These data suggest that frequent HD is an additional dialytic alternative that should be considered for the pediatric patient, although a great deal more study of this approach to therapy is necessary in children.

Nutritional Management of Children on Hemodialysis

The nutritional goal for children undergoing chronic HD is to optimize their growth and development, while avoiding exacerbation of their underlying fluid and electrolyte disturbances and uremia. An individual child's prescribed intake is based on an analysis of RKF and nutritional needs. Malnutrition, which plays a role in the poor growth of children with CKD, may result from inadequate dietary intake resulting from uremic anorexia and dysgeusia and prescribed nutrient restrictions (289,290). Monitoring the nutritional status of the child on HD is, in turn, a crucial element of patient management. Parameters to monitor have been published in the KDOQI Nutrition Guidelines for CKD, and in addition to traditional measurements of height, weight, and serum albumin, the nPCR has emerged as an accurate marker of nutritional status in the adolescent HD patient (61,291).

The dietary protein and caloric intake of each child should be sufficient to allow a positive nitrogen balance associated with an increase in lean body mass and stature. An increase in dietary energy intake without sufficient protein intake may result in obesity without increasing a child's lean body mass. In contrast, an increase in the dietary protein intake without sufficient energy intake will increase the amount of protein used for energy needs rather than increasing lean body mass and, therefore, will increase the urea generation rate. The concept of protein-energy wasting (PEW), defined as a state of decreased body protein mass and fuel reserves (body protein and fat mass), is common in ESKD and multifactorial in nature with contributions from hormonal imbalances, low nutrient intake, low RKF, inadequate dialysis dose, chronic inflammation, and metabolic acidosis (292). Whereas adult PEW is well defined, there is no accepted pediatric definition of PEW (293,294). A multidisciplinary approach has been suggested to gauge an individual pediatric patient's overall nutritional status by incorporating dietary intake, anthropometric parameters, and for adolescents on HD, nPCR (293).

The dietary needs of children with CKD are not the same as the National Research Council's Food and Nutrition Board's recommended nutrient intakes (RNIs) because these recommendations are for populations of healthy children. For example, the needs of children on HD are affected by the catabolic effects of HD, including the loss of amino acids in the dialysate. Protein intake must be sufficient to allow an increase in muscle mass and maximize growth while minimizing urea generation. An ongoing assessment of the balance of dietary protein intake and urea removal can be gained through the use of UKM, which can calculate the nPCR in patients undergoing maintenance HD (270). Pediatric data demonstrate algebraic nPCR approximation equations to be accurate, and in adolescents, a low nPCR (less than 1 g/kg/d) is a sensitive and specific means by which to predict impending weight loss over the next 3 months (276,295).

The KDOQI pediatric guidelines recommend a caloric requirement equivalent to that of healthy children and an initial dietary protein intake to meet the recommended dietary allowance (RDA) for chronologic age with an additional increment of 0.1 g/kg/d when receiving HD (61,291). The usual dietary requirements for protein and calories may, however, be most accurately estimated in terms of stature because this measure is independent of fluid balance or the amount of body fat. In one report, a positive nitrogen balance was attained in children receiving a diet that provided 0.3 g of protein per 1 cm of statural height with an energy intake of 10 kcal/cm (270). Intradialytic parenteral nutrition (IDPN) may also have a role in treatment of severe protein-energy malnutrition in children receiving HD (273,274,296,297). IDPN is composed of a 70% dextrose solution and a 15% amino acid solution and is prescribed to provide 1.2 to 1.4 g protein per kilogram of patient weight each treatment. In addition, patients may receive IV lipids. In two pediatric studies, patient's nutrition status as measured by nPCR increased monthly with IDPN, with no change in their dialysis dose (273,274).

Children receiving HD have a pattern of lipid abnormalities similar to that seen in familial endogenous hypertriglyceridemia or type IV hyperlipidemia (298,299) with a prevalence of 39% to 65% (300). In children with ESKD, the lipid profile consists of elevated triglycerides, triglyceride-rich lipoproteins, and apolipoprotein C3, as well as decreased levels of cholesteryl ester transfer protein and high-density lipoproteins (HDLs). There is also enhanced hepatic synthesis of serum very low-density and reduced conversion of intermediate-density lipoproteins to low-density lipoproteins (LDLs) (300). The significance of these lipid abnormalities in children with ESKD is unclear, but such abnormalities may increase the risk of atherosclerosis in a patient population already at risk for CVD, and it is the recommendation of the American Heart Association

Expert Panel on Population and Prevention Science that prevention of CVD in high-risk pediatric patients (including dialysis patients) is warranted (301). Although the basis for the lipid abnormalities has not been completely ascertained, possible contributing factors include a high fat content in the diet and decreased lipoprotein lipase and hepatic triglyceride lipase activities. In addition, carnitine levels are decreased in children treated with HD as compared with healthy controls (296,302–304). Carnitine, a low molecular weight molecule that transports fatty acids from the cytoplasm to the mitochondria for oxidation, may be lost in the dialysate.

Treatment of lipid abnormalities is first directed at therapeutic lifestyle changes. The role of pharmacologic lipid-lowering agents, such as statins, in children on HD has not been determined. However, supplementation with L-carnitine has been suggested as a potential treatment. Although one short-term trial of IV L-carnitine (5 mg/kg during dialysis) resulted in a marked decrease in triglyceride levels and an increase in HDL cholesterol concentration, two more recent studies failed to confirm these findings (302,304,305).

Water-soluble vitamins are removed during HD making supplementation with these vitamins, especially vitamins B_6, C, and folate, necessary. Restriction of water intake is necessary to prevent interdialytic volume overload. A child's fluid restriction is generally the sum of insensible losses, residual urine output, and an amount that can be safely accumulated and ultrafiltered after a 2- to 3-day interdialytic period. The sodium intake of most children is restricted to help maintain the desired fluid restriction and avoid hypertension. In contrast to older children, infants with minimal urine output or with large urinary sodium losses from dysplastic renal syndromes who are receiving low-sodium formulas are at risk for hyponatremia. The accumulation of water over an interdialytic period coupled with very low sodium content in the formula may result in dilutional hyponatremia.

HEMODIALYSIS FOR NEONATES AND INFANTS

Although all pediatric HD requires specialized nursing and medical expertise, HD for neonates and infants is an especially complicated procedure. Few infants receive HD as maintenance RRT; the 2011 NAPRTCS report reveals that only 70 out of 927 children less than 1 year of age received HD as their initial dialysis modality since 1992 (6). Therefore, little evidence base exists to guide the provision of maintenance HD for infants (306).

As noted earlier, neonatal-sized blood tubing is available to minimize the blood volume of the extracorporeal circuit. Neonatal tubing is one-fourth the diameter of standard tubing, so the blood pump flow rate must be quadrupled to deliver the same blood volume per minute (e.g., a Q_B of 160 mL/min on the dialysis machine yields an actual blood flow of 40 mL/min through the dialyzer when neonatal tubing is used). Even with smaller neonatal tubing, the extracorporeal volume usually comprises greater than 10% of patient blood volume in infants less than 8 kg. Therefore, the circuit should be primed with 5% albumin when performing HD treatments in infants less than 8 kg in size. Circuit priming with PRBCs diluted with albumin or saline to a hematocrit of 35% should be considered in small infants expected to receive a prolonged course of maintenance HD to prevent anemia resulting from repeated red blood cell loss in the circuit.

Adequate urea clearance can be achieved with blood pump flow rates of 30 to 50 mL/min, flows which generally require a 7-Fr or

8-Fr dual-lumen HD catheter, but catheter choice and anatomic insertion site will need to be made on a case-by-case basis in the small infant (116,307).

Current volumetric HD machines produce an ultrafiltration accuracy of 50 to 100 mL, which is acceptable for most pediatric patients but is not tolerable for neonates. Digital scales, which are accurate to within 10 g, can be placed under an infant warmer and help guide ultrafiltration during a neonatal HD treatment. A newer product, the Newcastle infant dialysis and ultrafiltration system (Nidus), has been shown to be effective in both the pediatric intensive care unit and outpatient intermittent HD setting for babies weighing less than 8 kg. (**FIGURE 37.2**) This device generates higher dialysis clearances than PD and delivers more precise ultrafiltration control than either PD or conventional HD (308).

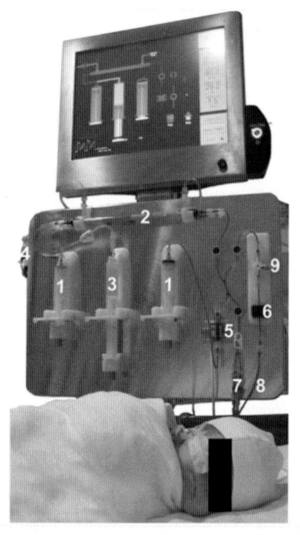

FIGURE 37.2 **1.** Two operating syringes, **2.** High-flux polysulfone 0.045 m² filter, **3.** Heparin syringe, **4.** Pumped dialysate, **5.** Pressure transducer, **6.** Air-detector, **7.** Heparinized saline "dummy", **8.** Infant line, **9.** Blood sampling site. [From Coulthard MG, Crosier J, Griffiths C, et al. Haemodialysing babies weighing <8 kg with the Newcastle infant dialysis and ultrafiltration system (Nidus): comparison with peritoneal and conventional haemodialysis. *Pediatr Nephrol* 2014;29(10):1873–1881.]

Complications of Hemodialysis in Children: Access Infection

Of the 8,060 courses of dialysis registered to 6,300 pediatric patients reviewed in the 2011 NAPRTCS dialysis report, 42% were HD courses, and 78.7% of those were via a percutaneous catheter as the HD access. When change of modality was the reason for termination of HD, 7% were due to excessive infection and 12.6% were due to access failure (6). A study of HD patients aged 12 to <18 years old identified in the 2000 ESRD Clinical Performance Measure Project found that of 418 patients, 58% had a central venous catheter. Patients in this study with a catheter had an adjusted relative risk of hospitalization due to infection of 4.74 [95% confidence interval (CI) 2.02 to 11.14] compared to those with an AVF or AVG (309). Despite a clear understanding that central catheters are associated with an increased risk of infection as compared to AVF or AVG, recent literature continues to show that catheters are the predominant vascular access in pediatric dialysis (263).

In 2011, the Centers for Disease Control and Prevention (CDC) published Guidelines for the Prevention of Intravascular Catheter-Related Infections, recommending the use >0.5% chlorhexidine solution to clean the exit site and application of prophylactic antibiotic ointment or cream at the catheter exit site (310). More recently, investigators examined the efficacy of chlorhexidine solutions and a 5% povidone-iodine solution on the incidence of central venous catheter–related infections in children on HD. Although the numbers were small, 14 catheters in the povidone-iodine group and 13 in the chlorhexidine group, the investigators found that 10 exit-site infections and 5 blood stream infections occurred in the povidone-iodine group as compared to only 1 exit site and 1 blood stream infection in the chlorhexidine group, $p = 0.008$ and $p = 0.06$, respectively (311). While the push remains for AVFs or AVGs over central venous catheters, when caring for those patients with catheters, one must be diligent about hand hygiene and exit-site care in order to prevent infections in this at risk population. The Standardizing Care to Improve Outcomes in Pediatric ESRD (SCOPE) quality collaborative is a multicenter, pediatric initiative that is currently aiming to define best practice in terms of infection prevention in the pediatric HD population (218).

⬡ ADDITIONAL CLINICAL ISSUES IN THE PEDIATRIC DIALYSIS PATIENT

Anemia Management

The most recent KDOQI guidelines confirmed that anemia in a child with CKD is defined as a hemoglobin (Hgb) below the normal range for age/gender [i.e., <5th percentile based on National Health and Nutrition Examination Survey (NHANES) II reference data]. In turn, the KDIGO guidelines recommend that the evaluation for anemia in children with CKD should be initiated for an Hgb <11 g/dL in children <5 years, <11.5 g/dL in children 5 to 12 years, and <12.0 g/dL in those 12 to 15 years; adult values apply to those >15 years (<13.0 for males; <12.0 for females) (312). The factors contributing to the anemia associated with CKD in children are similar to those in adults and include erythropoietin deficiency, decreased erythrocyte survival, inhibition of erythropoiesis, and increased blood loss (313–316). The average red blood cell life span is reduced from a normal value of 120 days to a mean of 80 days in uremic individuals. This shortened life span is in part due to intestinal losses and to losses related to the HD procedure (e.g., anticoagulation, blood lost in HD tubing, repeated blood tests). Intestinal blood loss in 12 children undergoing chronic HD was reported as 11.1 ± 2.3 mL/m^2/d. Extraintestinal blood losses were 8.3 ± 5.1 mL/m^2 per dialysis treatment. In this same group of children, the erythrocyte life span was 80% of normal (316).

Erythropoiesis-Stimulating Agents

Before the availability of ESAs, essentially all children on HD were transfusion dependent; now, virtually all children treated with ESAs have little or no transfusion requirement (317). Similarly, a child being treated with CPD typically required a red blood cell transfusion every 1.5 to 5 months to maintain a hematocrit of 22% to 25% before the availability of ESAs (318). With the advent of ESAs, the need for transfusions has been essentially eliminated, and Hgb levels can be maintained at near-normal levels. Currently, an ESA is used by more than 90% of children being treated with dialysis (6). Correction of anemia with ESAs may be associated with the development or exacerbation of hypertension, making careful monitoring of BP and aggressive treatment of hypertension mandatory. It is noteworthy that the USRDS report revealed that only 29% of children (less than 20 years) who initiated chronic dialysis in 2012 were receiving an ESA at dialysis initiation; however, the reported mean Hgb was 10.5 g/dL, suggesting that greater attention to anemia management is occurring in the patient with CKD before dialysis (1).

ESAs may be administered through the IV, SC, or IP routes. Subcutaneously administered ESAs, particularly epoetin-α, may have a longer half-life than intravenously administered drug, with the sustained lower level being more physiologic and cost-effective, and with a potentially greater erythropoietic effect. However, as a practical matter (including issues of pain and convenience), 85% of children on HD receive an ESA by the IV route during their regular HD sessions and 95% children on CPD receive SC ESAs (6). A small number of CPD patients (less than 3% in the NAPRTCS registry) receive IP ESAs (6). Epoetin-α is well absorbed from the peritoneal cavity when administered in a small volume (e.g., 50 mL) of dialysis fluid during a prolonged dwell (319,320). In one study, children were changed from SC to IP ESA administration and maintained their hematocrit levels with an ESA dose that was not significantly greater than the SC dose (321). In an evaluation of the pharmacokinetics of IP dosing, a history of repeated peritonitis was associated with lower peritoneal absorption (321). The small volume of dialysate also has the potential of compromising dialysis clearance. In the United States, most children on dialysis (87% of children on CPD, 90% on HD) receive erythropoietin-α as a result of reimbursement policies; the remainder are receiving darbepoetin-α (6). Darbepoetin-α administered intravenously once per week has been shown to be as effective as shorter acting ESAs administered three times per week with a pharmacokinetic profile that is similar to that found in adult dialysis patients (322,323).

Although ESA requirements vary among children due to underlying disease, treatment modality, and route of administration, the most marked variation in dosing is based on age. Infants may require significantly higher doses, as high as 350 to 450 U/kg/wk, to achieve their target Hgb (6,312,324). In one multicenter European trial in HD patients aged 2 to 21 years, the median weekly maintenance epoetin dose varied from 136 U/kg in those older than 15 years to 321 U/kg in children younger than 5 years (317). The higher ESA requirement in infants may be related to nonhematopoietic binding and elimination, expanding

blood volume with rapid growth, or a greater percentage of blood volume lost with phlebotomies and dialysis losses (324–327). Analysis of data from the International Pediatric Peritoneal Dialysis Network (IPPN) has shown that although weight-related dosing is inversely related to age, the weekly ESA dose normalized to BSA is age independent: 4,208 U/m^2 BSA in this analysis of children on CPD (120).

In addition to the influential issues above, the most important cause of ESA hyporesponsiveness is insufficient iron stores. Additional causes include latent blood loss, hyperparathyroidism, and infection or inflammation (328). In patients with severe hyperparathyroidism who are hyporesponsive to ESAs (329), the poor response may be due to inhibition of erythropoiesis by circulating parathyroid hormone (PTH) or to osteitis fibrosa resulting in decreased marrow space for erythropoiesis. Uremia may be an inflammatory state *per se*, altering both iron transport and erythropoietin receptor expression (328). The most frequent form of infection in children undergoing CPD is peritonitis. The effect of a peritonitis episode on erythropoiesis may persist beyond the period of evident infection. In one center, the hematocrit remained at least 20% below baseline 4 weeks following the infection in association with 50% of peritonitis episodes. Whereas the hematocrit had returned to baseline by 8 weeks, some patients required an increase in the ESA dose (330). The blunting of erythropoiesis by peritonitis or other inflammatory processes results from decreased erythropoietin levels, the inhibitory effects of circulating cytokines on marrow activity, and a decreased ability to mobilize iron from the reticuloendothelial system (RES) (331,332). Elevated levels of hepcidin that occur in the setting of inflammation likely play a key role in iron homeostasis by impairing iron absorption across the gastrointestinal tract and by restricting release of iron from the RES by binding to ferroportin (333,334). Pure red cell aplasia (PRCA) due to circulating anti-ESA antibodies is an uncommon cause for ESA resistance, but it has been reported in pediatric patients (335–337).

The optimum Hgb level for children being treated with dialysis (HD or CPD) and ESAs has not been determined. The issues to be considered in choosing a target in adult dialysis patients include QOL, with the suggestion that higher Hgb levels may be associated with improvement of some QOL parameters, and concerns about potential adverse cardiovascular outcomes with higher Hgb levels (338–340). There may well be an additional adverse effect associated with the administration of higher doses of ESAs, in addition to an effect related to the Hgb level *per se* (341,342). Data from the IPPN has revealed the risk of patient mortality to be significantly increased in association with a weekly ESA dose of $> 6,000$ U/m^2/wk versus a lower dose, even when correcting for the Hgb value (120). In children, there is no definitive evidence for benefit or harm associated with a given level of Hgb for an individual child. Most of the demonstrated benefits accrue with the change from severe anemia to an Hgb level greater than 10 g/dL. Certainly, the risk of requiring a transfusion increases with an Hgb <10 g/dL and the prevention of transfusion is a primary goal of ESA treatment. As stated in the most recent KDOQI update on anemia management, there are no studies to support targeting pediatric Hgb levels greater than the targets set for adults with CKD (11 to 12 g/dL); accordingly, the pediatric practitioner will have to consider whether an individual child is likely to have an incremental benefit to QOL, school performance, or exercise tolerance with a higher Hgb level (341,342).

In one of the few studies that has evaluated the impact of anemia management in children with ESKD, the outcome of 1,942 pediatric dialysis patients enrolled in the NAPRTCS registry from 1992 to 2001 was reviewed to determine if there was an association between anemia (defined as a hematocrit less than 33%) 30 days after dialysis initiation and subsequent morbidity and mortality (343). Overall, 67.8% of patients were anemic at the start of dialysis with a decrease from 79.7% of children in 1992 to 50.6% in 2000. Anemic HD or CPD patients were hospitalized for more days in the first year of dialysis than those with a hematocrit of 33% or more. Importantly, after adjusting for age, treatment modality, etiology of ESKD, as well as iron and ESA use, patients with a hematocrit less than 33% had a 52% greater risk of death compared with those with a hematocrit in the range of 33% to less than 36%. In addition, there was an 81% increased risk of death for those with a hematocrit 27% to 30% or less, and an 80% increased risk for those with a hematocrit less than 27%. There was no difference in the risk of death for those with a hematocrit 30% to 33% or 36% or more (343).

In a second study, Amaral et al. (344) reviewed data from the CMS's ESRD Clinical Performance Measures Project to evaluate the correlation between average Hgb level achieved in adolescent HD patients, hospitalization, and mortality. In this assessment of 677 patients, an Hgb level of 11 to 12 g/dL (vs. less than 10 g/dL) was associated with a decrease in mortality risk of 69%. No statistically significant difference in risk between Hgb categories with respect to hospitalization was found (344). Most recently, a report from the IPPN found a relationship between Hgb <11 g/dL as compared to a higher Hgb and an increased risk of mortality (120).

Despite the apparent benefits of Hgb >11.0 g/dL, this target has not been consistently achieved historically. An analysis of data in a prior USRDS report compared the anemia management of children (0 to 19 years) and adults on dialysis between 1996 and 2000 (345). The mean annual Hgb was calculated. In each year, 54.1% of children on HD had a mean annual Hgb of less than 11 g/dL, whereas 39.3% of adults were anemic. In children treated with CPD, low mean Hgb levels were found in 69.5% of patients as compared to 55.1% of adults (345). Children also used less IV iron than adults in this time period. More recently, treatment outcomes have improved, and in 2005, more than 75% of all prevalent pediatric dialysis patients had an Hgb of >11 g/dL (346).

Iron Supplementation

The goal of iron supplementation during ESA treatment is to maintain sufficient iron stores for optimal erythropoiesis without the development of hemosiderosis. In the past, children on HD were multiply transfused and eventually became iron overloaded. Now that children are no longer regularly transfused, the blood and iron losses associated with CKD and dialysis are not replaced, and children have a net iron loss, prompting the need for iron supplementation. In a NAPRTCS report from 2001, after 12 months on dialysis, 77% of pediatric HD patients and 84% of CPD patients were receiving oral iron. The most recent report from 2011, however, reported that only 29% of those on HD and 77% on CPD were receiving enteral iron (6,103). Oral iron supplementation is often associated with poor adherence secondary to gastrointestinal intolerance and rarely is it sufficient to maintain the iron stores necessary for erythropoiesis, especially in patients who receive HD. Therefore, it is now recognized that most HD patients and some CPD patients receive IV iron on a regular or maintenance

basis: in one report from 2011, 52% of HD and 12% of CPD patients (6). In part, this is related to the fact that there is limited gastrointestinal iron absorption in patients with ESKD who have relative, but not absolute iron deficiency, possibly as a result of elevated hepcidin levels. Intestinal iron absorption is also inversely related to the body's iron stores (347).

Current recommendations (primarily based on data in adult patients) are to treat with iron to maintain a transferrin saturation (TSAT) of at least 20% and a serum ferritin of greater than 100 ng/mL in those on CPD, greater than 200 ng/mL for adult HD patients and greater than 100 ng/mL for pediatric HD patients (348). The age-related differences in the recommendations pertaining to serum ferritin during HD are merely the result of the lack of pediatric data available on the subject; in children with CKD, a TSAT <20% has been shown to be predictive of iron deficiency, whereas the ferritin value has been less predictive (349–352). Caution is advised when the serum ferritin level is greater than 500 ng/mL (341), highlighting the need to evaluate such patients for their Hgb level, ESA responsiveness, and the likely impact of their clinical status on iron availability (e.g., inflammatory block vs. functional iron deficiency) before considering additional iron therapy (341,353). As noted earlier, due to a poor response to oral iron, the IV route is recommended for HD patients, whereas the oral route alone may be sufficient for some CPD patients (341). IV iron treatment includes both repleting iron stores (with a short course of a series of iron doses) and maintaining iron stores with regular IV iron administration. Trials of maintenance IV iron dosing have demonstrated decreased ESA requirements in both children and adult patients receiving HD (354–357).

Three formulations of IV iron are currently in use: iron dextran, ferric sodium gluconate, and ferric saccharate (iron sucrose). Iron dextran was used extensively in the United States until the other formulations became available. Although iron dextran was relatively safe, there were anaphylactic-like reactions consisting of dyspnea, wheezing, abdominal cramps, and hypotension occasionally associated with its use. Whereas data on the incidence of anaphylactic-like reactions in children is sparse, review of the adult HD patient experience has demonstrated that 4.7% of patients experience adverse events attributable to iron dextran (358). The other forms of IV iron, ferric gluconate and iron sucrose, are associated with fewer serious adverse effects and have been given in multiple doses to pediatric dialysis patients safely (357,359,360). Therefore, they have replaced iron dextran in most adult and pediatric dialysis programs (361). In a prospective multicenter trial, ferric gluconate was shown to be safe and effective in children when administered at doses of 1.5 to 3 mg/kg dosed intermittently to treat iron deficiency or on a maintenance schedule to avoid iron deficiency (357,362). Iron sucrose has been shown to be safe and effective on a maintenance schedule using 0.5 to 2.0 mg/kg/dose every 2 weeks in HD patients and every 4 weeks in CPD patients (359). A newer iron preparation, ferric pyrophosphate, is administered per the dialysate of HD patients and was recently approved for clinical use (363). Pediatric trials with this medication should begin in late 2015.

Growth Retardation

Before the use of recombinant human growth hormone (rhGH), severe growth retardation was almost universally present in children with ESKD. The impact of growth retardation on adult height is greatest for those children with ESKD during infancy and puberty, the periods of most rapid growth. Recent publications have provided evidence for the significant negative impact that growth retardation may have on the QOL experienced by adults with childhood onset ESKD (364,365). Several factors may contribute to the poor growth of children with impaired kidney function, including protein and calorie malnutrition, metabolic acidosis, renal osteodystrophy, endocrine abnormalities, and the accumulation of uremic toxins. Although some of these factors are improved by dialysis, many persist despite aggressive dialytic therapy (366).

A number of endocrine abnormalities are present in CKD that may contribute to poor growth. These endocrine alterations include abnormalities of vitamin D metabolism, alterations of the GH axis, hypothyroidism, and peripheral insulin resistance. Alterations in GH secretion and the activity of insulin-like growth factor-1 (IGF-1) are particularly important (366). IGF-1 stimulates the clonal expansion of chondrocytes and collagen formation in the long-bone growth plates. The bioactivity of IGF-1 is limited in uremic children through an increase in IGF-1–binding proteins. Treatment with rhGH may accelerate growth by increasing IGF-1 levels to supraphysiologic levels with a resultant increase in its bioactivity (366–370).

The treatment of children who have developed ESKD with rhGH has been extensively reviewed elsewhere, and the therapy has proven to be safe and effective (367,371). Although rhGH improves the growth of children undergoing CPD and HD, the response may be blunted after the initial year of treatment (367,372–375). There is also evidence that the impact of therapy may be greatest in those patients who are treated before the development of ESKD, in part related to differences in the severity of alterations in IGF-binding protein concentrations and GH receptor density (375,376). Most importantly, when all other factors associated with growth retardation in children receiving HD or CPD (i.e., acidosis, hyperphosphatemia, secondary hyperparathyroidism, sodium losses, and poor nutrition) are being aggressively and successfully treated and poor growth persists, rhGH therapy is indicated. The KDOQI nutrition guidelines recommend the initiation of rhGH treatment in children with a height standard deviation score (SDS) more negative than −2.0 or a height velocity more negative than −2.0 SDS (61,377). Similarly, a consensus committee recommended that rhGH therapy be considered in children with CKD whose height SDS was less than −1.88 or whose height velocity SDS was less than −2 (**FIGURE 37.3**) (366). Nevertheless, for reasons that are not clear, a minority of growth-retarded patients with CKD/ESKD receive rhGH therapy. In the 2011 NAPRTCS annual report, the mean height SDS for patients initiating CPD was −1.71; however, only 10% of patients were treated with rhGH at 1 month, increasing to 20% at 1 year, and 25% at 2 years postdialysis initiation (6). Children treated with HD had an initial mean height SDS −1.4, and 10% were receiving rhGH at 1 month, increasing to 12% at 1 year and 16% at 2 years (6). Equally impressive and concerning is data from the USRDS which demonstrates that 37.2% of pediatric HD patients are more than 2 SD below the standardized mean height for their age, gender, or race/ethnicity, but only 14.6% of this group receive rhGH (**FIGURE 37.4**) (378). Clearly, greater attention to this issue should be encouraged.

Chronic Kidney Disease–Associated Mineral and Bone Disorder: Calcium and Phosphorus Homeostasis

The metabolic abnormalities that may arise in children treated with chronic dialysis are common to all children with CKD and include elevated body phosphate stores, insufficient 1-α-hydroxylation of 25-hydroxy-cholecalciferol, and resultant inadequate intestinal absorption of calcium. In fact, children being treated with dialysis may experience progression of the bone disease that starts before dialysis. Data collected from the IPPN registry of 890 children treated with CPD showed that 15% had symptoms or radiologic evidence of mineral and bone disorder (MBD) at the start of dialysis including 44% with intact parathyroid hormone (iPTH) levels above the K/DOQI target. Of note, an iPTH >500 pg/mL was associated with impaired growth (379). In turn, aggressive medical management with vitamin D analogs, calcium supplements, oral dietary phosphorus binders, and diets with reduced phosphate content are all essential components of the effective prevention and/or management of renal bone disease in children with ESKD.

Treatment with Vitamin D, Vitamin D Analogs, and Calcimimetics

Vitamin D deficiency is common in the general population, and the majority of children on dialysis are vitamin D insufficient or deficient necessitating supplementation with vitamin D_2 (ergocalciferol) or D_3 (cholecalciferol) (183,380–382). The KDOQI guidelines recommend screening and supplementation to replete stores for 25-hydroxyvitamin D levels <30 ng/mL. As a consequence of decreased 1,25-dihydroxyvitamin D and depressed serum ionized calcium concentrations, there is an increase in fibroblast growth factor-23 (FGF-23) and iPTH levels in children with ESKD. The resultant renal osteodystrophy may impede growth and lead to long-term bony abnormalities. Therefore, supplementation with vitamin D or an analog is an essential component of the treatment of children being treated with HD or CPD (383). The optimal iPTH level to avoid suppressing growth with adynamic bone disease or worsening renal osteodystrophy during rhGH treatment has been debated; however, the most recent opinion from the KDOQI working group for Bone Metabolism and Disease in Children has recommended iPTH values of 200 to 300 pg/mL for patients on dialysis (183). Observational data from the IPPN has suggested that an iPTH value of 100 to 300 pg/mL should be targeted in children on CPD (379).

Oral calcitriol, which has been the mainstay of treatment, has been shown to be effective in controlling renal bone disease in children receiving CPD (384). In addition to stimulating intestinal calcium absorption, calcitriol directly suppresses the parathyroid gland growth and iPTH synthesis (385,386). IV forms of the vitamin D analogs, calcitriol and paricalcitol, are also currently available to treat the secondary hyperparathyroidism associated with ESKD (387,388). In a placebo-controlled trial in pediatric HD patients, IV paricalcitol was shown to decrease iPTH levels without significantly increasing serum calcium, phosphorus, or calcium–phosphorus product (389). Paricalcitol has the advantage in many patients of suppressing the parathyroid glands with less effect on intestinal calcium absorption (388). In a single-center crossover trial comparing calcitriol to paricalcitol in pediatric HD patients, there was no difference in the mean calcium–phosphorus product between the agents; however, there was a greater incidence of hypercalcemia and a calcium–phosphorus product greater than 70 mg^2/dL^2 during calcitriol treatment (390). Doxercalciferol (Hectorol) is also available as an oral and a parenteral preparation and has been shown to treat secondary hyperparathyroidism; however, there

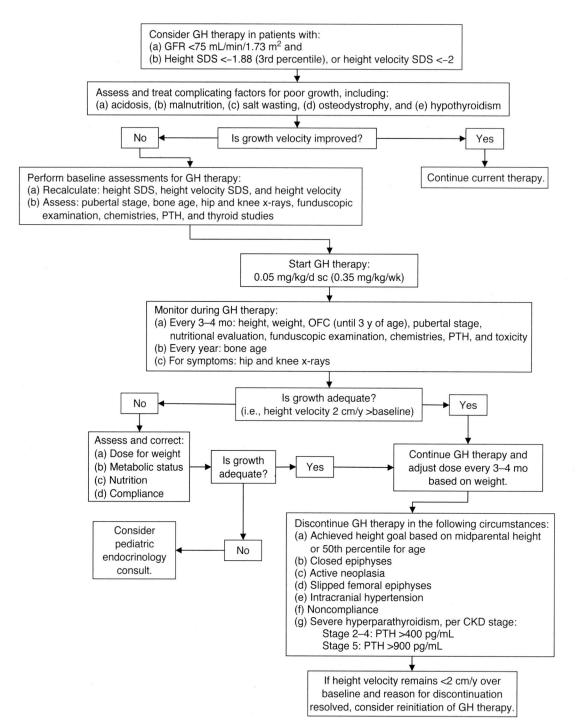

FIGURE 37.3 Algorithm for evaluation and treatment of growth failure in children with chronic renal insufficiency (CRI). GH, growth hormone; GFR, glomerular filtration rate; SDS, standard deviation score; PTH, parathyroid hormone; OFC, occipitofrontal circumference; CKD, chronic kidney disease. (From Mahan JD, Warady BA. Assessment and treatment of short stature in pediatric patients with chronic kidney disease consensus statement. *Pediatr Nephrol* 2006;21:917–930.)

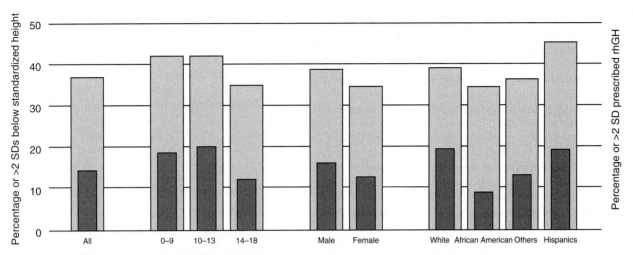

FIGURE 37.4 Percentage of children more than 2 standard deviation (SD) below standardized height, by age, gender, and race/ethnicity (*gray bars*) and percentage of these children with recombinant human growth hormone (rhGH) prescription (*black bars*). (From United States Renal Data System. *USRDS 2007 Annual Report: Atlas of Chronic Kidney Disease and End-Stage Renal Disease in the United States.* Bethesda, MD: National Institutes of Health, National Institute of Diabetes and Digestive and Kidney Diseases, 2007.)

are currently limited data on its use in children (183). Calcitriol or analogs are utilized by 73% of CPD patients (3% IV) and 71% of HD patients (46% IV) after 1 year of dialysis in the NAPRTCS registry (6). Finally, calcimimetic agents (e.g., cinacalcet hydrochloride), which suppress iPTH without increasing calcium by enhancing the activity of the calcium-sensing receptor (CaSR) of the parathyroid gland, are efficacious and have been approved for treatment in adults (391). Anecdotal reports of the efficacy of this agent in children have been published and a formal multicenter study in pediatric patients in currently being conducted (392,393). Of note, there is the potential for adverse effects of this treatment as the CaSR is also located in the growth plate (183).

Phosphate Binders

Hyperphosphatemia may lead to extraskeletal metastatic calcifications. Prevention requires dietary phosphate restriction, administration of intestinal phosphate binders, and supplementation with vitamin D analogs. The KDOQI pediatric bone guidelines recommend a target phosphorus level of 4 to 6 mg/dL for children aged 1 to 12 years and of 3.5 to 5.5 mg/dL for adolescents, whereas the KDOQI nutrition guidelines target a normal phosphorus level for age in view of the contribution of hyperphosphatemia to CVD (61). To minimize the risk of soft tissue (including vascular) calcification, KDOQI also recommends that phosphate binders and vitamin D analogs be adjusted in children to maintain a calcium–phosphate product less than 65 mg^2/dL^2 for children aged 1 to 12 years and less than 55 mg^2/dL^2 for adolescents (183). Of note, in the 2007 USRDS report, there was an association noted between a low calcium–phosphorus product and abnormal height: 76.9% of those with calcium × phosphorus less than 30.8 had heights more than 2 SDs below the mean for age (378).

Calcium-containing phosphate binders have replaced aluminum-based binders in pediatric patients because of the development of osteomalacia, anemia, and severe neurologic complications associated with aluminum exposure (394). However, when high

doses of calcium-containing phosphate binders are required to maintain the serum phosphate level within normal limits, hypercalcemia may be seen especially in the setting of adynamic bone disease. When calcium carbonate is used as a phosphate binder, there is significant absorption of the ingested calcium. In addition to adversely affecting bone, the role of an elevated serum calcium or an elevated calcium–phosphate product in the progression of vascular calcification has been demonstrated and very likely is a factor in the cardiovascular morbidity and mortality described in children with CKD/ESKD (395). Hypercalcemia may be averted by the use of a different form of calcium (e.g., calcium acetate), by decreasing the dialysate calcium content, and by adding or replacing the calcium-based binder with polymeric forms of phosphate binders such as sevelamer (396–399).

In a randomized crossover trial comparing sevelamer with calcium acetate in children, there was equivalent phosphorus control with the two agents without a change in the overall calcium level (400). However, there was a higher incidence of hypercalcemia during calcium acetate treatment. Metabolic acidosis was more frequent during treatment with sevelamer. Interestingly, the levels of total cholesterol and LDL cholesterol were both significantly lower during sevelamer therapy, as has been seen in adults (395,401). The use of sevelamer carbonate in children on dialysis has been associated with an increase in the serum bicarbonate level (402). Both forms of sevelamer have also been used to pretreat breast milk and reduce its phosphorus content (403).

In addition to the use of non–calcium-containing phosphate binders, decreased doses of vitamin D analogs or low-calcium dialysate help to control the serum calcium level. Traditionally, the dialysate calcium concentration in HD has been 3.0 to 2.5 mEq/L, producing a positive calcium balance during an HD treatment. The use of physiologic, low-calcium (2 to 2.5 mEq/L) dialysate will produce a negative calcium balance during the dialysis treatment (404). Similarly, low-calcium (with or without low magnesium) dialysate is available for CPD (405).

Blood Pressure Management

Hypertension is a significant problem in children with ESKD as it contributes to acute and long-term cardiovascular events. As such, the KDOQI guidelines on hypertension have recommended target BPs of less than the 90% for gender, age, and height for pediatric patients (406,407). Irrespective of the dialysis modality used (e.g., HD or CPD), children with ESKD develop hypertension due to varying degrees of intravascular volume expansion, elevated activity of the renin-angiotensin system, increased sympathetic tone, and elevated serum calcium levels with resultant increased peripheral vascular resistance (408–410). The relative contributions of the sympathetic nervous system, renin and volume overload can be determined in part by the BP response to ultrafiltration. BP should improve with ultrafiltration when hypertension is due to volume overload (409). One caveat is that the BP may increase during HD in those patients in whom BP is controlled with antihypertensive medications that are cleared by the dialysis treatment. In patients with primarily sympathetic overactivity or renin-mediated hypertension, the BP will not decrease and may actually increase with ultrafiltration during the dialysis treatment (408–410). Children with CKD/ESKD as a result of glomerular disease, chronic or recurrent pyelonephritis, or reflux nephropathy are most likely to have renin-mediated hypertension.

Minimization of intravascular volume expansion (overhydration) requires both a decrease in the intake of salt and water—the former is the most important area of focus as effective removal of fluid typically occurs on dialysis. The first approach to hypertension control in a HD patient should always be a reassessment of the patient's dry weight. Correction of overhydration will ameliorate hypertension for most patients (409). However, ultrafiltration of large volumes of fluid during HD may result in increased dialytic morbidity, including cramps, nausea, vomiting, and fatigue. These symptoms may be decreased with the use of "sodium modeling" techniques and NIVM of the hematocrit. The initial approach to the management of children with suspected renin-mediated hypertension in terms of antihypertensive agents is the use of ACEI and angiotensin II (A-II) receptor blockers, with close monitoring for the development of hyperkalemia. In some cases, nephrectomies are needed to achieve BP control. Apart from ACEIs/A-II blockers in those patients with renin-mediated hypertension, there is no single ideal or recommended type of antihypertensive medication for children receiving chronic dialysis (406,407,409). Use of a vasodilator will increase the incidence of intradialytic symptoms of intravascular depletion such as hypotension and cramps and therefore may limit ultrafiltration capacity.

Despite the availability of antihypertensive agents with multiple physiologic targets of action and an understanding of many of the factors contributing to the elevated BP values, BP remains poorly controlled in children treated with chronic dialysis, although recent reports with patients receiving frequent HD have provided evidence of a reversal of this trend (57,162,411,412). Information on children in the NAPRTCS dialysis database who had been treated with dialysis between 1992 and 2004 was retrospectively analyzed to determine the frequency of BPs greater than or equal to 95th percentile (162). Uncontrolled hypertension (95% or more) was present at baseline in 56.9% of patients, systolic hypertension alone in 7.3%, diastolic in 16.9%, and both systolic and diastolic hypertension in 33.2%. Hypertension at baseline was more common in those on HD (65.1%) when compared to those on CPD (52.9%). Hypertensive children were also younger, more likely to be African American, and to have an acquired kidney disease (162). The prevalence of uncontrolled hypertension decreased from 56.9% at baseline to 51% at 1 year and 48% at 2 years of follow-up (162). Similarly, an analysis of 71 children treated in 10 dialysis centers demonstrated hypertension (BP greater than or equal to the 95th percentile) in 59% of patients and prehypertension (BP between the 90th and 95th percentiles) in 15.5%. Only 25.3% of patients had a normal BP (412). Clearly, greater attention to this issue is mandatory if the incidence of CVD is to decrease. To that end, in the most recent NAPRTCS dialysis registry report, 63% of children on CPD and 68% of those on HD were on antihypertensive medication at the initiation of dialysis (6).

Educational Needs

School attendance is an important factor contributing to the development of children, in terms of providing the occasion to both interact with peers and to develop their academic skills. Therefore, the impact of school on a child's QOL can be significant. Therefore, the goal of any pediatric dialysis program is to ensure that children attend school regularly. There is generally greater school attendance in children treated with CPD (e.g., 78% full-time attendance in children aged 6 to 12 years on CPD vs. 53% in those on HD) (413). A greater proportion of children treated with in-center HD attend school part-time (28%) and may require supplementation of schoolwork with tutoring due to the timing of the HD sessions (413). Of note, some of the data on school attendance are confounded by the increasing trend among well children in some parts of the country to be home schooled. Young children may benefit from placement in an early intervention program as well.

Neurophysiologic and Cognitive Deficits

Early research into the neurocognitive development of children with CKD revealed substantial risk for delays in infants and young children (414). Polinsky et al. (415) evaluated 85 pediatric patients with ESKD; 72% of whom had been diagnosed with ESKD in the first year of life. They found the head circumference to be more than 2 SD below the mean in 62% of patients and that most patients demonstrated some form of developmental delay. Whereas similar findings were noted by Rotundo et al. (416) and McGraw and Haka-Ikse (417), attention to the prevention of malnutrition and elimination of aluminum-containing phosphate binders from the medical regimen led to more positive neurocognitive outcomes as documented by Warady et al. and Lederman et al. (418–421). Although an earlier initiation of RRT should lead to a lower prevalence of neurocognitive delay in at-risk children with CKD, only recently has a standardized approach been developed to evaluate neurocognitive functioning in children with CKD (414). In the most recent data pertaining to the long-term neurocognitive follow-up of children who initiated dialysis at <16 months of age as well as the patient's siblings, Johnson and Warady (422) found that younger age at transplant and fewer months on dialysis were associated with better neurocognitive outcomes.

Intradialytic seizures have been described in 7% to 16% of children receiving chronic HD treatment and may be more common in children with a prior history of seizures (423). Because some anticonvulsant medications are removed by HD, additional intradialytic dosing may be necessary to prevent seizures during the dialysis treatment. Anticonvulsant therapy has been prescribed to 14% and 8% of the HD and PD populations, respectively, in the NAPRTCS registry (6).

Finally, it is imperative that health care providers for children with ESKD be aware of the support services available to their patients so that referral to early intervention programs designed to improve specific developmental areas such as motor functions, language abilities, and social-emotional skills can occur when deemed necessary.

Health-Related Quality of Life

As most children are surviving with ESKD into adulthood, provision of optimal dialysis requires attention to the pediatric patient's psychologic status and HRQOL (424). Early research into the HRQOL of pediatric patients with ESKD, occurring over 20 years ago, demonstrated that although pediatric patients with ESKD have some developmental and psychosocial issues that are similar to those of children with other chronic illnesses, they also have challenges that are specifically related to ESKD (425–429). Obstacles common to most chronically ill children include physical changes related to illness, the need to take many medications and undergo medical treatment, and time away from school and peers, which can lead to perceived differences and isolation. Additional challenges include maintaining a restricted dietary and fluid regimen, chronic dependence on medical equipment to sustain life, very obvious physical changes associated with transplantation and the use of steroids and calcineurin inhibitors, and the knowledge that they will live their whole lives with the recurrent cycle of dialysis and transplantation. To better understand this important issue, pediatric studies have begun to use specific instruments to assess the pediatric ESKD patient's HRQOL. Most of these studies demonstrate that pediatric patients with ESKD and their parents report worse HRQOL than healthy peers, and patients receiving dialysis report a worse HRQOL than patients with a renal transplant (59,430). The standardized measures of HRQOL are no longer research tools alone, and their use is essential to identify areas for interventions as part of clinical care. Therefore, the CMS mandates that all dialysis patients in the United States have an HRQOL assessment at least annually (431–433), and there are pediatric-specific, validated HRQOL tools that can be utilized (59,431,434,435).

School attendance is an important part of childhood development. As noted earlier, ESKD, and especially in-center HD, imparts significant constraints and restrictions on this activity, which may have a significant negative impact on normal psychosocial development. The medical requirements for HD, which include receipt of HD in an HD center multiple times throughout the week during school hours, may isolate the child with ESKD from their healthy peers. Such interruptions in the normal daily life of a child are a likely primary cause for the relatively low self-esteem and low rates of independent living, close interpersonal relationships, and employment reported in adult survivors of pediatric ESKD (436,437). Studies of adolescent and young adult patients with ESKD have previously reported lower employment rates and greater concern about body image than a similarly aged cohort of diabetic patients. Therefore, a goal of any pediatric dialysis program is to ensure that children attend school regularly and have access to normal socialization. A cohort of adult Dutch patients (32 to 52 years) who had started RRT at <15 years was assessed for long-term QOL and social outcomes. As compared the general Dutch population, QOL in the areas of general health, vitality, and physical problems was most affected, particularly in those individuals currently being treated with dialysis. Interestingly, these patients scored better than the general population in the emotional and mental health domains. However, compared to the general population, they were less likely to work full-time (61.8% vs. 81.0% of the general population) and less likely to have completed high school. There was a nonsignificant difference in the frequency of being married or living with a partner (67.4% vs. 74.4% of the general population) (438). A similar survey was conducted in the United Kingdom to evaluate the impact of CKD from infancy in a group of young adults (439). Forty-one young adults who had CKD from infancy and required RRT in childhood were compared to the general population. At the time of survey, 12.5% of the patients were being treated with dialysis, and 85.5% had a functioning transplant. Half of the patients had significant comorbidities, including heart disease, neurologic involvement, or underlying syndromes. The employment rate was comparable to the general population, and educational attainment of the patients was similar to their parents (439). The patients did not differ from the general population in their perceptions of limitations due to physical health, emotional problems, vitality, emotional well-being, or pain. However, they did have reduced scores for physical and social functioning and the general perception of their health. Lower scores were associated with the presence of comorbidities, being on dialysis at the time of the survey, and short stature (439).

◆ LONG-TERM OUTCOMES AND PATIENT MORTALITY

An analysis of children in the NAPRTCS dialysis registry from 1992 to 2006 showed an overall patient survival of 95%, 90%, and 86% at 12, 24, and 36 months, respectively, with the lowest survival estimates for those younger than 12 months at the initiation of dialysis: 83%, 74%, and 66% at 12, 24, and 36 months, respectively (440). The most frequent cause of death was infection, followed by cardiopulmonary events. The most recent report describes an overall improvement in survival by era with the overall 24-month survival improving from 92.9% for those initiating dialysis in 1992 to 1994 to 96.9% for those who started dialysis in 2007 to 2010 (440). Similar improvements in 12-month survival by era are described in the most recent USRDS report (**Figure 37.5**) (1). In 2007 to 2011, the 1-year-adjusted all-cause mortality was 35 per 1,000 patient-years, a decrease of 22.2% from 2002 to 2006. The decrease was shown across age-groups and treatment modalities. However, the mortality of the youngest patients (85 per 1,000 patient-years) and those treated with HD remains highest (57 per 1,000 patient-years) (1). It is most striking to compare the expecting remaining lifetime in years for various populations of children aged less than 15 years: 23.7 years for patients on dialysis, 63.0 years for those with a functioning transplant, and 72.3 years in the general population (1). This remarkable data emphasizes the need to pursue transplantation in virtually every pediatric patient who receives chronic dialysis therapy.

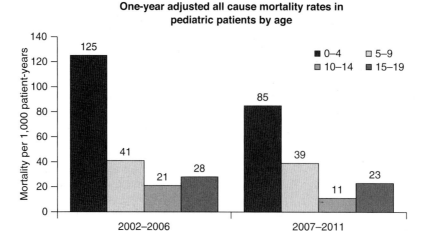

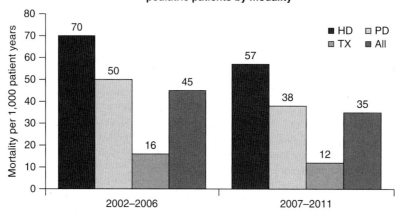

FIGURE 37.5 One-year-adjusted all-cause mortality rates (per 1,000 patient-years) in pediatric dialysis patients by age (*upper panel*) and treatment modality (*lower panel*); comparison of patients who initiated dialysis in 2002 to 2006 versus 2007 to 2011. HD, hemodialysis; PD, peritoneal dialysis; TX, transplant. (Charts from United States Renal Data System. *USRDS 2014 Annual Data Report: End-Stage Renal Disease in the United States*. Bethesda, MD: National Institutes of Health, National Institute of Diabetes and Digestive and Kidney Diseases, 2014.)

REFERENCES

1. United States Renal Data System. *USRDS 2014 Annual Data Report: Epidemiology of Kidney Disease in the United States*. Bethesda, MD: National Institutes of Health, National Institute of Diabetes and Digestive and Kidney Diseases, 2014.
2. Harambat J, van Stralen KJ, Kim JJ, et al. Epidemiology of chronic kidney disease in children. *Pediatr Nephrol* 2012;27(3):363–373.
3. Hoffman JI. Congenital heart disease: incidence and inheritance. *Pediatr Clin North Am* 1990;37(1):25–43.
4. Dores GM, Devesa SS, Curtis RE, et al. Acute leukemia incidence and patient survival among children and adults in the United States, 2001-2007. *Blood* 2012;119(1):34–43.
5. Alexander SR, Honda M. Continuous peritoneal dialysis for children: a decade of worldwide growth and development. *Kidney Int* 1993;43(40):S65–S74.
6. North American Pediatric Renal Trials and Collaborative Studies. *Annual Dialysis Report*. Rockville, MD: EMMES Corp, 2011.
7. Wiggelinkhuizen J. Peritoneal dialysis in children. *S Afr Med J* 1971; 45(38):1047–1054.
8. Putiloff P. Materials for the study of the laws of growth of the human body in relation to the surface areas of different systems: the trial on Russian subjects of planographic anatomy as a means for exact anthropometry; one of the problems of anthropology. Paper presented at: Meeting of the Siberian Branch of the Russian Geographic Society, 1884.
9. Wegner G. Chirurgische Bemerkungen umlautuber die peritoneal Humlautohle, mit besonder Berucksichigung der Ovariotomie [in German]. *Arch Klin Chir* 1887;20:51.
10. Esperanca M, Collins D. Peritoneal dialysis efficiency in relation to body weight. *J Pediatr Surg* 1966;1:162–69.
11. Gruskin A, Lerner G, Fleischmann L. Developmental aspects of peritoneal dialysis kinetics. In: Fine RN, ed. *Chronic Ambulatory Peritoneal Dialysis (CAPD) and Chronic Cycling Peritoneal Dialysis (CCPD) in Children*. Norwell, MA: Martinus Nijhoff, 1987:33–45.
12. Kohaut EC. The effect of dialysate volume on ultrafiltration in young patients treated with CAPD. *Int J Pediatr Nephrol* 1986;7(1):13–16.
13. Schaefer F, Haraldsson B, Haas S, et al. Estimation of peritoneal mass transport by three-pore model in children. *Kidney Int* 1998;54(4):1372–1379.
14. Fischbach M, Haraldsson B. Dynamic changes of the total pore area available for peritoneal exchange in children. *J Am Soc Nephrol* 2001;12(7): 1524–1529.
15. Rippe B, Stelin G. Simulations of peritoneal solute transport during CAPD. Application of two-pore formalism. *Kidney Int* 1989;35(5):1234–1244.
16. Nolph K. Peritoneal anatomy and transport physiology. In: Drukker W, Parsons FM, Maher JF, eds. *Replacement of Renal Function by Dialysis*. 2nd ed. Dordrecht, The Netherlands: Martinus Nijhoff, 1983:440–456.

17. Mactier RA, Khanna R, Twardowski ZJ, et al. Role of peritoneal cavity lymphatic absorption in peritoneal dialysis. *Kidney Int* 1987;32(2):165–172.

18. Fischbach M, Warady BA. Peritoneal dialysis prescription in children: bedside principles for optimal practice. *Pediatr Nephrol* 2009;24(9):1633–1642.

19. Haraldsson B. Assessing the peritoneal dialysis capacities of individual patients. *Kidney Int* 1995;47(4):1187–1198.

20. Morgenstern B, Pyle WK, Gruskin A, et al. Transport characteristics of the pediatric peritoneal membrane. *Kidney Int* 1984;24:259.

21. Geary DF, Harvey EA, Balfe JW. Mass transfer area coefficients in children. *Perit Dial Int* 1994;14(1):30–33.

22. Warady BA, Alexander SR, Hossli S, et al. Peritoneal membrane transport function in children receiving long-term dialysis. *J Am Soc Nephrol* 1996;7(11):2385–2391.

23. Bouts AH, Davin JC, Groothoff JW, et al. Standard peritoneal permeability analysis in children. *J Am Soc Nephrol* 2000;11(5):943–950.

24. Fischbach M, Zaloszyc A, Schaefer B, et al. Optimizing peritoneal dialysis prescription for volume control: the importance of varying dwell time and dwell volume. *Pediatr Nephrol* 2014;29(8):1321–1327.

25. Morgenstern BZ. Equilibration testing: close, but not quite right. *Pediatr Nephrol* 1993;7(3):290–291.

26. Kohaut EC, Waldo FB, Benfield MR. The effect of changes in dialysate volume on glucose and urea equilibration. *Perit Dial Int* 1994;14(3):236–239.

27. de Boer AW, van Schaijk TC, Willems HL, et al. The necessity of adjusting dialysate volume to body surface area in pediatric peritoneal equilibration tests. *Perit Dial Int* 1997;17(2):199–202.

28. Rippe B, Stelin G, Haraldsson B. Computer simulations of peritoneal fluid transport in CAPD. *Kidney Int* 1991;40(2):315–325.

29. Rippe B. A three-pore model of peritoneal transport. *Perit Dial Int* 1993;(13 Suppl 2):S35–S38.

30. La Milia V, Pozzoni P, Virga G, et al. Peritoneal transport assessment by peritoneal equilibration test with 3.86% glucose: a long-term prospective evaluation. *Kidney Int* 2006;69(5):927–933.

31. Pyle W. *Mass Transfer in Peritoneal Dialysis*. Austin, TX: University of Texas, 1987.

32. Kohaut E, Alexander S. Ultrafiltration in the young patient on CAPD. In: Moncrief J, Popovich R, eds. *CAPD Update*. New York, NY: Masson, 1981:221–226.

33. Balfe J, Hanning R, Vigneux A. A comparison of peritoneal water and solute movement in younger and older children on CAPD. In: Fine R, Schaefer F, Mehls O, eds. *CAPD in Children*. New York, NY: Springer, 1985:14–19.

34. Schaefer F, Fischbach M, Heckert K. Hydrostatic intraperitoneal pressure in children on peritoneal dialysis. *Perit Dial Int* 1996;16(Suppl 2):S79.

35. Rippe B. Is intraperitoneal pressure important? *Perit Dial Int* 2006;26(3):317–319, discussion 411.

36. Mactier RA, Khanna R, Moore H, et al. Kinetics of peritoneal dialysis in children: role of lymphatics. *Kidney Int* 1988;34(1):82–88.

37. Schröder CH, Reddingius RE, van Dreumel JA, et al. Transcapillary ultrafiltration and lymphatic absorption during childhood continuous ambulatory peritoneal dialysis. *Nephrol Dial Transplant* 1991;6(8):571–573.

38. Chelamcharla M, Leypoldt JK, Cheung AK. Dialyzer membranes as determinants of the adequacy of dialysis. *Semin Nephrol* 2005;25(2):81–89.

39. Leypoldt JK, Cheung AK. Removal of high-molecular-weight solutes during high-efficiency and high-flux haemodialysis. *Nephrol Dial Transplant* 1996;11(2):329–335.

40. Schoumacher R, Chevalier RL, Gomez RA, et al. Enhanced clearance of vancomycin by hemodialysis in a child. *Pediatr Nephrol* 1989;3(1):83–85.

41. Hakim RM, Fearon DT, Lazarus JM. Biocompatibility of dialysis membranes: effects of chronic complement activation. *Kidney Int* 1984;26(2):194–200.

42. Zaoui PM, Stone WJ, Hakim RM. Effects of dialysis membranes on β-2-microglobulin production and cellular expression. *Kidney Int* 1990;38(5):962–968.

43. Martinez-Miguel P, de Sequera P, Albalate M, et al. Evaluation of a polynephron dialysis membrane considering new aspects of biocompatibility. *Int J Artif Organs* 2015;38(1):45–53.

44. Memoli B. Cytokine production in haemodialysis. *Blood Purif* 1999;17(2–3):149–158.

45. Memoli B, Marzano L, Bisesti V, et al. Hemodialysis-related lymphomononuclear release of interleukin-12 in patients with end-stage renal disease. *J Am Soc Nephrol* 1999;10(10):2171–2176.

46. Sawires HK, Mohamed WA, Schaalan MF. High-flux and low-flux dialysis membranes and levels of intercellular adhesion molecule-1 and vascular cell adhesion molecule-1 in children with chronic kidney failure. *Iran J Kidney Dis* 2012;6(5):366–372.

47. Bereket G, Fine RN. Pediatric renal transplantation. *Pediatr Clin North Am* 1995;42(6):1603–1628.

48. Fine RN. Renal transplantation for children—the only realistic choice. *Kidney Int Suppl* 1985;17:S15–S17.

49. Goldstein SL. Advances in renal replacement therapy as a bridge to renal transplantation. *Pediatr Transplant* 2007;11(5):463–470.

50. Smith JM, Stablein DM, Munoz R, et al. Contributions of the Transplant Registry: the 2006 annual report of the North American Pediatric Renal Trials and Collaborative Studies (NAPRTCS). *Pediatr Transplant* 2007;11(4):366–373.

51. Baum M, Powell D, Calvin S, et al. Continuous ambulatory peritoneal dialysis in children: comparison with hemodialysis. *N Engl J Med* 1982;307(25):1537–1542.

52. Quinn RR, Hux JE, Oliver MJ, et al. Selection bias explains apparent differential mortality between dialysis modalities. *J Am Soc Nephrol* 2011;22(8):1534–1542.

53. Warady BA, Neu AM, Schaefer F. Optimal care of the infant, child, and adolescent on dialysis: 2014 update. *Am J Kidney Dis* 2014;64(1):128–142.

54. Watson AR, Hayes WN, Vondrak K, et al. Factors influencing choice of renal replacement therapy in European paediatric nephrology units. *Pediatr Nephrol* 2013;28(12):2361–2368.

55. Geary DF, Piva E, Tyrrell J, et al. Home nocturnal hemodialysis in children. *J Pediatr* 2005;147(3):383–387.

56. Fischbach M, Terzic J, Menouer S, et al. Intensified and daily hemodialysis in children might improve statural growth. *Pediatr Nephrol* 2006;21(11):1746–1752.

57. Warady B, Fischbach M, Geary D, et al. Frequent hemodialysis in children. *Adv Chronic Kidney Dis* 2007;14:297–303.

58. Warady BA, Alexander SR, Watkins S, et al. Optimal care of the pediatric end-stage renal disease patient on dialysis. *Am J Kidney Dis* 1999;33(3):567–583.

59. Goldstein SL, Graham N, Burwinkle T, et al. Health-related quality of life in pediatric patients with ESRD. *Pediatr Nephrol* 2006;21(6):846–850.

60. Park KS, Hwang YJ, Cho MH, et al. Quality of life in children with end-stage renal disease based on a PedsQL ESRD module. *Pediatr Nephrol* 2012;27(12):2293–2300.

61. Kidney Disease Outcomes: Quality Initiative Work Group. KDOQI clinical practice guideline for nutrition in children with CKD. *Am J Kidney Dis* 2009;53(Suppl 2):S1.

62. Palmer RA, Quinton WE, Gray JE. Prolonged peritoneal dialysis for chronic renal failure. *Lancet* 1964;1(7335):700–702.

63. Palmer RA, Newell JE, Gray EJ, et al. Treatment of chronic renal failure by prolonged peritoneal dialysis. *N Engl J Med* 1966;274(5):248–254.

64. Tenckhoff H, Schechter H. A bacteriologically safe peritoneal access device. *Trans Am Soc Artif Intern Organs* 1968;14:181–187.

65. Boen ST, Mion CM, Curtis FK, et al. Periodic peritoneal dialysis using the repeated puncture technique and an automatic cycling machine. *Trans Am Soc Artif Intern Organs* 1964,10.409–414.

66. Tenckhoff H, Meston B, Shilipetar G. A simplified automatic peritoneal dialysis system. *Trans Am Soc Artif Intern Organs* 1972;18:436–440.

67. Counts S, Hickman R, Garbaccio A, et al. Chronic home peritoneal dialysis in children. *Trans Am Soc Artif Intern Organs* 1973;19:157–163.

68. Hickman O. Nine years experience with chronic peritoneal dialysis in childhood. *Dial Transplant* 1978;7:803.

69. Brouhard BH, Berger M, Cunningham RJ, et al. Home peritoneal dialysis in children. *Trans Am Soc Artif Intern Organs* 1979;25:90–94.

70. Baluarte HJ, Grossman MS, Polinsky MD, et al. Experience with intermittent home peritoneal dialysis (IHPD) in children. *Pediatr Res* 1980;(14):994.

71. Lorentz WB Jr, Hamilton RW, Disher B, et al. Home peritoneal dialysis during infancy. *Clin Nephrol* 1981;15(4):194–197.

72. Potter D, McDaid T, Ramirez J. Peritoneal dialysis in children. In: Adkins R, Thomson N, Farrell P, eds. *Peritoneal Dialysis*. New York, NY: Churchill Livingstone, 1981:356–361.

73. Popovich R, Moncrief J, Dechered J, et al. The definition of a novel portable/wearable equilibrium dialysis technique. *Trans Am Soc Artif Intern Organs* 1976;5:64.

74. Balfe J, Irwin M. Continuous ambulatory peritoneal dialysis in children. In: Legrain M, ed. *Continuous Ambulatory Peritoneal Dialysis*. Amsterdam, The Netherlands: Excerpta Medica, 1980:131–136.

75. Oreopoulos D, Katirtzoglou A, Arbus G, et al. Dialysis and transplantation in young children. *BMJ* 1979;1(6178):1628–1629.

76. Kohaut EC. Continuous ambulatory peritoneal dialysis: a preliminary pediatric experience. *Am J Dis Child* 1981;135(3):270–271.

77. Eastham E, Kirplani H, Francis D, et al. Pediatric continuous ambulatory peritoneal dialysis. *Arch Dis Child* 1982;57:677–680.

78. Guillot M, Clermont MJ, Gagnadoux MF, et al. Nineteen months' experience with continuous ambulatory peritoneal dialysis (CAPD) in children: main clinical and biological results. In: Gahl G, Kessel M, Nolph KD, eds. *Advances in Peritoneal Dialysis*. Amsterdam, The Netherlands: Excerpta Medica, 1981:203–207.

79. Price C, Suki W. Newer modifications of peritoneal dialysis: options in the treatment of patients with renal failure. *Am J Nephrol* 1980;1(2):97–104.

80. von Lilien T, Salusky IB, Boechat I, et al. Five years' experience with continuous ambulatory or continuous cycling peritoneal dialysis in children. *J Pediatr* 1987;111:513–518.

81. Fine R, Ho M. The role of APD in the management of pediatric patients: a report of the North American Pediatric Renal Transplant Cooperative Study. *Semin Dial* 2002;15:427–429.

82. Verrina E, Edefonti A, Gianoglio B, et al. A multicenter experience on patient and technique survival in children on chronic dialysis. *Pediatr Nephrol* 2004;19(1):82–90.

83. Twardowski Z, Nolph K, Khanna R, et al. Peritoneal equilibration test. *Perit Dial Bull* 1987;7:378–383.

84. Verrina E, Cappelli V, Perfumo F. Selection of modalities, prescription, and technical issues in children on peritoneal dialysis. *Pediatr Nephrol* 2009;24(8):1453–1464.

85. Warady B, Andrews W. Peritoneal dialysis access. In: Geary D, Schaefer F, eds. *Comprehensive Pediatric Nephrology*. Philadelphia, PA: Mosby Elsevier, 2008:823–834.

86. Haggerty S, Roth S, Walsh D, et al. Guidelines for laparoscopic peritoneal dialysis access surgery. *Surg Endosc* 2014;28(11):3016–3045.

87. Hagen S, Lafranca J, Steyerberg E, et al. Laparoscopic versus open peritoneal dialysis catheter insertion: a meta-analysis. *PLoS One* 2013;8(2): e56351.

88. Xie H, Zhang W, Cheng J, et al. Laparoscopic versus open catheter placement in peritoneal dialysis patients: a systematic review and meta-analysis. *BMC Nephrol* 2012;13:69.

89. Strippoli GF, Tong A, Johnson D, et al. Catheter type, placement and insertion techniques for preventing peritonitis in peritoneal dialysis patients. *Cochrane Database Syst Rev* 2004;(4):CD004680.

90. Gokal R, Alexander S, Ash S, et al. Peritoneal catheters and exit-site practices toward optimum peritoneal access: 1998 update. (Official report from the International Society for Peritoneal Dialysis). *Perit Dial Int* 1998;18(1):11–33.

91. Washburn KK, Currier H, Salter KJ, et al. Surgical technique for peritoneal dialysis catheter placement in the pediatric patient: a North American survey. *Adv Perit Dial* 2004;20:218–221.

92. Daschner M, Gfrorer S, Zachariou Z, et al. Laparoscopic Tenckhoff catheter implantation in children. *Perit Dial Int* 2002;22(1):22–26.

93. Flanigan M, Gokal R. Peritoneal catheters and exit-site practices toward optimum peritoneal access: a review of current developments. *Perit Dial Int* 2005;25(2):132–139.

94. Katyal A, Mahale A, Khanna R. Antibiotic prophylaxis before peritoneal dialysis catheter insertion. *Adv Perit Dial* 2002;18:112–115.

95. Warady BA, Bakkaloglu S, Newland J, et al. Consensus guidelines for the prevention and treatment of catheter-related infections and peritonitis in pediatric patients receiving peritoneal dialysis: 2012 update. *Perit Dial Int* 2012;32(Suppl 2):S32–S86.

96. Crabtree JH. Development of surgical guidelines for laparoscopic peritoneal dialysis access: down a long and winding road. *Perit Dial Int* 2015;35(3):241–244.

97. Sieniawska M, Roszkowska-Blaim M, Warchol S. Preliminary results with the swan neck presternal catheter for CAPD in children. *Adv Perit Dial* 1993;9:321–324.

98. Twardowski ZJ, Prowant BF, Pickett B, et al. Four-year experience with swan neck presternal peritoneal dialysis catheter. *Am J Kidney Dis* 1996;27(1):99–105.

99. Chadha V, Jones LL, Ramirez ZD, et al. Chest wall peritoneal dialysis catheter placement in infants with a colostomy. *Adv Perit Dial* 2000;16:318–320.

100. Warchol S, Roszkowska-Blaim M, Sieniawska M. Swan neck presternal peritoneal dialysis catheter: five-year experience in children. *Perit Dial Int* 1998;18(2):183–187.

101. Warchol S, Ziolkowska H, Roszkowska-Blaim M. Exit-site infection in children on peritoneal dialysis: comparison of two types of peritoneal catheters. *Perit Dial Int* 2003;23(2):169–173.

102. Yerram P, Gill A, Prowant B, et al. A 9-year survival analysis of the presternal Missouri swan-neck catheter. *Adv Perit Dial* 2007;23:90–93.

103. Neu AM, Ho PL, McDonald RA, et al. Chronic dialysis in children and adolescents. The 2001 NAPRTCS annual report. *Pediatr Nephrol* 2002;17(8):656–663.

104. Lerner GR, Warady BA, Sullivan EK, et al. Chronic dialysis in children and adolescents. The 1996 annual report of the North American Pediatric Renal Transplant Cooperative Study. *Pediatr Nephrol* 1999;13(5):404–417.

105. Phan J, Stanford S, Zaritsky JJ, et al. Risk factors for morbidity and mortality in pediatric patients with peritoneal dialysis catheters. *J Pediatr Surg* 2013;48(1):197–202.

106. Neu A, Kohaut E, Warady B. Current approach to peritoneal access in North American children: a report of the Pediatric Peritoneal Dialysis Study Consortium. *Adv Perit Dial* 1995;11:289–292.

107. Reissman P, Lyass S, Shiloni E, et al. Placement of a peritoneal dialysis catheter with routine omentectomy: does it prevent obstruction of the catheter? *Eur J Surg* 1998;164(9):703–707.

108. Lewis M, Webb N, Smith T, et al. Routine omentectomy is not required in children undergoing chronic peritoneal dialysis. *Adv Perit Dial* 1995;11:293–295.

109. Warady B, Sullivan E, Alexander S. Lessons from the peritoneal dialysis patient database: a report of the North American Pediatric Renal Transplant Cooperative Study. *Kidney Int* 1996;53:S68–S71.

110. Sliman GA, Klee KM, Gall-Holden B, et al. Peritoneal equilibration test curves and adequacy of dialysis in children on automated peritoneal dialysis. *Am J Kidney Dis* 1994;24(5):813–818.

111. Schaefer F, Langenbeck D, Heckert K, et al. Evaluation of peritoneal solute transfer by the peritoneal equilibration test in children. *Adv Perit Dial* 1992;8:410–415.

112. Warady BA, Jennings J. The short PET in pediatrics. *Perit Dial Int* 2007;27(4):441–445.

113. Cano F, Sanchez L, Rebori A, et al. The short peritoneal equilibration test in pediatric peritoneal dialysis. *Pediatr Nephrol* 2010;25(10):2159–2164.

114. Warady B. The peritoneal equilibration test (PET) in pediatrics. *Contemp Dial Nephrol* 1994:21–41.

115. Blake P, Burkart JM, Churchill DN, et al. Recommended clinical practices for maximizing peritoneal dialysis clearances. *Perit Dial Int* 1996;16(5):448–456.

116. National Kidney Foundation. K/DOQI clinical practice guidelines and clinical practice recommendations for 2006 updates. Hemodialysis adequacy, peritoneal dialysis adequacy and vascular access. *Am J Kidney Dis* 2006;48:S1–S322.

117. Rocco MV, Jordan JR, Burkart JM. Changes in peritoneal transport during the first month of peritoneal dialysis. *Perit Dial Int* 1995;15(1): 12–17.

118. Rocco M. Body surface area limitations in achieving adequate therapy in peritoneal dialysis patients. *Perit Dial Int* 1996;16:617–622.

119. Johnson D, Mudge D, Blizzard S, et al. A comparison of peritoneal equilibration tests performed 1 and 4 weeks after PD commencement. *Perit Dial Int* 2004;24(5):460–465.

120. Borzych-Duzalka D, Bilginer Y, Ha IS, et al. Management of anemia in children receiving chronic peritoneal dialysis. *J Am Soc Nephrol* 2013;24(4):665–676.

121. Schaefer F, Klaus G, Mehls O. Peritoneal transport properties and dialysis dose affect growth and nutritional status in children on chronic peritoneal dialysis. Mid-European Pediatric Peritoneal Dialysis Study Group. *J Am Soc Nephrol* 1999;10(8):1786–1792.

122. Fried L. Higher membrane permeability predicts poorer patient survival. *Perit Dial Int* 1997;17(4):387–389.

123. Churchill DN, Thorpe KE, Nolph KD, et al. Increased peritoneal membrane transport is associated with decreased patient and technique survival for continuous peritoneal dialysis patients. The Canada-USA (CANUSA) Peritoneal Dialysis Study Group. *J Am Soc Nephrol* 1998;9(7):1285–1292.

124. Rönnholm KA, Holmberg C. Peritoneal dialysis in infants. *Pediatr Nephrol* 2006;21(6):751–756.

125. White CT, Gowrishankar M, Feber J, et al. Clinical practice guidelines for pediatric peritoneal dialysis. *Pediatr Nephrol* 2006;21(8):1059–1066.

126. Fischbach M, Stefanidis CJ, Watson AR. Guidelines by an ad hoc European committee on adequacy of the paediatric peritoneal dialysis prescription. *Nephrol Dial Transplant* 2002;17(3):380–385.

127. Burkart JM, Schreiber M, Korbet SM, et al. Solute clearance approach to adequacy of peritoneal dialysis. *Perit Dial Int* 1996;16(5):457–470.

128. Dufek S, Holtta T, Fischbach M, et al. Pleuro-peritoneal or pericardio-peritoneal leak in children on chronic peritoneal dialysis—a survey from the European Paediatric Dialysis Working Group. *Pediatr Nephrol* 2015;30(11):2021–2027.

129. Fischbach M, Terzic J, Menouer S, et al. Impact of fill volume changes on peritoneal dialysis tolerance and effectiveness in children. *Adv Perit Dial* 2000;16:321–323.

130. Rusthoven E, van der Vlugt ME, van Lingen-van Bueren LJ, et al. Evaluation of intraperitoneal pressure and the effect of different osmotic agents on intraperitoneal pressure in children. *Perit Dial Int* 2005;25(4):352–356.

131. Fischbach M, Terzic J, Becmeur F, et al. Relationship between intraperitoneal hydrostatic pressure and dialysate volume in children on PD. *Adv Perit Dial* 1996;12:330–334.

132. Fischbach M, Terzic J, Laugel V, et al. Measurement of hydrostatic intraperitoneal pressure: a useful tool for the improvement of dialysis dose prescription. *Pediatr Nephrol* 2003;18(10):976–980.

133. Fischbach M, Terzic J, Provot E, et al. Intraperitoneal pressure in children: fill-volume related and impacted by body mass index. *Perit Dial Int* 2003;23(4):391–394.

134. Warady BA, Watkins SL, Fivush BA, et al. Validation of PD Adequest 2.0 for pediatric dialysis patients. *Pediatr Nephrol* 2001;16(3):205–211.

135. Verrina E, Amici G, Perfumo F, et al. The use of the PD Adequest mathematical model in pediatric patients on chronic peritoneal dialysis. *Perit Dial Int* 1998;18:322–328.

136. Fischbach M, Terzic J, Menouer S, et al. Effects of automated peritoneal dialysis on residual daily urinary volume in children. *Adv Perit Dial* 2001;17:269–273.

137. Feber J, Scharer K, Schaefer F, et al. Residual renal function in children on haemodialysis and peritoneal dialysis therapy. *Pediatr Nephrol* 1994;8(5):579–583.

138. Canada-USA (CANUSA) Peritoneal Dialysis Study Group. Adequacy of dialysis and nutrition in continuous peritoneal dialysis: association with clinical outcomes. *J Am Soc Nephrol* 1996;7(2):198–207.

139. Lutes R, Perlmutter J, Holley JL, et al. Loss of residual renal function in patients on peritoneal dialysis. *Adv Perit Dial* 1993;9:165–168.

140. Li PK, Chow KM, Wong TY, et al. Effects of an angiotensin-converting enzyme inhibitor on residual renal function in patients receiving peritoneal dialysis. A randomized, controlled study. *Ann Intern Med* 2003;139(2):105–112.

141. Suzuki H, Kanno Y, Sugahara S, et al. Effects of an angiotensin II receptor blocker, valsartan, on residual renal function in patients on CAPD. *Am J Kidney Dis* 2004;43(6):1056–1064.

142. Phakdeekitcharoen B, Leelasa-nguan P. Effects of an ACE inhibitor or angiotensin receptor blocker on potassium in CAPD patients. *Am J Kidney Dis* 2004;44(4):738–746.

143. Ha IS, Yap HK, Munarriz RL, et al. Risk factors for loss of residual renal function in children treated with chronic peritoneal dialysis. *Kidney Int* 2015;88(3):605–613.

144. Paniagua R, Amato D, Vonesh E, et al. Effects of increased peritoneal clearances on mortality rates in peritoneal dialysis: ADEMEX, a prospective, randomized, controlled trial. *J Am Soc Nephrol* 2002;13(5):1307–1320.

145. Lo WK, Lui SL, Chan TM, et al. Minimal and optimal peritoneal Kt/V targets: results of an anuric peritoneal dialysis patient's survival analysis. *Kidney Int* 2005;67(5):2032–2038.

146. Lo W, Bargman J, Burkart J, et al. Guideline on targets for solute and fluid removal in adult patients on chronic peritoneal dialysis. *Perit Dial Int* 2006;26(5):520–522.

147. Holtta T, Ronnholm K, Jalanko H, et al. Clinical outcome of pediatric patients on peritoneal dialysis under adequacy control. *Pediatr Nephrol* 2000;14(10–11):889–897.

148. McCauley L, Champoux S, Parvex P, et al. Enhanced growth in children on peritoneal dialysis (PD): dialysis dose, nutrition, and metabolic control. *Perit Dial Int* 2000;20(Suppl 1):S89.

149. Champoux S. Enhanced growth in children on peritoneal dialysis (PD): dialysis dose, nutrition, and metabolic control. *Perit Dial Int* 2001;21(Suppl 1):S86.

150. Chadha V, Blowey DL, Warady BA. Is growth a valid outcome measure of dialysis clearance in children undergoing peritoneal dialysis? *Perit Dial Int* 2001;21(Suppl 3):S179–S184.

151. van der Voort JH, Harvey EA, Braj B, et al. Can the DOQI guidelines be met by peritoneal dialysis alone in pediatric patients? Dialysis Outcomes Quality Initiative. *Pediatr Nephrol* 2000;14(8–9):717–719.

152. Centers for Medicare & Medicaid Services. *Annual Report, End Stage Renal Disease Clinical Performance Measures Project.* Baltimore, MD: U.S. Department of Health and Human Services, Centers for Medicare & Medicaid Services, Office of Clinical Standards & Quality, 2005.

153. Wühl E, Fusch C, Schärer K, et al. Assessment of total body water in paediatric patients on dialysis. *Nephrol Dial Transplant* 1996;11(1):75–80.

154. Morgenstern B, Nair K, Lerner G, et al. Impact of total body water errors on Kt/V estimates in children on peritoneal dialysis. *Adv Perit Dial* 2001;17:260–263.

155. Mendley SR, Majkowski NL, Schoeller DA. Validation of estimates of total body water in pediatric dialysis patients by deuterium dilution. *Kidney Int* 2005;67(5):2056–2062.

156. Mellits D, Cheek D. The assessment of body water and fatness from infancy to adulthood. *Monogr Soc Res Child Dev* 1970;35:12–26.

157. Morgenstern BZ, Mahoney DW, Warady BA. Estimating total body water in children on the basis of height and weight: a reevaluation of the formulas of Mellits and Cheek. *J Am Soc Nephrol* 2002;13(7):1884–1888.

158. Morgenstern BZ, Wuhl E, Nair KS, et al. Anthropometric prediction of total body water in children who are on pediatric peritoneal dialysis. *J Am Soc Nephrol* 2006;17(1):285–293.

159. Gehan EA, George SL. Estimation of human body surface area from height and weight. *Cancer Chemother Rep* 1970;54(4):225–235.

160. Heimburger O, Stenvinkel P, Berglund L, et al. Increased plasma lipoprotein (a) in continuous ambulatory peritoneal dialysis is related to peritoneal transport of proteins and glucose. *Nephron* 1996;72(2):135–144.

161. Mitsnefes MM, Daniels SR, Schwartz SM, et al. Severe left ventricular hypertrophy in pediatric dialysis: prevalence and predictors. *Pediatr Nephrol* 2000;14(10–11):898–902.

162. Mitsnefes M, Stablein D. Hypertension in pediatric patients on long-term dialysis: a report of the North American Pediatric Renal Transplant Cooperative Study (NAPRTCS). *Am J Kidney Dis* 2005;45(2):309–315.

163. Fusshoeller A, Plail M, Grabensee B, et al. Biocompatibility pattern of a bicarbonate/lactate-buffered peritoneal dialysis fluid in APD: a prospective, randomized study. *Nephrol Dial Transplant* 2004;19(8):2101–2106.

164. Schmitt CP, von Heyl D, Rieger S, et al. Reduced systemic advanced glycation end products in children receiving peritoneal dialysis with low glucose degradation product content. *Nephrol Dial Transplant* 2007;22(7):2038–2044.

165. McIntyre CW. Update on peritoneal dialysis solutions. *Kidney Int* 2007;71(6):486–490.

166. Canepa A, Perfumo F, Carrea A, et al. Nutritional status in children receiving chronic peritoneal dialysis. *Perit Dial Int* 1996;16(Suppl 1):S526–S531.

167. Salusky IB, Fine RN, Nelson P, et al. Nutritional status of children undergoing continuous ambulatory peritoneal dialysis. *Am J Clin Nutr* 1983;38(4):599–611.

168. Scolnik D, Balfe JW. Initial hypoalbuminemia and hyperlipidemia persist during chronic peritoneal dialysis in children. *Perit Dial Int* 1993;13(2):136–139.

169. Ruley EJ, Bock GH, Kerzner B, et al. Feeding disorders and gastro-esophageal reflux in infants with chronic renal failure. *Pediatr Nephrol* 1989;3(4):424–429.

170. National Research Council. *Recommended Dietary Allowances*. 10th ed. Washington, DC: National Academy Press, 1989:1–284.

171. Balfe J, Vigneaux A, Williamson J, et al. The use of CAPD in the treatment of children with end-stage renal disease. *Perit Dial Bull* 1981;1:35–38.

172. Edefonti A, Paglialonga F, Picca M, et al. A prospective multicentre study of the nutritional status in children on chronic peritoneal dialysis. *Nephrol Dial Transplant* 2006;21(7):1946–1951.

173. Drachman R, Niaudet P, Dartois AM, et al. Protein losses during peritoneal dialysis in children. In: Fine R, Schaerer K, Mehls O, et al, eds. *CAPD in Children*. New York, NY: Springer, 1985:78–83.

174. Kopanati S, Baum M, Quan A. Peritoneal protein losses in children with steroid-resistant nephrotic syndrome on continuous-cycler peritoneal dialysis. *Pediatr Nephrol* 2006;21(7):1013–1019.

175. Quan A, Baum M. Protein losses in children on continuous cycler peritoneal dialysis. *Pediatr Nephrol* 1996;10(6):728–731.

176. Wassner SJ, Abitbol C, Alexander S, et al. Nutritional requirements for infants with renal failure. *Am J Kidney Dis* 1986;7(4):300–305.

177. London GM, Guérin AP, Marchais SJ, et al. Arterial media calcification in end-stage renal disease: impact on all-cause and cardiovascular mortality. *Nephrol Dial Transplant* 2003;18(9):1731–1740.

178. Siirtola A, Virtanen SM, Ala-Houhala M, et al. Diet does not explain the high prevalence of dyslipidaemia in paediatric renal transplant recipients. *Pediatr Nephrol* 2008;23(2):297–305.

179. Cano F, Azocar M, Delucchi M, et al. Nitrogen balance studies and Kt/V urea in children undergoing chronic peritoneal dialysis. *Adv Perit Dial* 2004;20:245–250.

180. Meireles C, Price S, Pereira A, et al. Nutrition and chronic renal failure in rats: what is an optimal dietary protein? *J Am Soc Nephrol* 1999;10(11):2367–2373.

181. Balfe J. Intraperitoneal amino acids in children receiving chronic peritoneal dialysis. *Perit Dial Int* 1996;16(Suppl 1):S515–S516.

182. Taylor GS, Patel V, Spencer S, et al. Long-term use of 1.1% amino acid dialysis solution in hypoalbuminemic continuous ambulatory peritoneal dialysis patients. *Clin Nephrol* 2002;58(6):445–450.

183. National Kidney Foundation. K/DOQI clinical practice guidelines for bone metabolism and disease in children with chronic kidney disease. *Am J Kidney Dis* 2005;46(Suppl 1):S1–S122.

184. Warady BA, Kriley M, Alon U, et al. Vitamin status of infants receiving long-term peritoneal dialysis. *Pediatr Nephrol* 1994;8(3):354–356.

185. Kriley M, Warady BA. Vitamin status of pediatric patients receiving long-term peritoneal dialysis. *Am J Clin Nutr* 1991;53(6):1476–1479.

186. Pereira AM, Hamani N, Nogueira PC, et al. Oral vitamin intake in children receiving long-term dialysis. *J Ren Nutr* 2000;10(1):24–29.

187. Parrott K. Plasma vitamin A levels in children on CAPD. *Perit Dial Bull* 1987;7:90–92.

188. Warady BA, Borum P, Stall C, et al. Carnitine status of pediatric patients on continuous ambulatory peritoneal dialysis. *Am J Nephrol* 1990;10(2):109–114.

189. Murakami R, Momota T, Yoshiya K, et al. Serum carnitine and nutritional status in children treated with continuous ambulatory peritoneal dialysis. *J Pediatr Gastroenterol* 1990;11(3):371–374.

190. Belay B, Esteban-Cruciani N, Walsh CA, et al. The use of levo-carnitine in children with renal disease: a review and a call for future studies. *Pediatr Nephrol* 2006;21(3):308–317.

191. Tamura T, Vaughn WH, Waldo FB, et al. Zinc and copper balance in children on continuous ambulatory peritoneal dialysis. *Pediatr Nephrol* 1989;3(3):309–313.

192. Zlotkin SH, Rundle MA, Hanning RM, et al. Zinc absorption from glucose and amino acid dialysis solutions in children on continuous ambulatory peritoneal dialysis (CAPD). *J Am Coll Nutr* 1987;6(4):345–350.

193. Warady BA, Weis L, Johnson L. Nasogastric tube feeding in infants on peritoneal dialysis. *Perit Dial Int* 1996;16(Suppl 1):S521–S525.

194. Warady BA, Kriley M, Belden B, et al. Nutritional and behavioural aspects of nasogastric tube feeding in infants receiving chronic peritoneal dialysis. *Adv Perit Dial* 1990;6:265–268.

195. Brewer ED. Growth of small children managed with chronic peritoneal dialysis and nasogastric tube feedings: 203-month experience in 14 patients. *Adv Perit Dial* 1990;6:269–272.

196. Rees L, Mak RH. Nutrition and growth in children with chronic kidney disease. *Nat Rev Nephrol* 2011;7(11):615–623.

197. Coleman JE, Watson AR, Rance CH, et al. Gastrostomy buttons for nutritional support on chronic dialysis. *Nephrol Dial Transplant* 1998;13(8):2041–2046.

198. Ellis EN, Yiu V, Harley F, et al. The impact of supplemental feeding in young children on dialysis: a report of the North American Pediatric Renal Transplant Cooperative Study. *Pediatr Nephrol* 2001;16(5):404–408.

199. Kamen RS. Impaired development of oral-motor functions required for normal oral feeding as a consequence of tube feeding during infancy. *Adv Perit Dial* 1990;6:276–278.

200. Lapeyraque AL, Haddad E, Andre JL, et al. Sudden blindness caused by anterior ischemic optic neuropathy in 5 children on continuous peritoneal dialysis. *Am J Kidney Dis* 2003;42(5):E3–E9.

201. Dufek S, Feldkoetter M, Vidal E, et al. Anterior ischemic optic neuropathy in pediatric peritoneal dialysis: risk factors and therapy. *Pediatr Nephrol* 2014;29(7):1249–1257.

202. Di Zazzo G, Guzzo I, De Galasso L, et al. Anterior ischemic optical neuropathy in children on chronic peritoneal dialysis: report of 7 cases. *Perit Dial Int* 2015;35(2):135–139.

203. Parekh RS, Flynn JT, Smoyer WE, et al. Improved growth in young children with severe chronic renal insufficiency who use specified nutritional therapy. *J Am Soc Nephrol* 2001;12(11):2418–2426.

204. Roodhooft AM, Van Hoeck KJ, Van Acker KJ. Hypophosphatemia in infants on continuous ambulatory peritoneal dialysis. *Clin Nephrol* 1990;34(3):131–135.

205. Harvey E, Secker D, Braj B, et al. The team approach to the management of children on chronic peritoneal dialysis. *Adv Renal Replace Ther* 1996;3(1):3–13.

206. Verrina E, Honda M, Warady BA, et al. Prevention of peritonitis in children on peritoneal dialysis. *Perit Dial Int* 2000;20(6):625–630.

207. Hisano S, Miyazaki C, Hatae K, et al. Immune status of children on continuous ambulatory peritoneal dialysis. *Pediatr Nephrol* 1992;6(2):179–181.

208. Warady BA, Campoy SF, Gross SP, et al. Peritonitis with continuous ambulatory peritoneal dialysis and continuous cycling peritoneal dialysis. *J Pediatr* 1984;105(5):726–730.

209. Watson AR, Vigneux A, Bannatyne RM, et al. Peritonitis during continuous ambulatory peritoneal dialysis in children. *CMAJ* 1986;134(9):1019–1022.

210. Levy M, Balfe J. Optimal approach to the prevention and treatment of peritonitis in children undergoing continuous ambulatory and continuous cycling peritoneal dialysis. *Semin Dial* 1994;7:442–449.

211. Warady BA, Schaefer FS. Peritonitis. In: Warady BA, Fine RN, Schaefer FS, et al, eds. *Pediatric Dialysis*. Dordrecht, The Netherlands: Kluwer Academic Publishers, 2004:393–413.

212. United States Renal Data System. *USRDS 2013 Annual Data Report: Atlas of Chronic Kidney Disease and End-Stage Renal Disease in the United States*. Bethesda, MD: National Institutes of Health, National Institute of Diabetes and Digestive and Kidney Diseases, 2013.

213. Kingwatanakul P, Warady BA. *Staphylococcus aureus* nasal carriage in children receiving long-term peritoneal dialysis. *Adv Perit Dial* 1997;13:281–284.

214. Oh J, von Baum H, Klaus G, et al. Nasal carriage of *Staphylococcus aureus* in families of children on peritoneal dialysis. European Pediatric Peritoneal Dialysis Study Group (EPPS). *Adv Perit Dial* 2000;16:324–327.

215. Warady BA, Schaefer F, Holloway M, et al. Consensus guidelines for the treatment of peritonitis in pediatric patients receiving peritoneal dialysis. *Perit Dial Int* 2000;20(6):610–624.

216. Auron A, Simon S, Andrews W, et al. Prevention of peritonitis in children receiving peritoneal dialysis. *Pediatr Nephrol* 2007;22(4):578–585.

217. Holloway M, Mujais S, Kandert M, et al. Pediatric peritoneal dialysis training: characteristics and impact on peritonitis rates. *Perit Dial Int* 2001;21(4):401–404.

218. Neu AM, Miller MR, Stuart J, et al. Design of the standardizing care to improve outcomes in pediatric end stage renal disease collaborative. *Pediatr Nephrol* 2014;29(9):1477–1484.

219. Prestidge C, Ronaldson J, Wong W, et al. Infectious outcomes following gastrostomy in children receiving peritoneal dialysis. *Pediatr Nephrol* 2015;30(5):849–854.

220. Warady BA, Feneberg R, Verrina E, et al. Peritonitis in children who receive long-term peritoneal dialysis: a prospective evaluation of therapeutic guidelines. *J Am Soc Nephrol* 2007;18(7):2172–2179.

221. Schaefer F, Feneberg R, Aksu N, et al. Worldwide variation of dialysis-associated peritonitis in children. *Kidney Int* 2007;72(11):1374–1379.

222. Piraino B, Bailie GR, Bernardini J, et al. Peritoneal dialysis-related infections recommendations: 2005 update. *Perit Dial Int* 2005;25(2):107–131.

223. Stefanidis CJ, Shroff R. Encapsulating peritoneal sclerosis in children. *Pediatr Nephrol* 2013;21.

224. Warady BA. Sclerosing encapsulating peritonitis: what approach should be taken with children? *Perit Dial Int* 2000;20(4):390–391.

225. Araki Y, Hataya H, Tanaka Y, et al. Long-term peritoneal dialysis is a risk factor of sclerosing encapsulating peritonitis for children. *Perit Dial Int* 2000;20(4):445–451.

226. Hoshii S, Honda M, Itami N, et al. Sclerosing encapsulating peritonitis in pediatric peritoneal dialysis patients. *Pediatr Nephrol* 2000;14(4):275–279.

227. Vidal E, Edefonti A, Puteo F, et al. Encapsulating peritoneal sclerosis in paediatric peritoneal dialysis patients: the experience of the Italian Registry of Pediatric Chronic Dialysis. *Nephrol Dial Transplant* 2013;28(6):1603–1609.

228. Kolff W, Berk H, ter Welle M, et al. The artificial kidney: a dialyzer with great area. *Acta Med Scand* 1944;117:121–134.

229. Andrus F. Use of Visking sausage casing for ultrafiltration. *Proc Soc Exp Biol Med* 1919;27:127–128.

230. Mateer FM, Greenman L, Danowski TS. Hemodialysis of the uremic child. *AMA Am J Dis Child* 1955;89(6):645–655.

231. Morse TS. Synthetic arteriovenous shunts for hemodialysis in children. *J Pediatr Surg* 1970;5(1):23–31.

232. Hickman RO, Scribner BH. Application of the pumpless hemodialysis system to infants and children. *Trans Am Soc Artif Intern Organs* 1962;8:309–314.

233. Alexander S, Cochat P. Notes on the history of dialysis therapy in children. In: Warady B, Schaefer F, Alexander S, eds. *Pediatric Dialysis*. 2nd ed. New York, NY: Springer, 2004:3–16.

234. Hicks CW, Canner JK, Arhuidese I, et al. Mortality benefits of different hemodialysis access types are age dependent. *J Vasc Surg* 2015;61(2):449–456.

235. Bourquelot P, Cussenot O, Corbi P, et al. Microsurgical creation and follow-up of arteriovenous fistulae for chronic haemodialysis in children. *Pediatr Nephrol* 1990;4(2):156–159.

236. Bourquelot P, Raynaud F, Pirozzi N. Microsurgery in children for creation of arteriovenous fistulas in renal and non-renal diseases. *Ther Apher Dial* 2003;7(6):498–503.

237. Harlander-Locke M, Jimenez JC, Lawrence PF, et al. Bovine carotid artery (Artegraft) as a hemodialysis access conduit in patients who are poor candidates for native arteriovenous fistulae. *Vasc Endovascular Surg* 2014;48(7–8):497–502.

238. Goldstein SL, Allsteadt A, Smith CM, et al. Proactive monitoring of pediatric hemodialysis vascular access: effects of ultrasound dilution on thrombosis rates. *Kidney Int* 2002;62(1):272–275.

239. Goldstein S, Smith C, Currier H. Noninvasive interventions to decrease hospitalization and associated costs for pediatric patients receiving hemodialysis. *J Am Soc Nephrol* 2003;14(8):2127–2131.

240. Sheth RD, Brandt ML, Brewer ED, et al. Permanent hemodialysis vascular access survival in children and adolescents with end-stage renal disease. *Kidney Int* 2002;62(5):1864–1849.

241. Briones L, Diaz Moreno A, Sierre S, et al. Permanent vascular access survival in children on long-term chronic hemodialysis. *Pediatr Nephrol* 2010;25(9):1731–1738.

242. Wartman SM, Rosen D, Woo K, et al. Outcomes with arteriovenous fistulas in a pediatric population. *J Vasc Surg* 2014;60(1):170–174.

243. North American Pediatric Renal Trials and Collaborative Studies. *2007 Annual Report*. Rockville, MD: EMMES Corp, 2007.

244. Ramage I, Bailie A, Tyerman K, et al. Vascular access survival in children and young adults receiving long-term hemodialysis. *Am J Kidney Dis* 2005;45(4):708–714.

245. Goldstein SL, Macierowski CT, Jabs K. Hemodialysis catheter survival and complications in children and adolescents. *Pediatr Nephrol* 1997;11(1):74–77.

246. Sharma A, Zilleruelo G, Abitbol C, et al. Survival and complications of cuffed catheters in children on chronic hemodialysis. *Pediatr Nephrol* 1999;13(3):245–248.

247. Richard HM III, Hastings GS, Boyd-Kranis RL, et al. A randomized, prospective evaluation of the Tesio, Ash split, and Opti-flow hemodialysis catheters. *J Vasc Interv Radiol* 2001;12(4):431–435.

248. Sheth RD, Kale AS, Brewer ED, et al. Successful use of Tesio catheters in pediatric patients receiving chronic hemodialysis. *Am J Kidney Dis* 2001;38(3):553–559.

249. Stalter KA, Stevens GF, Sterling WA Jr. Late stenosis of the subclavian vein after hemodialysis catheter injury. *Surgery* 1986;100(5):924–927.

250. Centers for Medicare & Medicaid Services. *ESRD Basic Technical Surveyor Training Interpretive Guidance, Interim Final Version 1.1*. Baltimore, MD: Centers for Medicare & Medicaid Services, 2008.

251. Hothi DK, Stronach L, Harvey E. Home haemodialysis. *Pediatr Nephrol* 2013;28(5):721–730.

252. Muller D, Geary D. Intensified hemodialysis in children. In: Warady B, Schaefer F, Alexander S, eds. *Pediatric Dialysis*. New York, NY: Springer, 2012:329–344.

253. Goldstein SL, Silverstein DM, Leung JC, et al. Frequent hemodialysis with NxStage system in pediatric patients receiving maintenance hemodialysis. *Pediatr Nephrol* 2008;23(1):129–135.

254. Steuer RR, Leypoldt JK, Cheung AK, et al. Hematocrit as an indicator of blood volume and a predictor of intradialytic morbid events. *ASAIO J* 1994;40(3):M691–M696.

255. Steuer RR, Leypoldt JK, Cheung AK, et al. Reducing symptoms during hemodialysis by continuously monitoring the hematocrit. *Am J Kidney Dis* 1996;27(4):525–532.

256. Jain SR, Smith L, Brewer ED, et al. Non-invasive intravascular monitoring in the pediatric hemodialysis population. *Pediatr Nephrol* 2001;16(1):15–18.

257. Michael M, Brewer ED, Goldstein SL. Blood volume monitoring to achieve target weight in pediatric hemodialysis patients. *Pediatr Nephrol* 2004;19(4):432–437.

258. Patel HP, Goldstein SL, Mahan JD, et al. A standard, noninvasive monitoring of hematocrit algorithm improves blood pressure control in pediatric hemodialysis patients. *Clin J Am Soc Nephrol* 2007;2(2):252–257.

259. Mahoney CA, Arieff AI. Uremic encephalopathies: clinical, biochemical, and experimental features. *Am J Kidney Dis* 1982;2(3):324–336.

260. Nissenson AR, Weston RE, Kleeman CR. Mannitol. *West J Med* 1979;131(4):277–284.

261. Visweswaran P, Massin EK, Dubose TD Jr. Mannitol-induced acute renal failure. *J Am Soc Nephrol* 1997;8(6):1028–1033.

262. Sadowski RH, Allred EN, Jabs K. Sodium modeling ameliorates intradialytic and interdialytic symptoms in young hemodialysis patients. *J Am Soc Nephrol* 1993;4(5):1192–1198.

263. Valentini RP, Geary DF, Chand DH. Central venous lines for chronic hemodialysis: survey of the Midwest Pediatric Nephrology Consortium. *Pediatr Nephrol* 2008;23(2):291–295.

264. Hothi DK, Harvey E. Anticoagulation in children on hemodialysis. In: Nisenson AR, Fine RN, eds. *Handbook of Dialysis Therapy*. 4th ed. Philadelphia, PA: Saunders Elsevier, 2008:1280–1294.

265. Goldstein SL. Adequacy of dialysis in children: does small solute clearance really matter? *Pediatr Nephrol* 2004;19(1):1–5.

266. Smye SW, Evans JH, Will E, et al. Paediatric haemodialysis: estimation of treatment efficiency in the presence of urea rebound. *Clin Phys Physiol Meas* 1992;13(1):51–62.

267. Gotch FA, Sargent JA. A mechanistic analysis of the National Cooperative Dialysis Study (NCDS). *Kidney Int* 1985;28(3):526–534.

268. Evans JH, Smye SW, Brocklebank JT. Mathematical modelling of haemodialysis in children. *Pediatr Nephrol* 1992;6(4):349–353.

269. Borah MF, Schoenfeld PY, Gotch FA, et al. Nitrogen balance during intermittent dialysis therapy of uremia. *Kidney Int* 1978;14(5):491–500.

270. Grupe WE, Harmon WE, Spinozzi NS. Protein and energy requirements in children receiving chronic hemodialysis. *Kidney Int Suppl* 1983;15:S6–S10.

271. Kaysen GA, Chertow GM, Adhikarla R, et al. Inflammation and dietary protein intake exert competing effects on serum albumin and creatinine in hemodialysis patients. *Kidney Int* 2001;60(1):333–340.

272. Tom A, McCauley L, Bell L, et al. Growth during maintenance hemodialysis: impact of enhanced nutrition and clearance. *J Pediatr* 1999;134(4):464–471.

273. Goldstein SL, Baronette S, Gambrell TV, et al. nPCR assessment and IDPN treatment of malnutrition in pediatric hemodialysis patients. *Pediatr Nephrol* 2002;17(7):531–534.

274. Orellana P, Juarez-Congelosi M, Goldstein SL. Intradialytic parenteral nutrition treatment and biochemical marker assessment for malnutrition in adolescent maintenance hemodialysis patients. *J Ren Nutr* 2005;15(3):312–317.

275. Goldstein SL, Sorof JM, Brewer ED. Natural logarithmic estimates of Kt/V in the pediatric hemodialysis population. *Am J Kidney Dis* 1999;33(3):518–522.

276. Goldstein SL. Hemodialysis in the pediatric patient: state of the art. *Adv Renal Replace Ther* 2001;8(3):173–179.

277. Goldstein S, Brewer E. Logarithmic extrapolation of a 15-minute postdialysis BUN to predict equilibrated BUN and calculate doublepool Kt/V in the pediatric hemodialysis population. *Am J Kidney Dis* 2000;36(1):98–104.

278. Goldstein S, Sorof J, Brewer E. Evaluation and prediction of urea rebound and equilibrated Kt/V in the pediatric hemodialysis population. *Am J Kidney Dis* 1999;34(1):49–54.

279. Sharma A, Espinosa P, Bell L, et al. Multicompartment urea kinetics in well-dialyzed children. *Kidney Int* 2000;58(5):2138–2146.

280. Marsenic OD, Pavlicic D, Peco-Antic A, et al. Prediction of equilibrated urea in children on chronic hemodialysis. *ASAIO J* 2000;46(3):283–287.

281. Brem AS, Lambert C, Hill C, et al. Clinical morbidity in pediatric dialysis patients: data from the Network 1 Clinical Indicators Project. *Pediatr Nephrol* 2001;16(11):854–847.

282. Goldstein S, Brem A, Warady B, et al. Comparison of single-pool and equilibrated Kt/V values for pediatric hemodialysis prescription management: analysis from the Centers for Medicare & Medicaid Services Clinical Performance Measures Project. *Pediatr Nephrol* 2006;21(8):1161–1166.

283. Lockridge RS, Kjellstrand CM. Nightly home hemodialysis: outcome and factors associated with survival. *Hemodial Int* 2011;15(2):211–218.

284. Pierratos A. Daily nocturnal home hemodialysis. *Kidney Int* 2004;65(5):1975–1986.

285. Chertow GM, Levin NW, Beck GJ, et al. In-center hemodialysis six times per week versus three times per week. *N Engl J Med* 2010;363(24):2287–2300.

286. Rocco MV, Daugirdas JT, Greene T, et al. Long-term effects of frequent nocturnal hemodialysis on mortality: the Frequent Hemodialysis Network (FHN) Nocturnal Trial. *Am J Kidney Dis* 2015;66(3):459–468.

287. Hothi DK, Harvey E, Piva E, et al. Calcium and phosphate balance in adolescents on home nocturnal haemodialysis. *Pediatr Nephrol* 2006;21(6):835–841.

288. Fischbach M, Terzic J, Menouer S, et al. Daily on line haemodiafiltration promotes catch-up growth in children on chronic dialysis. *Nephrol Dial Transplant* 2010;25(3):867–873.

289. Simmons J, Wilson C, Potter D, et al. Relation of calorie deficiency to growth failure in children on hemodialysis and the growth response to calorie supplementation. *N Engl J Med* 1971;285(12):653–656.

290. Conley S, Rose G, Robson A, et al. Effects of dietary intake and hemodialysis on protein turnover in uremic children. *Kidney Int* 1980;17(6):837–846.

291. Srivaths PR, Wong C, Goldstein SL. Nutrition aspects in children receiving maintenance hemodialysis: impact on outcome. *Pediatr Nephrol* 2009;24(5):951–957.

292. Mastrangelo A, Paglialonga F, Edefonti A. Assessment of nutritional status in children with chronic kidney disease and on dialysis. *Pediatr Nephrol* 2014;29(8):1349–1358.

293. Paglialonga F, Felice Civitillo C, Groppali E, et al. Assessment of nutritional status in children with chronic kidney disease. *Minerva Pediatr* 2010;62(3):295–306.

294. Abraham AG, Mak RH, Mitsnefes M, et al. Protein energy wasting in children with chronic kidney disease. *Pediatr Nephrol* 2014;29(7):1231–1238.

295. Juarez-Congelosi M, Orellana P, Goldstein SL. Normalized protein catabolic rate versus serum albumin as a nutrition status marker in pediatric patients receiving hemodialysis. *J Ren Nutr* 2007;17(4):269–274.

296. Zachwieja J, Duran M, Joles JA, et al. Amino acid and carnitine supplementation in haemodialysed children. *Pediatr Nephrol* 1994;8(6):739–743.

297. Krause I, Shamir R, Davidovits M, et al. Intradialytic parenteral nutrition in malnourished children treated with hemodialysis. *J Ren Nutr* 2002;12(1):55–59.

298. Asayama K, Ito H, Nakahara C, et al. Lipid profiles and lipase activities in children and adolescents with chronic renal failure treated conservatively or with hemodialysis or transplantation. *Pediatr Res* 1984;18(8):783–788.

299. Van Gool S, Van Damme-Lombaerts R, Cobbaert C, et al. Lipid and lipoprotein abnormalities in children on hemodialysis and after renal transplantation. *Transplant Proc* 1991;23(1 Pt 2):1375–1377.

300. Khurana M, Silverstein DM. Etiology and management of dyslipidemia in children with chronic kidney disease and end-stage renal disease. *Pediatr Nephrol* 2015;30(12):2073–2084.

301. Kavey RE, Allada V, Daniels SR, et al. Cardiovascular risk reduction in high-risk pediatric patients: a scientific statement from the American Heart Association Expert Panel on Population and Prevention Science; the Councils on Cardiovascular Disease in the Young, Epidemiology and Prevention, Nutrition, Physical Activity and Metabolism, High Blood Pressure Research, Cardiovascular Nursing, and the Kidney in Heart Disease; and the Interdisciplinary Working Group on Quality of Care and Outcomes Research. *Circulation* 2006;114(24):2710–2738.

302. Gusmano R, Oleggini R, Perfumo F. Plasma carnitine concentrations and dyslipidemia in children on maintenance hemodialysis. *J Pediatr* 1981;99(3):429–432.

303. Gloggler A, Bulla M, Puchstein C, et al. Plasma and muscle carnitine in healthy and hemodialyzed children. *Child Nephrol Urol* 1988;9(5):277–282.

304. Gloggler A, Bulla M, Furst P. Effect of low dose supplementation of L-carnitine on lipid metabolism in hemodialyzed children. *Kidney Int* 1989;27:S256–S258.

305. Verrina E, Caruso U, Calevo MG, et al. Effect of carnitine supplementation on lipid profile and anemia in children on chronic dialysis. *Pediatr Nephrol* 2007;22(5):727–733.

306. Ulinski T, Cochat P. Maintenance hemodialysis during infancy. In: Warady B, Schaefer F, Alexander S, eds. *Pediatric Dialysis*. 2nd ed. New York, NY: Springer, 2004:321–328.

307. Sadowski RH, Harmon WE, Jabs K. Acute hemodialysis of infants weighing less than five kilograms. *Kidney Int* 1994;45(3):903–936.

308. Coulthard MG, Crosier J, Griffiths C, et al. Haemodialysing babies weighing <8 kg with the Newcastle infant dialysis and ultrafiltration system (Nidus): comparison with peritoneal and conventional haemodialysis. *Pediatr Nephrol* 2014;29(10):1873–1881.

309. Fadrowski JJ, Hwang W, Frankenfield DL, et al. Clinical course associated with vascular access type in a national cohort of adolescents who receive hemodialysis: findings from the Clinical Performance Measures and US Renal Data System projects. *Clin J Am Soc Nephrol* 2006;1(5):987–992.

310. O'Grady NP, Alexander M, Burns LA, et al. Guidelines for the prevention of intravascular catheter-related infections, 2011. *Am J Infect Control* 2011;39(4 Suppl 1):S1–S34.

311. Paglialonga F, Consolo S, Biasuzzi A, et al. Reduction in catheter-related infections after switching from povidone-iodine to chlorhexidine for the exit-site care of tunneled central venous catheters in children on hemodialysis. *Hemodial Int* 2014;18(Suppl 1):S13–S18.

312. Kidney Disease: Improving Global Outcomes. KDIGO clinical practice guideline for anemia in chronic kidney disease. *Kidney Int* 2012;2(4):279–335.

313. Eschbach JW. The anemia of chronic renal failure: pathophysiology and the effects of recombinant erythropoietin. *Kidney Int* 1989;35(1):134–148.

314. Eschbach JW, Korn D, Finch CA. 14C cyanate as a tag for red cell survival in normal and uremic man. *J Lab Clin Med* 1977;89(4):823–828.

315. Meytes D, Bogin E, Ma A, et al. Effect of parathyroid hormone on erythropoiesis. *J Clin Invest* 1981;67(5):1263–1269.

316. Muller-Wiefel DE, Sinn H, Gilli G, et al. Hemolysis and blood loss in children with chronic renal failure. *Clin Nephrol* 1977;8(5):481–486.

317. Scigalla P. Effect of recombinant human erythropoietin treatment on renal anemia and body growth of children with end-stage renal disease. The European Multicenter Study Group. *Contrib Nephrol* 1991;88:201–214.

318. Alexander SR. Pediatric uses of recombinant human erythropoietin: the outlook in 1991. *Am J Kidney Dis* 1991;18(4 Suppl 1):42–53.

319. Kausz AT, Watkins SL, Hansen C, et al. Intraperitoneal erythropoietin in children on peritoneal dialysis: a study of pharmacokinetics and efficacy. *Am J Kidney Dis* 1999;34(4):651–656.

320. Reddingius RE, Schroder CH, Monnens LA. Intraperitoneal administration of recombinant human erythropoietin in children on continuous ambulatory peritoneal dialysis. *Eur J Pediatr* 1992;151(7):540–542.

321. Huang TP, Lin CY. Intraperitoneal recombinant human erythropoietin therapy: influence of the duration of continuous ambulatory peritoneal dialysis treatment and peritonitis. *Am J Nephrol* 1995;15(4):312–317.

322. De Palo T, Giordano GM, Palumbo F, et al. Clinical experience with darbepoietin alfa (NESP) in children undergoing hemodialysis. *Pediatr Nephrol* 2004;19:337–340.

323. Lerner G. The pharmacokinetics of novel erythropoiesis stimulating protein (NESP) in pediatric patients with chronic renal disease. *J Am Soc Nephrol* 2000;11:282A.

324. Koshy SM, Geary DF. Anemia in children with chronic kidney disease. *Pediatr Nephrol* 2008;23(2):209–219.

325. Port RE, Kiepe D, Van Guilder M, et al. Recombinant human erythropoietin for the treatment of renal anaemia in children: no justification for bodyweight-adjusted dosage. *Clin Pharmacokinet* 2004;43(1):57–70.

326. Port RE, Mehls O. Erythropoietin dosing in children with chronic kidney disease: based on body size or on hemoglobin deficit? *Pediatr Nephrol* 2009;24(3):435–437.

327. Warady BA, Silverstein DM. Management of anemia with erythropoietic-stimulating agents in children with chronic kidney disease. *Pediatr Nephrol* 2014;29(9):1493–1505.

328. Bamgbola OF. Pattern of resistance to erythropoietin-stimulating agents in chronic kidney disease. *Kidney Int* 2011;80(5):464–474.

329. Rao DS, Shih MS, Mohini R. Effect of serum parathyroid hormone and bone marrow fibrosis on the response to erythropoietin in uremia. *N Engl J Med* 1993;328(3):171–175.

330. Hymes LC, Hawthorne SM, Chavers BM. Impaired response to recombinant human erythropoietin therapy in children with peritonitis. *Dial Transplant* 1994;23:462–469.

331. Bargman JM, Nong Y, Silverman ED. The effect of in vivo erythropoietin on cytokine mRNA in CAPD patients. *Adv Perit Dial* 1994;10:129–134.

332. Stevens JM, Winearls CG. Serum from continuous ambulatory peritoneal dialysis patients with acute bacterial peritonitis inhibits in vitro erythroid colony formation. *Am J Kidney Dis* 1994;24(4):569–574.

333. Atkinson MA, White CT. Hepcidin in anemia of chronic kidney disease: review for the pediatric nephrologist. *Pediatr Nephrol* 2012;27(1):33–40.

334. Young B, Zaritsky J. Hepcidin for clinicians. *Clin J Am Soc Nephrol* 2009;4(8):1384–1387.

335. Macdougall IC, Roger SD, de Francisco A, et al. Antibody-mediated pure red cell aplasia in chronic kidney disease patients receiving erythropoiesis-stimulating agents: new insights. *Kidney Int* 2012;81(8):727–732.

336. Mattison P, Upadhay K, Wilcox JE, et al. Anti-erythropoietin antibodies followed by endogenous erythropoietin production in a dialysis patient. *Pediatr Nephrol* 2010;25(5):971–976.

337. Casadevall N, Nataf J, Viron B, et al. Pure red-cell aplasia and antierythropoietin antibodies in patients treated with recombinant erythropoietin. *N Engl J Med* 2002;346(7):469–475.

338. NKF-DOQI clinical practice guidelines for the treatment of anemia of chronic renal failure. National Kidney Foundation-Dialysis Outcomes Quality Initiative. *Am J Kidney Dis* 1997;30(4 Suppl 3):S192–S240.

339. Drueke TB, Locatelli F, Clyne N, et al. Normalization of hemoglobin level in patients with chronic kidney disease and anemia. *N Engl J Med* 2006;355(20):2071–2084.

340. Singh AK, Szczech L, Tang KL, et al. Correction of anemia with epoetin alfa in chronic kidney disease. *N Engl J Med* 2006;355(20):2085–2098.

341. KDOQI clinical practice guidelines and clinical practice recommendations for anemia in chronic kidney disease. *Am J Kidney Dis* 2006;47(5 Suppl 3):S11–S145.

342. KDOQI clinical practice guideline and clinical practice recommendations for anemia in chronic kidney disease: 2007 update of hemoglobin target. *Am J Kidney Dis* 2007;50(3):471–530.

343. Warady BA, Ho M. Morbidity and mortality in children with anemia at initiation of dialysis. *Pediatr Nephrol* 2003;18(10):1055–1062.

344. Amaral S, Hwang W, Fivush B, et al. Association of mortality and hospitalization with achievement of adult hemoglobin targets in adolescents maintained on hemodialysis. *J Am Soc Nephrol* 2006;17(10):2878–2885.

345. Chavers BM, Roberts TL, Herzog CA, et al. Prevalence of anemia in erythropoietin-treated pediatric as compared to adult chronic dialysis patients. *Kidney Int* 2004;65(1):266–273.

346. Excerpts from the United States Renal Data Systems 2002 annual report: atlas of end-stage renal disease in the United States. *Am J Kidney Dis* 2003;41(4 Suppl 2):v–ix, S7–254.

347. Milman N. Iron absorption measured by whole body counting and the relation to marrow iron stores in chronic uremia. *Clin Nephrol* 1982;17(2):77–81.

348. National Kidney Foundation. K/DOQI clinical practice guidelines and clinical practice recommendations for anemia in chronic kidney disease. *Am J Kidney Dis* 2006;47:S1–S146.

349. Frankenfield DL, Neu AM, Warady BA, et al. Adolescent hemodialysis: results of the 2000 ESRD Clinical Performance Measures Project. *Pediatr Nephrol* 2002;17(1):10–15.

350. Greenbaum LA, Pan CG, Caley C, et al. Intravenous iron dextran and erythropoietin use in pediatric hemodialysis patients. *Pediatr Nephrol* 2000;14(10–11):908–911.

351. Morris KP, Watson S, Reid MM, et al. Assessing iron status in children with chronic renal failure on erythropoietin: which measurements should we use? *Pediatr Nephrol* 1994;8:51–56.

352. Tenbrock K, Muller-Berghaus J, Michalk D, et al. Intravenous iron treatment of renal anemia in children on hemodialysis. *Pediatr Nephrol* 1999;13(7):580–582.

353. Coyne DW, Kapoian T, Suki W, et al. Ferric gluconate is highly efficacious in anemic hemodialysis patients with high serum ferritin and low transferrin saturation: results of the Dialysis Patients' Response to IV Iron with Elevated Ferritin (DRIVE) Study. *J Am Soc Nephrol* 2007;18:9765–9984.

354. Fudin R, Jaichenko J, Shostak A, et al. Correction of uremic iron deficiency anemia in hemodialyzed patients: a prospective study. *Nephron* 1998;79(3):299–305.

355. Morgan HE, Gautam M, Geary DF. Maintenance intravenous iron therapy in pediatric hemodialysis patients. *Pediatric Nephrol* 2001;16(10):779–783.

356. Warady BA, Kausz A, Lerner G, et al. Iron therapy in the pediatric hemodialysis population. *Pediatr Nephrol* 2004;19(6):655–661.

357. Warady BA, Zobrist RH, Wu J, et al. Sodium ferric gluconate complex therapy in anemic children on hemodialysis. *Pediatr Nephrol* 2005;20(9):1320–1327.

358. Fishbane S, Ungureanu VD, Maesaka JK, et al. The safety of intravenous iron dextran in hemodialysis patients. *Am J Kidney Dis* 1996;28(4):529–534.

359. Goldstein SL, Morris D, Warady BA. Comparison of the safety and efficacy of 3 iron sucrose iron maintenance regimens in children, adolescents, and young adults with CKD: a randomized controlled trial. *Am J Kidney Dis* 2013;61(4):588–597.

360. Horl WH. Iron therapy for renal anemia: how much needed, how much harmful? *Pediatr Nephrol* 2007;22(4):480–489.

361. St. Peter W, Obrador G, Roberts T, et al. Trends in intravenous iron use among dialysis patients in the United States (1994-2002). *Am J Kidney Dis* 2005;46:650–660.

362. Warady B, Zobrist RH, Finan E, et al. Sodium ferric gluconate complex maintenance therapy in children on hemodialysis. *Pediatr Nephrol* 2006;21:553–560.

363. Fishbane SN, Singh AK, Cournoyer SH, et al. Ferric pyrophosphate citrate (Triferic) administration via the dialysate maintains hemoglobin and iron balance in chronic hemodialysis patients. *Nephrol Dial Transplant* 2015;30(12):2019–2026.

364. Broyer M, Le Bihan C, Charbit M, et al. Long-term social outcome of children after kidney transplantation. *Transplantation* 2004;77:1033–1037.

365. Rosenkranz J, Reichwald-Klugger E, Oh J, et al. Psychosocial rehabilitation and satisfaction with life in adults with childhood-onset of end-stage renal disease. *Pediatr Nephrol* 2005;20:1288–1294.

366. Mahan JD, Warady BA. Assessment and treatment of short stature in pediatric patients with chronic kidney disease: a consensus statement. *Pediatr Nephrol* 2006;21(7):917–930.

367. Fine RN, Kohaut EC, Brown D, et al. Growth after recombinant human growth hormone treatment in children with chronic renal failure: report of a multicenter randomized double-blind placebo- controlled study. Genentech Cooperative Study Group. *J Pediatr* 1994;124:374–382.

368. Fine R. Growth hormone treatment of children with chronic renal insufficiency, end-stage renal disease and following renal transplantation-update 1997. *Pediatr Endocrinol* 1997;10(4):361–370.

369. Warady BA. Growth retardation in children with chronic renal insufficiency. *J Am Soc Nephrol* 1998;9(12 Suppl):S85–S89.

370. Warady BA, Jabs K. New hormones in the therapeutic arsenal of chronic renal failure. Growth hormone and erythropoietin. *Pediatr Clin North Am* 1995;42(6):1551–1577.

371. Fine R, Ho M, Tejani A, et al. Adverse events with rhGH treatment of patients with chronic renal insufficiency and end-stage renal disease. *J Pediatr* 2003;142:539–545.

372. Haffner D, Schaefer F, Nissel R, et al. Effect of growth hormone treatment on the adult height of children with chronic renal failure. German Study Group for Growth Hormone Treatment in Chronic Renal Failure. *N Engl J Med* 2000;343(13):923–930.

373. Schaefer F, Wuhl E, Haffner D, et al. Stimulation of growth by recombinant human growth hormone in children undergoing peritoneal or hemodialysis treatment. German Study Group for Growth Hormone Treatment in Chronic Renal Failure. *Adv Perit Dial* 1994;10:321–326.

374. Tönshoff B, Mehis O, Heinrich U, et al. Growth-stimulating effects of recombinant human growth hormone in children with end-stage renal disease. *J Pediatr* 1990;116(4):561–566.

375. Wühl E, Haffner D, Nissel R, et al. Short dialyzed children respond less to growth hormone than patients prior to dialysis. German Study Group for Growth Hormone Treatment in Chronic Renal Failure. *Pediatr Nephrol* 1996;10(3):294–298.

376. Tonshoff B, Mehls O. Growth retardation in children with chronic renal insufficiency: current aspects of pathophysiology and treatment. *J Nephrol* 1995;8:133–142.

377. National Kidney Foundation. KDOQI clinical practice guidelines for nutrition in chronic renal failure. *Am J Kidney Dis* 2000;35 (Suppl 2):S105–S136.

378. United States Renal Data System. *USRDS 2007 Annual Data Report: Atlas of End-Stage Renal Disease in the United States.* Bethesda, MD: National Institutes of Health, National Institute of Diabetes and Digestive and Kidney Diseases, 2007.

379. Borzych D, Rees L, Ha IS, et al. The bone and mineral disorder of children undergoing chronic peritoneal dialysis. *Kidney Int* 2010;78(12):1295–1304.

380. Kidney Disease Outcomes Quality Initiative Work Group. KDOQI clinical practice guideline for nutrition in children with CKD: 2008 update. Executive summary. *Am J Kidney Dis* 2009;53(3 Suppl 2):S11–S104.

381. Dibas BI, Warady BA. Vitamin D status of children receiving chronic dialysis. *Pediatr Nephrol* 2012;27(10):1967–1973.

382. Kidney Disease: Improving Global Outcomes CKD-MBD Work Group. KDIGO clinical practice guideline for the diagnosis, evaluation, prevention and treatment of chronic kidney disease-mineral bone disorder (CKD-MBD). *Kidney Int* 2009;76:S1–S130.

383. Klaus G, Watson A, Edefonti A, et al. Prevention and treatment of renal osteodystrophy in children on chronic renal failure: European guidelines. *Pediatr Nephrol* 2006;21:151–159.

384. Salusky IB, Coburn JW, Brill J, et al. Bone disease in pediatric patients undergoing dialysis with CAPD or CCPD. *Kidney Int* 1988;33(5):975–982.

385. Delmez JA, Tindira C, Grooms P, et al. Parathyroid hormone suppression by intravenous 1,25-dihydroxyvitamin D. A role for increased sensitivity to calcium. *J Clin Invest* 1989;83(4):1349–1355.

386. Szabo A, Merke J, Beier E, et al. 1,25(OH)2 vitamin D3 inhibits parathyroid cell proliferation in experimental uremia. *Kidney Int* 1989;35(4):1049–1056.

387. Andress DL. Intravenous versus oral vitamin D therapy in dialysis patients: what is the question? *Am J Kidney Dis* 2001;38(5 Suppl 5):S41–S44.

388. Sprague S, Lerma E, McCormmick D, et al. Suppression of parathyroid hormone secretion in hemodialysis patients: comparison of paricalcitol with calcitriol. *Am J Kidney Dis* 2001;38(5 Suppl 5):S51–S56.

389. Greenbaum L, Benador N, Goldstein S, et al. Intravenous paricalcitol for treatment of secondary hyperparathyroidism in children on hemodialysis. *Am J Kidney Dis* 2007;49(6):814–823.

390. Seeherunvong W, Nwobi O, Abitbol C, et al. Paricalcitol versus calcitriol treatment for hyperparathyroidism in pediatric hemodialysis patients. *Pediatr Nephrol* 2006;21:1434–1439.

391. Strippoli G, Tong A, Palmer S, et al. Calcimimetics for secondary hyperparathyroidism in chronic kidney disease patients. *Cochrane Database Syst Rev* 2006;(18):CD006254.

392. Muscheites J, Wigger M, Drueckler E, et al. Cinacalcet for secondary hyperparathyroidism in children with end-stage renal disease. *Pediatr Nephrol* 2008;23(10):1823–1829.

393. Silverstein DM, Kher KK, Moudgil A, et al. Cinacalcet is efficacious in pediatric dialysis patients. *Pediatr Nephrol* 2008;23(10):1817–1822.

394. Sedman A, Wilkening G, Warady B, et al. Encephalopathy in childhood secondary to aluminum toxicity. *J Pediatr* 1984;105:836–838.

395. Chavers BM, Li S, Collins AJ, et al. Cardiovascular disease in pediatric chronic dialysis patients. *Kidney Int* 2002;62(2):648–653.

396. Amin N. The impact of improved phosphorus control: use of sevelamer hydrochloride in patients with chronic renal failure. *Nephrol Dial Transplant* 2002;17(2):340–345.

397. Mactier RA, Van Stone J, Cox A, et al. Calcium carbonate is an effective phosphate binder when dialysate calcium concentration is adjusted to control hypercalcemia. *Clin Nephrol* 1987;28(5):222–226.

398. Mai ML, Emmett M, Sheikh MS, et al. Calcium acetate, an effective phosphorus binder in patients with renal failure. *Kidney Int* 1989;36(4):690–695.

399. Salusky I, Goodman W, Sahney S, et al. Sevelamer controls parathyroid hormone-induced bone disease as efficiently as calcium carbonate without increasing serum calcium levels during therapy with active vitamin D sterols. *J Am Soc Nephrol* 2005;16:2501–2508.

400. Pieper AK, Haffner D, Hoppe B, et al. A randomized crossover trial comparing sevelamer with calcium acetate in children with CKD. *Am J Kidney Dis* 2006;47(4):625–635.

401. Chertow G, Burke S, Raggi P, et al. Sevelamer attenuates the progression of coronary and aortic calcification in hemodialysis patients. *Kidney Int* 2002;62(1):245–252.

402. Gonzalez E, Schomberg J, Amin N, et al. Sevelamer carbonate increases serum bicarbonate in pediatric dialysis patients. *Pediatr Nephrol* 2010;25(2):373–375.

403. Raaijmakers R, Houkes LM, Schroder CH, et al. Pre-treatment of dairy and breast milk with sevelamer hydrochloride and sevelamer carbonate to reduce phosphate. *Perit Dial Int* 2013;33(5):565–572.

404. Slatopolsky E, Weerts C, Lopez-Hilker S, et al. Calcium carbonate as a phosphate binder in patients with chronic renal failure undergoing dialysis. *N Engl J Med* 1986;315(3):157–161.

405. Osorio A, Seidel FG, Warady BA. Hypercalcemia and pancreatitis in a child with adynamic bone disease. *Pediatr Nephrol* 1997;11(2):223–225.

406. National High Blood Pressure Education Program Working Group on High Blood Pressure in Children and Adolescents. The fourth report on the diagnosis, evaluation, and treatment of high blood pressure in children and adolescents. *Pediatrics* 2004;114:555–576.

407. National Kidney Foundation. K/DOQI clinical practice guidelines on hypertension and antihypertensive agents in chronic kidney disease. *Am J Kidney Dis* 2004;22:S1–S290.

408. Converse RL Jr, Jacobsen TN, Toto RD, et al. Sympathetic overactivity in patients with chronic renal failure. *N Engl J Med* 1992;327(27):1912–1918.

409. Zucchelli P, Zuccala A. Control of blood pressure in patients on haemodialysis. In: Cameron S, Davison A, Grunfeld J, et al, eds. *Oxford Textbook of Clinical Nephrology*. Oxford, United Kingdom: Oxford University Press, 1992:1458–1467.

410. Zucchelli P, Santoro A, Zuccala A. Genesis and control of hypertension in hemodialysis patients. *Semin Nephrol* 1988;8(2):163–168.

411. Goldstein S, Silverstein D, Leung J, et al. Frequent hemodialysis with NxStage system in pediatric patients receiving maintenance hemodialysis. *Pediatr Nephrol* 2007;23:129–135.

412. Van DeVoorde R, Barletta G, Chand D, et al. Blood pressure control in pediatric hemodialysis: the Midwest Pediatric Nephrology Consortium Study. *Pediatr Nephrol* 2007;22:547–553.

413. North American Pediatric Renal Trials and Collaborative Studies. NAPRTCS: 2011 annual dialysis report. https://web.emmes.com/study/ped/annlrept/annualrept2011.pdf. Accessed August 17, 2016.

414. Gerson AC, Butler R, Moxey-Mims M, et al. Neurocognitive outcomes in children with chronic kidney disease: current findings and contemporary endeavors. *Ment Retard Dev Disabil Res Rev* 2006;12(3):208–215.

415. Polinsky MS, Kaiser BA, Stover JB, et al. Neurologic development of children with severe chronic renal failure from infancy. *Pediatr Nephrol* 1987;1(2):157–165.

416. Rotundo A, Nevins TE, Lipton M, et al. Progressive encephalopathy in children with chronic renal insufficiency in infancy. *Kidney Int* 1982;21(3):486–491.

417. McGraw ME, Haka-Ikse K. Neurologic-developmental sequelae of chronic renal failure in infancy. *J Pediatr* 1985;106(4):579–583.

418. Warady BA. Neurodevelopment of infants with end-stage renal disease: is it improving? *Pediatr Transplant* 2002;6(1):5–7.

419. Ledermann S, Scanes M, Fernando O, et al. Long-term outcome of peritoneal dialysis in infants. *J Pediatr* 2000;136(1):24–29.

420. Madden SJ, Ledermann SE, Guerrero-Blanco M, et al. Cognitive and psychosocial outcome of infants dialysed in infancy. *Child Care Health Dev* 2003;29(1):55–61.

421. Warady BA, Belden B, Kohaut E. Neurodevelopmental outcome of children initiating peritoneal dialysis in early infancy. *Pediatr Nephrol* 1999;13(9):759–765.

422. Johnson RJ, Warady BA. Long-term neurocognitive outcomes of patients with end-stage renal disease during infancy. *Pediatr Nephrol* 2013;28(8):1283–12891.

423. Glenn CM, Astley SJ, Watkins SL. Dialysis-associated seizures in children and adolescents. *Pediatr Nephrol* 1992;6(2):182–186.

424. McDonald S, Craig J. Long-term survival of children with end-stage renal disease. *N Engl J Med* 2004;350:2654–2662.

425. Brownbridge G, Fielding DM. Psychosocial adjustment to end-stage renal failure: comparing haemodialysis, continuous ambulatory peritoneal dialysis and transplantation. *Pediatr Nephrol* 1991;5:612–662.

426. Brownbridge G, Fielding D. Psychosocial adjustment and adherence to dialysis treatment regimes. *Pediatr Nephrol* 1994;8:744–749.

427. Fukunishi I, Honda M. School adjustment of children with end-stage renal disease. *Pediatr Nephrol* 1995;9:553–557.

428. Fukunishi I, Kudo H. Psychiatric problems of pediatric end-stage renal failure. *Gen Hosp Psychiatry* 1995;17:32–36.

429. Rosenkranz J, Bonzel K, Bulla M, et al. Psychosocial adaptation of children and adolescents with chronic renal failure. *Pediatr Nephrol* 1992;6:459–463.

430. McKenna A, Keating L, Vigneux A, et al. Quality of life in children with chronic kidney disease—patient and caregiver assessments. *Nephrol Dial Transplant* 2006;21:1899–1905.

431. Goldstein SL, Graham N, Warady BA, et al. Measuring health-related quality of life in children with ESRD: performance of the generic and ESRD-specific instrument of the Pediatric Quality of Life Inventory (PedsQL). *Am J Kidney Dis* 2008;51(2):285–297.

432. Centers for Medicare & Medicaid Services. Medicare and Medicaid programs: conditions for coverage for end-stage renal disease facilities. http://www.cms.gov/Regulations-and-Guidance/Legislation/CFCsAndCoPs/Downloads/ESRDfinalrule0415.pdf. Accessed August 17, 2016.

433. Neul SK, Minard CG, Currier H, et al. Health-related quality of life functioning over a 2-year period in children with end-stage renal disease. *Pediatr Nephrol* 2013;28(2):285–293.

434. Gerson A, Hwang W, Fiorenza J, et al. Anemia and health-related quality of life in adolescents with chronic kidney disease. *Am J Kidney Dis* 2004;44(6):1017–1023.

435. Gerson A, Riley A, Fivush B, et al. Assessing health status and health care utilization in adolescents with chronic kidney disease. *J Am Soc Nephrol* 2005;16(5):1427–132.

436. Reynolds JM, Morton MJ, Garralda ME, et al. Psychosocial adjustment of adult survivors of a paediatric dialysis and transplant programme. *Arch Dis Child* 1993;68(1):104–110.

437. Morton MJ, Reynolds JM, Garralda ME, et al. Psychiatric adjustment in end-stage renal disease: a follow up study of former paediatric patients. *J Psychosom Res* 1994;38(4):293–303.

438. Tjaden LA, Vogelzang J, Jager KJ, et al. Long-term quality of life and social outcome of childhood end-stage renal disease. *J Pediatr* 2014;165(2):336.e1–342.e1.

439. Mekahli D, Ledermann S, Gullett A, et al. Evaluation of quality of life by young adult survivors of severe chronic kidney disease in infancy. *Pediatr Nephrol* 2014;29(8):1387–1393.

440. North American Pediatric Renal Trials and Collaborative Studies. NAPRTCS 2006 annual report: renal transplantation, dialysis, chronic renal insufficiency. https://web.emmes.com/study/ped/annlrept/annlrept2006.pdf. Accessed August 17, 2016.

CHAPTER 38

Acute Dialysis in Children

Susan R. Mendley

Renal replacement therapy (RRT) options for the pediatric patient include the full spectrum of modalities available for adults—peritoneal dialysis (PD), intermittent hemodialysis (HD), and continuous renal replacement therapy (CRRT) (1–4). Historically, PD had been preferred because peritoneal access is easier to achieve than vascular access and the technique is simpler to perform, not requiring specialized equipment or a need for highly trained personnel. However, advances in vascular access placement techniques, availability of pediatric-sized catheters, and improvements in CRRT machines and associated equipment (dialyzers and blood lines) have increased the use of CRRT for management of pediatric acute kidney injury (AKI) (2,3). The incidence of AKI requiring RRT is lower in hospitalized children than in adults, so prospective randomized studies comparing treatment modalities for management of pediatric AKI are lacking. The choice of RRT continues to be strongly influenced by the physician's experience and the technical expertise available at each hospital.

ACUTE KIDNEY INJURY IN CHILDREN

A full picture of the incidence and outcome of AKI in children is made more complicated by the use of varying definitions: the Pediatric Risk, Injury, Failure, Loss, End-Stage Renal Disease (pRIFLE) (5), the AKI network (6), and the Kidney Disease: Improving Global Outcomes (KDIGO) (7) assessments. The incidence of AKI in a large pediatric study varied from 37% to 51% depending upon the definition; capture rates and stages of AKI differed between methods (8). However, AKI, by any definition, was associated with higher mortality and longer length of stay. Furthermore, pediatric intensive care unit (PICU) patients showed increasing mortality with greater severity of AKI irrespective of definition.

The causes of AKI in children differ substantially from those in adults and between industrialized and developing countries (9,10). Common causes of AKI in referral centers in industrialized countries include complications of cardiac surgery, treatment of malignancies, and nephrotoxins (11,12). Additional causes common to both settings include hemolytic uremic syndrome, sepsis with multiorgan dysfunction, ischemia, glomerulonephritis, and congenital kidney disease (9,13,14). In a larger referral center, two decades of observation showed neonates and infants were commonly affected and had higher mortality than older children (15). Several comprehensive reviews on pediatric AKI are available (16–19).

Conservative management of the child with AKI includes careful fluid resuscitation, if intravascular volume depletion is present. Once euvolemia has been restored, if oligoanuria is present, maintenance of fluid balance is attempted through the use of diuretics and fluid restriction. Additional measures include diet modification (restriction of potassium and phosphorus, using specialized formula in infants) to minimize development of metabolic disturbances and the use of medications (sodium polystyrene, sodium bicarbonate, and phosphate binders) to correct electrolyte disturbances. Conservative measures, however, are often not sufficient to allow optimal management particularly with prolonged and severe AKI when fluid restriction often compromises the ability to provide appropriate nutrition, which is essential for recovery (20).

INDICATIONS FOR RENAL REPLACEMENT THERAPY

The indications for initiation of RRT in pediatric AKI are similar to those in adults. The indications include (a) oligoanuria requiring fluid and/or electrolyte removal to optimize nutritional and medical support; (b) hypervolemia complicated by congestive heart failure, pulmonary edema, or severe hypertension despite diuretic therapy and fluid restriction; (c) hyperkalemia refractory to medical management or associated with cardiac involvement as evidenced by electrocardiogram changes; (d) metabolic acidosis refractory to medical management with sodium bicarbonate or limited by sodium overload; (e) symptomatic uremia with pericarditis, neuropathy, or encephalopathy; (f) tumor lysis syndrome or severe hyperuricemia; and (g) toxic ingestions (21). Furthermore, RRT in children is used for specific nonkidney disease indications including inborn errors of metabolism with hyperammonemia or unremitting acidosis and toxic ingestions (22–24). These rare conditions require prompt recognition and emergency resuscitation to allow nephrologists to provide rapid, efficient clearance of accumulated metabolites and toxins (see below).

Fluid overload is recognized to be an independent risk factor for mortality in pediatric patients in PICU settings (25,26). Single-center and multicenter retrospective studies have supported the observation that survivors of AKI are more likely to have a lesser degree of volume overload at the time of initiation of CRRT (27–29). This has led some pediatric centers to develop protocols for initiation of CRRT when patients become 10% fluid volume overloaded or at initiation of mechanical ventilation regardless of glomerular filtration rate (GFR) (30–32).

⬡ PERITONEAL DIALYSIS

PD offers several advantages for the care of the pediatric patient with AKI. Technically, it is a simple procedure that does not require specialized personnel. Nurses in PICUs can be trained to perform the procedure with an acceptably low infection rate. Currently available automated cycler devices permit frequent dialysis exchanges without repeatedly opening the circuit, further lowering the infection risk. Fluid and solute removal occur gradually, making the procedure well tolerated in the hemodynamically compromised child and eliminating the risk of hypotension or dialysis disequilibrium (33–35). From a practical standpoint, placement of a PD catheter is technically easier than placement of vascular access, which can be particularly challenging in the small infant (36) (**TABLE 38.1**).

TABLE 38.1	Causes of Acute Kidney Injury in Children	
Etiologies of Acute Kidney Injury	Referral Center in Developing Country	Tertiary Center in Industrialized Country
	n (%)	*n* (%)
Hemolytic uremic syndrome	25 (31)	5 (3)
Glomerulonephritis	18 (23)	—
Intrinsic kidney disease	—	64 (44)
Urinary obstruction	7 (9)	—
Postoperative sepsis	14 (18)	49 (34)
Ischemic and prerenal	14 (18)	—
Organ and bone marrow transplant	—	19 (13)
Miscellaneous	2 (3)	9 (6)
Total	80	146

Adapted from Flynn JT. Causes, management approaches, and outcome of acute renal failure in children. *Curr Opin Pediatr* 1998;10(2):184–189, with permission.

PD provides particularly efficient solute and fluid removal in the youngest patients. Peritoneal membrane surface area correlates with body surface area rather than with body mass; this ratio is most favorable in infants and young children who can thus achieve large peritoneal clearance (37,38). Use of PD also avoids the need for anticoagulation and blood exposure through priming of a blood circuit. Because PD is the preferred mode of dialysis for children with chronic kidney disease, initiating the therapy in the acute setting can facilitate the transition to chronic dialysis. This form of dialysis is less expensive to perform and requires a smaller initial capital investment than other CRRTs (see subsequent text) (1).

PD has been used to manage volume overload and AKI after cardiac surgery in infants with some success (39–41). However, not all studies demonstrate benefit from PD or superiority over CRRT (42,43).

PD, however, is not appropriate for all patients. It is contraindicated in those with abdominal wall defects (e.g., bladder exstrophy, omphalocele, and gastroschisis) and diaphragmatic lesions (e.g., diaphragmatic hernia and surgical defects). It cannot be used immediately after abdominal surgery. The presence of a ventriculoperitoneal shunt is a relative contraindication because of the risk of ascending infection should peritonitis develop; many pediatric nephrologists choose another modality in that setting. PD may not be successful after extensive abdominal surgery because adhesions can cause failure of dialysate drainage, which is manifested as slow outflow rates or poor ultrafiltration.

In clinical situations in which rapid removal of solute (e.g., hyperkalemia), toxin (ingestion), or metabolite (e.g., ammonia) is required, PD does not provide an optimal response. The gradual nature of the treatment, which is advantageous in uremia, will limit the rapid response those emergencies require. Furthermore, in states of acute volume overload with pulmonary edema or congestive heart failure, the ultrafiltration provided by PD may not be rapid or predictable enough to prevent clinical deterioration or mortality (42). Nonetheless, in life-threatening emergencies, PD may be the most accessible and familiar dialysis modality available and can be used until alternate modalities can be arranged (24,44).

Peritoneal Dialysis Catheters

Neonatal and pediatric sizes of most adult catheter configurations are available. These include acute "temporary" catheters and chronic catheters appropriate for operative placement. Acute catheters can be placed percutaneously at the bedside after filling the abdomen with dialysate, as is done in adults (36,45). This permits dialysis therapy to be initiated quickly even in patients too unstable for surgery. Before placement of the dialysis catheter, a Foley catheter should be inserted to empty the bladder and decrease the risk of bladder perforation.

Temporary catheters have several disadvantages: Percutaneous placement can result in injury to an abdominal viscus; bowel and bladder perforations are recognized complications (46). Older catheters were stiff, and even after successful placement, they could cause bowel injury; this often necessitated immobilizing the child while the catheter was in place. Newer more flexible catheters perform better (45). In addition, temporary catheters are uncuffed and, therefore, carry a much greater risk of dialysate leakage at the exit site and subsequent infection. The risk of catheter complications increases significantly after 6 days of use, and it is usually impossible to predict renal recovery at the initiation of PD (47). Therefore, many nephrologists prefer an operatively placed catheter that is used immediately.

The Tenckhoff catheter, although designed as a chronic catheter, is often used in the acute setting (47,48). The catheter can be placed in the intensive care unit or in an operating suite; laparoscopic placement may have advantages (49). There is an increased risk of leakage at the exit site when the catheter is used immediately after placement, and strategies to limit that complication are described in the subsequent text.

Data from the North American Pediatric Renal Transplant Cooperative Study (NAPRTCS) do not suggest that one type of chronic catheter design is superior to the others. However, data do suggest a downward (caudally) oriented exit site is preferable because this has been associated with a reduced risk of peritonitis in chronic dialysis (50,51). In infants, it is preferable to position the exit site above the diaper area to reduce the risk of fecal contamination. Similarly, in children with ostomies, it is preferred that the dialysis catheter be positioned on the contralateral side to maximize the distance between the ostomy and the catheter exit site, thereby minimizing the risk of exit-site contamination and infection. Omental obstruction resulting in poor outflow is common especially in small children; therefore, many advocate performing an omentectomy at the time of the original surgery to avoid outflow obstruction (52–55). This issue, however, remains controversial because other authors do not believe that it is necessary (56). Intraoperatively, should any hernial defects be noted, they should be repaired to minimize this potential complication of PD.

Peritoneal Dialysis Solutions

Acute pediatric PD is usually performed using the commercially available lactate-based dialysis solution. Calcium concentrations (1.25 and 1.75 mM) are chosen based on the need for calcium-based phosphorus binders and vitamin D supplements, but that choice may be less relevant in the acute setting. Lactate-based dextrose solutions have the disadvantages of low pH and glucose absorption with prolonged dwells. Low pH can contribute to pain on inflow and impaired phagocytic activity resulting in increased risk for infection (57). More biocompatible PD solutions, such as neutral-pH low-glucose degradation product solution (58) and bicarbonate-based solution (59), have been tested in children. Short-term and intermediate-term safety has been demonstrated in chronic PD. A comparison of bicarbonate and lactate PD solution in adults with AKI showed improved serum bicarbonate, lactate, and pH with the former solution (60). There are no similar data in children.

Because peritoneal surface area in children is large relative to body surface area, glucose absorption during PD can, unfortunately, prove to be too efficient (38). Such glucose absorption during prolonged dwells dissipates the osmotic gradient between plasma water and dialysate leading to suboptimal ultrafiltration, hyperglycemia, hyperinsulinemia, and hyperlipidemia (61,62). Short dwells are used to limit glucose absorption. Alternative osmotic agents such as amino acids may prove useful, at least permitting nutritional benefit from the enhanced absorption. Combined amino acid–glucose-based dialysate has been used in children for acute PD (63). There are no data on icodextrin use in acute PD in children, although it has been studied in chronic PD patients (64).

Dialysis Prescription Considerations

Acute PD is usually initiated with small volumes to limit leakage around a new catheter. Small fill volumes of approximately 10 to 20 mL/kg are often the starting range, although poor drainage, slow

clearance, and inadequate ultrafiltration may limit the effectiveness of low-volume therapy. Fill volumes are gradually increased over many days to a goal of 40 to 50 mL/kg, as tolerated. Short exchange times (45 to 90 minutes) may be used to overcome the limitations of low fill volume and to facilitate ultrafiltration by limiting glucose absorption (65). Even shorter dwell times are possible; however, they are less efficient because a larger proportion of time is spent filling and draining leaving less time for actual dialysis (66).

Although efficient peritoneal glucose absorption may necessitate high dextrose concentrations for infants and small children to achieve ultrafiltration with long dwell times, short exchanges usually provide acceptable or even excessive ultrafiltration using 1.5% dextrose. Therefore, frequent dialysis exchanges for adequate clearance may result in unpredictable fluid removal in small children; careful reassessment of volume status and supplemental fluid, either enteral or parenteral, must be provided to prevent intravascular volume depletion that, in turn, may impair renal recovery.

PD can be performed manually or with an automated cycler. Low-volume manual PD exchanges use a Y-type connector, one limb of which is attached to the inflow line and dialysate bag and the other limb is attached to the drain line and bag to avoid repeatedly opening the catheter connection. A commercially available product (Gesco Dialy-Nate Set) is available as a closed system which permits repeated small exchanges by using an in-line graduated measuring device inserted between the dialysate bag and inflow tubing; this allows more precise measurement of fill volumes and infrequent opening of the dialysis circuit to limit potential contamination. An automated cycling PD machine can be programmed for short dwell treatments appropriate for acute PD; this method also limits opening the catheter circuit to once a day, which decreases the risk of contamination. Currently available cyclers that permit very low volume exchanges (beginning at 60 mL) and low-volume tubing (to decrease the dead space or recirculation volume) facilitate therapy in infants and small children.

Complications of Peritoneal Dialysis

The most common complications of acute PD are catheter malfunction and infection. Catheter malfunction includes dialysate leakage, inflow problems, and outflow problems. Leakage can be external, occurring around the exit site or the incision used to insert the catheter, or internal, resulting in a hernia. Risk factors for external leaks include use of a stiff temporary catheter, frequent catheter manipulation, malnourishment, and initiation of PD with large fill volumes immediately after catheter placement. Strategies to minimize the risk of leakage include use of small fill volumes, minimal catheter manipulation, and two purse-string sutures to seal the peritoneum around the catheter and to seal the posterior rectus sheath opening (67). Temporary discontinuation of PD and use of smaller fill volumes is the initial approach to catheter leaks, but surgical repair is sometimes required. Three retrospective reviews of pediatric acute PD found an increased rate of complications with temporary catheters compared with Tenckhoff catheters (1,47,68).

Obstruction to dialysate flow or excessively slow flow is a frequent catheter complication. Inflow obstruction is usually due to a mechanical blockage: a kink in the catheter, clamp on the catheter, or the presence of blood clot or fibrin. Addition of heparin to the dialysate at a concentration of 250 to 1,000 U/L may diminish fibrin and blood clots. Outflow obstruction is more common and is usually a greater impediment to successful therapy. Catheter entrapment or occlusion by omentum can limit flow and may require reoperation for omentectomy; many surgeons, therefore, perform this at the time of catheter placement. Intra-abdominal adhesions may prevent free flow of dialysate throughout the abdomen, and poor outflow will be noted. Catheter migration can occur and result in painful inflow of dialysate and poor outflow; this may be correctable using a stylet under fluoroscopy or it may require laparoscopic repositioning. Constipation and intestinal distention often limit outflow and should be managed with stool softeners, enemas, or laxatives (avoiding magnesium and phosphorus) (69).

Infectious complications may involve the exit site, tunnel, and/or peritoneum. In the acute setting, an exit-site infection is essentially a surgical wound infection and should be managed as such with parenteral antibiotics. The risk for dialysate leakage and contamination of the peritoneal space is high. Peritonitis is a serious complication of acute PD. It presents a large inflammatory burden to already debilitated, catabolic patients. Resistant organisms and fungi are a greater risk in the intensive care setting where patients are often already receiving antibiotic therapy. Frequent surveillance cell counts and cultures are advisable in this setting because the typical features of fever, abdominal pain, and cloudy effluent may be difficult to discern. Empiric broad-spectrum antibiotic therapy is often required until culture results are available. Intravenous or intraperitoneal therapies are appropriate, depending on the severity of the infection; combined therapy has been used in debilitated patients. Risk factors for developing peritonitis include use of a temporary catheter for more than 3 days, leakage around the exit site, age younger than 2 years, and poor dialysis technique (46).

Hernias are more often a complication of chronic PD, resulting from dialysis performed in an upright posture and increased intra-abdominal pressure. However, a diaphragmatic defect (pleuroperitoneal fistula) can result in hydrothorax even at initiation of dialysis, compromising ventilation and preventing adequate dialysis drainage. A patent processus vaginalis can cause a hydrocele or genital edema. Although these hernias could be corrected surgically, in the acute setting, one is more likely to turn to an alternate modality of dialysis.

Acute PD can cause metabolic complications, most often resulting from glucose absorption. Hyperglycemia may occur and require insulin therapy. Hypertriglyceridemia can result from glucose absorption and be difficult to distinguish from the effects of hyperalimentation. There is spontaneous loss of albumin into dialysate, which can cause hypoalbuminemia; this loss is dramatically increased if peritonitis complicates therapy (46). Lactic acidosis secondary to lactate absorption from the dialysate can occur in small children, but most patients see an improvement in acidosis with initiation of PD. Hyponatremia is common, particularly in very young patients. It is exacerbated by the administration of hypotonic fluids; hypernatremia can develop with excessive ultrafiltration and insufficient free water intake.

⬡ HEMODIALYSIS

Acute HD can be safely and effectively performed in infants and children of all sizes (70–73). It requires highly trained personnel, specialized equipment, and a well-functioning vascular access. Acute HD is often preferred in situations requiring rapid removal of fluid, solute, or toxins (e.g., hyperammonemic coma or other inborn errors of metabolism, ingestion, or hyperkalemia) (21,22,74–77). In fact, HD treatments in small children can be strikingly efficient because body water space (V) is small relative to the potential clearance that one can provide with standard or high-flux dialyzers and typical blood flows (Q_B) (78). Improvements in HD machinery and availability of size-appropriate equipment (blood lines, dialyzers, and vascular access) have facilitated the use of HD in infants and small children. However, the ability to perform HD is contingent on vascular access, which is a challenge in infants and small children.

Technical Considerations

Although the principles of HD are the same in children as in adults, there are several technical aspects unique to children.

Personnel

Skilled dialysis nurses with pediatric experience are required to perform acute HD in children. A nurse-to-patient ratio of 1:1 is needed to provide focused continuous attention to small patients. Keen observation skills and an awareness of age-dependent norms for vital signs are necessary to assess pediatric HD patients and intervene appropriately. Children who are ill are often unable to communicate their distress verbally. Warning signs of decompensation such as agitation or poor perfusion must be recognized quickly. Normal blood pressure in small children is much lower than in adults, leaving little margin for error and hypotension may develop precipitously (79).

Hemodialysis Machines

Technologic improvements in the design of HD machines that have benefited children include the incorporation of volumetric ultrafiltration controllers and blood pumps capable of being calibrated for neonatal, infant, and pediatric blood lines. The blood pump must be able to accurately deliver blood-flow rates within the range 20 to 300 mL/min, appropriate for neonates through older adolescents. The presence of an accurate volumetric ultrafiltration controller is also essential because even small errors in ultrafiltration volume of a few hundred milliliters can result in symptomatic fluid overload or intravascular volume depletion and hypotension.

Extracorporeal Circuit–Blood Lines

In infants and small children, the extracorporeal circuit volume may represent a significant fraction of total blood volume, and severe hypotension can occur at initiation of the treatment. The typical extracorporeal circuit for adult patients may exceed 150 mL; neonatal, infant, and pediatric blood lines are available to limit the circuit volume for some manufacturers. Low demand has caused many manufacturers to withdraw pediatric-specific dialysis supplies. In some cases, the blood pump must be calibrated for the chosen blood line for accurate blood flow. Neonatal lines may not be compatible with available volumetric dialysis machines. However, even using low-volume bloodlines and dialyzers, the total circuit volume cannot always be reduced to less than 10% of the patient's blood volume, particularly in the case of newborns and small infants. When the circuit volume exceeds 10% of the patient's blood volume or when the patient is severely anemic, the circuit can be primed with blood to maintain hemodynamic stability (71). Packed red blood cells may be diluted 1:1 with normal saline to decrease the hematocrit to approximately 35%, thereby decreasing the viscosity and risk for clotting. Blood priming carries its own particular risks. The greatest concern is that of potential antigen exposure, which will complicate future renal transplantation in patients who do not regain renal function. The risk of sensitization to antigens is multiplied by the number of HD treatments required, because each will require a separate blood prime. In addition, a blood prime is a potential infectious exposure, and young children may acquire cytomegalovirus infection as a result. Furthermore, even if the primed blood circuit is infused at a low blood-flow rate (20 to 50 mL/min), it represents a rapid rate of blood transfusion. This may result in a transfusion reaction or hypocalcemia from citrate infusion. Finally, the potassium load associated with transfusion of packed red blood cells may produce sudden hyperkalemia with cardiac arrhythmias, which may not be corrected quickly enough by HD. This risk is diminished by washing packed red blood cells before the procedure. At the end of an HD treatment which began with a blood prime, the blood circuit is not returned to the patient.

Dialyzers

A wide variety of dialyzers have been used in children; no pediatric data suggest an advantage of one type of membrane. Extrapolating from studies in adults suggesting a benefit of biocompatible membranes on survival and recovery of AKI (80–82), these dialyzers have become standard in children. A more significant challenge is finding dialyzers of sufficiently small volume, surface area, and ultrafiltration coefficient (Kuf). Choices in dialyzers with surface area less than 0.4 m² are limited, and availability changes often. Small priming volume is an advantage when dialyzing infants and small children because it may allow one to avoid priming the circuit with blood. Dialyzers with relatively large surface area may be advantageous when rapid clearance is needed, but in most cases, clearance will be determined by the blood flow that one can achieve throughout the treatment, rather than the surface area or KoA of the dialyzer. In practice, all standard and high-flux dialyzers have a higher Kuf than is needed for adequate ultrafiltration in small children. Earlier, this was a great concern because small errors in setting the dialysis machine transmembrane pressure (TMP) could result in large ultrafiltration errors and hypotension. In addition, because pediatric vascular access is generally of small caliber, one finds high venous pressures that, in turn, result in greater TMP. This concern has been alleviated by the widespread use of machines with volumetric ultrafiltration controllers. However, during isovolemic HD (or even during modest ultrafiltration) with a high-flux dialyzer, backfiltration of dialysate is to be anticipated; this can be avoided by increasing the ultrafiltration rate sufficient to reverse negative TMP and infusing saline through the treatment (**TABLE 38.2**).

Vascular Access

Obtaining a well-functioning vascular access remains a challenge in small patients. Vascular access for acute HD is usually established by percutaneous placement of a double-lumen catheter. Whether a temporary or permanent (tunneled) dialysis catheter is chosen depends on one's estimate of the duration of dialysis therapy needed. This is often merely an approximation; patients typically begin urgent dialysis therapy with a temporary catheter, and a tunneled catheter is placed electively. Double-lumen catheters are available in sizes from 7 Fr to 14 Fr and come in various lengths; manufacturers and availability of the smallest catheters change frequently. Single-lumen catheters of 5 Fr and smaller are used for neonates. **TABLE 38.2** provides guidelines for catheter selection based on patient size. Ideally, the catheter should offer low resistance to blood flow and, therefore, should be a stiff catheter

TABLE 38.2	**Vascular Access Recommendations for the Pediatric Patient**	
Patient Size	**Catheter Size**	**Access Site**
Neonate	Umbilical artery catheter 3.5–5.0 Fr OR Umbilical vein catheter 5.0–8.5 Fr OR 5.0 Fr single lumen OR 7.0 Fr dual lumen	Umbilical vessels Femoral vein
5–15 kg	7–8 Fr dual lumen	Femoral/subclavian/ internal jugular vein
16–30 kg	9–11 Fr dual lumen	Internal jugular/femoral/ subclavian vein
>30 kg	10–12 Fr dual or triple lumen	Internal jugular/femoral/ subclavian vein

Adapted from Bunchman and Donckerwolcke (83) and Hacbarth et al. (84).

with a short length but large internal diameter (85). Broviac catheters, often already placed in oncology patients, are inappropriate because of their flexibility, length, and small lumen size. Acute dialysis catheters can be placed in the femoral vein, subclavian vein, or internal jugular vein; the choice depends on the size of the patient and the availability of central venous sites. Femoral catheters are technically easier to insert and are not associated with the risks of pneumothorax and pneumomediastinum or hemothorax and hemomediastinum. However, there is an increased risk of infection when left in place for more than a few days and patients are confined to bed. Catheters placed in the subclavian vein or internal jugular vein should have their tips positioned at the junction of the superior vena cava and right atrium to allow adequate blood flow and minimize recirculation. They may be left in place for several weeks, although a tunneled catheter would be a better choice for such a duration of dialysis.

In an infant, vessel size may make placement of even a small-caliber double-lumen catheter impossible, and one may be obliged to place single-lumen catheters in two sites. In the newborn, HD can be performed through small single-lumen catheters placed in the umbilical artery and vein. Small-caliber catheters increase the risk of hemolysis from sheer stress and can cause wide swings in access pressures affecting ultrafiltration and compromising the overall success of the treatment.

Dialysis Prescription

There are no prospective trials to assist clinicians in determining the adequacy of acute HD therapy in children with AKI. Because the spectrum of diseases causing AKI is different from that in adults, extrapolation from that literature may be difficult. Therefore, the duration, frequency, and efficiency of the HD treatments are a matter of judgment aided by an understanding of kinetic modeling and of the modifiable variables (blood flow, dialysate flow). Often, a single metabolic derangement (e.g., intoxication, hyperammonemia) defines the length and efficiency of the treatment. Nonetheless, when children are dialyzed for advanced uremia with standard dialyzers, the urea clearances that are achieved may be sufficient to cause true disequilibrium or seizures (which are a more common complication in children than in adults) (86,87). Blood-flow rate for the first few treatments may be decreased to target urea clearance of 2 to 3 mL/kg/min, and treatment length will usually be shortened to 1.5 to 2 hours to avoid precipitous falls in blood urea nitrogen (BUN) (86). Single-pool Kt/V for a first treatment in a uremic child should probably not exceed 0.6. Short daily treatments are often the most appropriate way to initiate HD therapy without patient discomfort or instability. Subsequent treatments are lengthened to 3 to 4 hours or longer if needed, and higher urea clearance rates can be targeted (blood-flow rates of 4 to 5 mL/kg/min). Smaller blood vessels and catheters cause higher venous resistance than in adults, and this will eventually limit blood flow, perhaps as low as 25 to 100 mL/min.

Acute HD treatments in children should only be performed with bicarbonate-based dialysate. Otherwise, small patients will be presented with a disproportionately large acetate load, and their small muscle mass will be inadequate to metabolize it. Dialysate flow rates range from 300 to 900 mL/min, as in adults. For treatments using low blood flows and dialyzers of low KoA, dialysate flow rates are not rate limiting for clearance and the lower range will be sufficient.

Ultrafiltration is targeted to the patient's clinical situation. If severe volume overload is present, rapid ultrafiltration may be appropriate. Otherwise, one attempts to limit total fluid removal per session to 5% of the patient's body weight (71). Critically ill patients in intensive care units often require large volumes of medications, feedings, and blood products resulting in ongoing fluid overload and hemodynamic instability with HD treatments. Close monitoring of blood pressure, ideally by an arterial line, is required. If isolated ultrafiltration without dialysate is planned in an infant or small child, hypothermia may develop because the dialysis circuit acts as a radiator that is relatively large for the patient's total blood volume.

Some form of anticoagulation is generally needed when performing HD in children particularly because the blood-flow rates are often slow, increasing the risk of clotting. Systemic heparinization is used most commonly with doses scaled to body size and then adjusted according to activated clotting times (ACTs). A loading dose of 10 to 30 U/kg is given at the start followed by a maintenance dose of 10 to 20 U/kg/hr. ACTs are followed at the bedside when machines and trained personnel are available, and the heparin dose is titrated to keep the ACT between 150 and 200 seconds (88).

There are alternative strategies for maintaining circuit patency in children at high risk for bleeding complications including (a) saline flushes without other anticoagulation, (b) regional heparinization with protamine reversal, (c) low-dose heparin, and (d) regional citrate anticoagulation. There is little published experience on the use of these other anticoagulation strategies in pediatric HD patients, and many nephrologists rely on saline flushes and avoid the use of anticoagulation (88). However, the volume of saline used to flush the circuit increases the treatment ultrafiltration and may be poorly tolerated in small child. Heparin-induced thrombocytopenia has been reported in children receiving dialysis, although the largest pediatric experience comes from patients on extracorporeal life-support systems after cardiac repair; argatroban, danaparoid, and hirudin have been used successfully for anticoagulation in this setting (89–92). See Chapter 4 for further details regarding anticoagulation on HD.

Dialysis Prescription for Nonkidney Disease Indication–Hyperammonemia and Other Inborn Errors of Metabolism

Prescription considerations are somewhat different when children are being dialyzed for nonkidney disease indications such as intoxications, hyperammonemia, or other inborn errors of metabolism. In this situation, rapid clearance from the blood is paramount (74); therefore, it is essential to have a well-functioning vascular access because blood-flow rates as high as 10 to 15 mL/kg/min may be needed (75,77). Dialysis disequilibrium is not a concern in this situation because patients are not uremic. These children are critically ill and are often intravascularly volume depleted because there is often a preceding history of lethargy, poor intake, and vomiting. In addition, because their kidney function is normal, they continue to produce urine. Careful monitoring of intravascular volume status and electrolyte balance is required. Supplemental intravenous fluids should be provided as needed, and pressor support may be required to tolerate the dialysis procedures. Dialysate potassium and bicarbonate must be adjusted to avoid creating hypokalemia and metabolic alkalosis, and one should avoid high-calcium dialysate. Phosphorus levels can be expected to fall, and supplementation may be required (76–77). Metabolite levels are monitored and dictate the duration, efficiency, and frequency of HD sessions, but prolonged and repeated sessions are often required (93). Rebound and ongoing production of metabolites following HD should be anticipated. CRRTs have also been used successfully alone and in conjunction with HD to control the hyperammonemia and other inborn errors of metabolism (94–97).

Hemodialysis for Management of Toxic Ingestions

Initial management of toxic ingestions involves gastric decontamination measures, administration of antidotes if available, and supportive care (98). Certain drugs and toxins have been shown to be effectively removed by extracorporeal therapies (99). HD may be beneficial for removal of small molecular weight compounds (e.g., lithium, salicylates) that are not highly protein bound and that have a small volume of distribution. In addition, HD allows correction of metabolic disturbances that may result from the ingestion. For toxins with a large volume of distribution in which one anticipates a rebound following acute HD, addition of continuous hemofiltration or continuous HD has been reported to be effective (21,100). For toxins that are highly protein bound, hemofiltration may still be of benefit to remove free drug once the protein is saturated (101). Charcoal hemoperfusion has also been shown to be effective in removing certain drugs that are protein bound (e.g., phenytoin, phenobarbital, theophylline, carbamazepine). Published reports on the use of hemoperfusion in pediatrics are limited but suggest that the procedure can be safely performed in children (101–103). As with HD, the volume of the extracorporeal circuit is of concern and should not exceed 10% of the child's blood volume to ensure hemodynamic stability. See Chapter 36 for further detail regarding hemoperfusion and its indications. Case reports suggest that high-efficiency HD may be an effective alternative therapy to charcoal hemoperfusion for removal of certain drugs (e.g., vancomycin, carbamazepine) (104,105). Potential complications associated with charcoal hemoperfusion such as thrombocytopenia, coagulopathy, hypocalcemia, and hypothermia can also be avoided using high-efficiency HD.

Selected Complications of Hemodialysis in Infants and Children

Hemodynamic instability is one of the most common complications occurring on dialysis. Risk factors in the pediatric patient include (a) hypotension due to multiple organ dysfunction syndrome (MODS), (b) excessive ultrafiltration, (c) extracorporeal circuit volume exceeding 10% of the patient's blood volume in the absence of a blood prime, and (d) removal of vasopressors by dialysis. Under normal conditions, children have lower blood pressures than adults and a narrower margin to development of hypotension. Intradialytic hypotension may develop abruptly; therefore, volume removal must be closely monitored during treatments.

As mentioned earlier, overly rapid urea clearance is more likely to occur in small children and in those with high BUN or prolonged azotemia. It may precipitate osmolar shifts and symptomatic disequilibrium with nausea, vomiting, headache, and even seizures and coma. Strategies to limit clearance (as mentioned earlier) for the first few treatments in children with long-standing uremia are usually advisable.

Dialyzer reactions are infrequent but potentially fatal when they occur; therefore, prompt recognition and management are essential. Mild forms include itching, urticaria, wheezing, flushing, cough, and emesis, whereas severe reactions include dyspnea and hypotension. Various inciting agents have been implicated including ethylene oxide, bradykinin (with the AN69 membrane), contaminated dialysate, and heparin (106–108). If suspected, dialysis should immediately be terminated and the blood not returned to the patient (see Chapter 1).

Additional potential complications include bleeding, infection, air embolus, and thrombosis. Those with a catheter in the subclavian or internal jugular vein are also at risk for developing the superior vena cava syndrome given the placement of a relatively large diameter catheter into a small vessel.

⬡ CONTINUOUS RENAL REPLACEMENT THERAPIES

CRRT offers several advantages over the other forms of RRT including more gradual and predictable, yet more efficient, correction of hypervolemia and uremia. However, as with HD, a well-functioning vascular access is mandatory, and some form of anticoagulation is typically needed (see Chapter 10). With the development of more sophisticated CRRT machines, it is possible to provide precise ultrafiltration control, thermal control, and a variety of blood-flow rates appropriate for infants through adolescents. The machines offer a wide range of therapeutic options: slow continuous ultrafiltration (SCUF), continuous venovenous hemofiltration (CVVH), continuous venovenous hemodialysis (CVVHD), or continuous venovenous hemodiafiltration (CVVHDF), with some machines having the added flexibility for use in conventional HD (109). Additional improvements have included the development of pediatric blood lines and hemofilters and hemodialyzers. CRRT can now be safely and effectively performed in infants and children, and it has become the preferred mode of therapy in many tertiary care pediatric hospitals in the industrialized world (3,10,27,110). Prospective registry data on CRRT in infants and children is now available, providing valuable insights into practice patterns and outcomes (111). The recognition that fluid overload is an independent risk factor for mortality in children with AKI has spurred earlier use of CRRT to manage diuretic-resistant hypervolemia (28,29).

The use of CRRT in pediatrics extends beyond therapy for AKI. Phosphorus clearance through CRRT is superior to HD and is frequently employed in tumor lysis syndrome in children with Burkitt lymphoma and acute lymphoblastic leukemia (112,113). It may be used alone or as an adjunct to HD in cases of toxic ingestions, and inborn errors of metabolism where rebound of solute is anticipated (74,95,97,114–116). In addition, it is used as an adjunctive therapy with extracorporeal membrane oxygenation (ECMO) (see below) (117–119).

Slow Continuous Ultrafiltration

SCUF is shown to be beneficial in clinical situations such as postoperative congenital heart repair in which isolated fluid removal is required (120). Significant volume overload (usually considered greater than 10% body weight) is a risk factor for mortality in AKI and after bone marrow transplant (BMT), encouraging earlier initiation of CRRT, although SCUF is usually not described separately in those reports (14,16,17,27–29). Ultrafiltration volumes must be carefully monitored to prevent excessive fluid and solute loss. Furthermore, hypothermia may occur in small children if warmed dialysate or replacement fluid is not used. In-line blood warmers are available for some machines, but they may add significantly to the volume of the extracorporeal circuit.

Continuous Arteriovenous Hemofiltration

Continuous arteriovenous hemofiltration (CAVH) has been used successfully in the management of pediatric AKI and in the management of fluid overload and azotemia in oliguric children following surgical repair of congenital heart disease (42,120–124). It is tolerated well in hemodynamically unstable children and offers the advantages of technical simplicity, low priming volume, and gentle fluid removal. However, it requires both arterial and venous vascular access. In the neonate, this may be accomplished by cannulating the umbilical vessels or the femoral vessels, whereas in an older child, arterial access can be obtained through the radial artery. Reasonable blood-flow rates have been reported with mean arterial pressures greater than 40 mm Hg (83). However, because the circuit is driven by the patient's arterial blood pressure, the blood-flow rate and ultrafiltration rate may vary as the blood pressure fluctuates, which in turn increases the risk for clotting. Some form of anticoagulation is, therefore, necessary to maintain circuit patency. Incorporation of a pump into the circuit to provide more consistent blood flow (pump-assisted CAVH) has been reported to be beneficial in patients with low blood pressures (125,126). If needed, dialysis can be added for better metabolic control (continuous arteriovenous HD or hemodiafiltration).

Continuous Venovenous Hemofiltration/Hemodialysis/Hemodiafiltration

The development of more sophisticated CRRT machines that are suitable for use in small children makes CVVH, CVVHD, and CVVHDF the more common choice for initial management of pediatric AKI; venovenous forms of CRRT are the most common of the continuous modalities used in children (3,27). With the venovenous forms of CRRT, one avoids the need for arterial catheter placement and its associated risks of bleeding, thrombosis, and limb ischemia with potential impaired future limb growth. Incorporation of a blood pump into the circuit increases the extracorporeal circuit volume and complexity of the procedure, but it also allows consistency in blood-flow rate which stabilizes clearance and ultrafiltration (127). Fluid or blood warmers provide thermal control and the addition of integrated balances and tightly calibrated pumps allows for greater confidence in monitoring ultrafiltration (83,128). Newer machines are also equipped with software programs to assist in troubleshooting problems at the bedside, a particularly beneficial feature for the intensive care unit staff providing therapy. Nonetheless, currently available machines are not designed to provide sufficient precision in ultrafiltration and replacement solutions for children under 10 kg, and clinicians must be vigilant for unintended volume overload or depletion. A truly miniaturized CRRT device for neonates is still in development (129).

Vascular Access and Extracorporeal Circuit

As with HD, a well-functioning venous vascular access is critical. See section "Hemodialysis" of this chapter for a review of issues related to pediatric vascular access. An analysis of catheter size in CRRT showed that circuit survival was significantly worse for the smallest catheters (5 Fr, 7 Fr, and 9 Fr, although not 8 Fr) and better when the catheter was placed in the internal jugular vein (84). There did not seem to be a difference in circuit survival when comparing larger catheters (10 to 12 Fr).

As in HD, whenever possible, the blood lines and hemofilter or hemodialyzer should be selected to keep the extracorporeal circuit volume less than 10% of the patient's blood volume or a blood prime may be necessary. Some systems offer flexibility in choosing blood lines and hemofilters. However, even with this flexibility, the circuit volume may still exceed 10% of the patient's blood volume and a blood prime may be necessary (83). Risks associated with use of a blood prime are reviewed in detail in section "Hemodialysis" and include potential antigen exposure, potential infectious exposure, transfusion reaction, hyperkalemia, and citrate overload with hypocalcemia. Washing red blood cells diminishes excess potassium but does not remove concerns of rapid antigen exposure or electrolyte disturbance. Furthermore, use of a blood prime in conjunction with an AN-69 membrane may result in the bradykinin release syndrome. Brophy et al. (130) described this potentially fatal syndrome in two children beginning CRRT with an AN-69 hemofilter. Symptoms of hypotension, tachycardia, vasodilatation, and anaphylaxis typically begin within minutes of CRRT initiation and resolve with discontinuation of CRRT. It is important to be cognizant of this potential complication as it is may be preventable. On the basis of the theory that exposure of blood to the AN-69 hemofilter in an acidotic milieu results in the generation of bradykinin, prevention strategies have been proposed. One strategy, zero-balance ultrafiltration, entails circulating the blood prime through the CRRT machine with a customized, electrolyte-balanced replacement solution to normalize potassium, calcium, and pH prior to initiating therapy (131). Another strategy involves buffering the packed red blood cells with tromethamine (THAM) and bicarbonate to correct the pH closer to physiologic (7.3 to 7.6) before priming the circuit (132). If the CRRT procedure is interrupted for a short time, the blood prime may be recirculated. However, the circuit pH and electrolyte composition should be rechecked before resuming the CRRT treatment. If clotting or deterioration in the circulated blood occurs, a new blood prime should be performed. Finally, larger infants and toddlers may tolerate a normal saline prime and simultaneous direct transfusion of blood into the patient at therapy initiation (130).

Anticoagulation

Anticoagulation strategies are evenly divided between heparin and citrate, but individual centers have marked preferences (133). There is no difference in circuit life, although there are more bleeding episodes associated with heparin use. In large series, 7% to 12% of treatments were performed without anticoagulation because of bleeding concerns. This practice is associated with shorter circuit life (133,134).

Heparin anticoagulation is more often used in infants and children less than 10 kg (134). Heparin doses are adjusted for body weight as for HD and then titrated as per the ACT or activated partial thromboplastin time (aPTT). A loading dose of 10 to 50 U/kg is administered at the start, followed by a maintenance dose of 10 to 20 U/kg/h. ACT levels are monitored postfilter and the heparin dose adjusted to keep the ACT between 150 and 220 seconds or the aPTT 1.5 to 2 times control (83). Potential complications associated with heparin use include risk of bleeding, heparin-induced thrombocytopenia, and allergic reactions.

Regional citrate anticoagulation offers the advantage of anticoagulating the extracorporeal circuit but not the patient and, therefore, reduces the risk of hemorrhage. Citrate exhibits its effect by chelating calcium, a necessary cofactor for the coagulation cascade. Citrate is infused into the arterial limb of the circuit at a rate that results in a postfilter ionized calcium level of 0.35 to 0.45 mmol/L and a systemic calcium infusion is administered postfilter or through a separate vascular access at a rate that maintains a systemic ionized calcium level of 1.1 to 1.3 mmol/L (135,136). Placement of a triple-lumen dialysis catheter can be advantageous when citrate anticoagulation is used because the third port can be used for calcium infusion. Calcium-free dialysate is preferable because calcium present in dialysate may chelate with citrate on the surface of the hemofilter membrane resulting in a higher citrate requirement to achieve adequate anticoagulation. Monitoring is much easier than with heparin and consists of following the postfilter ionized calcium and systemic ionized calcium. Citrate use can, however, result in several metabolic complications; therefore, close monitoring of serum electrolytes is also required. Generally, these metabolic derangements can be anticipated, allowing appropriate interventions to be made in a timely fashion. Metabolic alkalosis is the major disturbance that arises as citrate is metabolized into bicarbonate. Children are particularly prone to the development of metabolic alkalosis because the rate of citrate infusion is proportional to the blood-flow rate, which is relatively higher in small children as compared with adults. Management requires adjustment of the bicarbonate concentration in the dialysate. In one pediatric series, metabolic alkalosis was noted in every patient who required more than 7 days of CRRT (136). Additional metabolic complications include hypomagnesemia resulting from citrate chelation of magnesium and hypernatremia resulting from the sodium content of the citrate solution. Two citrate preparations are currently available: trisodium citrate (4% sodium citrate) and anticoagulant citrate dextrose-A (ACD-A; sodium citrate, anhydrous citrate, and dextrose) that differ in their sodium and dextrose content. ACD-A contains 2.45% dextrose and can result in hyperglycemia, particularly in infants. Trisodium citrate solution is more likely to result in hypernatremia. "Citrate lock," another potential risk, manifests by a rising total serum calcium associated with falling ionized calcium and results from citrate accumulation, when the rate of infusion exceeds the clearance and metabolism. Caution with the use of citrate is, therefore, required in the presence of liver disease and frequent blood transfusions. Overall regional citrate is a successful anticoagulation strategy in children with comparable circuit survival time (133) and decreased nursing time compared with the use of heparin (136).

Alternative strategies for maintaining patency of the CRRT circuit are similar to those used in HD and include (a) use of saline flushes and no anticoagulation, (b) regional heparinization with protamine reversal postfilter, (c) low molecular weight heparin, (d) prostacyclin, and (e) use of other anticoagulants such as hirudin and argatroban. Regional heparinization with protamine reversal has been problematic because of difficulty achieving good control over the degree of anticoagulation and because of the potential risk of hypotension and anaphylaxis associated with protamine (83). There are no data to guide the use of low molecular weight heparin or hirudin in children on CRRT. However, the successful use of argatroban in two neonates undergoing extracorporeal life-support therapy (ECMO) has been reported (137).

Solutions

Dialysate solutions specifically designed for use with CRRT are commercially available with a bicarbonate buffer. PD fluid is not a desirable choice for dialysate with CRRT. Studies in adults and children have shown improved hemodynamic stability and lower lactate levels when a bicarbonate-based solution is used as compared to lactate solutions (138).

While commercially manufactured solutions are approved by the U.S. Food and Drug Administration (FDA) as dialysate, most centers use them as replacement solution in CVVH or for both fluids when CVVHDF is performed (139). Standard intravenous fluids such as lactated Ringer's and normal saline with or without other supplemental electrolytes are sometimes infused simultaneously or alternated with commercial dialysate when severe metabolic alkalosis occurs. However, if lactated Ringer's or normal saline are used alone as replacement solutions in small patients, one can anticipate metabolic perturbation because of the nonphysiologic pH and electrolyte composition of the solutions. Custom-made solutions prepared by hospital pharmacists have been used with the goal of tailoring the electrolyte replacement to individual patient needs, but they lack regulated quality control standards, are time-consuming to prepare, and carry the well-recognized risk of formulation error (139). Replacement fluid can be administered either prefilter or postfilter. Hemodilution from prefilter replacement could theoretically decrease the risk of filter clotting in children requiring slow blood-flow rates, but comparative data to support this are lacking.

Prescription Considerations

Descriptive data are available on typical blood-flow rate (Q_B), dialysate flow rate (Q_D), and ultrafiltration rate for pediatric patients receiving CRRT (27,134). Data regarding the adequacy of CRRT for pediatric AKI do not exist. Prescription guidelines are, therefore, based on experience and extrapolation from the adult literature. Although the blood-flow rate for adults receiving CRRT is significantly lower than that required for HD, the blood-flow rate required for small children on CRRT is comparable to that required for HD to maintain circuit patency. It typically ranges from 3 to 5 mL/kg/min, although reported ranges are much wider and the lowest Q_B delivered by most machines (20 to 30 mL/min) results in very large flow rates in the smallest patients (83,128,134). Dialysate and replacement fluid flow rates, on the other hand, generally range from 35 to 50 mL/kg/h and is similar to the rate of 2 to 3 L/1.73 m^2/h used for adults. Data regarding a safe rate of fluid removal on CRRT are lacking. There are no prospective pediatric data indicating that one modality (CVVH vs. CVVHD vs. CVVHDF) is superior to another. Small molecular weight solutes are removed equally well with continuous hemofiltration and continuous HD; larger molecular weight solutes are cleared better with hemofiltration than HD.

However, due to small patient size and relatively large Q_B, clearance can be very efficient by all modalities.

CRRT is utilized for nonkidney disease indications as well. Current practice in many PICUs is to consider initiating therapy based upon degree of volume overload rather than waiting for severe electrolyte disturbance. CRRT is the preferred mode of clearance in the tumor lysis syndrome because it permits efficient phosphate removal without rebound and it can be sustained while cell lysis is ongoing (92,112,140). It provides efficient urate clearance as well. CRRT has been combined with acute HD in the management of hyperammonemia from inborn errors of metabolism to prevent rebound at the end of HD treatment (94,95).

Selected Complications

Although CRRT seems to be better tolerated hemodynamically than intermittent HD, hypotension still occurs, particularly at the initiation of therapy if the extracorporeal circuit volume is large relative to the patient's circulating blood volume, or when excessive fluid is removed. Unpredictable and excessive fluid removal is a concern when pediatric CRRT is performed using ad hoc or adaptive machinery: Medication infusion pumps used to measure dialysate flow and ultrafiltration are unreliable at high flow rates (83,128,141). Currently available sophisticated CRRT machines contain integrated, precise scales or pumps that reduce errors in fluid balance, although there remains concern for excessive volume removal or overload in neonates. A blood prime can reduce hemodynamic instability, yet the use of a blood prime in association with an AN-69 hemofilter membrane may result in the potentially fatal yet potentially preventable bradykinin release syndrome discussed in section "Vascular Access and Extracorporeal Circuit" (130). Rapid transfusion of the blood prime at CRRT initiation can cause hypocalcemia, hyperkalemia, or transfusion reaction. Other risks of blood priming are discussed earlier in the chapter.

In addition to solute and electrolyte losses on CRRT, data in children and neonates indicate that amino acid losses on CRRT can also be significant, contributing to negative nitrogen balance (142). Therefore, to maintain a positive nitrogen balance, nutritional supplementation adjusted to provide higher protein intake (up to 3 to 4 g/kg/d) may be required. The potential catabolic complications of pediatric CRRT require further research.

CVVH can provide extremely efficient clearance in a small child, rivalling endogenous renal function. Critical medications which may have had dose adjustments applied for kidney disease may then circulate at ineffectively low levels. Vasopressor clearance can be corrected based upon measured blood pressure, but antibiotics or antineoplastic agents may be erroneously underdosed in this situation. Pediatric pharmacokinetic guidelines have not been developed, and one often extrapolates from adult studies (where clearance and circuit volume are in a very different relationship than in children) (143). Finally, if CRRT is paused for any reason, the pharmacokinetic extrapolations may no longer be valid. Repeated reevaluation of medication dosing in relation to CRRT efficiency and clinical response is required.

Dialysis disequilibrium generally does not occur with continuous therapies because solute removal occurs more slowly, thereby avoiding the development of rapid osmolar shifts and risk for the disequilibrium syndrome (144).

Hypothermia occurs more commonly when adaptive machinery is used for pediatric CRRT. Newer machines are available with an integrated fluid warmer or a blood warmer. Additional risks associated with CRRT relate to the need for anticoagulation to maintain circuit patency and include (a) hemorrhage if heparin is used, (b) metabolic alkalosis if regional citrate is used (see section "Anticoagulation" for more complete discussion on potential complications associated with citrate use), and (c) blood loss through circuit clotting if anticoagulation therapy is not administered. Finally, there are also risks associated with placing and maintaining vascular access. This is reviewed in the subsection regarding complications of pediatric HD.

Continuous Renal Replacement Therapy and Extracorporeal Life-Support Therapy

The use of ECMO for management of children with cardiac and respiratory failure has become more widespread. Hypervolemia and AKI are well-recognized complications during ECMO (145). CRRT has become an important adjunctive therapy in this setting when diuretic therapy alone is insufficient for fluid removal. CRRT can be performed simultaneously with ECMO in critically ill children (118–120,146–149). A hemofilter can be incorporated into the ECMO circuit without the need for additional vascular access or the need for additional anticoagulation (96,97). While some centers will use only a dialyzer and permit pressure-driven ultrafiltration, use of a CRRT machine allows more precise volume control and chemical clearance by hemofiltration, continuous HD, or hemodiafiltration. The CRRT circuit is placed in line with the ECMO circuit before the oxygenator (150–152). Consideration should be given to positioning of the hemofilter within the ECMO circuit with regard to blood recirculation and shunting away from the oxygenator, although the blood flow through the CRRT circuit is a small fraction of the flow within the overall ECMO circuit (150).

Continuous Renal Replacement Therapy and Cardiopulmonary Bypass

Hemofiltration has also been beneficial for fluid removal in children receiving cardiopulmonary bypass (153). In a novel extension of hemofiltration in this setting, Journois et al. (154) reported initial experience with high-volume zero-balanced hemofiltration (5 L/m^2) in 10 children during the rewarming phase of cardiopulmonary bypass in an attempt to decrease the inflammatory response to cardiopulmonary bypass. The authors attributed the improved outcome (less blood loss, fever, and ventilatory support) to the removal of proinflammatory mediators during the rewarming phase.

⬡ SUMMARY

Nephrologists have the tools to provide all forms of RRT to infants and children. However, despite these advances, the mortality rate from AKI in children remains high, likely in part the result of the severity of the underlying disease process (10,155). While no prospective data exist comparing the three treatment modalities for management of pediatric AKI, the Pediatric CRRT Registry has gathered more complete data on pediatric experience with CRRT from which prescription guidelines may emerge. At present, however, the choice of modality for RRT in children continues to be made at the bedside based upon the best institutional experience.

⬡ REFERENCES

1. Flynn JT. Choice of dialysis modality for management of pediatric acute renal failure. *Pediatr Nephrol* 2002;17(1):61–69. doi:10.1007/s004670200011.
2. Warady BA, Bunchman T. Dialysis therapy for children with acute renal failure: survey results. *Pediatr Nephrol* 2000;15(1–2):11–13.
3. Goldstein SL. Overview of pediatric renal replacement therapy in acute kidney injury. *Semin Dial* 2009;22(2):180–184. doi:10.1111/j.1525-139X.2008.00551.x.
4. Walters S, Porter C, Brophy PD. Dialysis and pediatric acute kidney injury: choice of renal support modality. *Pediatr Nephrol* 2009;24(1):37–48. doi:10.1007/s00467-008-0826-x.
5. Akcan-Arikan A, Zappitelli M, Loftis LL, et al. Modified RIFLE criteria in critically ill children with acute kidney injury. *Kidney Int* 2007;71(10):1028–1035.
6. Mehta RL, Kellum JA, Shah SV, et al. Acute kidney injury network: report of an initiative to improve outcomes in acute kidney injury. *Crit Care* 2007;11(2):R31.
7. Kidney Disease: Improving Global Outcomes. KDIGO clinical practice guideline for acute kidney injury. *Kidney Int* 2012;2(1):1–141.
8. Sutherland SM, Byrnes JJ, Kothari M, et al. AKI in hospitalized children: comparing the pRIFLE, AKIN, and KDIGO definitions. *Clin J Am Soc Nephrol* 2015;10(4):554–561. doi:10.2215/CJN.01900214.
9. Hui-Stickle S, Brewer ED, Goldstein SL. Pediatric ARF epidemiology at a tertiary care center from 1999 to 2001. *Am J Kidney Dis* 2005;45(1):96–101. doi:10.1053/j.ajkd.2004.09.028.
10. Bunchman TE, McBryde KD, Mottes TE, et al. Pediatric acute renal failure: outcome by modality and disease. *Pediatr Nephrol* 2001;16(12):1067–1071. doi:10.1007/s004670100029.
11. Lex DJ, Tóth R, Cserép Z, et al. A comparison of the systems for the identification of postoperative acute kidney injury in pediatric cardiac patients. *Ann Thorac Surg* 2014;97(1):202–210. doi:10.1016/j.athoracsur.2013.09.01.
12. Moffett BS, Goldstein SL. Acute kidney injury and increasing nephrotoxic-medication exposure in noncritically-ill children. *Clin J Am Soc Nephrol* 2011;6(4):856–863. doi:10.2215/CJN.08110910.
13. Flynn JT. Causes, management approaches, and outcome of acute renal failure in children. *Curr Opin Pediatr* 1998;10(2):184–189.
14. Ball EF, Kara T. Epidemiology and outcome of acute kidney injury in New Zealand children. *J Paediatr Child Health* 2008;44(11):642–646. doi:10.1111/j.1440-1754.2008.01373.x.
15. Williams DM, Sreedhar SS, Mickell JJ, et al. Acute kidney failure: a pediatric experience over 20 years. *Arch Pediatr Adolesc Med* 2002;156(9):893–900.
16. Radhakrishnan J, Kiryluk K. Acute renal failure outcomes in children and adults. *Kidney Int* 2006;69(1):17–19.
17. Barletta GM, Bunchman TE. Acute renal failure in children and infants. *Curr Opin Crit Care* 2004;10(6):499–504. doi:00075198-200412000-00013.
18. Fortenberry JD, Paden ML, Goldstein SL. Acute kidney injury in children: an update on diagnosis and treatment. *Pediatr Clin North Am* 2013;60(3):669–688. doi:10.1016/j.pcl.2013.02.006.
19. Basu RK, Devarajan P, Wong H, et al. An update and review of acute kidney injury in pediatrics. *Pediatr Crit Care Med* 2011;12(3):339–347. doi:10.1097/PCC.0b013e3181fe2e0b.
20. Bunchman TE. Treatment of acute kidney injury in children: from conservative management to renal replacement therapy. *Nat Clin Pract Nephrol* 2008;4(9):510–514. doi:10.1038/ncpneph0924.
21. Darracq MA, Cantrell FL. Hemodialysis and extracorporeal removal after pediatric and adolescent poisoning reported to a state poison center. *J Emerg Med* 2013;44(6):1101–1107. doi:10.1016/j.jemermed.2012.12.018.
22. Tsai IJ, Hwu WL, Huang SC, et al. Efficacy and safety of intermittent hemodialysis in infants and young children with inborn errors of metabolism. *Pediatr Nephrol* 2014;29(1):111–116. doi:10.1007/s00467-013-2609-2.
23. Fleming GM, Walters S, Goldstein SL, et al. Nonrenal indications for continuous renal replacement therapy: a report from the prospective pediatric continuous renal replacement therapy registry group. *Pediatr Crit Care Med* 2012;13(5):e299–e304. doi:10.1097/PCC.0b013e31824fbd76.
24. Bunchman TE. The complexity of dialytic therapy in hyperammonemic neonates. *Pediatr Nephrol.* 2015;30(5):701–702. doi:10.1007/s00467-014-2998-x.

25. Sutherland SM, Zappitelli M, Alexander SR, et al. Fluid overload and mortality in children receiving continuous renal replacement therapy: the prospective pediatric continuous renal replacement therapy registry. *Am J Kidney Dis* 2010;55(2):316–325. doi:10.1053/j.ajkd.2009.10.048.

26. Bridges BC, Askenazi DJ, Smith J, et al. Pediatric renal replacement therapy in the intensive care unit. *Blood Purif* 2012;34(2):138–148. doi:10.1159/000342129.

27. Goldstein SL, Somers MJ, Baum MA, et al. Pediatric patients with multi-organ dysfunction syndrome receiving continuous renal replacement therapy. *Kidney Int* 2005;67(2):653–658.

28. Foland JA, Fortenberry JD, Warshaw BL, et al. Fluid overload before continuous hemofiltration and survival in critically ill children: a retrospective analysis. *Crit Care Med* 2004;32(8):1771–1776.

29. Gillespie RS, Seidel K, Symons JM. Effect of fluid overload and dose of replacement fluid on survival in hemofiltration. *Pediatr Nephrol* 2004;19(12):1394–1399. doi:10.1007/s00467-004-1655-1.

30. Michael M, Kuehnle I, Goldstein SL. Fluid overload and acute renal failure in pediatric stem cell transplant patients. *Pediatr Nephrol* 2004;19(1):91–95. doi:10.1007/s00467-003-1313-z.

31. DiCarlo JV, Alexander SR, Agarwal R, et al. Continuous veno-venous hemofiltration may improve survival from acute respiratory distress syndrome after bone marrow transplantation or chemotherapy. *J Pediatr Hematol Oncol* 2003;25(10):801–805.

32. Flores FX, Brophy PD, Symons JM, et al. Continuous renal replacement therapy (CRRT) after stem cell transplantation. A report from the prospective pediatric CRRT registry group. *Pediatr Nephrol* 2008;23(4):625–630. doi:10.1007/s00467-007-0672-2.

33. Flynn JT, Kershaw DB, Smoyer WE, et al. Peritoneal dialysis for management of pediatric acute renal failure. *Perit Dial Int* 2001;21(4):390–394.

34. Passadakis PS, Oreopoulos DG. Peritoneal dialysis in patients with acute renal failure. *Adv Perit Dial* 2007;23:7–16.

35. Bonilla-Félix M. Peritoneal dialysis in the pediatric intensive care unit setting. *Perit Dial Int* 2009;29(Suppl 2):S183–S185.

36. Bunchman TE. Acute peritoneal dialysis access in infant renal failure. *Perit Dial Int* 1996;16(Suppl 1):S509–S511.

37. Esperanca M, Collins D. Peritoneal dialysis efficiency in relation to body weight. *J Pediatr Surg* 1966;1:162–169.

38. Mendley SR, Majkowski NL. Peritoneal equilibration test results are different in infants, children, and adults. *J Am Soc Nephrol* 1995;6(4):1309–1312.

39. Kwiatkowski DM, Menon S, Krawczeski CD, et al. Improved outcomes with peritoneal dialysis catheter placement after cardiopulmonary bypass in infants. *J Thorac Cardiovasc Surg* 2015;149(1):230–236. doi:10.1016/j.jtcvs.2013.11.040.

40. Lin MC, Fu YC, Fu LS, et al. Peritoneal dialysis in children with acute renal failure after open heart surgery. *Acta Paediatr Taiwan* 2003;44(2):89–92.

41. Sasser WC, Dabal RJ, Askenazi DJ, et al. Prophylactic peritoneal dialysis following cardiopulmonary bypass in children is associated with decreased inflammation and improved clinical outcomes. *Congenit Heart Dis* 2014;9(2):106–115. doi:10.1111/chd.12072.

42. Fleming F, Bohn D, Edwards H, et al. Renal replacement therapy after repair of congenital heart disease in children. A comparison of hemofiltration and peritoneal dialysis. *J Thorac Cardiovasc Surg* 1995;109(2):322–331. doi:10.1016/S0022-5223(95)70394-2.

43. Ryerson LM, Mackie AS, Atallah J, et al. Prophylactic peritoneal dialysis catheter does not decrease time to achieve a negative fluid balance after the Norwood procedure: a randomized controlled trial. *J Thorac Cardiovasc Surg* 2015;149(1):222–228. doi:10.1016/j.jtcvs.2014.08.011.

44. Picca S, Dionisi-Vici C, Bartuli A, et al. Short-term survival of hyperammonemic neonates treated with dialysis. *Pediatr Nephrol* 2015;30(5):839–847. doi:10.1007/s00467-014-2945-x.

45. Auron A, Warady BA, Simon S, et al. Use of the multipurpose drainage catheter for the provision of acute peritoneal dialysis in infants and children. *Am J Kidney Dis* 2007;49(5):650–655.

46. Day RE, White RH. Peritoneal dialysis in children. Review of 8 years' experience. *Arch Dis Child* 1977;52(1):56–61.

47. Chadha V, Warady BA, Blowey DL, et al. Tenckhoff catheters prove superior to cook catheters in pediatric acute peritoneal dialysis. *Am J Kidney Dis* 2000;35(6):1111–1116.

48. Lewis MA, Nycyk JA. Practical peritoneal dialysis—the Tenckhoff catheter in acute renal failure. *Pediatr Nephrol* 1992;6(5):470–475.

49. Daschner M, Gfrörer S, Zachariou Z, et al. Laparoscopic Tenckhoff catheter implantation in children. *Perit Dial Int* 2002;22(1):22–26.

50. Furth SL, Donaldson LA, Sullivan EK, et al. Peritoneal dialysis catheter infections and peritonitis in children: a report of the North American Pediatric Renal Transplant Cooperative Study. *Pediatr Nephrol* 2000;15(3–4):179–182.

51. Warady BA, Sullivan EK, Alexander SR. Lessons from the peritoneal dialysis patient database: a report of the North American Pediatric Renal Transplant Cooperative Study. *Kidney Int Suppl* 1996;53:S68–S71.

52. Washburn KK, Currier H, Salter KJ, et al. Surgical technique for peritoneal dialysis catheter placement in the pediatric patient: a North American survey. *Adv Perit Dial* 2004;20:218–221.

53. Clark KR, Forsythe JL, Rigg KM, et al. Surgical aspects of chronic peritoneal dialysis in the neonate and infant under 1 year of age. *J Pediatr Surg* 1992;27(6):780–783.

54. Orkin BA, Fonkalsrud EW, Salusky IB, et al. Continuous ambulatory peritoneal dialysis catheters in children. *Arch Surg* 1983;118(12):1398–1402.

55. Conlin MJ, Tank ES. Minimizing surgical problems of peritoneal dialysis in children. *J Urol* 1995;154(2 Pt 2):917–919.

56. Lewis M, Webb N, Smith T, et al. Routine omentectomy is not required in children undergoing chronic peritoneal dialysis. *Adv Perit Dial* 1995;11:293–295.

57. Liberek T, Topley N, Jörres A, et al. Peritoneal dialysis fluid inhibition of phagocyte function: effects of osmolality and glucose concentration. *J Am Soc Nephrol* 1993;3(8):1508–1515.

58. Nau B, Schmitt CP, Almeida M, et al. BIOKID: randomized controlled trial comparing bicarbonate and lactate buffer in biocompatible peritoneal dialysis solutions in children. *BMC Nephrol* 2004;5:14.

59. Haas S, Schmitt CP, Arbeiter K, et al. Improved acidosis correction and recovery of mesothelial cell mass with neutral-pH bicarbonate dialysis solution among children undergoing automated peritoneal dialysis. *J Am Soc Nephrol* 2003;14(10):2632–2638.

60. Thongboonkerd V, Lumlertgul D, Supajatura V. Better correction of metabolic acidosis, blood pressure control, and phagocytosis with bicarbonate compared to lactate solution in acute peritoneal dialysis. *Artif Organs* 2001;25(2):99–108.

61. Ramos JM, Heaton A, McGurk JG, et al. Sequential changes in serum lipids and their subfractions in patients receiving continuous ambulatory peritoneal dialysis. *Nephron* 1983;35(1):20–23.

62. Mak RH, DeFronzo RA. Glucose and insulin metabolism in uremia. *Nephron* 1992;61(4):377–382.

63. Vande Walle J, Raes A, Dehoorne J, et al. Combined amino-acid and glucose peritoneal dialysis solution for children with acute renal failure. *Adv Perit Dial* 2004;20:226–230.

64. Rusthoven E, Krediet RT, Willems HL, et al. Peritoneal transport characteristics with glucose polymer-based dialysis fluid in children. *J Am Soc Nephrol* 2004;15(11):2940–2947.

65. Wood EG, Lynch RE, Fleming SS, et al. Ultrafiltration using low volume peritoneal dialysis in critically ill infants and children. *Adv Perit Dial* 1991;7:266–268.

66. Fischbach M. Peritoneal dialysis prescription for neonates. *Perit Dial Int* 1996;16(Suppl 1):S512–S514.

67. Alexander SR, Tank ES. Surgical aspects of continuous ambulatory peritoneal dialysis in infants, children and adolescents. *J Urol* 1982;127(3):501–504.

68. Wong SN, Geary DF. Comparison of temporary and permanent catheters for acute peritoneal dialysis. *Arch Dis Child* 1988;63(7):827–831.

69. Stonehill WH, Smith DP, Noe HN. Radiographically documented fecal impaction causing peritoneal dialysis catheter malfunction. *J Urol* 1995;153(2):445–446.

70. Maxvold NJ, Smoyer WE, Gardner JJ, et al. Management of acute renal failure in the pediatric patient: hemofiltration versus hemodialysis. *Am J Kidney Dis* 1997;30(5 Suppl 4):S84–S88.

71. Donckerwolcke RA, Bunchman TE. Hemodialysis in infants and small children. *Pediatr Nephrol* 1994;8(1):103–106.

72. Sadowski RH, Harmon WE, Jabs K. Acute hemodialysis of infants weighing less than five kilograms. *Kidney Int* 1994;45(3):903–906.

73. Bock GH, Campos A, Thompson T, et al. Hemodialysis in the premature infant. *Am J Dis Child* 1981;135(2):178–180.

74. McBryde KD, Kershaw DB, Bunchman TE, et al. Renal replacement therapy in the treatment of confirmed or suspected inborn errors of metabolism. *J Pediatr* 2006;148(6):770–778.

75. Rutledge SL, Havens PL, Haymond MW, et al. Neonatal hemodialysis: effective therapy for the encephalopathy of inborn errors of metabolism. *J Pediatr* 1990;116(1):125–128.

76. Wiegand C, Thompson T, Bock GH, et al. The management of life-threatening hyperammonemia: a comparison of several therapeutic modalities. *J Pediatr* 1980;96(1):142–144.

77. Donn SM, Swartz RD, Thoene JG. Comparison of exchange transfusion, peritoneal dialysis, and hemodialysis for the treatment of hyperammonemia in an anuric newborn infant. *J Pediatr* 1979;95(1):67–70.

78. Sargent JA, Gotch FA. Mathematic modeling of dialysis therapy. *Kidney Int Suppl* 1980;10:S2–S10.

79. Knight F, Gorynski L, Bentson M, et al. Hemodialysis of the infant or small child with chronic renal failure. *ANNA J* 1993;20(3):315–323.

80. Hakim RM, Wingard RL, Parker RA. Effect of the dialysis membrane in the treatment of patients with acute renal failure. *N Engl J Med* 1994;331(20):1338–1342. doi:10.1056/NEJM199411173312003.

81. Himmelfarb J, Tolkoff Rubin N, Chandran P, et al. A multicenter comparison of dialysis membranes in the treatment of acute renal failure requiring dialysis. *J Am Soc Nephrol* 1998;9(2):257–266.

82. Schiffl H, Lang SM, Konig A, et al. Biocompatible membranes in acute renal failure: prospective case-controlled study. *Lancet* 1994;344(8922):570–572.

83. Bunchman TE, Donckerwolcke RA. Continuous arterial-venous diahemofiltration and continuous veno-venous diahemofiltration in infants and children. *Pediatr Nephrol* 1994;8(1):96–102.

84. Hackbarth R, Bunchman TE, Chua AN, et al. The effect of vascular access location and size on circuit survival in pediatric continuous renal replacement therapy: a report from the PPCRRT registry. *Int J Artif Organs* 2007;30(12):1116–1121.

85. Jenkins RD, Kuhn RJ, Funk JE. Clinical implications of catheter variability on neonatal continuous arteriovenous hemofiltration. *ASAIO Trans* 1988;34(2):108–111.

86. Arieff AI. Dialysis disequilibrium syndrome: current concepts on pathogenesis and prevention. *Kidney Int* 1994;45(3):629–635.

87. Grushkin CM, Korsch B, Fine RN. Hemodialysis in small children. *JAMA* 1972;221(8):869–873.

88. Geary DF, Gajaria M, Fryer-Keene S, et al. Low-dose and heparin-free hemodialysis in children. *Pediatr Nephrol* 1991;5(2):220–224.

89. Potter KE, Raj A, Sullivan JE. Argatroban for anticoagulation in pediatric patients with heparin-induced thrombocytopenia requiring extracorporeal life support. *J Pediatr Hematol Oncol* 2007;29(4):265–268.

90. Neuhaus TJ, Goetschel P, Schmugge M, et al. Heparin-induced thrombocytopenia type II on hemodialysis: switch to danaparoid. *Pediatr Nephrol* 2000;14(8–9):713–716.

91. Saxon BR, Black MD, Edgell D, et al. Pediatric heparin-induced thrombocytopenia: management with danaparoid (Orgaran). *Ann Thorac Surg* 1999;68(3):1076–1078.

92. Agha-Razii M, Amyot SL, Pichette V, et al. Continuous veno-venous hemodiafiltration for the treatment of spontaneous tumor lysis syndrome complicated by acute renal failure and severe hyperuricemia. *Clin Nephrol* 2000;54(1):59–63.

93. Rajpoot DK, Gargus JJ. Acute hemodialysis for hyperammonemia in small neonates. *Pediatr Nephrol* 2004;19(4):390–395.

94. Lai YC, Huang HP, Tsai IJ, et al. High-volume continuous venovenous hemofiltration as an effective therapy for acute management of inborn errors of metabolism in young children. *Blood Purif* 2007;25(4):303–308.

95. Falk MC, Knight JF, Roy LP, et al. Continuous venovenous haemofiltration in the acute treatment of inborn errors of metabolism. *Pediatr Nephrol* 1994;8(3):330–333.

96. Schaefer F, Straube E, Oh J, et al. Dialysis in neonates with inborn errors of metabolism. *Nephrol Dial Transplant* 1999;14(4):910–918.

97. Picca S, Dionisi-Vici C, Abeni D, et al. Extracorporeal dialysis in neonatal hyperammonemia: modalities and prognostic indicators. *Pediatr Nephrol* 2001;16(11):862–867.

98. Tenenbein M. Recent advancements in pediatric toxicology. *Pediatr Clin North Am* 1999;46(6):1179–1788, vii.

99. Bunchman TE, Ferris ME. Management of toxic ingestions with the use of renal replacement therapy. *Pediatr Nephrol* 2011;26(4):535–541. doi:10.1007/s00467-010-1654-3.

100. Meyer RJ, Flynn JT, Brophy PD, et al. Hemodialysis followed by continuous hemofiltration for treatment of lithium intoxication in children. *Am J Kidney Dis* 2001;37(5):1044–1047.

101. Papadopoulou ZL, Novello AC. The use of hemoperfusion in children. Past, present, and future. *Pediatr Clin North Am* 1982;29(4):1039–1052.

102. Chavers BM, Kjellstrand CM, Wiegand C, et al. Techniques for use of charcoal hemoperfusion in infants: experience in two patients. *Kidney Int* 1980;18(3):386–389.

103. Donmez O, Cetinkaya M, Canbek R. Hemoperfusion in a child with amitriptyline intoxication. *Pediatr Nephrol* 2005;20(1):105–107. doi:10.1007/s00467-004-1654-2.

104. Bunchman TE, Valentini RP, Gardner J, et al. Treatment of vancomycin overdose using high-efficiency dialysis membranes. *Pediatr Nephrol* 1999;13(9):773–774.

105. Schuerer DJ, Brophy PD, Maxvold NJ, et al. High-efficiency dialysis for carbamazepine overdose. *J Toxicol Clin Toxicol* 2000;38(3):321–323.

106. Pearson F, Bruszer G, Lee W, et al. Ethylene oxide sensitivity in hemodialysis patients. *Artif Organs* 1987;11(2):100–103.

107. Bommer J, Wilhelms OH, Barth HP, et al. Anaphylactoid reactions in dialysis patients: role of ethylene-oxide. *Lancet* 1985;2(8469–8470):1382–1385.

108. Verresen L, Fink E, Lemke HD, et al. Bradykinin is a mediator of anaphylactoid reactions during hemodialysis with AN69 membranes. *Kidney Int* 1994;45(5):1497–1503.

109. Abdeen O, Mehta RL. Dialysis modalities in the intensive care unit. *Crit Care Clin* 2002;18(2):223–247.

110. Hayes LW, Oster RA, Tofil NM, et al. Outcomes of critically ill children requiring continuous renal replacement therapy. *J Crit Care* 2009;24(3):394–400.

111. Askenazi DJ, Goldstein SL, Koralkar R, et al. Continuous renal replacement therapy for children ≤10 kg: a report from the prospective pediatric continuous renal replacement therapy registry. *J Pediatr* 2013;162(3):587–592.e3. doi:10.1016/j.jpeds.2012.08.044.

112. Sakarcan A, Quigley R. Hyperphosphatemia in tumor lysis syndrome: the role of hemodialysis and continuous veno-venous hemofiltration. *Pediatr Nephrol* 1994;8(3):351–353.

113. Saccente SL, Kohaut EC, Berkow RL. Prevention of tumor lysis syndrome using continuous veno-venous hemofiltration. *Pediatr Nephrol* 1995;9(5):569–573.

114. Shah M, Quigley R. Rapid removal of vancomycin by continuous veno-venous hemofiltration. *Pediatr Nephrol* 2000;14(10–11):912–915.

115. Wong KY, Wong SN, Lam SY, et al. Ammonia clearance by peritoneal dialysis and continuous arteriovenous hemodiafiltration. *Pediatr Nephrol* 1998;12(7):589–591.

116. Castillo F, Nieto J, Salcedo S, et al. Treatment of hydrops fetalis with hemofiltration. *Pediatr Nephrol* 2000;15(1–2):14–16.

117. Bunchman TE. Extracorporeal therapies in pediatric organ dysfunction: extracorporeal membrane oxygenation and continuous renal replacement therapy. *Pediatr Crit Care Med* 2007;8(4):405–406. doi:10.1097/01.PCC.0000269384.28300.31.

118. Sell LL, Cullen ML, Whittlesey GC, et al. Experience with renal failure during extracorporeal membrane oxygenation: treatment with continuous hemofiltration. *J Pediatr Surg* 1987;22(7):600–602.

119. Heiss KF, Pettit B, Hirschl RB, et al. Renal insufficiency and volume overload in neonatal ECMO managed by continuous ultrafiltration. *ASAIO Trans* 1987;33(3):557–560.

120. Zobel G, Stein JI, Kuttnig M, et al. Continuous extracorporeal fluid removal in children with low cardiac output after cardiac operations. *J Thorac Cardiovasc Surg* 1991;101(4):593–597.

121. Ronco C, Parenzan L. Acute renal failure in infancy: treatment by continuous renal replacement therapy. *Intensive Care Med* 1995;21(6):490–499.

122. Paret G, Cohen AJ, Bohn DJ, et al. Continuous arteriovenous hemofiltration after cardiac operations in infants and children. *J Thorac Cardiovasc Surg* 1992;104(5):1225–1230.

123. Zobel G, Rödl S, Urlesberger B, et al. Continuous renal replacement therapy in critically ill patients. *Kidney Int Suppl.* 1998;66:S169–S173.

124. Latta K, Krull F, Wilken M, et al. Continuous arteriovenous haemofiltration in critically ill children. *Pediatr Nephrol* 1994;8(3):334–337.

125. Ellis EN, Pearson D, Belsha CW, et al. Use of pump-assisted hemofiltration in children with acute renal failure. *Pediatr Nephrol* 1997;11(2):196–200.

126. Chanard J, Milcent T, Toupance O, et al. Ultrafiltration-pump assisted continuous arteriovenous hemofiltration (CAVH). *Kidney Int Suppl* 1988;24:S157–S158.

127. Yorgin PD, Krensky AM, Tune BM. Continuous venovenous hemofiltration. *Pediatr Nephrol* 1990;4(6):640–642.

128. Bunchman TE, Maxvold NJ, Kershaw DB, et al. Continuous venovenous hemodiafiltration in infants and children. *Am J Kidney Dis* 1995;25(1):17–21.

129. Ronco C, Garzotto F, Brendolan A, et al. Continuous renal replacement therapy in neonates and small infants: development and first-in-human use of a miniaturised machine (CARPEDIEM). *Lancet* 2014;383(9931):1807–1813.

130. Brophy PD, Mottes TA, Kudelka TL, et al. AN-69 membrane reactions are pH-dependent and preventable. *Am J Kidney Dis* 2001;38(1):173–178.

131. Hackbarth RM, Eding D, Gianoli Smith C, et al. Zero balance ultrafiltration (Z-BUF) in blood-primed CRRT circuits achieves electrolyte and acid-base homeostasis prior to patient connection. *Pediatr Nephrol* 2005;20(9):1328–1333.

132. Elton CD, Gain EA, Moonie G. A clinical study on the use of T.H.A.M. for buffering A.C.D. blood prior to use in extracorporeal bypass procedures. *Can Anaesth Soc J* 1963;10:419–427.

133. Brophy PD, Somers MJ, Baum MA, et al. Multi-centre evaluation of anticoagulation in patients receiving continuous renal replacement therapy (CRRT). *Nephrol Dial Transplant* 2005;20(7):1416–1421.

134. Symons JM, Chua AN, Somers MJ, et al. Demographic characteristics of pediatric continuous renal replacement therapy: a report of the prospective pediatric continuous renal replacement therapy registry. *Clin J Am Soc Nephrol* 2007;2(4):732–738.

135. Mehta RL, McDonald BR, Aguilar MM, et al. Regional citrate anticoagulation for continuous arteriovenous hemodialysis in critically ill patients. *Kidney Int* 1990;38(5):976–981.

136. Bunchman TE, Maxvold NJ, Brophy PD. Pediatric convective hemofiltration: Normocarb replacement fluid and citrate anticoagulation. *Am J Kidney Dis* 2003;42(6):1248–1252.

137. Kawada T, Kitagawa H, Hoson M, et al. Clinical application of argatroban as an alternative anticoagulant for extracorporeal circulation. *Hematol Oncol Clin North Am* 2000;14(2):445–457, x.

138. Barenbrock M, Hausberg M, Matzkies F, et al. Effects of bicarbonate- and lactate-buffered replacement fluids on cardiovascular outcome in CVVH patients. *Kidney Int* 2000;58(4):1751–1757.

139. Barletta JF, Barletta GM, Brophy PD, et al. Medication errors and patient complications with continuous renal replacement therapy. *Pediatr Nephrol* 2006;21(6):842–845.

140. Jaing TH, Hsueh C, Tain YL, et al. Tumor lysis syndrome in an infant with Langerhans cell histiocytosis successfully treated using continuous arteriovenous hemofiltration. *J Pediatr Hematol Oncol* 2001;23(2):142–144.

141. Jenkins R, Harrison H, Chen B, et al. Accuracy of intravenous infusion pumps in continuous renal replacement therapies. *ASAIO J* 1992;38(4):808–810.

142. Maxvold NJ, Smoyer WE, Custer JR, et al. Amino acid loss and nitrogen balance in critically ill children with acute renal failure: a prospective comparison between classic hemofiltration and hemofiltration with dialysis. *Crit Care Med* 2000;28(4):1161–1165.

143. Nehus EJ, Mizuno T, Cox S, et al. Pharmacokinetics of meropenem in children receiving continuous renal replacement therapy: validation of clinical trial simulations. *J Clin Pharmacol* 2016;56(3):291–297.

144. Bunchman TE, Hackbarth RM, Maxvold NJ, et al. Prevention of dialysis disequilibrium by use of CVVH. *Int J Artif Organs* 2007;30(5):441–444.

145. Roy BJ, Cornish JD, Clark RH. Venovenous extracorporeal membrane oxygenation affects renal function. *Pediatrics* 1995;95(4):573–578.

146. Chen H, Yu RG, Yin NN, et al. Combination of extracorporeal membrane oxygenation and continuous renal replacement therapy in critically ill patients: a systematic review. *Crit Care* 2014;18(6):675. doi:10.1186/s13054-014-0675-x.

147. Santiago MJ, Lopez-Herce J, Urbano J, et al. Continuous renal replacement therapy in children after cardiac surgery. *J Thorac Cardiovasc Surg* 2013;146(2):448–454. doi:10.1016/j.jtcvs.2013.02.042.

148. Cavagnaro F, Kattan J, Godoy L, et al. Continuous renal replacement therapy in neonates and young infants during extracorporeal membrane oxygenation. *Int J Artif Organs* 2007;30(3):220–226.

149. Selewski DT, Cornell TT, Blatt NB, et al. Fluid overload and fluid removal in pediatric patients on extracorporeal membrane oxygenation requiring continuous renal replacement therapy. *Crit Care Med* 2012;40(9):2694–2699. doi:10.1097/CCM.0b013e318258ff01.

150. Yorgin PD, Kirpekar R, Rhine WD. Where should the hemofiltration circuit be placed in relation to the extracorporeal membrane oxygenation circuit? *ASAIO J* 1992;38(4):801–803.

151. Santiago MJ, Sanchez A, Lopez-Herce J, et al. The use of continuous renal replacement therapy in series with extracorporeal membrane oxygenation. *Kidney Int* 2009;76(12):1289–1292.

152. Jacobs R, Honore PM, Spapen HD. Intertwining extracorporeal membrane oxygenation and continuous renal replacement therapy: sense or nonsense? *Crit Care* 2015;19:145. doi:10.1186/s13054-015-0860-6.

153. Journois D. Hemofiltration during cardiopulmonary bypass. *Kidney Int Suppl* 1998;66:S174–S177.

154. Journois D, Pouard P, Greeley WJ, et al. Hemofiltration during cardiopulmonary bypass in pediatric cardiac surgery. Effects on hemostasis, cytokines, and complement components. *Anesthesiology.* 1994;81(5):1181–1189, discussion 26A–27A.

155. Gong WK, Tan TH, Foong PP, et al. Eighteen years experience in pediatric acute dialysis: analysis of predictors of outcome. *Pediatr Nephrol* 2001;16(3):212–215.

CHAPTER 39

Depurative Modality Options

**Tushar Chopra, Iheanyichukwu Ogu, Rafia Chaudhry,
Thomas A. Golper, and Gerald Schulman**

This chapter discusses the therapeutic options for the management of patients with end-stage kidney disease (ESKD), exclusive of kidney transplantation. The decision begins with an understanding of the implications of patients arriving at the threshold of needing treatment for ESKD. This is discussed in the section of life plans and treatment options. The next step involves the education of the patients, their families, and health care providers. In particular, recent trends suggest that a greater proportion of patients may start their treatment with peritoneal dialysis. An appreciation of the benefits of peritoneal dialysis is required. In addition, particularly for elderly patients or those with serious comorbid conditions, an important consideration is to offer the option of conservative management. The role of conservative management is included. The indications and contraindications for the depurative therapies are also discussed in this chapter. Finally, the reasons for transferring from one method of renal replacement therapy to another is discussed at the end of the chapter.

LIFE PLANNING

A patient facing ESKD must understand that no matter how successful his or her therapy (dialysis and/or transplantation), life span is less than if ESKD were not present. Therefore, it is imperative for the patient, in conjunction with his or her advisors (medical and nonmedical), to establish some form of life plan with ESKD. Early in the course of the disease, education will be important: that education coming from the patient's research on the subject and that provided by the health care team. The strategy in developing a life plan is to live well and extend life with ESKD. To do so, one must recognize a possible distinction between quantity and quality of life. Of course, one prefers both, and an organized plan is the best way to achieve that goal. A life plan is a roadmap to such success and does so by anticipating risks and considering options. Thus, decisions

become structured along the lines of the life plan. For example, a living donor for transplantation may not be available for a year, but ESKD is now. Rather than create an arteriovenous fistula (AVF), a permanent use of the vessels, consider short-term peritoneal dialysis (PD). In 15 years when the transplant is no longer functional, those vessels may be used for fistula creation, and hemodialysis (HD) can be performed with the access that offers the best chance of healthy HD. The life plan leverages all modalities over the lifetime and would emphasize the right therapy at the right time for this individual. During the education process leading to the life plan, all therapies should be presented in a positive light. Patients highly motivated and intensely engaged in their care may disparage in-center dialysis. That is not a healthy approach. All therapies must be respected as they may unexpectedly be necessary. So while discussions take place, the nephrologist should make sure that all therapies are included in a positive light. Crucial to this understanding is the recognition that transition points will inevitably occur. These are not therapy or human failures. They are events that make us change our approach. An example is an incapacitating stroke in a self-care dialysis patient who is now dependent on a helper, usually to in-center dialysis or to the rare skilled nursing facility that performs PD. This is not a "failure" to either the patient or therapy. It represents a transition point and should be described as such in the life plan's attempt at anticipating risk. So the Life Plan is frequently revisited, and adjustments to it become a standard operation.

OPTIONS WHEN FACING LOSS OF KIDNEY FUNCTION

As chronic kidney disease (CKD) progresses, patients may die from other causes or survive to face either death from their kidney disease or seek renal replacement therapy. It takes repeated observations over time and familiarity to at least reasonably predict outcomes in this setting. More and more observations on such outcomes are being published including updated guidelines as to how best approach the decision involved (1). This becomes particularly relevant as the population ages bringing numerous comorbidities into the CKD arena. Herein, we describe a practical and successful approach to the decision making on clinical options for patients, families, and physicians as ESKD approaches.

There are several components to the decision-making processes, but first up are the team members. The patient and family with the nephrologist are the obvious participants, but also variably important are the referring physician(s), especially the primary care physician, friends, coreligionists or spiritual leaders, other patients, and CKD education team. The latter could be a designated group, a staff nurse, a nurse practitioner, a physician assistant, a dietitian, a technician, or a home dialysis trainer. Oftentimes, this may be just the physician using visit discussions, written and/or online materials, or videos provided by kidney organizations or dialysis providers. The key here is to individualize the education to suit the patient and family's unique situation, including economic status, education, discipline, and overall stability. This cannot succeed without the knowledge of these conditions by the attending nephrologist(s), hence the previous comment on familiarity. Repetition helps, even when initially rejected as consuming too much time.

For the education process to succeed for the unique situation for that patient, the nephrologist must offer, or have at immediate access, all services needed for an integrated ESKD care system. For what is available in 2015 that includes conservative care, in-center dialysis, home dialysis, and transplantation (**FIGURE 39.1**). Some of those services may be indirectly provided by referral or specifically and directly provided by the attending nephrologist.

◆ PATIENT PERSONAL CHARACTERISTICS

Occasional patients facing ESKD are completely unaware of their disease and have no preparation for the shock facing them. In those situations, salvage approaches are required with an increasingly popular approach to urgent start PD (further discussion in the following text). However, even patients unaware of their situation can be rapidly educated to the point of at least making some informed decisions. Easiest of all is to simply insert a central venous catheter (CVC) and initiate HD. However, this often sets the stage for complacency where in-center HD with the CVC becomes permanent. We strongly urge the rejection of this approach unless a life-threatening need can only be addressed by the CVC. So in this

situation, the patient's personal characteristics have an immediate and dramatic influence on decisions.

Far more often however is the case where the patient has been seeing a physician and often a nephrologist for months. It is in this setting that some of the most rewarding aspects of delivering chronic care are experienced. Learning about the patient, the family, life style choices, health status, needs, wants, and desires all contribute to advising patients about their options. Education status may play a role but is often for secondary to psychosocial and economic issues. Fear is not unique to any groups. Explanations and instilling confidence can often overcome fear. Throughout this process of probing, provoking, listening, and addressing, patients, families, and the physician all acquire knowledge such that more informed advice is given and decisions made.

It is through this process that a sequence of decisions is made. Without the knowledge of the physician about the patient and the patient about the options, unsatisfactory decisions are likely to result. The first decision is whether to actively pursue some form of renal replacement therapy versus letting nature take its course with progressive kidney failure and ultimate death from it. Not embarking on replacement therapy is called undergoing conservative care. It is imperative that the physicians involved in the care and decision making emphasize that there is no abandonment of care. Depending on the patient's and family's preferences, the primary care provider under conservative care could well be the nephrologist. This is just one of the many shared decisions. In any case, all of the care providers must be prepared to acknowledge that abandonment is not going to occur at any level.

Too often, this first decision is never formally addressed, and assumptions are made about renal replacement therapy. We consider this a serious mistake both ethically and practically. Without a complex ethical argument, informing/discussing conservative care is mandatory simply because it is an option, and no options are withheld in this setting. Practically, it is important because it empowers patients about a choice, and if they are making a choice to pursue renal replacement therapy (versus death from kidney failure), then they are committing to the attempt to succeed at the renal replacement therapy.

The second decision is a derivative of the first. Having decided to pursue renal replacement therapy will then lead to deciding on preemptive transplantation versus dialysis. Often, this decision is out of the hands directly of the patient and physician due to availability of a donor kidney. Nonetheless, the decision step is important for the same reason, as in the first decision. It requires an education, understanding, and commitment, all critical attributer for success. Because of health conditions, transplantation may be eliminated, but the understanding of why that is so is helpful and educational going forward with dialysis and the subsequent decisions.

If transplantation is not an immediate option, then the third decision is what type of dialysis will be performed. This third decision is then dialysis at home versus dialysis at a center. While independence often dominates this decision, other important factors contribute. Here again, knowledge about the patient is beneficial. Patients have fears about self-care, may have other dominating obligations at home, or may prefer to be around other patients with similar conditions. That can work the other way as well because the sicker ESKD patients are often dialyzed in-center. Nonetheless, the third decision of dialyzing at home or in-center is an important shared decision requiring thoughtful knowledge and understanding.

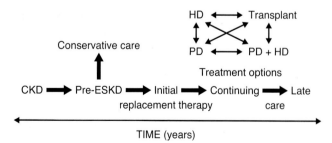

FIGURE 39.1 Integrated care across chronic kidney disease continuum.

TABLE 39.1	Some Reasons for Selecting Home Hemodialysis versus Peritoneal Dialysis

Training time needed (1–8 wk)
Cosmetics of the dialysis access
Actual treatment schedule
Portability
Fear of needles
Perceived complexity
Space
Need or availability of a helper

TABLE 39.2	Transition Points in Dialysis	
PD Transfer to HD	**HD Transfer to PD**
Recurrent infection	Recurrent volume excess
Catheter malfunction	Angio access failure
Ultrafiltration failure	Hypercoagulable
Solute removal failure	Malnutrition
Psychological burnout	Hypertension
Activity of daily living failure	Loss of transportation
Overwhelming comorbidities	
Peritoneal membrane disrupting surgery	
Uncontrolled diabetes	
Excessive obese weight gain	
Hypotension	
Malnutrition	

PD, peritoneal dialysis; HD, hemodialysis.

Because there are only limited in-center PD programs, for these purposes, we will consider in-center dialysis to mean HD. Thus, if the third decision is in-center dialysis, by virtue of the aforementioned assumption, that implies HD. However, if the third decision is to perform home dialysis, then the fourth decision is HD versus PD. Some of the reasons for selecting either of these options are listed in **TABLE 39.1**. Our dialysis program varies at any time between one-quarter to one-third of all patients dialyze at home, so our experience with this decision process is vast. While it would be ideal if all aspects of the two therapies would be considered in this decision, that is typically not what occurs, despite our best efforts to make it so. The overriding factor tends to be the time necessary for training. By virtue of its simplicity and less severe immediate complications, PD takes 1/2 to 1/8 of the training time than does home HD. Furthermore, HD generally requires another person so that training time commitments involve two people. Thus, at least in our program and we suspect in many others, patients choosing to dialyze at home tend to make PD the fourth decision. We do not prefer PD over home HD except in special circumstances such as very poor options for angio access, and in marginally stable patients who do not have a helper for home HD. The fourth decision can be made in a short time frame when circumstances dictate. PD can still be a viable option in this urgent setting. Small-volume supine exchanges can be performed either in the home training unit or hospital while the catheter implant heals.

The fifth and final decision in our options process is what type of home HD or PD is preferred. Our HD options include nocturnal three to six times per week, daytime thrice weekly, traditional flows and times, and short frequent HD which averages 5.2 times weekly, generally for about 2.5 hours. It is with these varieties of HD that the greater difference in training time is noted. In New Zealand, some HD training may last for many months, whereas in our program, 2 to 3 months. Rarely is this training on specific technique but more likely to concern preparation for complications. For nocturnal, especially when performed more than thrice weekly, and for short frequent HD, because of the frequency, complications are less frequent and often never observed during training. Hence, the duration of training tends to be far less than training for traditional thrice-weekly HD. The decision on frequency of HD depends on many factors such as status of access, hemodynamic stability, psychosocial factors, availability of a helper, time to set up and take down the equipment, and many more. We try to determine this at the time of the fourth decision, so factors of the fifth decision impact on the fourth decision. For PD, a helper is less often needed and manual exchange techniques are generally learned within 2 weeks. Cycler techniques can be learned in this same time frame, and in the United States, 80% of PD patients utilizes a cycler in what is termed automated PD. As in the varieties of home HD, the varieties of PD are often determined as part of the fourth decision, home HD versus PD.

The last point to be made regarding dialysis options is the flexibility to accept that in a dialysis patient's lifetime, there will be transitions from one therapy to another. These are almost inevitable and should be truly considered transitions of therapy rather than a failure of a patient or the therapy. We refer to these transitions points as moving in either direction and as guides to selecting and utilizing the right therapy for that patient at that point in time (**TABLE 39.2**).

ROLE OF EDUCATION AND CONSERVATIVE CARE

Section: Role of Education

The commencement of maintenance dialysis is a major life-altering event (2), and a patient-centered approach which involves a partnership among nephrologist and other health care providers, patients, and their families should be established to ensure that decisions respect patients' wants, needs, and preferences and that patients have the education and support they need to make decisions and participate in their own care. Clinical guidelines recommend that treatment option for CKD include the preference of a fully informed patient (3).

However, data from observational studies and the United States Renal Data System suggest that patients with CKD may not be presented with adequate information on treatment option or given sufficient time in which to discuss management alternatives with their family or caregivers (3). Incomplete presentation of treatment option and poor education are responsible for the inconsistencies noted in most studies about the preferred and actual modality of patients' treatment choice (2).

Patient and Family Education

Most CKD patients at baseline generally do not have sophisticated knowledge about their kidney disease or modalities of management of ESKD. This also causes a significant amount of worry. Finkelstein et al. (4) in their study about perceived knowledge among patients about CKD and ESKD therapies noted that 23% patients reported having extensive knowledge, while 35% reported no knowledge about their disease. Also, 43% reported having no knowledge of HD, 57% had no knowledge of chronic ambulatory PD, 66% had no knowledge of automated PD, and 56% had no knowledge of transplant. A total of 35% of patients had no knowledge of therapeutic modality for ESKD.

From the 2012 United States Renal Data System, 114,813 incident ESKD patients began renal replacement therapy with 98,954 starting HD, 9,175 PD, and 2,803 receiving a preemptive kidney transplant—this data has remained relatively stable over the past years. The United States Renal Data System (Wave 2) Study surveyed patients shortly after they initiated renal replacement therapy, with either of HD or PD, to determine who took the lead in deciding on the mode of dialysis. Among the patients who received HD, 53% had physicians taking the lead, 17% patients, and 30% had a joint decision. Of the patients undergoing PD, physicians led in 17%, patients in 36%, and joint decision in 48%. Thus, of all the patients undergoing PD, 84% had contributed substantially to the decision, whereas of all patients undergoing HD, only 47% contributed to the decision.

Mehrotra et al. (2) examined the effect of pre-ESKD processes on the selection of renal replacement therapy among incident ESKD patients (2). Of the 1,365 eligible patients, 93% was undergoing maintenance HD and 7% were undergoing PD, and of the 427 who completed the study, 94 % were on maintenance HD and 6% on PD. In this study, they found that 70% of incident HD patients reported that chronic PD was not offered as an option for renal placement therapy. However, they noted that there was a strong relationship between the probabilities of presentation of PD as a treatment option to the selection of PD as a treatment modality.

Patient education has multiple benefits. It allows an informed choice of renal replacement therapy, improves patient–doctor relationship, and also enhances compliance (5). Studies have suggested that education of CKD patients can delay the onset of dialysis and improve outcomes after they start dialysis (4). Also, provision of educational programs for patients with CKD can increase the percentage of patients who will start dialysis with less expensive self-care as opposed to traditional facility-based, standard care dialysis, and significantly reduce urgent dialysis which might impact on patient survival given that the mortality rate in emergent situation is high.

With a CKD, patient education is not just nice to have—it is fundamental to long-term survival. The content and depth of patient education should be guided by current best practices. To achieve improved outcomes, we must emphasize predialysis and dialysis education and ensure that it is designed to empower patients (6).

Nephrologist Education

Providing education about therapy options to patients with CKD/ESKD is uniformly accepted as important; however, there appears to be a problem in its delivery (7). There is a significant relationship between the timing of presentation to the length of time the patient knew of his or her kidney failure and the duration of predialysis nephrologist care (2). Research on nephrologist–patient communication suggests that nephrologist provides information on treatment option over an extended period of time but increases the amount of detail about specific treatment when the patient requires renal replacement therapy (3). This approach reduces the amount of time available to patient to make decision and means that information

provision may coincide with the time patients are symptomatic and cognitively impaired to make informed decision about their treatment. The value of education and an appreciation for the timing for its occurrence are clear (7); thus, nephrologists should be educated to be aware of this challenge that limit effective communication with patients and work in a timely manner so that patients' knowledge of ESKD is improved.

In terms of modality selection when patients approach ESKD, nephrologists have reported that patient choice is the most important factor in choosing a dialysis therapy, yet there exists a disparity in knowledge of the different treatment options (4). For example, there has been a renewed interest in home HD, but as Jayanti et al. (8) showed, despite the interest and belief in this therapy among providers, home HD is still not available to a majority of patients. Suboptimal patient preparation pathways, lack of appropriately trained personnel, and physician unwillingness were some of the key barriers to widespread adoption of this therapy resulting in the disconnect between belief and practice of home HD. Adequate exposure of physicians during their fellowship to the various modalities of dialysis will give them the capacity to educate patient on treatment options and also care for them, and as Jayanti et al. (8) noted, a generation of nephrologists may lose out to the training opportunities in this field if knowledge of home-based dialysis is not made an integral part of the training curriculum.

Other Provider Education

Given the complexity of CKD, patients approaching ESKD are often managed by a multidisciplinary team—primary care provider, nurses, dietitians, social workers, and other medical specialist (cardiologist, endocrinologists, etc.). Encounter with these providers has a potential effect on a patient's knowledge, belief, and attitude about CKD, ESKD, and treatment modalities.

The recognition of early CKD and referral to a nephrologist is an obligation providers have to these patients. Timing of referral of patients with CKD to a nephrology service affects their outcomes. The majority of patients with kidney disease are referred close to the time of initiation of renal replacement therapy, which contributes to poor patient outcomes on renal replacement therapy (e.g., the use of central venous catheters vs. AVFs). There are now several measures that have proven efficacy for slowing progression of CKD and a number of treatments that are effective at preventing and reversing the morbidity of CKD that patients will benefit from if they are referred early to nephrologists. Also, timely referral can allow informed decision to be made about renal replacement therapy.

Other providers who are directly involved in provision of ESKD treatment modalities should have a purposeful education about renal replacement therapies as inexperienced staff might present negative views about treatment modalities. A synchronized education of these providers leads to a consistent message transmitted to patients about the various treatment modalities (7).

Role of Conservative Care
Definition

Conservative care or nondialytic treatment is a viable option in the integrated management of patients with advanced CKD. It includes treatment of anemia, bone mineral metabolism disorders, hyperkalemia, metabolic acid–base abnormalities, hypertension, and protein-energy malnutrition associated with CKD. Conservative care also pays careful attention to psychological, social, and spiritual support to the patient as well as their families. Furthermore, it

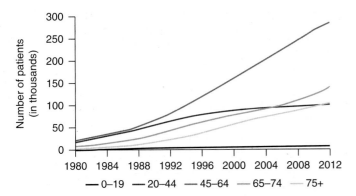

FIGURE 39.2 Prevalent end-stage kidney disease cases in the U.S. population, 1980 to 2012, per United States Renal Data System annual report 2014. United States Renal Data System. Mortality. In: *USRDS 2014 Annual Data Report: Atlas of End-Stage Renal Disease in the United States.* Bethesda, MD: National Institutes of Health, National Institute of Diabetes and Digestive and Kidney Diseases, 2014:145–152.

involves advanced care planning and adopting palliative care principles to improve symptom burden and functional status to maximize quality of life (QOL) prior to death.

It is crucial to learn about the statistics of CKD in the elderly.

Incidence and Prevalence of Chronic Kidney Disease and End-Stage Kidney Disease in the Elderly

Important subsets of CKD population are the elderly. They are the fastest growing CKD subset. The percentage prevalence of all CKD in the National Health and Nutrition Examination Survey (NHANES) population with age 60 years and older is 33.2%, compared to 8.9% in the 40- to 59-year-old subset during 2007 to 2012. Of these, the percentage prevalence of CKD with estimated glomerular filtration rate (eGFR) <60 mL/min/1.73 m^2 is 22.7% in the age group >60 years of age compared to 2.3% in 40- to 59-year-old subset (9).

The elderly is also highly represented in the prevalent and incident cases of ESKD. The prevalence of ESKD increases in all age groups, with a sharp increase in ages 45 years and older (**FIGURE 39.2**) (9).

The incident cases of ESKD per year was steadily rising for age 45 years and older, with an impressive rise for age 65 years and older

initially, followed by a flat trend in recent years (**FIGURE 39.3A**). The ESKD incidence rates have slightly declined among older age groups: For ages 65 to 74 years, the incidence rates are lower than before, and in age group 75 years and older, a downward trend is noted (**FIGURE 39.3B**) (9).

Other factors leading to increased diagnoses of CKD in the elderly are their longevity, inherent risk of CKD, normal aging process with expected loss of eGFR, and better access to care.

Survival Statistics in the Elderly Chronic Kidney Disease Population

It is also known that the prognosis of geriatric patients on dialysis is poor. The expected remaining lifetime years of the prevalent ESKD patients age 65 and older is limited to 4.6 years compared to 15.5 years of the general U.S. population (**FIGURE 39.4A**) (10). The adjusted as well as unadjusted mortality rates are 2 to 3 times higher in prevalent dialysis patients 65 years and older compared to that of age-matched patients with cancer, congestive heart failure (CHF), diabetes mellitus (DM), and other comorbid conditions shown in **FIGURE 39.4B** (9).

Who Should Be Offered Conservative Care?

The decision whether the benefits of conservative care would outweigh the burden associated with dialysis needs to be personalized for each patient. Nephrologists need to lead realistic discussions with patients and their families about survival and the burden of dialysis. Difficult situations can arise, but the crux of medical ethics supports what is right for the patient. Providers have to lead a patient-centered shared decision making and communicate a recommendation to the patient and his or her family. It is important to recognize that patient "autonomy" does not overshadow other ethical principles. However, there are certain well-defined situations with CKD, acute kidney injury (AKI), or ESKD where conservative care would be appropriate to offer. These are the elderly frail individuals with significant comorbidities or nursing home residents, patients with nonkidney terminal disease, profound neurologic impairment/persistent vegetative state, if the patient/proxy declines dialysis, and how the nephrologist answers the question, "Would you be surprised if your patient died within 12 months?" (11).

A Incident Cases

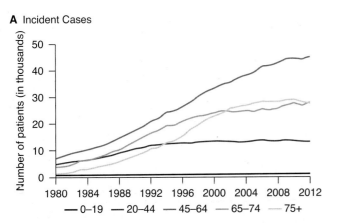

B Incidence Rates

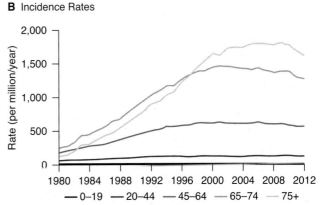

FIGURE 39.3 Trends in (**A**) ESRD incident cases, in thousands, and (**B**) adjusted end-stage kidney disease incidence rate, per million/year, by *age group*, in the U.S. population, 1980 to 2012. United States Renal Data System. Mortality. In: *USRDS 2014 Annual Data Report: Atlas of End-Stage Renal Disease in the United States.* Bethesda, MD: National Institutes of Health, National Institute of Diabetes and Digestive and Kidney Diseases, 2014:145–152.

| Ages | ESRD patients, 2012 | | | | | | General U.S. population, 2010 | | |
| | Dialysis | | | Transplant | | | | | |
	All	M	F	All	M	F	All	M	F
0–14	22.3	23.2	21.3	61.0	60.1	62.5	72.9	70.5	75.3
15–19	19.9	20.6	19.0	48.7	47.9	50.0	59.5	57.1	61.7
20–24	17.0	17.7	16.1	44.7	44.0	45.9	54.7	52.4	56.9
25–29	14.9	15.5	14.1	40.7	40.0	41.8	50.0	47.8	52.0
30–34	13.4	13.8	12.7	36.8	36.1	37.9	45.2	43.1	47.2
35–39	12.0	12.3	11.5	32.8	32.1	33.9	40.5	38.5	42.4
40–44	10.5	10.6	10.2	28.9	28.2	30.0	35.9	33.9	37.7
45–49	8.9	9.0	8.7	25.1	24.4	26.2	31.4	29.6	33.2
50–54	7.6	7.6	7.6	21.6	20.9	22.7	27.2	25.4	28.8
55–59	6.5	6.4	6.5	18.3	17.7	19.3	23.1	21.5	24.5
60–64	5.5	5.4	5.6	15.4	14.8	16.4	19.1	17.7	20.3
65–69	4.6	4.5	4.8	12.9	12.4	13.8	15.5	14.2	16.5
70–74	3.9	3.8	4.1	10.8	10.4	11.5	12.1	11.0	12.9
75–79	3.3	3.2	3.5	9.1	8.7	9.7	9.1	8.2	9.7
80–84	2.7	2.6	2.9	a	a	a	6.5	5.8	6.9
85+	2.2	2.1	2.4	a	a	a	3.4	3.0	3.5
Overall	6.6	6.6	6.6	18.6	18.0	19.5	22.2	20.7	23.4

A

FIGURE 39.4 A: Expected remaining lifetime (years) of the general U.S. population, prevalent dialysis patients, and transplant patients, by sex and age–*USRDS 2014 Annual Data Report: Epidemiology of End-stage Renal Disease in the United States*, Mortality. *(continued)*

	1996	2008	2009	2010	2011	2012
Unadjusted						
ESRD	337	264	257	247	241	223
Dialysis	354	298	291	281	277	258
Transplant	97	72	75	74	72	66
General Medicare						
Cancer	150	115	113	111	109	109
Diabetes	93	74	71	71	71	72
CHF	205	196	183	189	188	191
CVA/TIA	156	133	125	129	127	128
AMII	149	155	146	153	153	163
Adjusted						
ESRD	350	263	255	246	240	223
Dialysis	364	290	284	275	270	252
Transplant	133	94	93	94	89	83
General Medicare						
Cancer	144	106	105	102	100	99
Diabetes	87	66	63	63	62	64
CHF	166	145	137	138	137	143
CVA/TIA	130	106	100	101	100	103
AMI	131	131	122	127	125	137

B

FIGURE 39.4 *(Continued)* **B:** Unadjusted and adjusted mortality rates in the end-stage kidney disease and comorbidity-specific Medicare populations, age 65 and older (per 1,000 patient-years), by calendar year—*USRDS 2014 Annual Data Report: Epidemiology of End-stage Renal Disease in the United States*, Mortality. United States Renal Data System. Mortality. In: *USRDS 2014 Annual Data Report: Atlas of End-Stage Renal Disease in the United States*. Bethesda, MD: National Institutes of Health, National Institute of Diabetes and Digestive and Kidney Diseases, 2014:145–152.

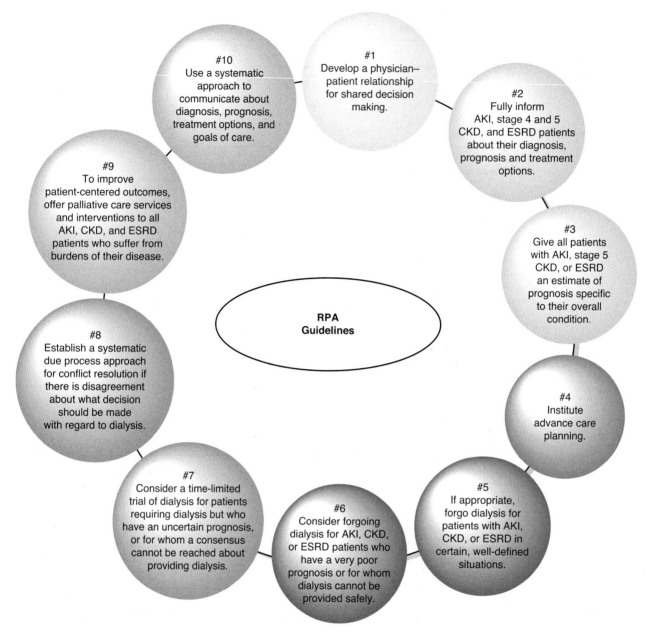

FIGURE 39.5 Revised Renal Physicians Association guidelines.

There is evidence supporting that predialysis functional status declines after initiating dialysis in elderly nursing home patients with a mortality rate approaching 58% in the first year (12). Hence, offering supportive care to an elderly nursing home patient with significant comorbidities and poor functional status would be appropriate. This data cannot be extrapolated to a cognitively intact elderly patient seen in an ambulatory clinic. The evidence for conservative management in this patient population is summarized in the following section.

The Renal Physicians Association (RPA) has published guidelines about shared decision making, informing patients, facilitating advanced care planning, making decisions withhold or discontinue dialysis, conflict resolution, and provisions for palliative care in the comprehensive management of a patient with kidney disease. The revised recommendations are summarized in **FIGURE 39.5** (11).

What Is the Current Evidence for Conservative Management?

Extensive literature survey supports that mostly elderly dialysis patients live longer than those managed without dialysis (**FIGURE 39.6**) (13).

Currently, only cohort studies are available addressing the role of conservative management. It would be challenging to conduct a randomized controlled trial. The key issues in this prospective studies at the differences in start time for the dialysis group, rate of decline in kidney function, definitions of comorbidities, functional scoring, presence or absence of a dedicated conservative care clinic, health care system, and quality-of-life information.

Literature Survey: Survival in Elderly ESRD Patients

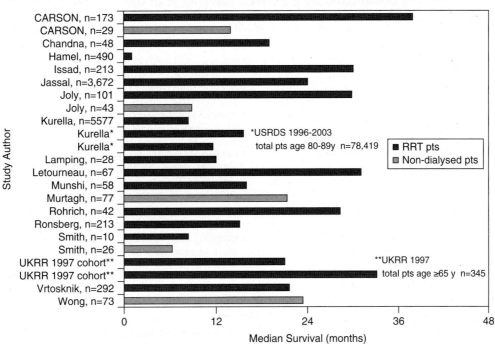

FIGURE 39.6 Summary graph of survival of elderly patients with end-stage kidney disease. [Adapted from Carson RC, Juszczak M, Davenport A, et al. Is maximum conservative management an equivalent treatment option to dialysis for elderly patients with significant comorbid disease? *Clin J Am Soc Nephrol* 2009;4(10):1611–1619.]

Median survival with conservative management ranges from 6.3 to 23.4 months based on current data. This wide range in survival is due to differences in patient characteristics in the cohort studies. For example, the studies with the longest survival recruited patients with the youngest median age (14).

Three cohort studies showed a survival advantage for dialysis patients compared to conservative management. They are summarized as follows in **TABLE 39.3**.

Carson et al. (13) followed 202 elderly ESKD patients in a prospective study who were offered either conservative management or renal replacement therapy. Although the authors demonstrated a survival benefit in the renal replacement therapy group, but the conservative care group patients were 4 times more likely to die at home or under hospice care. The renal replacement therapy group spent majority of their extended survival time either admitted in the hospital or in an outpatient dialysis unit. The conservative care group survived more than a year and had similar hospital free days as the renal replacement therapy group. Yes, this study demonstrated prolonged survival time in the renal replacement therapy group, but whether that time was "quality time" for the patient and their family members is unknown (13).

Joly et al. (15) followed 144 elderly ESKD patients prospectively from 1989 to 2000. They demonstrated a large survival benefit in the renal replacement therapy group compared to the conservative management (28.9 months vs. 8.9 months). The conservative management group had more socially isolated patients, diabetics, lower Karnofsky scores, and late referrals compared to renal replacement therapy group. Hence, it is not surprising that they have a shorter survival time compared to the renal replacement therapy group (15).

Chandna et al. (16) looked at a retrospective cohort of 844 patients with stage 5 CKD (CKD 5). They demonstrated a median survival benefit in the renal replacement therapy group compared to the conservative management group. However, the conservative management group had higher percentage of elderly more than 75 years of age with significant comorbidities. After adjusting for age and comorbidities among elderly more than 75 years of age in a subgroup analysis, the statistical difference between the two groups disappeared (16).

Murtagh et al. (17) and Smith et al. (18) have demonstrated almost identical findings in their cohort studies. Dialysis did not demonstrate a significant survival benefit compared to conservative management in the elderly with significant comorbidities, especially ischemic heart disease (17). See **TABLE 39.4** for details.

Cohort studies in which dialysis did not demonstrate a significant survival benefit compared to conservative management are as follows (14).

SYMPTOM BURDEN AND QUALITY OF LIFE AS AN OUTCOME

Limited observational data is available regarding symptom burden and quality of life in the elderly patients with advanced CKD. A systematic review identified six studies addressing symptom burden and/or QOL. Memorial Symptom Assessment Scale Short Form (MSAS-SF) and modified version of Patient Outcome Scale Symptoms were more frequently utilized tools to assess symptom burden. Average number of symptoms reported was 6.8 to 17 in patients undergoing conservative management. QOL was assessed by three small studies where both the conservative management group and the comparison group had similar impairment of QOL (14).

TABLE 39.3	Cohort Studies Demonstrating a Survival Advantage in the Renal Replacement Therapy Group Compared to Conservative Management	
	Patient Characteristics	**Results and Comments**
Carson et al. (13) Prospective cohort study N = 202 elderly	Age > or = 70 y divided into **MCM** n = 29 Age = 83 y CCI = 7.4 DM: 13.8% **RRT** n = 173 Age = 75 y CCI = 7.4 DM: 29.5%	Median survival was 37.8 mo for RRT patients and 13.9 mo for MCM patients (p <0.01). RRT patients had higher rates of hospitalization [0.069 (95% CI 0.068 to 0.070) versus 0.043 (95% CI 0.040 to 0.047) hospital days/patient-days survived] compared with MCM patients. MCM patients were 4 times more likely to die at home or in a hospice (odds ratio 4.15, 95% CI 1.67 to 10.25). MCM had older patients with a modest size group compared to RRT. Interestingly, MCM group survived more than 1 year and were more likely to die in their home or hospice compared to RRT group who spent a greater proportion of days in the hospital.
Chandna et al. (16) Retrospective cohort study N = 844 elderly	**MCM** n = 155 Age = 77.5 y >75 y = 68.4% High comorbidity: 49.7% **RRT** n = 689 Age = 58.5 y >75 y = 11.2% High comorbidity: 17.3%	Median survival from entry into CKD 5 was less in the MCM than in RRT group (21.2 vs. 67.1 mo: p <0.001). A subgroup analysis of age 75 years and older was performed after correcting for comorbidity scores, diabetes, and age. The survival benefit in the RRT group was no longer statistically significant.
Joly et al. (15) Prospective cohort study N = 144	**MCM** Age 84 y Late referral: 51.4% DM: 21.6% Social isolation: 43% **RRT** Age 83.2 y Late referral: 28.9% DM: 6.5% Social isolation: 14.7%	Median survival was strikingly larger in the RRT group of 28.9 mo vs. 8.9 mo in the MCM group: p <0.0001.

MCM, maximum conservative management; RRT, renal replacement therapy; CCI, Charlson Comorbidity Index; DM, diabetes mellitus; CI, confidence interval.
From O'Connor NR, Kumar P. Conservative management of end-stage renal disease without dialysis: a systematic review. *J Palliat Med* 2012;15(2):228–235.

Brown et al. (19) studied survival, symptom burden, and QOL as an outcome in a cohort of 467 pre-ESKD patients. One hundred twenty-two patients opted for conservative management, whereas 92 (34%) out of the 273 predialysis clinic comparison group opted for dialysis. The patients in the conservative management group had higher mean age (82 years), dementia, and comorbidities compared to the comparison group (predialysis). They utilized MSAS-SF and Medical Outcomes Study Short Form 36-Item Health Survey (SF-36) to assess symptom burden and QOL. The response rate for the SF-36 for was 56% in the conservative management group and 51% in the predialysis group. The response rate for the MSAS-SF was 45.5 % in the conservative management group and 49% in the predialysis group.

In the conservative group, 57% had stable or improvement in symptom burden toward the end of 12 months and QOL remained stable or improved in 58% of the conservative management group. The response rates for the two surveys were roughly 50% in both groups. However, they did not resurvey the predialysis clinic

TABLE 39.4	Cohort Studies Demonstrating a No Survival Advantage in the Renal Replacement Therapy Group Compared to Conservative Management	
	Patient Characteristics	**Results and Comments**
Murtagh et al. (17) Retrospective cohort study N = 129 Elderly >75 years	**MCM** n = 52 Median age: 83 y DM: = 25% **RRT** n = 77 Median age: 79.6 y DM: = 23.4%	Median survival from first known date of GFR <15: 18 mo in MCM group vs. 19.6 mo in RRT group This modest survival benefit is reduced with growing comorbidities and ceases to exist in patients with ischemic heart disease.
Smith et al. (18) Prospective cohort study	**MCM** N = 32	**RRT** N = 10	Median survival was 6.3 mo in CM vs. 8.3 mo in RRT group.

MCM, maximum conservative management; RRT, renal replacement therapy; DM, diabetes mellitus; GFR, glomerular filtration rate; CM, conservative management.

A Stepwise Decline in Function with Intercurrent Events in Progressive CKD

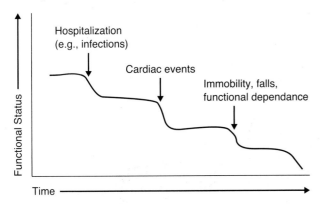

B Frailty and Dementia

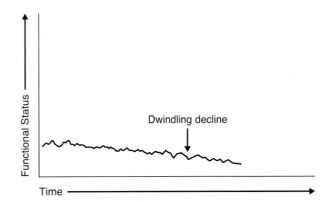

C Terminal Illness

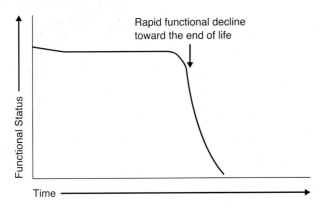

FIGURE 39.7 Chronic illness trajectories. [Adapted from Murray SA, Kendall M, Boyd K, et al. Illness trajectories and palliative care. *BMJ* 2005;330(7498): 1007–1011.]

patients who opted for dialysis, which may have biased the results. This study reinforces that patients on conservative management can survive more than a year and their symptom can be managed fairly to maintain a QOL.

Concept of Chronic Illness Trajectories to Envision a Clinical Course

Understanding chronic illness trajectories may help nephrologists formulate a care plan addressing the multifaceted needs of the patients and their families. Three kinds of chronic illness trajectories are described: a stepwise decline in functional status in progressive organ failure (CKD), frailty and dementia, and terminal illness.

A stepwise functional decline can occur with each sentinel event. These events could be hospitalizations related to cardiovascular events, infections, vascular access, comorbid conditions, or the primary disease. Each of these events provides a unique opportunity for the nephrologist to reassess the "global picture" and involve the renal palliative care team, if indicated.

Frailty and dementia has been described in the elderly CKD patients. They demonstrate a dwindling low functional status leading to death over a prolonged period.

Lastly, the progressive CKD stage 5 patients managed with conservative care can maintain a steady functional status trajectory, until the last few months of life where a precipitous decline occurs. However, palliative care and hospice services are available during this time frame (20). See **FIGURE 39.7** for details.

How to Prognosticate Survival?

The nephrologist also needs to be well equipped with prognostication tools to predict outcomes.

Charlson Comorbidity Index (CCI): Developed in 1987 to predict 1-year mortality among internal medicine patients based on age and comorbidities. It has been validated in 268 dialysis patients over 3-year period in the university hospital to predict patient outcomes. The CCI is strongly predicted admission rates, hospitalization days, inpatient costs, and mortality. Patients with the CCI >8 had the highest mortality of 0.49 per patient-year (21).

Surprise Question (SQ): Cohen et al. (22) developed a short-term prognostic model utilizing prospective data from dialysis clinics in Northeast United States. The derivation cohort had 512 patients, and the validation cohort had 514 in which providers answered an SQ, "Would you be surprised if this patient died in the next 6 months?" A robust area under the curve (AUC) for a 6-month survival in the derivation cohort. It was 0.87 [95% confidence interval (CI) 0.82 to 0.92] in the derivation cohort and 0.80 (95% CI 0.73 to 0.88) in the validation cohort (22). Revised RPA guidelines have developed an integrated prognostic tool that includes patient's age, serum albumin, comorbidities, and the response of the clinician to the SQ. It is available online at http://touchcalc.com/sq (11).

French Renal Epidemiology and Information Network (REIN) developed a 6-month mortality prognostic score in 2,500 dialysis patients more than 75 years of age; a point system scoring was allocated to nine risk factors (**FIGURE 39.8**). They found an overall 6-month mortality of 19%, and age was not associated with mortality (23).

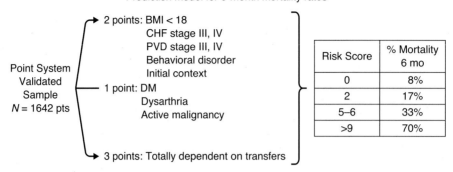

FIGURE 39.8 French Renal Epidemiology and Information Network. BMI, body mass index; PVD, peripheral vascular disease.

RPA guidelines recommend conservative care as an option in elderly CKD 5 patients with two or more of the following predictors of poor survival are present such as high Co-morbidities score of modified Charlson Comorbidity Index > or = 8; poor functional status (Karnofsky performance score < 40); poor nutritional status (serum albumin <2.5g/dl) and if the answer to the surprise question ("Would you be surprised if your patient died within the next year?) is "no". (see **FIGURE 39.5**, Step #6) (11).

CCI: Charlson Comorbidity Index.

Components of Conservative Care or "Active Medical Management"

Conservative care in CKD patients involves advanced care planning, continuing medical management, treatment of symptom burden, patient and family support, and timely hospice referral.

Advanced care planning should be available to all patients, especially if they have CKD stage 4. It involves a patient-focused discussion with the patient and his or her family members. This can be used as an opportunity to name a health care proxy, discuss patient's wishes at the end of life, prognosticate clinical course, determine functional age, and strengthen a doctor–patient relationship.

Continue predialysis medical care such as diet, anemia management, fluid balance, electrolyte and acid–base disturbances, bone mineral disorders, and blood pressure control. Some treatments are modified, such as, if fluid restriction needs to be liberalized, the patient can undergo ultrafiltration to help with fluid balance.

Regardless of the stage of CKD, every patient should receive palliative care. The application of palliative care principles to patients with CKD is called "renal palliative care" (**FIGURE 39.9**). It involves a multidisciplinary team consisting of nephrologists, palliative care specialists, senior renal nurses, counselors, social workers, and hospice workers. They personalize treatment plans, formulate goals, assess functional status, and control symptom burden from ESKD and/or from comorbid conditions, for example, diabetes. They also provide support to the family and the patient with hospice referral, community nurses, social services, and outpatient clinic visits (24,25).

Summary

- Conduct discussions which are patient-centered and incorporate shared decision making between the patient and his or her family to tailor treatment options based on his or her preferences and goals.

- Discuss the risks and benefits of each treatment and provide prognosis to all patients to help understand clinical course.
- Identify patients who would benefit from conservative care.
- Recognize observational data demonstrating an equal survival benefit among elderly frail patients when treated with conservative management or renal replacement therapy.
- Incorporate advanced care planning and palliative care early.

◆ INDICATIONS AND CONTRAINDICATIONS FOR SPECIFIC THERAPIES

While the first and foremost indication and decision to opt for any particular dialysis modality should be patient preference and lifestyle, there are special circumstances where a particular therapy may be indicated or contraindicated.

Home versus In-Center Dialysis

The decision to perform home dialysis (home HD or PD) versus in-center dialysis is often made to offer better lifestyle and flexibility to patients. A few crucial prerequisites must be met to allow patients to dialyze at home. For all home therapies, adequate physical

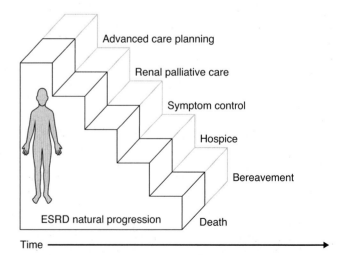

FIGURE 39.9 Patient-centered integrated model of care for end-stage kidney disease.

space has to be available to dedicate to dialysis supplies whether it is peritoneal dialysate bags or home HD set up and dialysate. House pets and small children must be barred from the room during PD exchanges and HD access cannulation.

Also, certain comorbidities or the need for significant assistance may limit the patient's ability to dialyze at home. An extreme example would be patients with advanced cardiac failure on a left ventricular assist device (LVAD), who may only be eligible to dialyze in-center at a dialysis facility qualified to manage such complicated patients. Tracheostomy patients are also candidates for in-center HD. Many dialysis facilities now have a policy to accept them.

Inability to participate in self-care is a relative contraindication to home therapies, including PD and home HD. The presence of a reliable caregiver may allow exceptions to be made. Significant others may be willing to provide the care, particularly in PD patients. No doubt, this care places a burden on the caregivers that nevertheless they may be willing to undertake. If they do so, a "Plan B" should be in place to spell the caretaker if that person needs a break or develops an illness, called "respite." Plan B for infirm patients might be the creation of an AVF [or even an arteriovenous graft (AVG) in patients >75 to 80 years old] if the family elects to support the PD treatment. The same approach could be used for an intact patient on PD who becomes enfeebled. Because the patient will be treated with PD, there is time to make provision for an angioaccess. This permits the patient to be transitioned to HD either temporarily, to provide relief to the caregiver, or in certain cases permanently.

Psychosis is also a contraindication particular to home HD and PD and would fall under the category of inability to perform sustained, adequate self-care. Uncontrolled psychosis may be a contraindication to any form of dialysis. Other barriers to home HD such as inability or fear of performing cannulation by caregivers can often be overcome with training. It must be noted that as opposed to PD where the patient may be trained to perform therapy independently, home HD requires a caregiver to assist the patient for safety reasons.

Peritoneal Dialysis versus Hemodialysis

PD is a slower, continuous therapy when compared to intermittent HD and may offer hemodynamic advantages in patients with low blood pressures, increased incidence of intradialytic hypotension, and geriatric populations. PD is also the preferred modality of choice for infants and children.

Any patient who prefers PD as the modality of choice, and has no contraindications, should be strongly encouraged to pursue PD. PD may be especially beneficial and particularly indicated in patients with significant residual renal function, where incremental dialysis can be started. The practice of incremental dialysis prescription allows maximizing benefit from the residual renal function, slowly increasing the dialysis dose in an incremental manner over time. This can also be done with HD, especially short daily HD; however, PD just lends itself easier to do this. This sequence of HD initiation may eventually translate into access preservation and possibly offer a mortality benefit for a patient by preserving dialysis access, maximizing options of later treatments, and in turn likely increasing the number of years they can survive on dialysis.

There are a few absolute contraindications to performing PD but many relative contraindications or at least special circumstances where PD can be done with close guidance and special training.

Previous major abdominal surgery may result in excessive scarring and fibrosis. Adhesions may cause PD catheter malfunction

due to kinking and obstruction. Morbid obesity may also be a relative contraindication, and individualized decisions must be made in these cases. Part of the challenge in morbid obesity is PD catheter hygiene and concerns with exit-site infections. One way around this particular situation may be a presternal exit site. A colostomy, ileostomy, nephrostomy, or ileal conduit are also relative contraindications due to anatomic manipulation, adhesions, and possibly increased risk of contamination and peritonitis. However, in such circumstances, a presternal catheter may be an option in the highly motivated patient. Severe diverticular disease may be another relative contraindication.

PD can be performed in special populations with support from nephrologists and staff. In Canada, staff-assisted PD assists maximizes support to these special populations to perform therapy at home, especially for automated PD with cyclers. These populations include the elderly, diabetics, polycystic kidney disease, patients with cirrhosis, and patients with previous abdominal surgeries.

In cases with frequent and recurrent peritonitis, patients should be retrained frequently to eliminate faulty technique and observed closely for future episodes of peritonitis. If this continues to be a recurring or life-threatening issue, certain individuals may have to be transitioned to HD, either home HD or in-center, where dialysis staff would be able to provide treatment care.

Other more common circumstances, which would be limiting to HD, may be limited vascular access. In patients with limited arteriovenous (AV) access options, that is, AVFs and AVGs, PD should be considered and preferred over use of tunneled catheters due to increased incidence of infections and mortality.

In-center HD usually or typically becomes the dialysis modality of choice in urgent or "crash start" situations. This is often with patients who develop AKI and progress to ESKD, or advanced CKD patients who progress to ESKD with no planned access or prior health care.

However, it must be kept in mind that inability to train in performing PD exchanges initially due to uremia may be a relative contraindication to PD, and once the patient is improved on intermittent HD, he or she may be able to transition to PD if this is the patient's preferred modality of choice. An alternative approach would be urgent start PD, where a PD catheter would be placed in the hospital and patient is dialyzed in the hospital or PD unit until he or she is clinically improved from the uremia and able to train for home PD. Urgent start PD is a specialized procedure, and care must be taken to institute the protocol for it. A bowel regimen must be introduced immediately, and the importance of clean bowels emphasized both prior to PD catheter placement, and postoperatively as well. Following placement of the PD catheter, low-volume exchanges (500 to 1,000 mL/exchange depending on the patient's body size) can be initiated in a supine position. Many patients will do well with every 2-hour exchanges with 1.5% dextrose solution to begin. If the patient wishes to ambulate, he or she must do so "empty," that is, after the abdominal cavity has been drained completely.

Again, as discussed earlier, ESKD care has multiple ongoing transition points and decisions, and transitioning from one kind of therapy to another is not always to be considered "therapy failure" and in fact may reflect changing patient preferences that dictate these choices on a continuum.

Short Daily versus In-Center Thrice-Weekly versus Long Dialysis (Nocturnal)

The variation in manner of delivery of HD between short daily, thrice-weekly in-center and long dialysis (nocturnal) is largely

TABLE 39.5	Peritoneal Dialysis: Absolute and Relative Contraindications

Contraindications

Previous major abdominal surgery with intra-abdominal adhesions limiting dialysate flow

Ileostomy, colostomy, nephrostomy

Severe diverticular disease

Inability to participate in self-care (physically or mentally) and lack of assistance

Mechanical defects not amenable to surgery that may affect PD or increase infections (omphalocele, large irreparable hernia, bladder exstrophy)

Loss of peritoneal function

Relative Contraindications

Severe malnutrition

Morbid obesity (especially in short individuals)

Intra-abdominal foreign body (<4 mo)

Peritoneal leaks and diaphragmatic defects

Intolerance to PD volumes needed for adequate PD

Inflammatory or ischemic bowel disease

Severe diverticular disease or frequent diverticulitis

Abdominal wall or skin infection

PD, peritoneal dialysis.
From the National Kidney Foundation. Measurement of peritoneal dialysis dose. In: *NFK-DOQI Clinical Practice Guidelines for Peritoneal Dialysis Adequacy.* New York, NY: National Kidney Foundation, 1997;S80–S82.

impacted by patient preference. There are other factors that may impact the decision toward one therapy or the other.

ESKD and dialysis has been associated with low conception rates and poor pregnancy outcomes, and it is important to discuss these aspects with patients. Longer treatments and more frequent weekly dialysis may impact better pregnancy-related outcomes. Hence, while a switch in modality is not required for pregnancy, increased treatment times and frequency may be beneficial.

Long dialysis, that is, nocturnal therapy offers better phosphorous control, as it allows mobilization of phosphorous from various body compartments including bones and increased phosphorus removal per treatment due to increased session length. This allows patients to liberalize their diets and decreases the pill burden of phosphate binders. In addition, patients who are actively working and choose not to opt for a home dialysis therapy can benefit from utilizing nocturnal HD, which allows them to have their full next day (TABLE 39.5).

MODALITY TRANSFERS

The initial decision to choose a particular dialysis modality is not immutable. During their course of depurative therapy for ESKD, patients may change modalities. The patients' characteristics that govern their suitability have been described previously. Transition occurs between all renal replacement therapies (TABLE 39.6). Transitions to and from transplantation are straightforward: A kidney becomes available or fails, respectively. The rest of this section discusses the reasons for transition between the artificial modalities.

The causes of modality transfers have been described (26–31). The causes of transfer from PD to HD include multiple episodes of

TABLE 39.6	Switching Modalities
Initial Modality	**Transition**
Hemodialysis (HD)	
In-center HD	Home HD, peritoneal dialysis, transplantation, conservative management
Home HD	In-center HD, peritoneal dialysis, transplantation, conservative management
Peritoneal dialysis	In-center HD, home HD, transplantation, conservative management
Transplantation	In-center HD, home HD, peritoneal dialysis, conservative management

peritonitis, loss of adequacy of the peritoneal membrane resulting in poor solute exchange or ultrafiltration failure, leakage including PD fluid causing pleural effusions through diaphragm defects, and social problems. HD patients transfer to PD due to exhaustion of access sites, cardiovascular instability, intractable hypotension, and personal choice (TABLE 39.2).

Implications of Transition

The long-term effects of switching modalities have been examined. A retrospective study or 223 HD patients and 194 PD patients examined the outcome in patients who switched modalities (29). TABLE 39.7 shows the reasons for transferring.

The survival of patients initially receiving PD and switched to HD was better than patients who remained on PD. Patients who switched from PD to HD did not have an improved survival. However, patients who began on PD but later switched to HD had lower mortality than those HD patients who never were on PD. It is known that residual renal function is better preserved in patients who start on PD compared to patients initiated on HD (32–34). Preserved residual renal function enhances solute clearance, and this may confer a survival benefit (35). These findings support a role for integrated care.

Switching from PD to HD often occurs within the first 2 years of therapy and is frequently associated with episodes of peritonitis but does not always result in increased mortality (30). Patients in another study comparing survival of patients who switched from PD to HD to those who remained on PD, it was found that technique failure had an increased risk of mortality that was attributed to episodes of fatal peritonitis (31). An added risk factor was the use of central venous catheters for HD. However, if patients survived more than 60 months after technique failure, there was no adverse effect of switching to HD.

TABLE 39.7	Reasons for Transfer	
From HD to PD (*n* = 35)	**From PD to HD (*n* = 32)**
• Peritonitis/exit-site infection 50%	• Cardiovascular problems 40%
• Access problems 25%	• Adequacy and/or ultrafiltration problems 25%
• Personal choice 23%	• Social problems 14%
• Blood pressure problems 12%	• Extraperitoneal leakage of dialysis fluid 11%

HD, hemodialysis; PD, peritoneal dialysis.

Integrated renal care management includes patients receiving treatments of HD, PD, as well as transplantation for ESKD. A study comparing the outcome of 1,067 maintained on PD to 43 patients transferred to PD following a failed transplant and 245 patients transferred from HD to PD revealed no differences in survival between the three groups (36).

It is reassuring that patients can change modalities if necessary and that their outcomes are favorable. Of course, an individual patient's outcome will be determined by the reason that a patient has to transition to an alternative modality. A need for a colostomy, although not an absolute contraindication to PD, might make HD an attractive option. A patient with severe CHF and hypotension on HD may be better treated by PD. However, the outcome of an individual patient depends on comorbid conditions. For patients who must transfer from PD to HD, plans to create an AVF or AVG should be a priority to minimize the length of time that a central venous catheter is required.

 SUMMARY

There have multiple studies comparing survival between HD and PD (37–44). The conclusions of these studies are conflicting with some favoring HD, others favoring PD, and some showing no differences between the modalities. The statistical methods in these studies differ. In balancing the diverse findings, the experience of the centers that render care is most important. The choice of treatment should ultimately be decided on the lifestyle requirements of the patient. The home therapies offer the most schedule flexibility. In-center thrice-weekly nocturnal HD allows the patient to work. Home HD requires a partner to assist with the treatments. In-center HD is appropriate for those who do not have a partner or who are unwilling or cannot perform PD.

 REFERENCES

1. Renal Physicians Association. Clinical practice guidelines on shared decision-making in the appropriate initiation and withdrawal from dialysis. Renal Physicians Association/American Society of Nephrology Working Group. *J Am Soc Nephrol* 2000;11(9):2 p following 1788.

2. Mehrotra R, Marsh D, Vonesh E, et al. Patient education and access of ESRD patients to renal replacement therapies beyond in-center hemodialysis. *Kidney Int* 2005;68:378–390.

3. Morton RL, Tong A, Howard K, et al. The views of patients and carers in treatment decision making for chronic kidney disease: systematic review and thematic synthesis of qualitative studies. *BMJ* 2010;340:c112. doi:10.1136/bmj.c112.

4. Finkelstein FO, Story K, Firanek C, et al. Perceived knowledge among patients cared for by nephrologists about chronic kidney disease and end-stage renal disease therapies. *Kidney Int* 2008;74:1178–1184.

5. Golper T. Patient education: can it maximize the success of therapy? *Nephrol Dial Transplant* 2001;16(Suppl 17):20–24.

6. Alt M, Schatell D. Shifting to chronic care model saves life. *Nephrol News Issues* 2008;22:28, 30, 32.

7. Golper TA, Saxena AB, Piraino B, et al. Systematic barriers to the effective delivery of home dialysis in the United State: a report from the Public Policy/Advocacy Committee of the North America Chapter of the International Society for Peritoneal Dialysis. *Am J Kidney Dis* 2011;58(6):879–885.

8. Jayanti A, Morris J, Stenvinkel P, et al. Home hemodialysis: beliefs, attitudes, and practice patterns. *Hemodialysis Int* 2014;18:767–776.

9. United States Renal Data System. *USRDS 2014 Annual Data Report: Epidemiology of Kidney Disease in the United States*. Bethesda, MD: National Institutes of Health, National Institute of Diabetes and Digestive and Kidney Diseases, 2014.

10. United States Renal Data System. Mortality. In: *USRDS 2014 Annual Data Report: Epidemiology of End-stage Renal Disease in the United States*. Bethesda, MD: National Institutes of Health, National Institute of Diabetes and Digestive and Kidney Diseases, 2014:145–152.

11. Moss AH. Revised dialysis clinical practice guideline promotes more informed decision-making. *Clin J Am Soc Nephrol* 2010;5(12):2380–2383.

12. Tamura MK, Covinsky KE, Chertow GM. Functional status of elderly adults before and after initiation of dialysis. *N Engl J Med* 2009;361(16):1539–1547.

13. Carson RC, Juszczak M, Davenport A, et al. Is maximum conservative management an equivalent treatment option to dialysis for elderly patients with significant comorbid disease? *Clin J Am Soc Nephrol* 2009; 4(10):1611–1619.

14. O'Connor NR, Kumar P. Conservative management of end-stage renal disease without dialysis: a systematic review. *J Palliat Med* 2012;15(2): 228–235.

15. Joly D, Anglicheau D, Alberti C, et al. Octogenarians reaching end-stage renal disease: cohort study of decision-making and clinical outcomes. *J Am Soc Nephrol* 2003;14:1012–1021.

16. Chandna SM, Da Silva-Gane M, Marshall C, et al. Survival of elderly patients with stage 5 CKD: comparison of conservative management and renal replacement therapy. *Nephrol Dial Transplant* 2011;26(8):1608–1614.

17. Murtagh FE, Marsh JE, Donohoe P, et al. Dialysis or not? A comparative survival study of patients over 75 years with chronic kidney disease stage 5. *Nephrol Dial Transplant* 2007;22(7):1955–1962.

18. Smith C, Da Silva-Gane M, Chandna S, et al. Choosing not to dialyse: evaluation of planned non-dialytic management in a cohort of patients with end-stage renal failure. *Nephron Clin Pract* 2003;95(2):c40–c46. doi:10.1159/000073708.

19. Brown MA, Collett GK, Josland EA, et al. CKD in elderly patients managed without dialysis: survival, symptoms, and quality of life. *Clin J Am Soc Nephrol* 2015;10(2):260–268.

20. Murray SA, Kendall M, Boyd K, et al. Illness trajectories and palliative care. *BMJ* 2005;330(7498):1007–1011.

21. Beddhu S, Bruns FJ, Saul M, et al. A simple comorbidity scale predicts clinical outcomes and costs in dialysis patients. *Am J Med* 2000;108: 609–613.

22. Cohen LM, Ruthazer R, Moss AH, et al. Predicting six-month mortality for patients who are on maintenance hemodialysis. *Clin J Am Soc Nephrol* 2010;5(1):72–79.

23. Couchoud C, Labeeuw M, Moranne O, et al. A clinical score to predict 6-month prognosis in elderly patients starting dialysis for end-stage renal disease. *Nephrol Dial Transplant* 2009;24(5):1553–1561.

24. Crail S, Walker R, Brown M; for the Renal Supportive Care Working Group. Renal supportive and palliative care: position statement. *Nephrology (Carlton)* 2013;18(6):393–400.

25. Swidler M. Considerations in starting a patient with advanced frailty on dialysis: complex biology meets challenging ethics. *Clin J Am Soc Nephrol* 2013;8(8):1421–1428.

26. Van Biesen W, Dequidt C, Vijit D, et al. Analysis of the reasons for transfers between hemodialysis and peritoneal dialysis and their effect on survivals. *Adv Perit Dial* 1998;14:90–94.

27. Schreiber M. XVIth Annual Conference on Peritoneal Dialysis. *Perit Dial Int* 1996;16:S66.

28. Burkart J. XVIth Annual Conference on Peritoneal Dialysis. *Perit Dial Int* 1996;16:S36.

29. Van Biesen W, Dequidt C, Vanholder R, et al. The impact of healthy start peritoneal dialysis on the evolution of residual renal function and nutrition parameters. *Adv Perit Dial* 2002;18:44–48.

30. Jaar BG, Plantinga LC, Crews DC, et al. Timing, causes, predictors and prognosis of switching from peritoneal dialysis to hemodialysis: a prospective study. *BMC Nephrol* 2009;10:3.

31. Pajek J, Hutchison AJ, Bhutani S, et al. Outcomes of peritoneal dialysis patients and switching to hemodialysis: a competing risks analysis. *Perit Dial Int* 2014;34:289–298.

32. Churchill D, Taylor D, Keshaviah P. Adequacy of dialysis and nutrition in continuous peritoneal dialysis: association with clinical outcomes. *J Am Soc Nephrol* 1996;7:198–207.

33. Lameire N, Vanholder R, Veyt D, et al. A longitudinal, five year survey of urea kinetic parameters of CAPD patients. *Kidney Int* 1992;42:426–532.
34. Rottembourg J. Residual renal function and recovery of renal function in patients treated by CAPD. *Kidney Int* 1993;43(Suppl 40):S106–S110.
35. Iest C, Vanholder R, Ringoir S. Loss of residual renal function in patients on regular hemodialysis. *Int J Artif Organs* 1989;12:154–159.
36. Najafi I, Hosseini M, Atabac S, et al. Patient outcome in primary peritoneal dialysis patients versus those transferred from hemodialysis and transplantation. *Int Urol Nephrol* 2012;44:1237–1242.
37. Port F, Wolfe R, Bloembergen W, et al. The study of outcomes for CAPD versus hemodialysis patients. *Perit Dial Int* 1996;16:628–633.
38. Bloembergen W, Port F, Mauger E, et al. A comparison of mortality between patients treated with hemodialysis and peritoneal dialysis. *J Am Soc Nephrol* 1995;6:177–183.
39. Bloembergen W, Port F, Mauger E, et al. A comparison of cause of death between patients treated with hemodialysis and peritoneal dialysis. *J Am Soc Nephrol* 1995;6:184–191.
40. Maiorca R, Cancarini G, Brunori G, et al. Morbidity and mortality of CAPD and hemodialysis. *Kidney Int* 1993;43(Suppl 40):S4–S15.
41. Foley R, Parfrey P, Harnett J, et al. Mode of dialysis therapy and mortality in end-stage renal disease. *J Am Soc Nephrol* 1998;9:267–276.
42. Khan I, Campbell MK, Cantarovich D, et al. Survival on renal replacement therapy in Europe: is there a 'center effect'? *Nephrol Dial Transplant* 1996;11:300–307.
43. Vonesh E, Moran J. Mortality in end-stage renal disease: a reassessment of differences between patients treated with hemodialysis and peritoneal dialysis. *J Am Soc Nephrol* 1999;10:354–365.
44. Fenton S, Schaubel D, Desmeules M, et al. Hemodialysis versus peritoneal dialysis: a comparison of adjusted mortality rates. *Am J Kidney Dis* 1997;30:334–342.

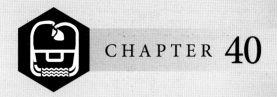

CHAPTER **40**

Choosing the Best Dialysis Option in the Patient with Acute Kidney Injury and in the Intensive Care Unit

Ami M. Patel and Beje Thomas

Acute kidney injury (AKI) occurs commonly in the intensive care unit (ICU) inflicting up to a third of the patients (1). The incidence of patients requiring renal replacement therapy (RRT) in the ICU is about 5% to 6% (2). It is well known that AKI is associated with increased mortality, and patients with AKI and multiorgan failure have mortality rates more than 50% (2,3). The use of RRT in AKI has been independently associated with even higher risk of death with mortality rates reaching as high as 75% (3–6). Over the past decade, dialysis-requiring AKI has increased about 10% per year, and the number of deaths associated with it has more than doubled (7). As many as 40% of survivors of AKI are left with stage 3 or greater chronic kidney disease, and approximately 5% remained dialysis dependent at 90 days (2,8,9).

With the lack of effective pharmacologic treatments, the care of the patient with AKI is limited to supportive management, in which RRT plays an integral role. There has been a significant evolution of RRT with the advent of continuous renal replacement therapy (CRRT). Initially, CRRT was offered as a therapy of last resort in the most critically ill patients who were hemodynamically intolerant of intermittent hemodialysis (IHD). As CRRT gained popularity as the dominant form of RRT in the ICU, it has been used for the broader application of extracorporeal blood purification (ECBP) during critical illness. The role of CRRT has been expanded for nonrenal indications, such as a tool for anti-inflammatory therapy and volume control (10).

The goals of this chapter are to characterize different forms of RRTs in the ICU, review the evidence-based literature on the application and the use of RRT in the ICU, and describe the role of RRT in specific disease conditions commonly confronted in the ICU.

 TECHNICAL ASPECTS OF RENAL REPLACEMENT THERAPY IN THE INTENSIVE CARE UNIT

This section of the chapter discusses different modalities of RRT in the ICU and review through the calculations for clearance. Also, it reviews forms of anticoagulation for CRRT, dialysis solution, dialysis access, and other technical aspects.

Modes of Renal Replacement Therapy

There are multiple options for RRT that can be used in the treatment of AKI in the ICU. These include conventional IHD; various modalities of CRRT; "hybrid" modalities that combine features of IHD and CRRT, which are known as prolonged intermittent renal replacement therapy (PIRRT); and peritoneal dialysis (PD). **TABLE 40.1** summarizes solute clearance and prescription for each therapy.

Intermittent Hemodialysis

Traditionally, nephrologists have used IHD to treat AKI in the ICU. Solute clearance is mainly through diffusion, and volume is removed via ultrafiltration. The principal advantages of IHD include rapid removal of solute and volume, making it ideal for certain clinical scenarios such as drug intoxication and management of severe hyperkalemia. The major disadvantage of IHD is the risk of hypotension, which occurs in approximately 20% to 30% of hemodialysis sessions (11,12). The rapid solute removal and shift in electrolytes can exacerbate hemodynamic instability, causing IHD to be intolerable in critically ill patients. For adequacy, the target Kt/V is 1.2 per treatment or urea reduction ratio greater than 0.7. IHD and PD are discussed in greater detail in other sections of this book.

TABLE 40.1	Typical Dialysis Prescription for Various Modalities[a]						
Type of Therapy	Solute Transport	Duration (h)	Replacement Fluid (mL/h)	Blood Flow (mL/min)	Dialysate Flow (mL/h)	Ultrafiltrate Flow (mL/h)
CVVH	Convection	24	500–4,000	100–300	0	500–4,000
CVVHD	Diffusion	24	–	100–300	500–4,000	0–350
CVVHDF	Convection and diffusion	24	500–4,000	100–300	500–4,000	500–4,000
PIRRT (<12 h) or SLED	Diffusion mostly	6–10	–	100–250	200–400	0–1,000
PIRRT (>12 h)	Diffusion mostly	~20	–	100–300	100–200	0–350
IHD	Diffusion mostly	3–4	–	200–450	400–800	0–1,500

[a]Rates of flow are typical in clinical practice.

CVVH, continuous venovenous hemofiltration; CVVHD, continuous venovenous hemodialysis; CVVHDF, continuous venovenous hemodiafiltration; PIRRT, prolonged intermittent renal replacement therapy; SLED, sustained low-efficiency dialysis; IHD, intermittent hemodialysis.

From Teo BW, Messer JS, Paganini EP, et al. Slow continuous therapies. In: Daugirdas JT, Blake PG, Ing TS, eds. *Handbook of Dialysis*. 4th ed. Philadelphia, PA: Lippincott Williams & Wilkins, 2007:219–251; Tolwani A. Continuous renal-replacement therapy for acute kidney injury. *N Engl J Med* 2012;367(26):2505–2514.

Prolonged Intermittent Renal Replacement Therapy

This category is also known as extended daily dialysis (EDD). The common form of PIRRT is sustained low-efficiency dialysis (SLED), which uses the same dialysis machine as for IHD, but the therapy is delivered at reduced blood and dialysate flow rate over a longer duration of time, usually over 6 to 10 hours. Typical blood-flow rate is around 200 to 300 mL/min with dialysate flow rate around 200 to 400 mL/min. Also, PIRRT can be delivered longer than SLED with duration around 20 hours. In this situation, blood flow is around 150 mL/min with dialysate flow around 100 mL/min. The major benefits of SLED are the reduced cost and staff time while providing solute removal equivalent to CRRT. Also, SLED may be routinely performed without anticoagulation. In one study, the weekly cost to the hospital was $1,431 for SLED; $2,607 for CRRT with heparin; and $3,089 for CRRT with citrate (13).

Continuous Renal Replacement Therapy

CRRT was developed in the 1980s specifically for the treatment of critically ill patients with AKI who could not tolerate conventional IHD due to hemodynamic instability or when IHD could not control volume and metabolic derangements. The slower clearance and volume removal through CRRT make it the preferred modality in the ICU patient requiring vasopressors. CRRT allows for greater volume removal with better hemodynamic tolerance in patients who have high obligate fluid intake such as more than 4 L/d. Disadvantages for CRRT include the higher cost, increased nursing support, frequent clotting, and risk of underdosing of antibiotics and other medications (**Table 40.2**). Medication dosing in CRRT is not well studied.

The blood circuit for CRRT is commonly a venovenous circuit through a double-lumen, large-bore catheter. There are four options for CRRT: continuous venovenous hemodialysis (CVVHD), continuous venovenous hemofiltration (CVVH), continuous venovenous hemodiafiltration (CVVHDF), and slow continuous ultrafiltration (SCUF) (14,15). **Figure 40.1** shows the circuit components in the various forms of CRRT. **Table 40.1** summarizes typical dialysis prescription for different forms of CRRT. The usual blood flow is around 200 to 300 mL/min. Increasing blood flow from 100 or 150 mL/min to 200 or 300 mL/min helps increase the efficiency of clearance and reduce the risk of clotting (16).

Continuous Venovenous Hemodialysis

The primary means of solute clearance is through diffusion. The dialysate flow is slower in comparison to IHD and runs in the opposite direction to the faster moving blood flow in a counter-current course, allowing for maximal saturation of solutes of the outflow dialysis. Solute removal occurs by concentration gradient between blood and dialysate compartment across a semipermeable biosynthetic membrane otherwise known as the hemodiafilter. Substances such as urea, creatinine, and potassium diffuse down their concentration gradient from the blood to dialysate compartment during hemodialysis, while other solutes, such as bicarbonate, move from the dialysate to blood compartment. The rate of removal of solute through diffusion depends on the size. Smaller molecules diffuse more easily, and larger molecules diffuse slowly and are not as easily removed (14,15).

Continuous Venovenous Hemofiltration

The primary means of solute clearance is through convection. As the blood flows through the hemodiafilter, transmembrane pressure gradient between the blood and ultrafiltrate compartment forces plasma water to be filtered across the hemodiafilter (or also

TABLE 40.2	Advantages and Disadvantages of Continuous Renal Replacement Therapy	
Advantages	**Disadvantages**
Better hemodynamic stability	Not for intoxication and severe hyperkalemia
Capable of greater clearance over time	Expensive
Better volume control for high obligate fluid intake	Increased nursing support
Less effects on intracranial pressure	Increased clearance of antibiotics and medications
	Hypophosphatemia and other electrolyte disturbance
	Frequent clotting
	Limit patient mobility
	Bleeding complication with anticoagulation
	Nutrient losses

From Tolwani A. Continuous renal-replacement therapy for acute kidney injury. *N Engl J Med* 2012;367(26):2505–2514; and Clark EG, Bagshaw SM. Unnecessary renal replacement therapy for acute kidney injury is harmful for renal recovery. *Semin Dial* 2015;28(1):6–11.

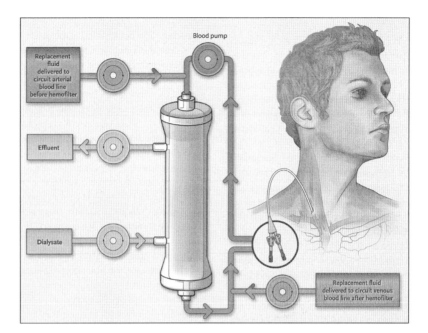

FIGURE 40.1 Circuit components in continuous renal replacement therapy. [Reprinted with permission from Tolwani A. Continuous renal-replacement therapy for acute kidney injury. *N Engl J Med* 2012;367(26):2505–2514.]

known as hemofilter). The small-sized solutes (such as urea and electrolytes) are removed in the same concentration as the plasma. The volume removed in the ultrafiltrate is replenished by a replacement (or substitution) fluid to prevent excessive fluid removal and volume depletion, thereby diluting the concentration of the plasma solutes. The replacement fluid is infused into the blood compartment either prefilter (also known as predilution), postfilter (also known as postdilution), or both. The rate of solute removal depends on the size of hemofilter pores and the convective force, which allows for larger molecules to be removed in contrast to hemodialysis (14,15).

The downside of using only postfilter replacement is the increased rate of clotting as the blood filters through the hemofilter and becomes increasingly concentrated at the end of the hemofilter with the removal of the ultrafiltrate. Therefore, replacement fluid is usually infused either as all prefilter or as a combination of prefilter and postfilter to reduce the risk of clotting. Common percentages for replacement fluid is 100% prefilter, 70% prefilter with 30% postfilter, and 50% prefilter with 50% postfilter. As the percentage of replacement fluid is increased postfilter, the risk of clotting rises, which can be ascertained by calculating the filtration fraction. Filtration fraction above 25% indicates a greater risk for clotting, and these calculations are described further in the next section of this chapter. On the other hand, when replacement fluid is given prefilter, the blood entering the filter will become diluted, reducing the maximum solute clearance. For instance, if prefilter replacement fluid is infusing at 40 mL/min and blood flow is at rate of 200 mL/min, the dilution factor will be 200/240 = 83% or there is a 17% dilution. Depending on the solute and dialysis prescription, prefilter replacement reduces clearance by 15% to 20% (17). On a milliliter for milliliter basis, CVVHD is more efficient, removing small-sized solutes in comparison to CVVH with prefilter replacement. However, middle-sized molecule solutes (500 Da to 60 kDa) such as β_2-microglobulin are cleared more effectively with CVVH due convective clearance.

Continuous Venovenous Hemodiafiltration

This combines both CVVHD and CVVH, which is usually with prefilter replacement therapy. There are several types of CRRT machines available, and depending on the machine, it can provide different modalities.

Slow Continuous Ultrafiltration

This is used commonly in patients who need only volume removal but not solute clearance. There is no dialysis or replacement fluid in this mode of therapy; only ultrafiltrate is removed at a slow rate using a hemofilter.

Dialysate Solution

Dialysate and replacement solutions are very similar, and many of the dialysate solutions are being used as replacement fluid off-label. These solutions contain potassium, calcium, magnesium, and glucose in physiologic ranges. There are additional solutions such as varying potassium and calcium baths, which are available for special circumstances. For hyperkalemia, one can use 0 to 2 mEq/L potassium bath. As for the anion buffer, acetate, lactate, citrate, and bicarbonate have all been used, but bicarbonate is preferred (14). Lactate-based solutions are unfavorable because it can cause hyperlactatemia in critically ill patients with liver dysfunction and may be associated with higher episodes of hypotension in comparison to bicarbonate-based (15,18). Acetate-based dialysate fluid has been implicated with contributing to intradialytic hypotension with IHD. Acetate can induce production of nitric oxide, a vasodilator (19). However, recent study showed that acetate-containing solution does not seem to affect hemodynamics because lower amount of acetate is delivered in comparison to the amount delivered in IHD (15,20). Popular dialysate solutions have predominant concentration bicarbonate with low concentration of lactate, usually around 3 mmol/L. Lower levels of bicarbonate are recommended with citrate anticoagulation to avoid severe metabolic alkalosis since citrate is metabolized by liver to bicarbonate.

Vascular Access

Vascular access is absolutely necessary for RRT. However, it must be kept in mind that with ICU patients with AKI, there is the possibility of long-term dialysis, so maintaining the vasculature is important for future dialysis access. There are primarily three forms of access: dialysis catheters (DCs), arteriovenous fistula (AVF), and arteriovenous graft (AVG). In the various modes of CRRT, the DC is preferred. There is limited data on DCs used in the ICU as most of the data is actually from studies looking at central venous catheters (CVCs) and access in end-stage kidney disease (ESKD) patients. It is questionable if this data is applicable as there are significant differences between the catheters and a patient in the ICU versus a patient in the dialysis unit.

Blood flow through the catheter is a significant factor in determining the dialysis dose provided. This is particularly important in IHD since blood flow tends to be higher in comparison to CRRT, in which dosing is more dependent on the effluent volume. DC dysfunction as defined in various studies as a low blood flow of <150 to 200 mL/min with inadequate dialysis dose delivery and blood flow reduction of more than 20% even after attempts to maintain patency of the DC (21). Early DC dysfunction is usually due to improper catheter placement technique such as cannulating the wrong vessel, catheter tip malposition, or kinking of the catheter. Late DC dysfunction is usually due to thrombosis intrinsic (obstructive thrombosis of the catheter lumen) or extrinsic (thrombosis or stenosis of the blood vessel) to the catheter. The majority of DC catheter dysfunction occurs in the first 10 days but increases the longer the catheter remains inside (21,22). Countermeasures that can be used to increase the blood flow after catheter placement include repositioning the patient, flushing the line with saline, using an anticoagulation (citrate or heparin) dwell in the DC, and reversing the lines. Of course, accurate placement of the DC is important, and this has improved with the use of ultrasound guidance to image the targeted vessel throughout the procedure and x-ray to confirm placement. If all measures fails, then replacing the DC might be the only alternative to provide an adequate dialysis dose. This can be done over a guidewire.

Another complication of DC is infection, which is defined by two separate cultures separated by 120 minutes that grow the same phenotypic organism. One culture is drawn from the peripheral blood and the other from the CVC. The rates of catheter infections have dramatically declined due to various methods aimed at preventing CVC infections in the ICU. These methods include adequate hand hygiene, barrier precautions, prompt removal of catheter when it is no longer necessary, and advancements in dressings. There is a need for large randomized trials before the routine use of antimicrobial locks or antimicrobial catheters can be recommended (22,23).

The options of dialysis access site are the internal jugular (IJ) vein, the subclavian vein, and the femoral vein. The most recent Kidney Disease: Improving Global Outcomes (KDIGO) AKI guidelines present an ungraded recommendation for which vessels to use. In descending order from most to least desired site, right IJ vein, femoral vein, left IJ vein, and lastly, the subclavian veins. The reason for the left IJ vein and both subclavian veins are less desirable are due to the increased risk of the development of central vein stenosis (24). Traditionally, femoral vein access has been attributed to greater infection risk and to restrict patient mobility (23). This has more recently come under scrutiny. Parienti et al. (25) performed one of the first randomized controlled trials on catheter site insertion. They found that the risk for a catheter-related blood stream infection was lower for femoral lines if the body mass index (BMI) was <24.2 and for the IJ if BMI was >28. A meta-analysis reported that outside of patients with a high BMI that there was no significant increase in infection rates between the subclavian or IJ veins versus the femoral vein. The meta-analysis also stated that there was no difference in the deep vein thrombosis rates (26). Both of these conclusions of no significant difference in infectious or thrombosis rates were reported by a recent Cochrane review (27).

The catheter site does also play a role in catheter dysfunction rates and the dose of dialysis delivered to a patient. In the multicenter Cathedia Study, which included 736 patients, there were similar rates of first DC dysfunction between the IJ (11.1%) and femoral (10.3%) veins. It is important to note the side of the DC affected dysfunction rates: the right IJ was 6.6%, the femoral veins 10.3 %, and the left IJ was 19.5%. In regard to dialysis dose, if the desired blood flow is less than 200 mL/min, there is negligible difference between the IJ and femoral veins; however, if the blood flow is over 200 mL/min, the right IJ vein is preferred (28). Remember, the right IJ vein is the most direct and straight route to the superior vena cava (22).

In summary, the first choice of access should be the right IJ vein; remember, an advantage of IJ access is that the patient will be able to mobilize easier (24). The femoral veins should be considered particularly in patients with a lower BMI (<24), high likelihood of long-term dialysis, and if emergent dialysis is needed with inexperienced operator or no ultrasound available. The left IJ vein should be considered if the right IJ and femoral veins are not optimal choices. The subclavian vein is the last resort with the right side being preferable (23).

Anticoagulation

The CRRT extracorporeal circuit's patency and filter lifespan are of critical importance to ensure that there is adequate solute clearance and filtration. A major hindrance to this is clotting in the extracorporeal circuit leading to a discontinuation of therapy (29). It has been shown that when 24 hours of CRRT are prescribed on average without anticoagulation, the patient receives therapy for about 16 to 18 hours. This interrupted treatment results in a higher cost, unnecessary blood loss, and an increased strain on nursing. Hence, prevention of clotting by various methods including anticoagulation is required for the patient on CRRT. In regard to anticoagulation, it is usually necessary for the patient on CRRT, and this is a distinct disadvantage of this modality of RRT. Studies have shown 5% to 50% of patients on anticoagulation with CRRT have bleeding complications. The desired anticoagulant should have certain qualities including providing optimal anticoagulation with minimal systemic side effects including bleeding. It should be readily available, able to be monitored, reversible, and inexpensive (30–32). In this section, we will discuss both nonanticoagulant and anticoagulant strategies to prevent clotting of the CRRT extracorporeal circuit.

The patient's clinical status, characteristics of the extracorporeal circuit, and blood flow all affect the coagulation pathophysiology of the patient. The clinical status can have a procoaguable effect from the pathologic presence of proteins as in antiphospholipid syndrome or secondary to overt inflammation as in sepsis. It is thought that once blood comes into contact with the extracorporeal circuit, there is stimulation of the coagulation system. This includes activation of the intrinsic and extrinsic coagulation systems with thrombin generation, monocytes, and platelets. In an inflamed state, there is diminished activity of the endogenous anticoagulation system with decreased antithrombin, protein C, and tissue factor plasminogen inhibitor. This is due to decreased production and even direct lysis of anticoagulants. Once the clotting starts, usually there is fibrinolysis, but this is impaired as well with the increased activity of plasminogen activator inhibitor. The endothelium's antithrombogenic properties are also lost due to inflammation and oxidative stress. Other causes of clotting are blood flow stasis, hemoconcentration, turbulent blood flow, and contact between blood and air (30,32).

Vascular access obviously affects blood flow. We have gone into further detail elsewhere about vascular access but will briefly review the type and location of access. There is no significant difference in filter life when comparing the IJ and femoral sites (33,34). However, there is less infectious risk and recirculation with an internal IJ. Femoral catheters tend to kink more particularly in the obese patient. IJ catheters can generate high access pressures when a patient is agitated or coughing. There is some data that show the right side for both catheters are associated with less catheter dysfunction (34). The actual catheter itself should optimally be short and have a wide inner diameter. In addition, staff managing the CRRT extracorporeal circuit should respond to pump alarms in a timely manner, be able to recognize when a catheter is kinked, and properly rinse the filter to minimize the blood-air contact which initiates clotting (32). We will discuss filtration fraction later in this chapter.

We will primarily discuss the use of heparin and citrate for anticoagulation. There are other potential agents available that are not routinely used. These include heparinoids and platelet-inhibiting agents. We will not cover these agents in this section.

Unfractionated Heparin Anticoagulation

Unfractionated heparin (UFH) is the most commonly used anticoagulant. UFH's mechanism potentiates the effects of antithrombin III by a thousandfold, inhibiting thrombin activity and factor Xa. The half-life of UFH is about 90 minutes to 3 hours depending on kidney function. UFH has advantages including physician familiarity, reversibility with protamine, relative short half-life, and ease of monitoring. There are significant disadvantages such as dosing variability, heparin-induced thrombocytopenia (HIT), heparin resistance, and risk of hemorrhage. The incidence of bleeding has a wide range of 10% to 50%. UFH when used is usually as a bolus of 2,000 to 5,000 IU at 30 IU/kg. This is followed by a continuous infusion in the arterial arm of 5 to 10 IU/kg/h to maintain an activated partial thromboplastin time (aPTT) of 34 to 45 seconds or an aPTT of 1.5 to 2.0 times the normal level (31,35).

The reversal agent or antagonist for UFH is protamine. When used in CRRT, protamine is given postfilter at a ratio of 100 between prefilter heparin (IU) and protamine (mg). The protamine–heparin complex is released into the body and broken down by the reticuloendothelial system. The side effects of protamine include hypotension, thrombocytopenia, leukopenia, cardiac depression, and anaphylaxis. Regional anticoagulation using heparin with protamine reversal is cumbersome due to the difficulty in calculating how much protamine is actually necessary. There is also variability in prolonging filter life. Therefore, heparin anticoagulation is commonly applied without the use of protamine. Low molecular weight heparin (LMWH) is not used routinely for CRRT anticoagulation. This is due to an increased risk of bleeding, cost with need to monitor anti-Xa activity, and risk of HIT, and lack of clearance in kidney disease (31). However, even if one is able to perform anti Xa monitoring, it is not entirely reliable in predicting bleeding complications (10).

Heparin-Induced Thrombocytopenia

Once there is a suspicion for HIT, all heparinoids should be stopped as soon as possible and replaced with alternative anticoagulation. Thrombocytopenia occurs in up to 60% critically ill patients, and when

CRRT is initiated, a drop in platelet count by as much as 50% has been reported. The diagnosis of HIT is based on detection of platelet factor 4 antibodies (10,36,37). Another functional assay used as a diagnostic test is the serotonin releases assay. The alternative anticoagulation used in the clinical setting of HIT with CRRT is a direct thrombin inhibitor. The preferred direct thrombin inhibitor of choice in renal dysfunction without liver failure is argatroban and in those with liver failure, bivalirudin. These agents would treat both the procoagulable state of HIT and provide anticoagulation for the CRRT. An alternative anticoagulation strategy to prevent HIT is to avoid heparin-based agents all together and use citrate anticoagulation (37–39).

Citrate Anticoagulation

Citrate has multiple advantages, namely, avoidance of systemic anticoagulation and no association with HIT. It has been shown to have better filter survival times and less bleeding when compared to heparinoids (40–42). Disadvantages of citrate anticoagulation are metabolic abnormalities, increased complexity, and the lack of universal availability. Citrate solutions and protocols have been reviewed recently. Citrate prevents clotting in CRRT by chelating ionized calcium in the extracorporeal circuit. Calcium is required for multiple steps in the coagulation cascade. There is also thought to be additional antihemostatic and anti-inflammatory properties of citrate. Citrate is infused in the arterial limb (prefilter) of the CRRT proportional to the blood flow. Citrate itself is not measured, but instead, the postfilter ionized calcium is used. The citrate infusion is titrated so that the postfilter ionized calcium is <0.35 mmol/L. This level of ionized calcium is associated with optimal anticoagulation in the extracorporeal circuit and correlates with a citrate concentration of 4 to 6 mmol/L (40,42,43). Citrate has a low molecular weight, high sieving coefficient, and high diffusion/convective clearance so that a major portion of the citrate–calcium complexes is lost in the effluent (44). This would lead to systemic hypocalcemia if not for the calcium infusion postfilter to replace the lost calcium. Calcium chloride or calcium gluconate is used for the calcium infusion. Citrate–calcium complexes that are not lost in the effluent but instead return to the systemic circulation are metabolized to bicarbonate by the skeletal muscle, kidney, and liver. Each citrate–calcium complex yield three molecules of bicarbonate and returns the ionized calcium to the patient (40,42).

Metabolic Abnormalities with Citrate Anticoagulation

The most common metabolic complications of regional citrate anticoagulation are hypocalcemia and metabolic alkalosis (45). We will discuss monitoring of electrolytes in the next section. Intravenous infusion of calcium postfilter is given and adjusted on an ongoing basis to prevent hypocalcemia. In general, with blood-flow rates of about 200 mL/min and effluent rates of 25 to 30 mL/kg/h, calcium supplementation starts at 2 to 3 mmol/h. One has to be cognizant of the replacement fluid/dialysate containing calcium as this could affect the rate of citrate and calcium infusions. The goal for the systemic ionized calcium is 0.9 to 1.2 mmol/L. The other possible etiology of hypocalcemia with citrate infusion is ineffective metabolism and subsequent citrate accumulation seen in liver failure or tissue hypoperfusion (shock). If citrate is not metabolized, then calcium is not released from the citrate–calcium complex. The solutions for this include reducing the citrate infusion, enhancing citrate removal in the effluent (by increasing the replacement fluid or dialysate rate), and switching from citrate- to bicarbonate-based replacement fluid or dialysate. Hypercalcemia also occurs with citrate anticoagulation if there is an excessive replacement with intravenous calcium (40,42).

Another effect of inadequate citrate metabolism is anion gap metabolic acidosis. The management of this is similar as mentioned previously for hypocalcemia in the same clinical setting. Metabolic acidosis is also caused by an imbalance of buffer (citrate and bicarbonate) being delivered to the patient and that being lost in the effluent. One can increase the amount of buffer by increasing the citrate infusion rate or by decreasing the loss in the effluent by reducing the replacement fluid or dialysate rates. Other options are intravenous bicarbonate infusion or increasing the amount of bicarbonate in the replacement fluid or dialysate.

Metabolic alkalosis as we have mentioned is the second most common complication. This is usually secondary to an excess buffer load or not appropriately matching the CRRT solutions with citrate. An excess buffer load is a result of a higher blood-flow rate, which subsequently infuse citrate at a higher rate. One option is to reduce the amount of citrate entering the circuit by decreasing blood flow or by aiming for a higher ionized calcium goal (i.e., lower citrate level). The other option is to increase the citrate lost in the effluent by increasing the replacement or dialysate flow rates. An important caveat is that there are other sources of citrate in the intensive care setting. Citrate is the preservative for blood products, and so the patient receiving multiple transfusions is also receiving an increased amount of citrate. Another example is acetone in total parenteral nutrition. The other mechanism of metabolic alkalosis is inappropriately high bicarbonate in the replacement fluid or dialysate in a patient receiving citrate. The conversion of the citrate that reaches systemic circulation to bicarbonate must be accounted for when considering the replacement fluid or dialysate. For instance, when starting a patient on citrate who was not previously on anticoagulation with CRRT, one must lower the bicarbonate in the CRRT fluids being used. Another approach to prevent metabolic alkalosis is to use hyperchloremic solutions such as normal saline pre- or postfilter (40,42,45).

Other electrolytes potentially affected include magnesium and sodium. Magnesium is also chelated by citrate but usually does not need replacement as magnesium is found in the dialysate or the replacement fluids. Hypernatremia can result from not adjusting to the sodium load that occurs with citrate anticoagulation. To prevent hypernatremia, it is important to reduce the sodium concentration in the dialysate or the replacement fluids. Hyponatremia is seen if there is an excess of hypotonic fluid being given to the patient or a technical error where the citrate has not been given (45).

Citrate Toxicity and Monitoring

Citrate accumulation and toxicity risks include the patient with liver dysfunction, with severe tissue hypoperfusion (shock), or a large citrate load (multiple blood products). The liver is the main site of metabolism for citrate. Clinically, this is seen with worsening metabolic acidosis and hypocalcemia potentially leading to hypotension and arrhythmias. Typically, electrolytes are monitored frequently when a patient is on CRRT by as much as every 4 to 6 hours. More frequent monitoring could be required for the patient with an increased risk for citrate toxicity (40,42). Citrate itself is not routinely measured but instead the ratio of total-to-ionized calcium (calcium ratio) is used as a surrogate for the citrate level. The accumulation of citrate results in an increased infusion of calcium postfilter leading to a disproportionate rise in total calcium as compared to ionized calcium. The critical cutoff for the calcium ratio is >2.5 indicating that the patient is at increased risk for metabolic complications and citrate toxicity (46). Management of citrate

accumulation and toxicity revolves around reducing exposure and increasing the clearance of citrate. This can be done by reducing the blood-flow rate and amount of citrate infused aiming again for higher calcium targets. On the other hand, the clinician can increase clearance by increasing convective or dialysis forces (43).

In high-risk patients, such as those with liver failure, citrate may be used but with caution. Liver indices are not always reliable in predicting metabolic clearance. Better predictors of the liver's ability to metabolize citrate include a prothrombin time ≥33 seconds and a lactic acid level ≥3.4 mmol/L (47,48). Laboratory monitoring should be more frequent as much as every 2 hours and should include the calcium ratio and the pH. We have mentioned citrate toxicity management by decreasing the exposure and increasing the clearance of citrate in this section already. Other available measures to manage metabolic acidosis and hypocalcemia are the systemic infusion of bicarbonate and/or calcium as needed. If acidosis is present, we advise to correct the calcium first as bicarbonate infusion can result in a further drop in ionized calcium level (43).

In summary in deciding which modality of anticoagulation to use for CRRT, it is best to consider the time interval it will be required for, the bleeding risk of the individual patient, and the therapeutic agents available. The clinician must also be aware of the intensity of monitoring and the use of resources required with anticoagulation in CRRT. In the patient that cannot have anticoagulation, it is possible to maintain CRRT with other strategies as we have described (49).

Clearance for Continuous Renal Replacement Therapy

The "dose" of RRT administered is determined by the effluent flow, which comprises of ultrafiltrate in CVVH, the spent dialysate in CVVHD, and both in CVVHDF. It is commonly reported as the effluent flow rate in milliliters per kilogram per body weight. The recommended effluent flow dose is at least 20 to 25 mL/kg of body weight per hour in order to achieve adequate solute clearance (14,50,51). There are often frequent interruptions in CRRT such as procedures and clotting of hemofilter; therefore, effluent flow may need to be increased to account for lost time. In addition, clotting and protein deposition on hemofilter can reduce actual solute clearance (14).

Calculations

$$K = Q_E \times C_E / C_B \qquad (40.1)$$

Where K is the clearance, Q_E is the effluent rate, C_E is the effluent concentration, and C_B is the blood concentration. K is expressed in mL/min (**EQUATION 40.1**) (52).

$$Q_E = Q_d + Q_R + Q_{net} \qquad (40.2)$$

$$Q_{uf} = Q_R + Q_{net} \qquad (40.3)$$

where Q_d is dialysate fluid rate, Q_R is replacement fluid rate, Q_{net} is the net fluid removal rate, and Q_{uf} is the total ultrafiltration volume. All are reported in mL/min. The effluent rate, which is also known as "dose" of CRRT, can be expressed in mL/h or as mL/kg/h. The recommended "dose" of RRT is at least 20 to 25 mL/kg/h (**EQUATIONS 40.2 and 40.3**) (50–53).

$$\sigma = C_E / C_B \qquad (40.4)$$

where σ is the sieving coefficient. For small molecules, the sieving coefficient approximates to 1. Using urea as the solute, equilibrium is achieved between C_E and C_B since the effluent rate is much smaller

TABLE 40.3	Sieving Coefficient of Different Molecules in Continuous Renal Replacement Therapy^a	
Molecule	**Molecular Weight (Da)**	**Sieving Coefficients**
Urea	60	1.0
Creatinine	113	1.0
Vitamin B$_{12}$	1,355	1.0
Albumin	65,000	<0.01
Myoglobin	17,000	0.58

^{a}The sieving coefficient depends on multitude of factors, including dialysis prescription, characteristics of the molecule, and characteristics of the hemodiafilter membrane. The sieving coefficient is for the AN69 ST membrane for the Prismaflex sets.

than the blood-flow rate and the solute size for urea is small (60 Da) (**Equation 40.4**). For instance, effluent rate is usually ranging 17 to 50 mL/min versus blood-flow rate around 200 to 300 mL/min. Therefore, the sieving coefficient for urea is 1. Another determinant of the sieving coefficient is the pore size of the hemodiafilter. **Table 40.3** shows an example of the sieving coefficient of different molecules (54).

$$\text{Dilution factor} = Q_B / (Q_B + Q_R) \quad (40.5)$$

Diluting factor is used in calculating K for CVVH with prefilter replacement, which reduces the maximum solute clearance per unit volume of replacement fluid in comparison to postfilter replacement (**Equation 40.5**). With the infusion of prefilter replacement fluid, the blood entering the hemofilter becomes diluted and as a result, the effluent has a lower concentration of solutes than plasma (52).

$$FF = Q_{uf} / Q_p \quad (40.6)$$

$$Qp = (1 - \text{hematocrit}) (Q_B) \quad (40.7)$$

$$FF = Q_{uf} / (1 - \text{hematocrit}) (Q_B) \quad (40.8)$$

where FF is filtration fraction, Q_p is plasma flow expressed in mL/min, and Q_B is blood flow expressed in mL/min (**Equations 40.6 to 40.8**).

FF is the ratio of the ultrafiltrate to the plasma flow entering the hemofilter (**Figure 40.2**). The goal filtration fraction is <25% to reduce the chances of clotting. When FF is ≥25%, there is a greater chance of clotting. Raising the blood flow or reducing the ultrafiltration rate decreases the risk of clotting. Conversely, lowering the blood flow or increasing the ultrafiltration rate increases the risk of clotting. Furthermore, adding prefilter replacement lowers the filter fraction because the prefilter replacement fluid dilutes the plasma

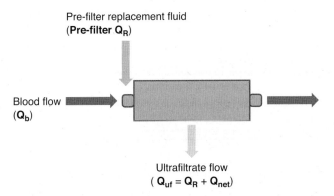

FIGURE 40.2 Determinants of filtration fraction.

flow entering the hemofilter (49). To calculate FF, the prefilter replacement fluid is added to the denominator (**Equation 40.9**).

$$FF = Q_{uf} / [(1 - \text{hematocrit}) (Q_B) + \text{prefilter } Q_R] \quad (40.9)$$

Example 1: Continuous Venovenous Hemodialysis

70-kg patient with CVVHD at Q_B 100 mL/min, Q_d 1,500 mL/h. Net fluid removal by CVVHD was 2 L. Hematocrit is 30%; C_E/C_B or σ for urea = 1.

$$K = Q_E \times C_E / C_B \qquad Q_E = Q_d + Q_R + Q_{net}$$
$$= 1,500 \text{ mL/h} + 0 + 83 \text{ mL/h}$$
$$= 1,583 \text{ mL/h}$$

$$K = (1,583 \text{ mL/h}) (1) = 26 \text{ mL/min}$$

"Dose" is (1,583 mL/h) / 70 kg = 23 mL/kg/h

$$FF = Q_{uf} / [(1 - \text{hematocrit}) (Q_B)]; Q_{uf} = Q_R + Q_{net}$$

$$Q_{uf} = 0 + 2 = 2 \text{ L/d or } 1.4 \text{ mL/min}$$

$$FF = 1.4 \text{ mL/min} / (1 - 0.3) (100 \text{ mL/min}) = 0.02 \text{ or } 2\%$$

Example 2: Continuous Venovenous Hemofiltration with Postfilter Replacement

70-kg patient with CVVH at Q_B 100 mL/min, Q_R 1,500 mL/h (postfilter). Net fluid removal by CVVH was 0. Hematocrit is 30%; C_E/C_B or σ for urea = 1.

$$K = Q_E \times C_E / C_B \qquad Q_E = Q_d + Q_R + Q_{net}$$
$$= 1,500 \text{ mL/h} + 0 + 0$$
$$= 1,500 \text{ mL/h}$$

$$K = (1,500 \text{ mL/h}) (1) = 25 \text{ mL/min}$$

"Dose" is (1,500 mL/h) / 70 kg = 21 mL/kg/h

$$FF = Q_{uf} / (1 - \text{hematocrit}) (Q_B); Q_{uf} = Q_R + Q_{net}$$

$$Q_{uf} = 1,500 \text{ mL/h} + 0 = 1500 \text{ mL/h or } 25 \text{ mL/min}$$

$$FF = 25 \text{ mL/min} / [100 \text{ mL/min} \times (1 - 0.3)] = 0.36 \text{ or } 36\%$$

Example 3: Continuous Venovenous Hemofiltration with Prefilter Replacement

70-kg patient with CVVH at Q_B 100 mL/min, Q_R 1,500 mL/h (prefilter). Net fluid removal by CVVH was 0. Hematocrit is 30%; C_E/C_B or σ for urea = 1.

$$K = Q_E \times C_E / C_B \qquad Q_E = Q_d + Q_R + Q_{net}$$
$$= 1,500 \text{ mL/h} + 0 + 0$$
$$= 1,500 \text{ mL/h}$$

Use dilution factor = $Q_B / (Q_B + Q_R)$

Therefore, $K = [Q_E \times C_E/C_B] \times [Q_B / (Q_B + Q_R)]$

$$K = (1,500 \text{ mL/h}) \times 1 \times (6,000 \text{ mL/h}) / (6,000 \text{ mL/h} + 1,500 \text{ mL/h}) = 1,200 \text{ mL/h or } 20 \text{ mL/min or } 17 \text{ mL/kg/h}$$

$$FF = Q_{uf} / [(1 - \text{hematocrit}) (Q_B) + \text{prefilter } Q_R]; Q_{uf} = Q_R + Q_{net}$$

$$Q_{uf} = 1,500 \text{ mL/h} + 0 = 1,500 \text{ mL/h or } 25 \text{ mL/min}$$

$$FF = 25 \text{ mL/min} / [100 \text{ mL/min} \times (1 - 0.3) + 25 \text{ mL/min}] = 0.26 \text{ or } 26\%$$

Example 4: Continuous Venovenous Hemodiafiltration

70-kg patient with CVVHDF at Q_B 100 mL/min, Q_R 1,500 mL/h (prefilter), Q_d 1,500 mL/h. Net fluid removal by CVVHDF was 0. Hematocrit is 30%; C_E/C_B or σ for urea = 1.

Total K = K for CVVH + K for CVVHD

K for CVVH = 1,200 mL/h or 20 mL/min or 17 mL/kg/h (see Example 3)

K for CVVHD = $Q_E \times C_E / C_B$ = (1,500 mL/h + 0) × 1 = 1,500 mL/h or 25 mL/min or 21 mL/kg/h (refer to Example 1)

Total K = 1,200 mL/h + 1,500 mL/h = 2,700 mL/h or 45 mL/min or 38 mL/kg/h

FF = Q_{uf} / [(1 − hematocrit) (Q_B) + prefilter Q_R]

Q_{uf} = Q_R + Q_{net} = 1,500 mL/h + 0 = 1,500 mL/h or 25 mL/min

FF = 25 mL/min / [(1 − 0.3) × 100 mL/min + 25 mL/min] = 0.26 or 26%

CLINICAL ISSUES OF RENAL REPLACEMENT THERAPY IN THE INTENSIVE CARE UNIT

There has been substantial advancement in regard to the optimal dosing of RRT through large multicenter, randomized clinical trials. However, the optimal timing of initiation of dialysis remains elusive, and the preferred modality of RRT in the ICU is somewhat controversial. This section of the chapter reviews through the literature discussing the issues surrounding the clinical applications of RRT in the ICU.

Indications for and Timing of Initiation of Renal Replacement Therapy

When first introduced into clinical practice in the 1940 to 1950s, RRT was mainly used to treat late and severe symptoms of kidney disease. Studies published during the 1960s to 1970s showed a worse mortality if RRT was started when blood urea nitrogen (BUN) exceeded 163 to 200 mg/dL versus BUN 93 to 150 mg/dL (55–57). The concept of "prophylactic" dialysis for AKI was first introduced by Teschan et al. (58) more than 50 years ago. They recommended starting dialysis before obvious clinical symptoms or biochemical derangements occur and they theorized that postponing dialysis can cause "retention of dialyzable substances which interfere with the functions of many cells and tissues," resulting in irreversible damage (58). However, it is difficult to conclude the benefits of preemptive dialysis from older studies since many were observational studies, the study population was younger compared to current, and

lastly, many would consider what was claimed to be early start with BUN ranging 90 to 150 mg/dL as rather late for initiation.

The indications for and optimal timing of initiation of RRT in patients with AKI has remained uncertain. There is little debate about initiation of RRT when there is severe volume overload, hyperkalemia, refractory metabolic acidosis, and overt uremic manifestations such as pericarditis. However, when there is no classic indication for RRT initiation, it is debatable whether starting dialysis "preemptively" will improve outcome. Some of the reasons to start dialysis preemptively are to improve volume control, restore acid–base homeostasis quicker, avoid situations for emergent "rescue" dialysis, and remove small middle-sized molecules. **TABLE 40.4** outlines conventional, preemptive, and nonrenal indications for RRT.

In this regard, it is worth reviewing key recent studies investigating the role of preemptive dialysis. Using the data from the Program to Improve Care in Acute Renal Disease (PICARD) cohort, which was a multicenter observational retrospective study, Liu et al. (59) analyzed 243 patients who required dialysis for AKI and subdivided the group by the level of BUN when dialysis was initiated. The higher degree of azotemia group was defined as BUN >76 mg/dL, and lower azotemia group was BUN ≤76 mg/dL. After multivariate adjustment for comorbid diseases and for propensity for initiation of RRT, late RRT was associated with a twofold risk of death at 60 days since the diagnosis of AKI (59). In another study, Vaara et al. (60) examined 239 patients who were started on RRT in the ICU using the prospective observational cohort from the Finnish Acute Kidney Injury Study Group. Patients were divided into those who were started on RRT for classic indications versus preemptive initiation. The classic group was further subdivided into delayed, which meant RRT was initiated >12 hours since the indication, versus urgent, which meant that RRT was initiated <12 hours. The crude 90-day mortality rate was 68% for the classic-delayed group, 39% for classic-urgent, and 30% for the preemptive group. The crude 90-day mortality rate was 49.3% for the non-RRT match equivalent to the preemptive group. Although initial studies reported decreased mortality with earlier initiation of renal support, the results are obscured by multiple limitations such as nonrandomization of groups and probable differences in the indications for initiation. More importantly, these studies did not include the analysis of patients with AKI who did not receive RRT because they either recovered renal function or died (60).

There are a few small-sized randomized controlled trials investigating the optimal timing of RRT. Study by Bouman et al. (61) was a prospective study of 106 critically ill patients with AKI randomized into three groups: early low-volume CVVH at average dose 20 mL/kg/h, early high-volume CVVH at average dose 48 mL/kg/h, and late low-volume CVVH at average dose 19 mL/kg/h. Early group started CVVH within 12 hours of oliguria after optimization of

TABLE 40.4	Indications for Renal Replacement Therapy	
Conventional Indications	**Preemptive**[a]	**Nonrenal Indications**[a]
Hyperkalemia	Azotemia	Sepsis/removal of cytokines
Diuretic-resistant volume overload	Disrupted fluid balance	Increased intracranial pressure
Refractory acidosis	Restoration of acid–base homeostasis	Acute respiratory distress syndrome
Uremic manifestations (e.g., pericarditis)	Increased catabolic states (e.g., rhabdomyolysis and tumor lysis)	
Oliguria/anuria	Electrolyte abnormalities	
Some drug intoxication		

[a]Preemptive and nonrenal indications for renal replacement therapy are controversial and are opinion-based.

hemodynamics or measured creatinine clearance <20 mL/min on a 3-hour timed collection. The late group started CVVH when BUN was >112 mg/dL, hyperkalemia (K >6.5 mEq/L), or presence of pulmonary edema. There was no observed difference in 28-day survival (74.3%, 68.8%, 75%, respectively, $p = 0.8$) and renal recovery rate. Of the 36 patients who were randomized to the late low-volume group, 4 recovered kidney function and 2 died. This finding suggests that preemptive RRT may be unnecessary in some patients. Nevertheless, the study was underpowered to detect survival differences, and the overall high survival rate of these patients suggests that the study population is not representative of an average ICU.

Another study was an open label, randomized controlled trial of 208 patients with severe AKI in Western India. Patients were randomized to either early-start with serum creatinine >7 mg/dL or BUN 70 mg/dL versus usual-start for clinical indications as determined by the treating nephrologists (62). For the usual-start group, the mean starting BUN was 101 mg/dL and creatinine 10.4 mg/dL. There was no difference in-hospital mortality or risk of chronic dialysis at 3 months. Early-start group had 90-day mortality of 21% versus 12% for the usual-start, with relative risk ratio of 1.67 [95% confidence interval (CI) 0.88 to 3.17, $p = 0.2$]. Overall, dialysis dependence was reported in about 5% of the patients. The time to renal recovery of kidney function was significantly longer in the early-start group by 2 days. Limitations of the study include small sample size and that the study group was not representative of a typical ICU population. About half of the study population had tropical infections and obstetric complications. However, it is worth noting that 17% of patients in the usual-start group recovered kidney function before initiation of RRT (62).

Meta-analysis of 15 studies by Karvellas et al. (63) concluded that early initiation of RRT in ICU patients with AKI may have a favorable impact on survival. It should be recognized that the findings of this study were based on prospective and retrospective studies of varying quality and heterogeneity and that there were only two randomized controlled trials. Observational data showing improved outcomes may reflect inclusion of patients with a lesser degree of organ injury, whose outcomes would have been better regardless of treatment strategy. Some patients with severe AKI recovered kidney function, and if these patients were included in

the "late" group, then the mortality for late group would be less. Furthermore, the argument that initiation of RRT early during the ICU stay is associated with increased survival may not be related to timing of initiation but rather due to the characteristics of patients who develop AKI early in the ICU stay compared to those who develop AKI several days or weeks after ICU admission. In addition, several of these studies used BUN as a surrogate marker for the duration of AKI (63). Yet, BUN is an imperfect surrogate marker for time and uremia because urea generation is not constant between patients or even within an individual patient over time.

While in some patients, preemptive RRT may improve outcome, it has been argued that a strategy of early initiation of RRT might expose patients to the risk of dialysis in those who would recover renal function with conservative therapy alone and may subject patients to further renal damage, delaying renal recovery (64). Repeated episodes of transient intradialytic hypotension can prolong AKI and reduce the chance of renal recovery (65). Although IHD may have higher likelihood of hemodynamic instability (65), episodes of hypotension can also occur with CRRT and SLED (2,66). Additionally, blood contact with dialyzer membrane may incite an inflammatory response that can exacerbate AKI, but this inflammatory stimulus was mostly caused by cellulose dialyzer membranes, which are now infrequently used (67).

Other potential risks of preemptive but unnecessary RRT in patients who would have had renal recovery are shown in **Table 40.5**. Patients are exposed to the risk of complications related to vascular access, subtherapeutic levels of essential medications, and electrolyte derangements. Medication dosing in AKI during RRT has been inadequately examined in particular for CRRT and SLED (64). Limited knowledge about proper dosing of antibiotics for CRRT can lead to suboptimal levels of antibiotics, which are potentially lifesaving in septic shock. Another complication of RRT is depletion of essential nutrients and electrolytes such as phosphorus. Hypophosphatemia is a common occurrence in patients on CRRT and has been linked to prolong recovery from critical illness (68).

Based on the available data and literature, there is no consensus about the optimal timing and initiation of dialysis. It is advised to initiate RRT when life-threatening changes in fluid, electrolytes, and acid–base balance occur (69). However, most nephrologists

TABLE 40.5	**Risks of Renal Replacement Therapy**
Risks	**Examples**
Hemodynamic instability	Hypotension, arrhythmias
Access-related complications	Bleeding, thrombosis, hemothorax, pneumothorax, air embolus, arteriovenous fistula formation
Electrolyte disturbances	Hypophosphatemia, hypokalemia, hypocalcemia
Anticoagulation-related complications	Bleeding, heparin-induced thrombocytopenia, citrate-induced alkalosis, and hypocalcemia
Impair renal recovery	
Dialyzer reaction	Anaphylaxis
Subtherapeutic levels of essential medications	Antibiotics, antiepileptic drugs
Depletion of micronutrients	Amino acids and proteins, vitamins, and trace mineral
Limit patient mobility	
Hypothermia	

From Clark EG, Bagshaw SM. Unnecessary renal replacement therapy for acute kidney injury is harmful for renal recovery. *Semin Dial* 2015;28(1):6–11; and Finkel KW, Podoll AS. Complications of continuous renal replacement therapy. *Semin Dial* 2009;22(2):155–159.

will initiate RRT before the overt complications of AKI occur while considering age, severity of illness, presence of other organ dysfunction, and degree of kidney disease. Our capacity to predict which AKI will worsen and need RRT and which AKI will improve obviating the need for RRT is relatively poor. The clinical decision to start RRT should be based on the overall clinical context, presence of modifiable conditions by RRT, and the trends of laboratory values rather than single BUN and creatinine levels alone (69). Currently, Initiation of Dialysis EArly versus Late in Intensive Care Unit (IDEAL-ICU) study and Artificial Kidney Initiation in Kidney Injury (AKIKI) are two multicenter randomized controlled trials conducted in France investigating the impact of the timing of RRT initiation on outcome (70,71).

Fluid Overload

Fluid overload is a common indication for initiating RRT. Several observational studies have demonstrated that the degree of fluid accumulation in critically ill patients with AKI is linked to adverse outcomes including mortality (72–74). Furthermore, it has been reported that fluid overload at time of RRT initiation has been associated with increased mortality and decreased renal recovery (75,76). Possible explanations for these associations include failure to recognize AKI due to creatinine dilution, direct tissue edema leading to impaired renal perfusion, and increased risk of other complications such as prolonged ventilator-dependent respiratory failure and sepsis (77). It is unknown whether fluid overload is the result of more severe kidney disease or that fluid overload contributes to the cause of kidney disease. Also, higher volume administration may be suggestive of a more severe inflammatory state with greater vasodilation and capillary leak. Future studies are necessary to determine whether fluid overload is directly causing adverse outcomes or merely it is a confounding sign of illness severity (77).

After initial resuscitation, it is important to avoid unnecessary fluid buildup to limit later requirements of fluid removal. Patients should be evaluated routinely for fluid overload, and the rate and final goal of fluid removal must be carefully assessed and frequently reassessed. The rate of removal depends on severity of fluid overload and its complications, expected fluid intake, estimated vascular refilling, and hemodynamic tolerance to fluid removal from the intravascular space. There is no consensus in the method to evaluate fluid balance. The most commonly used methods to calculate fluid balance are monitoring changes in body weight relative to baseline and tallying daily fluid balance. Fluid overload is often defined as greater than 10% increase in body weight relative to baseline. Bioimpedance analysis and relative blood volume monitor may assist in estimating the amount of fluid removal, but these techniques are not commonly utilized (10,78). While there are tools such as pulse pressure variations and passive leg raising to help predict the hemodynamic tolerance to fluid removal, these tools are not perfect. Often, a fluid removal trial (reverse fluid challenge) is the only option left to determine the hemodynamic tolerance of fluid removal with RRT.

The impact of different CRRT fluid management strategies on outcomes has not been studied well. Michael et al. (79) investigated patients retrospectively who developed AKI after stem cell transplantation and showed that maintaining euvolemia with aggressive use of diuretics and early initiation of RRT was associated with increased survival. In the absence of randomized control trials, whether correcting fluid overload with CRRT improve outcomes remains uncertain.

Modality of Renal Replacement Therapy

As mentioned previously, there are multiple modalities that can be used in the treatment of AKI, which include conventional IHD, various modalities of CRRT, PIRRT, and PD. The optimal modality of RRT in ICU has been the subject of ongoing controversy. Among ICU patients treated with RRT, CRRT is the most common initial modality used. In the observational multinational study, Beginning and Ending Supportive Therapy for the Kidney (BEST Kidney), 80% of the patients with AKI in the ICU were initially treated with CRRT, followed by intermittent RRT in 16.9%, and PD and SCUF in 3.2% (2).

Intermittent Renal Replacement Therapy versus Continuous Renal Replacement Therapy

The impact of RRT modality in ICU patients with AKI on long-term kidney function is unknown, and there does not appear to be an effect on mortality. In comparison to conventional CRRT, IHD may hinder renal recovery by conferring greater hemodynamic instability (34). Removing relatively large volume of fluid in short period of time can cause hypotension and secondary renal ischemia. On the other hand, CRRT allows for more gradual removal of fluid and solutes and has been associated with greater hemodynamic stability. A retrospective cohort study of 2,004 patient pairs by Wald et al. (34) revealed that the risk of chronic dialysis was significantly lower among patients who received CRRT initially versus IHD with hazard ratio 0.75 (95% CI 0.65 to 0.87). This relation was stronger among patients with preexisting chronic kidney disease and heart failure (34). Likewise, Uchino et al. (80) analyzed recovery of kidney function in 1,218 patients who received RRT in the BEST study. Although hospital survival was lower in CRRT group (35.8 vs. 51.9%, $p < 0.0001$), dialysis independence at hospital discharge was more common in CRRT group (85.5 vs. 66.2%, $p < 0.0001$) (80). Another study by Bell et al. (81) from the Swedish Intensive Care Nephrology Group (SWING) reported on outcomes in 2,202 patients from 32 ICU in Sweden who underwent RRT. Mortality at 90 days was around 50% for both groups. Of patients who survived, there was a higher proportion of patients in IHD group who were dialysis dependent compared to CRRT group, 16.5% versus 8.3%, respectively (81). The major limitation of these studies relates to the possibility of residual confounding and, in particular, baseline factors that may have influenced the initial selection of RRT modality according to treatment intention (81).

Currently, randomized controlled trials has not shown that CRRT is superior to IHD in terms of survival and renal survival. There are only few small-sized randomized controlled trials that have investigated the optimal modality. One of the most notable is the Hemodiafe Study by Vinsonneau et al. (82), which was a randomized controlled trial of 360 patients across 21 ICUs in France to either IHD versus CVVHDF. Patients were well matched with regard to severity of illness, with more than 85% of patients requiring vasopressor support and more than 95% ventilator dependence. There was no significant difference in mortality at 60 days with mortality rate of 68% in IHD group versus 67% in CVVHDF ($p = 0.98$). There was no difference in hemodynamic intolerance, number of ICU and hospital days, and renal recovery. After discharge from the ICU, 6 of 61 (10%) patients remained dependent on dialysis in the IHD group compared with 4 of 61 (7%) patients in the CVVHDF ($p = 0.5$). After hospital discharge, only one patient from CVVHDF remained dependent on dialysis. Of note, the average treatment time for IHD in this study was 5.2 hours, which is longer than typical IHD treatment, and IHD was prescribed about three times a week (82).

Another study is the Stuivenberg Hospital Acute Renal Failure (SHARF) study by Lins et al. (83), which was a multicenter randomized controlled trial of 316 ICU patients in Belgium with AKI to either IHD versus CVVH. Patients underwent IHD (or IRRT) daily with each session lasting about 4 to 6 hours. In-hospital mortality was 62.5% in IHD group versus 58.1% in the CVVH group ($p = 0.43$). There was no significant difference in renal recovery and ICU and hospital days (83). A recent meta-analysis by Bagshaw et al. (84), involving nine randomized controlled trials with 1,403 patients, showed that the initial RRT modality did not seem to affect mortality or renal recovery. However, the authors identified numerous issues related to study design, conduct, and quality. They concluded that further high-quality studies, which are suitably powered are needed to address this issue (84).

PIRRT have become an increasingly used modality of RRT in the ICU that theoretically offers advantages of both IHD and CRRT in the ICU. SLED is becoming popular due to the lower cost, and it is the mode of RRT in the ICU of hospital centers without the capabilities of CRRT. The available studies have shown that SLED and CRRT have similar outcomes (85,86). The hemodynamic stability is similar in both groups. The correction of acidosis is faster, and less heparin is required with SLED (85). Study by Schwenger et al. (86) is a prospective, single-center randomized clinical trial of 232 patients in a surgical ICU, who were randomized to either 12-hour SLED versus 24-hour predilutional CVVH. The target dose of CVVH was 35 mL/kg/h. The 90-day mortality rate was similar between groups with 49.6% in SLED versus 55.6% in CVVH groups ($p = 0.43$). In this study, hemodynamic stability did not differ between groups during the treatment. Interestingly, SLED group had significantly fewer days of mechanical ventilation (17.7 ± 19.4 vs. 20.9 ± 19.8, $p = 0.047$) and fewer ICU days (19.6 ± 20.1 vs. 23.7 ± 21.9, $p = 0.04$). The SLED group required fewer blood transfusions (1,375 ± 2,573 mL vs. 1,976 ± 3,316 mL, $p = 0.02$) and had a considerable reduction in nursing time and support for RRT ($p < 0.001$) which resulted in lower costs (86).

Although many consider CRRT as the preferred therapy in the ICU (87), the predominance of the available evidence does not support a benefit of CRRT over IHD or PIRRT (4,82,84,88–90). Studies suggesting decreased renal recovery raise concern that episodes of intradialytic hypotension can impair recovery of kidney function; however, it should be recognized that the studies showing these findings are predominantly reported in observational studies (34,80,81) and that many of the published randomized trials have not observed this (4,82–84,88).

Hemofiltration versus Hemodialysis

Many clinicians prefer hemofiltration with the preconception that convection can remove middle-sized cytokines and reduce systemic inflammatory response; however, clinical studies have not shown significant and sustained reduction of cytokine concentration or improvement in clinical outcome with hemofiltration. The clearance of cytokines through high-volume CVVH is marginal in comparison to the greater endogenous production. Also, anti-inflammatory mediators are probably cleared, which can theoretically worsen the overall inflammatory state (14,53). The role of hemofiltration in sepsis is discussed in greater detail in the next section of this chapter.

The OMAKI (Optimal Mode of RRT of AKI) study by Wald et al. (91) randomized 78 ICU patients to either CVVH or CVVHD. Both modalities were delivered at 35 mL/kg/h. Mortality (54% CVVH; 55% CVVHD) and dialysis dependence in survivors (24% CVVH; 19% CVVHD) at 60 days were similar. Interestingly, there was a trend toward reduced vasopressor requirements among CVVH group during the first week of treatment (91). Recent meta-analysis by Friedrich et al. (92) concluded that there was no significant clinical benefit of hemofiltration on mortality, RRT dependence, vasopressor use, and organ dysfunction compared to hemodialysis. However, it is important to point out that this study showed that filter survival time was reduced by one-third, on average of 7 hours, with CVVH in comparison to CVVHD. There was a 50% increase in the number of filters despite the use of heparin and predominantly prefilter replacement. Combined with its higher fluid requirements to achieve similar small molecule clearance (need 15% to 20% more) and frequent filter clotting suggest that hemofiltration may consume more resources than hemodialysis (92).

Peritoneal Dialysis

High-volume PD can be an acceptable alternative to IHD and CRRT in the treatment of AKI in the ICU especially in low-resource regions. Because local renal hemodynamics are better preserved without extracorporeal circulation, there is a theoretical benefit of increased renal recovery with PD. PD may be more physiologic with less inflammation provoked than extracorporeal circulation with exposure to synthetic surfaces of the dialyzer. In the acute setting, PD is often delivered via a flexible catheter and with the use of a cycler. The minimum standardized Kt/V urea should be at least 1.7 per week. The most commonly described complication related to acute PD is peritonitis, which can reach as high as 40%, followed by mechanical complication (93). In a single-center study in Brazil by Ponce et al. (94), peritonitis occurred in 12% after mean of 5 days of therapy and 7% had mechanical complication of catheter.

There are limited studies examining the impact of acute PD on clinical outcomes. Study by Gabriel et al. (95) randomized 120 patients with AKI to high-volume PD (daily Kt/V = 0.65) with IHD (Kt/V = 1.2 per session) provided six times per week. Hospital mortality, renal recovery, and metabolic control were similar in both groups. The PD regimen consisted of 2-L exchanges with 30 to 60 minutes of dwell time, resulting in total PD fluid of 36 to 44 L/d and 18 to 22 exchanges per day (95). These findings are in contrast to study by Phu et al. (96), which randomized 70 patients to high-volume PD versus CVVH. PD regimen was 2-L exchanges with 30-minute dwell time (∼70 L/d). Majority of the study patients suffered from severe malaria and other sepsis. The mortality rate was 47% in the PD group compared to 15% in CVVH group ($p = 0.005$). CVVH group had a faster resolution of acidosis. It was postulated that the poor outcome in the PD group was attributed to accelerated growth of malarial parasite due to the presence of high splanchnic blood glucose resulting from the glucose-enriched PD fluid (96). Meta-analysis by Chionh et al. (93) concluded that there was no difference in mortality between PD and ECBP in AKI. There is a need for well-designed studies in this area.

Intensity of Renal Replacement Therapy

There are multiple randomized controlled trials that have provided guidance for dialysis dosing in AKI in the ICU. Initial studies have shown improvement in mortality with higher intensity dosing for CRRT (97). One of the major landmark studies is the United States–based Veterans Affairs/National Institutes of Health Acute Renal Failure Trial Network (ATN) study, which randomized 1,124 patients in the ICU with AKI to high- and low-intensity dosing of

RRT. This study categorized the critically ill patients by the Sequential Organ Failure Assessment (SOFA) score to hemodynamically stable and hemodynamically unstable groups (50). The hemodynamically stable group was randomized to IHD three times a week versus six times a week. The hemodynamically unstable group was randomized to either CVVHDF at 35 mL/kg/h versus 20 mL/kg/h or SLED six versus three times a week. The single-pool Kt/V was aimed for 1.2 to 1.4. The rate of death from any cause by day 60 was 53.6% with intensive therapy and 51.5% with less-intensive therapy [odds ratio (OR) 1.09, 95% CI 0.86 to 1.40, $p = 0.47$]. There was no significant difference between the two groups in the RRT duration, renal recovery, and recovery of nonrenal organ failure. Dialysis independence at day 60 in those who survived was around 34% for both groups ($p = 0.75$) (50). Second large study was the Randomized Evaluation of Normal versus Augmented Level (RENAL) Replacement Therapy, which randomized 1,508 patients across 35 ICUs in Australia to postdilution CVVHDF 40 mL/kg/h versus 25 mL/kg/h (51). The 90-day mortality was 44.7% in high-intensity and 44.7% in the low-intensity group. The dialysis dependence at 90 days was reported in 6.8% of survivors in high-intensity versus 4.4% in intensity group (OR 1.59, 95% CI 0.86 to 2.92, $p = 0.14$). There was no difference in renal recovery, ventilator-dependent days, ICU, and hospital days (51).

There are limited studies investigating dialysis dosing in PIRRT. In the ATN study, less than 5% of the treatments were SLED treatments (50). A study by Faulhaber-Walter et al. (98) conducted a prospective randomized control trial of standard versus intensified extended dialysis in patients with AKI in ICU in a single-center tertiary center. A total of 156 patients with AKI requiring RRT were randomly assigned to receive standard dialysis [dosed to maintain plasma urea levels between 120 and 150 mg/dL (20 to 25 mmol/L)] or intensified dialysis [dosed to maintain plasma urea levels <90 mg/dL (<15 mmol/L)]. No differences between intensified and standard treatment were observed for survival by day 14 (70.4% vs. 70.7%) or day 28 (55.6% vs. 61.3%), or for renal recovery in survivors by day 28 (60.0% vs. 63.0%) (98).

Meta-analysis of 12 randomized or quasi-randomized clinical trials by Van Wert et al. (99) showed no difference in high versus low intensity therapy. High-intensity therapy groups included effluent rates of >30 mL/kg/h, or at least six sessions per week of IHD or SLED compared to standard-dosage therapies which included CRRT with effluent flow rates of <30 mL/kg/h or two to four sessions per week of IRRT (99). The prescribed dose of CRRT should be higher to account for loss time on CRRT due to interruptions. In the ATN study, the dose delivered was 89% of that prescribed for higher intensity treatment (50). In contrast, another study reported that patients received only 68% of their prescribed dose of CRRT (100). The reported prescribed clearance overestimated the actual delivered clearance by 24% (52). This gap was related to decrease in filter function by assessing the FUN/BUN ratio (where FUN is filtrate urea nitrogen). To assess adequacy of CRRT, solute clearance should be measured rather than estimated by the effluent volume. The other major interruptions were related to filter clotting, disconnection for procedures, and change in patient clinical status (52). Study by Overberger et al. (101) showed that IHD and CRRT were the most popularly used modalities of RRT, with SLED and other "hybrid" treatments used in fewer than 10% of patients. IHD was most commonly provided on a thrice-weekly or every-other-day schedule, with only infrequent assessment of the delivered dosage of therapy. Majority of the practitioners did not routinely monitor Kt/V and did not dose CRRT on the basis of patient weight (101).

For IHD or PIRRT, the recommended minimum dose of dialysis is Kt/V of 1.3 per treatment (corresponding to urea reduction ratio >0.7) scheduled three times per week (69). For CRRT, the recommended effluent volume, which is the dialysis dose, is at least 20 to 25 mL/kg/h. In order to ensure the target dose, CRRT dose should be prescribed at 25 to 30 mL/kg/h to account for the interruptions in treatment. The dose of dialysis should be assessed frequently and adjusted to achieve electrolytes, acid-base, solute, and fluid balance (69).

⬢ RENAL REPLACEMENT THERAPY FOR SPECIAL CIRCUMSTANCES

Respiratory Failure

Acute respiratory distress syndrome (ARDS) is common in the ICU, and it is characterized by alveolar damage resulting in increased permeability of the alveolar–capillary barrier and accumulation of extravascular fluid. Mortality is high with patients with ARDS, in the range of 25% to 40%, and the predominant causes of death are sepsis and multiorgan failure rather than hypoxemia (102). AKI occurs frequently in patients with ARDS, with reported incidence around 44% in one study (103), and the presence of AKI raises the risk of mortality to approximately 60% (102). Patients with ARDS are susceptible to fluid retention, which occur through multiple mechanisms. The increased thoracic pressures caused by the positive end-expiratory pressure from the ventilator results in decreased renal perfusion and activation of water- and sodium-retaining hormonal systems (104). Greater fluid retention worsens interstitial edema in the lung parenchyma, compromising lung function and hypoxia. In addition, injured lungs from mechanical ventilation stimulate cytokine release, which can exacerbate AKI, which then reduces cytokine clearance further, resulting in a vicious cycle (102,105,106).

Lung-protective ventilation using low tidal volumes around 6 mL/kg is the mainstay of therapy to improve clinical outcomes (10,107), which can be viewed as "kidney-protective ventilation" (10). In addition, measures aimed to reduce fluid and inflammatory mediators may help improve outcome with ARDS. With fluid overload and ARDS, CRRT may be used to diminish pulmonary edema and allow for less intense ventilator settings, shielding the lung from further injury. Patients are often left with a combined respiratory and metabolic acidosis as a result of permissive hypercapnia from using low tidal volume and kidney disease that often occurs in these patients. In these situations, CRRT can help restore acid–base balance (10).

There is conflicting evidence whether CRRT has beneficial effects beyond fluid removal and metabolic control such as improvement in gas exchange or cytokine removal resulting in enhanced recovery of ARDS. Several studies have shown improvement in outcome with CRRT including the use of high-volume hemofiltration (105,108–110), while other studies have shown unimpressive results (111). A study by Vesconi et al. (109) is a prospective, multicenter observational study comparing more intensive (CRRT ≥35 mL/kg/h, IRRT ≥6 sessions/wk) or less intensive (CRRT <35 mL/kg/h, IRRT <6 sessions/wk). Although there was no difference in mortality, shorter duration of mechanical ventilation was observed among survivors in the more intensive group in addition to shorter ICU stay (109). Timing of dialysis is another matter of debate. A study by Han et al. (105) showed that early initiation of CRRT, defined as within 12 hours of presentation of ARDS, is associated with improvement in oxygenation and shorter duration of mechanical ventilation compared to late initiation of CRRT after 48 hours. However, study by Hoste et al.

(111) observed no improvement in oxygenation in 37 patients with ARDS who received CVVHDF with zero fluid balance. This finding suggests that the benefits seen with CRRT in patients with ARDS may be related to reestablishing fluid balance rather than removing inflammatory mediators.

Since clearance of complement and cytokine depends mainly on adsorption and less on convective force (112,113), there may be a role for cytokine-adsorbing hemofilter in the treatment of ARDS. A study by Matsuda et al. (114) showed that there were decreased levels of cytokines and improved survival rate in patients with ARDS complicated by renal failure who were treated with cytokine-adsorbing hemofilter. Further studies are needed to validate the efficacy of cytokine-adsorbing hemofilters.

In cases of severe but reversible cardiopulmonary failure, extracorporeal membrane oxygenation (ECMO) and pumpless CO$_2$ removal systems (PECLA) are utilized to support lung-protective ventilation strategies and to improve CO$_2$ removal and respiratory acidosis. ECMO is associated with high incidence of AKI, reaching to 70% to 85%, and those patients who require RRT have even higher risk of mortality, independent of confounding variables. Fluid overload occurs frequently in patients who are on ECMO and is a common indication to initiate RRT in addition for metabolic control. Cumulative fluid overload is associated with increased mortality, prolonged mechanical ventilation, and ICU stay (75,76). Improvement in fluid balance is associated with enhanced pulmonary function and earlier weaning of ECMO. CRRT is the most common modality used for RRT in ECMO because of its ability to make rapid changes to fluid removal while maintaining hemodynamics. Although fluid overload at time of CRRT initiation was associated with increased mortality, correction of fluid overload did not appear to improve survival (115). In patients who required CRRT, prolonged ECMO duration and higher mortality were observed, but this association may reflect underlying higher severity of illness (116).

There are three principal methods to provide CRRT for patients on ECMO: (a) incorporate an in-line hemofilter, (b) incorporate a traditional CRRT device into the ECMO circuit, and (c) perform CRRT through venous access independent of ECMO circuit (117). In the first scenario, the in-line hemofilter is typically inserted after the pump, which provides forward blood flow to the hemofilter, and before the oxygenator, which can help trap air clot in case of complications (**FIGURE 40.3**). The blood after passing through the hemofilter is returned to the proximal limb of the ECMO circuit, creating a shunt. Because of an existence of a shunt, an ultrasonic probe is attached to arterial return line to measure the actual flow delivered to the patient. The hemofilter blood-flow rate is calculated by subtracting the flow delivered to the patient from the total ECMO blood-flow rate. The hemofilter blood-flow rate can be adjusted by using a stopcock or other flow-restricting device; however, this can result in turbulent flow, increasing the risk of hemolysis and thrombus. Because the hemofilter is designed for high pressure system, it does not work well for diffusion. It is primarily uses convection as its primary means of clearance. The amount of replacement fluid is controlled by an intravenous infusion pump, which is integrated into the circuit. The disadvantages of this circuit are the inaccuracy of fluid removal and absence of pressure monitoring, which can lead to delayed detection of clotting or rupture of filter (117).

In the second scenario, the CRRT machine is usually connected to the venous limb of the roller-head ECMO circuit before the pump (**FIGURE 40.4**). The blood returns from the CRRT to the ECMO circuit near the venous CRRT connection and before the ECMO (117). If the ECMO pump is centrifugal, it is necessary to

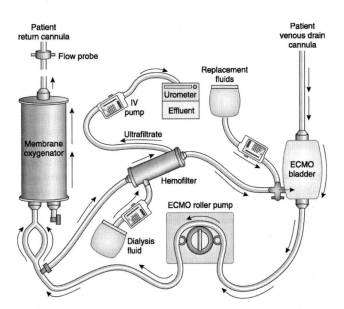

FIGURE 40.3 Using an in-line hemofilter during extracorporeal membrane oxygenation. Renal replacement therapy using an in-line hemofilter during extracorporeal membrane oxygenation (ECMO). As blood comes from the patient via the venous drain cannula, it goes through the ECMO bladder to the ECMO pump, to the membrane oxygenator, and back to the patient via a return cannula. Blood is shunted from the circuit to the in-line hemofilter and returned to the ECMO pump. Fluid (ultrafiltrate) can be controlled using an intravenous (IV) pump. Replacement or dialysis fluid can be used for solute clearance and/or to achieve metabolic control. [Reprinted with permission from Askenazi DJ, Selewski DT, Paden ML, et al. Renal replacement therapy in critically ill patients receiving extracorporeal membrane oxygenation. *Clin J Am Soc Nephrol* 2012;7(8):1328–1336.]

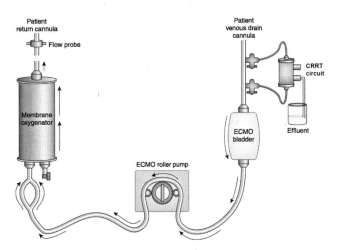

FIGURE 40.4 Incorporating renal replacement machine during extracorporeal membrane oxygenation. Renal replacement therapy (RRT) using RRT machine during extracorporeal membrane oxygenation (ECMO). If the ECMO circuit uses a roller pump, a proportion of the circuit blood comes from the patient via the venous drain cannula and enters the RRT machine where replacement, dialysis, and ultrafiltration occur. Blood from the RRT machine then goes back to the ECMO bladder to the ECMO pump, the membrane oxygenator, and back to the patient via a return cannula. If a centrifugal pump is used, the RRT machine must be connected after the ECMO bladder to prevent air entrapment. [Reprinted with permission from Askenazi DJ, Selewski DT, Paden ML, et al. Renal replacement therapy in critically ill patients receiving extracorporeal membrane oxygenation. *Clin J Am Soc Nephrol* 2012;7(8):1328–1336.]

integrate the CRRT machine after the pump because of the risk of air entrapment. The reconnection of the return blood from CRRT device should be before the oxygenator to trap air or clots before it return to the patients. Additional anticoagulation is not necessary since the ECMO circuit is heparinized. Furthermore, the life span of CRRT that is part of the ECMO circuit is longer than when it is independent. Also, integration of CRRT provides more accurate assessment of fluid removal (116). The pressure alarms for CRRT may need to be adjusted when incorporating into ECMO. Typically, the access pressure alarms are negative; however, when CRRT is operating in series with ECMO, the positive pressure at the entry point of the CRRT machine will create pressures close to zero or positive. Some machines (including Gambro, Prismaflex, and the Braun Diapact) allow clinicians to adjust alarm while other machines (including NxStage, Fresenius 2008K, and older Gambro Prisma) do not have these capabilities. Alternatively, flow restrictors can be used to reduce the pressure the CRRT circuit; however, this can increase risk for hemolysis and thrombosis (117).

Since ECMO requires high blood flow to support the circuit, it requires a large-diameter cannula, which poses additional risk to patients. In recent years, studies have looked into low-flow CO_2 removal using a hollow-fiber gas exchanger (**FIGURE 40.5**) (118,119). Conventional CRRT can be used by integrating it into a series after the roller pump (118). Blood flow typically ranges from 300 to 500 mL/min. In a small observational study of 10 ICU patients with ARDS and multiorgan failure by Forster et al. (118), low-flow CO_2 removal improved respiratory acidosis (average reduction of 17.3 mm Hg pCO_2) with a concomitant rapid correction of arterial pH and improvement of hemodynamics with reduction of vasopressors. Low-flow CO_2 did not affect systemic oxygenation, which would require ECMO in settings of severe hypoxia (118). Although not as effective as ECMO, low-flow CO_2 removal can help reduce tidal volume and potentially benefit patients with severe cases of ARDS.

Sepsis

Sepsis is the leading cause of death in the ICU, especially when complicated by AKI (120). Cytokine and other inflammatory mediators play a role in the pathogenesis of septic shock and sepsis-related

AKI (121). There is correlation between high levels of cytokines and mortality (122). The role of EBCP in removing cytokines and other inflammatory mediators to impact clinical outcomes remain uncertain. Depending on the pore size of the dialyzer membrane, majority of the cytokines that are cleared are water-soluble with midrange molecular weights ranging 5 to 51 kDa (33). **TABLE 40.6** shows the convective removal of selected cytokines and mediators. Since hemofiltration is considered the preferred modality for middle molecule clearance, some experts have argued that CRRT using convective clearances such as CVVH or CVVHDF should be used at higher prescribed doses of 30 to 35 mL/kg/h in the setting of septic AKI (123). However, traditional CVVH has not been shown to significantly reduce plasma cytokine levels and influence clinical outcomes (124). Earlier studies demonstrated an initial reduction in cytokine levels after starting CVVH followed by increase in cytokine levels to baseline within hours (125,126). The initial reduction is attributed to adsorption of cytokines to the hemofilter membrane, which then becomes saturated. Currently, exact timing of RRT has not been defined for sepsis-related AKI, and recent studies have not shown any clinical benefit of early CRRT initiation (124,127). Early application of CVVH at standard dosing of 25 mL/kg/h resulted in greater severity of organ failure in one randomized study of 80 ICU patients (124). A recent retrospective review of 120 ICU patients found no difference in dialysis requirement and mortality in "early" versus "late" start CRRT for septic shock and AKI (127).

There are four main techniques investigated for cytokine removal in sepsis: high-volume hemofiltration, high-cutoff techniques, combined plasma filtration adsorption, and polymyxin B hemoperfusion. There is suggestion that early short-term, high-volume hemofiltration may be a therapeutic value in the treatment of intractable septic shock. Hemodynamic and metabolic response improved in a small prospective study involving 20 patients with refractory septic shock who underwent 4 hours of 35 L of ultrafiltrate, followed by CVVH for 4 days (128). However, other studies utilizing high-volume hemofiltration, as defined as an effluent rate greater than 50 mL/kg/h, failed to show promising results in sepsis (108,129). In the hIgh VOlume in Intensive caRE (IVOIRE) study, 140 ICU patients with catecholamine-dependent septic shock and AKI were randomized to high-volume hemofiltration at 70 mL/

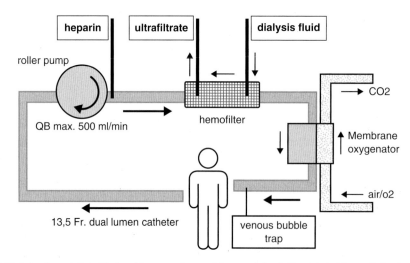

FIGURE 40.5 Implementation of hollow-filter gas exchanger into a renal circuit. [Reprinted with permission from Forster C, Schriewer J, John S, et al. Low-flow CO_2 removal integrated into a renal-replacement circuit can reduce acidosis and decrease vasopressor requirements. *Crit Care* 2013;17(4):R154.]

TABLE 40.6 Sieving Coefficient of Inflammatory Mediators		
Mediator	**Molecular Weight (Da)**	**Sieving Coefficient**
AA mediators	600	0.5–0.91
Bradykinin	1,100	—
Endothelin	2,500	0.19
C3a/C5a	11,000	0.11–0.77
Factor D	24,000	—
MDS	600–30,000	—
LPS	67,000	—
LPS fragments	>1,000–20,000	—
TNF-α (trimer)	17,000 (54,000)	0.0–0.2
sTNFr	30,000–50,000	<0.1
IL-1	17,500	0.07–0.42
IL-1ra	24,000	0.28–0.45
IL-6	22,000	—
IL-8	8,000	0.0–0.48
IL-10	18,000	0.0
INF-γ	20,000	—

AA, arachidonic acid; MDS, myocardial depressant substances; LPS, lipopolysaccharide; TNF-α, tumor necrosis factor-α; sTNFr, soluble tumor necrosis factor receptor; IL, interleukin; INF, interferon.
From Schetz M. Non-renal indications for continuous renal replacement therapy. *Kidney Int* 1999;56:S88–S94, with permission.

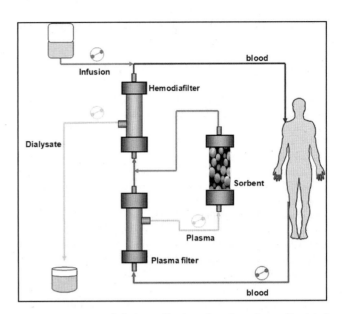

FIGURE 40.6 Coupled plasma filtration adsorption schema. [Reprinted with permission from Livigni S, Bertolini G, Rossi C, et al. Efficacy of coupled plasma filtration adsorption (CPFA) in patients with septic shock: a multicenter randomised controlled clinical trial. *BMJ Open* 2014;4(1):e003536.]

kg/h versus standard-volume hemofiltration at 35 mL/kg/h for 96 hours. High-volume hemofiltration failed to improve mortality, hemodynamic profile, or organ function (129). Investigators have also shown that even extra high-volume hemofiltration with doses reaching up to 85 mL/kg/h had no impact on mortality and renal outcomes in sepsis (130). Finally, a recent meta-analysis by Clark et al. (131) of four randomized controlled trials using high-volume hemofiltration, including 470 patients, showed no difference in mortality in addition to renal recovery, vasopressor reduction, and ICU stay. There are complications that can occur with high-volume hemofiltration such as electrolyte abnormalities, excessive antibiotic removal, and micronutrient depletion (131). Based on these findings, no specific recommendations regarding the use of high-volume hemofiltration can be supported for sepsis and septic AKI.

In recent years, high-cutoff membranes with larger pore size have been introduced to remove greater amount of cytokines (132,133). Treatment using high-cutoff membranes has shown enhanced immune cell function and survival in animal models of sepsis (134). In a pilot study by Morgera et al. (135), high-cutoff hemofiltration using a hemofilter with a cutoff point of about 60 kDa had a beneficial effect on reducing norepinephrine requirement in septic patients and was superior to conventional hemofiltration in clearing interleukin-6 and interleukin-1 receptor antagonist in septic patients. Although high-cutoff hemofiltration has shown greatest cytokine removal in terms of sieving and clearance in comparison to all other approaches, it is associated with greater plasma protein losses including albumin (132,135). Additional studies are needed to determine the efficacy of high-cutoff hemofiltration in sepsis.

Another therapy is coupled plasma filtration and adsorption (CPFA), which allows for removal of large soluble inflammatory mediators. In contrast to high-volume high filtration which removes molecules less than 45 kDa, plasma filtration removes below 900 kDa (123). This extracorporeal circuit consists of a plasma filter, a resin cartridge, and a high-flux dialyzer (**FIGURE 40.6**). The plasma filter separates plasma from blood and then the plasma passes through a synthetic resin cartridge for adsorption. Once the blood is reconstituted, it passes through another filter to remove fluid and small molecular weight toxins. Thus, CPFA and CRRT can function in series. The minimum volume of plasma treated per day should be 10 L, corresponding to a blood flow of 150 mL/min and a filtration fraction of 12% (136). In a small pilot study, CPFA was associated with decreased levels of vasopressors and improved immune function of leukocytes in sepsis (137). In an Italian multicenter study conducted by Livigni et al. (136), 192 ICU patients with septic shock were randomized to CPFA versus standard care. CPFA was performed daily for 5 days, lasting at least 10 h/d (136). The investigators found no statistical difference in hospital mortality (47.3% controls, 45.1% CPFA; *p* = 0.76), occurrence of new organ failures, or ICU-free days for first 30 days. The study was terminated early on the grounds of futility. One possible reason for a negative result was that nearly half of the patients randomized to the CPFA group were found to be undertreated. This indicates the poor feasibility of delivering this therapy. Majority of the centers encountered frequent clotting despite using heparin or citrate anticoagulation to maintain circuit patency. Also, the therapy was expensive. A subgroup analysis showed that those who received CPFA dose >0.18 L/kg/d had a lower mortality compared with controls (OR 0.36, 95% CI 0.13 to 0.99) (136).

A novel therapy undergoing investigation is polymyxin B direct hemoperfusion (PMX-DHP), which was developed in Japan in the 1990s. Polymyxin B is adsorbed to a polystyrene fiber in a hemoperfusion device that is used to bind and remove circulating endotoxin, which stimulate cytokine release in gram-negative sepsis (138,139). Typical treatment course requires two PMX cartridges, administered 24 hours apart. Each treatment is 2-hour session at a blood-flow rate of approximately 100 mL/min through the circuit, using a standard IHD machine as a blood pump (140). Meta-analysis by Cruz et al. (141) reviewed 28 trials using PMX-DHP for severe sepsis, largely conducted in Europe and Japan, with a total cohort of 978 patients. Although there was heterogeneity among trials, PMX-DHP was associated with improvement in hemodynamics with overall mean arterial pressure increase by 19 mm Hg (95% CI 15 to 22 mm Hg; $p < 0.001$), significantly lower mortality risk (risk ratio 0.53, 95% CI 0.43 to 0.6), and improved oxygenation (PaO_2/Fio_2 ratio) (142). More recently in 2009, Early Use of Polymyxin B Hemoperfusion in Abdominal Sepsis (EUPHAS) is a prospective multicenter randomized controlled trial of 64 ICU patients in Italy with severe sepsis or septic shock who underwent emergent surgery for intra-abdominal infection that compared addition of two sessions of PMX-DHP versus standard therapy. The investigators demonstrated that PMX-DHP was associated with improved blood pressure, reduced organ failure, and improved survival. The absolute risk of death at 28 days improved significantly from 53% in the conventional group to 32% in the PMX-DHP group (adjusted HR 0.36, 95% CI 0.16 to 0.80) (142). The Evaluating the Use of Polymyxin B Hemoperfusion in a Randomized controlled trial of Adults Treated for Endotoxemia and Septic shock (EUPHRATES) trial (ClinicalTrials.gov identifier: NCT01046669) is currently enrolling patients in North America to investigate the safety and efficacy of polymyxin B hemoperfusion in patients with septic shock (140).

At the current level of evidence, the clinical significance of cytokine removal using blood purification technique is unknown (132). High-volume hemofiltration and CPFA have not been associated with significant improvement in clinical outcome in recent trials. Preliminary studies using polymyxin B hemoperfusion has a positive effect on arterial pressure, gas exchange, and mortality, and recent randomized controlled trials hopefully will provide definite conclusions regarding its role in sepsis.

Lactic Acidosis

Lactic acidosis occurs commonly in ICU patients with AKI who are treated with RRT, and it is associated with higher mortality. Up to one-third of the ICU patients have severe lactic acidosis as defined as serum lactate concentration >5 mmol/L and pH <7.35 (143). Lactic acidosis can be classified based on the presence (type A) or absence (type B) of tissue hypoxia. The kidney is the major lactate-consuming organ following the liver. Approximately 25% to 30% of the exogenous lactate is removed by the kidneys primarily through lactate metabolism rather than excretion. While acidosis inhibits hepatic lactic metabolism, the renal contribution to lactate removal increases from 16% at a pH of 7.45 to 44% at a pH of 6.75 to compensate for the hepatic loss of lactic metabolism. Even in the setting of reduced renal blood flow and endotoxemia, the kidney continues to remove lactate from circulation (144).

Initiating RRT for solely due to lactic acidosis with stable serum pH is controversial. Although RRT provides a means to correct severe acidemia from lactic acidosis, RRT is often futile in cases of severe lactic acidosis since many of these patients already have high mortality. After starting RRT, the decreased lactate levels may be related to improvement of clinical situation rather than clearance of lactate by RRT. In addition, even though lactate is cleared through RRT, its clearance is much lower than the mass quantity of lactate

produced in severe lactic acidosis. For instance, study by Levraut et al. (145) showed that the median lactate clearance using bicarbonate-buffered CRRT was only 24.2 mL/min compared to median endogenous clearance of 1,379 mL/min, thereby RRT accounted for <3% of the total body clearance. One should note that this study of lactate clearance was performed using relatively low level of RRT dosing with CVVHDF at Q_B 100 mL/min and Q_d 1,000 mL/h. Further studies are needed examining lactate clearance using different modalities and dosing of RRT. In general, lactate-buffered replacement solution should be avoided to prevent exacerbating hyperlactatemia, and bicarbonate-buffered solution is preferred to restore acid–base balance (144).

Liver Failure and Extracorporeal Liver Assist Devices

AKI occurs frequently in hospitalized patients with decompensated cirrhosis, reportedly around 20% (146). The common etiologies are prerenal azotemia, acute tubular necrosis (ATN), and hepatorenal syndrome (HRS). The pathophysiology in cirrhosis is distinguished by the development of splanchnic vasodilatation causing decreased effective circulating volume, which stimulates the renin-angiotensin-aldosterone system, sympathetic system, and nonosmotic release of antidiuretic hormone. This contributes to hypoperfusion of the kidneys and sodium retention, leading to ascites that is refractory to diuretics and ultimately HRS (147). Mortality in patients with cirrhosis who develop AKI is high especially when RRT is required. Often, these patients are in the ICU due to sepsis and multiorgan failure. CRRT is often employed over intermittent dialysis because many of these patients have hypotension that require ionotropic support and are susceptible for worsening hypotension with fluid removal.

Due to the extremely high mortality associated with AKI in ICU patients with liver failure, the role of RRT is controversial. Dialysis in patients with HRS who are not transplant candidates are unlikely to prolong length or quality of life. One study by Wong et al. (148) reported that the mortality rate was 94% in patients with liver failure who did not receive transplant, and half of these patients died within 8 days of receiving RRT. Discussions about goals of care should occur with the family early on especially when the patient is not considered a transplant candidate and/or the patient has developed severe shock with multiorgan failure, unlikely to survive. In situations where it is unclear if the patient may have renal recovery, a trial of RRT may be offered with the understanding that overall survival in patients with irreversible liver failure without the prospect for liver transplantation is still poor (147).

Extracorporeal liver assist devices (ELADs) can provide temporary liver support in patients as a bridge to liver transplantation or hepatic recovery. In general, ELADs can be categorized into biologic devices, which incorporate either whole animal livers or bioreactors with hepatocytes which provide excretory and synthetic liver function, and nonbiologic devices, which provide no synthetic functions but utilizes EBCP to remove endogenous hepatotoxins. Bioartificial livers currently remain experimental and are not discussed further in this chapter (149).

Recently, nonbiologic ELADs using albumin-based dialysis have been implemented to remove protein-bound substances such as bile acids that accumulate in patients with liver failure. These therapies include single pass albumin dialysis (SPAD), molecular absorbent recirculating system (MARS), and the fractionated plasma separation and adsorption (Prometheus). Since 1993, over 400 patients with liver failure have been treated with MARS worldwide.

Treatment with MARS and other extracorporeal blood detoxification therapies result in significant removal of bilirubin, bile acids, tryptophan, short- and middle-chain fatty acids, aromatic amino acids, and ammonia. In addition, nitric oxide, renin, and aldosterone concentration have been reduced after treatment with MARS (150). Clearance rates for albumin-bound substances vary between 10 and 60 mL/min. Studies have shown the use of albumin-based dialysis has been associated with improvement in hepatic encephalopathy, reduction in intracranial pressure (ICP), decreased level of bilirubin, and increased sodium level (149,151). While few studies showed improved hemodynamics, renal function, and urine output (151,152), others have noted disappointing renal and hemodynamic outcomes with the use of albumin-based dialysis (148,153). In addition, worsening coagulopathy and decrease in platelets were observed in patients with MARS (154). The major downsides of these studies are that all were small scale and none included renal outcomes or survival as their primary endpoint. Larger scale studies are necessary to determine the utility of these modalities.

Both SPAD and MARS are modified dialysis modalities that use albumin-containing dialysate. Toxin-rich blood passes along one side of a semipermeable membrane (that is not permeable to albumin), while albumin-enriched dialysate flows in the opposite direction, allowing for passage of unbound and bound toxins down their osmotic gradient. In SPAD, the albumin-rich dialysate is discarded after circulating through the dialyzer and then replenished, whereas in MARS, it is regenerated by using low-flux dialysis and two different absorbers to wash away or bind the toxins off the albumin.

The MARS system consists of three circuits: blood circuit, albumin dialysate circuit, and a bicarbonate-based dialysate circuit (**Figure 40.7**). The albumin dialysate circuit is interposed in between the blood and bicarbonate-based dialysate circuits. The MARS monitor (Teraklin AG, Rostock, Germany) has a single roller pump that pumps the albumin dialysate. This circuit is coupled to either a standard dialysis machine or CRRT machine. Using the standard venous dual-lumen central catheter, the blood leaves the patient and enters the hollow fibers of the MARSFlux filter (Teraklin AG, Rostock, Germany), which is a high-flux polysulfone membrane that is impermeable to albumin. The blood bathes in the albumin dialysate, allowing for exchange for protein-bound substances between the blood circuit and albumin dialysate circuit. Simultaneously, the water-soluble solutes that are nonprotein bound such as uremic toxins diffuse from the blood into the albumin circuit. Thus,

the "spent" albumin dialysate leaving the MARS filter is saturated with albumin-bound liver toxins and water-soluble uremic toxins and is then pumped through the hollow fibers of a second dialyzer of either a standard HD or CRRT machine. The "spent" albumin dialysate is bathed in a fresh bicarbonate dialysate, allowing for diffusion of water-soluble uremic toxins into the bicarbonate dialysate circuit. The albumin dialysate leaves the second dialyzer and passes through two sequential columns, charcoal and then an anionic resin, both which help regenerate the albumin (149). The albumin circuit contains about 600 mL of 20% human serum albumin, and because the albumin is constantly regenerated, no additional albumin is required for the circuit. The duration of MARS treatment is typically 6 to 8 hours, and single treatment does not typically exceed 10 hours given the possible risk of albumin becoming a culture medium for bacteria. UFH can be prescribed to prevent the filter from clotting (1,000 to 2,000 IU heparin for priming followed by 250 to 500 IU/h continuous infusion). Both the blood and albumin pump speeds are around 150 to 200 mL/min. The dialysate flow rate can be set <300 mL/min if CRRT is used or 300 to 500 mL/min if a standard HD machine is used (149,150).

In the case of Prometheus, an albumin-permeable polysulfone filter (AlbuFlow) is utilized. Due to the high sieving coefficient, albumin (68 kDa) easily passes from blood into the secondary circuit. The filtered plasma with albumin-bound toxins flows through one or two adsorbers, which remove the liver toxin, and the purified plasma is returned to the blood side of the albumin filter and back to the patients. A traditional hemodialysis machine can be incorporated in series with the circuit to remove water-soluble toxins (155,156).

MARS and other extracorporeal blood detoxification therapies can be effective in treating patients with fulminant hepatic failure who are awaiting liver transplant or spontaneous liver recovery. Large multicenter controlled trials are necessary to confirm whether these therapies alter the natural course of liver failure including renal and survival outcomes. In addition to its role in patients with liver failure, MARS has been approved by the U.S. Food and Drug Administration for overdose and poisoning as of June 2005. MARS have been used in patients poisoned by paracetamol or *Amanita phalloides* who present with liver failure. ELADs have also been used to promote clearance of drugs that are highly protein bound such as phenytoin, theophylline, and calcium channel blockers (157).

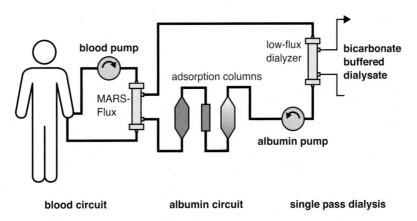

FIGURE 40.7 Schematic drawing of the molecular adsorbent recirculating system (MARS). (Reprinted with permission from Mitzner SR, Stange J, Klammt S, et al. *J Am Soc Nephrol* 2001;12:S75–S82.)

Renal Replacement in Neurotrauma

Patients with ESKD on renal replacement therapy regardless of it being PD or hemodialysis have an increased incidence of intracranial, extradural, and subdural hemorrhage (158). Those patients with increased ICP particularly when on dialysis have a mortality of 80% (159). It is important for the patient to have the appropriate dialysis prescription to help improve a patient's outcome.

An acute brain hemorrhage is a space-occupying lesion in the cranium leading to brain injury. The brain tissue at the center of the injury is most at risk for apoptosis and necrosis. As ICP increases, brain perfusion is hindered, and the physiologic response is for the systolic blood pressure (SBP) to be elevated. In management of this elevated SBP to maintain cerebral perfusion, the BP is only decreased by 15% to 30 % in the first 24 hours (158). Hemodialysis's adverse effects include an elevating ICP with increased cerebral edema or decreased cerebral perfusion with ultrafiltration (160,161).

When hemodialysis is started, there is a rapid clearance of urea from the plasma in the first hour. As this urea is cleared from the plasma, a gradient develops between the brain and the plasma because urea is slow to move out of the brain down its gradient into the plasma. The result is a low serum osmolality versus brain osmolality. Water will go down this osmolality gradient and enter the brain causing cerebral edema. It is important to be aware that the transport of water is much faster than that of urea (158).

There are three parts of the hemodialysis prescription to focus on to prevent worsening cerebral edema. These are the urea clearance and the concentration of sodium and bicarbonate in the dialysate. The clearance of urea is dependent on diffusion and can be slowed by using a dialysis filter with a smaller surface area, slowing the blood and dialysate flow, and reducing the duration of dialysis. Daily hemodialysis would help as the predialysis urea would be lower so there would be less of a drop in urea concentration each session (162). Serum sodium also affects osmolality. In the patient with elevated ICP, the sodium prescription should be 5 to 10 mEq/L higher than the serum concentration. This is to offset drop in serum osmolality with the rapid loss of urea by increasing serum sodium concentration temporarily thereby raising serum osmolality. The concentration of bicarbonate in the dialysate is supraphysiologic, and so there is a rapid rise in bicarbonate during dialysis. Once the bicarbonate is in the plasma, it is converted to water and carbon dioxide, both of which can rapidly cross cell membranes. This carbon dioxide enters brain tissue causing an intracellular acidosis and increase in osmolality drawing water in and worsening cerebral edema. This can be prevented by using a lower bicarbonate bath of 30 to 32 mEq/L when there is an elevated ICP (158). Most neurotrauma units try to maintain a cerebral perfusion pressure (CPP) of 60 mm Hg. This can be affected by hypotension a frequent complication of routine hemodialysis. Strategies to combat this include increasing dialysate concentration of sodium (about 10 mEq/L above the serum sodium concentration), potassium, and calcium. Another method is cooling the dialysate (163).

If CRRT is available, it is the optimal modality of RRT in the patient with an elevated ICP. There are slower rates of change of urea, bicarbonate, sodium, and other electrolytes decreasing the risk of worsening cerebral edema. CRRT also is associated with less hypotension as compared to intermittent HD (163). In regard to anticoagulation if using CRRT, systemic anticoagulation is avoided. Regional anticoagulation with citrate is possible and can be considered. Obviously, the safest method would be to optimize all other nonanticoagulant-based strategies in the setting of a cerebral hemorrhage (31,164).

⬢ REFERENCES

1. Ostermann M, Chang RW. Acute kidney injury in the intensive care unit according to RIFLE. *Crit Care Med* 2007;35(8):1837–1843, 1852.
2. Uchino S, Kellum JA, Bellomo R, et al. Acute renal failure in critically ill patients: a multinational, multicenter study. *JAMA* 2005;294(7):813–818.
3. Brivet FG, Kleinknecht DJ, Loirat P, et al. Acute renal failure in intensive care units—causes, outcome, and prognostic factors of hospital mortality; a prospective, multicenter study. French Study Group on Acute Renal Failure. *Crit Care Med* 1996;24(2):192–198.
4. Mehta RL, McDonald B, Gabbai FB, et al. A randomized clinical trial of continuous versus intermittent dialysis for acute renal failure. *Kidney Int* 2001;60(3):1154–1163.
5. Metcalfe W, Simpson M, Khan IH, et al. Acute renal failure requiring renal replacement therapy: incidence and outcome. *QJM* 2002; 95(9):579–583.
6. Elseviers MM, Lins RL, Van der Niepen P, et al. Renal replacement therapy is an independent risk factor for mortality in critically ill patients with acute kidney injury. *Crit Care* 2010;14(6):R221.
7. Hsu RK, McCulloch CE, Dudley RA, et al. Temporal changes in incidence of dialysis-requiring AKI. *J Am Soc Nephrol* 2013;24(1):37–42.
8. Ponte B, Felipe C, Muriel A, et al. Long-term functional evolution after an acute kidney injury: a 10-year study. *Nephrol Dial Transplant* 2008;23(12):3859–3866.
9. Gallagher M, Cass A, Bellomo R, et al. Long-term survival and dialysis dependency following acute kidney injury in intensive care: extended follow-up of a randomized controlled trial. *PLoS Med* 2014; 11(2):e1001601.
10. Ronco C, Ricci Z, De Backer D, et al. Renal replacement therapy in acute kidney injury: controversy and consensus. *Crit Care* 2015;19(1):146.
11. Selby NM, McIntyre CW. A systematic review of the clinical effects of reducing dialysate fluid temperature. *Nephrol Dial Transplant* 2006;21(7):1883–1898.
12. Sherman RA, Daugirdas JT, Ing TS. Complications during hemodialysis. In: Sherman RA, Daugirdas JT, Ing TS, eds. *Handbook of Dialysis*. 4th ed. Philadelphia, PA: Lippincott Williams & Wilkins, 2007: 158–164.
13. Berbece AN, Richardson RM. Sustained low-efficiency dialysis in the ICU: cost, anticoagulation, and solute removal. *Kidney Int* 2006; 70(5):963–968.
14. Tolwani A. Continuous renal-replacement therapy for acute kidney injury. *N Engl J Med* 2012;367(26):2505–2514.
15. Teo BW, Messer JS, Paganini EP, et al. Slow continuous therapies. In: Daugirdas JT, Blake PG, Ing TS, eds. *Handbook of Dialysis*. 4th ed. Philadelphia, PA: Lippincott Williams & Wilkins, 2007:219–251.
16. Clark WR, Turk JE, Kraus MA, et al. Dose determinants in continuous renal replacement therapy. *Artif Organs* 2003;27(9):815–820.
17. Brunet S, Leblanc M, Geadah D, et al. Diffusive and convective solute clearances during continuous renal replacement therapy at various dialysate and ultrafiltration flow rates. *Am J Kidney Dis* 1999;34(3): 486–492.
18. Barenbrock M, Hausberg M, Matzkies F, et al. Effects of bicarbonate- and lactate-buffered replacement fluids on cardiovascular outcome in CVVH patients. *Kidney Int* 2000;58(4):1751–1757.
19. Amore A, Cirina P, Mitola S, et al. Acetate intolerance is mediated by enhanced synthesis of nitric oxide by endothelial cells. *J Am Soc Nephrol* 1997;8(9):1431–1436.
20. Abe M, Maruyama N, Matsumoto S, et al. Comparison of sustained hemodiafiltration with acetate-free dialysate and continuous venovenous hemodiafiltration for the treatment of critically ill patients with acute kidney injury. *Int J Nephrol* 2011;2011:432094.
21. Crosswell A, Brain MJ, Roodenburg O. Vascular access site influences circuit life in continuous renal replacement therapy. *Crit Care Resusc* 2014;16(2):127–130.
22. Mrozek N, Lautrette A, Timsit JF, et al. How to deal with dialysis catheters in the ICU setting. *Ann Intensive Care* 2012;2(1):48.
23. Clark EG, Barsuk JH. Temporary hemodialysis catheters: recent advances. *Kidney Int* 2014;86(5):888–895.

24. Khwaja A. KDIGO clinical practice guidelines for acute kidney injury. *Nephron Clin Pract* 2012;120(4):c179–c184.

25. Parienti JJ, Thirion M, Megarbane B, et al. Femoral vs jugular venous catheterization and risk of nosocomial events in adults requiring acute renal replacement therapy: a randomized controlled trial. *JAMA* 2008;299(20):2413–2422.

26. Marik PE, Flemmer M, Harrison W. The risk of catheter-related bloodstream infection with femoral venous catheters as compared to subclavian and internal jugular venous catheters: a systematic review of the literature and meta-analysis. *Crit Care Med* 2012;40(8):2479–2485.

27. Ge X, Cavallazzi R, Li C, et al. Central venous access sites for the prevention of venous thrombosis, stenosis and infection. *Cochrane Database Syst Rev* 2012;(3):CD004084.

28. Parienti JJ, Megarbane B, Fischer MO, et al. Catheter dysfunction and dialysis performance according to vascular access among 736 critically ill adults requiring renal replacement therapy: a randomized controlled study. *Crit Care Med* 2010;38(4):1118–1125.

29. Lyndon WD, Wille KM, Tolwani AJ. Solute clearance in CRRT: prescribed dose versus actual delivered dose. *Nephrol Dial Transplant* 2012;27(3):952–956.

30. Oudemans-van Straaten HM. Hemostasis and thrombosis in continuous renal replacement treatment. *Semin Thromb Hemost* 2015;41(1):91–98.

31. Tolwani AJ, Wille KM. Anticoagulation for continuous renal replacement therapy. *Semin Dial* 2009;22(2):141–145.

32. Dunn WJ, Sriram S. Filter lifespan in critically ill adults receiving continuous renal replacement therapy: the effect of patient and treatment-related variables. *Crit Care Resusc* 2014;16(3):225–231.

33. Lehner GF, Wiedermann CJ, Joannidis M. High-volume hemofiltration in critically ill patients: a systematic review and meta-analysis. *Minerva Anestesiol* 2014;80(5):595–609.

34. Wald R, Shariff SZ, Adhikari NK, et al. The association between renal replacement therapy modality and long-term outcomes among critically ill adults with acute kidney injury: a retrospective cohort study. *Crit Care Med* 2014;42(4):868–877.

35. Hirsh J, Anand SS, Halperin JL, et al. Mechanism of action and pharmacology of unfractionated heparin. *Arterioscler Thromb Vasc Biol* 2001;21(7):1094–1096.

36. Ferreira JA, Johnson DW. The incidence of thrombocytopenia associated with continuous renal replacement therapy in critically ill patients. *Ren Fail* 2015;37:1232–1236.

37. Gupta S, Tiruvoipati R, Green C, et al. Heparin induced thrombocytopenia in critically ill: diagnostic dilemmas and management conundrums. *World J Crit Care Med* 2015;4(3):202–212.

38. Bhatt VR, Aryal MR, Armitage JO. Nonheparin anticoagulants for heparin-induced thrombocytopenia. *N Engl J Med* 2013;368(24):2333–2334.

39. Treschan TA, Schaefer MS, Geib J, et al. Argatroban versus Lepirudin in critically ill patients (ALicia): a randomized controlled trial. *Crit Care* 2014;18(5):588.

40. Tolwani A, Wille KM. Advances in continuous renal replacement therapy: citrate anticoagulation update. *Blood Purif* 2012;34(2):88–93.

41. Lanckohr C, Hahnenkamp K, Boschin M. Continuous renal replacement therapy with regional citrate anticoagulation: do we really know the details? *Curr Opin Anaesthesiol* 2013;26(4):428–437.

42. Morabito S, Pistolesi V, Tritapepe L, et al. Regional citrate anticoagulation for RRTs in critically ill patients with AKI. *Clin J Am Soc Nephrol* 2014;9(12):2173–2188.

43. Bouchard J, Madore F. Role of citrate and other methods of anticoagulation in patients with severe liver failure requiring continuous renal replacement therapy. *NDT Plus* 2009;2(1):11–19.

44. Mariano F, Morselli M, Bergamo D, et al. Blood and ultrafiltrate dosage of citrate as a useful and routine tool during continuous venovenous haemodiafiltration in septic shock patients. *Nephrol Dial Transplant* 2011;26(12):3882–3888.

45. Fall P, Szerlip HM. Continuous renal replacement therapy: cause and treatment of electrolyte complications. *Semin Dial* 2010;23(6):581–585.

46. Bakker AJ, Boerma EC, Keidel H, et al. Detection of citrate overdose in critically ill patients on citrate-anticoagulated venovenous haemofiltration: use of ionised and total/ionised calcium. *Clin Chem Lab Med* 2006;44(8):962–966.

47. Saner FH, Treckmann JW, Geis A, et al. Efficacy and safety of regional citrate anticoagulation in liver transplant patients requiring post-operative renal replacement therapy. *Nephrol Dial Transplant* 2012;27(4):1651–1657.

48. Schultheiss C, Saugel B, Phillip V, et al. Continuous venovenous hemodialysis with regional citrate anticoagulation in patients with liver failure: a prospective observational study. *Crit Care* 2012;16(4):R162.

49. Joannidis M, Oudemans-van Straaten HM. Clinical review: patency of the circuit in continuous renal replacement therapy. *Crit Care* 2007;11(4):218.

50. Palevsky PM, Zhang JH, O'Connor TZ, et al. Intensity of renal support in critically ill patients with acute kidney injury. *N Engl J Med* 2008;359(1):7–20.

51. Bellomo R, Cass A, Cole L, et al. Intensity of continuous renal-replacement therapy in critically ill patients. *N Engl J Med* 2009;361(17):1627–1638.

52. Claure-Del Granado R, Macedo E, Chertow GM, et al. Effluent volume in continuous renal replacement therapy overestimates the delivered dose of dialysis. *Clin J Am Soc Nephrol* 2011;6(3):467–475.

53. Tolwani A. Continuous renal-replacement therapy for acute kidney injury. *N Engl J Med* 2013;368(12):1160–1161.

54. Gambro. Improving the hemocompatibility of the extracorporeal device. http://www.gambro.com/PageFiles/6052/Prismaflex%20sets%20with%20AN69ST%20membrane,%20Produktdatablad.pdf?epslanguage=en. Accessed September 3, 2015.

55. Parsons FM, Hobson SM, Blagg CR, et al. Optimum time for dialysis in acute reversible renal failure. Description and value of an improved dialyzer with large surface area. *Lancet* 1961;1(7169):129–134.

56. Fischer RP, Griffen WO Jr, Reiser M, et al. Early dialysis in the treatment of acute renal failure. *Surg Gynecol Obstet* 1966;123(5):1019–1023.

57. Kleinknecht D, Jungers P, Chanard J, et al. Uremic and non-uremic complications in acute renal failure: evaluation of early and frequent dialysis on prognosis. *Kidney Int* 1972;1(3):190–196.

58. Teschan PE, Baxter CR, O'Brien TF, et al. Prophylactic hemodialysis in the treatment of acute renal failure. *Ann Intern Med* 1960;53:992–1016.

59. Liu KD, Himmelfarb J, Paganini E, et al. Timing of initiation of dialysis in critically ill patients with acute kidney injury. *Clin J Am Soc Nephrol* 2006;1(5):915–919.

60. Vaara ST, Reinikainen M, Wald R, et al; for the FINNAKI Study Group. Timing of RRT based on the presence of conventional indications. *Clin J Am Soc Nephrol* 2014;9(9):1577–1585.

61. Bouman CS, Oudemans-Van Straaten HM, Tijssen JG, et al. Effects of early high-volume continuous venovenous hemofiltration on survival and recovery of renal function in intensive care patients with acute renal failure: a prospective, randomized trial. *Crit Care Med* 2002;30(10):2205–2211.

62. Jamale TE, Hase NK, Kulkarni M, et al. Earlier-start versus usual-start dialysis in patients with community-acquired acute kidney injury: a randomized controlled trial. *Am J Kidney Dis* 2013;62(6):1116–1121.

63. Karvellas CJ, Farhat MR, Sajjad I, et al. A comparison of early versus late initiation of renal replacement therapy in critically ill patients with acute kidney injury: a systematic review and meta-analysis. *Crit Care* 2011;15(1):R72.

64. Clark EG, Bagshaw SM. Unnecessary renal replacement therapy for acute kidney injury is harmful for renal recovery. *Semin Dial* 2015;28(1):6–11.

65. Jansen MA, Hart AA, Korevaar JC, et al. Predictors of the rate of decline of residual renal function in incident dialysis patients. *Kidney Int* 2002;62(3):1046–1053.

66. Lima EQ, Silva RG, Donadi EL, et al. Prevention of intradialytic hypotension in patients with acute kidney injury submitted to sustained low-efficiency dialysis. *Ren Fail* 2012;34(10):1238–1243.

67. Gutierrez A, Alvestrand A, Wahren J, et al. Effect of in vivo contact between blood and dialysis membranes on protein catabolism in humans. *Kidney Int* 1990;38(3):487–494.

68. Finkel KW, Podoll AS. Complications of continuous renal replacement therapy. *Semin Dial* 2009;22(2):155–159.

69. Kidney Disease: Improving Global Outcomes Acute Kidney Injury Work Group. KDIGO clinical practice guideline for acute kidney injury. *Kidney Int Suppl* 2012;2:1–138.

70. Barbar SD, Binquet C, Monchi M, et al. Impact on mortality of the timing of renal replacement therapy in patients with severe acute kidney injury in septic shock: the IDEAL-ICU study (initiation of dialysis early versus delayed in the intensive care unit): study protocol for a randomized controlled trial. *Trials* 2014;15:270.

71. Gaudry S, Hajage D, Schortgen F, et al. Comparison of two strategies for initiating renal replacement therapy in the intensive care unit: study protocol for a randomized controlled trial (AKIKI). *Trials* 2015;16:170.

72. Bouchard J, Soroko SB, Chertow GM, et al. Fluid accumulation, survival and recovery of kidney function in critically ill patients with acute kidney injury. *Kidney Int* 2009;76(4):422–427.

73. Grams ME, Estrella MM, Coresh J, et al. Fluid balance, diuretic use, and mortality in acute kidney injury. *Clin J Am Soc Nephrol* 2011;6(5):966–973.

74. Vaara ST, Korhonen AM, Kaukonen KM, et al. Fluid overload is associated with an increased risk for 90-day mortality in critically ill patients with renal replacement therapy: data from the prospective FINNAKI study. *Crit Care* 2012;16(5):R197.

75. Sutherland SM, Zappitelli M, Alexander SR, et al. Fluid overload and mortality in children receiving continuous renal replacement therapy: the prospective pediatric continuous renal replacement therapy registry. *Am J Kidney Dis* 2010;55(2):316–325.

76. Heung M, Wolfgram DF, Kommareddi M, et al. Fluid overload at initiation of renal replacement therapy is associated with lack of renal recovery in patients with acute kidney injury. *Nephrol Dial Transplant* 2012;27(3):956–961.

77. Butcher BW, Liu KD. Fluid overload in AKI: epiphenomenon or putative effect on mortality? *Curr Opin Crit Care* 2012;18(6):593–598.

78. Chen H, Wu B, Gong D, et al. Fluid overload at start of continuous renal replacement therapy is associated with poorer clinical condition and outcome: a prospective observational study on the combined use of bioimpedance vector analysis and serum N-terminal pro-B-type natriuretic peptide measurement. *Crit Care* 2015;19:135.

79. Michael M, Kuehnle I, Goldstein SL. Fluid overload and acute renal failure in pediatric stem cell transplant patients. *Pediatr Nephrol* 2004;19(1):91–95.

80. Uchino S, Bellomo R, Kellum JA, et al. Patient and kidney survival by dialysis modality in critically ill patients with acute kidney injury. *Int J Artif Organs* 2007;30(4):281–292.

81. Bell M, SWING, Granath F, et al. Continuous renal replacement therapy is associated with less chronic renal failure than intermittent haemodialysis after acute renal failure. *Intensive Care Med* 2007;33(5):773–780.

82. Vinsonneau C, Camus C, Combes A, et al. Continuous venovenous haemodiafiltration versus intermittent haemodialysis for acute renal failure in patients with multiple-organ dysfunction syndrome: a multicentre randomised trial. *Lancet* 2006;368(9533):379–385.

83. Lins RL, Elseviers MM, Van der Niepen P, et al. Intermittent versus continuous renal replacement therapy for acute kidney injury patients admitted to the intensive care unit: results of a randomized clinical trial. *Nephrol Dial Transplant* 2009;24(2):512–518.

84. Bagshaw SM, Berthiaume LR, Delaney A, et al. Continuous versus intermittent renal replacement therapy for critically ill patients with acute kidney injury: a meta-analysis. *Crit Care Med* 2008;36(2):610–617.

85. Kielstein JT, Kretschmer U, Ernst T, et al. Efficacy and cardiovascular tolerability of extended dialysis in critically ill patients: a randomized controlled study. *Am J Kidney Dis* 2004;43(2):342–349.

86. Schwenger V, Weigand MA, Hoffmann O, et al. Sustained low efficiency dialysis using a single-pass batch system in acute kidney injury—a randomized interventional trial: the REnal Replacement Therapy Study in Intensive Care Unit PatiEnts. *Crit Care* 2012;16(4):R140.

87. Ronco C, Bellomo R. Dialysis in intensive care unit patients with acute kidney injury: continuous therapy is superior. *Clin J Am Soc Nephrol* 2007;2(3):597–600.

88. Augustine JJ, Sandy D, Seifert TH, et al. A randomized controlled trial comparing intermittent with continuous dialysis in patients with ARF. *Am J Kidney Dis* 2004;44(6):1000–1007.

89. Uehlinger DE, Jakob SM, Ferrari P, et al. Comparison of continuous and intermittent renal replacement therapy for acute renal failure. *Nephrol Dial Transplant* 2005;20(8):1630–1637.

90. Pannu N, Klarenbach S, Wiebe N; for the Alberta Kidney Disease Network. Renal replacement therapy in patients with acute renal failure: a systematic review. *JAMA* 2008;299(7):793–805.

91. Wald R, Friedrich JO, Bagshaw SM, et al. Optimal Mode of clearance in critically ill patients with Acute Kidney Injury (OMAKI)—a pilot randomized controlled trial of hemofiltration versus hemodialysis: a Canadian Critical Care Trials Group project. *Crit Care* 2012;16(5):R205.

92. Friedrich JO, Wald R, Bagshaw SM, et al. Hemofiltration compared to hemodialysis for acute kidney injury: systematic review and meta-analysis. *Crit Care* 2012;16(4):R146.

93. Chionh CY, Soni SS, Finkelstein FO, et al. Use of peritoneal dialysis in AKI: a systematic review. *Clin J Am Soc Nephrol* 2013;8(10):1649–1660.

94. Ponce D, Berbel MN, Regina de Goes C, et al. High-volume peritoneal dialysis in acute kidney injury: indications and limitations. *Clin J Am Soc Nephrol* 2012;7(6):887–894.

95. Gabriel DP, Caramori JT, Martim LC, et al. High volume peritoneal dialysis vs daily hemodialysis: a randomized, controlled trial in patients with acute kidney injury. *Kidney Int* 2008;73(Suppl 108):S87–S93.

96. Phu NH, Hien TT, Mai NT, et al. Hemofiltration and peritoneal dialysis in infection-associated acute renal failure in Vietnam. *N Engl J Med* 2002;347(12):895–902.

97. Ronco C, Bellomo R, Homel P, et al. Effects of different doses in continuous veno-venous haemofiltration on outcomes of acute renal failure: a prospective randomised trial. *Lancet* 2000;356(9223):26–30.

98. Faulhaber-Walter R, Hafer C, Jahr N, et al. The Hannover Dialysis Outcome study: comparison of standard versus intensified extended dialysis for treatment of patients with acute kidney injury in the intensive care unit. *Nephrol Dial Transplant* 2009;24(7):2179–2186.

99. Van Wert R, Friedrich JO, Scales DC, et al; for the University of Toronto Acute Kidney Injury Research Group. High-dose renal replacement therapy for acute kidney injury: systematic review and meta-analysis. *Crit Care Med* 2010;38(5):1360–1369.

100. Venkataraman R, Kellum JA, Palevsky P. Dosing patterns for continuous renal replacement therapy at a large academic medical center in the United States. *J Crit Care* 2002;17(4):246–250.

101. Overberger P, Pesacreta M, Palevsky PM, et al. Management of renal replacement therapy in acute kidney injury: a survey of practitioner prescribing practices. *Clin J Am Soc Nephrol* 2007;2(4):623–630.

102. Liu KD, Matthay MA. Advances in critical care for the nephrologist: acute lung injury/ARDS. *Clin J Am Soc Nephrol* 2008;3(2):578–586.

103. Darmon M, Clec'h C, Adrie C, et al. Acute respiratory distress syndrome and risk of AKI among critically ill patients. *Clin J Am Soc Nephrol* 2014;9(8):1347–1353.

104. Annat G, Viale JP, Bui Xuan B, et al. Effect of PEEP ventilation on renal function, plasma renin, aldosterone, neurophysins and urinary ADH, and prostaglandins. *Anesthesiology* 1983;58(2):136–141.

105. Han F, Sun R, Ni Y, et al. Early initiation of continuous renal replacement therapy improves clinical outcomes in patients with acute respiratory distress syndrome. *Am J Med Sci* 2015;349(3):199–205.

106. Murugan R, Karajala-Subramanyam V, Lee M, et al. Acute kidney injury in non-severe pneumonia is associated with an increased immune response and lower survival. *Kidney Int* 2010;77(6):527–535.

107. Malhotra A. Low-tidal-volume ventilation in the acute respiratory distress syndrome. *N Engl J Med* 2007;357(11):1113–1120.

108. Zhang JC, Chu YF, Zeng J, et al. Effect of continuous high-volume hemofiltration in patients with severe acute respiratory distress syndrome. *Zhonghua Wei Zhong Bing Ji Jiu Yi Xue* 2013;25(3):145–148.

109. Vesconi S, Cruz DN, Fumagalli R, et al. Delivered dose of renal replacement therapy and mortality in critically ill patients with acute kidney injury. *Crit Care* 2009;13(2):R57.

110. Garzia F, Todor R, Scalea T. Continuous arteriovenous hemofiltration countercurrent dialysis (CAVH-D) in acute respiratory failure (ARDS). *J Trauma* 1991;31(9):1277–1285.

111. Hoste EA, Vanholder RC, Lameire NH, et al. No early respiratory benefit with CVVHDF in patients with acute renal failure and acute lung injury. *Nephrol Dial Transplant* 2002;17(12):2153–2158.

112. De Vriese AS, Colardyn FA, Philippe JJ, et al. Cytokine removal during continuous hemofiltration in septic patients. *J Am Soc Nephrol* 1999;10(4):846–853.

113. Gasche Y, Pascual M, Suter PM, et al. Complement depletion during haemofiltration with polyacrylonitrile membranes. *Nephrol Dial Transplant* 1996;11(1):117–119.

114. Matsuda K, Moriguchi T, Oda S, et al. Efficacy of continuous hemodiafiltration with a cytokine-adsorbing hemofilter in the treatment of acute respiratory distress syndrome. *Contrib Nephrol* 2010;166:83–92.

115. Selewski DT, Cornell TT, Blatt NB, et al. Fluid overload and fluid removal in pediatric patients on extracorporeal membrane oxygenation requiring continuous renal replacement therapy. *Crit Care Med* 2012;40(9):2694–2699.

116. Chen H, Yu RG, Yin NN, et al. Combination of extracorporeal membrane oxygenation and continuous renal replacement therapy in critically ill patients: a systematic review. *Crit Care* 2014;18(6):675.

117. Askenazi DJ, Selewski DT, Paden ML, et al. Renal replacement therapy in critically ill patients receiving extracorporeal membrane oxygenation. *Clin J Am Soc Nephrol* 2012;7(8):1328–1336.

118. Forster C, Schriewer J, John S, et al. Low-flow CO(2) removal integrated into a renal-replacement circuit can reduce acidosis and decrease vasopressor requirements. *Crit Care* 2013;17(4):R154.

119. Burki NK, Mani RK, Herth FJ, et al. A novel extracorporeal CO(2) removal system: results of a pilot study of hypercapnic respiratory failure in patients with COPD. *Chest* 2013;143(3):678–686.

120. Martin GS, Mannino DM, Eaton S, et al. The epidemiology of sepsis in the United States from 1979 through 2000. *N Engl J Med* 2003;348(16):1546–1554.

121. Zarjou A, Agarwal A. Sepsis and acute kidney injury. *J Am Soc Nephrol* 2011;22(6):999–1006.

122. Zhou F, Peng Z, Murugan R, et al. Blood purification and mortality in sepsis: a meta-analysis of randomized trials. *Crit Care Med* 2013;41(9):2209–2220.

123. Honore PM, Jacobs R, Joannes-Boyau O, et al. Septic AKI in ICU patients. Diagnosis, pathophysiology, and treatment type, dosing, and timing: a comprehensive review of recent and future developments. *Ann Intensive Care* 2011;1(1):32.

124. Payen D, Mateo J, Cavaillon JM, et al. Impact of continuous venovenous hemofiltration on organ failure during the early phase of severe sepsis: a randomized controlled trial. *Crit Care Med* 2009;37(3):803–810.

125. Bellomo R, Tipping P, Boyce N. Continuous veno-venous hemofiltration with dialysis removes cytokines from the circulation of septic patients. *Crit Care Med* 1993;21(4):522–526.

126. Bellomo R, Tipping P, Boyce N. Tumor necrosis factor clearances during veno-venous hemodiafiltration in the critically ill. *ASAIO Trans* 1991;37(3):M322–M323.

127. Shum HP, Chan KC, Kwan MC, et al. Timing for initiation of continuous renal replacement therapy in patients with septic shock and acute kidney injury. *Ther Apher Dial* 2013;17(3):305–310.

128. Honore PM, Jamez J, Wauthier M, et al. Prospective evaluation of short-term, high-volume isovolemic hemofiltration on the hemodynamic course and outcome in patients with intractable circulatory failure resulting from septic shock. *Crit Care Med* 2000;28(11):3581–3587.

129. Joannes-Boyau O, Honore PM, Perez P, et al. High-volume versus standard-volume haemofiltration for septic shock patients with acute kidney injury (IVOIRE study): a multicentre randomized controlled trial. *Intensive Care Med* 2013;39(9):1535–1546.

130. Zhang P, Yang Y, Lv R, et al. Effect of the intensity of continuous renal replacement therapy in patients with sepsis and acute kidney injury: a single-center randomized clinical trial. *Nephrol Dial Transplant* 2012;27(3):967–973.

131. Clark E, Molnar AO, Joannes-Boyau O, et al. High-volume hemofiltration for septic acute kidney injury: a systematic review and meta-analysis. *Crit Care* 2014;18(1):R7.

132. Atan R, Crosbie DC, Bellomo R. Techniques of extracorporeal cytokine removal: a systematic review of human studies. *Ren Fail* 2013;35(8):1061–1070.

133. Atan R, Crosbie D, Bellomo R. Techniques of extracorporeal cytokine removal: a systematic review of the literature. *Blood Purif* 2012;33(1–3):88–100.

134. Haase M, Bellomo R, Morgera S, et al. High cut-off point membranes in septic acute renal failure: a systematic review. *Int J Artif Organs* 2007;30(12):1031–1041.

135. Morgera S, Slowinski T, Melzer C, et al. Renal replacement therapy with high-cutoff hemofilters: impact of convection and diffusion on cytokine clearances and protein status. *Am J Kidney Dis* 2004;43(3):444–453.

136. Livigni S, Bertolini G, Rossi C, et al. Efficacy of coupled plasma filtration adsorption (CPFA) in patients with septic shock: a multicenter randomised controlled clinical trial. *BMJ Open* 2014;4(1):e003536.

137. Ronco C, Brendolan A, Lonnemann G, et al. A pilot study of coupled plasma filtration with adsorption in septic shock. *Crit Care Med* 2002;30(6):1250–1255.

138. Kushi H, Miki T, Sakagami Y, et al. Hemoperfusion with an immobilized polymyxin B fiber column decreases macrophage and monocyte activity. *Ther Apher Dial* 2009;13(6):515–519.

139. Cantaluppi V, Assenzio B, Pasero D, et al. Polymyxin-B hemoperfusion inactivates circulating proapoptotic factors. *Intensive Care Med* 2008;34(9):1638–1645.

140. Klein DJ, Foster D, Schorr CA, et al. The EUPHRATES trial (Evaluating the Use of Polymyxin B Hemoperfusion in a Randomized controlled trial of Adults Treated for Endotoxemia and Septic shock): study protocol for a randomized controlled trial. *Trials* 2014;15:218.

141. Cruz DN, Perazella MA, Bellomo R, et al. Effectiveness of polymyxin B-immobilized fiber column in sepsis: a systematic review. *Crit Care* 2007;11(2):R47.

142. Cruz DN, Antonelli M, Fumagalli R, et al. Early use of polymyxin B hemoperfusion in abdominal septic shock: the EUPHAS randomized controlled trial. *JAMA* 2009;301(23):2445–2452.

143. De Corte W, Vuylsteke S, De Waele JJ, et al. Severe lactic acidosis in critically ill patients with acute kidney injury treated with renal replacement therapy. *J Crit Care* 2014;29(4):650–655.

144. Bellomo R. Bench-to-bedside review: lactate and the kidney. *Crit Care* 2002;6(4):322–326.

145. Levraut J, Ciebiera JP, Jambou P, et al. Effect of continuous venovenous hemofiltration with dialysis on lactate clearance in critically ill patients. *Crit Care Med* 1997;25(1):58–62.

146. Garcia-Tsao G, Parikh CR, Viola A. Acute kidney injury in cirrhosis. *Hepatology* 2008;48(6):2064–2077.

147. Belcher JM. Is there a role for dialysis in patients with hepatorenal syndrome who are not liver transplant candidates? *Semin Dial* 2014;27(3):288–291.

148. Wong F, Raina N, Richardson R. Molecular adsorbent recirculating system is ineffective in the management of type 1 hepatorenal syndrome in patients with cirrhosis with ascites who have failed vasoconstrictor treatment. *Gut* 2010;59(3):381–386.

149. Tan HK. Molecular adsorbent recirculating system (MARS). *Ann Acad Med Singapore* 2004;33(3):329–335.

150. Mitzner SR, Stange J, Klammt S, et al. Extracorporeal detoxification using the molecular adsorbent recirculating system for critically ill patients with liver failure. *J Am Soc Nephrol* 2001;(12 Suppl 17):S75–S82.

151. Mitzner SR, Klammt S, Peszynski P, et al. Improvement of multiple organ functions in hepatorenal syndrome during albumin dialysis with the molecular adsorbent recirculating system. *Ther Apher* 2001;5(5):417–422.

152. Mitzner SR, Stange J, Klammt S, et al. Improvement of hepatorenal syndrome with extracorporeal albumin dialysis MARS: results of a prospective, randomized, controlled clinical trial. *Liver Transpl* 2000;6(3):277–286.

153. Lavayssiere L, Kallab S, Cardeau-Desangles I, et al. Impact of molecular adsorbent recirculating system on renal recovery in type-1 hepatorenal syndrome patients with chronic liver failure. *J Gastroenterol Hepatol* 2013;28(6):1019–1024.

154. Olin P, Hausken J, Foss A, et al. Continuous molecular adsorbent recirculating system treatment in 69 patients listed for liver transplantation. *Scand J Gastroenterol* 2015;50(9):1127–1134.

155. Rifai K, Manns MP. Review article: clinical experience with Prometheus. *Ther Apher Dial* 2006;10(2):132–137.

156. Rifai K, Ernst T, Kretschmer U, et al. Prometheus—a new extracorporeal system for the treatment of liver failure. *J Hepatol* 2003;39(6):984–990.

157. Wittebole X, Hantson P. Use of the molecular adsorbent recirculating system (MARS) for the management of acute poisoning with or without liver failure. *Clin Toxicol (Phila)* 2011;49(9):782–793.

158. Davenport A. Changing the hemodialysis prescription for hemodialysis patients with subdural and intracranial hemorrhage. *Hemodial Int* 2013;(17 Suppl 1):S22–S27.

159. Lin CM, Lin JW, Tsai JT, et al. Intracranial pressure fluctuation during hemodialysis in renal failure patients with intracranial hemorrhage. *Acta Neurochir Suppl* 2008;101:141–144.

160. Davenport A. Continuous renal replacement therapies in patients with acute neurological injury. *Semin Dial* 2009;22(2):165–168.

161. Davenport A. Can modification of renal replacement therapy improve the outcome of patients with systemic inflammatory response syndrome? *Blood Purif* 2006;24(3):317–318.

162. Davenport A. Practical guidance for dialyzing a hemodialysis patient following acute brain injury. *Hemodial Int* 2008;12(3):307–312.

163. Nongnuch A, Panorchan K, Davenport A. Brain-kidney crosstalk. *Crit Care* 2014;18(3):225.

164. Davenport A. Management of acute kidney injury in neurotrauma. *Hemodial Int* 2010;14(Suppl 1):S27–S31.

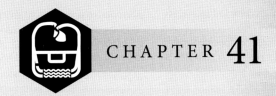

CHAPTER 41

Preparing Dialysis Patients for Renal Transplantation

Feras F. Karadsheh, Matthew R. Weir, Charles B. Cangro, and Beje Thomas

Kidney transplantation is now regarded as the treatment of choice for end-stage kidney disease (ESKD). Kidney transplantation has saved over a million life-years in the United States during the last 25 years, with 4.4 life-years saved per transplant recipient (1). A successful kidney transplant reduces the risk of dying for patients when compared with maintenance dialysis and improves the quality of life. Multiple studies comparing patients who have undergone transplantation with those remaining on the waiting list have clearly shown that renal transplantation confers a survival advantage (2–6). This survival benefit was seen in all age groups including the elderly and among African Americans and diabetic patients.

KIDNEY TRANSPLANT TYPES AND THE WAIT LIST

Kidney transplantation procedures can be divided into several types based on the living status of the donor and the potential relationship between donor and recipient. The two major groups include deceased donor renal transplants and living renal transplants. Deceased donor renal transplants are further divided into standard criteria (donor <50 years old), expanded criteria living donor (donor >60 years old or 50 to 60 years old with two of the following, history of hypertension, terminal creatinine >1.5, or died of a stroke), and donation after cardiac death. Living-related transplants may related or unrelated. Deceased donor renal transplantation remains the most common transplant procedure. It is important to note the type of transplant a patient receives has an important impact on patient survival, allograft organ survival, and time spent waiting for transplantation.

There are currently 123,175 people waiting for lifesaving organ transplants in the United States. Of these, 101,170 await kidney transplants. Nearly 3,000 new patients are added to the kidney waiting list each month. (7). However, the number of available organs has been outpaced by the increasing number of patients listed resulting in longer wait times. Patients who entered the waiting list after 2002 had a median waiting time of more than 3 years (8). Approximately 12 people die each day while waiting for a transplant (4). It is no surprise then that patients who have a preemptive transplant (one done before the initiation of dialysis) or spend less than 1 year on the waiting list have shown to have an improved survival following transplantation (9–11). In particular, the faster the elderly patient is transplanted, the greater the survival benefit as they are more prone to have issues arise and die on the wait list (12). Over the last decade, there have been only marginal increases in the number of deceased donors. In 2006, there were 8,024 deceased donors. This increased to 11,163 in 2013 and to 13,124 in 2014 in part due to expanding the criteria for acceptable donors (7,13). In regard to living donors, the volume of living donation in transplantation peaked in 2006 (1). Recently, there has been a decline of about 13% per year and is more pronounced among blacks, males, younger adults, siblings, and parents (13,14). In absolute numbers, in 2005, there were 6,500 living donations compared to 5,733 in 2013 (7,8).

The United Network for Organ Sharing (UNOS), which is the agency that governs transplant policy and organ distribution, recently in December of 2014 revised the system that matches kidneys from deceased donors with patients needing transplantation. This aimed to extend the length of functioning transplants, to increase the likelihood of receiving a transplant for candidates who are difficult to match, and to make better use of available kidneys through increasing organ usage and reducing the need for repeat transplants. Now, UNOS will calculate the transplant waiting time from the date the patient begins dialysis, even if he or she started dialysis before being accepted for listing at a transplant center (15). This new system gave priority to candidates whom are sensitized and have difficulty finding a human leukocyte antigen (HLA)-compatible donor

685

and allows patients expected to live longer to receive kidneys likely to function longer.

The former standard criteria/expanded criteria donor has been replaced by the Kidney Donor Profile Index (KDPI). The KDPI is calculated as a percentage; it describes how long a deceased donor kidney is expected to function compared to all the kidneys donated in the previous year in the United States. For instance, if a donor kidney has a KDPI score of 85%, then that kidney is expected to have a shorter functional life than 85% of kidneys harvested the year before (i.e., the lower the number, the better). Roughly, a KDPI score of 0% to 20% has a graft survival of about 11 years, 21% to 85% of 9 years, and 86% to 100% of about 6 years. Expanded criteria donor kidneys are thought to be the equivalent of a KDPI score of 85% or higher (15). The group of patients that would be recommended to sign for a kidney with a KDPI of >85% would be a high-risk patient that might not be expected to survive long without a transplant (15).

Transplant candidates are also risk stratified based on their estimated posttransplant survival score. This is calculated using recipient age, diabetes status, history of previous transplantation, and duration on dialysis. Those patients in the top 20th percentile will receive kidneys with a KDPI score of <20%. This is longevity matching so providing kidney allografts expected to survive posttransplant for a longer time with individuals expected to live longer. There is concern this will bias against older recipients (15).

TRANSPLANT OUTCOMES

In deceased donor transplantation, the 1-year allograft survival rates have gradually improved over the last decade and have reached 92% recently. This is not dramatically different from the 96.6% 1-year graft survival for all living donor transplants (13). The truly important differences between deceased donor renal transplantation and living donor renal transplantation emerge with the examination of the long-term graft survival rates. With deceased donor renal transplantation, there is a substantial fall in graft survival over time. By 5 years, deceased donor allograft survival has decreased to 72.1%, whereas living donor transplant graft survival remains at 84% (13). The results of renal transplantation using kidneys from living unrelated donors such as spouses are similar to those results obtained with living-related donors. With both deceased donor and living donor transplantation, there is a significant effect of HLA matching on allograft survival, particularly in long-term graft survival (**TABLE 41.1**). Five-year allograft survival of a zero-mismatched HLA deceased donor organ is 75%, whereas a six-antigen mismatched deceased donor organ has a 5-year survival of 66% (8). This can be contrasted with a two haplotype matched or

(zero antigen mismatch) living donor transplant that has a 5-year survival of 84% (8). In addition to the benefits of living donor renal transplantation on allograft survival, there is a substantial benefit on patient survival as well. Patients who received deceased donor transplants in the last decade had a 10-year survival of 62.4%. This is in contrast to a 78% 10-year patient survival for recipients of living donor transplants (13). The benefits of living donor transplantation for dialysis patients can perhaps best be appreciated by noting that the outcome for both patient and allograft survival with any category of living donor transplant is superior to even well-matched deceased donor transplantation. In addition, patients able to undergo living donor transplantation can have this procedure scheduled on an elective basis and are able to avoid a prolonged period on the transplant waiting lists.

Historically, the increasing size of the wait list and wait times led to the use of the previously mentioned expanded criteria donor kidneys. Elderly patients receiving these expanded criteria organs have been shown to have improved survival compared with patients who remain on the transplant waiting list (16). These transplants do, however, have a shortened allograft survival compared with kidneys obtained from standard criteria donors.

COMBINED KIDNEY TRANSPLANT PROCEDURES

The kidney transplantation can be combined with other organs, heart, lung, liver, pancreas, and bone marrow. An extensive review of all the combined organ transplants is beyond the scope of this chapter and is reviewed elsewhere in the literature. However, we will focus on the combined pancreas and kidney transplant.

Combined kidney and pancreas transplantation for patients with ESKD and type 1 diabetes has been widely available over the past 15 years. Dialysis patients who have previously received a deceased donor or living donor kidney transplant are also potential candidates for a solitary pancreas transplant. The primary indications for pancreas transplant are type 1 diabetic or a type 2 diabetic with a progressive secondary diabetic complications or a brittle diabetic. The major benefits of kidney and pancreas transplantation are an improved quality of life, freedom from insulin therapy, the potential of avoiding additional secondary complications, and a normalization of fasting glucose with a decrease in the incidence of hypoglycemic episodes (17–19). The results of studies of secondary complications of diabetic patients undergoing pancreas transplantation are difficult to interpret in light of the fact that most of these patients have had diabetes for up to two decades. Successful pancreas transplantation is associated with normalization of serum insulin responses and a normalization of glycosylated hemoglobin. Glucose counterregulation associated with hypoglycemia improves after pancreas transplantation. The symptom recognition of hypoglycemia is restored, and dangerous episodes of hypoglycemia can be avoided. Diabetic neuropathy has been shown to be stabilized, and in some instances, autonomic and peripheral diabetic neuropathy improves (20). At present, there has been no clear benefit in halting the progression of the advanced diabetic retinopathy following pancreas transplantation. Recurrent diabetic nephropathy in the transplant kidney is prevented by pancreas transplantation and native kidney diabetic nephropathy may improve (21). In addition, some data suggest that combined kidney and pancreas transplantation may be associated with improved patient survival compared with diabetic patients who undergo kidney transplantation alone.

TABLE 41.1	**Five-Year Kidney Allograft Survival Related To Human Leukocyte Antigen Mismatch**	
Mismatch	**Cadaveric Donor Survival**	**Living Donor Survival**
0	72%	79%
1	69%	76%
3	65%	71%
6	59%	87%

Although the potential for significant improvement in outcome for diabetic patients with kidney disease exists, the combined kidney–pancreas transplantation procedure has an increased morbidity compared with kidney transplantation alone. Surgical complications are increased with a significant incidence of wound problems, intra-abdominal infections, recurrent urinary tract infections, and primary technical failure of the pancreas allograft. In addition, successful kidney and pancreas transplantation requires a more aggressive antirejection immunosuppression strategy and results in the increased risk of infection associated with this procedure (22,23). The decision to undergo kidney and pancreas transplantation is perhaps best made by the patient in conjunction with the patient's nephrologist in consultation with a transplant center experienced in pancreas transplantation.

MEDICAL EVALUATION OF THE PATIENT WITH END-STAGE KIDNEY DISEASE

Organ transplantation improves the duration of life for the patient with ESKD (5). This result is in part due to the selection process of healthier individuals but is also related to other issues such as progression of atherosclerotic cardiovascular disease (5). However, in the perioperative period, the relative risk of death is greater in the transplant recipient compared with the same patient remaining on dialysis. Only at the point of 3 to 4 months posttransplantation does the relative risk of death equalize between the patients remaining on dialysis and those receiving a kidney transplant. It is for this reason that a very thorough medical evaluation of each patient must be performed pretransplant to ensure that the recipient is medically and nutritionally stable to undergo the rigors of an elective surgical procedure and be capable of tolerating not only the medications but also various treatments during the posttransplantation course (Table 41.2).

The leading causes of death posttransplantation are cardiovascular (24,25). Hence, management strategies for patients with incipient or existing cardiovascular disease remain most important. In addition, issues relating to lung disease, malignancy, preexisting viral infections, and risk for recurrent kidney disease also play an important role in stratifying the risk among candidates and may require specific therapy before transplantation and may influence the strategy for donor selection and even immunosuppression.

Cardiovascular Disease

Cardiovascular disease is the leading cause of death and graft loss after renal transplantation (26). Almost half of deaths with graft function that occur within 30 days of transplantation are due to cardiovascular disease, primarily myocardial infarction (27). Risk stratification before transplantation is critical to avoid perioperative mortality and minimize the risk for long-term morbidity and mortality (28,29). The presence or absence and the extent of

cardiovascular disease may also play a role in the decision whether to undergo elective transplantation.

Although there is a large body of literature evaluating cardiovascular risk of nontransplant populations having elective surgery (30), there is limited study of transplant populations despite the fact that they have a substantial increased risk for cardiovascular disease (24,25).

The surgical risk of patients undergoing kidney transplantation is considered intermediate (1% to 5%) (31). All patients' evaluation should start with detailed history, careful physical examination, electrocardiogram (ECG), and chest radiograph.

In 2012, the American Heart Association (AHA) and the American College of Cardiology (ACC) Foundation published their recommendations for evaluation and management for kidney transplant candidates. In addition to ECG, patients with three or more coronary artery risk factors (Table 41.3) with no active cardiac disease should be considered for noninvasive stress testing (32). The most recent European Renal Best Practice (ERBP) (33) Guidelines on the Management and Evaluation of the Kidney Donor and Recipient published in 2013 recommended performing a standard exercise tolerance test and cardiac ultrasound in asymptomatic high risk patients.

However, to this date, the optimal noninvasive test remains unclear (5).

Most of the available data on the effectiveness of noninvasive screening techniques come from studies examining either dipyridamole, thallium, or sestamibi scintigraphy (34,35), or dobutamine echocardiography (36,37). Myocardial perfusion determination with stress single photon emission computed tomographic (SPECT) imaging has proved to be helpful. If negative, 97% of patients are cardiovascular event-free with 42 months follow-up (38). Although most of the available data with these screening techniques have been in patients without ESKD, some well-defined studies have looked at patients being screened for transplantation (34–37).

Dobutamine stress echocardiography and thallium myocardial perfusion scan both have moderate sensitivity and specificity among kidney transplant candidates (32) and might even have lower accuracy for coronary artery disease (CAD) detection in dialysis patients compared to the general population (39). One systematic review suggested that dobutamine stress echocardiography is superior to myocardial perfusion scintigraphy in detecting CAD in patients who are potential kidney transplant recipients (40). In the non-ESKD population, some investigators have suggested that dobutamine echocardiography was more specific for detecting CAD than dipyridamole sestamibi scanning, whereas the sensitivities of the two tests were very similar (41). However, direct comparisons between these two screening modalities in patients with ESKD are lacking.

TABLE 41.2	Contraindications to Transplantation

Active infection
Recent or current malignancy
Severe uncorrectable nonrenal disease
Active substance abuse
Severe psychiatric illness
Pregnancy

TABLE 41.3	Coronary Artery Disease Risk Factors

Diabetes mellitus
Prior cardiovascular disease
More than 1 year on dialysis
Left ventricular hypertrophy
Age more than 60 years
Smoking
Hypertension
Dyslipidemia

Echocardiography by itself is considered a reasonable test for assessing the left ventricular function in kidney transplant candidates (32). However, hemodialysis patients undergo regular hemodynamic changes that also may affect echocardiographic findings (42). Myocardial contrast echocardiography (MCE) was recently identified as a safe and uncomplicated bedside technique with good accuracy for ruling out the presence of a significant coronary artery stenosis in patients with ESKD. MCE may help along with other methods to select candidates for coronary revascularization ESKD patients (43,44).

CT scan is also not recommended for the diagnosis of CAD in dialysis patients because the correlation between coronary calcification and luminal diameter in dialysis patients is less certain than in the general population, since vascular calcification in this population is often the result of medial calcification rather than atherosclerosis (45). Stress cardiac magnetic resonance imaging (MRI) was established as valuable tool for the diagnosis and management of ischemic heart disease (46); however, experience with cardiac MRI in dialysis patients is very limited. In summary, all of these noninvasive tests are less than perfect in predicting angiographically documented coronary disease or cardiovascular events. Many still support coronary angiography as the gold standard (47).

Now, with the median waiting time for a kidney transplant is more than 3 years and can even be several years for some patients, the question of the need to repeat cardiac testing done at the time of listing or the frequency of performing such tests becomes vital. Again, to this date, there are no clear guidelines exit and most centers have their own protocols. The AHA and the ACC Foundation suggest that the usefulness of periodically screening asymptomatic kidney transplantation candidates for myocardial ischemia while on the transplant waiting list to reduce the risk of major adverse cardiac events is uncertain (32). However, an annual ECG is reasonable in all patients waiting for a transplant, and for ESKD patients with moderate aortic stenosis, an annual echocardiogram is also reasonable (32).

National Kidney Foundation Kidney Disease Outcomes Quality Initiative (NKF/KDOQI) guidelines from 2005 for CAD in dialysis patients recommend for kidney transplantation candidates with normal cardiac stress testing at listing, an annual testing in those with diabetes mellitus or known CAD, testing every 2 years in those classified as "high risk," and testing every 3 years in others (48) (Table 41.4). For the optimal cardiac testing method, NKF/KDOQI recommend exercise or pharmacologic stress echocardiographic or nuclear imaging tests (48).

So far, we reviewed the recommendations for initial cardiac testing and follow-up while on the waiting list. As for intervention, the AHA and the ACC Foundation recommend cardiology referral for patients with angina, patients with ejection fraction (EF) less than 50%, patients with ischemic left ventricular dilatation, and patients with established exercise-induced hypotension (Table 41.4). Patients who appear to have critical lesions should undergo revascularization or angioplasty, stenting, and so forth before transplantation. One study demonstrated that patients randomized to revascularization before transplantation had fewer posttransplant cardiovascular disease events compared with patients managed medically (49). These findings suggest that, in particular, diabetic patients and those with high risk for severe CAD should undergo elective revascularization before rather than after renal transplantation. However, this study was small and, therefore, cannot be generally extrapolated to the whole ESKD population group in large part

TABLE 41.4 Summary of Suggested Cardiac Evaluation for Kidney Transplant Candidates

Test	At the Time of Listing	Frequency While on the Waiting List
ECG	All patients	Annual
CXR	All patients	N/A
Noninvasive stress test	Patients with three or more coronary artery risk factors[a]	• Annual for DM, known CAD • Every 2 years for high risk patients • Every 3 years for all other patient
Cardiology referral for percutaneous angiography	Patients with: • Angina • Ejection fraction less than 50% • Ischemic left ventricular dilatation • Established exercise induced hypotension	

ECG, electrocardiogram; CXR, chest x-ray; DM, diabetes mellitus; CAD, coronary artery disease.
[a]Refer to **Table 41.3**.

because morbidity and mortality are increased in dialysis patients who undergo coronary artery bypass surgery compared with non-ESKD patients (50). The decision to perform coronary revascularization before transplantation should be considered in patients who meet the criteria for general population. In some asymptomatic transplant candidates, the risk of coronary revascularization may outweigh the risk of transplantation. These risks must be weighed by the multidisciplinary transplantation team on a case-by-case basis (32). For the choice of the optimal method for coronary revascularization in patients awaiting kidney transplant, coronary artery bypass grafting (CABG) appears to be superior to percutaneous coronary intervention (PCI) in diabetic candidates with multivessel CAD (51).

Perioperatively, patients already taking β-adrenergic blockers before renal transplantation should continue the medication perioperatively and postoperatively. For patients not on β-blockers but who have high cardiac risk (Table 41.3), it should be considered for initiating β-blockers preoperatively and to be continued postoperatively if no contraindication exists.

In regard to antiplatelets therapy, aspirin therapy should be continued indefinitely after renal transplantation in patients with known CAD, following the same ACC/AHA guidelines for general population with CAD.

Congestive heart failure is an important clinical consideration as part of the kidney transplant evaluation. Fifty percent of hemodialysis patients have a history of volume overload at some point during their clinical course during dialysis (52), and as many as 20% may have decreased systolic function on echocardiogram (53). However, it is important to note that many patients have left ventricular hypertrophy and diastolic dysfunction with impaired lusitropy. This interferes with ventricular filling during diastole and can ultimately lead to output failure. The rationale for treatment is entirely different depending on ventricular function. Those with systolic heart failure will require preload and afterload reduction, whereas those with diastolic dysfunction will need antihypertensive agents, especially those that slow heart rate and facilitate ventricular relaxation (53). There are no overt contraindications to transplantation in patients with left ventricular hypertrophy or ventricular dysfunction unless the EF is less than 20%. An analysis by Wali et al. (54) indicated that one important factor that reduced the likelihood of improvement in ventricular function posttransplantation was increasing time on dialysis. Consequently, an echocardiogram is an important part of the evaluation. On a positive note, renal transplantation improves ventricular function in most patients with EFs in the 20% to 40% range (54,55).

Reversible causes of myocardial dysfunction should also be identified and treated. Problems related to alcohol abuse, anemia, and hypertension need to be considered. Reversible ischemia also may impair ventricular function.

Cerebral vascular disease is also an important consideration that must be considered as part of the pretransplant evaluation. The increasing age and prevalence of hypertension and diabetes as a cause of ESKD with the associated macrovascular disease increases the likelihood of cerebral vascular disease. Patients with audible bruits or prior histories of transient ischemic attack (TIA) or stroke should have carotid artery Dopplers and consideration for carotid endarterectomy if significant disease is noted. Data from studies in the general population indicate that prophylactic surgery may be effective in selected patients, especially in those with a surgical risk of less than 3% and a greater than 60% diameter reduction on ultrasound or in those patients whose surgical risk is slightly higher, but have more substantial stenoses in the presence of contralateral internal carotid artery stenosis of greater than 75% (56). In addition, whether patients with cerebral vascular disease are symptomatic or not, aspirin prophylaxis should be considered, although there are no data on transplant patients to support its use. In the presence of chronic atrial fibrillation, anticoagulation should be considered for guideline as in the general population (57).

Patients with polycystic kidney disease as a cause of ESKD with a family history of intracranial aneurysms or with a previous episode of intracranial bleeding should undergo computed tomography (CT) scan or MRI to evaluate the presence of intracranial aneurysm (58). Those aneurysms greater than 10 mm should be considered for prophylactic surgical removal to prevent bleeding (59).

Peripheral vascular disease is common in patients with ESKD (60). Its presence may help identify patients who need more careful evaluation of potential CAD or cerebral vascular disease. Because the renal transplant is connected to the iliac vessels, it is important to know the status of vasculature. Disruption of compromised iliac flow with a kidney transplant could render more distal vascular beds to impair blood supply. Some patients may require reconstructive surgery of aortoiliac disease before or at the time of renal transplantation. Consequently, in high-risk patients, lower extremity noninvasive testing should be considered followed by angiography if there is any question concerning the adequacy of the circulation.

In summary, atherosclerotic cardiovascular disease involving the heart, brain, and peripheral vasculature is one of the most important aspects of the pretransplant evaluation. Careful evaluation of all risk factors, adequacy of treatment, and provision of optimal medical management is necessary. In addition, preoperative evaluation of all possible areas of vascular compromise should be rigorously pursued and surgically corrected if indicated.

Cancer

In the past decade, malignancy has become one of the three major causes of death after transplantation. Malignancies are responsible for 1% to 4% of all deaths in the dialysis population and 9% to 12% of deaths in the renal transplant population (61). Kidney transplant recipients have a 3- to 12-fold increased risk of developing nonlymphoid or solid organ cancers when compared to the general population (62). Consequently, careful pretransplant screening is important to rule out preexisting malignancy prior to transplant. The most important cancers to screen for pretransplant are those that occur with greater frequency in the general population including cancers of the lung, prostate, breast, and cervix, which will be discussed later in greater detail (63). What is not known is whether pretransplant screening may have a benefit in reducing the incidence of posttransplant malignancies. The recommendations for cancer screening in the posttransplant period are mostly extrapolated from the general populations and are consistent with screening guidelines in the general population, with the exception of cervical, skin, colorectal, and renal cancers (64).

Patients with prior episodes of cancer have a waiting period before transplantation because most forms of immunosuppression will likely inhibit surveillance mechanisms that would otherwise counteract the development of a malignancy (**TABLE 41.5**). The Cincinnati Transplant Tumor Registry indicates that 54% of recurrences occur in patients who underwent transplantation within 2 years of treatment, whereas 33% of recurrences occurred in patients 2 to 5 years before transplantation (63). Only 13% of recurrences occurred in patients treated more than 5 years before transplantation. These statistics provide some general consideration in terms of the duration of wait between the time of treatment for cancer and transplantation. Other reports also provide some suggestions (65).

Lung cancer is the leading cause of cancer deaths (66). Screening chest x-ray film and a possible low-dose CT of the lung may be appropriate in high-risk patients with a family history who are smokers. Preferably, every patient who smokes should be made to stop before transplantation.

The overall age of male transplant recipients has risen, and it is important to consider yearly evaluation of prostate-specific antigen (PSA) and digital rectal examination before transplantation,

TABLE 41.5	Recommended Tumor-Free Intervals before Transplantation	

Malignancy	Time
Basal cell	None
In situ cervical	None
In situ bladder	None
Clark's level 1 melanoma	None
Duke's A colon	None
In situ lobular breast	None
Prostate	2 y
Uterine	2 y
Lymphoma	2 y
Breast	2–5 y
Invasive cervical	2–5 y
Colorectal	2–5 y

particularly for those older than 50 years (67). This may also be even more important in the African American population in which there is a higher incidence of prostate cancer (68). If identified, it should be treated before transplantation. In the Cincinnati Transplant Tumor Registry, 40% of prostate cancer recurrences occurred within 2 years of treatment (69). However, it should be noted that the death rate associated with remaining on dialysis is often higher than death due to prostate cancer. Some investigators have developed a nomogram, based on PSA, to evaluate this risk (70), so that one can decide on an appropriate time period to delay transplantation.

The overall incidence of cervical cancers in women who received a kidney transplant is at least 2 to 3 times greater than the age- and gender-matched population. For women, a pelvic examination with cervical evaluation and manual examination of the uterus should be part of every workup and should be continued on an annual basis while on the waiting list of a transplant. In regard to human papillomavirus (HPV), studies are currently underway to determine the efficacy of HPV vaccination in women with advanced stage chronic kidney disease (CKD) and ESKD (71).

Cancer of the breast is the most common form of *in situ* cancer in female patients with ESKD after nonmelanoma skin cancer and cancer of the uterine cervix (72). Interestingly, renal transplant recipients appear to have a lower relative risk of breast cancer than the general population. The explanation for this may be due to improved screening or previously unidentified effects of the immunosuppression (73). Factors associated with an increased risk of recurrence posttransplantation include prior nodal involvement, bilateral disease, inflammatory carcinoma, and prior bone metastases (63). Most clinicians would recommend a waiting period of 2 years after treatment and preferably longer (5 years) for most patients given the fact that the recurrence rate may be as high as 23% and mortality associated with it is substantial (63). Biennial mammographic screening for breast cancer is standard practice in the general population. (64). Kidney Disease: Improving Global Outcomes (KDIGO) workgroup did not make a recommendation for or against mammographic screening. However, the European Best Practice Guidelines Expert Group recommended following the guidelines established for the general population (71).

Renal cell cancer is more common in the population with ESKD than in the general population, particularly in younger patients and those with ESKD from toxic, infectious, or obstructive uropathies (74). In addition, uroepithelial malignancies need to be screened for if there is any evidence of abnormalities in urinary sediment. High-risk patients may deserve an abdominal CT scan as part of their pretransplant workup.

Cutaneous malignancy is the most common form of cancer posttransplantation, particularly squamous cell carcinoma (63). Renal transplant patients have a 60- to 250-fold increased risk of developing a nonmelanoma skin cancer, which includes squamous cell carcinoma, basal cell carcinoma, Kaposi's sarcoma, Merkel cell carcinoma, and adnexal tumors (75). There is a high recurrent rate of nonmelanoma skin cancers that occur over time after renal transplantation despite timely removal of lesions. However, this is rarely a cause of death.

Although the incidence of colorectal cancer in dialysis patients is not increased compared with the general population (76), it remains a common cancer; therefore, screening colonoscopy should be considered in all patients older than 50 years, as would be standard for the general population (72). Kidney transplant recipients

appear to have a risk for colorectal cancer comparable to those in the general population 10 to 20 years older, so consideration can be given to routine screening starting at age 40 or 5 years after transplantation (77). Patients with previously treated colon cancer should wait at least 5 years before renal transplantation because the recurrence rate diminishes with time, and mortality from recurrent colon cancer after renal transplantation is very high (63).

Lymphoproliferative disorders are more common in patients with ESKD than the general population (74) and may be substantially higher in renal transplant patients if they are exposed to the Epstein-Barr virus (EBV) *de novo* in the posttransplantation period (78). There is a question as to whether or not prophylactic treatment with acyclovir would be capable of suppressing EBV infection and the likelihood of EBV-associated posttransplantation lymphoproliferative disease (79,80). To date, published reports supporting the potential efficacy of antiviral agents have been retrospective and have been limited by the use of either historical or no specific controls (81). In general, complete medical history and physical examination coupled with standard laboratory screening and judicious use of imaging techniques in higher risk patients should be considered as part of the standard workup. Individual determination of time to wait posttreatment of cancer before transplantation should be made on a case-by-case basis. In general, waiting at least 5 years is preferred for most previously treated cancers.

Pulmonary Disease

Anticipating respiratory complications posttransplantation in the patient with ESKD is no different than would be seen for patients without ESKD facing elective surgery. The primary focus should be elimination of smoking and evaluation of pulmonary function if there is a history of chronic obstructive pulmonary disease or other forms of lung disease that interferes with oxygenation. All patients should be screened with a careful history and physical examination and a chest x-ray film. As mentioned previously, specific focus should be addressed on the smoker because studies in the general population indicate that smokers were 5.5 times more likely to develop pulmonary complications postsurgery compared with those who did not smoke (82).

Endocrine Disease

The endocrine evaluation of a dialysis patient should primarily focus on issues surrounding diabetes, obesity, and ESKD-related bone disease. Diabetes is the leading cause of ESKD, so the proportion of patients on dialysis awaiting a transplant with diabetes is substantial. Patients with diabetes, which is most commonly type 2, have advanced risk for atherosclerotic cardiovascular disease and death (83). Consequently, all diabetic patients need careful focus on evaluation of vascular beds pretransplantation. Retinopathy, neuropathy, autonomic dysfunction, and associated complications from diabetes persist and/or progress during dialytic therapy. Despite greater likelihood of progression of complications of the diabetes posttransplantation, survival is demonstrably improved for diabetic patients with renal transplantation compared with remaining on dialysis (5).

Pancreas transplantation as discussed earlier may also be an appropriate strategy for a patient with type 1 diabetes who requires renal replacement therapy (84). With improving techniques and immunosuppression, pancreas transplantation has become an accepted therapy for patients with type 1 diabetes with patient survival rates exceeding 90% and rates of insulin independence of more than 80% at 1 year (85–87).

In the ESKD population, a higher body mass index (BMI) is associated with a reduced mortality among dialysis patients (88–90). The average cutoff for BMI for a potential transplant recipient at most transplant centers is 30 to 40. Obesity is associated with increased morbidity and mortality posttransplantation (91). Obese patients have higher rates of delayed graft function, suffer from more surgical complications and wound infections, and will frequently require prolonged hospitalization (88,92,93). Some investigators even suggest obesity is associated with increased graft failure (89), although others disagree (92). Posttransplant diabetes mellitus is more common in obese patients, and some transplant centers even suggest that increased risk of acute rejection and graft loss occurs in obese patients (91,94). In regard to weight loss prior to transplantation, transplant centers generally recommend weight loss through lifestyle and dietary changes. It is important to note that BMI should not only be looked at alone but also the overall body habitus of the patient should be taken into consideration. If a patient does not have central obesity or has a high muscle mass with a high BMI, they might not necessarily need weight loss prior to listing (95). In regard to mode of dialysis and obesity, peritoneal dialysis has not been shown to lead to greater weight gain or limit the opportunity for transplantation compared to patients on hemodialysis (96). Bariatric surgery is not routinely recommended but should be considered on a case-by-case basis particularly with recent advancements in surgical technique (95).

Pretransplant planning for the treatment of metabolic bone disease is important because preemptive strategies may prevent the development of pathologic fractures (97). However, a meta-analysis of clinical trials indicated that vitamin D and bisphosphonate therapy helps bone mineral density but did not reveal evidence of reduction in fractures (98). Patients with ESKD can suffer from high-turnover bone disease because of secondary hyperparathyroidism, low-turnover bone disease resulting from osteomalacia, or variance of both (99,100). Patients may also have dialysis-related amyloid bone disease. Renal transplantation is an effective treatment for most causes of low-turnover bone disease and for dialysis-related amyloid bone disease. However, persistence of hyperparathyroidism after successful renal transplantation is common (101). Therefore, parathyroid hormone (PTH) levels should be checked pretransplant and posttransplantation, and surgical removal may be necessary. However, since the advent of cinacalcet therapy (102), the need for parathyroidectomy has become less common.

Gastrointestinal Disease

The primary gastrointestinal issues in the patient with ESKD revolve around the presence or absence of diverticulosis or diverticulitis or other forms of colonic disease; peptic ulcer disease; gallbladder disease; or chronic liver disease, usually resulting from major hepatitis viruses or gallbladder disease.

Colon disease resulting from diverticulosis or diverticulitis is not uncommon in the patient with ESKD; in many cases, it is due to sedentary lifestyle and the medications predisposing to constipation (103). Although posttransplantation colonic perforation is a morbid and mortal consequence (104), it is unknown how to best diagnose and treat it preemptively. Patients with severe diverticulosis may require partial colectomy pretransplant. However, there is no accepted standard in terms of how to approach this problem. Patients with polycystic kidney disease have an even greater risk for colonic perforation posttransplantation, as high as 5%, which is substantially more than the 0.5% to 2% that is seen in patients with

ESKD receiving renal transplantation, resulting from nonacquired polycystic kidney disease (non-APKD) (105).

Peptic ulcer disease can be a serious complication posttransplantation (106,107). The perioperative use of corticosteroids and infections such as herpes virus, cytomegalovirus (CMV), or Candida markedly increase the risk for gastritis and gastrointestinal hemorrhage. Prior history of peptic ulcer disease should prompt physicians to perform upper gastrointestinal endoscopy and fecal occult blood testing. During endoscopy, screening for *Helicobacter pylori* should be planned (108). With the advent of proton pump inhibitors, the risk of serious complications of gastrointestinal hemorrhage posttransplantation has markedly improved (109). Patients with a history of peptic ulcer disease have a threefold greater incidence of ulceration posttransplantation compared with those patients without a history of peptic ulcer disease (107). However, progressive screening and proton pump inhibitor use largely mitigates this risk.

All patients should have pretransplant screening for gallstones. If evident, the patient should have an elective cholecystectomy pretransplant since there is an increased risk of posttransplant complications, including cholangitis.

Liver disease is a significant cause of late morbidity and mortality among renal transplant recipients (110). In fact, death from liver failure has been reported in anywhere from 8% to 28% of renal transplant recipients (111). Chronic posttransplant liver disease is usually related to viral hepatitis, primarily hepatitis B virus (HBV) and hepatitis C virus (HCV). Serum transaminases should be routinely followed pretransplantation, and if persistently abnormal, a liver biopsy should be obtained. The primary use of the liver biopsy is to screen for cirrhosis and active hepatitis. Renal transplant recipients should be routinely screened for HBV surface antigen and HCV. Patients who are HBV surface antigen positive will also have circulating HBV antigen or serologic evidence of acute viral replication (HBV DNA) and are at increased risk of progressive liver disease posttransplantation compared to seronegative patients (112,113). All patients who are HBV surface antigen negative should receive the recombinant HBV vaccine. Although chronic dosing of lamivudine may help control viral replication in these patients, drug resistance likely limits the long-term effectiveness of this therapy (114,115).

Current guidelines recommend the use of nucleoside analogs (NA) in HBV surface antigen–positive patients preemptively before immunosuppressive therapy, regardless of baseline HBV DNA levels and for 12 months after its cessation. Lamivudine can be used only in patients with low HBV DNA (<2,000 IU/mL) and when a finite and short duration of immunosuppression is scheduled; otherwise, the candidates should be treated with a newer generation NA (116).

HCV-related liver disease is a substantial problem for hemodialysis patients because of its frequency and increased risk of death and graft failure compared to seronegative patients (117–119). Roughly 10% to 20% of hemodialysis patients are positive for HCV. Up to 50% of the cases of liver disease posttransplantation can be attributed to HCV infection (117,118). All transplant candidates should be screened for anti-HCV radioimmunoassay with confirmation testing by radioimmunoblot assay (RIBA). If positive, serum should be tested for HCV RNA to confirm current HCV infection. Serum transaminases can be followed, but a liver biopsy should be strongly considered. Patients with cirrhosis on liver biopsy should, in most instances, remain on dialysis because of an unacceptable increased risk for progressive liver failure posttransplantation (120). One exception is patients with cirrhosis but with a hepatic portal venous gradient below 10, a kidney transplant alone in this situation may be safely performed (121). Without evidence of cirrhosis, the presence of HCV antibody *per se* should not be a contraindication to transplantation because survival after transplantation is markedly higher than that of HCV patients who remain on chronic HD (122). Patients who are HCV RNA positive may benefit from a course of interferon-α before transplantation (123–126). Ribavirin is contraindicated in the setting of late-stage kidney disease. Thus, it would be preferable for ESKD and kidney transplant patients to have an interferon/ribavirin-free regimen. This is possible with the advent of direct-acting antivirals (DAAs). These drugs are more tolerable and avoid many of the side effects and drug interactions as compared to interferon/ribavirin. However, there presently is no recommended dosage for patients with an eGFR <30 mL/min, ideally an ESKD patient would be transplanted and would have enough renal function to dose DAA. The management of both hepatitis B and C should be done in conjunction with a hepatologist (127). This is also potentially useful to expedite a hepatitis C positive patient's transplant as they can accept a hepatitis C positive kidney and then be treated afterward.

The goal of pretransplantation treatment is to decrease the risk of progressive liver disease and prevent the development of posttransplant HCV-associated renal disease (126). Interestingly, HCV is also associated with an increased incidence of glomerulonephritis and diabetes posttransplantation (128).

The role of immunosuppression on the progression of fibrosis in cases of HCV infection is uncertain in kidney transplant recipients. Actually, there is some evidence that cyclosporine inhibits the replication of HCV *in vitro* (129). It has been routine over the last decade to give HCV-positive transplant candidates HCV-positive donor kidneys (130). Most reported experiences do not suggest that there is any increased risk of progressive liver disease to the recipient in the short term (131). However, long-term observation will ultimately be necessary to demonstrate the safety of this practice. It is important to note that waiting times on the transplantation list are reduced if HCV-positive kidneys are used in HCV-infected recipients (131).

Infections

An important part of the pretransplant evaluation in the dialysis patient is to eliminate infection that may persist posttransplantation and that may become more difficult to treat or possibly become life threatening. A careful history and physical examination are important to identify possible sites of infection such as at the site of hemodialysis or peritoneal dialysis access. Peritoneal fluid should be cultured. A serologic evaluation of past viral exposures is important and may help in the design of proper posttransplantation prophylaxis treatment as well as guide decisions with regard to transplantation of a kidney from an infected donor. Transplant candidates should receive immunizations for known infections that are prevalent before transplantation, such as HBV and any childhood immunizations, that may have been missed. Seroscreening for CMV, EBV, and all the hepatitis viruses is routinely recommended. However, it is not possible to exclude possible infection with other unusual pathogens such as syphilis, strongyloidiasis, toxoplasma, or herpes. Seroscreening for HIV and tuberculin testing should also be routine.

CMV infection, until the development of effective anti-CMV drugs, was a morbid and mortal event that could occur in the transplant recipient. The incidence of CMV disease is generally less than 5% for recipients who do not have antibodies to CMV and who receive kidneys from donors who are antibody negative (132,133). However, the incidence of primary CMV disease among antibody-negative recipients of CMV-positive kidneys is high, on the order of 50% to 75% without specific and effective prophylactic regimens (132,133). This drops to 15% to 35% when using a prophylactic regimen (134). CMV disease in antibody-positive recipients receiving either positive or negative donor kidneys is approximately 25% to 40% (106,107). Therefore, this illness is frequent in the posttransplant patient and will require careful assessment of the amount of immunosuppression because this directly influences the incidence and severity of CMV disease.

A meta-analysis of controlled clinical trials demonstrated that specific antiviral agents (acyclovir or ganciclovir) were effective in preventing CMV infection in solid organ transplant recipients (135). However, it is important to note that this regimen is associated with side effects and can be expensive. Therefore, judicious and appropriate screening, pretransplantation can help identify those patients who will derive greatest benefit from the investment in prophylactic therapy. There is a concern that ganciclovir- and valganciclovir-resistant CMV strains can develop in patients receiving prophylaxis, which could undermine this therapeutic strategy (136).

Patients with ESKD are at greater risk for mycobacterial disease. This is frequently asymptomatic despite the fact that up to a third of patients with ESKD may be anergic. Purified protein derivative (PPD) testing is recommended so that isoniazid prophylaxis can be used, and performance of a chest x-ray examination can be helpful to rule out the likelihood of active infection. There is no evidence that prophylaxis with isoniazid reduces the incidence of reactivation of tuberculosis after transplantation (137). Despite this, many centers require pretransplant and/or posttransplant isoniazid prophylaxis for patients with a positive PPD skin test.

Peritoneal dialysis patients must be carefully screened for occult tunnel track or peritoneal fluid infections. In particular, *Staphylococcus epidermidis* may cause an occult peritonitis that can flourish once immunosuppression is started posttransplantation. Clinical studies indicate that patients on peritoneal dialysis more frequently develop infections within the first month posttransplantation compared with patients on hemodialysis. More often than not, these sites are located in the abdominal cavity, the surgical wound, or in the peritoneal fluid. Peritoneal dialysis patients with active infections should have transplantation delayed, if at all possible, if they have a history of active or recent peritonitis to ensure that proper therapy can be employed. Documentation of clearing of the infection is appropriate.

Careful evaluation of the dentition is appropriate pretransplantation in all dialysis patients. Periodontal infections and active periodontitis could worsen posttransplantation because of the use of immunosuppressive agents, particularly cyclosporine because it induces gingival hyperplasia (138). Although there are no controlled clinical trials demonstrating that treatment of periodontal disease reduces the likelihood of recurrence posttransplantation, it is appropriate to consider strategies to care for active disease processes before using medications that will stimulate gingival growth and could cover up underlying infectious processes.

Pulmonary infections posttransplantation are an important concern. Some studies suggest that renal transplant recipients develop pneumococcal infections at a rate of approximately 1% per year (139). Pneumococcal immunization is currently recommended for all chronic dialysis patients (140). It is particularly important for those who have been previously splenectomized. Annual immunization with influenza vaccine is also currently recommended for all chronic dialysis patients (140). However, there are no good studies to indicate that influenza is more severe when it occurs in an immunosuppressed transplant patient compared with a dialysis patient. Most childhood vaccinations should be employed pretransplantation, if they have never been received.

Patients who are HIV positive and have a strong desire for transplantation may be evaluated for transplantation. Data from several large prospective multicenter cohort studies have shown that solid organ transplantation in carefully selected HIV-infected individuals is safe (141). Newer approaches for immunosuppression have made transplantation feasible, and HIV is no longer an absolute contraindication for solid organ transplantation (142,143).

Genitourinary Disease

The patient with ESKD needs a careful examination of the genitourinary tract for a number of important reasons. There may be abnormalities in the drainage system that lead to the original renal dysfunction, such as bladder disease, stones, prostatic disease, or urethral strictures. These underlying abnormalities would need to be identified and corrected before the same urinary tract is used for drainage for the transplanted kidney. For this reason, a careful history and physical examination are needed. Routine recommendation for a voiding cystourethrogram (VCUG) should be considered in patients with a history of genitourinary abnormalities. Up to 25% of pretransplant VCUGs are abnormal in patients with ESKD (144). Most of the time, the abnormalities are minor and do not require surgical correction. Among younger individuals, the likelihood of congenital abnormalities is greater, whereas in older individuals, prostatic hypertrophy either from benign growth or from malignancy is a possibility. In addition, bladder cancer is 1.4 to 4.8 times more common in dialysis patients than in the general population (74). Therefore, any abnormalities on urinalysis should be carefully followed up with either a VCUG or cystoscopy. Urine cytology may also be helpful.

A neurogenic bladder is also an important problem that should be identified pretransplant. Although there are many causes, the most common are due to neurogenic issues usually related to diabetes. Patients may require intermittent catheterization or urinary diversion. In addition, patients with small bladders may need a bladder augmentation procedure or bladder stretching.

Patients with a history of urinary tract infections or stones need careful evaluation to ensure that there are no structural abnormalities that could predispose them to recurrence of these infections posttransplantation. Patients with bladder diverticula, large stones, or infected cysts, such as patients with polycystic kidney disease, may benefit from either unilateral or bilateral nephrectomy to reduce the likelihood of recurrent infection.

Other causes for a nephrectomy could include the identification of a renal cell carcinoma on ultrasound, oversized kidneys resulting from polycystic kidney disease that could impair placement of a new allograft, or possibly an inability to control blood pressure.

Recurrent Kidney Disease

It is important to identify the cause of ESKD in patients being evaluated for a kidney transplant. Almost all causes of kidney disease can recur in the kidney transplant with few exceptions such as polycystic kidney disease, Alport's syndrome, or toxic nephropathies

resulting from drug ingestion. The risk of recurrence for certain kidney diseases can be substantial and possibly lead to graft loss. In those patients who do have recurrent kidney disease, the risk of graft failure is 1.9 times higher than for patients without recurrent disease (145). In large part, the physician's assessment of the risk of recurrence is difficult because many patients progress to ESKD without proper identification of the cause. In addition, the incidence of recurrent disease may depend on the length of follow-up, and sometimes the ability to diagnose recurrent disease from chronic allograft nephropathy may be difficult. Registry data are being collected to provide a timely understanding about their risk (146).

Recurrent glomerulonephritis is most commonly seen with focal segmental glomerulosclerosis (FSGS), immunoglobulin A (IgA) nephropathy, and membranoproliferative glomerulonephritis (MPGN). Other glomerulonephritides such as membranous glomerulonephritis, Wegener's granulomatosis, and hemolytic uremic syndrome (HUS) can also recur (TABLE 41.6) (117).

FSGS recurs in 30% of patients, and, of those that do recur, 40% to 50% will lose their grafts (147,148). Those patients with rapid progression to original ESKD with FSGS are at greatest risk. African Americans and patients with younger age at onset of disease are more likely to have recurrence (149). The strongest predictor, however, is recurrence in a previous transplant. Podocyte effacement is the primary pathologic manifestation of FSGS posttransplant (150). Recently, lots of effort have been put into identifying a factor that is implicated in the pathogenesis of native and recurrent FSGS. FSGS is not viewed as a contraindication to renal transplantation because it is a heterogeneous disease process, and it is impossible to predict who would not be an ideal candidate.

IgA nephropathy can also recur frequently (20% to 40%) (151). Although graft failure can occur in 6% to 33% of patients with recurrent disease (152), a shorter interval between onset and the development of ESKD with IgA nephropathy appears to correlate with the likelihood of recurrence (152). It is also more common to recur in recipients of living related transplants. However, donor source has not affected graft survival in patients with ESKD who

TABLE 41.6	**Recurrence of Glomerulonephritis after Renal Transplantation**	
Disease	**Histologic Recurrence (%)**	**Graft Loss with Recurrence (%)**
Focal segmental glomerulosclerosis	20–40	40–50
IgA nephropathy	20–40	6–33
Membranoproliferative		
Type I	20–30	30–40
Type II	80–90	10–20
Membranous nephropathy	10–20	0–50
Anti-GBM nephritis	10–25	Rare
Henoch-Schönlein purpura	15–35	Rare
Hemolytic uremic syndrome	10–25	10–40
Lupus nephritis	Rare	Rare

IgA, immunoglobulin A; GBM, glomerular basement membrane.

underwent transplantation resulting from IgA nephropathy. Graft loss because of recurrent IgA nephropathy is not a contraindication for retransplantation because good long-term graft survival is observed after repeat renal transplantation.

Henoch-Schönlein purpura recurs in 15% to 35% of patients but rarely causes graft failure (153). It usually recurs in individuals with disease that has been recently active. However, occasionally, it can recur in patients who have had no evidence of disease for several years. Most data suggest that a shorter duration of original disease makes recurrence more likely (153). However, only 11% of graft failure can be attributed to recurrent disease despite the fact that histologic evidence of recurrence is common (153).

Patients with MPGN have recurrence rates of 20% to 30% (154). Graft loss may be seen in 40% of patients (154). In patients with type 2 MPGN, the risk of recurrence is approximately 80%; however, graft loss is less common than in type 1 MPGN occurring in approximately 10% to 20% of patients with recurrence (154). It is important to differentiate these idiopathic forms of MPGN from that which occurs secondary to HCV infection. It is also important to differentiate MPGN from chronic rejection by careful histologic evaluation, including immunofluorescence and electron microscopy.

Less common glomerulonephritides include membranous glomerulonephritis, which occurs in 10% to 20% of patients (155). Graft loss may be as high as 50% if patients are followed up for more than 10 years (155). There are no readily identifiable risk factors to determine the likelihood of recurrence.

HUS can recur in 10% to 25% of patients. However, it can be primary (without obvious cause) or secondary (related to the use of calcineurin inhibitors such as cyclosporine or tacrolimus) (156). It has even been reported with the use of antilymphocyte globulin and OKT3 monoclonal antibody (157,158). The older the age of onset of HUS, the shorter the interval for recurrent HUS posttransplantation and the shorter the interval between HUS onset and ESKD. The use of living donors should be contraindicated in these patients because it increases the risk for recurrence (155). The risk for graft failure is substantial. It may be as high as 50% (155). It is reported to be more than 5 times higher than for patients without posttransplant HUS. Strategies to provide necessary immunosuppression, particularly with the need for deceased donors in these patients, are important because most transplant centers would prefer not to use calcineurin inhibitors. Some centers have suggested that the use of prophylactic antiplatelet therapy may help reduce the chances of recurrence. However, there are no data to support this effort.

Antiglomerular basement membrane (anti-GBM) disease may recur in 10% to 25% of patients, although histologic recurrence may be seen in approximately 50% of patients. Anti-GBM antibodies should be documented as undetectable in the pretransplant workup to minimize the likelihood of recurrence.

Patients with ESKD resulting from Wegener's granulomatosis may also experience a recurrence rate as high as 15% to 50% (159). Data from small uncontrolled studies indicate that patients with recurrent disease can be successfully treated with cyclophosphamide (159). Most centers would recommend waiting until the disease is quiet before transplantation, although there are no data to indicate optimal timing of renal transplantation in patients with this disease process.

Patients with ESKD resulting from systemic lupus erythematosus (SLE) have a low risk of recurrence, perhaps less than 10% (160). However, a recent review indicates it is not rare (161). It is generally recommended that patients not have any evidence of clinical disease before transplantation. It is preferable that the serologic parameters such as complements and antinuclear anti-DNA antibody be normal or at least stable before transplantation. Recurrence that results in graft failure is unusual, and there does not appear to be any effect of prior SLE on patient or graft survival (160).

Unusual causes of ESKD such as oxalosis, cystinosis, Fabry's disease, and sickle cell disease can recur. Oxalosis is the most important with regard to its recurrence rate, and preferably, the patient should receive a simultaneous liver transplant at the time of the kidney transplant to reduce the likelihood that hyperoxalosis will destroy the transplanted graft.

Amyloidosis can recur in the kidney in approximately one-third of patients posttransplantation (162). If patients have severe multiorgan involvement with amyloidosis, transplantation should be generally discouraged because their survival is low. However, with primary injury to the kidneys, transplantation should not be precluded. More often than not, the outcome of transplantation appears to be determined by the severity of systemic disease affecting survival rather than recurrence in the allograft leading to graft dysfunction.

Because diabetes is the most common cause of ESKD, it is important to note that both type 1 and type 2 diabetes can recur within the transplanted kidney. For type 1 diabetes patients, this explains the rationale behind simultaneous pancreas and kidney transplantation. In the patients with type 2 diabetes, careful attention should be focused on blood pressure, cholesterol, and glycemic control. In addition, therapeutic strategies incorporating drugs that block the renin-angiotensin system should be used. Although no studies have indicated effects on graft survival using this approach, it has certainly been demonstrated to be effective in patients with type 2 diabetes and kidney disease without kidney transplantation.

Coagulopathies

Patients with a history of recurrent graft clotting on dialysis or deep vein thrombosis should have special attention focused on their clotting studies. Limited studies have attempted to determine the prevalence of coagulation abnormalities among kidney transplant candidates. Patients with SLE may have antiphospholipid antibodies, which may manifest as a lupus anticoagulant, and may have increased thrombotic risk (163). Other clotting abnormalities may also occur. Unfortunately, they may increase the risk for perioperative graft thrombosis. Consequently, a proactive approach is necessary to screen high-risk patients for coagulation abnormalities and to use prophylaxis to prevent clotting.

Psychosocial

A complete psychosocial evaluation should be performed on all prospective transplant recipients at the time of their initial evaluation. The importance of this evaluation is to be sure that there are not psychosocial barriers to transplantation or potential problems with compliance or chemical dependency that could interfere with the complicated medical regimen of posttransplantation. As part of the initial evaluation, the family and social support available to a candidate should be established. Transplant patients require frequent follow-up clinic visits, trips to the laboratory, hospital, and pharmacy. What mechanism does the patient have to get to and from clinic appointments and other locations? What will be the cost of travel to the patient? Does the patient drive, and if not, how will he or she get to and from clinic and local laboratory for blood draws?

Identification of those members of the patient's closest contacts who are willing to help the recipient over the long haul is essential. The magnitude of this commitment should not be underestimated, especially when patients are old and have multiple comorbid conditions. Patients may wait years for a deceased donor transplant, so the social support available to each candidate should be updated frequently, perhaps as often as their cardiac status is reviewed. An elderly type 2 diabetic patient who initially was counting on his or her spouse to assist posttransplant will require a much higher level of assistance from the posttransplant team if his or her significant other suffer a major change in health and is no longer available. A significant change in a patient's social support network should not remove him or her from the transplant waiting list; however, early awareness and contingencies need to be identified.

At the time of initial evaluation, an extensive review of a patient's employment history, finances, and insurance coverage should be undertaken. Transplant social workers are the best members of the health care team to assist each patient select what choices will be the best interest (164). According to the UNOS, the first-year billed charges for a kidney transplant are more than $262,000. Should a patient continue to work and maintain benefits or seek disability? Transplant social workers are uniquely positioned to perform biopsychosocial assessments of individual candidates and identify barriers that individual will face in returning to full employment after transplantation (165). The answer must be individualized for each patient and can best be considered with the help of an experienced transplant social worker.

Language and cultural barriers should be evaluated. If a patient does not speak English, who will accompany the recipient to clinic visits and be available to take phone instruction when the posttransplant team calls with medication changes? Optimal care requires a competent translator accompany the patient to every clinic visit.

Reversible medical causes of cognitive impairment could be identified with a dementia workup such as evaluating thyroid function and obtaining thiamin, vitamin B$_{12}$, and folate levels. In particular, alcohol and drug abuse must be identified and treated. Underreporting of individuals with substance abuse is common, as patients believe it will mean they will be denied transplantation. Substance abuse may lead to graft loss because of noncompliance (166,167), but if change is undertaken and documented, such patients can be successfully transplanted. Those at greater risk for relapse should be willing to submit to unannounced testing for substance abuse and be able to demonstrate continued abstinence.

Mental illness is common in patients with ESKD. Depression is the most common psychiatric illness in patients with ESKD (168). The stress of a transplant and concern about the viability of the transplant could lead many patients into significant depression that could interfere with the maintenance of proper medical care. Consequently, susceptible individuals should be identified pretransplant so that careful support systems can be used during the transplantation course (169,170).

In the past, mental retardation was considered a contraindication for organ transplantation (171). The concern was that such patients would not be able to comply with the posttransplant medical regimen and so would be doomed to rejection and graft loss. A recent review on the accessibility and success of organ transplantation on patients with mental retardation documented 1- and 3-year survival rates of 100% and 90%, respectively (172). Good compliance with posttransplant regimens was noted and attributed to the presence of supportive family members and caregivers.

Well-managed schizophrenia is generally not considered a transplantation contraindication. Patients who are not well controlled deserve an opportunity for proper treatment before transplantation. Bipolar patients can be successfully transplanted and do well. If a bipolar patient is maintained on lithium pretransplant, the psychiatrist may wish to try alternative medications to control the disease while the patient is on dialysis. Long-term exposure to lithium can lead to nephrogenic diabetes insipidus in 20% of patients who take this medication. Before transplantation, the goal should be to determine if a non–lithium-based regime could control the patient's bipolar disease. Bipolar patients who can only be managed on lithium can be continued on this medication posttransplant if no other reasonable alternative medication controls the illness. Although lithium is nephrotoxic at high serum concentrations, its toxic effects can be significantly reduced if serum drug levels are kept within therapeutic range. Patients who receive renal transplants have frequent blood draws to monitor immunosuppressant levels, and this requirement facilitates the frequent monitoring of lithium levels. Bipolar transplant recipients who were only controlled on lithium pretransplant can be maintained on the regimen, questioned frequently about nocturia, and monitored for a concentrating defect. Monitoring of lithium levels will minimize the detrimental effects on the kidney and will offer the recipient the best quality of life and control of the bipolar disorder. Those patients who receive a renal transplant require lithium and develop a concentrating defect may be candidates for treatment with amiloride.

In summary, a careful examination of psychosocial issues is imperative before transplantation because noncompliance is the third leading cause of graft failure (173). Moreover, a poor home situation and financial or social problems could interfere with proper delivery of care and may lead to an adverse outcome posttransplantation.

◆ MANAGEMENT OF PATIENTS ON THE CADAVERIC KIDNEY WAITING LIST

How should the health status of dialysis patients on the UNOS deceased donor kidney waiting list be followed up? Unfortunately, evidence-based guidelines describing the best mechanism to manage the health and psychosocial well-being of patients on the deceased donor renal transplant waiting list have never been published. Knowledge about the correct management of patients on the waiting list for deceased donor kidney transplantation is in its infancy (174). Recognition of the significant death rate and the demonstration that the length of time on the waiting list is an independent determinant of long-term posttransplant prognosis has prompted intense interest in this subject (175).

The Clinical Practice Guidelines Committee of the American Society of Transplantation published the results of a survey, which polled transplant centers in the United States and asked how they managed patients on the deceased donor transplant waiting list (176). Sixty-seven percent (192 of 287) of centers polled responded to the survey. Despite a lack of evidence-based guidelines for the management of dialysis patients awaiting renal transplantation, certain important points merit discussion. During the months and years that a patient is maintained on hemodialysis awaiting a renal transplant, many things may change including demographics, psychosocial support, general medical condition, and cardiovascular status. A regular review and update of these aspects of a patient's condition should be undertaken to ensure the continued preparedness for transplantation.

The transplant procedure has been described as an urgent surgery performed on an elective population. When a kidney becomes available, time is of the essence. The patient must be easily contacted, and a mechanism to transport the patient to the transplant center must be readily available. Patients undergoing maintenance hemodialysis must be continually reminded to update their telephone numbers and addresses with the transplant center. It should be pointed out to the patient that his or her diligence in this regard will benefit the patient greatly. Notifying the transplant center when a listed patient is going on a prolonged vacation, temporarily residing at an alternative location, or when changing residence will ensure that the patient can be promptly contacted when an organ becomes available. Delay in physically having the patient in the operating room leads to prolonged cold ischemia time, which increases the risk for delayed graft function, may increase the risk of early acute rejection, and overall negatively affects graft survival (177,178).

Many important psychosocial issues change for patients on maintenance hemodialysis. Unfortunately, these issues can be viewed as being of secondary importance compared with the general and more specifically cardiovascular health of potential recipients on the waiting list. Nevertheless, a patient's employment status, marital status, state of residence, insurance coverage, and psychological support mechanisms can all change while on hemodialysis and on the waiting list. Although it is unlikely that any of these issues would directly prevent a patient from receiving a kidney transplant, these issues are important. For example, patients who stop working, graduate from school, relocate to a nearby state, or suffer the loss of spousal support as a result of death or divorce might find themselves nearly destitute in the posttransplant period as they face various challenges. These include the financial cost of medications, repeat hospitalizations, and professional fees during the months and years following transplantation. Currently, maintenance medications for a renal transplant patient approach $15,000 per year. Few, if any, are able to cover these costs out-of-pocket. As a result, every patient should be reminded, while on the waiting list, to seek advice about how changes in psychosocial issues could alter benefits, insurance, and prescription coverage and thereby affect posttransplant life. Dialysis patients on the waiting list and transplant centers should maintain a routine dialogue about such issues. Patients should seek advice from social workers and financial counselors at their transplant center or dialysis unit when contemplating major life changes, such as changing jobs, seeking early retirement, seeking disability, and moving to another state. Ideally, individuals would have all the appropriate information to make the best decision before irreversible loss of coverage or benefits occur.

Ensuring that a patient, who might be on dialysis for several years before transplantation, is medically fit to undergo surgery is a daunting task for many transplant centers. At this time, given the lack of evidence-based data from studies of this population, the recommendation is to follow age-appropriate health maintenance and screening guidelines for colon, prostate, breast, and uterine malignancy (174,179).

Dialysis patients are catabolic, are at risk for malnutrition, suffer recurrent life-threatening infections, and, most significantly of all, live with the atherogenic burden of CKD (180–183).

Strict medical guidelines for the initial listing of patients with renal insufficiency are standard at most transplant centers. Once a patient is listed, however, the frequency with which a patient on dialysis is reevaluated and the integrity of the cardiovascular reserve to permit a safe surgical procedure varies widely (184–186).

Given the importance of appropriate cardiovascular clearance and the often asymptomatic deterioration of cardiovascular function on dialysis, many centers surveyed responded that they closely followed up patients on the waiting list. Most centers (79%) indicated that they screened patients on an annual basis. Of these, 40% employed nuclear perfusion scanning, 33% used exercise thallium scanning, 31% employed dobutamine echocardiography, and only 15% required coronary angiography (176). Unfortunately, these diagnostic studies are less reliable among patients with ESKD. Noninvasive testing for CAD among asymptomatic patients with ESKD is of limited value (187). Unfortunately, the frequency of follow-up assessments required and long-term studies comparing this with gold standard angiographic evidence are lacking. Dobutamine stress echocardiography has a sensitivity of 75% and a specificity of only 71%, compared with angiography when evaluating lesions of greater than 70% stenosis (188). Dipyridamole and thallium imaging has a sensitivity of only 37% and a specificity of only 73% in this population. It does not clearly predict cardiac prognosis among patients with ESKD (189). Efforts to facilitate communication and to educate patients, primary care physicians, local subspecialists (especially cardiologists), dialysis social workers, and dialysis center staff about the importance of updating the transplant center about changes in demographic, psychosocial, and health issues must be stressed. Most importantly, patients themselves, their nephrologists, and the pretransplant coordinators should work in concert and communicate frequently and freely to maximize preparedness at all times. It has been suggested that regular contact between the patient, nephrologist, and transplant centers, perhaps during site visits to dialysis centers by members of the transplant center team, could serve to educate patients, maintain motivation, diminish a sense of hopelessness, and offer time to reevaluate living donor options.

⬡ REFERENCES

1. Rana A. Gruessner A, Agopian VG, et al. Survival benefit of solid-organ transplant in the United States. *JAMA Surg* 2015;150:252–259. doi:10.1001/jamasurg.2014.2038.
2. Schnuelle P, Lorenz D, Trede M, et al. Impact of renal cadaveric transplantation on survival in end-stage renal failure: evidence for reduced mortality risk compared with hemodialysis during long-term follow-up. *J Am Soc Nephrol* 1998;9:2135–2141.
3. Port FK, Wolfe RA, Mauger EA, et al. Comparison of survival probabilities for dialysis patients versus cadaveric renal transplant recipients. *JAMA* 1993;270:1339–1343.
4. Ojo AO, Port FK, Wolfe RA, et al. Comparative mortality risks of chronic dialysis and cadaveric transplantation in black end-stage renal disease patients. *Am J Kidney Dis* 1994;24:59–64.
5. Wolfe RA, Ashby VB, Milford EL, et al. Comparison of mortality in all patients on dialysis, patients on dialysis awaiting transplantation, and recipients of a first cadaveric transplant. *N Engl J Med* 1999;341:1725–1730.
6. Meier-Kriesche HU, Ojo AO, Port FK, et al. Survival improvement among patients with end-stage renal disease: trends over time for transplant recipients and wait-listed patients. *J Am Soc Nephrol* 2001;12:1293–1296.
7. National Kidney Foundation. *Organ Donation and Transplantation Statistics.* New York, NY: National Kidney Foundation, 2014.
8. U.S. Department of Health and Human Services, Health Resources and Services Administration. *2006 OPTN/SRTR Annual Report: Transplant Data 1996-2005.* Washington, DC: U.S. Department of Health and Human Services, 2006.
9. Meier-Kriesche HU, Port FK, Ojo AO, et al. Effect of waiting time on renal transplant outcome. *Kidney Int* 2000;58:1311–1317.

10. Matas AJ, Payne WD, Sutherland DE, et al. 2,500 Living donor kidney transplants: a single-center experience. *Ann Surg* 2001;234:149–164.
11. Vats AN, Donaldson L, Fine RN, et al. Pretransplant dialysis status and outcome of renal transplantation in North American children: a NAPRTCS study. *Transplantation* 2000;69:1414–1419.
12. Schold J, Srinivas TR, Sehgal AR, et al. Half of kidney transplant candidates who are older than 60 years now placed on the waiting list will die before receiving a deceased-donor transplant. *Clin J Am Soc Nephrol* 2009;4:1239–1245.
13. OPTN/SRTR 2012 Annual Data Report. Introduction. *Am J Transplant* 2014;14(Suppl 1):8–10.
14. Rodrigue JR, Schold JD, Mandelbrot DA. The decline in living kidney donation in the United States: random variation or cause for concern? *Transplantation* 2013;96:767–773.
15. Israni AK, Salkowski N, Gustafson S, et al. New national allocation policy for deceased donor kidneys in the United States and possible effect on patient outcomes. *J Am Soc Nephrol* 2014;25:1842–1848.
16. Savoye E, Tamarelle D, Chalem Y, et al. Survival benefits of kidney transplantation with expanded criteria deceased donors in patients aged 60 years and over. *Transplantation* 2007;84:1618–1624.
17. Osei K, Henry ML, O'Dorisio TM, et al. Physiological and pharmacological stimulation of pancreatic islet hormone secretion in type I diabetic pancreas allograft recipients. *Diabetes* 1990;39:1235–1242.
18. Robertson RP, Diem P, Sutherland DE. Time-related, cross-sectional and prospective follow-up of pancreatic endocrine function after pancreas allograft transplantation in type 1 (insulin-dependent) diabetic patients. *Diabetologia* 1991;34(Suppl 1):S57–S60.
19. Katz H, Homan M, Velosa J, et al. Effects of pancreas transplantation on postprandial glucose metabolism. *N Engl J Med* 1991;325:1278–1283.
20. Navarro X, Sutherland DE, Kennedy WR. Long-term effects of pancreatic transplantation on diabetic neuropathy. *Ann Neurol* 1997;42:727–736.
21. Fioretto P, Steffes MW, Sutherland DE, et al. Reversal of lesions of diabetic nephropathy after pancreas transplantation. *N Engl J Med* 1998;339:69–75.
22. Cheung AH, Sutherland DE, Gillingham KJ, et al. Simultaneous pancreas-kidney transplant versus kidney transplant alone in diabetic patients. *Kidney Int* 1992;41:924–929.
23. Sollinger HW, Odorico JS, Knechtle SJ, et al. Experience with 500 simultaneous pancreas-kidney transplants. *Ann Surg* 1998;228:284–296.
24. Kasiske BL, Guijarro C, Massy ZA, et al. Cardiovascular disease after renal transplantation. *J Am Soc Nephrol* 1996;7:158–165.
25. Ojo AO, Hanson JA, Wolfe RA, et al. Long-term survival in renal transplant recipients with graft function. *Kidney Int* 2000;57:307–313.
26. Collins A, Foley RN, Herzog C, et al. U.S. Renal Data System 2012 annual report. *Am J Kidney Dis* 2013;61:A7, e1–e476.
27. Yeo FE, Villines TC, Bucci JR, et al. Cardiovascular risk in stage 4 and 5 nephropathy. *Adv Chronic Kidney Dis* 2004;11:116–133.
28. Hedayati SS, Szczech LA. The evaluation of underlying cardiovascular disease among patients with end-stage renal disease. *Adv Chronic Kidney Dis* 2004;11:246–253.
29. Fishbane S. Cardiovascular risk evaluation before kidney transplantation. *J Am Soc Nephrol* 2005;16:843–845.
30. Goldman L. Multifactorial index of cardiac risk in noncardiac surgery: ten-year status report. *J Cardiothorac Anesth* 1987;1:237–244.
31. Windecker S, Kolh P, Alfonso F, et al. 2014 ESC/EACTS guidelines on myocardial revascularization: the Task Force on Myocardial Revascularization of the European Society of Cardiology (ESC) and the European Association for Cardio-Thoracic Surgery (EACTS). Developed with the special contribution of the European Association of Percutaneous Cardiovascular Interventions (EAPCI). *Eur Heart J* 2014;35:2541–2619.
32. Lentine KL, Costa SP, Weir MR, et al. AHA/ACCF/ASTS/AST/NKF 2012 cardiac disease evaluation and management among kidney and liver transplantation candidates. *Circulation* 2012;126:617–663.
33. European Renal Best Practice Transplantation Guideline Development Group. ERBP guideline on the management and evaluation of the kidney donor and recipient. *Nephrol Dial Transplant* 2013;28(Suppl 2): ii1–ii71.
34. Dahan M, Viron BM, Faraggi M, et al. Diagnostic accuracy and prognostic value of combined dipyridamole-exercise thallium imaging in hemodialysis patients. *Kidney Int* 1998;54:255–262.
35. Brown JH, Vites NP, Testa HJ, et al. Value of thallium myocardial imaging in the prediction of future cardiovascular events in patients with end-stage renal failure. *Nephrol Dial Transplant* 1993;8:433–437.
36. Herzog CA, Marwick TH, Pheley AM, et al. Dobutamine stress echocardiography for the detection of significant coronary artery disease in renal transplant candidates. *Am J Kidney Dis* 1999;33:1080–1090.
37. Bates JR, Sawada SG, Segar DS, et al. Evaluation using dobutamine stress echocardiography in patients with insulin-dependent diabetes mellitus before kidney and/or pancreas transplantation. *Am J Cardiol* 1996;77:175–179.
38. Patel AD, Abo-Auda WS, Davis JM, et al. Prognostic value of myocardial perfusion imaging in predicting outcome after renal transplantation. *Am J Cardiol* 2003;92:146–151.
39. Herzog CA. Kidney disease in cardiology. *Nephrol Dial Transplant* 2007;22:43–46.
40. Wang LW, Fahim MA, Hayen A, et al. Cardiac testing for coronary artery disease in potential kidney transplant recipients. *Cochrane Database Syst Rev* 2011;(12):CD008691.
41. Smart SC, Bhatia A, Hellman R, et al. Dobutamine-atropine stress echocardiography and dipyridamole sestamibi scintigraphy for the detection of coronary artery disease: limitations and concordance. *J Am Coll Cardiol* 2000;36:1265–1273.
42. Chiu DYY, Green D, Abidin N, et al. Echocardiography in hemodialysis patients: uses and challenges. *Am J Kidney Dis* 2014;64:804–816.
43. Sobkowicz B, Tomaszuk-Kazberuk A, Kralisz P, et al. Application of myocardial contrast echocardiography for the perfusion assessment in patients with end-stage renal failure—comparison with coronary angiography. *Am J Nephrol* 2008;28:929–934.
44. Tomaszuk-Kazberuk A, Sobkowicz B, Malyszko J, et al. Real-time myocardial contrast echocardiography as a useful tool to select candidates for coronary revascularization among patients with end-stage renal disease—a 3-year follow-up study. *Adv Med Sci* 2011;56(2):207–214.
45. Hart A, Weir MR, Kasiske BL. Cardiovascular risk assessments in kidney transplantation. *Kidney Int* 2015;87(3):527–534. doi:10.1038/ki.2014.335.
46. Al Sayari S, Kopp S, Bremerich J. Stress cardiac MR imaging: the role of stress functional assessment and perfusion imaging in the evaluation of ischemic heart disease. *Radiol Clin North Am* 2015;53(2):355–367.
47. De Lima JJ, Sabbaga E, Vieira ML, et al. Coronary angiography is the best predictor of events in renal transplant candidates compared with noninvasive testing. *Hypertension* 2003;42:263–268.
48. Kidney Disease Outcomes Quality Initiative Workgroup. K/DOQI clinical practice guidelines for cardiovascular disease in dialysis patients. *Am J Kidney Dis* 2005;45(4 Suppl 3):S1–S153.
49. Manske CL, Wang Y, Rector T, et al. Coronary revascularisation in insulin-dependent diabetic patients with chronic renal failure. *Lancet* 1992;340:998–1002.
50. Liu JY, Birkmeyer NJ, Sanders JH, et al. Northern New England Cardiovascular Disease Study Group. Risks of morbidity and mortality in dialysis patients undergoing coronary artery bypass surgery. *Circulation* 2000;102:2973–2977.
51. Farkouh ME, Domanski M, Sleeper LA, et al; and the FREEDOM Trial Investigators. Strategies for multivessel revascularization in patients with diabetes. *N Engl J Med* 2012;367:2375–2384.
52. Longenecker JC, Coresh J, Klag MJ, et al. Validation of comorbid conditions on the end-stage renal disease medical evidence report: the CHOICE study. Choices for Healthy Outcomes in Caring for ESRD. *J Am Soc Nephrol* 2000;11:520–529.
53. Parfrey PS, Foley RN, Harnett JD, et al. Outcome and risk factors for left ventricular disorders in chronic uraemia. *Nephrol Dial Transplant* 1996;11:1277–1285.
54. Wali RK, Wang GS, Gottlieb SS, et al. Effect of kidney transplantation on left ventricular systolic dysfunction and congestive heart failure in patients with end-stage renal disease. *J Am Coll Cardiol* 2005;45:1051–1060.

55. Foley RN, Parfrey PS, Kent GM, et al. Serial change in echocardiographic parameters and cardiac failure in end-stage renal disease. *J Am Soc Nephrol* 2000;11:912–916.

56. Biller J, Feinberg WM, Castaldo JE, et al. Guidelines for carotid endarterectomy: a statement for healthcare professionals from a Special Writing Group of the Stroke Council, American Heart Association. *Circulation* 1998;97:501–509.

57. Matcher DB, McCrory DC, Barnett HJM, et al. American College of Physicians. Guidelines for medical treatment for stroke prevention. *Ann Intern Med* 1994;121:54–55.

58. Chapman AB, Rubinstein D, Hughes R, et al. Intracranial aneurysms in autosomal dominant polycystic kidney disease. *N Engl J Med* 1992;327:916–920.

59. Wiebers DO. Unruptured intracranial aneurysms—risk of rupture and risks of surgical intervention. *N Engl J Med* 1998;339:1724–1733.

60. Sung RS, Althoen M, Howell TA, et al. Peripheral vascular occlusive disease in renal transplant recipients: risk factors and impact on kidney allograft survival. *Transplantation* 2000;70:1049–1054.

61. U.S. Renal Data System. Causes of death. In: *USRDS 1999 Annual Data Report*. Bethesda, MD: National Institute of Diabetes, Digestive and Kidney Diseases, 1999:89–100.

62. Apel H, Walschburger-Zorn K, Häberle L, et al. De novo malignancies in renal transplant recipients: experience at a single center with 1882 transplant patients over 39 yr. *Clin Transplant* 2013;27:E30–E36.

63. Penn I. Evaluation of transplant candidates with pre-existing malignancies. *Ann Transplant* 1997;2:14–17.

64. Chapman JR, Webster AC, Wong C. Cancer in the transplant recipient. *Cold Spring Harb Perspect Med* 2013;3:a015677.

65. Girndt M, Kohler H. Waiting time for patients with history of malignant disease before listing for organ transplantation. *Transplantation* 2005;80:S167–S170.

66. United States Preventive Services Task Force. Screening for lung cancer. In: *Guide to Clinical Preventive Services*. Baltimore, MD: Williams & Wilkins, 1996:135–139.

67. Konety BR, Tewari A, Howard RJ, et al. Urologic Society for Transplantation and Vascular Surgery. Prostate cancer in the post-transplant population. *Urology* 1998;52:428–432.

68. U.S. Preventive Task Force. Screening for prostate cancer. In: *Guide to Clinical Preventive Services*. 2nd ed. Baltimore, MD: Williams & Wilkins, 1996:119–134.

69. Penn I. The effect of immunosuppression on pre-existing cancers. *Transplantation* 1993;55:742–747.

70. Secin FP, Carver B, Kattan MW, et al. Current recommendations for delaying renal transplantation after localized prostate cancer treatment: are they still appropriate? *Transplantation* 2004;78:710–712.

71. Asch WS, Bia MJ. Oncologic issues and kidney transplantation: a review of frequency, mortality, and screening. *Adv Chronic Kidney Dis* 2014;21:106–113.

72. Brunner FP, Landais P, Selwood NH. European Dialysis and Transplantation Association-European Renal Association. Malignancies after renal transplantation: the EDTA-ERA registry experience. *Nephrol Dial Transplant* 1995;10(Suppl 1):74–80.

73. Stewart T, Tsai SC, Grayson H, et al. Incidence of de-novo breast cancer in women chronically immunosuppressed after organ transplantation. *Lancet* 1995;346:796–798.

74. Maisonneuve P, Agodoa L, Gellert R, et al. Cancer in patients on dialysis for end-stage renal disease: an international collaborative study. *Lancet* 1999;354:93–99.

75. Hope CM, Coates PT, Carroll RP. Immune profiling and cancer post transplantation. *World J Nephrol* 2015;4(1):41–56.

76. Saidi RF, Dudrick PS, Goldman MH. Colorectal cancer after renal transplantation. *Transplant Proc* 2003;35:1410–1412.

77. Park JM, Choi MG, Kim SW, et al. Increased incidence of colorectal malignancies in renal transplant recipients: a case control study. *Am J Transplant* 2010;10:2043–2050.

78. Ellis D, Jaffe R, Green M, et al. Epstein-Barr virus-related disorders in children undergoing renal transplantation with tacrolimus-based immunosuppression. *Transplantation* 1999;68:997–1003.

79. Birkeland SA, Andersen HK, Hamilton-Dutoit SJ. Preventing acute rejection, Epstein-Barr virus infection, and post-transplant lymphoproliferative disorders after kidney transplantation: use of aciclovir and mycophenolate mofetil in a steroid-free immunosuppressive protocol. *Transplantation* 1999;67:1209–1214.

80. Darenkov IA, Marcarelli MA, Basadonna GP, et al. Reduced incidence of Epstein-Barr virus-associated posttransplant lymphoproliferative disorder using preemptive antiviral therapy. *Transplantation* 1997;64:848–852.

81. Green M, Michaels MG. Epstein–Barr virus infection and posttransplant lymphoproliferative disorder. *Am J Transplant* 2013;13:41–54.

82. Bluman LG, Mosca L, Newman N, et al. Preoperative smoking habits and postoperative pulmonary complications. *Chest* 1998;113:883–889.

83. Friedman EA. Management choices in diabetic end-stage renal disease. *Nephrol Dial Transplant* 1995;10(Suppl 7):61–69.

84. Gaston RS, Basadonna G, Cosio FG, et al. Transplantation in the diabetic patient with advanced chronic kidney disease: a task force report. *Am J Kidney Dis* 2004;44:529–542.

85. Gruessner AC, Sutherland DE. Analysis of United States (US) and non-US pancreas transplants as reported to the International Pancreas Transplant Registry (IPTR) and to the United Network for Organ Sharing (UNOS). *Clin Transpl* 1998;1:53–73.

86. Becker BN, Brazy PC, Becker YT, et al. Simultaneous pancreas-kidney transplantation reduces excess mortality in type 1 diabetic patients with end-stage renal disease. *Kidney Int* 2000;57:2129–2135.

87. Ojo AO, Meier-Kriesche HU, Hanson JA, et al. The impact of simultaneous pancreas-kidney transplantation on long-term patient survival. *Transplantation* 2001;71:82–90.

88. Leavey SF, Strawderman RL, Jones CA, et al. Simple nutritional indicators as independent predictors of mortality in hemodialysis patients. *Am J Kidney Dis* 1998;31:997–1006.

89. Meier-Kriesche HU, Arndorfer JA, Kaplan B. The impact of body mass index on renal transplant outcomes: a significant independent risk factor for graft failure and patient death. *Transplantation* 2002;73:70–74.

90. Winkelmayer WC, Lorenz M, Kramar R, et al. C-reactive protein and body mass index independently predict mortality in kidney transplant recipients. *Am J Transplant* 2004;4:1148–1154.

91. Meier-Kriesche HU, Vaghela M, Thambuganipalle R, et al. The effect of body mass index on long-term renal allograft survival. *Transplantation* 1999;68:1294–1297.

92. Massarweh NN, Clayton JL, Mangum CA, et al. High body mass index and short- and long-term renal allograft survival in adults. *Transplantation* 2005;80:1430–1434.

93. Pirsch JD, Armbrust MJ, Knechtle SJ, et al. Obesity as a risk factor following renal transplantation. *Transplantation* 1995;59:631–633.

94. Modlin CS, Flechner SM, Goormastic M, et al. Should obese patients lose weight before receiving a kidney transplant? *Transplantation* 1997;64:599–604.

95. Pham PT, Danovitch GM, Pham PC. Kidney transplantation in the obese transplant candidates: to transplant or not to transplant? *Semin Dial* 2013;26:568–577.

96. Lievense H, Kalantar-Zadeh K, Lukowsky LR, et al. Relationship of body size and initial dialysis modality on subsequent transplantation, mortality and weight gain of ESRD patients. *Nephrol Dial Transplant* 2012;27:3631–3638.

97. Ahn HJ, Kim HJ, Kim YS, et al. Risk factors for changes in bone mineral density and the effect of antiosteoporosis management after renal transplantation. *Transplant Proc* 2006;38:2074–2076.

98. Palmer SC, Strippoli GF, McGregor DO. Interventions for preventing bone disease in kidney transplant recipients: a systematic review of randomized controlled trials. *Am J Kidney Dis* 2005;45:638–649.

99. Sakhaee K, Gonzalez GB. Update on renal osteodystrophy: pathogenesis and clinical management. *Am J Med Sci* 1999;317:251–260.

100. Massari PU. Disorders of bone and mineral metabolism after renal transplantation. *Kidney Int* 1997;52:1412–1421.

101. Tajima A, Ishikawa A, Ohta N, et al. Parathyroid function after kidney allografting. *Transplant Proc* 1996;28:1629–1630.

102. Lindberg JS, Culleton B, Wong G, et al. Cinacalcet HCl, an oral calcimimetic agent for the treatment of secondary hyperparathyroidism in hemodialysis and peritoneal dialysis: a randomized, double-blind, multicenter study. *J Am Soc Nephrol* 2005;16:800–807.

103. Pirenne J, Lledo-Garcia E, Benedetti E, et al. Colon perforation after renal transplantation: a single-institution review. *Clin Transplant* 1997;11:88–93.

104. Stelzner M, Vlahakos DV, Milford EL, et al. Colonic perforations after renal transplantation. *J Am Coll Surg* 1997;184:63–69.

105. Lederman ED, Conti DJ, Lempert N, et al. Complicated diverticulitis following renal transplantation. *Dis Colon Rectum* 1998;41:613–618.

106. Reese J, Burton F, Lingle D, et al. Peptic ulcer disease following renal transplantation in the cyclosporine era. *Am J Surg* 1991;162:558–562.

107. Troppmann C, Papalois BE, Chiou A, et al. Incidence, complications, treatment, and outcome of ulcers of the upper gastrointestinal tract after renal transplantation during the cyclosporine era. *J Am Coll Surg* 1995;180:433–443.

108. Teenan RP, Burgoyne M, Brown IL, et al. Helicobacter pylori in renal transplant recipients. *Transplantation* 1993;56:100–103.

109. Skála I, Marecková O, Vítko S, et al. Prophylaxis of acute gastroduodenal bleeding after renal transplantation. *Transpl Int* 1997;10:375–378.

110. Weir MR, Kirkman RL, Strom TB, et al. Liver disease in recipients of long-functioning renal allografts. *Kidney Int* 1985;28:839–844.

111. Pereira BJ, Levey AS. Hepatitis C virus infection in dialysis and renal transplantation. *Kidney Int* 1997;51:981–999.

112. Fairley CK, Mijch A, Gust ID, et al. The increased risk of fatal liver disease in renal transplant patients who are hepatitis Be antigen and/or HBV DNA positive. *Transplantation* 1991;52:497–500.

113. Fabrizi F, Martin P, Dixit V, et al. HBsAg seropositive status and survival after renal transplantation: meta-analysis of observational studies. *Am J Transplant* 2005;5:2913–2921.

114. Jung YO, Lee YS, Yang WS, et al. Treatment of chronic hepatitis B with lamivudine in renal transplant recipients. *Transplantation* 1998;66:733–737.

115. Fontaine H, Thiers V, Chretien Y, et al. HBV genotypic resistance to lamivudine in kidney recipients and hemodialyzed patients. *Transplantation* 2000;69:2090–2094.

116. Cholongitas E, Tziomalos K, Pipili C. Management of patients with hepatitis B in special populations. *World J Gastroenterol* 2015;21(6):1738–1748.

117. Pereira BJG, Wright TL, Schmid CH, et al. The impact of pretransplantation hepatitis C infection on the outcome of renal transplantation. *Transplantation* 1995;60:799–805.

118. Cosio FG, Sedmak DD, Henry ML, et al. The high prevalence of severe early post-transplant renal allograft pathology in hepatitis C positive recipients. *Transplantation* 1996;62:1054–1059.

119. Fabrizi F, Martin P, Dixit V, et al. Hepatitis C virus antibody status and survival after renal transplantation: meta-analysis of observational studies. *Am J Transplant* 2005;5:1452–1461.

120. Mathurin P, Mouquet C, Poynard T, et al. Impact of hepatitis B and C virus on kidney transplantation outcome. *Hepatology* 1999;29:257–263.

121. Campos S, Parsikia A, Zaki RF, et al. Kidney transplantation alone in ESRD patients with hepatitis C cirrhosis. *Transplantation* 2012;94:65–66.

122. Ingsathit A, Kamanamool N, Thakkinstian A, et al. Survival advantage of kidney transplantation over dialysis in patients with hepatitis C: a systematic review and meta-analysis. *Transplantation* 2013;95:943–948.

123. Izopet J, Rostaing L, Moussion F, et al. High rate of hepatitis C virus clearance in hemodialysis patients after interferon-alpha therapy. *J Infect Dis* 1997;176:1614–1617.

124. Casanovas-Taltavull T, Baliellas C, Benasco C, et al. Efficacy of interferon for chronic hepatitis C virus-related hepatitis in kidney transplant candidates on hemodialysis: results after transplantation. *Am J Gastroenterol* 2001;96:1170–1177.

125. Kamar N, Ribes D, Izopet J, et al. Treatment of hepatitis C virus infection (HCV) after renal transplantation: implications for HCV-positive dialysis patients awaiting a kidney transplant. *Transplantation* 2006;82:853–856.

126. Terrault NA, Adey DB. The kidney transplant recipient with hepatitis C infection: pre- and posttransplantation treatment. *Clin J Am Soc Nephrol* 2007;2:563–575.

127. Bunchorntavakul C, Maneerattanaporn M, Chavalitdhamrong D. Management of patients with hepatitis C and renal disease. *World J Hepatol* 2015;7(2):213–225.

128. Bloom RD, Rao V, Weng F, et al. Association of hepatitis C with posttransplant diabetes in renal transplant patients on tacrolimus. *J Am Soc Nephrol* 2002;13:1374–1380.

129. Aguirre Valadez J, García Juárez I, Rincón Pedrero R, et al. Management of chronic hepatitis C virus infection in patients with end-stage renal disease: a review. *Ther Clin Risk Manag* 2015;11:329–338.

130. Kiberd BA. Should hepatitis C-infected kidneys be transplanted in the United States? *Transplantation* 1994;57:1068–1072.

131. Mandal AK, Kraus ES, Samaniego M, et al. Shorter waiting times for hepatitis C virus seropositive recipients of cadaveric renal allografts from hepatitis C virus seropositive donors. *Clin Transplant* 2000;14:391–396.

132. Jassal SV, Roscoe JM, Zaltzman JS, et al. Clinical practice guidelines: prevention of cytomegalovirus disease after renal transplantation. *J Am Soc Nephrol* 1998;9:1697–1708.

133. Sagedal S, Nordal KP, Hartmann A, et al. A prospective study of the natural course of cytomegalovirus infection and disease in renal allograft recipients. *Transplantation* 2000;70:1166–1174.

134. Eid AJ, Razonable RR. New developments in the management of cytomegalovirus infection after solid organ transplantation. *Drugs* 2010;70:965–981.

135. Couchoud C. Cytomegalovirus prophylaxis with antiviral agents for solid organ transplantation. *Cochrane Database Syst Rev* 2000;(2):CD001320.

136. Limaye AP, Corey L, Koelle DM, et al. Emergence of ganciclovir-resistant cytomegalovirus disease among recipients of solid-organ transplants. *Lancet* 2000;356:645–649.

137. Apaydin S, Altiparmak MR, Serdengecti K, et al. Mycobacterium tuberculosis infections after renal transplantation. *Scand J Infect Dis* 2000;32:501–505.

138. Margiotta V, Pizzo I, Pizzo G, et al. Cyclosporin- and nifedipine-induced gingival overgrowth in renal transplant patients: correlations with periodontal and pharmacological parameters, and HLA-antigens. *J Oral Pathol Med* 1996;25:128–134.

139. Linnemann CC Jr, First MR. Risk of pneumococcal infections in renal transplant patients. *JAMA* 1979;241:2619–2621.

140. Rangel MC, Coronado VG, Euler GL, et al. Vaccine recommendations for patients on chronic dialysis. The Advisory Committee on Immunization Practices and the American Academy of Pediatrics. *Semin Dial* 2000;13:101–107.

141. Harbell J, Terrault NA, Stock P. Solid organ transplants in HIV-infected patients. *Curr HIV/AIDS Rep* 2013;10(3):217–225.

142. Roland ME, Stock PG. Solid organ transplantation is a reality for patients with HIV infection. *Curr HIV/AIDS Rep* 2006;3:132–138.

143. Ciuffreda D, Pantaleo G, Pascual M. Effects of immunosuppressive drugs on HIV infection: implications for solid-organ transplantation. *Transpl Int* 2007;20:649–658.

144. Kabler RL, Cerny JC. Pre-transplant urologic investigation and treatment of end stage renal disease. *J Urol* 1983;129:475–478.

145. Hariharan S, Adams MB, Brennan DC, et al. Recurrent and de novo glomerular disease after renal transplantation: a report from Renal Allograft Disease Registry (RADR). *Transplantation* 1999;68:635–641.

146. Hariharan S, Savin VJ. Recurrent and de novo disease after renal transplantation: a report from the Renal Allograft Disease Registry. *Pediatr Transplant* 2004;8:349–350.

147. Artero M, Biava C, Amend W, et al. Recurrent focal glomerulosclerosis: natural history and response to therapy. *Am J Med* 1992;92:375–383.

148. Toth CM, Pascual M, Williams WW Jr, et al. Recurrent collapsing glomerulopathy. *Transplantation* 1998;65:1009–1010.

149. Stephanian E, Matas AJ, Mauer SM, et al. Recurrence of disease in patients retransplanted for focal segmental glomerulosclerosis. *Transplantation* 1992;53:755–757.

150. Alachkar N, Wei C, Arend LJ, et al. Podocyte effacement closely links to suPAR levels at time of posttransplantation focal segmental glomerulosclerosis occurrence and improves with therapy. *Transplantation* 2013;96(7):649–656.

151. Briggs JD, Jones E. European Renal Association-European Dialysis and Transplant Association. Recurrence of glomerulonephritis following renal transplantation. Scientific Advisory Board of the ERA-EDTA Registry. *Nephrol Dial Transplant* 1999;14:564–565.

152. Freese P, Svalander C, Norden G, et al. Clinical risk factors for recurrence of IgA nephropathy. *Clin Transplant* 1999;13:313–317.

153. Meulders Q, Pirson Y, Cosyns JP, et al. Course of Henoch-Schonlein nephritis after renal transplantation. Report on ten patients and review of the literature. *Transplantation* 1994;58:1179–1186.

154. Andresdottir MB, Assmann KJ, Hoitsma AJ, et al. Renal transplantation in patients with dense deposit disease: morphological characteristics of recurrent disease and clinical outcome. *Nephrol Dial Transplant* 1999;14:1723–1731.

155. Couchoud C, Pouteil-Noble C, Colon S, et al. Recurrence of membranous nephropathy after renal transplantation. Incidence and risk factors in 1614 patients. *Transplantation* 1995;59:1275–1279.

156. Ducloux D, Rebibou JM, Semhoun-Ducloux S, et al. Recurrence of hemolytic-uremic syndrome in renal transplant recipients: a meta-analysis. *Transplantation* 1998;65:1405–1407.

157. Franz M, Regele H, Schmaldienst S, et al. Post-transplant hemolytic uremic syndrome in adult retransplanted kidney graft recipients: advantage of FK506 therapy? *Transplantation* 1998;66:1258–1262.

158. Hebert D, Sibley RK, Mauer SM. Recurrence of hemolytic uremic syndrome in renal transplant recipients. *Kidney Int Suppl* 1986;19:S51–S58.

159. Doutrelepont JM, Abramowicz D, Florquin S, et al. Early recurrence of hemolytic uremic syndrome in a renal transplant recipient during prophylactic OKT3 therapy. *Transplantation* 1992;53:1378–1379.

160. Nachman PH, Segelmark M, Westman K, et al. Recurrent ANCA-associated small vessel vasculitis after transplantation: a pooled analysis. *Kidney Int* 1999;56:1544–1550.

161. Goral S, Ynares C, Shappell SB, et al. Recurrent lupus nephritis in renal transplant recipients revisited: it is not rare. *Transplantation* 2003;75:651–656.

162. Ward MM. Outcomes of renal transplantation among patients with end-stage renal disease caused by lupus nephritis. *Kidney Int* 2000;57:2136–2143.

163. Heering P, Hetzel R, Grabensee B, et al. Renal transplantation in secondary systemic amyloidosis. *Clin Transplant* 1998;12:159–164.

164. Fisher MS. Psychosocial evaluation interview protocol for pretransplant kidney recipients. *Health Soc Work* 2006;31:137–144.

165. Monroe J, Raiz L. Barriers to employment following renal transplantation: implications for the social work professional. *Soc Work Health Care* 2005;40:61–81.

166. Stone JH, Amend WJ, Criswell LA. Antiphospholipid antibody syndrome in renal transplantation: occurrence of clinical events in 96 consecutive patients with systemic lupus erythematosus. *Am J Kidney Dis* 1999;34:1040–1047.

167. Rundell JR, Hall RC. Psychiatric characteristics of consecutively evaluated outpatient renal transplant candidates and comparisons with consultation-liaison inpatients. *Psychosomatics* 1997;38:269–276.

168. Kimmel PL, Thamer M, Richard CM, et al. Psychiatric illness in patients with end-stage renal disease. *Am J Med* 1998;105:214–221.

169. Watnick S, Kirwin P, Mahnensmith R, et al. The prevalence and treatment of depression among patients starting dialysis. *Am J Kidney Dis* 2003;41:105–110.

170. Christensen AJ, Ehlers SL, Raichle KA, et al. Predicting change in depression following renal transplantation: effect of patient coping preferences. *Health Psychol* 2000;19:348–353.

171. Collins TL, Wayne Holden E, Scheel JN. Cognitive functioning as a contraindication to organ transplant surgery dilemmas encountered in medical decision making. *Kidney Int* 1996;3:413–422.

172. Martens MA, Jones L, Reiss S. Organ transplantation, organ donation and mental retardation. *Pediatr Transplant* 2006;10:658–664.

173. Kimmel PL, Peterson RA, Weihs KL, et al. Psychologic functioning, quality of life, and behavioral compliance in patients beginning hemodialysis. *J Am Soc Nephrol* 1996;7:2152–2159.

174. Matas AJ, Kasiske B, Miller L. Proposed guidelines for re-evaluation of patients on the waiting list for renal cadaver transplantation. *Transplantation* 2002;73:811–812.

175. Ojo AO, Hanson JA, Meier-Kriesche H, et al. Survival in recipients of marginal cadaveric donor kidneys compared with other recipients and wait-listed transplant candidates. *J Am Soc Nephrol* 2001;12:589–597.

176. Danovitch GM, Hariharan S, Pirsch JD, et al. Management of the waiting list for cadaveric kidney transplants: report of a survey and recommendations by the Clinical Practice Guidelines Committee of the American Society of Transplantation. *J Am Soc Nephrol* 2002;13:528–535.

177. Tullius SG, Reutzel-Selke A, Nieminen-Kelha M, et al. Contribution of donor age and ischemic injury in chronic renal allograft dysfunction. *Transplant Proc* 1999;31:1298–1299.

178. Cecka JM, Shoskes DA, Gjertson DW. Clinical impact of delayed graft function for kidney transplantation. *Transplant Rev* 2001;15:67.

179. Sox HC Jr. Preventive health services in adults. *N Engl J Med* 1994;330:1589–1595.

180. Rostand SG. Coronary heart disease in chronic renal insufficiency: some management considerations. *J Am Soc Nephrol* 2000;11:1948–1956.

181. Danovitch GM. The epidemic of cardiovascular disease in chronic renal disease: a challenge to the transplant physician. *Graft* 1999;2(Suppl):S108–S112.

182. Levey AS, Beto JA, Coronado BE, et al. Controlling the epidemic of cardiovascular disease in chronic renal what do we know? What do we need to learn? Where do we go from here? National Kidney Foundation Task Force on Cardiovascular Disease. *Am J Kidney Dis* 1998;32:853–906.

183. Braun WE, Marwick TH. Coronary artery disease in renal transplant recipients. *Cleve Clin J Med* 1994;61:370–385.

184. Middleton RJ, Parfrey PS, Foley RN. Left ventricular hypertrophy in the renal patient. *J Am Soc Nephrol* 2001;12:1079–1084.

185. Gallon LG, Leventhal JR, Kaufman DB. Pretransplant evaluation of renal transplant candidates. *Semin Nephrol* 2002;22:515–525.

186. Scandling JD. Kidney transplant candidate evaluation. *Semin Dial* 2005;18:487–494.

187. Schmidt A, Stefenelli T, Schuster E, et al. Informational contribution of noninvasive screening tests for coronary artery disease in patients on chronic renal replacement therapy. *Am J Kidney Dis* 2001;37:56–63.

188. Schweitzer EJ, Wilson J, Jacobs S, et al. Increased rates of donation with laparoscopic donor nephrectomy. *Ann Surg* 2000;232:392–400.

189. Marwick TH, Steinmuller DR, Underwood DA, et al. Ineffectiveness of dipyridamole SPECT thallium imaging as a screening technique for coronary artery disease in patients with end-stage renal failure. *Transplantation* 1990;49:100–103.

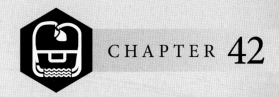

CHAPTER 42

The Geriatric Dialysis Patient

Yusra Cheema and Wendy Weinstock Brown

The dialysis population in the United States continues to grow, and the elderly constitute the most rapidly expanding segment of this population. Care of the elderly patient with kidney disease is particularly challenging, both because of the increased number of comorbid conditions that tend to be present and because these conditions are superimposed on the anatomic and physiologic changes seen with normal aging (1,2). Many elderly patients do not tolerate rapid changes in volume or electrolytes, and many have impaired or atypical responses to medications; stress; intercurrent illness; and changes in diet, mobility, and environment (2–9). Importantly, age alone should not be a contraindication to renal replacement therapies, especially as not all individuals age biologically at the same rate (6,10–14).

This chapter discusses the incidence, prevalence, and demographics of kidney failure in the elderly; summarizes morbidity and mortality in these individuals; reviews causes of kidney failure in the elderly; and addresses special issues in the elderly kidney failure patient including timing of dialysis initiation, modality choice, dialysis access considerations, and comorbid conditions such as cognitive impairment and depression.

DEMOGRAPHIC CHARACTERISTICS OF THE GERIATRIC POPULATION WITH END-STAGE KIDNEY DISEASE

Incidence and Prevalence of End-Stage Kidney Disease in the Elderly

When the Medicare end-stage kidney disease (ESKD) program was funded in 1973, individuals receiving dialysis comprised the healthiest, most motivated, and youngest segment of the population with kidney failure. The advent of systematic funding of ESKD care in the United States widened the availability of renal replacement therapies

and rendered committees judging "Who Shall Live and Who Shall Die" obsolete. Renal replacement therapies have now become available to all segments of the population, including the elderly (15).

Patients older than 65 years represent a rapidly growing segment of the population with ESKD in North America, Europe, Australia, and Japan (10,16–19). This is particularly notable among octogenarians and nonagenarians (FIGURE 42.1). In the United States, from 1995 to 2004, there was a greater than 60% increase in incident dialysis patients 80 years and older, such that in 2004, approximately 28,000 individuals in this age-group initiated dialysis (21). In more recent years, incident cases of ESKD in those aged 75 years and older appear to have plateaued, but the incidence rate remains highest in this age-group (21). However, these oldest old comprise a fraction of the elderly hemodialysis (HD) population; in 2011 to 2012, there were 56,000 incident patients with ESKD 65 years or older, representing 50% of the incident U.S. dialysis population.

Despite higher mortality rates and lower life expectancy, the rise in the elderly dialysis population in the United States is seen in prevalent as well as incident HD patients. In 2012, there were 244,324 individuals age 65 years and older prevalent in the ESKD program compared with 166,695 patients in 2004. This comprises 38% of prevalent patients with ESKD (includes individuals with a functioning transplant) and 44% of prevalent dialysis patients. The very elderly (over age 75 years) on dialysis numbered more than 94,000 (21% of the dialysis population). Although the rise in the total number of dialysis patients in the United States is apparent in all age-groups, with the prevalent dialysis population increasing from 335,000 in 2004 to 450,000 in 2012, the largest proportional increase (50%) is seen among individuals 75 years and older (FIGURE 42.2) (20).

As with younger patients, there remains a disproportionate, *albeit* far less marked, overrepresentation of ethnic minorities in the elderly U.S. population with ESKD. Although African Americans comprise

701

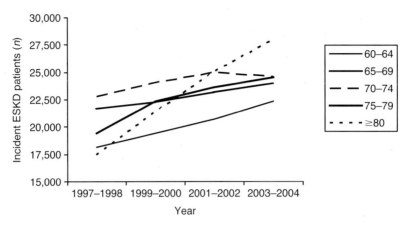

FIGURE 42.1 Incident cases with end-stage kidney disease (ESKD) in the United States among individuals aged 60 years or older (20).

35.5% of the incident population with ESKD younger than 65 years, they comprise only 22.8% of the population with ESKD 65 years and older and just 17.3% of octogenarians and nonagenarians. A similar pattern is seen for those of Hispanic ethnicity (both African American and non–African American Hispanics), where the proportion of incident Hispanic dialysis patients declines as the population ages from more than 17% in individuals younger than 65 years to 11% among individuals aged 70 to 75 years and fewer than 9% among those 80 years and older (20). The reasons for this demographic shift are not known.

Causes of End-Stage Kidney Disease in the Elderly

Similar to the population as a whole, the most common causes of ESKD in the elderly are diabetes and hypertension. Among individuals 50 to 69 years old, diabetes is the primary cause in 50% and hypertension in 23%. In contrast, hypertension is reported as the primary cause in 38% of incident dialysis patients 70 years and older and in 46% of patients 80 years and older (**FIGURE 42.3**). This

pattern is similar for prevalent dialysis patients (**FIGURE 42.3**). Notably, diabetes is increasingly the primary cause of incident ESKD in individuals both older and younger than 70 years (20). Unfortunately, due to the reluctance to biopsy elderly patients, even in the presence of common indications for biopsy including nephrotic-range proteinuria and unexplained kidney failure, elderly patients with treatable causes of kidney failure may go underdiagnosed and therefore untreated (17,22–24). This may explain the high prevalence of hypertension as the primary cause of kidney failure as this diagnosis is often indicated in the absence of other known causes. Critically, elderly patients with atypical presentations of ESKD should be evaluated for treatable causes of kidney disease just as younger patients are.

Mortality in End-Stage Kidney Disease in the Elderly

Although mortality is higher in the elderly ESKD population compared to their younger counterparts, elderly individuals with ESKD

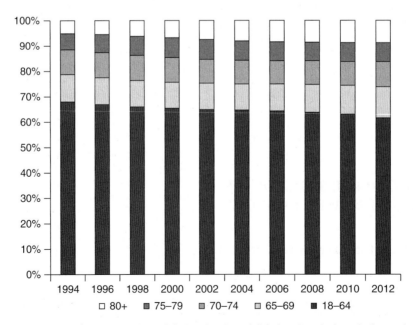

FIGURE 42.2 Prevalence rates of elderly hemodialysis and peritoneal dialysis patients in the United States from 2003 to 2012 as a proportion of the adult dialysis population.

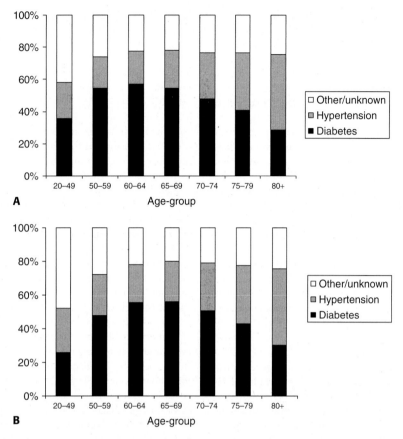

FIGURE 42.3 The primary cause of end-kidney renal disease (ESKD) among incident **(A)** and prevalent **(B)** dialysis patients in 2004. (From United States Renal Data System. *Annual Data Report: Atlas of End-Stage Renal Disease in the United States.* Bethesda, MD: National Institute of Diabetes, Digestive and Kidney Diseases, 2006.)

do surprisingly well on dialysis. In 2003, median survival was 16 months for individuals aged 80 to 84 years but dropped to less than a year for those 85 years and older. This compared with median survival of 24 months among individuals aged 65 to 79 years initiating dialysis in the United States (25). More recent data from the Dialysis Outcomes and Practice Patterns Study (DOPPS) demonstrates a median survival of 3 years for those patients starting dialysis after age 75 years compared to 6 years for those aged 45 to 74 years old (26).

This pattern is similar in other countries, and, with careful management, many elderly dialysis patients accommodate well to ESKD and maintain reasonably good quality of life (27–30). In Italy, patients initiating dialysis at age 65 years or older (mean 71.3 years) had a survival rate of 82.7% at 1 year and 62.3% at 2 years (31). In Spain, dialysis patients aged 65 to 85 years had the same mortality rate as the age-matched general population (32). A German study of 76 patients starting dialysis after age 80 years reported 1-year survival of 87% and 3-year survival of 52%. They noted improved outcomes linked with duration of predialysis nephrology care (33). In the very elderly dialysis population in Japan, the median survival in those 80 to 84 years old, 85 to 89 years old, and >90 years old was 3 years, 2.5 years, and 0.9 years, respectively (19). In a retrospective analysis from the United Kingdom, patients starting dialysis after age 80 years had 1-year survival of 78.5%, whereas the median time to death for those who pursued maximum conservative therapy for their advanced kidney disease was 6 months. However, these results may have been skewed by some selection bias (34). Röhrich et al.

(35) note that in their practice, there has been a progressive increase in mean survival time for patients who begin treatment when older than 80 years, from 22.7 months before 1990 to 28.3 months after 1990; they opine that this is due to improvements in dialysis techniques, diet, and anemia therapy. Despite these outcomes, a survey of physicians in the United Kingdom conducted in 1996 showed that a previously healthy octogenarian would not be referred for dialysis by 68% of primary care physicians or accepted for dialysis by 28% of nephrologists (36). Given the growth in the elderly dialysis population, it appears that these practices are changing.

Dialysis Modality

Elderly individuals initiating dialysis in the United States overwhelmingly receive HD. Compared to incident patients with ESKD younger than 65 years where 82.8%, 10.0%, and 3.8% initiated renal replacement therapy with HD, peritoneal dialysis (PD), and transplant, respectively, patients with ESKD 65 years and older had rates of 89.8%, 5.8%, and 0.9%, respectively, in 2012. This trend is most marked in the oldest patients with ESKD, where only 4.8% initiated renal replacement therapy with PD (21).

◆ INDICATIONS FOR INITIATION OF DIALYSIS

Chronic Dialysis

The decision to initiate dialysis in the elderly is multifaceted, requiring careful weighing of advantages and disadvantages associated with this lifesaving modality. Unfortunately, many patients are not referred to nephrologists with sufficient time for careful decision making for initiating dialysis or determination of the optimal modality should the patient decide to initiate dialysis therapy. Non-nephrologist physicians may not be aware that elderly patients are candidates for dialysis therapy and may not recognize the severity of their kidney dysfunction, potentially leading to late referral. After adjusting for comorbid conditions, Mignon et al. (37) found that the increased mortality observed in the elderly in the first 3 months of dialysis correlated with late referral. It has been questioned whether earlier initiation of dialysis in the elderly may reduce this excess early mortality, but studies have not been conclusive. Meta-analyses certainly do not support the idea of initiating HD at a higher glomerular filtration rate (GFR), but there may be benefit to starting peritoneal dialysis earlier (24,38,39).

Determining when to initiate dialysis in elderly patients can be challenging due to problems of assessing kidney function in this population and the overlapping symptoms of uremia with other chronic or acute conditions common in the elderly. Decreased protein intake and loss of muscle mass lead to maintenance of the serum creatinine values despite an approximately 10% decrease in GFR per decade after the age of 40 years (40). Estimating equations, such as the Modification of Diet in Renal Disease (MDRD) study equation, are developed to accommodate this age-related change in creatinine generation (41,42). Although used widely, the MDRD equation tends to overestimate GFR in the elderly and recently has been shown to be less accurate than the newer Chronic Kidney Disease-Epidemiology Collaboration (CKD-epi) and Berlin Initiative Study (BIS) equations (43). In addition, GFR-estimating equations cannot account for accelerated muscle loss that may occur with very frail or sick patients and therefore tend to overestimate actual GFR in such patients. Cystatin C, a filtration marker that is not generated from muscle, has been posited to be a better marker than creatinine, especially in the elderly. However, we now know that there are non-GFR determinants of cystatin C levels, making its utility as a sole filtration marker similar to that of serum creatinine. The most accurate GFR estimation equations in the elderly appear to be those that include both serum cystatin C and creatinine measurements (43).

In addition, symptoms often attributed to uremia are commonly seen in other chronic conditions in the elderly. Porush and Faubert (16) evaluated the signs and symptoms present before initiation of maintenance dialysis in 118 elderly patients. The most common symptoms were anorexia and weight loss (61%), generalized weakness (58%), encephalopathy (49%), and nausea and vomiting (41%), many of which are seen in other diseases. Some potential indications for a trial of dialysis in the elderly are listed in **TABLE 42.1**. There are several reasons why nephrologists may not initiate dialysis in an elderly person. In particular, it may be appropriate not to

initiate dialysis in patients with dementia given the need for cooperation to safely deliver adequate dialysis.

Acute Dialysis

The effect of age as an independent risk factor for development, mortality, and prognosis in acute kidney injury (AKI) has been well established (44–51). In a study of critically ill patients, there was a 20% greater rate of AKI in those patients greater than 75 years compared with the age-group of 18 to 54 years (52). An analysis of Medicare data showed that for the years 1992 to 2001, the overall incidence rate of AKI was 23.8 cases per 1,000 discharges, with rates increasing by approximately 11% per year. Older age, male gender, and African American race were strongly associated ($p < 0.0001$) with AKI (53). Subsequent data has demonstrated a further increase in incidence of AKI across all ages and races from 2000 to 2009 (52). As advanced age is a strong risk factor, this increase in AKI to some extent is explained by the overall growth in the elderly population (44,51). Other contributing factors include higher incidence of comorbidities such as hypertension, cardiovascular disease, and chronic kidney disease (CKD), in addition to exposures such as surgery, sepsis, and nephrotoxic medications (44,45,54).

In addition to age, prognosis in AKI appears related to the presence of comorbid conditions, cause of the acute illness, oliguria, requirement for dialysis, and number of nephrotoxic events (44,45,47,54–57). In the analysis of Medicare patients described earlier, the in-hospital mortality rates were 15% and 33% in discharges with AKI diagnostic codes as the principal and secondary diagnosis, respectively, compared to 5% without a diagnosis code for AKI. Death within 90 days of hospital admission was 35% and 49% in discharges with AKI as the principal and secondary diagnosis, respectively, compared to 13% in discharges without AKI (46). Among cases of AKI, mortality was greatest in the oldest patients (52,58). In critically ill patients with AKI, in-hospital mortality was 24% versus 13.9% when comparing the oldest patients (>75 years) to the youngest (<54 years). This trend continued to the 90-day point with mortality rates of 35.7% versus 17.2% in the oldest versus youngest groups (52). In terms of renal recovery, a meta-analysis of 17 studies demonstrated advancing age to be a negative predictor of renal recovery (59). Kane-Gill et al. (52) noted an overall renal recovery rate at 90 days of 31%, but patients aged 18 to 54 had a 15.8% higher rate of recovery compared with those over age 75 years.

There is frequently reluctance to initiate dialysis in an elderly individual with AKI and multiple medical or psychosocial disorders because of the fear of committing the patient to chronic long-term dialysis or because of ethical concerns (60). In fact, despite the highest incidence of AKI, patients over age 75 years are least likely to receive renal replacement therapy (RRT) (52). However, while elderly survivors of AKI seem to require more time for total recovery and recover function less completely, dialysis should not be automatically withheld. These patients should be involved in a shared decision-making process with the nephrologist and a trial of dialysis should be considered following a discussion of overall prognosis, comorbidities, functional status, and perceived risks and benefits of RRT (45,60–62).

CHOOSING A RENAL REPLACEMENT THERAPY MODALITY

Hemodialysis versus Peritoneal Dialysis

As in younger populations, factors affecting the selection modality for treatment of ESKD in the elderly include patient or physician preference, availability of trained personnel, proximity to a dialysis

TABLE 42.1	Indications for a Trial of Dialysis in the Elderly

Uremia
Potentially reversible acute renal failure
Unexplained dementia or cognitive impairment
Unexplained worsening of congestive heart failure
Personality change
Irritability, irascibility, or newly subdued demeanor
Adult failure to thrive
Change in sense of well-being

center, concurrent illnesses or comorbid conditions, and specific contraindications to a particular modality. Potential advantages of PD in the elderly include better preservation of renal function, avoidance of large volume or electrolyte shifts leading to improved cardiovascular stability, allowance of a more liberal diet, avoidance of vascular access, decreased transportation time, and ease of travel and holiday times (63). Patients who tolerate HD poorly because of cardiovascular disease or difficulty with vascular access also may do better with PD (64,65), whereas HD may be a better choice for patients with inguinal or abdominal hernias, diverticulitis, compromised peritoneal surface area secondary to abdominal surgery or adhesions, abdominal aortic aneurysm, morbid obesity, or physical or psychosocial inability to perform PD (9). Many patients find PD more compatible with an independent lifestyle and desire active participation in their treatment, whereas others find the responsibility of self-care overwhelming. There may be age bias in this selection process (66).

There are conflicting reports as to the survival advantage of one modality over another in elderly patients. In a small European study of patients older than 70 years, the annual mortality rates in PD versus HD were similar (26.1 vs. 26.4 deaths per 100 person-years) (67). However, other analyses in the United States have suggested increased mortality rates for those on PD, particularly among the elderly and those with diabetes (68–70). A study of 1,041 patients beginning HD and PD in 81 dialysis clinics in 19 U.S. states showed an increased risk for mortality for PD patients after the first year of dialysis with no difference based on patient age (71). Recent large cohort studies have provided more clarity on the issue. In an analysis of all incident dialysis patients between 1996 and 2004 in the United States, Mehrotra et al. (72) demonstrated no significant difference in risk of death between those treated with HD or PD in the cohort of patients beginning dialysis after 2002. The increased mortality that had previously been seen in PD patients decreased over time, suggesting that advances in PD have seemingly closed this survival gap between HD and PD. In concordance with prior studies however, the subset of diabetic patients over age 65 years continued to have an increased risk of death with PD (72). In a large study of all incident dialysis patients in the United States, Weinhandl et al. (73) used a propensity-matching scheme to compare HD versus PD survival given the inability to have a true randomized trial. Their results support the finding of decreased survival with PD versus HD in patients >65 years of age, diabetics, and those with cardiovascular disease (73). It has been suggested that poor nutritional status in diabetic PD patients may account for increased mortality (74). Excess mortality for elderly PD patients is relevant in consideration of appropriate treatment modality and must be included in the equation along with considerations of comorbidity, quality of life, distance from center, and other issues.

Peritoneal Dialysis in the Elderly

In the United States, 8.1%, 6.4%, 5.9%, and 4.9% of dialysis patients aged 20 to 44 years, 45 to 64 years, 65 to 74 years, and older than 75 years are on PD compared to 49.7%, 60.2%, 70.0%, and 86.1% on HD (20). Other countries have a higher use of PD, likely in part, due to geographic and financial considerations. In Hong Kong, Mexico, and New Zealand, for example, 74%, 49%, and 33% of patients are on PD, respectively (20). In most countries, PD use decreases as patients age, especially for the older-than-75-year age-group; exceptions are New Zealand and Iceland, where 60% and 47% of patients aged 75 years or older were treated with PD as of 2004 (75). Worldwide use of home HD also decreases dramatically with age;

in-center HD is the predominant modality for dialysis patients older than 65 years (**FIGURE 42.4**) (75).

As a home-based modality, PD may help elderly patients with ESKD maintain independence (63). Additionally, in patients with excessive volume gains, hemodynamic instability, or limited vascular access options, PD may be the most desirable ESKD treatment modality for medical reasons. Unfortunately, many elderly patients may perceive limitations in their ability to perform PD; reasons include decreased strength and manual dexterity, vision problems, limitations in mobility, and anxiety. Another limitation, not often considered, is storage space for dialysate and potentially for a cycler; this may assume greater importance in the elderly who often have limited housing options. Finally, assistance from a family member or paramedical staff may be essential (76). Automated PD, such as continuous cyclic peritoneal dialysis (CCPD), or intermittent peritoneal dialysis (IPD) may be a good option for the elderly patient who requires assistance with dialysis, particularly when the assisting spouse or children work during the day (63,77–79).

A recent retrospective cohort study in France analyzed data from all incident PD patients between 2002 and 2010. In comparing those requiring assisted PD (PD performed with assistance of a health care technician, community nurse, or family member) versus self-care PD, they found a lower risk for transfer to HD (80). Those patients requiring assisted PD were generally older (mean age 78 years vs. 56 years), had a higher Charlson Comorbidity Index, and were found to have a higher risk of death attributed to the aforementioned differences between these groups. A cost analysis of this French system found PD, even when requiring assistance, a cheaper alternative to in-center HD (81). In Hong Kong, a comparison of elderly patients on assisted chronic ambulatory peritoneal dialysis (CAPD) and those performing self-care CAPD noted no difference in patient survival, technique survival, or peritonitis-free period between these groups. Two-year survival was 88% in the self-care group and 95% in the assisted group with technique survival rates of 84.7% and 80.9%, respectively (82). In a recent study in Toronto, Canada, when home care assistance was available, only 20% of the elderly population had contraindications to PD, and 59% of those eligible accepted it (83). These experiences suggest a role for assisted PD to safely and effectively increase utilization of PD among the elderly.

Home Hemodialysis in the Elderly

In recent years, there has been increased international interest in home HD as an alternative to both PD and in-center HD. Several nonrandomized studies have shown improved morbidity and mortality, although the magnitude of the advantages may differ on method of delivery (84–86). Home HD requires a high level of functional status and independence by the patient as well as appropriate physical space, support, and resources (84,86). Given the multiple comorbid conditions and common frail status, many elderly patients may not be eligible for this therapy.

In the United States in 2012, 0.4% of dialysis patients aged 65 to 74 years and 0.3% of patients aged 75 years and older chose home HD as their first modality; this is comparable to the very low level of home HD use in other age-groups in the United States (20). Worldwide, the proportion of individuals using home HD declines as the population ages (75,87). Agraharkar et al. (85) suggest that staff-assisted home HD may be an appropriate short-term option for debilitated or terminally ill patients, particularly when ambulance transportation is required. A financial analysis performed in 2002 revealed that staff-assisted home HD was less costly than either in-hospital HD or outpatient HD with ambulance transportation, with a week of

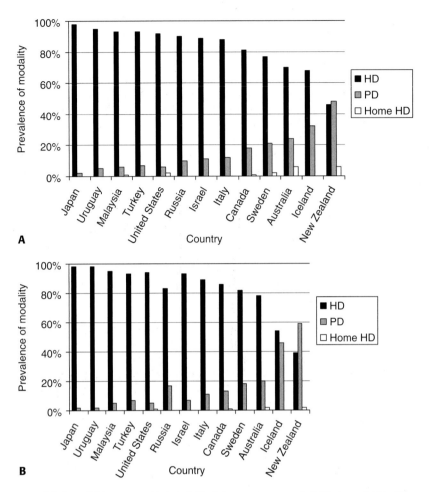

FIGURE 42.4 Dialysis modalities among elderly individuals by country among individuals aged 65 to 74 years **(A)** and older than 75 years **(B)**. HD, hemodialysis; PD, peritoneal dialysis. (From United States Renal Data System. *Annual Data Report: Atlas of End-Stage Renal Disease in the United States.* Bethesda, MD: National Institute of Diabetes, Digestive and Kidney Diseases, 2006.)

staff-assisted home HD costing $1,200 and a week of in-center HD with ambulance transportation costing $2,640 (United States).

Transplant as a Modality for Kidney Replacement in the Elderly

Although low, transplant rates among the elderly have been steadily rising. In 1990, only 1.9% of all transplants in incident ESKD patients occurred in those over the age of 65 years, while in 2002, this number had increased to 7.7%. According to 2012 United States Renal Data System (USRDS) data, 16.6% of incident ESKD patients receiving transplants were between the ages of 65 and 74 years, and 2% were 75 years or older (20).

Recent reports have recognized the benefits of kidney transplantation for carefully selected older patients (88–90). Although elderly transplant recipients have a higher mortality rate than younger patients, they also have a 41% lower risk of death than age-matched patients on the transplant waiting list (89,90). In a 2005 study, the expected survival for dialysis patients over the age of 70 years was 8.2 years for those who received a kidney transplant compared to 4.5 years for those that remained on the wait-list (91). Wolfe et al. (89) showed that the risk of death decreases below the waiting list group by 148 days after transplant in the elderly as compared to 95 days for patients aged 40 to 59 years. Owing to reduced

life expectancy in older adults, death with a functioning graft occurs in 50% of patients older than 65 years, and most grafts last throughout the life of the transplant patient (88,91,92).

Given the heterogeneous population of older patients with ESKD, it may be a challenge for medical providers to decide which patients to recommend for transplant evaluation. Decision to refer a patient for transplant evaluation should be made on an individual basis, independent of age (27,93–96). As in younger patients, kidney transplantation evaluation should be performed to identify conditions that may interfere with surgery, recovery, or the patient's survival after surgery. Advanced peripheral vascular disease and cardiac disease are the most common barriers to kidney transplantation in the elderly. In addition, smoking and obesity may be more important relative contraindications for the elderly (88).

As the population with ESKD has increased, the supply of kidneys has not met demand (88). Practices in the United States and internationally have evolved to meet this demand by creating the expanded criteria donors (ECD) list, a full description of which is beyond the scope of this chapter (88). Port et al.'s (97) analysis of U.S. kidney transplant recipients from 1995 to 2000 shows that it takes 1.5 years for patients to achieve better outcomes from ECD kidneys than from dialysis alone, and Ojo (98) demonstrates that an ECD kidney transplanted to recipients older than 65 years results in 3.8 years of projected additional life span. A recent study by Molnar et al. (99) demonstrated that ECD kidneys were significant predictors of mortality in nonelderly patients (<70 years old), but in the elderly population, there were similar patient and graft survival outcomes when comparing ECD versus non-ECD allografts. It is recommended to use ECD kidneys in older patients, especially those with diabetes, who are shown to have increased benefit from reduced waiting time and may have shorter life expectancies, thereby maximizing the benefit of ECD kidneys (88,89,100).

DIALYSIS TECHNICAL CONSIDERATIONS

Hemodialysis Vascular Access

Following the publication of the first National Kidney Foundation (NKF) Clinical Practice Guideline on vascular access in 2001 (101), the 2005 Fistula First initiative in the United States was promoted as a means to "substantially improve the health of Americans who need kidney dialysis or transplantation" (102). Although fistula rates in the United States increased subsequent to these campaigns, much of this rise is attributable to a precipitous drop in arteriovenous graft (AVG) use with a much more modest decline in catheter use. From 1997 to 2013, fistula prevalence increased from 24% to 68% with a decline in AVG use from 49% to 18% and catheter use from 27% to 15% (103). This has led to a call for a "catheter last" rather than just a "fistula first" strategy (104).

Despite success in increasing fistula prevalence, little progress has been made in reducing catheter use among incident HD patients. In an analysis of the DOPPS from 2012 to 2014, 67% of patients in the United States initiated HD with a catheter, 28% with a fistula, and 5% with an AVG (103). More concerning is the relatively low rate of conversion to use of a graft or fistula, particularly among the elderly. In a report from Centers for Medicare & Medicaid Services ESKD Clinical Performance Project, among individuals who initiated with a catheter, 59% were still catheter dependent, while 15% had transitioned to a fistula and 25% to a graft after 3 months. Critical within this report is that, in adjusted analyses, individuals younger than 50 years had a twofold increased likelihood of converting to arteriovenous fistula (AVF) use compared with patients older than 75 years [odds ratio (OR) 2.14, 95% confidence interval (CI) 1.40 to 3.28], whereas patients between 65 and 74 years of age were 39% more likely to convert to AVG use than continue to use a central venous catheter compared with patients older than 75 years (OR 1.39, 95% CI 1.01 to 1.92) (105).

In this section, the advantages, disadvantages, and special issues associated with permanent vascular access methods in the elderly HD patient are discussed.

Fistulas

Multiple recent studies have focused on the question of ideal HD vascular access in the elderly as there are notable differences in this population compared to younger counterparts. Because of the high prevalence of diabetes, chronic hypertension, and both atherosclerosis and arteriosclerosis, the vascular substrate for access creation is certainly less satisfactory than that in younger patients (106). Not surprisingly, fistulas are less prevalent and catheters are more prevalent in elderly U.S. dialysis patients (**FIGURE 42.5**).

Current Kidney Disease Outcome Quality Initiative (KDOQI) recommendations suggest that a fistula should be placed at least 6 months before the anticipated start of HD treatments. This time frame is suggested to allow for both initial access evaluation as well as additional time for revision to ensure that a working fistula is available at initiation of dialysis therapy (107). In general, a working fistula must have the following characteristics: blood flow adequate to support dialysis (generally greater than 600 mL/min); a diameter greater than 0.6 cm, with location accessible for cannulation and discernible margins to allow for repetitive cannulation; and a depth of approximately 0.6 cm (ideally, between 0.5 to 1.0 cm from the skin surface). Determination of whether a fistula is likely to function may take up to 2 months, and adequate maturity for cannulation as much as 4 months, particularly with upper arm access in individuals with small veins at baseline. Not unexpectedly, the primary failure rate of fistulas may be higher in elderly patients and further attempts at fistula creation may be needed, resulting in a longer duration from initial fistula creation to successful fistula use. It is easy to foresee that this process may take a year or more, even with a dedicated access team. Does this mean that fistula creation should occur even earlier in the elderly? On an individual patient level, it makes sense—the earlier the fistula creation, the more attempts can be made to obtain successful access. However, particularly in the elderly, the earlier a fistula is created, the more likely it is that a patient will die of other causes before requiring dialysis (108). The competing risk of death increases with increasing age; Lee et al. (109) found in a cohort of 3,418 elderly (>70 years old) CKD patients who had predialysis access created, 67% started dialysis within 2 years. However, when

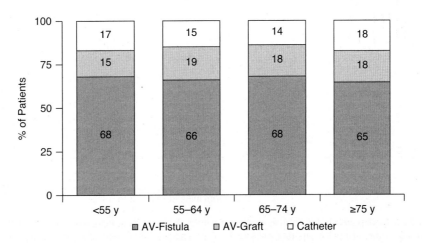

FIGURE 42.5 Vascular access use among a cross-section of U.S. prevalent patients by age. (From Pisoni RL, Zepel L, Port FK, et al. Trends in US vascular access use, patient preferences, and related practices: an update from the US DOPPS Practice Monitor with international comparisons. *Am J Kidney Dis* 2015;65:905–915.)

stratified further by age, 69% of those aged 70 to 74 years initiated dialysis within 2 years with only 12% dying before requiring dialysis, while for those over the age of 85, 21.9% died before requiring dialysis with 60% initiating dialysis within the 2-year follow-up period (109). Furthermore, a recent study evaluating the optimal timing of fistula placement in the elderly concluded that there appears to be little benefit of placing access more than 6 to 9 months prior to anticipated need to start dialysis. The likelihood of initiating dialysis with a functioning fistula increased with fistula creation greater than 3 to 6 months prior to starting dialysis but plateaued after the 6- to 9-month range. In addition, the number of interventional access procedures increased over time, greatest in those who had fistulas placed >12 months predialysis (110). In another study of individuals 75 years and older, the number of access surgeries needed to allow one elder to initiate dialysis with a functioning fistula ranged from 8 to 12 procedures when surgery was performed at a GFR of 25 mL/min/1.73 m^2 or lower to two to three surgeries at a threshold of 15 mL/min/1.73 m^2 within a 6-month time frame (108).

A large study of fistula placement in an elderly population retrospectively evaluated access success among 196 patients aged 65 years and older and 248 patients younger than 65 years (111). There was a 64.8% primary and 75.1% cumulative fistula patency at 1 year among patients 65 years and older. This was comparable to that seen in younger patients. However, fistulas in the elderly group were more likely to have maturation failure with a relative risk of 1.7 compared to the <65 group. It is notable that analysis by anatomic type showed better survival of radiocephalic fistulas in the younger cohort, which had been described previously (112).

Fistula success can be maintained in an elderly population. Although Leapman et al. (113) demonstrated only 40% patency rates at 1 year among patients 70 years or older, many others reported better results. Wing et al. (114) reported 80% 1-year fistula survival in individuals older than 65 years, whereas Berardinelli et al. (112)

described 78% 3-year patency for upper arm fistulas and 57% patency for forearm fistulas. Konner et al. (115) describe excellent 1-year primary access survival of first AVFs for nondiabetic patients 65 years and older (73% for women, 77% for men) and diabetic patients 65 years and older (78% women, 81% men) with use of either forearm AVFs or perforating vein or nonperforating vein fistulas at the elbow.

Grafts

Prosthetic grafts have a higher stenosis rate and a higher infection rate than AVFs (see Chapter 3) (106). The most common cause of graft loss is uncorrected stenosis with associated thrombosis (116). This is probably not different in the elderly. As in younger patients, it is vital to look for underlying cause(s) of thrombosis and try to correct them (16,106,117). Although KDOQI guidelines favor active access monitoring of AVGs, small studies have failed to show a consistent benefit in graft survival.

Tunneled Catheters

An indwelling central double-lumen cuffed catheter or twin single-lumen tunneled cuffed catheters may be the preferred intermediate or long-term access for some patients (118,119), in particular, those individuals who lack adequate vessels for fistula or graft creation, individuals with limited life expectancy, and individuals prone to steal syndrome with severe high-output heart failure unable to tolerate AVFs or grafts; these situations are all more common in the elderly than in younger patients.

One Strategy for Access in Geriatric Dialysis Patients

There are no clinical trials to guide therapeutic decisions for dialysis access in the elderly. Numerous studies have found that survival among incident dialysis patients with a functioning AVF is superior to that with a catheter or graft; however, survival with a graft is far superior to that with a catheter (**FIGURE 42.6**) (120). A large recent

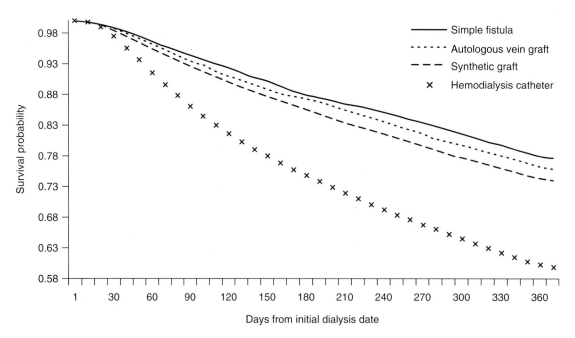

FIGURE 42.6 Survival probability by dialysis access type at initiation among Medicare recipients in 1995, 1996, and 1997: age 67 years and older, adjusted for age, race, sex, year, blood urea nitrogen (BUN), creatinine, albumin, diabetes, and time since access placement. [Xue JL, Dahl D, Ebben JP, et al. The association of initial hemodialysis access type with mortality outcomes in elderly Medicare ESRD patients. *Am J Kidney Dis* 2003;42(5):1013–1019.]

analysis of outcomes in elderly patients (>67 years old) based on predialysis access placement found no significant mortality difference between those patients who had a fistula placed as initial access versus those with AVG placement (121). When stratified further by age, it appeared there was a survival benefit for those ages 67 to 79 years with initial fistula placement compared with those with an AVG, but this disappeared in those greater than 80 years old. Importantly, of those with a fistula as their predialysis access, only 50.7% initiated dialysis with an AVF, the remainder required catheter placement. In those with an AVG as predialysis access, only 25.4% required conversion to catheter at time of dialysis initiation. This increased conversion to catheter use likely limits the prior benefits associated with "Fistula First" in the elderly. Another key variable as described by O'Hare et al. (108) is that many elderly individuals either do not progress to kidney failure or die before requiring dialysis. On the basis of clinical experience, observational data, and KDOQI guidelines, the authors favor the approach presented in TABLE 42.2 for individuals receiving care before kidney failure, taking into consideration life expectancy and expected time until dialysis will be required. This strategy should allow for at least one revision in the setting of primary access failure and allows the surgeons to progressively work their way up the arm. Finally, although a forearm access may not become usable for dialysis, often

---

TABLE 42.2	**Strategies for Vascular Access in Elderly Individuals with Stage 4 to 5 Chronic Kidney Disease**

For all patients
1. Nephrology referral by onset of stage 4 CKD (eGFR <30 mL/min/1.73 m^2)
2. Discussion of modality choice at onset of stage 4 CKD

For patients referred before need for renal replacement therapy
1. Ultrasonographic artery and vein mapping of both arms to facilitate a hemodialysis access plan
   a. If unsuccessful, contrast venography can be considered.
   b. Use very low volume of contrast and premedication.
2. Avoidance of venipuncture in the designated extremity based on vein mapping
3. Assessment of life expectancy (no tools available at this time to assist)
   a. Poor life expectancy (<2 y); place AV graft ~3–4 months before expected dialysis initiation, preferably a forearm loop graft in the nondominant arm
   b. Good life expectancy (≥2 y); place AV fistula at least 1 year before expected dialysis initiation, beginning with a forearm fistula if the vessels are viable

For incident or prevalent elderly dialysis patients with a catheter for access
1. Ultrasonographic artery and vein mapping of both arms or contrast venography to facilitate a hemodialysis access plan
2. Avoidance of venipuncture in the designated extremity based on vein mapping
3. Assessment of life expectancy (no tools available at this time to assist)
   a. Poor life expectancy (<1–2 y); place AV graft, preferably a forearm loop graft in the nondominant arm
   b. Good life expectancy (≥1–2 y); place AV fistula, beginning with a forearm fistula if the vessels are viable

CKD, chronic kidney disease; eGFR, estimated glomerular filtration rate; AV, arteriovenous.

---

times in the setting of inflow stenosis, early creation may facilitate more rapid maturation of an upper arm outflow vein, especially when anastomosed to the larger caliber upper arm brachial artery.

A similar approach can be taken in elderly individuals initiating dialysis with a catheter, especially as it was demonstrated in a *post hoc* analysis of Hemodialysis (HEMO) Study data that changing vascular access type from a catheter to a fistula or graft was associated with a substantially lower risk for mortality compared with continuous use of a catheter, whereas changing from a fistula or graft to a catheter was associated with more than a twofold greater death rate compared with patients who used a fistula or a graft throughout the study (122). A strategy for incident or prevalent elderly dialysis patients with a catheter for access is also summarized in TABLE 42.2. The rationale behind these time frames is that the median survival of an AVG for individuals initiating dialysis with a functioning graft is more than 1 year (123), indicating that in individuals with limited life expectancy, it may be a beneficial trade-off to have higher initial success rates as seen with grafts than higher long-term access survival rates seen with a fistula.

Peritoneal Dialysis Access and Performance

Catheter Survival

In the early days of CAPD experience (1982), Ponce et al. (124) found decreased 2-year peritoneal catheter survival (67% vs. 78%) and increased pericatheter dialysate leakage (42.3% vs. 26.9%) in patients older than 60 years compared with younger patients. They hypothesized that the difference was secondary to "loose abdominal walls." Because more than 90% of dialysate leaks occurred within the first week of insertion (catheters were used immediately) and leakage resolved if the catheter was not used for 1 to 2 weeks, catheters are usually inserted 2 to 3 weeks before use, with temporary HD if necessary, until the insertion site is completely healed. If it is necessary to use the catheter earlier, small frequent exchanges are employed with the patient in the supine position, gradually increasing in volume once integrity has been established (10).

Contrary to earlier findings, recent studies support the finding that catheter survival is either equivalent or improved in older versus younger patients (65,125,126). Kim et al. (127), in a retrospective multiyear comparison of peritoneal catheter survival with arteriovenous access, found greater long-term peritoneal access than arteriovenous access patency, particularly in diabetic patients and the elderly. Gentile (125) observed fewer catheter-related complications in elderly patients than in younger patients.

Peritonitis

Several large studies reveal no differences in peritonitis rates between young and old PD patients (10,65,125,126,128–130). Nissenson et al. (126), in a large two-center study, reported that after 1 year of CAPD, 60% of patients younger than 60 years were free of peritonitis versus 65% of the patients older than 60 years. At 3 years, the figures were 38% and 46%, respectively, and at 7 years, 30% and 38%. Nolph et al. (128) found an increased incidence of peritonitis in bedridden patients, although there was no increase in exit-site and tunnel infection rates or catheter replacements. A recent study evaluated first year outcomes in incident peritoneal dialysis patients and reported the highest rate of peritonitis among those aged 55 to 65 years old (43 per 100 patient-years) with lower rates in those younger than 55 and older than 65 years (131). See Chapter 37 for further discussion of peritonitis in CAPD patients.

Exit-Site and Tunnel Infections

There is little difference in exit-site infection rates (10,128), tunnel infections (65,128), or dialysate drainage pain in young versus elderly CAPD patients (10,132).

Adequacy

Poor adequacy may be related to poor drainage. This may be commonly caused by constipation in the elderly and can be treated with laxatives or catheter reinsertion. There are no reports as to differences in membrane characteristics by age.

Automated Peritoneal Dialysis

The use of automated or assisted PD can facilitate the use of this therapy even in patients with apraxia, cognitive difficulties, or even a person with disability treated either at home or at a nursing home.

SPECIAL SITUATIONS IN THE ELDERLY DIALYSIS PATIENT

Compliance with Therapy

There are little data evaluating compliance with dialysis prescriptions and lifestyle among the elderly. Recently, however, a recent large retrospective study of over 180,000 HD patients found that missed treatments were more frequent among younger patients (133). Avram et al. (134) describe a positive correlation between increased age and lower intradialytic weight gain, lower serum creatinine, and lower urea generation rate for both HD and PD patients, whereas McKevitt et al. (135) noted that dialysis patients aged 60 years and older demonstrated good compliance with potassium restriction, fair to good compliance for serum phosphorus, and fair to poor compliance with fluid restriction. Many factors may influence compliance among the elderly. These include cognitive impairment, visual impairment, depression, and social support. Therefore, individualized approaches to compliance and social support for the elderly dialysis patient, including evaluation of physiologic and psychosocial factors are essential for dialysis success (135–137).

Infection

Abnormalities of Immune Function with Aging

The altered immune status of uremia (138,139) is complicated in many elderly patients by similar changes in the immune system that may occur with aging, including increased susceptibility to infection and malignancy (140), and abnormalities in lymphocyte function and cell-mediated and humoral immunity (141,142). Whether there is a specific interaction with age, such that the double hit of uremia and aging synergistically enhances the risk of infection, is unknown. Whereas an older Israeli study found that infection was the most common cause of death in patients beginning dialysis at age 80 years or older, USRDS data reveal that, among prevalent U.S. dialysis patients aged 75 years and older, cardiovascular disease was 4 times more often the cause of death than infection from 2010 to 2012 (20,143).

Manifestations of Infection in the Elderly

In addition to changes in immune responsiveness, the presentation of infection in elderly patients is often subtle (see Chapter 37). The elderly patient may not manifest fever or leukocytosis, and even severe processes like acute abdomens may have less apparent manifestations. Similarly, elderly dialysis patients may manifest occult infection in subtle ways, including anorexia, apparent depression,

vague feelings of malaise, apparent development of dementia, or decreased ability to cope with the usual activities of daily living. Occasionally, the only indication of infection is an increase in predialysis blood urea nitrogen (BUN) levels without any apparent change in clinical status (144). Notably, urinary tract infections are common in the elderly but may be overlooked as a potential source in dialysis patients (145,146). Successful treatment of infection is generally associated with a return to the previous level of function.

Nutrition
Nutrition and Outcomes

It is particularly important to emphasize adequate nutrition in the older dialysis patient. The presence of protein-energy wasting and serum albumin levels have been shown to be independent predictors of mortality in dialysis patients (147). Both serum albumin and prealbumin predict hospitalization and mortality due to infection (148). Whether reduced nutritional indices are a marker of infection or indicate individuals predisposed to infection is unknown, although Kalantar-Zadeh and Kopple (149) postulate the existence of a "malnutrition inflammation complex syndrome" in maintenance dialysis patients with protein-energy malnutrition that predisposes to illness and infection and leads to poor quality of life and increased morbidity and mortality.

Strategies to Enhance Nutrition in Elderly Dialysis Patients

Some causes of nutritional impairment and strategies to enhance good nutrition in elderly dialysis patients are listed in TABLE 42.3 (150). Many of these strategies are self-explanatory. Patients who are disabled or living alone may benefit from programs such as meals-on-wheels, which deliver one or two prepared meals per day to the patient's home and can accommodate a prescribed diet. Home assistance

TABLE 42.3	Nutrition in Elderly Dialysis Patients	
Challenges	**Strategies**
Dialysis associated	
• Loss of nutrients by dialysis	Multivitamin formulated for dialysis
• Catabolism	High protein diet and supplements
Common comorbid conditions	
• Impaired absorption	Assess medications
• Gastroparesis	Promotility agents
• Dentition	Dental care
• Constipation	Bowel regimen (sorbitol, lactulose, senna)
Food security	
• Low income	Meals on wheels, and so forth
• Access to food	Involve friends and family in care
• Food preparation	Common dining Home services
Other	
• Anorexia	Assess and treat depression
• Dysgeusia	Adequate dialysis Megestrol and other appetite stimulants Consider reducing dietary restrictions, zinc supplementation

services that provide aides to prepare meals, shop for groceries, and/ or provide companionship can be very helpful. Patients with poor intake may benefit from liberalized diets at the expense of permitting higher potassium and/or phosphate levels. The benefit of oral intradialytic nutritional supplementation remains controversial, but more recent observational data demonstrate an association between protein supplementation and reduced mortality, irrespective of serum albumin levels (151). Patients with diabetic gastroparesis may benefit from metoclopramide, 5 to 10 mg orally administered 30 minutes before meals. Zinc deficiency can occur in dialysis patients and may be associated with dysgeusia; supplementation may enhance the taste of food (152). Megestrol acetate can stimulate appetite in selected patients (153). Good oral hygiene is also very important. It is difficult for elderly patients to eat properly if they have sore gums, poor dentition, or poorly fitting dentures. Depression and constipation, both of which inhibit appetite, must also be treated. Finally, a thorough review of the patient's medication list may reveal a large number of prescribed pills. Consolidating or eliminating unnecessary and less necessary medications may be associated with improved appetite.

Pruritus

Pruritus is one of the most common and distressing cutaneous symptoms of CKD. CKD-associated pruritus may be difficult to differentiate from pruritus caused by nonrenal comorbidities frequently associated with CKD, such as liver and thyroid disease (154). In the Japanese Dialysis Outcomes Practice Patterns Study (JDOPPS) (1999–2008), pruritus was associated with a 22% higher mortality risk; unlike prior studies, this effect was not attenuated after adjusting for sleep quality measures, likely indicating that the systemic adverse effects of pruritus are not completely mediated by sleep abnormalities (155). Pruritus was also associated with significantly lower mental and physical quality of life scores. In the JDOPPS, older age was a modest but significant risk factor for dialysis-associated pruritus.

First-line treatments include topical therapies such as emollients, particularly those with a high water content, capsaicin creams, and potentially bath oil containing polidocanol. Other topical therapies include bathing less frequently using tepid rather than hot water and increasing ambient humidity with vaporizers or humidifiers. Many systemic medications, including antihistamines (diphenhydramine or hydroxyzine), gabapentin, and opioid (κ-receptor) agonists, have been successfully used to treat CKD-associated pruritus, but the sedative effects of these medications may cause confusion in elderly patients.

Chronic Pain and Pain Management

Chronic pain and management of that pain is a major problem in the elderly dialysis patient. As expected, pain is a common symptom experienced by dialysis patients, relating both to underlying medical conditions like osteoarthritis common in all elderly individuals and also related to conditions more common in CKD, including bone pain in hyperparathyroidism, frequent medical procedures, neuropathy, and cramping related to the dialysis procedure itself (156).

The dialysis population is likely both understudied and undertreated for chronic pain. Reasons for this may include severity of comorbid conditions as well as a justified concern with use of certain medications in dialysis patients. This often results in worsened quality of life and life expectancy. Chronic pain has also been associated with increased likelihood of abbreviated HD sessions and hospitalizations (157). Two recent studies focused specifically on pain in HD patients. A Canadian study found that chronic pain was present in more than

50% of HD patients and that approximately 20% had multiple causes of pain (158). Most remarkable was that pain management was described as ineffective in 75%, and almost 30% of patients were not receiving any analgesic therapy. A second study evaluated the efficacy of the analgesic ladder published by the World Health Organization for the treatment of pain in dialysis and found that adequate analgesia could be obtained in 96% of patients with a stepwise escalation of analgesic therapies but critically noted that pain management was significantly more difficult in the elderly (159). Both these studies used multiple classes of medications for pain management.

On the basis of this limited literature, several items can be extracted: (a) pain is common in ESKD and affects quality of life; (b) pain may be multifactorial; (c) pain control can be accomplished in ESKD with minimal side effects; (d) pain can and should be measured in ESKD and serial assessments can assist treatment; and (e) although there are few absolute contraindications to pain medications in ESKD, there are many precautions in their use. In particular, medications should be dosed appropriate for kidney function and titrated as tolerated.

Bleeding Risk and Anticoagulation Therapy

Despite limited data, major bleeding events are felt to be fairly common in dialysis patients, particularly in the elderly (see Chapter 5). Chester et al. (28) found evidence of gastrointestinal bleeding in 22% of elderly HD patients older than 70 years compared with 7% of younger controls, whereas Porush and Faubert (16) found that gastrointestinal bleeding accounts for 18% of hospital admissions in elderly dialysis patients. The potential causes of increased bleeding risk are manifold but are most notable for (a) platelet dysfunction in uremia; (b) nonsteroidal anti-inflammatory drug and aspirin use for pain management; (c) heparin use during HD; (d) systemic absorption of heparin from catheter-locking solutions; and (e) use of anticoagulation therapies, including warfarin, aspirin, and clopidogrel, to treat comorbid conditions.

Despite the frequency with which anticoagulation therapies are used in the dialysis population, little is truly known about their safety, efficacy, and appropriate use. Warfarin remains the most commonly used agent for systemic anticoagulation, although multiple antiplatelet agents are also in use, in particular aspirin and clopidogrel. Newer anticoagulants such as direct thrombin inhibitors have not been studied in dialysis populations and are not recommended for use currently (160). In the general population, warfarin is indicated for use in individuals with deep venous thromboses, pulmonary embolus, and other severe thrombotic disease; however, its most common use is for stroke prophylaxis in atrial fibrillation. Although current practice favors use of warfarin for thromboembolism prevention in the elderly with atrial fibrillation, recent data stress the bleeding risks. Among individuals between ages 65 and 80 years, risk of major bleeding is 4.7 episodes per 100 person-years, whereas for those aged 80 years and older, the risk is 13.1 per 100 person-years; this risk is highest at initiation of anticoagulation therapy (161). Dialysis patients have reasons to be both at increased bleeding risk as well as increased thrombosis risk, making treatment decisions in atrial fibrillation particularly challenging. In the absence of randomized trials, meta-analyses of retrospective and observational studies provide the best clues to date. In trials chiefly looking at maintaining access patency (for which anticoagulation with warfarin has proved unsuccessful to date), major bleeding episode rates associated with warfarin ranged from 10 to 54 events per patient-year (162). These rates are approximately twice as high as those of HD patients receiving either no warfarin or subcutaneous heparin alone and far exceed rates seen in the elderly nondialysis population. DOPPS data in patients with atrial fibrillation demonstrated an increased risk of stroke in those dialysis patients on warfarin (compared to dialysis patients with atrial fibrillation without anticoagulation) across all age-groups but more so in those over 75 years old (160). A cost–utility analysis used this and other published data to estimate the utility of using aspirin, warfarin, or neither for thromboembolism prophylaxis in dialysis patients with atrial fibrillation. Aspirin and warfarin both prolonged survival compared with no treatment (0.06 and 0.15 quality-adjusted life-years, respectively). Aspirin was associated with an incremental cost-effectiveness ratio of $82,100 per quality-adjusted life-year, whereas warfarin provided additional benefits at an additional cost of $88,400 for each quality-adjusted life-year gained relative to aspirin (163). This study did not specifically examine the elderly. Given the available data, it is not clear that the benefit of anticoagulation for stroke prevention in dialysis patients with atrial fibrillation outweighs the risk; the decision to anticoagulate remains a very individualized one, particularly in the elderly.

Dementia, Depression, and Neuropathies

Cognitive Impairment and Dementia

Cognitive impairment describes a spectrum of mental function extending from subtle alterations to severe dementia and loss of executive functions (see Chapter 33). The two most common causes of dementia in adults are Alzheimer's disease and vascular dementia. The prevalence of dementia in North America was estimated at 6.9% in 2010 with incidence rates ranging from 3.1 per 1,000 patient-years in individuals aged 60 to 64 years to as high as 175 per 1,000 patient-years among individuals 95 years or older (164). About 60% to 80% of these cases are related to Alzheimer's disease, whereas most non-Alzheimer's cases are related to vascular causes. Although more subtle than overt dementia, mild cognitive impairment that does not meet the definition for dementia is also a major public health problem, with a prevalence in individuals aged 65 years and older of 20% or higher (165).

Several studies have examined cognition in HD patients. One investigation found that 70% of patients demonstrated significant cognitive impairment (166). Additionally, dialysis patients had significantly more brain atrophy and cerebrovascular lesions than age-matched controls (167). Murray et al. (168) evaluated 338 prevalent HD patients aged 55 years and older from Minnesota and diagnosed 73% with either moderate or severe cognitive impairment, 14% with mild impairment, and only 13% with no cognitive impairment. In further evaluation of a subset of this cohort, these researchers noted an association between time of testing and cognitive performance, such that cognitive performance during the dialysis procedure itself was inferior to that just before dialysis or on the day between dialysis sessions (169). Another study in a cohort of prevalent HD patients in Boston found that despite relatively well-preserved scores on the Mini Mental State Examination, cognitive impairment was prominent and primarily subcortical in nature; this pattern is consistent with small vessel cerebrovascular disease (170).

Accordingly, several studies have found that dialysis patients are at greater risk for covert or silent ischemic brain disease, defined as infarcts on cranial imaging that are not associated with a clinical syndrome consistent with an acute stroke. These silent infarcts are common in older adults in the general population, and their presence predicts incident dementia, additional strokes, and cognitive and physical decline (171–173). Dialysis patients are particularly high risk, with 5 times greater prevalence in HD patients compared to those without kidney disease (174). Dialysis patients

with subclinical infarcts also have a fourfold increased risk of acute vascular events compared to those without subclinical infarcts in adjusted analyses (175). Similar findings were recently noted in a PD population in Korea, where there was a 68.4% prevalence of silent ischemic brain disease. This high prevalence is striking given that this population was relatively young (mean age of 48 years) and nondiabetic and compared with a prevalence of 17.5% in an age- and sex-matched nondialysis hypertensive control population (176).

In summary, cognitive impairment in dialysis patients impacts both quality of life and the ability to make crucial social, economic, and health-related decisions that affect physical and emotional well-being, including obtaining a kidney transplant. Newer data even suggest an association between decreased cognitive function (particularly executive function and memory) and increased mortality in dialysis patients (177). Because of the complexity of medical and dietary regimens among dialysis patients, clinicians must recognize individuals who will experience difficulty with treatment plans and choices. Whether the dialysis process itself contributes to cognitive impairment, possibly by inducing cerebral ischemia or cerebral edema through intravascular volume loss and fluid shifts, or the high prevalence of cognitive impairment reflects the very high burden of comorbid conditions, including diabetes and cardiovascular disease, is currently unknown (178).

Depression

In recent years, more attention has been paid to the relatively common comorbidity of depression in dialysis patients. It has been estimated that almost 40% of dialysis patients exhibit depressive symptomatology (179). Multiple studies and meta-analyses in recent years have looked at the impact of depression on outcomes in dialysis patients. Although it is challenging to differentiate depression as a cause versus a situational consequence of medical comorbidity, several large studies have demonstrated an association between presence of depressive symptoms and increase in mortality of up to 50% among dialysis patients (179). In one study of patients on a transplant waiting list, depression was associated with worse dialysis compliance (180), and in another study of HD patients, the number of depressive symptoms was directly associated with lower quality of life (181). Although therapy has not been adequately explored, one small Korean study suggests that the combination of antidepressant medication and supportive psychotherapy can successfully treat depression and improve nutritional status in chronic HD patients with depression (182). Unfortunately, there are very little data focusing specifically on elderly dialysis patients and no adequately powered trials looking at depression treatment and outcomes in this population.

Cardiovascular Disease

A full discussion of cardiovascular disease in the geriatric dialysis population is beyond the scope of this chapter and is discussed in Chapters 16 and 17. Of note, elderly individuals may have more autonomic dysfunction and thereby diminished ability to tolerate ultrafiltration during the HD procedure (183). See Chapter 18 for particular problems with dialysis hypotension and selection of the proper dialysate. The elderly represent a dialysis group that is particularly fragile in this regard and may benefit from techniques to minimize intradialytic hypotension including avoidance of low-calcium baths, cool dialysate, and midodrine and consideration of PD.

As in HD patients, volume status and fluid intake must be monitored in PD patients, and patients must be educated about the importance of adjusting their PD prescription to allow for fluid losses from sources such as diarrhea, vomiting, fever, or perspiration.

If hypotension is secondary to poor cardiovascular status, performing small frequent exchanges with a cycler and keeping the abdominal cavity empty during the day may be considered. Meticulous attention to weight gain or loss and adequate salt intake are also important.

SPECIAL SITUATIONS IN THE ELDERLY PERITONEAL DIALYSIS PATIENT

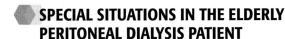

There is a higher incidence of inguinal hernias, fluid leaks, and vascular ischemia of the lower extremities in older PD patients as compared with younger patients (10,184).

Hernias

Inguinal or abdominal hernias may be aggravated by decreased abdominal muscle tone. Kyphosis in the elderly patient may be associated with widening of the diaphragm and subsequent development of a hiatal hernia (10). Hernias may be aggravated by the stress of carrying 2 L or more fluid in the abdominal cavity. Hernias should be repaired, as in a younger patient. If surgical repair is not feasible, it may be possible to continue PD by doing small volume exchanges with a cycler while the patient is recumbent.

Back Pain

Back pain and musculoskeletal disorders in elderly PD patients may be related to decreased abdominal muscle tone, preexisting back pain or lumbar disk disease, obesity, or weight of dialysate in the abdominal cavity (185). Patients may benefit from exercises to strengthen back and abdominal muscles that do not increase intra-abdominal pressure and from training in body mechanics—for example, squatting to pick up an object rather than bending over. If back pain continues to be a problem, patients can learn to perform low-volume exchanges with a cycler at night while keeping the abdominal cavity empty during the day (186). If back pain persists despite these measures, the patient may need to switch to HD.

Constipation

Constipation is more common in elderly patients and is a particularly important problem in elderly PD patients because it may interfere mechanically with dialysate drainage. Recommendations include the use of sorbitol or other nonstimulant cathartics, adequate fluid intake, and avoidance of medications that interfere with bowel function.

DIALYSIS IN A NURSING HOME SETTING

As the dialysis population ages and becomes more debilitated, more patients may require skilled nursing care on a temporary or permanent basis (187). In 1997, 0.4% to 0.6% of nursing home patients were on dialysis, and in 1999, it was reported that more than 4.8% of dialysis patients lived in nursing homes (90% HD and 10% PD) (188,189). Patients with ESKD in nursing homes have many concomitant chronic diseases, with higher rates of diabetes mellitus, coronary artery disease, cardiovascular disease, peripheral vascular disease, and amputations compared to the noninstitutionalized population with ESKD. They also have a high rate of physical and cognitive impairments. A recent meta-analysis demonstrated an 80% decline in functional status for ESKD patients in a nursing home setting by 12 months after dialysis initiation; cognitive function declined by 90% over the same time frame. Although many of the included studies were small and observational in nature, the 1-year survival rate from nursing home admission for dialysis patients ranged 26% to 42% (187).

Nursing homes can aid patients by reducing hospitalization time and providing rehabilitation programs, social stimulation, and comprehensive care. However, there are significant challenges to caring for patients with ESKD in a nursing home, including difficulties with transportation and multiple chronic diseases that require specialized knowledge for appropriate management requiring consultation with specialists. Therefore, many nursing homes refuse to admit patients with ESKD because of the extra challenge of caring for them (188). In the early 1990s, Schleifer (190) found that almost half of 197 nursing homes contacted in the Philadelphia area accepted patients with ESKD, 19% of whom were treated with PD and the rest with HD, 18% of the nursing homes refused patients with ESKD, and 34% had never been asked; current data are not known. Reasons given for not accepting patients with ESKD included lack of nurse training, transportation problems, inadequate physician coverage, administrative objection, and financial concerns.

Nursing home residents have several modality options: in-center HD, staff-assisted "home" HD in the nursing home, or PD. In-center HD has the advantage of providing treatment in a specialized facility with trained technicians. However, time spent away from the nursing home may interfere with rehabilitation, social interaction, and meals, and transportation to dialysis facilities may be uncomfortable, inconvenient, and costly. USRDS data from 2004 indicate that 44% of dialysis patients in nursing homes are unable to ambulate necessitating either ambulance or wheelchair-accessible transportation to get to dialysis facilities (189).

Staff-assisted home HD is less commonly used than in-center HD because it requires nursing home investment, training of nursing home staff, and partnerships with a nephrology unit. Reddy et al. (189) conducted a study of 271 staff-assisted home HD patients and assessed patient survival from entry into the nursing home program. Results showed that survival was 82% at 1 month, 64% at 3 months, 38% at 6 months, and 26% at 12 months, with a median survival of 4.1 months, compared to median survival of 3.4 years for the general HD population.

PD is a good option for use in nursing homes that are willing to take on the responsibility of delivering the dialysis. Carey et al. (191) developed an educational program to train personnel in 10 community-based extended care facilities to care for PD patients who required temporary or permanent placement. Over a 5-year period, 1-month, 6-month, and 1-year patient survival rates were 90%, 50%, and 40%, respectively, with short-term rehabilitation patients having significantly better survival than long-term nursing home residents. In a study by Anderson et al. (192), technique survival rates were 94%, 86% and 79%, at 1 month, 6 months, and 1 year, respectively. Peritonitis rates were slightly higher than in noninstitutionalized patients (10.4 per 100 patient-months vs. 7.4 per 100 patient-months) but overall were comparable with National CAPD Registry data. A Toronto-based group recently published their experience instituting PD programs at three local nursing homes. They found peritonitis rates similar to the community at 1 episode every 40.3 treatment months, mean patient survival of 34.4 months, and a 5.3% transfer rate to HD (193).

ETHICAL ISSUES IN ELDERLY DIALYSIS PATIENTS

As the dialysis population expands, ages, and becomes more infirm, and the societal cost of the Medicare ESKD program continues to grow (194), many ethical dilemmas arise.

Access to End-Stage Kidney Disease Treatment

Do elderly dialysis patients have equal access to treatment or is age a reason for denial of treatment (194–196)? Up until quite recently, most discussions focused on age discrimination in initiation of dialysis. Most essayists on the subject were fond of quoting Berlyne's letter regarding dialysis age discrimination in the United Kingdom (197), and other reports have noted ESKD treatment age inequality in other European countries (32,198). In a survey of French nephrologists nearly two decades ago, 90% refused patients 75 years and older if they were not independent and did not have a supportive family (24). However, there are increasing questions about the appropriateness of biomedicalization at the end of life, as it relates to dialysis and other medical interventions. These are fitting given the success of the medical interventions to extend life but often in the absence of independence and quality of life. Consideration should also be made to the allocation of scarce financial resources, the constant pressure to reduce health care costs, and the national debt (194,199–204). Given its disproportionate consumption of Medicare dollars, dialysis will most certainly be a target for health care reform in coming years. Whether access to RRT will once again be limited by age criteria remains to be seen (204). Societal expectations will have a clear impact on these decisions. While less than 5% of patients with CKD in the United States elect not to start dialysis, this number is approximately 15% in United Kingdom and Canada.

Decisions to initiate dialysis should be made on an individual patient basis and ought to consider treatment goals, physiologic and chronologic age, and equitable access in addition to allocation of resources and cost (205). Appropriateness of the therapy should be reevaluated with major changes in the medical condition of the individual. Solutions to these difficult ethical questions will never be easy, and they require the utmost respect for the individual, great compassion for the patient and family, and a considerate health care provider.

Quality of Life and Rehabilitation

Elderly patients with ESKD seem to segregate into two populations. The first group of elderly patients adjusts to dialysis very well and seems satisfied with the lifestyle. Some of these patients appear to enjoy the increased social interaction of thrice-weekly visits to the dialysis unit. Some investigators have found an unusually high level of life satisfaction among the elderly dialysis patients (206), and others note that older patients frequently appear satisfied with a lifestyle that might be unacceptable to a younger patient (28,207). On the contrary, the second group of patients has more comorbidity and less functional capacity. These are the patients who have higher rates of depression. A survey of Canadian patients, mean age 68 years old, with ESKD reported that 60.7% regretted their decision to start dialysis after a mean of 27 months of treatment (208). This is also reflected in the increasing rate of death following withdrawal of dialysis, currently representing the second leading cause of death after cardiovascular disease in patients with ESKD (208).

There is a wide variability reported in the quality of life assessments in elderly dialysis patients. This may not be surprising given that the elderly dialysis population is heterogeneous, and the assessments themselves are subjective. Different outcomes reported in various studies may reflect differences in physician and patient–family treatment goals, patient selection, rehabilitation needs, support services, and attitude. A recent study of Canadian elderly dialysis patients found that although elderly dialysis patients' mental health and satisfaction with their lives is often as good as or better than those of younger dialysis patients and their peers, they

have higher rates of depression and impaired physical functioning (209). Loos et al. (210) reported that older patients with ESKD have a lower quality of life than elderly patients with chronic disease but without ESKD; however, predialysis care of older patients with severe CKD improved quality of life.

A high quality of life and good emotional and mental state may be related to independence and lack of symptoms. (63). Indeed, geriatric dialysis patients suffer from as much as 50% decreased functional capacity compared to age-matched healthy subjects (211). In a study of nursing home residents initiating dialysis, only 13% maintained their predialysis level of functional status after 12 months (212). It has therefore been suggested that rehabilitative programs may be able to maintain or improve quality of life and increase level of functioning. This was recently demonstrated in a report of the first 3 years of an inpatient geriatric HD rehabilitation program in Toronto. In the 164 patients cared for, 69% were ultimately discharged home and 82% met at least one of their rehabilitation goals (213).

Special attention should be given to the quality of life and well-being of the caregiver for these elderly dialysis patients. Belasco et al. (214) surveyed elderly and nonelderly dialysis patients and their caregivers in Brazil and concluded that while all caregivers had lower scores in most dimensions (including functional capacity, physical capacity, and mental health), caregivers of elderly patients had significantly decreased mental health scores compared to caregivers of younger patients. Caregivers of elderly HD patients had lower social aspect, pain and vitality scores, and had more weekly hours of care; caregivers of elderly PD patients had lower overall scores than HD patients and suffered from lower Mental Component Summary and Karnofsky Index scores. They recommended that professionals provide training and counseling to caregivers, starting from the beginning of dialysis treatment (214).

Discontinuation of Dialysis

Withdrawal from dialysis has been a cause of death in dialysis patients ever since the availability of dialysis for chronic uremia. In recent years, there have been more formalized recommendations from the ESKD Working Group funded by the Robert Wood Johnson Foundation, and consensus guidelines have been published by the Renal Physicians Association/American Society of Nephrology (215). Currently, withdrawal from dialysis is the second leading cause of death amongst patients with ESKD over the age of 75 years (20).

Patients who do withdraw from dialysis therapy should be offered care to provide a "good death; that is, one that is free from pain, brief, peaceful, occurring in the presence of loved ones, and at the place of one's choice" (216). There are several barriers to good end-of-life care in dialysis patients. TABLE 42.4 describes barriers and proposed solutions. Nephrologists and dialysis units need to incorporate end-of-life care from other disciplines and work with local palliative care and hospice services. Although hospice enrollment of ESKD patients has been increasing, these services remain underutilized for dialysis patients. This is in part related to the fact that hospice services often refuse patients who continue dialysis therapy and also due to an overall lack of education of patients on palliative and hospice options on the part of the dialysis providers.

A recent study compared do not resuscitate (DNR) orders and rates of withdrawal from 208 dialysis facilities in France, Germany, Italy, Japan, Spain, the United Kingdom, and United States who

TABLE 42.4	**Barriers and Solutions to Good Palliative Care for Patients with Chronic Kidney Disease and to Hospice Care for Dialysis Patients**

Barriers	Solutions
Doctors are uncomfortable and do not discuss end-of-life issues with patients and family.	Train doctors on communication skills and "breaking bad news."
Patients have not told their physician and family what their wishes are.	Advanced care planning (breaking bad news skills)
Patients and family have fears and misperceptions about end-of-life care and hospice.	Education and discussion surrounding these issues
Patients and family do not have a clear understanding of their prognosis.	Frank discussions of prognosis (breaking bad news skills)
Poor system management, particularly pain	Emphasis on symptom management in nephrology practice and dialysis units Better training in fellowship Research into best practices
Patient and family lack knowledge concerning withholding and withdrawal of dialysis.	Patients and family should have a clear understanding from the earliest contacts concerning the option of withholding and withdrawal of dialysis and what they may expect if they choose either option
Renal team: lack of knowledge about hospice	Educate on national and local coverage issues.
Local hospice: lack of knowledge about ESKD-specific issues	Awareness of local hospice services, establish relationship with local hospice services Education of local hospice
CMS national policy: confusion on the meaning of coverage in ESKD and "related" diagnosis section of the hospice manual	Work with CMS to clarify this confusion. Consider change in regulations through Congress.
CMS regional coverage: lack of uniformity on interpretation of national coverage rules in ESKD	Work with CMS to develop uniformity in local coverage decision.

ESRD, end-stage kidney disease; CMS, Centers for Medicare & Medicaid Services.
From Germain MJ, Cohen LM, Davison SN. Withholding and withdrawal from dialysis: what we know about how our patients die. *Semin Dial* 2007;20(3):195–199.

were participating in the DOPPS (217). The United States had the highest rate of DNR (7.5%) and rate of withdrawal from HD (3.5 per 100 patient-years). There was a small increased risk for DNR status with age (OR of 1.16 per 10 years, $p = 0.03$).

Although decisions to withhold or withdraw dialysis are very difficult and have generated a complex legal and ethical literature (218,219), consideration of established ethical principles may make decisions somewhat easier (**TABLE 42.5**).

Self-determination and Autonomy

The first issue to be considered is whether the patient is competent to make a decision to withdraw a life-sustaining technology. Is there evidence of dementia or psychiatric disorder, or is the patient's judgment clouded by depression, pain, medication, or metabolic derangement? Can the patient understand the choices involved and consequences of any decision? If the patient is truly competent, then he or she has the right to make an informed decision regarding medical care (218,220); recent survey data suggest that ESKD patients want to be involved in this process and have conversations

with their nephrologists about prognosis and end-of-life care (221). The American College of Physicians Ethics Manual (222) suggests that if the patient is not competent, the order of priority for decision making should be advance directives, substituted judgments, and the best interests of the patient.

Since 1991, the Patient Self-Determination Act has given adults the capacity to make medical decisions for themselves and the right to make decisions today about health care treatment they would want to receive in the future; it is now widely recommended that HD patients be encouraged to write advance directives. In a survey of dialysis units in London and Ontario, only 50% of HD patients had considered their wishes in regard to cardiopulmonary resuscitation (CPR), mechanical ventilation, and withdrawal of dialysis (223). In a survey of Canadian patients, only 38% had completed an advanced directive (208). Physicians and other dialysis staff need to be familiar with the concepts and legal ramifications of advance directives, durable powers of attorney, and living wills and be willing and able to discuss them when indicated. The patient's family or significant other may be asked to assist in the decision making and must know they are basing that decision on the patient's best interests, on prior advance directives made by the patient when competent, or on knowledge of what the patient would have wished given the circumstances (218,224).

Understanding the dynamics of the patient–family relationship may also be necessary. Decisions may be made for various reasons, including the best interest of the patient, financial interest, guilt because of the family member's limited contact with the patient, or a misunderstanding of role and process. If the caretaker or physician is uncomfortable with the decision to withhold or withdraw dialysis, he or she may wish to refer the patient to another physician.

TABLE 42.5	**Ethical Principles for Withholding and/or Withdrawing Dialysis**

Self-determination/autonomy
Benefit versus burden
Futile therapy
Conflict between physician and family

Benefit versus Burden

Is the patient likely to benefit from dialysis? In this situation, age is not an appropriate independent criterion (218). Each patient must be evaluated individually for medical and psychological suitability for dialysis and whether dialysis is technically possible. Recently, some have recommended use of prognostic calculators to aid in this assessment. The "surprise" question has been demonstrated to be quite powerful in mortality prediction—"Would you be surprised if Mr. X died within the next 6 months?"—especially when combined with serum albumin levels and age (225).

A nephrologist is not ethically or legally obligated to offer dialysis if treatment would not benefit the patient. Hirsch et al. (226) suggest that dialysis is inappropriate for patients with poor prognoses, including those with multiple organ system failure; nonuremic dementia; metastatic, refractory malignancy; or irreparable and debilitating neurologic disease. When dialysis is appropriate, the patient and/or family member may believe that dialysis poses a burden to the patient that outweighs potential benefit, either because of the process or because of its impact on quality of life (218,224). Understanding why the patient and/or family considers dialysis burdensome is important because it may be possible to modify treatment or even initiate dialysis on a trial basis for a patient who fears dialysis but does not actually know what it is like. Also, the patient's environment or support system can perhaps be adjusted in a way that makes dialysis more tolerable or desirable.

Can Dialysis be a Futile Therapy?

Dialysis may be viewed as a futile therapy—prolonging death rather than sustaining life. For example, a patient may be facing imminent death from terminal cancer or may be comatose with irreversible brain damage. Removing a life support such as dialysis would not "cause" the patient's death but rather allow it to occur naturally. Kilner (218) refers to this as *passive facilitating*.

Conflict between Physician and Family

When the physician and family cannot agree on the best course of action for a patient, several options are available. These options may include review by an ethics committee or the courts or transfer of the patient to another physician or hospital. It is generally preferable for these discussions to remain among medical staff, patient, and family rather than resorting to the courts. Ethics committees provide a forum for discussion rather than dictate medical decisions (222).

Adequate and clear communication is the most important factor in resolving conflicts regarding terminal care, not only between physician and family but also among all the health professionals involved in the care of the patient. Roberts et al. (227), in a study of the impact of withdrawal of dialysis on surviving relatives, noted that the relatives were most disappointed when physicians failed to tell the truth; were too optimistic; continued dialysis too long; and/or were unwilling to discuss withdrawal, alternatives, and implications.

Cardiopulmonary Resuscitation

A study of CPR performed in an HD unit in Montreal, Canada, between August 1997 and December 2004 showed an incidence rate of 0.012% with a 30-day survival of 79% (228). As expected, CPR during dialysis treatment is associated with better outcomes due to likelihood of electrolyte disturbances that are more readily correctable. On the contrary, survival at 6 months for hospitalized dialysis patients undergoing CPR has been estimated at a dismal 3% (229). When dialysis patients were surveyed regarding their attitudes toward CPR in multiple studies, 65% to 87% of patients reported that they would request CPR (229). Perceptions and preferences tended to be similar to those of nondialysis elderly patients. Poor health status and increasing illness severity seemed to influence likelihood to decline resuscitation. Age was not a factor in decisions to refuse respiratory support or dialysis, although older dialysis patients were more likely to have thought about it. Ultimately, most dialysis patients would like to take part in shared medical decision making with their nephrologist and are open to discussions regarding end-of-life care (208).

⬡ REFERENCES

1. Radecki SE, Nissenson AR. Dialysis for chronic renal failure: comorbidity and treatment differences by disease etiology. *Am J Nephrol* 1989;9(2):115–123.
2. Williams AJ, Nicholl J, el Nahas AM, et al. Continuous ambulatory peritoneal dialysis and haemodialysis in the elderly. *Q J Med* 1990;74(274):215–223.
3. Brown WW, Davis BB, Spry LA, et al. Aging and the kidney. *Arch Intern Med* 1986;146(9):1790–1796.
4. Hutteri H, Locking-Cusolito H. Retirement to renal failure: the management of the elderly dialysis patient. *J CANNT* 1992;2(1):14–16.
5. Brown WW. Introduction. Proceedings from the International Conference: geriatric nephrology and urology: interdisciplinary perspectives. *Am J Kidney Dis* 1990;16:273–274.
6. Oreopoulos D. Opinion: how can the care of elderly dialysis patients be improved? *Semin Dial* 1992;5:24–25.
7. Bower J. Opinion: how can the care of elderly patients be improved? *Semin Dial* 1992;5:26–28.
8. Boag J. The impact of aging on dialysis: human and technical considerations. *Dial Transplant* 1992;21(3):124–127.
9. Ross C, Rutsky EA. Dialysis modality selection in the elderly patient with end-stage renal disease: advantages and disadvantages of peritoneal dialysis. *Adv Perit Dial* 1990;6(Suppl 1):2–5.
10. Macias-Nunez J, Cameron J. Treatment of end-stage renal disease in the elderly. In: Cameron J, Davison AM, Grünfeld J-P, et al, eds. *Oxford Textbook of Clinical Nephrology*. London, United Kingdom: Oxford University Press, 1992:1621–1635.
11. Brown WW. Dialysis and transplantation in the elderly. In: Morley J, ed. *Geriatric Care*. St. Louis, MO: G.W. Manning & Associates, 1992:345–352.
12. DeLuca L, Cardella CJ. Opinion: how can the care of elderly dialysis patients be improved? *Semin Dial* 1992;5:28–29.
13. Mooradian AD. Biological and functional definition of the older patient: the role of biomarkers of aging. *Oncology (Huntingt)* 1992;6(Suppl 2): 39–44.
14. Oreopoulos D. The aging kidney. *Adv Perit Dial* 1990;6(Suppl):2–5.
15. Blagg CR. The early history of dialysis for chronic renal failure in the United States: a view from Seattle. *Am J Kidney Dis* 2007;49(3): 482–496.
16. Porush J, Faubert RF. Chronic renal failure. In: Porush JG, Faubert RF, eds. *Renal Disease in the Aged*. Boston, MA: Little, Brown and Company, 1991:285–313.
17. Barbanel C. Renal diseases and dialysis in elderly patients. *Contrib Nephrol* 1989;71:95–99.
18. Disney A. Demography and survival of patients receiving treatment for chronic renal failure in Australia and New Zealand: report on dialysis and renal transplantation treatment from the Australia and New Zealand Dialysis and Transplant Registry. *Am J Kidney Dis* 1995;25(1): 165–175.
19. Hatakeyama S, Murasawa H, Hamano I, et al. Prognosis of elderly Japanese patients aged ≥80 years undergoing hemodialysis. *ScientificWorldJournal* 2013;2013:693514.

20. United States Renal Data System. *USRDS 2013 Annual Data Report: Atlas of Chronic Kidney Disease and End-Stage Renal Disease in the United States.* Bethesda, MD: National Institutes of Health, National Institute of Diabetes and Digestive and Kidney Diseases, 2013.

21. United States Renal Data System. *USRDS 2014 Annual Data Report: An Overview of the Epidemiology of Kidney Disease in the United States.* Bethesda, MD: National Institutes of Health, National Institute of Diabetes and Digestive and Kidney Diseases, 2014.

22. Glickman J, Kaiser DL, Bolton K. Aetiology and diagnosis of chronic renal insufficiency in the aged: the role of renal biopsy. In: Macias-Nuñez JF, Cameron JS, eds. *Renal Function and Disease in the Elderly.* London, United Kingdom: Butterworths, 1987:485–508.

23. Levison S. Renal disease in the elderly: the role of the renal biopsy. *Am J Kidney Dis* 1990;16(4):300–306.

24. Mignon F, Michel C, Mentre F, et al. Worldwide demographics and future trends of the management of renal failure in the elderly. *Kidney Int Suppl* 1993;41:S18–S26.

25. Kurella M, Covinsky KE, Collins AJ, et al. Octogenarians and nonagenarians starting dialysis in the United States. *Ann Intern Med* 2007;146(3):177–183.

26. Canaud B, Tong L, Tentori F, et al. Clinical practices and outcomes in elderly hemodialysis patients: results from the Dialysis Outcomes and Practice Patterns Study (DOPPS). *Clin J Am Soc Nephrol* 2011;6(7):1651–1662.

27. Capelli J. Haemodialysis and the elderly patient. In: Michelis M, Davis B, eds. *Geriatric Nephrology.* New York, NY: Field, Rich and Associates, 1986:129–134.

28. Chester AC, Rakowski TA, Argy WP Jr, et al. Hemodialysis in the eighth and ninth decades of life. *Arch Intern Med* 1979;139(9):1001–1005.

29. Ponticelli C, Graziani G, Cantaluppi A, et al. Dialysis treatment of end-stage renal disease in the elderly. In: Macias-Nuñez J, Cameron JS, eds. *Renal Function and Disease in the Elderly.* London, United Kingdom: Butterworths, 1987:509–528.

30. Lamping DL, Constantinovici N, Roderick P, et al. Clinical outcomes, quality of life, and costs in the North Thames Dialysis Study of elderly people on dialysis: a prospective cohort study. *Lancet* 2000;356(9421):1543–1550.

31. Giuseppe P, Mario S, Barbara PG, et al. Elderly patients on dialysis: epidemiology of an epidemic. *Nephrol Dial Transplant* 1996;11(Suppl 9): 26–30.

32. Rotellar E, Lubelza RA, Rotellar C, et al. Must patients over 65 be haemodialysed? *Nephron* 1985;41:152–156.

33. Leimbach T, Kron J, Czerny J, et al. Hemodialysis in patients over 80 years. *Nephron* 2015;129:214–218.

34. Isaacs A, Burns A, Davenport A. Is dialysis a viable option for the older patient? Outcomes for patients starting dialysis aged 80 years or older. *Blood Purif* 2012;33:257–262.

35. Röhrich B, von Herrath D, Asmus G, et al. The elderly dialysis patient: management of the hospital stay. *Nephrol Dial Transplant* 1998;13 (Suppl 7):69–72.

36. Parry RG, Crowe A, Stevens JM, et al. Referral of elderly patients with severe renal failure: questionnaire survey of physicians. *BMJ* 1996;313(7055):466.

37. Mignon F, Siohan P, Legallicer B, et al. The management of uraemia in the elderly: treatment choices. *Nephrol Dial Transplant* 1995;10(Suppl 6): 55–59.

38. Susantitaphong P, Altamimi S, Ashkar M, et al. GFR at initiation of dialysis and mortality in CKD: a meta-analysis. *Am J Kidney Dis* 2012; 59(6):829–840.

39. Crews D, Scialla JJ, Boulware LE, et al. Comparative effectiveness of early versus conventional timing of dialysis initiation in advanced CKD. *Am J Kidney Dis* 2014;63(5):806–815.

40. Rowe J, Andres R, Tobin J. Age-adjusted normal standards for creatinine clearance in man. *Ann Intern Med* 1976;84:567–569.

41. Levey AS, Coresh J, Greene T, et al. Using standardized serum creatinine values in the Modification of Diet in Renal Disease Study equation for estimating glomerular filtration rate. *Ann Intern Med* 2006;145(4): 247–254.

42. Levey AS, Bosch JP, Lewis JB, et al. A more accurate method to estimate glomerular filtration rate from serum creatinine: a new prediction equation. *Ann Intern Med* 1999;130:461–470.

43. Lopes M, Araujo LQ, Passos MT, et al. Estimation of glomerular filtration rate from serum creatinine and cystatin C in octogenarians and nonagenarians. *BMC Nephrol* 2013;14(265):2–9.

44. Pascual J, Orofino L, Liaño F, et al. Incidence and prognosis of acute renal failure in older patients. *J Am Geriatr Soc* 1990;38(1):25–30.

45. Pascual J, Orofino L, Burgos J. Acute renal failure in the elderly. *Geriatr Nephrol Urol* 1992;2:51–61.

46. Gentric A, Cledes J. Immediate and long-term prognosis in acute renal failure in the elderly. *Nephrol Dial Transplant* 1991;6(2):86–90.

47. Groeneveld AB, Tran DD, van der Meulen J, et al. Acute renal failure in the medical intensive care unit: predisposing, complicating factors and outcome. *Nephron* 1991;59(4):602–610.

48. Hsu RK, McCulloch CE, Dudley RA, et al. Temporal changes in incidence of dialysis-requiring AKI. *J Am Soc Nephrol* 2013;24(1):37–42.

49. Hsu CY, McCulloch CE, Fan D, et al. Community-based incidence of acute renal failure. *Kidney Int* 2007;72:208–212.

50. Cartin-Ceba R, Kashiouris M, Plataki M, et al. Risk factors for development of acute kidney injury in critically ill patients: a systematic review and meta-analysis of observational studies. *Crit Care Res Pract* 2012;2012:691013.

51. Feest TG, Round A, Hamad S. Incidence of severe acute renal failure in adults: results of a community based study. *BMJ* 1993;306(6876):481–483.

52. Kane-Gill SL, Sileanu FE, Murugan R, et al. Risk factors for acute kidney injury in older adults with critical illness: a retrospective cohort study. *Am J Kidney Dis* 2015;65:860–869.

53. Xue J, Daniels F, Star RA, et al. Incidence and mortality of acute renal failure in Medicare beneficiaries, 1992 to 2001. *J Am Soc Nephrol* 2006;17(4):1135–1142.

54. Corwin HL, Bonventre JV. Factors influencing survival in acute renal failure. *Semin Dial* 1989;2:220–225.

55. Macias-Nunez JF, Sanchez Tomero J. Acute renal failure in old people. In: Macias-Nunez JF, Cameron JS, eds. *Renal Functions and Disease in the Elderly.* London, United Kingdom: Butterworths, 1987:461–484.

56. Sonnenblick M, Slotki IN, Friedlander Y, et al. Acute renal failure in the elderly treated by onetime peritoneal dialysis. *J Am Geriatr Soc* 1988;36(11):1039–1044.

57. Spiegel DM, Ullian ME, Zerbe GO, et al. Determinants of survival and recovery in acute renal failure patients dialyzed in intensive-care units. *Am J Nephrol* 1991;11(1):44–47.

58. Pascual J, Orofino L, Liaño F, et al. Prognosis of acute renal failure among elderly patients. *J Am Geriatr Soc* 1991;39(1):102–103.

59. Schmitt R, Coca S, Kanbay M, et al. Recovery of kidney function after acute kidney injury in the elderly: as systematic review and meta-analysis. *Am J Kidney Dis* 2008;52:262–271.

60. Dahlberg J, Schaper A. Acute renal failure in octogenarians. *Wis Med J* 1989;88(12):19–23.

61. Macias-Nunez JF, Lopez-Novoa JM, Martinez-Maldonado M. Acute renal failure in the aged. *Semin Nephrol* 1996;16(4):330–338.

62. Moss AH. Revised dialysis clinical practice guideline promotes more informed decision-making. *Clin J Am Soc Nephrol* 2010;5:2380–2383.

63. Ho-dac-Pannekeet MM. PD in the elderly—a challenge for the (pre) dialysis team. *Nephrol Dial Transplant* 2006;21(Suppl 2):ii60–ii62.

64. Capuano A, Sepe V, Cianfrone P, et al. Cardiovascular impairment, dialysis strategy and tolerance in elderly and young patients on maintenance haemodialysis. *Nephrol Dial Transplant* 1990;5(12):1023–1030.

65. Maiorca R, Cancarini GC, Camerini C, et al. Modality selection for the elderly: medical factors. *Adv Perit Dial* 1990;6(Suppl):18–25.

66. Nissenson AR. Chronic peritoneal dialysis in the elderly. *Geriatr Nephrol Urol* 1991;1:3–12.

67. Harris S, Lamping DL, Brown EA, et al. Clinical outcomes and quality of life in elderly patients on peritoneal dialysis versus hemodialysis. *Perit Dial Int* 2002;22(4):463–470.

68. Winkelmayer WC, Glynn RJ, Mittleman MA, et al. Comparing mortality of elderly patients on hemodialysis versus peritoneal dialysis: a propensity score approach. *J Am Soc Nephrol* 2002;13(9):2353–2362.

69. Vonesh EF, Moran J. Mortality in end-stage renal disease: a reassessment of differences between patients treated with hemodialysis and peritoneal dialysis. *J Am Soc Nephrol* 1999;10(2):354–365.

70. Maitra S, Jassal SV, Shea J, et al. Increased mortality of elderly female peritoneal dialysis patients with diabetes—a descriptive analysis. *Adv Perit Dial* 2001;17:117–121.

71. Jaar BG, Coresh J, Plantinga LC, et al. Comparing the risk for death with peritoneal dialysis and hemodialysis in a national cohort of patients with chronic kidney disease. *Ann Intern Med* 2005;143(3): 174–183.

72. Mehrotra R, Chiu YW, Kalantar-Zadeh K, et al. Similar outcomes with hemodialysis and peritoneal dialysis in patients with end-stage renal disease. *Arch Intern Med* 2011;171:110–118.

73. Weinhandl ED, Foley RN, Gilbertson DT, et al. Propensity-matched mortality comparison of incident hemodialysis and peritoneal dialysis patients. *J Am Soc Nephrol* 2010;21:499–506.

74. Chung SH, Lindholm B, Lee HB. Influence of initial nutritional status on continuous ambulatory peritoneal dialysis patient survival. *Perit Dial Int* 2000;20(1):19–26.

75. United States Renal Data System. *USRDS 2006 Annual Data Report: Atlas of End-Stage Renal Disease in the United States.* Bethesda, MD: National Institute of Diabetes, Digestive and Kidney Diseases, 2006.

76. Michel C, Bindi P, Viron B. CAPD with private home nurses: an alternative treatment for elderly and disabled patients. *Adv Perit Dial* 1990;6(Suppl):331–335.

77. Diaz-Buxo J, Adcock A, Nelms M, et al. Experience with continuous cyclic peritoneal dialysis in the geriatric patient. *Adv Perit Dial* 1990;6(Suppl):61–64.

78. Diaz-Buxo J. The place for cycler-assisted peritoneal dialysis in geriatric patients: comparison with hemodialysis. *Geriatr Nephrol Urol* 1993;3:7–13.

79. Mattern WD, Morris CR, Heffley DL. A three-year experience with CCPD in a university-based dialysis and transplantation program. *Clin Nephrol* 1988;30(Suppl 1):S49–S52.

80. Lobbedez T, Verger C, Ryckelynck JP, et al. Is assisted peritoneal dialysis associated with technique survival when competing events are considered? *Clin J Am Soc Nephrol* 2012;7:612–618.

81. Benain JP, Faller B, Briat C, et al. Cost of dialysis in France. *Nephrol Ther* 2007;3:96–106.

82. Dimkovic N, Oreopoulos DG. Assisted peritoneal dialysis as a method of choice for elderly with end-stage renal disease. *Int Urol Nephrol* 2008;40:1143–1150.

83. Oliver MJ, Quinn RR, Richardson EP, et al. Home care assistance and the utilization of peritoneal dialysis. *Kidney Int* 2007;71(7):673–678.

84. Kumar VA, Ledezma ML, Rasgon SA. Daily home hemodialysis at a health maintenance organization: three-year experience. *Hemodial Int* 2007;11(2):225–230.

85. Agraharkar M, Barclay C, Agraharkar A. Staff-assisted home hemodialysis in debilitated or terminally ill patients. *Int Urol Nephrol* 2002;33:139–144.

86. Tennankore KK, Chan CT, Curran SP. Intensive home haemodialysis: benefits and barriers. *Nat Rev Nephrol* 2012;8:515–522.

87. MacGregor MS, Agar JW, Blagg CR. Home haemodialysis-international trends and variation. *Nephrol Dial Transplant* 2006;21(7): 1934–1945.

88. Morrissey PE, Yango A. Renal transplantation: older recipients and donors. *Clin Geriatr Med* 2006;22(3):687–707.

89. Wolfe R, Ashby VB, Milford EL, et al. Comparison of mortality in all patients on dialysis, patients on dialysis awaiting transplantation, and recipients of a first cadaveric transplant. *N Engl J Med* 1999;341: 1725–1730.

90. Rao PS, Merion RM, Ashby VB, et al. Renal transplantation in elderly patients older than 70 years of age: results from the scientific registry of transplant recipients. *Transplantation* 2007;83(8):1069–1074.

91. Hod T, Goldfarb-Rumyantzev AS. Clinical issues in renal transplantation in the elderly. *Clin Tranplant* 2015;29:167–175.

92. Oniscu G, Brown H, Forsythe J. How old is old for transplantation? *Am J Transplant* 2004;4:2067–2074.

93. Doyle SE, Matas AJ, Gillingham K, et al. Predicting clinical outcome in the elderly renal transplant recipient. *Kidney Int* 2000;57(5): 2144–2150.

94. Saudan P, Berney T, Leski M, et al. Renal transplantation in the elderly: a long-term, single-centre experience. *Nephrol Dial Transplant* 2001;16(4):824–828.

95. Cameron JS. Renal transplantation in the elderly. *Int Urol Nephrol* 2000;32(2):193–201.

96. Basu A, Greensteein SM, Clemetson S, et al. Renal transplantation in patients above 60 years of age in the modern era: a single center experience with a review of the literature. *Int Urol Nephrol* 2000;32(2): 171–176.

97. Port F, Bragg-Gresham JL, Metzger RA, et al. Donor characteristics associated with reduced graft survival: an approach to expanding the pool of kidney donors. *Transplantation* 2002;74(9):1281–1286.

98. Ojo AO. Expanded criteria donors: process and outcomes. *Semin Dial* 2005;18(6):463–468.

99. Molnar MZ, Streja E, Kovesdy CP, et al. Age and the associations of living donor and expanded criteria donor kidneys with kidney transplant outcomes. *Am J Kidney Dis* 2012;9:841–848.

100. Delmonico FL, Burdick JF. Maximizing the success of transplantation with kidneys from older donors. *N Engl J Med* 2006;354(4):411–413.

101. III. NKF-K/DOQI clinical practice guidelines for vascular access: update 2000. *Am J Kidney Dis* 2001;37(1 Suppl 1):S137–S181.

102. Centers for Medicare & Medicaid Services. CMS launches breakthrough initiative for major improvement in care for kidney patients: safe vascular access through collaborative Fistula First initiative. https://www.cms.gov/Newsroom/MediaReleaseDatabase/Press-releases/2005-Press-releases-items/2005-03-17.html. Accessed April 2015.

103. Pisoni RL, Zepel L, Port FK, et al. Trends in US vascular access use, patient preferences, and related practices: an update from the US DOPPS Practice Monitor with international comparisons. *Am J Kidney Dis* 2015;65:905–915.

104. Lacson E Jr, Lazarus JM, Himmelfarb J, et al. Balancing fistula first with catheters last. *Am J Kidney Dis* 2007;50(3):379–395.

105. Wasse H, Hopson S, McClellan W. Predictors of delayed transition from central venous catheter use to permanent vascular access among ESRD patients. *Am J Kidney Dis* 2007;49(2):276–283.

106. Schwab S. Opinion: what can be done to preserve vascular access for dialysis? *Semin Dial* 1991;4:152–153.

107. National Kidney Foundation. *New Diagnosis Codes for Chronic Kidney Disease to be Based on National Kidney Foundation's KDOQI Guidelines.* New York, NY: National Kidney Foundation. https://.kidney.org/news/newsroom/newsreleases/0267. Accessed April 2015.

108. O'Hare AM, Bertenthal D, Walter LC, et al. When to refer patients with chronic kidney disease for vascular access surgery: should age be a consideration? *Kidney Int* 2007;71(6):555–561.

109. Lee T, Thamer M, Zhang Y, et al. Outcomes of elderly patients after predialysis vascular access creation. *J Am Soc Nephrol* 2015;26:3133–3140.

110. Hod T, Patibandla BK, Vin Y, et al. Arteriovenous fistula placement in the elderly: when is the optimal time? *J Am Soc Nephrol* 2015;26: 448–456.

111. Lok CE, Oliver MJ, Su J, et al. Arteriovenous fistula outcomes in the era of the elderly dialysis population. *Kidney Int* 2005;67(6):2462–2469.

112. Berardinelli L, Vegeto A. Lessons from 494 permanent accesses in 348 haemodialysis patients older than 65 years of age: 29 years of experience. *Nephrol Dial Transplant* 1998;13(Suppl 7):73–77.

113. Leapman SB, Boyle M, Pescovitz MD, et al. The arteriovenous fistula for hemodialysis access: gold standard or archaic relic? *Am Surg* 1996;62(8):652–657.

114. Wing A, Brunner FP, Brynger H. Combined report on regular dialysis and transplantation in Europe, IX 1978. *Proc Eur Dial Transplant Assoc Eur Ren Assoc* 1979;13:2–52.

115. Konner K, Hulbert-Shearon TE, Roys EC, et al. Tailoring the initial vascular access for dialysis patients. *Kidney Int* 2002;62(1):329–338.

116. Windus DW, Jendrisak MD, Delmez JA. Prosthetic fistula survival and complications in hemodialysis patients: effects of diabetes and age. *Am J Kidney Dis* 1992;19(5):448–452.

117. Valji K, Bookstein JJ, Roberts AC, et al. Pharmacomechanical thrombolysis and angioplasty in the management of clotted hemodialysis grafts: early and late clinical results. *Radiology* 1991;178(1):243–247.

118. Prabhu N, Kerns SR, Sabatelli FW, et al. Long-term performance and complications of the Tesio twin catheter system for hemodialysis access. *Am J Kidney Dis* 1997;30(2):213–218.

119. Shusterman NH, Kloss K, Mullen JL. Successful use of double-lumen, silicone rubber catheters for permanent hemodialysis access. *Kidney Int* 1989;35(3):887–890.

120. Xue JL, Dahl D, Ebben JP, et al. The association of initial hemodialysis access type with mortality outcomes in elderly Medicare ESRD patients. *Am J Kidney Dis* 2003;42(5):1013–1019.

121. DeSilva RN, Patibandla BK, Vin Y, et al. Fistula first is not always the best strategy for the elderly. *J Am Soc Nephrol* 2013;24:1297–1304.

122. Allon M, Daugirdas J, Depner TA, et al. Effect of change in vascular access on patient mortality in hemodialysis patients. *Am J Kidney Dis* 2006;47(3):469–477.

123. Tordoir JM, Bode AS, van Loon MM. Preferred strategy for hemodialysis access creation in elderly patients. *Eur J Vasc Endovasc Surg* 2015;49:738–743.

124. Ponce SP, Pierratos A, Izatt S, et al. Comparison of the survival and complications of three permanent peritoneal dialysis catheters. *Perit Dial Bull* 1982;2:82–86.

125. Gentile D. Peritoneal dialysis in geriatric patients: a survey of clinical practices. *Adv Perit Dial* 1990;6(Suppl):29–32.

126. Nissenson AR, Diaz-Buxo JA, Adcock A, et al. Peritoneal dialysis in the geriatric patient. *Am J Kidney Dis* 1990;16(4):335–338.

127. Kim YS, Yang CW, Jin DC, et al. Comparison of peritoneal catheter survival with fistula survival in hemodialysis. *Perit Dial Int* 1995;15(2):147–151.

128. Nolph K, Lindblad A, Novak J, et al. Experiences with the elderly in the National CAPD Registry. *Adv Perit Dial* 1990;6(Suppl):33–37.

129. Gokal R. CAPD in the elderly—European and U.K. experience. *Adv Perit Dial* 1990;6(Suppl):38–40.

130. Segoloni G, Salomone M, Piccoli GB. CAPD in the elderly: Italian multicenter study experience. *Adv Perit Dial* 1990;6(Suppl):41–46.

131. Pulliam J, Li NC, Maddux F, et al. First-year outcomes of incident peritoneal dialysis patients in the United States. *Am J Kidney Dis* 2014;64(5):761–769.

132. Holley JL, Bernardini J, Piraino B. Risk factors for tunnel infections in continuous peritoneal dialysis. *Am J Kidney Dis* 1991;18(3):344–348.

133. Chan KE, Thadani RI, Maddux FW. Adherence barriers to chronic dialysis in the United States. *J Am Soc Nephrol* 2014;25:2642–2648.

134. Avram MR, Pena C, Burrell D, et al. Hemodialysis and the elderly patient: potential advantages as to quality of life, urea generation, serum creatinine, and less interdialytic weight gain. *Am J Kidney Dis* 1990;16(4):342–345.

135. McKevitt M, Jones JF, Lane DA, et al. The elderly on dialysis: some considerations in compliance. *Am J Kidney Dis* 1990;16(4):346–350.

136. Kaiser FE. Principles of geriatric care. *Am J Kidney Dis* 1990;16(4):354–359.

137. King K. Strategies for enhancing compliance in the dialysis elderly. *Am J Kidney Dis* 1990;16(4):351–353.

138. Lim WH, Kireta S, Russ GR, et al. Uremia impairs blood dendritic cell function in hemodialysis patients. *Kidney Int* 2007;71(11):1122–1131.

139. Chonchol M. Neutrophil dysfunction and infection risk in end-stage renal disease. *Semin Dial* 2006;19(4):291–296.

140. Franceschi C, Monti D, Barbieri D, et al. Successful immunosenescence and the remodelling of immune responses with ageing. *Nephrol Dial Transplant* 1996;11(Suppl 9):18–25.

141. Delafuente JC. Immunosenescence. Clinical and pharmacologic considerations. *Med Clin North Am* 1985;69(3):475–486.

142. Gillis S, Kozak R, Durante M, et al. Immunological studies of aging. Decreased production of and response to T cell growth factor by lymphocytes from aged humans. *J Clin Invest* 1981;67(4):937–942.

143. Morduchowicz G, Winkler J, Derazne E, et al. Renal replacement therapy in the ninth decade of life. *Geriatr Nephrol Urol* 1992;2:147–149.

144. Tinetti ME, Schmidt A, Baum J. Use of the erythrocyte sedimentation rate in chronically ill, elderly patients with a decline in health status. *Am J Med* 1986;80(5):844–848.

145. Baldassare J, Kaye D. Special problems of urinary tract infection in the elderly. *Med Clin North Am* 1991;75:375–390.

146. Marketos SG, Papanayiotou C, Dontas AS. Bacteriuria and nonobstructive renovascular disease in old age. *J Gerontol* 1969;24(1):33–36.

147. Leinig CE, Moraes T, Ribeiro S, et al. Predictive value of malnutrition markers for mortality in peritoneal dialysis patients. *J Ren Nutr* 2011;21(2):176–183.

148. Chertow GM, Goldstein-Fuchs DJ, Lazarus JM, et al. Prealbumin, mortality, and cause-specific hospitalization in hemodialysis patients. *Kidney Int* 2005;68(6):2794–2800.

149. Kalantar-Zadeh K, Kopple JD. Relative contributions of nutrition and inflammation to clinical outcome in dialysis patients. *Am J Kidney Dis* 2001;38(6):1343–1350.

150. Wolfson M. Nutrition in elderly dialysis patients. *Semin Dial* 2002;15(2):113–115.

151. Weiner DE, Tighiouart H, Ladik V, et al. Oral intradialytic nutritional supplement use and mortality in hemodialysis patients. *Am J Kidney Disease* 2014;63(2):276–285.

152. Jern NA, VanBeber AD, Gorman MA, et al. The effects of zinc supplementation on serum zinc concentration and protein catabolic rate in hemodialysis patients. *J Ren Nutr* 2000;10(3):148–153.

153. Karcic E, Philpot C, Morley JE. Treating malnutrition with megestrol acetate: literature review and review of our experience. *J Nutr Health Aging* 2002;6(3):191–200.

154. Patel TS, Freedman BI, Yosipovitch G. An update on pruritus associated with CKD. *Am J Kidney Dis* 2007;50(1):11–20.

155. Kimata N, Fulle DS, Saito A, et al. Pruritus in hemodialysis patients: results from the Japanese Dialysis Outcomes and Practice Patterns Study. *Hemodial Int* 2014;18(3):657–667.

156. Meyer KB, Espindle DM, DeGiacomo JM, et al. Monitoring dialysis patients' health status. *Am J Kidney Dis* 1994;24(2):267–279.

157. Weisbord SD, Mor MK, Sevick MA, et al. Associations of depressive symptoms and pain with dialysis adherence, health resource utilization, and mortality in patients receiving chronic hemodialysis. *Clin J Am Soc Nephrol* 2014;9:1594–1602.

158. Davidson S. Pain in hemodialysis patients: prevalence, cause, severity and management. *Am J Kidney Dis* 2003;42(6):1239–1247.

159. Barakzoy AS, Moss AH. Efficacy of the world health organization analgesic ladder to treat pain in end-stage renal disease. *J Am Soc Nephrol* 2006;17(11):3198–3203.

160. Krüger T, Brandenburg V, Schliepe G, et al. Sailing between Scylla and Charybdis: oral long-term anticoagulation in dialysis patients. *Nephrol Dial Transplant* 2013;28(3):534–541.

161. Hylek EM, Evans-Molina C, Shea C, et al. Major hemorrhage and tolerability of warfarin in the first year of therapy among elderly patients with atrial fibrillation. *Circulation* 2007;115(21):2689–2696.

162. Elliott M, Zimmerman D, Holden R. Warfarin anticoagulation in hemodialysis patients: a systematic review of bleeding rates. *Am J Kidney Dis* 2007;50(3):433–440.

163. Quinn RR, Naimark DM, Oliver MJ, et al. Should hemodialysis patients with atrial fibrillation undergo systemic anticoagulation? A cost-utility analysis. *Am J Kidney Dis* 2007;50(3):421–432.

164. Sosa-Ortiz AL, Acosta-Castillo I, Prince MJ. Epidemiology of dementias and Alzheimer's disease. *Arch Med Res* 2012;43(8):600–608.

165. Lopez OL, Jagust WJ, DeKosky ST, et al. Prevalence and classification of mild cognitive impairment in the Cardiovascular Health Study Cognition Study: part 1. *Arch Neurol* 2003;60(10):1385–1389.

166. Elias MF, Dore GA, Davey A. Kidney disease and cognitive function. *Contrib Nephrol* 2013;179:42–57.

167. Fazekas G, Fazekas F, Schmidt R, et al. Brain MRI findings and cognitive impairment in patients undergoing chronic hemodialysis treatment. *J Neurol Sci* 1995;134(1–2):83–88.

168. Murray AM, Tupper DE, Knopman DS, et al. Cognitive impairment in hemodialysis patients is common. *Neurology* 2006;67(2):216–223.

169. Murray AM, Pederson SL, Tupper DE, et al. Acute variation in cognitive function in hemodialysis patients: a cohort study with repeated measures. *Am J Kidney Dis* 2007;50(2):270–278.

170. Pereira AA, Weiner DE, Scott T, et al. Subcortical cognitive impairment in dialysis patients. *Hemodial Int* 2007;11(3):309–314.

171. Vermeer SE, Prins ND, den Heijer T, et al. Silent brain infarcts and the risk of dementia and cognitive decline. *N Engl J Med* 2003;348(13):1215–1222.

172. Bernick C, Kuller L, Dulberg C, et al. Silent MRI infarcts and the risk of future stroke: the cardiovascular health study. *Neurology* 2001;57(7):1222–1229.

173. Vermeer SE, Hollander M, van Dijk EJ, et al. Silent brain infarcts and white matter lesions increase stroke risk in the general population: the Rotterdam Scan Study. *Stroke* 2003;34(5):1126–1129.

174. Nakatani T, Naganuma T, Uchida J, et al. Silent cerebral infarction in hemodialysis patients. *Am J Nephrol* 2003;23(2):86–90.

175. Naganuma T, Uchida J, Tsuchida K, et al. Silent cerebral infarction predicts vascular events in hemodialysis patients. *Kidney Int* 2005;67(6):2434–2439.

176. Kim CD, Lee HJ, Kim DJ, et al. High prevalence of leukoaraiosis in cerebral magnetic resonance images of patients on peritoneal dialysis. *Am J Kidney Dis* 2007;50(1):98–107.

177. Drew DA, Weiner DE, Tighiouart H, et al. Cognitive function and all-cause mortality in maintenance hemodialysis patients. *Am J Kidney Dis* 2015;65(2):303–311.

178. Elsayed E, Weiner DE. In the literature: cognitive impairment in hemodialysis patients. *Am J Kidney Dis* 2007;49(2):183–185.

179. Farrokhi F, Abedi N, Beyene J, et al. Association between depression and mortality in patients receiving long-term dialysis: a systematic review and meta-analysis. *Am J Kidney Disease* 2014;63(4):623–635.

180. Akman B, Uyar M, Afsar B, et al. Adherence, depression and quality of life in patients on a renal transplantation waiting list. *Transpl Int* 2007;20(8):682–687.

181. Zimmermann R, Camey SA, Mari Jde J. A cohort study to assess the impact of depression on patients with kidney disease. *Int J Psychiatry Med* 2006;36(4):457–468.

182. Koo JR, Yoon JY, Joo MH, et al. Treatment of depression and effect of antidepression treatment on nutritional status in chronic hemodialysis patients. *Am J Med Sci* 2005;329(1):1–5.

183. Zucchelli P, Sturani A, Zuccalà A, et al. Dysfunction of autonomic nervous system in patients with end-stage renal failure. *Contrib Nephrol* 1985;45:69–81.

184. Nissenson A, Gentile DE, Soderblom RE, et al. Peritoneal dialysis in the elderly. In: Oreopoulos D, ed. *Geriatric Nephrology*. Dordrecht, The Netherlands: Martinus Nijhof, 1986:147–156.

185. Homodraka-Mailis A. Pathogenesis and treatment of back pain in peritoneal dialysis patients. *Perit Dial Bull* 1983;3(Suppl 3):S41–S43.

186. Twardowski ZJ, Khanna R, Nolph KD, et al. Intraabdominal pressures during natural activities in patients treated with continuous ambulatory peritoneal dialysis. *Nephron* 1986;44(2):129–135.

187. Hall RK, O'Hare AM, Anderson RA, et al. End-stage renal disease in nursing homes: a systematic review. *J Am Med Dir Assoc* 2013;4:242–247.

188. Tong E, Nissenson A. Dialysis in nursing homes. *Semin Dial* 2002;15(2):103–106.

189. Reddy NC, Korbet SM, Wozniak JA, et al. Staff-assisted nursing home haemodialysis: patient characteristics and outcomes. *Nephrol Dial Transplant* 2007;22(5):1399–1406.

190. Schleifer C. Peritoneal dialysis in nursing homes. *Adv Perit Dial* 1990;6(Suppl):86–91.

191. Carey HB, Chorney W, Pherson K, et al. Continuous peritoneal dialysis and the extended care facility. *Am J Kidney Dis* 2001;27(3):580–587.

192. Anderson JE, Kraus J, Sturgeon D. Incidence, prevalence, and outcomes of end-stage renal disease patients placed in nursing homes. *Am J Kidney Dis* 1993;21(6):619–627.

193. Taskapan H, Tam P, Leblanc D, et al. Peritoneal dialysis in the nursing home. *Int Urol Nephrol* 2010;42:545–551.

194. Fox R, Swazey JP. Social and ethical problems in the treatment of end-stage renal disease patients. In: Narins E, ed. *Controversies in Nephrology and Hypertension*. New York, NY: Churchill Livingstone, 1984:45–70.

195. Wetle T. Age as a risk factor for inadequate treatment. *JAMA* 1987;258(4):516.

196. Rothenberg LS. Withholding and withdrawing dialysis from elderly ESRD patients: part 1—a historical view of the clinical experience. *Geriatr Nephrol Urol* 1992;2(2):109–117.

197. Berlyne GM. Over 50 and uremic equals death. The failure of the British National Health Service to provide adequate dialysis facilities. *Nephron* 1982;31(3):189–190.

198. Kjellstrand CM, Logan GM. Racial, sexual and age inequalities in chronic dialysis. *Nephron* 1987;45(4):257–263.

199. Klahr S. Rationing of health care and the end-stage renal disease program. *Am J Kidney Dis* 1990;16(4):392–395.

200. Cassel CK. Issues of age and chronic care: another argument for health care reform. *J Am Geriatr Soc* 1992;40(4):404–409.

201. Pawlson LG, Glover JJ, Murphy DJ. An overview of allocation and rationing: implications for geriatrics. *J Am Geriatr Soc* 1992;40(6):628–634.

202. Cummings NB. Ethical issues in geriatric nephrology: overview. *Am J Kidney Dis* 1990;16(4):367–371.

203. Lamm RD. High technology health care. *Am J Kidney Dis* 1990;16(4):378–383.

204. Andersen MJ, Friedman AN. The coming fiscal crisis: nephrology in the line of fire. *Clin J Am Soc Nephrol* 2013;8:1252–1257.

205. Brodeur D. Ethical principles in geriatric nephrology. *Am J Kidney Dis* 1990;16(4):372–374.

206. Westlie L, Umen A, Nestrud S, et al. Mortality, morbidity, and life satisfaction in the very old dialysis patient. *Trans Am Soc Artif Intern Organs* 1984;30:21–30.

207. Tonkin-Crine S, Okamoto I, Leydon GM, et al. Understanding by older patients of dialysis and conservative management for chronic kidney failure. *Am J Kidney Dis* 2015;65(3):443–450.

208. Davison SN. End-of-life care preferences and needs: perceptions of patients with chronic kidney disease. *Clin J Am Soc Nephrol* 2010;5:195–204.

209. Kutner NG, Jassal SV. Quality of life and rehabilitation of elderly dialysis patients. *Semin Dial* 2002;15(2):107–112.

210. Loos C, Briançon S, Frimat L, et al. Effect of end-stage renal disease on the quality of life of older patients. *J Am Geriatr Soc* 2003;51(2):229–233.

211. Sterky E, Stegmayr BG. Elderly patients on haemodialysis have 50% less functional capacity than gender- and age-matched healthy subjects. *Scand J Urol Nephrol* 2005;39(5):423–430.

212. Kurella Tamura M, Covinsky KE, Chertow GM, et al. Functional status of elderly adults before and after initiation of dialysis. *N Engl J Med* 2009;361:1539–1547.

213. Li M, Porter E, Lam R, et al. Quality improvement through the introduction of interdisciplinary geriatric hemodialysis rehabilitation care. *Am J Kidney Dis* 2007;50(1):90–97.

214. Belasco A, Barbosa D, Bettencourt AR, et al. Quality of life of family caregivers of elderly patients on hemodialysis and peritoneal dialysis. *Am J Kidney Dis* 2006;48(6):955–963.

215. Renal Physicians Association. *Shared Decision-Making in the Appropriate Initiation of and Withdrawal from Dialysis*. 2nd ed. Rockville, MD: Renal Physicians Association, 2010.

216. Germain MJ, Cohen LM, Davison SN. Withholding and withdrawal from dialysis: what we know about how our patients die. *Semin Dial* 2007;20(3):195–199.

217. Fissell RB, Bragg-Gresham JL, Lopes AA, et al. Factors associated with "do not resuscitate" orders and rates of withdrawal from hemodialysis in the international DOPPS. *Kidney Int* 2005;68(3):1282–1288.

218. Kilner JF. Ethical issues in the initiation and termination of treatment. *Am J Kidney Dis* 1990;15(3):218–227.

219. Thorsteindottir B, Swetz KM, Albright RC. The ethics of chronic dialysis for the older patient; time to reevaluate the norms. *Clin J Am Soc Nephrol* 2015;10:2094–2099.

220. Rodin GM, Chmara J, Ennis J, et al. Stopping life-sustaining medical treatment: psychiatric considerations in the termination of renal dialysis. *Can J Psychiatry* 1981;26(8):540–544.

221. Singh P, Germain MJ, Cohen L, et al. The elderly patient on dialysis: geriatric considerations. *Nephrol Dial Transplant* 2014;29(5):990–996.

222. American College of Physicians. American College of Physicians ethics manual. Third edition. *Ann Intern Med* 1992;117(11):947–960.

223. Tigert J, Chaloner N, Scarr B, et al. Development of a pamphlet: introducing advance directives to hemodialysis patients and their families. *J CANNT* 2005;15(1):20–24.

224. Tobe SW, Senn JS. The End-Stage Renal Disease Group. Foregoing renal dialysis: a case study and review of ethical issues. *Am J Kidney Dis* 1996;28(1):147–153.

225. Moss AH, Ganjoo J, Sharma S, et al. Utility of the "surprise" question to identify dialysis patients with high mortality. *Clin J Am Soc Nephrol* 2008;3:1379–1384.

226. Hirsch D, West ML, Cohen AD, et al. Experience with not offering dialysis to patients with poor prognosis. *Am J Kidney Dis* 1994;23:463–466.

227. Roberts JC, Snyder R, Kjellstrand CM. Withdrawing life support—the survivors. *Acta Med Scand* 1988;224(2):141–148.

228. Lafrance J, Nolin L, Senécal L, et al. Predictors and outcome of cardiopulmonary resuscitation (CPR) calls in a large haemodialysis unit over a seven-year period. *Nephrol Dial Transplant* 2006;21(4):1006–1012.

229. Hijazi F, Holley JL. Cardiopulmonary resuscitation and dialysis: outcome and patients' views. *Semin Dial* 2003;16(1):51–53.

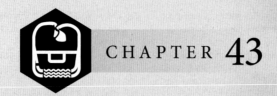

CHAPTER 43

Current Outcomes for Dialysis Patients and Improving Quality of Care for Dialysis Patients

Brent W. Miller

Dialysis has evolved from a mostly failed attempt to keep patients with acute kidney injury alive until recovery of kidney function in the 1940s to a small-scale attempt to keep relatively young and healthy patients with chronic kidney disease alive in the 1960s to the widespread, lifesaving, and life-preserving therapy it is today for a broad spectrum of patients with kidney failure.

Despite this positive trajectory, the current state of dialysis therapy still produces insufficient gains in quality of life, morbidity, and mortality. Furthermore, the cost of this therapy has attracted aggressive scrutiny so that any improvement in medical outcomes must also be cost-neutral or even save money (1).

This chapter reviews the current state of dialysis outcomes, potential outcome measurements other than mortality and quality processes that may improve the patient experience, and the involvement of regulatory bodies and payers in outcome measurement.

 CURRENT OUTCOME DATABASES

United States Renal Data System

In 1988, the National Institute of Diabetes and Digestive and Kidney Diseases (NIDDK) awarded a contract for formation of a national end-stage kidney disease (ESKD) registry. This resulted in the formation of the United States Renal Data System (USRDS) (2). When an incident patient begins dialysis treatment in the United States, a Centers for Medicare & Medicaid Services (CMS) 2728 Medical Evidence Report is completed and submitted to the appropriate End-Stage Renal Disease (ESRD) Network (see following text). A similar process occurs when a dialysis patient dies with CMS 2746 ESRD Death Notification Form. This data is then blindly combined with other CMS data such as Medicare part A, B and D claims from care of dialysis patients.

An annual report based on this data is published and readily available online in many formats. Researchers with expertise can purchase the database and separately analyze the data for their own academic purposes.

The accuracy and integrity of the USRDS data, while widely assumed, has only been examined cursorily. Two studies in 1992 demonstrated a >90% accuracy of most data points obtained from patients (3,4). However, other studies raise concerns. In one study on erythropoiesis-stimulating agent (ESA) use in 8,033 patients at the Department of Veteran Affairs, the sensitivity of accuracy for predialysis ESA use recorded on the 2728 form was 57% (5). Another study of 1,105 incident dialysis patients showed a sensitivity of 0.59 in reporting the 17 comorbid conditions on the 2728 form with significant underreporting (6). Finally, the inaccuracy of the Death Notification Form was demonstrated during the Hemodialysis (HEMO) trial where the major source of misclassification was the frequent use of "unknown cause of death" and "other heart conditions" on the Death Notification Form (7).

Dialysis Outcomes and Practice Patterns Study

The Dialysis Outcomes and Practice Patterns Study (DOPPS) is an international, prospective, observational study beginning in 1996 and divided in multiple time periods ("phases") that examines multiple patient outcomes (8). Over 200,000 patient-years patients in over 600 hemodialysis centers have been included in the data analysis in the first five phases, and the annual reports are available in a variety of formats and online. In 2013, peritoneal dialysis collection began for Peritoneal Dialysis Outcomes and Practice Patterns Study (PDOPPS) (9).

Large Dialysis Organizations

In the United States, over 60% of patients undergo dialysis therapy in outpatient facilities owned and operated by one of two large corporations. With the introduction of computers and large-scale database management software, hundreds of millions of data points can be analyzed regarding ESKD (10). These databases can be used to measure various clinical outcomes and suggesting where and how clinical attention may be needed (11–13).

The recruitment of the Large Dialysis Organization (LDOs) to perform structured, nonclassically randomized trials, so-called "large pragmatic trials" may help answer clinical questions in a more timely and less costly manner than the current NIDDK process. The first of these trials in dialysis will examine the effect of 4.25 hours of hemodialysis versus usual care in incident hemodialysis patients (14,15).

GOVERNMENT MEASURES

End-Stage Renal Disease Quality Incentive Program

In 2008, the United States Congress passed the Medicare Improvements for Patients and Providers Act, which directed the Secretary of Health and Human Services to establish quality incentives for

providers of dialysis (1). The incentive chosen was avoidance of a payment reduction from CMS of up to 2%.

New quality targets are chosen each year according to a deliberate process with some public input (**TABLE 43.1**). Although the inclusion of quality measurements, better patient care, and safety and implementation of best clinical practices has been widely praised, the particular choices of quality measures have been controversial. From a global perspective of caring for a complex patient, intense concentration on a few specific measures may distract from other important functions of the dialysis center and clinician. Second, some of the measures chosen have questionable scientific rationale and could potentially harm patients or at best have no effect if implemented aggressively. For example, in 2012, avoiding a hemoglobin less than 10 g/dL has no basis in literature, and earlier studies demonstrated that the use of ESA may have harmful side effects (16). Furthermore, urea reduction ratio (URR) as an absolute measure

---

TABLE 43.1	Summary of End-Stage Renal Disease Quality Incentive Program Performance Measures to Avoid Payment Reductions in Years 2012–2018						
2012	**2013**	**2014**	**2015**	**2016**	**2017**	**2018**
Hemoglobin >12 g/dL	Hemoglobin >12 g/dL	Hemoglobin >12 g/dL	Hemoglobin >12 g/dL	Hemoglobin >12 g/dL		
Urea reduction ratio ≥65%	Urea reduction ratio ≥65%	Urea reduction ratio ≥65%	Urea Kt/V	Urea Kt/V	Urea Kt/V	Urea Kt/V
Hemoglobin <10 g/dL		% of arteriovenous fistulas and catheters	% of arteriovenous fistulas and catheters	% of arteriovenous fistulas and catheters	% of arteriovenous fistulas and catheters	% of arteriovenous fistulas and catheters
			National Healthcare Safety Network (NHSN) reporting to Center for Disease Control and Prevention (CDC)	Bloodstream infections in hemodialysis patients	Bloodstream infections in hemodialysis patients	Bloodstream infections in hemodialysis patients
			Administration of Patient Experience of Care Survey	Administration of Patient Experience of Care Survey	Administration of Patient Experience of Care Survey	Administration of Patient Experience of Care Survey
			Serum calcium and phosphorus reporting	Hypercalcemia	Hypercalcemia	Hypercalcemia
			ESA dose reporting	ESA dose reporting	ESA dose and hemoglobin reporting	ESA dose and hemoglobin reporting
				Serum phosphorus reporting	Serum phosphorus reporting	Serum phosphorus reporting
					Standardized readmission ratio	Standardized readmission ratio
						Pain assessment and follow-up
						Clinical depression screening and follow-up
						Health care personnel influenza vaccination

For further details and explanations see www.cms.gov. ESA, erythropoiesis-stimulating agent.

of dialysis adequacy had been abandoned by most practitioners by 2012 because of its lack of considering ultrafiltration, dialysis time, residual kidney function, and the other 12 dialysis treatments during the month in addition to marginal evidence that small solute clearance alone corrects the uremic syndrome. To put it bluntly, ESKD patients were not suffering and dying in 2012 for lack of hemoglobin values between 10 and 12 g/dL and a URR ≤65%.

Dialysis Facility Compare

Utilizing electronic data derived from Medicare claims and electronic data submitted directly from dialysis centers (Consolidated Renal Operations in a Web-enabled Network or CROWNWeb), CMS annually gives each dialysis facility a "star rating" from 1 to 5 based on the attainment of certain measurable outcomes. These ratings are posted online and also required to be visible in each dialysis center.

While trying to attain the laudable goal of providing dialysis patients a system to judge their care similar to the way they would choose a restaurant or buy a pair of shoes, the current methodology has raised concerns. First, the system does not measure attained outcomes but rather separates each variable along a curve. Thus, there will always be 10% of dialysis centers with a 1-star rating and 10% of facilities with a 5-star rating regardless of the actual metrics obtained. Second, as providers aggressively react to the few metrics, the separation between a 1-star rating and a 5-star rating may be clinically insignificant. For example, the difference in Kt/V values and hypercalcemia percentages are a few percentage points in the high 90s. Lastly, some physicians may overreact to the metrics with unintended consequences.

End-Stage Renal Disease Networks

In 1978, the United States Congress authorized the establishment of ESRD Network Organizations to support the ESKD program. Currently as of 2015, there are 18 networks with contracts awarded by CMS. The ESRD Network Organization is responsible in its geography for collecting data for the ESKD program, improving the quality of care, addressing patient grievances, and providing technical support to patients, dialysis providers, and other health care professionals and organizations involved in the care of ESKD patients. However, even the well-intentioned programs of the ESRD Networks can go awry such as the Fistula First Initiative which had some unintended consequences of patients likely having catheters in place longer while waiting for multiple fistula surgeries and maturation (17,18).

Randomized Controlled Trials in Dialysis

Given the multiple clinical issues in patients with kidney failure requiring dialysis therapies, the field would seem a frequent target of innovative clinical studies. Alas, this has not been the case and, furthermore, patients on dialysis or even with moderate chronic kidney disease are often excluded from other trials with diverse disease states.

Additionally, many of the interventions suggested by numerous observational studies in ESKD patients have been shown to not be effective when rigorously and formally tested. Applying conclusions broadly from nonrandomized trials has led to errors in clinical practice. One prominent example of this was the Canada-USA (CANUSA) study in peritoneal dialysis where the failure to account for the impact of residual renal function over time led to recommendations of targeting of Kt/V urea >2.1 in thousands of patients

who were previously doing fine and potentially led to more glucose exposure and an early technique failure (19,20).

Despite the lack of many ongoing or planned clinical trials to improve care to the ESKD patient, there is a recognition of the continued scope of the problem. In 2012, the U.S. Food and Drug Administration announced an innovation challenge with ESKD and received 32 proposals from which 3 were selected including a vascular access device, an implantable artificial kidney, and a wearable artificial kidney (21).

Clinical Guidelines

The combination of outcome measurement and expert opinion has led to the formation of various guidelines for managing ESKD patients (**TABLE 43.2**). While these well-meaning endeavors can lead to a standardization of therapy and particularly attention on substandard performance, unintended consequences can potentially lead to worse outcomes. One of the better known examples of this is the KDOQI anemia management guidelines (22).

Roles of Medical Director in Outcomes

Over the last decade, the legal responsibilities of the nephrologist who assumes the role of the medical director of the dialysis center have been better defined. The quality of care and continuous improvement in the quality of care is one of these tasks. To succeed in this role, more endpoints need to be considered than the quality incentive program (QIP) or 5-star measures and a more vigorous process enacted than simply reviewing computer-generated laboratory and spreadsheet summaries provided monthly by the corporate management.

An entire field of study has evolved in dialysis about continuous quality improvement (CQI), quality assurance (QA), and quality assurance process improvement (QAPI) (23). Much of this attention has focused on the high infection rate and its concomitant morbidity and mortality in ESKD.

The medical director should act as the leader of a multidisciplinary team at the local level to address specific patient-focused problems in the dialysis center. Monthly meetings of this group

TABLE 43.2	**Various Dialysis Clinical Practice Guidelines**
Guideline Name	**Author Organization**
Kidney Disease Outcomes Quality Initiative (KDOQI)	National Kidney Foundation
Kidney Disease Improving Global Outcomes (KDIGO)	KDIGO
Renal Physicians Association (RPA) Clinical Practice Guidelines	RPA
Center for Disease Control and Prevention (CDC) Guidelines	CDC
Canadian Society of Nephrology Guidelines	Canadian Society of Nephrology
The British Renal Association	The Renal Association
Kidney Health Australia–Caring for Australasians with Renal Impairment (KHA-CARI) Guidelines	KHA and Australian and New Zealand Society of Nephrology
European Best Practice Guidelines	European Renal Association and European Dialysis and Transplantation Association

seem most effective with attendance monitored and minutes of the meeting being taken. The process should be data-driven with measureable outcomes and relevant, feasible performance criteria. A rudimentary understanding of quality improvement principles such as Pareto analysis, Deming principles, and the use of fishbone diagrams may help. One author suggests a mnemonic of "SMART:" specific, measurable, achievable, realistic and timely, while the Institute of Medicine has suggested safe, effective, patient-centered, timely, and equitable (24,25).

What Are the Desired Outcomes in Dialysis Therapy?

The intersection of a serious chronic disease state, an immense economic burden borne largely by one payer and a provision of the majority of dialysis therapy by two large multinational corporations has focused the attention of outcomes on a small number of measures that shift the focus away from an individual patient. Nissenson (26) has proposed shifting the focus back to the patient and what each patient's goals are for their dialysis therapy within a reasonable framework of clinical medicine. This type of action seems to have as much a chance as succeeding as any bold national proposal. In my practice, this is often expressed to the patient as my desire to turn the disaster of kidney failure into an annoyance of dialysis therapy rather than a new disaster.

 REFERENCES

1. Medicare Improvements for Patients and Providers Act of 2008 §113, 122, 42 USC §§1320b-14, 1396u-5(a) (2010).
2. Collins AJ, Foley RN, Gilbertson DT, et al. United States Renal Data System public health surveillance of chronic kidney disease and end stage renal disease. *Kidney Int Suppl* 2015;5:2–7.
3. Completeness and reliability of USRDS data: comparisons with the Michigan Kidney Registry. *Am J Kidney Dis* 1992;20(5 Suppl 2):84–88.
4. United States Renal Data System. How good are the data? USRDS data validation special study. *Am J Kidney Dis* 1992;20(5 Suppl 2):68–83.
5. Fischer JF, Stroupe KT, Hynes DM, et al. Validation of erythropoietin use data on Medicare's End-Stage Renal Disease Medical Evidence Report. *J Rehab Res Dev* 2010;47:751–762.
6. Longenecker JC, Coresh J, Klag MJ, et al. Validation of comorbid conditions on the End-Stage Renal Disease Medical Evidence Report: the CHOICE study. Choices for Healthy Outcomes in ESRD. *J Am Soc Nephrol* 2000;11:520–529.
7. Rocco MV, Yan G, Gassman J, et al. Comparison of causes of death using HEMO study and HCFA end-stage renal disease death notification classification systems. *Am J Kidney Dis* 2002;39:146–153.
8. Pisoni RL, Gillespie BW, Dickinson DM, et al. Dialysis Outcomes and Practice Patterns Study (DOPPS): design, data elements, and methodology. *Am J Kidney Dis* 2004;44(5 Suppl 2):7–15.
9. Perl J, Davies S, Lambie M, et al. The Peritoneal Dialysis Outcomes and Practice Patterns Study (PDOPPS): unifying efforts to inform practice and improve global outcomes in peritoneal dialysis [published online ahead of print November 2, 2015]. *Perit Dial Int.* doi:103747/pdi.2014.00288.
10. Krishnan M, Wilfehrt HM, Lacson E Jr. In data we trust: the role and utility of provider databases in the policy process. *Clin J Am Soc Nephrol* 2012;7:1891–1896.
11. Lacson E Jr, Wang W, Lazarus JM, et al. Hemodialysis facility–based quality-of-care indicators and facility-specific patient outcomes. *Am J Kidney Dis* 2009;54:490–497.
12. Pun PH, Horton JR, Middleton JP. Dialysate calcium concentration and the risk of sudden cardiac arrest in hemodialysis patients. *Clin J Am Soc Nephrol* 2013;8:797–803.
13. Karnik JA, Young BS, Lew NL, et al. Cardiac arrest and sudden death in dialysis units. *Kidney Int* 2001;60:350–357.
14. A cluster-randomized, pragmatic trial of hemodialysis session duration (TiME). https://clinicaltrials.gov/ct2/show/study/NCT02019225. Accessed April 30, 2016.
15. Johnson KE, Neta G, Dember LM, et al. Use of PRECIS ratings in the National Institutes of Health (NIH) Health Care Systems Research Collaboratory. *Trials* 2016;17:32.
16. Singh AK, Szczech L, Tan KL, et al. Correction of anemia with epoetin alfa in chronic kidney disease. *N Engl J Med* 2006;355:2085–2098.
17. Lacson E Jr, Lazarus JM, Himmelfarb J, et al. Balancing fistula first with catheters last. *Am J Kidney Dis* 2007;50:379–395.
18. Wish JB. Catheter last, fistula not-so-first. *J Am Soc Nephrol* 2015; 26:5–7.
19. Canada-USA (CANUSA) Peritoneal Dialysis Study Group. Adequacy of dialysis and nutrition in continuous peritoneal dialysis: association with clinical outcomes. *J Am Soc Nephrol* 1996;7:198–207.
20. Bargman JM, Thorpe KE, Churchill DN; and the CANUSA Peritoneal Dialysis Study Group. Relative contribution of residual renal function and peritoneal clearance to adequacy of dialysis: a reanalysis of the CANUSA study. *J Am Soc Nephrol* 2001;12:2158–2162.
21. U.S. Food and Drug Administration. Innovation challenge: end-stage renal disease. http://www.fda.gov/AboutFDA/CentersOffices/Officeof MedicalProductsandTobacco/CDRH/CDRHInnovation/Innovation Pathway/ucm286140.htm. Accessed April 30, 2016.
22. Coyne D. Influence of industry on renal guideline development. *Clin J Am Soc Nephrol* 2007;2:3–7.
23. U.S. Department of Health and Human Services, Health Resources and Services Administration. *Quality Improvement.* Rockville, MD: Health Resources and Services Administration, 2011.
24. Doran GT. There's a S.M.A.R.T. way to write management's goals and objectives. *Manage Rev* 1981;70:35–36.
25. Institute of Medicine. *Crossing the Quality Chasm: A New Health System for the 21st Century.* Washington, DC: National Academies Press, 2001.
26. Nissenson AR. Improving outcomes for ESRD patients: shifting the quality paradigm. *Clin J Am Soc Nephrol* 2014;9:430–434.

CHAPTER **44**

The Business of Nephrology

Robert Provenzano

When Medicare was established in 1965, it did not provide coverage for individuals with end-stage kidney disease (ESKD). At that time, kidney failure was considered a fatal disease, as treatment was not available outside a limited number of academic centers. In 1972, Congress passed the Social Security Amendments of 1972. Under this Act, Congress extended coverage to individuals who were younger than 65 years old, had ESKD, and had worked long enough to qualify for Social Security. This coverage became effective July 1, 1973 (1).

At that time, a typical "nephrologist" (as most did not formally train in nephrology but rather had "an interest" and served as a local expert) was on staff at one hospital, rounded in one dialysis facility, and saw office patients in one clinic. He or she was in solo practice or at most shared a small practice with one or two others. There were no thoughts of running their "business" as they were making a good living with robust reimbursement for their much needed, unique skills; slowly but surely this all changed. Reimbursement, in real and adjusted dollars, began to decrease as patient numbers and costs rapidly exceeded projections and nephrologists responded consistent with their training: They worked harder, saw more patients, and rounded at more hospitals and more dialysis facilities, trying to maintain their lifestyles and incomes. The most recent Renal Physicians Association (RPA) Benchmarking survey reports all nephrologists are now on staff at more than one hospital, 27% at four to six hospitals, and 85% round at four or more dialysis facilities in addition to 68% seeing patients in more than three offices (clinics). The average number of ESKD they care for has increased year over year and now stands at 68 patients per nephrologist (2). How this has impacted patient care, safety, quality, or satisfaction can be debated, but to be sure things would need to change as this model was and is unsustainable. This workload is now compounded by recent and expanding regulatory requirements

including meaningful use (MU), physician quality reporting system (PQRS), and electronic medical record (EMR) requirements.

BUSINESS AS USUAL

The majority of physicians have little to no formal training in business or business principles. As mentioned earlier, this was not necessary or relevant to running a successful practice. With robust reimbursement for skills learned in medical school and honed in residency and fellowship training, most practices had no business structures. Practices consisted of what I call a *Marcus Welby* (3) structure, front office staff answering phones, checking patients in and out, and medical assistants placing patients in rooms and billing staff. There were no business processes, protocols, measures of practice success, nor the expertise needed to keep abreast of the increasingly complex billing and coding requirements. Governance structure often rested with the most senior rather than most capable physician and rarely did nonphysician business savvy employees participate. Data collection, either on patient-centric information or on basic business metrics, was nonexistent. Inefficiency was the standard. Patient care was rendered one on one, by the physician, delivered to each patient as they were seen. Little focus on education, prevention, or population health was present. Marketing was by reputation alone or word of mouth and was more often based on who you were rather than your capabilities. Your "success" in the eyes of a hospital administrator was solely predicated on your ability to admit as many patients as possible. From a purely business perspective—this is a receipt for disaster, one that has now come due.

CHANGING TIDE

As noted above, since 1972 when Congress passed the Social Security Amendments allowing for coverage of ESKD for all patient services irrespective of age, the number of patients and costs incurred in their care has increased dramatically. Most recent United States Renal Data System (USRDS) data reports that ESKD patients make up 1% of Medicare beneficiaries and consume 5.6% of all Medicare dollars (4). Anemic reimbursement updates over the past 20 years have resulted in ESKD provider consolidation that successfully drove economies of scale in a fee-for-service (FFS) world (5). Although there have been substantial and complex changes in reimbursement under this model, most recently moving to a partially bundled payment model, the end result was business survival favored large integrated providers with the top two now representing over 70% of all ESKD patients in the United States. Predictably, their market power influences payers: Centers for Medicare and Medicaid Services (CMS) and legislators, in ways not available/accessible to the average nephrologist. These realities are influencing the business of the practice nephrology in ways never envisioned before.

If the previous paragraph represents the "macrocosm" of the business of nephrology, the "microcosm" of nephrology (nephrology practices) has also been impacted by the economic impact of legislation passed to influence rising overall health costs. In 2008, Congress passed the Patient Protection and Affordable Care Act (PPACA) (6). This legislation was a game changer for all of health care impacting how hospitals, insurers, and health care providers rendered care and ran their businesses. Forgoing the dominant FFS payment model for a value-based reimbursement (VBR) model, this legislation, as yet unproven in its benefits, has placed disproportional burdens on medical practices challenging the practice models, or lack thereof, on which they were built.

The PPACA granted a windfall of power to hospitals via accountable care organizations (ACOs). ACOs, population risk vehicles, have driven hospital consolidation into mega-health care systems to mitigate this risk. Physicians, faced with little to no ability to compete in this space, quickly became hospital employed, primary care first, followed by high-revenue subspecialists (oncology, cardiology, orthopedics) all who recently saw their outpatient procedure reimbursement gutted, destroying practice models that had sustained them for years. The hospital strategy is to create seamless care models over wide geographies and manage risk by serving large populations while controlling and directing physician care, hoping to link this to higher care quality and therefore—value.

Although one may quibble over the details or the wisdom of this approach, given how the PPACA is constructed, this scenario is predictably rapidly gaining ground.

Given these realities, the practice of nephrology, or better stated, the business of practicing nephrology must rapidly digest this information and access its business options to survive.

◆ ACCESSING YOUR BUSINESS

The first step in the process of remaining competitive in a changing reimbursement environment is to better understand your business. **TABLE 44.1** provides some critical questions you should ask yourself. But basically, you need to do a SWOT (strengths, weaknesses, opportunities, threat) analysis (7). Although beyond the scope of this chapter, a SWOT analysis is a simple, powerful, and insightful business tool. Block off time, without distraction, to list as many ideas for each category as you can.

There are several items that you will identify in your SWOT analysis worth focusing on; a few high-level items are discussed here.

One item is the practices' internal business structure. How is your practice managed? What is the governance structure? How are

TABLE 44.1	Accessing Your Business

What services do you provide?
Where do your business/referrals come from?
What or who is your competition?
What are the risks facing you?
What are your payment sources?
Do you know your costs?
What is your hospital planning?
Are you growing?

decisions made, and by whom? Who operationalizes change within the practice? Is it measured? Without a strong governance structure, the ability to rapidly implement change is limited and will negatively impact any meaningful and necessary change.

What business reports are available? How often are they produced? Who produces them? What information are they providing to you? Do you have business partners? Hospitals, dialysis providers, large primary care provider groups? Are you nurturing these relationships?

Understanding the importance of these questions will be critical for the practice to be credible to outsider providers, in recruiting new physicians, to make decisions quickly and nimbly, and to develop and implement process changes in how clinical services are provided.

Another item to consider is, where do your business/patient referrals come from? In the past, direct relationships with referral sources ruled. That pattern has been rapidly eroded. For the most part, your primary care referral sources no longer round in the hospital, a major source of patient referrals; rather, they outsource this work to hospitalists to better focus on their outpatient patient care. Hospitalists remain a moving target with high turnover, making development of a referral relationship with them challenging; often, there is a generational separation from you, and they tend to be looking for very specific renal services from your practice. Are you meeting that need? Also, direct relationships with insurers/payers are becoming more common and are often tied to risk contracts.

In the broadest sense, you should determine exactly what services you offer. **TABLE 44.2** lists a few. Importantly, do you know what it costs to provide these services? If you do not know what it costs you to deliver, let us say, CKD stage 4 care, in your office, how can you negotiate payment from insurers? Or how can you render

TABLE 44.2	Services Offered

Chronic kidney disease (CKD) care
Kidney stones
ESKD care (peritoneal, in-center, home, nocturnal)
AKI management
Hypertension
Glomerulonephritis management
Apheresis
Management of CKD/AKI in pregnancy
Management of autoimmune disorders
Vascular access services
Ultrasound services
Laboratory services

ESKD, end-stage kidney disease; AKI, acute kidney injury.

that service more economically? Developing a list of services and understanding their costs will serve you well in measuring, marketing, and reporting outcomes.

According to the RPA's (2) 2014 Benchmarking survey, 40% to 50% of a nephrologist's income comes from ESKD care and medical directorships, 30% from hospital work, and the remainder from the office. Each of these "business lanes" needs to be separately analyzed for growth, profitability, and sustainability.

The following sections describe details on nephrology-specific business care lanes that can be a focus of your practice analysis with conclusions drawn specifically to the VBR future for all of health care.

PRACTICE CLINICAL AND BUSINESS STRUCTURES

Nephrology practices are structured in three clinical and four business domains. The clinical domains include hospital services, dialysis services, and office/clinic practice. The business domains include these three plus ancillary nephrology services. Ancillary services traditionally include research, laboratory services, dialysis facility joint ventures or direct ownership, real estate, and vascular access centers, each with their own unique reimbursement and business challenges and are beyond the scope of this chapter. The ability of practices to participate in ancillary services varies from practice to practice and is heavily weighted on practice size, patient density, financial resources, and the practice leaderships' desire to expand into other areas.

The financial viability of the four business domains has historically been predicated on FFS and therefore high patient volumes and market share. Each domain existed in isolation resulting in the fragmented delivery of renal services and, excepting ESKD, had little quality oversight and was innately inefficient.

As mentioned earlier, the PPACA is influencing all of these domains and must be considered in your business planning moving forward.

FINANCIAL MODELS

The best example of a mature business/economic model of renal care is that of ESKD. For greater than 30 years, a focus on ESKD care has created precise financial models. Ease of identifying patients with ESKD, incident rates, defined payment for treatment, known hospitalization, and mortality rates have all allowed this medical industry to prosper and grow. Much less focus and data exists for CKD patients who have been, for all intents and purposes, an FFS payment model. Valid arguments have been made that without viable financial models for CKD patients, providers, out of financial necessity, will continue to apply disproportional resources to ESKD. The PPACA changed the focus in all of health care, targeting health care value rather than care volume. This game changing concept was best summed up by then CMS director, Donald Berwick, in his "triple aim of care": improvement in the health of populations, improvement in the experience of care, and reducing health care costs (8). This creates an incentive to move the FFS CKD payment system to a value care model that may be linked to the totality of renal care potentially inclusive of ESKD care.

Creating a "value-based" model around kidney disease offers us an opportunity to uniquely offer to patients the benefits of Dr. Berwick's triple aim of care. Unfortunately, our kidney care systems remain fragmented, and this creates real barriers that must first be surmounted to move forward in a meaningful way. Additionally, the capital investments necessary for this metamorphosis to occur is out of reach of most practices, necessitating the consideration of strategic partnerships for participation in this model of care. The reality remains though, that the future of the practice/business of nephrology will be linked to this expectation and any considerations of altering your practices' business model must take this seriously.

END-STAGE KIDNEY DISEASE CARE

ESKD care is, for the most part, provided by organized for-profit and not-for-profit providers in partnership with nephrologists (clinical care, medical directorships, and/or joint venture relationships). The greatest proportion of the practice income emanates for ESKD care, and therefore, much attention should be paid here as this income stream is under threat.

Medical directors fee contributes substantially to the practices' income. CMS estimates that the roles and responsibilities contracted for these services consume approximately 25% of a nephrologist's time. Therefore, the number of agreements one can provide will be under scrutiny, and this fact should be considered in their allocation within the practice.

Nephrologists are currently paid on an FFS model for incremental monthly clinical care (one visit, two to three visits, and four visits per month); this changed from the traditional monthly capitated payment not tied to frequency of visits in 2005 (9). The greater the number of patients under your care and the more efficiently you can deliver that care, the more financially successful the practice. This very model incentivizes increasing the volume of ESKD patients rather than delivering "upstream" value-based care that may negatively impact ESKD incident rates. Although it may seem counterintuitive, achieving and maintaining high ESKD patient volume is critical in a VBR model as more patients buffer the practices' ability to accept risk contracts. Therefore, continued efforts at growth must not be ignored.

However, providing ESKD services in an economically viable manner include careful analysis of the number of patients, the number of dialysis facilities served, the geographic placement of these facilities, and travel time to each (**TABLE 44.3**). This "process of care" is under increased pressure as payments are now starting to be tied to risk models (see the following text), and the ability of physicians to render care personally is in question. Use of physician extenders to provide the noncomprehensive care visits and field questions from dialysis care staff frees the nephrologists' time to focus on other practice business needs and should be considered. Recall, the ESKD population under the practices' care has a specific quantifiable income *and* cost. These should be determined and monitored as a business metric.

TABLE 44.3	End-Stage Kidney Disease Considerations

Patient number
Facility number
Geographic distribution/windshield time
Risk contract exposure
Use of extenders
Cost of delivering care

END-STAGE KIDNEY DISEASE SEAMLESS CARE ORGANIZATIONS

End-stage kidney disease seamless care organizations (ESCOs) are the first disease-specific ACO model designed by CMS to identify, test, and evaluate new ways to improve care for Medicare beneficiaries with ESKD (10). This "award" is predicated on the "bet" that the ACO model of care will be successful and seems reasonable given the knowledge gained by the ESKD care community in the demonstration projects and special needs programs for the past 10 years. Challenges remain in the details for risk/payment in ESCO, but the broad strategy has been accepted. ESCOs must have more than 350 Medicare beneficiaries; they must entail a joint venture between a dialysis provider and nephrologists (with the option to include a third Medicare provider/supplier). Savings versus a historical benchmark will shared with CMS (with up to 75% going to the ESCO) predicated on defined quality measures. This is the first economic model that substantially puts the nephrologist in a position of impacting care delivery. Directing care from more expensive sites of service [hospital, emergency room (ER), dialysis clinic] to less expensive venues, when appropriate (nephrology offices), may deliver savings.

These provocative economic models set the stage for not only a closer more collaborative relationship between dialysis providers, nephrologists, and hospitals on ESKD patients but also, and more importantly, the critical opportunity to focus upstream to influence care and management of transitional CKD patients (CKD stage 4/5) as impacting/improving these patients care [education, arteriovenous fistula (AVF) placement, conservative management, home modalities] may positively influence the risk and outcomes of incident ESKD patients in an ESCO.

HOSPITAL SERVICES

Fully approximately 30% of a nephrology practice income is earned via hospital-rendered care (2). The number of services a practice provides (**TABLE 44.1**) and business considerations (**TABLES 44.2** and **44.4**) enhances the volume of care they are invited to provide in the hospital setting. Under the current FFS payment system, patients with advanced CKD present to the hospital with other immediate critical health problems. They may develop acute kidney injury (AKI) and recover or have an accelerated progression to ESKD. One of the largest sources of incident ESKD patients continues to emanate from the hospital. Similarly, hospitalized patients with previously undiagnosed CKD are newly identified and require care in nephrologists' offices following discharge. While the FFS diagnosis-related group (DRG) payment models are defined and predictable, there are no strong incentives to identify at risk patients and apply processes of care to avoid AKI, move the patients efficiently through the hospital stay, or ensure proper handoffs and follow-up posthospitalization to decrease readmissions. Nephrologists receive FFS payment incenting them to freely admit patients and accept daily payments. To be fair, there are many regulatory barriers that prevent alignment of incentives among care providers adding to this problem. One of the intents of accountable care organizations (below) is to align incentive toward a value-based system rather than FFS. This, along with ESCOs could go a long way to improve this fragmented system and must be considered in your business model. This alignment allows your practice to take a leadership role within the hospital to help develop newer care models focused on integrated kidney care. Nephrologists are in a pivotal role with the ability to bridge fragmented care linking dialysis facilities, hospitals, and their practices.

ACCOUNTABLE CARE ORGANIZATIONS

The PPACA created risk vehicles known as accountable care organizations (ACOs) (6). The stated goal is alleviating regulatory barriers to encourage an integrated system of care, thereby delivering higher care value. By doing so, Congress has thrust health care into a full-risk model of care placing hospitals/hospital systems in a unique position of responsibility for the cost and outcomes of all patients within their networks. This has resulted in rapid and significant mergers and acquisitions of hospitals into mega-systems of care. Although this may address the problem of care fragmentation, it does not address the operational realities of assembling all the pieces necessary to deliver value. To accomplish this, it became necessary for hospitals/ACOs to seek out relationships with physicians in a manner not seen since health maintenance organizations (HMOs) of the 1980s. Through employment of care networks, primary care and relevant subspecialties were assembled into care panels to integrate care based on disease avoidance, early disease identification, or specific models of care for those with chronic disorders.

Hospitals'/ACOs' initial focus on primary care physician employment to secure a patient base was followed by arrangements with higher revenue-generating subspecialists (cardiology, oncology, and others). Nephrologists do not fall into this high revenue-generating category and therefore have not been a high target. Nephrologists have reasonable concern that system "savings" generated by this model of care may not trickle down to them given the perceived impact they have on overall ACO revenues. ESCOs offer a more reasonable renal risk model with stronger alignments than general ACOs will or can. Nevertheless, this process is still ongoing and as yet unproven in its overall impact on economic value or improvement in population health.

It is critical to mention at this point that to effectively deliver health care "value," ACOs must first ensure patient volume to offset risk; this reality is also true of ESCOs. This has resulted in aggressive marketing campaigns to consolidate/grow hospital networks. Additionally, the PPACA has created incentives to blur the lines between insurers and traditional brick and mortar hospitals with both morphing into the other. How this process matures remains unknown and will need to be monitored closely but must be carefully considered as hospitals are exerting much pressure on physicians to service their patients and the high cost of ESKD patients is on their radar.

CHRONIC KIDNEY CARE

Outpatient (office-based) CKD care, patients identified with CKD by their primary care providers are referred to nephrologists for diagnosis and treatment plans, remains mired in an FFS payment system that has been eroded yearly based on real inflation-based dollars (**FIGURE 44.1**). Previous attempts at "disease management"

TABLE 44.4	Hospital Services

Number of hospital(s) served?
Nephrology services offered?
Cost of your services?
Your position in hospital/partnerships?
What are your hospitals plans? ACO? Pay for performance?

ACO, accountable care organization.

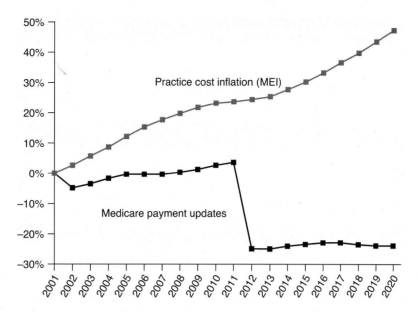

FIGURE 44.1 Disparity over time of practice cost inflation versus Medicare payment updates. (Data from 2011 Medicare Trustees Report, with adjustments based on 2012 Medicare physician payment schedule Final Rule. Prepared by American Medical Association, Economic and Health Policy Research, January 2012.)

of CKD care have failed for a variety of reasons: poor alignment of incentives across the care continuum, regulatory barriers, underpowered EMR, and analytics to name a few (11). Although FFS payment models for outpatient care are defined, the reimbursement does not sustain the costs of providing that care. This creates financial incentives that favor cross subsidization of office CKD care with income from hospital and ESKD care. Therefore, transition of patients to ESKD and liberal use of hospital care remains lucrative, and prevention of ESKD or hospital avoidance is not, clearly poorly aligned physician incentives.

The challenge for providers of kidney care is how to unite these three foci of care in a manner that improves patient outcomes and provides an attractive financial model for the practice and other stakeholders.

In the short term, the volume model can be sustained only by finding more efficient ways to manage increased patient volumes and to improve practice business efficiencies. You must challenge your current delivery model. The American Society of Nephrology (ASN) recently reported on nephrology manpower data suggests a shortage of nephrologists in the market (12). I would posit that there are plenty of nephrologists but with poor clinical deployment. Expanded use of physician extenders in the ESKD space coupled with their use in the office can improve outcomes and lower costs. A nephrologist can see new patients, determine the working diagnosis and treatment plan, and then turn the ongoing care and management to their physician assistant or advanced practice nurse under the guidance of defined CKD guidelines. This obviously frees up the nephrologists time to spend in more critical areas of the practice. This model of care is starting to gain traction and has been successful. In the long term, the economics of CKD will be more closely, if not entirely, tied to broader care models through ACOs, ESCOs, or other yet undetermined economic vehicles.

If one accepts that ESCOs or other risk models will be the economic future of kidney care, then several issues must be addressed in preparation.

REDEFINING KIDNEY CARE DELIVERY

If one accepts the triple aim of care as earlier referenced and espoused by CMS, then three points will help guide you in the process of practice restructure:

- Allocate resources to deliver population-level care in your areas of core competency.
- Leverage economies of scope and scale to allow these same resources to fund care.
- Develop and implement key programs to further improve outcomes.

Restructuring/retooling how a practice delivers quality kidney care, development and implementation of predictable, incremental CKD processes of care (CKD stages 3, 4, and 5), measurement, aggregating and reporting of quality metrics, development of robust integrated EMR systems, and challenging the "minds-set" of all nephrologists will all be necessary.

Structural changes will include processes allowing patients to be seen within 72 hours of hospital discharge, ER avoidance strategies, the capacity to see new/urgent outpatient referrals in a timely fashion, and developing robust business metrics, such as how much does it cost to deliver CKD, ESKD, and hospital care? (**FIGURE 44.2**)

These changes are critical to remain viable in a value-based care system and must be addressed. If a practice does not have the resources or expertise to provide answers, outsourcing your back office management to professionals will add great value to your practice as well as allow you to focus both on care and strategic goals going forward.

Additionally, hospital care will no longer be a passive process. Rather, avoiding unnecessary hospitalizations and readmissions, moving patients through their hospital stay in an efficient manner, and creating a posthospital care process will become critical.

Lastly, relationships with providers are evolving. Hospital via ACOs and dialysis providers via ESCOs will be looking for practices sensitive to value-based care. They are aware of the changes required in broader care models and are taking steps to partner with

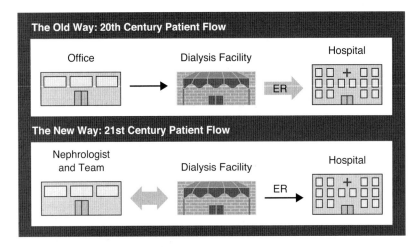

FIGURE 44.2 Patient flow. Arrow size represents volume of patients.

forward thinking nephrologists in meaningful ways. Practices must consider these strategic partnerships as business opportunities.

Focused goals will include presenting healthier incident patients to dialysis providers, determining who actually benefits from dialysis (elderly vs. conservative CKD management) and which method of dialysis is suited for which patient. Dialysis facility care models will be more intense and specific. Low-hanging opportunities in vascular care, diabetes management, immunization, and so on will have direct financial implications.

 CONCLUSION

The "business of nephrology" does not and can no longer exist in isolation. Rather, the financial viability of practices will necessarily be linked to broader risk pools that may include ESKD. A level of practice sophistication with a broad focus and strategy including strategic partnerships will drive the economic future of kidney care. Practices large enough to accept risk will have an advantage; smaller practices are aligning in legal vehicles, independent practice associations (IPAs), or merging to maintain relevance; and many practices are now looking to divest their practices to dialysis providers or hospital systems to fully align incentives. Ultimately, each practice must determine the best business strategies to make upfront capital investments to reap any longer term, as yet, poorly defined, economic returns.

Services, cost, data, process, and patient satisfaction will drive CKD care in the future. Practices' viability will be determined by developing CKD stage-specific, focused clinical processes with the ability to track, aggregate, analyze, and report outcomes.

Practices will need to take into consideration integrated care requirements including rapid patient assessments and reporting, timely follow-up posthospitalization, ER strategies, efficient use of physician extenders, as well as care models driven by predictive analytics.

Applying high-level practice management will allow your practice to become the business that it is. Revenue cycle management, accounts receivable, denial rates, coding and auditing, personnel management, and credentialing must all be performed in the most economical manner with measurable returns.

Despite a shift to value-driven care, volume of care is still a necessity to weather the financial costs incurred for this transition. Delivering high-volume, high-quality care while moving to value care requires efficiencies in care previously not required.

It remains too early to judge the success or failure of these new economic models, but early results from pioneer ACOs have shown some added value, defined as improved selected clinical metrics and financial savings. Additionally, nephrologists have always led in the delivery of value-based care, and although much will need to change, integrating the delivery of kidney care into a broader risk pool may prove economically attractive for many practices.

REFERENCES

1. Social Security. DI 11052.001 Initial end-stage renal disease Medicare cases. https://secure.ssa.gov/poms.nsf/lnx/0411052001. Published May 31, 2011. Accessed June 15, 2016.
2. Renal Physicians Association. RPA Benchmarking Survey 2014. http://www.renalmd.org. Accessed June 15, 2016 .
3. Beaulieu-Volk D. Marcus Welby didn't know everything: what to appreciate about healthcare today. http://www.fiercehealthcare.com/practices/marcus-welby-didn-t-know-everything-what-to-appreciate-about-healthcare-today. Accessed June 15, 2016.
4. United States Renal Data System. *USRDS 2014 Annual Data Report: Atlas of Chronic Kidney Disease and End-Stage Renal Disease in the United States.* Ann Arbor, MI: United States Renal Data System.
5. Neumann ME. What's next for dialysis providers? *Nephrology News & Issues.* July 16, 2015. http://www.nephrologynews.com/a-quiet-year-for-consolidation-among-largest-dialysis-providers/. Accessed June 15, 2016.
6. U.S. Department of Health and Human Services. Patient Protection and Affordable Care Act; exchange and insurance market. Standards for 2015 and beyond. https://www.federalregister.gov/articles/2014/05/27/2014-11657/patient-protection-and-affordable-care-act-exchange-and-insurance-market-standards-for-2015-and-beyond. Published May 27, 2014. Accessed June 15, 2016.
7. How to conduct SWOT analysis in healthcare organizations. http://pestleanalysis.com/swot-analysis-in-healthcare/. Accessed June 15, 2016.
8. Berwick DM, Nolan TW, Whittington J. The triple aim: care, health, and cost. *Health Aff (Millwood)* 2008;27(3):759–769.
9. U.S. Department of Health & Human Services. MANUALIZATION of payment for outpatient ESRD-related services. https://www.cms.gov/Regulations-and-Guidance/Guidance/Transmittals/downloads/R1456CP.pdf. Published February 22, 2008. Accessed June 15, 2016.
10. Centers for Medicare & Medicaid Services. Comprehensive ESRD care model. http://innovation.cms.gov/initiatives/comprehensive-esrd-care/. Accessed July 8, 2014.
11. Rocco M. Disease management programs for CKD patients: the potential and pitfalls. *Am J Kidney Dis* 2009;53(3 Suppl 3):S56–S63.
12. Masselink L, Salsberg E, Wu X, et al. *2015 ASN Nephrology Fellows Survey Report.* Washington, DC: American Society of Nephrology, 2016. https://www.asn-online.org/education/training/workforce/. Accessed June 15, 2016.